Prostate Cancer

To all our patients and their supporters, who have struggled so hard and from whom we have learnt so much.

Prostate Cancer
Principles and Practice

Edited by

Roger S Kirby, MD, FRCS (Urol)
Institute of Urology, University College London, London, UK

Alan W Partin, MD
The Brady Urological Institute, The Johns Hopkins Medical Institute, Baltimore, Maryland, USA

Mark R Feneley, MD, FRCS (Urol), FRCS (Eng)
Institute of Urology, University College London, London, UK

J Kellogg Parsons, MD, MHS
Division of Urology, University of California, San Diego, California, USA

Foreword by Peter T Scardino, MD

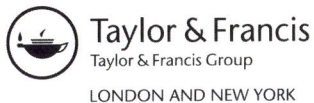

Taylor & Francis
Taylor & Francis Group

LONDON AND NEW YORK

© 2006 Taylor & Francis, an imprint of The Taylor & Francis Group
Taylor & Francis Group is the Academic Division of Informa plc

First published in the United Kingdom in 2006 by Taylor & Francis, an imprint of the Taylor & Francis Group, 2 Park Square, Milton Park, Abingdon, Oxon OX14 4RN

Tel: +44 (0)20 7017 6000
Fax: +44 (0)20 7017 6699
Email: info.medicine@tandf.co.uk
Website: http://www.tandf.co.uk/medicine

Although every effort has been made to ensure that all owners of copyright material have been acknowledged in this publication, we would be glad to acknowledge in subsequent reprints or editions any omissions brought to our attention.

Although every effort has been made to ensure that drug doses and other information are presented accurately in this publication, the ultimate responsibility rests with the prescribing physician. Neither the publishers nor the authors can be held responsible for errors or for any consequences arising from the use of information contained herein. For detailed prescribing information or instructions on the use of any product or procedure discussed herein, please consult the prescribing information or instructional material issued by the manufacturer.

A CIP record for this book is available from the British Library.

Library of Congress Cataloging-in-Publication Data
Data available on application

ISBN 1-84184-458-6
ISBN 978-1-84184-458-9

Distributed in North and South America by
Taylor & Francis
2000 NW Corporate Blvd
Boca Raton, FL 33431, USA

Within Continental USA
Tel: 800 272 7737; Fax: 800 374 3401
Outside Continental USA
Tel: 561 994 0555; Fax: 561 361 6018
Email: orders@crcpress.com

Distributed in the rest of the world by
Thomson Publishing Services
Cheriton House
North Way
Andover, Hampshire SP10 5BE, UK
Tel: +44 (0)1264 332424
Email: salesorder.tandf@thomsonpublishingservices.co.uk

Composition by Phoenix Photosetting, Chatham, Kent, UK
Printed and bound in Great Britain by CPI, Bath

Contents

SECTION 1: Introduction

SECTION 2:   Pathology of prostate cancer

SECTION 3:   Etiology of prostate cancer

SECTION 4:   Molecular mechanisms of prostate carcinogenesis

SECTION 5: Clinical diagnosis and staging of prostate cancer

SECTION 6: Treatment of early stage prostate cancer

SECTION 7: Treatment of locally advanced and metastatic prostate cancer

Contributors

Neil A Abrahams, MD
Assistant Professor, Department of Pathology and Microbiology, University of Nebraska Medical Center, Omaha, Nebraska, USA

Aamir Ahmed, PhD
Senior Research Fellow, Prostate Cancer Research Center, Institute of Urology and Nephrology, University College London, London, UK

Michele Albert, MD
Brigham and Women's Hospital and Dana Farber Cancer Institute, Department of Radiation Oncology, Boston, Massachusetts, USA

Peter C Albertsen, MD, MS
Professor of Surgery (Urology), University of Connecticut Health Center, Farmington, Connecticut, USA

Mohamad E Allaf, MD
Senior Resident in Urology, Brady Urological Institute, The Johns Hopkins Medical Institutions, Baltimore, Maryland, USA

Andrew J Armstrong, MD
Medical Oncology Fellow, Sidney Kimmel Comprehensive Cancer Center at Johns Hopkins, Baltimore, Maryland, USA

William J Aronson, MD
Professor of Urology, Veterans Administration Greater Los Angeles Healthcare System, UCLA School of Medicine, California, USA

Carlos Arroyo, MD
Resident in Urology, Department of Urology, Institute Montsouris, Paris, University Rene Descartes, Paris, France

Vasily J Assikis, MD
Assistant Professor of Oncology and Urology, Winship Cancer Institute, Emory University, Atlanta, Georgia, USA

Alberto G Ayala, MD
Department of Pathology & Microbiology, University of Nebraska Medical Center, University Medical Centre, Omaha, Nebraska, USA

George Bakale, PhD
Senior Research Associate, University Hospitals of Cleveland, Case University School of Medicine, Department of Radiology, Division of Nuclear Medicine, Cleveland, Ohio, USA

Steven P Balk, MD
Associate Professor, Cancer Biology Program, Division of Hematology-Oncology, Beth Israel Deaconess Medical Center and Harvard Medical School, Boston, Massachusetts, USA

Lionel L Bañez MD
Staff Scientist, Department of Surgery, Center for Prostate Disease Research, Uniformed Services University of the Health Sciences, Bethesda, Maryland, USA

Albaha Barqawi
Walter Reed Army Medical Center, Washington, District of Columbia, USA

Eric Barret, MD
Senior Urologist, Department of Urology, Institute Montsouris, Paris; University Rene Descartes, Paris, France

George Bartsch, MD
Chairman, Department of Urology, University of Innsbruck, Austria

Clair Beard, MD
Assistant Professor in Radiation Oncology, Brigham and Women's Hospital and Dana Farber Cancer Institute, Department of Radiation Oncology, Boston, Massachusetts, USA

Kathleen W Beekman, MD
Lecturer, University of Michigan Comprehensive Cancer Center, Ann Arbor, Michigan, USA

Andreas Berger, MD
Assistant Professor, Department of Urology, University of Innsbruch, Austria

Jeetesh Bhardwa, MDBhB, MRCS (Eng)
Clinical Assistant in Urology, The London Clinic, London, UK

Isabelle Bisson, PhD
Post-doctoral Research Assistant, Prostate Cancer Research Center, Institute of Urology and Nephrology, University College London, London, UK

Peter Boyle, MD
Director, International Agency for Research on Cancer (IARC), Lyon, France

Michael K Brawer, MD
Director, NW Prostate Institute, Seattle, Washington, USA

Alberto Briganti, MD
Resident in Training, Department of Urology, University Vita Salute San Raffaele, Milan, Italy

James D Brooks, MD
Assistant Professor, Department of Urology, Stanford University School of Medicine, Stanford, California, USA

James A Brown, MD, FACS
Fellow, Vattikuti Urology Institute, Henry Ford Hospital, Detroit, Michigan, USA

Mick D Brown, PhD
Scientific Team Leader, MRC/ProMPT Prostate Cancer Research Collaborative, CRUK Paterson Institute, Christie Hospital, Manchester, UK

Glenn Bubley
Associate Professor of Medicine, Harvard Medical School; Director of GenitoUrinary Oncology, Beth Israel Deaconess, Boston, Massachusetts, USA

Grant Buchanan, PhD
Research Fellow, Dame Roma Mitchell Cancer Research Laboratories, University of Adelaide and Hanson Institute, Adelaide, Australia

Fiona C Burkhard, MD
Staff member, Department of Urology, University Hospital of Bern, Bern, Switzerland

Jason Bylund, MD
Resident, Division of Urology, Department of Surgery, Department of Molecular and Cellular Biochemistry, The Markey Cancer Center, University of Kentucky Medical Center, Lexington, Kentucky, USA

Henning Cammann, PhD
Institute for Medical Informatics, Charité University Medicine Berlin, Germany

Edith Canby-Hagino, MD
Instructor, Department of Urology, The University of Texas Health Science Center at San Antonio, Texas, USA

Eduardo I Canto, MD
Professor, Scott Department of Urology, Houston, Texas, USA

Michael Carducci, MD
Associate Professor of Oncology and Urology; Co-Leader, Prostate Cancer Program; Co-Director, Translational Drug Development, Kimmel Cancer Center, Johns Hopkins Baltimore, Maryland, USA

Peter R Carroll, MD
Professor and Chair, Department of Urology, University of California, San Francisco, California, USA

H Ballentine Carter, MD
Professor of Urology, Brady Urological Institute, The Johns Hopkins Medical Institutions, Baltimore, Maryland, USA

William J Catalona, MD
Professor, Departments of Urology and the Robert H Lurie Comprehensive Cancer Center, Feinberg School of Medicine, Northwestern Memorial Hospital, Chicago, Illinois, USA

Xavier Cathelineau, MD
Senior Urologist, Department of Urology, Institute Montsouris, Paris; University Rene Descartes, Paris, France

Jamie A Cesaretti, MD, MS
Assistant Professor, Mount Sinai School of Medicine, New York, New York, USA

Arul M Chinnaiyan, MD, PhD
Associate Professor of Pathology and Urology, University of Michigan, Ann Arbor, Michigan, USA

Gerald W Chodak, MD FACS
Midwest Urology Research Foundation, Chicago, Illinois, USA

Noel W Clarke, MBBS (Lond), ChM, FRCS(Urol)
Consultant Urologist, Christie and Hope Hospitals, Manchester; Principal Investigator, Manchester arm MRC/ProMPT Prostate Cancer Research Collaborative, Manchester, UK

Donald S Coffey, PhD
Professor of Urology, Pathology, Oncology,
Pharmacology, and Molecular Sciences, The Brady
Urological Institute, The Johns Hopkins Medical
Institutions, Baltimore, Maryland, USA

Timothy S Collins, MD
Medical Oncology Fellow, Duke University Medical
Center, Durham, North Carolina, USA

Robert A Cormack, MD
Physicist, Brigham and Women's Hospital and Dana
Farber Cancer Institute, Department of Radiation
Oncology, Boston, Massachusetts, USA

Jonathan P Coxon, MD
Research Fellow, Department of Urology, St George's
Hospital, London, UK

E David Crawford, MD
Professor of Surgery and Radiation Oncology; Head,
Urologic Oncology, University of Colorado Health
Sciences Center, Colorado, USA

Jeremy Crew, MA, MD, FRCS (Urol)
Consultant Urologist, The Churchill Hospital, Oxford,
Oxfordshire, UK

Anthony V D'Amico, MD, PhD
Professor and Chief of Genitourinary Radiation
Oncology, Brigham and Women's Hospital, Dana Farber
Cancer Institute, Harvard Medical School, Boston,
Massachusetts, USA

Jane Dawoodi, RGN, DN
Urology Specialist Nurse, London Clinic, London, UK

David P Dearnaley, MA, FRCP, FRCR, MD
Professor and Honorary Consultant in Clinical
Oncology, Head of Urology Unit, Royal Marsden
Hospital, Sutton, Surrey, UK

Serdar Deger, MD
Department of Urology, Charite University Medicine
Berlin, Berlin, Germany

Jeffrey Demanes, MD
Radiation Oncologist, California Endocurietherapy
Center, Oakland, California, USA

Theodore L DeWeese, MD
Professor of Radiation Oncology, Urology and
Oncology; Chair, Department of Radiation Oncology
and Molecular Radiation Sciences, Johns Hopkins
University School of Medicine, Baltimore, Maryland,
USA

P Anthony di Sant'Agnese, MD
Professor, Department of Pathology and Laboratory
Medicine, University of Rochester Medical Center,
Rochester, New York, USA

Robert Djavan, MD, PhD
Professor of Urology; Vice Chairman, Department of
Urology; Director Prostate Disease Center; Co-Director
Ludwig Bolzman Institute for Prostatic Disease,
Department of Urology, University of Vienna, Vienna,
Italy

John F Donohue, FRCSI (Urol)
Fellow, Department of Urology, Memorial Sloan-
Kettering Cancer Center, New York, New York, USA

Zach S Dovey, MD
Resident Medical Officer, Department of Uro-oncology,
Cromwell Hospital, London, UK

Brian J Duggan, MD, FRCS (Urol)
Urology Fellow, Monash Medical Centre, Melbourne,
Australia

William D Dunsmuir, FRCS (Urol)
Consultant Urologist, Ashford and St Peters' Hospitals
NHS Trust, Chertsey, UK

James A Eastham, MD
Associate Professor, Memorial Sloan-Kettering Cancer
Center, New York, New York, USA

Mario Eisenberger, MD
R Dale Hughes Professor of Oncology and Urology,
Sidney Kimmel Comprehensive Cancer Center at Johns
Hopkins, Baltimore, USA

Lars Ellison, MD
Assistant Professor, Department of Urology, University
of California, Davis, California, USA

Jonathan I Epstein, MD
Professor of Pathology, Urology and Oncology, Reinhard
Professor of Urological Pathology; Director of Surgical
Pathology, The Johns Hopkins Hospital, Baltimore,
Maryland, USA

Hywel Evans, MA, MBBS, FRCS, FRCR
Consultant Radiologist, Frimley Park Hospital NHS
Foundation Trust, Frimley, Surrey, UK

Peter F Faulhaber, MD
Associate Professor, Case University School of Medicine,
Department of Radiology, Division of Nuclear Medicine,
University Hospitals of Cleveland, Cleveland, Ohio,
USA

Steven J Feigenberg, MD
Assistant Professor, Department of Radiation Oncology,
Fox Chase Cancer Center, Philadelphia, Pennsylvania,
USA

**Mark R Feneley, MD (Cantab), FRCS (Urol),
FRCS (Eng)**
Senior Lecturer in Urological Oncological Surgery,
Institute of Urology, University College London;
Honorary Consultant Urologist, University College
Hospital, London, UK

John M Fitzpatrick, MCh, FRCSI, FC Urol(SA), FRCS Glas, FRCS
Professor of Surgery, Mater Misercordiae Hospital and Conway Institute, University College Dublin, Dublin, Ireland

Charlotte Foley, MRCS
Specialist Registrar in Urology, Institute of Urology and Nephrology, Middlesex Hospital, London, UK

Yan Kit Fong
Ludwig Bolzman Institute for Prostatic Disease, Department of Urology, University of Vienna, Vienna, Italy

Yves Fradet, MD, FRCSC
Professor of Surgery and Urology, Chairman, Department of Surgery, University Laval, Quebec, Canada

Stephen J Freedland, MD
Assistant Professor of Surgery (Urology), Pathology, and Epidemiology, Veterans Administration Medical Center, Durham, Duke University School of Medicine, Durham, North Carolina, USA

A Alex Freeman, BSc, MBBS, MD, MRCPath
Consultant Urological Pathologist, University College Hospital NHS Foundation Trust; Honorary Senior Lecturer, Institute of Urology, University College, London, UK

Marc Galiano, MD
Department of Urology, Institute Montsouris, Paris; Universite Rene Descartes, Paris, France

Razvan Galalae, MD
Radiation Oncologist, Kiel University, Kiel, Germany

Peter H Gann, MD, ScD
Professor, Department of Preventive Medicine and The Robert H Lurie Comprehensive Cancer Center, Feinberg School of Medicine, Northwestern University, Chicago, Illinois, USA

Marc Garnick, MD
Chief Medical Officer, Praecis Pharmaceuticals Inc.; Clinical Professor of Medicine, Harvard Medical School, Beth Israel Deaconess Medical Center, Boston, Massachusetts, USA

Daniel George, MD
Associate Professor of Medicine and Surgery, Duke University Medical Center, Durham, North Carolina, USA

Howard L Geyer, MD, PhD
Assistant Professor, Department of Neurology, Albert Einstein College of Medicine, Yeshiva University, New York, New York, USA

Edward Giovannucci, MD, ScD
Professor of Nutrition and Epidemiology, Harvard School of Public Health; Associate Professor of Medicine, Brigham and Women's Hospital, Harvard Medical School, Boston, Massachusetts, USA

Martin Gleave, MD, FRCSC
Director, Clinical Research, Prostate Center, Vancouver General Hospital, Vancouver, Canada

S Larry Goldenberg, MD
Head of UBC Prostate Clinic, Vancouver General Hospital, Vancouver, Canada

Leonard G Gomella, MD
Professor and Chairman, Department of Urology, Kimmel Cancer Center, Thomas Jefferson University, Philadelphia, Pennsylvania, USA

Jose Gonzalez, MD
Urologist, William Beaumont Hospital, Department of Radiation Oncology, Royal Oak Michigan, Michigan, USA

Norman W Greenberg, PhD
Principal, Norman Greenberg's Lab, Clinical Resarch Division, Fred Hutchinson Cancer Research Center, Seattle, Washington, USA

Gary Gustafson, MD
William Beaumont Hospital, Department of Radiation Oncology, Royal Oak Michigan, Michigan, USA

Misop Han, MD, MS
Assistant Professor, Northwestern Memorial Hospital, Department of Urology, Chicago, Illinois, USA

David M Hartke, MD
Resident, Department of Urology, Case Western Reserve University School of Medicine, University Hospitals of Cleveland, Cleveland, Ohio, USA

Ashok K Hemal, MD, MCh, FACS
Professor, Department of Urology, All India Institute of Medical Sciences, Ansari Nagar, New Delhi, India

Mitchell Hollander, MD
Urologist, William Beaumont Hospital, Department of Radiation Oncology, Royal Oak Michigan, Michigan, USA

Jeffrey M Holzbeierlein
Assistant Professor of Urology, University of Kansas Hospital, Kansas, USA

Wolfgang Horninger
Associate Professor of Urology, Head of Prostate Cancer Center, Department of Urology, Innsbruck Medical University, Innsbruck, Austria

Eric M Horwitz, MD
Clinical Director and Associate Professor, Department of Radiation Oncology, Fox Chase Cancer Center, Philadelphia, Pennsylvania, USA

Hedvig Hricak, MD, DrMedSc
Chairman, Department of Radiology, Carroll and Milton Petrie Chair; Professor of Radiology, Weill Medical College of Cornell University, Memorial Sloan-Kettering Cancer Center, New York, New York, USA

Jiaoti Huang, MD, PhD
Associate Professor, Department of Pathology and
Laboratory Medicine, University of Rochester Medical
Center, Rochester, New York, USA

Peter A Humphrey, MD, PhD
Professor of Pathology and Immunology, Washington
University School of Medicine, St Louis, Missouri, USA

Mark D Hurwitz, MD
Assistant Professor in Radiation Oncology, Brigham and
Women's Hospital and Dana Farber Cancer Institute,
Department of Radiation Oncology, Boston,
Massachusetts, USA

William Isaacs, MD
The Johns Hopkins University School of Medicine,
Department of Urology, Baltimore, USA

Salma K Jabbour, MD
Chief Resident, Department of Radiation Oncology and
Molecular Radiation Sciences, Johns Hopkins University
School of Medicine, Baltimore, Maryland, USA

Andrew Jackson, MD
Assistant Research Professor, Genitourinary Cancer
Immunotherapy Program, Division of Urology,
Department of Surgery, Duke University Medical Center,
Durham, North Carolina, USA

Thomas L Jang, MD, MPH
Department of Urology, Feinberg School of Medicine,
Northwestern University, Chicago, Illinois, USA

William Jonas, MD
Fellow, Winship Cancer Insitute, Emory University,
Atlanta, Georgia, USA

Klaus Jung, MD
Professor, Department of Urology, Charité Hospital of
Humbolt University, Berlin, Germany

Daniel Kahn, MD
Associate Professor, University of Iowa Department of
Radiology; Chief, Nuclear Medicine Section, Veterans
Administration Medical Center, Iowa City, Iowa, USA

Johnny Kao, MD
Assistant Professor, Mount Sinai School of Medicine,
New York, New York, USA

Michael Kattan, PhD
Chair, Department of Quantitative Health Sciences, The
Cleveland Clinic Foundation, Cleveland, Ohio, USA

Vincent Khoo, MBBS, FRACR, FRCR, MD
Consultant in Clinical Oncology, Royal Marsden
Hospital, London, UK

Michael Kirby, MBBS, LRCP, MRCS, FRCP
Director, Hertfordshire Primary Care Research Network,
Letchworth, Hertfordshire, UK

Roger S Kirby, MD, FRCS (Urol)
Professor, Directory, The Prostate Centre, London;
Visiting Professor of Urology, St. Georges Hospital,
Healthcare Trust, London; Honorary Professor, Institute
of Urology, University College London, London, UK

David Kirk, DM, FRCS
Consultant Urologist, Gartnavel General Hospital,
Glasgow; Honorary Professor, University of Glasgow,
Glasgow, UK

Adam P Klausner, MD
Assistant Professor of Urology, Department of Urology,
University of Virginia and Medical College of Virginia,
Charlottesville, Virginia, USA

Eric A Klein, MD
Head, Section of Urologic Oncology, Glickman
Urological Institute, Cleveland; Professor of Surgery,
Cleveland Clinic Lerner College of Medicine, Cleveland
Clinic Foundation, Cleveland, Ohio, USA

Helmut Klocker, MD
Professor, Research Laboratory of the Department of
Urology, Innsbruck Medical University, Innsbruck,
Austria

Laurence Klotz, MD
Professor, Department of Surgery, University of Toronto,
Toronto; Chief, Division of Urology, Sunnybrook and
Women's Health Sciences Center, Toronto, Ontario,
Canada

Badrinath R Konety, MD
Assistant Professor, University of Iowa Departments of
Urology and Epidemiology, Iowa; Chief, Section of
Urology, Veterans Administration Medical Center, Iowa
City, Iowa, USA

Natasha Kyprianou, PhD
Professor of Urology, Molecular Biology and Pathology,
Division of Urology, University of Kentucky Medical
Center, Lexington, Kentucky, USA

John S Lam, MD
Clinical Instructor in Urology, Department of Urology,
David Geffen School of Medicine at University of
California-Los Angeles, Los Angeles, California, USA

Paul H Lange, MD, FACS
Professor and Chair, Department of Urology, University
of Washington, Seattle, Washington, USA

Robin J Leach, PhD
Professor, Department of Cellular and Structural
Biology, The University of Texas Health Science Center
at San Antonia, Texas, USA

Dan Leibovici, MD
Senior Urologist, Department of Urology, Assef-Harofeh
Medical Center, Zerifin, Israel

Herbert Lepor, MD
Professor and Martin Spatz Chairman, Department of Urology, New York University School of Medicine, New York, New York, USA

Daniel W Lin, MD
Assistant Professor, University of Washington, Washington, USA

Sarah Linstrom, MD
Department of Radiation Sciences, Oncology, University of Umeå, Umeå, Sweden

Massimo Loda, MD
Associate Professor of Pathology, Harvard Medical School, Dana Farber Cancer Institute, Brigham and Women's Hospital, Boston, Massachusetts, USA

Stefan A Loening, MD, FRCPR
Professor, Head, Department of Urology, Charité University Medicine Berlin, Germany

Gregory T MacLennan, MD
Associate Professor of Pathology, Urology and Oncology, Department of Pathology, University Hospitals of Cleveland, Case University School of Medicine, Department of Radiology, Division of Nuclear Medicine, Cleveland, Ohio, USA

John H Makari,
Chief Resident, The George Washington University, Washington, District of Columbia, USA

Kozhaya N Mallah, MD
Internal Medicine Residency Program, Saint Michael's Medical Center, Newark, New Jersey, USA

Murugesan Manoharan, MD
Assistant Professor of Urology, University of Miami School of Medicine, Miami, Florida, USA

Michael J Manyak, MD, FACS
Vice President of Medical Affairs, Cytogen Corporation, Princeton, New Jersey, USA

Susan Ruth Marengo, PhD
Associate Professor, Departments of Urology, Pathology, Cancer Center; Director, Jim and Eilleen Dicke Research Laboratory, Case Western Reserve University, Cleveland, Ohio, USA

Paul D Maroni, MD
Resident in Urology, University of Colorado and Denver Health Sciences Center, Colorado, USA

Alvaro A Martinez, MD, FACR
William Beaumont Hospital, Department of Radiation Oncology, Royal Oak Michigan, Michigan, USA

John R Masters, PhD, FRCPath
Professor, Experimental Pathology, Prostate Cancer Research Center, Institute of Urology, University College London, London, UK

David McLeod, MD
Residency Program Director and Director, Urologic Oncology, Walter Reed Army Medical Center, Washington, District of Columbia, USA

Alan K Meeker, PhD
Assistant Professor, Department of Pathology, Division of Genitourinary Pathology, The Sidney Kimmel Comprehensive Cancer Center at Johns Hopkins Medical Institutions, Baltimore, Maryland, USA

Maxwell Meng, MD
Department of Urology, University of California San Francisco Comprehensive Cancer Center School of Medicine, San Francisco, California, USA

Mani Menon, MD, FACS
Raj and Padma Vattikuti Distinguished Chair, Professor, Department of Urology, Case Western Reserve University School of Medicine, Cleveland, Ohio; Director, Vattikuti Urology Institute, Henry Ford Hospital, Detroit, Michigan, USA

David Miller, MD
Health Services Research Fellow, Department of Urology, University of Michigan Urology Center, Ann Arbor, Michigan, USA

Leslie Moffat, BSc, MB, MBA, FRCS (Ed & Glas), FACS, FRCP (Ed),
Senior Lecturer, University of Aberdeen, Department of Urology, Aberdeen Royal Infirmary, Aberdeen, UK

Francesco Montorsi, MD
Associate Professor, Department of Urology, University Vita Salute San Raffaele, Milan, Italy

Alvaro Morales, MD, FRCSC, FACS
Emeritus Professor, Director, Centre of Advanced Urological Research, Queen's University, Kingston, Ontario, USA

Camille Motta, PhD
Professor, Department of Medical Information, Praecis Pharmaceuticals Inc., Waltham, Massachusetts, USA

Judd W Moul, MD, FACS
Professor and Chief, Division of Urologic Surgery, Duke University Medical Center, Durham, North Carolina, USA

Mark A Moyad, MD, MPH
Phil F Jenkins Director of Complimentary Medicine, Urologic Oncology, Clinical Cancer Researcher/ Consultant, University of Michigan, Ann Arbour, Michigan, USA

Robert P Myers, MD
Consultant, Department of Urology, Mayo Clinic, Rochester, Minnesota, USA

A Dennis Nelson, PhD
President, MIMVista Corporation, Cleveland, Ohio, USA

Joel B Nelson, MD
Professor and Chairman, Department of Urology, Pittsburgh, Pennsylvania, USA

Donald Newling
Medical Director (Urology), AstraZeneca plc, Macclesfield, Cheshire, UK

Nils Nuernberg, MD
Radiation Oncologist, Kiel University, Kiel, Germany

Grenville M Oades
Specialist Registrar in Urology, Glasgow, UK

Wilhelm Oberaigner, MD
Director, Tyrol Cancer Registry, Austria

Lincol Olsen,
Resident, Department of Urology, University of Kansas Hospital, Kansas, USA

Jonathan R Osborn, MB ChB MSc MRCS
Research Fellow, Midwest Urology Research Foundation, Chicago, Illinois, USA

Ajay Pahuja, MS, FRCS (Ed)
Senior House Officer Urology, Ashford and St Peters' Hospitals NHS Trust, Chertsey, UK

Christopher Parker, BA, MRCP, MD, FRCP
Senior Lecturer and Honorary Consultant in Clinical Oncology, Academic Urology Unit, Institute of Cancer Research and Royal Marsden Hospital, Sutton, Surrey, UK

J Kellogg Parsons, MD, MHS
Assistant Professor of Surgery/Urology, Division of Urology, University of California, San Diego, California, USA

Alan W Partin, MD
David Hall McConnell Professor and Director, The Brady Urological Institute, The Johns Hopkins Medical Institute, Baltimore, Maryland, USA

Uday Patel, MRCP, FRCR
Consultant Radiologist, St George's Hospital and Medical School, London, UK

Alexandre Pelzer, MD
Assistant Professor, Department of Urology, University of Innsbruck, Austria

David F Penson, MD, MPH
Associate Professor of Urology and Preventive Medicine, Keck School of Medicine, University of Southern California, Los Angeles, California, USA

Louis L Pisters, MD
Associate Professor, The University of Texas M.D. Anderson Cancer Center, Houston, Texas, USA

Elizabeth A Platz, ScD, MPH
Associate Professor of Epidemiology, Johns Hopkins Bloomberg School of Public Health; The James Buchanan Brady Urological Institute; The Sidney Kimmel Comprehensive Cancer Center, Johns Hopkins Medical Institutions, Baltimore, Maryland, USA

Alan Pollack, MD
Chairman and Professor, The Gerald E Hanks Endowed Chair in Radiation Oncology, Department of Radiation Oncology, Fox Chase Cancer Center, Philadelphia, Pennsylvania, USA

Kati P Porkka, PhD
Post-doctoral Fellow, Institute of Medical Technology, University of Tampere and Tampere University Hospital, Tampere, Finland

Marcus L Quek, MD
Urologic Oncology Fellow, Keck School of Medicine, University of Southern California, Los Angeles, California, USA

Jowad Raja, MBChB, MRCS, FRCR
Specialist Registrar, Radiology, St. Georges Hospital NHS Trust, London, UK

Navin Ramachandran, MBBS
Registrar in Radiology, St George's Hospital, London, UK

J Robert Ramey, MD
Resident, Department of Urology, Kimmel Cancer Center, Thomas Jefferson University, Philadelphia, Pennsylvania, USA

Charlotte Rees, BSc, MEd, PhD, CPsychol
Senior Lecturer in Medical Education, Peninsula Medical School, Universities of Exeter and Plymouth, Devon, UK

Robert E Reiter, MD
Professor of Urology, Department of Urology; Co-Director, Prostate Cancer Program; Associate Director, Genitourinary Oncology Program Area, Jonsson Comprehensive Cancer Center, David Geffen School of Medicine at University of California-Los Angeles, Los Angeles, California, USA

Martin I Resnick, MD
Lester Persky Professor and Chairman, Department of Urology, Case Western Reserve University School of Medicine, University Hospitals of Cleveland, Cleveland, Ohio, USA

Patrizio Rigatti, MD
Professor and Chairman, Department of Urology, University Vita Salute San Raffaele, Milan, Italy

Chris Robertson, MD
Statistician, International Agency for Research on Cancer (IARC), Lyon, France

Mark Rochester, MA, MD, MRCS
Specialist Registrar in Urological Surgery, Norfolk and Norwich University Hospital, Norwich, Norfolk, UK

Rodney Rodriguez, MD
Radiation Oncologist, California Endocurietherapy Center, Oakland, California, USA

Francois Rozet, MD
Senior Urologist, Department of Urology, Institute Montsouris, Paris; University Rene Descartes, Paris, France

Mark Rubin, MD
Associate Professor of Pathology, Harvard Medical School, Brigham and Women's Hospital, Boston, Massachusetts, USA

Andrea Salonia, MD
Fellow, Department of Urology, University Vita Salute San Raffaele, Milan, Italy

Jack A Schalken, PhD
Professor of Experimental Urology, Department of Urology, Radboud University Nijmegen Medical Centre, Nijmegen, The Netherlands

Paul Schellhammer, MD
Program Director, Virginia Prostate Center; Professor of Urology, Eastern Virginia Medical School, Norfolk, Virginia, USA

Howard Scher, MD
D Wayne Calloway Chair in Urologic Oncology, Attending Physician and Chief, Genitourinary Oncology Service, Department of Medicine, Sidney Kimmel Center for Prostate and Urologic Cancers, Memorial Sloan-Kettering Cancer Center, New York, New York, USA

Dieter Schonitzer, MD
Chairman, Institute of Transfusion Medicine, University of Innsbruck, Austria

Fritz H Schröder
Professor and Chair, Department of Urology, Erasmus University, Rotterdam, The Netherlands

Martin Schumacher, MD
Staff member, Department of Urology, University Hospital of Bern, Bern, Switzerland

William A See, MD
Professor and Chairman, Department of Urology, Medical College of Wisconsin, Milwaukee, Wisconsin, USA

Gianluca Severi, MD
Statistician, International Agency for Research on Cancer (IARC), Lyon, France

Jonathan W Simons, MD
Director, Winship Cancer Institute, Emory University, Atlanta, Georgia, USA

Kevin M Slawin, MD
Resident, Scott Department of Urology, Houston, Texas, USA

D Bruce Sodee, MD
Professor of Radiology/Nuclear Medicine, University Hospitals of Cleveland, Case Western Reserve, Cleveland, Ohio, USA

Mark Soloway, M.D.
Professor and Chairman, Department of Urology, University of Miami Miller School of Medicine, Miami, Florida, USA

Danny Y Song, MD
Assistant Professor of Radiation Oncology, Urology and Oncology, Department of Radiation Oncology and Molecular Medicine, Johns Hopkins University School of Medicine, The Sidney Kimmel Comprehensive Cancer Center, Baltimore, Maryland, USA

Shiv Srivastava, PhD
Co-Director and Scientific Director, Center for Prostate Disease Research; Professor of Surgery, Department of Surgery, Uniformed Services University of the Health Sciences, Bethesda, Maryland, USA

Thomas A Stamey
University of Stanford, Faculty of Medicine, Stanford, California, USA

William D Steers, MD
Hovey Dabney Professor and Chair, Department of Urology, University of Virginia School of Medicine, Charlottesville, Virginia, USA

Carsten Stephan, MD
Resident, Department of Urology, Charite Hospital, Berlin, Germany

Richard G Stock, MD
Professor and Chairman of Radiation Oncology, Mount Sinai School of Medicine, New York, New York, USA

Nelson N Stone, MD
Clinical Professor of Urology and Radiation Oncology, Mount Sinai School of Medicine, New York, New York, USA

Urs E Studer, MD
Chairman and Professor, Department of Urology, University Hospital of Bern, Bern, Switzerland

Brent W Sutherland, PhD
Post-doctoral Fellow, Norm Greenberg's Lab, Clinical Resarch Division, Fred Hutchinson Cancer Research Center, Seattle, Washington, USA

Anatasias Tahmatzopoulos
Post-Doctoral Fellow, Division of Urology, Department of Surgery, Department of Molecular and Cellular Biochemistry, The Markey Cancer Center, University of Kentucky Medical Center, Lexington, Kentucky, USA

Clare M Tempany, MD
Professor of Radiology, Harvard Medical School;
Director of Clinical MRI, Department of Radiology,
Brigham and Women's Hospital and Dana Farber
Cancer Institute, Departments of Radiation Oncology
and Radiology, Boston, Massachusetts, USA

Ian M Thompson, MD
Chair, Department of Urology, The University of Texas
Health Science Center at San Antonio, Texas, USA

J Brantley Thrasher
Professor and William L Valk Chair, Department of
Urology, University of Kansas Hospital, Kansas, USA

Wayne D Tilley, PhD
Chair, Dame Roma Mitchell Chair in Cancer Research
Laboratories, University of Adelaide and Hanson
Institute, Adelaide, Australia

Bruce J Trock, PhD,
Director of Epidemiology, Brady Urological Institute;
Associate Professor of Urology, Epidemiology,
Oncology, and Environmental Health Sciences, Johns
Hopkins School of Medicine, Baltimore, Maryland,
USA

Natalie Tschan
Department of Urology, University Hospital of Bern,
Bern, Switzerland

Guy Vallancien, MD
Professor, Department of Urology, Institute Montsouris,
Paris; University Rene Descartes, Paris, France

Carlos Vargas, MD
William Beaumont Hospital, Department of Radiation
Oncology, Royal Oak Michigan, Michigan, USA

Robert W Veltri, PhD
Associate Professor, Department of Urology, Brady
Urological Institute, Baltimore, Maryland, USA

Johannes Vieweg, MD, FACS
Associate Professor of Urology, Associate Professor of
Immunology, Vice Chief of Research, Division of
Urology, Duke University Medical Center, Durham,
North Carolina, USA

Arnauld Villers, MD, PhD
Professor in Urology, Service d'Urologie, Hopital Huriez,
Centre Hospitalier Regional University, Lille, France

Tapio Visakorpi, MD, PhD
Professor of Cancer Genetics, Institute of Medical
Technology, University of Tampere, and Tampere
University Hospital, Tampere, Finland

Alessandro Volpe, MD
Fellow, Division of Urology, Department of Surgical
Oncology, Sunnybrook and Women's College Health
Sciences Center, Toronto, Ontario, Canada

Eugene V Vykhovanets, MD, PhD
Postdoctoral Fellow, Jim and Eilleen Dicke Research
Laboratory, Department of Urology, Case Western
Reserve University, Cleveland, Ohio, USA

Patrick C Walsh
University Distinguished Service Professor of Urology,
The James Buchanan Brady Urological Institute, Johns
Hopkins Medical Institutions, Baltimore, Maryland, USA

Sinead E Walsh, BSc
Post graduate student,
Mater Misercordiae Hospital and Conway Institute,
University College Dublin, Dublin, Ireland

R William G Watson, BSc, Phd
Senior Lecturer, Mater Misercordiae Hospital and
Conway Institute, University College Dublin, Dublin,
Ireland

John T Wei, MD, MS
Associate Professor, Director, Division of Clinical
Research and Quality Assurance, University of Michigan
Urology Center, Ann Arbor, Michigan, USA

Brian Wells, MD, FRCPsch
Consultant Psychiatrist, The Prostate Centre, London, UK

Richard D Williams, MD
Professor and Head, Rubin Flock Chair, Department of
Urology, University of Iowa, Iowa City, Iowa, USA

Ulrich Karl Friedrich Witzsch, MD
Professor and Chair E Becht, Chief of Urology,
Krankenhaus Nordwest Hospital for urology and child
urology, Frankfurt, Germany

Jianfeng Xu, MD, Dr PH
Professor of Public Health and Cancer Biology; Director,
Program for Genetic and Molecular Epidemiology of
Cancer; Associate Director, Center for Human
Genomics, Wake Forest University School of Medicine,
Winston-Salem, North Carolina, USA

Jorge L Yao, MD
Assistant Professor, Department of Pathology and
Laboratory Medicine, University of Rochester Medical
Center, Rochester, New York, USA

Alexandre R Zlotta, MD
Associate Professor of Urology, Department of Urology,
Erasme Hospital, University Clinics of Brussels, Belgium

Foreword

By any measure, prostate cancer is a major public health problem throughout the developed world. Already the leading cause of internal cancer in men, the number of new cases per year is expected to increase substantially in coming decades. The age-specific incidence rate is rising and screening is becoming more prevalent. No cancer increases in incidence with age more rapidly than prostate cancer, and the male population is aging steadily. Some epidemiologists have predicted that the number of new cases per year in the United States will rise from 230,000 in 2005 to 350,000 by 2025.

Despite widespread misperception, prostate cancer is no "toothless lion". This year we expect some 30,000 deaths from this disease in North America and the same number in Europe. About 3.5% of all male deaths are from prostate cancer, making the lifetime risk that a man will die of this disease about 1 in 28. This compares to the lifetime risk of dying in an automobile accident about 1 in 4,000 or in a commercial airline accident about 1 in 100,000.[1]

Nearly every aspect of this disease generates controversy within the medical profession and consternation among patients and their families. While dietary fat as been repeatedly associated with the risk of developing or dying of prostate cancer, there is no compelling evidence that dietary alterations or any micronutrients can prevent or modify the course of the disease. Deficiencies of certain vitamins, minerals or micronutrients have been associated with an increased risk as well, but no prospective studies have yet demonstrated a benefit for any dietary supplement except in individuals deficient at baseline. Chemoprevention may indeed be possible with hormonally active agents such as 5-alpha reductase inhibitors, but the only trial reported also found an absolute increase in the risk of high grade cancers with finasteride compared to placebo. Further studies may clarify the issue, dismissing the high grade cancers as an artifact of over detection in the smaller, finasteride-treated prostates. But these drugs do have sexual side effects that make them less attractive than a vitamin supplement, for example, and it is not clear who would benefit – all men or only those at substantially increased risk.

Diagnosis and staging are no less controversial. While annual screening with PSA and DRE will almost always detect a cancer before it becomes metastatic, the benefits of screening large populations remain unproven. The PSA test has dramatically altered the stage at diagnosis in the US, where the mortality rate from prostate cancer, corrected for age, has decreased more than 25% since 1992. Nevertheless, the PSA test has been criticized for its lack of specificity[2] and for over detection of innocuous cancers which may not cause symptoms or early demise within a man's remaining lifespan.

After diagnosis, treatment decisions are hampered by the difficulties in staging the disease. Prostate cancers are most often detected by multiple, "systematic" needle biopsies rather than targeted biopsy of a palpable nodule or a lesion visible by imaging. Once detected, the size, location and extent of the lesion, as well as its grade, are difficult to determine with precision. Clinicians widely believe that biopsy results underestimate the extent of the cancer, and they lack confidence in imaging, despite real progress in the quality of endorectal magnetic resonance imaging and spectroscopy. Their recommendations for treatment, therefore, arise from a profound sense of uncertainty about the precise nature of the cancer they are treating. Few prostate cancers detected today are metastatic at diagnosis, yet physicians hesitate to omit bone scans and computed tomography scans for fear of missing a metastatic site.[3]

In this atmosphere it is no wonder treatment decisions are so difficult for patients and their physicians. Thanks to the efforts of investigators from Sweden, we now have convincing evidence that treatment alters the natural history of the disease, answering Whitmore's classic question: "is treatment possible when necessary?" In a prospective randomized trial surgery reduced the risk of metastases and of death from prostate cancer and prolonged overall survival compared to watchful waiting.[4] Definitive therapy with surgery or radiation controls most early stage cancers and many high grade or locally advanced tumors.[5] Nevertheless, every effective treatment modality carries some risk of serious adverse effects on sexual, urinary and bowel function. "Watchful waiting" – simply ignoring the disease until the appearance of symptoms – has few advocates today, but there is growing interest in "active monitoring" or "deferred therapy," postponing definitive treatment until there are clear signs of progression.[6] This approach avoids the immediate impact of treatment on quality of life, but raises patients' anxiety about the sudden development of metastases and the need for more aggressive therapy, with greater morbidity, when progressive growth of the local tumor is recognized. Do we really have a way to identify local progression before the risk of metastases increases significantly?

For the patient who chooses active rather than deferred therapy, which treatment is best: radical prostatectomy, external beam irradiation, brachytherapy or some combination? While most agree that brachytherapy alone should be reserved for low risk cancers, the indications for other approaches overlap, leaving patients and their physicians in a quandary. We simply do not have data to document the relative benefits and risks of each form of therapy, as there have been few comparative trials. Not only do the treatments differ in timing of onset and degree of risk of side effects, but the likelihood of cancer control and the rate of complications and side effects depend as much on the specific technique employed and the expertise of the treating physician as on the method of therapy chosen.[7] Furthermore, local therapy continues to evolve, periodically refined by improvements in technology (laparoscopic and robotic assisted prostatectomy, intensity modulated and proton beam irradiation therapy). Evaluating and comparing outcomes in this dynamic setting is challenging.

Advanced prostate cancer responds, often dramatically, to androgen deprivation therapy, but the timing and nature of hormonal therapy remain steeped in controversy. Few advocate androgen deprivation for localized cancer, and all agree that such therapy is essential for symptomatic metastases, but the use of hormones as adjuvant therapy before and after local therapy, the time to intervene in men with a rising PSA after definitive local therapy, and the benefits of continuous versus intermittent therapy are not settled.

Only recently has chemotherapy (docetaxel) been shown to prolong life in men with hormone refractory prostate cancer. Studies are just being initiated to determine the benefits of chemotherapy earlier in the course of the disease – for rising PSA only and as adjuvant therapy for high risk cancers after surgery. Combination chemotherapy has not yet been proven superior to docetaxel as a single agent, but, again, studies are underway.

Novel techniques for systemic therapy emerge regularly, faster than clinical trials can fully evaluate them. The first hint that immunotherapy may prolong survival appeared this past year. Biological agents that target angiogenesis, bone metastases, the androgen receptor or other signaling pathways, and tumor antigens are all in clinical trials.

This is an exciting time for those who have long labored in the field of prostate cancer, and this new, comprehensive textbook fully captures that excitement. Authored by the world's leading authorities in prostate cancer biomedical research and clinical care, each chapter delivers a clear, concise, authoritative view of the state-of-the-science. Every controversy in the modern understanding and management of prostate cancer is thoroughly covered. Drs. Kirby, Partin, Feneley and Parsons, and the authors they have chosen, have produced a gem. Their timing is perfect. This elegant text will efficiently bring students of this disease up to date, clarify issues for seasoned investigators, and provide the practicing physician with a reliable, contemporary guide to the modern management of this common, controversial cancer.

Peter T Scardino, MD
Memorial Sloan-Kettering Cancer Center
New York, New York, USA

REFERENCES

1. Scardino PT and Kelman JK. Dr. Peter Scardino's Prostate Book. New York: Avery Press, 2005.

2. Stamey TA, Caldwell M, McNeal JE, Nolley R, Hemenez M, Downs J. The prostate specific antigen era in the United States is over for Prostate Cancer: What happened in the last 20 years? Journal of Urology 2004; 172:1297–1301.

3. Cooperberg MR, Lubeck DP, Grossfeld GD, Mehta SS, Carroll PR. Contemporary Trends in Imaging Test Utilization for Prostate Cancer Staging: Data from the Cancer of the Prostate Strategic Urologic Research Endeavor. Journal of Urology 2002; 168:491–495.

4. Bill-Axelson A, Holmberg L, Ruutu M, Haggman M, Andersson SO, Bratell S, Spangberg A, Busch C, Nordling S, Garmo H, Palmgren J, Adami HO, Norlen BJ, Johansson JE; Scandinavian Prostate Cancer Group Study No. 4. Radical prostatectomy versus watchful waiting in early prostate cancer. N Engl J Med 2005; 352:1977–84.

5. Ohori M, Scardino PT. Localized prostate cancer. Curr Probl Surg 2002: 39:833–957.

6. Patel MI, DeConcini DT, Lopez-Corona E, Ohori M, Wheeler T, Scardino PT. An analysis of men with clinically localized prostate cancer who deferred definitive therapy. J Urol 2004: 171:1520-1524.

7. Begg CB, Riedel ER, Bach PB, Kattan MW, Schrag D, Warren JL, Scardino PT. Variations in morbidity after radical prostatectomy. N Engl J Med 2002: 346:1138–1144.

Preface

Although there are a number of admirable books on prostate cancer already available, nearly all of them reflect the views of a relatively small number of individuals or institutions. By contrast, when we conceived *Prostate Cancer: Principles and Practice* we employed a different approach. We met in Baltimore to draw up a list of the great and the good in prostate cancer, we noted their specific area of expertise and we wrote to invite them to contribute. Fortunately nearly everyone we asked accepted readily, and that is why the author list of this volume reads like a "Who's Who" of prostate cancer and constitutes a state-of-the-art account of the problem.

Cancer of the prostate continues to challenge the medical profession and to sufferers in a number of ways. Why is the disease so prevalent and what is its molecular and genetic basis? Can it be prevented and what are the optimum ways to diagnose and stage the disorder? How can we distinguish the "tigers", which may be rapidly fatal, from the "pussy cats" which pose little or no threat to the sufferer? Which treatment option should be selected for which individual? All of these crucial issues, and very many more, are addressed in this volume, which represents the most definitive text on this subject to date.

Although in truth we have to concede that many of these questions remain either equivocal or unanswered, a number of the issues are now being clarified. It will certainly be some time before the scourge of prostate malignancy is comprehensively defeated. In the meantime we sincerely hope that the up-to-date information presented in this book will serve to inform the healthcare professionals in both urology and oncology, and perhaps in family practice. As a consequence it should help them care more effectively for the very many current and future sufferers of prostate cancer as well as to provide much needed support for their families and loved ones.

Roger S Kirby, Alan W Partin, Mark R Feneley and
J Kellogg Parsons

Acknowledgments

We would like to thank Alan Burgess and Rupal Malde at Taylor and Francis; Dee McLean, medical artist; and the team at Naughton Project Management, in particular Kathy Syplywczak.

Introduction

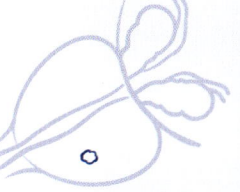

Prostate cancer: the last twenty years

1

Thomas A Stamey

To a large extent, the modern history of prostate cancer is intrinsically related to serum prostate-specific antigen (PSA)[1] and to the recognition of the great utility of the Gleason histologic grading system.[2,3] We reported in 1987 that preoperative serum PSA was proportional to the size of the *palpable* cancer on digital rectal examination.[1] Cancer volume was accurately measured in histologic sections of the prostate cut at 3 mm intervals, as were all other histologic variables, the most important of which was an assessment of the Gleason grade in the largest cancer. Dr Gleason spent 2 days with Dr McNeal and I at Stanford in those early years to make sure we fully understood the merits of his new and powerful five-point grading system, and Drs McNeal and Gleason later co-authored a paper on prostate cancer.[3] We showed in 1999 that for every 10% increase in Gleason grades 4 and 5 (Figure 1.1) in the largest cancer of the radical prostatectomy specimen, we lost 10% cures on follow-up as measured by a postoperative, rising serum PSA.[4] To my knowledge, no patient whose prostate contained only Gleason grades 1, 2, or 3 cancer has ever died from prostate cancer.

These observations mean that an accurate, unequivocal estimate of the amount of Gleason grade 4/5 cancer in biopsies, and especially in radical prostatectomy specimens, is the key to advising patients about the chances of a cure from prostate cancer. Perhaps more importantly for this book, Gleason grade 4/5 cancer is also the key to directing future research at the molecular level in prostate cancer. Both clinicians and basic scientists need to recognize that Gleason grade 4/5 cancer is not a late development in the histologic history of prostate cancer; in fact, it occurs in 30% to 40% of radical prostatectomies at Stanford in which the largest cancer in the prostate is less than 0.5 mL in volume.

Because almost all untreated radical prostatectomies at Stanford and at the Palo Alto Medical Clinic since 1983 have been examined quantitatively in 3-mm step-sections in the Department of Urology by John McNeal (an expert pathologist who has devoted his professional career exclusively to the histologic study of prostate cancer), we believe these observations are valid.

However, any reader of the chapters that follow in this book needs to recognize that a highly significant, unexpected change has occurred in the natural morphology of prostate cancer in the past 20 years, at least in the United States, and probably in other countries as well that have experienced such extensive PSA screening.[5] At Stanford, from 1983 to 1988 92% of radical prostatectomies were performed for palpable cancers on digital rectal examination; in the recent

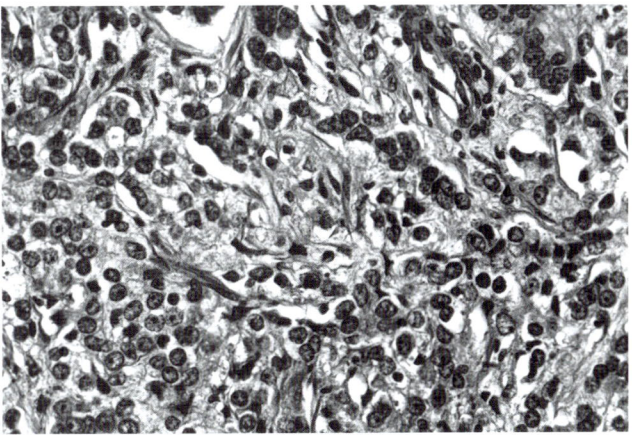

Fig. 1.1

An example of an undifferentiated Gleason grade 4/5 cancer from a radical prostatectomy specimen.

5-year period ending 7/1/2004 only 17% of cancers were palpable. Of the six histologic cancer variables that are routinely measured quantitatively in every radical prostatectomy, *only* prostate weight now correlates with preoperative serum PSA in the most recent 5-year period ending July 2004 (i.e., benign prostatic hyperplasia [BPH]: Pearson correlation 0.246, $P < 0.001$).[5] In the earlier 5-year period, August, 1983–December, 1988 PSA related strongly to almost all morphologic variables: the volume of the largest cancer, the amount of capsular penetration, positive lymph nodes, seminal vesicle invasion, and the percentage of the largest cancer that was Gleason grade 4/5.[5] Importantly, prostate weight (BPH) in this period was also strongly related to preoperative serum PSA with similar coefficients as in the more recent 5-year period, clearly indicating how strongly serum PSA has been related to the amount of BPH since the very inception of measurements for serum PSA.[5] Moreover, the recent work by Roehrborn et al[6] on the placebo control arm of the Proscar long-term efficacy and safety study (PLESS), which included men with six negative sextant biopsies and enlarged prostates followed for several years with serial magnetic resonance imaging (MRI) studies of the prostate to measure accurately the volume of the prostate, shows clearly that serum PSA between 2 and 10 ng/mL is caused by BPH. In fact, if you tell these investigators that a man's serum PSA is 3.6, they will tell you the size of his prostate.

In our 20-year morphologic analysis of the relationship of preoperative serum PSA to cancer volume in the prostate,[5] it is important to recognize that prostate weight has a highly significant and strong correlation with preoperative serum PSA across *all four 5-year periods*, even though the size of the cancer continuously decreases.[5] This means that we have been carrying out biopsies of prostates in the past 20 years largely because of PSA liberated from BPH. This being so, why do we find so much cancer on biopsy at almost any level of serum PSA? It is because prostate cancer is age related and highly ubiquitous in whites and African Americans in the United States; it begins in men in both races in their 20s and increases steadily with each passing decade until 80% have cancer in their 70s.[7] When we biopsy men because of PSA driven by BPH between 2 and 10 ng/mL of PSA and sometimes between 10 and 20 ng/mL, for the most part their PSA is related to BPH. It is interesting and important that the correlations and p-values for serum PSA and prostate weight are virtually identical and highly significant across all four 5-year periods ending in 2003.[5]

As I have studied the list of outstanding authors and the interesting titles of their research efforts in this book, there must be several authors within these pages who hold the key in their laboratory records that could lead to a new marker specific for prostate cancer. Since for every 10% increase in Gleason grade 4/5 within the index (largest) cancer in the peripheral zone of the prostate, we lose 10% of cures after radical prostatectomy,[4] there cannot be any question as to what a new prostate cancer serum marker must be based on: the amount of Gleason grade 4/5 in the largest peripheral zone cancer. It is true that 20% of the time the index cancer is located in the transition zone where it originates in BPH nodules; however, these cancers usually liberate very large amounts of PSA into the serum (for the same reason that BPH nodules liberate PSA into the serum), and are much more easily cured even when there are much higher levels of serum PSA than peripheral zone cancers of similar size.

Since virtually all men get prostate cancer (starting as early as the third decade of life in 8% of men[7]), any useful serum marker must be proportional to the volume of Gleason grade 4/5 cancer based on the fact that for every 10% increase in grade 4/5, we lose 10% of cures by radical prostatectomy.[4] The superb research talent chosen for Section 4 on the Molecular Mechanisms of Prostate Carcinogenesis of this book should continually search their laboratory records for *any* possibility of a new serum marker that might be proportional to the amount of grade 4/5 cancer in the prostate, whether this potential is for new genes or proteins. It will not be easy. Unfortunately, all we need to ask ourselves is how many serum cancer markers available today are proportional to the amount of cancer within the organ of origin; the answer is virtually none. Nevertheless, we urgently need something to stop the wholesale overdiagnosis of prostate cancer based on serum PSA and its tragic consequences of over-treatment, at least in the United States.

We who are responsible for patients should never forget that the death rate for prostate cancer in the United States is only 226 per 100,000 men over 65 years of age, or 0.226%.[8] This death rate can be placed in proper perspective by comparing it to the death rate from lung cancer caused by smoking, which is at least 80%, approximately 350 times greater than the death rate from prostate cancer. For those who like to point out to their patients that prostate cancer is the second leading cause of cancer death in the United States, they should include the 350 times greater risk of death from lung cancer.

REFERENCES

1. Stamey TA, Yang N, Hay AR, et al. Prostate-specific antigen as a serum marker for adenocarcinoma of the prostate. New Engl J Med 1987;317:909–916.

2. Gleason DF. Histologic grading of prostatic adenocarcinoma. In: Tannenbaum M (ed), Urologic pathology: the prostate. Philadelphia: Lea & Febiger, 1977, p 181.

3. McNeal JE, Gleason DF. Classification de Gleason des adenocarcinomes prostatiques. An Path 1991; 11: 163–168.

4. Stamey TA, McNeal JE, Yemoto CM, et al. Biological determinants of cancer progression in men with prostate cancer. J Am Med Assoc 1999;281:1395–400.

5. Stamey TA, Caldwell M, McNeal JE, et al. The PSA era in the United States is over for prostate cancer: What happened in the past 20 years? J Urol 2004;172:1297–1301.

6. Roehrborn CG, McConnell J, Bonilla J, et al. Serum prostate specific antigen is a strong predictor of future prostate growth in men with benign prostatic hyperplasia. J Urol 2000;163:13–20.

7. Sakr WA, Grignon DJ, Haas GP, et al. Age and racial distribution of prostatic intraepithelial neoplasia. Eur Urol 1996; 30:138–144 [Note: Despite the author's emphasis on dysplasia in the title of this paper, he carefully tabulated prostate cancers in 525 accidental deaths on the streets of Detroit (314 African Americans and 211 whites). It is a key paper illustrating the increasing ubiquity of prostate cancer starting in men in their 20s.].

8. National Cancer Institute. SEER Cancer Statistics Review 1973–1997 http://seer.cancer.gov/publications/csr1973_1997/prostate.pdf (accessed February, 2001).

Genetic epidemiology 2

Peter H Gann, Thomas L Jang, William J Catalona

OVERVIEW

The realization that genetic factors play a role in determining a man's risk of developing prostate cancer is at least 50 years old; however, the epidemiological search for the specific genetic variants responsible has only begun recently (Figure 2.1). In this review, we summarize the knowledge gained initially during the premolecular era, and then the surge of new information since the mid-1990s resulting from the application of rapidly emerging technologies in molecular genetics. All genetic variants that affect prostate cancer risk lie along a continuum of penetrance, which can be defined as the probability of an individual experiencing the disease phenotype during a specified time interval, given a particular genotype. It is useful to divide the discussion of genetic factors into those with relatively high and low penetrance, however, because the behavior of variants at either end of the spectrum produce different patterns of occurrence within populations and, therefore, lend themselves to different methodological approaches. Our focus here is on germline variants; other chapters in this volume discuss somatic gene variants that might contribute to prostate carcinogenesis through acquired mechanisms alone. We also focus on genetic determinants of etiology rather than prognosis, although the two are related; good discussions on genetic determinants of prostate cancer aggressiveness can be found in the literature.[1,2]

The relative importance of genes versus environmental factors in prostate cancer etiology is a

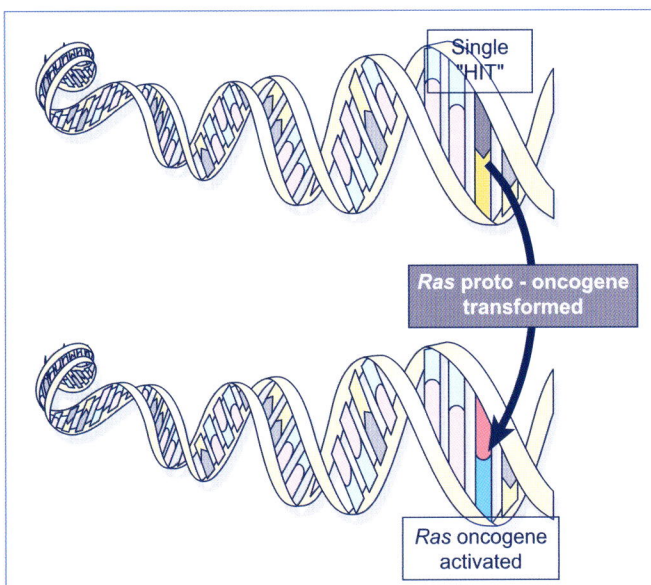

Fig. 2.1
An example of a genetic mutation causing cancer. A single "hit" may transform the Ras proto-oncogene to its activated form.

matter of common misunderstanding. We will argue that there is evidence to suggest that both genetic and environmental factors are very important in prostate cancer; indeed, the interaction of genes and the environment is most likely at play in most individual cases of the disease, and is the basis for the wide variation in penetrance itself. The ubiquity of these interactions means that for any group of prostate cancer cases, such as those occurring in the US, the sum total of cases attributable to individual risk factors can greatly exceed 100%. A recent study of monozygotic versus dizygotic twins estimated that 42% of prostate cancer cases are attributable to hereditable factors, a figure that was among the highest for any cancer site.[3] However, two important points must be noted: 1) 42% represents the sum total contribution of all genetic variants, not just one or two; and 2) the principle of interacting causes means that all or most of these 42% of cases equally could be said to have been caused by environmental factors, in that without the presence of both the genetic variant and the environmental exposure, the case would not have occurred. In fact, epidemiologists long ago observed by studying migrants that prostate cancer risk appears to be unusually sensitive to changes in environment. Among Japanese-American immigrants, for example, the risk of prostate cancer already begins to approach the risk for US-born Japanese Americans, even among men who migrated after the onset of adulthood.[4]

PREMOLECULAR STUDIES

Observant clinicians were the first to report the existence of family clustering in prostate cancer during the 1950s.[5] Subsequent case-control studies and later cohort studies performed before the prostate-specific antigen (PSA) era found relatively consistent elevations in risk for men with first-degree relatives who had prostate cancer compared with those who did not, with relative risks ranging from about 2.0 to 3.0.[6] The diagnosis of prostate cancer in a close relative before the age of 65 years increases the relative risk reported in meta-analyses to 4.3 (95% confidence interval [CI]: 2.9–6.3), and presence of multiple affected relatives increases relative risk to approximately 4.6 (95% CI: 2.7–8.0). Excess risk for men with second-degree relatives only is much smaller and perhaps nondetectable. However, among men with three or more affected first-degree relatives, risk has been estimated to increase 11-fold,[7] an impressive figure that approaches those seen for cigarette smoking and lung cancer. Similar risk estimates for family history are seen in men of European, Asian, and African ancestry. Besides age and race, family history has long been one of the few reliably established risk factors for prostate cancer. Genetic epidemiologists have

classified prostate cancer according to the degree of family clustering as hereditary, familial, or sporadic. These categories become important in selecting families for gene discovery studies, as discussed below. Commonly used criteria for hereditary prostate cancer (HPC) require at least three affected first-degree relatives or prostate cancer in three consecutive generations or at least two first-degree relatives affected before 55 years of age. Approximately 5% to 10% of all cases in the US can be classified as hereditary, and are most likely to be caused by high-penetrance genetic variants that exhibit mendelian patterns in extended pedigrees. Familial cases, which have affected relatives but do not meet the more stringent hereditary criteria, account for about 10% to 20% of all cases. Sporadic cases, defined as those with no affected relatives, form the remainder and thus make up about 75% to 85% of all cases seen in a typical population.

TWIN STUDIES

To assess whether this clustering was due to hereditary or environmental influences, several important twin studies comparing the concordance of cancer in monozygotic and dizygotic twins have been carried out. If the concordance for cancer is higher among monozygotic twins (who share all genes) than among dizygotic twins (who, on average, share 50% of their segregating genes), a genetic etiology is suggested. However, if the concordance is similar for both types of twins, then shared environmental influences are likely important.

Gronberg et al[8] combined data from the Swedish Twin and Swedish Cancer Registries to identify 458 prostate cancers among 4840 male twin pairs. Proband concordance rates of 19% and 4% were found for monozygotic and dizygotic pairs, respectively. In a later study, Page et al[9] identified a total of 1009 prostate cancer cases among a cohort of 31,848 veteran twins and likewise found that the proband concordance for prostate cancer was substantially higher among monozygotic twin pairs (27%) than among dizygotic twin pairs (7.1%). In the study of 44,788 pairs of twins from Sweden, Denmark, and Finland mentioned above, Lichtenstein et al[3] estimated that 42% (95% CI: 29–50%) of the risk of developing prostate cancer may be explained by heritable factors. This was the largest degree of heritability observed for any major cancer site; for example, breast cancer heritability was estimated as 27%. It is important to re-emphasize, however, that these results might not apply to non-Scandinavian populations, that the calculations assumed no gene–environment interaction—which can make the genetic contribution appear larger—and that a high degree of heritability can occur due to the cumulative effects of many weakly penetrating genes as well as the effects of a few powerful ones. Furthermore, concordance rates in twin studies are dependent on the timing and method of prostate cancer ascertainment.[3,8,9]

SEGREGATION ANALYSES

To assess the specific genetic mode of inheritance of prostate cancer within families, numerous segregation analyses have been performed. Most of the currently available data suggest that the familial aggregation of prostate cancer can be explained best by mendelian autosomal dominant inheritance.[10-14] However, evidence for X-linked,[15] non-mendelian[16] (multiple genes each having low penetrance), and recessive[14,15] modes of inheritance have also been reported.

The first segregation analysis, performed in 1992 by Carter et al,[10] provided important insight into characteristics of genes involved in hereditary prostate cancer. They evaluated 691 families affected by prostate cancer ascertained through 740 consecutive probands undergoing radical prostatectomy for clinically localized prostate cancer at Johns Hopkins. The study provided evidence that familial clustering of prostate cancer among those with early onset may be attributed to autosomal dominant inheritance of a rare, yet highly penetrant allele (q = 0.0030), with carriers having an 88% cumulative risk of disease by age 85 years compared with only 5% for noncarriers. Furthermore, this inherited form of prostate cancer accounted for 43% of early onset disease (age ≤ 55 years) but, overall, was responsible for a small proportion of prostate cancer occurrence (9% by age 85 years).

Findings from this study were corroborated by later segregation analyses of prostate cancer that reported disease allele frequencies ranging from 0.4%[13] to 1.7%,[11] moderate-to-high life-time penetrance in gene carriers varying from 63%[11] to 97%,[13] and a relatively small proportion of all prostate cancers that were attributable to the high-risk allele (8%[13] to 16%[12] by the age of 85 years).

Recently, Gong et al[16] reported that a multifactorial model (in which the risk of prostate cancer within families was determined by both genetic and environmental factors) explained their data better than did the mendelian models. Their model suggested that multiple genes, each having low penetrance, may be responsible for most inherited prostate cancer susceptibility, and that the contribution of rare highly penetrant mutations was small.

Ideally, interpretation of these patterns of family clustering would rapidly lead to the discovery of disease-causing genes and pathways, as well as to refined predictions for genetic counseling. Unfortunately, the genetic causes of prostate cancer have proved to be far more complex for several important reasons:

1. Variable, often low penetrance—only genetic variants with relatively high penetrance are strong enough to produce obvious family clustering. As a result of interaction with other genes and environmental factors, the other variants will produce non-mendelian patterns or no apparent clustering at all.
2. Late age at onset of prostate cancer—some men with genetic predisposition do not live long enough to develop detectable disease, even though hereditary cases (as defined above) are diagnosed a mean of 5 to 6 years earlier than sporadic cases.[17]
3. Phenocopies—genetic and nongenetic cases are essentially indistinguishable, and family clustering can easily occur without genetic factors.[18] This problem is currently exacerbated by the widespread use of PSA screening, which can cause apparent clustering simply through similar patterns of healthcare utilization.
4. Genetic heterogeneity—as discussed below, we now know that there are at least several relatively high-penetrance genes that could affect prostate cancer risk, and an unknown but greater number of low penetrance genes. Thus, the particular set of genetic factors involved will vary from family to family and population to population. Even families with the right combinations of weak low penetrance genes can exhibit clustering.

With these concepts as background, the next two sections discuss the results and methods so far used in the search for genetic determinants of prostate cancer risk in the era of molecular genetics.

HIGH-PENETRANCE GENETIC VARIANTS

Positional cloning strategies using genome-wide scans and linkage analyses allow for the localization of disease genes using mapping techniques with only limited information about the intrinsic biochemical defect or the function of the gene.[19] Thus far, genome scans and linkage analyses for prostate cancer susceptibility genes have identified 10 chromosomal loci and 5 specific genes that have been confirmed in at least one independent study; these loci are summarized in Table 2.1.

Linkage refers to the propensity for two or more genetic markers to pass together through generations. The closer two loci are on a given chromosome, the more likely they will exhibit linkage. The likelihood of a marker being linked to a disease locus is measured by the "likelihood of linkage" score (LOD score), which refers to the log 10 of an odds ratio for being linked to a disease versus being unlinked. For example, a LOD score of 3 suggests a 10^3:1 (or 1000:1) odds that the marker is linked to the disease locus. A LOD score of 3 generally suggests true linkage in simple mendelian disorders, whereas a score below –2 is convincing evidence against linkage. For complex diseases that exhibit genetic heterogeneity, such as prostate cancer, lower LOD scores are accepted as evidence of linkage. It is also possible to calculate LOD scores for multiple loci concurrently

Table 2.1 Hereditary prostate cancer susceptibility loci (confirmed in independent populations)

Locus	Candidate gene	Initial report by	Number of families	HLOD[a]
13q12-13	BRCA2	Thorlacius et al, 1996[110]	21	–
1q24-25 (HPC1)	RNASEL	Smith et al, 1996[23]	91	5.43
1q42.2-43 (PCAP)		Berthon et al, 1998[32]	47	2.2
Xq27-28 (HPCX)		Xu et al, 1998[42]	360	2.57[b]
1p35-36 (CAPB)		Gibbs et al, 1999[45]	12	3.65[b]
20q11-q13 (HPC20)		Berry et al, 2000[49]	162	3.02
2q37-38, 12p13-p12, 15q26, 16p13, 16q23-24		Suarez et al, 2000[48]	504 sibpairs	2.92, 2.0, 1.71, 2.81, 3.15
17p13	HPC2/ELAC2	Tavtigian et al, 2001[60]	33	4.53
8p22-p23	MSR1	Xu et al, 2001[55]	159	1.84
22q12	CHEK2	Dong et al, 2003[65]	149	

[a]LOD score refers to the log 10 of an odds ratio for being linked to a disease versus being unlinked. For example a LOD score of 3 suggests a 10^3:1 (or 1000:1) odds that the marker is linked to the disease locus. HLOD refers to a heterogeneity LOD score, which assumes genetic heterogeneity (more than one causal locus) exists.

[b]Two-point LOD score, which to the likelihood between only two loci at one time; all other LOD scores are multipoint, which are likelihood scores for multiple loci concurrently.

(multipoint LOD), instead of calculating likelihood scores between only two loci at one time.[20,21]

Parametric linkage analyses predicate that a disease phenotype with a known model of inheritance is caused by a single locus, and thus assumes a classic mendelian inheritance pattern. However, as previously mentioned, several modes of inheritance (dominant, recessive, X-linked, non-mendelian) for prostate cancer have been suggested, and so it is important to interpret findings from parametric analyses in conjunction with nonparametric linkage (NPL) analyses, where knowledge of a specific genetic model is not required. This approach identifies chromosomal locations that are shared by affected individuals by comparing the observed versus the expected sharing of chromosomal segments among affected relatives.[20-22]

1q24-25 (HPC1)

The first prostate cancer susceptibility locus, designated *HPC1* (hereditary prostate cancer 1), was mapped to chromosome 1 in 1996 by collaborators from the US and Sweden. In this study, Smith et al[23] used a linkage analysis of 91 families with a high-risk of prostate cancer to demonstrate striking evidence of linkage in the 1q24-25 region. A multipoint LOD score of 5.43 ($10^{5.43}$:1 or 270,000:1 odds in favor of linkage) was observed for markers mapping to this region. *HPC1* was suggested to account for 34% of prostate cancers in the 91 families studied. Furthermore, later studies[24,25] indicated that individuals linked to this locus tend to develop prostate cancer at an early age (younger than 65 years).

Despite convincing evidence of linkage in the initial report[23] and confirmation in some subsequent studies,[25-29] other investigators did not find evidence of linkage at the 1q24-25 locus.[30-32] Furthermore, linkage was found to be much less common across high-risk families than the 34% originally proposed. Goode et al[29], Eeles et al,[31] and Xu et al[25] estimated that 2.6%, 4%, and 6% of families, respectively, were linked to 1q24-25 in their respective studies of 150, 136, and 772 high-risk prostate cancer families. These conflicting findings provided the first signs that the identification of prostate cancer susceptibility genes might prove more challenging than originally suspected. Lessons learned from this difficulty are discussed below.

Interestingly, recent analyses have identified a specific gene at 1q24-25 (ribonuclease L [*RNASEL*]) that is mutated in some high-risk families.[33,34] Research on *RNASEL*, which has functions related to inflammatory response, is actively ongoing; however, it appears thus far that the specific mutation(s) in the gene responsible for altered risk is not clear, and it is likely that other susceptibility genes exist at or near the 1q24-25 locus.[35]

1q42.2-43 (PCAP)

In 1998, investigators reported evidence for a second prostate cancer susceptibility locus on the long arm of chromosome 1 (1q42.2-43) designated *PCAP* (predisposing for cancer of the prostate). In this study, Berthon et al[32] studied 47 European families (37 French and 10 German) with a high incidence of prostate cancer and estimated that 50% of the families linked to the

PCAP locus. Similarly as for the *HPC1* locus, these investigators noted that individuals linked to *PCAP* developed early-onset disease. These results were challenged by Gibbs et al,[36] who, in a study of 152 American families, estimated that *PCAP* accounted for only 4% to 9% of familial cancers. In later reports, Whittemore et al[37] and Berry et al,[38] in studies of 97 and 144 HPC families using three and six markers, respectively, both found negative parametric and nonparametric LOD scores for 1q42.3-43, suggesting no linkage. More recently, however, Goddard et al[39] and Cancel-Tassin et al[40] reported evidence of linkage to the *PCAP* locus in their respective studies of 254 and 64 families.

Xq27-28 (HPCX)

An X-linked model of inheritance for prostate cancer has been suggested by previous studies that showed a higher risk of prostate cancer in men with affected brothers compared with those with affected fathers.[15,41] This is now supported by the identification of a prostate cancer susceptibility locus on the X chromosome (Xq27-28), termed *HPCX*. Xu et al[42] studied 360 prostate cancer families from North America, Sweden, and Finland. Subjects were stratified into two categories based on the presence or absence of male-to-male transmission in order to reduce a possible source of genetic heterogeneity. For families without a male-to-male transmission, a two-point LOD score of 4.6 was observed for markers at Xq27-28. Furthermore, the *HPCX* locus accounted for approximately 16% of prostate cancers in this study. *HPCX* linkage has been confirmed independently in some studies but not others.[43,44]

1p36 (CAPB)

In 1999, Gibbs et al[45] localized another putative prostate cancer susceptibility locus known as *CAPB* (cancer of the prostate and brain) to chromosome 1p36. Strong evidence of linkage (overall two-point LOD score = 3.22) at this locus was seen in a subset of 12 families (out of 141 studied) with a history of prostate cancer and primary brain cancer, in which loss of heterozygosity at 1p36 frequently occurs.[46] No evidence for linkage was seen in either early or late age of onset families without a history of brain cancer. Later studies have produced conflicting results. Berry et al[38] studied 13 HPC families with brain and prostate cancers and did not find evidence for linkage. Badzioch et al[47] found evidence of linkage to 1p36 in families with early-onset prostate cancer, although no association with other cancers was noted. Finally, Suarez et al reported nonsignificant but positive LOD scores in three markers mapping to the *CAPB* locus in 13 families with a history of prostate and brain cancer.[48]

20q13 (HPC20)

Berry et al[49] found evidence for linkage (multipoint NPL score = 3.02) to chromosome 20q13 (*HPC20*) in a genome-wide search on 162 North American families with HPC. Approximately 12% of all families in this study were linked to *HPC20*. These results were later independently questioned[50] and confirmed[51] by other investigators. Recently, a linkage analysis from a very large pooled set of 1234 multiplex families failed to detect any sign of linkage at this locus, indicating that *HPC20* probably does not play a significant role in hereditary prostate cancer.[52]

16q23

Given the problems inherent in collecting samples from multiple generations of men at risk for prostate cancer, study designs involving sibships are becoming increasingly attractive. In 2000, Suarez et al reported an analysis of 504 brothers from 230 sibships and found evidence for linkage at several sites, on chromosomes 2q, 12p, 15q, 16p, and 16q. Evidence for a suppressor gene at 16q23.2 was particularly strong.[48] A subsequent replication study from the same group using 49 families (45 of which were new) provided strong support for the existence of a susceptibility locus on 16p. Though evidence for a susceptibility locus on 16q was weakened in this study, the region immediately proximal to 16q23 continued to reflect increased allele sharing among affected family members.[53] In a new genome scan using a different sample of affected sib pairs (259 brothers), the same investigators used finer mapping and replicated the previous findings of a very strong linkage signal for susceptibility at 16q23[54](Figure 2.2).

8p22-23 (MSR1)

Following the earlier observation by Smith et al[23] of possible linkage at 8p and the frequent detection of loss of heterozygosity at this site in sporadic cancers, Xu et al reported evidence of linkage at 8p22-23 in 159 HPC families.[55] The same association was found in a study of 57 Swedish HPC families.[56] Subsequently, Xu et al reported that several mutations in the macrophage scavenger receptor gene (*MSR1*) located at 8p22 co-segregated with prostate cancer.[57] The association between *MSR1* variants and prostate cancer has been supported in some[58] but not all reports.[59]

17p11 (HPC2/ELAC2)

After an initial genome-wide scan in eight large Utah pedigrees suggested linkage at a locus on chromosome

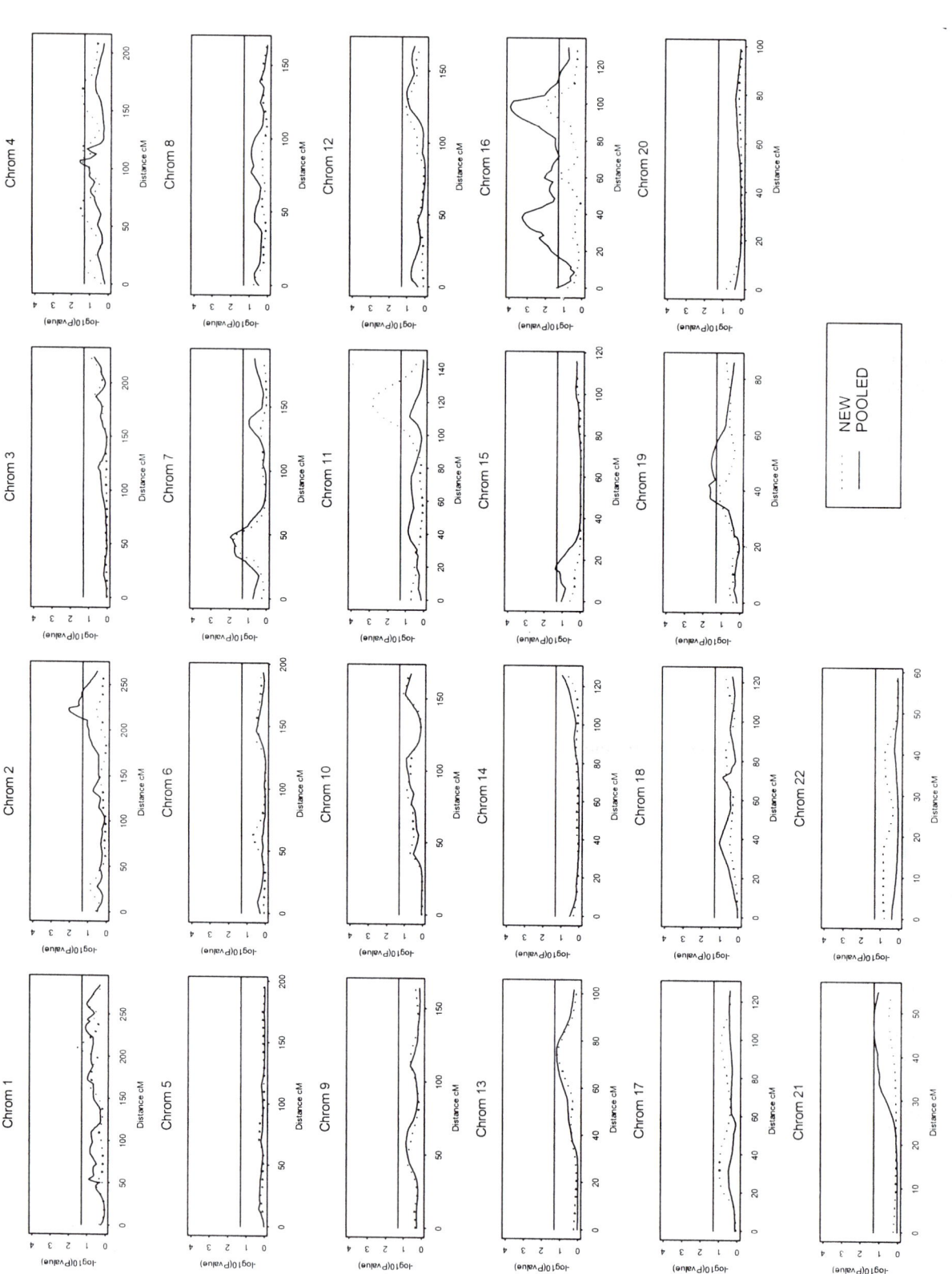

Fig. 2.2
P-values from genome-wide scans for new set of 259 brothers from families with two or more brothers with prostate cancer (*dotted lines*), and pooled results including 594 previously studied brothers from similar families. Tick-marks across horizontal axes indicate marker locations in centimorgans (cM). Horizontal solid line indicates where p = 0.05; thus peaks above these lines have p < 0.05.

Reproduced with permission from Witte JS, Suarez BK, Thiel B, et al. Genome-wide scan of brothers: replication and fine mapping of prostate cancer susceptibility and aggressiveness loci. Prostate 2003;57:298–308.

17, Tavtigian et al[60] performed finer mapping and eventually cloned a putative prostate cancer susceptibility gene at 17p11, which was named *HPC2/ELAC2*. Two missense mutations—a relatively common serine-to-leucine change at codon 217 and a rare alanine-to-threonine change at codon 541—were implicated. These results were replicated in one other study,[61] but not in two others.[62,63] More recently, a large population-based case control study in the Seattle–Puget Sound area reported that men who were homozygous for both the Ser217Leu and the Ala541Thr variants had a relative risk (measured as odds ratio [OR]) of 1.84 (95% CI: 1.11–3.05) compared with those with wild type.[64] This is an example of variant–variant interaction within a single gene, a phenomenon that adds another order of magnitude of complexity to the problem of identifying heritable factors for prostate cancer. In the same study,[64] when tumor aggressiveness was considered, a single 217Leu allele conferred a significantly elevated risk (OR = 1.36) for localized cancer with Gleason <8, and two 217Leu alleles was associated with even higher risk (OR = 1.75). If these results for the Seattle–Puget Sound area can be extrapolated to the entire US population, it would mean that 15% of all non-aggressive cases and 10% of total cases could be attributed to the Ser217Leu genotype in *HPC2/ELAC2*.

22q (CHEK2)

A very interesting relationship between prostate cancer risk and the *CHEK2* gene has just been described. The protein CHEK2 is activated in response to DNA damage, whereupon it prevents cellular entry into mitosis most likely via phosphorylation of BRCA1 and P53. Truncation and missense mutations in *CHEK2* have been observed in patients with Li-Fraumeni syndrome, a highly penetrant multisite cancer syndrome typically related to *P53* dysfunction, and in women with familial breast cancer without *BRCA1/2* mutations. Dong et al were the first to evaluate *CHEK2* in relation to prostate cancer risk, finding several mutations more commonly in both sporadic and familial cases compared to controls.[65] Confirmatory evidence for an association with a truncation mutation (1100delC) and a missense mutation of isoleucine to threonine (Ile157Thr) was soon reported in two small family-based studies from Finland and Poland.[66,67] Further work on *CHEK2* in prostate cancer is certainly needed, especially since the Ile157Thr variant may be as prevalent as 5% in some populations.

17q12-21/13q12-13 (BRCA1 AND BRCA2)

Co-occurrence of breast and prostate cancer in families has been observed for years. Following cloning of

BRCA1 and *BRCA2*, it was reported that male carriers of mutations in these genes had 3-fold and 7-fold increased risk of developing prostate cancer, respectively.[68,69] Loss-of-heterozygosity at these loci is relatively common in prostate cancer. Gayther et al analyzed the entire coding regions of *BRCA1* and *BRAC2* in 38 multiplex prostate cancer families in the UK.[70] They found no association with any *BRCA1* variants, but two families with early-onset disease had deletion mutations in *BRCA2*. Other studies have also reported associations between *BRCA2* variants and prostate cancer risk; therefore, *BRCA2* qualifies as a putative susceptibility gene. In a large cohort study involving 1539 Icelandic women with breast cancer, a significantly increased risk of prostate cancer in all male relatives, including first- and second-degree relatives, was noted.[71] However, in study populations without a strong family history of breast cancer, *BRCA1* and *BRCA2* were not found to significantly contribute to prostate cancer risk.[72]

FAILURE TO REPLICATE—WHY?

The identification of multiple loci and genes implicated in heritable prostate cancer, and the lack of consistent replication of findings across studies, suggests the degree of challenge that investigators face in this area. We have already mentioned how genetic heterogeneity and phenocopies complicate the search for high-penetrance prostate cancer genes. As this new field rapidly matures, at least five important lessons have been learned:

1. Very large pedigrees enriched with many cases are especially valuable in overcoming the phenocopy problem, since in these families heritable cases are more likely to dominate relative to sporadic ones. For example, a study using Mormon pedigrees with a mean of 10.7 affected men per family obtained the first strong replication of linkage at *HPC1*.[73]
2. Earlier analyses based solely on parametric models, which require specifying the correct mode of transmission for high-penetrance alleles, can be wrong due to model misspecification, given the variety of ways in which prostate cancer genes can be transmitted. Therefore, nonparametric analyses, which do not require specification of a transmission model, are becoming more popular.
3. Early studies were often unable to restrict analysis to a set of cases with homogeneous etiology. It is now appreciated that identifying subsets (stratification) of cases might be essential in detecting genetic signals. Subsets can be formed based on age at diagnosis, tumor aggressiveness, mode of transmission, and concurrent phenotype (such as brain cancer in the case of *CAPB*). A study by Goddard et al provides an excellent example.[39] These investigators re-examined a set of sib pairs that had not shown linkage at

HPC1[53]; this time their analysis included adjustment for age at diagnosis, Gleason score, male-to-male transmission and number of affected first degree relatives. The results now showed a LOD score of 3.25 ($P = 0.00012$) at *HPC1*.

4. Studies must be large if they are going to detect small effects due to variant–variant interaction or effects within restricted subsets. For example, Gillanders et al combined four study populations comprising a total of 426 families to conduct the largest genome-wide scan for prostate cancer susceptibility to date.[74]

5. Estimating the proportion of disease attributable to a given genotype requires studies that are at least partially population-based, otherwise selection biases can over- or underestimate the contribution of the genotype to the wider public health burden.

LOW-PENETRANCE GENETIC VARIANTS

Notwithstanding the importance of high-penetrance genes in prostate cancer, there are several reasons to assume that low-penetrance variants will contribute more to the overall genetic burden in prostate cancer, and will, therefore, have a greater impact on public health. Relative risk refers to the strength or power of a genetic variant to affect the likelihood of an individual getting disease, and is analogous to the concept of penetrance; i.e., high-penetrance genes confer high relative risk, low-penetrance genes confer low relative risk. To understand the impact of a variant on a population, however, we have to consider attributable risk, which is affected not only by the relative risk but by the prevalence of the variant in the population. This means that a low-penetrance genotype with a relative risk of only 1.5 but a prevalence of 40% can account for 17% of all cases, far more than are attributable to a genotype with a relative risk of 10 but a prevalence of only 0.05% (1 per 200).

Now that the human genome has been entirely sequenced and mapped, more attention is turning to the amount of genetic variation within specific genes and loci. Although the degree to which genes are polymorphic varies, a surprising amount of variation within populations is observed in apparently normal functioning genes. Disregarding hot spots where variation is especially intense, the human genome is estimated to contain single nucleotide polymorphisms (SNPs) or simple sequence repeats (SSRs) at 1 out of every 1000 bases in the human genome.[75,76] The SNP library maintained by the SNP Consortium, a collaboration of 14 major pharmaceutical companies and the Wellcome Trust, as well as members of the Human Genome Project, currently contains over 1.4 and 2.1 million SNPs in public and private databases,

respectively.[76] Very recently, investigators can use either family-based or non-family-based (i.e., standard case-control studies of unrelated subjects) study designs to identify low-penetrance variants. However, it has been shown that case-control studies with unrelated subjects (sometimes referred to as "association studies" in the genetics literature) are more powerful for detection of small low-penetrance effects, and also have the advantage of more power for the evaluation of gene–environment interactions, which, of course, are heavily implicated in low-penetrance situations virtually by definition.[77]

Investigators also can use either genomic or candidate gene strategies to find significant genotypes amidst this enormous amount of variation. Genomic strategies, which are commonly used in the linkage analysis and positional cloning studies discussed above, involve high-density SNP or SSR maps covering the entire genome. Association of one or more of these anonymous markers with disease in a case-control or family-based study could mean that the marker is in linkage with a causal variant nearby. For reasons that will be discussed later in this section, this approach has several problems that have limited its use for studying low-penetrance genetic susceptibility to prostate cancer. Thus, nearly all of the results to date come from case-control studies and candidate gene approaches. Table 2.2 summarizes the major characteristics and findings of some of these studies, organized by type of biological mechanism. The search for candidate genes stems from existing models regarding important causal pathways in prostate carcinogenesis. This gives an overview of activity in this rapidly expanding field; a more comprehensive review can be found elsewhere.[78]

ANDROGEN SYNTHESIS, METABOLISM, AND ACTION

The evidence implicating androgen action in the development and progression of prostate cancer is diverse and abundant; so, not surprisingly, the most intense search for causal genetic polymorphisms has been in this area. Despite early studies showing increased risk for prostate cancer among men with shorter CAG or GGN repeats in exon 1 of the androgen receptor gene (*AR*), several studies have failed to replicate this finding. It is noteworthy that the biological plausibility of an effect due to short CAG length is unusually strong, given that an inherited androgen deficiency disorder (Kennedy syndrome) exists in which the primary defect is long CAG repeats, and that transfection of prostate cells in vitro with short CAG *AR* increases the rate of AR transcription. Moreover, African-American men, who have one of the highest incidence rates for prostate cancer in the world, have on average shorter CAG lengths in *AR*.

Table 2.2 Low-penetrance genetic polymorphisms most widely evaluated for association with prostate cancer risk to date

Group	Gene	Polymorphism(s)*	Evidence for function?	Reference
Androgen synthesis/action	AR	CAG, GGN repeats	Kennedy syndrome, in vitro (CAG)	
	SRD5A2	$(TA)_n$, Val89Leu, Ala49Thr	In vitro (Ala49Thr, Val89Leu), x-section* (Ala49Thr)	
	CYP17	T→C 5' promoter		
	HSD3B1	Asn367Thr		111
	HSD3B2	$(TG)_n(TA)_n(CA)_n$ repeat 3' UTR C→G		111, 112
	PSA	−158 bp G→A ARE1 −4643 bp G→A −5412 bp C→T	In vitro (−4643, −5412), x-section	82
Xenobiotic metabolism	CYP1A1	Ile462Val	In vitro	83
	CYP2D6	G_A exon 3/intron 4	X-section, "poor drug metabolizer" phenotype	84
	CYP3A4	−287 bp A→G 5' regulatory	In vitro, drug challenges negative	87, 113
	NAT1	−1088 bp T→A, −1095 C→A (23 other alleles)	Slow/rapid acetylator phenotype established	90
	NAT2	Ala197Gly (M12 allele +25 other alleles)	Slow/very slow/rapid acetylator phenotypes	85
	GSTM1	GSTM1-0 (null)		
	GSTT1	GSTT1-0 (null)		
	GSTP1	$(ATAAA)_n$ repeat, Ile105Val	In vitro (Ile105Val)	114, 115
DNA repair	XRCC1	Arg399Gln	In vitro	100
	XPD	312Asn/Asn	Increased DNA adducts in tissue	
	hOGG1	−11657 bp A→G		99
Insulin/IGF system	INS	+1127 bp T→C 3' UTR	In vitro	97
	IGF1	$(CA)_n$ promoter		98
	IGFBP3	−202bp C→A promoter	X-section*	98
Vitamin D	VDR	polyA, Bsm1, Taq1 (linked)		96
Inflammation	MIC1	His6Asp		102

Amino acids: Ala, alanine; Arg, argenine; Asn, asparagine; Asp, aspartate; Gln, glutamine; Gly, glycine His; histidine; Ile, isoleucine; Leu, leucine; Thr, threonine; Val, valine. Bases: A, adenine; C, cytosine; G, guanine; T, thymine.

AR, androgen receptor; ARE1, androgen response element 1 in promoter region; SRD5A2, 5α-reductase, type II; CYP17, 17α-hydroxylase; hOGG1, 8-oxoguanine DNA glycosylase; HSD3B, 3β-hydroxysteroid dehydrogenase; CYP, cytochrome P450; MIC1, Macrophage-inhibitory cytokine-1; NAT, N-acetyltransferase; GST, glutathione S-transferase; UTR, untranslated region; VDR, vitamin D receptor; XPD, xeroderma pigmentosum group D; XRCC1, X-ray repair cross complementing protein 1.

*X-section refers to cross-sectional studies of genotype–phenotype relationships in human populations.

The gene *SRD5A2* encodes for 5α-reductase type II, the enzyme responsible for conversion of testosterone to dihydrotestosterone (DHT) in the prostate. Men with a rare inactivating mutation in *SRD5A2* have largely undeveloped prostates. Despite some laboratory evidence that TA dinucleotide repeat length in an untranslated region of the gene affects enzyme activity, case-control studies on prostate cancer risk have proved conflicting. A similar situation has occurred for the Val89Leu polymorphism, which replaces valine with leucine at codon 89. Based on functional activity assays and higher prevalence of Val89Leu among low-risk Asian populations, there is biological plausibility for this variant being protective; however, once again association studies have not been consistent. A third variant, an alanine-to-threonine substitution at codon 49, is more common in African-American and Hispanic men and also appears to increase enzyme activity five-fold in vitro. Initial studies indicate that the Ala49Thr variant could be associated with elevated prostate cancer risk in these racial/ethnic groups, although the allele frequency is still only 2% to 3% and thus could not explain a large proportion of cases. Interestingly, 5α-reductase inhibitors such as finasteride bind with 11.7-fold lower affinity to the Ala49Thr variant enzyme than to wild type, indicating that this polymorphism could play a significant role in modifying drug response.[79]

Polymorphic variants in several other genes in the androgen synthesis/metabolic pathway have been discovered, including *HSD3B2*, *CYP17*, and *CYP19*; however, no consistent associations with prostate cancer risk have been observed, and, in the case of the *CYP17A2* allele (a T→C substitution in the 5′ promoter region), studies show both positive and inverse associations. There are many other candidate genes in the androgen system, such as *SHBG* and *HSD17B3*, whose variants are yet to be studied.

PSA is an androgen response gene in the prostate, and its polymorphic variants could influence risk of prostate cancer diagnosis through alteration of PSA levels in blood or through direct effects on tumor growth. Xue et al reported that men who were homozygous for the G allele at position −158 (located within an androgen response element in a promoter region) had a significantly elevated risk of advanced prostate cancer,[80] and that men with a homozygous A/A genotype had higher serum PSA levels. However, subsequent studies failed to confirm both the risk association for the −158G/A variant as well as the association with serum PSA.[81,82] More thorough sequencing of the PSA gene suggests that discrepant results for −158G/A could have occurred if this variant was in linkage disequilibrium with a truly important variant in some but not all study populations, and that several other SNPs or haplotypes in *PSA* are associated with serum PSA levels and are functionally active when inserted into cultured prostate cells.[82]

XENOBIOTIC METABOLISM

Several genes encoding enzymes involved in metabolism of drugs and environmental chemicals have polymorphisms that have been evaluated for their association with prostate cancer risk. These enzymes can activate, detoxify, or promote excretion of foreign compounds involved in carcinogenesis. *CYP1A1*, which plays an important role in activation of carcinogens such as the polycyclic aromatic hydrocarbons found in cigarette smoke and dioxins, is polymorphic in exon 7. One study so far has reported an elevated risk of prostate cancer (OR = 2.6) in men homozygous for the valine allele compared with men homozygous for isoleucine.[83] *CYP2D6* encodes an enzyme that catalyzes the metabolism of several important drugs but also activates tobacco-specific nitrosamines. It is known that polymorphisms near the junction of exon 3 and intron 4 in this gene cause functionally reduced capacity to metabolize certain drugs—a phenotype that is seen in about 5% to 10% of the white population. Three studies that genotyped the *CYP2D6-B* allele at this location or classified men based on poor-versus-extensive metabolizor phenotype have failed to provide convincing results for an effect on risk.[84–86] *CYP3A4* codes for an abundant enzyme involved in metabolizing many drugs, but also involved in the oxidation of

testosterone. Rebbeck et al reported that men carrying a G allele in the 5′ regulatory region of this gene were more likely to have late-stage disease at diagnosis,[87] and hypothesized that in these men reduced oxidation shunts more testosterone towards formation of the more potent DHT. A subsequent study reported a similar association for the G allele in African-American cases, but other work indicated that this allele did not decrease enzyme amount or activity.[88,89]

The *N*-acetyltransferases NAT1 and NAT2 catalyze the activation or deactivation of a variety of heterocyclic amines and arylamine carcinogens. Slow and fast acetylation phenotypes are observed in conjunction with over 50 alleles identified so far in these genes. Two relatively small case control studies conducted thus far reported no associations for *NAT2* genotypes; a third study in Japan found increased risk associated with homozygosity for the *NAT2*10* allele, which is linked to rapid acetylation.[85,86,90] Glutathione S-transferases detoxify numerous genotoxic compounds through conjugation with glutathione. Variants in *GSTM1*, *GSTT1*, and *GSTP1* have been studied in relation to prostate cancer risk. Homozygous deletions of *GSTM1* and *GSTT1* are relatively common, and these men are hypothesized to be more susceptible to tumor formation. Case-control results so far, however, do not demonstrate any consistent associations between *GSTM* or *GSTT* null (deleted) status and prostate cancer risk[83,91]; in fact, one study found a significant reduction in risk in men with deleted *GSTT1*.[92] *GSTP1* is particularly interesting because its expression is nearly always lost in prostate cancer compared with normal tissue; however, studies of three variant alleles in this gene have all been negative.[86,93]

VITAMIN D RECEPTOR

An array of evidence supports the hypothesis that vitamin D metabolites, acting through the vitamin D receptor (VDR), reduce prostate cancer risk. Three polymorphisms in *VDR* have been studied thus far—Taq1, BsmI, and Poly-A. None of these variants appears to be functionally significant, and all three are in various degrees of linkage disequilibrium in different populations. Although early studies reported significant positive risk associations with the T allele at Taq1 and the long Poly-A allele, several subsequent studies of these loci and BsmI have been negative.[94–96]

OTHER GENES AND PATHWAYS

Candidate prostate cancer susceptibility genes with low penetrance might also be found in other pathways, including the insulin-like growth factor (IGF)/insulin, DNA repair, and inflammatory response systems. The data are sparse thus far. Ho et al reported a three-fold increase in prostate cancer risk among men with homozygous C/C genotype at a noncoding site on the insulin gene (*INS*).[97] Another recent study found no association with risk for a (CA)$_n$ dinucleotide repeat in the promoter region of the IGF1 gene and a single nucleotide polymorphism in the promoter region (–202) of the IGFBP3 gene.[98] Three genes involved in DNA repair—*XRCC1*, *XPD*, and *hOGG1*—have been studied in relation to prostate cancer risk. Xu et al observed that two variants in *hOGG1* were associated with risk; while Rybicki et al recently reported a positive risk association for the Asn312Asn genotype in *XPD* (xeroderma pigmentosa group D gene).[99,100] The latter association was much stronger in men who also had the Gln399Gln genotype in *XRCC1*, indicating a gene–gene interaction. Interestingly, another study suggests that the Arg399Arg genotype in *XRCC1* is associated with elevated risk among men with low dietary intake of vitamin E and lycopene.[101] *CHEK2*, another DNA damage response gene, in prostate cancer is discussed above as it is sufficiently to be associated with family clustering.

Recently, the role of inflammation in prostate carcinogenesis is receiving greater attention; a population-based case control study in Sweden found that an amino acid substitution (histidine to aspartic acid at codon 6) in the macrophage-inhibitory cytokine-1 (MIC1) gene, which regulates macrophage activity, was associated with reduced risk in both familial and sporadic cases.[102]

METHODOLOGIC PROBLEMS

The search for low-penetrance genetic variants that affect prostate cancer risk, which was begun in the mid-1990s, has produced largely null and inconsistent results. The amount of variation in the human genome is greater than had been anticipated, and too many early studies might have obtained null results because the wrong polymorphism in the gene was selected for study. Systematic evaluation of genetic variation in the source population prior to performing risk estimation is preferable to haphazard selection of genotypes based on what has been reported in the literature or even in SNP libraries.[103] Better prioritization of SNPs and SSRs based on functional significance will help, although direct laboratory testing of functional significance for each variant constitutes a major bottleneck. Cross-sectional studies of genotype–phenotype associations and emphasis on missense coding and promoter regions can also help. Haplotyping, which can now be done routinely using computational methods, will improve the chances of focusing on the relevant variants in a given study population and reduce the amount of effort wasted studying equivalent genotypes. Hinds et al

recently reported and made publicly available by far the densest map of the human genome ever produced, based on sequencing of nearly 1.6 million SNPs in 71 Americans of European, African-American, and Chinese ancestry.[104] Failure to account for linkage differences between populations is troublesome, in that a locus linked to a disease-causing gene in one population may not be linked in another, and in some cases can even produce opposite risk effects (protective and harmful) for the same allele, as was the case for *CYP17A2*.[105] Importantly, there is now recognition that small "main effect" risks require much larger study populations and will often require consideration of gene–gene, variant–variant, or gene–environment interactions (i.e., modified effects) in order to be detected. Too few studies thus far have had high-quality environmental data for studying interactions. To illustrate, a large case control study in Seattle that conducted detailed in-person interviews found a small risk for prostate cancer (OR = 1.4) among smokers, and a positive trend with pack-years of exposure.[106] These investigators recently observed that the risk due to smoking appears to be modified by *GSTM1* genotype; among men who were *GSTM1* null, they found a linear trend for prostate cancer risk with pack-years of smoking (P_{trend} = 0.007).[107] Prospective cohort studies generally provide more valid environmental data than case control studies, although the latter can provide more extensive data, and are less time and cost-consuming.

Second-order and certainly higher order interactions require study populations that are too large for any single institution to assemble. Ironically, although cross-classification of subjects by multiple genotypes or environmental exposure makes it more likely that gene effects will be detected, the public health impact of these gene effects inevitably becomes smaller. The chief benefit of discovering low-penetrance genetic effects, in fact, probably lies in verification of targets and pathways for preventive or therapeutic intervention, rather than in the clinical diagnostic or risk stratification possibilities.

Early studies in this field were also constrained by methodological problems such as use of prevalent as opposed to incident cases, casual selection of controls, and possible confounding due to ethnicity (population stratification). Particular attention should be paid in data analysis to the problem of false-positive results, since the number of genotype combinations and their interactions that can be tested is staggering. The fraction of false-positive findings in studies of the association between a genetic variant and a complex disease has been estimated to exceed 95%.[108] Wacholder et al have recently proposed using the false-positive report probability (FPRP), an intriguing approach that incorporates a defined level of plausibility with the study findings to help determine if a particular result is noteworthy or not.[109]

A LOOK TO THE FUTURE

The study of the genetic determinants of prostate cancer risk is in its infancy, and many important lessons have been learned about how to design studies commensurate with the enormous complexity of the topic. Many signs indicate that the next generation of studies will be more powerful and sophisticated. Technological advances leading to faster, cheaper genotyping and expanding SNP libraries will permit denser mapping and higher information content in pedigree studies. Improved understanding of the biology of prostate cancer will inform decisions about relevant genes and pathways that require testing. In a striking example that also illustrates the importance of gene-gene interaction, Xu et al recently conducted a linkage analysis that focused on two tumor suppressor genes—*PTEN* and *CDKN1B*—that have been demonstrated to affect prostate cancer risk in animal models, including compound knockout models indicating strong joint effects.[109a] With fine mapping of both chromosome 10 and 12, no linkage was observed in either the *PTEN* region (10q23-24) or the *CDKN1B* region (12p11-13) alone; however, the strongest

evidence for linkage was observed for allele-sharing precisely at *both* loci (P = 0.0002). The probability surface for this bellwether analysis is shown in Figure 2.3. Finally, genetic epidemiologists themselves are responding to the challenge by forming multi-institutional collaborations that can overcome the statistical power limitations of previous studies on both high and low penetrance gene effects. The International Consortium for Prostate Cancer Genetics (ICPCG) includes investigators from over 20 institutions in North America, Europe, and Australia and has collected DNA from over 1700 multiplex prostate cancer families. Using this resource, investigators have confirmed linkage for *HPC1* in 772 families[25] and reported an important failure to replicate linkage for *HPC20* based on analysis of 1234 families.[52] Another significant resource for high penetrance studies is deCODE genetics, a private company capable of linking genotype, medical records and genealogical data on over 100,000 residents of Iceland (www.decode.com). For low penetrance genes, the most significant collaborative development is the Breast and Prostate Cancer and Hormone-related Gene Variants Cohort Consortium (BPC3 Study) launched by the US National Cancer Institute (NCI) in 2003. The BPC3 combines subjects

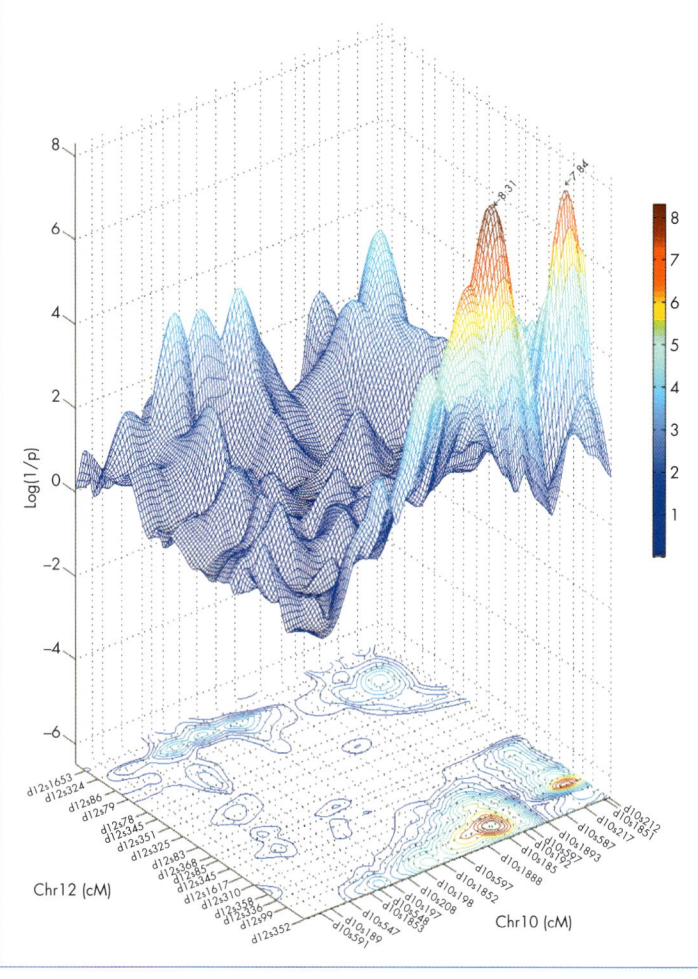

Fig. 2.3

Linkage results for interaction between loci on chromosomes 10 and 12, including regions containing the genes *PTEN* and *CDKN1B* respectively. In a collection of 188 hereditary prostate cancer families, the strongest linkage signals were detected at the precise loci (10q23-24 and 12p11-13) closest to these candidate tumor suppressor genes, implying highest risk among individuals who have altered alleles at both sites. This is evidence for a gene-gene effect, which is supported by knockout animal models.

Reproduced with permission from Xu J, Langefeld CD, Zheng SL, et al. Interaction effect of PTEN and CDKN1B chromosomal regions on prostate cancer linkage. Hum Genet 2004;115:255–262.

and samples from 10 separate epidemiological cohorts totaling 8,850 men with prostate cancer. This project will test the assumption that pooling data and samples across cohorts will allow us to identify crucial gene-gene and gene-environment interactions.

Given the mixed results obtained so far in the search for prostate cancer susceptibility genes, it is premature to recommend widespread use of genetic testing based on specific genes or loci. Men with family histories of prostate cancer, however, are often in need of expert counseling in order to understand their risks and the steps they can take to mitigate them.

REFERENCES

1. Witte JS, Goddard KA, Conti DV, et al. Genomewide scan for prostate cancer-aggressiveness loci. Am J Hum Genet 2000;67:92–99.
2. Neville PJ, Conti DV, Krumroy LM, et al. Prostate cancer aggressiveness locus on chromosome segment 19q12-q13.1 identified by linkage and allelic imbalance studies. Genes Chromosomes. Cancer 2003;36:332–339.
3. Lichtenstein P, Holm NV, Verkasalo PK, et al. Environmental and heritable factors in the causation of cancer—analyses of cohorts of twins from Sweden, Denmark, and Finland. N Engl J Med 13 2000;343:78–85.
4. Shimizu H, Ross RK, Bernstein L, et al. Cancers of the prostate and breast among Japanese and white immigrants in Los Angeles County. Br J Cancer 1991;63:963–966.
5. Morganti G, Gianferrari L, Cresseri A, et al. Clinico-statistical and genetic research on neoplasms of the prostate. Acta Genet Stat Med 1956;6:304–305.
6. Johns LE, Houlston RS. A systematic review and meta-analysis of familial prostate cancer risk. BJU Int 2003;91:789–794.
7. Steinberg GD, Carter BS, Beaty TH, et al. Family history and the risk of prostate cancer. Prostate 1990;17:337–347.
8. Gronberg H, Damber L, Damber JE. Studies of genetic factors in prostate cancer in a twin population. J Urol Nov 1994;152:1484–1487; [discussion 1487–1489].
9. Page WF, Braun MM, Partin AW, et al. Heredity and prostate cancer: a study of World War II veteran twins. Prostate 1997;33:240–245.
10. Carter BS, Beaty TH, Steinberg GD, et al. Mendelian inheritance of familial prostate cancer. Proc Natl Acad Sci USA 1992;89:3367–3371.
11. Gronberg H, Damber L, Damber JE, et al. Segregation analysis of prostate cancer in Sweden: support for dominant inheritance. Am J Epidemiol 1997;146:552–557.
12. Schaid DJ, McDonnell SK, Blute ML, et al. Evidence for autosomal dominant inheritance of prostate cancer. Am J Hum Genet 1998;62:1425–1438.
13. Verhage BA, Baffoe-Bonnie AB, Baglietto L, et al. Autosomal dominant inheritance of prostate cancer: a confirmatory study. Urology 2001;57:97–101.
14. Cui J, Staples MP, Hopper JL, et al. Segregation analyses of 1,476 population-based Australian families affected by prostate cancer. Am J Hum Genet 2001;68:1207–1218.
15. Monroe KR, Yu MC, Kolonel LN, et al. Evidence of an X-linked or recessive genetic component to prostate cancer risk. Nat Med 1995;1:827–829.
16. Gong G, Oakley-Girvan I, Wu AH, et al. Segregation analysis of prostate cancer in 1,719 white, African-American and Asian-American families in the United States and Canada. Cancer Causes Control 2002;13:471–482.
17. Bratt O. Hereditary prostate cancer: clinical aspects. J Urol Sep 2002;168:906–913.
18. Keetch DW, Humphrey PA, Smith DS, et al. Clinical and pathological features of hereditary prostate cancer. J Urol 1996;155:1841–1843.
19. Ellsworth DL, Manolio TA. The emerging importance of genetics in epidemiologic research II. Issues in study design and gene mapping. Ann Epidemiol 1999;9:75–90.
20. Nupponen NN, Carpten JD. Prostate cancer susceptibility genes: many studies, many results, no answers. Cancer Metastasis Rev 2001;20:155–164.
21. Karayi MK, Neal DE, Markham AF. Current status of linkage studies in hereditary prostate cancer. BJU Int 2000;86:659–669.
22. Ott J. Complex traits on the map. Nature 1996;379:772–773.
23. Smith JR, Freije D, Carpten JD, et al. Major susceptibility locus for prostate cancer on chromosome 1 suggested by a genome-wide search. Science 1996;274:1371–1374.
24. Gronberg H, Isaacs SD, Smith JR, et al. Characteristics of prostate cancer in families potentially linked to the hereditary prostate cancer 1 (HPC1) locus. JAMA 1997;278:1251 1255.
25. Xu J. Combined analysis of hereditary prostate cancer linkage to 1q24-25: results from 772 hereditary prostate cancer families from the International Consortium for Prostate Cancer Genetics. Am J Hum Genet 2000;66:945–957.
26. Cooney KA, McCarthy JD, Lange E, et al. Prostate cancer susceptibility locus on chromosome 1q: a confirmatory study. J Natl Cancer Inst 1997;89:955–959.
27. Hsieh CL, Oakley-Girvan I, Gallagher RP, et al. Re: prostate cancer susceptibility locus on chromosome 1q: a confirmatory study. J Natl Cancer Inst 1997;89:1893–1894.
28. Gronberg H, Smith J, Emanuelsson M, et al. In Swedish families with hereditary prostate cancer, linkage to the HPC1 locus on chromosome 1q24-25 is restricted to families with early-onset prostate cancer. Am J Hum Genet 1999;65:134–140.
29. Goode EL, Stanford JL, Chakrabarti L, et al. Linkage analysis of 150 high-risk prostate cancer families at 1q24-25. Genet Epidemiol 2000;18:251–275.
30. McIndoe RA, Stanford JL, Gibbs M, et al. Linkage analysis of 49 high-risk families does not support a common familial prostate cancer-susceptibility gene at 1q24-25. Am J Hum Genet 1997;61:347–353.
31. Eeles RA, Durocher F, Edwards S, et al. Linkage analysis of chromosome 1q markers in 136 prostate cancer families. The Cancer Research Campaign/British Prostate Group U.K. Familial Prostate Cancer Study Collaborators. Am J Hum Genet 1998;62:653–658.
32. Berthon P, Valeri A, Cohen-Akenine A, et al. Predisposing gene for early-onset prostate cancer, localized on chromosome 1q42.2-43. Am J Hum Genet 1998;62:1416–1424.
33. Carpten J, Nupponen N, Isaacs S, et al. Germline mutations in the ribonuclease L gene in families showing linkage with HPC1. Nat Genet 2002;30:181–184.
34. Rokman A, Ikonen T, Seppala EH, et al. Germline alterations of the RNASEL gene, a candidate HPC1 gene at 1q25, in patients and families with prostate cancer. Am J Hum Genet 2002;70:1299–1304.
35. Casey G, Neville PJ, Plummer SJ, et al. RNASEL Arg462Gln variant is implicated in up to 13% of prostate cancer cases. Nat Genet 2002;32:581–583.
36. Gibbs M, Chakrabarti L, Stanford JL, et al. Analysis of chromosome 1q42.2-43 in 152 families with high risk of prostate cancer. Am J Hum Genet 1999;64:1087–1095.
37. Whittemore AS, Lin IG, Oakley-Girvan I, et al. No evidence of linkage for chromosome 1q42.2-43 in prostate cancer. Am J Hum Genet 1999;65:254–256.
38. Berry R, Schaid DJ, Smith JR, et al. Linkage analyses at the chromosome 1 loci 1q24-25 (HPC1), 1q42.2-43 (PCAP), and 1p36 (CAPB) in families with hereditary prostate cancer. Am J Hum Genet 2000;66:539–546.
39. Goddard KA, Witte JS, Suarez BK, et al. Model-free linkage analysis with covariates confirms linkage of prostate cancer to chromosomes 1 and 4. Am J Hum Genet 2001;68:1197–1206.
40. Cancel-Tassin G, Latil A, Valeri A, et al. PCAP is the major known prostate cancer predisposing locus in families from south and west Europe. Eur J Hum Genet 2001;9:135–142.
41. Narod SA, Dupont A, Cusan L, et al. The impact of family history on early detection of prostate cancer. Nat Med 1995;1:99–101.

42. Xu J, Meyers D, Freije D, et al. Evidence for a prostate cancer susceptibility locus on the X chromosome. Nat Genet 1998;20:175–179.

43. Schleutker J, Matikainen M, Smith J, et al. A genetic epidemiological study of hereditary prostate cancer (HPC) in Finland: frequent HPCX linkage in families with late-onset disease. Clin Cancer Res 2000;6:4810–4815.

44. Peters MA, Jarvik GP, Janer M, et al. Genetic linkage analysis of prostate cancer families to Xq27-28. Hum Hered 2001;51:107–113.

45. Gibbs M, Stanford JL, McIndoe RA, et al. Evidence for a rare prostate cancer-susceptibility locus at chromosome 1p36. Am J Hum Genet 1999;64:776–787.

46. Smith JS, Alderete B, Minn Y, et al. Localization of common deletion regions on 1p and 19q in human gliomas and their association with histological subtype. Oncogene 1999;18:4144–4152.

47. Badzioch M, Eeles R, Leblanc G, et al. Suggestive evidence for a site specific prostate cancer gene on chromosome 1p36. The CRC/BPG UK Familial Prostate Cancer Study Coordinators and Collaborators. The EU Biomed Collaborators. J Med Genet 2000;37:947–949.

48. Suarez BK, Lin J, Burmester JK, et al. A genome screen of multiplex sibships with prostate cancer. Am J Hum Genet 2000;66:933–944.

49. Berry R, Schroeder JJ, French AJ, et al. Evidence for a prostate cancer-susceptibility locus on chromosome 20. Am J Hum Genet 2000;67:82–91.

50. Bock CH, Cunningham JM, McDonnell SK, et al. Analysis of the prostate cancer-susceptibility locus HPC20 in 172 families affected by prostate cancer. Am J Hum Genet 2001;68:795–801.

51. Zheng SL, Xu J, Isaacs SD, et al. Evidence for a prostate cancer linkage to chromosome 20 in 159 hereditary prostate cancer families. Hum Genet 2001;108:430–435.

52. Schaid DJ, Chang BL. Description of the international consortium for prostate cancer genetics, and failure to replicate linkage of hereditary prostate cancer to 20q13. Prostate 2005;63:276–290.

53. Suarez BK, Lin J, Witte JS, et al. Replication linkage study for prostate cancer susceptibility genes. Prostate 2000;45:106–114.

54. Witte JS, Suarez BK, Thiel B, et al. Genome-wide scan of brothers: replication and fine mapping of prostate cancer susceptibility and aggressiveness loci. Prostate 2003;57:298–308.

55. Xu J, Zheng SL, Hawkins GA, et al. Linkage and association studies of prostate cancer susceptibility: evidence for linkage at 8p22-23. Am J Hum Genet 2001;69:341–350.

56. Wiklund F, Jonsson BA, Goransson I, et al. Linkage analysis of prostate cancer susceptibility: confirmation of linkage at 8p22-23. Hum Genet 2003;112:414–418.

57. Xu J, Zheng SL, Komiya A, et al. Common sequence variants of the macrophage scavenger receptor 1 gene are associated with prostate cancer risk. Am J Hum Genet 2003;72:208–212.

58. Miller DC, Zheng SL, Dunn RL, et al. Germ-line mutations of the macrophage scavenger receptor 1 gene: association with prostate cancer risk in African-American men. Cancer Res 2003;63:3486–3489.

59. Wang L, McDonnell SK, Cunningham JM, et al. No association of germline alteration of MSR1 with prostate cancer risk. Nat Genet 2003;35:128–129.

60. Tavtigian SV, Simard J, Teng DH, et al. A candidate prostate cancer susceptibility gene at chromosome 17p. Nat Genet 2001;27:172–180.

61. Rebbeck TR, Walker AH, Zeigler-Johnson C, et al. Association of HPC2/ELAC2 genotypes and prostate cancer. Am J Hum Genet 2000;67:1014–1019.

62. Vesprini D, Nam RK, Trachtenberg J, et al. HPC2 variants and screen-detected prostate cancer. Am J Hum Genet 2001;68:912–917.

63. Xu J, Zheng SL, Carpten JD, et al. Evaluation of linkage and association of HPC2/ELAC2 in patients with familial or sporadic prostate cancer. Am J Hum Genet 2001;68:901–911.

64. Stanford JL, Sabacan LP, Noonan EA, et al. Association of HPC2/ELAC2 polymorphisms with risk of prostate cancer in a population-based study. Cancer Epidemiol Biomarkers Prev 2003;12:876–881.

65. Dong X, Wang L, Taniguchi K, et al. Mutations in CHEK2 associated with prostate cancer risk. Am J Hum Genet 2003;72:270–280.

66. Seppala EH, Ikonen T, Mononen N, et al. CHEK2 variants associate with hereditary prostate cancer. Br J Cancer 2003;89:1966–1970.

67. Cybulski C, Huzarski T, Gorski B, et al. A novel founder CHEK2 mutation is associated with increased prostate cancer risk. Cancer Res 2004;64:2677–2679.

68. Ford D, Easton DF, Bishop DT, et al. Risks of cancer in BRCA1-mutation carriers. Breast Cancer Linkage Consortium. Lancet 1994;343:692–695.

69. Tonin P, Ghadirian P, Phelan C, et al. A large multisite cancer family is linked to BRCA2. J Med Genet 1995;32:982–984.

70. Gayther SA, de Foy KA, Harrington P, et al. The frequency of germ-line mutations in the breast cancer predisposition genes BRCA1 and BRCA2 in familial prostate cancer. The Cancer Research Campaign/British Prostate Group United Kingdom Familial Prostate Cancer Study Collaborators. Cancer Res 2000;60:4513–4518.

71. Tulinius H, Egilsson V, Olafsdottir GH, et al. Risk of prostate, ovarian, and endometrial cancer among relatives of women with breast cancer. BMJ 1992;305:855–857.

72. Langston AA, Stanford JL, Wicklund KG, et al. Germ-line BRCA1 mutations in selected men with prostate cancer. Am J Hum Genet 1996;58:881–884.

73. Neuhausen SL, Farnham JM, Kort E, et al. Prostate cancer susceptibility locus HPC1 in Utah high-risk pedigrees. Hum Mol Genet 1999;8:2437–2442.

74. Gillanders EM, Xu J, Chang BL, et al. Combined genome-wide scan for prostate cancer susceptibility genes. J Natl Cancer Inst 18 2004;96:1240–1247.

75. Sachidanandam R, Weissman D, Schmidt SC, et al. A map of human genome sequence variation containing 1.42 million single nucleotide polymorphisms. Nature 2001;409:928–933.

76. Venter JC, Adams MD, Myers EW, et al. The sequence of the human genome. Science 2001;291:1304–1351.

77. Risch N. Genetic Analysis Workshop II: multiple-locus segregation analysis incorporating linkage markers. Genet Epidemiol 1984;1:207–211.

78. Coughlin SS, Hall IJ. A review of genetic polymorphisms and prostate cancer risk. Ann Epidemiol Apr 2002;12:182–196.

79. Makridakis NM, Ross RK, Pike MC, et al. Association of mis-sense substitution in SRD5A2 gene with prostate cancer in African-American and Hispanic men in Los Angeles, USA. Lancet 1999;354:975–978.

80. Xue W, Irvine RA, Yu MC, et al. Susceptibility to prostate cancer: interaction between genotypes at the androgen receptor and prostate-specific antigen loci. Cancer Res 2000;60:839–841.

81. Wang LZ, Sato K, Tsuchiya N, et al. Polymorphisms in prostate-specific antigen (PSA) gene, risk of prostate cancer, and serum PSA levels in Japanese population. Cancer Lett 2003;202:53–59.

82. Cramer SD, Chang BL, Rao A, et al. Association between genetic polymorphisms in the prostate-specific antigen gene promoter and serum prostate-specific antigen levels. J Natl Cancer Inst 2003;95:1044–1053.

83. Murata M, Shiraishi T, Fukutome K, et al. Cytochrome P4501A1 and glutathione S-transferase M1 genotypes as risk factors for prostate cancer in Japan. Jpn J Clin Oncol 1998;28:657–660.

84. Febbo PG, Kantoff PW, Giovannucci E, et al. Debrisoquine hydroxylase (CYP2D6) and prostate cancer. Cancer Epidemiol Biomarkers Prev 1998;7:1075–1078.

85. Agundez JA, Martinez C, Olivera M, et al. Expression in human prostate of drug- and carcinogen-metabolizing enzymes: association with prostate cancer risk. Br J Cancer 1998;78:1361–1367.

86. Wadelius M, Autrup JL, Stubbins MJ, et al. Polymorphisms in NAT2, CYP2D6, CYP2C19 and GSTP1 and their association with prostate cancer. Pharmacogenetics 1999;9:333–340.

87. Rebbeck TR, Jaffe JM, Walker AH, et al. Modification of clinical presentation of prostate tumors by a novel genetic variant in CYP3A4. J Natl Cancer Inst 1998;90:1225–1229.

88. Paris PL, Kupelian PA, Hall JM, et al. Association between a CYP3A4 genetic variant and clinical presentation in African-American prostate cancer patients. Cancer Epidemiol Biomarkers Prev 1999;8:901–905.

89. Amirimani B, Walker AH, Weber BL, et al. RESPONSE: re: modification of clinical presentation of prostate tumors by a novel genetic variant in CYP3A4. J Natl Cancer Inst 1999;91:1588–1590.

90. Fukutome K, Watanabe M, Shiraishi T, et al. N-acetyltransferase 1 genetic polymorphism influences the risk of prostate cancer development. Cancer Lett 1999;136:83–87.

91. Autrup JL, Thomassen LH, Olsen JH, et al. Glutathione S-transferases as risk factors in prostate cancer. Eur J Cancer Prev 1999;8:525–532.

92. Rebbeck TR, Walker AH, Jaffe JM, et al. Glutathione S-transferase-mu (GSTM1) and -theta (GSTT1) genotypes in the etiology of prostate cancer. Cancer Epidemiol Biomarkers Prev 1999;8:283–287.

93. Harries LW, Stubbins MJ, Forman D, et al. Identification of genetic polymorphisms at the glutathione S-transferase Pi locus and association with susceptibility to bladder, testicular and prostate cancer. Carcinogenesis 1997;18:641–644.

94. Taylor JA, Hirvonen A, Watson M, et al. Association of prostate cancer with vitamin D receptor gene polymorphism. Cancer Res 1996;56:4108–4110.

95. Ingles SA, Haile RW, Henderson BE, et al. Strength of linkage disequilibrium between two vitamin D receptor markers in five ethnic groups: implications for association studies. Cancer Epidemiol Biomarkers Prev 1997;6:93–98.

96. Ma J, Stampfer MJ, Gann PH, et al. Vitamin D receptor polymorphisms, circulating vitamin D metabolites, and risk of prostate cancer in United States physicians. Cancer Epidemiol Biomarkers Prev 1998;7:385–390.

97. Ho GY, Melman A, Liu SM, et al. Polymorphism of the insulin gene is associated with increased prostate cancer risk. Br J Cancer 2003;88:263–269.

98. Li L, Cicek MS, Casey G, et al. No association between genetic polymorphisms in IGF-I and IGFBP-3 and prostate cancer. Cancer Epidemiol Biomarkers Prev 2004;13:497–498.

99. Xu J, Zheng SL, Turner A, et al. Associations between hOGG1 sequence variants and prostate cancer susceptibility. Cancer Res 2002;62:2253–2257.

100. Rybicki BA, Conti DV, Moreira A, et al. DNA repair gene XRCC1 and XPD polymorphisms and risk of prostate cancer. Cancer Epidemiol Biomarkers Prev 2004;13:23–29.

101. van Gils CH, Bostick RM, Stern MC, et al. Differences in base excision repair capacity may modulate the effect of dietary antioxidant intake on prostate cancer risk: an example of polymorphisms in the XRCC1 gene. Cancer Epidemiol Biomarkers Prev 2002;11:1279–1284.

102. Lindmark F, Zheng SL, Wiklund F, et al. H6D polymorphism in macrophage-inhibitory cytokine-1 gene associated with prostate cancer. J Natl Cancer Inst 2004;96:1248–1254.

103. Freedman ML, Pearce CL, Penney KL, et al. Systematic evaluation of genetic variation at the androgen receptor locus and risk of prostate cancer in a multiethnic cohort study. Am J Hum Genet 2005;76:82–90.

104. Hinds DA, Stuve LL, Nilsen GB, et al. Whole-genome patterns of common DNA variation in three human populations. Science 18 2005;307:1072–1079.

105. Makridakis NM, Reichardt JK. Molecular epidemiology of hormone-metabolic loci in prostate cancer. Epidemiol Rev 2001;23:24–29.

106. Plaskon LA, Penson DF, Vaughan TL, et al. Cigarette smoking and risk of prostate cancer in middle-aged men. Cancer Epidemiol Biomarkers Prev 2003;12:604–609.

107. Agalliu A. Paper presented at: InterProstate SPORE Meeting; February 2005; Houston.

108. Colhoun HM, McKeigue PM, Davey Smith G. Problems of reporting genetic associations with complex outcomes. Lancet 2003;361:865–872.

109. Wacholder S, Chanock S, Garcia-Closas M, et al. Assessing the probability that a positive report is false: an approach for molecular epidemiology studies. J Natl Cancer Inst 2004;96:434–442.

110. Thorlacius S, Olafsdottir G, Tryggvadottir L, et al. A single BRCA2 mutation in male and female breast cancer families from Iceland with varied cancer phenotypes. Nat Genet 1996;13:117–119.

111. Chang BL, Zheng SL, Hawkins GA, et al. Joint effect of HSD3B1 and HSD3B2 genes is associated with hereditary and sporadic prostate cancer susceptibility. Cancer Res 2002;62:1784–1789.

112. Devgan SA, Henderson BE, Yu MC, et al. Genetic variation of 3 beta-hydroxysteroid dehydrogenase type II in three racial/ethnic groups: implications for prostate cancer risk. Prostate 1997;33:9–12.

113. Westlind A, Lofberg L, Tindberg N, et al. Interindividual differences in hepatic expression of CYP3A4: relationship to genetic polymorphism in the 5'-upstream regulatory region. Biochem Biophys Res Commun 1999;259:201–205.

114. Debes JD, Yokomizo A, McDonnell SK, et al. Gluthatione-S-transferase P1 polymorphism I105V in familial and sporadic prostate cancer. Cancer Genet Cytogenet 2004;155:82–86.

115. Ho GY, Knapp M, Freije D, et al. Transmission/disequilibrium tests of androgen receptor and glutathione S-transferase pi variants in prostate cancer families. Int J Cancer 20 2002;98:938–942.

Risk factors for prostate cancer: diet and lifestyle studies

3

Edward Giovannucci, Elizabeth A Platz

INTRODUCTION

The role that diet and lifestyle factors play in prostate carcinogenesis remains controversial. Nonetheless, several lines of evidence suggest that lifestyle could have a large influence on prostate cancer occurrence or progression. First, large interpopulation differences in rates of prostate cancer incidence or mortality are observed, which probably cannot be explained solely by genetic differences among these populations.[1] Studies have demonstrated strong correlations between per capita measures of various foods or nutrients and prostate cancer mortality.[2,3] Although the specificity of these associations may be questioned, they do indicate that some dietary component or pattern influences prostate cancer. Second, rates of prostate cancer have been shown to increase with changing lifestyle patterns within populations, and migrating populations tend to take on the prostate cancer experience of the new country.[4] Third, although the results have not been entirely consistent, numerous epidemiologic studies have correlated specific dietary factors with risk of prostate cancer. Factors that have been shown to increase risk include higher intake of red and processed meat and dairy products, and those that decrease risk include higher intake of tomato products, which contain the carotenoid lycopene, and selenium, and supplemental intake of vitamin E.

A fourth line of supportive evidence is that some hormonal factors, including insulin-like growth factor 1 (IGF1) have been shown to influence prostate cancer risk. While IGF1 concentrations have a strong genetic component, they can also be influenced by nutritional patterns, so, at least in principle, it may be possible to influence risk of prostate cancer by nutritional means through the IGF1 axis. Other factors, including obesity, physical inactivity, occupation, environmental contaminants, cigarette smoking, vasectomy, sexually transmitted infections, or prostatitis have been studied as risk factors for prostate cancer, though evidence remains controversial.

In this chapter, we review demographic patterns of prostate cancer and population-based studies of diet and lifestyle in the etiology of prostate cancer. Before doing so, it may be useful to summarize a number of complexities regarding prostate cancer. In addition to typical considerations in studying cancer epidemiology—such as study size limitations, bias from various study designs, measurement error in exposure assessment—some unique features of prostate cancer render it particularly difficult to study. First, prostate cancer displays a wide array of aggressive biologic potential, and the intensity of screening and use of diagnostic procedures largely determines the number and spectrum of cancers diagnosed. For example, widespread prostate-specific antigen (PSA) screening in the US has reduced the age of diagnosis, substantially increased the pool of cancers diagnosed, and lowered the stage of diagnosis. Whether the indolent cancers diagnosed through PSA have the same risk factors as aggressive cancers is unknown. Second, the natural history of prostate cancer may be particularly long, with putative precursor lesions quite prevalent in early adulthood, but the average age of mortality from prostate cancer occurs quite late in life. Third, some evidence suggests heterogeneity of risk factors between early and later onset prostate cancers. Finally, the etiology of prostate cancer is likely to be multifactorial, and exposures could have divergent effects on various mechanisms. For example, obesity is associated with lower testosterone levels, higher estrogen and leptin levels, and perhaps higher free IGF1 levels. These particular complexities of prostate cancer are likely to add to the heterogeneity in results.

DEMOGRAPHIC PATTERNS

Demographic patterns of prostate cancer may provide some insight into its etiology. Many hypotheses have been generated by the marked variation in prostate cancer mortality rates around the world, which is more than 30-fold.[5] Developed or "Westernized" countries tend to have much higher prostate cancer rates than do developing countries.[1] The lowest rates of this cancer occur in the Far East and on the Indian subcontinent, whereas the highest rates occur in Western Europe, Australia, and North America. In Northern Europe (e.g., Sweden, Norway, and Denmark), prostate cancer morality rates are approximately double those in Southern Europe (e.g., Greece).[5] Adjusting the rates to the World Health Organization world standard population, the mortality rate for prostate cancer was approximately 1 per 100,000 men annually in China compared with 17.9 per 100,000 for men in the US in the year 2000.[1] In addition, the prostate incidence rate in China is 2.9 per 100,000 men contrasted with 107.8 and 185.4 per 100,000 men in the US for white and black men, respectively.[1] Whereas some of the disparity in prostate cancer incidence rates among countries is likely due to differences in medical practice leading to differential rates of detection of subclinical tumors, such as PSA screening, the pronounced variation in mortality rates supports the importance of factors that influence promotion and progression.

Prostate cancer ranks as the third most common cause of cancer death in the US. In 2003, 28,900 men died of prostate cancer, accounting for 10% of all cancer deaths in men. Prostate cancer is the most commonly diagnosed cancer in men in the US, accounting for an estimated 220,900 new cases in 2003 or 33% of all cancer diagnoses in men.[5] The high mortality rate clearly establishes prostate cancer as a formidable disease, but it is interesting to note that the incidence rate highly exceeds the mortality rate. In fact, even with the extensive screening for PSA in the US, many prostate cancers are missed. Thus, a relatively small proportion of prostate cancer ultimately progresses to mortality, due to a combination of relatively slow growth rates in many of them, relatively late age at onset, and competing causes of death.

From the early 1970s to the late 1980s, which is prior to the introduction of PSA screening, prostate cancer incidence rates were on the rise,[6] and, with the introduction of widespread screening for PSA in the early to mid-1990s, the prostate cancer incidence rate soared.[7] Meanwhile, after decades of a stable or slightly increasing mortality rate, the prostate cancer mortality rate has declined more recently. These patterns illustrate that in the current PSA era in the US, prostate cancer incidence and mortality are not well correlated. While it is obvious that one must have a prostate cancer to die from it, the factors that increase risk of prostate cancer incidence may differ from those that influence its progression. Traditionally, epidemiologists have focused on incidence rather than mortality for studying etiologic factors, because of concerns that mortality is "contaminated" by factors that influence survival, such as early detection, screening, and medical treatment. However, for prostate cancer, while these concerns for mortality cannot be ignored, incidence may be even more problematic and prone to bias because it is largely related to screening practices. In addition, small, incidental prostate cancers diagnosed may not provide clues to the factors related to progression, which may ultimately be most important to identify. Risk factors for endpoints such as fatal or metastatic cancer may be most important to identify.

RACE AND ETHNICITY

Although this chapter is focused on modifiable lifestyle factors, racial and ethnic variation in prostate cancer incidence and mortality rates may provide some important etiologic clues. In the US, racial variation is pronounced. African Americans have the highest prostate cancer incidence rate (standardized to 2000 US population age standard, 1992–1999: 275.3 per 100,000 men annually) and mortality rate (75.1 per 100,000 men annually) among any racial or ethnic group in the US. For comparison, the incidence and mortality rates are 1.6 (172.9 per 100,000 men) and 2.3 (32.9 per 100,000 men) times that for whites, respectively. In addition, a greater proportion of African-American men present with distant metastases (18%, compared with 10% for whites), and stage-specific survival is slightly poorer compared with whites (5-year survival for distant stage: 33% for whites versus 30% for African Americans).[6] Prostate cancer incidence and mortality rates for Asian/Pacific Islander, American Indian/Alaskan Native, or Hispanic are substantially lower than those for white Americans.[5]

The differences in rates among the racial groups have generated a number of explanatory hypotheses, but none have been confirmed. The contributions of genetic, hormonal, and lifestyle factors remain a controversial area. In a study of highly educated health professionals of relatively high socioeconomic status, risk of prostate cancer remained elevated in African Americans even after adjusting for purported dietary and lifestyle risk factors.[8] This suggests either a role of inherent factors, or that the racial differences are accounted for by yet unidentified lifestyle factors, or a combination of these. Given the high rates of prostate cancer in African-Americans, it is of interest to examine rates among men of African descent elsewhere in the world. Among the highest prostate cancer rates are found on Caribbean islands, including Trinidad and Tobago, which has the highest mortality rate among 45 countries evaluated[5] and Jamaica (high incidence rate).[9] In comparison, prostate cancer incidence and mortality rates in African countries such as Nigeria appear to be substantially lower than in these islands.[10] However, whether cancer incidence and mortality information is sufficiently comprehensive in African countries to make valid comparisons is questionable. Nonetheless, the evidence is suggestive that factors related to industrialization or economic development contribute to higher incidence and mortality rates of prostate cancer in men of African descent.

The markedly lower prostate cancer rate in Asian populations has generated some hypotheses focused on dietary differences, such as the large consumption of soybean products in many Asian populations. These are discussed below.

NUTRITION

ENERGY INTAKE AND OBESITY

Experience with other cancers common in Western countries, such as breast and colon cancer, have pointed to the importance of energy balance (caloric intake minus expenditure). In addition, animal studies consistently show that diets with restricted total energy reduce tumor burden relative to *ad libitum* feeding, including for prostate cancer.[11–13] However, energy intake and energy balance have not yielded clear associations for prostate cancer. Energy balance is probably more relevant than absolute energy intake, which is related to factors such as body size and physical activity. Unfortunately, true energy balance is almost impossible to study in epidemiologic studies, but several surrogates may be informative. These include adult height, body mass index (BMI), and energy intake.

Attained height reflects factors that characterize the growth phase of adolescence, including marked changes in circulating concentrations of steroid hormones, growth hormone, and IGF1. Inadequate energy intake, acting largely through these hormones, reduces attained adult height. Populations that have shorter average heights have lower rates of prostate cancer incidence and mortality. It is plausible that a relative energy restriction during the growth period could account in part or largely for the international patterns for prostate cancer. During puberty, the prostate gland is responsive to the changing balance of hormonal factors, and it develops

and matures to adult size. Precursor lesions are highly prevalent in men shortly after adolescence, so it is likely that many important early events in prostate cancer occur during the growth phase. Within Western populations, height has been shown to be positively associated with total prostate cancer in some studies,[14–22] although several do not support such an association.[23] Height may not be a consistent risk factor in all populations because the relative importance of nutritional and genetic factors may vary across populations. Possibly, energy restriction is more prevalent and extreme in populations in developing countries than within individuals in a developed country population.

If excessive energy intake in adulthood increased the risk of prostate cancer, one may expect that obesity would be associated with increased prostate cancer risk. However, no consistent association of high BMI with prostate cancer is supported in the literature.[23] Prospective studies have reported conflicting results, with some showing a positive relation for BMI or body weight and prostate cancer risk, but most are not supportive.[23] The prospective Cancer Prevention Study II showed a 34% higher risk of prostate cancer death for a very high BMI (>35 kg/m^2) compared with normal BMI (<25 kg/m^2).[24] Case-only studies suggest that risk of more aggressive prostate cancer in men who had clinically organ-confined disease is greater with higher BMI.[25,26] Thus, obesity could be related to the progression rate, and possibly mortality from prostate cancer, but does not appear related appreciably to increased incidence.

Energy intake has been evaluated in relation to prostate cancer risk in more than 20 epidemiologic studies, but findings have not been consistent.[27] However, energy intake is not a straightforward variable to consider in epidemiologic studies. For example, men with higher physical activity will require a higher energy intake to maintain energy balance. A recent large prospective study showed a positive association between energy intake and advanced prostate cancer in leaner men, but not in overweight and obese men.[28] The findings that men who remain lean despite higher energy intake suggest a specific metabolic profile that is related to a higher risk of prostate cancer progression.

Thus, epidemiologic studies suggest a complex pattern for energy balance and prostate cancer risk. It is possible that energy restriction during the growth period is important in lowering risk, and could possibly explain the lower prostate rates in less developed countries. However, obesity in adulthood has not been a consistent risk factor. Rather, one study suggests that a metabolic profile reflective of high energy intake with the maintenance of relative leanness is associated with an increased risk. Whether this reflects a hormonal pattern, such as high androgen and/or IGF1 levels, needs to be determined.

MACRONUTRIENT COMPOSITION

As discussed above, energy balance is likely to be important for prostate carcinogenesis. However, its precise role, when in the lifespan it is most relevant, and how it may interact with specific metabolic profiles needs to be better understood. Many hypotheses have been raised to explain the international differences in prostate cancer rates. Fat intake, particularly from animal sources (e.g., saturated fat), has been hypothesized to be a modifiable risk factor for prostate cancer.[2,3] However, many studies that have examined factors such as dietary fat, particularly earlier studies, have not always distinguished between independent effects of fat, or the fact that fat is a major contributor of total calories.

Diets in Western countries, where the prostate cancer rates are high, are high in animal fat (and related types of fat, such as saturated fat), protein, meat, and processed carbohydrates, and low in plant foods such as legumes. To date, dietary fat has been emphasized, but because of various methodologic limitations, definitive results have not been yielded. Nonetheless, a link between dietary fat or higher fat foods (especially foods from animals, such as meat and dairy) and prostate cancer has been further supported in case-control studies conducted in several different populations and often after adjusting for potentially confounding factors.[29] Findings for dietary fat and prostate cancer from prospective cohort studies, which are less prone to bias, are not consistent. Some studies have not supported an association,[30-32] whereas others have supported an association for total fat or fat from animal products,[14] mainly for advanced prostate cancer.[33] Some studies noted stronger relations for fat and advanced disease (e.g., extra-prostatic extension, metastasis, and death), with relative risks in the order of 1.6 to 2.9 between high and low intake categories.[20,33-35] These studies suggest that diet influences late stages of carcinogenesis in the prostate.

Some evidence, though not consistent, has suggested that higher intake of α-linolenic acid, an omega-3 polyunsaturated fatty acid, increases risk of prostate cancer.[33,36-38] In addition to meat and dairy fat, this fatty acid is found in vegetable oils such as soy and canola, and in leafy green vegetables in small amounts. A recent study found that α-linolenic acid from plant sources, in addition to that from animal sources, was associated with an increased risk of advanced prostate cancer.[38] However, the long-chain marine omega-3 fatty acids (eicosapentaenoic acid [EPA] and docosahexaenoic acid [DHA]) found in fatty fish, such as salmon, which are formed from α-linolenic acid, have been either unrelated or inversely associated with risk of prostate cancer.[29] The essential fatty acid linoleic acid, an omega-6 fatty acid found in vegetable and soy oils, and a precursor to arachidonic acid, has not been consistently associated with prostate cancer risk.

It is possible that the frequent associations observed with animal fat in many (though not all) studies is not related directly to fat, but to other components in foods that are the main sources of animal fat. Besides being sources of fat, red meat and processed meat are sources of high quality protein, iron, as well as added nitrites and byproducts of cooking, such as heterocyclic amines. Across countries, it is not surprising that total meat intake is also positively correlated with prostate cancer mortality.[2,3] In some cohort studies consumption of red meat is associated with a higher risk of prostate cancer,[14,33,39-41] particularly for processed or cured meats.[41,42] However, not all studies are supportive. In contrast to red meat, fish is either unrelated to risk or perhaps even protective.[43,44] Besides marine omega-3 fatty acids, fatty fish is essentially the only substantial natural dietary source (unfortified) of vitamin D (see below).

Perhaps among the most consistent dietary findings for prostate cancer has been a positive association with milk consumption. Countries with greater per capita consumption of milk have higher prostate cancer mortality rates.[2,3] A recent meta-analysis method estimated the combined odds ratio between milk consumption and prostate cancer from 11 case-control studies published between 1984 and 2003. The combined odds ratio was 1.68 (95% confidence interval [CI] = 1.34–2.12) for high versus low consumption, and it varied little by study stratification for various factors.[45] In addition, prospective cohort[46-48] studies have shown positive associations between calcium intake and prostate cancer risk, especially for advanced disease. Milk is high in high-quality protein and minerals, which increase IGF1 levels.[49] Milk is also high in calcium, which has been hypothesized independently to increase risk because calcium supplements have also been shown to increase risk of prostate cancer.[46,48] The association with milk does not appear to be due primarily to its fat composition.

In summary, although the roles of energy and macronutrients remain unresolved, it appears that high consumption of certain food groups (including red meat, processed meat, and dairy products) may be associated with an increased risk of advanced prostate cancer. Of note, such diets contribute concentrated energy, high-quality protein, minerals, heme iron, certain fatty acids, and factors such as heterocyclic amines and nitrites. Many of these factors may stimulate a growth-promoting environment that could increase risk for prostate cancer. Which are the most relevant factors needs to be determined.

FRUITS, VEGETABLES, LEGUMES, AND MICRONUTRIENTS

Fruits and vegetables contain a wide spectrum of phytochemicals, some of which may protect against prostate cancer. The putative beneficial compounds include antioxidants, essential vitamins and minerals, and nonessential but bioactive compounds. However, higher intake of total fruits and vegetables has generally not been associated with lower prostate cancer risk in most studies,[32] though there have been some exceptions.[50,51] Although the evidence does not support that total intake of fruits and vegetables is associated with a reduced risk of prostate cancer, three botanical families are of interest. Inverse associations are supported for tomato-based foods,[52,53] brassicas (the cabbage family), and allium vegetables (including garlic and onions).[54-56] Each of these groups is characterized by some phytochemicals that have putative anticancer benefits. The potential benefit from tomatoes and tomato products has been attributed at least in part to lycopene, a strong antioxidant in vitro.[57] Besides lycopene, other antioxidants of interest are vitamin E and selenium. These are discussed in detail in Chapter 4.

Brassica or cruciferous vegetables include broccoli, Brussels sprouts, and cabbage. This botanical group has generated interest because these vegetables are high in glucosinolates—compounds that induce phase I and II detoxification enzymes. These enzymes may protect against carcinogens, although which carcinogens are important for prostate cancer remains unclear. Several studies have found that men with higher intakes of brassicas may have a lower risk of prostate cancer.[50,51,56,58,59] Not all studies have supported this hypothesis.

In many Asian countries, consumption of soy products is high. The lower rate of prostate cancer in Asian countries has helped generate the hypothesis that higher intake of soy beans and related products lowers risk of prostate cancer. This hypothesis has also been supported by the presence of common soy phytoestrogens, including genistein and daidzein, which are known to induce growth arrest and apoptosis, to inhibit hormone metabolizing enzymes (such as 5α-reductase and 17β-hydroxysteroid dehydrogenase), and to have antioxidant properties.[60] Despite the appeal of this hypothesis, many important exogenous and endogenous factors may contribute to differences between Asian and non-Asian populations, and relatively few studies have considered phytoestrogens or soy intake in relation to risk for prostate cancer. A large case-control study based in a multiethnic population showed an inverse association between soy food intake and risk of prostate cancer,[51] but other studies have not supported the soy hypothesis.[31,61] Interestingly, some studies have suggested inverse associations between intake of legumes in general (primarily not soybeans) and risk of prostate cancer, including ecologic (for prostate cancer mortality r = −0.59),[3] cohort,[52,56] and case-control.[50,51,55] A potential beneficial role of legumes deserves further investigation.

A final micronutrient that warrants discussion is vitamin D because the metabolically active component $1,25(OH)_2$ vitamin D_3 inhibits proliferation and induces differentiation of prostatic epithelial cells[62] and may be particularly important for preventing prostate cancer metastasis.[63] However, perhaps because $1,25(OH)_2$ vitamin D_3 is tightly homeostatically regulated and is not substantially influenced by dietary vitamin D (except in deficiency states), studies generally do not support an association between dietary or supplemental intake of vitamin D and prostate cancer risk.[32,46,64,65] In addition, sunlight exposure is probably the biggest contributor to vitamin D levels. Interestingly, in a case-control study conducted in the UK, where vitamin D deficiency is relatively common, childhood sunburn frequency, regular foreign holidays, sunbathing score, and higher exposure to UV radiation were associated with a reduced risk of prostate cancer.[66] Studies of circulating vitamin D are summarized in Chapter 4.

LIFESTYLE FACTORS

PHYSICAL ACTIVITY

Physical activity could influence the levels of various hormones hypothesized to affect prostate cancer. Whether physical activity influences prostate cancer risk remains unsettled. The epidemiologic literature is quite mixed on the matter, probably for a number of reasons, including the difficulty in accurately assessing physical activity, potentially different roles of moderate and high intensity exercise, when in the lifespan physical activity is assessed, and what stage of prostate cancer is considered. Three studies showed that greater physical activity in young adulthood may be associated with increased risk later in life,[67-69] whereas a higher level of physical activity later in elderly men has been found to decrease risk of advanced prostate cancer.[70,71] These important methodological issues need to be addressed in future studies.

CIGARETTE SMOKING

Generally, cigarette smoking has not been considered an important risk factor for prostate cancer incidence. However, in the literature, there are reports of higher risk of metastatic or fatal prostate cancer in smokers.[30,72-78] The risk of advanced prostate cancer may be greater for recent smoking rather than cumulative exposure.[78] Supporting a role of cigarette smoking for prostate cancer progression are studies that show smokers with a higher stage or grade at the time of diagnosis[25,79-82] and with poorer survival.[83] The mechanisms whereby smoking may influence prostate cancer progression is unclear, but it is possible that carcinogens in cigarette smoke cause mutations in relatively non-aggressive prostate cancers making them more aggressive.

ALCOHOL DRINKING

From approximately 60 epidemiologic studies that have evaluated alcohol consumption in relation to risk of prostate cancer, it can be concluded that alcohol intake is probably not a strong risk factor for prostate cancer incidence or mortality.[84] However, heavy alcohol drinkers, particularly those with potentially deleterious patterns (i.e., binge drinkers), may be at modestly higher risk of prostate cancer.[85] Moderate drinking, which may have some health benefits, probably is not a major factor, either beneficial or deleterious, in prostate cancer risk.

SEXUAL ACTIVITY

Sexual activity may plausibly be related to prostate cancer risk through some causal and some indirect mechanisms. For example, men with low androgenicity may experience a low sexual drive; if androgenicity is related to prostate cancer risk (see Chapter 68), then sexual activity may be indirectly (noncausally) associated with risk. If exposure to sexually transmitted agents (as discussed below) enhances risk, then sexual activity, at least to the extent it is associated with transmitted diseases, could increase risk. Most epidemiologic studies reporting on sexual activity are case-control studies, in which sexual activity is based on reporting after the diagnosis in cases, which may cause biased results. In a meta-analysis, men with prostate cancer were more likely to report slightly greater past sexual activity; associations with sexually transmitted diseases was stronger than for overall sexual activity.[86] However, two recent studies, one a case-control study[87] and the other a prospective study[88] found that men reporting more ejaculations in the past had a lower risk of prostate cancer. Whether reduced ejaculation may causally increase risk of prostate cancer is speculative at present but deserves some consideration.

MEDICATIONS USE AND MEDICAL PROCEDURES

ASPIRIN AND NONSTEROIDAL ANTI-INFLAMMATORY DRUGS

Aspirin and nonsteroidal anti-inflammatory drugs (NSAIDs) could plausibly decrease prostate cancer risk by inhibiting cyclooxygenase (COX) enzymes. Overall, prospective and case-control studies suggest a weak inverse association between regular use of aspirin or NSAIDs and risk of total or advanced prostate cancer, although associations have been relatively modest (about 15–25% reduction in risk) for most studies[89–93] except two that found strong inverse associations of 0.35[94] and 0.45.[95] These latter two studies were case-control studies, so differential likelihood of participation of cases and controls by use of aspirin and NSAIDs and differential accuracy in recall between cases and controls could have inflated the apparent benefit. A recent meta-analysis confirmed a modest reduction in risk associated with aspirin use.[96] Although the benefits of anti-inflammatory agents in the prevention of prostate cancer may be relatively modest, additional well-designed prospective studies are warranted.

VASECTOMY

Whether vasectomy causally increases prostate cancer is controversial, particularly since a biological basis underlying this relation remains unclear. A meta-analysis reported a summary relative risk for 22 studies of 1.37 (95% CI = 1.15–1.62) for ever having had a vasectomy; the summary relative risk was 1.22 (95% CI = 0.90–1.64) for the five prospective studies considered.[97] The risk of prostate cancer was greater for a longer time since vasectomy.[97] Some have argued that detection bias or confounding may account for the positive results.[98,99]

INFECTION AND THE RESPONSE TO INFECTION

SEXUALLY TRANSMITTED INFECTIONS

A recent meta-analysis reported statistically significant summary estimates from 23 case-control studies of 1.44 for any history of sexually transmitted infection (STI), 2.30 for syphilis, and 1.34 for gonorrhea.[86] Although suggestive of a link between STIs and prostate cancer, all of these studies ascertained STI history retrospectively, which raises concern about differential accuracy in report of past STI. It is possible that cases are more likely to report a history of STI than controls, who may be less invested in the study. However, positive associations with prostate cancer have been reported for circulating antibodies against various STIs, providing some support of this hypothesis. The role of STIs and other infections in the etiology of prostate cancer remains unresolved, but it is a promising area.

PROSTATITIS

Clinical prostatitis is a common urologic condition with multiple, often unclear causes. In some cases of prostatitis, if not most, bacterial infections may be the underlying cause.[100] A meta-analysis of 11 case-control studies reported a statistically significant summary estimate for prostate cancer of 1.57 in men ever having had prostatitis compared with those without this diagnosis.[101] These studies potentially suffer from recall bias, variable quality confirmation of prostatitis, inability to classify type of prostatitis or to detect asymptomatic prostatitis, and prostate cancer detection bias due to enhanced surveillance in men with prostatitis.[101] Because of the suggestive evidence, and the strong biologic plausibility that chronic inflammation would increase cancer risk, this area deserves further study.

FUTURE RESEARCH

Understanding the epidemiology of prostate cancer has promise in providing leads that can be ultimately formulated into preventive strategies. However, unraveling the relationship between diet and lifestyle factors and prostate carcinogenesis remains a major challenge. The study of this malignancy has not produced consistent results, probably due to a number of factors as summarized in the Introduction. Nevertheless, several areas hold promise for primary prevention. These include energy imbalance and dietary macronutrient composition, inflammation, and micronutrients and phytochemicals as potentially protective agents.

The reasons explaining higher risk in African-Americans, lower risk in Asian populations, and higher risk in Western countries, especially those in Northern Europe, remain unexplained. Energy imbalance, intake of red meat and dairy products, and low intake of soy products and fish could contribute to higher risk in some populations. Hormonal and genetic factors may also play a role. The increasing prevalence of overweight and obesity has drawn much interest into their influence on health. For prostate cancer, energy balance may be important but questions remain regarding the relative importance of factors early and late in life. The relationship with obesity has been not clear, and how individual metabolic differences in processing energy influence risk needs to be studied.

In recent years, increasing interest has centered on the role of chronic intraprostatic inflammation in prostate carcinogenesis, largely because of pathologic studies. Inflammation merits attention because of the recognition of the potential significance of proliferative inflammatory atrophy lesions in the prostate,[102] and because of the potential in targeting inflammation for intervention. Specifically, the identification of potential infectious agents could lead to treatments that may ultimately decrease the risk of prostate cancer. Some evidence already suggests a potential benefit of aspirin use, albeit modest, on prostate cancer incidence or progression. Many nonspecific and selective COX2 inhibitors should be evaluated in relation to risk of prostate cancer.

A third promising area concerns the potential use of micronutrients, antioxidants, and phytochemicals as potential nutritional or chemopreventive agents. A number of candidates exist, though the evidence is not yet compelling for them. Among the most promising candidates include selenium, α- and γ-tocopherol (vitamin E), lycopene, marine omega-3 fatty acids, vitamin D, and components in cruciferous vegetables, legumes, and allium vegetables. Of note, current epidemiologic evidence for many of these is based primarily on food sources of these (e.g., tomato products for lycopene, oily fish for omega-3 fatty acids). For items that have other established health benefits, or at least that are unlikely to be harmful, it may be reasonable to make prudent recommendations indicating potential benefits on prostate cancer risk based on the best available data. Intervention studies must be conducted before recommendations may be made about use of concentrated forms of putative protective agents in pills (e.g., lycopene as the active agent in tomatoes).

REFERENCES

1. Parkin DM, Whelan SL, Ferlay J, et al. Cancer Incidence in Five Continents. Lyon: International Agency for Research on Cancer, IARC Scientific Publications No. 155, 2003.

2. Armstrong B, Doll R. Environmental factors and cancer incidence and mortality in different countries, with special reference to dietary practices. Int J Cancer 1975;15:617–31.

3. Rose DP, Boyar AP, Wynder EL. International comparisons of mortality rates for cancer of the breast, ovary, prostate, and colon, and per capita food consumption. Cancer 1986;58:2263–2271.

4. Shimizu H, Ross RK, Bernstein L, et al. Cancers of the prostate and breast among Japanese and white immigrants in Los Angeles county. Br J Cancer 1991;63:963–966.

5. American Cancer Society. Cancer Facts & Figures, 2003. Atlanta, GA, 2003.

6. Jemal A, Murray T, Samuels A, et al. Cancer Statistics, 2003. CA Cancer J Clin Med 2003;53:5–26.

7. Potosky AL, Miller BA, Albertsen PC, et al. The role of increasing detection in the rising incidence of prostate cancer. J Am Med Assoc 1995;273:548–552.

8. Platz EA, Rimm EB, Willett WC, et al. Racial variation in prostate cancer incidence and in hormonal system markers among male health professionals. J Natl Cancer Inst 2000;92:2009–2017.

9. Glover Jr FE, Coffey DS, Douglas LL, et al. The epidemiology of prostate cancer in Jamaica. J Urol 1998;159:1984–1986.

10. Ahluwalia B, Jackson MA, Jones GW, et al. Blood hormone profiles in prostate cancer patients in high-risk and low-risk populations. Cancer 1981;48:2267–2273.

11. Kritchevsky D. Caloric restriction and experimental carcinogenesis. Toxicol Sci 1999;52 (suppl):13–16.

12. Thompson HJ, Jiang W, Zhu Z. Mechanisms by which energy restriction inhibits carcinogenesis. Adv Exp Med Biol 1999;470:77–84.

13. Mukherjee P, Sotnikov AV, Mangian HJ, et al. Energy intake and prostate tumor growth, angiogenesis, and vascular endothelial growth factor expression. J Natl Cancer Inst 1999;91:512–523.

14. Le Marchand L, Kolonel LN, Wilkens LR, et al. Animal fat consumption and prostate cancer: a prospective study in Hawaii. Epidemiology 1994;5:276–282.

15. Andersson SO, Baron J, Wolk A, et al. Early life risk factors for prostate cancer: a population-based case-control study in Sweden. Cancer Epidemiol Biomarkers Prev 1995;4:187–192.

16. Andersson SO, Baron J, Bergström R, et al. Lifestyle factors and prostate cancer risk: a case-control study in Sweden. Cancer Epidemiol Biomarkers Prev 1996;5:509–513.

17. Andersson SO, Wolk A, Bergström R, et al. Body size and prostate cancer: a 20-year follow-up study among 135 006 Swedish construction workers. J Natl Cancer Inst 1997;89:385–389.

18. Giovannucci E, Rimm EB, Stampfer MJ, et al. Height, body weight, and risk of prostate cancer. Cancer Epidemiol Biomarkers Prev 1997;6:557–563.

19. Herbert PR, Ajani U, Cook N, et al. Adult height and incidence of total malignant neoplasms and prostate cancer: the Physicians' Health Study [abstract]. Am J Epidemiol 1996;143:S78.

20. Hayes RB, Ziegler RG, Gridley G, et al. Dietary factors and risks for prostate cancer among blacks and whites in the United States. Cancer Epidemiol Biomarkers Prev 1999;8:25–34.

21. Lund Nilsen TI, Vatten LJ. Anthropometry and prostate cancer risk: a prospective study of 22,248 Norwegian men. Cancer Causes Control 1999;10:269–275.

22. Habel LA, Van Den Eeden SK, Friedman GD. Body size, age at shaving initiation, and prostate cancer in a large, multiracial cohort. Prostate 2000;43:136–143.

23. Nomura AM. Body size and prostate cancer. Epidemiol Rev 2001;23:126–131.

24. Calle EE, Rodriguez C, Walker-Thurmond K, et al. Overweight, obesity, and mortality from cancer in a prospectively studied cohort of U.S. adults. N Engl J Med 2003;348:1625–1638.

25. Spitz MR, Strom SS, Yamamura Y, et al. Epidemiologic determinants of clinically relevant prostate cancer. Int J. Cancer 2000;89:259–264.

26. Rohrmann S, Roberts WW, Walsh PC, et al. Family history of prostate cancer and obesity in relation to high-grade disease and extraprostatic extension in young men with prostate cancer. Prostate 2003;55:140–146.

27. Platz E. Energy imbalance and prostate cancer. J Nutr 2002;132 (suppl):3471S–3481S.

28. Platz EA, Michaud DS, Willett WC, et al. Interrelation of energy intake and body size with metastatic/fatal prostate cancer. Proc Am Assoc Cancer Res 2002;43:933–934.

29. Kushi L, Giovannucci E. Dietary fat and cancer. Am J Med 2002;113:63S–70S.

30. Hsing AW, McLaughlin JK, Schuman LM, et al. Diet, tobacco use, and fatal prostate cancer: results from the Lutheran Brotherhood Cohort Study. Cancer Res 1990;50:6836–6840.

31. Severson RK, Nomura AMY, Grove JS, et al. A prospective study of demographics, diet, and prostate cancer among men of Japanese ancestry in Hawaii. Cancer Res 1989;49:1857–1860.

32. Chan JM, Pietinen P, Virtanen M, et al. Diet and prostate cancer risk in a cohort of smokers, with a specific focus on calcium and phosphorus (Finland). Cancer Causes Control 2000;11:859–867.

33. Giovannucci E, Rimm EB, Colditz GA, et al. A prospective study of dietary fat and risk of prostate cancer. J Natl Cancer Inst 1993;85:1571–1579.

34. West DW, Slattery ML, Robison LM, et al. Adult dietary intake and prostate cancer risk in Utah: a case-control study with special emphasis on aggressive tumors. Cancer Causes Control 1991;2:85–94.

35. Whittemore AS, Kolonel LN, Wu AH, et al. Prostate cancer in relation to diet, physical activity, and body size in blacks, whites, and Asians in the United States and Canada. J Natl Cancer Inst 1995;87:652–661.

36. Groff JL, Gropper SS. Advanced Nutrition and Human Metabolism. Belmont, CA: Wadsworth, 2000.

37. Schuurman AG, van den Brandt PA, Dorant E, et al. Association of energy and fat intake with prostate carcinoma risk: results from the Netherlands Cohort Study. Cancer 1999;86:1019–1027.

38. Leitzmann MF, Stampfer MJ, Michaud DS, et al. Dietary intake of omega-3 and omega-6 fatty acids and the risk of prostate cancer. Am J Clin Nutr 2004;80:204–216.

39. Gann PH, Hennekens CH, Sacks FM, et al. Prospective study of plasma fatty acids and risk of prostate cancer. J Natl Cancer Inst 1994;86:281–286.

40. Veierod MB, Laake P, Thelle DS. Dietary fat intake and risk of prostate cancer: a prospective study of 25,708 Norwegian men. Int J Cancer 1997;73:634–638.

41. Michaud DS, Augustsson K, Rimm EB, et al. A prospective study on intake of animal products and risk of prostate cancer. Cancer Causes Control 2001;12:557–567.

42. Schuurman AG, van den Brandt PA, Dorant E, et al. Animal products, calcium and protein and prostate cancer risk in the Netherlands Cohort Study. Br J Cancer 1999;80:1107–1113.

43. Terry P, Lichtenstein P, Reychting M, et al. Fatty fish consumption and risk of prostate cancer. Lancet 2001;357:1764–1766.

44. Augustsson K, Michaud DS, Rimm EB, et al. A prospective study of intake of fish and marine fatty acids and prostate cancer. Cancer Epidemiol Biomarkers Prev 2003;12:64–67.

45. Qin LQ, Xu JY, Wang PY, et al. Milk consumption is a risk factor for prostate cancer: meta-analysis of case-control studies. Nutr Cancer 2004;48:22–27.

46. Giovannucci E, Rimm EB, Wolk A, et al. Calcium and fructose intake in relation to risk of prostate cancer. Cancer Res 1998;58:442–447.

47. Chan JM, Stampfer MJ, Ma J, et al. Dairy products, calcium, and prostate cancer risk in the Physicians' Health Study [comment]. Am J Clin Nutr 2001;74:549–554.

48. Rodriguez C, McCullough ML, Mondul AM, et al. Calcium, dairy products, and risk of prostate cancer in a prospective cohort of United States men. Cancer Epidemiol Biomarkers Prev 2003;12:597–603.

49. Giovannucci E, Pollak M, Liu Y, et al. Nutritional predictors of insulin-like growth factor I and their relationships to cancer in men. Cancer Epidemiol Biomarkers Prev 2003;12:84–89.

50. Cohen JH, Kristal AR, Stanford JL. Fruit and vegetable intakes and prostate cancer risk. J Natl Cancer Inst 2000;92:61–68.

51. Kolonel LN, Hankin JH, Whittemore AS, et al. Vegetables, fruits, legumes and prostate cancer: a multiethnic case-control study. Cancer Epidemiol Biomarkers Prev 2000;9:795–804.

52. Mills PK, Beeson WL, Phillips RL, et al. Cohort study of diet, lifestyle, and prostate cancer in Adventist men. Cancer 1989;64:598–604.

53. Giovannucci E, Rimm EB, Liu Y, et al. A prospective study of tomato products, lycopene, and prostate cancer risk. J Natl Cancer Inst 2002;94:391–398.

54. Hsing AW, Chokkalingam AP, Gao YT, et al. Allium vegetables and risk of prostate cancer: a population-based study. J Natl Cancer Inst 2002;94:1648–1651.

55. Key TJA, Silcocks PB, Davey GK, et al. A case-control study of diet and prostate cancer. Br J Cancer 1997;76:678–687.

56. Schuurman AG, Goldbohm A, Dorant E, et al. Vegetable and fruit consumption and prostate cancer risk: a cohort study in the Netherlands. Cancer Epidemiol Biomarkers Prev 1998;7:673–680.

57. Sies H, Stahl W. Vitamins E and C, β-carotene, and other carotenoids as antioxidants. Am J Clin Nutr 1995;62:1315S–1321S.

58. Kristal AR, Lampe JW. Brassica vegetables and prostate cancer risk: a review of the epidemiologic evidence. Nutr Cancer 2002;42:1–9.

59. Giovannucci E, Rimm EB, Liu Y, et al. A prospective study of cruciferous vegetables and prostate cancer. Cancer Epidemiol Biomarkers Prev 2003;12:1403–1409.

60. Morrissey C, Watson RW. Phytoestrogens and prostate cancer. Curr Drug Targets 2003;4:231–241.

61. Villeneuve PJ, Johnson KC, Kreiger N, et al. The Canadian Cancer Registries Epidemiology Research Group. Risk factors for prostate cancer: results from the Canadian National Enhanced Cancer Surveillance System. Cancer Causes Control 1999;10:355–367.

62. Peehl DM, Skowronski RJ, Leung GK, et al. Antiproliferative effects of 1,25-dihydroxyvitamin D_3 on primary cultures of human prostatic cells. Cancer Res 1994;54:805–810.

63. Sung V, Feldman D. 1,25-Dihydroxyvitamin D_3 decreases human prostate cancer cell adhesion and migration. Mol Cell Endocrinol 2000;164:133–143.

64. Chan JM, Giovannucci E, Andersson S-O, et al. Dairy products, calcium, phosphorus, vitamin D, and risk of prostate cancer. Cancer Causes Control 1998;9:559–566.

65. Kristal AR, Cohen JH, Qu P, et al. Associations of energy, fat, calcium, and vitamin D with prostate cancer risk. Cancer Epidemiol Biomarkers Prev 2002;11:719–725.

66. Luscombe CJ, Fryer AA, French ME, et al. Exposure to ultraviolet radiation: association with susceptibility and age at presentation with prostate cancer. Lancet 2001;358:641–642.

67. Polednak AP. College athletics, body size, and cancer mortality. Cancer 1976;38:382–387.

68. Whittemore AS, Paffenbarger Jr RS, Anderson K, et al. Early precursors of site-specific cancers in college men and women. J Natl Cancer Inst 1985;74:43–51.

69. Paffenbarger Jr RS, Hyde RT, Wing AL. Physical activity and incidence of cancer in diverse populations: a preliminary report. Am J Clin Nutr 1987;45:312–317.

70. Lee IM, Paffenbarger Jr RS, Hsieh CC. Physical activity and risk of prostatic cancer among college alumni. Am J Epidemiol 1992;135:169–179.

71. Giovannucci E, Leitzmann M, Spiegelman D, et al. A prospective study of physical activity and prostate cancer in male health professionals. Cancer Res 1998;58:5117–5122.

72. Hsing AW, McLaughlin JK, Hrubec Z, et al. Tobacco use and prostate cancer: 26-year follow-up of US veterans. Am J Epidemiol 1991;133:437–441.

73. Hiatt RA, Armstrong MA, Klatsky AL, et al. Alcohol consumption, smoking, and other risk factors and prostate cancer in a large health plan cohort in California (United States). Cancer Causes Control 1994;5:66–72.

74. Adami HO, Bergström R, Engholm G, et al. A prospective study of smoking and risk of prostate cancer. Int J Cancer 1996;67:764–768.

75. Coughlin SS, Neaton JD, Sengupta A. Cigarette smoking as a predictor of death from prostate cancer in 348,874 men screened for the Multiple Risk Factor Intervention Trial. Am J Epidemiol 1996;143:1002–1006.

76. Rodriguez C, Tatham LM, Thun MJ, et al. Smoking and fatal prostate cancer in a large cohort of adult men. Am J Epidemiol 1997;145:466–475.

77. Cerhan JR, Torner JC, Lynch CF, et al. Association of smoking, body mass, and physical activity with risk of prostate cancer in the Iowa 65+ Rural Health Study (United States). Cancer Causes Control 1997;8:229–238.

78. Giovannucci E, Rimm EB, Ascherio A, et al. Smoking and risk of total and fatal prostate cancer in United States health professionals. Cancer Epidemiol Biomarkers Prev 1999;8:277–282.

79. Daniell HW. A worse prognosis for smokers with prostate cancer. J Urol 1995;154:153–157.

80. Roberts WW, Platz EA, Walsh PC. Association of cigarette smoking with extraprostatic prostate cancer in young men. J Urol 2003;169:512–516.

81. Kobrinsky NL, Klug MG, Hokanson PJ, et al. Impact of smoking on cancer stage at diagnosis. J Clin Oncol 2003;21:907–913.

82. Pickles T, Liu M, Berthelet E, et al. The effect of smoking on outcome following external radiation for localized prostate cancer. Prostate Cohort Outcomes Initiative. J Urol 2004;171:1543–1546.

83. Oefelein MG, Resnick MI. Association of tobacco use with hormone refractory disease and survival of patients with prostate cancer. J Urol 2004;171:2281–2284.

84. Dennis L. Meta-analysis for combining relative risks of alcohol consumption and prostate cancer. Prostate 2000;42:56–66.

85. Platz EA, Leitzmann MF, Rimm EB, et al. Alcohol intake, drinking patterns, and risk of prostate cancer in a large prospective cohort study. Am J Epidemiol 2004;159:444–453.

86. Dennis LK, Dawson DV. Meta-analysis of measures of sexual activity and prostate cancer. Epidemiology 2002;13:72–79.

87. Giles GG, Severi G, English DR, et al. Sexual factors and prostate cancer. BJU Int 2003;92:211–216.

88. Leitzmann MF, Platz EA, Stampfer MJ, et al. Ejaculation frequency and subsequent risk of prostate cancer. JAMA 2004;291:1578–1586.

89. Habel LA, Zhao W, Stanford JL. Daily aspirin use and prostate cancer risk in a large, multiracial cohort in the US. Cancer Causes Control 2002;13:427–434.

90. Leitzmann MF, Stampfer MJ, Ma J, et al. Aspirin use in relation to risk of prostate cancer. Cancer Epidemiol Biomarkers Prev 2002;11:1108–1111.

91. Norrish AE, Jackson RT, McRae CU. Non-steroidal anti-inflammatory drugs and prostate cancer progression. Int J Cancer 1998;77:511–515.

92. Bucher C, Jordan P, Nickeleit V, et al. Relative risk of malignant tumors in analgesic abusers. Effects of long-term intake of aspirin. Clin Nephrol 1999;51:67–72.

93. Irani J, Ravery V, Pariente JL, et al. Effect of nonsteroidal anti-inflammatory agents and finasteride on prostate cancer risk. J Urol 2002;168:1985–1988.

94. Nelson JE, Harris RE. Inverse association of prostate cancer and non-steroidal anti-inflammatory drugs (NSAIDS): results of a case-control study. Oncol Rep 2000;7:169–170.

95. Roberts RO, Jacobson DJ, Girman CJ, et al. A population-based study of daily nonsteroidal anti-inflammatory drug use and prostate cancer. Mayo Clin Proc 2002;77:219–225.

96. Mahmud S, Franco E, Aprikian A. Prostate cancer and use of nonsteroidal anti-inflammatory drugs: systematic review and meta-analysis. Br J Cancer 2004;90:93–99.

97. Dennis LK, Dawson DV, Resnick MI. Vasectomy and the risk of prostate cancer: a meta-analysis examining vasectomy status, age at vasectomy, and time since vasectomy. Prostate Cancer Prostatic Dis 2002;5:193–203.

98. Skegg D. Vasectomy and prostate cancer: is there a link? NZ Med J 1993;106:242–243.

99. Howards SS, Peterson HB. Vasectomy and prostate cancer: Chance, bias, or a causal relationship. J Am Med Assoc 1993;269:913–914.

100. Roberts RO, Lieber MM, Rhodes T, et al. Prevalence of a physician-assigned diagnosis of prostatitis: the Olmsted County Study of Urinary Symptoms and Health Status Among Men. Urology 1998;51:578–584.

101. Dennis LK, Lynch CF, Torner JC. Epidemiologic association between prostatitis and prostate cancer. Urology 2002;60:78–83.

102. De Marzo AM, Marchi VL, Epstein JI, et al. Proliferative inflammatory atrophy of the prostate: implications for prostatic carcinogenesis. Am J Pathol 1999;155:1985–1992.

Molecular epidemiology of prostate cancer

4

Elizabeth A Platz, Edward Giovannucci

INTRODUCTION

In molecular epidemiologic studies of prostate cancer, the association of biomarkers of exposure measured in blood or other tissues is evaluated in relation to incidence or mortality. These biomarkers capture aspects of diet, environmental contaminants, and factors for which concentrations are partially inherently determined. In summarizing the evidence for these biomarkers, studies of large size and that used sound designs and methods for assessing the biomarkers are highlighted. Possible methodologic explanations for inconsistencies in findings among studies are advanced. Finally, direction for future molecular epidemiologic investigations on the causes and prevention of prostate cancer is given.

BIOMARKERS OF DIET

Collecting self-reported usual diet allows for the estimation of intake and ranking of individuals on their intake of major macro- and micronutrients (details on the association of intake of foods and nutrients with prostate cancer is reviewed in Chapter 66). However, some nutrients are not well captured by self-report because the amounts in food depend on levels in the soil in which the food was grown; and also because of person-to-person variability in bioavailability due to inherent factors or differences in other diet components that affect uptake. Measurement of biomarkers may better account for absorption and reflect better the opportunity for dietary constituents to influence prostate carcinogenesis. The most studied dietary biomarkers in relation to prostate cancer are plasma lycopene; plasma and toenail selenium; plasma vitamin E; plasma vitamin D; and plasma, erythrocyte, and adipose fatty acids. Despite their common use, for the most part, the correlation between biomarker levels in these tissues and in the prostate is unknown.

LYCOPENE

Following publication in the mid-1990s of a possible protective effect of tomatoes on the risk of prostate cancer in a large prospective cohort study, a number of investigators have evaluated the association of plasma concentrations of lycopene and prostate cancer. Lycopene, a carotenoid that is an efficient free radical scavenger,[1] was targeted as the explanatory constituent of tomatoes because they are the major food source of lycopene in the US diet. Lycopene imparts the red color to tomatoes, and also to pink grapefruit and watermelon, but the amount consumed and absorbed from these foods in the US is minor relative to tomatoes.

When taken together, case-control studies nested in prospective cohorts[2-4] support inverse associations for prostate cancer overall, local disease, and advanced disease on the order of a 25% to 50% lower risk in the top versus bottom quantile of plasma lycopene. A decreasing dose-response has not been observed; however, the benefit seems to be limited to the top quartile, the cut-point for which has varied among studies. A study nested in the CLUE II cohort observed a nonstatistically significant odds ratio (OR) of total prostate cancer for plasma lycopene that was weaker in magnitude than in other cohorts reporting inverse associations.[5] In the CARET trial of current and former smokers, men in the second and third, but not the fourth, quantile of plasma lycopene had a reduced risk of prostate cancer.[6] A prospective study not showing an association[7] had very low mean lycopene (13.4 µg/dL) compared with studies showing inverse associations (18.7–38.8 µg/dL). In a prostate-specific antigen (PSA) era cohort study, the inverse association for plasma lycopene and prostate cancer was limited to older men.[4] Prostate cancer in older men may be more likely the result of cumulative oxidative damage and nongenetic mechanisms over life, whereas prostate cancer in younger men may have a greater genetic predisposition. Plasma levels of the carotenoids α-carotene, β-carotene, β-cryptoxanthin, lutein/zeaxanthin[2,3,5–10] and vitamin A[2,3,5,7,11,12] have not been consistently related to prostate cancer.

Overall, molecular epidemiologic data indicate that a higher circulating lycopene concentration is probably associated with a lower risk of prostate cancer. Because lycopene is a potent antioxidant in vitro, the major hypothesized mechanism is the reduction in oxidative damage via the quenching of free radicals—a mechanism that could apply to all stages of prostate cancer. Another mechanism of action that has been suggested is suppression of expression of genes involved in hormone and growth factor production.[13] Although studies have considered confounding, favorable dietary and lifestyle patterns that are not accounted for cannot be ruled out as an explanation. Importantly, further work is needed to determine whether the observed benefit is due to lycopene or other tomato-specific constituents. Lycopene does reach the prostate and has been found to be present at the highest concentration compared with other tissues.[14] However, a study in a rodent model of prostate carcinogenesis found that whole-tomato powder was much more effective in decreasing prostate cancer mortality than was pure lycopene.[15]

SELENIUM

Although an anticancer effect of selenium has been hypothesized for many decades, excitement about the potentially protective effect of selenium against prostate cancer arose primarily from a secondary finding from a trial of selenium in the prevention of recurrent skin cancer.[16] Study subjects had a prior skin cancer and were living in regions with low soil selenium. Skin cancer risk was not reduced in the group receiving the selenium supplement versus the placebo group, but those who received selenium did have a 63% lower risk of prostate cancer. Selenium was selected for testing in that trial because it is essential for the activity of glutathione peroxidase,[17] making it an indirect antioxidant. Selenium also exhibits antiproliferative and proapoptotic activity, and may be important for DNA stability.[18,19]

Because the selenium content of food depends on geographical source, and its intestinal absorption and distribution depends on the presence of metals that compete for uptake,[20] dietary selenium intake may not adequately assess selenium stores. Selenium content in blood and toenails is a good marker of bioavailable selenium. Several prospective studies support inverse associations between selenium level in toenail clippings[21–23] or plasma[24–26] and prostate cancer incidence or mortality of 50% to 60% across extreme quantiles. No such association was observed in the CARET trial (plasma)[27] or in a UK population-based case-control study (fingernail).[28] Four cohort studies[21,22,25,26] suggested a threshold effect for selenium, although where the threshold occurred varied, with some suggesting an association only in the top versus bottom quantile and in others suggesting an equal benefit in all quantiles compared with the bottom. The threshold effect is consistent with the skin cancer trial[29] in which the reduced prostate cancer risk in the selenium group was present only in men with low baseline serum selenium.

In the Physicians' Health Study, an inverse association was present for advanced, but not local, prostate cancer overall, but, when examined according to whether the study was from the pre-PSA era or the PSA era, the association was inverse for both local and advanced prostate cancer in the pre-PSA era and inverse only for advanced disease in the PSA era.[26] Other studies observed inverse associations that were stronger for advanced disease than for local disease[24] or that were present for both local and advanced disease.[23] Because screening for elevated PSA concentrations can lead to the detection of small, clinically insignificant disease, even local disease diagnosed in the PSA era may have a less aggressive phenotype than local disease diagnosed in the pre-PSA era. The changed nature of the cases with PSA screening may account for some differences in findings for selenium by stage.

The inverse association in the Physicians' Health Study also was limited to cases with a baseline plasma PSA of more than 4 ng/mL, possibly suggesting that selenium influences prostate cancer progression, rather than development. A similar inference could be made from the skin cancer trial; the decrement in prostate cancer cases in the selenium group compared with the placebo group occurred early in the trial. Such short-term exposure would not be expected to influence prostate cancer development given that by middle age a substantial proportion of men already have occult disease. However, if selenium does influence progression, the observation of fewer cases is compatible with a short-term exposure inhibiting small tumors from becoming large enough to be detectable by screening.

A prospective study in Finland, a country with low selenium intake during the study follow-up, showed no association between serum selenium and prostate cancer.[30] Participants had circulating levels almost three times lower than in other studies. Beginning in 1984 in Finland, fertilizers were fortified with selenium and, despite increases in blood selenium, over the next decades prostate cancer incidence rates continued to rise while mortality did not change much. Why US studies indicate a benefit with selenium, whereas Finnish data[30] are not supportive is unclear.

Resolving the potential influence of selenium as a preventive agent against prostate cancer is a top priority and is being evaluated in the SELECT trial.[31] The trial is of middle-aged men, and so the inferences drawn will be relevant to prostate cancer progression in the PSA era. Selenium has been shown to accumulate in prostate tissue after short-term administration of L-selenomethionine,[32] although the correlation between intraprostatic and toenail or plasma concentrations is yet to be defined.

VITAMIN E

Interest in vitamin E as a prostate cancer chemoprevention agent arose from findings of the Alpha Tocopherol Beta Carotene (ATBC) Trial on lung cancer in male Finnish smokers. In a secondary analysis, men randomized to the α-tocopherol supplement had statistically significant 32% and 41% reductions in prostate cancer incidence and mortality, respectively.[33] Risk decreased early in the trial, suggesting that vitamin E influences prostate cancer progression.[33] Tocopherol isomers, found in nuts and vegetable oils, exhibit antioxidant properties and may be proapoptotic.[34]

Overall, plasma concentrations of total, α-, and γ-tocopherols have not been shown to significantly influence prostate cancer risk in nested case-control studies.[2,3,7] Two exceptions are an inverse association for α-tocopherol (across extreme quintiles: OR = 0.64) and γ-tocopherol (OR = 0.25) in the CLUE II cohort,[5,22] and an inverse association for α-tocopherol (OR = 0.59), but not γ-tocopherol in the CARET trial.[6] Some prospective studies suggest an inverse association of higher circulating α-tocopherol concentrations in cigarette smokers,[3,6,12] in particular for more advanced prostate cancer, whereas, no association with baseline α-tocopherol was found in men not randomized to α-tocopherol in the ATBC trial of smokers.[35]

The SELECT trial is investigating α-tocopherol along with selenium.[31] Attention to the effects of specific tocopherol isomers and their interrelations is essential. Supplementation with α-tocopherol appears to diminish plasma level of γ-tocopherol,[36] which has a greater capacity to detoxify NO· than α-tocopherol.[37] In addition, alternative biological actions of vitamin E should be considered, such as the possible suppression of aromatase expression.[13]

VITAMIN D

Schwartz and Hulka hypothesized that vitamin D protects against prostate cancer based on their correlational study showing that US states with higher ultraviolet radiation tend to have lower prostate cancer mortality rates.[38] Cholecalciferol (vitamin D_3) is derived from ultraviolet light conversion of 7-dehydrocholesterol in the skin, but also from fortified milk products, breakfast cereals, and vitamin supplements. Cholecalciferol is converted in the liver to 25-hydroxyvitamin D_3—$25(OH)D_3$—which is converted in the kidney to 1,25-dihydroxyvitamin D_3—$1,25(OH)_2D_3$. The latter is a steroid hormone that augments calcium absorption from the bowel, and also plays a role in the control of proliferation and differentiation of prostate epithelial cells.[39]

Vitamin D sufficiency is assessed clinically by plasma concentration of $25(OH)D_3$. Perhaps because circulating $1,25(OH)_2D_3$ level is so tightly homeostatically regulated, five of six nested case-control studies do not support an association between $1,25(OH)_2D_3$ and prostate cancer,[40-44] the exception being an inverse association in a US study.[45] Only one[46] of eight studies[40-45,47] supports an inverse association for $25(OH)D_3$. In that Finnish study, more than half of the participants were clinically deficient in vitamin D, whereas in the other studies most men were replete, suggesting that only deficiency increases prostate cancer risk. A large prospective study consisting of three Nordic countries, showed a U-shaped association for $25(OH)D_3$: the lowest and highest quintiles had higher risks of prostate cancer compared with the middle.[47] Although at odds at face value, these findings are consistent with vitamin D deficiency increasing prostate cancer risk; the authors hypothesized that low $25(OH)D_3$ results in low intraprostatic $1,25(OH)_2D_3$, and high $25(OH)D_3$ results in $1,25(OH)_2D_3$ inactivation by 24-hydroxylase and thus lower intraprostatic $1,25(OH)_2D_3$.[47]

A possible explanatory mechanism for the apparent benefit of vitamin D on prostate cancer comes from experiments showing that $1,25(OH)_2D_3$ decreases the invasiveness of cells derived from prostate cancer metastases by reducing expression of cell adhesion integrins.[48] Thus, vitamin D is predicted to especially influence risk of metastatic disease. In three prospective studies,[41,45,46] in which all or most cases were detected in the pre-PSA era, vitamin D metabolites were suggestively more strongly inversely associated with advanced disease. Plasma $1,25(OH)_2D_3$ also was suggestively inversely associated with advanced prostate cancer, albeit based on few cases, in a prospective PSA era study.[43] More work is needed to discern effect of vitamin D on metastasis.

FATTY ACIDS

Polyunsaturated fatty acids are divided into omega-3 (precursor is α-linolenic acid) and omega-6 (precursor is linoleic acid). Eicosapentaenoic acid (EPA) and docosahexaenoic acid (DHA) are omega-3 fatty acids found in oily fish. Arachidonic acid, a precursor for prostaglandin synthesis, is an omega-6 fatty acid. In epidemiologic studies α-linolenic acid and omega-3 fatty acids, especially EPA and DHA, protect against cardiovascular disease,[49] and in vitro and in animal models these inhibit cancer growth, whereas linoleic acid enhances cancer cell growth. Biomarkers include fatty acids in plasma, erythrocytes, and adipose tissue.

Two nested case-control studies suggested a positive association between plasma α-linolenic acid concentration and prostate cancer risk,[50,51] although another did not.[52] In a small case-control study, men in the top three quartiles of erythrocyte and adipose α-linolenic acid had a nonstatistically significant higher prostate cancer risk.[53] Serum linoleic acid has not been associated with an increased risk of prostate cancer, and some studies are compatible with an inverse association.[50-52,54] However, higher levels of erythrocyte and adipose linoleic acid were associated with a nonstatistically significant higher risk of prostate cancer in a small case-control study.[53] Circulating concentrations of arachidonic acid, EPA, and DHA have not been associated with prostate cancer.[50-52] However, in case-control studies, men with higher erythrocyte and adipose EPA and DHA levels had a lower risk.[53,55]

Explanations are unknown for why experimental studies suggest that α-linolenic acid should protect against prostate cancer whereas some molecular epidemiologic studies suggest it increases risk. Only a small percentage of α-linolenic acid is converted to DHA and EPA and so the study of other metabolites may be relevant. Clearly more work is needed, including how variation in the fatty acid content of prostate epithelial cell membranes influences cell function and signaling, and on the correlation between fatty acid biomarkers and prostate tissue concentrations.

ENVIRONMENTAL CONTAMINANTS

Biomarkers of environmental contaminants have not been widely studied in relation to prostate cancer. Areas needing more investigation are cadmium, pesticides, and other contaminants that may affect hormone signaling. Cadmium is a metal that experimentally promotes prostate cancer cell growth and tumorigenesis and can signal through the androgen and estrogen receptors.[56] Toenail cadmium level was not positively associated with prostate cancer in a cohort without an occupational or environmental source of cadmium exposure.[57] Cadmium is unlikely to be a major risk factor for prostate cancer because of very low population exposure; however, biomarker studies in exposed men are needed. Many organochlorine pesticides and polychlorinated biphenyls (PCBs) are banned in the US, but persist in the environment. In a small hospital-based case-control study, a suggestion of a higher risk of prostate cancer with higher serum total PCBs, oxychlordane, and PCB 180 levels was suggested.[58]

FACTORS PARTIALLY INHERENTLY DETERMINED

SEX STEROID HORMONES

ANDROGENS

Androgens influence the development, maturation, and the maintenance of the prostate, affecting both proliferation and differentiation of the luminal epithelium. Whether normal range androgen concentrations are associated with risk of prostate cancer is unclear. Among the many prospective studies that assessed the association of circulating sex steroid hormones with prostate cancer,[59-62] only the Physicians' Health Study, in which most cases were diagnosed in the pre-PSA era, observed what had been hypothesized: testosterone and androstanediol glucuronide, a metabolite of dihydrotestosterone, were positively associated and estradiol and sex hormone binding globulin (SHBG) were inversely associated with prostate cancer. However, these associations emerged only after mutual statistical adjustment of the hormones and SHBG.[63] In the Baltimore Longitudinal Study of Aging, clinically low bioavailable testosterone (molar ratio of total testosterone to SHBG) measured several times over decades was associated with a lower prostate cancer risk; risk in the top three quartiles was equally as elevated.[62]

In four prospective studies, evidence for a higher risk of prostate cancer for a higher ratio of testosterone to either dihydrotestosterone or androstanediol glucuronide was present.[60,64-66] A meta-analysis of prospective studies conducted up to 1999 did not find case-control differences in concentrations, except possibly for slightly higher androstanediol glucuronide in the cases.[67] None of the studies included in the meta-analysis, except that by Gann et al[63] adjusted for SHBG or mutually for hormones, which might account for the overall lack of case-control differences in hormone levels. However, mutual adjustment in recent studies did not alter the lack of association of hormones with prostate cancer.[60,61,66]

A PSA era prospective study showed that men with higher plasma total and free testosterone concentrations had a lower risk of high-grade and a higher risk of low-grade prostate cancer,[61] findings consistent with clinical studies of nonmetastatic prostate cancer.[68-71] Given that lower grade reflects the maintenance of the normal functional tissue architecture, increased androgenic stimulation may prevent the dedifferentiation of the prostate epithelium in the nascent tumor. Alternatively, a reduction in intraprostatic dihydrotestosterone may allow a less differentiated phenotype to emerge. A higher detection rate of small, well-differentiated tumors because of greater PSA elevations in men with higher circulating androgens cannot be ruled out as an explanation for these findings, however.

The elevated risk of high-grade prostate cancer with lower testosterone is possibly supported by the Prostate Cancer Prevention Trial. Men were randomized to finasteride—a drug that inhibits 5α-reductase type 2, the enzyme catalyzing the conversion of testosterone to dihydrotestosterone in the prostate—or placebo for 7 years. The proportion of prostate cancers that were high grade was higher in the finasteride (35.9%) than in the placebo group (20.7%) despite a 24% reduction in prostate cancer prevalence in the finasteride group.[72] Whether finasteride enhances the development of high-grade disease merely produces pathologic artifactm or differential detection of high-grade cases, is under investigation.

ESTROGENS

Estrogens have been postulated to protect against prostate cancer via inhibition of prostate epithelial cell growth, but conversely to increase risk by eliciting inflammation in concert with androgens[73] or by the production of mutagenic metabolites.[74] Two prospective studies suggested that men in the low quantile of circulating estradiol are at increased risk of prostate cancer.[60,63] Another study suggested that higher estrogen levels are associated with higher prostate cancer risk.[75] Complicating interpretation of the findings, estradiol can be produced from testosterone intraprostatically by aromatase expressed in stroma.[76]

The role of androgens and estrogens in the etiology of prostate cancer remains complex. More work is needed on the action of androgens on the differentiation versus growth of prostate adenocarcinoma and the effects of estrogens jointly with androgens and independently on risk of prostate cancer.

INSULIN-LIKE GROWTH FACTOR AXIS

Insulin-like growth factor 1 (IGF1) is a peptide hormone that promotes growth in adolescence and childhood and is correlated with adult lean body mass.[77] It promotes proliferation and inhibits apoptosis in normal prostate and tumor cells in vitro.[78,79] Insulin-like growth factor 1 is produced in the liver, but also in other tissues including the prostate, and it circulates bound to binding proteins, the most prevalent of which is insulin-like growth factor binding protein 3 (IGFBP3). In the prostate, IGFBP3 promotes apoptosis via the retinoid X receptor[80] and may mediate growth

inhibition by 1,25(OH)$_2$D$_3$.[81] Insulin-like growth factor binding protein 3 can be cleaved by PSA[82] reducing its proapoptotic activity.

A positive association between plasma IGF1 level and prostate cancer is supported by several studies,[83–90] with a summary adjusted OR of 1.49 (95% CI = 1.14–1.95) comparing high to low IGF1 in a meta-analysis[91] (exclusive of subsequent publications[90,92]). The findings for IGFBP3 are not consistent; in some studies in which IGFBP3 was adjusted for IGF1 an inverse association was suggested overall[84,87,89,92] or at least in a subset of men.[86] In the meta-analysis, the summary adjusted OR for IGFBP3 was 0.95 (95% CI = 0.70–1.28),[91] contrary to the hypothesis of a protective effect of IGFBP3.

In a continuation of the Physicians' Health Study through 1995, IGF1 adjusted for IGFBP3 was no longer associated with prostate cancer overall, but was limited to cases that were of advanced stage at diagnosis (C or D) and were in the pre-PSA era.[92] These findings were echoed in a continuation of the Northern Sweden Health and Disease Cohort; IGF1 was more strongly positively associated with advanced than local disease in a population largely not PSA screened.[90] In a PSA era cohort study, a slightly increased risk of prostate cancer was observed in men in the highest quartile of IGF1 and in the highest quartile of IGFBP3; these associations were attenuated and no longer statistically significant after mutual statistical adjustment,[93] a finding that was comparable to those for nonadvanced disease in the Stattin et al study.[90]

The dichotomy in findings for IGFBP3 suggests that the associations for IGFBP3 in the literature are unlikely to be due solely to chance; other explanation(s) is likely, whether biological or methodological. One possible explanation for the differences in the direction of association with prostate cancer may be related to the forms of IGFBP3 (e.g., intact, fragments, glycosylated, phosphorylated) detected by commercial enzyme-linked immunosorbent assay (ELISA) kits. The extent of measurement error may have varied among studies and possibly within studies that have measured IGFBP3 in batches across time. Work is needed to uncover the variant patterns of association of IGF1 and IGFBP3 by nature of the prostate cancer case, early versus late stage, in the pre-PSA and PSA eras.

INSULIN AND GLUCOSE

Insulin and glucose are growth factors in vitro, but elevated concentrations result in lower androgen levels, at least in men with severe diabetes mellitus type 2, possibly as a result of the detrimental effect of hyperglycemia on the Leydig cells.[94] Therefore, if androgens are related to risk, it would be expected that longer-term poor insulin and glucose control in severe diabetics would be associated with a lower risk of prostate cancer. In contrast, hyperinsulinemia appears to increase risk of colon cancer, and could also be associated with a high risk of prostate cancer.

Studies on circulating insulin and glucose concentrations and measures of insulin resistance and the risk of prostate cancer have not been consistent.[86,95–100] For example, in a case-control study of Chinese men in which most of the cases were symptomatic at diagnosis, risk of prostate cancer was higher in men with insulin resistance than in men without,[96] yet in a prospective study of US men with repeated measures of fasting insulin over decades, no association was observed with prostate cancer.[97] More work is needed to uncover the relationship of insulin and glucose with prostate cancer at elevated levels and across the normal range, as well as by stage and grade of prostate cancer.

LEPTIN

Leptin, a peptide hormone produced by adipocytes, contributes to the control of body weight by modulating energy utilization.[101] Obese individuals become leptin resistant and exhibit elevated plasma leptin.[102] Findings for circulating leptin concentrations and prostate cancer have not been consistent.[95,103–106] Energy imbalance is emerging as a possible contributor to the progression of prostate cancer to metastasis and death.[107,108] Biomarkers of energy imbalance, such as leptin and adiponectin along with insulin and IGF1, need to be investigated in detail.

IMMUNE RESPONSE TO INFECTION AND OTHER SOURCES OF TISSUE DAMAGE

Chronic inflammation leading to hyperproliferation to replace damaged tissue contributes to the development of infection-associated cancers of the liver and stomach, and also colon cancer in patients with inflammatory bowel disease. If the inflammation–carcinogenesis model is relevant for the prostate, given the prevalence of prostate cancer, intraprostatic inflammation and regenerative lesions should be highly prevalent. Indeed, inflammatory infiltrates are frequent in prostate specimens.[109–111] Inflammatory infiltrates in regions of atrophy (called proliferative inflammatory atrophy lesions) are also frequent. These atrophic lesions, which exhibit low apoptosis and high proliferation, may be regenerative lesions, possibly the consequence of infection or cell trauma resulting from oxidant damage, hypoxia, or autoimmunity.[112]

Two classes of biomarkers pertinent to the inflammation hypothesis have been investigated for prostate cancer: antibodies against sexually transmitted infections (STIs) and circulating levels of cytokines produced by the innate or adaptive immune response. Molecular epidemiologic studies focusing on other possible contributors to or sequelae of the inflammatory response are needed.

ANTIBODIES AGAINST SEXUALLY TRANSMITTED INFECTIONS

Molecular epidemiologic studies evaluating the seroprevalence of antibodies against STIs provide indirect evidence for the role of inflammation in prostate carcinogenesis. Unlike studies of self-reported history of STIs, antibody studies are not susceptible to reporting bias. A small number of studies have reported positive associations of antibodies against syphilis,[113] human papillomavirus (HPV),[114,115] and human herpesvirus 8 (HHV8)[116] with prostate cancer. The putative biological mechanisms underlying these associations are likely varied. For example, HPV encodes oncogenic sequences,[117] whereas HHV8 encodes viral interleukin 6 (IL6) that shows homology to human IL6.[118] However, not all antibody studies are confirmatory, including for HPV[119] and *Chlamydia trachomatis*.[114]

Because prostate cancer is so common, to account for anything but a small portion of cases, a candidate infection must be common, such as cytomegalovirus (CMV). One study found that CMV antibody seroprevalence was higher in prostate cancer cases than in benign prostatic hyperplasia (BPH) controls.[120] Inadequate clearance of CMV-infected cells might lead to a chronic inflammatory response.

Although some of these infectious agents have been detected in the prostate or in semen, the presence of circulating antibodies against these agents does not imply that the prostate was or is infected. New approaches to the study of infection and prostate cancer risk are needed, including candidate agents beyond classic STIs.

CYTOKINES

Both the innate and adaptive immune responses are relevant to the chronic inflammation—prostate cancer hypothesis. Aberrant signaling by cytokines involved in the innate response (interleukins 1β, 6, 8 [IL1β, IL6, IL8], tumor necrosis factor-α [TNFα]) may allow an infection to persist and constantly stimulate inflammation. Of particular importance is the T-cell component of the adaptive immune response, especially the balance between T_H1 (favors cell mediated response) and T_H2 (favors humoral response) cells, the major producers of cytokines. The activation of the T_H2 response blocks the T_H1 response and vice versa. Thus, factors that tilt the T helper cell response away from T_H1 and towards T_H2, whether through decreased production of cytokines by T_H1 cells (interferon-γ

[IFNγ], IL12, IL2) or increased production of cytokines by T_H2 cells (IL4, IL10) would tend to produce chronic inflammation. A poor T_H1 response to infection initially might allow the agent to persist with a continued nonproductive T-cell presence, both of which might continue to cause tissue damage.

Clinical studies have documented elevated levels of plasma IL6[121] and C-reactive protein,[122] a component of the innate immune response produced by the liver in response to elevated circulating IL6, in metastatic or hormone refractory prostate cancer. These elevations are likely a response to the disease or tumor derived. The only prospective study, which used plasma samples collected years prior to prostate cancer diagnosis, did not show an association between C-reactive protein and prostate cancer.[123] Molecular epidemiologic studies of some cytokines and related proteins may not be useful because of large intra-individual variability and lack of correspondence between circulating and intraprostatic concentrations. Despite the limited epidemiologic evidence for links between inflammation and infectious agents and prostate cancer, the pathology and basic science studies support the continued study in populations, which will necessitate the development of more accurate and reliable biomarkers of intraprostatic inflammation.

METHODOLOGIC ISSUES IN THE MOLECULAR EPIDEMIOLOGY OF PROSTATE CANCER

Biomarkers in theory improve the measurement of exposure by quantifying internal dose. Nevertheless, a number of methodologic issues should be considered when drawing inferences from molecular epidemiologic studies of prostate cancer. It should be considered whether:

1. The measurement of biomarker is concurrent in time with prostate cancer leading to reverse causation.
2. The biomarker is not capturing the etiologically relevant moment.
3. The extent of exposure is not adequately reflected by a single measurement of the biomarker.
4. The biomarker does not reflect the intraprostatic level.
5. Biomarkers consist of a small number of components of large, complex, interrelated pathways.
6. There is limited variability in the biomarker range.

With the exception of the first issue, the bias that results from these measurement issues is to attenuate any real association. These measurement issues may explain some of the null biomarker studies in the prostate cancer literature for which there were compelling hypotheses.

The design of investigations of biomarkers and prostate cancer must take into account: 1) the enrichment of case pool with early lesions now that the PSA test is widely used for screening in the US, which may reduce the ability to detect association with biomarkers of factors postulated to influence progression to clinically apparent disease; and 2) undetected prostate cancer in the controls, which will produce a bias (modest-to-moderate depending on the sample size and strength of the "true" association), which attenuates associations in case-control and nested case-control studies. To avoid the latter bias, some investigators have restricted the controls to very low PSA, the net effect of which is to eliminate from the controls not just men with occult prostate cancer, but those with BPH and prostatitis, whereas the case group would still include men with BPH and prostatitis. This lack of comparability might result in the inadvertent study of risk factors for benign conditions, not cancer and, therefore, in molecular epidemiologic studies, a better approach is to ensure that the cases and controls have an equal opportunity to have an occult prostate cancer detected.

FUTURE DIRECTIONS

The molecular epidemiology of prostate cancer continues to evolve. Inconsistencies in findings among studies of varying design and in different populations abound. Careful consideration of the methodologic issues in the study of biomarkers of diet, environmental contaminants, and partially inherently determined factors during the design and inferential phases of studies and when comparing findings among studies may help to avoid or at least clarify some of the inconsistencies.

Two of the most promising findings, for selenium and vitamin E, in molecular epidemiology studies are largely consistent with secondary findings from clinical trials; these nutrients are currently being tested in chemoprevention trials. Biomarker studies should continue investigating lycopene, vitamin D, α-linolenic acid, and omega-3 fatty acids in detail. Molecular epidemiologic research is needed immediately to clarify the relation of adiposity, energy intake, and physical activity and their correlates hormonal and metabolic perturbations to prostate cancer risk. Robust methods to measure biomarkers of these factors are essential, as is evaluating the timing of exposure through life. The role of chronic intraprostatic inflammation merits immediate attention because of the recent recognition of the potential significance of proliferative inflammatory atrophy lesions and because inflammation is a rational target for prevention and intervention. Future biomarker studies must take an integrated approach by considering both the causes and consequences of the inflammatory response. Easy to measure, reliable biomarkers of intraprostatic inflammation are needed.

REFERENCES

1. Di Mascio P, Kaiser S, Sies H. Lycopene as the most efficient biological carotenoid singlet oxygen quencher. Arch Biochem Biophys 1989;274:532–538.
2. Hsing AW, Comstock GW, Abbey H, et al. Serologic precursors of cancer. Retinol, carotenoids, and tocopherol and risk of prostate cancer. J Natl Cancer Inst 1990;82:941–946.
3. Gann PH, Ma J, Giovannucci E, et al. Lower prostate cancer risk in men with elevated plasma lycopene levels: results of a prospective analysis. Cancer Res 1999;59:1225–1230.
4. Wu K, Erdman JW Jr, Schwartz SJ, et al. Plasma and dietary carotenoids, and the risk of prostate cancer: a nested case-control study. Cancer Epidemiol Biomarkers Prev 2004;13:260–269.
5. Huang HY, Alberg AJ, Norkus EP, et al. Prospective study of antioxidant micronutrients in the blood and the risk of developing prostate cancer. Am J Epidemiol 2003;157:335–344.
6. Goodman GE, Schaffer S, Omenn GS, et al. The association between lung and prostate cancer risk, and serum micronutrients: results and lessons learned from beta-carotene and retinol efficacy trial. Cancer Epidemiol Biomarkers Prev 2003;12:518–526.
7. Nomura AM, Stemmermann GN, Lee J, et al. Serum micronutrients and prostate cancer in Japanese Americans in Hawaii. Cancer Epidemiol Biomarkers Prev 1997;6:487–491.
8. Giovannucci E, Ascherio A, Rimm EB, et al. Intake of carotenoids and retinol in relation to risk of prostate cancer. J Natl Cancer Inst 1995;87:1767–1776.
9. Cohen JH, Kristal AR, Stanford JL. Fruit and vegetable intakes and prostate cancer risk. J Natl Cancer Inst 2000;92:61–68.
10. Vogt TM, Mayne ST, Graubard BI, et al. Serum lycopene, other serum carotenoids, and risk of prostate cancer in US blacks and whites. Am J Epidemiol 2002;155:1023–1032.
11. Reichman ME, Hayes RB, Ziegler RG, et al. Serum vitamin A and subsequent development of prostate cancer in the first National Health and Nutrition Examination Survey Epidemiologic Follow-up Study. Cancer Res 1990;50:2311–2315.
12. Eichholzer M, Stahelin HB, Gey KF, et al. Prediction of male cancer mortality by plasma levels of interacting vitamins: 17-year follow-up of the prospective Basel study. Int J Cancer 1996;66:145–150.
13. Siler U, Barella L, Spitzer V, et al. Lycopene and vitamin E interfere with autocrine/paracrine loops in the Dunning prostate cancer model. FASEB J 2004;18:1019–1021.
14. Clinton SK, Emenhiser C, Schwartz SJ, et al. *cis-trans* lycopene isomers, carotenoids, and retinol in the human prostate. Cancer Epidemiol Biomarkers Prev 1996;5:823–833.
15. Boileau TW, Liao Z, Kim S, et al. Prostate carcinogenesis in N-methyl-N-nitrosourea (NMU)-testosterone-treated rats fed tomato powder, lycopene, or energy-restricted diets. J Natl Cancer Inst 2003;95:1578–1586.
16. Clark LC, Combs Jr GF, Turnbull BW, et al. Effects of selenium supplementation for cancer prevention in patients with carcinoma of the skin. A randomized controlled trial. Nutritional Prevention of Cancer Study Group. J Am Med Asso 1996;276:1957–1963.
17. Combs GF Jr, Combs SB. The nutritional biochemistry of selenium. Annu Rev Nutr 1984;4:257–280.
18. Waters DJ, Shen S, Cooley DM, et al. Effects of dietary selenium supplementation on DNA damage and apoptosis in canine prostate. J Natl Cancer Inst 2003;95:237–241.
19. Karunasinghe N, Ryan J, Tuckey J, et al. DNA stability and serum selenium levels in a high-risk group for prostate cancer. Cancer Epidemiol Biomarkers Prev 2004;13:391–397.
20. Chow CK. Nutritional influence on cellular antioxidant defense systems. Am J Clin Nutr 1979;32:1066–1081.
21. Yoshizawa K, Willett WC, Morris SJ, et al. A study of prediagnostic selenium level in toenails and the risk of advanced prostate cancer. J Natl Cancer Inst 1998;90:1219–1224.
22. Helzlsouer KJ, Huang H-Y, Alberg AJ, et al. Association between α-tocopherol, γ-tocopherol, selenium and subsequent prostate cancer. J Natl Cancer Inst 2000;92:2018–2023.
23. van den Brandt PA, Zeegers MP, Bode P, et al. Toenail selenium levels and the subsequent risk of prostate cancer: a prospective cohort study. Cancer Epidemiol Biomarkers Prev 2003;12:866–871.
24. Nomura AMY, Lee J, Stemmermann GN, et al. Serum selenium and subsequent risk of prostate cancer. Cancer Epidemiol Biomarkers Prev 2000;9:883–887.
25. Brooks JD, Metter EJ, Chan DW, et al. Plasma selenium level before diagnosis and the risk of prostate cancer development. J Urol 2001;166:2034–2038.
26. Li H, Stampfer MJ, Giovannucci EL, et al. A prospective study of plasma selenium levels and prostate cancer risk. J Natl Cancer Inst 2004;96:696–703.
27. Goodman GE, Schaffer S, Bankson DD, et al. Predictors of serum selenium in cigarette smokers and the lack of association with lung and prostate cancer risk. Cancer Epidemiol Biomarkers Prev 2001;10:1069–1076.
28. Allen NE, Morris JS, Ngwenyama RA, et al. A case-control study of selenium in nails and prostate cancer risk in British men. Br J Cancer 2004;90:1392–1396.
29. Clark LC, Dalkin B, Krongrad A, et al. Decreased incidence of prostate cancer with selenium supplementation: results of a double-blind cancer prevention trial. Br J Urol 1998;81:730–734.
30. Knekt P, Aromaa A, Maatela J, et al. Serum selenium and subsequent risk of cancer among Finnish men and women. J Natl Cancer Inst 1990;82:864–868.
31. Klein EA, Thompson IM, Lippman SM, et al. SELECT: the selenium and vitamin E cancer prevention trial. Urol Oncol 2003;21:59–65.
32. Sabichi AL, Lee JJ, Taylor RJ, et al. Selenium accumulates in prostate tissue of prostate cancer patients after short term administration of L-selenomethionine. Proc Am Assoc Cancer Res 2002;43:1007–1008.
33. Heinonen OP, Albanes D, Virtamo J, et al. Prostate cancer and supplementation with alpha-tocopherol and beta-carotene — incidence and mortality in a controlled trial. J Natl Cancer Inst 1998;90:440–446.
34. Sigounas G, Anagnostou A, Steiner M. dl-α-tocopherol induces apoptosis in erythroleukemia, prostate, and breast cancer cells. Nutr Cancer 1997;28:30–35.
35. Hartman TJ, Albanes D, Pietinen P, et al. The association between baseline vitamin E, selenium, and prostate cancer in the Alpha-Tocopherol, Beta-Carotene Cancer Prevention Study. Cancer Epidemiol Biomarkers Prev 1998;7:335–340.
36. Huang HY, Appel LJ. Supplementation of diets with alpha-tocopherol reduces serum concentrations of gamma- and delta-tocopherol in humans. J Nutr 2003;133:3137–3140.
37. Cooney RV, Franke AA, Harwood PJ, et al. γ-Tocopherol detoxification of nitrogen dioxide: superiority to α-tocopherol. Proc Natl Acad Sci 1993;90:1771–1775.
38. Schwartz GG, Hulka BS. Is vitamin D deficiency a risk factor for prostate cancer? (Hypothesis). Anticancer Res 1990;10:1307–1311.
39. Peehl DM, Skowronski RJ, Leung GK, et al. Antiproliferative effects of 1,25-dihydroxyvitamin D$_3$ on primary cultures of human prostatic cells. Cancer Res 1994;54:805–810.
40. Braun MM, Helzlsouer KJ, Hollis BW, et al. Prostate cancer and prediagnostic levels of serum vitamin D metabolites (Maryland, United States). Cancer Causes Control 1995;6:235–239.
41. Gann PH, Ma J, Hennekens CH, et al. Circulating vitamin D metabolites in relation to subsequent development of prostate cancer. Cancer Epidemiol Biomarkers Prev 1996;5:121–126.
42. Nomura AM, Stemmermann GN, Lee J, et al. Serum vitamin D metabolite levels and the subsequent development of prostate cancer. Cancer Causes Control 1998;9:425–432.

43. Platz EA, Leitzmann MF, Hollis BW, et al. Plasma 1,25-dihydroxy- and 25-hydroxyvitamin D and subsequent risk of prostate cancer. Cancer Causes Control 2004;15:255–265.

44. Jacobs ET, Giuliano AR, Martinez ME, et al. Plasma levels of 25-hydroxyvitamin D, 1,25-dihydroxyvitamin D and the risk of prostate cancer. J Steroid Biochem Mol Biol 2004;89–90:533–537.

45. Corder EH, Guess HA, Hulka BS, et al. Vitamin D and prostate cancer: a prediagnostic study with stored sera. Cancer Epidemiol Biomarkers Prev 1993;2:467–472.

46. Ahonen MH, Tenkanen L, Hakama M, et al. Prostate cancer risk and prediagnostic serum 25-hydroxyvitamin D levels (Finland). Cancer Causes Control 2000;11:847–852.

47. Tuohimaa P, Tenkanen L, Ahonen M, et al. Both high and low levels of blood vitamin D are associated with a higher prostate cancer risk: a longitudinal, nested case-control study in the Nordic countries. Int J Cancer 2004;108:104–108.

48. Sung V, Feldman D. 1,25-Dihydroxyvitamin D3 decreases human prostate cancer cell adhesion and migration. Mol Cell Endocrinol 2000;164:133–143.

49. Harper CR, Jacobson TA. Beyond the Mediterranean diet: the role of omega-3 fatty acids in the prevention of coronary heart disease. Prev Cardiol 2003;6:136–146.

50. Gann PH, Hennekens CH, Sacks FM, et al. Prospective study of plasma fatty acids and risk of prostate cancer. J Natl Cancer Inst 1994;86:281–286.

51. Harvei S, Bjerve KS, Tretli S, et al. Prediagnostic level of fatty acids in serum phospholipids: omega-3 and omega-6 fatty acids and the risk of prostate cancer. Int J Cancer 1997;71:545–551.

52. Mannisto S, Pietinen P, Virtanen MJ, et al. Fatty acids and risk of prostate cancer in a nested case-control study in male smokers. Cancer Epidemiol Biomarkers Prev 2003;12:1422–1428.

53. Godley PA, Campbell MK, Gallagher P, et al. Biomarkers of essential fatty acid consumption and risk of prostatic carcinoma. Cancer Epidemiol Biomarkers Prev 1996;5:889–895.

54. Laaksonen DE, Laukkanen JA, Niskanen L, et al. Serum linoleic and total polyunsaturated fatty acids in relation to prostate and other cancers: A population-based cohort study. Int J Cancer 2004;111:444–450.

55. Norrish AE, Jackson RT, Sharpe SJ, et al. Men who consume vegetable oils rich in monounsaturated fat: their dietary patterns and risk of prostate cancer (New Zealand). Cancer Causes Control 2000;11:609–615.

56. Martin MB, Voeller HJ, Gelmann EP, et al. Role of cadmium in the regulation of AR gene expression and activity. Endocrinology 2002;143:263–275.

57. Platz EA, Helzlsouer KJ, Hoffman SC, et al. Prediagnostic toenail cadmium and zinc and subsequent prostate cancer risk. Prostate 2002;52:288–296.

58. Ritchie JM, Vial SL, Fuortes LJ, et al. Organochlorines and risk of prostate cancer. J Occup Environ Med 2003;45:692–702.

59. Hsing AW. Hormones and prostate cancer: what's next? Epidemiol Rev 2001;23:42–58.

60. Chen C, Weiss NS, Lewis SK, et al. Endogenous sex hormones and prostate cancer risk: a case-control study nested with the Carotene and Retinol Efficiency Trial. Cancer Epidemiol Biomarkers Prev 2003;12:1410–1416.

61. Platz EA, Leitzmann M, Rifai N, et al. Sex steroid hormones and the androgen receptor gene CAG repeat and subsequent risk of prostate cancer in the PSA era. Cancer Epidemiol Biomarkers Prev 2005;14:1262–1269.

62. Parsons JK, Carter HB, Landis P, et al. Higher serum free testosterone is associated with an increased risk of prostate cancer: results from the Baltimore Longitudinal Study on Aging. J Urol 2004;171:116.

63. Gann PH, Hennekens CH, Ma J, et al. Prospective study of sex hormone levels and risk of prostate cancer. J Natl Cancer Inst 1996;88:1118–1126.

64. Nomura A, Heilbrun LK, Stemmermann GN, et al. Prediagnostic serum hormones and the risk of prostate cancer. Cancer Res 1988;48:3515–3517.

65. Hsing AW, Comstock GW. Serological precursors of cancer: serum hormones and risk of subsequent prostate cancer. Cancer Epidemiol Biomarkers Prev 1993;2:27–32.

66. Dorgan JF, Albanes D, Virtamo J, et al. Relationships of serum androgens and estrogens to prostate cancer risk: results from a prospective study in Finland. Cancer Epidemiol Biomarkers Prev 1998;7:1069–1074.

67. Eaton NE, Reeves GK, Appleby PN, et al. Endogenous sex hormones and prostate cancer: a quantitative review of prospective studies. Br J Cancer 1999;80:930–934.

68. Schatzl G, Madersbacher S, Thurridl T, et al. High-grade prostate cancer is associated with low serum testosterone levels. Prostate 2001;47:52–58.

69. Schatzl G, Madersbacher S, Haitel A, et al. Associations of serum testosterone with microvessel density, androgen receptor density and androgen receptor gene polymorphism in prostate cancer. J Urol 2003;169:1312–1315.

70. Hoffman MA, DeWolf WC, Morgentaler A. Is low serum free testosterone a marker for high grade prostate cancer? J Urol 2000;163:824–827.

71. Zhang PL, Rosen S, Veeramachaneni R, et al. Association between prostate cancer and serum testosterone levels. Prostate 2002;53:179–182.

72. Thompson I, Goodman P, Tangen C, et al. The influence of finasteride on the development of prostate cancer. N Engl J Med 2003;349:215–224.

73. Naslund MJ, Strandberg JD, Coffey DS. The role of androgens and estrogens in the pathogenesis of experimental nonbacterial prostatitis. J Urol 1988;140:1049–1053.

74. Yager JD. Endogenous estrogens as carcinogens through metabolic activation. J Natl Cancer Inst Monogr 2000:27;67–73.

75. Barrett-Connor E, Garland C, McPhillips JB, et al. A prospective, population-based study of androstenedione, estrogens, and prostatic cancer. Cancer Res 1990;50:169–173.

76. Risbridger GP, Bianco JJ, Ellem SJ, et al. Oestrogens and prostate cancer. Endocr Relat Cancer 2003;10:187–191.

77. Severson RK, Grove JS, Nomura AMY, et al. Body mass and prostatic cancer: a prospective study. BMJ 1988;297:713–715.

78. Cohen P, Peehl DM, Rosenfeld RG. The IGF axis in the prostate. Hormone Metab Res 1994;26:81–84.

79. Cohen P, Peehl DM, Lamson G, et al. Insulin-like growth factors (IGFs), IGF receptors, and IGF-binding proteins in primary cultures of prostate epithelial cells. J Clin Endocrinol Metab 1991;73:401–407.

80. Liu B, Lee HY, Weinzimer SA, et al. Direct functional interactions between insulin-like growth factor-binding protein-3 and retinoid X receptor-a regulate transcriptional signaling and apoptosis. J Biol Chem 2000;275:33607–33613.

81. Boyle BJ, Zhao XY, Cohen P, et al. Insulin-like growth factor binding protein-3 mediates 1 alpha,25-dihydroxyvitamin d^3 growth inhibition in the LNCaP prostate cancer cell line through p21/WAF1. J Urol 2001;165:1319–1324.

82. Koistinen H, Paju A, Koistinen R, et al. Prostate-specific antigen and other prostate-derived proteases cleave IGFBP-3, but prostate cancer is not associated with proteolytically cleaved circulating IGFBP-3. Prostate 2002;50:112–118.

83. Mantzoros CS, Tzonou A, Signorello LB, et al. Insulin-like growth factor 1 in relation to prostate cancer and benign prostatic hyperplasia. Br J Cancer 1997;76:1115–1118.

84. Chan JM, Stampfer MJ, Giovannucci E, et al. Plasma insulin-like growth factor-I and prostate cancer risk: a prospective study. Science 1998;279:563–566.

85. Wolk A, Mantzoros CS, Andersson SW, et al. Insulin-like growth factor I and prostate cancer risk: a population-based, case-control study. J Natl Cancer Inst 1998;90:911–915.

86. Stattin P, Bylund A, Rinaldi S, et al. Plasma insulin-like growth factor-I, insulin-like growth factor-binding proteins, and prostate cancer risk: a prospective study. J Natl Cancer Inst 2000;92:1910–1917.

87. Harman SM, Metter EJ, Blackman MR, et al. Serum levels of insulin-like growth factor I (IGF-I), IGF-II, IGF-binding protein-3, and prostate-specific antigen as predictors of clinical prostate cancer. J Clin Endocrinol Metab 2000;85:4258–4265.

88. Khosravi J, Diamandi A, Mistry J, et al. Insulin-like growth factor-I (IGF-I) and IGF-binding protein-3 in benign prostatic hyperplasia and prostate cancer. J Clin Endocrinol Metab 2001;86:694–699.

89. Chokkalingam A, Pollak M, Fillmore C, et al. Insulin-like growth factors and prostate cancer: a population-based case-control study in China. Cancer Epidemiol Biomarkers Prev 2001;10:421–427.

90. Stattin P, Rinaldi S, Biessy C, et al. High levels of circulating insulin-like growth factor-I increase prostate cancer risk: a prospective study in a population-based nonscreened cohort. J Clin Oncol 2004;22:3104–3112.

91. Renehan AG, Zwahlen M, Minder C, et al. Insulin-like growth factor (IGF)-I, IGF binding protein-3, and cancer risk: systematic review and meta-regression analysis. Lancet 2004;363:1346–1353.

92. Chan JM, Stampfer MJ, Ma J, et al. Insulin-like growth factor-I (IGF-1) and IGF binding protein-3 as predictors of advanced-stage prostate cancer. J Natl Cancer Inst 2002;94:1099–1109.

93. Platz EA, Pollak M, Leitzmann MF, et al. Plasma insulin-like growth factor-1 and binding protein-3 and subsequent risk of prostate cancer in the PSA era. Cancer Causes Control 2005;16:255–262.

94. Andò S, Rubens R, Rottiers R. Androgen plasma levels in male diabetics. J Endocrinol Invest 1984;7:21–24.

95. Hsing AW, Chua S, Gao YT, et al. Prostate cancer risk and serum levels of insulin and leptin: a population-based study. J Natl Cancer Inst 2001;93:783–789.

96. Hsing AW, Gao YT, Chua S, et al. Insulin resistance and prostate cancer risk. J Natl Cancer Inst 2003;95:67–71.

97. Hubbard JS, Rohrmann S, Landis PK, et al. Association of prostate cancer risk with insulin, glucose, and anthropometry in the Baltimore longitudinal study of aging. Urology 2004;63:253–258.

98. Gapstur SM, Gann PH, Colangelo LA, et al. Postload glucose concentration and 27-year prostate cancer mortality (United States). Cancer Causes Control 2001;12:763–772.

99. Thune I, Lund E. Physical activity and the risk of prostate and testicular cancer: a cohort study of 53,000 Norwegian men. Cancer Causes Control 1994;5:549–556.

100. Lund Nilsen TI, Johnsen R, Vatten LJ. Socio-economic and lifestyle factors associated with the risk of prostate cancer. Br J Cancer 2000;82:1358–1363.

101. Friedman JM. The function of leptin in nutrition, weight, and physiology. Nutr Rev 2002;60:S1–S14.

102. Chu NF, Spiegelman D, Yu J, et al. Plasma leptin concentrations and four year weight gain among US men. Int J Obes 2001;25:346–353.

103. Lagiou P, Signorello LB, Trichopoulos D, et al. Leptin in relation to prostate cancer and benign prostatic hyperplasia. Int J Cancer 1998;76:25–28.

104. Stattin P, Soderberg S, Hallmans G, et al. Leptin is associated with increased prostate cancer risk: a nested case-referent study. J Clin Endocrinol Metab 2001;86:1341–1345.

105. Chang S, Hursting SD, Contois JH, et al. Leptin and prostate cancer. Prostate 2001;46:62–67.

106. Stattin P, Kaaks R, Johansson R, et al. Plasma leptin is not associated with prostate cancer risk. Cancer Epidemiol Biomarkers Prev 2003;12:474–475.

107. Platz EA, Leitzmann MF, Michaud DS, et al. Interrelation of energy intake, body size, and physical activity with prostate cancer in a large prospective cohort study. Cancer Res 2003;63:8542–8548.

108. Calle EE, Rodriguez C, Walker-Thurmond K, et al. Overweight, obesity, and mortality from cancer in a prospectively studied cohort of U.S. adults. N Engl J Med 2003;348:1625–1638.

109. Schatteman PH, Hoekx L, Wyndaele JJ, et al. Inflammation in prostate biopsies of men without prostatic malignancy or clinical prostatitis: correlation with total serum PSA and PSA density. Eur Urol 2000;37:404–412.

110. Gerstenbluth RE, Seftel AD, MacLennan GT, et al. Distribution of chronic prostatitis in radical prostatectomy specimens with up-regulation of bcl-2 in areas of inflammation. J Urol 2002;167:2267–2270.

111. Di Silverio F, Gentile V, De Matteis A, et al. Distribution of inflammation, pre-malignant lesions, incidental carcinoma in histologically confirmed benign prostatic hyperplasia: A retrospective analysis. Eur Urol 2003;43:164–175.

112. De Marzo AM, Marchi VL, Epstein JI, et al. Proliferative inflammatory atrophy of the prostate: implications for prostatic carcinogenesis. Am J Pathol 1999;155:1985–1992.

113. Hayes RB, Pottern LM, Strickler H, et al. Sexual behaviour, STDs and risks for prostate cancer. Br J Cancer 2000;82:718–725.

114. Dillner J, Knekt P, Boman J, et al. Sero-epidemiological association between human-papillomavirus infection and risk of prostate cancer. Int J Cancer 1998;75:564–567.

115. Hisada M, Rabkin CS, Strickler HD, et al. Human papillomavirus antibody and risk of prostate cancer. JAMA 2000;2000:340–341.

116. Hoffman LJ, Bunker CH, Pellett PE, et al. Elevated seroprevalence of human herpesvirus-8 among men with prostate cancer. J Infect Dis 2004;189:15–20.

117. Munger K, Howley PM. Human papillomavirus immortalization and transformation functions. Virus Res 2002;89:213–228.

118. Deng H, Song MJ, Chu JT, et al. Transcriptional regulation of the interleukin-6 gene of human herpesvirus 8 (Kaposi's sarcoma-associated herpesvirus). J Virol 2002;76:8252–8264.

119. Rosenblatt KA, Carter JJ, Iwasaki LM, et al. Serologic evidence of human papillomavirus 16 and 18 infections and risk of prostate cancer. Cancer Epidemiol Biomarkers Prev 2003;12:763–768.

120. Geder L, Rapp F. Herpesviruses and prostate carcinogenesis. Arch Androl 1980;4:71–78.

121. Twillie DA, Eisenberger MA, Carducci MA, et al. Interleukin-6: a candidate mediator of human prostate cancer morbidity. Urology 1995;45:542–549.

122. Latif Z, McMillan DC, Wallace AM, et al. The relationship of circulating insulin-like growth factor 1, its binding protein-3, prostate specific antigen and C-reactive protein with disease stage in prostate cancer. Br J Urol 2002;89:396–399.

123. Platz EA, De Marzo AM, Erlinger TP, et al. No association between pre-diagnostic plasma C-reactive protein concentration and subsequent prostate cancer. Prostate 2004;59:393–400.

Applications of gene array technology to prostate cancer

5

Bruce J Trock

INTRODUCTION

Cancer development and progression represent a continuum of biological behavior driven by altered patterns of gene expression. Characterizing the critical gene targets associated with tumor subtypes or different points along the continuum has become the goal of molecular taxonomy of tumors. Molecular classification includes identification of stages or risk factors in the carcinogenic process, genetic signatures that confer the malignant phenotype to provide a biomarker for early detection or diagnosis, prediction of prognosis and response to specific therapies, and identification of fundamental mechanisms that can be targeted for prevention or treatment. Until recently, these studies were done using a candidate gene approach, wherein genes of interest were investigated one at a time. However, cancer phenotypes involve multiple genetic alterations, and not every case with the same phenotype will exhibit the same set of perturbed genes. Consequently, classification of the determinants of biological behavior may require the ability to evaluate *patterns* of synchronized genetic events.

For prostate cancer, there is a particular need for improved methods to classify clinical subtypes and elucidate underlying mechanisms. While it is the most common non-skin cancer among men, etiologic pathways providing targets for prevention have yet to be conclusively established. Serum prostate-specific antigen (PSA) has proven to be one of the most successful biomarkers of early detection, yet it has poor specificity, and established cutpoints miss a substantial proportion of cancers.[1] Furthermore, there is evidence that a nontrivial proportion of cancers detected by PSA testing would never cause clinically significant disease during a man's remaining lifetime.[2] Because prostate cancer treatment can produce significant morbidity, and conventional prognostic factors (stage, PSA, and Gleason score) exhibit a fairly narrow range in most cases diagnosed today, there is a great need for new prognostic factors that can aid treatment decisions. Metastatic prostate cancer, while initially responsive to hormone ablation, eventually progresses to a hormone refractory state, for which there is no effective systemic therapy. Identification of a pattern of co-regulated genes associated with hormone independence could provide targets for new therapies.

Gene expression (DNA) microarrays represent a dramatic advance in our ability to perform molecular classification studies by measuring the expression of thousands or tens of thousands of genes or gene sequences in a single tumor sample. This provides the ability to identify clusters of genes that discriminate different tumor phenotypes or elements of common pathways involved in tumor progression. This approach has already led to identification of novel prostate cancer biomarkers[3–5] and may provide new approaches to the problems described above.

DNA MICROARRAYS

A DNA microarray is a platform for measuring the level of expression of thousands of different messenger RNA (mRNA) transcripts in a biological specimen such as tumor tissue. The microarray is a glass slide, nylon membrane, or other solid matrix to which strands of complementary DNA (cDNA) or oligonucleotides (short sequences of single strand DNA) have been affixed in specified positions. These cDNA or oligonucleotide "spots" are referred to as probes; they represent the specific genes or gene sequences that one would like to assay in the tumor specimen. The mRNA is extracted from the cells of interest and from a reference sample and each is reverse-transcribed in the presence of a different colored fluorescent tag (typically red and green, respectively). The resulting labeled cDNA samples (targets) are pooled and then hybridized to the probes on the array, which is then illuminated with a laser. The intensity of the fluorescence emitted from the target bound to each probe is proportional to the relative expression of that gene in the tissue of interest. If a particular gene probe is more highly expressed in the sample of interest (e.g., tumor) than the reference sample, red fluorescence will predominate. Conversely, if the gene is underexpressed relative to the reference sample, green fluorescence will predominate. If tumor and reference sample have similar levels of expression of the gene of interest, the spot will appear yellow (Figure 5.1). The fluorescence signal is captured using a detector, typically a confocal microscope, and converted using an image analysis algorithm to a ratio of intensities of the fluorescence from the tumor tissue relative to the reference sample.

STATISTICAL ANALYSIS OF MICROARRAY DATA

Microarrays result in "high-dimensional" data, that is, data wherein the number of variables (gene probes) is many times larger than the number of patients (samples). For example, it is not uncommon for a study to measure expression of more than 20,000 genes on only 30 patients.[6] In such a setting the conventional multivariable analysis methods such as logistic regression are not appropriate. With such a large volume of data, and many sources of experimental and biological variability, careful consideration of study design and analysis are critical to discern true signal within the large amount of noisy data. Addressing these issues is beyond the scope of this chapter, but excellent reviews of these problems are available that clearly explain the concepts of microarray data analysis in nonstatistical terms and that highlight potential pitfalls to be aware of when reading the literature,[7,8] as well as a more detailed exposition (useful to both nonstatisticians and statisticians) can be found in the excellent text by Simon et al.[9]

The analysis problems of microarray data primarily fall into three categories: class discovery, class comparison, and class prediction problems. *Class discovery* problems attempt to identify gene profiles that can uncover previously unknown subtypes (classes) among a particular group of tumors or patients—for example, identification of distinct prognostic subgroups within categories of Gleason score and stage,[10] or identification of androgen-regulated genes.[11] Typically, class discovery analyses use some form of cluster analysis such as k-means clustering, self-organizing maps, and hierarchical clustering. These methods attempt to find clusters of patients with similar profiles of gene expression. These methods are referred to as unsupervised, because the clusters are determined without using any information from the samples (other than gene expression data) that might indicate the class in which the patient belongs. A point of caution with cluster analysis is that clusters will almost always be identified, even in random data with no true distinct classes. Therefore, clusters that purport to define new subtypes should be validated by 1) comparing the probability that any distinct clusters exist versus no

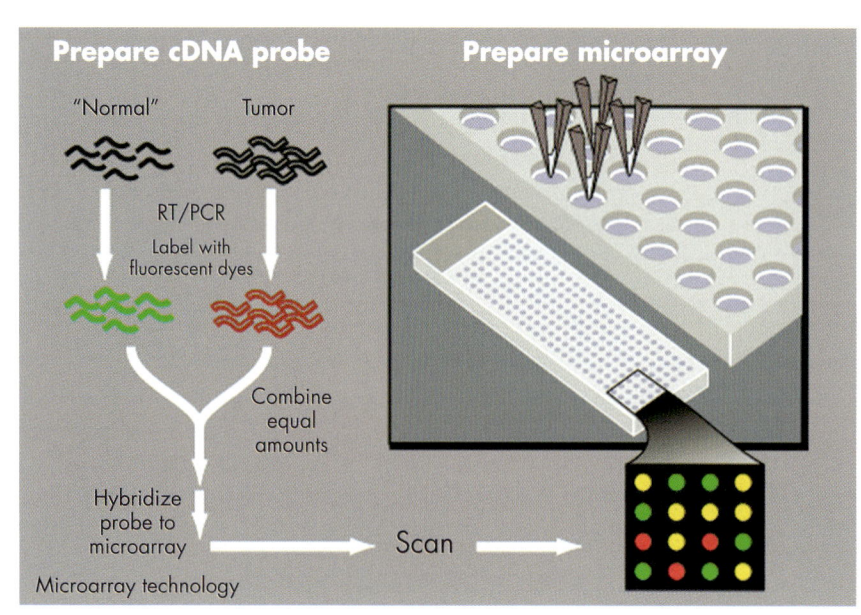

Figure 5.1

Hybridization and fluorescent labeling of tumor sample on complementary DNA (cDNA) microarray. (From National Human Genome Research Institute: Talking Glossary of Genetic Terms. http://www.nhgri.nih.gov/glossary.cfm?key=microarray%20technology)

clusters; and 2) evaluating the reproducibility of the clusters identified.[12]

Class comparison problems attempt to identify gene expression profiles that discriminate samples from two or more predefined classes, such as tumor versus benign,[5] localized versus metastatic tumor, or androgen sensitive versus androgen independent.[13] These methods are referred to as supervised, because the comparison is between classes that are already determined. These approaches typically use traditional statistical methods (such as t-tests) for comparing expression one gene at a time between groups, then apply adjustments to control the probability of false positives or false discovery inherent in comparing thousands of genes among samples (subjects) that typically number less than 100.[9]

Class prediction problems similarly seek gene expression profiles that discriminate among predefined classes, but the focus is on developing a model or prediction rule to predict the class for a new observation. This type of problem arises when the objective is to define a molecular signature that can predict future patient outcomes, such as early detection, prognosis (e.g., recurrence after prostatectomy),[14] or response to a specific therapy. These analyses typically begin with an initial data reduction, or feature selection step to reduce the number of candidate genes, then employ a multivariate model or nonparametric classification algorithm to identify groups of genes that best predict class membership. Such methods (which are also considered as supervised analysis) include forms of discriminant analysis, support vector machines, nearest neighbor classification, neural networks, and classification trees. Because of the large number of predictor variables (genes) relative to samples, there is strong possibility that random patterns in the data will influence the prediction model, resulting in a model that predicts very well in the original data set but does not adequately predict new observations. This problem, referred to as overfitting, results in estimates of the error rate for the model that are overly optimistic, i.e., models that appear to predict with minimal or no errors. To provide an accurate estimate of the error rate to be expected when the model is used to predict future patient events, rigorous validation methods are used, such as bootstrapping, cross-validation, or splitting data into training and validation samples.[9]

Regardless of the type of problem to be evaluated with microarray data, fundamental aspects of study design are just as relevant as in more traditional biomedical research. Calculation of study power, i.e., the number of samples (patients) necessary to detect a given difference in expression ratio between tumor and normal samples, is infrequently performed prior to conducting a microarray experiment. Without such calculations, adjusted for false discovery rate,[15] it is difficult to interpret whether lack of significance for a given gene represents lack of biological relevance or insufficient sample size. Microarray studies often depend on convenience samples, producing a sample population that cannot validly be referred back to a clinical population of interest. Microarray technology provides unparalleled opportunity for hypothesis generation, however, it is important whenever possible to base the study on an underlying biological or clinical hypothesis. Because the large number of predictors (genes) allows the potential for selecting genes that actually predict random or nonrelevant variability in the data (overfitting), extraneous sources of variation that differ between classes must be strictly controlled; for example, patients from different classes should be enrolled from the same populations, chips used for different classes should be from the same batch, and samples from different classes should use similar methods for sample handling and processing, array hybridization, signal detection, and data preprocessing. If the samples are from cell cultures, then additional variation can arise from differences in culture conditions. The validity of the analysis can be strengthened if sample sets from multiple populations can be analyzed together (subject to the above control measures within each population), since it is very unlikely that the above sources of bias will occur similarly across different populations. Finally, it is important that gene expression profiles identified through microarray analysis be considered within a specific context of clinical or biological relevance (e.g. as a biomarker for early detection), and that validation should occur within that context.

APPLICATION OF DNA MICROARRAYS TO PROSTATE CANCER

DNA microarrays have been used to study the entire continuum of the prostate cancer process, from characterizing prostatic changes associated with aging to identifying potential targets for therapy of advanced cancer. Genes identified to be abnormally over- or underexpressed can be validated in independent samples using real time polymerase chain reaction (RT-PCR), and immunohistochemistry to determine if gene expression (mRNA production) correlates with protein level.

ETIOLOGY AND MALIGNANT PHENOTYPE

The ACI/Seg rat provides a model for spontaneous prostate cancer associated with aging, although lesions occur in the ventral prostate, whereas the dorsolateral prostate is the rat homolog of the peripheral zone in humans. Since the dorsolateral prostate has not been well studied in this rat model, a study was conducted to evaluate genetic changes associated with aging in the prostate. Comparison of whole prostate tissue (epithelial and stromal cells combined) in 6- and 18-month old rats revealed 187 genes with significant up- or downregulation in the older prostates. These were categorized into functional processes, with the most significant changes in genes associated with oxidative stress, inflammation, modulation of apoptosis, tissue remodeling, and energy metabolism.[16] Several of the genes identified represent interacting pathways, for example *oxidative stress* (increased: ceruloplasmin; decreased: superoxide dismutase), *apoptosis/stress response* (increased: NF-kappa-B, mitogen activated protein kinase kinase kinase, HSP70), *inflammatory response* (increased: interleukin 6 [IL6] signal transducer, IL6 receptor). These data suggest that normal aging prior to even microscopic prostate cancer is associated with changes in a number of pathways known to be associated with increased prostate cancer risk. Potential limitations in this study include the use of only three rats in each of the two age groups, and the use of unsupervised clustering to identify aberrant gene expression.

A number of studies have compared gene expression in prostate tumor versus normal tissue, or in prostatic intraepithelial neoplasia (PIN) versus invasive cancer. One of the most clinically significant of the genes identified as being differentially expressed in tumor versus normal or benign prostate encodes α-methylacyl-CoA racemase (AMACR), an enzyme involved in β-oxidation of dietary branched-chain fatty acids, such as those found in dairy and red meat.[3,4,17] This may have etiologic significance since dairy and red meat have been associated with increased prostate cancer risk, and β-oxidation is a source of oxidative stress.[4] Validation of the microarray results with immunohistochemistry demonstrated that *AMACR* is overexpressed in more than 95% of primary prostate cancers, compared with less than 4% of normal or benign tissues.[3,4] Further validation of these results in a number of subsequent studies has led to the use of *AMACR* in the differential diagnosis of prostate cancer, which is especially useful with small biopsy samples where discrimination between atypia and frank cancer may be difficult.[18] A novel meta-analysis approach was recently used to compare microarray data for prostate cancer versus benign prostatic hyperplasia (BPH) tissue in four independent studies, representing 41 benign tissues and 61 prostate cancers. The transmembrane serine protease *hepsin* was found in all four studies to be highly overexpressed in prostate cancer.[19] Hepsin is also overexpressed in ovarian cancer, but its functional significance is unknown. Recently, it was shown to promote disorganization of the basement membrane in a mouse model of prostate cancer, and may facilitate metastasis,[20] although studies in humans have shown

inconsistent associations with prognosis.[21,22] Other genes overexpressed in all studies included that encoding fatty acid synthase and *AMACR*, while *SPARCL-1*, which encodes an extracellular matrix protein and possible tumor suppressor, and the gene for integrin-α_1 were consistently underexpressed.[19] Extremely low or absent levels of the SPARCL-1 product, known also as hevin or MAST9, have been observed in metastatic prostate cancer,[23] suggesting it may participate in a lethal phenotype; this gene is also downregulated in non-small cell lung cancer and colon cancer.[24]

Perhaps surprisingly, there was little overlap between the genes abnormally expressed in the meta-analysis and those in the study of the aging rat prostate. The genes encoding fatty-acid synthase and integrin-α_1, the primary genes overlapping both studies, exhibited expression changes opposite to those observed in the rat model.[16] Possible reasons for the lack of overlap include the following: 1) prostate cancer cases and benign tissue controls have similar age distributions and small numbers, thus limiting evaluation of age-associated changes; 2) prominent changes with aging include mechanisms associated with risk of cancer initiation events while those in comparisons of similarly aged tumor and benign reflect the phenotype of clinical malignancy, which may be dominated by progression; 3) human tissue lesions were chosen to avoid obvious areas of inflammation; 4) lack of correspondence between aging in the dorsolateral rat prostate and human prostate cancer phenotype; or 5) lack of overlap in the cDNAs comprising the arrays in the cancer versus aging studies.

One potential problem in comparing tumor versus normal or tumor versus PIN is that whole tissue samples represent a mixture of tumor or epithelial cells, stroma, and inflammatory cells, and the relative proportions differ by histology. To overcome this, Ashida et al used laser capture microdissection to isolate pure subpopulations of tumor, PIN, and normal epithelial cells from Japanese men undergoing radical prostatectomy. In a comparison of normal versus PIN or prostate cancer they identified 21 genes upregulated and 63 genes downregulated, while a comparison of PIN versus prostate cancer identified 40 upregulated and 98 downregulated genes.[6] Among all significantly upregulated genes, only 3 were included in those consistently found in the meta-analysis performed by Rhodes[19] (genes for AMACR, fatty acid synthase, and death-associated protein); notably absent was the gene encoding hepsin. Seven downregulated genes matched those in the meta-analysis, including three among the 10 most significant genes from the meta-analysis (*Meis 1*, genes encoding Down syndrome critical region 1, and gap junction protein-α_1). Ashida et al attributed the relatively low degree of overlap between their study and the meta-analysis to over-estimation of upregulation or downregulation as an artifact of contamination with stromal cells or noncancer epithelial cells in the whole tissue samples used in the four studies from the meta-analysis.[6]

ANDROGEN REGULATION

Androgen regulation was one of the first aspects of prostate cancer to be investigated using DNA microarrays. Microarray analysis of androgen-regulated genes may identify coordinated expression patterns indicative of biochemical pathways or functions associated with prostate cancer progression, particularly development of androgen independence. Most studies of androgen regulation have used LNCaP cells with and without androgen supplementation with synthetic androgen R1881[25-27] or dihydrotestosterone (DHT).[11] These studies found 262 to 692 genes either overexpressed or underexpressed by two-fold or more after androgen stimulation for periods ranging from 0.5 to 72 hours. Nelson found that genes associated with fatty acid or cholesterol metabolism were strongly upregulated, including seladin1, which codes for a protein that protects cells from oxidative stress and amyloid-β peptide-induced apoptosis. They also found significant upregulation of genes associated with cellular transport or trafficking, including 25-fold upregulation of the gene for FK506 binding protein 5 (*FKBP5*), an immunophilin involved in protein folding and trafficking.[25] *FKBP5* was also the most highly upregulated gene (>20-fold) in another study.[27] Also upregulated in this group was ankylosis progressive homolog (*ANKH*), a gene shown to induce calcium phosphate deposition and joint destruction when mutated in mice, which could suggest a role in the destructive effects of prostate cancer metastasis to bone. Among genes associated with proliferation and differentiation, inhibitor of differentiation 2 (*ID2*) was upregulated, which counteracts the anti-growth effects of Rb and p16.[25]

A novel group of androgen-regulated genes involves the endoplasmic reticulum (ER) stress response, known as the unfolded protein response (UPR). This stress response is triggered by accumulation in the ER of proteins whose aberrant folding prevents their normal trafficking or secretion to lysosomes. In response, the genes encoding molecular chaperones and folding enzymes in the ER are transcriptionally activated, including those for oxygen regulated protein 150 (*ORP150*), protein disulfide isomerase-related (*PDIR*), N-myc downstream regulated gene 1 (*NDRG1*), and homocysteine-inducible, endoplasmic reticulum stress-inducible ubiquitin-like domain member 1 (*HERPUD1*). The function of the latter is unknown; it is strongly upregulated by thapsigargin and may be involved in the cellular survival response to stress.[26] Another study also found prominent androgen-

regulated changes in genes associated with protein trafficking and secretory vesicle formation, and included that for the stress-associated endoplasmic reticulum protein 1 (*SERP1*).[27] Because androgens have been shown to induce oxidative stress,[28] and also activate hypoxia-inducible factor 1,[29] and both redox changes and hypoxia can trigger the UPR,[30] the ER stress response may represent a protective response to androgen-induced cellular stress.[26]

A comparison of gene expression across four studies that all examined changes in LNCaP cells with extended time courses of androgen stimulation found that only 13 genes were up- or downregulated in all four studies.[11] These included the genes for FK506 binding protein 5, matrix metalloproteinase 16, N-myc downstream regulated gene 1, hect domain and RLD 3, RAB4 member RAS oncogene family, C-terminal binding protein 1, phosphoinositide-3-kinase, regulatory subunit 3 (p55, gamma), leukemia inhibitory factor receptor, cyclin-dependent kinase 8, PSA, fibronectin 1, seladin1/24-dehydrocholesterol reductase, and human fetal butyrlcholinesterase. Velasco, whose study identified the largest number of androgen-regulated genes (692), enumerated a number of possible reasons for the small degree of overlap among the studies: use of R1881 versus DHT; inclusion of only a single untreated control versus inclusion of untreated control with each time point of androgen treatment; and use of cDNA spotted arrays versus Affymetric GeneChips. The largest overlap (113 genes) was between the two studies that used Affymetrix GeneChips.[11,28]

AGGRESSIVE PHENOTYPE

Clinical behavior of prostate cancers is traditionally predicted by factors such as preoperative PSA, Gleason score on biopsy or surgical specimen, and tumor stage. These clinicopathologic factors are phenotypes that represent the collective effect of a constellation of genes. Thus, identification of gene-expression changes associated with the aggressive phenotype can provide insights into the mechanisms that determine tumor behavior. Singh used an Affymetrix U95AV2 array with 12,600 genes and expressed sequence tags (ESTs) to evaluate genotype–phenotype associations in 52 prostate tumors. Twenty-nine genes were significantly correlated with Gleason score (15 upregulated and 14 downregulated), but none correlated significantly with PSA, extraprostatic extension (EPE), surgical margin status, or perineural invasion.[31] Upregulated genes included those encoding N-sulfoglucosamine sulfohydrolase, cholecystokinin, NADH dehydrogenase 1 alpha subcomplex 6, and downregulated genes included *SPARC*, and the genes encoding insulin-like growth factor binding protein 3, and collagen type 1 alpha 2. Lapointe and colleagues identified 41 genes significantly associated with high Gleason grade, including four also identified by Singh[31] (*SPARC*, genes encoding collagen type 1 alpha 2, biglycan, and ATP-binding cassette subfamily C member 5), and one associated with the transition from PIN to prostate cancer in the study by Ashida[6] (chondroitin sulfate proteoglycan). However, unlike the findings in the Singh study, they also found 11 genes to be associated with high tumor stage, including two associated with the transition from PIN in the Ashida study[6] (coagulation factor V and inhibitor of DNA binding 2).[10]

A number of genes were downregulated in a comparison of 20 metastatic tumor samples with 16 primary tumors. These included genes in the following functional groups: 1) cell growth/cell death: *TRAIL* and sel-1 suppressor of lin-12 like (*SEL1L*), connective tissue growth factor 3 (*CTFG3*); 2) cell adhesion: lumicam (*LUM*), integrin β1D, hevin, thrombospondin 1; 3) inflammation/immunity: small inducible cytokine A2; 4) phosphatase/kinase: *PTEN*; and 5) transcription: activating transcription factor 3 (*ATF3*) and FBJ murine osteosarcoma viral oncogene homolog B.[32] Among these, *ATF3* had been previously identified as downregulated in the transition from PIN to prostate cancer, but *LUM* and *SEL1L* were noted to be upregulated from PIN to cancer.[6] This study used two "normal" reference standards: pooled normal adjacent tissue and pooled normal tissue from prostates without apparent pathology. Most genes downregulated in metastatic tissue were only apparent using the latter standard. It was not clear whether any primary and metastatic tissues came from the same patients. A subsequent report from this same study identified EZH2 as the gene upregulated to the greatest degree in metastatic relative to primary prostate cancer.[33] EZH2 did not correlate significantly with Gleason score, stage, or surgical margin status. Fifty-five genes were significantly upregulated and 480 were significantly downregulated in metastatic compared with primary tumor. Other strongly upregulated genes included *MEN1* and the gene encoding ATP-binding cassette subfamily C member 5 (previously correlated with high Gleason Grade[10,31]).

PROGNOSIS

The stage-shift in prostate cancer diagnosis that has accompanied the adoption of PSA testing has resulted in a narrower range of adverse prognostic features, so that most men are diagnosed with low-to-intermediate risk of recurrence. Within strata defined by established prognostic features, there is still uncertainty in clinical outcome, particularly in the intermediate risk category. Classification by gene expression patterns may identify subgroups of biological behavior that would not be captured by established clinical or prognostic factor phenotypes. Because comparison of tumor versus

normal microarrays showed upregulation of *hepsin* and *PIM1* in tumors, Dhanasekaran evaluated these in multivariable models of PSA recurrence in 78 men with clinically localized prostate cancer. Both were inversely associated with PSA recurrence, i.e., absent or low expression increased risk of recurrence, with hazard ratios of 2.9 and 4.5, respectively.[32] However, these analyses were based on multiple samples from each patient, and the analysis did not account for this lack of independence, so it is difficult to interpret this result. In a subsequent report this same group showed *EZH2* to be the strongest predictor of recurrence in a multivariable survival model, with a hazard ratio of 4.6. This analysis also does not appear to have accounted for multiple specimens from each patient.[33] Singh studied 21 men (8 of whom recurred) with the Affymetrix U95AV2 array, with 12,600 genes and ESTs, and did not find any single genes significantly associated with recurrence. However, a k-nearest neighbor analysis (class prediction) identified a five-gene model that predicted recurrence better than Gleason score; a total of 11 genes were significant predictors of recurrence. The model with the top five genes included those encoding inositol 1,4,5-triphosphate receptor type 3, sialyltransferase 1 (upregulation associated with recurrence), and PDGFR-beta, chromogranin A, and *HOXC6* (downregulation associated with recurrence). Sample size was insufficient for multivariable analysis to determine whether this model provided additional prognostic information beyond that available from established prognostic factors.[14,31]

Henshall used the larger Eos-Hu03 Affymetrix array (59,619 probesets) in 72 radical prostatectomy patients (17 of whom recurred) and identified 266 probesets with significant associations with recurrence. A novel survival analysis approach was used for initial identification of prognostic genes, allowing fullest use of the time to recurrence data. Of these, the strongest predictor was the transient receptor potential cation channel subfamily 8 (trp-p8), a putative calcium channel protein. Downregulation of trp-p8 increased risk of recurrence 3.8-fold in a univariate analysis; it remained significant in multivariable analysis but the hazard ratio was not provided. Also among the 10 top-ranked genes were those encoding seladin-1, leukotriene B4 12-hydroxydehydrogenase, and RALBP1 associated Eps domain containing 2. The only gene among the top-ranked 10 that is expressed primarily in the prostate was *trp-p8*.[34] Proteins in the trp family regulate influx of calcium through the plasma membrane. This is triggered by depletion of intracellular calcium following activation by hormones or growth factors that stimulate inositol 1,4,5-triphosphate. Since apoptosis in response to androgen-deprivation is linked to increased intracellular calcium, it is possible that trp-p8 may play a role in protecting prostate cancer from apoptosis by depleting calcium stores.[35] None of 11 genes identified by Singh[31] as significant predictors of recurrence overlapped with the 266 prognostic probesets identified by Henshall. This may be due to: 1) larger array used by Henshall (trp-p8 was not included in the array used by Singh); and 2) use of a survival analysis approach for initial identification of candidate genes allowing use of all patient survival times, maximizing statistical information content.[34]

RESPONSE TO THERAPY AND PREVENTION

Studying genetic changes that occur in response to therapeutic or preventive treatments, and those associated with treatment failure can identify new therapeutic targets or strategies. For prostate cancer this usually requires working with in-vitro or xenograft models since disseminated disease is rarely biopsied. Development of androgen independence was evaluated with the CWR22 androgen-dependent, and CWR22-R androgen-independent xenograft models using the UniGEM 1.0 expression array with 9792 genes. The CWR22 model most closely resembles human disease with initial strong response to androgen deprivation, followed by eventual emergence of an androgen-independent state, the CWR22-R xenograft.[36] Using a cutoff of greater than 2.5-fold change in expression, 24 genes were upregulated and 120 genes were downregulated after 20 days of androgen deprivation. The specific genes with expression changes varied over time—71% of genes downregulated at day 8 remained downregulated at day 20; in contrast, only 27% of genes upregulated at day 8 remained upregulated at day 20. The downregulated genes represented functional pathways such as: 1) cell cycle (including cdc2, cyclin B1, cyclin D2, M-phase phosphoprotein); 2) protein degradation/cleavage (including cathepsin K, ubiquitin-specific protease 11, peptidase-β); and 3) metabolism/respiration (including glyceraldehyde-3-phosphate dehydrogenase, lactate dehydrogenase, α-enolase). Genes in the apoptotic pathway did not appear to be affected. Among the 122 genes with reduced expression at any time after androgen deprivation, 94 exhibited similar levels in CWR22-R as in CWR22 at baseline, suggesting that acquisition of androgen independence requires cells to re-enter the cell-cycle.[36] In contrast, 28 genes reduced after androgen deprivation continued to exhibit reduced levels in proliferating CWR22-R tumors, suggesting that expression of these genes depends on transcription of androgen receptor (AR). These included the genes encoding hsp40-3, FGF9, ubiquitin specific protease 11, mitochondrial processing peptidase-β, α-tubulin, and protein phosphatase 1 subunit 10. This was confirmed by administering androgens to CWR22-R mice, which caused all 28 genes to increase to levels approaching baseline CWR22 levels, indicating that decreases in

these genes upon androgen deprivation reflected a true reduction in activity of androgen-responsive genes, rather than phenotypic changes associated with growth arrest. Finally, genes upregulated in CWR22-R compared with CWR22 included those for syndecan-I, FK506 binding protein 5, laminin receptor α-integrin 6, and thyroid hormone receptor-α.[36]

Estramustine is commonly used for treatment of hormone refractory disease. Changes in gene expression in hormone-resistant PC-3 cells after treatment with 4 μmol/L estramustine for 6, 36 or 72 hours were examined using the Affymetrix U133A array with 22,215 probes. Expression changes greater than 2-fold were exhibited by 726 genes after treatment. Cluster analysis and grouping by biological function identified downregulated genes to be mostly associated with cell proliferation (TGFβ2, TGFβR2, and the genes encoding activating transcription factor 5, S-phase kinase-associated protein 2, cyclin E2) and signal transduction and transcription (ERK and the gene for mitogen-activated protein kinase kinase kinase 2; while upregulated genes involved ion transport (the gene for potassium inwardly-rectifying channel subfamily J member 15), cell shape/cytoskeleton (genes for keratin 17, human 56k cystoskeletal type II keratin [KRT6A], connective tissue growth factor), apoptosis/cell-cycle arrest (GADD34, and the genes encoding interleukin 1α, interleukin 24, cyclin G2).[37]

Genistein is the major isoflavone in soy, which is of interest as possibly contributing to the low prostate cancer risk of men in Asia. A number of studies have shown that genistein and other soy isoflavones modulate androgen-mediated pathways, and induce growth arrest and apoptosis in prostate cancer cells. LNCaP cells were exposed to genistein at levels consistent with human dietary exposure (1, 5, and 25 μM), and the Affymetrix U133A array was used to compare expression in control and treated cells. A concentration-dependent pattern was observed with the number of genes down- or upregulated being 22 and 8 (1 μM), 15 and 21 (5 μM), and 243 and 108 (25 μM), respectively. A large number of androgen-regulated genes were affected. Among genes normally upregulated by androgen that were downregulated more than 2-fold by genistein were those encoding PSA, kallikrein 2, NKX3.1, aldehyde dehydrogenase 1 member A3 (ALDH1A3), Ca/calmodulin dependent protein kinase kinase 2β (CAMKK2), and serine threonine kinase 39 (STK39/SPAK). However, at typical dietary levels (5 μM) only the genes for the following were downregulated by more than 2-fold: v-maf fibrosarcoma oncogene homolog, transmembrane protease serine 2, and transmembrane prostate androgen induced RNA. Genes that were normally downregulated by androgen that were upregulated by genistein included those for BRCA1-associated RING domain 1 (CDK8) and dopa decarboxylase (DDC), but only the gene encoding butyrylcholinesterase (*BCHE*) was upregulated at the 5 µM dose. The fact that genistein produced changes in the opposite direction to the normal response to androgens is consistent with a risk-lowering effect. Genistein strongly upregulated genes associated with DNA damage response, such as *clusterin* and *JUN*, and genes associated with the peroxisome proliferator-activated receptor-α (PPAR-α) pathway, such as that encoding malic enzyme 1 (ME1), but only at the 25 µM dose. A novel finding was that *IGF1R* was downregulated by genistein, suggesting potential inhibition of the IGF1 pathway that has been linked to increased prostate cancer risk. Expression changes of key genes altered by genistein were confirmed with real-time PCR.[38]

CONCLUSIONS

Application of expression microarrays to prostate cancer research offers the possibility of genome-wide searches to identify not just individual gene targets, but important functional pathways and complimentary mechanisms affecting prostate cancer clinical behavior. However, there is a critical need, especially at this relatively early stage in the application of microarrays to prostate cancer, to call for rigorous attention to study design, data analysis methods, and development of standardized protocols. The technological advance represented by the microarray will not by itself overcome the difficulty of moving a biomarker to clinical usage that has bedeviled biomarkers previously studied by the candidate gene approach. Despite thousands of studies of molecular biomarkers for prostate cancer, only one (PSA) is routinely used by clinicians. Reasons for this lack of translation relate primarily to inconsistent results among studies, stemming from differences in patient populations, sample handling, processing, assay methods, cutpoints for positive tests, and inadequate statistical analysis. Similar problems are already apparent in microarray studies. As the examples above indicate, there is a relatively small degree of overlap in top-ranked genes identified among multiple studies of the same aspect of prostate cancer. Some of the reasons for this include overfitting, i.e., false-positive identification of altered expression resulting from inadequate patient numbers, different (and poorly described) patient populations, different probesets on the arrays, and variation in microarray procedures, including sample handling, hybridization, normalization, and definition of altered expression. While it is unrealistic to expect standardization of all methods, there is a need for greater consistency in reporting standards at a minimum. Despite the tremendously valuable access to supplementary data routinely provided by web-sites linked to electronic publications, data on the patient

samples are still inadequate for clinical correlation studies. It is often impossible to tell if multiple samples come from different patients or the same patients, especially for tumor versus normal samples, or primary versus metastases. Furthermore, because microarray studies based on human material are essentially population studies, it is important to take account of other factors, particularly for prognostic marker studies. Established prognostic factors for prostate cancer, such as Gleason score, are phenotypes that represent a constellation of genes. Therefore, any potentially prognostic genes identified through microarray analyses should be examined to determine their independent prognostic contribution after accounting for correlation with established prognostic factors in a multivariable model. As with most cancer biomarker studies it is often difficult to differentiate between causal genetic changes and those that are the consequence of progression. Consequently, novel alterations identified by expression microarrays need to be replicated using transgenic or knockout models. Microarrays represent an enormously powerful tool to identify etiologic mechanisms, individualize treatment, develop novel targeted therapies, and define new preventive strategies. By allowing researchers to view synchronized pathways and co-regulated genes, microarrays, and the complimentary applications of proteomics and transcriptomics, have the potential to bring about a paradigm shift in the study of cancer biology.

REFERENCES

1. Thompson IM, Goodman PJ, Tangen CM, et al. The influence of finasteride on the development of prostate cancer. N Engl J Med 2003;349:215–224

2. Etzioni R, Penson DF, Legler JM, et al. Overdiagnosis due to prostate-specific antigen screening: lessons from U.S. prostate cancer incidence trends. J Natl Cancer Inst 2002;94:981–990.

3. Rubin MA, Zhou M, Dhanasekaran SM, et al. alpha-Methylacyl coenzyme A racemase as a tissue biomarker for prostate cancer. JAMA 2002; 287:1662–1670.

4. Luo J, Zha S, Gage WR, et al. Alpha-methylacyl-CoA racemase: a new molecular marker for prostate cancer. Cancer Res 2002;62:2220–2226.

5. Luo J, Duggan DJ, Chen Y, et al. Human prostate cancer and benign prostatic hyperplasia: molecular dissection by gene expression profiling. Cancer Res 2001;61:4683–4688.

6. Ashida S, Nakagawa H, Katagiri T, et al. Molecular features of the transition from prostatic intraepithelial neoplasia (PIN) to prostate cancer: genome-wide gene-expression profiles of prostate cancers and PINs. Cancer Res 2004;64:5963–5972.

7. Quackenbush J. Computational analysis of microarray data. Nat Rev Genet 2001;2:418–427.

8. Simon R. Diagnostic and prognostic prediction using gene expression profiles in high-dimensional microarray data. Br J Cancer 2003;89:1599–1604.

9. Simon RM, Korn EL, McShane LM, et al. Design and analysis of DNA microarray investigations. New York: Springer, 2003.

10. Lapointe J, Li C, Higgins JP, et al. Gene expression profiling identifies clinically relevant subtypes of prostate cancer. Proc Natl Acad Sci 2004;101:811–816.

11. Velasco AM, Gillis KA, Li Y, et al. Identification and validation of novel androgen-regulated genes in prostate cancer. Endocrinology 2004;145:3913–3924.

12. McShane LM, Radmacher MD, Freidlin B, et al. Methods for assessing reproducibility of clustering patterns observed in analyses of microarray data. Bioinformatics 2002;18:1462–1469.

13. Bisoffi M, Klima I, Gresko E, et al. Expression profiles of androgen independent bone metastatic prostate cancer cells indicate up-regulation of the putative serine-threonine kinase GS3955. J Urol 2004;172:1145–1150.

14. Febbo PG, Sellers WR. Use of expression analysis to predict outcome after radical prostatectomy. J Urol 2003;170:S11–20.

15. Yang MC, Yang JJ, McIndoe RA, et al. Microarray experimental design: power and sample size considerations. Physiol Genomics 2003;16:24–28.

16. Reyes I, Reyes N, Iatropoulos M, et al. Aging-associated changes in gene expression in the ACI rat prostate: implications for carcinogenesis. Prostate 2004; [Epub ahead of print]:1–18.

17. Xu J, Stolk JA, Zhang X, et al. Identification of differentially expressed genes in human prostate cancer using subtraction and microarray. Cancer Res 2000;60:1677–1682.

18. Zhou M, Aydin H, Kanae H, et al. How often does α-methylacyl-CoA racemase contribute to resolving an atypical diagnosis on prostate needle biopsy beyond that provided by basal cell markers. Am J Surg Path 2004;28:239–243.

19. Rhodes DR, Barrette TR, Rubin MA, et al. Meta-analysis of microarrays: interstudy validation of gene expression profiles reveals pathway dysregulation in prostate cancer. Cancer Res 2002;62:4427–4433.

20. Klezovitch O, Chevillet J, Mirosevich J, et al. Hepsin promotes prostate cancer progression and metastasis. Cancer Cell 2004;6:185–195.

21. Stephan C, Yousef GM, Scorilas A, et al. Hepsin is highly over expressed in and a new candidate for a prognostic indicator in prostate cancer. J Urol 2004;171:187–191.

22. Rhodes DR, Sanda MG, Otte AP, et al. Multiplex biomarker approach for determining risk of prostate-specific antigen-defined recurrence of prostate cancer. J Natl Cancer Inst 2003;95:661–668.

23. Nelson PS, Plymate SR, Wang K, et al. Hevin, an antiadhesive extracellular matrix protein, is down-egulated in metastatic prostate adenocarcinoma. Cancer Res 1998;58:232–236.

24. Isler SG, Schenk S, Bendik I, et al. Genomic organization and chromosomal mapping of SPARC-like 1, a gene down regulated in cancers. Int J Oncol 2001;18:521–526.

25. Nelson PS, Clegg N, Arnold H, et al. The program of androgen-responsive genes in neoplastic prostate epithelium. Proc Natl Acad Sci 2002;99:11890–11895.

26. Segawa T, Nau ME, Xu LL, et al. Androgen-induced expression of endoplasmic reticulum (ER) stress response genes in prostate cancer cells. Oncogene 2002;21:8749–8758.

27. DePrimo SE, Diehn M, Nelson JB, et al. Transcriptional programs activated by exposure of human prostate cancer cells to androgen. Genome Biol 2002;3:RESEARCH0032 (Epub).

28. Ripple MO, Henry WF, Rago RP, et al. Prooxidant-antioxidant shift induced by androgen treatment of human prostate carcinoma cells. J Natl Cancer Inst 1997;89:40–48.

29. Mabjeesh NJ, Willard MT, Frederickson CE, et al. Androgens stimulate hypoxia-inducible factor 1 activation via autocrine loop of tyrosine kinase receptor/phosphatidylinositol 3′-kinase/protein kinase B in prostate cancer cells. Clin Cancer Res 2003;9:2416–2425.

30. Ma Y, Hendershot LM. The role of the unfolded protein response in tumour development: friend or foe? Nat Rev Cancer 2004;4:966–977.

31. Singh D, Febbo PG, Ross K, et al. Gene expression correlates of clinical prostate cancer behavior. Cancer Cell 2002;1:203–209.

32. Dhanasekaran SM, Barrette TR, Ghosh D, et al. Delineation of prognostic biomarkers in prostate cancer. Nature 2001;412:822–826.

33. Varambally S, Dhanasekaran SM, Zhou M, et al. The polycomb group protein EZH2 is involved in progression of prostate cancer. Nature. 2002;419:624–629.

34. Henshall SM, Afar DE, Hiller J, et al. Survival analysis of genome-wide gene expression profiles of prostate cancers identifies new prognostic targets of disease relapse. Cancer Res 2003;63:4196–203.

35. Tsavaler L, Shapero MH, Morkowski S, et al. Trp-p8, a novel prostate-specific gene, is up-regulated in prostate cancer and other malignancies and shares high homology with transient receptor potential calcium channel proteins. Cancer Res 2001;61:3760–3769.

36. Amler LC, Agus DB, LeDuc C, et al. Dysregulated expression of androgen-responsive and nonresponsive genes in the androgen-independent prostate cancer xenograft model CWR22-R1. Cancer Res 2000;60:6134–141.

37. Hong X, Li Y, Hussain M, et al. Gene expression profiling reveals novel targets of estramustine phosphate in prostate cancer cells. Cancer Lett 2004;209:187–195.

38. Takahashi Y, Lavigne JA, Hursting SD, et al. Using DNA microarray analyses to elucidate the effects of genistein in androgen-responsive prostate cancer cells: identification of novel targets. Mol Carcinog 2004;41:108–119.

Topographic anatomy of prostate, seminal vesicles, vas deferens, and ejaculatory ducts

6

Ajay Pahuja, Jeetesh Bhardwa, Jowad Raja, Navin Ramachandran,
W D Dunsmuir, Roger S Kirby

THE PROSTATE

The prostate is the largest accessory gland of the male reproductive system. The healthy adult prostate is about the size of a chestnut, somewhat conical in shape, and generally measures about 20 mL in volume, though it can grow up to five or six times that size with increasing age. It is shaped like an inverted pyramid and lies between the urinary bladder and the pelvic floor. The prostate is a fibromuscular organ that is incompletely enveloped by the prostatic capsule and surrounds the prostatic urethra (Figure 6.1). It lies behind the inferior border of the symphysis pubis and pubic arch and anterior to the rectal ampulla, through which it may be palpated digitally. The superior portion of the prostate is known as the base, while the inferior portion is known as the apex. The prostate provides about 30% of the volume of seminal fluid (60% comes from the seminal vesicle).

The prostatic urethra traverses the whole length of the gland, entering its base (vesicular surface) near the anterior border, which is largely contiguous with the bladder neck above it, and exiting from the front of the narrowed blunt apex at the level of the urogenital diaphragm to become the membranous urethra (Figure 6.2).

ANATOMICAL LIMITS

- Superiorly, the prostate is limited by the preprostatic sphincter and the bladder neck.
- Inferiorly, the prostate is limited by the external (striated) sphincter.

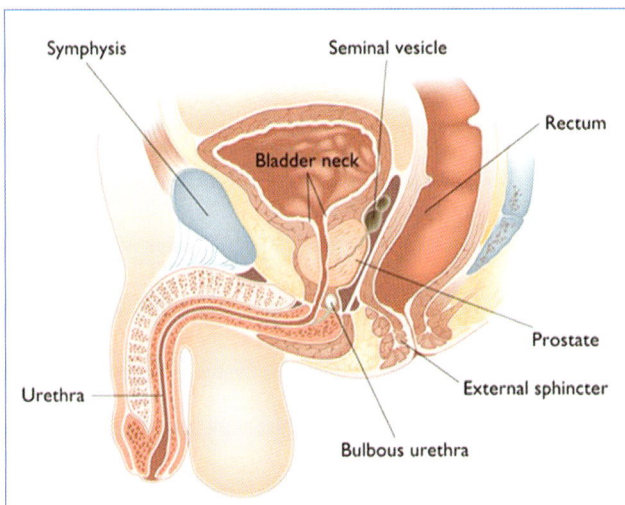

Fig. 6.1
Mid-sagittal section showing structures adjacent to prostate.

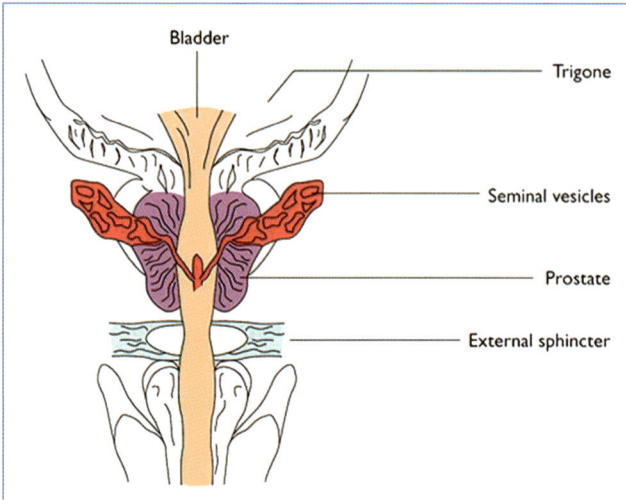

Fig. 6.2
Mid coronal section showing the relationship of the prostate and the verumontanum to the external striated sphincter. In TURP, the resection is always done proximal to the veru, this ensures the spincter is not damaged and continence is preserved.

- Inferolaterally, the prostate is limited by the levator prostatae muscle, which is a part of the levator ani muscle.
- Anteriorly, the pubic bone limits the prostate, to which the prostate is connected inferiorly by the tough puboprostatic ligaments.
- Posteriorly, the prostate is separated from the rectum by the rectovesical fascia (Denonvilliers' fascia).

The ejaculatory ducts pierce the posterior surface of the prostate just below the bladder and pass obliquely through the prostate for about 2 cm to open either side of the verumontanum in the prostatic urethra. The verumontanum is located just proximal to the external striated sphincter.

SURFACES

The prostate is referred to as having an anterior, posterior, and two inferolateral surfaces.

The anterior convex surface lies 2 cm behind the symphysis pubis, separated from it by the extraperitoneal fat and venous plexus in the retropubic space (known as the cave of Retzius). The fibrous sheath of the prostate is attached to the posterior aspect of the inferior border of the pubic bones by the condensations of the pelvic fascia known as the puboprostatic ligaments. These lie on either side of the midline and fix the apex of the prostate to the pubis.[1-3]

The posterior surface is nearly flat transversely and convex vertically, with a midline depression that is normally felt on rectal examination referred to as the median sulcus. Along with the seminal vesicles and the ampulla of the vasa, it is separated from the rectum by a layer of a surgically important fascia, the Denonvillers' fascia. This fascia is derived from two layers of pelvic peritoneum in the retrovesical space. The two ejaculatory ducts pierce the posterior surface in the depression near its superior aspect. The ducts pass obliquely through the gland for about 2 cm to open into the prostatic urethra at the colliculus seminalis or verumontanum, one on either side of the prostatic utricle just proximal to the striated external urinary sphincter.

The inferolateral surfaces of the prostate meet anteriorly with the convex anterior surface and rest on the pubococcygeal portion of the levator ani and its overlying endopelvic fascia. The levator ani muscles have an almost vertical orientation, funneling inferiorly to surround the rectum and bracket the striated urethral sphincter and middle and apical portions of the prostate.[4]

ZONAL ANATOMY

The lobar concept of the prostate anatomy as suggested by Lowsley[5] is no longer helpful and, therefore, not used. The agreed consensus is to accept McNeal's view of the zonal anatomy of the prostate. The concept of zonal anatomy first suggested by McNeal[6,7,8] in 1968 was later confirmed by Blacklock and Bouskill.[9] This divides the prostate into three distinct zones (Figure 6.3). The ventral fibromuscular zone is not a glandular region and is, therefore, considered by some not to be a true part of the prostate gland, but it is an anatomical part of the prostate organ and can be considered as a fourth zone.

PERIPHERAL ZONE

The peripheral zone (PZ) constitutes about 70% of the glandular portion of the prostate. It forms the lateral and the posterior part of the prostate. It is funnel shaped, and its distal part constitutes the apex of the prostate while the proximal part opens up to receive the inferior portion of the wedge shaped central zone. Most prostatic cancers arise from this zone. It is here that most attention is paid to while undertaking transrectal ultrasound (TRUS) biopsies of the prostate with a view

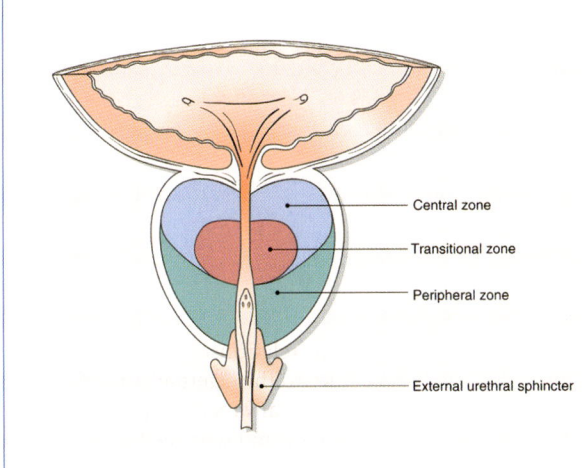

Central zone

Transitional zone

Peripheral zone

External urethral sphincter

Fig. 6.3
This figure demonstrates the zonal anatomy of the prostate.

to establishing whether or not a patient has a diagnosis of prostate cancer.

CENTRAL ZONE

The central zone (CZ) constitutes about 25% of the prostate gland. It is wedge shaped, and it has its broad base just below the bladder neck and its narrow apex lying at the verumontanum. The ejaculatory duct runs in the middle of the central zone. The central zone also has a broad base at its proximal part to accommodate the proximal segment of the urethra. The funnels of both the central and peripheral zone are incomplete anteriorly where they are embedded into the fibromuscular stroma.

TRANSITION ZONE

The transition zone (TZ) only comprises about 5% to 10% of the prostate gland. It is actually two independent smaller lobes that can be imagined as clasping the urethra at the point of its angulation just distal to the preprostatic sphincter and touching it.

VENTRAL FIBROMUSCULAR ZONE

The ventral fibromuscular zone is not a glandular structure. As such it is not regarded as part of the prostate gland, but it can be considered a part of the prostate organ. It constitutes about one third the size of the entire prostate organ and, as such, is the largest single component of it. It envelopes the transition zone and provides an anchor for the central and peripheral zones.

RADIOLOGIC ANATOMY

The prostate can be imaged by ultrasound, computed tomography (CT), and magnetic resonance imaging

(MRI). Transabdominal ultrasound is largely obsolete to image the prostate gland, however, TRUS is widely used and provides detailed imaging.

Using CT, the prostate gland is inadequately seen, although a well-defined fat plane separates it from the levator ani muscle. At the base and apex its relations are largely unclear. The peripheral zone may occasionally show enough contrast enhancement to become radiologically distinct from the remainder of the gland. In the majority, zonal anatomy cannot be reliably distinguished with CT.

In comparison, using TRUS the zonal divisions are readily apparent. The PZ is seen as a hyperechoic structure, whereas the central and transitional zones are of lower echogenicity and not seen as clearly separate structures. These non-PZ glandular portions are sometimes collectively termed the inner gland. The seminal vesicles are seen separate and distinct from the prostate gland. These are of lower echogenicity and lie superoposterior to the gland. The neurovascular bundles and apical anatomy can be seen on TRUS, but the dorsal vein complex does present difficulty.

Overall, MRI demonstrates prostate anatomy most accurately. T_2-weighted sequences will demonstrate zonal anatomy. On T_1-weighted sequences, the gland appears of uniform low signal. The PZ and seminal vesicles show high signal on T_2-weighted images. The CZ and TZ demonstrate low signal, and the two zones are not easily differentiated. The neurovascular bundles, located at the posterolateral position (5 o'clock and 7 o'clock positions) are easily defined, as is the apex. (Figure 6.4)

All the modalities discussed above can contribute to staging of prostate cancer. Computed tomography has poor sensitivity and specificity for assessment of local disease staging and extracapsular spread. The benefit of CT is identifying nodal status and distal disease. With TRUS, tumors are seen as hypoechoic areas. These are easier to identify in the PZ but largely sonographically invisible within the CZ or TZ. Approximately 60% to

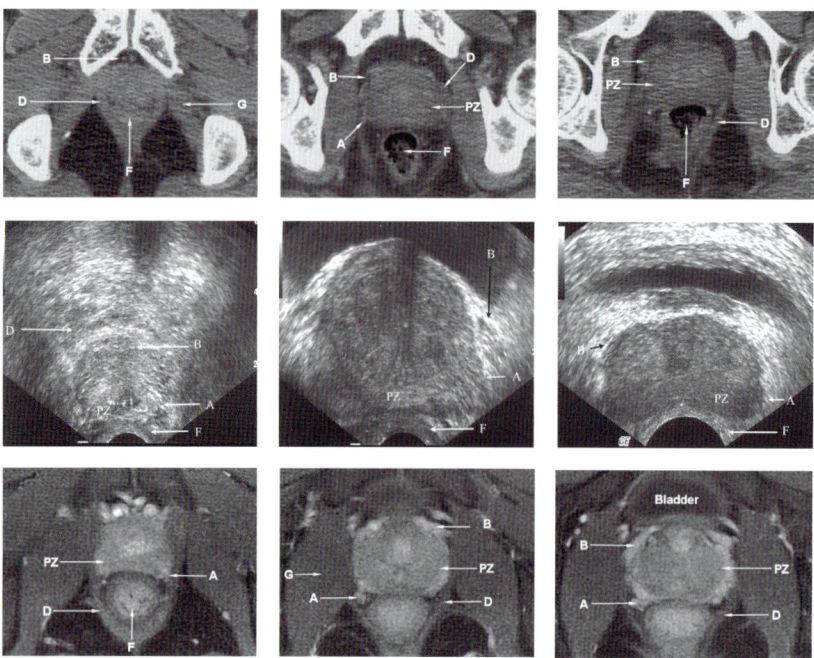

Fig. 6.4

The above images are comparisons of the images obtained in the axial plane using CT, TRUS and MRI (top, middle and bottom respectively) at the apex, midzone and base (left to right) of the prostate. The peripheral zone is well demonstrated with both TRUS and MRI, but is less easily appreciated with CT. For either open or laparoscopic prostatectomy, two of the key surgical landmarks are the neurovascular bundles and the deep and superficial venous plexi, and these structures are both well demonstrated using MRI, with TRUS also useful in this regard. CT poorly demonstrates the local peri-prostatic anatomy. Key: Neurovascular bundles (A), prostatic venous plexus (B), prostatic fascia (C), levator ani (D), seminal vesicles (E), rectum (F), obturator internus (G), peripheral zone (PZ).

70% of PZ tumors are hypoechoic, the remainder being isoechoic and so invisible by TRUS. Moreover, hypoechogenicity is not specific for cancer, and several benign disorders and post-biopsy appearance can look similar. The positive predictive value (PPV) in detection of tumors is reported as 9% when other screening tests are normal.[10,11] The PPV is higher if both prostate-specific antigen (PSA) and DRE are abnormal. Local extension may be identified on TRUS as irregularity of the prostate capsule or periprostatic fat planes, neurovascular bundles, or seminal vesicle enlargement (Figure 6.5).

On MRI, tumor is more consistently visualized than TRUS. The majority of tumors will demonstrate lower signal on T_2-weighted images compared with surrounding normal intermediate signal peripheral zones. Sensitivity in the TZ is lower due to the normally heterogeneous signal returned for benign prostatic hyperplasia (BHP).

Signs of extracapsular extension on MRI include irregular bulging of the prostate, focal capsular thickening, asymmetry, or direct involvement of the neurovascular bundles. Capsular involvement most commonly occurs adjacent to the neurovascular bundles at the site of neural perforation of the capsule, at the posterolateral aspect of the prostate. Involvement of

seminal vesicles is suggested by the inability to visualize the ejaculatory duct and low signal in the seminal vesicles on T_2-weighted sequences. The reported sensitivity for tumor detection in the peripheral zone is 92% (Figures 6.6 and 6.7).

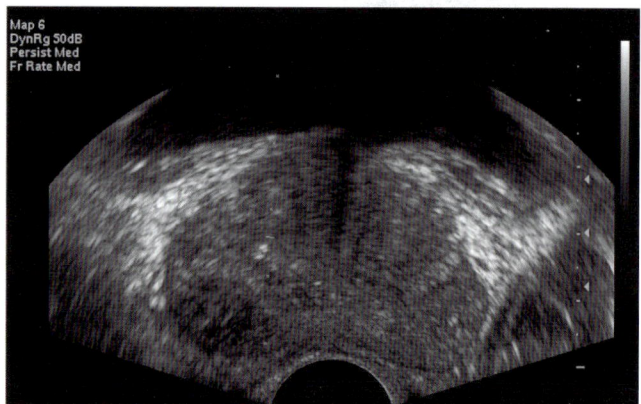

Fig. 6.5

This TRUS image shows a lesion in the right peripheral zone (on the left side of the image), demonstrating low echogenicity. Appearances are consistent with a carcinoma, however ultrasound has a poor specificity and biopsy confirmation is required for all suspected cases.

As well as staging, imaging can provide valuable information regarding surgical planning. The areas where positive surgical margins are more likely are the apex, the posterolateral aspects, and the base of the gland. Magnetic resonance imaging will provide more detailed pathology in these regions than any other modality (Table 6.1).

Table 6.1 Comparing sensitivity versus specificity in the detection of extracapsular spread		
	TRUS (%)	**MRI (%)**
Sensitivity	23–58	67–80
Specificity	81–95	50–97

MRI, magnetic resonance imaging; TRUS, transrectal ultrasound.[12,13]

THE PROSTATIC CAPSULE AND ITS FASCIAL COVERINGS

The prostate gland is incompletely enveloped in a thin fibrous capsule (the true capsule or the anatomical capsule). It is not a discrete structure but forms the outer non-glandular portion of the prostatic parenchyma. It may lie so near in some areas that a distinct capsular covering may not be demonstrated histologically.[14] Microscopically, it is an integral part of the prostate gland and cannot be separated from it. No clear capsule separates the prostate from the striated urethral sphincter at the apex and the bladder neck at the base. The true capsule is enclosed within a loose sheath derived from the pelvic fascia called the prostatic sheath popularly known as the false or the signal capsule.

The false capsule and the surrounding fibroareolar tissue form a dense condensation and are collectively called the periprostatic fascia, which extends from the anterior surface of the prostate to the posterolateral area, where it encases the neurovascular bundle before it becomes part of the rectovesical septum, which separates the bladder, seminal vesicles, and prostate from the rectum.[15] The superficial branch of the dorsal vein lies outside the periprostatic fascia in the retropubic fat and drains into the dorsal venous complex inside the periprostatic fascia.

A thin layer of connective tissue sweeps down from the lateral pelvic sidewall and covers the bladder and prostate. This tissue is known as the endopelvic, or pelvic, fascia. The parietal pelvic fascia covers the levator ani musculature, and the visceral pelvic fascia covers the bladder and prostate. The convergence of these two leaves forms a white line (the tendinous arch) and superiorly forms the puboprostatic ligaments.[16] During radical prostatectomy, the endopelvic fascia is incised just lateral to this white line. After incision, a remnant levator fascia remains attached to the prostate and is called the lateral pelvic fascia. The lateral pelvic fascia

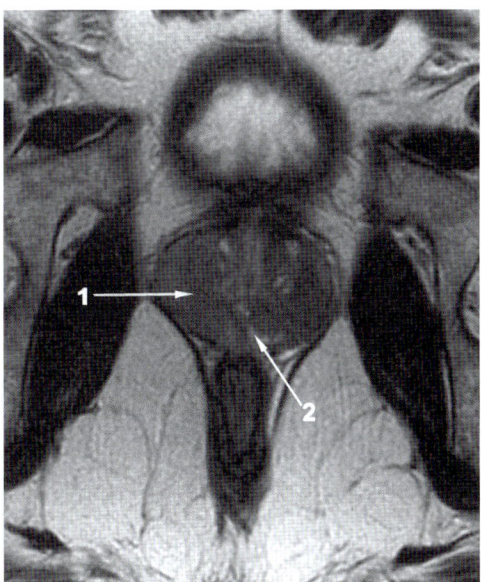

Fig. 6.6
This is a T2 weighted axial MRI image through the prostate showing extensive infiltration of the peripheral zone with low signal tumour (1), leaving only a small region of normal relatively high signal peripheral zone (2) posteriorly. The identification of pathology in the peripheral zone relies largely on the contrast between normal and abnormal tissue. This image illustrates the potenial difficulty in identifying tumour if the gland is diffusely involved.

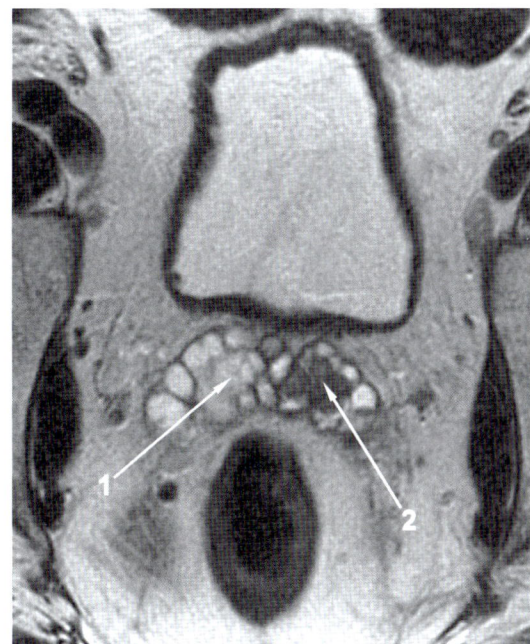

Fig. 6.7
This T2 weighted axial MRI image through the seminal vesicles shows the contrast between normal high signal (1) and infiltrated low signal (2) seminal vesicle. MRI demonstrates involvement of the seminal vesicles more clearly than the other imaging modalities, although TRUS also has an important role.

covers the neurovascular bundle, which lies posterolateral to the prostate.

The posterior surfaces of the prostate and seminal vesicles are separated from the anterior rectal wall by a rather light, but usually definite, fibrous layer of tissue—the Denonvilliers' fascia. It covers the entire posterior surface of the prostate from the apex upwards over the surface of the seminal vesicles to the beginning of the peritoneal cavity at the rectovesical pouch. It serves as a surgical landmark for operations that involve reflection of the rectal wall from the surface of the prostate.

ARTERIAL SUPPLY

The primary arterial supply to the prostate comes from the prostatovesical artery that descends inferiorly along the bladder base. The origin of this artery is variable, but it most commonly arises from the anterior division of the internal iliac artery.[11] The prostatovesical artery further divides into the inferior vesical artery and the prostatic artery to supply the prostate. The prostatic artery divides at the base of the prostate into a larger posterolateral branch supplying most of the gland and the smaller anterior branch supplying only the anterolateral portion. The inferior portion of the prostate receives some blood from the prostatovesical branch of the internal pudendal artery. The prostate, seminal vesicle, and the vas deferens are also supplied by small accessory arteries from the middle rectal artery.[17]

Within the prostate, two groups of arteries (urethral and capsular branches) follow a fairly regular pattern of distribution.[18] The urethral branches provide the principal arterial supply to the prostate. These are the 5- and 7-o'clock arterial vessels that are frequently responsible for the significant bleeding encountered during transurethral resection of the prostate.[19] The capsular branches run along the posterolateral surface of the prostate in the lateral pelvic fascia, and along with the cavernous nerves, form the neurovascular bundle of Walsh, which is the visible landmark and aids in identification of the microscopic cavernous nerves.[20]

VENOUS DRAINAGE

The veins that drain the prostate form the prostatic venous plexus known as Santorini's plexus. This lies within the periprostatic fascia on the anterior surface of the gland.[21] Prostate parenchymal veins, as well as veins draining all deep pelvic structures, intercommunicate with the prostatic venous plexus.

The deep dorsal vein of the penis penetrates the urogenital diaphragm; it then emerges beneath the symphysis pubis between the puboprostatic ligaments on the anterior aspect of the prostate to join the prostatic venous plexus. At this level, the prostatic venous plexus divides into three major branches, the superficial branch and the right and left lateral plexus. The superficial branch is centrally located and travels between the puboprostatic ligaments as visualized during laparoscopic or retropubic surgery[18,22] (Figure 6.8). The majority of the venous blood drains directly into the prostatic plexus and, thence, to the vesical veins; these in turn drain into the internal iliac veins.

The internal iliac veins communicate with the internal vertebral venous plexus, and this vertebral route is thought to be responsible for the dissemination of prostatic cancer cells to the vertebral bodies.[23]

NERVE SUPPLY

The prostate receives its nerve supply from the prostatic nerve plexus, which in itself is part of the pelvic autonomic plexus. The prostatic plexus receives parasympathetic (cholinergic) input from S2–4, while it receives sympathetic (noradrenergic) fibers from the presacral nerves T10–L2 (Figure 6.9). The nerves to the prostate travel outside its capsule and Denonvilliers' fascia until they perforate the capsule at the point of entry into the prostate.

The branches to the membranous urethra and corpora cavernosa also travel outside the prostate capsule in the lateral pelvic fascia posterolaterally between the prostate and rectum and follow the branches of the capsular artery.

The neurovascular bundle that supplies part of the prostate and penis runs within the periprostatic fascia at the junction of the lateral and posterior portions of the endopelvic (lateral pelvic) fascia. It is separated from the prostate by a distance of 1.5 mm at the base and 3 mm at the apex. Although it is closely applied to the prostate because of its posterolateral position, the neurovascular bundle can be dissected from the gland by entering the periprostatic fascia laterally.[24] These nerves need to be spared during urologic pelvic procedures to prevent iatrogenic erectile dysfunction.[24,25]

The cavernous nerves supplying innervation to the coporal bodies travel dorsolaterally in the lateral pelvic fascia and continue laterally on the surface of the membranous urethra. Walsh described the standard approach to nerve sparing, which entails the retrograde removal of the prostate after initial transaction of the membranous urethra.[26] Therefore, by incising the lateral pelvic fascia in a vertical fashion to the level of the membranous urethra and avoiding excessive lateral traction, damage to the cavernous nerves can be minimized and potency spared.

LYMPHATIC DRAINAGE

The lymph capillaries from either side of the prostate join to from the periprostatic lymphatic network, which lies within the prostatic sheath. Vessels from the ejaculatory ducts and the prostatic urethra contribute to the network.[15] Most major lymphatic vessels leave the prostate with the branches of the prostatic artery in the prostatic pedicle. These vessels are important conduits for metastatic spread of prostatic carcinoma. The major route of lymphatic drainage occurs along the prostatic artery in the vascular pedicle to the obturator and internal iliac nodes. The obturator and internal iliac nodes are particularly important to urologists as they are the initial site for lymphatic metastasis of prostate cancer. Secondary lymphatic drainage occurs to the external iliac nodes and less commonly to the sacral nodes.

SEMINAL VESICLES

The seminal vesicles are paired, thin-walled sac-shaped glands each about 5 cm long and somewhat pyramidal, the base being directed up and posterolaterally. They are essentially a single coiled tube with irregular diverticula; the coils and the diverticula are connected by fibrous tissue. The diameter of the tube is 3 to 4 mm and its uncoiled length varies from 10 to 15 cm. They lie obliquely just superior to the prostate on the posterior surface of the bladder next to the ampulla of the ductus deferentia. Their upper ends are widely separated and their lower ends are close together.

The anterior surface contacts the posterior aspect of the bladder, extending from near the entry of the ureter to the prostate base. The posterior surface is related to the rectum, separated from it by the rectovesical fascia. The main arterial supply to the seminal vesicle is from the inferior vesical and middle rectal arteries, and its venous drainage is through veins draining into the internal iliac veins by way of the prostatic plexus.

The secretions of the seminal vesicles comprise 60% of the ejaculate. Its contents are released by contraction of the smooth-muscle wall at ejaculation, which is under the control of the autonomic nervous system. It was formerly believed that the seminal vesicles just served as storage space for accumulated sperm. However, today the opinion prevails that their main function is to provide a fluid that, together with that of the prostate gland, activates the vigorous movement of the sperm cells after ejaculation

EJACULATORY DUCTS AND VASA DEFERENTIA

The ejaculatory ducts are delicate, paired, collagenous tubes measuring 4 to 8 mm in diameter with a 2 mm lumen. The ejaculatory ducts (approx 2.5 cm long) arise near the neck of the bladder and run close together as they pass anteroinferiorly through the posterior surface of the prostate and terminate by opening into the prostatic part of the urethra as separate slit-like orifices on the seminal colliculus at the side of prostatic utricle.

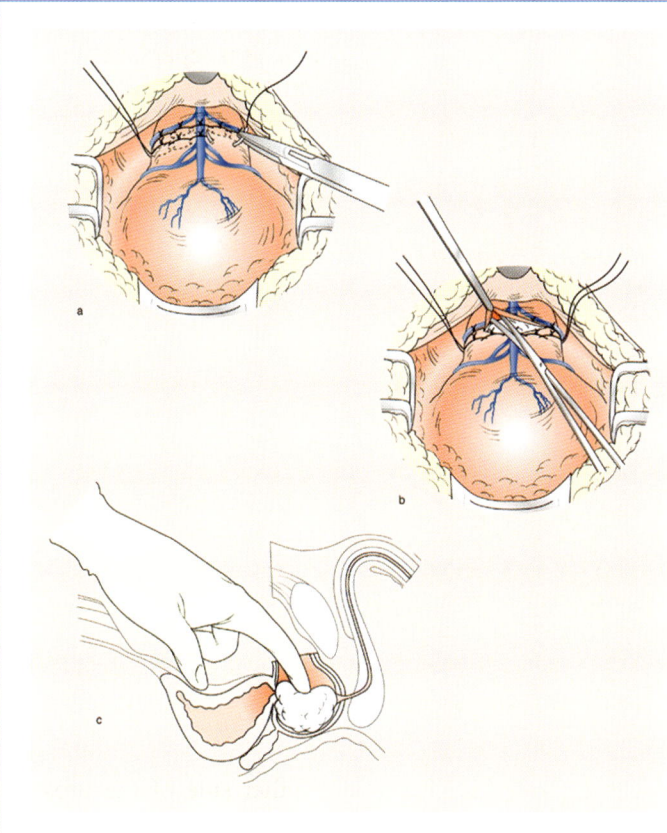

Fig. 6.8
A knowledge of anatomy is very important as surgery is shown in a simple retropubic prostectomy.

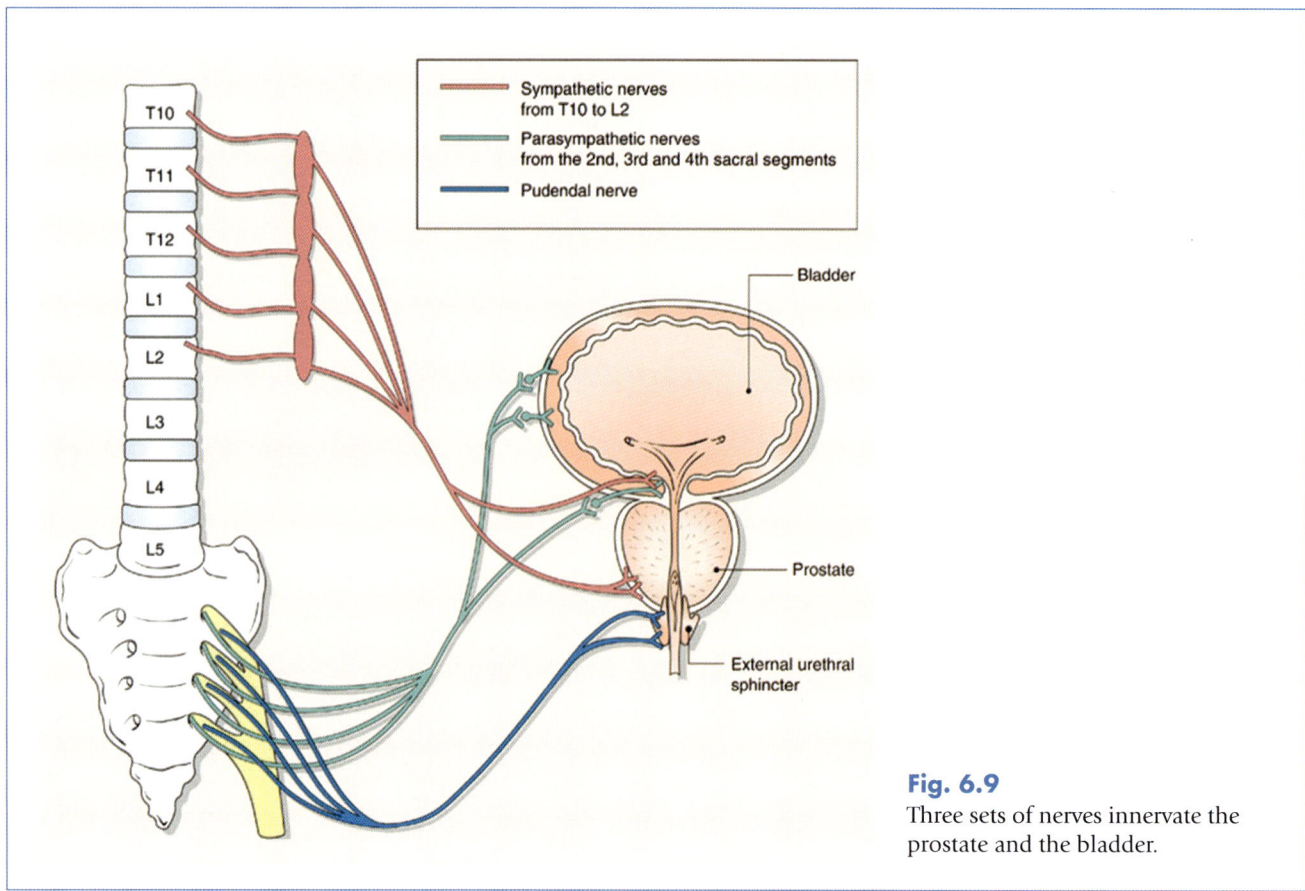

Fig. 6.9
Three sets of nerves innervate the prostate and the bladder.

There are three distinct anatomic regions to the ejaculatory duct: 1) the proximal, largely extraprostatic portion; 2) the middle intraprostatic segment; and 3) a distal segment that empties into the verumontanum in the urethra. There is no muscular sphincter in the region where the ejaculatory ducts join the verumontanum, but smooth muscle fibers may be found at their termination to help prevent reflux.

The vas deferens is the conduit that transports mature sperm from the epididymis to the ejaculatory duct and the urethra. It begins at the cauda epididymis and is very tortuous as it leaves the lower part of the tail of the epididymis, but it gradually becomes less twisted as it ascends behind the testis. It assumes its position in the posterior portion of the cord before passing through the inguinal canal. At the internal ring, it passes lateral to the epigastric vessels. It then passes downward and backward on the lateral wall of the pelvis and crosses the ureter in the region of the ischial spine.[2] It then travels behind the bladder and widens and becomes tortuous to form the ampulla of the vas deferens. Here it approaches the opposite vas and joins the duct of the seminal vesicle to become the ejaculatory duct. The artery to the vas is usually a small vessel from the superior vesical artery, and its venous drainage is into the internal iliac veins. Cutting the vas deferens (vasectomy) is a common method of (essentially permanent) male sterilization.

SMOOTH AND STRIATED MUSCLE SPHINCTERS

Knowledge of the anatomy of the sphincters is necessary to preserve urinary continence during surgery. While voluntary control of voiding begins with relaxation of the striated sphincter in the membranous urethra, smooth-muscle components of the bladder neck and prostate contribute to continence in men.[27] The preprostatic sphincter is composed of muscle elements from the bladder. These muscles encircle the urethra and travel along and insert into the urethra more distally. The preprostatic sphincter and the vesical neck musculature (commonly called the internal sphincter) form a single sphincteric complex and provide resistance to urinary leakage and retrograde ejaculation. A passive prostatic sphincter is located distal to the verumontanum and is related closely to the striated muscle elements of the prostatomembranous sphincter[28]

The voluntary external sphincter mechanism consists of two separate muscular components. One is an intramural prostatomembranous sphincter and the other is the extramural, periurethral striated sphincter. The prostatomembranous striated sphincter may be divided into a prostatic striated sphincter and a membranous urethral sphincter. Fibers of the membranous striated sphincter encircle the urethra and insert broadly over the surface of the prostatic fascia near the apex and play an important role in regaining continence after radical prostatectomy.[29,30]

REFERENCES

1. Steiner MS. The puboprostatic ligament and the male urethral suspensory mechanism, An anatomic study. Urology 1994;44:530–534.

2. Snell RS. Clinical Anatomy, 7th ed. Lippincott, Wiliams and Wilkins, 2004, p. 377.

3. Albers DD, Faulkner KK, Cheathem WN, et al. Surgical anatomy of the pubovesical (puboprostatic) ligaments. J Urol 1973;109:388.

4. Brooks JD, Chao WM, Kerr J. Male pelvic anatomy reconstructed from visible human data set. J Urol 1998;159:868–872.

5. Lowsley OS. The development of the human prostate gland with reference to the development of other structures at the neck of the urinary bladder. Am J Anat 1912;13:299–346.

6. McNeal JE. Regional morphology and pathology of the prostate. Am J of Clin Path 1968;49:347–357.

7. McNeal JE. Anatomy of the prostate: An historical survey of divergent views. Prostate 1980;1:3.

8. McNeal JE. Normal and pathologic anatomy of the prostate. Urology 1981;17(Suppl):11.

9. Blacklock NJ, Bouskill J. The zonal anatomy of the prostate in man and in the rhesus monkey. Urol Res 1977;5:163–167.

10. Babaian R, Mettlin C, Kane R, Murphy GP, Lee F, Drago VR, et al. The relationship of PSA to DRE and TRUS. Cancer 1992;69:1195–1200.

11. Coley CM, Barry MJ, Fleming C, Mulley AG. Early detection of prostate cancer. Part 1. Prior probability and effectiveness of tests. The American College of Physicians. Ann Intern Med 1997;126:394–406.

12. May F, Treumann T, Dettmar P, Hartung R, Breul J. Limited value of endorectal magnetic resonance imaging and transrectal ultrasonography in the staging of clinically localized prostate cancer. BJU Int. 2001 Jan;87(1):66–9.

13. Bates TS, Gillat DA, Cavanagh PM. A comparision of endorectal MRI and TRUS in the local staging of prostate cancer with histopathological correlation. BJU 1997;79(6):927–932.

14. Tobin CE, Benjamin JA. Anatomical and surgical restudy of Denonvillers' fascia. Surg Gynecol Obst 1945;80:373.

15. Hinman F Jr. Atlas of Urosurgical Anatomy. Philadelphia: WB Saunders, 1993

16. Myers RP: Practical pelvic anatomy pertinent to radical retropubic prostatectomy. AUA Update Ser 1994;XIII:26–31.

17. Williams PL, Bannister LH, Berry MM, et al. Gray's Anatomy, 38th ed. London: Churchill-Livingstone, 1995, p.1838.

18. Walsh PC. Radical retropubic prostatectomy. In: Walsh PC, Retik AB, Stamey TA, Vaughan ED Jr (eds): Campbell's Urology, vol 3, 6th ed. Philadelphia: WB Saunders, 1992, pp. .

19. Flocks RH. The arterial distribution within the prostate gland: Its role in transurethral prostatic resection. J Urol 1937;37:524–548.

20. Walsh PC, Donker PJ. Impotence following radical prostatectomy: insight into etiology and prevention. J Urol 1982;128:492–497.

21. Myer RP. Gross and Applied Anatomy of the Prostate. In Kantoff PW, Carroll P, D'Amico A: Prostate Cancer, chapter 1. Philadelphia: Lippincott Williams & Wilkins, 2002, pp 3–15.

22. Reiner WG, Walsh PC. An anatomical approach to the surgical management of the dorsal vein and Santorini's plexus during radical retropubic surgery. J Urol 1979;121:198–200.

23. Romanes GJ. Cunningham's Textbook of Anatomy, 12th ed. Oxford: Oxford University Press, 1981

24. Lepor H, Gregerman M, Crosby R, et al. Precise localization of the autonomic nerves from the pelvic plexus to the corpora cavernosa: A detailed anatomical study of the adult male pelvis. J Urol 1985;133:207.

25. LeDuc IE. The anatomy of the prostate and the pathology of benign hypertrophy. J Urol 1939;42:1217.

26. Walsh PC, Lepor H, Eggleston JC. Radical prostatectomy with preservation of sexual function; anatomical and pathological considerations. Prostate 1983;4:473.

27. Oelrich TM. The urethral sphincter muscle in the male, Am J Anat 1980;158:229–246.

28. Light JK, Rapoll E, Wheeler TM. The striated urethral sphincter: muscle fibre types and distribution in the prostatic capsule. Br J Urol 1997;79:539.

29. Burnett AL, Mostwin JL. In situ anatomical study of the male urethral sphincteric complex: relevance to continence preservation following major pelvic surgery, J Urol 1998;160:1301.

30. Myers RP, Goellner JR, Cahill DR. Prostate shape, external striated urethral sphincter and radical prostatectomy: the apical dissection. J Urol 1987;138:543.

Prostate physiology and function 7

Eugene V Vykhovanets, Susan Ruth Marengo

INTRODUCTION

Sperm experimentally removed from the epididymis can fertilize ova, indicating that the secretions of the accessory sex glands are not essential for fertility. However, under natural conditions fertility has not been optimized through genetics, management, or advanced reproductive technology and the secretions of the accessory sex glands are likely to play a larger role in maximizing the male's fertility. The functions of the secretions of the accessory sex glands include: 1) dilution of the sperm; 2) flushing of urine and bacteria from urethra; 3) provision of buffering and energy sources for the spermatozoa; 4) maintenance of the sperm in a reversibly quiescent state; 5) protection from the female immune system; and 6) if present, the chemical components for formation and dissolution of the seminal clot. This review will focus on the human prostate, but because rats and mice are used as models for investigating prostatic physiology and pathology, these species will be included where appropriate.

COMPARISON OF ANATOMY BETWEEN THE RAT AND HUMAN PROSTATE

The reader is referred to several previously published studies for detailed discussions of the anatomy and histology of the rodent prostate.[1-6] Unlike the human prostate, which is arranged in zones, the rodent prostate is clearly divided into three or four lobes (Figure 7.1). The ventral lobe is the largest and rests on the ventral surface of the bladder. There has been discussion as to whether the dorsal and lateral lobes are actually one pair of lobes or two,[3,5] however,

because of their small size, they are frequently studied as a single unit. The dorsal lobe can be observed by reflection of the bladder, while the lateral lobes curve between the two other lobes. The final lobe is the coagulating gland or anterior prostate, which lies within the curve of the seminal vesicles. It secretes transglutaminase, which crosslinks the seminal vesicle secretions to form the copulatory plug.[7] Because experimental and spontaneous prostatic tumors generally arise in the dorsal/lateral lobes of mice and rats,[8-10] it has been hypothesized that this lobe is analogous to the peripheral zone in the human. However, definitive biochemical and anatomical evidence supporting this hypothesis are not available.

Histologically, the two most obvious differences between the human and rat prostates are the differences in the amount of stroma and neuroendocrine cells (endocrine–paracrine, amine precursor uptake and decarboxylation [APUD]). The rodent prostate has a much higher ratio of epithelium to stroma, and the smooth muscle is largely limited to thin sheaths enveloping the ductules and acini.[4,11] In humans, the smooth muscle infiltrates the entire stroma and accounts for 22% of the gland's area. In both rodents and humans, smooth muscle cells express androgen receptors. The reader is referred to the review by Farnsworth[12] for a detailed discussion of prostatic stromal physiology. Unlike human prostates, the normal rat prostate appears to lack APUD cells.[13]

IMMUNOLOGICAL ASPECTS OF PROSTATE PHYSIOLOGY

Given the high incidence of prostatitis[14] and the potential role of inflammation in prostatic hyperplasia

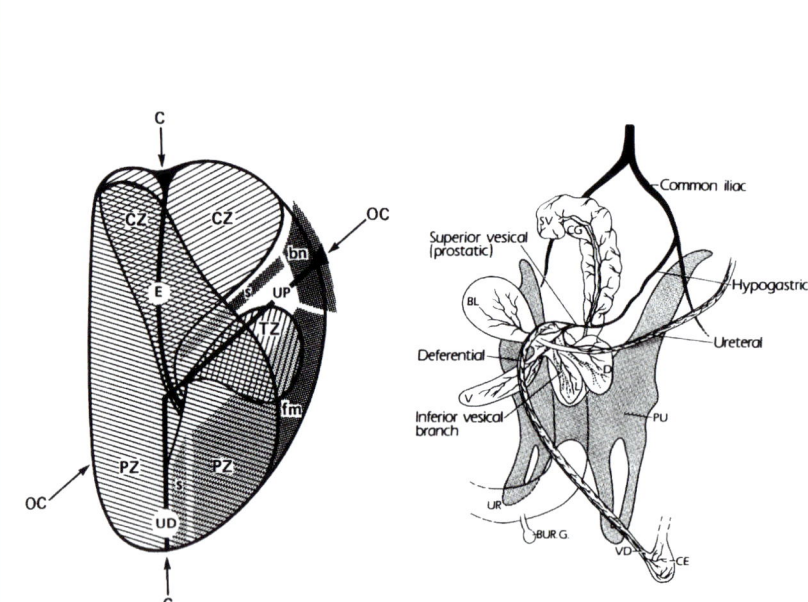

Fig. 7.1

Comparison of the gross anatomy of the human prostate *(left)* and rat prostate *(right)*. (BL, bladder; bn, bladder neck; Bur G, bulbourethral gland; C, Coronal plane; CG, coagulating gland; CZ, central zone; D, distal lobe of the prostate; E, ejaculatory ducts; fm, anterior fibromuscular stroma; L, lateral lobe of the prostate; OC, oblique coronal plane; PU, pubis; PZ, peripheral zone; s, preprostatic and distal striated urethral sphincters; SV, seminal vesicles; TZ, transition zone; UD, distal urethra; UP, proximal urethral segment; UR, urethra; V, ventral lobe of the prostate.)

Adapted from Price H, McNeal JE, Stamey TA. Evolving patterns of tissue composition in benign prostatic hyperplasia as a function of specimen size. Hum Pathol 1990;21:578–585 and Jesik CJ, Holland JM, Lee C. An anatomic and histologic study of the rat prostate. Prostate 1982;3:81–97. Reprinted with permission of John Wiley & Sons, Inc.

and cancer,[15,16] the immunology of the prostate merits some discussion. The prostatic fluid contributes several immunosuppressive components to the ejaculate, which probably serve to protect the sperm from the female's immunosurveillance system (Figure 7.2). Thus, the prostate finds itself in the unusual position of having to protect itself from invading microorganisms ascending the urethra and at the same time producing and storing a variety of immunosuppressive substances.

Using a mechanical isolation procedure and flow cytometry, we characterized the lymphocyte populations in the healthy Sprague-Dawley rat dorsal/lateral prostate.[17] Approximately 90% of the prostatic lymphocytes are found within the dorsal/lateral lobe. Like the human prostate,[18] the proportion of B cells

(CD45RA$^+$) in the rat prostate is very low, and the proportion of T cells ($\alpha\beta$TCR$^+$) is unremarkable (Figure 7.3A). We also determined the proportions of natural killer (NK) cells (CD161a$^+$, $\alpha\beta$TCR$^-$), which are key members of the immunosurveillance system. Natural killer cells kill virally-infected and tumor cells by both antibody-dependent and natural cytotoxic mechanisms. The prostate has high proportions of both NK and NK-T cells (CD161a$^+$, $\alpha\beta$TCR$^+$; Figure 7.3B). Natural killer-T cells are involved in modulating autoimmune diseases, and it has been speculated that some forms of prostatitis are due to autoimmune reactions.[19,20] In rats and mice, injection of prostatic proteins induces prostatitis and the formation of autoantibodies to prostatein and prostatic acid phosphatase.[21,22] Levels of CD161a$^+$ cells

THE PROSTATE'S IMMUNOLOGICAL BALANCING ACT

PROSTATIC SECRETIONS ASSIST IN PROTECTING SPERM & SEMINAL PROTEINS FROM THE FEMALE'S IMMUNOSURVEILLANCE SYSTEM

Prostasomes:
- ↓ Lymphocyte proliferation
- ↓ Complete Phagocytosis
- ↓ Compliment mediated lysis
- ↑ Replenish CD59 on sperm surface

Prostate Binding Protein:
- ↓ Natural killer cell activity
- ↓ T cell cytotoxicity

Prostatic Acid Phosphatase::
- ↓ Natural killer cell and neutrophil activity

THE PROSTATE MUST PROTECT ITSELF FROM PATHOGENS ASCENDING THE URETHRA & PREVENT AUTOIMMUNE REACTIONS AGAINST SECRETORY PROTEINS "LEAKED" BASALATERALLY

Natural Killer Cells: ↑ Innate immunity

CD8+ Cytotoxic T cells: ↑ Acquired immunity

Balanced ratio of autoreactive : regulatory T cells

PGE$_2$:
- ↑ Vasodilation
- ↓ T cell proliferation & activity
- ↑ Th2 responses

TGFβ's
- ↓ T & B cell proliferation & expression of Ig's
- ↓ IFNγ by natural killer cells
- ↓ Acquired immunity
- ↑ Levels of professional & regulatory cells

Fig. 7.2

The prostate's immunological balancing act. Proposed functions of prostatic secretions in protecting the sperm from the female's immunosurveillance system, the gland from autoimmune reactions by the male's immunosurveillance system, and the gland from infection from pathogens ascending the urethra. (IFNγ, interferon-γ; PAP, prostatic acid phosphatase; PBP, prostatic-binding protein; PGE$_2$, prostaglandin E$_2$; PSA, prostate-specific antigen; TGFβ, transforming growth factor-β.)

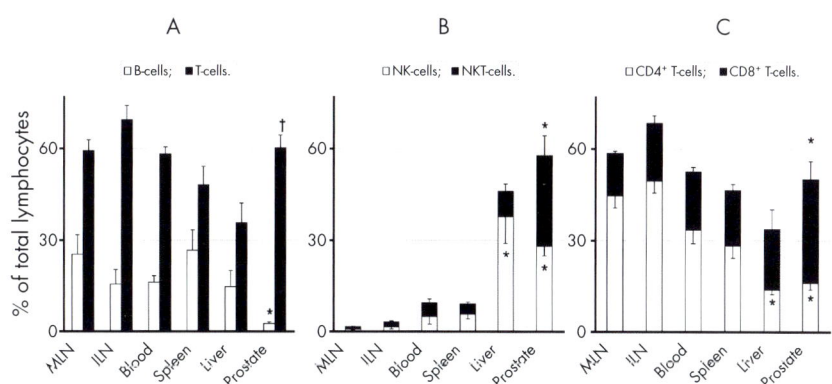

Fig. 7.3
Tissue distribution of the intraprostatic lymphocyte subsets within the total population of lymphocytes. A. Percent distribution of B cells (CD45RA⁺) and T cells (αβTCR⁺). B. Percent distribution of natural killer (NK) cells (CD161a⁺, αβTCR⁻) and NKT-cells (CD161a⁺, αβTCR⁺). White and black bars together present all CD161a-bearing NK-like cells in tissues studied. C. Percent distribution of helper-inducer (CD4⁺, αβTCR⁺) and cytotoxic (CD8⁺, αβTCR⁺) T cells. White and black bars together present all αβTCR⁺ T cells in tissues studied. Cell distributions are expressed as the percentage of total lymphocytes for each tissue (mean ± SD).
*$P < 0.05$ compared with all other tissues; †$P < 0.005$ compared with liver and ILN. Three experiments were performed (n = 6 rats, each prostate was analyzed individually). Antibodies (from BD/Pharmigen; San Diego, CA) and labels for flow cytometry: CD45RA (OX33, Cy-Chrome), αβTCR (R73, PerCP), CD161a (10/78, PE), CD4 (OX35, FITC), CD8a (OX8-biotin, SAv-APC). (MLN: mesenteric lymph nodes. ILN: iliac lymph nodes.)

have not been studied in the human prostate, largely because of the NK marker's sensitivity to enzymatic isolation.[23] Like other tissues that are exposed to the environment, and the human prostate,[24] the rat prostate has a ratio of CD4⁺ cells (helper/inducer cells) to CD8⁺ cells (cytotoxic cells) of less than 1 (Figure 7.3C). The roles these subsets play in protecting the prostate from environmental insults, and how they modulate the development of chronic prostatic inflammation or other prostatic diseases, remains to be determined.

During inflammation, a variety of oxidative molecules, cytokines, and growth factors are released. These molecules can affect both the intended target, e.g. other inflammatory cells, bacteria and infected cells, or bystander targets such as the epithelium and stroma. T-cells can stimulate prostatic stromal cell proliferation with interleukins 2 and 7 (IL2, IL7) and interferon-γ (IFNγ).[25] Theoretically, there is the possibility of paracrine crosstalk between the inflammatory cells and the prostate. Interferon-γ can stimulate the stromal production of IL15,[26] which, in turn, can stimulate inflammatory processes. Interleukin 17 can stimulate production of IL6 and IL8 by the stroma,[27] and these interleukins can then further stimulate inflammation.

The prostate contains constitutively high levels of prostaglandin E₂ (PGE₂) and transforming growth factors-β (TGFβ). Both PGE₂ and TGFβ have several context specific functions, including the capability to suppress or alter immune functions.[28,29] Expression of cyclooxygenase 2, which is the rate limiting enzyme for prostaglandin synthesis, is limited to the smooth muscle and basal epithelial cells in the noncancerous human prostate.[30] Despite its name, it is the seminal vesicles and not the prostate that are the primary source of prostaglandins in men with healthy prostates.[30] The rat prostate does not express cyclooxygenase.[31] In the healthy human prostate, TGFβ acts as a paracrine factor for crosstalk between the stroma (produces most of the TGFβ) and epithelium (TGFβ receptors, a little TGFβ).[32] In the rat ventral lobe, the stroma is the primary source of TGFβ.[33] The role of PGE₂ and TGFβ in the normal prostate is not well defined despite their high concentrations. It has been postulated that they have a role in inhibiting prostatic inflammation.

IONIC COMPOSITION

The composition of human prostatic fluid and that of other mammalian species has been detailed by Amuller[34] and Setchel et al.[35] Little is known about the biochemical composition of rat prostatic fluid. In humans, the prostate contributes about 0.5 to 1 mL to the total ejaculate (2–6 mL, 40–240 million sperm/mL[36,37]). Due to the high concentration of citric acid (≈91 mM), the pH is slightly acidic (6.5). Compared with plasma and interstitial fluid, human prostate secretions contain extremely high levels of divalent cations (including Ca²⁺, Zn²⁺ and Mg²⁺), roughly equivalent amounts of Na⁺, and relatively low amounts of Cl⁻ and HCO₃⁻. Protein averages about 24 mg/mL. The most prevalent sugar is inositol (8.2 mM), and levels of glucose are low (0.9 mM). Virtually no fructose is present in the prostatic fluid.

ZINC AND CITRATE

Normal prostatic epithelial cells contain about 10 times more citrate and 3 to 5 times more zinc than a "typical" mammalian cell.[38,39] Human plasma contains approximately 90 to 110 nmol/g of citrate and 1 μg/g of zinc. In contrast, levels of citrate in the normal prostate are 8 mmol/g (8000 nmol/g) of citrate and 209 μg/g of zinc. In humans, citrate is concentrated in the peripheral zone,[39] while in the rat citrate is concentrated in both the lateral and ventral lobes.[38,40] The zonal distribution of zinc in the human prostate is not well defined. In the rat, concentrations are high in the lateral lobe and very low in the ventral lobes.[38,41]

Most of the zinc in the interstitial fluid, cytoplasm, mitochondria, and prostatic fluid is loosely bound to carriers, and it is the high concentration of these carriers that allow the prostate to concentrate zinc.[38,42] Citrate is the primary carrier; other carriers include aspartate, calcium, cysteine, histidine, and metallothionine. Most of the transfer of zinc between compartments is accomplished by a carrier donating its zinc to a membrane-bound transporter such as Zrt/Irt-like protein 1, which in turn releases free zinc in the next compartment (in this case, the cytosol) where it can again be bound to a carrier.[42,43] Because of its key roles in the tricarboxylic acid (TCA) cycle and fatty acid synthesis, the metabolism of most tissues is designed to conserve citrate. The prostate produces citrate for secretion by short-circuiting the TCA cycle. Zinc binds m-aconitase, and inhibits citrate's oxidation to isocitrate.[44] A citrate-stimulated sodium aspartate pump is used to transport aspartate into the mitochondria, where it can be transaminated to oxaloacetate, a downstream intermediate of the TCA cycle (Figure 7.4).[45,46] Citrate enters the prostatic lumen by several mechanisms including replacement of Cl⁻ as the primary anion for the luminal sodium transporter[45] and an electrogenic citrate–potassium transporter.[47] Citrate secretion is positively regulated by prolactin, which increases m-aspartate aminotransferase activity while decreasing that of m-aconitase.[48] Secretion is negatively regulated by testosterone, which increases m-aconitase activity and citrate oxidation.[46,49] Of interest to this audience is the observation that even early stages of prostate cancer show decreased secretion/increased oxidation of citrate.[39]

Citrate is the primary anion within semen.[50] In addition to its function as a pH buffering agent,[50] it probably acts to buffer the sperm against changes in calcium levels[51] and as a scavenger of free radicals.[52] Zinc is able to bind and inhibit the proteolytic activity of prostate-specific antigen (PSA) and other seminal proteases.[53] It may also act as a bactericide and fungicide.[54] Both free and protein bound zinc can bind to sperm, especially over the acrosome.[55,56] Treating sperm with the diethyldithiocarbamate, a zinc specific chelator that can cross the plasmalemma, inhibits sperm motility, whereas EDTA, which cannot, does not affect motility.[57] Additionally, high levels of zinc in the seminal fluid or on spermatozoa is correlated with lower progressive forward motility.[58]

POLYAMINES

Polyamines play a crucial but, as yet, poorly defined role in progression from the G_1 to the S phase of the cell cycle.[53,59] Ornithine decarboxylase (ODC) catalyzes the rate-limiting step in polyamine synthesis, and its activity in most nonproliferating tissues is low and strictly regulated. However, in humans and rats (but not mice) prostatic levels of both ODC and polyamines are high.[60,61] This is puzzling given that only 0.14% to 1.7% of the cells in the prostate are proliferating at any given time and that organ turnover is estimated to be 1.5 to 2 years.[62-64] The expression of ODC is localized to the luminal epithelium.[65] In humans, spermine accounts for approximately 90% of the total polyamines, with

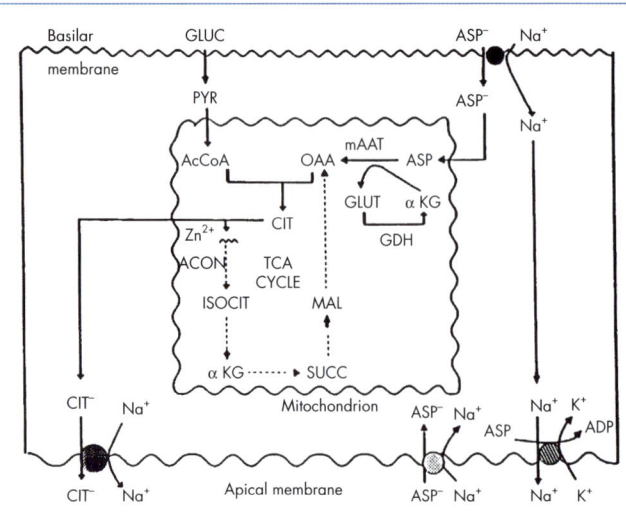

Fig. 7.4
Aspartate transport and citrate production in prostate luminal epithelial cells. The low affinity L-aspartate transporter, Na⁺K⁺ ATPase, and a citrate transporter are represented at the apical membrane. The high affinity L-aspartate transporter and glucose transporters are represented in the basal membrane. (ACON, aconitase; ASP, aspartate; CIT, citrate; GDH, glutamate dehydrogenase; GLUC, glucose; ISOCIT, isocitrate; mAAT, m-aspartate aminotransferase; OAA, oxaloacetate; PYR, pyruvate; SUCC, succinate). Reproduced with permission from Lao L, Franklin RB, Costello LC. High-affinity L-aspartate transporter in prostate epithelial cells that is regulated by testosterone. Prostate 1993;22:53–63.

putrescine, or spermidine accounting for most of the rest.[60,61] In the rat, spermidine is the most abundant polyamine.[66] In contrast to ODC activity in the ventral prostate, ODC activity in the dorsal/lateral lobe of the prostate of pubertal rats or androgen-supplemented castrates parallels that of proliferation and does not decrease with age.[67,68]

The role of polyamines in the seminal fluid is not well understood. Spermine binds to the outer acrosomal membrane and the midpiece.[69] It has a biphasic effect on several events necessary for capacitation and the acrosome reaction (calcium uptake, phospholipase C activity, acrosomal fusion, and acrosomal exocytosis) with millimolar concentrations inhibiting and micromolar concentrations promoting these events. It's been postulated that during ejaculation spermine binds to the spermatozoa at high levels and that this helps to maintain quiescence.[69] As the sperms ascend the female tract, levels of bound spermine decrease until they can promote, or at least not inhibit, capacitation and the acrosome reaction. Polyamines have also been postulated to play roles in seminal clot formation, sperm motility or metabolism, or to act as bactericides.[35,70]

PROSTASOMES

Human prostatic fluid is unique in that it contains an enormous number of 150 to 200 nm vesicles called prostasomes.[71-73] They are covered by a trilaminar membrane that has an unusually high proportion of cholesterol and sphingomyelin and a low proportion of phosphatidylcholine[74] resulting in a highly ordered, very fluid membrane.[75] The vesicular fluid contains very high levels of calcium, plus zinc, selenium, ATP, ADP, GDP, chromogranin B, neuropeptide Y, and vasoactive intestinal polypeptide. Prostasomes also contain a surprising number and variety of proteins.[76] Some of these, such as aminopeptidase and dipeptidyl peptidase IV, are transferred to the sperm.[77,78] Following ejaculation, the low pH of the vagina (pH 5.0), promotes fusion of the prostasomes along the length of the sperm.[72] Through fusion or transfer, the prostasome donates cholesterol, calcium, proteins, and assorted lipids to the sperm.[72,73,75,77,79] These transfers are believed to stabilize the membrane and modulate the acrosome reaction.[72,73] Prostasomes have been reported to stimulate sperm motility,[80,81] increase sperm membrane fluidity,[75] and act as bactericidal agents.[72]

It is likely that prostasomes play a role in the immunoprotection of sperm by proteinaceous and nonproteinaceous mechanisms.[73] Prostasomes contain human cationic antimicrobial protein, which is a component of the innate immune system and could protect the sperm from vaginal microbes or help protect the prostate from microbes ascending the urethra.[19] Prostasomes are able to inhibit phagocytosis of latex beads by macrophages, neutrophils, and monocytes.[73] They also help prevent oxidative damage by binding to polymorphoneutrophils and inhibiting NADPH-oxidase activity, which in turn prevents the release of hydrogen peroxide (H_2O_2).[82] One proposed mechanism for this is the insertion of 16-doxyl-steric acid into polymorphoneutrophil plasmalemmas, which increases their rigidity.[83] Prostasomes carry several glycosylphosphatidylinositol (GPI)-anchored immunomodulatory proteins such as CD59 (membrane attack complex inhibitor), CD55 (decay accelerating factor), and CD46 (membrane cofactor protein), which are able to inhibit complement mediated cell lysis.[84-86] At least one of these, CD59 is transferred to the sperm[86] and may serve to replenish endogenous CD59 lost during storage in the epididymis, ejaculation, or incubation in the vaginal fluids. Prostasomes also contain C3-step and C9-step inhibitors of the complement cascade[85] and are able to inhibit mitogen-stimulated lymphocyte proliferation.[87]

INOSITOL

Human and rat prostatic fluid have high concentrations of myo-inositol.[88-90] The rat prostate can concentrate inositol from the plasma,[88,89] and the ventral lobe can synthesize myo-inositol from glucose.[91] Ejaculated human sperm do not metabolize inositol.[91] In somatic cells, inositol can act as an osmotic agent, and it has been speculated that it may have a similar function in spermatozoa.[92,93]

PROTEINS

The prostatic secretions contain a variety of growth factors, proteases, phosphatases, and binding proteins.[6] In humans, the primary secreted proteins are PSA, prostatic acid phosphatase (PAP) and β-microseminoprotein.[94,95] In the rat, the primary secreted proteins are prostatic-binding protein (PBP; 30–50%[96]) and cystatin-related protein (5–10%[97]). The following discussion will be limited to the major secretory products or those proteins being exploited for diagnostic or experimental use.

KALLIKREINS

The prostatic epithelium secretes two members of the human kallikrein family of serum proteases: PSA (kallikrein 3) and kallikrein 2.[95,98-100] Both PSA and kallikrein 2 are 33 kDa single-chain glycoproteins. Prostate-specific antigen has chymotrypsin-like activity whereas kallikrein 2 has trypsin-like activity. Levels of kallikrein 2 are only about 1% of those of PSA, and, like PSA, it is expressed in several tissues and by both sexes. In the normal prostate, the majority of PSA is secreted apically, and serum levels of PSA are negligible. As cancerous cells dedifferentiate, a higher proportion of PSA is secreted basally into the blood stream, thus making it available for diagnostic and follow-up purposes. An analogous protein has not been found in the rat prostate.

Prostate-specific antigen is initially secreted as a zymogen that is activated by kallikrein 2.[101] In situ, PSA's activity is inhibited by complex formation with protein C inhibitor and zinc.[53,102,103] In humans, ejaculated sperm are coated with semenogelen from the seminal vesicles, which immobilizes the sperm and causes coagulation of the ejaculate. Within 5 to 20 minutes, PSA enzymatically dissolves the clot, freeing the sperm so that they can enter the cervical crypts and begin their ascent up the female reproductive tract (Figure 7.5).[102–104] Prostate-specific antigen also activates seminal α2-macroglobulin, a nonspecific protease inhibitor, which then is able to bind to sperm.[105] Even in the healthy prostate, a little PSA and kallikrein 2 are secreted basally. Both have been shown to cleave several insulin-like growth factor binding proteins (IGFBPs).[106] Cleaved IGFBPs are unable to bind IGF1, which is then able to bind to its receptors and stimulate proliferation of the prostatic epithelium and stroma.[107,108] Prostate-specific antigen is also able to cleave and activate latent TGFβ₂[109] growth factor, which potentially has far-reaching effects on the vascular, epithelial, and stromal compartments.[110,111]

PROSTATIC ACID PHOSPHATASE

The structure and properties of PAP in the human prostate have been reviewed by Moss et al,[112] and Chu et al.[113] Prostatic acid phosphatase is a member of the nonspecific orthophosphate monoesterase family and has maximal activity at a pH similar to that of the vagina. Being a general phosphatase it dephosphorylates serine, threonine, and tyrosine.[114] It is also able to inhibit neutrophil and NK cell activity, so it may also have immunoprotective functions.[115] Following the identification of PAP (isoform 2a) in the serum of patient's with PCa,[116] PAP was utilized for the detection of disseminated prostatic carcinoma (capsular extravasation, or metastasis) using enzymatic and, later, immunologic assays. However, due to methodological difficulties and the failure of PAP to be detectable in the serum until after dissemination of the disease, PAP has largely been replaced by PSA.[112] The epithelium of the ventral prostate of the rat also produces an acid phosphatase that has approximately 75% identity to the human protein, but is not inhibited by tartrate.[112,117,118]

PSP94/β-INHIBIN/β-MICROSEMINOPROTEIN

The protein known as β-inhibin, β-microseminoprotein, or PSP94 is a nonglycoslyated heterodimer consisting of α- and β-subunits of approximately 18 kDa and is related to the TGFβ/immunoglobulin-binding superfamily.[119,120] It is expressed by the epithelia of both rat and human prostates.[94,121] It is usually thought of as a hormone because it is secreted by the ovaries and testis to inhibit the secretion of follicle-stimulating hormone (FSH).[120] Beta-inhibin is readily detected in the linings of the reproductive, respiratory, gastrointestinal, and urinary tracts, especially in the mucosal cells.[122] It may play a role in modulating the mucus characteristics of the tract. It is also present in human seminal fluid and binds to ejaculated sperm.[123]

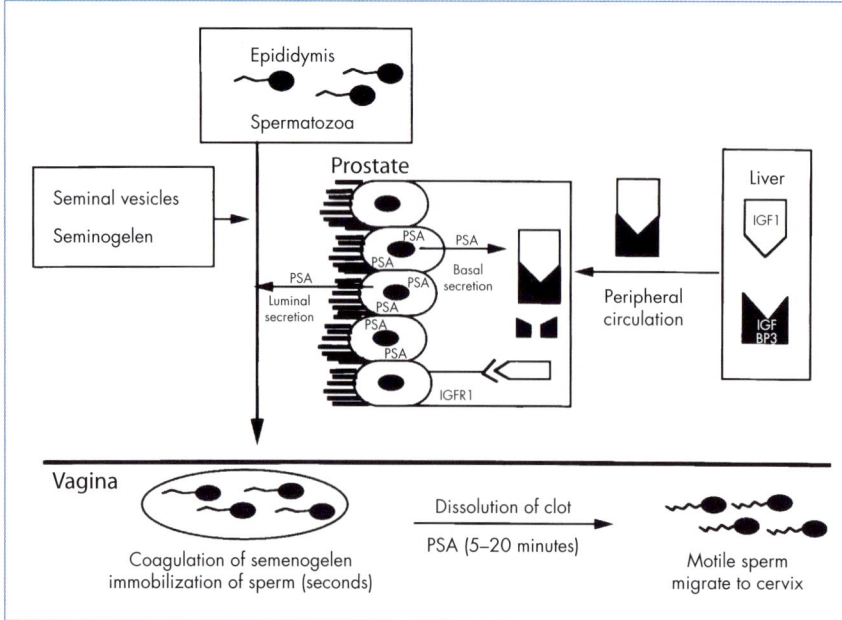

Fig. 7.5

Proposed functions of prostate-specific antigen (PSA). IGF1, insulin-like growth factor 1; IGFBP3, insulin-like growth factor binding protein 3; IGFR1, insulin-like growth factor receptor 1. Adapted from Malm J, Lilja H. Biochemistry of prostate specific antigen, PSA. Scand J Clin Lab Invest Suppl 1995;221:15–22. Reproduced with permission from Marengo SR. Prostate physiology and regulation. In Resnick MI, Thompson IM (eds): Advanced therapy of prostate disease. Hamilton: BC Decker Inc, 2000, pp 92–117.

PROSTATIC-BINDING PROTEIN AND PROBASIN

Prostatic-binding protein, also known as prostatein and estramustine-binding protein, is a member of the uteroglobin superfamily of proteins and is a serine protease.[124–126] Structurally, it is a tetramer composed of two dimers: C1-C3 and C1-C2.[127] The C2 peptide contains the steroid-binding capabilities. In the rat, PBP is the major secretory protein of the prostate, accounting for approximately 20% of the secreted protein, and its expression is limited to the ventral lobe of the prostate.[126,128] In contrast, in humans, PBP is a minor prostatic secretory product and is expressed in a variety of organs including the liver, and colon.[129,130] Its function has not been intensely investigated although it is assumed to regulate the availability, metabolism, or uptake of steroids. Additionally, PBP has been shown to have substantial immunosuppressive capabilities as it is able to inhibit mitogen-induced proliferation of mononuclear lymphocytes, the human mixed lymphocyte reaction, and the production of IL2 and its receptors.[131] Experimentally, PBP has been used as a differentiation marker[128,132] and as a tool for studying the androgen receptor promoter.[133]

Probasin is a 20 kDa, single chain, highly basic (pI ≈11.5) nonhistone protein found in the prostatic secretions, prostatic epithelial granules, and nuclei.[112,134] The differential localization within the cell appears to be due to multiple transcripts.[135] The primary site of expression is the dorsal/lateral prostate, although small amounts are also expressed in the ventral prostate.[136,137] Based on sequence identity, probasin is a member of the ligand-binding family,[135] which includes such members as retinol binding protein, and α2-macroglobulin. In research, it has been exploited as a marker of androgen-dependent differentiation of the dorsal/lateral prostate,[132,138] elucidation of androgen regulation of gene expression,[139–141] and determining how environmental toxins can activate androgen-regulated genes.[142] Probasin's promoter has been utilized to target androgen-dependent gene expression to the prostate in transgenic mice[143,144] and to drive the targeted expression of apoptotic agents such as Bax.[145]

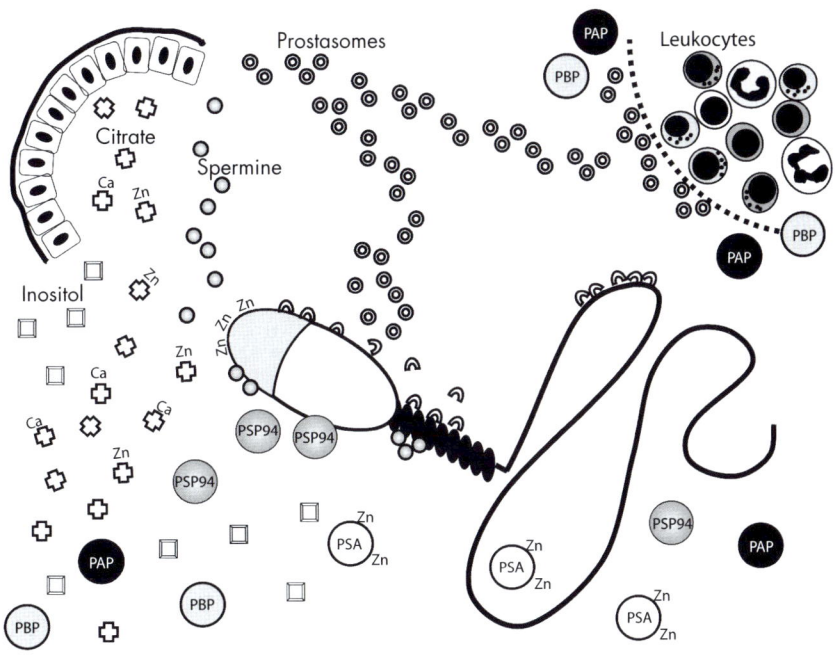

Fig. 7.6

Proposed functions of the prostatic secretions to the seminal fluid. Citrate *(crosses)* buffers against changes in pH and calcium concentrations; citrate also chelates zinc. Zinc inhibits the proteolytic activity of PSA; zinc also binds to sperm and may inhibit premature motility. Spermine *(small gray spheres)* binds to acrosomal membrane and the midpiece; high concentrations promote sperm quiescence while low concentrations foster capacitation and the acrosome reaction. Inositol *(squares)* is an osmotic agent. Prostasomes *(double circles)* fuse to the sperm and transfer calcium, cholesterol, enzymes, and immunoprotective proteins to the sperm; prostasomes also directly inhibit leukocyte activity and the complement cascade providing another layer of immunoprotection in the female tract. Prostate specific antigen (PSA) liberates the sperm from the seminogelen clot. Prostatic acid phosphatase (PAP) inhibits neutrophil and natural killer cell activity. Prostatic binding protein/prostatein/ estramustine binding protein (PBP) inhibits leukocyte activity. PSP94/β-inhibin /β-microseminoprotein (PSP94) binds to sperm and regulates mucus characteristics.

CONCLUSIONS

As can be deduced from this review, relatively little is known about normal prostatic function (summarized in Figure 7.6) or the mechanisms regulating the gland's function and growth (see other chapters, this volume). In addition to having a fairly obscure function, the prostate is extremely unusual in that it is the only organ in the human body in which aberrant proliferation or inflammation is guaranteed to develop if one lives long enough. Additionally, the near-universal development of some form of prostatic pathology in senior males is limited to humans. Unlike the skin and colon, the prostate is relatively protected from environmental assault and has a very low rate of turnover. Is there a basic regulatory mechanism in the prostatic housekeeping machinery that that goes awry as men age? What are the physiologic differences between the transitional zone and peripheral zone that cause one zone to be highly predisposed to benign disease while the other demonstrates almost no benign disease but develops cancer instead? If truly effective preventative or curative therapies are to be developed, it is essential that future research be directed towards understanding the prostate's basic physiology, development, and regulatory pathways.

REFERENCES

1. Brandes D. The fine structure and histochemistry of prostatic glands in the relation to sex hormones. Int Rev Cytol 1966;20:207–276.
2. Price D. Comparative aspects of development and structure in the prostate. In Vollmer EP (ed.): Biology of the Prostate and Related Tissues. Bethesda, Md: U.S. Department of Health, Education, and Welfare, 1963, p 1–27.
3. Jesik CJ, Holland JM, Lee C. An anatomic and histologic study of the rat prostate. Prostate 1982;3:81–97.
4. Flickinger CJ. The fine structure of the interstitial tissue of the rat prostate. Am J Anat 1972;134:107–126.
5. Gunn SA, Gould TC. A correlative anatomical and functional study of the dorsolateral prostate of the rat. Anat Rec 1957;128:41–53.
6. Marengo SR. Prostate physiology and regulation. In Resnick MI, Thompson IM (eds): Advanced Therapy of Prostate Disease. Hamilton: BC: Decker Inc, 2000, pp 92–117.
7. Lin HJ, Luo CW, Chen YH. Localization of the transglutaminase cross-linking site in SVS III, a novel glycoprotein secreted from mouse seminal vesicle. J Biol Chem 2002;277:3632–3639.
8. Greenberg NM, DeMayo F, Finegold MJ, et al. Prostate cancer in a transgenic mouse. Proc Natl Acad Sci USA 1995;92:3439–3443.
9. Leav I, Ho S-M, Ofner P, et al. Biochemical alterations in sex hormone-induced hyperplasia and dyplasia of the dorsolateral prostates of Noble rats. J Natl Cancer Inst 1988;80:1045–1053.
10. Pollard M. The Lobund-Wistar rat model of prostate cancer. J Cell Biochem Suppl 1992;16H:84–88.
11. Cunha GR, Hayward SW, Dahiya R, et al. Smooth muscle-epithelial interactions in normal and neoplastic development. Acta Anat 1996;155:63–72.
12. Farnsworth WE. Prostate stroma: physiology. Prostate 1999;38:60–72.
13. Angelsen A, Mecsei R, Sandvik AK, et al. Neuroendocrine cells in the prostate of the rat, guinea pig, cat and dog. Prostate 1997;33:18–25.
14. Roberts RO, Lieber MM, Bostwick DG, et al. A review of clinical and pathological prostatitis syndromes. Urology 1997;49:809–821.
15. Platz EA, De Marzo AM. Epidemiology of inflammation and prostate cancer. J Urol 2004;171:S36–40.
16. Gerstenbluth RE, Seftel AD, MacLennan GT, et al. Distribution of chronic prostatitis in radical prostatectomy specimens with up-regulation of bcl-2 in areas of inflammation. J Urol 2002;167:2267–2270.
17. Vykhovanets EV, Resnick MI, Marengo SR. The healthy rat prostate contains high levels of natural killer like cells and unique subsets of CD4+ helper-inducer T-cells: Implications for chronic prostatic inflammation. J Urol 2005;173:1004–1010.
18. Bostwick DG, de la Roza G, Dundore P, et al. Intraepithelial and stromal lymphocytes in the normal human prostate. Prostate 2003;55:187–193.
19. Andersson E, Sorensen OE, Frohm B, et al. Isolation of human cationic antimicrobial protein-18 from seminal plasma and its association with prostasomes. Hum Reprod 2002;17:2529–2534.
20. Alexander RB, Brady F, Ponniah S. Autoimmune prostatitis: evidence of T cell reactivity with normal prostatic proteins. Urology 1997;50:893–899.
21. Rivero V, Carnaud C, Riera CM. Prostatein or steroid binding protein (PSBP) induces experimental autoimmune prostatitis (EAP) in NOD mice. Clin Immunol 2002;105:176–184.
22. McNeel DG, Nguyen LD, Disis ML. Identification of T helper epitopes from prostatic acid phosphatase. Cancer Res 2001;61:5161–5167.
23. Curry MP, Norris S, Golden-Mason L, et al. Isolation of lymphocytes from normal adult human liver suitable for phenotypic and functional characterization. J Immunol Methods 2000;242:21–31.
24. Steiner GE, Newman ME, Paikl D, et al. Expression and function of pro-inflammatory interleukin IL-17 and IL-17 receptor in normal, benign hyperplastic, and malignant prostate. Prostate 2003;56:171–182.
25. Kramer G, Steiner GE, Handisurya A, et al. Increased expression of lymphocyte-derived cytokines in benign hyperplastic prostate tissue, identification of the producing cell types, and effect of differentially expressed cytokines on stromal cell proliferation. Prostate 2002;52:43–58.
26. Handisurya A, Steiner GE, Stix U, et al. Differential expression of interleukin-15, a pro-inflammatory cytokine and T-cell growth factor, and its receptor in human prostate. Prostate 2001;49:251–262.
27. Schroder FH. Endocrine treatment of prostate cancer. In Walsh PC, Retik AB, Vaughan ED Jr, Wein AJ (eds): Campbell's Urology. Philadelphia: WB Saunders, 1998, pp 2627–2644.
28. Letterio JJ, Roberts AB. Regulation of immune responses by TGF-beta. Annu Rev Immunol 1998;16:137–161.
29. Tilley SL, Coffman TM, Koller BH. Mixed messages: modulation of inflammation and immune responses by prostaglandins and thromboxanes. J Clin Invest 2001;108:15–23.
30. Kirschenbaum A, Klausner AP, Lee R, et al. Expression of cyclooxygenase-1 and cyclooxygenase-2 in the human prostate. Urology 2000;56:671–676.
31. McKanna JA, Zhang MZ, Wang JL, et al. Constitutive expression of cyclooxygenase-2 in rat vas deferens. Am J Physiol 1998;275:227–233.
32. Lee C, Sintich SM, Mathews EP, et al. Transforming growth factor-beta in benign and malignant prostate. Prostate 1999;39:285–290.
33. Nemeth JA, Sensibar JA, White RR, et al. Prostatic ductal system in rats: tissue-specific expression and regional variation in stromal distribution of transforming growth factor-beta 1. Prostate 1997;33:64–71.
34. Aumuller G. Morphologic and regulatory aspects of prostatic function. Anat Embryol 1989;179:519–531.
35. Setchell BP, Maddocks S, Brooks DE. Anatomy, vasculature, innervation, and fluids of the male reproductive tract. In Knobil E, Neill JD (eds): The Physiology of Reproduction, 2nd ed. New York: Raven Press, 1994, pp 1063–1175.
36. Sigman M, Howards SS. Male infertility. In Walsh PC, Retik AB, Vaughan ED, Wein AJ (eds): Campbell's Urology. 7th ed. Philadelphia: WB Saunders, 1998, pp 1287–1330.
37. Harper MJK. Gamete and zygote transport. In Knobil E, Neill JD (eds): The Physiology of Reproduction. New York: Raven Press, 1994, pp 123–187.
38. Costello LC, Franklin RB. Novel role of zinc in the regulation of prostate citrate metabolism and its implications in prostate cancer. Prostate 1998;35:285–296.

39. Costello LC, Franklin RB. The intermediary metabolism of the prostate: a key to understanding the pathogenesis and progression of prostate malignancy. Oncology 2000;59:269–282.

40. Lowry M, Liney GP, Turnbull LW, et al. Quantification of citrate concentration in the prostate by proton magnetic resonance spectroscopy: zonal and age related differences. Magn Reson Med 1996;36:352–358.

41. Sorensen MB, Stoltenberg M, Juhl S, et al. Ultrastructure localization of zinc ions in the rat prostate: an autometallographic study. Prostate 1997;31:125–130.

42. Guan Z, Kukoyi B, Feng P, et al. Kinetic identification of a mitochondrial zinc uptake transport process in prostate cells. J Inorg Biochem 2003;97:199–206.

43. Franklin RB, Ma J, Zou J, et al. Human ZIP1 is a major zinc uptake transporter for the accumulation of zinc in prostate cells. J Inorg Biochem 2003;96:435–442.

44. Costello LC, Liu Y, Franklin RB, et al. Zinc inhibition of mitochondrial aconitase and its importance in citrate metabolism of prostate epithelial cells. J Biol Chem 1997;272:28875–28881.

45. Costello LC, Lao L, Franklin R. Citrate modulation of high-affinity aspartate transport in prostate epithelial cells. Cell Mol Biol 1993;39:515–524.

46. Lao L, Franklin RB, Costello LC. High-affinity L-aspartate transporter in prostate epithelial cells that is regulated by testosterone. Prostate 1993;22:53–63.

47. Mycielska ME, Djamgoz MB. Citrate transport in the human prostate epithelial PNT2-C2 cell line: electrophysiological analyses. J Physiol 2004;559:821–833.

48. Liu Y, Costello LC, Franklin RB. Prolactin specifically regulates citrate oxidation and m-aconitase of rat prostate epithelial cells. Metabolism 1996;45:442–449.

49. Costello LC, Liu Y, Franklin RB. Testosterone stimulates the biosynthesis of m-aconitase and citrate oxidation in prostate epithelial cells. Mol Cell Endocrinol 1995;112:45–51.

50. Kavanagh JP. Sodium, potassium, calcium, magnesium, zinc, citrate and chloride content of human prostatic and seminal fluid. J Reprod Fertil 1985;75:35–41.

51. Magnus O, Abyholm T, Kofstad J, et al. Ionized calcium in human male and female reproductive fluids: relationships to sperm motility. Hum Reprod 1990;5:94–98.

52. Gavella M, Lipovac V, Vucic M, et al. Evaluation of ascorbate and urate antioxidant capacity in human semen. Andrologia 1997;29:29–35.

53. Janne J, Alhonen L, Pietila M, et al. Genetic approaches to the cellular functions of polyamines in mammals. Eur J Biochem 2004;271:877–894.

54. Mardh PA, Colleen S. Antimicrobial activity of human seminal fluid. Scand J Urol Nephrol 1975;9:17–23.

55. Stoltenberg M, Sorensen MB, Danscher G, et al. Autometallographic demonstration of zinc ions in rat sperm cells. Mol Hum Reprod 1997;3:763–767.

56. Sansone G, Martino M, Abrescia P. Binding of free and protein-associated zinc to rat spermatozoa. Comp Biochem Physiol 1991;99C:113–117.

57. Sorensen MB, Stoltenberg M, Danscher G, et al. Chelation of intracellular zinc ions affects human sperm cell motility. Mol Hum Reprod 1999;5:338–341.

58. Sorensen MB, Bergdahl IA, Hjollund NH, et al. Zinc, magnesium and calcium in human seminal fluid: relations to other semen parameters and fertility. Mol Hum Reprod 1999;5:331–337.

59. Pegg AE, Shantz LM, Coleman CS. Ornithine decarboxylase: structure, function, and translational regulation. Biochem Soc Trans 1994;22:846–852.

60. Russell DH. Polyamines and prostatic function. In: The Prostatic Cell: Structure and Function. New York: Alan R Liss, 1981, pp 207–224.

61. Sheth AR, Moodbidri SB. Significance of polyamines in reproduction. Adv. Sex Horm Res 1977;3:51–74.

62. Kyprianou N, Huacheng TU, Jacobs SC. Apoptotic versus proliferation activities in human benign prostatic hyperplasia. Hum Pathol 1996;27:668–675.

63. Neomoto R, Kawamura H, Miyakawa I, et al. Immunohistochemical detection of proliferating cell antigen PCNA/cyclin in human prostate adenocarcinoma. J Urol 1993;149:165–169.

64. Berges RR, Vukanovic J, Epstein JI, et al. Implication of cell kinetic changes during the progression of human prostatic cancer. Clin Cancer Res 1995;1:473–480.

65. Blackshear PJ, Manzella JM, Stumpo DJ, et al. High level, cell-specific expression of ornithine decarboxylase transcripts in rat genitourinary tissues. Mol Endo 1989;3:68–78.

66. Shain SA, Moss AL. Aging in the AXC rat: differential effects of chronic testosterone treatment on restoration of diminished prostate L-ornithine decarboxylase and S-adenosyl-L-methionine decarboxylase activities. Endocrinology 1981;109:1184–1191.

67. Robertson FM, Gilmour SK, Beavis AJ, et al. Flow cytometric detection of ornithine decarboxylase activity in epidermal cell subpopulations. Cytometry 1990;11:832–836.

68. Schultz JJ, Shain SA. Effect of aging on AXC/SSh rat ventral and dorsolateral prostate S-adenosyl-L-methionine decarboxylase and L-ornithine decarboxylase messenger ribonucleic acid content. Endocrinology 1988;122:120–126.

69. Breitbart H, Rubinstein S, Lax Y. Regulatory mechanisms in acrosomal exocytosis. Rev Reprod 1997;2:165–174.

70. Schipper RG, Romijn JC, Cuijpers VM, et al. Polyamines and prostatic cancer. Biochem Soc Trans 2003;31:375–380.

71. Ronquist G, Brody I. The prostasome: its secretion and function in man. Biochem Biophys Acta 1985;822:203–218.

72. Arienti G, Carlini E, Saccardi C, et al. Role of human prostasomes in the activation of spermatozoa. J Cell Mol Med 2004;8:77–84.

73. Kravets FG, Lee J, Singh B, et al. Prostasomes: current concepts. Prostate 2000;43:169–174.

74. Arvidson G, Ronquist G, Wikander G, et al. Human prostasomes membranes exhibit very high cholesterol/phospholipid ratios yielding high molecular ordering. Biochem Biophys Acta 1989;984:167–173.

75. Carlini E, Palmerini CA, Cosmi VC, et al. Fusion of sperm with prostasomes: effects on membrane fluidity. Arch Biochem Biophys 1997;343:6–12.

76. Utleg AG, Yi EC, Xie T, et al. Proteomic analysis of human prostasomes. Prostate 2003;56:150–161.

77. Arienti G, Polci A, Carlini E, et al. Transfer of CD26/dipeptidylpeptidase IV (E.C. 3.5.4.4) from prostasomes to sperm. FEBS Letts 1997;410:343–346.

78. Arienti G, Carlini E, Verdacchi R, et al. Prostasome to sperm transfer of CD13/aminopeptidase N (EC 3.4.11.2). Biochim Biophys Acta 1997;1336:533–538.

79. Arienti G, Carlini E, Verdacchi R, et al. Transfer of aminopeptidase activity from prostasomes to sperm. Biochem Biophys Acta 1997;1336:269–274.

80. Fabiani R, Johansson L, Lundkvist O, et al. Prolongation and improvement of prostasome promotive effect on sperm forward motility. Eur J Obstet Gynecol Reprod Biol 1995;58:191–198.

81. Fabiani R, Johansson L, Lundvist O, et al. Promotive effect by prostasomes on normal human spermatozoa exhibiting no forward motility due to buffer washings. Eur J Obstet Gynecol Reprod Biol 1994;57:181–188.

82. Saez F, Motta C, Boucher D, et al. Prostasomes inhibit the NADPH oxidase activity of human neutrophils. Mol Hum Reprod 2000;6:883–891.

83. Saez F, Motta C, Boucher D, et al. Antioxidant capacity of prostasomes in human semen. Mol Hum Reprod 1998;4:667–672.

84. Rooney IA, Heuser JE, Atkinson JP. GPI-anchored complement regulatory proteins in seminal plasma. An analysis of their physical condition and the mechanisms of their binding to exogenous cells. J Clin Invest 1996;97:1675–1686.

85. Kitamura M, Namiki M, Matsumiya K, et al. Membrane cofactor protein (CD46) in seminal plasma is a prostasome-bound form with complement regulatory activity and measles virus neutralizing activity. Immunology 1995;84:626–632.

86. Rooney IA, Atkinson JP, Krul ES, et al. Physiologic relevance of the membrane attack complex inhibitory protein CD59 in human seminal plasma: CD59 is present on extracellular organelles

(prostasomes), binds cell membranes, and inhibits complement-mediated lysis. J Exp Med 1993;177:1409–1420.

87. Kelly RW, Holland P, Skibinski G, et al. Extracellular organelles (prostasomes) are immunosuppressive components of human semen. Clin Exp Immunol 1991;86:550–556.

88. Lewin LM, Sulimovici S. The distribution of radioactive myoinositol in the reproductive tract of the male rat. J Reprod Fert 1975;43:355–358.

89. Lewin LM, Yannai Y, Sulimovici S, et al. Studies on the metabolic role of myo-inositol: distribution of radioactive myo-inositol in the male rat. Biochem J 1976;156:375–380.

90. Lewin LM, Beer R. Prostatic secretion as the source of myo-inositol in human seminal fluid. Fertil Steril 1973;24:666–670.

91. Brown-Woodman PD, Marley PB, Morris S, et al. Origin of glycerylphosphorylcholine, inositol, N-acetylaminosugar, and prostaglandins in human seminal plasma and their effects on sperm metabolism. Arch Androl 1980;4:149–155.

92. Lang F, Busch GL, Ritter M, et al. Functional significance of cell volume regulatory mechanisms. Physiol Rev 1998;78:247–306.

93. Yeung CH, Anapolski M, Depenbusch M, et al. Human sperm volume regulation. Response to physiological changes in osmolality, channel blockers and potential sperm osmolytes. Hum Reprod 2003;18:1029–1036.

94. Abrahamsson PA, Lilja H. Three predominant prostatic proteins. Andrologia 1990;22:122–131.

95. Balk SP, Ko YJ, Bubley GJ. Biology of prostate-specific antigen. J Clin Oncol 2003;21:383–391.

96. Heyns W, De Moor P. Prostatic binding protein: a steroid-binding protein secreted by the rat prostate. J Steroid Biochem 1977;7:987–991.

97. Winderickx J, Hemschoote K, De Clercq N, et al. Tissue-specific expression and androgen regulation of different genes encoding rat prostatic 22-kilodalton glycoproteins homologous to human rat cystatin. Mol Endocrinol 1990;4:657–667.

98. Clements JA. The human kallikrein gene family: a diversity of expression and function. Mol Cell Endocrinol 1994;99:C1–C6.

99. Rittenhouse HG, Finlay JA, Mikolajczyk SD, et al. Human kallikrein 2 (hK2) and prostate-specific antigen (PSA): two closely related, but distinct, kallikreins in the prostate. Crit Rev Clin Lab Sci 1998;35:275–368.

100. Diamandis EP, Yousef GM. Human tissue kallikreins: a family of new cancer biomarkers. Clin Chem 2002;48:1198–1205.

101. Takayama TK, Fujikawa K, Davie EW. Characterization of the precursor of prostate-specific antigen. J Biol Chem 1997;272:21582–21588.

102. Kise H, Nishioka J, Kawamura J, et al. Characterization of semenogelin II and its molecular interaction with prostate-specific antigen and protein C inhibitor. Eur J Biochem 1996;238:88–96.

103. Robert M, Gibbs BF, Jacobson E, et al. Characterization of prostate-specific antigen proteolytic activity on its major physiological substrate, the sperm motility inhibitor precursor/semenogelin I. Biochemistry 1997;36:3811–3819.

104. Malm J, Lilja H. Biochemistry of prostate specific antigen, PSA. Scand J Clin Lab Invest Suppl 1995;221:15–22.

105. Birkenmeier G, Usbeck E, Schafer A, et al. Prostate-specific antigen triggers transformation of seminal alpha-2-macroglobulin (alpha-2-M) and its binding to alpha-2-macroglobulin receptor/low-density lipoprotein receptor-related protein (alpha-2-M-R/LRP) on human spermatozoa. Prostate 1998;36:219–225.

106. Rehault S, Monget P, Mazerbourg S, et al. Insulin-like growth factor binding proteins (IGFBPs) as potential physiological substrates for human kallikreins hK2 and hK3. Eur J Biochem 2001;268:2960–2968.

107. Djavan B, Waldert M, Seitz C, et al. Insulin-like growth factors and prostate cancer. World J Urol 2001;19:225–233.

108. Grimberg A, Cohen P. Role of insulin-like growth factors and their binding proteins in growth control and carcinogenesis. J Cell Physiol 2000;183:1–9.

109. Dallas SL, Zhao S, Cramer SD, et al. Preferential production of latent transforming growth factor beta-2 by primary prostatic epithelial cells and its activation by prostate-specific antigen. J Cell Physiol 2004:[Epub ahead of print].

110. Huang X, Lee C. Regulation of stromal proliferation, growth arrest, differentiation and apoptosis in benign prostatic hyperplasia by TGF-beta. Front Biosci 2003;8:740–749.

111. Wong YC, Wang YZ. Growth factors and epithelial-stromal interactions in prostate cancer development. Int Rev Cytol 2000;199:65–116.

112. Moss DW, Raymond FD, Wile DB. Clinical and biological aspects of acid phosphatase. Crit Rev Clin Lab Sci 1995;32:431–467.

113. Chu TM, Wang MC, Lee C-L, et al. Prostatic acid phosphate in human prostate cancer. In: Chu TM (ed): Biochemical Markers for Cancer. New York: Marcel Dekker, 1982, pp 117–136.

114. Lee H, Chu TM, Lee CL. Endogenous protein substrates for prostatic acid phosphatase in human prostate. Prostate 1991;19:251–263.

115. Mukhopadhyay NK, Saha AK, Smith W, et al. Inhibition of neutrophil and natural killer cell function by human seminal fluid acid phosphatase. Clin Chim Acta 1989;182:31–40.

116. Gutman AB, Gutman EB. An acid phosphatase occurring in the serum of patients with metastasizing carcinoma of the prostate gland. J Clin Invest 1938;17:473–478.

117. Terracio L, Rule A, Salvato J, et al. Immunofluorescent localization of an androgen-dependent isoenzyme of prostatic acid phosphatase in rat ventral prostate. Anat Rec 1985;213:131–139.

118. Roiko K, Janne OA, Vihko P. Primary structure of rat secretory acid phosphatase and comparison to other acid phosphatases. Onocogene 1990;89:223–229.

119. Liang ZG, Kamada M, Koide SS. Structural identity of immunoglobulin binding factor and prostatic secretory protein of human seminal plasma. Biochem Biophys Res Commun 1991;180:356–359.

120. Vale W, Bilezikjian LM, Rivier C. Reproductive and other roles of inhibins and activins. In Knobil E, Neill JD (eds): The Physiology of Reproduction, 2nd ed. New York: Raven Press, 1994, pp 1861–1878.

121. Risbridger GP, Thomas T, Gurusinghe CJ, et al. Inhibin-related proteins in rat prostate. J Endocrinol 1996;149:93–99.

122. Weiber H, Andersson C, Murne A, et al. Beta microseminoprotein is not a prostate-specific protein. Its identification in mucous glands and secretions. Am J Pathol 1990;137:593–603.

123. Ito Y, Tsuda R, Kimura H. Ultrastructural localizations of beta-microseminoprotein, a prostate-specific antigen, in human prostate and sperm: comparison with gamma-seminoprotein, another prostate-specific antigen. J Lab Clin Med 1989;114:272–277.

124. Baker ME. Amino acid sequence homology between rat prostatic steroid binding protein and rabbit uteroglobin. Biochem Biophys Res Commun 1983;114:325–330.

125. Yu JX, Chao L, Chao J. Prostasin is a novel human serine proteinase from seminal fluid. J Biol Chem 1994;269:18843–18848.

126. Forsgren B, Bjork P, Carlstrom K, et al. Purification and distribution of a major protein in rat prostate that binds estramustine, a nitrogen mustard derivative of estradiol-17 beta. Proc Natl Acad Sci USA 1979;76:3149–3153.

127. Parker MG, White R, Hurst H, et al. Prostatic steroid-binding protein. J Biol Chem 1983;258:12–15.

128. Takeda H, Suematsu N, Mizuno T. Transcription of prostatic steroid binding protein (PSBP) gene is induced by epithelial-mesenchymal interaction. Development 1990;110:273–281.

129. Bjork P, Forsgren B, Gustafsson JA, et al. Partial characterization and "quantification" of human prostatic estramustine-binding protein. Cancer Res 1982;42:1935–1942.

130. Yu JX, Chao L, Chao J. Molecular cloning, tissue-specific expression, and cellular localization of human prostasin mRNA. J Biol Chem 1995;270:13483–13489.

131. Maccioni M, Riera CM, Rivero V. Identification of rat prostatic steroid binding protein (PSBP) as an immunosuppressive factor. J Reprod Immunol 2001;50:133–49.

132. Prins GS, Woodham C, Lepinske M, et al. Effects of neonatal estrogen exposure on prostatic secretory genes and their correlation with androgen receptor expression in the separate prostate lobes of the adult rat. Endocrinology 1993;132:2387–2398.

133. Claessens F, Rushmere NK, Davies P, et al. Sequence-specific binding of androgen-receptor complexes to prostatic binding protein genes. Mol Cell Endocrinol 1990;74:203–212.

134. Matuo Y, Nishi N, Negi T, et al. Isolation and characterization of androgen-dependent non-histone chromosomal protein from dorsolateral prostate of rats. Biochem Biophys Res Commun 1982;109:334–340.

135. Spence AM, Sheppard PC, Davie JR, et al. Regulation of a bifunctional mRNA results in synthesis of secreted and nuclear probasin. Proc Natl Acad Sci USA 1989;86:7843–7847.

136. Matuo Y, Nishi N, Muguruma Y, et al. Localization of prostatic basic protein ("Probasin") in the rat prostates by use of monoclonal antibody. Biochem Biophys Res Commun 1985;130:293–300.

137. Matuo Y, Nishi N, Negi T, et al. Difference in androgen-dependent change of non-histone proteins between dorsolateral and ventral prostates of rats. Biochem Biophys Res Commun 1982;107:209–216.

138. Matuo Y, Nishi N, Tanaka Y, et al. Changes of an androgen-dependent nuclear protein during functional differentiation and by dedifferentiation of the dorsolateral prostate of rats. Biochem Biophys Res Commun 1984;118:467–473.

139. Wilson EM, Viskochil DH, Bartlett RJ, et al. Model systems for studies on androgen-dependent gene expression in the rat prostate. Prog Clin Biol Res 1981;75A:351–380.

140. Rennie PS, Bruchovsky N, Leco KJ, et al. Characterization of two cis-acting DNA elements involved in the androgen regulation of the probasin gene. Mol Endocrinol 1993;7:23–36.

141. Reid KJ, Hendy SC, Saito J, et al. Two classes of androgen receptor elements mediate cooperativity through allosteric interactions. J Biol Chem 2001;276:2943–2952.

142. Martin MB, Voeller HJ, Gelmann EP, et al. Role of cadmium in the regulation of AR gene expression and activity. Endocrinology 2002;143:263–275.

143. Kasper S, Sheppard PC, Yan Y, et al. Development, progression, and androgen-dependence of prostate tumors in probasin-large T antigen transgenic mice: a model for prostate cancer. Lab Invest 1998;78:i–xv.

144. Greenberg NM, DeMayo FJ, Sheppard PC, et al. The rat probasin gene promoter directs hormonally and developmentally regulated expression of a heterologous gene specifically to the prostate in transgenic mice. Mol Endrocrinol 1994;8:230–239.

145. Andriani F, Nan B, Yu J, et al. Use of the probasin promoter ARR2PB to express Bax in androgen receptor-positive prostate cancer cells. J Natl Cancer Inst 2001;93:1314–1324.

146. Price H, McNeal JE, Stamey TA. Evolving patterns of tissue composition in benign prostatic hyperplasia as a function of specimen size. Hum Pathol 1990;21:578–585.

Neuroanatomy and neuroregulation of the prostate

8

William D Steers, Adam P Klausner

OVERVIEW

Understanding prostatic innervation is of paramount importance for elucidating the basis of lower urinary tract symptoms (LUTS) associated with benign prostatic hyperplasia (BPH). Recognition that neurotransmitter blockade or reduced innervation to prostate tissues can reduce prostate volume underscores the crucial role of neural input in prostate growth and possibly development of malignancy. Decreasing the dynamic, nerve-controlled component of obstruction in BPH is the basis for treating LUTS with α-adrenoceptor antagonists.[1–3] The focus on prostate pharmacology has heightened interest in prostate innervation.[4–11] Nerves direct prostatic smooth muscle contraction, secretion, and the growth of the gland.[12] Neural input affects the secretion rate and the composition of prostatic fluid. The effects of drugs on emission and ejaculation have arisen with the development of survey instruments assessing these aspects of sexual function.

The physiologic responses of the prostate to neural stimulation resemble those of other exocrine glands. Circulating hormones influence growth, elicit contraction of the prostate (oxytocin)[13,14] and regulate innervation (androgens).[15–19] Neural input and neurotransmitters have been implicated in the growth of the prostate. Despite experiments showing that α-adrenergic mechanisms trigger apoptosis and kinases leading to cell proliferation,[20,21] long-term administration does not reduce prostate volume, alter prostate-specific antigen (PSA), or induce histologic changes. Nerves also transmit the discomfort of prostatitis and may even be involved in its pathogenesis.[22] The prostate possesses a rich afferent innervation. Prostate afferents contain neuropeptides that can trigger inflammatory responses. Conversely, secretory products, cytokines, and growth factors such as nerve growth factor (NGF) and basic fibroblast growth factor (bFGF) produced in the prostate can influence nerves in addition to prostate growth and development.[23–26] Given these observations, the clinician should be aware of the relevant neuroanatomy, physiology, and neuropharmacology of this accessory sex gland.

NEUROANATOMY

The prostate receives input from the parasympathetic and sympathetic nervous systems.[27–37] These pathways merge in the prostatic plexus, regarded as that portion of the pelvic plexus lying adjacent to the posteriolateral prostatic capsule (Figure 8.1). Nerves enter the prostate coursing posterior with the ejaculatory ducts.[27,28] Some axons travel medially over the base of the prostate to supply the central zone. Others fan out to penetrate the capsule. Nerves course within the prostatorectal fascia of Denonvilliers with the arterial sheet. In addition, some branches enter the prostate near the apex from the neurovascular bundle. After entering the prostate from these portals, axons branch and lie adjacent to walls of ducts and acini or course through stroma. Whether any of these nerves branch to supply the prostatic urethra is uncertain, but could have important implications for development of LUTS or continence after prostate surgery. It is tempting to speculate that this richness in innervation implies significant functional importance.

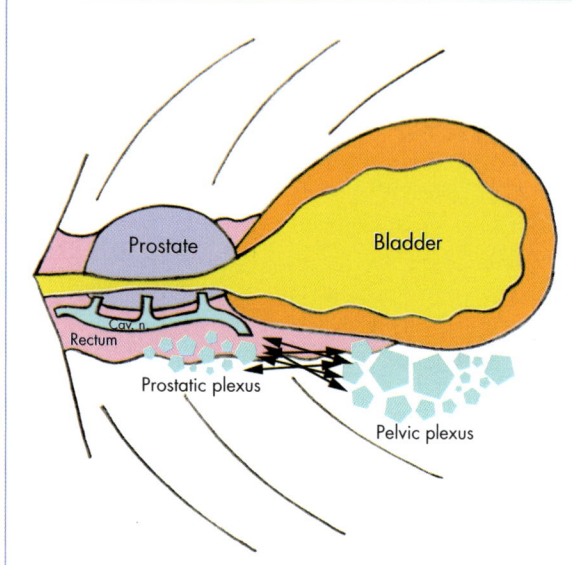

Fig. 8.1

Gross innervation of the prostate. Schematic representation of the gross innervation of the prostate depicting relationships to adjacent tissues. Nerve pathways to the prostate merge in the prostatic plexus, which lies adjacent to the posterior-lateral prostatic capsule. The cavernous nerve (Cav. n.) forms as a condensation of fibers from the prostatic plexus and runs between the layers of Denonvilliers' fascia in the groove between the posterolateral prostate and the anterior rectum. Nerve fibers penetrate the prostate medially at the base to supply the central zone. Other fibers penetrate the capsule and the prostatic apex.

SYMPATHETIC INNERVATION

Sympathetic nerves provide the predominant efferent neural input to the prostate. Sympathetic preganglionics reside within the thoracolumbar spinal cord from T10 to L2. Based on combined labeling/tracing studies in the rat, nearly 80% of the prostate's innervation is derived from sympathetic outflow while 21% to 33% originates from parasympathetic pathways.[35] In the cat, nearly two thirds of the neurons in the pelvic plexus supplying the prostate are noradrenergic.[9] The remaining cholinergic nerves may also receive sympathetic preganglionic input. Labeled neurons from the prostate in the inferior mesenteric and chain ganglia are exclusively noradrenergic. Some chain fibers travel in the pelvic nerve as well or branch to coalesce with the hypogastric nerve to supply the prostate.[9] Sympathetic preganglionics synapse on pelvic and prostatic ganglion cells in the prostatic plexus.

PARASYMPATHETIC INNERVATION

Although controversial, some believe the prostate receives some parasympathetic innervation[35] originating in the sacral (S2–S4) spinal cord and conveyed by the pelvic nerve (Figure 8.2). Preganglionic axons originating in the parasympathetic nucleus (SPN) located in the intermediolateral cell column travel in the pelvic nerve and synapse on ganglion cells within the body and capsule of the prostate. Some ganglion cells reside near the bladder neck.[29,30,37,38] Postganglionic fibers project from these neurons to cellular targets within the prostate. Whether most of the cholinergic fibers are sympathetic in origin is debatable.

AFFERENT NERVES

Peripheral afferents from the prostate travel to the central nervous system (CNS) in the hypogastric and pelvic nerves, and correspondingly, to the thoracolumbar and sacral dorsal root ganglia (DRG).[9,35] A duality of sensory innervation is most apparent when assessing patterns of referred prostate pain. Suprapubic and groin discomfort correspond to referred pain from T12 to L2 levels conveyed from the prostate by hypogastric nerves,[39] whereas perineal pain reflects input from the pelvic nerve (S2–S4). Fine subepithelial terminals that freely end within the epithelium with few synaptic vesicles but abundant mitochondria may represent sensory nerve endings.[27] Specialized Pacinian-like sensory endings, although described in neonatal and fetal prostates, are rare in adults and limited to the prostatic capsule.[28] Prostatic afferents transmit the sensations of pain or contraction, and may relay information necessary for reflex phenomena such as emission and ejaculation. Afferents can also release substances within the prostate that affect immune mechanisms, vascular permeability or smooth muscle tone.

CENTRAL SITES

Studies using retrograde viral tracers that cross synapses, and are, therefore, used to identify neurons in the CNS, indicate that prostatic innervation may be part of a large neural network that interacts with neurons belonging to micturition reflex pathways and sexual function.[36] Many of the sites in the brain and spinal cord labeled following prostatic injection match those identified following injection of viral tracers into the penis or bladder/urethra[40] with one exception. In contrast to previous studies, little or no labeling of

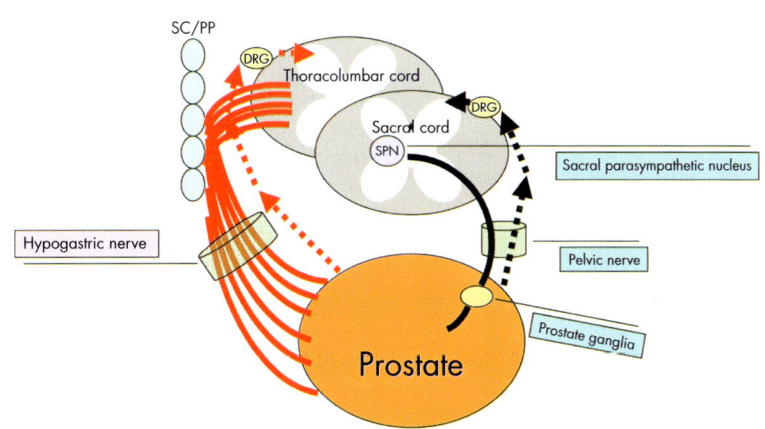

Fig. 8.2
Adrenergic, cholinergic, and non-adrenergic non-cholinergic (NANC) innervation of the prostate. The prostate receives sensory and motor input from the hypogastric and pelvic nerves. Sensory nerves *(dotted lines)* whose cell bodies are in the thoracolumbar and sacral dorsal root ganglia (DRG) contain pituitary adenylate cyclase activating peptide (PACAP), substance P (SP), calcitonin gene-related peptide (CGRP), vasoactive intestinal polypeptide (VIP), and nitric oxide synthase (NOS). Sympathetic nerves *(red)* supply the majority of the prostate (about 80%) and contain either norepinephrine (NE) or acetylcholine (ACh). Norepinephrine cells also contain neuropeptide Y (NY). Preganglionic sympathetics synapse directly on ganglia of the sympathetic chain (SC) or on ganglia of the prostatic plexus (PP) prior to supplying the prostate. Parasympathetic pathways *(black)* are much less abundant in the prostate (about 20–30%) and preganglionic fibers originate in the sacral parasympathetic nucleus (SPN) in the intermediolateral cell column (IMLCC) of the sacral spinal cord and synapse directly on ganglia within the prostate. Cholinergic efferent neurons in these parasympathetics contain ACh, VIP and NOS.

parasympathetic nerves in the intermediolateral cell column has been described by one group.[41] These discrepancies are likely due to methodological differences. In addition to the expected labeling in autonomic centers and sensory receiving areas of the dorsal horn at the sacral and thoracolumbar levels, prostate-labeled neurons can be found in Barrington's nucleus (micturition center), raphe magnus, reticular formation, A5, A7, periaqueductal gray, red nucleus, and subcoeruleus. The physiologic significance of these associations is unclear but raises the possibility that the function of the prostate or prostatic urethra is intimately linked to that of the bladder/urethra and penis.

IMMUNOHISTOCHEMISTRY

Histochemical findings provide insight into the function of prostatic nerves. Adrenergic, cholinergic nerves, and nerves containing nonadrenergic, noncholinergic (NANC) transmitter and/or mediator-forming enzymes have been demonstrated in prostates from humans and other mammals[10,11,29–31,38,42–45] (Box 8.1). Cell bodies for neurons are abundant in the periurethral region in the capsule and near the base of the seminal vesicle.[29,37] Neuronal perikarya are often found near the base or within the capsule as opposed to

nerve trunks, which are abundant around the lateral aspect of the prostatic capsule.[32] It is crucial for surgeons to note that nerves near the lateral aspect of the seminal vesicle are just a few millimeters from the neurovascular bundle supplying the penis.

Box 8.1 Neurotransmitter phenotypes in the prostate
Acetylcholine
Bombesin*
Calcitonin gene-related peptide (CGRP)*
Carbon monoxide (CO)
Galanin*
Leu-enkephalin (l-ENK)*
Met-enkephalin (m-ENK)*
Neuropeptide Y (NPY)*
Nitric oxide (NO)
Norephinephrine
Peptide histidine isoleucine (PHI)*
Pituitary adenylate cyclase activating peptide (PACAP)*
Somatostatin*
Substance P (SP)*
Vasoactive intestinal polypeptide (VIP)*
*Neuropeptides

NORADRENERGIC NERVES

Noradrenergic nerves are identified by glyoxylic acid fluorescence (all monoamines detected) or more specifically by tyrosine hydroxylase (TH) immunostaining. Data from fetuses and young men reveal that many stromal nerves follow the vasculature branching to form a moderately dense noradrenergic plexus around veins and arteries.[7,8,46] Noradrenergic nerve fibers course along smooth muscle bundles in the capsule and form a dense network in stromal smooth muscle. These fibers are prominent around the prostatic ducts, especially near their openings into the posterior urethra. Branching varicose noradrenergic axons lie beneath the epithelium of the prostatic acini.[47] This contrasts with data showing no TH-immunoreactive terminals in relation to acinar epithelium.[11]

CHOLINERGIC NERVES

Cholinergic fibers have been identified using acetylcholinesterase (AChE) histochemistry and more recently by very specific vesicular acetylcholine transporter (VAChT) immunohistochemistry. Cell bodies that are positive for AChE are found in the dorsal capsule, and AChE-positive nerves, although less numerous than adrenergic fibers, are distributed to the fibromuscular stroma, around acini and ducts, and around blood vessels.[6,11,44,47,48] Axons that are positive for AChE and VAChT can also be demonstrated near the base of the epithelium.[11,48] Staining reveals cholinergic neurotransmitters in smooth muscle surrounding acini.[41]

NEUROPEPTIDES

Among the first NANC neuropeptides shown to occur in prostate were vasoactive intestinal polypeptide (VIP) and opium-related peptides met- and leu-enkephalin (m-ENK and l-ENK).[43,49] Further investigations have revealed numerous other peptides in the human prostate[7,8,11,29,30,46,50–54] (see Box 8.1). In general, cholinergic and noradrenergic fibers are more numerous than peptidergic fibers. The distribution of these neuropeptides may vary with the region of the prostate.[30] The proximal central prostate contains more peptidergic fibers than the anterior capsule, which exceeds the distal central zones, which in turn is greater

than the peripheral zone (Figure 8.3). However, much of this data is derived from aging prostates and is not consistent with other data showing uniform density of noradrenergic and cholinergic fibers in the central and peripheral zones.[38,47] Furthermore, density of innervation may vary with hormonal status and cell type content (smooth muscle versus glands). Therefore, temporal regional differences should be interpreted cautiously.

Some nerves in the prostate stain for nitric oxide synthase (NOS) or heme oxygenase (HO), suggesting that they respectively manufacture nitric oxide and carbon monoxide.[5–8,11,46,55] Confocal microscopy reveals that NOS and HO are not present in the same nerve terminals.[11] Nitric oxide synthase is expressed by both sensory and motor neurons.

Many neurotransmitters coexist in prostatic neurons.[7,11,31–35] Moreover, the relative abundance of nerves, their distribution, and their transmitter phenotype vary with species. Neuropeptides are found in TH-staining, noradrenergic perikarya and also in non-noradrenergic neurons. In the prostate, noradrenergic neurons contain ATP, whereas cholinergic fibers express neuropeptide Y (NPY) and possibly vasoactive intestinal peptide (VIP).[6] Nerves containing NPY are limited to the stroma while VIP fibers surround acini.[29] In the human prostate, NPY-immunoreactive nerves were similarly distributed as VIP- and NOS-immunoreactive fibers, and were found in rich amounts.[11] Vasoactive intestinal peptide and NOS tend to be found more commonly in non-noradrenergic (presumably cholinergic) neurons.[7,11]

Calcitonin gene-related peptide (CGRP) and substance P (SP) are detected exclusively in sensory nerves supplying the prostate of the cat.[9] However, in human fetal prostates these two neuropeptides can be expressed by both TH-positive and TH-negative neurons in the pelvic plexus.[7] In the fetal prostate, TH and NOS are colocalized in prostatic ganglion cells.[7] In the adult human prostate, NOS immunoreactivity is rare in noradrenergic neurons and found in a few cholinergic fibers.[6,11] In nerves of the prostatic stroma, NOS- and TH-immunoreactivities are similarly, but not identically, distributed, and in coarse nerve trunks single NOS- and TH-immunoreactive fibers are easily separable by confocal laser scanning microscopy.[11] Also, TH/nNOS fibers are not found in prostate epithelium. These discrepancies in sensory peptide localization and NOS coexpression may be explained by differences between transmitter expression by fetal versus adult neurons.

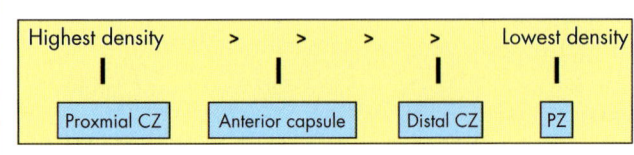

Fig. 8.3
Relative density of peptidergic innervation of the prostate according to zonal anatomy. (CZ, central zone. PZ, peripheral zone.)

Nerves that are immunoreactive to CGRP, considered to represent sensory nerves, are few compared with other phenotypes characterized. Terminals immunoreactive to NOS and CGRP have similar profiles, but the immunoreactivities are not colocalized.[11] Pituitary adenylate cyclase activating peptide (PACAP), presumably in pelvic afferents, is expressed by nerves supplying the prostate.[11]

The location of urethral and prostatic nerves, especially sensory, may be relevant for designing therapies for BPH. Thermotherapy for BPH appears to destroy these prostatic nerves or alter neurotransmitter receptor function.[56,57] Relief of symptoms may rely on relative denervation or reduced neurotransmission. Thick fibers coursing along the urethra could also be a potential target of ablative or thermal BPH treatments.

NEUROPHYSIOLOGY AND NEUROPHARMACOLOGY

The dual innervation of the prostate by sympathetic and parasympathetic nerves implies that each division possesses separate and opposing functions. However, this dichotomy does not exist in the prostate. Stimulation of the pelvic nerve in the dog produces subtle contraction of the prostate, while hypogastric nerve stimulation evokes a profound contraction and secretion.[58] Contraction of the prostatic capsule also occurs during hypogastric nerve stimulation contributing to "urethral" resistance. In contrast to secretion, contractile responses are primarily mediated by noradrenergic rather than cholinergic mechanisms. The contractile response to hypogastric nerve stimulation results from the release of norepinephrine from noradrenergic nerves supplying smooth muscle within the prostatic stroma and capsule.

The role of parasympathetic nerves is unclear. Cholinomimetic drugs contract the prostate capsule but the contraction is only 10% to 15% of that of α-agonists. Although pelvic afferents undoubtedly transmit pain, the pelvic nerve might also contribute to contraction and possibly secretion via cholinergic nerves. In the dog,

it was suggested that the function of cholinergic nerves in the stroma was to suppress norepinephrine release from adrenergic terminals.[61] Alternatively, these responses may be due to noradrenergic sympathetic chain fibers running within the pelvic nerve. Some viral tracing studies tend to show a parasympathetic input. A reassessment of parasympathetic cholinergic input to the prostate is needed. Placed in the context of sexual behavior, excitation and parasympathetic input triggering erection may heighten prostatic tone. Parasympathetic cholinergic input also contracts the prostatic vas deferens. However, not until a thoracolumbar spinal cord reflex initiates a sympathetic discharge does emission occur. Watanabe et al[62] investigated the importance of somatic nerves and found that pudendal nerve stimulation failed to alter either secretion or contraction of the dog prostate. Destruction of the sacral cord such as in myelomeningocele patients is associated with smaller prostates and lower PSA.[63] This indirectly supports some role for parasympathetic input in humans.

PROSTATIC SECRETION

The neurophysiology of innervation of the prostate closely resembles that of the sweat glands. Hypogastric stimulation (sympathetic) increases secretion.[64–68] Yet this secretion is blocked by the muscarinic agonist atropine,[66–68] implying that sympathetic cholinergic nerves control exocrine function (see reviews[27,31,69]). This secretory role of cholinergic nerves is consistent with the close proximity of these fibers to acini[11,47] and autoradiographic demonstration of muscarinic receptors on glandular but not stromal elements in the prostate.[70–72]

Pharmacologic data has substantiated physiological observations using nerve stimulation (Table 8.1). Muscarinic agonists including pilocarpine and urecholine induce prostatic secretion.[27,64–66,73] This secretion is mediated by muscarinic receptors located on prostatic acini.[70–72] Anti-muscarinics such as atropine completely block secretory responses to these agonists as well as hypogastric nerve-evoked secretion. Despite

Table 8.1 Responses of prostate smooth muscle or glands to neurotransmitters or neuroendocrine substance			
Substance	**Muscle**	**Gland**	**Growth**
Acetylcholine	Contraction (weak)	Secretion (strong)	+?
Norepinephrine	Contraction (strong)	Secretion (weak)	+
Vasoactive intestinal polypeptide (VIP)	Relaxation or inhibition of contraction (weak)	Increases acetylcholine-mediated secretion	+ invasion CA
Neuropeptide Y (NPY)	Relaxation or inhibition of contraction (weak)	–	?
Nitric oxide (NO)	Relaxation	–	?

this observation, a decrease in ejaculate volume is rarely a complaint of men on anticholinergics.

There are five molecular and three pharmacologically characterized muscarinic receptor subtypes.[74] The M_1 receptor is expressed in the prostate.[75,76] However, some cell lines from prostatic cancer express the M_3 receptor subtype.[76] Moreover, M receptor subtype expression varies by species. Although some species express M_1 receptor on epithelium, the stroma expresses M_2 to a lesser degree. In addition to acetylcholine, other neurotransmitters may participate in secretion.[77]

Exogenous VIP augments both pilocarpine- and hypogastric-evoked secretion in the dog, possibly through preganglionic mechanisms within the ganglia.[78] Nevertheless, in the rat, VIP alone fails to evoke prostatic secretion.[79] Therefore, VIP, probably released from cholinergic nerves, appears to be modulatory rather than a principal mediator of prostatic secretion. Nitric oxide inhibits secretion and reduces contractile action. Because acetylcholine, NO, and VIP coexist in prostatic nerves, their combined role in secretion has been proposed.[11] Nitric oxide alone has no consistent effect in the prostate.[12] Vasoactive intestinal peptide raises cyclic adenosine monophosphate (cAMP) in prostatic acini.[59] This rise in cAMP following exposure to VIP can be ameliorated by NPY, which supports the notion of interaction between transmitters released from nerves.[80]

Alpha-adrenergic agonists can also elicit prostatic secretion.[68,73] Thus, in the dog, phenylephrine increased epidermal growth factor (EGF) secretion four-fold. This effect was blocked by α-adrenoceptor antagonists, but not by the muscarinic receptor agonist atropine.[79] The response to α-adrenergic agonists is likely due to an emptying of ductal contents during contraction,[73] because adrenergic nerves surround prostatic ducts, not acini. The effects of both adrenergic and cholinergic agonists are due to direct stimulation of prostatic tissue because the actions of those drugs are unchanged after removal of the pelvic ganglia.[73] Transmitters released from prostatic nerves may alter the composition of prostatic secretions.[68,73,81,82] The concentration of sodium in prostatic secretions is essentially the same as that in plasma. In contrast, sodium and potassium concentrations in neurally evoked prostatic secretions exceed those in plasma. In carbachol-stimulated secretions, the protein concentration and prostatic acid phosphatase activity were reduced compared to noradrenaline- or phenylephrine-stimulated secretion.[73]

Nerves maintain the functional integrity of glandular tissue. Several studies have shown that denervation reduces prostatic weight and causes atrophy of acini.[83–85] Chemical sympathectomy decreases the weight of the prostate and glands appear dilated.[86,87] Moreover, patients with spinal myelopathy are less likely to develop prostate cancer.[88] Similarly, spinal cord injury reduces prostate size, lowers mRNA for the androgen receptor and reduces PSA.[89] Blockade of the α₁-receptor with doxazosin also induces apoptosis in the prostate and reduces cell proliferation in culture.[20,21] But long-term follow-up of men on this drug fails to show reduction in PSA.[22] The botulinum toxin, which prevents neurotransmitter release, causes long-term shrinkage of prostate in rats and men with reduction in PSA. Neuroendocrine cells in the prostate synthesize neurotransmitter-like substances capable of altering cellular proliferation and differentiation.[90,91] Loss of neural input to these cells does not alter their content. Therefore, neural input, aside from a direct influence on secretion, may play a role in the growth of the prostate.

Androgens affect neural morphology, number, and autonomic receptor function.[15–19] Castration reduces the size and neurotransmitter content in TH ganglion cells supplying the prostate. Castration reduces muscarinic receptor expression in the prostate independent from its direct reduction of glandular tissue.[16] Castration decreases the volume of prostatic secretion but not secretory composition.[73]

PROSTATIC SMOOTH MUSCLE CONTRACTION

As mentioned above, prostate smooth muscle contraction during seminal emission results from release of norepinephrine from noradrenergic nerves receiving hypogastric input (see Table 8.1). However, noradrenergic nerves are also considered responsible for maintaining prostatic smooth muscle tone,[92] and approximately 50% of the total urethral pressure in BPH patients may be due to α-adrenoceptor-mediated muscle tone.[93,94] It is conceivable that a global increase in sympathetic tone leads to increased urethral resistance and prostatic tone. Therefore, it is not surprising to find voiding symptoms or painful ejaculation in young anxious men.

Noradrenaline stimulates contraction-mediating α-adrenoceptors localized to predominately prostatic stroma. Although both α_1 and α_2 receptors can be identified in the human prostate,[71,95] the contractile properties are mediated primarily by α_1-adrenoceptors.[71,96–101] Many clinical investigations have confirmed that α₁-adrenoceptor blockade relieves LUTS, both of storage and voiding types, in BPH patients.[2,3,102,103] However, the inability to identify "uroselective" or "prostate selective" α-adrenoceptor agonists in clinical trials despite autoradiographic, molecular biological, and pharmacologic observations, suggests the actions of these agents on prostate function may be at sites separate from the prostate.[3] All three high-affinity α₁-adrenoceptor subtypes found in molecular cloning studies have been identified in prostatic stromal tissue.[3] The α_{1A}-adrenoceptor was found to be the most predominant, representing about 60% to 85% of the α_1-adrenoceptor population.

The α_{1A}-adrenoceptor was reported to mediate the contractile response of the human prostate in vitro.[104,105] However, there is some variability in expression. Differentiated responses to α-subtype drugs have been reported in men and correlate with the α_{1A} to α_{1b} ratio in the specimens.[106]

In addition to norepinephrine released from noradrenergic nerves, other transmitters may influence the contractility of prostatic smooth muscle and offer potential mechanisms for reducing urethral resistance and prostatic tone in disorders such as BPH. Relaxation of norepinephrine-contracted prostatic tissue can be prevented by NOS inhibition.[11,57] Similar to its effect on the urethra, exogenous NO relaxes prostatic tissues. Consistent with animal data is the finding that phosphodiesterase type 5 (PDE5) inhibitors that raise cGMP increase urine flow rates in men with BPH. Nitric oxide may play a role in controlling smooth muscle tone in the prostate; it may also be associated with inflammatory disorders of the prostate, mimicking findings in the bladder. ATP contracts prostate tissues via P_{2x1} receptors on stroma.[107] Lastly, angiotensin II enhances norepinephrine release in rat prostates, implying that the renin–angiotensin system can influence prostate tone. These observations raise the possibility that new pharmacologic therapies may be forthcoming for LUTS due to BPH.

SUMMARY

The recognition that the innervation of the prostate has an important role in prostatic symptoms and growth has focused attention on the neuroanatomy and neuropharmacology of this organ. The prostate receives input from sympathetic and possibly parasympathetic nerves. In contrast to other genitourinary tissues, postganglionic cholinergic sympathetics are responsible for secretion, while postganglionic noradrenergic sympathetics mediate contraction in this organ. Whether parasympathetic nerves and their diverse neurotransmitters within prostatic nerves exert any physiologic effects remains to be unraveled. Nonadrenergic, non-cholinergic nerves are likely to be modulatory with a potential role for NO in both contractile and secretory functions. These observations may lead to new classes of drugs such as long-acting PDE5 inhibitor for the treatment of LUTS due to BPH.

The precise role of nerves on prostatic growth and their role in BPH symptoms or male pelvic pain syndrome awaits further study. While the concept of stromal–epithelial interaction has been firmly established in the prostate, evidence is mounting that nerves influence these cellular interactions. The application of botulinum toxin is proof of the principle that abolishing neural input to the prostate reduces LUTS almost to the degree seen with surgery. Growth factors and other substances produced by the prostate are likely to influence neural growth, morphology, and transmitter expression, and function in an autocrine/paracrine-line fashion. Exploitation of these findings to further enhance BPH therapy is likely.

REFERENCES

1. Lepor H. The role of alpha blockade in the treatment of BPH. In Lepor H, Rawson RK (eds): Prostatic Diseases, Saunders, Philadelphia 1993, pp 170–183.
2. Eri L, Tveter KJ. Alpha-blockade in the treatment of symptomatic benign prostatic hyperplasia. J Urol 1995;154:923–934.
3. Andersson KE, Lepor H, Wyllie M. Prostate α_1 adrenoceptor and uroselectivity. Prostate 1977;30:202–216.
4. Andersson KE. The pharmacology of the lower urinary tract smooth muscles and penile erectile tissues. Pharmacol Rev 1993;5:253–308.
5. Burnett A, Takeda M, Maguire M, et al. Characterization and localization of nitric oxide synthase in the human prostate. Urol 1995;45:435–439.
6. Dixon J, Jen P, Gosling J. The distribution of vesicular acetylcholine transporter and NPY in and nitric oxide in the human genitourinary organs. Neurourol Urodynam 2000;19:185–194.
7. Jen P, Dixon J, Gosling J. Co-localisation of tyrosine hydroxylase, nitric oxide synthase and neuropeptides in neurons of the human postnatal male pelvic ganglia. J Auton Nerv Sys 1996;59:41–50.
8. Jen P, Dixon J, Gerahart J, et al. Nitric oxide synthase and tyrosine hydroxylase are co-localized in nerves supplying the postnatal human male genitourinary organs. J Urol 1996;155:1171–1121.
9. Danuser H, Springer J, Katofiasc M, et al. Extrinsic innervation of the cat prostate gland; a combined tracing and immunohistochemical study. J Urol 1997;157:1018–1024.
10. Hedlund P, Larsson B, Alm P, et al. Nitric oxide synthase-containing nerves and ganglia in the dog prostate: a comparison with other transmitters. Histochem J 1996;28:635–642.
11. Hedlund P, Ekstrom P, Larsson B, et al. Heme oxygenase and NO synthase in the human prostate— relation to adrenergic, cholinergic and peptide containing nerves. J Auton Nerv Sys 1997;63:115–126.
12. Isaacs J, Steinberg G. A guide to the physiology of the prostate. Cont Urol 1990;9:54–66.
13. Bodanzky M, Sharaf H, Roy J, et al. Contractile activity of vasotocin, oxytocin, and vasopressin on mammalian prostate. Euro J Pharmacol 1992;216:311–313.
14. Sharaf H, Foda HD, Said SI, et al. Oxytocin and related peptides elicit contractions of prostate and seminal vesicle. Ann NY Acad Sci 1992;652:474–477.
15. Partanen M, Hervonen A. The effect of long-term castration on the histochemically demonstrable catecholamines in the hypogastric ganglion of the rat. J Auton Nerv Sys 1979;1:139–147.
16. Shapiro E, Miller A, Lepor H. Down regulation of the muscarinic cholinergic receptor of the rat prostate following castration. J Urol 1985;134:179–182.
17. Melvin J, Hamill R. The major pelvic ganglion: androgen control of postnatal development. J Neurosci 1987;7:1607–1612.
18. Hamill R, Schroeder B. Hormonal regulation of adult sympathetic neurons: the effects of castration on neuropeptide Y, norepinephrine, and tyrosine hydroxylase activity. J Neurobiol 1990;21:731–742.
19. Regunathan S, Nassir Y, Sundaram K, et al. Expression of I_2-imidazoline sites in rat prostate. Effect of castration and aging. Biochem Pharmacol 1996;51:455–459.
20. Wu Y, Kawabe K. Effects of norepinephrine and alpha-1 adrenergic blockade on cultured stromal cell from benign prostatic hyperplasia. Jap J Urol 1993;84:2152–2157.
21. Kyprianou N, Litvak J, Borkowski A, et al. Induction of apoptosis by doxazosin targeting alpha-1 blockade in benign prostatic hyperplasia. J Urol 1997;157:1086A.

22. Hellstrom W, Schmidt R, Lue T, et al. Neuromuscular dysfunction in nonbacterial prostatitis. Urol 1987;30:183–188.

23. Harper G, Barde Y, Burnstock G, et al. Guinea pig prostate is a rich source of nerve growth factor. Nature l979;279:160–162.

24. Collins A, Robinson E, Neal D. Benign prostatic stromal cells are regulated by basic fibroblast growth factor and transforming growth factor beta 1. J. Endocrinol 1996;151:315–322.

25. Paul A, Grant E, Habib F. The expression and localization of beta nerve growth factor in benign and malignant human prostate tissue: relationship to neuroendocrine differentiation. Br J Cancer 1996;74:1990–1996.

26. Story M, Hopp K, Meier D. Regulation of basic fibroblast growth factor expression by transforming growth factor beta in cultured human prostate stromal cells. Prostate 1996;28:219–226.

27. Elbadawi A, Goodman D. Autonomic innervation of accessory male genital glands. In Spring-Mills E, Hafez E (eds): Male Accessory Sex Glands. Elsevier-North-Holland, Amsterdam, Biomedical Press, 1980.

28. Gosling J. Autonomic innervation of the prostate. In Hinman F (ed): Benign Prostatic Hypertrophy. New York: Springer Verlag, 1983, pp 349–360.

29. Higgins J, Gosling J. Studies on the structure and intrinsic innervation of normal human prostate. Prostate 1989;2:5–16.

30. Crowe R, Chapple C, Burnstock G. The human prostate gland: a histochemical and immunohistochemical study of neuropeptides, serotonin, dopamine beta-hydroxylase and acetylcholinesterase in autonomic nerves and ganglia. Br J Urol 1991;68:53–61.

31. Dail WG. Autonomic innervation of male reproductive genitalia. In CA Maggi (ed): The Autonomic Nervous System, vol 6. London: Harwood Academic Publishers, 1993, pp 69–101.

32. Benoit G, Merlaud L, Meduri G, et al. Anatomy of the prostatic nerves. Surg Radiolog Anat 1994;16:23–29.

33. Setchell B, Maddocks S, Brooks D. Anatomy, Vasculature, Innervation, and Fluids of the Male Reproductive Tract. New York: Raven Press, 1994.

34. Vaalasti A. Autonomic innervation of the human male accessory sex glands. In Riva A, Testa Riva F: Ultrastructure of Male Urogenital Glands: Prostate, Seminal Vesicles, Urethral, and Bulbourethral Glands. Kluwer Academic Pub, New York, 1994, pp 187–196.

35. Kepper M, Keast J. Immunohistochemical properties and spinal connections of pelvic autonomic neurons that innervate the rat prostate gland. Cell Tissue Res 1995;281:533–542.

36. Marson L, Orr R. Identification of rat spinal neurons that innervate the prostate comparison of hypogastric and pelvic inputs using transneuronal tracing with pseudorabies virus. Soc Neurosci 1996;22:1051 [Abstract].

37. Dixon J, Jen P, Gosling J. A double-label immunohistochemical study of intramural ganglia from the human male urinary bladder neck. J Anat 1997;190:125–134.

38. Gosling J, Thompson S. A neurohistochemical and histological study of peripheral autonomic neurons of the human bladder neck and prostate. Urol Int 1977;32:269.

39. Plancarte R, Amescua C, Patt RB, et al. Superior hypogastric plexus block for pelvic cancer pain. Anesthesiology 1990;73:236–239.

40. Vizzard MA, Erickson VL, Card JP, et al. Transneuronal labeling of neurons in the adult rat brainstem and spinal cord after injection of pseudorabies virus into the urethra. J Comp Neurol 1995;355:629–640.

41. Nadelhaft I, Miranda-Sousa AJ, Vera PL. Separate urinary bladder and prostate neurons in the central nervous system of the rat: simultaneous labeling with two immunohistochemically distinguishable pseudorabies viruses. BMC Neurosci 2002;3:8.

42. Baumgarten H, Falck B, Holstein A, et al. Adrenergic innervation of the human testis, epididymis, ductus deferens and prostate: a fluorescence microscopic and fluorometric study. Zeitschrift Fur Zellforschung Und Mikroskopische Anatomie 1968;90:81–95.

43. Alm P, Allumets J, Hakanson R, et al. Peptidergic (vasoactive intestinal peptide) nerves in the genitourinary tract. Neurosci 1977;2:751–754.

44. Dunzendorfer U, Jonas D, Weber W. The autonomic innervation of the human prostate. Histochemistry of acetylcholinesterase in the normal and pathologic states. Urol Res 1976;4:29–32.

45. Yokoyama R, Inokuchi T, Satoh H, et al. Distribution of tyrosine hydroxylase (TH)-like, neuropeptide Y (NPY)-like immunoreactive and acetylcholinesterase (ACHE)-positive nerve fibers in the prostate gland of the monkey (*Macacus fuscatus*). Kurume Med J 1990;37:1–8.

46. Jen P, Dixon J. Development of peptide-containing nerves in the human fetal prostate gland. J Anat 1995;187:169–179.

47. Vaalasti A, Hervonen A. Autonomic innervation of the human prostate. Inv Urol 1980;17:293–297.

48. Shirai M, Sasaki K, Rikimaru A. A histochemical investigation of the distribution of adrenergic and cholinergic nerves in the human male genital organs. Tohoku J Exp Med 1973;111:281–291.

49. Vaalasti A, Linnoila I, Hervonen A. Immunohistochemical demonstration of VIP, [Met^5]- and [Leu^5]-enkephalin immunoreactive nerve fibers in the human prostate and seminal vesicles. Histochem 1980;66:89–98.

50. Gu J, Polak JM, Probert L, et al. Peptidergic innervation of the human male genital tract. J Urol 1983;130:386–391.

51. Aumuller G, Jungblut T, Malek B, et al. Regional distribution of opioidergic nerves in human and canine prostate. Prostate 1989;14:279–288.

52. Sasaki A, Yoshinaga K. Immunoreactive somatostatin in male reproductive system in humans. J Clin Endocrin Metab 1989;68:996–999.

53. Lange W, Unger J. Peptidergic innervation within the prostate gland and seminal vesicle. Urol Res 1990;18:337–340.

54. Tainio H. Peptidergic innervation of the human prostate, seminal vesicle and vas deferens. Acta Histochem 1995;97:113–119.

55. Takeda M, Tang R, Shapiro E, et al. Effects of nitric oxide on human and canine prostates. Urology 1995;45:440–446.

56. Perichino M, Bozzo W, Puppo P, et al. Does transurethral thermotherapy induce long-term alpha blockade? An immunohistochemical study. Eur Urol 1993;23:299–301.

57. Arai Y, Jukuzawa S, Terai A, et al. Transurethral microwave thermotherapy for benign prostatic hyperplasia—relation between clinical response and prostate histology. Prostate 1996;28:84–88.

58. Eckhardt C. Untersuchungen uber die Erection des Penis beim Hunde. Beitrage zur Anatomie und Physiologie 1863;3:123–166.

59. Langley JN, Anderson HK. The innervation of the pelvis and adjoining viscera. Part IV. The internal generative organs. J Physiol (Lond) 1895;19:122–130.

60. Learmonth, JR. A contribution to the neurophysiology of the urinary bladder in man. Brain 1931;54:147–176.

61. Arver S, Sjostrand N. Functions of adrenergic and cholinergic nerves in canine effectors of seminal emission. Acta Physiol Scand 1982;115:67–77.

62. Watanabe H, Shima M, Kojima M, et al. Dynamic study of nervous control on prostatic contraction and fluid excretion in the dog. J Urol 1988;140:1567–1570.

63. Pannek J, Berges RR, Cubick G, et al. Prostate size and PSA serum levels in male patients with spinal cord injury. Urology 2003;62:845–848.

64. Farrell J, Lyman Y. A study of the secretory nerves and the action of certain drugs on, the prostate gland. Am J Phys 1937;118:64–70.

65. Farnsworth W, Lawrence M. Regulation of prostate secretion in the rat. Am J Physiol 1965;373–376.

66. Smith E, Lebeaux M. The mediation of the canine prostatic secretion provoked by hypogastric nerve stimulation. Inv Urol 1970;7:313–318.

67. Smith E, Lebeaux M. The composition of nerve induced canine prostatic secretion. Inv Urol 1971;8:100–103.

68. Bruschini H, Schmidt R, Tanagho E. Neurologic control of prostatic secretion in the dog. Inv Urol 1978;15:288–290.

69. Smith ER. The canine prostate and its secretion. In Thomas JA, Singhai RL (ed): Molecular Mechanisms of Gonadal Hormone Action. Baltimore: University Park Press, 1975, pp 167–204.

70. Lepor H, Khuhar M. Characterization of muscarinic cholinergic receptor binding in the vas deferens, bladder, prostate and penis of the rabbit. J Urol 1984;132:392–396.

71. Hedlund H, Andersson K, Larsson B. Alpha-adrenoceptors and muscarinic receptors in the isolated human prostate. J Urol 1985;134:1291–1298.

72. James S, Chapple C, Phillips M, et al. Autoradiographic analysis of alpha-adrenoceptors and muscarinic cholinergic receptors in the hyperplastic human prostate. J Urol 1989;142:438–444.

73. Wang J, McKenna KE, Lee C. Determination of prostatic secretion in rats: effect of neurotransmitters and testosterone. Prostate 1991;18:289–301.

74. Eglen RM, Hegde SS, Watson N. Muscarinic receptor subtypes and smooth muscle function. Pharmacol Rev 1996;48:531–565.

75. Ruggieri M, Colton M, Wang P, et al. Human prostate muscarinic receptor subtypes. J Pharmacol Exp Therap 1995; 274:976–982.

76. Luthin GR, Wang P, Zhou H, et al. Role of m1 receptor-G protein coupling in cell proliferation in the prostate. Life Sci 1997;60:963–968.

77. Ventura S, Pennefather J, Mitchelson F. Cholinergic innervation and function in the prostate gland. Pharmacol Ther 2002;94:93–112.

78. Smith E, Miller T, Wilson M, et al. Effects of vasoactive intestinal peptide on canine prostatic contraction and secretion. Am Phys Soc 1984;R701–R708.

79. Jacobs SC, Story MT. Exocrine secretion of epidermal growth factor by rat prostate: effect of adrenergic agents, cholinergic agents and vasoactive intestinal polypeptide. Prostate 1988;13:79–87.

80. Solano R, Carmena M, Guijarro L, et al. Neuropeptide Y inhibits vasoactive intestinal polypeptide stimulated adenyl cyclase in rat ventral prostate. Neuropeptides 1994;27:31–37.

81. Smith E, Miller T, Pebler R. Transepithelial voltage changes during prostatic secretion in the dog. Am Phys Soc 1983;245:F470–F477.

82. Jacobs SC, Story MT. Autonomic control of acid phosphatase exocrine secretion by the rat prostate. Urol Res 1989;17:311–315.

83. Martinez-Pineiro L, Dahiya R, Nunes L, et al. Pelvic plexus denervation in rats causes morphologic and functional changes of the prostate. J Urol 1993;150:215–218.

84. Wang J, McKenna K, McVary K, et al. Requirement of innervation for maintenance of structural and functional integrity in the rat prostate. Biol Reprod 1991;44:1171–1176.

85. McVary KT, Razzaq A, Lee C, et al. Growth of the rat prostate gland is facilitated by the autonomous nervous system. Biol Reprod 1994;51:99–107.

86. Vaalast A, Alho AM, Tainio H. The effect of sympathetic denervation with 6-hydroxydopamine on the ventral prostate of the rat. Acta Histochem 1986;79:49–54.

87. Lamano-Carvalho TL, Favaretto AL, Petenusci SO, et al. Prepubertal development of rat prostate and seminal vesicle following chemical sympathectomy with guanethidine. Braz J Med Biol Res 1993;26:639–646.

88. Frisbie J, Binard J. Low prevalence of prostatic cancer among myelopathy patients. J Am Paraplegia Soc 1994;17:148–149.

89. Huang HFS, Li MT, Linsenmeyer T, et al. The effects of spinal cord injury on the status of messenger ribonucleic acid for TRPM2 and androgen receptor in the prostate of the rat. J Androl 1997;18:250–256.

90. di Saint'Agnese P, deMesy J, Churukian C, et al. Human prostatic endocrine-paracrine (APUD) cells. Distributional analysis with a comparison of serotonin and neuron-specific enolase immunoreactivity and silver strains. Arc Path Lab Med 1985;109:607–612.

91. De Mesy Jensen K, Di Sant'Agnese P. A review of the ultrastructure of human prostatic and urethral endocrine-paracrine cells and neuroendocrine differentiation in prostatic carcinoma. In Riva A, Testa Riva F, Motta. P (ed): Ultrastructure of the Male Urogenital Glands: Prostate, Seminal Vesicles, Urethral, and Bulbourethral Glands. Kluwer Academic, New York, 1997, pp 139–161.

92. Caine M, Raz S, Zeigler M. Adrenergic and cholinergic receptors in the human prostate, prostatic capsule and bladder neck. Br J Urol 1975;47:193–202.

93. Appell RA, England HR, Hussell AR, et al. The effect of epidural anesthesia on the urethral closure pressure profile in patients with prostatic enlargement. J Urol 1980;124:410–411.

94. Furuya S, Kumamoto Y, Yokoyama E, et al. Alpha-adrenergic activity and urethral pressure in prostatic zone in benign prostatic hypertrophy. J Urol 1982;128:836–839.

95. Lepor H, Shapiro E. Characterization of alpha$_1$-adrenergic receptors in human benign prostatic hyperplasia. J Urol 1984;132:1226–1229.

96. Hiebel J, Ruffolo R. The use of alpha-adrenoceptor antagonists in the pharmacological management of benign prostatic hypertrophy: an overview. Pharmacol Res 1996;33:145–160.

97. Shapiro E, Lepor H. Alpha2 adrenergic receptors in hyperplastic human prostate: identification and characterization using 3H-rauwolscine. J Urol 1986;135:1038–1043.

98. Lepor H, Gup DI, Bauman M, et al. Laboratory assessment of terazosin and alpha1 blockade in prostatic hyperplasia. Urology 1988;32:21–26.

99. Kitada S, Kumazawa J. Pharmacological characteristics of smooth muscle in benign prostatic hyperplasia and normal prostatic tissue. J Urol 1987;138:158–160.

100. Chapple CR, Aubrey ML, James S, et al. Characterisation of human prostatic adrenoceptors using pharmacology receptor binding and localization. Br J Urol 1989;63;487–496.

101. Gup D, Shapiro E, Buamann M, et al. Contractile properties of human prostate adenomas and the development of infravesical obstruction. Prostate 1989;15:105–114.

102. Chapple CR. Selective alpha 1-adrenoceptor antagonists in benign prostatic hyperplasia: rationale and clinical experience. Eur Urol 1996;129:144.

103. Jardin A, Andersson K-E, Caine M, et al. Alpha-blockers therapy in benign prostatic hyperplasia. In Cockett ATK, Khoury S, Aso Y, Chatelain C, Denis L, Griffiths K, Murphy C (ed): The Third International Consultation on Benign Prostatic Hyperplasia (BPH). Health Publication Ltd, Plymouth, UK. SCI 1996, pp 527–564.

104. Forray C, Bard JA, Wetzel JM, et al. The alpha 1-adrenergic receptor that mediates smooth muscle contraction in human prostate has the pharmacological properties of the cloned human a1c subtype. Mol Pharmacol 1994;45:703–708.

105. Marshall I, Burt RP, Chapple CR. Noradrenaline contractions of human prostate mediated by alpha 1A-(alpha 1c-) adrenoceptor subtype. Br J Pharmacol 1995;115:781–786.

106. Fabiani ME, Sourial M, Thomas WG, et al. Angiotensin II enhances noradrenaline release from sympathetic nerves of the rat prostate via a novel angiotensin receptor: implications for the pathophysiology of benign prostatic hyperplasia. J Endocrinol 2001;171:97–108.

107. Ventura S, Dewalagama RK, Lau LCL. Adenosine 5'triphosphate is an excitatory cotransmitter with noradrenaline to smooth muscle of the rat prostate. Br J Pharmacol 2003;138:1277–1284.

Androgens and the androgen receptor in normal prostate

9

Helmut Klocker

INTRODUCTION

The human prostate gland develops and grows under the influence of androgens, and in adulthood their permanent stimulation is required for tissue maintenance and function. The most important androgen acting in the prostate is dihydrotestosterone (DHT), which is produced from testosterone by 5α-reductase activity. In the cells, the effects of androgens are mediated through the androgen receptor, a ligand-activated transcription factor and member of the superfamily of nuclear receptors. It is expressed in the stromal cells and in the luminal secretory epithelial cells, whereas basal epithelial cells and neuroendocrine cells are largely receptor negative. Androgenic stimulation of prostate growth is targeted on the stromal compartment that in turn stimulates the epithelium through release of growth factors, so-called andromedins. In the adult prostate, androgens are involved in the terminal differentiation of the secretory epithelium and directly stimulate the expression of secreted proteins such as prostate-specific antigen (PSA) or kallikreins. Defects in the development of the prostate are found in subjects with loss-of-function mutations in the 5α-reductase type 2 enzyme or in the androgen receptor.

THE PROSTATE IS AN ANDROGEN-DEPENDENT ORGAN

Androgen hormones are the key regulators of male differentiation and are required for the development of the prostate, the seminal vesicles, the vas deferens, and the male external genital organs. In the adult prostate gland,

continuous androgenic stimulation is necessary for tissue homeostasis and the maintenance of secretory function. During early embryonic development testosterone leads to the development and stabilization of the Wolffian duct system and subsequent differentiation into the epididymis, vas deferens, and seminal vesicles. For development of the prostate the androgen DHT is required. Its formation is controlled by 5α-reductase that is expressed in the urogenital sinus and swellings, but not in the Wolffian duct (Quigley, 1998). A deficiency in type 2 5α-reductase activity—for example, due to mutation of the gene—leads to an incomplete form of male pseudohermaphroditism.[1] The prostate in affected males remains rudimentary and is composed exclusively of stromal cells.[2] This occurs despite normal serum testosterone levels demonstrating the dependency of the prostate on DHT and suggesting a possible role of this androgen in diseases of aberrant prostate growth. After birth, androgen levels decrease to almost undetectable levels and prostate growth ceases at a size of 1 to 2 g until androgens rise again during puberty. In parallel, the prostate gland grows to the adult size of approximately 20 g between 10 and 20 years of age.[3]

Maintenance of prostate tissue and function requires chronic stimulation with androgens. Androgen deprivation—for example, by castration—induces programmed cell death (apoptosis) in the androgen-dependent prostate cells and results in a rapid involution of the gland.[4,5] The different cell types of the prostate display different sensitivity to the induction of apoptosis in this process. Whereas the secretory luminal epithelial cells are the most sensitive, basal epithelial cells and stromal cells are less prone to androgen deprivation-induced cell death. Some time after androgen withdrawal, a rudimentary prostate composed mainly of stroma tissue is left. This process is reversible and restimulation with androgen induces rapid proliferation and growth of the gland to its adult size. Induction of programmed cell death by androgen withdrawal is the basis for the treatment of advanced prostate cancer.[6]

ANDROGENS AND ANDROGEN METABOLISM IN THE PROSTATE

At first sight, it is surprising that the prostate absolutely depends on DHT and that testosterone alone is not sufficient, despite this androgen working well in other organs. Dihydrotestosterone has a slightly higher affinity for the androgen receptor (AR), the intracellular mediator of androgen action and the AR-DHT complex is more stable than the AR-testosterone complex, however, this alone does not explain the different action. Testosterone entering the prostate tissue is rapidly converted to DHT and, therefore, the DHT concentration in the prostate is about 10 times higher than the concentration of testosterone.[7] Consequently, both the formation of DHT by 5α-reductase and the balance between synthesis and metabolism are critical to constantly maintain the required level of androgen in the prostate tissue. Experiments in rats revealed that a certain threshold of androgen concentration has to be exceeded for induction of prostate growth.[8] This threshold was two to three times lower for DHT compared with testosterone.[8,9] Some DHT is also produced in other peripheral organs, such as the skin, and is circulating in the blood; but its concentration is low, and, although it can readily diffuse into the prostate, its contribution to prostatic DHT is probably negligible, at least under normal physiological conditions. It may, however, play a role during endocrine treatment of prostate cancer or treatment of benign prostatic hyperplasia (BPH) by 5α-reductase inhibitors.[10]

There are two 5α-reductase isoenzymes that catalyze the irreversible conversion of testosterone to DHT (Table 9.1).[11,12] The type 1 enzyme is expressed in most tissues of the body where 5α-reductase activity is present and is the dominant form in skin and liver.[13] The predominant enzyme in the prostate and genital organs is type 2; the type 1 enzyme is also expressed, but at a lower level. The two enzymes are encoded by two separate genes on

chromosomes 5 and 2, respectively. They share a similar hydrophobicity pattern, although their amino-acid sequence shows only about 50% identity, and there are profound differences in their enzymatic properties with regard to pH-optimum and substrate affinity[14] (see Table 9.1). Both isoenzymes are highly hydrophobic and are associated with intracellular membranes. Solubilization requires the use of detergents, and the lipophilic environment influences enzymatic activity.[15] Genetic defects have been found only for the type 2 enzyme: men with pseudo-hermaphroditism due to 5α-reductase deficiency have mutations in this isotype.[16,17] The lack of virilization in these subjects demonstrate that the type 1 enzyme alone is not sufficient to provide enough DHT in the genital organs.

The type 1 5α-reductase enzyme is predominant in the sebaceous glands of the skin and has a role in acne and male baldness. Its overall function, however, is unclear, because a genetic deficiency of this enzyme has been not been discovered. The contribution of the 5α-reductase type 1 to DHT production in the human prostate is not yet clear. Based on selective inhibitor experiment it was concluded that it contributes approximately 20% to 30%.[18] Recent expression studies in prostate cancer tissue indicate downregulation of the type 2 and relative upregulation of expression of the type 1 enzyme suggesting an increased importance of the type 1 enzyme in the production of DHT in cancer[19,20]

The major source of androgenic hormones in the prostate is the testosterone supplied by the testis through the blood flow—approximately 10% originates from the adrenal gland, mainly from dehydroepiandrosterone and androstenedione and their sulfates (Figure 9.1). Adrenal androgens are themselves weak androgens and, in addition, can be converted to DHT in the prostate tissue.[21–23] This source of androgens is especially important in the situation of androgen withdrawal therapy, where adrenal androgens significantly contribute to residual androgenic stimulation in tumors of the prostate. On the other side, DHT is extensively metabolized in prostate tissue (see Figure 9.1). It is converted to several androstane derivatives, androsterone and androstanedion and further to androstane and androsterone glucuronides, which can be excreted.[24] The tight control of the androgen metabolism within the prostate secures a constant level of DHT that is not too sensitive to variations in testosterone supply.

One of the metabolites of DHT, 5α-androstane-3β,17β-diol (Adiol), has estrogenic activity and is considered the principal estrogenic steroid in the prostate.[25] It binds to and activates the estrogen receptors (ER) -α and -β, both of which are expressed in prostate tissue.[26,27] Whereas ERα expression is higher in stromal cells, ERβ is the predominating ER in epithelial cells. There is a reciprocal regulatory link between the androgen receptor and ERβ. Genistein-activated ERβ down regulates expression of AR and thus influences the sensitivity of prostate epithelial cells to androgenic

Table 9.1 Properties of 5α-reductase isoenzymes

	Type 1	Type 2
Gene	SRD5A1	SRD5A2
Chromosomal localization	5p15	2p23
pH optimum	6.5–9	5.5
K_M (μM)	10	0.4
Inhibition by finasteride	–	+
Inhibition by dutasteride	+	+

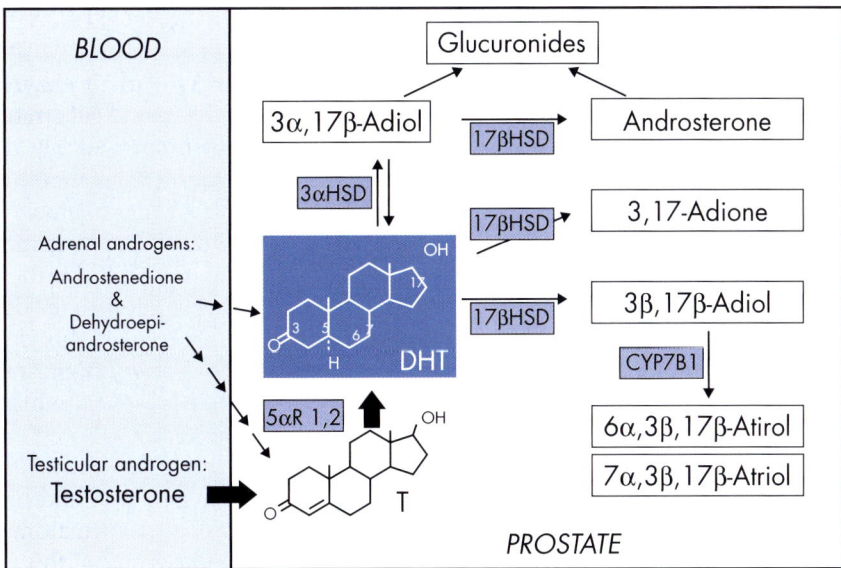

Fig. 9.1

Androgen metabolism in the prostate gland. The prostate is nourished though the blood circulation with the testicular androgen testosterone and the adrenal androgens androstenedione and dehydroepiandrosterone. The latter two contribute about 10% of total androgen supply. In the prostate cells, 5α-reductase (5αR) rapidly converts testosterone (T) to dihydrotestosterone (DHT), the pivotal androgen in the prostate gland. It is absolutely required for prostate development and growth and acts through activation of the androgen receptor. DHT is metabolized in prostate tissues to 3α,17β-androstanediol (3α,17β-Adiol), 3,17-androstanedione (3,17-Adione) and 3β,17β-androstanediol (3β,17β-Adiol) through the activities of different isoforms of hydroxysteroid dehydrogenase (HSD). 3α,17β-Androstanediol is further metabolized to androsterone and these two steroids are also glucuronidated. 3β,17β-Androstanediol, which has estrogenic activity and activates estrogen receptors, is further metabolized to 6α- and 7α- 3β, 17β androstanetriols (6α, 3β, 17β-Atriol, 7α, 3β, 17β-Atriol) by the cytochrome P450 CYP7B1.[24]

stimuli.[28] Under physiological conditions, one can expect Adiol to exert this effect by activating ERβ in epithelial prostate cells, thus representing a brake for overshooting androgenic stimulation.[25]

THE ANDROGEN RECEPTOR MEDIATES HORMONE EFFECTS AT THE CELLULAR LEVEL

The androgen receptor is a member of the superfamily of nuclear receptors (Figure 9.2).[29–31] It binds androgens with high affinity, becomes activated, and mediates the intracellular actions of androgens. Intracellular signal transmission involves a cascade of activation processes and interaction with other components of the cell's signaling network. The AR protein is composed of three functional domains: an N-terminal transactivation domain, a central DNA-binding domain built up of two zinc finger motifs, and a C-terminal ligand-binding domain.

After synthesis, the AR is associated with heat shock proteins in an inactive state. Binding of an androgen to the hormone-binding domain initiates a cascade of events that finally result in activation to a transcription factor that regulates the transcription of androgen-responsive genes. Activation includes dissociation of heat shock proteins, hyperphosphorylation, conformational changes, translocation into the nucleus, dimerization, and association with co-modulatory proteins.[32] Activated AR then interacts with the cellular transcription machinery and regulates transcription of genes through binding to androgen-responsive elements (AREs) in the promoters of androgen-responsive genes.[33] Gene regulation may be positive or negative depending on the promoter and cellular context.[34]

Besides through binding an androgenic hormone, AR can also be activated by ligand-independent processes through interaction with growth factor and regulatory signaling pathways. This route of activation becomes especially important in the situation of low androgen concentrations and plays a major role in generation of therapy resistance in prostate cancer.[35,36] Besides transcriptional regulatory effects, the androgen receptor also seems to have an additional, chromatin-independent activity that results in rapid activation of mitogen-activated kinases.[37] This nongenomic function is not well understood so far, but it may be important for androgen action in growth and differentiation.

The gene encoding the androgen receptor protein is located on the long arm of the X-chromosome at position Xq11-12 (see Figure 9.2).[38] Due to the X-chromosomal inheritance, males always receive their androgen receptor

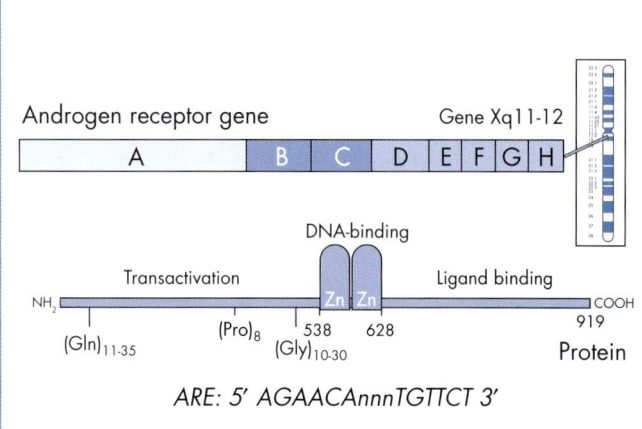

Fig. 9.2

The androgen receptor. Binding of androgens to the ligand-binding domain in the C-terminus induces a cascade of activation steps finally resulting in a transcriptionally active androgen receptor that regulates the transcription of genes by binding to target sequences in the chromatin, the so-called androgen responsive elements (AREs). This is done through the central DNA-binding domain of the receptor that consists of two zinc finger elements. The third domain, at the N-terminus, is mainly involved in the interaction with co-modulatory proteins and is called the transactivation domain. This domain contains two polymorphic amino-acid repeats encoded by triplet repeats in the AR gene that vary in size among individuals.

gene from their mother and are affected in case of an impaired-function mutation. In the first exon, encoding for the N-terminus of the receptor, there are two polymorphic triplet repeat regions encoding a glutamine and a glycine repeat, respectively, that vary in size. The lengths of these repeats have an influence on AR transcriptional activity and seem to be associated with prostate cancer risk and progression.[39] Pathological extension of the CAG (glutamine) repeat is the underlying cause of spinal and bulbar muscular atrophy.[40] The androgen receptor gene is a locus of frequent mutations (http//:www.mcgill.ca/androgendb). Several hundred mutations have been identified, most of them in male pseudohermaphroditism patients with various degrees of androgen insensitivity where the mutations result in partial or complete loss of AR function.[41,42] In contrast, in prostate cancer patients a number of gain-of-function mutations have been detected in tumor tissues that lead to

promiscuous receptors that are activated by non-androgen steroids and antiandrogens.[36,43]

ANDROGEN RECEPTOR FUNCTION AND GENE REGULATION

Regulation of prostate growth and function requires a close reciprocal interaction between the stromal and epithelial tissue components (Figure 9.3).[44,45] There is strong experimental evidence that androgens control the inductive function of the stroma to induce prostate growth. This is based on two observations: 5α-reductase activity was found predominantly in the stromal tissue of the prostate,[46,47] and, during fetal development, AR is expressed in the stroma at the time when prostate growth is initiated and only later appears in the epithelial cells of

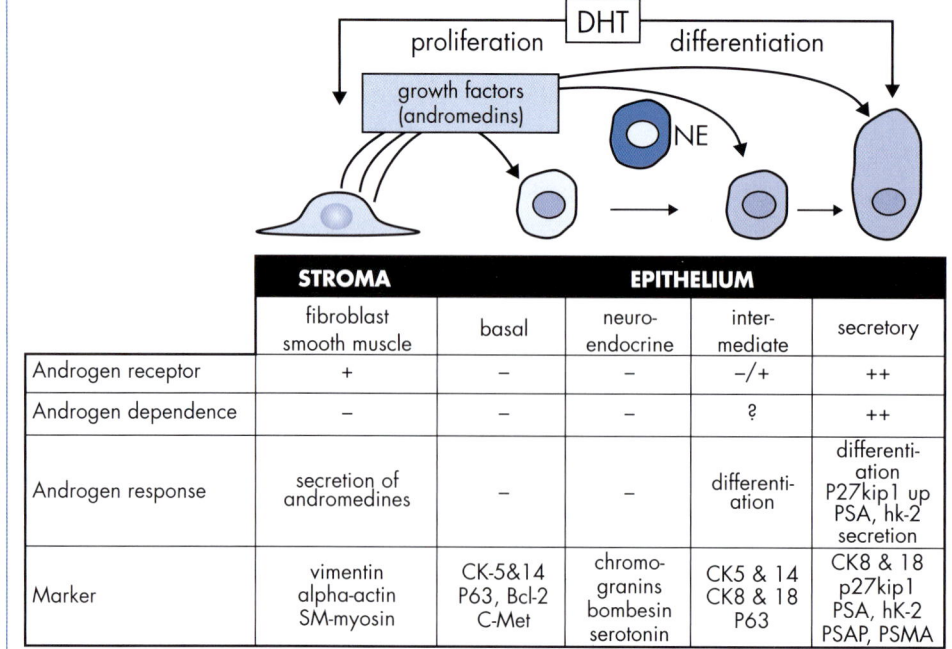

	STROMA	EPITHELIUM			
	fibroblast smooth muscle	basal	neuro-endocrine	inter-mediate	secretory
Androgen receptor	+	–	–	–/+	++
Androgen dependence	–	–	–	?	++
Androgen response	secretion of andromedines	–	–	differenti-ation	differenti-ation P27kip1 up PSA, hk-2 secretion
Marker	vimentin alpha-actin SM-myosin	CK-5&14 P63, Bcl-2 C-Met	chromo-granins bombesin serotonin	CK5 & 14 CK8 & 18 P63	CK8 & 18 p27kip1 PSA, hK-2 PSAP, PSMA

Figure 9.3

Androgen effects in different cells of the prostate gland. (DHT, dihydrotestosterone; 5-HT, 5-hydroxytryptamine (serotonin); NE, neuroendocrine cell; PSA, prostate-specific antigen.)

the prostate. In prenatal rodents, only the mesenchyme of the prostate contains AR; epithelial cells do not express AR before the end of the first postnatal week.[48–50] Moreover, recombination experiments by Cunha et al showed that AR in the stroma alone is sufficient for prostate tissue to respond to androgens and to induce prostatic morphogenesis and growth through paracrine action.[51]

The paracrine effects of androgen-stimulated mesenchyme cells on adjacent epithelial cells is mediated through the action of various growth factors.[52,53] Thus, androgens control prostate growth via activation of the AR in the stroma through that way orchestrating a network of autocrine and paracrine factors that function as andromedins, mediating androgen effects to the epithelial cells.[54,55]

The different cell types of the prostate express very different levels of androgen receptor. The highest protein levels are present in the secretory epithelial cells. In these cells the AR is a differentiation and survival factor. It enhances the stability of the cell cycle inhibitor p27kip1 and thus proliferation seems to be prevented, even in the presence of andromedins.[56,57] On the other hand, when persistent AR activation is interrupted by removal of androgens, the secretory epithelial cells undergo programmed cell death. The androgen receptor also regulates the expression of genes characteristic for differentiated secretory epithelial cells, such as those encoding PSA and kallikreins.[58]

Unlike the secretory cells, the basal epithelial cells express little or no AR and are insensitive to androgen withdrawal. This cell compartment is the reservoir for renewal of the epithelial cells of the prostate gland. According to the stem cell model, basal endothelial cell layers contain the stem cells that give rise to transient amplifying cells; these mature into an intermediate cell type that proliferates and finally migrates to the secretory luminal cell layer where it differentiates.[59] Androgen receptor expression turned-on during the differentiation process of the intermediate cells initiates terminal differentiation by inhibiting further proliferation and stimulating secretory function. Another cell type found in the epithelial compartment is the neuroendocrine cells that are interspersed in the epithelial cell layers.[60] They do not express the androgen receptor and are insensitive to androgen withdrawal. Neuroendocrine cells secrete a number of peptides, such as chromogranins, neuron-specific enolase, bombesin, calcitonin, somatostatin, and 5-hydroxytryptamine (5HT, serotonin) that exert paracrine effects on the surrounding cells. Finally, in the stromal cells AR is expressed in fibroblast as well as in smooth muscle cells; however, AR levels are lower than in secretory epithelial cells.[61] The AR in the stromal cells enhances expression and secretion of growth factors that have autocrine and paracrine effects and suppresses inhibitors such as transforming growth factor-β (TGFβ).[54,62–64]

Despite a clear picture of the actions of androgens and AR in the different cell types of prostate, we don't yet know many of the details of regulation of proliferation and differentiation and cell-type specific gene expression at the molecular level. High-throughput gene expression profiling and proteomics techniques that are now available to identify androgen-regulated genes and proteins should facilitate and enhance efforts in this direction. These techniques are broadly used now to elucidate androgen and AR action in prostate cancer and prostate cancer progression,[58,65–67] and they will also allow us to further our understanding of their effects in the normal prostate.

REFERENCES

1. Imperato-McGinley J, Zhu YS. Androgens and male physiology the syndrome of 5alpha-reductase-2 deficiency. Mol Cell Endocrinol 2002;198:51–59.

2. Imperato McGinley J, Sanchez RS, Spencer JR, et al. Comparison of the effects of the 5 alpha-reductase inhibitor finasteride and the antiandrogen flutamide on prostate and genital differentiation: dose-response studies. Endocrinology 1992;131:1149–1156.

3. Isaacs JT. Common characteristics of human and canine benign prostatic hyperplasia. In Kimball FA (ed): New approaches to the study of benign prostatic hyperplasia. New York: AR Liss Inc, 1984, pp 217–234.

4. Kyprianou N, Isaacs JT. Activation of programmed cell death in the rat ventral prostate after castration. Endocrinology 1988;122:552–562.

5. English HF, Kyprianou N, Isaacs JT. Relationship between DNA fragmentation and apoptosis in the programmed cell death in the rat prostate following castration. Prostate 1989;15:233–250.

6. Denmeade SR, Isaacs JT. Activation of programmed (apoptotic) cell death for the treatment of prostate cancer. Adv Pharmacol 1996;35:281–306.

7. Lamb JC, English H, Levandoski PL, et al. Prostatic involution in rats induced by a novel 5 alpha-reductase inhibitor, SK&F 105657: role for testosterone in the androgenic response. Endocrinology 1992;130:685–694.

8. Rittmaster RS, Magor KE, Manning AP, et al. Differential effect of 5alpha-reductase inhibition and castration on androgen-regulated gene expression in rat prostate. Mol Endocrinol 1991;5:1023–1029.

9. Wright AS, Douglas RC, Thomas LN, et al. Androgen-induced regrowth in the castrated rat ventral prostate: role of 5alpha-reductase. Endocrinology 1999;140:4509–4515.

10. Bartsch G, Rittmaster RS, Klocker H. Dihydrotestosterone and the concept of 5alpha-reductase inhibition in human benign prostatic hyperplasia. World J Urol 2002;19:413–425.

11. Russell DW, Wilson JD. Steroid 5 alpha-reductase: two genes/two enzymes. Annu Rev Biochem 1994;63:25–61.

12. Thigpen AE, Silver RI, Guileyardo JM, et al. Tissue distribution and ontogeny of steroid 5 alpha-reductase isozyme expression. J Clin Invest 1993;92:903–910.

13. Jenkins EP, Andersson S, Imperato-McGinley J, et al. Genetic and pharmacological evidence for more than one human steroid 5 alpha-reductase. J Clin Invest 1992;89:293–300.

14. Iehle C, Delos S, Guirou O, et al. Human prostatic steroid 5 alpha-reductase isoforms—a comparative study of selective inhibitors. J Steroid Biochem Mol Biol 1995;54:273–279.

15. Weisser H, Tunn S, Behnke B, et al. Effects of the sabal serrulata extract IDS 89 and its subfractions on 5 alpha-reductase activity in human benign prostatic hyperplasia. Prostate 1996;28:300–306.

16. Thigpen AE, Davis DL, Milatovich A, et al. Molecular genetics of steroid 5alpha-reductase 2 deficiency. J Clin Invest 1992;90:799–809.

17. Wilson JD, Griffin JE, Russell DW. Steroid 5alpha-reductase 2 deficiency. Endocrine Soc 1993;14:577–593.

18. Clark R, Hermann D, Gabriel H, et al. Effective suppression of dihydrotestosterone (DHT) by GI198745, a novel, dual 5 alpha reductase inhibitor. J Urol 1999;161:1037.

19. Thomas LN, Douglas RC, Vessey JP, et al. 5alpha-reductase type 1 immunostaining is enhanced in some prostate cancers compared

with benign prostatic hyperplasia epithelium. J Urol 2003;170:2019–2025.

20. Luo J, Dunn TA, Ewing CM, et al. Decreased gene expression of steroid 5 alpha-reductase 2 in human prostate cancer: implications for finasteride therapy of prostate carcinoma. Prostate 2003;57:134–139.

21. Labrie F, Dupont A, Simard J, et al. Intracrinology: the basis for the rational design of endocrine therapy at all stages of prostate cancer. Eur Urol 1993;24 Suppl 2:94–105.

22. Labrie C, Simard J, Zhao HF, et al. Stimulation of androgen-dependent gene expression by the adrenal precursors dehydroepiandrosterone and androstenedione in the rat ventral prostate. Endocrinology 1989;124:2745–2754.

23. Labrie C, Belanger A, Labrie F. Androgenic activity of dehydroepiandrosterone and androstenedione in the rat ventral prostate. Endocrinology 1988;123:1412–1417.

24. Isaacs JT. Testosterone and the prostate. In Nieschlag E, Behre HM (eds): Testosterone, 3rd ed. Cambridge: Cambridge Press; 2004, pp 347–374.

25. Weihua Z, Lathe R, Warner M, et al. An endocrine pathway in the prostate, ERbeta, AR, 5alpha-androstane-3beta,17beta-diol, and CYP7B1, regulates prostate growth. Proc Natl Acad Sci USA 2002;99:13589–13594.

26. Ito T, Tachibana M, Yamamoto S, et al. Expression of estrogen receptor (ER-alpha and ER-beta) mRNA in human prostate cancer. Eur Urol 2001;40:557–563.

27. Fixemer T, Remberger K, Bonkhoff H. Differential expression of the estrogen receptor beta (ERbeta) in human prostate tissue, premalignant changes, and in primary, metastatic, and recurrent prostatic adenocarcinoma. Prostate 2003;54:79–87.

28. Bektic J, Berger AP, Pfeil K, et al. Androgen receptor regulation by physiological concentrations of the isoflavonoid genistein in androgen-dependent LNCaP cells is mediated by estrogen receptor beta. Eur Urol 2004;45:245–51.

29. Mangelsdorf DJ, Thummel C, Beato M, et al. The nuclear receptor superfamily: the second decade. Cell 1995;83:835–839.

30. Tenbaum S, Baniahmad A. Nuclear receptors: structure, function and involvement in disease. Int J Biochem Cell Biol 1997;29:1325–1341.

31. Owen GI, Zelent A. Origins and evolutionary diversification of the nuclear receptor superfamily. Cell Mol Life Sci 2000;57:809–827.

32. Beato M, Truss M, Chavez S. Control of transcription by steroid hormones. Ann NY Acad Sci 1996;784:93–123.

33. McEwan IJ. Gene regulation through chromatin remodelling by members of the nuclear receptor superfamily. Biochem Soc Trans 2000;28:369–373.

34. Schneikert J, Peterziel H, Defossez PA, et al. Androgen receptor-Ets protein interaction is a novel mechanism for steroid hormone-mediated down-modulation of matrix metalloproteinase expression. J Biol Chem 1996;271:23907–23913.

35. Culig Z, Klocker H, Bartsch G, et al. Androgen receptors in prostate cancer. J Urol 2003;170:1363–1369.

36. Eder IE, Culig Z, Putz T, et al. Molecular biology of the androgen receptor: from molecular understanding to the clinic. Eur Urol 2001;40:241–251.

37. Peterziel H, Mink S, Schonert A, et al. Rapid signalling by androgen receptor in prostate cancer cells. Oncogene 1999;18:6322–6329.

38. Brown CJ, Goss SJ, Lubahn DB, et al. Androgen receptor locus on the human X chromosome: regional localization to Xq11-12 and description of a DNA polymorphism. Am J Hum Genet 1989;44:264–269.

39. Clark PE, Irvine RA, Coetzee GA. The androgen receptor CAG repeat and prostate cancer risk. Methods Mol Med 2003;81:255–266.

40. Walcott JL, Merry DE. Trinucleotide repeat disease. The androgen receptor in spinal and bulbar muscular atrophy. Vitam Horm 2002;65:127–147.

41. Hiort O, Holterhus PM. Androgen insensitivity and male infertility. Int J Androl 2003;26:16–20.

42. McPhaul MJ, Griffin JE. Male pseudohermaphroditism caused by mutations of the human androgen receptor. J Clin Endocrinol Metab 1999;84:3435–3441.

43. Culig Z, Klocker H, Bartsch G, et al. Androgen receptor mutations in carcinoma of the prostate: significance for endocrine therapy. Am J Pharmacogenomics 2001;1:241–249.

44. Verhoeven G, Swinnen K, Cailleau J, et al. The role of cell-cell interactions in androgen action. J Steroid Biochem Mol Biol 1992;41:487–494.

45. Cunha GR. Role of mesenchymal-epithelial interactions in normal and abnormal development of the mammary gland and prostate. Cancer 1994;74:1030–1044.

46. Bruchovsky N, Lieskovsky G. Increased ratio of 5 alpha-reductase: 3 alpha (beta)-hydroxysteroid dehydrogenase activities in the hyperplastic human prostate. J Endocrinol 1979;80:289–301.

47. Silver RI, Wiley EL, Davis DL, et al. Expression and regulation of steroid 5 alpha-reductase 2 in prostate disease. J Urol 1994;152:433–437.

48. Shannon JM, Cunha GR. Autoradiographic localization of androgen binding in the developing mouse prostate. Prostate 1983;4:367–373.

49. Shannon JM, Cunha GR. Characterization of androgen binding and deoxyribonucleic acid synthesis in prostate-like structures induced in the urothelium of testicular feminized (Tfm/Y) mice. Biol Reprod 1984;31:175–183.

50. Thompson TC, Cunha GR, Shannon JM, et al. Androgen-induced biochemical responses in epithelium lacking androgen receptors: characterization of androgen receptors in the mesenchymal derivative of urogenital sinus. J Steroid Biochem 1986;25:627–634.

51. Cunha GR, Young P, Brody J. Role of terine epithelium in the development of myometrial smooth muscle cells. Biology of Reproduction 1989;40:861–871.

52. Cunha GR. Growth factors as mediators of androgen action during male urogenital development. Prostate 1996;6:22–25.

53. Lee C. Cellular interactions in prostate cancer. Br J Urol 1997;79 Suppl 1:21–7.

54. Lu W, Luo Y, Kan M, et al. Fibroblast growth factor-10. A second candidate stromal to epithelial cell andromedin in prostate. J Biol Chem 1999;274:12827–12834.

55. Planz B, Wang Q, Kirley SD, et al. Regulation of keratinocyte growth factor receptor and androgen receptor in epithelial cells of the human prostate. J Urol 2001;166:678–683.

56. Waltregny D, Leav I, Signoretti S, et al. Androgen-driven prostate epithelial cell proliferation and differentiation in vivo involve the regulation of p27. Mol Endocrinol 2001;15:765–782.

57. Tsihlias J, Zhang W, Bhattacharya N, et al. Involvement of p27Kip1 in G1 arrest by high dose 5 alpha-dihydrotestosterone in LNCaP human prostate cancer cells. Oncogene 2000;19:670–679.

58. Waghray A, Feroze F, Schober MS, et al. Identification of androgen-regulated genes in the prostate cancer cell line LNCaP by serial analysis of gene expression and proteomic analysis. Proteomics 2001;1:1327–1338.

59. Schalken JA, van Leenders G. Cellular and molecular biology of the prostate: stem cell biology. Urology 2003;62:11–20.

60. di Sant'Agnese PA. Neuroendocrine cells of the prostate and neuroendocrine differentiation in prostatic carcinoma: a review of morphologic aspects. Urology 1998;51:121–124.

61. Kimura N, Mizokami A, Oonuma T, et al. Immunocytochemical localization of androgen receptor with polyclonal antibody in paraffin-embedded human tissues [see comments]. J Histochem Cytochem 1993;41:671–678.

62. Planz B, Aretz HT, Wang Q, et al. Immunolocalization of the keratinocyte growth factor in benign and neoplastic human prostate and its relation to androgen receptor. Prostate 1999;41:233–242.

63. Chung LW. The role of stromal-epithelial interaction in normal and malignant growth. Cancer Surv 1995;23:33–42.

64. Wikstrom P, Westin P, Stattin P, et al. Early castration-induced upregulation of transforming growth factor beta1 and its receptors is associated with tumor cell apoptosis and a major decline in serum prostate-specific antigen in prostate cancer patients. Prostate 1999;38:268–277.

65. Velasco AM, Gillis KA, Li Y, et al. Identification and validation of novel androgen-regulated genes in prostate cancer. Endocrinology 2004;145:3913–24.

66. Xu LL, Su YP, Labiche R, et al. Quantitative expression profile of androgen-regulated genes in prostate cancer cells and identification of prostate-specific genes. Int J Cancer 2001;92:322–8.

67. Eder IE, Haag P, Basik M, et al. Gene expression changes following androgen receptor elimination in LNCaP prostate cancer cells. Mol Carcinog 2003;37:181–91.

Growth factor signaling in the regulation of prostate growth

10

Jason Bylund, Anastasios Tahmatzopoulos, Natasha Kyprianou

INTRODUCTION

The regulation of prostate growth and survival is represented by a delicate balance between cell proliferation and apoptosis (programmed cell death). Loss of this growth equilibrium due to increased proliferation and/or reduced apoptosis ultimately results in aberrant, tumorigenic growth. In recent years there has been an explosion in our understanding of the mechanisms underlying this loss of regulatory control, and ongoing work promises to bring new preventive, diagnostic, and therapeutic insights for the management of prostate cancer.

Understanding the pathways governing normal and pathologic prostate growth regulation requires an appreciation of the androgen signaling axis and the critical role the androgen receptor (AR) plays in the development of hormone-refractory prostate cancer. In its early stages, prostate tumors are, like the normal prostate gland, androgen-dependent, relying primarily on AR signaling-mediated growth and survival of the luminal epithelial cells. Serum testosterone is converted to the active metabolic androgen 5α-dihydrotestosterone (DHT) by the 5α-reductase enzyme, which then binds to the AR in the cytoplasm. The DHT-AR complex is translocated into the nucleus, where it dimerizes and combines with androgen-response elements and other coactivators to affect cell growth. Prostate tumors retain the AR signaling pathways and thus are universally responsive, at least initially, to androgen ablation therapy. Although tumor regression occurs initially with androgen ablation, in the majority of patients, tumors eventually lose their sensitivity to antiandrogen therapy and

relapse to an androgen-independent state. Due to the emergence of androgen-independent prostate tumor epithelial cells, conventional treatments lose their efficacy as a means of increasing survival of patients with advanced disease. However, current advances in our understanding of the biochemical mechanisms underlying the development of androgen independence provide new insights into molecular targeting of hormone-refractory prostate cancer that would effectively increase patient survival. The challenge remains to fully exploit the apoptotic pathways towards identification of novel therapeutic modalities that will eliminate both the androgen-dependent as well as the androgen-independent prostate tumor cells, with minimum toxicity in the patient.

The molecular mechanisms that lead to the development of androgen-independent prostate cancer can be divided into two types: those that involve the AR and those that bypass it.[1] Mechanisms that involve the AR pathway include over-expression of the AR gene (*AR*), mutations of *AR* that allow for increased activation of the receptor by lower levels of androgens, or changes in the growth factors or coactivators involved in the pathway that allow androgen-independent activation of *AR* and its transcriptional regulatory elements.[2] A rapidly growing body of evidence documents an accumulation of molecular changes inducing gain-of-function in the *AR* signaling pathways during prostate cancer progression. Such changes render prostate cancer cells resistant to androgen ablation because of their acquired ability to activate novel *AR* signaling pathways for proliferation and survival without requiring physiological androgen ligand binding. Mechanisms that bypass the AR pathway altogether include increased expression of apoptosis regulators such as the BCL2 oncoprotein, which, as a potent apoptosis suppressor, can protect cells from the proapoptotic influence of antiandrogen therapy.[3]

Prostate cancer has a strong predilection for bone metastasis with other distant sites being only rarely involved. These lesions generally consist of multiple small nodules or diffuse lymphatic spread, as opposed to large metastatic deposits.[4] Compelling evidence documents the importance of angiogenesis in the development and osteoblastic nature of prostate cancer bone metastasis, and implicates the bone itself as an active facilitator of the metastatic process. The current understanding of the molecular mechanisms dictating prostate cancer cell survival, active proliferation, dissemination, and metastasis outside the realm of the normally imposed androgen regulatory axis provides promising therapeutic tools for the treatment of advanced disease.

A wide array of growth factors, along with their membrane and intracellular signaling effectors, are involved in dynamic interplay with the androgen signaling axis to maintain tissue homeostasis in the normal prostate. Better insights into the growth factor signaling pathways that regulate prostate growth may lead to the identification of molecular biomarkers that will allow early detection of prostate cancer and monitoring of disease progression or therapeutic response. Prostate-specific antigen (PSA) is a serine protease that has served as a serum marker used for prostate cancer screening as well as a means of monitoring disease progression or relapse following treatment for many years; limitations, however, surrounding the use of PSA as a predictive marker for prostate cancer have recently led to significant controversy. Criticisms include the low positive predictive value of increased PSA, lack of statistical mortality benefit due to screening, and the morbidity of prostate biopsy.[5] While extensive PSA testing has allowed clinicians to detect prostate cancer at an earlier stage, PSA levels do not distinguish indolent prostate tumors from more aggressive cancers. Ongoing efforts are focused on finding modalities that will allow the identification of the most aggressive prostate tumors, which would require more intense and selectively-targeted treatment approaches, while those cancers that may pose little or no risk of actual clinical morbidity or mortality could be treated more conservatively.[6]

Much progress has been made in the characterization of apoptosis regulatory signaling pathways, and the functional relationships these pathways have with the other growth regulatory mechanisms within the prostate in the normal and malignant state. Perhaps one of the most important regulators of prostate apoptosis is indirectly the AR itself. Removal of AR stimulation causes prostate cells to undergo apoptosis, which is why antiandrogen therapy has been such an effective treatment for prostate cancer. Other pathways that lead to the execution of the suicidal program of apoptotic cell death include the p53 tumor suppressor gene, which responds to DNA damage by monitoring genomic integrity and, to reduce the occurrence of perpetuated mutations, either inhibits entry into the cell cycle—enabling DNA repair—or triggers apoptosis. Thus, mutation of the p53 gene can lead to loss of its proapoptotic and tumor suppressor activity, increasing the cell's susceptibility to neoplastic growth. It appears p53 also can up-regulate *BAX* and down-regulate *BCL2*, thus modulating the ratio of these two factors, itself an important determinant of apoptosis. Transforming growth factor-β (TGFβ) is another growth factor that, among its other functions, serves as a regulator of prostate growth via its ability to inhibit cell proliferation and induce apoptosis.[7,8] Loss of TGFβ expression or of sensitivity to its effects jeopardizes both its anti-proliferative and proapoptotic functions, leading to increased proliferation of prostate epithelial cells. The BCL2 oncoprotein is a potent suppressor of apoptosis in a number of cellular systems and its overexpression has been associated with progression to hormone refractory prostate cancer.[9] The intracellular events that lead to the execution of a cell's apoptotic death are dictated by the caspase family of proteases via a cascade of sequential activation of initiator (such as caspase 1) and effector caspases (such as caspase 3 and caspase 9). The apoptotic action of caspases can, in turn, be modulated by another powerful "family" of adapter inhibitory apoptotic proteins (IAPs), which can bind the caspases and sequester their proteolytic activity.[7]

GROWTH FACTOR SIGNALING PATHWAYS IN NORMAL AND MALIGNANT PROSTATE

Increases in autocrine and paracrine growth-factor loops are among the most commonly reported changes correlated with progression of prostate cancer from localized and androgen-dependent to disseminated and androgen-independent. The progression from normal prostate function to malignant disease is marked by numerous changes at the molecular level, including the upregulation of positive growth factors, the deregulation of the cell cycle and apoptosis pathways, and downregulation of tumor suppressor genes (Box 10.1). These changes disrupt the homeostatic balance between cell proliferation and apoptosis and facilitate the acquisition of a highly aggressive, malignant phenotype by the prostate epithelial cells.

In this chapter we present an overview of the regulatory players controlling prostate growth, highlighting the contributions of the critical growth-factor signaling pathways, and examining their functional involvement in the malignant transformation and the development of androgen independence of prostate cancer cells, as well as their potential clinical significance as therapeutic targets for advanced prostate cancer and markers of tumor progression.

THE ANDROGEN RECEPTOR AXIS IN PROSTATE CANCER

The AR consists of an *N*-terminal transcriptional regulatory domain (AF1) that functions in the absence of the ligand, a DNA binding domain, a hinge region, and a *C*-terminal ligand-binding domain that is also associated with a second transcriptional regulatory function (AF2). In its unliganded state, the AR is sequestered with chaperones and is not concentrated in the nucleus. Upon ligand binding, a nuclear import signal is exposed and the receptor becomes concentrated in the nucleus, where it binds DNA and interacts with a constellation of transcriptional coregulators and transcription factors.[10,11] Recent evidence suggests that coactivators interacting with the AR as well as transcription factors that can bind directly to DNA could be involved in progression to decreased androgen dependence. Androgen receptors and coactivators are regulated by post-translational modifications such as phosphorylation, sumoylation, and methylation, as well

as acetylation.[12] Studies of HER2/NEU, a member of the epithelial growth factor (EGF) family of receptor tyrosine kinases, show that forced over-expression of HER2/NEU in androgen-dependent prostate cancer cells allows androgen ligand-independent growth. HER2/NEU also activated the AR pathway in the absence of ligand and synergized with low levels of androgen to "superactivate" the pathway. These findings indicate that, by modulating the response to low doses of androgen, a tyrosine kinase receptor may be able to restore AR function to prostate cancer cells, thus ultimately converting androgen-independent cells to their androgen-responsive state.[13] Such results, combined with evidence that the AR is upregulated in androgen-independent cancer cells, provide a strong rationale for therapeutic approaches that target the downregulation of AR to treat advanced prostate cancer, including heat shock protein 90 inhibitors, RNA interference, and ribozyme, antisense, and small-molecule approaches.[14]

GROWTH FACTOR SIGNALING PATHWAYS PROMOTING PROSTATE GROWTH: BEYOND THE ANDROGEN RECEPTOR AXIS

The normal human prostate is a tubular-alveolar gland composed of a well-developed stromal compartment (containing nerves, fibroblasts, infiltrating macrophages, endothelial cell capillaries, and smooth muscle cells) surrounding glandular acini composed of a two-layered epithelium (basal and secretory luminal cells). Most secretory luminal epithelial cells do not normally proliferate and are the terminally differentiated cells that perform the androgen-regulated functions of the prostate, such as PSA production. A growing number of factors and their signaling pathways that work closely to promote growth and proliferation of normal and abnormal prostate epithelial and surrounding stromal cells have been identified.

Since the landmark work of Huggins more than 60 years ago, androgens have been recognized for their crucial function in the regulation of prostate tumor growth.[15] Although the critical role of androgens in this capacity has been appreciated, in terms of their biological requirement for prostate cancer growth, the functional contribution of androgens and the AR axis to the development of hormone-refractory prostate cancer has been less well understood. While normal prostate epithelial cells grow in response to androgen stimulation of adjacent stroma tissue, prostate cancer cells appear to grow in direct response to androgens. Both the direct and indirect response to androgen is mediated through the production of growth factors that act in concordance with androgens to stimulate cell cycle progression—EGF, TGFα, TGFβ, keratinocyte growth factor (KGF), fibroblast growth factor (FGF), and

Table 10.1 Key growth and angiogenesis factors contributing to prostate cancer development and progression

Apoptosis inhibiting	bcl-2[9,100]
	Epidermal growth factor (EGF)[17,19]
	TGFα[18,19]
	Keratinocyte growth factor (KGF; FGF7)[73,101]
	Fibroblast growth factor 2 (FGF2)[71,72]
	Insulin-like growth factor 1 (IGF1)[33,36]
	Nerve growth factor (NGF)[102]
Apoptosis promoting, proliferation inhibiting	Transforming growth factor-β1 (TGFβ1)[46,48,103]
	Transforming growth factor-β receptor type II (TGFβRII)[51]
	P27[Kip1 104] Rb[105]
	PTEN[106]
Angiogenesis factors[64]	Vascular endothelial growth factor (VEGF)[62,64,86]
	Matrix metalloproteinases (MMPs)[64]
	FGF2[72]
	Interleukin 1β[107]
	IGF1[108]
	Nitric oxide[109]
	TGFβ[55]

insulin-like growth factor 1 (IGF1), as well as their cognate ligands, have been reported to be over-expressed in advanced prostate cancer, with the possibility that dysfunctional activation or inactivation of these growth factor pathways and their membrane signaling receptors is causal in driving progression to androgen independence.[16] In this section, we will examine the "protagonist" families of growth factors, their signaling effectors, and their mechanistic significance in the regulation of normal, benign, and malignant prostate growth.

EPIDERMAL GROWTH FACTOR AND TRANSFORMING GROWTH FACTOR-α

Epidermal growth factor and transforming growth factor-α are two structurally related growth factors that bind to the same 170 kDa transmembrane tyrosine kinase EGF receptor (EGFR or ERBB1).[17,18] The expression of EGF in the normal human prostate is confned to the basal cell layer of some benign glands, an expression pattern similar to that of the EGFR. In prostate cancer, however, there is increased expression of both EGF and EGFR in tumor cells compared with benign tissue.[19] In the rat prostate, castration results in a significant decrease in EGF mRNA within 24 hours, while exogenous administration of androgen to the castrated rats reverse the effect,[20] supporting the

potential crosstalk of EGF signaling with the androgen pathway. Expression of TGFα in the normal human prostate is detected predominantly in the stroma, suggesting a paracrine mode of regulation by this growth factor in the prostate gland, since the luminal prostate epithelial cells express high levels of receptor for TGFα. However, in prostatic adenocarcinomas coexpression of TGFα and the EGFR was detected in approximately 50% of the tumors, pointing to a switch from paracrine to autocrine regulation in these tumors.[21]

Several in-vitro and in-vivo experiments have suggested that anti-EGFR treatments may prove to be an alternative treatment modality in prostate cancer. Using a monoclonal anti-EGFR antibody, investigators found that the expression of the phosphorylated EGFR could be reduced, the proliferation of prostatic carcinoma cells could be inhibited, and sensitization to tumor necrosis factor could be achieved.[22] In a more recent in vivo study, administration of ZD1839 (Iressa), an inhibitor of the EGFR-associated tyrosine kinase, to mice with established prostate PC-3 and TSU-PR1 tumors resulted in 70% to 80% inhibition of growth and significant potentiation of cytotoxic treatment with various other chemotherapeutic agents.[23] Similar results were reported in a separate study of CWR22 xenografts in nude mice that showed significant growth inhibition in androgen-dependent and androgen-independent tumors. In the same study, co-administration of Iressa also markedly increased the antiproliferative effects of bicalutamide, carboplatin, and paclitaxel on these tumors.[24] Another study using the anti-EGFR antibody ImClone C225 (IMC-C225) revealed that in nude mice, cellular proliferation and angiogenesis in prostate tumors were inhibited, with a concomitant increase in apoptosis, and that these effects were enhanced by the administration of paclitaxel.[25]

The *ERBB2* oncogene that encodes the ERBB2 (HER2/NEU) protein, a tyrosine kinase receptor homologous to EGFR, has been reported to be amplified in human tumors, resulting in increased mRNA and protein expression, and established associations exist between ERBB2 over-expression and cancer progression.[26] In prostate cancer, HER2/NEU protein expression has been shown to increase in the progression towards androgen-independent disease,[27] although other reports indicate that this occurs only rarely.[28] While some studies showed efficacy in preclinical models of androgen-dependent prostate cancer,[29] clinical attempts to inhibit prostate cancer growth with a recombinant humanized antibody against the HER2/NEU receptor (trastuzumab, Herceptin) were disappointing in a recent Phase II trial.[30]

INSULIN-LIKE GROWTH FACTORS

The IGF axis consists of the growth factors IGF1 and IGF2, whose sequences are related to that of insulin, the two IGF receptors IGF1R and IGF2R, and at least six IGF-binding proteins, IGFBP1 to 6. The IGFBPs are produced by prostatic epithelial cells, and serve to modulate the activity of IGFs by adjusting the amount of free circulating IGF, which is normally less than 1%.[31] Insulin-like growth factors have been shown to be mitogenic, to protect cells from undergoing apoptosis, and also to be necessary for the acquisition of the transformed phenotype, both in vivo and in vitro and in several cell types, via activation of the IGF1R.[32,33] In the prostate, the stromally-produced IGFs act as paracrine growth factors in the normal prostatic epithelium, with an unchanged expression pattern in benign prostatic hyperplasia (BPH).

The intense investigational focus on the IGFs in prostate cancer is justified by evidence supporting a strong association between high plasma IGF1 levels with a significantly higher—as much as fourfold—relative risk of prostate cancer development.[34,35] With better understanding, IGF1 may prove to be a tool for prostate cancer risk assessment and reduction; for example, PSA or other screening of men with higher IGF1 levels at an earlier age could potentially allow earlier detection and treatment.[36]

Clinically, the most promising of the binding proteins appears to be IGFBP3, which binds more than 90% of the circulating IGFs and decreases in patients with prostate cancer, with a significant negative correlation with serum prostate specific antigen (PSA).[37] The well-known tumor marker PSA, a serine protease, has been shown to proteolytically cleave IGFBP3. The loss of the binding protein results in increased bioavailability of IGFs and may result in a potentiation of the growth effects of IGFs in patients with prostate cancer.[38] As IGF1 is able to activate the androgen receptor, resulting in the production of more PSA,[16] a positive feedback loop is created where PSA increases IGF availability, which increases the PSA production, etc. This "vicious cycle" may play a role in prostate cancer progression.

The use of the IGF axis as a therapeutic target has been explored somewhat with the use of IGF1R antisense oligonucleotides, which have been reported to inhibit the IGF axis with a resulting chemosensitization to cisplatin, mitoxantrone and paclitaxel in DU145 cells.[39]

THE NEGATIVE GROWTH FACTOR FAMILY: ACTIVATING APOPTOSIS AND INHIBITING PROLIFERATION

TRANSFORMING GROWTH FACTOR-β

The TGFβ superfamily is the most versatile considering the ability of its members to regulate proliferation, growth arrest, differentiation, and apoptosis of prostatic stromal and epithelial cells, as well as the formation of osteoblastic metastasis. The rationale for targeting TGFβ and its membrane receptors for therapeutic intervention stems from the fact that these proteins represent the most deregulated proximal component of the apoptotic signal transduction pathway in the prostate.

There are five TGFβ isoforms (TGFβ1–5), although only TGFβ1 to 3 are present in mammals.[40] Their effects are exerted through three different receptors, of which types I and II (TβRI and TβRII) are transmembrane serine/threonine kinases involved in signal transduction.[41] Type III (TβRIII) does not possess kinase activity but facilitates the binding of TGFβ to TβRII and TβRI. The TGFβ ligand binds to TβRII and then recruits TβRI to form a heterodimeric complex that ultimately results in inhibition of cell proliferation. Propagation of signaling to the nucleus is mediated through members of the Smad family, with Smad4 playing a key role in the transmission of signals to the nucleus.[42] The intracellular events leading to cell cycle arrest include suppression of retinoblastoma protein phosphorylation[43] and induction of the p27^{KIP1} and p15^{INK4} cyclin-cdk inhibitors.[44,45] Evidence also suggests that in prostate cancer caspase-1-mediated apoptosis and tumor suppression can be caused by activation of the TGFβ pathway.[46]

In the normal prostate, TGFβ is expressed in both epithelial and stromal cells.[47] The TGFβs have an inhibitory role on cellular proliferation in the normal prostate, and have been shown to induce apoptosis in prostate epithelial cells,[48] while causing inhibition of fibroblast growth in vitro.[49] Induced expression of TGFβ has been intimately linked with castration-induced apoptosis-mediated prostatic involution, and cell death of the luminal epithelial cells, an effect that is reversible by exogenous androgenic control.[8] Moreover, in vivo experimental evidence using the androgen-sensitive Dunning R3327 prostatic adenocarcinoma rat model, indicates that castration-induced androgen withdrawal alone or in combination with estrogen results in upregulation of TGFβ and its receptors, a change that temporally correlates with increased apoptosis among the prostate tumor epithelial cells.[50]

In prostate tumors, escape from the inhibitory effects of TGFβ seems to be mediated, at least in part, by a decrease in the expression of both TβRI and TβRII and genetic changes in the TβRI gene.[51,52] Paradoxically, it was also found that overexpression of TGFβ in prostatic neoplasms can induce growth, as TGFβ1-overexpressing prostate tumors (MATLyLu) were larger and produced more extensive metastatic disease in vivo.[53] A functional link with metastatic spread was recently established in studies using transgenic mice with a dominant negative TβRII mutant in their prostate, which exhibited increased metastatic spread of the primary tumors, although there was no change in the size of the neoplastic prostate.[54] Increased TGFβ1 expression in human prostate cancer specimens has been shown to correlate with angiogenesis, metastasis, and poor clinical outcome, especially when combined with decreased expression of TβRII.[55] Of particular clinical interest is evidence emerging from a recent study suggesting that pre- and postoperative plasma levels of TGFβ1 may have predictive value in prostate cancer progression after radical prostatectomy, as both levels were significantly elevated in patients with extracapsular extension and lymph node metastases.[56]

The pharmacologic exploitation of apoptosis induction in the development of effective therapeutic targeting for prostate cancer treatment dates back to the initial use of antiandrogen therapy, which was later shown to act by inducing apoptosis.[57] Efforts seeking effective treatment strategies for androgen-independent disease, focus on molecular targeting of apoptotic signaling components such as IAPs,[58] the FAS/TNFα receptor-mediated apoptotic signaling,[59] and the intracellular executioner of apoptosis, the caspase family.[60]

An attractive example of pharmacologic induction of apoptosis that has been recently explored is the newly-identified antitumor action of the commonly-used quinazoline α-adrenoceptor antagonists doxazosin and terazosin. Both in vitro and in vivo studies have demonstrated that these drugs, normally used in the treatment of BPH, may also play a significant role in the treatment of prostate cancer due to their andrenoceptor-independent induction of apoptosis.[61] This apoptotic effect is executed via upregulation of TGFβ in prostate cancer cells implying that activation of the TGFβ signaling pathway may account for the therapeutic effect. As this action appears to be independent of the androgen signaling axis, such drugs could potentially provide a powerful approach to the treatment of both androgen-dependent and -independent prostate cancer.

ANGIOGENESIS GROWTH FACTORS: MAINTAINING THE "OTHER" BALANCE IN THE CONTROL OF PROSTATE GROWTH

Angiogenesis became an established factor in tumor growth when the pioneering work of Folkman[62] showed that tumors need a blood supply to grow and metastasize, and are often able to recruit their own blood supply by over-expressing proangiogenic factors. The expression of these angiogenic factors results in a perturbation of the fine balance between endogenous angiogenesis inducers and inhibitors and produces the so-called "angiogenic switch" that allows for tumor growth beyond the 2 to 3 mm limit typical for avascular tumors.[63] A variety of factors with proangiogenic activity have been identified in prostate cancer, including vascular endothelial growth factor (VEGF), matrix metalloproteinases (MMPs), FGF2, FGF4, various

interleukins, cyclooxygenase 2 (COX2), IGF1, nitric oxide, and TGFβ.[64] The determination of microvessel density (MVD) after immunohistochemical tissue staining with specific anti-endothelial antibodies, such as the anti-von Willebrand Factor (Factor VIII-related antigen) antibody, and scoring the vessels under the microscope has been shown to be a valid predictor of disease-free survival and correlate with stage and grade in a number of studies,[65] although the results have not been uniform.[66]

Studies of the effects of the quinazoline-based α1-adrenoceptor antagonists have revealed new information about the regulation of angiogenesis. Long-term treatment with these drugs results in reduction of tissue vascularity in clinical prostate specimens. These findings provide new insight into the ability of this class of drugs to suppress the tumor growth and angiogenic response of human endothelial cells by interfering with VEGF and FGF2 action, while they highlight the potential therapeutic significance in using these drugs as antiangiogenic agents for the treatment of advanced prostate cancer.[67]

FIBROBLAST GROWTH FACTOR

The family of fibroblast growth factors includes 22 members and 4 receptors (FGFR1 to 4), which are produced as alternative splice variants that allow them to exhibit modified specificity for each FGFR isoform.[68,69] The FGFs contribute to development, wound healing, angiogenesis, and tumorigenesis. An important characteristic common to the members of this family is that they bind to heparin-like molecules in the extracellular matrix, where they are protected from degradation and form a growth factor reservoir for presentation to the cell receptors.[70] Fibroblast growth factor 1 (FGF-1; acidic FGF, aFGF) is expressed at low or undetectable levels in the adult prostate;[71] conversely, FGF2 (basic FGF, bFGF) is abundant in the prostate and is believed to be the main growth factor synthesized by fibroblasts, acting mainly in an autocrine fashion.[72] In BPH, FGF2 is overexpressed, correlating with increased stromal proliferation, and similar observations have been made for FGF7 (or keratinocyte growth factor, KGF).[73] FGF7 is the major FGF expressed in normal human prostate tissue and acts mainly as a paracrine stimulator of epithelial cell growth.[74]

In prostate cancer, tumor cells show increased immunoreactivity with FGF2 compared with benign epithelia, accompanied by increased serum levels of FGF2 in prostate cancer patients,[75] providing evidence for the theory that malignant cells become able to synthesize and respond to FGF2 independent of stromal cells due to exon switching of FGFR2.[76] In vitro, FGF2 enhances the motility of prostate cancer cells, which can be blocked by suramin, a growth factor antagonist.[77] Also, in vitro, stromal FGF7 mRNA has been shown to be expressed in 65% of prostate cancer cases and to be associated with hormone-insensitive tumors.[78] Androgen inducible growth factor (FGF8) is expressed in the cytoplasm of prostate cancer cells and increased levels correlate with higher Gleason score[79] and advanced stage[80] of prostate tumors, while its expression was uniformly absent in the normal prostate and BPH specimens. Furthermore, men with tumors exhibiting high levels of FGF8 mRNA expression have been shown to have significantly reduced survival compared to men with tumors expressing little or no FGF8 mRNA.[81]

VASCULAR ENDOTHELIAL GROWTH FACTOR

Vascular endothelial growth factor (VEGF, also known as VEGFA) is one of the most extensively studied angiogenic factors; it is a glycosylated protein that exists in at least 6 different isoforms as a result of alternative exon splicing ($VEGF_{121}$, $VEGF_{145}$, $VEGF_{183}$, $VEGF_{189}$, $VEGF_{206}$, and $VEGF_{165}$—the latter being the predominant isoform), each named after the number of amino acids it contains. VEGF exerts its actions via VEGFR1 (fms-like tyrosine kinase 1, FLT1) and VEGFR2 (kinase domain region, KDR; or fetal liver kinase 1, FLK1), receptor tyrosine kinases located on the cytoplasmic membrane of endothelial cells.[82] The expression of VEGF is primarily regulated by oxygen tension, with hypoxia resulting in induction of hypoxia-inducible factor 1 (HIF1), a key mediator of hypoxic responses.[83] However, other factors, including cytokines and other growth factors, can also mediate VEGF expression at the transcriptional, post-transcriptional and translational level. VEGF acts primarily as an endothelial cell mitogen[84] that induces proliferation and increases vascular permeability.[85] Furthermore, in vitro studies in prostate cancer cell lines suggest that VEGF may function directly as a stimulating autocrine growth factor in a VEGFR2-dependent manner.[86]

Both VEGF and VEGFR2 are expressed almost exclusively in the basal cell layer of benign glands. However, both markers are expressed in the vast majority of prostate cancer specimens.[87,88] Another study confirmed those findings, supporting the concept that upregulation of VEGF in prostate cancer, as opposed to benign glandular epithelium, contributes to tumor growth.[89] Increasing expression of VEGF also appears to be associated with dedifferentiation and the aggressive neuroendocrine phenotype.[90] In vivo studies using intraperitoneal administration of a monoclonal antibody against VEGF in nude mice, demonstrated an effective suppression of the growth of DU145 prostate tumor xenografts, via inhibition of tumor neovascularization.[91] Thalidomide, another angiogenesis inhibitor, was able to induce a PSA decline of more than 40% in 27% of patients with hormone-refractory prostate cancer in a Phase II clinical trial.[92] Several other antiangiogenic drugs are currently under clinical evaluation in prostate cancer, including suramin, which was shown to reduce PSA levels in 33% of patients and prolong the time to disease progression in a Phase III clinical trial.[93]

In view of the endothelial cell population present in the prostate, the role of hypoxia in controlling tumor angiogenesis must be considered. As the proliferating tumor cells outstrip the vascular supply, the tumor microenvironment becomes acidic and develops low oxygen tension and glucose levels. In response, HIF1 activity increases, mediating the transactivation of various angiogenic growth factors, including VEGF in both the endothelial and tumor epithelial cells.[94] In view of the critical part this hypoxic response plays in determining a tumor's ability to continue growth during the metastatic process, the hypoxia-response signaling system has become another appealing potential target for prostate cancer therapy.[95]

Antiangiogenic therapies offer an attractive management perspective in prostate cancer, because of its indolent clinical course and the low proliferation capacity of prostate tumor cells that renders them relatively resistant to standard chemotherapy regimens. This is particularly important in patients with bone metastasis, considering their contribution to the overall morbidity and mortality of the disease. Bone is reportedly the sole site of spread in approximately 80% of patients who develop clinical metastases,[96] and these lesions can produce the most debilitating complications of prostate cancer, such as severe pain, immobility, and hematopoietic and spinal cord compromise.[97] As current evidence suggests that the bone tissue itself is actively involved in facilitating the attraction, invasion, and proliferation of cancer cells, the concept of targeting the bone directly has emerged as a powerful therapeutic strategy.[98]

SUMMARY

The transition from normal prostate tissue to androgen-independent prostate cancer is a complex process. Recent advances in our molecular understanding of regulation of normal and abnormal prostate growth provided new insights into the dynamic crosstalk among the involved growth-factor signaling pathways. The pathways broadly classified in three categories—positive growth factors, negative growth factors, and angiogenesis factors—have been implicated in the regulation of prostate cancer development, progression, and metastasis. The diversity of the changes in autocrine and paracrine signaling in prostate cancer predicts that attempts to utilize a single receptor/ligand as a therapeutic target will not be clinically effective. To identify optimal targets for therapy, it will be necessary to identify the downstream signaling intermediates that are shared by these diverse growth factors and their receptors. Intracellular signaling may provide more effective targets; however, since redundancy is common in serving multiple cellular functions, one has to consider that inhibition of such complex pathways by these drugs might result in widespread mechanism-induced toxicities. Moreover, the problems associated with functional redundancy of growth factor receptors are inevitably complicated by the observation that receptor kinases (for some of the growth factors) are capable of intracellular signaling promiscuity by dimerization with other receptors or kinases. The success, however, already achieved in the effective targeting of positive growth factors such as EGF in prostate cancer cells, must be recognized. The striking example of the drug ZD1839 (Iressa), a selective inhibitor of the EGF receptor, provides compelling experimental and clinical evidence for the multiple potential uses of this drug, both as stand-alone therapy and in combination with either antiandrogen or more conventional chemotherapic agents for the treatment of prostate cancer (Figure 10.1). In clinical trials with androgen-dependent prostate cancer, Iressa could synergize with androgen ablation to slow prostate tumor growth and impede the transformation to androgen-independence. As illustrated in Figure 10.1, EGFR activation triggers a phosphorylation cascade involving multiple downstream factors that ultimately leads to upregulation of genes that promote cell proliferation. For those patients with advanced disease, such treatment should maintain efficacy since it acts independently of the androgen receptor pathway.[23-24]

Equally as important (for therapeutic purposes) as inhibiting the factors that induce cell growth and tumor progression is activating those negative growth factors that induce apoptosis. Within the context of its well-documented apoptosis regulatory actions in the prostate and the significance of its key receptor TβRII as a potential tumor suppressor, TGFβ provides an attractive candidate for such targeting. The idea is to restore TβRII expression in those prostate tumors that exhibit loss or inactivation of this critical signaling component of the TGFβ mechanism. As illustrated in Figure 10.1, one may appreciate the emerging therapeutic promise of the widely clinically used quinazoline-based adrenoceptor antagonists, such as terazosin and doxazosin, shown to induce apoptosis in malignant prostate cells, via an α1-adrenoceptor independent mechanism and by activating the TGFβ apoptotic signaling. The biological consequences may prove useful in the treatment and/or prevention of androgen-dependent as well as androgen-independent prostate cancer.[63]

The main obstacle to improving the survival of patients with advanced prostate cancer remains the lack of effective treatment approaches for androgen-

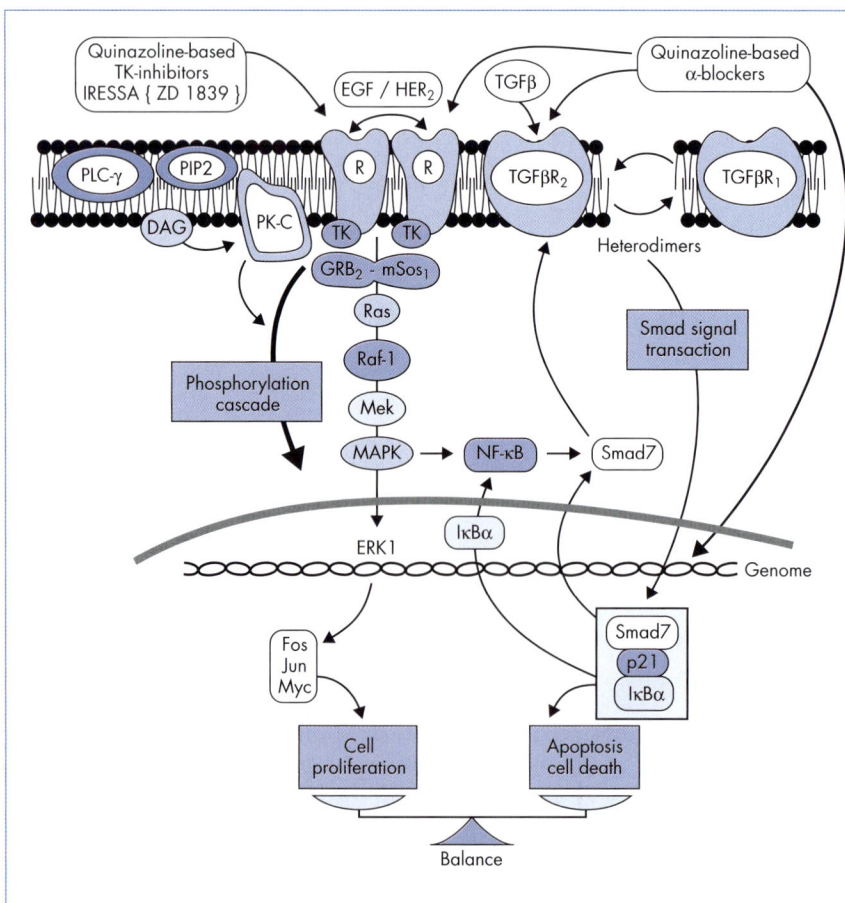

Figure 10.1

Therapeutic targeting of epidermal growth factor (EGF) and transforming growth factor-β (TGFβ) signaling pathways for prostate cancer. The two growth factor signaling pathways are critical in maintaining a balance between positive and negative growth factors, necessary for prostate homeostasis. Targeting the positive and negative growth factor signaling exploits the loss of such an imbalance that heavily characterizes prostate tumor growth. Drugs such as Iressa or certain quinazoline-based adrenoceptor antagonists, can potentially reverse the positive effect on growth or negative effect on apoptosis, respectively, and restore homeostatic equilibrium in the prostate.

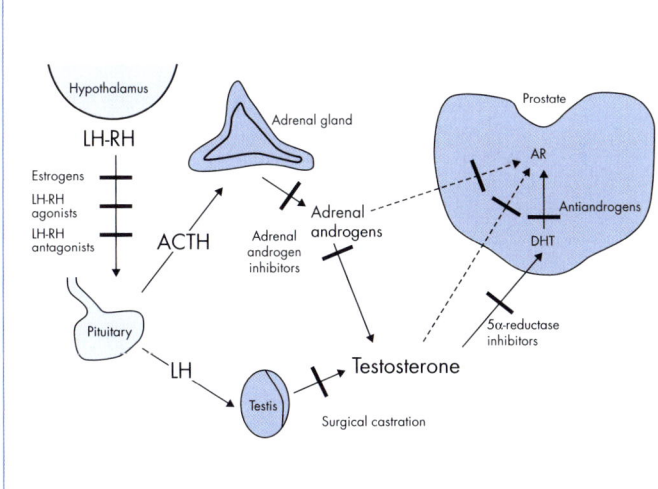

Figure 10.2

An overview of the current hormonally-based therapeutic strategies for prostate cancer treatment. In the early stages of prostate cancer, all tumors are essentially susceptible to hormonal therapy. At the cellular level, androgen deprivation leads to the apoptotic cell death of the androgen-dependent prostate epithelial tumor cells via one or more of the signaling pathways shown here. While debate still exists about the impact of these therapeutic approaches in increasing survival, one must recognize their critical importance as means of palliation and improving quality of life. Novel effective therapeutic strategies must be developed to effectively increase survival of patients with advanced prostate cancer. (ACTH, adrenocorticotrophic hormone; AR, androgen receptor; DHT, dihydrotestosterone; LH, luteinizing hormone; LH-RH, luteinizing hormone-releasing hormone.)

independent disease and an inability to pharmacologically prevent progression and metastasis to the bone and lymph nodes. Coordinated efforts on the identification of novel growth signaling pathways that contribute to prostate cancer progression and metastasis, greatly supported by the recent exciting evidence documenting a functional contribution of the hedgehog pathway in prostate cancer progression and metastasis,[99] will lead to the development of effective molecular targets for therapy as well as new markers of tumor progression.

REFERENCES

1. Debes J, Tindall D. Mechanisms of androgen-refractory prostate cancer. N Engl J Med 2004;351;15:1488–1490.

2. Feldman BJ, Feldman D. The development of androgen-independent prostate cancer. Nat Rev Cancer 2001;1:34–45.

3. Bruckheimer EM, Kyprianou N. Bcl-2 antagonizes the combined apoptotic effect of transforming growth factor-beta and dihydrotestosterone in prostate cancer cells. Prostate 2002;53:133–142.

4. Walsh PC, et al (ed). Campbell's Urology, 8th ed. Philadelphia: Saunders, 2002.

5. Murphy AM, McKiernan JM, Olsson CA. Controversies in prostate cancer screening. J Urol 2004;172:1822–1824.

6. Rubin MA. Using molecular markers to predict outcome. J Urol 2004;172:S18–21.

7. Bruckheimer EM, Kyprianou N. Apoptosis and cell cycle deregulation in prostate cancer. In Abel, Lalani (eds): Prostate Cancer: Clinical vs Scientific Aspects—Bridging the Gap. London: Imperial College Press, 2003, pp 511–549.

8. Kyprianou N, Isaacs JT. Expression of transforming growth factor-beta in the rat ventral prostate during castration-induced programmed cell death. Mol Endocrinol 1989;3:1515–1522.

9. McDonnell TJ, Troncoso P, Brisbay SM, et al. Expression of the protooncogene bcl-2 in the prostate and its association with emergence of androgen-independent prostate cancer. Cancer Res 1992;52:6940–6944.

10. McKenna NJ, O'Malley BW. Combinatorial control of gene expression by nuclear receptors and coregulators. Cell 2002;108:465–474.

11. Comuzzi B, Lambrinidis L, Rogatsch H, et al. The transcriptional co-activator cAMP response element-binding protein-binding protein is expressed in prostate cancer and enhances androgen- and anti-androgen-induced androgen receptor function. Am J Pathol 2003;162:233–241.

12. Poukka H, Karvonen U, Janne OA, et al. Covalent modification of the androgen receptor by small ubiquitin-like modifier 1 (SUMO-1). Proc Natl Acad Sci USA 2000;97:14145–14150.

13. Chen CD, Welsbie DS, Tran C, et al. Molecular determinants of resistance to antiandrogen therapy. Nat Med 2004;10:33–39.

14. Isaacs JT, Isaacs WB. Androgen receptor outwits prostate cancer drugs. Nat Med 2004;10:26–27.

15. Huggins C, Hodges CV. Studies on prostatic cancer: I. The effect of castration, of estrogen and of androgen injection on serum phosphatases in metastatic carcinoma of the prostate. Arch Surg 1941;43:209.

16. Culig Z, Hobisch A, Cronauer MV, et al, Androgen receptor activation in prostatic tumor cell lines by insulin-like growth factor-I, keratinocyte growth factor, and epidermal growth factor. Cancer Res 1994;54:5474–5478.

17. Carpenter G, Cohen S. Epidermal growth factor. J Biol Chem 1990;265:7709–7712.

18. Massague J, Transforming growth factor-alpha. A model for membrane-anchored growth factors. J Biol Chem 1990;265:21393–1396.

19. De Miguel P, Royuela, Bethencourt R, et al. Immunohistochemical comparative analysis of transforming growth factor alpha, epidermal growth factor, and epidermal growth factor receptor in normal, hyperplastic and neoplastic human prostates. Cytokine 1999;11:722–727.

20. Nishi N, Oya H, Matsumoto K, et al. Changes in gene expression of growth factors and their receptors during castration-induced involution and androgen-induced regrowth of rat prostates. Prostate 1996;28:139–152.

21. Cohen DW, Simak R, Fair WR, et al. Expression of transforming growth factor-alpha and the epidermal growth factor receptor in human prostate tissues. J Urol 1994;152:2120–2124.

22. Fong CJ, Sherwood ER, Mendelsohn J, et al. Epidermal growth factor receptor monoclonal antibody inhibits constitutive receptor phosphorylation, reduces autonomous growth, and sensitizes androgen-independent prostatic carcinoma cells to tumor necrosis factor alpha. Cancer Res 1992;52:5887–5892.

23. Sirotnak FM, Zakowski MF, Miller VA, et al. Efficacy of cytotoxic agents against human tumor xenografts is markedly enhanced by coadministration of ZD1839 (Iressa), an inhibitor of EGFR tyrosine kinase. Clin Cancer Res 2000;6:4885–4892.

24. Sirotnak FM, She Y, Lee F, et al. Studies with CWR22 xenografts in nude mice suggest that ZD1839 may have a role in the treatment of both androgen-dependent and androgen-independent human prostate cancer. Clin Cancer Res 2002;8:3870–3876.

25. Karashima T, Sweeney P, Slaton JW, et al. Inhibition of angiogenesis by the antiepidermal growth factor receptor antibody ImClone C225 in androgen-independent prostate cancer growing orthotopically in nude mice. Clin Cancer Res 2002;8:1253–1264.

26. Eccles SA. The role of c-erbB-2/HER2/neu in breast cancer progression and metastasis. J Mammary Gland Biol Neoplasia 2001;6:393–406.

27. Signoretti S, Montironi R, Manola J, et al. Her-2-neu expression and progression toward androgen independence in human prostate cancer. J Natl Cancer Inst 2000;92:1918–1925.

28. Lara PN Jr, Meyers FJ, Gray CR, et al. HER-2/neu is overexpressed infrequently in patients with prostate carcinoma. Results from the California Cancer Consortium Screening Trial. Cancer 2002;94:2584–2589.

29. Agus DB, Scher HI, Higgins B, et al. Response of prostate cancer to anti-Her-2/neu antibody in androgen-dependent and -independent human xenograft models. Cancer Res 1999;59:4761–4764.

30. Ziada A, Barqawi A, Glode LM, et al. The use of trastuzumab in the treatment of hormone refractory prostate cancer; phase II trial. Prostate 2004;60:332–337.

31. Baxter RC. Insulin-like growth factor binding proteins in the human circulation: a review. Horm Res 1994;42:140–144.

32. Macaulay VM. Insulin-like growth factors and cancer. Br J Cancer 1992;65:311–320.

33. Baserga R, Peruzzi F, Reiss K. The IGF-1 receptor in cancer biology. Int J Cancer 2003;107:873–877.

34. Chan JM, Stampfer MJ, Giovannucci E, et al. Plasma insulin-like growth factor-I and prostate cancer risk: a prospective study. Science 1998;279:563–566.

35. Stattin P, Rinaldi S, Biessy C, et al. High levels of circulating insulin-like growth factor-I increase prostate cancer risk: a prospective study in a population-based nonscreened cohort. J Clin Oncol 2004;22:3104–3112.

36. Djavan B, Waldert M, Seitz C, et al. Insulin-like growth factors and prostate cancer. World J Urol 2001;19:225–233.

37. Kanety H, Madjar Y, Dagan Y, et al. Serum insulin-like growth factor-binding protein-2 (IGFBP-2) is increased and IGFBP-3 is decreased in patients with prostate cancer: correlation with serum prostate-specific antigen. J Clin Endocrinol Metab 1993;77:229–233.

38. Cohen P, Graves HC, Peehl DM, et al. Prostate-specific antigen (PSA) is an insulin-like growth factor binding protein-3 protease found in seminal plasma. J Clin Endocrinol Metab 1992;75:1046–1053.

39. Hellawell GO, Ferguson DJ, Brewster SF, et al. Chemosensitization of human prostate cancer using antisense agents targeting the type 1 insulin-like growth factor receptor. BJU Int 2003;91:271–277.

40. Derynck R, Jarrett JA, Chen EY, et al. Human transforming growth factor-beta complementary DNA sequence and expression in normal and transformed cells. Nature 1985;316:701–705.

41. Wrana JL, Attisano L, Wieser R, et al. Mechanism of activation of the TGF-beta receptor. Nature 1994;370:341–347.

42. Heldin CH, Miyazono K, ten Dijke P. TGF-beta signalling from cell membrane to nucleus through SMAD proteins. Nature 1997;390:465–471.

43. Laiho M, DeCaprio JA, Ludlow JW, et al. Growth inhibition by TGF-beta linked to suppression of retinoblastoma protein phosphorylation. Cell 1990;62:175–185.

44. Hannon GJ, Beach D. p15INK4B is a potential effector of TGF-beta-induced cell cycle arrest. Nature 1994;371:257–261.

45. Polyak K, Kato JY, Solomon MJ, et al. p27Kip1, a cyclin-Cdk inhibitor, links transforming growth factor-beta and contact inhibition to cell cycle arrest. Gen Dev 1994;8:9–22.

46. Guo Y, Kyprianou N. Restoration of transforming growth factor beta signaling pathway in human prostate cancer cells suppresses tumorigenicity via induction of caspase-1-mediated apoptosis. Cancer Res 1999;59:1366–1371.

47. Perry KT, Anthony CT, Steiner MS. Immunohistochemical localization of TGF beta 1, TGF beta 2, and TGF beta 3 in normal and malignant human prostate. Prostate 1997;33:133–140.

48. Martikainen P, Kyprianou N, Isaacs JT. Effect of transforming growth factor-beta 1 on proliferation and death of rat prostatic cells. Endocrinology 1990;127:2963–2968.

49. Story MT, Hopp KA, Meier DA, et al. Influence of transforming growth factor beta 1 and other growth factors on basic fibroblast growth factor level and proliferation of cultured human prostate-derived fibroblasts. Prostate 1993;22:183–197.

50. Landstrom M, Eklov S, Colosetti P, et al. Estrogen induces apoptosis in a rat prostatic adenocarcinoma: association with an increased expression of TGF-beta 1 and its type-I and type-II receptors. Int J Cancer 1996;67:573–579.

51. Guo Y, Jacobs SC, Kyprianou N. Down-regulation of protein and mRNA expression for transforming growth factor-beta (TGF-beta1) type I and type II receptors in human prostate cancer. Int J Cancer 1997;71:573–579.

52. Kim IY, Ahn HJ, Zelner DJ, et al. Genetic change in transforming growth factor beta (TGF-beta) receptor type I gene correlates with insensitivity to TGF-beta 1 in human prostate cancer cells. Cancer Res 1996;56:44–48.

53. Steiner MS, Barrack ER. Transforming growth factor-beta 1 overproduction in prostate cancer: effects on growth in vivo and in vitro. Mol Endocrinol 1992;6:15–25.

54. Tu WH, Thomas TZ, Masumori N, et al. The loss of TGF-beta signaling promotes prostate cancer metastasis. Neoplasia 2003;5:267–277.

55. Wikstrom P, Stattin P, Franck-Lissbrant I, et al. Transforming growth factor beta1 is associated with angiogenesis, metastasis, and poor clinical outcome in prostate cancer. Prostate 1998;37:19–29.

56. Shariat SF, Kattan MW, Traxel E, et al. Association of pre- and postoperative plasma levels of transforming growth factor beta(1) and interleukin 6 and its soluble receptor with prostate cancer progression. Clin Cancer Res 2004;10:1992–1999.

57. Kyprianou N, Isaacs JT. Activation of programmed cell death in the rat ventral prostate after castration. Endocrinology 1988; 122:552–562.

58. Schimmer AD, Welsh K, Pinilla C, et al. Small-molecule antagonists of apoptosis suppressor XIAP exhibit broad antitumor activity. Cancer Cell. 200:5:25–35.

59. McEleny K, Coffey R, Morrissey C, et al. An antisense oligonucleotide to cIAP-1 sensitizes prostate cancer cells to fas and TNFalpha mediated apoptosis. Prostate 2004;59:419–425.

60. Liang H, Salinas RA, Leal BZ, et al. Caspase-mediated apoptosis and caspase-independent cell death induced by irofulven in prostate cancer cells. Mol Cancer Ther 2004;3:1385–1396.

61. Kyprianou N. Doxazosin and terazosin suppress prostate growth by inducing apoptosis: clinical significance. J Urol 2003;169:1520–1525.

62. Folkman J. Role of angiogenesis in tumor growth and metastasis. Semin Oncol 2002;29:S15–18.

63. Folkman J. Angiogenesis in cancer, vascular, rheumatoid and other disease. Nat Med 1995;1:27–31.

64. Nicholson B, Theodorescu D. Angiogenesis and prostate cancer tumor growth. J Cell Biochem 2004;91:125–150.

65. Borre M, Offersen BV, Nerstrom B, et al. Microvessel density predicts survival in prostate cancer patients subjected to watchful waiting. Br J Cancer 1998;78:940–944.

66. Rubin MA, Buyyounouski M, Bagiella E, et al. Microvessel density in prostate cancer: lack of correlation with tumor grade, pathologic stage, and clinical outcome. Urology 1999;53:542–547.

67. Keledjian K, Garrison JB, Kyprianou N. Doxazosin inhibits human vascular endothelial cell adhesion, migration, and invasion. J Cell Biochem 2005;94:374–388.

68. Ornitz DM, Itoh N. Fibroblast growth factors. Genome Biol 2001;2:reviews3005.1–3005.12.

69. Powers CJ, McLeskey SW, Wellstein A. Fibroblast growth factors, their receptors and signaling. Endocr Relat Cancer 2000;7:165–197.

70. Gospodarowicz D, Cheng J. Heparin protects basic and acidic FGF from inactivation. J Cell Physiol 1986;128:475–484.

71. Mydlo JH, Michaeli J, Heston WD, et al. Expression of basic fibroblast growth factor mRNA in benign prostatic hyperplasia and prostatic carcinoma. Prostate 1988;13:241–247.

72. Dow JK, deVere White RW. Fibroblast growth factor 2: its structure and property, paracrine function, tumor angiogenesis, and prostate-related mitogenic and oncogenic functions. Urology 2000;55:800–806.

73. Ropiquet F, Giri D, Lamb DJ, et al. FGF7 and FGF2 are increased in benign prostatic hyperplasia and are associated with increased proliferation. J Urol 1999;162:595–599.

74. Ittman M, Mansukhani A. Expression of fibroblast growth factors (FGFs) and FGF receptors in human prostate. J Urol 1997;157:351–356.

75. Cronauer MV, Hittmair A, Eder IE, et al. Basic fibroblast growth factor levels in cancer cells and in sera of patients suffering from proliferative disorders of the prostate. Prostate 1997;31:223–233.

76. Yan G, Fukabori Y, McBride G, et al. Exon switching and activation of stromal and embryonic fibroblast growth factor (FGF)-FGF receptor genes in prostate epithelial cells accompany stromal independence and malignancy. Mol Cell Biol 1993;13:4513–4522.

77. Pienta KJ, Isaacs WB, Vindivich D, et al. The effects of basic fibroblast growth factor and suramin on cell motility and growth of rat prostate cancer cells. J Urol 1991;145:199–202.

78. Leung HY, Mehta P, Gray LB, et al. Keratinocyte growth factor expression in hormone insensitive prostate cancer. Oncogene 1997;15:1115–1120.

79. Leung HY, Dickson C, Robson CN, et al. Over-expression of fibroblast growth factor-8 in human prostate cancer. Oncogene 1996;12:1833–1835.

80. Gnanapragasam VJ, Robinson MC, Marsh C, et al. FGF8 isoform b expression in human prostate cancer. Br J Cancer 2003;88:1432–1438.

81. Dorkin TJ, Robinson MC, Marsh C, et al. FGF8 over-expression in prostate cancer is associated with decreased patient survival and persists in androgen independent disease. Oncogene 1999;18:2755–2761.

82. Ferrara N, Gerber HP, LeCouter J. The biology of VEGF and its receptors. Nat Med 2003;9:669–676.

83. Semenza G. Signal transduction to hypoxia-inducible factor 1. Biochem Pharmacol 2002;64:993–998.

84. Ferrara N, Henzel WJ. Pituitary follicular cells secrete a novel heparin-binding growth factor specific for vascular endothelial cells. Biochem Biophys Res Com 1989;161:851–858.

85. Senger DR, Galli SJ, Dvorak AM, et al. Tumor cells secrete a vascular permeability factor that promotes accumulation of ascites fluid. Science 1983;219:983–985.

86. Jackson MW, Roberts JS, Heckford SE, et al. A potential autocrine role for vascular endothelial growth factor in prostate cancer. Cancer Res 2002;62:854–859.

87. Kollermann J, Helpap B. Expression of vascular endothelial growth factor (VEGF) and VEGF receptor Flk-1 in benign, premalignant, and malignant prostate tissue. Am J Clin Pathol 2001;116:115–121.

88. Ferrer FA, Miller LJ, Lindquist R, et al. Expression of vascular endothelial growth factor receptors in human prostate cancer. Urology 1999;54:567–572.

89. Ferrer FA, Miller LJ, Andrawis RI, et al. Angiogenesis and prostate cancer: in vivo and in vitro expression of angiogenesis factors by prostate cancer cells. Urology 1998;51:161–167.

90. Harper ME, Glynne-Jones E, Goddard L, et al. Vascular endothelial growth factor (VEGF) expression in prostatic tumours and its relationship to neuroendocrine cells. Br J Cancer 1996;74:910–916.

91. Borgstrom P, Bourdon MA, Hillan KJ, et al. Neutralizing anti-vascular endothelial growth factor antibody completely inhibits angiogenesis and growth of human prostate carcinoma micro tumors in vivo. Prostate 1998;35:1–10.

92. Figg WD, Dahut W, Duray P, et al. A randomized phase II trial of thalidomide, an angiogenesis inhibitor, in patients with androgen-independent prostate cancer. Clin Cancer Res 2001;7:1888–1893.

93. Small EJ, Meyer M, Marshall ME, et al. Suramin therapy for patients with symptomatic hormone-refractory prostate cancer: results of a randomized phase III trial comparing suramin plus hydrocortisone to placebo plus hydrocortisone. J Clin Oncol 2000;18:1440–1450.

94. Acker T, Plate K. Role of hypoxia in tumor angiogenesis—molecular and cellular angiogenic crosstalk. Cell Tissue Res 2003;314:145–155.

95. Anastasiadis AG, Bemis DL, Stisser BC, et al. Tumor cell hypoxia and the hypoxia-response system as a target for prostate cancer therapy. Curr Drug Targets 2003;4:191–196.

96. Scher HI, Chung LW. Bone metastases: improving the therapeutic index. Semin Oncol 1994;21:630–656.

97. Scher HI. Prostate carcinoma: Defining therapeutic objectives and improving overall outcomes. Cancer 2003;97:758–771.

98. Assikis VJ, Simons JW. Novel therapeutic strategies for androgen-independent prostate cancer: an update. Semin Oncol 2004;31:26–32.

99. Karhadkar SS, Bova GS, Abdallah N, et al. Hedgehog signalling in prostate regeneration, neoplasia and metastasis. Nature 2004;431:707–712.

100. Raffo AJ, Perlman H, Chen MW, et al. Overexpression of bcl-2 protects prostate cancer cells from apoptosis in vitro and confers resistance to androgen depletion in vivo. Cancer Res 1995;55:4438–4445.

101. Yan G, Fukabori Y, Nikolaropoulos S, et al. Heparin-binding keratinocyte growth factor is a candidate stromal-to-epithelial-cell andromedin. Mol Endocrinol 1992;6:2123–2128.

102. Djakiew D. Role of nerve growth factor-like protein in the paracrine regulation of prostate growth. J Androl 1992;13:476–487.

103. Bhowmick NA, Chytil A, Plieth D, et al. TGF-β signaling in fibroblasts modulates the oncogenic potential of adjacent epithelia. Science 2004, 303848–303851.

104. Nakayama K, Ishida N, Shirane M, et al. Mice lacking p27Kip1 display increased body size, multiple organ hyperplasia, retinal hyperplasia, and pituitary tumors. Cell 1996;85:733–736.

105. Day ML, Foster RG, Day KC, et al. Cell anchorage regulates apoptosis through the retinoblastoma tumor suppressor/E2F pathway. J Biol Chem 1997;27:8125–8128.

106. Sansal I, Sellers WR. The biology and clinical relevance of the PTEN tumor suppressor pathway. J Clin Oncol 2004;15;22:2954–2963

107. Voronov E, Shouval DS, Krelin Y, et al. IL-1 is required for tumor invasiveness and angiogenesis. Proc Natl Acad Sci USA 2003 4;100:2645–2650.

108. Wang Y, Sun Y. Insulin-like growth factor receptor-1 as an anti-cancer target: blocking transformation and inducing apoptosis. Curr Cancer Drug Targets 2002;2:191–207.

109. Wang J, Torbenson M, Wang Q, et al. Expression of inducible nitric oxide synthase in paired neoplastic and non-neoplastic primary prostate cell cultures and prostatectomy specimen. Urol Oncol 2003;21:117–122.

Pathology of prostate cancer

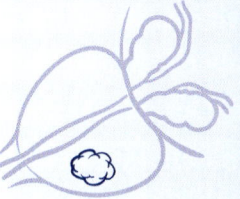

Histopathology of prostate cancer and pathologic staging

11

Jonathan I Epstein

GLEASON GRADE: OVERVIEW

The Gleason grading system is the most widely accepted grading system for prostate cancer.[1] The Gleason system is based on the glandular pattern of the tumor as identified at relatively low magnification (Figure 11.1). Cytologic features play no role in grading the tumor. Both the primary (predominant) and the secondary (second most prevalent) architectural patterns are identified and assigned a grade from 1 to 5, with 1 the most differentiated and 5 the least differentiated. When Gleason compared his grading system with survival rates, it was noted that in tumors with two distinct tumor patterns the observed number of deaths generally fell in between the number expected on the basis of the primary pattern and that based on the secondary pattern. Since both the primary and secondary patterns were influential in predicting prognosis, there resulted a Gleason score obtained by the addition of the primary and secondary grade patterns. If a tumor had only one histologic pattern, then for uniformity the primary and secondary patterns were given the same grade. Gleason scores range from 2 (1 + 1), which represents tumors uniformly composed of Gleason pattern 1 tumor, to 10 (5 + 5), which represents totally undifferentiated tumors. Gleason pattern 1 and pattern 2 tumors are composed of relatively circumscribed nodules of uniform, single, separate, closely packed, uniform medium-sized glands. Gleason pattern 3 tumor infiltrates in and amongst the non-neoplastic prostate, and the glands have marked variation in size and shape with smaller glands than seen in Gleason patterns 1 or 2. Gleason pattern 4 glands are no longer single and separate as seen in patterns 1 to 3. In Gleason pattern 4, one may also see large irregular cribriform glands as opposed to the smoothly circumscribed smaller nodules of cribriform Gleason pattern 3. Gleason pattern 5 tumor shows no glandular differentiation, composed of either solid sheets, cords, single cells, or solid nests of tumor with central comedonecrosis. Synonyms for Gleason score are "combined Gleason grade" and "Gleason sum."

The frequency and rate of grade progression is unknown. Tumor grade is on average higher in larger tumors.[2] However, this may be due to more rapid growth of high grade cancers. It has been demonstrated that some tumors are high grade when they are small.[3] Many studies addressing the issue of grade progression have a selection bias, because the patients have undergone a repeat transurethral resection or repeat biopsy due to symptoms of tumor progression.[4] The observed grade progression may be explained by a growth advantage of a tumor clone of higher grade that was present from the beginning but undersampled. In patients followed expectantly there is no evidence of grade progression within 1 to 2 years.[5]

RADICAL PROSTATECTOMY

PROCESSING

Whole mount sectioning of the prostate provides more esthetically pleasing sections for teaching and publication purposes. Whole mount sections do not provide more information than routine sections, but in some cases thicker slices of tissue used for whole mount processing will miss areas of extraprostatic extension (7–15%) and positive margins (12%) compared with

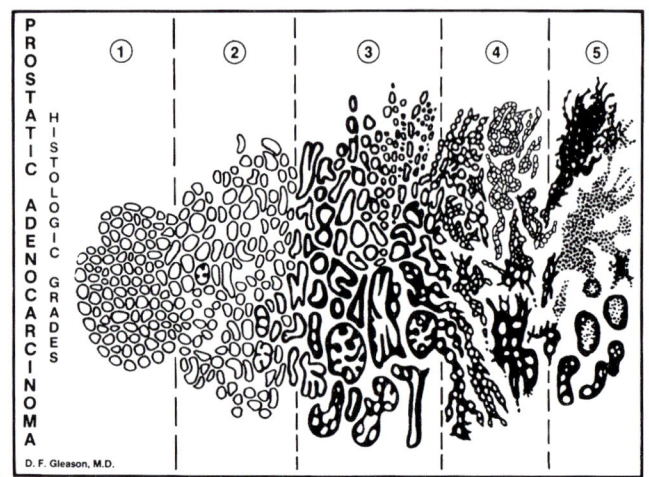

A

Fig. 11.1

Gleason grading system. *A,* Schematic diagram of Gleason grading system. *B,* Gleason pattern 2 carcinoma showing single, separate, relatively closely packed large glands. *C,* Gleason pattern 3 tumor showing discrete gland formation, yet smaller glands than seen in Gleason patterns 1 and 2. *D,* Irregular cribriform formation of Gleason pattern 4 tumor. *E,* Gleason pattern 5 with large solid nests of tumor with central comedonecrosis.

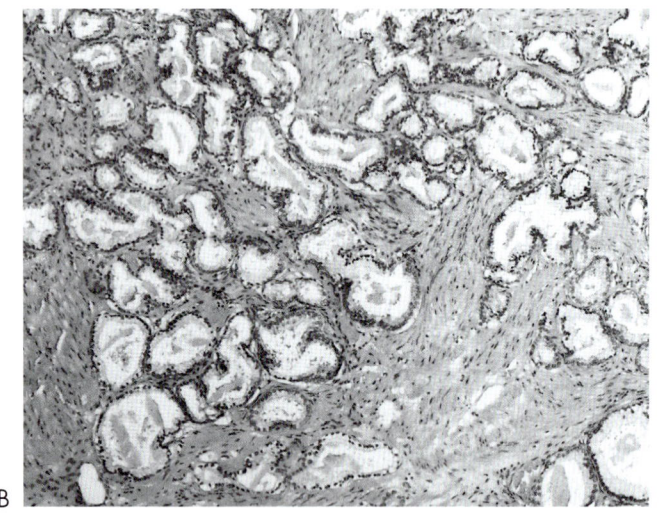

B

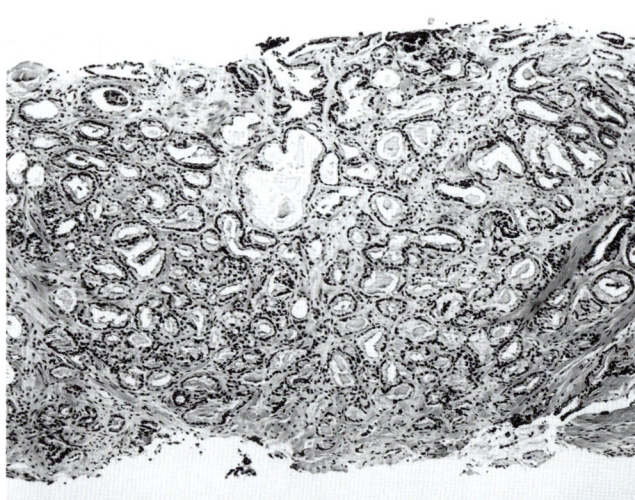

C

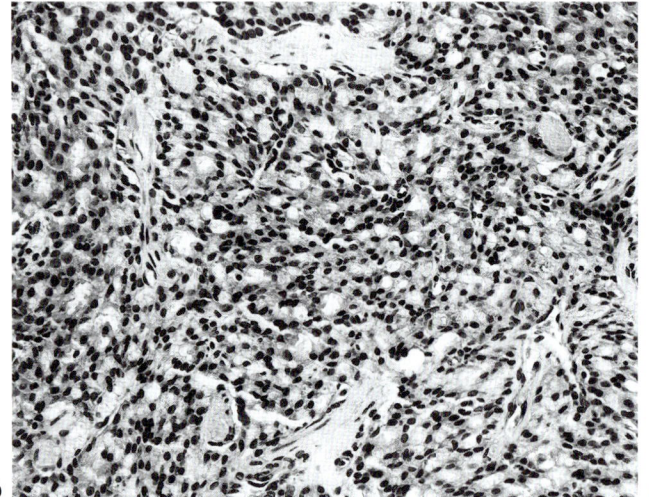

D

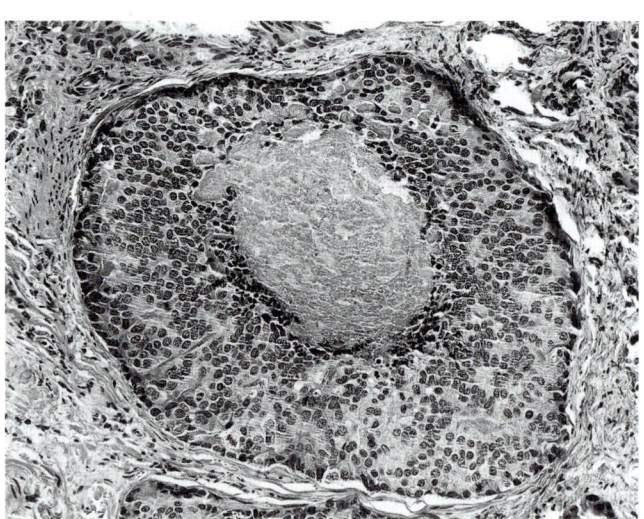

E

thinner routinely processed sections.[6,7] Processing radical prostatectomy specimens using whole mount sections also requires specialized processing techniques, storage facilities, materials and dedicated technicians. Furthermore, prostates processed with the whole mount technique require a greater fixation period resulting in a delay in the diagnosis. For all of the reasons stated above, the standard of care for pathologists is to process

radical prostatectomy specimens using routine rather than whole mount sectioning.

In a minority of institutions, the entire prostate is serially sectioned and submitted for histologic review. However, processing the entire radical prostatectomy specimen significantly increases the cost of specimen processing and can impose significant strains on a laboratory's resources. As a result, most pathologists have adopted various methods of partial sampling. A problem with partially sampled prostates is that sections are often submitted in a random fashion (i.e., four slices from the left and four slices from the right) without respect to gross findings or consideration as to the most likely location of the tumor. Pathologists should use one of several published methods for partially sampling radical prostatectomy specimens.[7,8] These methods differ depending on whether gross tumor is visualized. Sampling must take into account that in 15% to 25% of stage T1C tumors, the dominant lesion is primarily located within the transition zone anteriorly.[9,10]

Several techniques have been published as to how to obtain fresh prostate tissue for research purposes without compromising assessment of pathologic parameters. Doing so is not without difficulties as, once the prostate is incised in its fresh state, the more centrally located tissue tends to bulge beyond the plane of sectioning and the inked edge of the prostate gland retracts.[11–15]

TUMOR LOCATION

Multifocal adenocarcinoma of the prostate is present in more than 85% of prostates.[16] In many of these cases of bilateral and/or multifocal tumor the other tumors are small, low grade, and clinically insignificant. Consequently the distinction between pathological stages T2A and T2B is meaningless.

INTRAOPERATIVE PATHOLOGICAL ASSESSMENT OF PELVIC LYMPH NODES

The handling of lymphadenectomy specimens at the time of surgery is controversial and depends on the philosophy of the urologist. Some urologists will abort the radical prostatectomy in cases with positive lymph nodes identified at the time of surgery, since surgery will not be curative. With these urologists, the pathologist should try to optimize the identification of metastatic disease at the time of frozen section. It is not practical to freeze all of the pelvic lymph nodes, especially given the low likelihood of finding metastatic disease even on permanent sections. A more reasonable approach would be to preoperatively identify clinical parameters associated with such a low risk of lymph node metastases that frozen sections need not be performed. For example, in men with clinical stage T2, Gleason score less than 7 cancers on biopsy with serum prostate-specific antigen (PSA) levels of 4.1 to 10 ng/ml, the incidence of positive pelvic lymph nodes is less than 4%.[17] Keeping the same biopsy and serologic results, this risk drops to 1% for patients with stage T1C disease. In cases where the decision is made to go ahead with freezing the pelvic lymph nodes, the pathologist can freeze two or three small firm lymph nodes from each side, which will identify over half of small metastases.[18]

Other urologists will proceed with radical prostatectomy when positive lymph nodes are found intraoperatively, as long as patients are projected to have a long survival and might benefit in terms of local control. In patients who have positive lymph nodes, the best predictor of who will not benefit from radical prostatectomy is the presence of tumor with Gleason score 8 to10 on needle biopsy.[19] If these men undergo radical prostatectomy, they proceed to distant metastases in a short period of time, such that it is difficult to justify a radical prostatectomy for local control. In men with Gleason scores of 8 to 10 on needle biopsy, it is reasonable to recommend freezing all nodes or having these patients undergo laparoscopic lymph node dissection prior to radical prostatectomy. If nodes are positive in these cases, radical prostatectomy should not be performed. In men with Gleason score of less than 7 on needle biopsy, it is not necessary to freeze the lymph nodes, as the urologists would proceed with the radical prostatectomy for local control even if with positive nodes at the time of surgery (as these men have a reasonably long life expectancy).

ROUTINE PROCESSING OF LYMPH NODE SPECIMENS

One study found that in 6.5% of the cases the only lymph node metastasis was not in a grossly recognized lymph node but in presumed adipose tissue.[18] Some laboratories may routinely submit all of the adipose tissue from the pelvic lymphadenectomy specimens. However, given the current low frequency with which lymph node metastases are identified, one may modify this approach to submit all of the pelvic lymphadenectomy tissue only in cases with biopsy Gleason scores of greater than 6. In approximately 5% of radical prostatectomy specimens, periprostatic/periseminal vesicle lymph nodes are present; in 0.6% of all prostatectomy cases, metastatic disease can be found in these nodes. However, in 40% of the cases with metastases to these periprostatic/periseminal vesicle nodes, metastases are also present in pelvic nodes. For the rare case with metastases limited to periprostatic/periseminal vesicle nodes, there is an associated poor prognosis and these cases should be considered as having "N1" disease in the TNM staging classification.[20]

PROGNOSTIC PARAMETERS IN MEN WITH POSITIVE PELVIC LYMPH NODES

Although tumors within pelvic lymph nodes appear more dedifferentiated than the primary tumor, dedifferentiation is not an independent prognostic parameter.[21] There are conflicting studies as to whether the number of positive lymph nodes, largest metastasis, or perinodal extension independently correlates with prognosis,[19,22,23] such that the current practice is to report the number of lymph nodes involved by metastatic disease without further qualification.

DEFINITION OF SEMINAL VESICLE INVASION

Seminal vesicle invasion (SVI) is defined as tumor infiltrating the muscular coat of the seminal vesicle. It is controversial whether one can have SVI without extraprostatic extension (EPE).[24,25] Patients diagnosed as having SVI without EPE have a progression-free probability similar to men with EPE without SVI. In contrast, men with tumor having EPE and SVI have more than a 20% progression-free probability at 5 years. Although it could potentially be argued anatomically whether there is an intraprostatic portion of the seminal vesicle, the fact that invasion of these structures does not impart a worse prognosis than cases of EPE without SVI indicates that, functionally, these structures should not be designated as seminal vesicles. Most authorities restrict the diagnosis of SVI only for invasion of structures exterior to the prostate.

Possible routes of SVI are: 1) extension into soft tissue adjacent to the seminal vesicle and then into the seminal vesicle; 2) invasion via the sheath of the ejaculatory duct, penetrating the muscular wall of the ejaculatory duct, or extending up the ejaculatory duct wall into the seminal vesicle muscle wall; 3) direct invasion of the seminal vesicle; or 4) discontinuous metastases. There are conflicting studies as to whether the first or second method is most common. Metastases are the least common mode of spread.[26]

PROGNOSIS OF SEMINAL VESICLE INVASION

The finding of SVI in a radical prostatectomy specimen markedly diminishes the likelihood of cure. In contemporary series of men with positive seminal vesicles and negative pelvic lymph nodes, 5-year biochemical progression-free rates range from 5% to 60% (mean 34%).[24–32] Parameters reported to have prognostic significance in men with SVI include mechanism of SVI, grade, vascular invasion, extent of SVI, serum PSA levels, margins, tumor volume, and age. The one variable that appears significant in most studies is Gleason score, where the small number of patients with Gleason score 6 tumor and SVI have a relatively favorable prognosis.

EXTRAPROSTATIC EXTENSION

DEFINITION AND INCIDENCE

Histologically, the prostatic capsule is not well defined.[33] In some areas, there may appear to be a fibrous or fibromuscular band at the edge of the prostate although in other areas normal prostatic glands extend out to the edge of the prostate without any appearance that there is a capsule. Because the prostate lacks a discrete capsule, the term "extraprostatic extension" has replaced "capsular penetration" to describe tumor that has extended out of the prostate into periprostatic soft tissue. The term "capsular invasion" is also not recommended as it describes extension into a structure that is anatomically not well defined.

A study from the Cleveland Clinic Foundation documented a decrease from 81% to 36% in EPE with radical prostatectomies performed between 1987 and 1997.[34] The downward trend in extraprostatic extension was independent of the preoperative PSA level, clinical tumor stage, and biopsy Gleason score.

Because of the desmoplastic response associated with EPE, it can be difficult to judge whether the tumor has extended out of the gland or is within the fibrous tissue of the prostate. Pathologists often underdiagnose EPE, as some diagnose it only when tumor is seen in periprostatic adipose tissue.

LOCATION AND EXTENT

Extraprostatic extension preferentially occurs posteriorly and posterolaterally in stage T2 adenocarcinomas and often occurs via perineural invasion.[35] In transition zone cancers found in stage T1B and in some T1C tumors, EPE occurs anteriorly usually by direct stromal invasion without prominent perineural invasion.[35] The degree of EPE varies from only a few glands outside the prostate on one or two histological sections, termed "focal EPE," to cases with more extensive extraprostatic spread sometimes designated as "established EPE." More objective definitions for focal EPE have not been shown to superior in predicting prognosis.[36,37]

MARGINS OF RESECTION

DEFINITION

The pathological definition of positive margins of resection appears straightforward: "tumor extending to the surface of the prostate, which the surgeon has cut across." The difficulty with the practical application of this definition is that the prostate is surrounded by vital structures—the urogenital diaphragm distally, pelvic sidewall laterally, rectum posteriorly, and bladder neck superiorly—limiting the radical removal of the prostate. Consequently, in many sites the radical prostatectomy specimen is surrounded by less than a millimeter of periprostatic soft tissue. When tumor is not actually cut across and at the ink, close margins (<0.1 mm.) should not be designated as positive margins, as they are not associated with tumor that would be left within the patient or an increased risk of postoperative progression.[38,39]

ETIOLOGY

Capsular incision

One cause of a positive resection margin is transection of intraprostatic tumor (capsular incision). These cases should be designated as pathological stage T2X, denoting that elsewhere the tumor is organ-confined, yet one cannot determine whether there is EPE in the region of capsular incision as the edge of the prostate has been left in the patient. The percentage of positive margins resulting from capsular incision ranges from as low as 1.3% to as high as 71%.[40-45] One frequent site of capsular incision is posterolaterally, where less experienced surgeons inadvertently cut into the prostate in order to preserve the neurovascular bundle. The high incidence of capsular incision at the apex may, in large part, result from an artifact of how the apex is sectioned

and as a result of variations in pathologist's interpretation. If the apical margin is assessed as a shave (en face) margin, tumor may be seen admixed with benign glands and called capsular incision, whereas the margin would be negative for tumor if the apex had been processed as a perpendicular margin (Figure 11.2). Also, the histologic boundaries of the prostate in the region of the apex are extremely vague, with benign glands admixed with skeletal muscle. When tumor is seen extending to the inked edge of the tissue at the apex, it can be subjective as to whether the pathologist thinks that the tumor is still within the prostate (i.e., capsular incision) or shows a positive margin in an area of EPE. The approach that this author takes at the apex is that if tumor is seen extending to the inked edge of the prostate where benign prostate glands are not cut across, the assumption is that the surgeon is outside of the prostate and a diagnosis is rendered of a positive margin in an area of EPE.

Posteriorly, there is also the potential for overdiagnosis of capsular incision. In the posterior and posterolateral regions of the prostate, when tumor extends out of the prostate there is often an associated desmoplastic reaction, such even though EPE is present, it is uncommon to see tumor situated within adipose tissue. When tumor extends to the margin in an area of EPE associated desmoplasia, it may be misinterpreted as organ-confined cancer, since tumor

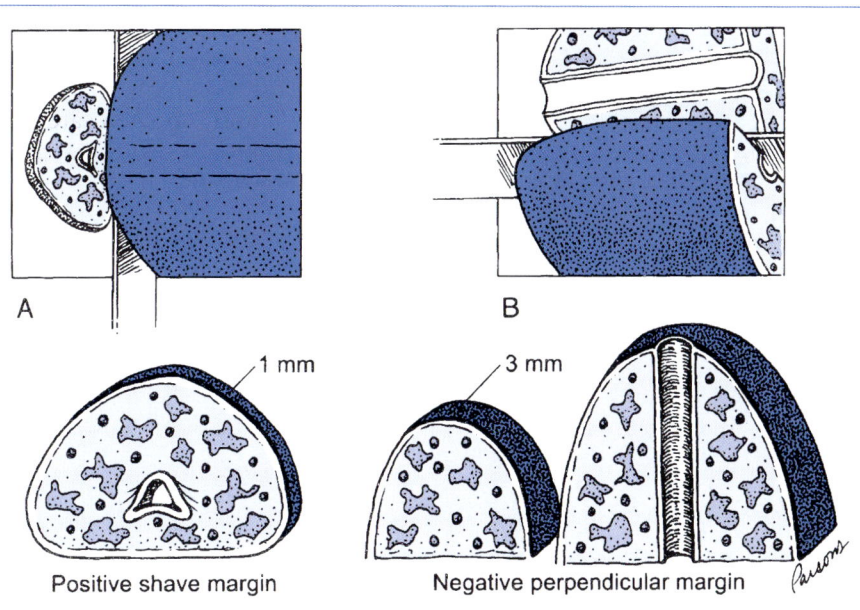

A

B

1 mm

3 mm

Positive shave margin   Negative perpendicular margin

Fig. 11.2

Different techniques of processing the apical margin in the same case where there is tumor at the apex. Small circles represent cancer. Larger irregular spaces represent benign glands. *A*, A shave margin of the apical margin consists of thin (1 mm) slice perpendicular to the urethra. The entire section is considered the margin, regardless if tumor extends to the inked edge of the section. The case would be signed out as showing a positive margin in an area of capsular incision, as both cancer and benign glands are at the margin, although as shown in part *B* the margins are truly negative.

B, Perpendicular margins consist of serial thicker (3 mm) slices parallel to the urethra. Only the inked edge of the section is considered the margin. The case would be signed out as showing organ-confined disease with negative margins and no capsular incision, as both benign glands and cancer do not extend to the inked edge of the section.

is not seen in fat, and overdiagnosed as capsular incision.

There are conflicting data regarding the prognostic significance of positive margins resulting from capsular incision, with most studies reporting lower progression.[29,44,46–50]

Non-iatrogenic causes of positive margins

Positive margins can result from a failure to widely excise tumor with EPE posterolaterally in the region of the neurovascular bundle.[35] Although with nerve sparing techniques some of the positive margins occur posterolaterally in the region of nerve sparing, it is uncommon (0–7%) for the sole positive margin to be in the area of the nerve preservation.[45,51,52] Failure to widely excise tumor showing EPE more commonly results from an attempt to preserve adjacent vital structures, where resection of additional tissue would result in unacceptable morbidity.

Artifactually positive margins

Because there is such a scant amount of flimsy connective tissue surrounding the prostate, which may be easily disrupted during the intraoperative or postoperative handling of the specimen, tumor may be artifactually seen at the inked edge of the gland.[38]

SITES OF POSITIVE SURGICAL MARGINS

Sites of positive margins tend to parallel sites of EPE, described above. It is uncommon for the bladder neck to be the sole site of a positive margin. Whereas positive margins in radical retropubic prostatectomy specimens most commonly occur apically and posteriorly, there is a relative increased risk of anterior and bladder neck positive margins in radical prostatectomies performed with the perineal approach.[45]

USE OF FROZEN SECTIONS TO ASSESS MARGINS

This author does not recommend performing frozen sections at the time of radical prostatectomy due to the high false positive and negative rates associated with the procedure.[53–56]

RELATIONSHIP OF MARGIN POSITIVITY TO PROGRESSION

Patients with positive margins have a significantly increased risk of progression compared with those with negative margins. In two of the studies the data are similar in that the progression-free probability at 5 years following radical prostatectomy ranges from 81% to 83% for margin-negative disease falling to 58% to 64% for margin-positive disease.[57,58] Multifocal and extensive positive margins are associated with a higher risk of progression compared with solitary and focally positive

margins, respectively.[44,45,52,59] Several studies have demonstrated that apically positive margins do not correlate independently with progression.[60–62] Usually when the bladder neck margin is involved, other areas show positive margins as well. A microscopic positive bladder-neck margin is not so adverse a finding such that it should not be designated as pathologic stage T4 disease.[63] However, a microscopic positive bladder-neck margin has a higher risk for biochemical progression than other locations..[60,64,65]

GRADE

GLEASON SCORES 2 TO 4

Gleason scores of 2 to 4 are rarely seen as the grade of the main tumor in radical prostatectomies performed for stages T1C or T2 disease. Tumors of this grade are typically seen in small multifocal incidental adenocarcinomas of the prostate, most commonly found within the transition zone on transurethral resection of the prostate (TURP).[66] Men with only Gleason scores 2 to 4 at radical prostatectomy are cured.[57]

GLEASON SCORES 5 TO 6

The prognosis of Gleason scores 5 to 6 at radical prostatectomy shows a spectrum in its biologic behavior depending on other variables, such as margin status and organ-confined status[57] (Table 11.1). It is important to recognize that for tumors with this grade the majority are cured regardless of whether they show EPE or positive margins.

GLEASON SCORE 7

Tumors with a Gleason score of 7 have a significantly worse prognosis than those with a Gleason score of 6[57,67] (see Table 11.1). Most studies document that a tumor with a Gleason score 4 + 3 has a worse prognosis than one with Gleason score 3 + 4.[67,68,69]

GLEASON SCORES 8 TO 10

Typically, men with tumors with Gleason scores of 8 to 10 have highly aggressive tumors and present at an advanced stage such that they are not amenable to localized therapy. Even in more recent series, 70% to 91% of men with Gleason score of 8 to 10 tumor do not present with organ-confined disease.[70–72] Overall, patients with Gleason scores 8 to 10 at radical prostatectomy have a 15% chance of having no evidence of disease at 15 years following surgery.[73] Although the numbers of men in each study is small and the follow-up fairly short, organ-confined tumors with Gleason scores of 8 to 10 have a better prognosis.[70,72,74–77]

Table 11.1 PSA progression Kaplan–Meier estimates of risk of progression with negative seminal vesicles and negative lymph nodes

Prostatectomy pathology	5 Years post-prostatectomy (%)	10 Years post-prostatectomy (%)
Gleason sum 2–4	0	4
Gleason sum 5–6	3	19
Gleason sum 7	25	50
Gleason sum 8–10	43	66
Organ-confined	0	17
Focal extraprostatic extension	10	33
Established extraprostatic extension	24	43
Margins negative	6	22
Margins positive	27	46
Gleason sum 5–6 (OC&MAR⁻)*	1	8
Gleason sum 5–6 (FEPE&MAR$^{+\backslash-}$) or (EEPE&MAR⁻)*	2	23
Gleason sum 5–6 (EEPE&MAR⁺)*	15	28
Gleason sum 7 (MAR⁻)	15	39
Gleason sum 7 (FEPE&MAR⁺)	36	36
Gleason sum 7 (EEPE&MAR⁺)	57	67

*Excluding tumors with Gleason pattern 4.

EEPE, established extra-prostatic extension; FEPE, focal extra-prostatic extension; MAR⁻, margins negative; MAR⁺, margins positive; MAR$^{+\backslash-}$, margins positive or negative; OC, organ-confined.

TERTIARY GLEASON PATTERN

Within radical prostatectomy specimens, as a result of the greater amount of tumor available for histological examination, a higher proportion of cases are found to contain more than two grades compared with needle biopsy. When a tumor contains tertiary high grades, the tumor should be graded routinely with a comment in the report noting the presence of the tertiary element.[78,79]

TUMOR VOLUME

In general, the size of a prostate cancer correlates with its extent.[80] Extraprostatic extension is uncommon in tumors of less than 0.5 mL. Tumors which are less than 4 mL uncommonly reveal lymph node metastases or seminal vesicle invasion. The location and grade of the tumor also modulate the effect of tumor volume.[66,80,81] Transition zone tumors extend out of the prostate at larger volumes than peripheral zone tumors, as a result of their lower grade and greater distance from the edge of the gland.

Measuring tumor volume in the prostate is not straightforward. Prostate cancers are not easily appreciated grossly, and they tend to have irregular shapes with infiltrative growth patterns. Although measuring tumor volume using a computer-assisted image analysis system is most accurate, this method is not feasible for routine clinical practice, and alternative simpler means of measuring tumor volume have been proposed.[82–86] There are conflicting studies as to whether tumor volume provides independent

information beyond that which is routinely recorded in a radical prostatectomy specimen, such that current practice does not mandate routine calculation of radical prostatectomy tumor volume.[62,84,87–92]

There is one situation where it is important to give some estimate of tumor volume at radical prostatectomy. As a consequence of screening for prostate cancer, radical prostatectomies increasingly harbor very small cancers.[93] The pathology report should note that these tumors are "small" or "minute" so that urologists can inform patients of their excellent prognosis.

VASCULAR AND PERINEURAL INVASION

Vascular invasion in radical prostatectomy specimens usually occurs in advanced tumors, but has been shown in most studies to be independently prognostic.[69,94–96] Perineural invasion is almost ubiquitously present in radical prostatectomy specimens containing cancer and, in general, has not been found to be predictive of progression.[94,96,97]

NEEDLE BIOPSY

PROCESSING

Prostate biopsies from different regions of the gland should be processed separately. Putting more than two biopsy specimens together in one jar (cassette) increases the loss of tissue at sectioning.[98] When atypia suspicious for cancer is found, a repeat biopsy should concentrate on the initial atypical site in addition to sampling the rest of the prostate.[99] This cannot be performed unless biopsies have been specifically designated as to their location (apex, mid, base: right vs. left). The normal histology at the base of the prostate is unique, and knowledge about biopsy location is helpful for the pathologist to avoid a misdiagnosis of high-grade prostatic intraepithelial neoplasia.[100] The location and extent of cancer may also be used by radiotherapists when planning brachytherapy.

CANCER LOCATION

Most clinically palpable prostate cancers diagnosed on needle biopsy are predominantly located posteriorly and posterolaterally.[16,101] In a few cases, large transition zone tumors may extend into the peripheral zone and become palpable. Nonpalpable cancers detected on needle biopsy are predominantly located peripherally, although 15% to 25% have tumor predominantly within the transition zone.[10]

GRADE

The Gleason grade on biopsy material has also been shown to correlate fairly well with that of the subsequent prostatectomy.[102–104] Undergrading of the needle biopsy is more a problem than overgrading, and, to some extent, is unavoidable due to sampling error. One way in which the practice of Gleason scoring can be improved is to not assign Gleason scores 2 to 4 for adenocarcinoma of the prostate on needle biopsy. The reasons for doing this are: 1) The vast majority of tumors graded as Gleason score 2 to 4 on needle biopsy, when reviewed by experts in urologic pathology, are graded as Gleason scores 5 to 6 or higher[103]; 2) there is poor reproducibility in the diagnosis of Gleason score 2 to 4 on needle biopsy even amongst urologic pathology experts[105]; 3) most importantly, assigning a Gleason score of 2 to 4 to adenocarcinoma on needle biopsies can adversely impact patient care, as clinicians may assume that low-grade cancers on needle biopsy do not need definitive therapy, when it has been shown that up to 55% of these cases can show extraprostatic extension at radical prostatectomy.[103] Both Gleason's data with 2911 patients and subsequent studies with long-term follow-up have demonstrated a good correlation between Gleason score and prognosis.[1,106]

It is recommended that a Gleason score be reported even when a minimal focus of cancer is present. The correlation between biopsy and prostatectomy Gleason score is equivalent or only marginally worse with minimal cancer on biopsy.[103,107,108] It is recommended that even in small cancers with one Gleason pattern that the Gleason score be reported. If only the pattern is reported, the clinician may misconstrue this as the Gleason score.

Although there is no data on tertiary patterns on needle biopsy material, in the setting of three grade patterns on biopsy where the highest grade is the least common, the highest grade is incorporated as the secondary pattern. The assumption is that a small focus of high-grade cancer on biopsy will correlate with a significant amount of high-grade cancer in the prostate, and that sampling artifact accounts for its limited nature on biopsy.

TUMOR EXTENT

Multiple techniques of quantifying the amount of cancer found on needle biopsy have been developed and studied, including measurement of: 1) the number of positive cores; 2) the total millimeters of cancer amongst all cores; 3) the percentage of each core occupied by cancer; 4) the total percentage of cancer in the entire specimen; and 5) the fraction of positive cores. There is no clear consensus as to the superiority of one technique over the other (reviewed in ref. 109). Extensive cancer on needle biopsy in general predicts for adverse prognosis. However, limited carcinoma on needle biopsy is not as predictive of a favorable prognosis due to sampling limitations. A feasible and rationale approach would be to have pathologists report the number of cores containing cancer, as well as one other system quantifying tumor extent (e.g., percentage, length).

PERINEURAL INVASION

Whereas almost all reports have noted an increased risk of EPE in the corresponding radical prostatectomy specimen, there are conflicting data as to whether perineural invasion (PNI) provides independent prognostication beyond that of needle biopsy grade and serum PSA levels (reviewed in ref. 109). It has also been demonstrated that the presence of PNI on the needle biopsy is associated with a significantly higher incidence of disease progression following radical prostatectomy and radiation.[109] As PNI is of prognostic significance and easy to assess histologically, its reporting on needle biopsy is recommended.

TRANSURETHRAL RESECTION

PROCESSING

A TURP specimen may contain more than a hundred grams of tissue, and it is often necessary to select a limited amount of tissue for histologic examination. Submission of eight cassettes will identify almost all stage T1B cancers and approximately 90% of stage T1A tumors.[110,111] In young men, submission of the entire specimen may be considered to ensure detection of all T1A tumors. Guidelines have been developed for whether additional sampling is needed following the initial detection of cancer in a TURP specimen.[112]

INCIDENCE AND LOCATION OF THE CANCER

When TURP is done without clinical suspicion of cancer, prostate cancer is incidentally detected in approximately 8% to 10% of the specimens. Cancers detected at TURP are often transition zone tumors, but they may also be of peripheral zone origin, particularly when they are large.[113,114] It is recommended that the extent of tumor is reported as percentage of the total specimen area. If the tumor occupies less than 5% of the specimen, it is stage T1A, and otherwise stage T1B. However, in the uncommon situation of less than 5% of cancer with Gleason score 7 or higher, patients are treated as if they had stage T1B disease.

CANCER PROGNOSIS

Although the risk of progression at 4 years with stage T1A cancer is low (2%), between 16% and 25% of men with untreated stage T1A prostate cancer and longer (8 to 10 years) follow-up have had clinically evident progression.[115] Stage T1B tumors are more heterogeneous in grade, location, and volume than are stage T2 carcinomas.[66] Stage T1B cancers tend to be lower grade and located within the transition zone as compared with palpable cancers.

DIFFERENTIAL DIAGNOSIS OF PROSTATE CANCER

The underdiagnosis of limited adenocarcinoma of the prostate on needle biopsy is one of the most frequent problems in prostate pathology. It is not uncommon to have several needle biopsy cores of prostatic tissue where there are only a few malignant glands, which may be difficult to diagnose. There are also numerous benign mimics of adenocarcinoma of the prostate.[116] In some of these cases, the use of antibodies to high-molecular-weight cytokeratin may resolve the diagnosis.[117,118] Benign glands contain basal cells and are labeled with these antibodies, whereas prostate cancer shows no staining. AMACR may be used as a confirmatory stain for prostatic adenocarcinoma, in conjunction with (H&E) morphology and a basal cell specific marker.[119] However, one must be cautious as some mimics of prostate cancer express AMACR and not all cancers on needle biopsy are positive for AMACR.

ADENOCARCINOMA WITH TREATMENT EFFECT

The histology of prostate cancer may be significantly altered following its treatment with total androgen blockade. For pathologists who have not seen a lot of these specimens it may be difficult to recognize hormone-treated cancer.[120-122] One of the problems with evaluating carcinomas that have been treated with hormone therapy is that the grade often appears artifactually higher. Evidence to support that the apparently higher grade is artifactual comes from evaluation of the pre-hormone therapy needle biopsies that often appear lower grade. Furthermore, the treated cancers are predominantly diploid and have low proliferation rates. There is controversy as to whether pathologists can accurately grade hormone-treated cancers taking into account the hormone effect. The majority of investigators believe that treated carcinomas cannot be assigned an accurate Gleason grade. However, if there are other areas of the tumor that do not show a pronounced hormone effect, these areas can be Gleason graded. It is controversial as to whether finasteride may cause similar changes to those seen with total androgen blockade.

After radiotherapy, recurrent/persistent adenocarcinoma may contain areas that look unaffected or may show cancer with treatment affect. When signing out post-radiotherapy biopsies, we diagnose them as "benign," "cancer without treatment effect" (a Gleason grade is assigned), or "cancer showing treatment effect" (no Gleason grade assigned). Biopsy pathology predicts prognosis with positive biopsies having a worse outcome than negative biopsies and cancers with treatment effect having an intermediate prognosis.[123]

SUBTYPES OF PROSTATE ADENOCARCINOMA

Mucinous adenocarcinoma of the prostate gland is one of the least common morphologic variants of prostatic carcinoma.[124-126] It has an aggressive biologic behavior and, like nonmucinous prostate carcinoma, has a propensity to develop bone metastases and increased serum PSA levels with advanced disease.

Between 0.4% and 0.8% of prostatic adenocarcinomas arise from prostatic ducts.[127,128] When prostatic duct adenocarcinomas arise in the large primary periurethral prostatic ducts, they may grow as an exophytic lesion into the urethra, most commonly in and around the verumontanum and give rise to either obstructive symptoms or hematuria. Tumors arising in the more peripheral prostatic ducts may present like ordinary (acinar) adenocarcinoma of the prostate and may be diagnosed on needle biopsy. Tumors are often underestimated clinically, since rectal exam and serum PSA levels may be normal. Most prostatic duct adenocarcinomas are advanced stage at presentation and have an aggressive course.

REFERENCES

1. Gleason DF, Mellinger GT, and the Veterans Administration Cooperative Urological Research Group. Prediction of prognosis for prostatic adenocarcinoma by combined histologic grading and clinical staging. J Urol 1974; 111;58–64.

2. McNeal JE, Villers AA, Redwine EA, et al. Histologic differentiation, cancer volume, and pelvic lymph node metastasis in adenocarcinoma of the prostate. Cancer 1990;66:1225–1233.

3. Epstein JI, Carmichael MJ, Partin AW. Small high grade adenocarcinomas of the prostate in radical prostatectomy specimens performed for non-palpable disease: pathogenic and clinical implications. J Urol 1994;151:1587–1592.

4. Cumming JA, Ritchie AW, Goodman CM, et al. De-differentiation with time in prostate cancer and the influence of treatment on the course of the disease. Br J Urol 1990;65:271–274.

5. Epstein JI, Walsh PC, Carter HB. Dedifferentiation of prostate cancer grade with time in men followed expectantly for stage T1c disease. J Urol 2001;166:1688–1691.

6. Cohen MB, Soloway MS, Murphy WM. Sampling of radical prostatectomy specimens: How much is adequate? Am J Clin Pathol 1994;101:250–252.

7. Hall GS, Kramer CE, Epstein JI. Evaluation of radical prostatectomy specimens: A comparative analysis of sampling methods. Am J Surg Pathol 1994;16:315–324.

8. Smith Sehdev AE, Pan CC, Epstein JI. Comparative analysis of sampling methods in nonpalpable (stage T1C) radical prostatectomy specimen. Hum Pathol 2001;32:494–499.

9. Carter HB, Sauvageot J, Walsh PC, et al. Prospective evaluation of men with stage T1C adenocarcinoma of the prostate. J Urol 1997;157:2206–2209.

10. Epstein JI, Walsh PC, Carmichael M, et al. Pathologic and clinical findings to predict tumor extent of nonpalpable (stage T1c) prostate cancer. JAMA 1994;271:368–374.

11. Bova GS, Fox WM, Epstein JI. Methods of radical prostatectomy specimen processing: A novel technique for harvesting fresh prostate cancer tissue and review of processing techniques. Mod Pathol 1993;6:201–207.

12. Egevad L, Engström K, Busch C. A new method for handling radical prostatectomies enabling fresh tissue harvesting, whole mount sections, and landmarks for alignment of sections. J Urologic Pathol 1998; 9:17–28.

13. Furman J, Murphy WM, Rice L, et al. Prostatectomy tissue for research. Balancing patient care and discovery. Am J Clin Pathol 1998:110:4–9.

14. Hoedemaeker RF, Ruitjer ETG, Ruizeveld-de Winter JA, et al. Processing radical prostatectomy specimens. A comprehensive and standardized protocol. J Urologic Pathol 1998:9:211–222.

15. Wheeler TM, Lebovitz RM. Fresh tissue harvest for research from prostatectomy specimens. The Prostate 1994;25:274–279.

16. Byar DP, Mostofi FK, and the Veterans Administrative Cooperative Urologic Research Groups. Carcinoma of the prostate; prognostic evaluation of certain pathologic features in 208 radical prostatectomies. Cancer 1972;30:5–13.

17. Partin AW, Kattan MW, Subong ENP, et al. Combination of prostate-specific antigen, clinical stage, and Gleason score to predict pathological stage of localized prostate cancer: A multi-institutional update. JAMA 1997;277:1445–1451.

18. Epstein JI, Oesterling JE, Eggleston JC, et al. Frozen section detection of lymph node metastases in prostatic carcinoma: Accuracy in grossly uninvolved pelvic lymphadenectomy specimens. J Urol 1986;136:1234–1237.

19. Sgrignoli AR, Walsh PC, Steinberg GD, et al. Prognostic factors in men with stage D1 prostate cancer: Identification of patients less likely to have prolonged survival after radical prostatectomy. J Urol 1994;152:1077–1081.

20. Kothari PS, Scardino PT, Ohori M, et al. Incidence, location, and significance of periprostatic and periseminal vesicle lymph nodes in prostate cancer. Am J Surg Pathol 2001;25:1429–1432.

21. Cheng L, Slezak J, Bergstralh EJ, et al. Dedifferentiation in the metastatic progression of prostate carcinoma. Cancer 1999;86:657–663.

22. Cheng L, Bergstralh EJ, Cheville JC, et al. Cancer volume of lymph node metastasis predicts progression in prostate cancer. Am J Surg Pathol 1998;22:1491–1500.

23. Steinberg GD, Epstein JI, Piantadosi S, et al. Management of stage D1 adenocarcinoma of the prostate: The Johns Hopkins Experience 1974 to 1987. J Urol 1990;144:1425–1432.

24. Debras B, Guillonneau B, Bougaran J. Prognostic significance of seminal vesicle invasion on the radical prostatectomy specimen. Eur Urol 1998;33:271–277.

25. Tefilli MV, Gheiler EL, Tiguert R, et al. Prognostic indications in patients with seminal vesicle involvement following radical prostatectomy for clinically localized prostate cancer. J Urol 1998;160:802–806.

26. Ohori M, Scardino PT, Lapin SL, et al. The mechanisms and prognostic significance of seminal vesicle involvement by prostate cancer. Am J Surg Pathol 1993;17:1252–1261.

27. Epstein JI, Partin AW, Potter SR, et al. Adenocarcinoma of the prostate invading the seminal vesicle: Prognostic stratification based on pathologic parameters. Urology 2000;56:283–288.

28. Catalona WJ, Smith DS. Cancer recurrence and survival rates after anatomic radical retropubic prostatectomy for prostate cancer: Intermediate-terms results. J Urol 1998:160:2428–2434.

29. D'Amico AV, Whittington R, Malkowicz B, et al. A multivariate analysis of clinical and pathological factors that predict for prostate specific antigen failure after radical prostatectomy for prostate cancer. J Urol 1995:154:131–135.

30. Trapasso JG, deKernion JB, Smith RB, et al. The incidence and significance of detectable levels of serum prostate specific antigen after radical prostatectomy. J Urol 1994;152:1821–1825.

31. Salomon L, Anastasiadis AG, Johnson CW, et al. Seminal vesicle involvement after radical prostatectomy: Predicting risk factors for progression. Urology 2003:62:304–309.

32. Sofer M, Savoi M, Kim SS, et al. Biochemical and pathological predictors of the recurrence of prostatic adenocarcinoma with seminal vesicle invasion. J Urol 2003; 169:154–156.

33. Ayala AG, Ro JY, Babaian R, et al. The prostatic capsule: Does it exist: Its importance in the staging and treatment of prostatic carcinoma. Am J Surg Pathol 1989;13:21–27.

34. Jhaveri F, Klein EA, Kupelian PA, et al. Declining rates of extracapsular extension after radical prostatectomy: Evidence of continued stage migration. J Clin Oncol 1999;17:3167–3172.

35. Villers A, McNeal JE, Redwine EA, et al. The role of perineural space invasion in the local spread of prostatic adenocarcinoma. J Urol 1989;142:763–768.

36. McNeal JE, Villers AA, Redwine EA, et al. Capsular penetration in prostate cancer. Am J Surg Pathol 1990;14:240–247.

37. Wheeler TM, Dillioglugil Ö, Kattan MW, et al. Clinical and pathological significance of the level and extent of capsular invasion in clinical stage T1-2 prostate cancer. Hum Pathol 1998;29:856–862.

38. Epstein JI. Evaluation of radical prostatectomy capsular margins of resection: The significance of margins designated as negative, closely approaching, and positive. Am J Surg Pathol 1990;14:626–632.

39. Epstein JI, Sauvageot J. Do close but negative margins in radical prostatectomy specimens increase the risk of postoperative progression? J Urol 1997;157:241–243.

40. Ackerman DA, Barry JM, Wicklund RA, et al. Analysis of risk factors associated with prostate cancer extension to the surgical margin and

pelvic node metastasis at radical prostatectomy. J Urol 1993;150:1845–1850.

41. Rosen MA, Goldstone L, Lapin S, et al. Frequency and location of extracapsular extension and positive surgical margins in radical prostatectomy specimens. J Urol 1992;148:331–337.

42. Stamey TA, Villers AA, McNeal JE, et al. Positive surgical margins at radical prostatectomy: Importance of the apical dissection. J Urol 1990;143:1166–1172.

43. Van Den Ouden D, Bentvelsen FM, Boevé ER, et al. Schröder: Positive margins after radical prostatectomy: Correlation with local recurrence and distant progression. Br J Urol 1993;72:489–494.

44. Watson RB, Civantos F, Soloway MS. Positive surgical margins with radical prostatectomy: Detailed pathological analysis and prognosis. Urology 1996;48:80–90.

45. Weldon VE, Tavel FR, Neuwirth H, et al. Patterns of positive specimen margins and detectable prostate specific antigen after radical perineal prostatectomy. J Urol 1995;153:1565–1569.

46. Barocas DA, Han M, Epstein JI, et al. Does capsular incision at radical retropubic prostatectomy affect disease-free survival in otherwise organ-confined prostate cancer? Urology 2001;58:746–751.

47. Freedland SJ, Aronson WJ, Presti JC, et al. Should a positive surgical margin following radical retropubic prostatectomy be pathological stage T2 or T3? Results from the search database. J Urol 2003;169:2142–2146.

48. Guillonneau B, El-Fettouh H, Baumert H, et al. Laparoscopic radical prostatectomy: Oncological evaluation after 1,000 cases at Montsouris Institute. J Urol 2003;169:1261–1266.

49. Kupelian P, Katcher J, Levin H, et al. Correlation of clinical and pathologic factors with rising prostate-specific antigen profiles after radical prostatectomy alone for clinically localized prostate cancer. Urology 1996;48:249–260.

50. Salomon L, Anastasiadis AG, Antiphon P, et al. Prognostic consequences of the location of positive surgical margins in organ-confined prostate cancer. Urol Int 2003;70:291–296.

51. Eggleston JC, Walsh PC. Radical prostatectomy with preservation of sexual function: pathological findings in the first 100 cases. J Urol 1985;134:1146–1148.

52. Epstein JI, Pizov G, Walsh PC. Correlation of pathologic findings with progression following radical retropubic prostatectomy. Cancer 1993;71:3582–3593.

53. Cangiano TG, Litwin MS, Naitoh J, et al. Intraoperative frozen section monitoring of nerve sparing radical retropubic prostatectomy. J Urol 1999;162:655–658.

54. Fromont G, Baumert H, Cathelineau X, et al. Intraoperative frozen section analysis during nerve sparing laparoscopic radical prostatectomy: Feasibility study. J Urol 2003;170:1843–1846.

55. Goharderakhshan RZ, Sudilovsky D, Carrol LA, et al. Utility of intraoperative frozen section analysis of surgical margins in region of neurovascular bundles at radical prostatectomy. Urology 2002;59:709–714.

56. Shah O, Melamed J, Lepor H. Analysis of apical soft tissue margins during radical retropubic prostatectomy. J Urol 2001;165:1943–1949.

57. Epstein JI, Partin AW, Sauvageot J, et al. Prediction of progression following radical prostatectomy: A multivariate analysis of 721 men with long-term follow-up. Am J Surg Pathol 1996;20:286–292.

58. Ohori M, Wheeler TM, Kattan MW, et al. Prognostic significance of positive surgical margins in radical prostatectomy specimens. J Urol 1995;154:1818–1824.

59. D'Amico A, Whittington R, Malkowicz SB, et al. An analysis of the time course of postoperative prostate-specific antigen failure in patients with positive margins: Implications on the use of adjuvant therapy. Urology 1996;47:538–547.

60. Blute ML, Bostwick DG, Bergstralh EJ, et al. Anatomic site-specific positive margins in organ-confined prostate cancer and its impact on outcome after radical prostatectomy. Urology 1997;50:733–739.

61. Fesseha T, Sakr W, Grignon D, et al. Prognostic implications of a positive apical margin in radical prostatectomy specimens. J Urol 1997;158:2176.

62. Ohori M, Abbas F, Wheeler TM, et al. Pathological features and prognostic significance of prostate cancer in the apical section determined by whole mount histology. J Urol 1999;161:500–504.

63. Yossepowitch O, Sircar K, Scardino PT, et al. Bladder neck involvement in pathological stage pT4 radical prostatectomy specimens is not an independent prognostic factor. J Urol 2002;168:2011–2015.

64. Aydin H, Tsuzuki T, Hernandez D, et al. Positive proximal (bladder neck) margin at radical prostatectomy confers a higher risk of biochemical progression 2004;63:551–555.

65. Obek C, Sadek S, Lai S, et al. Positive surgical margins with radical retropubic prostatectomy: anatomic site-specific pathological analysis and impact on prognosis. Urology 1999;54:682–688.

66. Christensen WN, Partin AW, Walsh PC, et al. Pathologic findings in clinical stage A2 prostate cancer. Relation of tumor volume, grade, and location to pathologic stage. Cancer 1990;65:1021–1027.

67. Chan TY, Partin AW, Walsh PC, et al. The prognostic significance of Gleason score 3+4 versus Gleason score 4+3 tumor at radical prostatectomy. Urology 2000;56:823–827.

68. Han M, Partin AW, Zahurak M, et al. Biochemical (prostate specific antigen) recurrence probability following radical prostatectomy for clinically localized prostate cancer. J Urol 2003;169:517–523.

69. Babaian RJ, Troncoso P, Bhadkamkar VA, et al. Analysis of clinicopathologic factors predicting outcome after radical prostatectomy. Cancer 2001;91:1414–1422.

70. Ohori M, Goad JR, Wheeler RM, et al. Can radical prostatectomy alter the progression of poorly differentiated prostate cancer? J Urol 1994;152:1843–1849.

71. Oefelein MG, Grayhack JT, McVary KT. Survival after radical prostatectomy of men with clinically localized high grade carcinoma of the prostate. Cancer 1995;76:2535–2542.

72. Perrotti M, Rabbani F, Russo P, et al. Early prostate cancer detection and potential for surgical cure in men with poorly differentiated tumors. Urology 1998;52:106–110.

73. Han M, Partin AW, Pound CR, et al. Long term biochemical disease-free and cancer-specific survival following anatomic radical retropubic prostatectomy: The 15-year Johns Hopkins Experience. Urol Clin N Am 2001;28:555–565.

74. Oefelein MG, Smith ND, Grayhack JT, et al. Long-term results of radical retropubic prostatectomy in men with high grade carcinoma of the prostate. J Urol 1997;158:1460–1465.

75. Mian BM, Troncoso P, Okihara K, et al. Outcome of patients with Gleason score 8 or higher prostate cancer following radical prostatectomy alone. J Urol 2002;167:1675–1680.

76. Rioux-Leclercq N, Chan DY, Epstein JI. Prediction of outcome after radical prostatectomy in men with organ-confined Gleason score 8 to 10 adenocarcinoma. Urology 2002;60:666–669.

77. Teffili MV, Gheiler EL, Tiguert R, et al. Should Gleason score 7 cancer be considered a unique grade category? Urology 1999;53:372–377.

78. Pan C-C, Potter SR, Partin AW, et al. The prognostic significance of tertiary Gleason patterns of higher grade in radical prostatectomy specimens: a proposal to modify the Gleason grading system Am J Surg Pathol 2000;24:563–569.

79. Mosse CA, Magi-Galuzi C, Tsuzuki T, et al. The prognostic significance of tertiary Gleason pattern 5 in radical prostatectomy specimens. Am J Surg Pathol 2004;28:394–398.

80. McNeal JE. Cancer volume and site of origin of adenocarcinoma of the prostate: Relationship to local and distant spread. Hum Pathol 1992;23:258–266.

81. Greene DR, Wheeler TM, Egawa S, et al. A comparison of the morphological features of cancer arising in the transition zone and in the peripheral zone of the prostate. J Urol 1991;146:1069–1076.

82. Humphrey PA, Vollmer RT. Percentage carcinoma as a measure of prostatic tumor size in radical prostatectomy tissues. Mod Pathol 1997;10:326–333.

83. Renshaw AA, Chang H, D'Amico AV. Estimation of tumor volume in radical prostatectomy specimens in routine clinical practice. Am J Clin Pathol 1997;107:704–708.

84. Renshaw AA, Richie JR, Loughlin KR, et al. Maximum diameter of prostatic carcinoma is a simple, inexpensive, and independent predictor of prostate-specific antigen failure in radical prostatectomy specimens. Am J Clin Pathol 1999;111:641–644.

85. Noguchi M, Stamey TA, McNeal JE, et al. Assessment of morphometric measurements of prostate carcinoma volume. Cancer 2000;89:1056–1064.

86. Chen ME, Johnston D, Reyes AO, et al. A streamlined three-dimensional volume estimation method accurately classifies prostate tumors by volume. Am J Surg Pathol 2003;27:1291–1301.

87. Carvalhal GF, Humphrey PA, Thorson P, et al. Visual estimate of the percentage of carcinoma is an independent predictor of prostate carcinoma recurrence after radical prostatectomy. Cancer 2000;89:1308–1314.

88. Epstein JI, Carmichael M, Partin AW, et al. Is tumor volume an independent predictor of progression following radical prostatectomy? A multivariate analysis of 185 clinical stage B adenocarcinomas of the prostate with 5 years of followup. J Urol 1993;149:1478–1481.

89. Manoharan M, Civantos F, Kim SS, et al. Visual estimate of percent of carcinoma predicts recurrence after radical prostatectomy. J Urol 2003; 170:1194–1198.

90. Palisaar R, Graefen M, Karakiewicz PI, et al. Assessment of clinical and pathologic characteristics predisposing to disease recurrence following radical prostatectomy in men with pathologically organ-confined prostate cancer. Eur Urol 2002;41:155–161.

91. Salomon L, Levrel O, Anastasiasdis AG, et al. Prognostic significance of tumor volume after radical prostatectomy: A multivariate analysis of pathological factors. Eur Urol 2003;43:39–44.

92. Stamey TA, McNeal JE, Yemoto CH, et al. Biological determinants of cancer progression in men with prostate cancer. JAMA 1999;281:1395–1400.

93. DiGiuseppe JA, Sauvageot J, Epstein JI. Increasing incidence of minimal residual cancer radical prostatectomy specimens. Am J Surg Pathol 1997;21:174–178.

94. Van Den Ouden D, Hop WCJ, Kranse R, et al. Tumour control according to pathological variables in patients treated by radical prostatectomy for clinically localized carcinoma of the prostate. Br J Urol 1997;79:203–211.

95. De la Taille A, Rubin MA, Buttyan R, et al. Is microvascular invasion on radical prostatectomy specimens a useful predictor of PSA recurrence for prostate cancer patients? Eur Urol 2000;38:79–84.

96. Ito K, Nakashima J, Mukai M, et al. Prognostic implication of microvascular invasion in biochemical failure in patients treated with radical prostatectomy. Urol Int 2003;70:297–302.

97. Maru N, Ohori M, Kattan MW, et al. Prognostic significance of the diameter of perineural invasion in radical prostatectomy specimens. Hum Pathol 2001;32:828–833.

98. Kao J, Upton M, Zhang P, et al. Individual prostate biopsy core embedding facilitates maximal tissue representation. J Urol 2002;168:496–499.

99. Allen EA, Kahane H, Epstein JI. Repeat biopsy strategies for men with atypical diagnoses on initial prostate needle biopsy. Urology 1998;52:803–807.

100. Srodon M, Epstein JI. Central zone histology of the prostate: A mimicker of high grade prostatic intraepithelial neoplasia. Hum Pathol 2002;33:518–523.

101. McNeal JE. Origin and development of carcinoma in the prostate. Cancer 1969;23:24–34.

102. Spires SE, Cibull ML, Wood DP Jr, et al. Gleason histologic grading in prostatic carcinoma. Correlation of 18-guage core biopsy with prostatectomy. Arch Pathol Lab Med 1994;118:705–708.

103. Steinberg DM, Sauvageot J, Piantadosi S, et al. Correlation of prostate needle biopsy and radical prostatectomy Gleason grade in academic and community settings. Am J Surg Pathol 1997;21:566–576.

104. Bostwick DG. Gleason grading of prostatic needle biopsies. Correlation with grade in 316 matched prostatectomies. Am J Surg Pathol 1994;18:796–803.

105. Allsbrook WC, Mangold KA, Yang X, et al. The Gleason grading system: an overview. J Urol Path 1999;10:141–157.

106. Sogani PC, Israel A, Lieberman PH, et al. Gleason grading of prostate cancer: A predictor of survival. Urology 1985;25:223–227.

107. Egevad L, Norlen BJ, Norberg M. The value of multiple core biopsies for predicting the Gleason score of prostate cancer. BJU Int 2001;88:716–721.

108. Rubin MA, Dunn R, Kambham N, et al. Should a Gleason score be assigned to a minute focus of carcinoma on prostate biopsy? Am J Surg Pathol 2000;24:1634–1640.

109. Epstein JI, Potter SR. The pathological interpretation and significance of prostate needle biopsy findings: implications and current controversies. J Urol 2001;166:402–410.

110. Murphy WM, Dean PJ, Brasfield JA, et al. Incidental carcinoma of the prostate. How much sampling is adequate? Am J Surg Pathol 1986;10:170–174.

111. Rohr LR. Incidental adenocarcinoma in transurethral resections of the prostate: partial versus complete microscopic examination. Am J Surg Pathol 1987;11:53–58.

112. McDowell PR, Fox WM, Epstein JI. Is submission of remaining tissue necessary when incidental carcinoma of the prostate is found on transurethral resection? Hum Pathol 1994;25:493–497.

113. Greene DR, Wheeler TM, Egawa S, et al. Relationship between clinical stage and histological zone of origin in early prostate cancer: morphometric analysis. Br J Urol 1991;68:499–509.

114. McNeal JE, Price HM, Redwine EA, et al. Stage A versus stage B adenocarcinoma of the prostate: morphological comparison and biological significance. J Urol 1988;139:61–65.

115. Epstein JI, Paull G, Eggleston JC, et al. Prognosis of untreated stage A1 prostatic carcinoma: A study of 94 cases with extended follow-up. J Urol 1986;136:837–839.

116. Epstein JI. Prostate Biopsy Interpretation, 3rd ed. New York: Lippincott William and Wilkins, 2002.

117. Kahane H, Sharp JW, Shuman GB, et al. Utilization of high molecular weight cytokeratin on prostate biopsies in an independent laboratory. Urology 1995;45:981–986.

118. Wojno KJ, Epstein JI. The utility of basal cell specific anti-cytokeratin antibody (34 beta E12) in the diagnosis of prostate cancer: a review of 228 cases. Am J Surg Pathol 1995;19:251–260.

119. Rubin MA, Zhou M, Dhanasekaran SM, et al. α-Methylacyl coenzyme A racemase as a tissue biomarker for prostate cancer. JAMA 2002;287:1662–1670.

120. Armas OA, Aprikian AG, Melamed J, et al. Clinical and pathobiological effects of neoadjuvant total androgen ablation therapy on clinically localized prostatic adenocarcinoma. Am J Surg Pathol 1994;18:979–991.

121. Smith DM, Murphy WM. Histologic changes in prostate carcinomas treated with Leuprolide (luteinizing hormone-releasing hormone effect). Distinction from poor tumor differentiation. Cancer 1994;73:1472–1477.

122. Vaillancourt L, Tâtu B, Fradet Y, et al. Effect of neoadjuvant endocrine therapy (combined androgen blockade) on normal prostate and prostatic carcinoma. A randomized study. Am J Surg Pathol 1996;20:86–93.

123. Crook J, Malone S, Perry G, et al. Postradiotherapy prostate biopsies: What do they really mean? Results for 498 patients. Int J Rad Onc Biol Phys 2000;48:355–367.

124. Ro JY, Grignon J, Ayala AG, et al. Mucinous adenocarcinoma of the prostate: Histochemical and immunohistochemical studies. Hum Pathol 1990;21:593–600.

125. Epstein JI, Lieberman P. Mucinous adenocarcinomas of the prostate gland. Am J Surg Pathol 1985;9:299–307.

126. Saito S, Iwaki H. Mucin-producing carcinoma of the prostate: review of 88 cases. Urology 1999;54:141–144.

127. Brinker DA, Potter SR, Epstein JI. Ductal adenocarcinoma of the prostate diagnosed on needle biopsy: correlation with clinical and radical prostatectomy findings and progression. Am J Surg Pathol 1999;23:1471–1479.

128. Christensen WN, Steinberg WN, Walsh PC, et al. Prostatic duct adenocarcinoma: Findings at radical prostatectomy. Cancer 1991;67:2118–2124.

Precursor lesions of prostatic adenocarcinoma

12

A Alex Freeman

INTRODUCTION

There is widespread acceptance that prostatic adenocarcinoma is preceded by a pre-invasive stage, where the atypical or malignant cells are confined within the boundaries of prostatic ducts/acini, analogous to the pre-invasive conditions seen in the cervix, gastrointestinal tract and skin. Terminology has varied greatly over the last 30 years, and "prostatic intraepithelial neoplasia" (PIN) is the term currently in use. Conversely, "atypical adenomatous hyperplasia" (commonly called "adenosis") was initially believed to be a precursor for prostatic carcinoma, but is now regarded as a proliferative lesion without established malignant potential.

This chapter concentrates on: 1) defining the criteria for the diagnosis of PIN; 2) discussing the evidence for its precursor status; 3) elucidating the difference between low-grade PIN (LGPIN) and high-grade PIN (HGPIN); 4) explaining the significance of these lesions in terms of clinical management.

The concept of a precursor lesion for prostatic carcinoma was first proposed by McNeal in the 1960s[1] and further characterized by several groups throughout the 1970s and 1980s.[2–8] A wide variety of terms have been used in the literature to describe the atypical cytological features seen in the cells of some acini in prostatic biopsies. These have included "atypical primary hyperplasia," "hyperplasia with malignant change," "intraductal dysplasia," "large acinar atypical hyperplasia," "atypia in hyperplasia," "duct-acinar dysplasia" and "prostatic dysplasia/atypical hyperplasia."

The term, "prostatic intraepithelial neoplasia" was first used in 1987,[9] conforming to the nomenclature applied to pre-invasive lesions in the testis and bladder and has gained widespread acceptance.

DEFINITION

Prostatic intraepithelial neoplasia is the term given to a lesion in which cytologically atypical cells are identified within a normal, hyperplastic or atrophic duct-acinar outline in the prostate. Thus, it requires the presence of cytological atypia in the context of a preserved duct-acinar architecture, in contrast to invasive carcinoma in which both architecture and cytology are abnormal.

SUBCLASSIFICATION

Prostatic intraepithelial neoplasia was initially classified into grades 1, 2 and 3[10] (Table 12.1) on the basis of:

- Cellular stratification
- Nuclear crowding
- Loss of polarity
- Increasing nuclear size and atypia
- Presence and increasing size of nucleoli.

However, it was quickly established that the inter-observer and intra-observer reproducibility for the diagnosis of PIN using a three-tiered classification system was low,[11] and the consensus was to simplify the classification into two grades (low-grade and high-grade). Currently, LGPIN equates to the previous grade 1 PIN, with HGPIN incorporating grades 2 and 3.[12] This simplified approach found subsequent clinical support in terms of detection of carcinoma on re-biopsy when controlled by a population whose initial biopsies were benign.[13] Figure 12.1 shows the criteria for HGPIN.

Table 12.1 Morphological features used for the subclassification of prostatic intraepithelial neoplasia

Grade	Stratification	Polarity	Nuclear size	Chromasia	Nucleoli
Grade 1	Minimal	Preserved	Mildly increased	Normal or mild focal hyperchromasia	Absent
Grade 2	Mild	Mild disarray	Moderately increased	Moderate, focal hyperchromasia	Few, small
Grade 3	Moderate	Marked disarray	Markedly increased	Marked extensive hyperchromasia	Multiple, prominent

ARCHITECTURAL PATTERNS

Four main architectural patterns of PIN are widely recognized: tufting, micropapillary, cribriform, and flat.[14] These are commonly seen in the same area, and in some cases even in a single acinus, and are thought to represent morphological variants of the same process. More unusual patterns of PIN have been reported in small numbers of cases, including signet ring, small cell (neuroendocrine), mucinous, and foamy types, and even "PIN with inverted nuclei."[15-16] These individual patterns of PIN do not have an established prognostic significance and are not routinely reported as part of the diagnostic process.

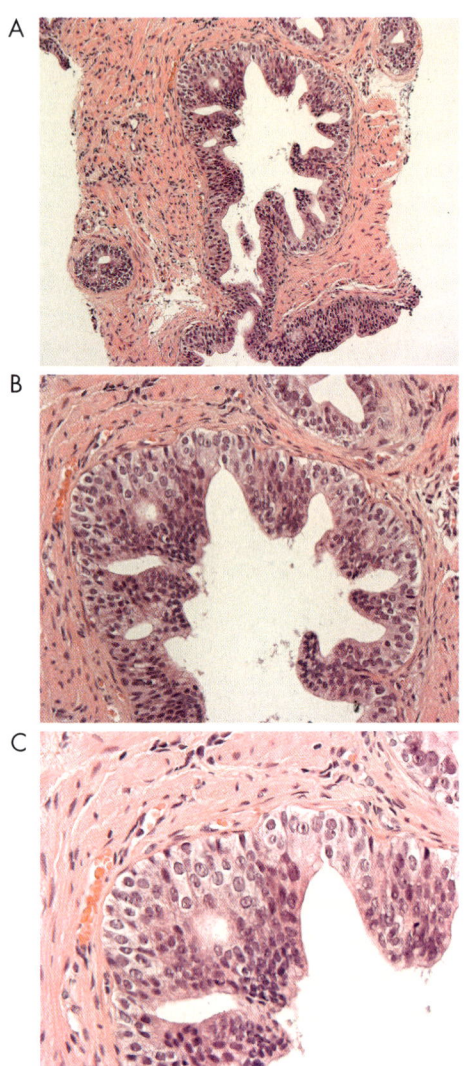

Fig. 12.1
Criteria for high-grade prostatic intraepithelial neoplasia (HGPIN). A prostatic acinus showing marked nuclear enlargement, nuclear stratification, and the presence of several prominent nucleoli required for the diagnosis of HGPIN. All are stained with hematoxylin and eosin (H&E) and are at the following magnifications: ×100 (A), ×200 (B), ×400 (C).

WHAT IS THE RELATIONSHIP WITH PROSTATIC CARCINOMA?

The evidence for PIN as a precursor lesion for prostatic carcinoma mostly relates to HGPIN, as LGPIN may be morphologically difficult to distinguish from benign lesions and the reproducibility of this diagnosis is low. However, this does not preclude the biological concept of an intermediary lesion between benign prostatic epithelium and HGPIN that is not reliably detected by current techniques.

EVIDENCE FOR A LINK BETWEEN PIN AND CARCINOMA

- Prostates with carcinoma show larger, more frequent foci of HGPIN, compared with prostates without carcinoma.[17]
- Prostates with multiple foci of carcinoma show more numerous areas of HGPIN compared with prostates with a small single area of carcinoma.
- Microscopic foci of carcinoma can be seen arising from HGPIN, showing a "transition" between the two lesions.[18]
- HGPIN is more commonly seen in the peripheral zone of the prostate, showing a marked spatial association with carcinoma.[17]
- There appears to be good correlation between the presence of peripheral zone HGPIN and high Gleason score peripheral zone carcinomas.[19]
- Some of the biological markers seen in carcinoma are also identified in HGPIN but are absent in benign acini, while other markers that are raised in carcinoma but normal in benign acini show intermediate levels of expression in HGPIN.[20]

EVIDENCE AGAINST A LINK BETWEEN PIN AND CARCINOMA

- HGPIN is recorded later than the presence of small foci of carcinoma in a recent autopsy study.[21]
- Although LGPIN is identified earlier than invasive carcinoma, the significance of this is unknown, and there is little convincing evidence linking LGPIN and carcinoma.[22]
- There is less correlation between HGPIN and transition zone carcinomas. These tumors are often of low Gleason grade, and may arise from another precursor lesion

GENETIC ALTERATIONS

Prostatic intraepithelial neoplasia has been found to be associated with progressive abnormalities of genotype and phenotype, intermediate between those of benign prostatic acini and those seen in carcinoma. These changes are more marked in HGPIN than LGPIN, suggesting that impairment of cell differentiation and regulation has a key role in prostatic carcinogenesis. High-grade PIN shows progressive loss or gain of a wide variety of biomarkers, including morphometric markers and markers of growth and differentiation, as well as alterations in oncogenes and tumor suppressor genes. Some of the identified changes are:

- Increased expression of α-methylacyl-CoA racemase (P504S) has been identified in HGPIN in 126/140 (90%) radical prostatectomy specimens.[23]
- Fluorescent in-situ hybridization (FISH) with probes for chromosomes 7, 8, 10 and 12 shows a high correlation in the pattern of genetic alterations in HGPIN and carcinoma in 75% of 57 radical prostatectomy specimens.[24]
- PIM-1, an oncogene whose protein product has serine/threonine kinase activity, shows increased expression in 97% of HGPIN and 68% of carcinomas in 121 radical prostatectomy specimens.[25]
- Human glandular kallikrein 2 (hK2) shows increased expression in HGPIN and carcinoma (compared with benign prostatic acini) in all of 2578 radical prostatectomy specimens.[26]
- Several genes show CpG island methylation in both HGPIN and prostatic carcinoma, including the gene coding for glutathione-S-transferase protein (GTSP1 gene), supporting a role for HGPIN as a precursor for carcinoma.[27]
- cDNA microarray studies show 21 upregulated and 63 downregulated genes in HGPIN and cancer compared with benign acini.[28]

MIMICS OF PROSTATIC INTRAEPITHELIAL NEOPLASIA

There are a variety of conditions that may result in stratification or increased nuclear size in prostatic acini, but that do not fulfill the criteria for a diagnosis of PIN. Therefore, true PIN lesions must be correctly distinguished from a range of benign mimics, as well as from variants of invasive prostatic carcinoma and from intraductal spread of a urothelial neoplasm:

1. Benign mimics (Figure 12.2):
   - Normal—central zone (CZ) acini; seminal vesicle/ejaculatory duct (SV)
   - Hyperplasia—basal cell hyperplasia (BCH); cribriform hyperplasia (CH)
   - Metaplasia—urothelial metaplasia (UM) in prostatic ducts.
2. Variants of prostatic carcinoma:
   - Cribriform acinar carcinoma
   - Hyperplastic acinar carcinoma
   - Ductal carcinoma (or intraduct spread of acinar carcinoma).
3. Others:
   - Urothelial carcinoma in situ (CIS) in prostatic ducts.

The morphological features helpful in distinguishing HGPIN from benign prostatic conditions are identified in Table 12.2).

A useful way of confirming PIN, and excluding invasive prostatic adenocarcinoma, is by identifying the presence of either a continuous or intermittent basal cell layer using immunohistochemical markers, such as pancytokeratins (LP34, 34βE12), CK5 or p63 (Figure 12.3).[29,30]

INCIDENCE OF PROSTATIC INTRAEPITHELIAL NEOPLASIA AT AUTOPSY

A study of 152 prostates obtained at autopsy in young to middle-aged adults showed the presence of PIN in 9% of individuals aged between 20 and 29 years, with the incidence rising to 20% at 30 to 39 years, and 44% at 40 to 49 years.[21] This contrasted with 0% showing small foci of carcinoma at 20 to 29 years, 28% at 30 to 39 years, and 34% at 40 to 49 years. In the majority of patients, the PIN was low grade. Five cases of HGPIN were identified, all in the 40 to 49 year age group, adjacent to foci of carcinoma. The findings of this study appear to suggest that the onset of HGPIN occurs only in individuals aged over 40 years, later than the onset of some cases of carcinoma. This raises the possibility that HGPIN might not be the only precursor lesion for prostatic carcinoma. A subsequent publication by the

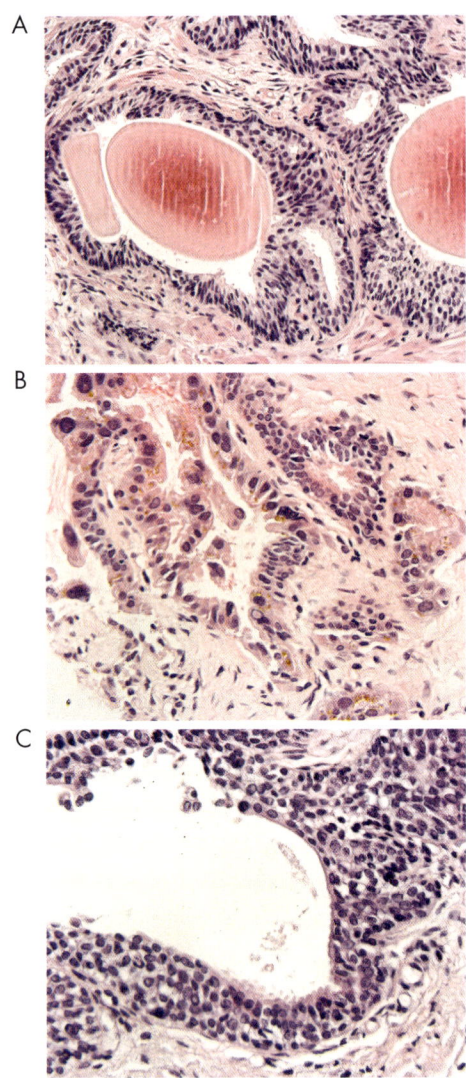

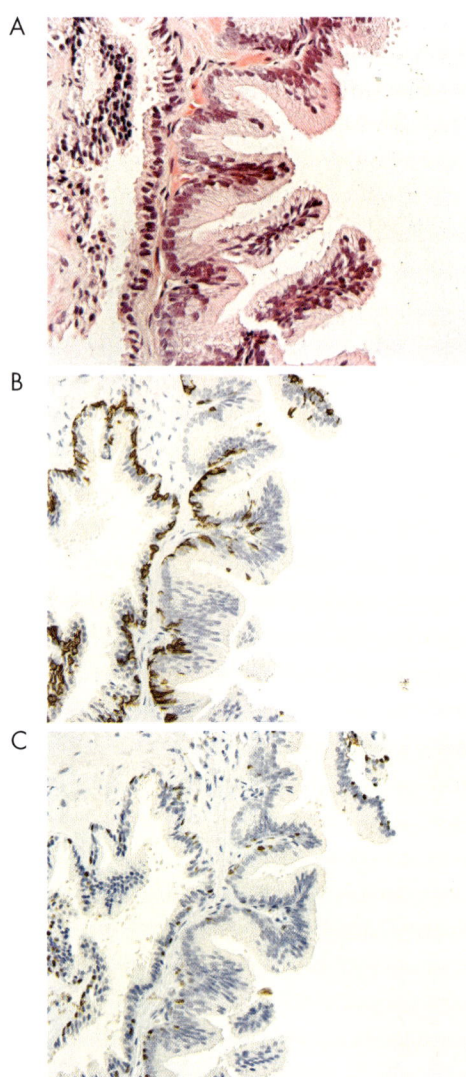

Fig. 12.2
Benign mimics of prostatic intraepithelial neoplasia (PIN).
A, Central zone acini (H&E, ×400). *B*, Ejaculatory duct epithelium (H&E, ×400). *C*, Urothelium growing along prostatic ducts (H&E, ×400).

Fig. 12.3
Basal cell markers in high-grade prostatic intraepithelial neoplasia (HGPIN). *A*, Staining with hematoxylin and eosin (H&E) (×400). *B*, Cytoplasmic staining of intermittant basal cells with CK5 (×400). *C*, Nuclear staining of basal cells with p63 (×400).

Table 12.2 Features used in the differential diagnosis of high-grade prostatic intraepithelial neoplasia

Condition	Acinar architecture	Atypia	Nucleoli	Basal cells
HGPIN	Normal	Present	Present, prominent	Continuous (intermittent)
CZ	Large square acini, lacunae	Absent	Absent	Present
SV	Normal (or small acini on cross-section)	Nucleomegaly, hyperchromasia (cytoplasmic yellow pigment)	Present, usually small	Present
BCH	Small rounded acini	Absent	Present, small (in basal cells)	Increased number
CH	Cribriform	Absent	Absent	Present
UM	Normal	Absent	Occasional, small	Present

BCH, basal cell hyperplasia; CH, cribriform hyperplasia; CZ, central zone; SV, seminal vesicle; UM, urothelial metaplasia.

same author has noted that HGPIN is more prevalent and extensive in Afro-Caribbean men compared with whites, and this difference may be detected as early as the third decade of life.[31]

PROSTATIC BIOPSY

INCIDENCE OF HGPIN

The identification of HGPIN rests on the presence of cytologically atypical cells with prominent nucleoli within a prostatic duct/acinus. There are no precise guidelines as to the amount of cytological atypia or the number or size of nucleoli required for HGPIN to be reliably diagnosed. As a result, there is significant inter-observer variation in the incidence of isolated HGPIN on biopsy reported from various institutions (from less than 1% to over 20%; Table 12.3).

There are several factors that may account for such a great variation in reported incidence: population group and ethnicity; prostatic biopsy sampling protocol; fixation and tissue processing methods; staining technique; number and size of nucleoli interpreted as "increased."

SIGNIFICANCE OF LGPIN

At low power, LGPIN may resemble HGPIN with regard to nuclear stratification and increased nuclear size, but typically lacks the prominent nucleoli that are seen in the latter. The well-established low reproducibility in the identification of LGPIN, even between experienced urologic pathologists, makes it an unreliable diagnosis.[41]

Furthermore, the presence of LGPIN on biopsy does not appear to confer an increased risk of subsequent prostatic carcinoma on re-biopsy compared with an individual with benign prostatic biopsies.[13] As a result of these pathological and clinical factors, most pathologists do not report the presence of LGPIN on prostatic biopsies.

RISK OF CANCER FOLLOWING RE-BIOPSY OF A PATIENT WITH ISOLATED HGPIN

The reason for reporting HGPIN on prostatic biopsy is to indicate to the urologist that the patient has an increased risk of concomitant prostatic carcinoma identified on re-biopsy. This prompts the urologist to re-biopsy within 3 to 6 months in most cases.

The percentage of patients in whom carcinoma is identified on re-biopsy is difficult to quantify accurately as these vary with study design, but reports in the literature have ranged from 14% to 79%.[42,48] However, the majority of studies in recent years show figures of between 23% and 35% (Table 12.4).

Morphologic features reported to strengthen the prognostic value of HGPIN in the prediction of concomitant invasive carcinoma include: the identification of adjacent atypical acini (PINATYP) and presence of HGPIN in multiple cores.[49,55,56] In both these situations, the predictive value for concomitant carcinoma is greater than that associated with isolated HGPIN in one core. In contrast, the prognostic significance of different architectural patterns of HGPIN remains controversial.

RE-BIOPSY TECHNIQUE

There is significant variation in clinical practice with regards to the timing, extent, and targeting of prostatic re-biopsy in patients identified with isolated HGPIN. This may in part account for the differences seen in the

Table 12.3 Incidence of isolated high-grade prostatic intraepithelial neoplasia on biopsy

Author	Year	Number of patients biopsied	Number (%) with isolated HGPIN on biopsy
Mettlin[32]	1991	2425	N/A (5.2)
Bostwick[33]	1995	200	N/A (16.5)
Cheville[34]	1997	1009	17 (1.5)
Wills[35]	1997	439	24 (5.5)
Renshaw[36]	1998	343	N/A (4.0)
Orozco[37]	1998	62,537	N/A (4.1)
Hoedemaker[38]	1999	1824	12 (0.7)
Kim[39]	2000	N/A	N/A (24.0)
Horninger[40]	2001	1474	70 (4.7)

N/A, not available.

Table 12.4 Incidence of cancer on re-biopsy of patients with isolated high-grade prostatic intraepithelial neoplasia (HGPIN)

Author	Year	Number of patients biopsied	Number with isolated HGPIN (number re-biopsied)	Number (%) with cancer on re-biopsy
Noguchi[43]	1999	218	7 (N/A)	2 (29)
Hoedemaeker[44]	1999	8763	12 (N/A)	0 (0)
Algaba[45]	1999	2807	126 (87)	25 (29)
Kamoi[46]	2000	611	63 (45)	10 (22)
Lujan Galan[47]	2000	N/A	41 (27)	11 (41)
Alsikafi[48]	2001	485	21 (N/A)	3 (14)
Kronz[49]	2001	N/A	346 (245)	79 (32)
Park[50]	2001	N/A	43 (N/A)	22 (50)
Lefkowitz[51]	2002	1223	119 (31)	8 (26)
San Francisco[52]	2003	387	49 (21)	5 (24)
Bishara[53]	2004	N/A	200 (132)	N/A (29)
Naya[54]	2004	1086	226 (47)	N/A (11)

N/A, not available.

figures for prostatic carcinoma identified on re-biopsy (see Table 12.4).

Several papers report experience of re-biopsy, using either identical sites to the original protocol or an extended technique, including additional sites in the anterior gland and transition zone (Table 12.5). However, there appears to be no consensus on the optimal regimen or timescale for re-biopsy for isolated HGPIN, and variation between institutions and individuals still exists.

TREATMENT

The morphological changes and treatment response seen in HGPIN following androgen deprivation or blockade have been examined. These have shown conflicting results, possibly explained by the difficulty in defining a matched control population. While some report a decrease in prevalence and extent of HGPIN in radical prostatectomy following androgen deprivation,[60,61] others have shown persistence of HGPIN following complete androgen blockade, with no significant decrease in extent after 3 or 6 months of treatment.[62]

CONCLUSION

High-grade prostatic intraepithelial neoplasia is the only precursor for prostatic carcinoma that is currently identifiable morphologically. Evidence for a relationship between HGPIN and prostatic carcinoma is supported by epidemiologic, morphologic, and biologic studies.

Isolated HGPIN diagnosed on prostatic biopsies is considered to be predictive of concomitant or subsequent invasive carcinoma. The reported strength of the association between HGPIN and concomitant cancer has varied over time and in different study populations (according to ethnicity and screening status). In a screening series including control patients, the additional risk apportioned specifically to the presence of HGPIN has fallen over time. In those screened prior to 1995, 51% of men showed invasive carcinoma on

Table 12.5 Correlation between detection of cancer and re-biopsy technique in patients with isolated high-grade prostatic intraepithelial neoplasia (HGPIN)

Author	Year	Number with HGPIN	Number re-biopsied; technique	Interval (months)	Cancer detected (%)
Langer[57]	1996	61	53; extended sites	N/A	28
Borboroglu[58]	2001	137*	100; extended sites	2	47
Roscigno[59]	2004	47	47; same sites	3–24	45

N/A, not available.

*This study grouped together HGPIN and atypical small acinar proliferation (ASAP).

re-biopsy, compared with 19% of those with initial benign biopsies. In contrast, only 28% of those screened between 1996 and 2000 had carcinoma on re-biopsy, compared with a control population risk of 24.5%.[41,63]

Consequently, although the majority of publications advocate clinical follow-up and re-biopsy of patients with isolated HGPIN, in the future, risk (and hence re-biopsy) may be stratified according to the population studied, patient age, serum prostate-specific antigen (PSA), and clinical findings.

REFERENCES

1. McNeal JE. Origin and development of carcinoma in the prostate. Cancer 1969;23:24–34.

2. Miller A, Seljelid R. Cellular dysplasia in the prostate. Scand J Urol Nephrol 1971;5:17–21.

3. Kastendieck H. Correlations between atypical primary hyperplasia and carcinoma of the prostate. Pathol Res Practice 1980; 169:366–387.

4. Mostofi FK. Precancerous lesions of the prostate, In Carter RL (ed): Precancerous States, New York: Oxford University Press, 1984 pp 304–316.

5. McNeal JE, Bostwick DG. Intraductal dysplasia: a premalignant lesion of the prostate. Hum Pathol 1986;17:64–71.

6. Kovi J, Mostofi FK, Heshmat MY, et al. Large acinar atypical hyperplasia and carcinoma of the prostate. Cancer 1988;61:555–561.

7. Kastendieck H, Helpap B. Prostatic "dysplasia / atypical hyperplasia." Terminology, histopathology, pathobiology and significance. Urology 1989;34:28–42.

8. McNeal JE, Leav I, Alroy J, et al. Differential lectin staining of the central and peripheral zones of the prostate and alterations in dysplasia. Am J Clin Pathol 1988;89:41–48.

9. Bostwick DG, Brawer MK. Prostatic intraepithelial neoplasia and early invasion in prostate cancer. Cancer 1987;59:788–794.

10. Bostwick DG. Prostatic intraepithelial neoplasia (PIN): current concepts. J Cell Biochem 1992;16:10–19.

11. Epstein JI, Grignon DJ, Humphrey PA, et al. Interobserver reproducibility in the diagnosis of prostatic intraepithelial neoplasia. Am J Surg Pathol 1995;19:873–886.

12. Drago JR, Mostofi FK, Lee F. Introductory remarks and workshop summary. Urology 1989;34:2–3.

13. Keetch DW, Humphrey PA, Stahl D, et al. Morphometric analysis and clinical follow-up of isolated prostatic intraepithelial neoplasia in needle biopsy of the prostate. J Urol 1995;154:347–351.

14. Bostwick DG, Amin MB, Dundore P, et al. Architectural patterns of high-grade prostatic intraepithelial neoplasia (PIN). Hum Pathol 1993;42:298–310.

15. Reyes AO, Swanson PE, Carbone JM, et al. Unusual histologic types of high-grade prostatic intraepithelial neoplasia. Am J Surg Pathol 1997;21:1215–1222.

16. Berman D, Yang J, Epstein J. Foamy gland high grade prostatic intraepithelial neoplasia. Am J Surg Pathol 2000;24:140–144.

17. Haggman MJ, Macoska JA, Wojno KJ, et al. The relationship between prostatic intraepithelial neoplasia and prostate cancer: critical issues. J Urol 1997;158:12–22.

18. McNeal JE, Villiers A, Redwine EA, et al. Microcarcinoma in the prostate: its association with duct-acinar dysplasia. Hum Pathol 1991;22:644–652.

19. Epstein JI. Relationship of dysplasia to prostate carcinoma. Semin Urol 1990;VIII:2–8.

20. Bostwick DG, Pacelli A, Lopez-Beltran A. Molecular biology of prostatic intraepithelial neoplasia. Prostate 1996;29:117–134.

21. Sakr WA, Haas GP, Cassin BF, et al. The frequency of carcinoma and intraepithelial neoplasia of the prostate in young male patients. J Urol 1993;150:379–385.

22. Goeman L, Joniau S, Ponette D, et al. Is low-grade prostatic intraepithelial neoplasia a risk factor for cancer? Prostatic Cancer Prostatic Dis 2003:6;305–310.

23. Wu CL, Yang XJ, Tretiakova M, et al. Analysis of alpha-methylacyl-CoA racemase (P504S) expression in high-grade prostatic intraepithelial neoplasia. Hum Pathol 2004;35:1008–1013.

24. Alcaraz A, Barranco MA, Corral JM, et al. High-grade prostate intraepithelial neoplasia shares cytogenetic alterations with invasive prostate cancer. Prostate 2001;47:29–35.

25. Valdman A, Fang X, Pang ST, et al. Pim-1 expression in prostatic intraepithelial neoplasia and human prostate cancer. Prostate 2004;60:367–371.

26. Darson MF, Pacelli A, Roche P, et al. Human glandular kallikrein 2 (hK2) expression in prostatic intraepithelial neoplasia and adenocarcinoma: a novel prostate cancer marker. Urology 1997;49:857–862.

27. Brooks JD, Weinstein M, Lin X, et al. CG island methylation near the GSTP1 gene in prostatic intraepithelial neoplasia. Cancer Epidemiol. Biomarkers Prev 1998;7:531–536.

28. Ashida S, Nakagawa H, Katagiri T, et al. Molecular features of the transition from prostatic intraepithelial neoplasia (PIN) to prostate cancer: genome-wide gene-expression profiles of prostate cancers and PINs. Cancer Res 2004;64:5963–5972.

29. Freeman A, Treurnicht K, Munson P, et al. A comparison of basal cell markers used in the prostate. Histopathology 2002;40:492–494.

30. Wu HH, Lapkus O, Corbin M. Comparison of 34beta E12 and p63 in 100 consecutive prostatic carcinomas diagnosed by needle biopsies. Appl Immunohistochem Mol Morphol 2004;12:285–289.

31. Sakr WA. Prostatic intraepithelial neoplasia: a marker for high-risk groups and a potential target for chemoprevention. Eur Urol 1999;35:474–478.

32. Mettlin C, Lee F, Drago J, et al. The American Cancer Society National Cancer Detection Project: findings on the detection of early prostate cancer in 2425 men. Cancer 1991;67:2949–2958.

33. Bostwick DG, Qian J, Frankel K. The incidence of high grade prostatic intraepithelial neoplasia in needle biopsies. J Urol 1995;154:1791–1794.

34. Cheville JC, Reznicek MJ, Bostwick DG. The focus of "atypical glands suspicious for malignancy" in prostatic needle biopsy specimens: incidence, histologic features and clinical follow-up of cases diagnosed in a community practice. Am J Clin Path 1997;108:633–640.

35. Wills ML, Hamper UM, Partin AW, et al. Incidence of high-grade prostatic intraepithelial neoplasia in sextant needle biopsy specimens. Urology 1997;49:367–373.

36. Renshaw AA, Santis WF, Richie JP. Clinicopathological characteristics of prostatic adenocarcinoma in men with atypical prostate needle biopsies. J Urol 1998;159:2018–2022.

37. Orozco R, O'Dowd G, Kunnel B, et al. Observations on pathology trends in 62,537 prostate biopsies obtained from urology private practices in the United States. Urology 1998;51:186–195.

38. Hoedemaeker RF, Kranse R, Rietbergen JB, et al. Evaluation of prostate needle biopsies in a population-based screening study: the impact of borderline lesions. Cancer 1999;85:145–152.

39. Kim SC, Weiser AC, Nadler RB, et al. The changing incidence of high grade prostatic intraepithelial neoplasia: clinical implications. J Urol 2000;163:279.

40. Horninger W, Volgger H, Rogatsch H, et al. Predictive value of total and percent free prostate specific antigen in high grade prostatic intraepithelial neoplasia lesions: results of the Tyrol Prostate Specific Antigen Screening Project. J Urol 2001;165:1143–1145.

41. Epstein JI, Grignon DJ, Humphrey PA, et al. Interobserver reproducibility in the diagnosis of prostatic intraepithelial neoplasia. Am J Surg Pathol 1995;19:873–886.

42. Aboseif S, Shinohara K, Weidner N, et al. The significance of prostatic intraepithelial neoplasia Br J Urol 1995;76:355–359.

43. Noguchi M, Yahara J, Koga H, et al. Necessity of repeat biopsies in men for suspected prostate cancer. Int J Urol 1999;6:7–12.

44. Hoedemaeker RF, Kranse R, Rietbergen JB, et al. Evaluation of prostate needle biopsies in a population-based screening study: the impact of borderline lesions. Cancer 1999;85:145–152.

45. Algaba F. Evolution of isolated high-grade prostate intraepithelial neoplasia in a Mediterranean patient population. Eur Urol 1999;35:496–497.

46. Kamoi K, Troncoso P, Babaian RJ. Strategy for repeat biopsy in patients with high-grade prostatic intraepithelial neoplasia. J Urol 2001;163:819–823.

47. Lujan Galan M, Paez Borda A, Romero Cajigal I, et al. Clinical significance of prostatic intraepithelial neoplasia. Arch Esp Urol 2000;53:227–229.

48. Alsikafi NF, Brendler CB, Gerber GS, et al. High grade prostatic intraepithelial neoplasia with adjacent atypia is associated with a higher incidence of cancer on subsequent needle biopsy than high grade prostatic intraepithelial neoplasia alone. Urology 2001;57:296–300.

49. Kronz JD, Allan CH, Shaikh AA, et al. Predicting cancer following a diagnosis of high grade prostatic intraepithelial neoplasia on needle biopsy Am J Surg Pathol 2001;25:1079–1085.

50. Park S, Shinohara K, Grossfeld GD, et al. Prostate cancer detection in men with prior high-grade prostatic intraepithelial neoplasia or atypical prostate biopsy. J Urol 2001;165:1409–1414.

51. Lefkowitz GK, Taneja SS, Brown J, et al. Follow up interval prostate biopsy after diagnosis of high grade prostatic intraepithelial neoplasia is associated with high likelihood of prostate cancer, independent of change in prostate specific antigen levels. J Urol 2002;168:1415–1418.

52. San Francisco IF, Olumi AF, Kao J, et al. Clinical management of prostatic intraepithelial neoplasia as diagnosed by extended needle biopsies. BJU Int 2003;91:350–354.

53. Bishara T, Ramnani DM, Epstein JI. High-grade prostatic intraepithelial neoplasia on needle biopsy: risk of cancer on repeat biopsy related to number of involved cores and morphologic pattern. Am J Surg Pathol 2004;28:629–633.

54. Naya Y, Ayala AG, Tamboli P, et al. Can the number of cores with high-grade prostatic intraepithelial neoplasia predict cancer in men who undergo repeat biopsy? Urology 2004;63:503–508.

55. Qian J, Wollan P, Bostwick DG. The extent and multicentricity of high-grade prostatic intraepithelial neoplasia in clinically localised prostatic adenocarcinoma. Hum Pathol 1997;28:143–148.

56. Kronz JD, Shaikh AA, Epstein JI. High-grade prostatic intraepithelial neoplasia with adjacent small atypical glands on prostate biopsy. Hum Pathol 2001;32:389–395.

57. Langer JE, Rovner ES, Coleman BG, et al. Strategy for repeat biopsy of patients with prostatic intraepithelial neoplasia detected by prostate needle biopsy. J Urol 1996;155:228–231.

58. Borboroglu PG, Sur RL, Roberts JL, et al. Repeat biopsy strategy in patients with atypical small acinar proliferation or high-grade prostatic intraepithelial neoplasia on initial prostate needle biopsy. J Urol 2001;166:866–870.

59. Roscigno M, Scattoni V, Freschi M, et al. Monofocal and plurifocal high-grade prostatic intraepithelial neoplasia on extended prostate biopsies: factors predicting cancer detection on extended repeat biopsy. Urology 2004;63:1105–1110.

60. Ferguson J, Zincke H, Ellison E, et al. Decrease of prostatic intraepithelial neoplasia following androgen deprivation therapy in patients with stage T3 carcinoma treated by radical prostatectomy. Urology 1994;44:91–95.

61. Bullock MJ, Srigley JR, Klotz LH, et al. Pathologic effects of neoadjuvant cyproterone acetate on non-neoplastic prostate, prostatic intraepithelial neoplasia and adenocarcinoma: a detailed analysis of radical prostatectomy specimens from a randomised trial. Am J Surg Pathol 2002;26:1400–1413.

62. van der Kwast TH, Labrie F, Tetu B. Persistence of high-grade prostatic intra-epithelial neoplasia under combined androgen blockade therapy. Hum Pathol 1999;30:1503–1507.

63. Gokden N, Roehl K, Humphrey PA. High-grade prostatic intraepithelial neoplasia in needle biopsy tissue as a risk factor for detection of adenocarcinoma: current level of risk in a screening population. United States and Canadian Academy of Pathology 2003; Abstract 689:152A.

Pathologic characteristics of soft tissue and osseous metastases

13

Neil A Abrahams, Alberto G Ayala

INTRODUCTION

Data from the National Cancer Institute (NCI) predicts that 232,090 new cases of prostate cancer will be diagnosed in 2005.[1,2] The estimated mortality is expected to reach 13% of the diagnosed population (30,350) placing a considerable burden on the overall diagnosis and management of cancer. Prostate cancer continues to be the forerunner in new cases of cancer diagnosed in the male population with an estimated 33% of new cancer and deaths projected for 2005. The alarming figure is not that prostate cancer is the leading cancer diagnosis in men, but that it is the leading cancer by almost double digits. In a far second and third place are lung cancer (13%) and colon and rectal cancer (10%).[1,3,4]

Of the one in six men expected to develop prostate cancer over a lifetime period,[2] 35% to 40% of these patients are expected to eventually experience a rise in serum prostate-specific antigen (PSA) signaling either local or metastatic spread.[5] Within the subgroup of patients with metastatic disease, bone metastases are considered the hallmark of advanced prostate cancer. The paradox with prostate cancer is that while the incidence of prostate cancer in both North America and Europe has increased, in part due to PSA screening, the mortality rate has remained fairly stable.[1,3,4,6] The low death rate indicates that many men are alive long after the initial diagnosis of prostate cancer, and a significant proportion of these patients, after a relatively long latency period, develop both soft tissue and osseous metastases.

While a discussion of metastatic prostate cancer could in itself fill an entire book, this chapter focuses on the pathologic and biologic aspects of soft tissue and osseous metastases. Predictors of advanced prostate cancer with distant spread including currently used standard pathologic parameters and novel biomarkers will be discussed. The varied morphologic appearance of metastatic prostate cancer within soft tissue and bone, with emphasis on ancillary confirmatory diagnostic techniques will be presented.

MOLECULAR BIOLOGY OF PROSTATE CANCER WITH IMPLICATION FOR METASTATIC SPREAD

Bone is by far the most frequent site of metastases from prostate cancer. Specific bone matrix proteins and their corresponding receptors localized on the surface of prostate cancer cells are intricately involved in the deposition of metastatic prostate cancer cells in bone. SPARC, also known as bone osteonectin, modulates cell-to-cell interactions and its expression is linked to invasive capability of tumors, promoting "invasiveness." Receptors located on the cell surface of prostate cancer cells that belong to the integrin family of adhesion receptors (subunits alpha-v) are responsible for the targeted bone metastases of prostate cancer. Vascular endothelial growth factor (VEGF) in turn is responsible, in part, for the activation of the integrin receptors and also plays a pivotal role in promoting angiogenesis of tumor metastases. Both VEGF and the corresponding receptors are expressed by prostate cancer.[7,8] The molecular biology of prostate cancer is discussed in more detail in Chapter 27 and 28.

PATTERN OF SPREAD OF PROSTATE CANCER

Prostate cancer is a disease that has a stepwise progression that begins with local extraprostatic spread and, ultimately, culminates with either bone and/or distant soft tissue involvement.[9] The most common route of extraprostatic extension is through the apex for transition zone carcinomas and through the superior neurovascular bundles for peripheral zone carcinomas.[10] The route of perineural spread, frequently observed along the posterolateral aspect of non-nerve sparing radical prostatectomies, has been identified as one of the paths of least resistance for local spread.[11] Ohori et al described three types of seminal vesicle and perivesicle soft tissue involvement by prostatic adenocarcinoma,[12] all three types of involvement are associated with a highly aggressive clinical course.

Metastatic spread of prostatic adenocarcinoma presents in a predictable sequence (Figure 13.1). In 1976, Viadana et al, in a seminal publication, presented the *"Cascade Hypothesis of the Metastatic Spread of Cancer"* with regards to cancers of the prostate and kidney.[13] While this publication received little attention, the hypothesis and facts presented have formed the basis of many future studies of metastatic prostate cancer. Briefly, they proposed that prostate cancer had a unique sequence of events that started with tumor being "seeded" in key metastatic sites, namely bone and lung, from where further dissemination occurred. In addition they proposed that the first key metastatic site was in fact bone (74%) and, from there, lung (54%) and liver (41%) would be the next affected.[13] This was one of the first studies that showed that the spread of prostate cancer was a systematic multistep process and not a random series of events.

ANGIOLYMPHATIC SPREAD

Metastatic spread of prostate cancer frequently begins with angiolymphatic invasion within the invaginated extraprostatic space (tissue surrounding the ejaculatory ducts).[14] This finding is invariably associated with regional lymph node metastases as well as being an independent predictor of disease progression.[15]

Angiolymphatic invasion is more likely to be found in high-grade (Gleason score >7), high-stage (pT3A–B) and high-volume cancers.[15–18]

LYMPH NODES

Elaborate lymphangiographic studies in the early 1980s demonstrated three routes of lymphatic drainage of the prostate: 1) along the superolateral aspect of the prostate into the internal iliac lymph nodes; 2) to presacral nodes; and 3) from the apex along the pudendal vessels into the internal iliac nodes. The internal iliac nodes ultimately drain into the common iliac and then into the lumbar nodes.[19] Subsequent imaging studies have corroborated these findings.[20]

In a series of 1589 patients with prostate cancer, 40% (631 patients) had evidence of nodal spread of disease at the time of death as evidenced by autopsy studies.[21] In order of frequency, the most frequently involved nodes are: para-aortic (80%); pelvic (50%); mediastinal (40%); inguinal (20%); and cervical, perigastric, mesenteric, periclavicular, and peripancreatic (10% or less).[21,22] In a different study on excised pelvic lymph nodes at the time of surgery, Golimbu et al found that the obturator and hypogastric nodes were the first to be affected, followed by the external iliac, common iliac, and presacral nodes.[23] Interestingly, in a small, albeit significant number of cases, the presacral nodes are involved.[24] These nodes are not part of a standard lymphadenectomy due to the increased morbidity surrounding their removal.[25–30]

Of note is the fact that the "gatekeeper" node, that is the node after which widespread dissemination occurs, is in fact the para-aortic node with simultaneous hematogenous dissemination being noticeably more frequent in tumors with para-aortic lymph node metastases (89%) compared with those with pelvic lymph node metastases (63%).[21]

BONE

The key site of distant spread of prostate cancer is the bone marrow and, more specifically, the lumbar vertebrae. While a long-standing hypothesis of the predilection of bone as the primary metastatic site has been "the seed and

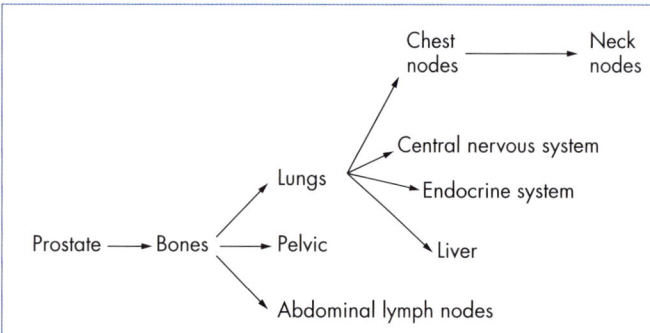

Fig. 13.1
Pathway for the spread of prostate cancer.

the soil" theory, whereby the ambiance within the bone marrow (the soil) makes for a fertile area for implantation of metastases (the seed),[31,32] newer and more clinically relevant studies (see Section 7) are relating bone metastases to molecular interactions between the cancer cells and target receptors. Despite these molecular developments, a constant question remains: why does prostate cancer go almost exclusively to the lumbar vertebrae? A theory that is widely accepted today is that proposed by Batson in 1940[33]: blood from the prostate enters a valveless venous system to the lower spine. Subsequent studies have indirectly validated this theory.[21]

The most frequent site of metastases is bone (Table 13.1), representing 67% to 90% of the cases.[21,34–36] There is a striking predilection for the vertebra (90%) with a distribution as follows: lumbar 97%, thoracic 66%, cervical 38% (thoracic and cervical metastases alone without lumbar involvement are 2% and 1% respectively).[21]

Outside of the spinal column, prostate cancer rarely metastasizes to the ribs, long bones, and skull.[21,34,36]

LUNG AND PLEURA

After the skeletal system, the lung is the next key metastatic site for prostate cancer. The incidence of lung metastases has been reported to be between 45% to 53%.[21,36] Interestingly, lung is rarely the sole metastatic site and concomitant bone and lymph node metastases are present in 53% of the cases.[34,36] Unpublished data from MD Anderson Cancer Center support the fact that the only instance in which lung is the primary and sole site of metastases is if the prostate cancer is of the ductal type (so called endometrioid prostate cancer). The pleura per se is involved in 21% of cases.[21]

LIVER

The liver has concomitant metastases from prostate cancer in 25% to 30% of the cases with synchronous

bone and lung involvement.[21,36] The liver is almost never involved as a single organ; reports vary but an incidence greater than 6% has not been reported.[34] In our experience, small cell carcinoma of the prostate frequently metastasizes to the liver.

ADRENAL GLAND AND KIDNEYS

The incidence of adrenal involvement from metastatic cancer ranges from 3% to 13%.[21,34] Kidney involvement is reported to be 14%.

INTRACRANIAL

The brain is involved in approximately 2% of the cases with meningeal involvement being more prevalent (6%).[21,34] Unusual sites of metastases such as the pituitary gland, optic canal, orbit, and chorial have been reported.[22,37–40]

OTHER SITES

Case reports and small series documenting metastatic prostate cancer in skin,[41,42] oral cavity,[43] stomach,[44,45] salivary glands,[46] spleen,[36] pancreas,[36] breast,[47] testis, penis[48] and ureter[49] are summarized in Table 13.2. Involvement of the rectum and bladder are considered as local and not distant spread.

Table 13.1 Pattern of spread of bone metastases of prostate cancer

Metastatic site in bone	Percentage*
Pelvis	76
Dorsal vertebra	73
Lumbar vertebra	63
Rib	57
Sacrum	47
Femur	28
Humerus	18
Sternum	14
Skull	7

*Data taken from Rana et al.[35]

Table 13.2 Pattern of spread of prostate cancer throughout the entire body

Metastatic site	Percentage
Bone	66–90
Lymph Nodes	68
Lung	45–49
Liver	25–36
Pleura	21
Adrenal gland	13–17
Kidney	3–11
Ureter	8
Pleura	8
Spleen	2–4
Pancreas	2–5
Heart	3
Skin	3
Central nervous system	2
Thyroid	2
Stomach	1

Data taken from studies by Bubendorf et al[21] and Saitoh et al.[34]

HISTOPATHOLOGY OF BONE METASTASES

While the vast majority of tumors that metastasize to bone cause osteolytic lesions, prostate cancer is one of the few cancers that invokes a predominantly osteoblastic reaction[7,50] (Figure 13.2). The importance of osteoblastic metastases is twofold: first, it is estimated that at least 30% of patients with advanced prostate cancer will experience an adverse skeletal event (pathologic fracture), and second, patients may experience elevated levels of PTH secondary to excessive osteoblastic activity causing entrapment of calcium within bone.[51] The clinical manifestations of prostate cancer metastases to bone include spinal cord compression and, if left untreated, subsequent paralysis.[51,52] The histologic parallel to the osteoblastic lesions identified with imaging studies is significant osteosclerosis with rare periosteal bone formation.[53] In a series by Roudier et al of 14 patients with prior androgen ablation, the metastatic deposits in bone displayed varying morphology.[54] The most frequent architectural growth pattern (71%) was tumor cells growing in solid sheets in a background devoid of medulla ossea and with pronounced blastic reaction of surrounding bone.[54] Less frequent patterns of deposit included microacinar, macroacinar, and cribriform patterns with comedonecrosis. At the cytologic level, the characteristic features of primary prostate cancer such as round-to-oval nuclei with open chromatin and prominent nucleoli are present. To date, there has been no study that has shown any relation between the primary Gleason grade and the morphology of the metastatic cancer. It goes without saying, however, that if the primary cancer within the prostate had significant undifferentiated small cell carcinoma features (neuroendocrine differentiation) then the metastases would be devoid of glandular features and resemble metastatic small cell carcinoma of the lung. Interestingly, the histopathologic effects of androgen deprivation on primary prostate cancer (cell shrinkage, pyknosis, and cytoplasmic vacuolization) were not recorded in the metastases of 14 patients receiving androgen ablation therapy.[54] Rarely, the metastatic foci may have a clear cell appearance reminiscent of metastatic renal cell carcinoma[54,55] or present as pure squamous carcinomas[56] in the setting of neoadjuvant hormonal and chemotherapy. Frequently, androgen-independent prostate cancer may present as bone metastases with pure small cell morphology, and, in these instances, correlation with the imaging studies to demonstrate an osteoblastic lesion is vital.

Immunohistochemically, variable expression of tumor metastases with PSA has been reported.[54,57–59] This is not a surprising finding for several reasons: first, the majority of these studies were based on patients with hormonal ablation therapy and, in this setting, the tumor cells are androgen independent and are unlikely to express PSA. However, the combination of PSA and PAP successfully identifies the tissue as prostate in over 90% of the cases; in addition, the more undifferentiated or anaplastic the prostate cancer is, the expression of PSA diminishes and the more likely the tumor will show the neuroendocrine differentiation, with corresponding positivity for chromogranin A, synaptophysin, and even

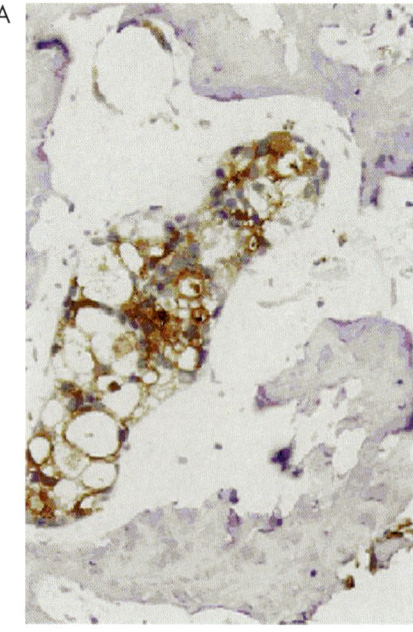
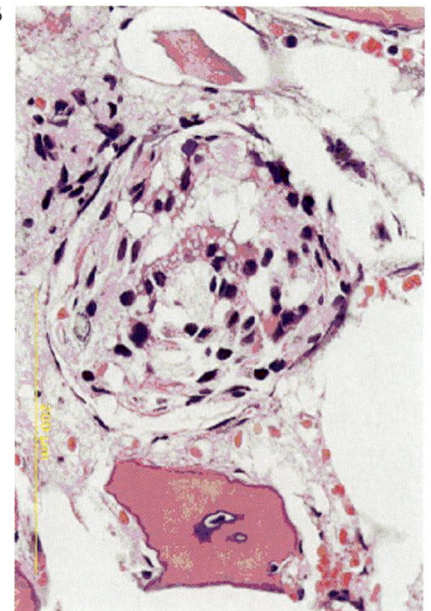

Fig. 13.2

Focus of metastatic prostate cancer in bone invoking an osteoblastic reaction. Immunohistochemical staining with prostate serum antigen (PSA) is positive.

thyroid transcription factor 1 (TTF1).[54,58–60] It should be noted that the positivity of metastatic small cell carcinoma for TTF1 is not an indicator of a primary lung cancer, as TTF1 has been reported as being positive in small cell carcinomas from several organs other than lung.[61] Cytokeratin markers such as keratin 34βE12 and cytokeratin 5/6 can be used to phenotypically exclude the metastases as of probable prostate origin. Both of these keratin markers are negative in primary and metastatic prostate cancer in our hands, although there is one controversial published report to the contrary.[62] An interesting paradox is the presence of squamous cell carcinoma in bone in patients with a known history of prostate cancer and several years of androgen ablation therapy.[56] In these cases, the immunohistochemical profile may be confusing, with up to 19% of the pure squamous carcinomas being positive for PAP or PSA as well as demonstrating diffuse strong positive staining with keratin 34βE12. Frequently, the association with a glandular component is present.[56] However, it should be emphasized that even in the setting of negative markers for prostate cancer (PSA and PAP) foci of metastatic squamous carcinoma in bone in patients with a history of prostate cancer and prior hormonal and/or chemohormonal ablation therapy should be considered as arising from the prostate.[63]

An increasing concern is the ability to detect micrometastases, which by standard imaging techniques is not possible, therefore, there has been an increasing interest in immunohistochemical and polymerase chain reaction detection of single prostate cancer cells within the circulating blood and in the bone marrow.[64,65]

HISTOPATHOLOGY OF LYMPH NODE METASTASES

The presence of prostate cancer within regional lymph nodes is an ominous sign of distant relapse. The morphology of lymph node metastases frequently resembles the primary organ and poses little diagnostic difficulties to the surgical pathologist. In addition these nodes are frequently removed at the time of radical prostatectomy. Often the tumor is located within the lymph node sinuses in a fused pattern reminiscent of Gleason pattern 4[9] with no stromal response of the surrounding tissue. We have observed lymph node metastases of prostate cancer in the setting of chemotherapy. In these cases, the only indication of a metastatic focus is an area of apparent scarring and fibrosis within the lymph node, and careful observation of this area reveals small neoplastic glands.[63] This is the only case, in our experience, in which the metastatic focus is surrounded by a stromal response. The presence of tumor within regional lymph nodes is associated in 60% to 70% of the cases with extranodal extension.[66]

Immunohistochemically, the tumor may demonstrate varying positivity for PSA, but, the combination of PSA and PAP invariably shows sufficient tumor cell positivity, at times with a luminal accentuation, to identify the tumor as of prostatic origin. Immunohistochemical profile with cytokeratins 7 and 20 may help in narrowing the differential of PSA⁻/PAP⁻ tumors. Prostate cancer has a CK7⁻/CK20⁻ profile in 81% of the cases.[67] Recently, newer antibodies for the detection of α-methylacyl coenzyme A racemase (AMACR) and p63 in combination have been marketed for diagnostic use in metastases.[68] While initially AMACR was promoted as being specific for prostatic carcinoma, the practical reality of the lack of specificity has hampered its diagnostic use.[68] More significant is the fact that AMACR has been found in benign prostatic acini, high-grade prostatic intraepithelial neoplasia (HGPIN) and, recently, even in papillary renal cell carcinoma, metastatic colorectal carcinoma and nephrogenic adenoma.[69,70]

HISTOPATHOLOGY OF LUNG AND SOFT TISSUE METASTASES

Pulmonary involvement without concomitant bone and/or lymph node involvement by metastatic prostate cancer is extremely rare. In our experience, the only time prostate cancer is found solely in the lung is when the primary morphology was of the ductal (endometrioid) type. As with all sites that contain metastatic prostate cancer, varying histologic features have been reported, however, one histologic appearance that is of importance from both a diagnostic and therapeutic stand point is the cases in which the metastatic prostate cancer resembles a carcinoid tumor.[71,72] In 13% of the cases of metastatic prostate cancer to the lung, the tumor has a distinct carcinoid-like morphology, with the tumor cells growing in a nested arrangement; however, the finely stippled chromatin pattern more reminiscent of neuroendocrine neoplasm is absent.[73] While the predominant histologic pattern is the microacinar with or without cribriform architecture (67%), the possibility for overlap with both primary neuroendocrine and epithelial carcinomas of the lung should be kept in mind. Invariably the metastatic tumor foci are positive for PSA and PAP and the majority are negative for chromogranin A and TTF1. Care should be taken when evaluating neuroendocrine markers since up to 40% of normal prostatic carcinomas can have focal neuroendocrine differentiation.[74,75] We recommend the interpretation of neuroendocrine markers in conjunction with PSA and PAP. Other subtle histologic features of metastatic tumors are the presence of necrosis, a lymphangitic distribution, mild nuclear pleomorphism, and prominent nucleoli.[73] A feature that, while infrequently present, has been of use to the authors is the presence of thin wispy intraluminal blue/basophilic mucin within the metastatic tumor deposits,[73] which is a strong association with neoplastic prostatic acini.[76] Other histologic patterns observed in lung metastases are the cribriform pattern with comedonecrosis (27%) and a tubulopapillary pattern(<5%).

Collectively, metastatic prostate cancer to all other organs and adjacent soft tissue is usually not biopsied for several reasons: first, a long protracted history of prostate cancer is known; and second, the systematic spread of prostate cancer to bones, lymph nodes, and lungs prior to any other organs raises the index of suspicion for subsequent metastases. If the lesion is biopsied the overwhelming majority of the cases show a glandular pattern with features reminiscent of prostatic primary (oval nuclei with prominent eosinophilic nucleoli) being present. One unique histopathologic presentation is gastric metastases that present with a signet ring morphology and even spread along the gastric wall in a similar fashion to primary gastric neoplasms (linitis plastica).[44] Once again careful review of the patient's history and inclusion of prostate immunomarkers will lead to the correct identification of a metastatic adenocarcinoma.

PREDICTORS OF METASTATIC PROSTATE CANCER

This section can be divided into three parts: 1) standard histopathologic predictors of distant spread; 2) bio-

Table 13.3 Histopathologic factors, tissue biomarkers and genetic markers predictive of disease progression in prostate cancer

Marker or factor	Comment
Histopathologic	
Gleason score	High Gleason scores (>7) correlate with increased risk of extracapsular extension, seminal vesicle invasion, and metastases.
Extraprostatic extension	Increase risk of distant spread.
Seminal vesicle invasion	Denotes a poor prognosis and early biochemical relapse.
Preoperative PSA	Does not by itself predict extraprostatic spread nor lymph node involvement. When used in combination with Gleason score in multivariate models is useful for predicting clinical stage.
Tumor volume	Together with high Gleason scores (Gleason 8–10) is an independent predictor of tumor progression.
Pathologic stage including margin status	pT3A, pT3B and pT4 tumors have increased risk of metastases and lymph node involvement. Margin status is not currently part of the TNM classification but has been shown to be an independent predictor of PSA progression.
Biomarkers	
DNA ploidy	Diploid tumors have a more favorable outcome than patients with aneuploid tumors.
p53 overexpression	Some groups have shown that overexpression of p53 correlates with adverse outcome and metastatic prostate cancer.
BCL2 overexpression	High levels of BCL2 are found in aggressive tumors that are androgen independent. Combined with overexpression of p53 can predict PSA recurrence in less than 5 years.
Ki67 proliferative index	Predicts tumor progression, biochemical recurrence and overall survival.
TGFβ1	Predictor of poor prognosis in prostate cancer with high levels enhancing metastases through induction of angiogenesis.
Gene expression markers	
AMACR	Characterized as a diagnostic marker of prostate cancer. May be useful if quantitated in predicting disease progression.
Caveolin 1	Candidate tumor suppressor gene. Serum factor is associated with metastases.
CDK1	Cell cycle marker that correlates with metastases and postsurgical recurrence.
E-Cadherin	Involved in cell-to-cell adhesion. Decreased levels are strongly associated with progression and metastases of prostate cancer.
EZH2	Highly expressed in metastatic prostate cancer.
MET	Hepatocyte growth factor receptor. Highly expressed in metastatic prostate cancer.
PSCA	Highly expressed in metastatic prostate cancer.
Chromosome 8q	Chromosomal marker most frequently associated with prostate cancer genesis and progression is 8q24, which contains the c-myc region.

AMACR, α-methylacyl-coenzyme A racemase; CDK1, cyclin-dependent kinase 1; EZH2, enhancer of zest homolog 2; PSA, prostate-specific antigen; PSCA, prostate stem cell antigen; TGFβ, transforming growth factor-β.

markers on prostatic adenocarcinoma; and 3) gene expression profiling that can be used to predict distant spread. Since these issues are dealt with in greater depth in separate chapters of this book (Section 4), a brief introduction is presented and summarized in Table 13.3.

HISTOPATHOLOGIC PREDICTORS OF METASTASES

Gleason score, tumor volume, pathologic stage, and overall TNM stage (including margin status) have all been correlated with disease progression.[77] Other factors such as DNA ploidy, perineural invasion, and angiolymphatic invasion have been shown to be adverse factors but are not widely accepted or individual prognostic parameters.[78]

TISSUE BIOMARKERS THAT PREDICT METASTASES

While there exists an endless number of biomarkers with varying degrees of correlation with disease progression, overexpression of p53, BCL2, Ki67 proliferative index and transforming growth factor-β (TGFβ) have been shown to be associated with high probability of recurrent and metastatic disease.[79]

GENE EXPRESSION PROFILING AND MOLECULAR MARKERS OF DISEASE PROGRESSION

Genomic and proteomic analysis of prostatic adenocarcinoma are continuously identifying novel markers associated with metastatic disease.[80] Markers that have been shown to be associated with recurrence include AMACR, Caveolin 1, CDK1, E-cadherin, enhancer of zeste homolog 2 (EZH2), MET, and prostate stem cell antigen (PSCA).[81]

SUMMARY

The prediction of prostate cancer progression and/or recurrence, involves multiple factors at the anatomic, cellular and biochemical level. The use of established nomograms, such as the "Partin tables" or the Kattan nomograms to predict outcome remains a robust method of channeling all available information into a single, predictive method that gives the most accurate possible outcome information.[82,83]

REFERENCES

1. Jemal A, Murray T, Ward E, et al. Cancer statistics, 2003. CA Cancer J Clin 2005;55:1–30.
2. Gloeckler Ries LA, Reichman ME, Lewis DR, et al. Cancer survival and incidence from the Surveillance, Epidemiology, and End Results (SEER) program. Oncologist 2003;8:541–552.
3. Parkin DM, Bray FI, Devesa SS. Cancer burden in the year 2000. The global picture. Eur J Cancer 2001;37(Suppl 8):S4–66.
4. Parkin DM. Global cancer statistics in the year 2000. Lancet Oncol 2001;2:533–543.
5. McMurtry CT, McMurtry JM. Metastatic prostate cancer: complications and treatment. J Am Geriatr Soc 2003;51:1136–1142.
6. Quaglia A, Parodi S, Grosclaude P, et al. Differences in the epidemic rise and decrease of prostate cancer among geographical areas in Southern Europe. An analysis of differential trends in incidence and mortality in France, Italy and Spain. Eur J Cancer 2003;39:654–665.
7. Roodman GD. Mechanisms of bone metastasis. N Engl J Med 2004;350:1655–1664.
8. De S, Chen J, Narizhneva NV, et al. Molecular pathway for cancer metastasis to bone. J Biol Chem 2003;278:39044–39050.
9. Humphrey P. Prostate Pathology, 1st ed. Chicago: ASCP Press, 2003.
10. McNeal JE, Haillot O. Patterns of spread of adenocarcinoma in the prostate as related to cancer volume. Prostate 2001;49:48–57.
11. Villers A, McNeal JE, Redwine EA, et al. The role of perineural space invasion in the local spread of prostatic adenocarcinoma. J Urol 1989;142:763–768.
12. Ohori M, Scardino PT, Lapin SL, et al. The mechanisms and prognostic significance of seminal vesicle involvement by prostate cancer. Am J Surg Pathol 1993;17:1252–1261.
13. Viadana E, Bross ID, Pickren JW. The metastatic spread of kidney and prostate cancers in man. Neoplasma 1976;23:323–332.
14. Fukuda H, Yamada T, Kamata S, et al. Anatomic distribution of intraprostatic lymphatics: implications for the lymphatic spread of prostate cancer—a preliminary study. Prostate 2000;44:322–327.
15. McNeal JE, Yemoto CE. Significance of demonstrable vascular space invasion for the progression of prostatic adenocarcinoma. Am J Surg Pathol 1996;20:1351–1360.
16. Pettaway CA, Pisters LL, Troncoso P, et al. Neoadjuvant chemotherapy and hormonal therapy followed by radical prostatectomy: feasibility and preliminary results. J Clin Oncol 2000;18:1050–1057.
17. Bahnson RR, Dresner SM, Gooding W, et al. Incidence and prognostic significance of lymphatic and vascular invasion in radical prostatectomy specimens. Prostate 1989;15:149–155.
18. Salomao DR, Graham SD, Bostwick DG. Microvascular invasion in prostate cancer correlates with pathologic stage. Arch Pathol Lab Med 1995;119:1050–1054.
19. Raghavaiah NV, Jordan WP Jr. Prostatic lymphography. J Urol 1979;121:178–181.
20. Flocks RH, Culp D, Porto R. Lymphatic spread from prostate cancer. J Urol 1959;81:194–196.
21. Bubendorf L, Schopfer A, Wagner U, et al. Metastatic patterns of prostate cancer: an autopsy study of 1,589 patients. Hum Pathol 2000;31:578–583.
22. Long MA, Husband JE. Features of unusual metastases from prostate cancer. Br J Radiol 1999;72:933–941.
23. Golimbu M, Morales P, Al-Askari S, et al. Extended pelvic lymphadenectomy for prostatic cancer. J Urol 1979;121:617–620.
24. Brossner C, Ringhofer H, Schatzl G, et al. Sacral distribution of prostatic lymph nodes visualized on spiral computed tomography with three-dimensional reconstruction. BJU Int 2002;89:44–47.
25. Weingartner K, Ramaswamy A, Bittinger A, et al. Anatomical basis for pelvic lymphadenectomy in prostate cancer: results of an autopsy study and implications for the clinic. J Urol 1996;156:1969–1971.
26. Winfield HN, Donovan JF, See WA, et al. Urological laparoscopic surgery. J Urol 1991;146:941–948.
27. McCullough DL, Prout GR Jr, Daly JJ. Carcinoma of the prostate and lymphatic metastases. J Urol 1974;111:65–71.
28. Lieskovsky G, Skinner DG, Weisenburger T. Pelvic lymphadenectomy in the management of carcinoma of the prostate. J Urol 1980;124:635–638.

29. McDowell GC 2nd, Johnson JW, Tenney DM, et al. Pelvic lymphadenectomy for staging clinically localized prostate cancer. Indications, complications, and results in 217 cases. Urology 1990;35:476–482.

30. Grossman IC, Carpiniello V, Greenberg SH, et al. Staging pelvic lymphadenectomy for carcinoma of the prostate: review of 91 cases. J Urol 1980;124:632–634.

31. Fidler IJ. The pathogenesis of cancer metastasis: the 'seed and soil' hypothesis revisited. Nat Rev Cancer 2003;3:453–458.

32. Fidler IJ. Seed and soil revisited: contribution of the organ microenvironment to cancer metastasis. Surg Oncol Clin N Am 2001;10:257–269, vii–viiii.

33. Batson O. The function of the vertebral veins and their role in the spread of metastases. Ann Surg 1940;112:138–149.

34. Saitoh H, Hida M, Shimbo T, et al. Metastatic patterns of prostatic cancer. Correlation between sites and number of organs involved. Cancer 1984;54:3078–3084.

35. Rana A, Chisholm GD, Khan M, et al. Patterns of bone metastasis and their prognostic significance in patients with carcinoma of the prostate. Br J Urol 1993;72:933–936.

36. Harada M, Iida M, Yamaguchi M, et al. Analysis of bone metastasis of prostatic adenocarcinoma in 137 autopsy cases. Adv Exp Med Biol 1992;324:173–182.

37. Losa M, Grasso M, Giugni E, et al. Metastatic prostatic adenocarcinoma presenting as a pituitary mass: shrinkage of the lesion and clinical improvement with medical treatment. Prostate 1997;32:241–245.

38. Patel N, Teh BS, Powell S, et al. Rare case of metastatic prostate adenocarcinoma to the pituitary. Urology 2003;62:352.

39. Perloff JJ, LeMar HJ Jr, Reddy BV, et al. Metastatic adenocarcinoma of the prostate manifested as a sellar tumor. South Med J 1992;85:1140–1141.

40. Couldwell WT, Chandrasoma PT, Weiss MH. Pituitary gland metastasis from adenocarcinoma of the prostate. Case report. J Neurosurg 1989;71:138–140.

41. Leonard GD, Zhuang SH, Dahut W. Prostate cancer metastatic to skin. Urology 2003;61:456–457.

42. Arita K, Kawashima T, Shimizu H. Cutaneous metastasis of prostate carcinoma. Clin Exp Dermatol 2002;27:64–65.

43. Piattelli A, Fioroni M, Rubini C. Gingival metastasis from a prostate adenocarcinoma: report of a case. J Periodontol 1999;70:441–444.

44. Ben-Izhak O, Lichtig C. Signet-ring cell carcinoma of the prostate mimicking primary gastric carcinoma. J Clin Pathol 1992;45:452–454.

45. Washington K, McDonagh D. Secondary tumors of the gastrointestinal tract: surgical pathologic findings and comparison with autopsy survey. Mod Pathol 1995;8:427–433.

46. Hrebinko R, Taylor SR, Bahnson RR. Carcinoma of prostate metastatic to parotid gland. Urology 1993;41:272–273.

47. Hajdu SI, Urban JA. Cancers metastatic to the breast. Cancer 1972;29:1691–1696.

48. Tu SM, Reyes A, Maa A, et al. Prostate carcinoma with testicular or penile metastases. Clinical, pathologic, and immunohistochemical features. Cancer 2002;94:2610–2617.

49. Hulse CA, O'Neill TK. Adenocarcinoma of the prostate metastatic to the ureter with an associated ureteral stone. J Urol 1989;142:1312–1313.

50. Charhon SA, Chapuy MC, Delvin EE, et al. Histomorphometric analysis of sclerotic bone metastases from prostatic carcinoma special reference to osteomalacia. Cancer 1983;51:918–924.

51. Clark PE, Torti FM. Prostate cancer and bone metastases: medical treatment. Clin Orthop 2003;415:S148–157.

52. Tazi H, Manunta A, Rodriguez A, et al. Spinal cord compression in metastatic prostate cancer. Eur Urol 2003;44:527–532.

53. Nguyen BD. Bilateral iliac metastases with sunburst pattern from prostate cancer. Clin Nucl Med 2003;28:931–932.

54. Roudier MP, True LD, Higano CS, et al. Phenotypic heterogeneity of end-stage prostate carcinoma metastatic to bone. Hum Pathol 2003;34:646–653.

55. de la Monte SM, Moore GW, Hutchins GM. Metastatic behavior of prostate cancer. Cluster analysis of patterns with respect to estrogen treatment. Cancer 1986;58:985–993.

56. Parwani AV, Kronz JD, Genega EM, et al. Prostate carcinoma with squamous differentiation: an analysis of 33 cases. Am J Surg Pathol 2004;28:651–657.

57. Stein BS, Vangore S, Petersen RO. Immunoperoxidase localization of prostatic antigens. Comparison of primary and metastatic sites. Urology 1984;24:146–152.

58. Roudier MP, Corey E, True LD, et al. Histological, immunophenotypic and histomorphometric characterization of prostate cancer bone metastases. Cancer Treat Res 2004;118:311–339.

59. Roudier MP, True LD, Vessella RL, et al. Metastatic conventional prostatic adenocarcinoma with diffuse chromogranin A and androgen receptor positivity. J Clin Pathol 2004;57:321–323.

60. Oesterling JE, Hauzeur CG, Farrow GM. Small cell anaplastic carcinoma of the prostate: a clinical, pathological and immunohistological study of 27 patients. J Urol 1992;147:804–807.

61. Ordonez NG. Value of thyroid transcription factor-1 immunostaining in distinguishing small cell lung carcinomas from other small cell carcinomas. Am J Surg Pathol 2000;24:1217–1223.

62. Yang XJ, Lecksell K, Gaudin P, et al. Rare expression of high-molecular-weight cytokeratin in adenocarcinoma of the prostate gland: a study of 100 cases of metastatic and locally advanced prostate cancer. Am J Surg Pathol 1999;23:147–152.

63. Abrahams NA, Pisters LL, McDonnell TJ, et al. Pathological characterization of residual prostate cancer following chemotherapy combined with hormonal ablation in the neoadjuavnt surgical model. Mod Pathol 2004;17:135A.

64. Moul JW, Merseburger AS, Srivastava S. Molecular markers in prostate cancer: the role in preoperative staging. Clin Prostate Cancer 2002;1:42–50.

65. Wood DP Jr., Banks ER, Humphreys S, et al. Sensitivity of immuno-histochemistry and polymerase chain reaction in detecting prostate cancer cells in bone marrow. J Histochem Cytochem 1994;42:505–511.

66. Cheng L, Pisansky TM, Ramnani DM, et al. Extranodal extension in lymph node-positive prostate cancer. Mod Pathol 2000;13:113–118.

67. Bassily NH, Vallorosi CJ, Akdas G, et al. Coordinate expression of cytokeratins 7 and 20 in prostate adenocarcinoma and bladder urothelial carcinoma. Am J Clin Pathol 2000;113:383–388.

68. Sanderson SO, Sebo TJ, Murphy LM, et al. An analysis of the p63/alpha-methylacyl coenzyme A racemase immunohistochemical cocktail stain in prostate needle biopsy specimens and tissue microarrays. Am J Clin Pathol 2004;121:220–225.

69. Zhou M, Chinnaiyan AM, Kleer CG, et al. Alpha-Methylacyl-CoA racemase: a novel tumor marker over-expressed in several human cancers and their precursor lesions. Am J Surg Pathol 2002;26:926–931.

70. Tretiakova MS, Sahoo S, Takahashi M, et al. Expression of alpha-methylacyl-CoA racemase in papillary renal cell carcinoma. Am J Surg Pathol 2004;28:69–76.

71. Ansari MA, Pintozzi RL, Choi YS, et al. Diagnosis of carcinoid-like metastatic prostatic carcinoma by an immunoperoxidase method. Am J Clin Pathol 1981;76:94–98.

72. Anton RC, Schwartz MR, Kessler ML, et al. Metastatic carcinoma of the prostate mimicking primary carcinoid tumor of the lung and mediastinum. Pathol Res Pract 1998;194:753–758.

73. Copeland JN, Amin MB, Humphrey PA, et al. The morphologic spectrum of metastatic prostatic adenocarcinoma to the lung: special emphasis on histologic features overlapping with other pulmonary neoplasms. Am J Clin Pathol 2002;117:552–557.

74. di Sant'Agnese PA. Neuroendocrine differentiation in carcinoma of the prostate. Diagnostic, prognostic, and therapeutic implications. Cancer 1992;70:254–268.

75. di Sant'Agnese PA. Neuroendocrine differentiation in human prostatic carcinoma. Hum Pathol 1992;23:287–296.

76. Ro JY, Grignon DJ, Troncoso P, et al. Mucin in prostatic adenocarcinoma. Semin Diagn Pathol 1988;5:273–283.

77. Bostwick DG, Foster CS. Predictive factors in prostate cancer: current concepts from the 1999 College of American Pathologists Conference on Solid Tumor Prognostic Factors and the 1999 World Health Organization Second International Consultation on Prostate Cancer. Semin Urol Oncol 1999;17:222–272.

78. Jorgensen T, Yogesan K, Skjorten F, et al. Histopathological grading and DNA ploidy as prognostic markers in metastatic prostatic cancer. Br J Cancer 1995;71:1055–1060.

79. Yossepowitch O, Trabulsi EJ, Kattan MW, et al. Predictive factors in prostate cancer: implications for decision making. Cancer Invest 2003;21:465–480.

80. Glinsky GV, Glinskii AB, Stephenson AJ, et al. Gene expression profiling predicts clinical outcome of prostate cancer. J Clin Invest 2004;113:913–923.

81. Kumar-Sinha C, Chinnaiyan AM. Molecular markers to identify patients at risk for recurrence after primary treatment for prostate cancer. Urology 2003;62 Suppl 1:19–35.

82. Partin AW, Yoo J, Carter HB, et al. The use of prostate specific antigen, clinical stage and Gleason score to predict pathological stage in men with localized prostate cancer. J Urol 1993;150:110–114.

83. Kattan MW, Eastham JA, Stapleton AM, et al. A preoperative nomogram for disease recurrence following radical prostatectomy for prostate cancer. J Natl Cancer Inst 1998;90:766–771.

Non-adenocarcinomatous cancers of the prostate

14

Peter A Humphrey

INTRODUCTION

The vast majority of prostate cancers are adenocarcinomas. Other histologic types of malignancies do arise within the prostate gland and include non-glandular epithelial cancers (carcinomas), neuroendocrine tumors (discussed in Chapter 15), prostatic stromal tumors, mesenchymal tumors, hematolymphoid tumors, and miscellaneous malignancies.[1–5] The 2004 World Health Organization (WHO) histologic classification of these primary non-adenocarcinomatous tumors of the prostate is presented in Box 14.1. Histologic diagnosis of these specific tumor types is critical, since this typing is of prognostic and therapeutic importance. In this chapter, the gross (macroscopic) and histopathologic features of non-adenocarcinomatous cancers of the prostate are presented, with clinicopathologic correlations. Tissue-based special studies of accepted, practical diagnostic utility will also be discussed.

NON-ADENOCARCINOMATOUS EPITHELIAL CANCERS

UROTHELIAL CARCINOMA

Urothelial (also known as transitional cell) carcinoma in the prostate is usually associated with a primary urinary bladder or urethral urothelial carcinoma. Prostatic urothelial carcinomas diagnosed in the absence of a bladder urothelial carcinoma are rare.[6–10] The mean incidence in nine series of 11,678 patients was 1.1% (range 0.2–3.5%) of all prostatic carcinomas.[2]

No gross features specific for prostatic urothelial carcinoma have been reported. Microscopically, prostatic urothelial carcinoma has a striking propensity for growth within prostatic ducts and acini. Rounded or elongated cylinders and plugs of solid tumor are characteristic profiles (Figure 14.1). Prostatic stromal invasion by urothelial carcinoma is typified by irregular solid nests and cords. Cytologically, urothelial carcinoma in the prostate is usually high nuclear grade with substantial nucleomegaly, nuclear pleomorphism, and nuclear hyperchromasia. The cytoplasm may have an eosinophilic "squamoid" appearance. Stromal sclerosis and inflammation are often pronounced. All these histologic findings can help point to a urothelial carcinoma rather than an adenocarcinoma. The immunophenotypic profile of prostatic urothelial

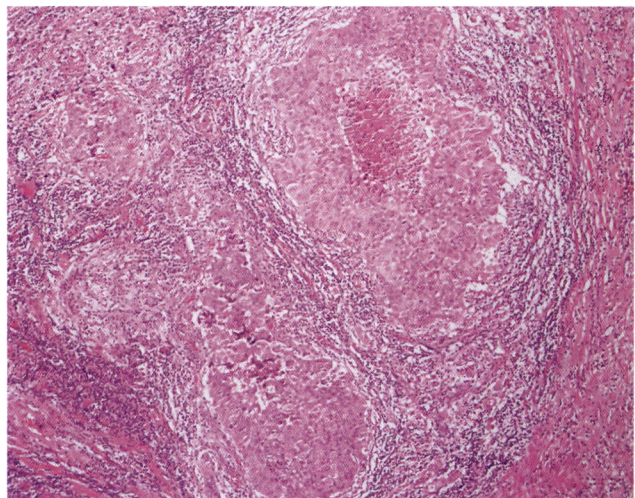

Fig. 14.1
Urothelial carcinoma in the prostate. Solid cylinders of tumor are present, with one cylinder showing central necrosis (comedo necrosis). Note the prominent lymphoid response.

performed. Three-tiered and four-tiered grading systems have been used.[7] The Gleason grading system should not be applied. For staging, the 2002 AJCC/UICC TNM staging manual should be used.[10] In staging, the distinction between prostatic urothelial carcinoma in situ (CIS) and stromal invasion, with or without an associated bladder carcinoma, is critical for prognosis.[11]

SQUAMOUS CELL AND ADENOSQUAMOUS CARCINOMAS

Squamous cell carcinoma and adenosquamous carcinomas that originate in the prostate are rare. The largest series is of 33 cases.[12] In this series, men with an average age of 68 years presented with bladder outlet obstruction and dysuria. The incidence is less than 1% of all prostate carcinomas.[13-16] Many cases of prostatic carcinoma with squamous differentiation are detected after radiation or hormonal therapy for prostatic adenocarcinoma. The time course for the appearance of squamous differentiation in the carcinoma varies from 3 months[17] to many years (up to 9) after therapy.[18] Squamous metaplasia and HPV infection do not appear to predispose to this development.[14] Prostatic squamous cell carcinoma has been shown to occur in association with prostatic schistosomiasis.[19]

Grossly, prostatic squamous cell carcinomas are usually large, measuring up to 6.5 cm in greatest dimension and often replacing a substantial portion of the prostate. Cut surfaces reveal a solid, firm, whitish yellow, white–gray, or gray–tan mass. Microscopically, pure squamous cell carcinoma is typified by infiltrating nests, strands, and sheets of polygonal cells with nuclear atypia, with squamous differentiation manifested as individual cell keratinization, intercellular bridges, and/or keratin pearl formation (Figure 14.2). The application of a three-tiered grading scheme, with well-, moderately, or poorly

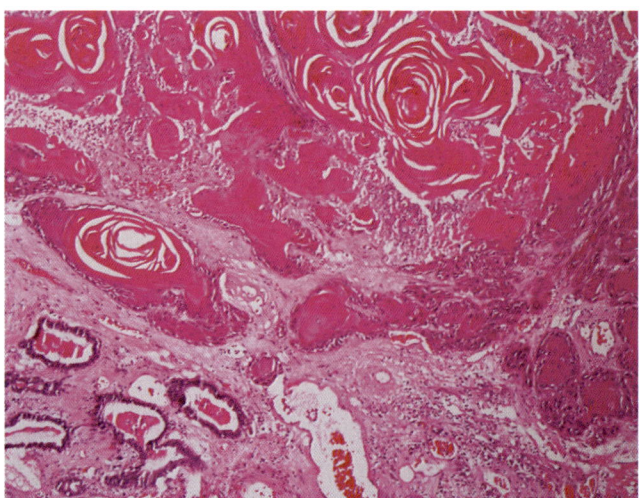

Fig. 14.2
Squamous cell carcinoma in the prostate. Abundant keratin production is evident.

carcinoma is useful in the differential diagnostic distinction from poorly-differentiated prostatic adenocarcinoma. The urothelial carcinoma cells are prostate-specific antigen (PSA) and prostatic acid phosphatase (PSAP) negative, and are frequently positive for the cytokeratins CK7 and CK20, high-molecular-weight cytokeratins bound by antibody 34βE12 (CK903),[6] and thrombomodulin.

Prostatic urothelial carcinoma may exhibit locally aggressive growth, with extension into the bladder and pelvis.[9] Lymph node, lung, and osteolytic (with a few osteoblastic) bone metastases have been identified.[9] Grading and pathologic staging have been inconsistently differentiated categories, is a reasonable approach. Prostatic squamous cell carcinoma and adenosquamous carcinoma, like pure adenocarcinomas, can spread along nerves, extend locally into periprostatic soft tissue, bladder, and seminal vesicles, and metastasize to lymph nodes and bone. In bone, however, the metastases are mainly osteolytic rather than osteoblastic.[14] Special studies are of limited use in diagnosis. The malignant squamous cells are most often negative for PSA and PSAP immunostains, and this correlates with the normal serum PSA and PSAP levels found in the vast majority of prostatic squamous cell carcinoma patients. The mean survival for prostatic squamous cell carcinoma is poor, at 6 to 24 months.[2,12]

BASAL CELL CARCINOMA

Basal cell carcinoma of the prostate includes malignant basaloid proliferations (basaloid carcinomas) and also neoplasms that resemble, to a certain degree, adenoid cystic carcinomas of the salivary glands.[20–25] A large number of terms have been utilized for these neoplasms such as adenoid basal cell tumor, adenoid cystic tumor, adenoid cystic-like tumor, basal cell carcinoma, and adenoid basal proliferation of uncertain significance. The difficulty in classification of these proliferations resides in the fact that they are rare, there is not agreement on histologic criteria, and follow-up is available for only a few cases. Basal cell carcinomas are extraordinarily rare, with only about 50 reported cases.[2,20] The gross features have been reported for fewer than 10 cases. In the largest series, the tumors were white and solid, sometimes with microcysts.[20] Microscopically, several growth arrangements may be evident including large basaloid nests with peripheral palisading and necrosis, a florid basal cell hyperplasia-like pattern, and an adenoid basal cell hyperplasia-like pattern (adenoid cystic carcinoma pattern).[1] Infiltrative permeation, extraprostatic extension, perineural invasion, necrosis, and stromal desmoplasia are characteristics of basal cell carcinoma that can help in the differential diagnostic distinction from basal cell hyperplasia. Immunohistochemical marker studies for BCL2 and Ki67 (for proliferation index) may also be of value in this separation.[24] Histologic grading of basal cell carcinoma is generally not done. Limited data on patient outcome have revealed a few cancer-specific deaths,[2,20] indicating that basal cell carcinoma of the prostate is a potentially aggressive neoplasm.

PROSTATIC SARCOMAS

Mesenchymal neoplasms are infrequently encountered in the prostate gland. Prostatic sarcomas are rare cancers, comprising 0.1% of all prostatic malignancies.[26] The most common sarcomas in the prostate are rhabdomyosarcomas in children and leiomyosarcoma

in adults.[27] Other sarcomas in the prostate are exceedingly rare.

RHABDOMYOSARCOMA

Rhabdomyosarcoma is the most common prostate cancer in children and adolescents.[26–36] The median age at diagnosis is 3.5 to 6.5 years, with a range of a few months to 68 years. Less than a dozen prostatic rhabdomyosarcomas have been reported in adults of the age 18 to 68 years.[30]

Grossly (and clinically), determination that a rhabdomyosarcoma is primary in the prostate rather than the bladder can be difficult to impossible, primarily due to the large size of these neoplasms and concurrent involvement of the bladder and prostate. Consequently, many series have lumped prostatic rhabdomyosarcomas as bladder–prostate rhabdomyosarcoma, lower urinary tract rhabdomyosarcoma, genitourinary rhabdomyosarcoma, or pelvic rhabdomyosarcoma.[26,28,29,31,32] For tumors of definite prostatic origin, the average size was 9 cm (range 6–20 cm).[27] They tend to be solid masses with a gelatinous appearance.[27,29] Microsopically, most are embryonal nonbotyroid rhabdomyosarcomas with a small percentage of cases being of the alveolar subtype.[36] The embryonal subtype is composed of diffuse sheets or nests of small rounded or elongated hyperchromatic cells with a moderate amount of eosinophilic cytoplasm. Condensation of cells along protrusions into adjacent cavities can create the compact, so-called "cambium layer." Cytologically, there is a range of differentiation, from primitive stellate or fusiform cells to "tadpole" and ribbon-like "strap" cells that have cross-striations indicative of skeletal muscle lineage. The alveolar subtype can show the classical alveolar structure of delicate anastomosing fibrous septa with tumor cells "floating" in the alveolar space and/or solid patterns. It is critical that, cytologically, these alveolar rhabdomyosarcomas be of high grade (Figure 14.3) with pleomorphic, hyperchromatic nuclei, coarse chromatin, and numerous mitotic figures. Treatment can lead to necrosis, fibrosis, and "maturation," where the tumor cells appear well-differentiated.[37] Immunohistochemical stains are of immense utility in confirming muscular differentiation, especially in neoplasms that are poorly-differentiated in hematoxylin and eosin (H&E) stained sections. Positivity for vimentin, muscle-specific actin, and desmin is the rule.[36] Specific, useful, markers of skeletal muscle differentiation include myoglobin, MyoD, and myogenin.[36] In most, but not all cases, light microscopy and immunostains are sufficient to establish the diagnosis of prostatic rhabdomyosarcoma. Genetic studies and electron microscopy can be helpful when histologic features do not fit with the immunohistochemical stain results.[36] Extremely useful, diagnostic genetic alterations are the characteristic t(2:13) and t(1:13) translocations found in about two thirds of

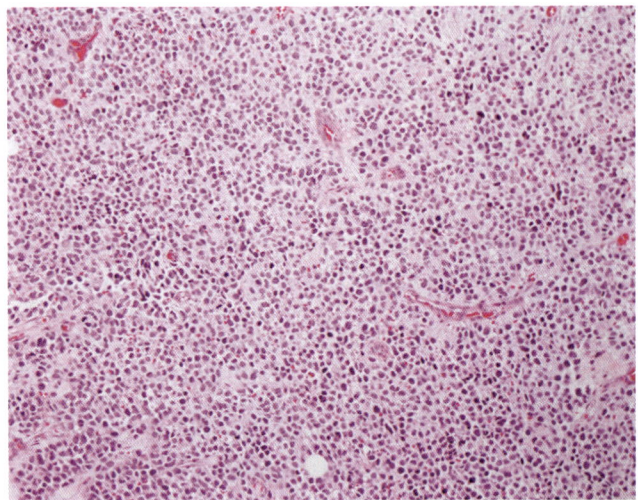

Fig. 14.3
Rhabdomyosarcoma of the prostate, alveolar subtype, with sheet-like growth. Reverse transcriptase polymerase chain reaction (PCR) and sequencing demonstrated the characteristic PAX3–FKHR gene fusion product in this case.

alveolar rhabdomyosarcoma cases.[36] These translocations, which fuse genes PAX3, or PAX7, and FKHR, can be detected by cytogenetics or reverse transcriptase polymerase chain reaction.[38] The latter technique can be performed using formalin-fixed, paraffin-embedded tissue. A diagnostic genetic alteration has thus far not been discovered in embryonal rhabdomyosarcomas.

Prostatic rhabdomyosarcoma is an aggressive neoplasm that exhibits direct, local extension into the bladder neck, posterior portion of the urethra, and perirectal/rectal tissues.[29] Lymph node metastases are fairly common, being seen in 20% to 40% of patients. Distant metastases are mainly to lungs, liver, and bone. In adults the disease is often lethal, and bony metastases are frequently osteolytic and generalized. Prognosis for rhabdomyosarcoma is related to histologic subtype, where embryonal rhabdomyosarcoma has an intermediate prognosis and alveolar rhabdomyosarcoma a poor prognosis.[34,39] TNM staging of childhood and prostatic rhabdomyosarcoma is also linked to prognosis.[34] The Intergroup Rhabdomyosarcoma Study uses a modified TNM staging system, where primary anatomic site of origin plays a role in stage assignment.[40] Bladder–prostate rhabdomyosarcomas are automatically stage 2 or 3, reflecting their worse prognosis compared with orbital, head and neck, and non-bladder–prostate genitourinary primaries.[40] It is not currently established that DNA content, P53 protein accumulation, or transcriptional expression profiles are of prognostic value.

LEIOMYOSARCOMA

Leiomyosarcoma is the most common sarcoma originating in the adult prostate, accounting for 30% of all prostatic sarcomas,[27] but is rare, with around 100 reported cases.[2] The mean age at diagnosis is approximately 57 years, with a range of 17 to 98 years. Patients typically present with urinary frequency, dysuria, urgency, retention, and nocturia.[41] Grossly, mean and median sizes of 9 and 5 cm, respectively, have been reported, with a size range of 2 to 24 cm.[27,41] The tumors are nodular and firm, and are frequently necrotic and cystic.[41] Microscopically, interlacing fascicles, bundles, and whorls of neoplastic spindle cells are found, with effacement of the normal prostatic tissue (Figure 14.4). Histologic grade is variable, with about one third being low grade (Broders's grade 1 of 4), with the remainder high grade (grade 3–4 of 4).[41] Higher-grade tumors are cellular, with marked nuclear pleomorphism, hyperchromasia, and macronuclei. Of substantial importance, mitotic figures are present, with a mean approaching one per high power field.[41] Necrosis is evident in half of cases, and, on average, half of the tumor is necrotic. By immunohistochemical staining, all tumor cells are vimentin positive, two thirds are actin positive, and weak desmin staining is seen in 20% of cases.[41] Leiomyosarcomas of the prostate are aggressive neoplasms, with most (10/11) patients suffering recurrence after surgical resection.[41] One half of the men developed distant metastases, with lung being the most common site for metastatic spread.[41] Average survival was 2 to 4 years after diagnosis.[27,41] There are no established pathologic prognostic factors (including grade, tumor size, and stage), although it has been suggested that low mitotic activity and ability to achieve complete surgical resection with negative margins may be predictive of survival.[35,41] Cytogenetic abnormalities involving chromosomes 2, 3, 9, 11, and 19 have been described in a single case,[42] but are currently not used for diagnosis.

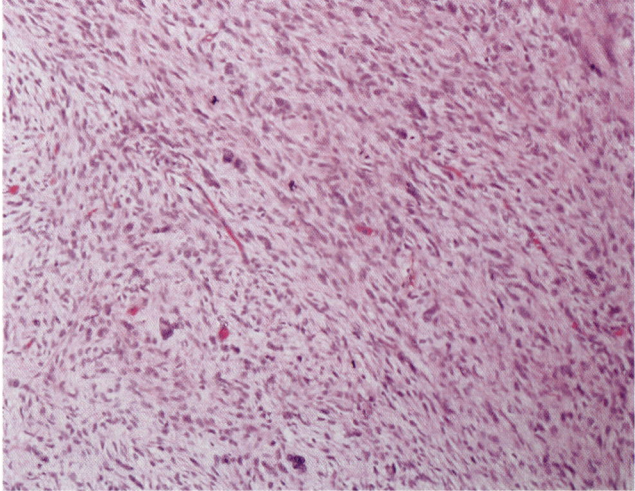

Fig. 14.4
Leiomyosarcoma of the prostate, with malignant spindle cells displaying cytologic atypia and mitotic activity.

OTHER SARCOMAS

Only a few cases of prostatic stromal sarcoma have been reported.[1,43] Sections show sheets of hypercellular atypical stroma.[1] The behavior of those stromal sarcomas is not well defined, although a few patients have suffered from metastatic disease.

Additional sarcomas primary in the prostate have mainly been the subject of case reports.[2] These include angiosarcoma, malignant peripheral nerve sheath tumor, malignant fibrous histiocytoma, synovial sarcoma, chondrosarcoma, osteosarcoma, Ewing's sarcoma/PNET, malignant rhabdoid tumors, malignant mesenchymoma, and ectomesenchymoma. A few sarcomas, mainly osteogenic sarcomas, have been reported to occur after radiation therapy.[44-48] Several cases of sarcoma emerging from prostatic phyllodes tumor have been reported.[49] Fibrosarcoma, fibromyosarcoma, myosarcoma, and spindle cell sarcoma are diagnostic terms applied to a few prostatic sarcomas in the older literature,[50] when immunohistochemistry and/or electron microscopy were not available for more precise characterization of tumor cell differentiation. Undifferentiated sarcoma or unclassified sarcoma does remain a viable diagnostic category for prostatic sarcomas not exhibiting any specific mesenchymal cell type differentiation after morphologic, immunophenotypic, and genotypic evaluations.

HEMATOLYMPHOID NEOPLASMS

Hematolymphoid neoplasms may involve the prostate, including leukemia, lymphoma, Hodgkin's disease, and multiple myeloma,[1-5,51-67] Leukemic infiltrates in the prostate are virtually always indicative of secondary spread, whereas about two thirds of prostatic lymphomas are secondary.[2] Leukemia and lymphoma commonly involve the prostate gland at post-mortem examination, but clinical manifestations of such infiltrates are rare, occurring in less than 1% of patients with lymphoma or leukemia. There are cases, however, where the initial clinical presentation of the leukemia or lymphoma was symptoms referable to the prostate. With or without a previous history of leukemia or lymphoma, prostatic involvement is usually clinically attributed to prostatitis, benign prostatic hyperplasia (BPH), or prostatic carcinoma.

LEUKEMIA

Leukemic infiltrates in the prostate are most often detected in transurethral resection of the prostate (TURP) chips or open prostatectomy specimens as an incidental finding in patients with obstruction and known leukemia.[53,68] While it is difficult to know for certain to what extent the leukemic infiltrates contribute to symptomatology, prostatic leukemic infiltrates may be a significant factor in development of acute retention of urine, but only in the presence of other factors such as BPH.[69]

There is little knowledge of the gross appearance of leukemic infiltrates in the prostate. A few reports of diffuse white parenchyma and white-to-yellow prostatic nodules exist.[69,70] Microscopically, the most common type of prostatic leukemic infiltrate is chronic lymphocytic lymphoma (CLL), followed in order by acute lymphoblastic lymphoma (ALL), acute AML, and CML. Growth in a diffuse sheet-like fashion, with replacement of benign prostatic parenchyma, can be observed. The proliferation is predominantly stromal-based, with dispersion around prostatic glands, which can be compressed and destroyed by the infiltrate. Rare cases (n = 5) of granulocytic sarcoma (chloroma) of the prostate, related to myelogenous leukemia or myeloproliferative disorder of the marrow, have been published.[71,72]

LYMPHOMA

Both primary and secondary lymphomas of the prostate have been recognized.[51,52,54-67] These are rare diseases in prostate, with less than 200 reported cases. Clinically, the mean age at presentation is around 57 years, with a wide age range of 5 to 89 years.[63,64] Patients present with obstructive symptoms, including urgency and frequency, sometimes with hematuria and retention.[63,64] Clinically, the main difference between patients with primary and secondary lymphoma of the prostate is that, by definition, patients with secondary lymphoma had their disease diagnosed in an extraprostatic site first (usually lymph nodes) or extraprostatic site involvement was discovered within 1 month of diagnosis of prostatic involvement.[62,63]

The few macroscopic descriptions of prostatic lymphoma in existence document large masses 6.5 cm in greatest dimension that often completely replaced the prostate and filled the entire pelvis.[73-77] Cut surfaces were homogenous, and variable in coloration, including yellow–brown, white, yellowish white, grayish pink, and grayish yellow. Gross extension into local, adjacent structures, especially the bladder, was frequently noted. Microscopically, there is usually a patchy, stromal, atypical lymphoid infiltrate (Figure 14.5), although the neoplasm can be extensive, obliterative, perivascular, or focal. For angiotropic or intravascular lymphomas (of which there are five reported cases) the tumor cells are confined to vascular lumens.[78] The neoplastic lymphoid cells can extend into prostatic epithelium in some cases, and, for the reported cases of prostatic mucosa-associated lymphoid tissue (MALToma), lymphoepithelial lesions were formed.

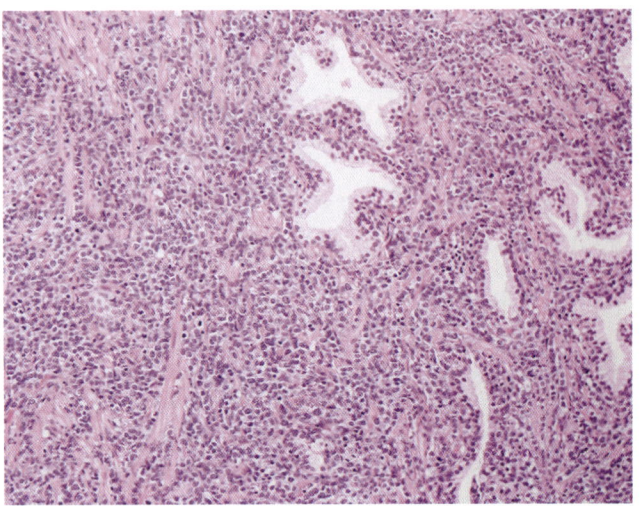

Fig. 14.5
Malignant lymphoma in the prostate, with destructive growth and preservation of only a few prostatic glands.

A wide variety of lymphoma types have been diagnosed in the prostate: 90% are B-cell lymphomas,[63] and the most common types are diffuse large lymphoma in 40% of all cases, and small lymphocytic lymphoma in 27% of cases. Other types include lymphoblastic lymphoma, Burkitt's lymphoma, monocytoid B-cell lymphoma, lymphomas of follicular center cell origin, and lymphomatoid granulomatosis.[63,64] Small lymphocytic lymphoma tends to be secondary, but otherwise no difference in histologic type can be discerned between primary and secondary lymphomas.[63] Admixed prostatic adenocarcinoma has been found in a few cases.[63,64,79] "Collision" between the lymphoma and adenocarcinoma has been depicted.[63]

Immunohistochemical stains and/or flow cytometry are needed as adjunctive tools to diagnose prostatic lymphoma, especially in the absence of previously diagnosed lymphoma. In the older literature some cases diagnosed as prostatic lymphoma prior to utilization of immunohistochemistry likely represented poorly differentiated carcinoma or sarcoma. The same diagnostic difficulty can be encountered today, as highlighted by a fairly recent case where biopsy misdiagnosis of a prostatic lymphoma as "anaplastic carcinoma" led to an unnecessary radical cystoprostatectomy.[80] The outcome for patients with prostatic lymphoma is generally unfavorable with a median survival of 23 to 28 months. Outcome did not differ according to histologic type,[63] except for prostatic angiotropic (intravascular) lymphoma, which has the most dismal prognosis of all.[64] Survival also did not differ based on whether the prostatic lymphoma was primary or secondary.

OTHERS

About 10 cases of Hodgkin's lymphoma and 6 cases of multiple myeloma have been detected in the prostate.[2]

MISCELLANEOUS TUMORS

Miscellaneous, extremely rare, primary malignancies involving the prostate include isolated case reports of perivascular epithelioid clear cell tumor (PEComa),[81] Wilms' tumor,[82] germ cell tumors including endodermal sinus (yolk sac) tumor,[83–85] seminoma,[86] and mixed malignant germ cell tumor.[87] Malignant melanoma can be detected in the prostate, although most cases represent spread from a cutaneous primary. Only a couple of cases of primary malignant melanoma have been published.[88,89]

METASTASES

Finally, one should recognize that malignancies from other anatomic sites can involve the prostate by direct extension or by metastatic spread (Table 14.1).[1,2,51,90] Overall, both are uncommon events. In two series of a total of 7436 autopsies, 346 (5% of cases) had a secondary tumor in the prostate.[51,90] Clinically, the neoplasm that most frequently involves the prostate by direct spread is urothelial carcinoma of the urinary bladder or urethra. Secondary metastatic spread is most often seen in patients with leukemia and lymphoma.[51] Solid tumors, even those that are well known for their capacity for widespread dissemination, such as melanoma and renal cell carcinoma, rarely metastasize to the prostate.[91] It is also rare for metastatic solid tumor deposits in the prostate to produce clinical symptoms, where TURP chips resected due to obstruction or biopsy disclosed clinically unsuspected metastatic tumor.[92–95]

Table 14.1 Secondary cancers of the prostate

Secondary cancer	% Prostates involved
Direct extension	
Bladder urothelial carcinoma	23
Colonic adenocarcinoma	Rare
Pelvic lymphoma	Rare
Metastatic spread	
Leukemia	14
Lymphoma	8
Germ cell tumor	2
Other carcinomas (thyroid, stomach, pancreas, kidney, lung)	0.6–1.5

REFERENCES

1. Tumours of the Prostate. In: Eble JN, Sauter G, Epstein JI, Sesterhenn IA (eds): Tumours of the Urinary System and Male Genital Organs. Lyon, France: IARC Press, 2004 pp 159–214.

2. Humphrey PA. Variants of Prostatic Carcinoma [Chapter 17] and Unusual Prostatic Neoplasms [Chapter 18]. In: Prostate Pathology. Chicago: ASCP Press, 2003, pp 390–454.

3. Epstein JI, Yang XJ. Transitional Cell Carcinoma [Chapter 15] and Mesenchymal Tumors and Tumor-like Conditions [Chapter 16]. In: Prostate Biopsy Interpretation, 3rd ed. Philadelphia:Lippincott Williams & Wilkins, 2002, pp 226–256.

4. Young RH, Srigley JR, Amin MB, et al. Variants of Prostatic Adenocarcinoma, Other Primary Carcinomas of Prostate, and Secondary Carcinomas [Chapter 5] and Miscellaneous Tumors of the Prostate [Chapter 6]. In: Tumors of the Prostate Gland, Seminal Vesicles, Male Urethra, and Penis, Third Series, Fascicle 28. Washington DC: Armed Forces Institute of Pathology, 2000, pp 217–288.

5. Bostwick DG, Dundore PA. Variants of Prostatic Carcinoma [Chapter 9], Urothelial Carcinoma [Chapter 11], Soft Tissue Tumors [Chapter 12], and Other Rare Malignant Tumors [Chapter 13]. In: Biopsy Pathology of the Prostate. London: Chapman & Hall Medical, 1997, pp 167–190, 205–210, 211–232.

6. Cheville JC. Urothelial carcinoma of the prostate. An immunohistochemical comparison with high grade prostatic adenocarcicoma and review of the literature. J Urol Pathol 1998;9:141–154.

7. Greene LF, O'Dea MJ, Dockerty MB. Primary transitional cell carcinoma of the prostate. J Urol 1976;116:761–763.

8. Goebbels R, Amberger L,Wernert N, et al. Urothelial carcinoma of the prostate. Appl Pathol 1985;3:242–254.

9. Nicolaisen GS, Williams RD. Primary transitional cell carcinoma of prostate. Urology 1984;24:544–549.

10. Greene FL, Page DL, Fleming ID, et al. Urethra. In: AJCC Cancer Staging Manual, 6th ed. New York: Springer Verlag, 2002, pp 341–343.

11. Cheville JC, Dundore PA, Bostwick DG, et al. Transitional cell carcinoma of the prostate. Clinicopathologic study of 50 cases. Cancer 1998;82:703–707.

12. Parwani AV, Kronz JD, Genega EM, et al. Prostate carcinoma with squamous differentiation: an analysis of 33 cases. Am J Surg Pathol 2004;28:651–657.

13. Sarma DP, Weilbaecher TG, Moon TD. Squamous cell carcinoma of prostate. Urology 1991;37:260–262.

14. Little NA, Wiener JS, Walther PJ, et al. Squamous cell carcinoma of the prostate: 2 cases of a rare malignancy and review of the literature. J Urol 1993;149:137–139.

15. Bennett RS, Edgerton EO. Mixed prostatic carcinoma. J Urol 1973;110:561–563.

16. Wernert N, Goebbels R, Bonkhoff H, et al. Squamous cell carcinoma of the prostate. Histopathology 1990;17:339–344.

17. Wang Q, Lin C-S, Unger PP. Squamous cell carcinoma arising in hormonally treated adenocarcinoma of the prostate. Int J Surg Pathol 1996;4:13–16.

18. Miller VA, Reuter V, Scher HL. Primary squamous cell carcinoma of the prostate after radiation seed implantation for adenocarcinoma. Urology 1995;46:111–113.

19. Al Adnani MS. Schistosomiasis, metaplasia and squamous cell carcinoma of the prostate: Histogenesis of the squamous cancer cells determined by localization of specific markers. Neoplasma 1985;32:613–622.

20. Iczkowski KA, Ferguson KL, Grier DD, et al. Adenoid cystic/basal cell carcinoma of the prostate. Am J Surg Pathol 2003;27:1523–1529.

21. Mastropasqua MG, Pruneri G, Renne G, et al. Basaloid cell carcinoma of the prostate. Virchows Archiv 2003;443:787–791.

22. Young RH, Frierson HF Jr, Mills SE, et al. Adenoid cystic-like tumor of the prostate gland. Am J Clin Pathol 1998;89:49–56.

23. Denholm SW, Webb JN, Howard G-CW, et al. Basaloid carcinoma of the prostate gland: Histogenesis and review of the literature. Histopathology 1992;20:151–155.

24. Yang XJ, McEntee M, Epstein JI. Distinction of basaloid carcinoma of the prostate from benign basal cell lesions by using immunohistochemistry for bcl-2 and Ki-67. Hum Pathol 1998;29:1447–1450.

25. Grignon DJ, Ro JY, Ordóñez NG, et al. Basal cell hyperplasia, adenoid basal cell tumor, and adenoid cystic carcinoma of the prostate gland: an immunohistochemical study. Hum Pathol 1988;19:1425–1433.

26. MacKenzie AR, Whitmore WF, Melamed MR. Myosarcomas of the bladder and prostate. Cancer 1968;22:833–844.

27. Smith BH, Dehner LP. Sarcoma of the prostate gland. Am J Clin Pathol 1972;58:43–50.

28. Merguerian PA, Agarwal S, Greenberg M, et al. Outcome analysis of rhabdomyosarcoma of the lower urinary tract. J Urol 1998;160:1191–1194.

29. Shapiro E, Strother D. Pediatric genitourinary rhabdomyosarcoma. J Urol 1992;148:1761–1768.

30. Waring PM, Newland RC. Prostatic embryonal rhabdomyosarcoma in adults. A clinicopathologic review. Cancer 1992;69:755–762.

31. Hays DM. Bladder/prostate rhabdomyosarcoma: results of multi-institutional trials of the Intergroup Rhabdomyosarcoma Study. Sem Surg Oncol 1993;9:520–523.

32. El-Sherbiny MT, El-Mekresh MH, El-Baz MA, et al. Paediatric lower urinary tract rhabdomyosarcoma: a single-centre experience of 30 patients. BJU Int 2000;86:260–267.

33. Dupree WC, Fisher C. Rhabdomyosarcoma of prostate in adult. Long-term survival and problem of histologic diagnosis. Urology 1982;19:80–82.

34. Wijnaendts LC, van der Linden JC, van Unnick AJ, et al. Histopathological classification of childhood rhabdomyosarcoma: relationship with clinical parameters and prognosis. Hum Pathol 1994;25:900–907.

35. Sexton WJ, Lance RE, Reyes AO, et al. Adult prostatic sarcoma. The M.D. Anderson Cancer Center Experience. J Urol 2001;166:521–525.

36. Parham DM. Pathologic classification of rhabdomyosarcomas and correlations with molecular studies. Mod Pathol 2001;14:506–514.

37. Coffin CM, Rulon J, Smith L, et al. Pathologic features of rhabdomyosarcoma before and after treatment: a clinicopathologic and immunohistochemical analysis. Mod Pathol 1997;10:1175–1187.

38. Barr FG, Chalten J, D'Cruz C, et al. Molecular assays for chromosomal translocations in the diagnosis of pediatric soft tissue sarcomas. JAMA 1995;273:553–557.

39. Newton WA, Gehan EA, Webber BL, et al. Classification of rhabdomyosarcomas and related sarcomas. Cancer 1995;76:1073–1085.

40. Wexler LH, Helman LJ. Pediatric soft tissue sarcoma. CA Cancer J Clin 1994;44:211–247.

41. Cheville JC, Dundore PA, Nascimento AG, et al. Leiomyosarcoma of the prostate. Report of 23 cases. Cancer 1995;76:1422–1427.

42. Limon J, Dal Cin Dal P, Sandberg AA. Cytogenetic findings in a primary leiomyosarcoma of the prostate. Cancer Genet Cytogenet 1986;22:159–167.

43. Gaudin PB, Rosai J, Epstein JI. Sarcomas and related proliferative lesions of specialized prostatic stroma. Am J Surg Pathol 1998;22:148–162.

44. Locke JR, Soloway MS, Evans J, et al. Osteogenic differentiation associated with x-ray therapy for adenocarcinoma of the prostate gland. Am J Clin Pathol 1976;85:375–378.

45. Nishiyam T, Ikarashi T, Terunuma M, et al. Osteogenic sarcoma of the prostate. Int J Urol 2001;8:199–201.

46. McKenzie M, MacLennan I, Kostashuk E, et al. Postradiation sarcoma after external beam radiation therapy for localized adenocarcinoma of the prostate: report of three cases. Urology 1999;53:1228.

47. Nghiem HV, Sommer FG, Moretto JC. MRI of radiation-induced prostate sarcoma. Clin Imaging 1995;19:54–56.

48. Terris MK. Transrectal ultrasound appearance of radiation-induced prostatic sarcoma. Prostate 1998;37:182–186.

49. Bostwick DG, Hossain D, Qian J, et al. Phyllodes tumor of the prostate: Long-term followup study of 23 cases. J Urol 2004;172:894–899.

50. Tefft M, Jaffe N. Sarcoma of the bladder and prostate in children. Cancer 1973;32:1161–1177.

51. Zein TA, Huben R, Lane W, et al. Secondary tumors of the prostate. J Urol 1985;133:615–616.

52. Sridhar KN, Woodhouse CRJ. Prostatic infiltration in leukaemia and lymphoma. Eur Urol 1983;9:153–156.

53. Melchior J, Valk WL, Foret JD, et al. The prostate in leukemia: evaluation and review of the literature. J Urol 1974,111:647–651.

54. Sarris A, Pimopoulos M, Pugh W, et al. Primary lymphoma of the prostate: good outcome with Doxorubicin-based combination chemotherapy. J Urol 1995;153:1852–1854.

55. Parks RW, Henry PG, Abram WP, et al. Primary non-Hodgkin's lymphoma of the prostate mimicking acute prostatitis. Br J Urol 1995;76:409.

56. Bell CRW, Napier MP, Morgan RJ, et al. Primary non-Hodgkin's lymphoma of the prostate gland: case report and review of the literature. Clin Oncol 1995;7:409–410.

57. Leung TW, Tung SY, Sze WK, et al. Primary non-Hodgkin's lymphoma of the prostate. Clin Oncol 1997;9:264–266.

58. Araki K, Kubota Y, Iijima Y, et al. Indolent behaviour of low-grade B-cell lymphoma of mucosa-associated lymphoid tissue involved in salivary glands, renal sinus and prostate. Scand J Urol Nephrol 1998;32:234–236.

59. Tomikawa S, Okumura H, Yoshida T, et al. Primary prostatic lymphoma of mucosa-associated lymphoid tissue. Intern Med 1998;37:628–630.

60. Tomura U, Ishikura H, Kon S-I, et al. Primary lymphoma of the prostate with features of low grade B-cell lymphoma of mucosa associated lymphoid tissue: a rare cause of urinary obstruction. J Urol 1999;162:496–497

61. Jhavar S, Agarwal JP, Naresh KN, et al. Primary extranodal mucosa associated lymphohoid tissue (MALT) lymphoma of the prostate. Leukemia and Lymphoma 2001;41:445–449.

62. Bostwick DG, Mann RB. Malignant lymphomas involving the prostate. A study of 13 cases. Cancer 1985;56:2932–2938.

63. Bostwick DG, Iczkowski KA, Amin MB, et al. Malignant lymphoma involving the prostate. Report of 62 cases. Cancer 1998;83:732–738.

64. Ferry JA, Young RH. Malignant lymphoma of the genitourinary tract. Curr Diagn Pathol 1997;4:145–169.

65. Doll DC, Weiss RB, Shah S. Lymphoma of the prostate presenting as benign prostatic hypertrophy. Southern Med J 1978;71:1170–1171.

66. Boe S, Nielsen H, Ryttov N. Burkitt's lymphoma mimicking prostatitis. J Urol 1981;125:891–892.

67. Cos LR, Rashid HA. Primary non-Hodgkin lymphoma of the prostate presenting as benign prostate hyperplasia. Urology 1984;23:176–179.

68. Wilber H, Taylor RJ. Prostatectomy in patients with leukemia. Urology 1981;18:580–581.

69. Dajani YF, Burke M. Leukemic infiltration of the prostate. A case study and clinicopathologic review. Cancer 1976;38:2442–2446.

70. Flaherty SA, Cope HE, Shecket HA. Prostatic obstruction as the presenting symptom of acute monocytic leukemia. J Urol 1940;44:488–497.

71. Chan YF, Granulocytic sarcoma (chloroma) of the kidney and prostate. Br J Urol 1990; 54:655–666.

72. Thalhammer F, Gisslinger H, Chott A, et al. Granulocytic sarcoma of the prostate as the first manifestation of a late relapse of acute myelogenous leukemia. Ann Hematol 1994;68:97–99.

73. Waller JI, Shullenberger WA. Lymphosarcoma of the prostate. J Urol 1949;62:480–487.

74. Ferguson RS, Stewart FW. Lymphosarcoma of the prostate. J Urol 1932;28:93–104.

75. Kirshbaum JD, Larkin HS, Culver H. Retothel sarcoma of the prostate gland; report of a case. J Urol 1943;50:597–607.

76. Kaufmann W, Wright AW. Lymphosarcoma of the prostate. With report of a case. Arch Surg 1941;43:1061–1075.

77. Rathbun ND, de Veer JA. Lymphosarcoma of the prostate. With report of a case. Mt Sinai Hos 1937–38;4:771–780.

78. DeGiuseppe JA, Nelson WG, Seifter EJ, et al. Intravascular lymphomatosis: A clinicopathologic study of 10 cases and assessment of response to chemotherapy. J Clin Oncol 1994;12:2573–2579.

79. Gros R, Richter S, Bechar L. Prostatic carcinoma with concomitant non-Hodgkin lymphoma: report of 2 cases. Urol Int 1984;39:121–122.

80. Kerbl K, Pauer W. Primary non-Hodgkin lymphoma of the prostate. Urology 1988;32:347–349.

81. Pan CC, Yang AK, Chiang H. Malignant perivascular epithelioid cell tumor involving the prostate. Arch Pathol Lab Med 2003;127:E96–E98.

82. Casiraghi O, Martinez-Madrigal F, Mostofi FK, et al. Primary prostatic Wilm's tumor. Am J Surg Pathol 1991;15:885–890.

83. Benson RC Jr, Segura JW, Carney JA. Primary yolk-sac (endodermal sinus) tumor of the prostate. Cancer 1978;41:1395–1398.

84. Dalla Palma PA, Dante S, Guazzieri S, et al. Primary endodermal sinus tumor of the prostate: report of a case. Prostate 1988;12:255–261.

85. Tay HP, Bidair M, Shabaik A, et al. Primary yolk sac tumor of the prostate in a patient with Kleinefelter's syndrome. J Urol 1995;153:1066–1069.

86. Hayman R, Patel A, Fisher C, et al. Primary seminoma of the prostate. Br J Urol 1995;76:273–274.

87. Michel F, Gattegno B, Roland J, et al. Primary nonseminomatous germ cell tumor of the prostate. J Urol 1986;135:597–599.

88. Berry NE, Reese L. Malignant melanoma which had its first clinical manifestations in the prostate gland. J Urol 1953;69:286–290.

89. Wang C-J, Chen Y-T, Shun C-T, et al. Primary malignant melanoma of the prostate. J Urol 1995; 154:1865.

90. Johnson DE, Chalbaud R, Ayala AG. Secondary tumors of the prostate. J Urol 1974;112:507–508.

91. Bates AW, Baithun SI. Secondary solid neoplasms of the prostate: a clinicopathologic series of 51 cases. Virchows Arch 2002;440:392–396.

92. Rub R, Jossiphov J, Avidor Y. Macroscopic hematuria as an initial manifestation of carcinoma of the colon. J Urol 1999;161:922.

93. Smedley KM, Brown C, Turner A. Ectopic ACTH-producing lung cancer presenting with prostatic metastasis. Postgrad Med J 1983;59:371–372.

94. Madersbacher S, Schatzl G, Susani M, et al. Prostatic metastasis of a small cell lung cancer in a young male. Eur Urol 1994;26:267–269.

95. Chibak RW, Haas R Jr, Koenen CT, et al. Metastatic renal cell carcinoma to the prostate gland: presentation as prostatic hypertrophy. J Urol 1980;123:991–992.

Neuroendocrine differentiation in prostate cancer

15

Jiaoti Huang, Jorge L Yao, P Anthony di Sant'Agnese

INTRODUCTION

The two major epithelial components of the benign prostate luminal secretory cells and basal cells, can be identified on routine light microscopy. There is a third minor component of neuroendocrine (NE) cells, which usually can only be identified by immunohistochemical staining for NE markers (chromogranin, synaptophysin, neuron-specific enolase) and NE products (Figure 15.1), or electron microscopy (Figure 15.2). Prostatic NE cells are intraglandular and intraductal cells with hybrid epithelial, neural, and endocrine characteristics. They express and secrete 5-hydroxytryptamine (5HT; serotonin) and numerous peptides/neuropeptides. Prostate NE cells are widely scattered throughout the prostate with only an occasional cell per gland or duct, but are most consistently found in the periurethral ducts and verumontanum. Among the different zones of the human prostate, the transition and peripheral zones have more abundant NE cells than the central zone, suggesting their potential involvement in benign prostatic

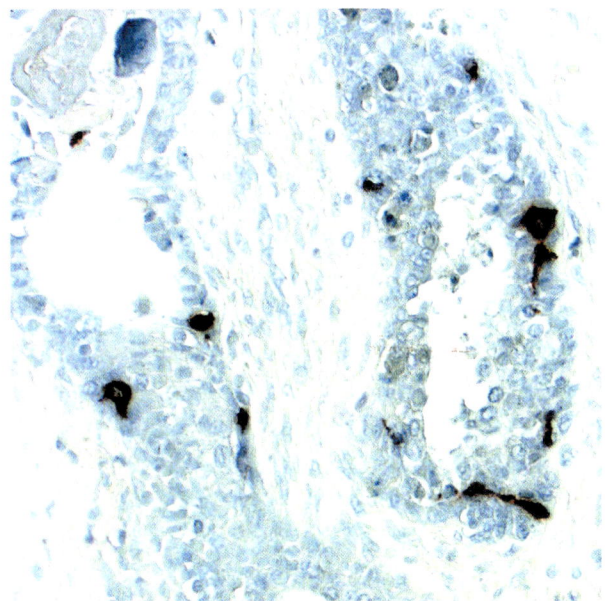

Fig. 15.1
Photomicrograph of neuroendocrine cells, identified by positive staining with chromogranin A, within normal prostate glands. Note dendritic processes. (Chromogranin A, ×100.)

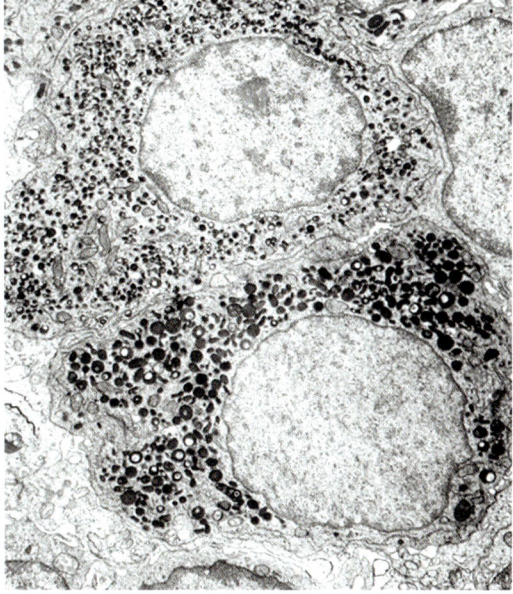

Fig. 15.2
Electronmicrograph of neuroendocrine cells from normal prostate. Note presence of secretory granules with varied appearance. (Transmission electron microscopy.)

hyperplasia and prostate cancer, respectively.[1] A small percentage of human prostates contain numerous NE cells.

The prostate NE cells are categorized into open and closed types. The open-type cells have an apical cytoplasmic process that extends to the lumen and has long specialized surface microvilli, while closed-type cells are surrounded by other epithelial cells and do not have direct contact with the lumen. Both types of NE cells have long, branching, dendrite-like processes, which extend between nearby epithelial cells. Ultrastructural studies have shown a wide range of neurosecretory granule morphologies considered to reflect the large number of known secretory products, including 5HT, histamine, chromogranin A and other members of the chromogranin family of peptides, calcitonin, calcitonin gene-related peptide, katacalcin, neuropeptide Y, vasoactive intestinal peptide (VIP), bombesin/gastrin releasing peptide (GRP), somatostatin, α-human chorionic gonadotropin (αHCG), parathyroid hormone-related protein (PTHrP), thyroid stimulating hormone-like peptide, cholecystokinin, adrenomedullin, and vascular endothelial growth factor (VEGF).[2] Some of these NE cell products have been detected in seminal fluid, raising the possibility that they may be actively secreted into the seminal fluid to regulate sperm function or female genital tract activity. Receptors for some of the NE products have been localized to the prostate epithelium and/or prostate cancer, including 5HT (5HT1a),[3,4] bombesin/GRP (GRPR),[5,6] neurotensin,[7] somatostatin (SSTR1–5),[8,9] cholecystokinin,[10] neuropeptide Y,[11] and calcitonin.[12] Hence, it is proposed that the NE cells may regulate the growth, differentiation, and secretory activity of the prostatic epithelium, possibly through a paracrine mechanism. The activity of the NE cells may be regulated by the neural network, the contents of the glandular lumen or endocrine, paracrine, or autocrine signals.

Neuroendocrine differentiation (NED) occurs in prostate cancer. Some carcinomas are completely differentiated along NE lines, such as carcinoid tumors and small cell carcinomas both of which are rare. Somewhat more common are mixed tumors of conventional adenocarcinoma with a component of small cell carcinoma. A recent report has proposed a category of large cell neuroendocrine carcinoma of the prostate.[13] The most common pattern is focal NED, which refers to the presence of scattered NE cells singly or in small nests in conventional prostatic adenocarcinomas.

TYPES OF NEUROENDOCRINE DIFFERENTIATION

SMALL CELL CARCINOMA AND CARCINOID TUMORS

Small cell carcinoma of the prostate is very rare, particularly in its pure form, and accounts for approximately one to two percent of all carcinomas of the prostate. They are aggressive tumors, which often present at an advanced local stage or as metastatic disease[14] and are occasionally associated with paraneoplastic syndromes.[15] Some small cell carcinomas represent recurrent tumors after hormonal therapy for conventional adenocarcinomas of the prostate.[16] Small cell carcinoma is often present as a component of mixed tumors along with conventional adenocarcinoma. Histologically, small cell carcinomas of the prostate are similar to the more common small cell carcinomas of the lung. They have a solid, sheet-like growth pattern, often with areas of tumor necrosis. Tumor cells are small, with fine chromatin pattern, scant cytoplasm, and nuclear molding. Mitotic figures are frequent and crush artifact can be seen (Figure 15.3).

The solid growth pattern of small cell carcinoma of the prostate is occasionally difficult to distinguish from Gleason grade 5 adenocarcinomas, and, in this situation, immunohistochemical evaluation may be useful. Small cell carcinomas are often positive for NE markers chromogranin A, synaptophysin, and neuron specific enolase (NSE), although one or more of these markers may be negative in any given case. Like small cell carcinomas of the lung, tumor cells often show a dotlike cytokeratin staining pattern and are often positive for TTF1. In contrast to prostatic

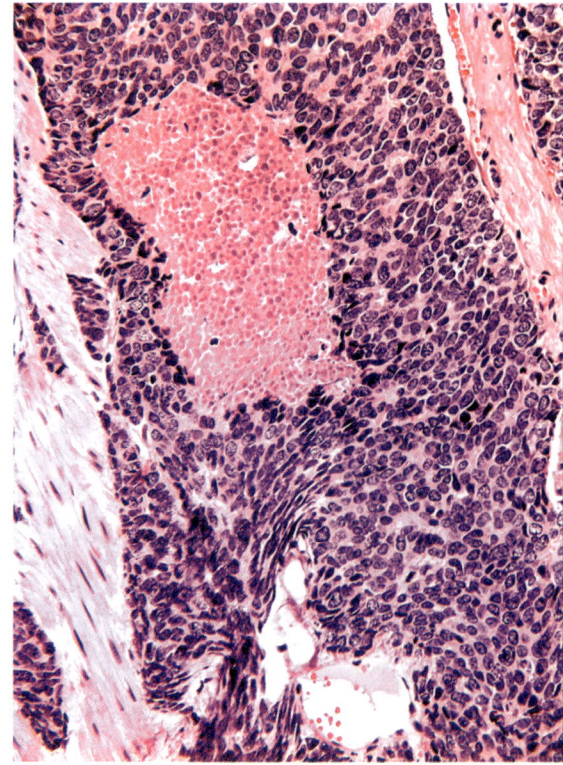

Fig. 15.3

Typical features of small cell carcinoma: sheet of small cells with nuclear molding, necrosis and crush artifact. (Hematoxylin and eosin, ×100.)

adenocarcinoma, tumor cells of small cell carcinoma are usually negative for androgen receptor and PSA, but exceptions exist.[15] It is important to keep in mind that the immunohistochemical profile varies from case to case, and that morphology remains the gold standard for pathological diagnosis.

The prognosis for small cell carcinomas is poor and the disease is usually rapidly fatal.[17] Hormonal therapy is ineffective in treating such tumors, while chemotherapy may have some value.[18]

Carcinoid tumors have also been reported in the prostate but are exceedingly rare. These tumors show complete NE differentiation and have morphologic features similar to carcinoid tumors of the lung or gastrointestinal (GI) tract. Compared with small cell carcinomas, the tumor cells have more abundant cytoplasm, rare mitotic figures, and no tumor necrosis. Similar to small cell carcinomas, carcinoid tumors often exist as a component of mixed tumors also containing conventional adenocarcinoma.[19]

FOCAL NEUROENDOCRINE DIFFERENTIATION IN PROSTATE CANCER

Neuroendocrine differentiation in prostate cancer generally refers to the presence of NE cells focally in an otherwise typical conventional adenocarcinoma. The NE cells are usually morphologically indistinguishable from the non-NE cancer cells and are identified by immunohistochemical study for NE markers (Figure 15.4) or electron microscopy (Figure 15.5). Chromogranin A is the most commonly used marker and is considered to be sensitive and specific. All carcinomas of the prostate have at least some NED when multiple generic NE markers and/or specific

peptides/neuropeptides are used and tissue preparation is controlled.[20] About 5% to 10% of prostatic carcinomas have rather extensive multifocal NED, and it is generally accepted that NE cells in prostate cancer are malignant since they are present in metastatic prostate cancers.[21] Compared with secretory epithelial cells, the malignant (and normal) NE cells usually do not express androgen receptor or prostate-specific antigen (PSA). In tumors (other that those that are entirely neuroendocrine), NE cells have been considered to be terminally differentiated and post-mitotic, as are normal NE cells.[22,23] However, a recent report suggests that the malignant NE cells may possess proliferative activity.[24]

The significance of NED as an independent prognostic factor in androgen-responsive prostate cancer is controversial. Some studies showed independent prognostic significance,[25,26] while many others did not.[27-32] There is more consistent evidence based on immunohistochemical and serologic studies that NE differentiation is a prognostic factor in androgen-independent prostate cancer.[33-35] Neuroendocrine differentiation increases in high-grade/high-stage tumors[27,36] particularly in androgen-deprived[37,38] and androgen-independent tumors,[33,39] although divergent findings have been reported.[40,41] Consistent with these findings, serum chromogranin A levels are increased in patients with advanced, androgen-independent cancers.[41,34,43] Measuring serum chromogranin A levels may be of value in prostate cancer patients with false-negative PSA or percent-free PSA,[44] and can be used to monitor treatment response.[45] In patients with advanced prostate cancer receiving hormonal therapy, an increase in the serum levels of chromogranin A may precede PSA elevation, signal treatment failure,[46] and correlate with bone metastasis.[47] Intermittent administration of complete

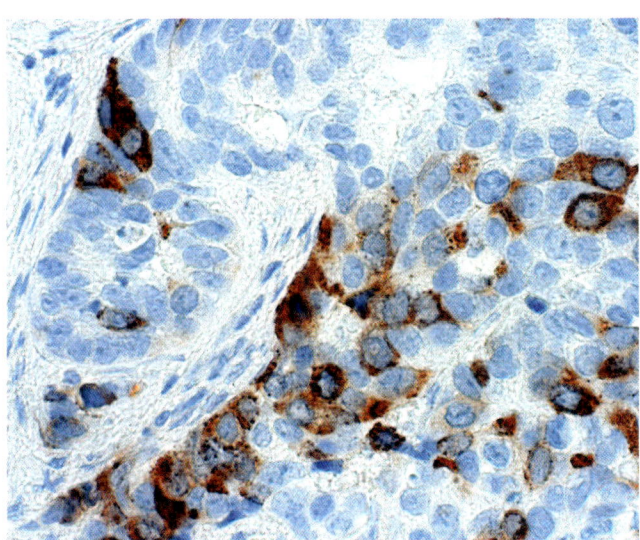

Fig. 15.4
Positive staining for chromogranin A in prostatic adenocarcinoma. (Chromogranin A, ×200.)

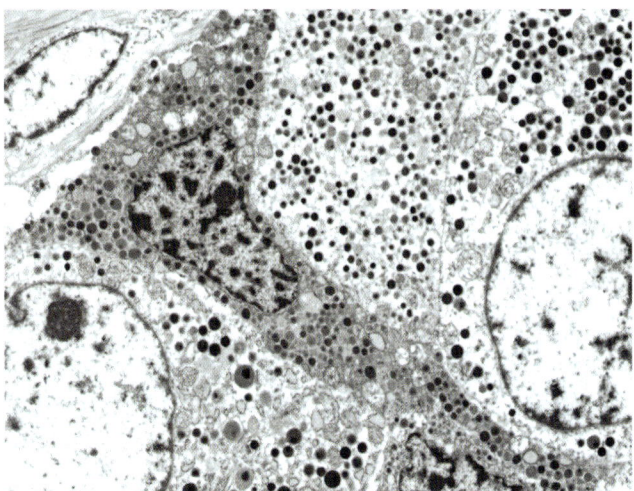

Fig. 15.5
Electronmicrograph of focus of neuroendocrine differentiation from the same prostatic adenocarcinoma shown in Figure 15.4. (Transmission electron microscopy.)

androgen deprivation therapy significantly inhibits the increase in serum chromogranin A levels compared with continuous therapy.[48] The serum levels of NSE may also have prognostic significance.[49,50] Other serum markers such as chromogranin B, secretoneurin, which is a proteolytic product of secretogranin II (chromogranin C), and gastrin-releasing peptide/ProGRP may serve as additional prognostic and/or diagnostic markers.[34,51,52]

MODELS OF NEUROENDOCRINE DIFFERENTIATION IN PROSTATE CANCER

Animal models of prostate cancer recapitulate human diseases and provide more evidence suggesting the importance of NED in prostate cancer. In a transgenic mouse model of prostate cancer (TRAMP), the degree of NED correlates with the degree of tumor differentiation, with the poorly differentiated tumors showing significantly more NED. Castration of TRAMP mice leads to aggressive and highly metastatic cancers in the majority of cases, reflecting androgen-independent growth. Neuroendocrine differentiation was detected in the majority of the primary and metastatic tumors in such animals.[53] Animal models of NE/small cell prostate carcinoma have also been established and should prove useful in studying the molecular mechanisms relating to the NE phenotype.[54,55] In xenograft models of human prostate cancer, NED increases markedly after castration[56,57] and precedes the emergence of increased cancer cell proliferation and progression to hormone-independent cancer.[24] Extensive NED is also seen in a mouse allograft model of androgen-independent prostate cancer.[58]

An androgen-dependent cell line, LNCaP cells, can be induced to show NED in vitro by androgen deprivation or agents that increase intracellular levels of cAMP. The NE phenotype is rapidly lost upon withdrawal of inducing agents.[59] These findings support the transdifferentiation model and suggest that the tumor NE cells may be derived from non-NE tumor cells. The caveat of this model is that NED of LNCaP cells is an "all or none" phenomenon and all cells acquire NE phenotype under appropriate culture conditions, while NED in human cancers is generally focal, making interpretation of the in-vitro findings problematic. Alternatively, some investigators believe that NE cells may be derived from the same stem cell or pluripotent cell that gives rise to luminal secretory cells.[60,61] A population of transiently proliferating/amplifying intermediate cells has been identified, which may be the common precursor for NE cells and other epithelial cells of the prostate.[62]

EXPERIMENTAL EVIDENCE

INDUCTION OF NEUROENDOCRINE DIFFERENTIATION AND NEUROENDOCRINE ACTIVITY

There is biochemical evidence that androgen deprivation may induce NE activity in prostate cancer. Androgen receptor may actively repress the NE phenotype,[63] providing an explanation for the emergence of the NE phenotype when androgen receptor (AR) signaling is inhibited, such as in hormonally-treated cancers or in LNCaP cells cultured in androgen-deprived media. Androgen and androgen receptor can regulate interleukin 6 (IL6) mediated LNCaP cell NED via directly modulating the IL6-PI3-kinase pathway.[64] Neutral endopeptidase 24.11 (NEP) is a cell surface enzyme expressed by prostatic epithelial cells and functions to cleave and inactivate a variety of neuropeptides. Downregulation of NEP after androgen deprivation may lead to increased activity of neuropeptides such as bombesin-like peptides and neurotensin. Interestingly, only androgen-deprived tumor cells respond to the growth-promoting effect of neurotensin.[65] The expression and catalytic activity of NEP are lost in androgen-independent but not androgen-dependent prostate cancer cell lines. In vivo, metastatic cancer cells from patients with androgen-independent prostate cancer commonly show lower levels of NEP than those from patients with androgen-dependent prostate cancer. Growth of androgen-independent cancer cells is inhibited by overexpression of NEP or incubation with recombinant NEP.[66]

The molecular mechanisms involved in NED have been extensively studied. Abrogation of fibroblast growth factor (FGF) signaling by expression of a truncated FGFR2iiib receptor in prostatic epithelium of transgenic mice promotes NED.[67] Interaction of insulin-like growth factor binding protein-related protein 1 (IGFBPrP) with a novel protein, neuroendocrine differentiation factor, results in NED of prostate cancer cells.[68] Neuroendocrine differentiation of LNCaP cells can be induced by agents increasing intracytoplasmic levels of cAMP,[59] IL6, or IL1,[69] or androgen deprivation.[63] Papaverine combined with prostaglandin E$_2$ (PGE2) synergistically induces NE differentiation of LNCaP cells.[70]

IL6-induced NED of LNCaP cells may be qualitatively different from that induced by agents such as epinephrine and forskolin, which cause rapid but reversible NE differentiation of LNCaP cells by increasing intracellular concentrations of cAMP. The process of IL6-induced NE differentiation takes more time and is permanent.[71] Although IL6 shares many biologic activities with other members of the gp130 cytokine family LIF and OSM, only IL6 induces NED of LNCaP cells.[72]

Neuroendocrine differentiation of LNCaP cells is accompanied by overexpression of an alpha-1H (Cav3.2) T-type calcium channel[73] and changes in intracytoplasmic calcium homeostasis.[74] Silibinin, a flavonoid antioxidant, induces G1 arrest and NED of LNCaP cells through increasing Rb level, decreasing Rb phosphorylation and inhibition of key cell cycle regulators.[75]

NEUROENDOCRINE DIFFERENTIATION AND PROLIFERATION

The function of NED in prostate cancer has been extensively studied. Results from a recent study using xenograft mice and in-vitro assays suggest that NE cells may induce ligand-independent androgen-receptor activation, thus promoting growth of LNCaP tumor cells in the absence of androgen.[76] Bombesin acts as a mitogen in prostate cancer and may do so through activation of the transcription factor Elk1 and the immediate early gene *FOS*.[77] In in-vitro assays, neuropeptides stimulate androgen-independent growth.[78] Calcitonin may play a role in the regulation of prostate cell growth.[79] Certain receptors for serotonin may be overexpressed in prostate cancer cells, particularly in high-grade tumors.[4] 5-Hydroxytryptamine receptor (5HT1A) agonists have been demonstrated to inhibit the growth of prostate cancer cells.[3]

NEUROENDOCRINE ACTION ON INVASION AND METASTASIS

Bombesin increases the expression of the proteolytic enzyme urokinase-type plasminogen activator (uPA) and plasminogen activator inhibitor 1 (PAI1) and also stimulates secretion and activation of matrix metalloprotease 9 (MMP9).[80] Neuropeptides stimulate the invasiveness of prostate cancer cell lines[81] and upregulate the activity of the type IV collagenase MMPs.[82] Matrix metalloproteases are associated with a variety of biologic activities, such as tumor invasion, metastasis, and angiogenesis. MT1-MMP protein and mRNA are expressed in androgen-independent PC-3, DU-145 and TSU-pr1 cells but not in the androgen-dependent LNCaP cells. Gastrin releasing peptide induces the expression of MT1-MMP protein in DU-145 cells and also increases Matrigel invasion by these cells.[83] High-grade tumors are more likely to express MMP9 and bombesin than low-grade tumors.[84] Calcitonin affects migration of certain prostate cancer cell lines and may play a role in metastases, especially to the bone.[79]

NEUROENDOCRINE ACTION ON APOPTOSIS RESISTANCE

Neuroendocrine differentiation may affect the apoptosis resistance of prostate cancer. The tissue levels of NSE correlate with BCL2, a major anti-apoptotic factor, and the BCL2-containing cancer cells are generally in close proximity to the NE cells,[85] suggesting that NE cells may confer apoptosis resistance to the neighboring cancer cells. Bombesin and calcitonin prevent apoptosis of prostate cancer cells in-vitro.[86] Neuroendocrine cells do not appear to undergo apoptosis[23,87] even though they are negative for BCL2.[88] They do express survivin, another anti-apoptotic factor,[89] providing a molecular basis for the hypothesis that NE cells may endure stressful conditions and escape from apoptosis during cancer therapy.

NEUROENDOCRINE ACTION ON ANGIOGENESIS

Neuroendocrine differentiation may promote neovascularization of prostate cancer. Prostatic NE cells are a major producer of VEGF.[90] Vasoactive intestinal peptide, which is produced by autonomic nerves and NE cancer cells of human prostate, stimulates NED and VEGF production in LNCaP cells.[91] In benign prostatic tissue, the level of expression of VEGF is low. All prostate cancers stain positively for VEGF, and staining intensity correlates with Gleason grade. Complete androgen block for 3 months before surgery decreases the level of VEGF and vascularization, except in the cell areas with NE features.[92] In radical prostatectomy specimens, there is a correlation between NE differentiation and neovascularization and both correlate with tumor grade and tumor stage. The number of NE cells was found to be the only predictor of neovascularization.[93] Another study reported similar results and, in addition, found expression of VEGF to be significantly correlated with increased microvessel density, high tumor stage, poor differentiation and shorter disease-free survival.[94] Bombesin stimulates expression of proangiogenic factors VEGF and IL8 in PC-3 cells, possibly through the NF-kappa B-dependent pathway.[95]

NEUROENDOCRINE DIFFERENTIATION AND FUTURE THERAPEUTIC IMPLICATIONS

Neuroendocrine differentiation is considered to be a feature of the androgen-independent state and promote progression of androgen-independent prostate cancer. Intervention therapy directed at blocking this NE differentiation may have beneficial effects in androgen-independent tumors. All-trans retinoic acid (ATRA) has been shown to slow prostate tumor cell proliferation, induce apoptosis and block the emergence of the neuroendocrine phenotype in TRAMP mice and TRAMP-derived C2N prostate tumor cells.[96]

Nonetheless, it is also possible that complete differentiation of cancer cells along the NE pathway may actually inhibit proliferation, providing a novel strategy for developing anti-prostate cancer therapy. The use of cell-permeant cAMP analogs to induce terminal differentiation in prostate cancer has been proposed as a therapeutic approach.[97] In LNCaP cells, different concentrations of IL6 have different effects on cell proliferation and NED. Long-term exposure of LNCaP cells to low concentrations of IL6 (5 ng/mL) results in the emergence of a LNCaP variant with more aggressive growth properties in vitro and in vivo.[98,99] LNCaP cells cultured in high concentrations of IL6 (100 ng/mL) for 2 weeks leads to permanent NED and significant loss of the proliferative potential.[71]

SUMMARY AND CONCLUSIONS

Neuroendocrine cells constitute a third type of prostatic epithelial cells (along with basal and secretory cells) and may play a role in the normal development and function of benign prostatic tissue. Neuroendocrine cells are also present in prostate cancers and their number and activity increase in high-grade and androgen-deprived cancers, particularly in those that are androgen independent. The origin of NE cells in prostate cancer is unclear, and they may be derived from transformed stem cells, from non-NE cancer cells through transdifferentiation, or from both. In-vitro and in-vivo evidence suggests that the products of the NE cells may contribute to the emergence of androgen-independent growth by acting on the receptors present in non-NE cancer cells in a paracrine fashion. Identification of the key molecules or pathways involved in NE differentiation or the crucial NE cell effectors that promote androgen-independent growth may provide novel targets that can be exploited to prevent the progression of prostate cancer to the hormone refractory state or androgen-independent growth.

REFERENCES

1. Santamaria L, Martin R, Martin JJ, et al. Stereologic estimation of the number of neuroendocrine cells in normal human prostate detected by immunohistochemistry. Appl Immunohistochem Mol Morphol 2002;10:275–281.

2. Huang J, di Sant'Agnese PA. Neuroendocrine differentiation in prostate cancer: an overview. In: Lamberts SWJ, Dogliotti L (eds): Advances in oncology: the expanding role of octreotide. Bristol, UK: BioScientifica Ltd, 2002, 243–262.

3. Abdul M, Anezinis PE, Logothetis CJ, et al. Growth inhibition of human prostatic carcinoma cell lines by serotonin antagonists. Anticancer Res 1994;14:1215–1220.

4. Dizeyi N, Bjartell A, Nilsson E, et al. Expression of serotonin receptors and role of serotonin in human prostate cancer tissue and cell lines. Prostate 2004;59:328–336.

5. Aprikian AG, Han K, Chevalier S, et al. Bombesin specifically induces intracellular calcium mobilization via gastrin-releasing peptide receptors in human prostate cancer cells. J Mol Endocrinol 1996;16:297–306.

6. Sun B, Halmos G, Schally AV, et al. Presence of receptors for bombesin/gastrin-releasing peptide and mRNA for three receptor subtypes in human prostate cancers. Prostate 2000;42:295–303.

7. Seethalakshmi L, Mitra SP, Dobner PR, et al. Neurotensin receptor expression in prostate cancer cell line and growth effect of NT at physiological concentrations. Prostate 1997;31:183–192.

8. Berruti A, Dogliotti L, Mosca A, et al. Effects of the somatostatin analog lanreotide on the circulating levels of chromogranin-A, prostate-specific antigen, and insulin-like growth factor-1 in advanced prostate cancer patients. Prostate 2001;47:205–211.

9. Dizeyi N, Konrad L, Bjartell A, et al. Localization and mRNA expression of somatostatin receptor subtypes in human prostatic tissue and prostate cancer cell lines. Urol Oncol 2002;7:91–98.

10. Petit T, Davidson KK, Lawrence RA, et al. Neuropeptide receptor status in human tumor cell lines. Anticancer Drugs 2001;12:133–136.

11. Magni P, Motta M. Expression of neuropeptide Y receptors in human prostate cancer cells. Ann Oncol 2001;12(Suppl 2):S27–29.

12. Wu G, Burzon DT, di Sant'Agnese PA, et al. Calcitonin receptor mRNA expression in the human prostate. Urology 1996;47:376–381.

13. Evans AL, Humphrey PA, Srigley JR. Large cell neuroendocrine carcinoma of the prostate. Mod Pathol 2004;17(Suppl 1):150A [abstract].

14. Erasmus CE, Verhagen WI, Wauters CA, et al. Brain metastasis from prostate small cell carcinoma: not to be neglected. Can J Neurol Sci 2002;29:375–377.

15. Kawai S, Hiroshima K, Tsukamoto Y, et al. Small cell carcinoma of the prostate expressing prostate-specific antigen and showing syndrome of inappropriate secretion of antidiuretic hormone: an autopsy case report. Pathol Int 2003;53:892–896.

16. Tanaka M, Suzuki Y, Takaoka K, et al. Progression of prostate cancer to neuroendocrine cell tumor. Int J Urol 2001;8:431–436.

17. Papandreou CN, Daliani DD, Thall PF, et al. Results of a phase II study with doxorubicin, etoposide, and cisplatin in patients with fully characterized small-cell carcinoma of the prostate. J Clin Oncol 2002;20:3072–3080.

18. Helpap B. Morphology and therapeutic strategies for neuroendocrine tumors of the genitourinary tract. Cancer 2002;95:1415–1420.

19. Ghannoum JE, DeLellis RA, Shin SJ. Primary carcinoid tumor of the prostate with concurrent adenocarcinoma: a case report. Int J Surg Pathol 2004;12:167–170.

20. Abrahamsson PA, Wadstrom LB, Alumets J, et al. Peptide-hormone- and serotonin-immunoreactive tumour cells in carcinoma of the prostate. Pathol Res Pract 1987;182:298–307.

21. Roudier MP, True LD, Higano CS, et al. Phenotypic heterogeneity of end-stage prostate carcinoma metastatic to bone. Hum Pathol 2003;34:646–653.

22. Bonkhoff H, Stein U, Remberger K. Endocrine-paracrine cell types in the prostate and prostatic adenocarcinoma are postmitotic cells. Hum Pathol 1995;26:167–170.

23. Bonkhoff H, Fixemer T, Hunsicker I, et al. Simultaneous detection of DNA fragmentation (apoptosis), cell proliferation (MIB-1), and phenotype markers in routinely processed tissue sections. Virchows Arch 1999;434:71–73.

24. Huss WJ, Gregory CW, Smith GJ. Neuroendocrine cell differentiation in the CWR22 human prostate cancer xenograft: association with tumor cell proliferation prior to recurrence. Prostate 2004;60:91–97.

25. Weinstein MH, Partin AW, Veltri RW, et al. Neuroendocrine differentiation in prostate cancer: enhanced prediction of progression after radical prostatectomy. Hum Pathol 1996;27:683–687.

26. Bollito E, Berruti A, Bellina M, et al. Relationship between neuroendocrine features and prognostic parameters in human prostate adenocarcinoma. Ann Oncol 2001;12(Suppl 2):S159–164.

27. Bohrer MH, Schmoll J. Immunohistochemical and morphometric studies on neuroendocrine differentiation of prostate carcinomas. Verh Dtsch Ges Pathol 1993;77:107–110.

28. Aprikian AG, Cordon-Cardo C, Fair WR, et al. Neuroendocrine differentiation in metastatic prostatic adenocarcinoma. J Urol 1994;151:914–919.

29. Noordzij MA, van der Kwast TH, et al. The prognostic influence of neuroendocrine cells in prostate cancer: results of a long-term follow-up study with patients treated by radical prostatectomy. Int J Cancer 1995;62:252–258.

30. Abrahamsson PA, Cockett AT, di Sant'Agnese PA. Prognostic significance of neuroendocrine differentiation in clinically localized prostatic carcinoma. Prostate Suppl 1998;8:37–42.

31. Segawa N, Mori I, Utsunomiya H, et al. Prognostic significance of neuroendocrine differentiation, proliferation activity and androgen receptor expression in prostate cancer. Pathol Int 2001;51:452–459.

32. Steineck G, Reuter V, Kelly WK, et al. Cytotoxic treatment of aggressive prostate tumors with or without neuroendocrine elements. Acta Oncol 2002;41:668–674.

33. Jiborn T, Bjartell A, Abrahamsson PA. Neuroendocrine differentiation in prostatic carcinoma during hormonal treatment. Urology 1998;51:585–589.

34. Ischia R, Hobisch A, Bauer R, et al. Elevated levels of serum secretoneurin in patients with therapy resistant carcinoma of the prostate. J Urol 2000;163:1161–1164.

35. Berruti A, Dogliotti L, Mosca A, et al. Circulating neuroendocrine markers in patients with prostate carcinoma. Cancer 2000;88:2590–2597.

36. Abrahamsson PA, Falkmer S, Falt K, Grimelius L. The course of neuroendocrine differentiation in prostatic carcinomas. An immunohistochemical study testing chromogranin A as an "endocrine marker." Pathol Res Pract 1989;185:373–380.

37. Ahlgren G, Pedersen K, Lundberg S, et al. Regressive changes and neuroendocrine differentiation in prostate cancer after neoadjuvant hormonal treatment. Prostate 2000;42:274–279.

38. Ismail AH, Altaweel W, Chevalier S, et al. Expression of vascular endothelial growth factor-A in human lymph node metastases of prostate cancer. Can J Urol 2004;11:2146–2150.

39. Hirano D, Okada Y, Minei S, et al. Neuroendocrine differentiation in hormone refractory prostate cancer following androgen deprivation therapy. Eur Urol 2004;45:586–592.

40. Kollermann J, Helpap B. Neuroendocrine differentiation and short-term neoadjuvant hormonal treatment of prostatic carcinoma with special regard to tumor regression. Eur Urol 2001;40:313–317.

41. Li GZ, Zeng L, Zhang J, et al. Impact of short-term neoadjuvant hormonal treatment on neuroendocrine differentiation in prostate carcinoma. Zhonghua Zhong Liu Za Zhi 2003;25:493–495.

42. Deftos LJ, Nakada S, Burton DW, et al. Immunoassay and immunohistology studies of chromogranin A as a neuroendocrine marker in patients with carcinoma of the prostate. Urology 1996;48:58–62.

43. Isshiki S, Akakura K, Komiya A, et al. Chromogranin A concentration as a serum marker to predict prognosis after endocrine therapy for prostate cancer. J Urol 2002;167:512–515.

44. Ahel MZ, Kovacic K, Tarle M. Cross-correlation of serum chromogranin A, %-F-PSA and bone scans in prostate cancer diagnosis. Anticancer Res 2001;21:1363–1366.

45. Zaky Ahel M, Kovacic K, Kraljic I, et al. Oral estramustine therapy in serum chromogranin A-positive stage D3 prostate cancer patients. Anticancer Res 2001;21:1475–1479.

46. Chuang CK, Wu TL, Tsao KC, et al. Elevated serum chromogranin A precedes prostate-specific antigen elevation and predicts failure of androgen deprivation therapy in patients with advanced prostate cancer. J Formos Med Assoc 2003;102:480–485.

47. Tarle M, Ahel MZ, Kovacic K. Acquired neuroendocrine-positivity during maximal androgen blockade in prostate cancer patients. Anticancer Res 2002;22:2525–2529.

48. Sciarra A, Monti S, Gentile V, et al. Variation in chromogranin A serum levels during intermittent versus continuous androgen deprivation therapy for prostate adenocarcinoma. Prostate 2003;55:168–179.

49. Kamiya N, Akakura K, Suzuki H, et al. Pretreatment serum level of neuron specific enolase (NSE) as a prognostic factor in metastatic prostate cancer patients treated with endocrine therapy. Eur Urol 2003;44:309–314.

50. Hvamstad T, Jordal A, Hekmat N, et al. Neuroendocrine serum tumour markers in hormone-resistant prostate cancer. Eur Urol 2003;44:215–221.

51. Angelsen A, Syversen U, Stridsberg M, et al. Use of neuroendocrine serum markers in the follow-up of patients with cancer of the prostate. Prostate 1997;31:110–7.

52. Yashi M, Nukui A, Kurokawa S, et al. Elevated serum progastrin-releasing peptide (31-98) level is a predictor of short response duration after hormonal therapy in metastatic prostate cancer. Prostate 2003;56:305–312.

53. Kaplan-Lefko PJ, Chen TM, Ittmann MM, et al. Pathobiology of autochthonous prostate cancer in a pre-clinical transgenic mouse model. Prostate 2003;55:219–237.

54. Garabedian EM, Humphrey PA, Gordon JI. A transgenic mouse model of metastatic prostate cancer originating from neuroendocrine cells (prostatic intraepithelial neoplasia). Proc Natl Acad Sci 1998;95:15382–15387.

55. Hu Y, Ippolito JE, Garabedian EM, et al. Molecular characterization of a metastatic neuroendocrine cell cancer arising in the prostates of transgenic mice. J Biol Chem 2002;277:44462–44474

56. Burchardt T, Burchardt M, Chen MW, et al. Transdifferentiation of prostate cancer cells to a neuroendocrine cell phenotype in vitro and in vivo. J Urol 1999;162:1800–1805.

57. Jongsma J, Oomen MH, Noordzij MA, et al. Different profiles of neuroendocrine cell differentiation evolve in the PC-310 human prostate cancer model during long-term androgen deprivation. Prostate 2002;50:203–215.

58. Masumori N, Tsuchiya K, Tu WH, et al. An allograft model of androgen independent prostatic neuroendocrine carcinoma derived from a large probasin promoter-T antigen transgenic mouse line. J Urol 2004;171:439–442.

59. Cox ME, Deeble PD, Lakhani S, et al. Acquisition of neuroendocrine characteristics by prostate tumor cells is reversible: implications for prostate cancer progression. Cancer Res 1999;59:3821–3830.

60. Bonkhoff H, Remberger K. et al. Differentiation pathways and histogenetic aspects of normal and abnormal prostatic growth: a stem cell model. Prostate 1996;28:98–106.

61. Rumpold H, Heinrich E, Untergasser G, et al. Neuroendocrine differentiation of human prostatic primary epithelial cells in vitro. Prostate 2002;53:101–108.

62. Schalken JA, van Leenders G. Cellular and molecular biology of the prostate: stem cell biology. Urology 2003;62:11–20.

63. Wright ME, Tsai MJ, Aebersold R. Androgen receptor represses the neuroendocrine transdifferentiation process in prostate cancer cells. Mol Endocrinol 2003;17:1726–1737.

64. Xie S, Lin HK, Ni J, et al. Regulation of interleukin-6-mediated PI3K activation and neuroendocrine differentiation by androgen signaling in prostate cancer LNCaP cells. Prostate 2004;60:61–67.

65. Sehgal I, Powers S, Huntley B, et al. Neurotensin is an autocrine trophic factor stimulated by androgen withdrawal in human prostate cancer. Proc Natl Acad Sci USA 1994;91:4673–4677.

66. Papandreou CN, Usmani B, Geng Y, et al. Neutral endopeptidase 24.11 loss in metastatic human prostate cancer contributes to androgen-independent progression. Nat Med 1998;4:50–57.

67. Foster BA, Evangelou A, Gingrich JR, et al. Enforced expression of FGF-7 promotes epithelial hyperplasia whereas a dominant negative FGFR2iiib promotes the emergence of neuroendocrine phenotype in prostate glands of transgenic mice. Differentiation 2002;70:624–632.

68. Wilson EM, Oh Y, Hwa V, et al. Interaction of IGF-binding protein-related protein 1 with a novel protein, neuroendocrine differentiation factor, results in neuroendocrine differentiation of prostate cancer cells. J Clin Endocrinol Metab 2001;86:4504–4511.

69. Albrecht M, Doroszewicz J, Gillen S, et al. Proliferation of prostate cancer cells and activity of neutral endopeptidase is regulated by bombesin and IL-1beta with IL-1beta acting as a modulator of cellular differentiation. Prostate 2004;58:82–94.

70. Shimizu T, Ohta Y, Ozawa H, et al. Papaverine combined with prostaglandin E2 synergistically induces neuron-like morphological changes and decrease of malignancy in human prostatic cancer LNCaP cells. Anticancer Res 2000;20:761–767.

71. Wang Q, Horiatis D, Pinski J. Interleukin-6 inhibits the growth of prostate cancer xenografts in mice by the process of neuroendocrine differentiation. Int J Cancer 2004;111:508–513.

72. Palmer J, Hertzog PJ, Hammacher A. Differential expression and effects of gp130 cytokines and receptors in prostate cancer cells. Int J Biochem Cell Biol 2004;36:2258–2269.

73. Mariot P, Vanoverberghe K, Lalevee N, et al. Overexpression of an alpha 1H (Cav3.2) T-type calcium channel during neuroendocrine

differentiation of human prostate cancer cells. J Biol Chem 2002;277:10824–10833.

74. Vanoverberghe K, Vanden Abeele F, Mariot P, et al. Ca^{2+} homeostasis and apoptotic resistance of neuroendocrine-differentiated prostate cancer cells. Cell Death Differ 2004;11:321–330.

75. Tyagi A, Agarwal C, Agarwal R. Inhibition of retinoblastoma protein (Rb) phosphorylation at serine sites and an increase in Rb-E2F complex formation by silibinin in androgen-dependent human prostate carcinoma LNCaP cells: role in prostate cancer prevention. Mol Cancer Ther 2002;1:525–532.

76. Jin RJ, Wang Y, Masumori N, et al. NE-10 neuroendocrine cancer promotes the LNCaP xenograft growth in castrated mice. Cancer Res 2004;64:5489–5495.

77. Xiao D, Qu X, Weber HC. GRP receptor-mediated immediate early gene expression and transcription factor Elk-1 activation in prostate cancer cells. Regul Pept 2002;109:141–148.

78. Jongsma J, Oomen MH, Noordzij MA, et al. Androgen-independent growth is induced by neuropeptides in human prostate cancer cell lines. Prostate 2000;42:34–44.

79. Ritchie CK, Thomas KG, Andrews LR, et al. Effects of the calciotrophic peptides calcitonin and parathyroid hormone on prostate cancer growth and chemotaxis. Prostate 1997;30:183–187.

80. Festuccia C, Guerra F, D'Ascenzo S, et al. In vitro regulation of pericellular proteolysis in prostatic tumor cells treated with bombesin. Int J Cancer 1998;75:418–431.

81. Hoosein NM, Logothetis CJ, Chung LW. Differential effects of peptide hormones bombesin, vasoactive intestinal polypeptide and somatostatin analog RC-160 on the invasive capacity of human prostatic carcinoma cells. J Urol 1993;149:1209–1213.

82. Sehgal I, Thompson TC. Neuropeptides induce Mr 92,000 type IV collagenase (matrix metalloprotease-9) activity in human prostate cancer cell lines. Cancer Res 1998;58:4288–4291.

83. Nagakawa O, Furuya Y, Fujiuchi Y, et al. Serum pro-gastrin-releasing peptide (31-98) in benign prostatic hyperplasia and prostatic carcinoma. Urology 2002;60:527–530.

84. Ishimaru H, Kageyama Y, Hayashi T, et al. Expression of matrix metalloproteinase-9 and bombesin/gastrin-releasing peptide in human prostate cancers and their lymph node metastases. Acta Oncol. 2002;41:289–296.

85. Segal NH, Cohen RJ, Haffejee Z, et al. BCL-2 proto-oncogene expression in prostate cancer and its relationship to the prostatic neuroendocrine cell. Arch Pathol Lab Med 1994;118:616–618.

86. Salido M, Vilches J, Lopez A. Neuropeptides bombesin and calcitonin induce resistance to etoposide induced apoptosis in prostate cancer cell lines. Histol Histopathol 2000;15:729–738.

87. Fixemer T, Remberger K, Bonkhoff H. Apoptosis resistance of neuroendocrine phenotypes in prostatic adenocarcinoma. Prostate 2002;53:118–123.

88. Xue Y, Verhofstad A, Lange W, et al. Prostatic neuroendocrine cells have a unique keratin expression pattern and do not express Bcl-2: cell kinetic features of neuroendocrine cells in the human prostate. Am J Pathol 1997;151:1759–1765.

89. Xing N, Qian J, Bostwick D, et al. Neuroendocrine cells in human prostate over-express the anti-apoptosis protein survivin. Prostate 2001;48:7–15.

90. Chevalier S, Defoy I, Lacoste J, et al. Vascular endothelial growth factor and signaling in the prostate: more than angiogenesis. Mol Cell Endocrinol 2002;189:169–179.

91. Collado B, Gutierrez-Canas I, Rodriguez-Henche N, et al. Vasoactive intestinal peptide increases vascular endothelial growth factor expression and neuroendocrine differentiation in human prostate cancer LNCaP cells. Regul Pept 2004;119:69–75.

92. Mazzucchelli R, Montironi R, Santinelli A, et al. Vascular endothelial growth factor expression and capillary architecture in high-grade PIN and prostate cancer in untreated and androgen-ablated patients. Prostate 2000;45:72–79.

93. Grobholz R, Boher MH, Siegsmund M, et al. Correlation between neovascularization and neuroendocrine differentiation in prostatic carcinoma. Pathol Res Pract 2000;196:277–284.

94. Borre M, Nerstrom B, Overgaard J. Association between immunohistochemical expression of vascular endothelial growth factor (VEGF), VEGF-expressing neuroendocrine-differentiated tumor cells, and outcome in prostate cancer patients subjected to watchful waiting. Clin Cancer Res 2000;6:1882–1890.

95. Levine L, Lucci JA 3rd, Pazdrak B, et al. Bombesin stimulates nuclear factor kappa B activation and expression of proangiogenic factors in prostate cancer cells. Cancer Res 2003;63:3495–3502.

96. Huss WJ, Lai L, Barrios RJ, et al. Retinoic acid slows progression and promotes apoptosis of spontaneous prostate cancer. Prostate 2004;61:142–152.

97. Bang YJ, Pirnia F, Fang WG, et al. Terminal neuroendocrine differentiation of human prostate carcinoma cells in response to increased intracellular cyclic AMP. Proc Natl Acad Sci USA 1994;91:5330–5334.

98. Hobisch A, Ramoner R, Fuchs D, et al. Prostate cancer cells (LNCaP) generated after long-term interleukin 6 (IL-6) treatment express IL-6 and acquire an IL-6 partially resistant phenotype. Clin Cancer Res 2001;7:2941–2948.

99. Steiner H, Godoy-Tundidor S, Rogatsch H, et al. Accelerated in vivo growth of prostate tumors that up-regulate interleukin-6 is associated with reduced retinoblastoma protein expression and activation of the mitogen-activated protein kinase pathway. Am J Pathol 2003;162:655–663.

New concepts in the molecular pathology of prostate cancer

16

Mark A Rubin, Arul M Chinnaiyan, Massimo Loda

THE ROLE OF MOLECULAR PATHOLOGY IN PREDICTING THE RISK OF ADVERSE OUTCOME

The prevalence of pathologic prostate cancer (PCA) is extremely high and increases with age. One in six men will be diagnosed with PCA during their lifetime. Prostate cancer is a leading cause of male cancer-related death, second only to lung cancer[1,2] and the American Cancer Society estimates that 230,110 American men will be diagnosed with PCA and 29,900 will die in 2004 representing 10% of all cancer deaths in men in the United States. Multiple factors contribute to the high incidence and prevalence of PCA. Risk factors include age, family history, and race. Environmental exposures also play a role. A single molecular test, the prostate-specific antigen (PSA) screening test, has impacted the detection of PCA and is directly responsible for a dramatic stage shift in many industrial countries. At time of initial diagnosis, 82% of PCA cases are clinically localized. A major limitation of the serum PSA test is a lack of PCA sensitivity and specificity, especially in the intermediate range of PSA detection (4–10 ng/ml). Elevated serum PSA levels can be detected in patients with nonmalignant conditions such as benign prostatic hyperplasia (BPH) or prostatitis. Therefore, PSA levels are not associated with tumor burden, and there is increasing evidence that PSA screening has led to the identification of insignificant prostate cancers.[3–5]

Thus, the clinical dilemma in the field of PCA today is that we are over-treating most men diagnosed with localized disease in the post-PSA screening era, yet inadequately treating those men diagnosed with metastatic PCA. The best example of this phenomenon comes from the Swedish studies on the natural history of PCA.[6–8] As demonstrated most recently by the randomized Scandinavian trial evaluating the benefit of prostatectomy over watchful waiting, surgery significantly decreased the incidence of metastatic PCA.[6] However, the study also suggests that 17 men need to be treated to benefit one man. With the population of males 65 years and older expected to increase from 14 million in year 2000 to 31 million by 2030,[9] it will be increasingly important to identify which men will die *with* PCA from those requiring intervention. Given the prevalence of the disease, the ease of diagnosis, the aging of the population, and the morbidity of treatment, the ability to distinguish aggressive from indolent forms of cancer is, therefore, critical.

Current methods of stratifying tumors to predict outcome are based on clinical factors. These factors include Gleason grade (a measure of the extent of glandular differentiation), PSA level, clinical stage (the extent of disease burden and spread), and, in some cases, other factors such as the percentage of biopsies that contain tumor cells. Nomograms and multifactorial staging schemes have been developed that aid in the prediction of freedom from biochemical relapse (PSA elevation) after local (surgical) and potentially curative therapy. While these clinical formulas are helpful, they are inaccurate in a large proportion of patients. Patients with high clinical risk factors are indeed at high risk of recurrence. The majority of patients, however, fall into low or intermediate clinical risk categories, yet these account for the majority of the recurrences observed. Most importantly, existing clinical predictors are not linked to the most meaningful clinical endpoint—PCA-specific death. That is, it is becoming increasingly clear that biochemical recurrence is *not* synonymous with death from disease. In many patients, PSA elevation is now recognized to be attributable to recurrent local disease (as opposed to metastasis) that would be amenable to further local therapy or perhaps requires no further therapy at all.

In order to improve on these clinical formulas and help determine responsiveness of prostate cancer to emerging medical therapies, understanding the molecular basis of prostate cancer is critical. The molecular oncology paradigm is based on the belief that the behavior of a tumor is ultimately dependent on certain key molecular characteristics. Therefore, the goal of molecular staging of prostate cancer is to identify genes involved in pathways relevant to prostate cancer pathogenesis and to utilize them as prognostic and/or predictive markers in both serum- and tissue-based assays. This chapter will cover some of the critical aspects of molecular staging of prostate cancer with an emphasis on some of the more recent emerging concepts.

GENETICS OF HEREDITARY PROSTATE CANCER

Currently, the evidence for a strong genetic component of prostate cancer is compelling. Observations made in the 1950s by Morganti et al suggested a strong familial predisposition for prostate cancer.[10] Strengthening the genetic evidence is a high frequency for prostate cancer in monozygotic compared with dizygotic twins in a study of twins from Sweden, Denmark, and Finland.[11] However, unlike the successful mapping and cloning of BRCA1 and BRCA2, which explain a large proportion of hereditary breast cancers, genes conferring susceptibility to prostate cancer have been more elusive. Work over the past decade using genome-wide scans in prostate cancer families has identified high-risk alleles, displaying either an autosomal dominant or X-linked mode of inheritance from at least seven candidate genetic loci (Table 16.1). From these loci, three candidate genes have emerged, HPC2/ELAC2 on 17p,[12,13] RNASEL on

1q25,[14] and MSR1 on 8p22-23.[15] While an initial attempt to confirm these findings was promising,[16] more recent reports find little evidence that ELAC2 is linked to hereditary or sporadic prostate cancer.[12,17–19] RNASEL (encoding ribonuclease L) is a ubiquitously expressed latent endoribonuclease involved in the mediation of the antiviral and proapoptotic activities of the interferon-inducible 2-5A system.[20,21] Work from several groups demonstrates that RNASEL mutations lead to decreased enzymatic activity rather than gene inactivation.[14,22–24] While approximately 13% of prostate cancer cases in the population have been reported to carry a mutation in this gene,[14] another study only found mutations in hereditary cases of prostate cancer.[25] Mutations in RNASEL predispose men to an increased incidence of prostate cancer, which in some cases appears to behave more aggressively and/or is diagnosed at an earlier age compared with non-RNASEL-linked cases.[26]

The other putative hereditary gene, MSR1, is a macrophage-specific receptor, which can bind polyanionic ligands including gram-negative and gram-positive bacteria. MSR1-knockout mice also have a reduced capacity to eradicate pathogens but no particular prostatic phenotype.[15]

It is clear, however, that these three genes do not account for the majority of hereditary prostate cancer cases. The discovery of highly penetrant prostate cancer genes has been particularly difficult for at least two main reasons. First, due to the advanced age of onset (median 60 years), identification of more than two generations to perform molecular studies on is difficult. Second, given the high frequency of prostate cancer, it is likely that cases considered to be hereditary during segregation studies actually represent phenocopies. Currently, it is not possible to distinguish sporadic (phenocopies) from hereditary cases in families with high rates of prostate cancer. In addition, hereditary prostate cancer does not occur in any of the known cancer syndromes and does not have any clinical (other than a somewhat early age of onset at times) or pathologic characteristics to allow researchers to distinguish it from sporadic cases.[27]

Table 16.1 Prostate cancer susceptibility loci identified by linkage analysis				
Susceptibility loci	**Locus**	**Mode**	**Putative gene**	**Reference**
HPC1	1q24-25	AD	RNASEL[14]	Smith et al.[206]
PCAP	1q42.2-43	AD	?	Berthon et al.[207]
CAPB	1p36	AD	?	Gibbs et al.[208]
HPCX	Xq27-28	X-linked/AR	?	Xu et al.[209]
HPC20	20q13	AD	?	Berry et al.[210]
HPC2	17p	AD	HPC2/ELAC2	Tavtigian et al.[13]
	8p22-23	AD	MSR1	Xu et al[15]

Mode, suggested mode of inheritance; AD, autosomal dominant; AR, autosomal recessive.

EARLY MOLECULAR ALTERATIONS IN PROSTATE CANCER PROGRESSION

Currently there are two candidate precursor lesions for prostate cancer: prostate intraepithelial neoplasia (PIN) and proliferative inflammatory atrophy (PIA). Much of the evidence that supports PIN as a potential precursor lesion is also true for PIA. It is also not clear whether these lesions can be seen along a spectrum or represent separate pathways. As PIN is covered elsewhere in more depth (see Chapter 12), we introduce the concept of PIA.

PROSTATE INTRAEPITHELIAL NEOPLASIA

Most authorities agree that PIN is a precursor lesion to prostatic adenocarcinoma. These lesions show morphologic features and molecular alterations characteristic of malignancy, including genetic instability, but occur within preexisting epithelia, and are confined within the basement membrane.[28-33]

PROLIFERATIVE INFLAMMATORY ATROPHY

Pathologists have long recognized focal areas of epithelial atrophy in the prostate.[34-36] Distinct from the diffuse atrophy seen after androgen deprivation, these focal areas of atrophy most often appear in the periphery of the prostate, where prostate cancers typically arise.[35,37-41] Epithelial atrophy may be associated with acute or chronic inflammation, contain proliferative epithelial cells, and may show morphologic transitions in continuity with high-grade PIN.[40,42] A direct transition from these atrophic lesion to carcinoma, with little or no recognizable PIN component, can also be observed.[36,43,44] Focal atrophy of the prostate exists as a spectrum of morphologies and can be quite extensive. Since these lesions have also been shown to have a high proliferation index,[37,40,41,45] they have been termed proliferative inflammatory atrophy lesions.[40] In support of PIA as a prostate cancer precursor, chromosome 8 gain, detected by fluorescence in situ hybridization (FISH) with a chromosome 8 centromere probe, was found in human PIA, PIN, and prostate cancer.[45,46] Others have recently documented rare p53 mutations in one variant of PIA,[47] and recent work from Nakayama et al shows that approximately 6% of PIA lesions show evidence of somatic methylation of the GSTP1 gene promoter.[48] The pi-class of glutathione S-transferase (GST), which plays a caretaker role by normally preventing stress-related damage, demonstrates hypermethlyation in a high percentage of invasive prostate cancers as well.[49-51] Thus, expression of this protective gene occurs early and persists throughout prostatic carcinogenesis. Focal atrophy lesions may arise either as a consequence of epithelial damage from infection, ischemia, or toxin exposure or as a direct consequence of inflammatory oxidant damage to the epithelium.[40] Regardless of the etiology of PIA, the epithelial cells in these lesions exhibit molecular signs of stress, expressing high levels of GSTP1, GSTA1, and cyclooxygenase 2 (COX2).[40,42,52,53] There is also mounting evidence that the atrophic luminal cells in PIA represent a form of intermediate epithelial cell[54] similar to cells postulated to be the targets of neoplastic transformation in the prostate.[55-58] Therefore, both PIA and high-grade PIN may represent steps along a pathway in the progression to invasive prostate cancer. However, it is not clear if they represent separate pathways or steps along the same pathway. On-going work sponsored by the National Cancer Institute is focusing on developing a consensus definition of PIA so that future studies can be optimally compared.

SERUM- AND TISSUE-BASED BIOMARKERS

Over the past 5 years there has been a dramatic increase in the number of putative prostate cancer biomarkers. In this section, we try to highlight some of the critical genes identified to date with emphasis on those genes specifically associated with prostate cancer (Table 16.2).

PROSTATE-SPECIFIC ANTIGEN

Prostate-specific antigen is a serine protease produced by the epithelial cells lining the acini and ducts of the prostate gland. Under normal conditions it is secreted into the lumens of prostatic ducts and can be detected in high concentrations in seminal plasma. Prostate-specific antigen expression, while highly restricted and confined mainly to benign and malignant prostatic luminal epithelial cells, can also be elevated in prostatitis, BPH, and after prostate manipulation, thus making this marker not absolutely cancer specific.

Pretreatment serum PSA is associated with clinical stage, Gleason grade, tumor volume, and pathological stage.[59] Serum PSA is currently used as a tumor marker for prostate cancer and also for the early detection, staging, and post-treatment follow-up of patients. Immunohistochemical staining for PSA is useful in the identification of metastatic tumors of unknown origin. Interestingly, prostate cancers with poor differentiation express lower amounts of immunologically detectable PSA compared with well differentiated tumors and behave more aggressively.[60]

Table 16.2 Selected genes associated with prostate cancer progression

Symbol	Gene name(s)	Locus	Functional role	Molecular alteration
KLK3	Kallikrein 3, Prostate specific antigen (PSA)	19q13	Serine protease	Unknown
FOLH1	Folate hydrolase, prostate-specific membrane antigen (PSMA)	11p11	Folate hydrolase, prostate cancer cell surface antigen	Elevated in advanced PCA
CDKN1B	Cyclin-dependent kinase inhibitor 1B (p27, Kip1)	12p13	Cyclin-dependent kinase inhibitor	Decreased in PIN and PCA
SKP2	S-phase kinase-associated protein 2 (p45)	5p13	Recognizes phosphorylated p27 and targets it for degradation	Overexpressed in some advanced PCA
CDH1	Cadherin 1, type 1, E-cadherin (epithelial)	16q22.1	Cell adhesion molecule	Downregulated with PCA progression
PTEN	Phosphatase and tensin homolog (mutated in multiple advanced cancers 1)	10q23.31	Tumor supressor gene	Mutations and haplotype insufficiency
AR	Androgen Receptor	Xq11.2-q12	Mediates survival, regeneration and differentiation processes in the normal prostate	mRNA overexpressed, amplified, and mutated in advanced prostate cancer
MYC	c-myc	8q24.21	Immediate-early response gene	Amplified in PCA
PSCA	Prostate Stem Cell Antigen	8q24.3	Stem cell/progenitor cell functions	Amplified in PCA
AMACR	alpha-methylacyl-CoA racemase	5p13.2-q11.1	β-Oxidation of branched-chain fatty acids	Overexpressed in PIN/PCA
FASN	Fatty Acid Syntase	17q25.3	Catalyzes the synthesis of palmitate from malonyl-CoA and acetyl-CoA	Overexpressed in PCA
HPN	hepsin	19q11-q13.2	Transmembrane protease, serine 1	Overexpressed in PIN/PCA
NKX3-1	NK3 transcription factor homolog A	8p21	Homeobox gene	Decreased with PCA progression
EZH2	Enhancer of zeste homolog 2	7q35-q36	Transcriptional repressor	Overexpressed in aggressive PCA and Breast Cancer
GST-pi	Glutathione S-transferase pi	11q13	Caretaker gene	Hypermethlyation
MTA1	Metastatis-associated 1	14q32.3	Transcription repressor	Overexpressed with PCA progression
TPD52	Tumor protein D52	8q21	Coiled-coil motif-bearing protein	Amplified in PCA
JAG1	Jagged 1 (Alagille syndrome)	20p12.1-p11.23	NOTCH receptor ligand	Overexpressed in PCA

PCA, prostate cancer; PIN, prostatic intraepithelial neoplasia.

PROSTATE SPECIFIC MEMBRANE ANTIGEN

Prostate-specific membrane antigen (PSMA) is a prostate cancer cell-surface antigen and constitutes an antigenic target in prostate cancer. Importantly, PSMA expression appears to be elevated in poorly differentiated, metastatic, and hormone-refractory carcinomas although it has been detected in nonprostatic tissues as well.[61] It is expressed at high density on the cell membrane of all prostate cancers, and, after antibody binding, the PSMA-antibody complex is rapidly internalized. Anti-PSMA monoclonal antibodies can be used to target delivery of highly cytotoxic agents to the cancer cells without affecting normal cells.[62,63] Prostate-specific membrane antigen is utilized as an immunoscintigraphic target using the antibody conjugate CYT-356 (ProstaScint; Cytogen, Princeton, NJ) and has been shown to have clinical value, particularly in detecting occult prostate cancer.[61]

THE CYCLIN DEPENDENT KINASE INHIBITOR P27

p27 is a cyclin-dependent kinase inhibitor (CKI) and a tumor suppressor gene. The p27 gene regulates progression of the cell cycle from G1 to S phase by predominantly binding to and inhibiting the cyclinE/CDK2 complex.[64] In the normal adult prostate, p27 protein is expressed primarily by secretory cells. Cells lacking p27 and expressing basal cell specific cytokeratin are present between the basal and luminal cells, and appear to be increased in prostate tissue previously subjected to androgen blockade and in benign prostatic hyperplasia (BPH). The lack of nuclear p27 expression in the suprabasal epithelial cells may, therefore, delineate a subcompartment of cells that proliferate in the absence of androgens.[56] Dysregulation of p27 expression may be a critical early event in the development of prostatic neoplasia. In addition, loss of expression of p27 by immunohistochemistry in invasive prostatic adenocarcinoma has been shown to be associated with poor prognosis independent of preoperative PSA levels and Gleason score.[65,66] p27 protein expression in the preoperative prostate needle biopsy has also been shown to be associated with subsequent radical prostatectomy, p27, Gleason grade, and pathological stage.[67]

S-phase kinase-associated protein 2 (Skp2) is a member of the F-box protein family, and specifically recognizes phosphorylated p27 and targets it for degradation. The oncogenic potential of *skp2* has been demonstrated by cotransfecting *skp2* and *RAS* (Gly12Val) into primary rat embryo fibroblasts. Transfected fibroblasts showed increase in colony formation in soft agar and tumor formation in nude mice.[68] In addition, transgenic mice expressing both *skp2* and *RAS* induce T-cell lymphomas with shorter latency and decreased survival when compared with *RAS* transgenic animals.[69]

skp2 expression inversely correlates with p27 gene expression in prostatic adenocarcinoma[70,71] and is overexpressed in a subset of highly proliferative androgen-independent prostate carcinomas metastatic to bone (M Loda and P Febbo, unpublished data). skp2 may, therefore, be a suitable therapeutic target in highly proliferative, androgen-independent prostate cancer.

E-CADHERIN

The long arm of chromosome 16 (16q22.1) is deleted in both primary and, more frequently, in some metastatic prostate cancer.[72,73] This region contains the *E-cadherin* gene. E-cadherin is found on the membrane of epithelial cells and functions as a Ca^{2+}-dependent epithelial cell adhesion molecule. Its intracellular domain binds directly to β-*catenin*, which links extracellular Wnt signals with transcription factors of the LEF/TCF family. In many carcinomas, cadherins are lost or downregulated. Decreased E-cadherin expression is associated with metastatic progression, while loss of E-cadherin determined by immunohistochemistry is a predictor of poor outcome and overall survival.[72]

Experimentally, expression of the E-cadherin protein suppresses while loss of expression enhances the invasiveness and motility of epithelial cells. E-cadherin appears to mediate both inhibition of invasion and proliferation via the induction of p27.[74] These findings link extracellular stimuli to the cell cycle machinery and suggest a role for E-cadherin and p27 in both invasion and metastasis.[75]

PHOSPHATASE AND TENSIN HOMOLOG, β-ALANYL-α-KETOGLUTARATE TRANSAMINASE, AND PHOSPHOINOSITOL-3 KINASE PATHWAY

Loss of phosphatase and tensin homolog (PTEN) expression occurs in three out of four of the most common prostate cancer cell lines[76] and a subset of hormone refractory prostatic adenocarcinoma.[77,78] PTEN mutations are less frequent in clinically localized tumors.[79] The tumor suppressor activity of PTEN is associated with its ability to antagonize phosphoinositol-3′ kinase (PI3K) signaling.[80] Loss-of-function of PTEN results in deregulated PI3K signaling, and constitutive activation of downstream targets including the β-alanyl-α-ketoglutarate transaminase/protein kinase B (AKT/PKB) serine/threonine kinase family, which promotes cell proliferation and survival.[81] In mouse models, inactivation of one PTEN allele and either haploinsufficiency or knock-out of p27 results in prostate carcinoma with complete penetrance within three months of age.[82]

Loss-of-function mutations in PTEN thus led to deregulated PI3K signaling, resulting in constitutive activation of downstream targets including the AKT serine/threonine kinase family.[81] Recent work from the Sellers laboratory demonstrates the critical role of the AKT/PI3K signaling pathway in prostate cancer progression. Transgenic mice expressing activated AKT1 only in the prostate (murine prostate-restricted AKT kinase activity transgenic expression model or MPAKT)[83] resulted in the activation of the p70[S6K] pathway and the induction of PIN similar in character to that observed in PTEN[+/−] mice. There is a marked overlap in the phenotype induced by activation of AKT and that resulting from loss of PTEN.[84-87] Importantly, mTOR inhibition in the MPAKT model induces epithelial cell apoptosis and the complete reversal of a neoplastic phenotype. Induction of cell-death requires the mitochondrial pathway as prostate-specific coexpression of BCL2 blocks apoptosis. Thus, there is an mTOR-dependent survival signal required downstream of AKT.[88] Emerging data suggests that the AKT/PTEN pathway may be altered in a significant percentage of advanced prostate cancers (Sellers et al, personal communication). Therefore, mTOR inhibitors may play a limited but critical role in treating prostate cancer.[89-91]

ANDROGEN RECEPTOR

Androgens, in concert with the androgen receptor (AR) mediate survival, regeneration, and differentiation processes in the normal prostate.[92] Huggins and Hodges realized in 1941 the critical role that androgens play in prostate cancer progression.[93] Clinically, it is well known that hormone ablation therapy leads to a rapid decrease in tumor volume followed by the regrowth of hormone-refractory prostate cancer. Understanding the role of the AR in prostate cancer progression has proven elusive. There have been a few recent observations suggesting how advanced tumors evade standard androgen ablation therapy. First, recent morphologic observations of metastatic prostate cancer demonstrate an extremely heterogeneous group of tumors.[94] Observations from autopsy series of hormone refractory metastatic prostate cancer reveal several histologic and molecular profiles.[95-97]

Proposed mechanisms of progression to androgen-independent growth include amplification of the AR gene,[98] mutations of the AR gene,[99] shortened numbers of CAG trinucleotide repeat sequences and recruitment of coactivators.[100-102] Immunohistochemical studies have demonstrated expression of AR in primary, advanced, and hormone-refractory prostate cancers, suggesting that disease progression is almost never associated with loss of AR expression. There is also considerable heterogeneity of AR expression in specimens and among patients, and the heterogeneity of AR expression increases with increasing Gleason grade.[103-105]

A recent study by Chen et al[106] supports strong evidence for upregulation of AR mRNA as the chief contributor to the development of hormone-refractory prostate cancer. The authors compared the gene expression profiles of isogenic hormone-sensitive and hormone-refractory xenografts. The analysis of the microarray data showed the AR gene to be three- to five-fold overexpressed. However, no differences were seen in the expression levels of any other genes tested. This observation is indeed surprising, and places the AR as the principal player in conferring androgen-resistant growth. The upregulation of the AR as seen by microarray was further confirmed by overexpressing AR in hormone-sensitive cell lines. Overexpression allowed growth of these cells in both an androgen-depleted environment and in the presence of the antiandrogen bicalutamide. Further, when these cells lines were implanted into castrated SCID mice, an early onset of tumor formation was seen compared with wild type. By use of short hairpin RNA (shRNA) against the AR, it was established that increased AR expression is required for tumor establishment in castrated xenograft models. The process of tumor establishment was shown to be ligand-dependent by overexpressing mutants of ligand binding domain (LBD). The rate of tumor progression was retarded when the LBD was mutated. They also showed that the action of AR is mediated by its binding to DNA and not merely by modulation of cytoplasmic processes. This was shown by disruption of nuclear targeting and use of a mutant DNA binding domain. Disruption of coupling to cytoplasmic proteins like Src, on the other hand, was shown to have no effect on the AR action. Hence, the authors suggested a ligand-dependent mass action model, where low levels of circulating androgens can bind to the overexpressed receptor leading to

nuclear-mediated alteration of gene expression, eventually resulting in tumor progression. They then tried to block the action of androgen using high concentrations of the antagonist bicalutamide. However, bicalutamide was seen to function as an agonist of hormone action by stimulating the expression of PSA. The same phenomenon was observed using other antagonists. In order to determine if bicalutamide acts as an agonist in the expression of PSA alone or in conjunction with other androgen-regulated genes, differences in gene expression patterns between AR-overexpressing and wild-type cells lines treated with bicalutamide were examined. This yielded a set of bicalutamide-induced androgen-sensitive genes expressed in the AR cell line. The expression of the same set of genes was also induced in response to low concentrations of synthetic androgen R1881. This shows that bicalutamide acts as a weak agonist. In order to investigate the reason for evolution of an agonistic response from well-established antagonists, chromatin immunoprecipitation experiments were carried out to identify the coactivator/co-repressor complexes that were recruited to androgen-regulated promoters upon treatment with the antagonist. It was seen that overexpression of the receptor led to the recruitment of a smaller subset of co-activators in response to antagonists.

This study indeed addresses a wide range of questions regarding the role of AR in the progression of cancer following therapy. The process is shown to be ligand-dependent and, therefore, the tumors are not strictly "hormone independent." Since AR is seen to be over expressed in all the xenograft models used in this study, the question arises as to why the level of AR increases following androgen ablation. Although amplification has been proposed as a method by which upregulation of AR expression occurs, the frequency of amplification seen is low to explain the observations made in this study. Moreover, overexpression of AR has been reported previously in the absence of amplification.[107,108] The potential role of AR is presented in Figure 16.1 and has recently been reviewed by Debes and Tindall.[109]

MYC

One of the most frequent genetic changes detected by means of comparative genomic hybridization (CGH) in hormone refractory prostate cancer is the gain of 8q and especially the 8q-qter region.[110,111] One potential target at the 8q24 region is the *MYC* gene. The *MYC* gene is an immediate-early response gene, which is activated by mitogenic stimuli, resulting in proliferation. Fluorescent in-situ hybridization analysis has identified high-level amplification of *MYC* in greater than 20% of recurrent and metastatic prostate cancers.[111,112] Amplification of *MYC* correlates with high level of MYC protein expression.[112] Furthermore, inhibition of MYC expression can mediate tumor regression in a prostate

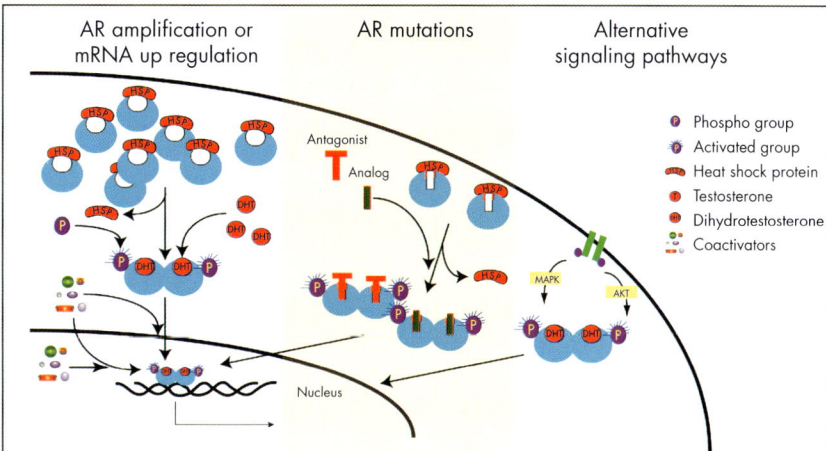

Fig. 16.1

Various mechanisms involving the androgen receptor (AR) have been proposed in order to explain the recurrence of prostate cancer following androgen ablation. Amplification of the AR gene is thought to cause upregulation of AR mRNA leading to activation of the AR-regulated genes by residual low concentrations of androgens. Mutations in the ligand-binding domain have been shown to alter the ligand specificity thereby allowing the binding of non-canonical ligands/antagonists, leading to the activation of the downstream gene expression. Unliganded androgen receptors have been proposed to activate gene expression when activated by phosphorylation by receptor tyrosine kinases. In addition, upregulation of coactivators has also been shown to increase the action of activated AR. The expression of the AR mRNA is upregulated in hormone refractory prostate cancer, leading to the activation of androgen-regulated genes. Upregulation of AR expression renders the receptor sensitive to low concentrations of ligand and also allows binding to antagonists of hormone action. The binding of the antagonist, however, results in agonistic response. The gene expression in this case is mediated by a limited medley of coactivator proteins.

cancer xenograft.[113] MYC can also cooperate with RAS to induce prostate cancer in various rat and murine model systems. Evaluation of case matched prostate cancer biopsies from patients undergoing androgen ablation suggests that levels of MYC expression increase following castration.[114] Bubendorf et al, using FISH on tissue microarrays, showed high-level *MYC* amplification in 11% of metastases from patients with hormone refractory disease, suggesting a role in metastatic progression.[115] Importantly, transgenic mice expressing human MYC in the mouse prostate developed murine prostatic intraepithelial neoplasia followed by invasive adenocarcinoma.[116] However, there may be other, currently unknown, target genes at the distal 8q locus, whose increased copy number is selected during cancer progression. One such candidate gene is that encoding prostate stem cell antigen (PSCA).

PROSTATE STEM CELL ANTIGEN

Prostate stem cell antigen may play a role in stem cell/progenitor cell functions such as self-renewal and/or proliferation. It is a prostate-specific cell surface protein that maps distal to *MYC* at the 8q24.2 locus. *PSCA* mRNA is expressed strongly in 80% of primary prostate cancers and is overexpressed in androgen-independent prostate cancer xenografts.[117] The protein is overexpressed in cancer compared with normal in 36%

of primary tumors and in 100% of bone metastases.[118] In addition, *PSCA* is co-amplified with *MYC*, and *PSCA* amplification correlates with overexpression.[119] Since it localizes to the surface of prostate cancer cells, and because of its almost exclusive expression in prostate, PSCA may in addition also represent an important therapeutic target. In fact, anti-PSCA antibodies that recognize PSCA expressed on the surface of live cells are efficiently internalized after antigen recognition, and kill tumor cells in vitro in an antigen-specific fashion upon conjugation with maytansinoid.[120]

ALPHA-METHYLACYL-COENZYME A RACEMASE

Alpha-methylacyl-coenzyme A racemase (AMACR) is an enzyme that plays an important role in bile acid biosynthesis and β-oxidation of branched-chain fatty acids.[121,122] In particular, this enzyme catalyzes the conversion of branched fatty acids from R to S configuration and allows them to undergo peroxisomal β-oxidation with the generation of hydrogen peroxide and potential procarcinogenic oxidative damage.[123,124] AMACR is upregulated in prostate cancer and, along with the loss of p63 and high-molecular-weight cytokeratins, is a useful marker of prostatic malignancy in prostate biopsies.[125–130] Interestingly, AMACR mRNA and protein expression is downregulated in hormone-refractory, metastatic prostate cancer. Thus, AMACR expression appears to be independent of androgen regulation and likely related inversely to tumor differentiation.[131] A recent study suggests that decreased AMACR expression in clinically localized prostate cancer is associated with prostate cancer specific death taking other clinical parameters into account.[132] Emerging work suggests that AMACR can be detected in the urine as a protein[133,134] or at the transcript level.[135] Finally, as AMACR is strongly expressed by prostate tumor cells, a novel approach has identified that men with prostate cancer develop a humoral immune response to AMACR that can be detected in the serum.[136] Currently AMACR is being used widely in conjunction with basal cell immunostains in the diagnosis of clinically challenging prostate cancer biopsies.[125,126,130,137–140]

FATTY ACID SYNTHASE

Fatty acid synthase (FAS) catalyzes the synthesis of palmitate from the condensation of malonyl-CoA and acetyl-CoA, thus playing an important role in energy homeostasis by converting excess carbon intake into fatty acids for storage. Fatty acids synthesis in tumor tissues occurs at very high rates.[141] In addition, almost all fatty acids derive from de novo synthesis despite adequate nutritional supply.[142–144]

Despite its apparently marginal physiologic role under normal conditions, FAS is overexpressed at both the protein and mRNA levels in prostate carcinoma.[145] Its high expression has also been associated with aggressive biologic behavior.[146] Interestingly, the highest levels of FAS expression are found in androgen-independent bone metastases.[147]

Fatty acid synthase has been shown to play a major role in the synthesis of phospholipids, primary components of cellular membranes.[148] Alterations in membrane lipid composition that may occur as a result of FAS overexpression can, therefore, have profound effects on many cellular processes such as signal transduction pathways.

Activation of the PI3K pathway occurs in the late phases of human prostate cancers.[149] In turn, PI3K activation increases FAS transcription at least in part through the activation of SREBPs in prostate cancer cell lines.[150] Importantly, in breast epithelial cells, HER2/NEU stimulates the FAS promoter through a PI3K-dependent pathway and mediates increased fatty acid synthesis, while pharmacologic inhibition of FAS preferentially induces apoptosis of HER2/NEU-overexpressing breast epithelial cells.[151] Since expression of HER2/NEU in prostate cancer increases with progression towards androgen independence,[152] and is (like FAS) highest in prostate cancer metastatic to bone, the oncogenic effects of PI3K activation may be mediated, at least in part, via the induction of FAS

expression. Finally, overexpression and enhanced activity of FAS would result in a significant improvement in redox balance despite hypoxic conditions.[153]

Fatty acid synthase inhibitors, such as C75 and the mycotoxin cerulenin, as well as RNA interference of FAS message, result in apoptosis of cancer cells[154,155] and decrease the size of prostate cancer xenographs that overexpress the enzyme.[156] The de-ubiquitinating enzyme ubiquitin-specific protease 2a (USP2a) interacts with and stabilizes FAS, thus providing post-transcriptional regulation. Interfering with USP2a, which is overexpressed in prostate cancer, results in decreased FAS protein levels and enhanced apoptosis in prostate cancer cells. Thus, the isopeptidase USP2a plays a critical role in prostate cancer cell survival through FAS stabilization and represents a therapeutic target in this disease.[157] Ubiquitin-specific protease 2a interference may circumvent the undesired effects of FAS inhibitors.[158]

HEPSIN

Hepsin, a cell surface serine protease, was determined to be overexpressed in localized and metastatic prostate cancer when compared with benign prostate or benign prostatic hyperplasia in several expression array experiments.[127,129,159,160] Hepsin expression is increased in PIN compared with the non-transformed adjacent cells, suggesting that dysregulation of hepsin is an early event in the development of prostate cancer.[127] There is lack of agreement as to whether hepsin is associated with prostate cancer progression.[161,162] However, hepsin may prove to be a valuable molecular biomarker for imaging of prostate cancer.[163]

NKX3.1

NKX3.1 is an androgen-regulated homeobox gene located at 8p21, expressed selectively in the prostate with lower levels also seen in the testis (Bieberich et al, 1996; He et al, 1997; Sciavolino et al, 1998; Korkmaz et al, 2000).[164–170] NKX3.1 is expressed early in mouse embryogenesis and targeted disruption in mice gives rise to aberrations in prostate ductal morphogenesis and secretory protein production (Bhatia-Gaur et al, 1999).[171] Although no mutations have been identified in this gene,[164] recent work suggests that decreased expression is associated with prostate cancer progression.[165] Given the possible role of NKX3.1 in prostate carcinogenesis, we studied its expression by immunohistochemistry. Our data indicate that NKX3.1 is specifically expressed in the nuclei of luminal cells of the prostate epithelium and that there is no significant change in NKX3.1 expression or distribution during prostate cancer progression.[170] However, NKX3.1 haploinsufficiency extends the proliferative stage of regenerating luminal cells, leading to epithelial hyperplasia.[172] Therefore, immunohistochemistry may not be quantitative enough to detect decreased expression occurring as a consequence of haploinsufficiency.

ENHANCER OF ZESTE HOMOLOG 2

Enhancer of zeste homolog 2 gene (EZH2), a member of the polycomb gene family, is a transcriptional repressor known to be active early in embryogenesis,[170,173,174] showing decreased expression as cells differentiate. Using cDNA microarray analysis, Varambally et al compared the gene expression patterns found in benign prostate tissue, organ-confined tumors, and androgen-independent metastatic prostate tumors and found that the polycomb group (PcG) protein EZH2 was among a group of transcripts whose increased expression distinguished metastatic tumors from those localized to the prostate.[175] In addition, RNA interference construct (RNAi)-mediated EZH2 knock-down leads to growth inhibition in cell culture, which potentially may be linked to alterations in the cell-cycle profile. These authors showed that the expression of both the EZH2 mRNA and protein progressively increase from benign, to organ-confined, to metastatic tumors, suggesting that increases in EZH2 precede the development of metastatic foci. These data raise the possibility that EZH2 protein levels might prove useful in predicting patient outcome after prostatectomy. Indeed, immunohistochemical analysis of the EZH2 protein in tissue microarrays predicted outcome independently of Gleason score, presurgical PSA, and stage.[172,175,176] If validated in larger datasets, these data could provide important additional information useful in patient stratification.[177]

TUMOR PROTEIN D52

The gene encoding tumor protein D52 (TPD52) was identified in the 8q21 amplicon as one of the most consistently overexpressed genes in prostate cancer.[178] The protein TPD52 is a coiled-coil motif-bearing protein, potentially involved in vesicle trafficking. Both mRNA and protein levels of TPD52 are highly elevated in prostate cancer tissues.[179,180] Array comparative genomic hybridization and amplification analysis using single nucleotide polymorphism arrays demonstrated increased DNA copy number in the region encompassing TPD52.[180] Fluorescence in situ hybridization on tissue microarrays confirmed TPD52 amplification in prostate cancer epithelia. Furthermore, our studies suggest that TPD52 protein levels may be regulated by androgens, consistent with the presence of androgen-response elements in the upstream promoter of TPD52.[180] These findings suggest that dysregulation of TPD52 by genomic amplification and androgen induction may play a role in prostate cancer progression.

METASTASIS ASSOCIATED PROTEIN 1

Expression of the metastasis-associated protein 1 (MTA1) has previously been found to be associated with progression to the metastatic state in various cancers.[181–184] DNA microarray found MTA1 to be selectively overexpressed in metastatic prostate cancer compared with clinically localized prostate cancer and benign prostate tissue.[185] These results were validated by demonstrating overexpression of MTA1 in metastatic prostate cancer by immunoblot analysis and by immunohistochemistry in a broad spectrum of prostate tumors with tissue microarrays.[185] Metastatic prostate cancer demonstrated significantly higher MTA1 protein expression compared with clinically localized prostate cancer.

JAGGED1

Recent studies suggest that NOTCH signaling can promote epithelial-mesenchymal transitions and augment signaling through AKT, an important growth and survival pathway in epithelial cells and prostate cancer in particular. Using a high throughput quantitative proteomic technique, Martin et al recently identified JAGGED1 (JAG1), a NOTCH receptor ligand, as a highly androgen-responsive gene product in the prostate cancer cell line LNCaP.[186] Work examining human tissues demonstrated that JAGGED1 is significantly more highly expressed in metastatic prostate cancer compared with localized prostate cancer or benign prostatic tissues, based on immunohistochemical analysis of JAGGED1 expression in human tumor samples from 154 men.[187] Furthermore, high JAGGED1 expression in a subset of clinically localized tumors was significantly associated with recurrence, independent of other clinical parameters. These findings support a model in which dysregulation of JAGGED1 protein levels plays a role in prostate cancer progression and metastasis and suggest that JAGGED1 may be a useful marker in distinguishing indolent and aggressive prostate cancer.

SIMULTANEOUS ASSESSMENT OF MULTIPLE BIOMARKERS

New technology makes it feasible to assess the status of tumors at a genome-wide level. Prostate cancer researchers have been very active in this arena. The following discussion reviews some of the emerging data from these studies.

GENE EXPRESSION PROFILING

Several methods of comparative gene expression have been described over the years, such as representational difference analysis (RDA) or serial analysis of gene expression (SAGE), each with its distinct advantages and disadvantages. The former identifies differences in gene expression in a sequence-independent manner but is not high throughput. The latter yields quantitative expression methods but is labor intensive and restricted in its source of information to a few tumors or cell lines. More recently, gene-expression profiling using either cDNA or oligonucleotide microarrays has been successfully applied in the molecular diagnostics of cancer.

The genetic basis of cancer including prostate cancer is indisputable. Although not proven, it is widely accepted that the heterogeneity in clinical behavior is either genetically determined or determined by a complex interaction of genetic and environmental factors. There is also increasing proof that prostate cancer can be genetically classified into different subtypes.[127,129,175,178,188,189] The implications of this are that, using genetic stratification, the clinical behavior of prostate cancer can be predicted.

The expression data obtained by microarray technology must be subjected to complex analytical methods. These include the use of supervised learning techniques for the identification of genes whose expression levels are predictive of rapid relapse following surgical resection, and the use of unsupervised learning methods (clustering) for the identification of previously unrecognized subgroups of tumors. It has been found that a gene expression signature of metastasis exists in a subset of primary tumors,[190] and the presence of that signature is predictive of eventual metastatic potential in prostate adenocarcinoma. These findings suggest that contrary to the prevailing model of metastasis development, the metastatic potential of primary tumors is encoded in the bulk of the primary tumor at the time of diagnosis.[188]

A general approach to cancer classification has been applied to a variety of tumor types including prostate cancer. As a result, efforts to develop a molecular taxonomy of cancer have yielded gene expression correlates of histologic grade and clinical outcome. Because these gene expression signatures are subtle, it is critical to attempt to validate these initial results in independent sets of samples and with different techniques.

PROTEOMICS

Recent achievements in genomics have created an infrastructure of biologic information. The enormous success of genomics promptly induced a subsequent explosion in proteomic technology, the emerging science for systematic study of proteins in complexes, organelles, and cells. Proteomics is developing powerful technologies to identify novel proteins, to quantify the differential expression of proteins under different states, to study aspects of protein–protein interaction, and, most importantly, to identify patterns of protein expression in tissues or sera, which would predict recurrence or response to therapy. The dynamic nature of protein expression, protein interactions, and protein modifications requires measurement as a function of time and cellular state. These types of studies require many measurements and, consequently, high throughput protein identification is essential. The most powerful, currently available technology to study protein expression in cells is mass spectrometry,[191] which allows for the characterization of extremely small samples (e.g., from laser capture microdissected material).

Analysis of tumors with expression array and genomic array technology can be compared and contrasted with the proteomic platform in biopsies, surgical specimens, and body fluids such as serum. Proteomics applied to serum samples can identify unique profiles that may be used for prognosis and diagnosis of prostate cancer.[192] The output of a proteomic platform is a protein profile that can differentiate benign from malignant[192] or provide prognostic/predictive information. One can also image the use of protein or expression array profiles to identify patients at highest risk for developing a disease state (e.g., prostate cancer) or even which patients would benefit from a treatment protocol.

GENOME-WIDE SCANNING

The power of comparative genomic hybridization (CGH) has been clearly proven as a tool to characterize chromosomal imbalances in neoplasias. Comparative genomic hybridization and, more recently, array-CGH can detect a number of recurrent regions of amplification or deletion. This has led to the identification of new chromosomal loci involved in the development and progression of tumors. While mutations in any of the classic oncogenes and tumor suppressor genes are not found in high frequency in primary prostate cancers, a large number of studies have identified nonrandom somatic genome alterations. Using CGH to screen the DNA of prostate cancer, the most common chromosomal alterations in prostate cancer are losses at 1p, 6q, 8p, 10q, 13q, 16q, and 18q; and gains at 1q, 2p, 7, 8q, 18q, and Xq.[111,193–195] The application of novel single nucleotide polymorphic allele (SNP) informatic platforms to a series of prostate cancer specimens specifically recognized regions of deletion on chromosomes 1p33-34, 3q27, 8p21, 10q23, 15q12 16q23-24, 17p13.[73] Loss of heterozygosity

(LOH) in prostate cancer localized to 1p, 8p21, 10q23 (the site of the tumor suppressor gene *PTEN*), 16q23 (the site of the tumor suppressor gene for E-cadherin), and 17p13 (the site of the p53 gene), had all been previously reported by multiple investigators.[196] Thus, when CGH data from different studies are combined, a pattern of nonrandom genetic aberrations appears. As is the case for array-CGH, SNP analysis allows investigators to study simultaneously multiple tumors for common regions of genetic loss.

Based on these technical developments, we have begun to characterize the prostate cancer genome on the latest SNP arrays. This latest generation of arrays contains probes for 120,000 SNPs. The SNP markers on this array are spaced across the genome with a mean intermarker distance of 9 kb. Thus, these arrays provide the highest resolution of any array-based genome mapping method yet tested.

Samples of androgen-dependent lymph node metastatic prostate cancer, androgen-independent metastatic prostate cancer, prostate cancer xenografts, and prostate cancer cell lines have been analyzed on the 11K platform and preliminary maps of LOH, gene amplification, and homozygous deletion have been developed. As shown previously,[73] the arrays robustly detect LOH, and we can again define distinct genetic subtypes of prostate cancer by organizing tumors through hierarchical clustering based on LOH. As shown in Figure 16.2, LOH inferred based on length of homozygous regions robustly separates tumor from normal (normal samples are in the middle and shown little-to-no inferred LOH). Moreover, two distinct tumor clusters can be seen (a major cluster on the left and one on the right). This clustering appears to be driven, at least in part, by differences on chromosome 2 and 8.

Homozygous deletion mapping has also been analyzed. While not as prevalent as LOH, 14 novel regions of homozygous deletion in this initial data set have been detected. Finally, gene amplification events can be detected: for example, high-level amplification of the AR in an androgen-independent prostate cancer xenograft was detected.

The genome-wide information obtained by both the SNP chip and array-CGH analysis of pure tumor samples can be merged with expression data obtained from corresponding frozen tumor material. Merging genomic and transcriptome signatures of solid tumors will begin to unravel patterns of activation or silencing of entire pathways essential for tumor initiation or progression. This will accomplish the ultimate goal of classifying tumors not only by traditional clinicopathologic parameters, but by molecular genetic means as well. One can speculate that targets will be identified for the subsequent synthesis of chemical compounds aimed at inactivation of pathways. Importantly, simple genomic analysis of paraffin-embedded tumors will eventually be indicative of the expression signature of a given tumor (e.g., LOH of the PTEN locus will reflect activation of the PI3K pathway, and such a tumor may be targeted with *AKT* inhibitors).

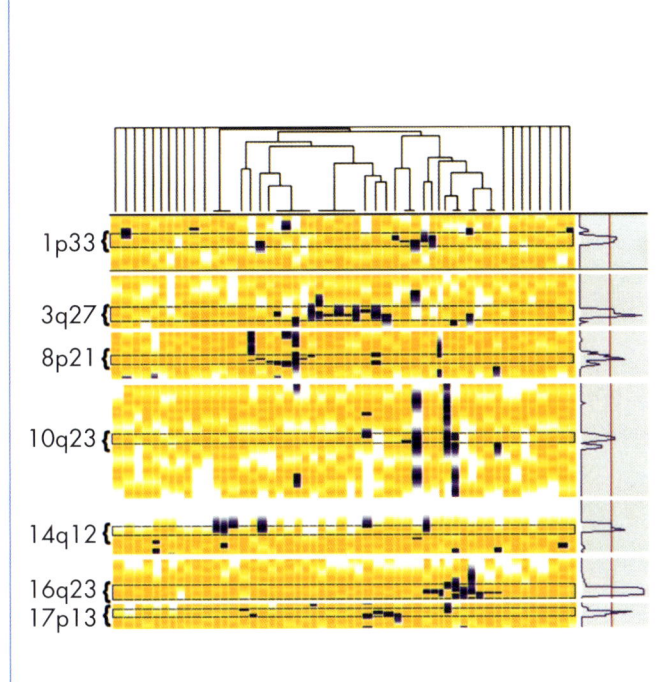

Fig. 16.2

Hierarchical clustering of prostate cancers based on loss of heterozygosity (LOH) similarity. In this study from Lieberfarb et al,[73] ligonucleotide arrays that detect single nucleotide polymorphisms were used to generate genome-wide loss of heterogeneity (LOH) maps from laser capture microdissected paraffin-embedded samples using as little as 5 ng of DNA. The allele detection rate from such samples was comparable with that obtained with standard amounts of DNA prepared from frozen tissues. A novel informatics platform, dChipSNP, was used to automate the definition of statistically valid regions of LOH, assign LOH genotypes to prostate cancer samples, and organize by hierarchical clustering prostate cancers based on the pattern of LOH. This organizational strategy revealed apparently distinct genetic subsets of prostate cancer. Each of the cancers was assigned a designation of retention of heterozygosity (RET), LOH, or uninformative for the seven regions of LOH detected in this data set. Hierarchical clustering of samples without clustering of regions was undertaken using the comparisons of LOH:LOH and LOH:RET, whereas RET:RET and uninformative loci were ignored. Tumor normal pairs are shown as *columns*, whereas the indicated regions of LOH and SNP alleles within them are shown as *rows*. Regions of LOH are indicated by *blue*, although regions of RET are indicated by *yellow*.

TECHNOLOGIES FOR THE DISCOVERY AND ASSESSMENT OF BIOMARKERS

The identification of candidate genes through proteomics and gene expression analysis requires other tools to help validate these biomarkers. The following discussion addresses some of the most commonly used tools.

TISSUE MICROARRAY TECHNOLOGY

Analysis of candidate biomarkers of response or prognosis has been done mostly at the tissue level by staining selected slides from individual cases. More recently, tissue microarray (TMA) technology has allowed for the placement of several hundred tissue samples into a single standard tissue block.[197] The advantage of this technology is that multiple tumors can be evaluated by immunohistochemistry or in-situ hybridization on a single slide. Test conditions are similar for all elements on the slide, providing more uniformity than standard experiments, while conservation of resource is maximized. One limitation of TMA technology is that, due to tumor (tissue) heterogeneity, sampling may miss areas of protein expression. By redundant sampling, one can minimize this problem.

There are screening arrays that are used for the evaluation and development of biomarkers. These TMAs tend to be small (100–200 samples) and are used to test new antibodies or work out the optimal test conditions. Larger outcome TMAs are used to evaluate putative biomarkers. The use of automated arrayers allows the production of multiple replicate blocks. This is ideal for studying large cohorts between multiple institutions (Figure 16.3).

LASER CAPTURE MICRODISSECTION

Laser capture microdissection (LCM) represents an important improvement on standard microdissection techniques, which are limited in the study of prostate cancer due to its heterogeneous nature.[194] Laser capture microdissection offers laser precision and can achieve transfer and isolation of single cells, from which DNA, RNA, and proteins can be extracted. Coupled with immunohistochemistry, it allows the isolation of nucleic acids from subpopulation of cells not identifiable by morphology alone.[199] It was developed by Emmert-Buck and colleagues at the National Cancer Institute (NCI).[200] Laser capture microdissection was born out of a need to isolate pure populations of tumor, normal, and dysplastic tissues as part of the Cancer Genome Anatomy Project (CGAP) (*http://cgap.nci.nih.gov*),[201,202] and it now

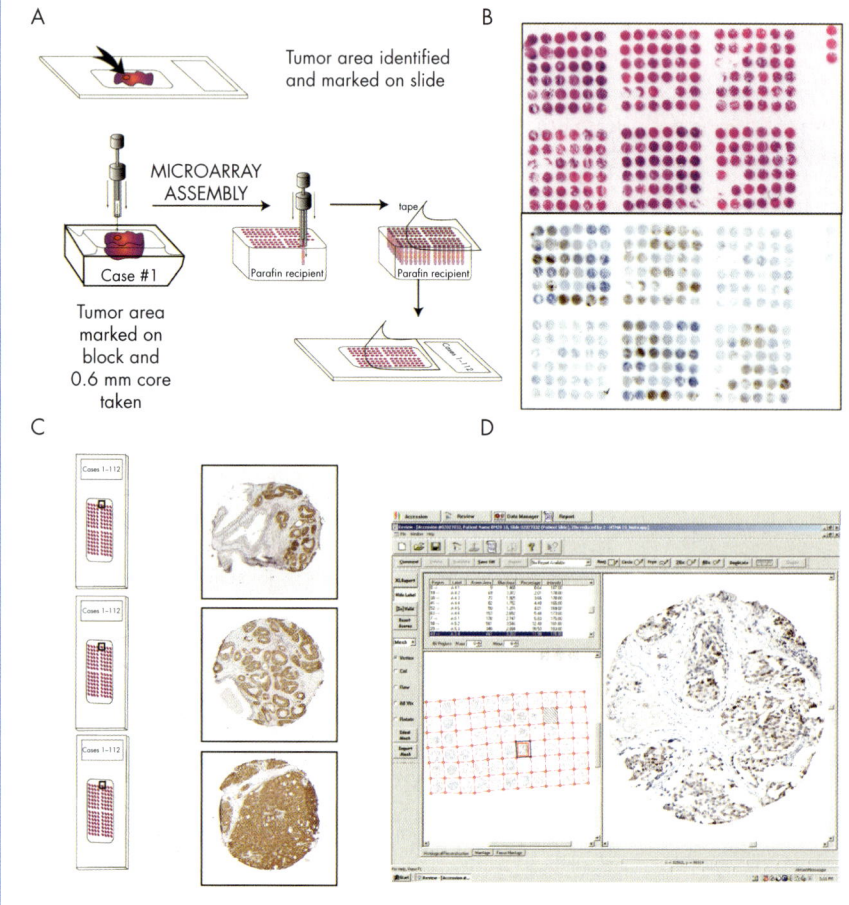

Fig. 16.3
Using tissue microarrays (TMAs) to validate candidate prostate cancer biomarkers. *A*, The construction of TMAs starts with the identification of prostate cancer (or other tissue of interest). This area is then biopsied from the standard paraffin block and placed into a recipient TMA. Four to five micrometer thick sections are cut off the surface of the array. *B*, The final slides can be stained using standard hematoxylin and eosin for visualization (top panel) or can be used for molecular analysis such as immunohistochemistry (bottom panel). *C*, Biomarkers such as α-methylacyl-coenzyme A racemase (see text for details) can then be evaluated. *D*, Several research groups have developed relational databases in order to coordinate the entry of molecular data for each TMA sample. In this example, quantitative evaluation of immunohistochemistry is being performed.

allows the investigator to ask questions regarding individual cells and the relationship between tumor cells and the surrounding stromal tissues.

BIOINFORMATICS

A rapidly emerging field, bioinformatics, is starting to alter the way research is being conducted. Using information from large databases, *in silico* studies can be conducted to discover and validate new candidate genes and pathways significant in areas such as the development of prostate cancer. Bioinformatics is the mainstay of analysis in experiments of expression profiling or large scale genomic analysis. Rhodes et al identified lists of significant prostate cancer-related genes by performing a meta-analysis on publicly available cDNA expression array datasets.[178] This study was also able to extrapolate prostate cancer-related pathways by piecing together data from multiple studies. This approach has now become available on an Internet-based web site (www.oncomine.org) that allows users to perform a meta-analysis on genes of interest and contains links to other websites that provide information regarding their genes of interest.[203] An example of how bioinformatics may be applied in this setting is presented in Figure 16.4. This meta-analysis demonstrates some of the most highly overexpressed genes in prostate cancer based on eight studies based on methods developed by Rhodes et al[178] (Setlur et al, unpublished data). When sifting through hundreds of genes, this approach allows researchers to concentrate on the most consistently altered genes.

Bioinformatics platforms for use in the internet-based evaluation of TMAs have already been developed.[204] Such applications need no special client software since any Java™-compliant browser will work. Encryption of the data passing between the client and the server allows for patient confidentiality to be maintained.

CLINICAL DATABASES

Although a clinical database may not seem related to molecular studies at first glance, it is becoming ever more apparent that annotated clinical information is vital in the area of biomarker development. One recent example comes from the field of lung cancer research where investigators identified that activating mutations in the epithelial growth factor receptor (EGFR) in a small set of lung cancers were associated with excellent clinical response to gefitinib (Iressa) therapy.[205] Without the annotation to clinical data, researchers would not have made this connection.

There is a large-scale effort underway in the US to develop a systematic nationwide collection of human tissue samples to help accelerate cancer research. This program is called the National Biospecimens Network (NBN), and currently pilot projects are being developed to explore the optimal way to set up the NBN. The pilot

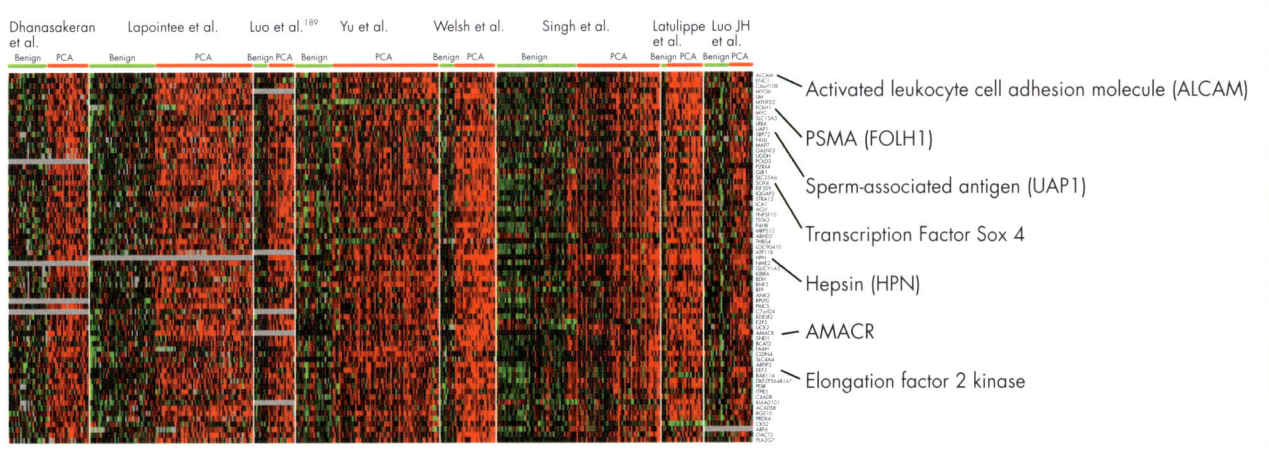

Fig. 16.4
A cohort of cross-validated overexpressed genes identified by meta-analysis of prostate cancer microarray data using a method described by Rhodes et al.[178] Eisen matrix representation of genes consistently differentially expressed between clinically localized prostate cancer *(red bar)* and benign prostate tissue *(green bar)* across eight independent microarray studies. *Each column* represents an individual sample (number of samples is in parentheses), and *each row* represents a specific gene. Within each study, the data were normalized so that the mean expression level of the genes in the benign prostate specimens equaled zero and the SD = 1. *Red* intensity level indicates degree of overexpression, *Green* intensity level indicates degree of under expression, whereas *black* indicates equal or higher expression than the mean benign sample (see scale). *Gray* signifies technically inadequate or not present in a particular study. There are 213 overexpressed genes and 420 underexpressed genes (not shown). Several genes are highlighted on the right including hepsin (HPN), α-methylacyl-coenzyme A racemase (AMACR), and prostate-specific membrane antigen (PSMA).

project from the NCI is being developed by the Prostate Cancer SPORE groups. The Prostate Cancer SPORE pilot project would link the 11 existing Prostate Cancer SPORE sites using state-of-the-art informatics. Tissue collection protocols and existing tissue resources would be electronically visible to research investigators using an internet-based tool. One of the key components of this pilot project will be to collect prostate biopsy samples from multiple sites as part of a prospective biomarker study. The value of these tissues will increase over time and as data from the analysis of each biomarker is added to the database. Critical issues related to this NBN pilot project include maintaining compliance with federal Health Insurance Portability and Accountability (HIPAA) regulations regarding patient confidentiality and protection of intellectual property associated with the research. One critical issue will be the governance of these finite samples so that all accredited researchers can gain assess.

CONCLUSION

Prostate cancer exhibits a wide range of biological behavior. Preoperative serum PSA, Gleason tumor grade, and stage are the most widely-used variables at present in predicting prognosis, relapse, and metastatic potential. In this chapter, we have discussed the technologies available for the discovery and assessment of biomarkers and many biomarkers that have been found to be relevant in the various stages of prostate cancer progression. The challenge ahead is to conclusively determine the role some of these genes play as prognostic and/or predictive markers utilizing large, retrospective, possibly multi-institutional databases with long-term follow-up. More importantly, such markers need to be applied to needle biopsy specimens in order to help guide therapy. Potential therapeutic targets are also beginning to emerge, identification of which may result in novel and more specific therapeutic modalities.

ACKNOWLEDGMENTS

This work was supported by grants from the NCI (RO1, PO1, SPORE in prostate cancer), the Gelb center for genito-urinary oncology at Dana Farber Cancer Institute, Prostate Cancer Foundation award to ML and MAR. The authors thank Sunita Setlur at the Brigham and Women's Hospital and Jianjun Yu at the University of Michigan for the preparation of Figures 16.1 and 16.4, respectively.

REFERENCES

1. Jemal A, Tiwari RC, Murray T, et al. Cancer statistics, 2004. CA Cancer J Clin 2004;54:8–29.
2. Weir HK, Thun MJ, Hankey BF, et al. Annual report to the nation on the status of cancer, 1975–2000, featuring the uses of surveillance data for cancer prevention and control. J Natl Cancer Inst 2003;95:1276–1299.
3. Stamey TA, Johnstone IM, McNeal JE, et al. Preoperative serum prostate specific antigen levels between 2 and 22 ng/ml correlate poorly with post-radical prostatectomy cancer morphology: prostate specific antigen cure rates appear constant between 2 and 9 ng/ml. J Urol 2002;167:103–111.
4. Klotz L. Active surveillance: an individualized approach to early prostate cancer. BJU Int 2003;92:657.
5. Barry MJ. Clinical practice. Prostate-specific-antigen testing for early diagnosis of prostate cancer. N Engl J Med 2001;344:1373–1377.
6. Holmberg L, Bill-Axelson A, Helgesen F, et al. A randomized trial comparing radical prostatectomy with watchful waiting in early prostate cancer. N Engl J Med 2002;347:781–789.
7. Johansson JE, Adami HO, Andersson SO, et al. High 10-year survival rate in patients with early, untreated prostatic cancer. Jama 1992;267:2191–2196.
8. Johansson JE, Holmberg L, Johansson S, et al. Fifteen-year survival in prostate cancer. A prospective, population-based study in Sweden. JAMA 1997;277:467–471.
9. Day JC. Population projections of the United States by a age, sex, and hispanic origin: 1995–2050. Washington, DC: U.S. Bureau of the Census, 1996.
10. Morganti G, Gianferrari L, Cresseri A, et al. Recherches clinico-statistiques et genetiques sur les neoplasies de la prostate. Acta Genet 1956;6:304–305.
11. Lichtenstein P, Holm NV, Verkasalo PK, et al. Environmental and heritable factors in the causation of cancer—analyses of cohorts of twins from Sweden, Denmark, and Finland. N Engl J Med 2000;343:78–85.
12. Rokman A, Ikonen T, Mononen N, et al. ELAC2/HPC2 involvement in hereditary and sporadic prostate cancer. Cancer Res 2001;61:6038–6041.
13. Tavtigian SV, Simard J, Teng DH, et al. A candidate prostate cancer susceptibility gene at chromosome 17p. Nat Genet 2001;27:172–180.
14. Carpten J, Nupponen N, Isaacs S, et al. Germline mutations in the ribonuclease L gene in families showing linkage with HPC1. Nat Genet 2002;30:181–184.
15. Xu J, Zheng SL, Komiya A, et al. Germline mutations and sequence variants of the macrophage scavenger receptor 1 gene are associated with prostate cancer risk. Nat Genet 2002;32:321–325.
16. Rebbeck TR, Walker AH, Zeigler-Johnson C, et al. Association of HPC2/ELAC2 genotypes and prostate cancer. Am J Hum Genet 2000;67:1014–1019.
17. Wang L, McDonnell SK, Elkins DA, et al. Role of HPC2/ELAC2 in hereditary prostate cancer. Cancer Res 2001;61:6494–6499.
18. Suarez BK, Gerhard DS, Lin J, et al. Polymorphisms in the prostate cancer susceptibility gene HPC2/ELAC2 in multiplex families and healthy controls. Cancer Res 2001;61:4982–4984.
19. Xu J, Zheng SL, Carpten JD, et al. Evaluation of linkage and association of HPC2/ELAC2 in patients with familial or sporadic prostate cancer. Am J Hum Genet 2001;68:901–911.
20. Zhou A, Paranjape J, Brown TL, et al. Interferon action and apoptosis are defective in mice devoid of 2′,5′-oligoadenylate-dependent RNase L. Embo J 1997;16:6355–6363.
21. Kerr IM, Brown RE. pppA2′p5′A2′p5′A: an inhibitor of protein synthesis synthesized with an enzyme fraction from interferon-treated cells. Proc Natl Acad Sci USA 1978;75:256–260.
22. Casey G, Neville PJ, Plummer SJ, et al. RNASEL Arg462Gln variant is implicated in up to 13% of prostate cancer cases. Nat Genet 2002;32:581–583.
23. Rokman A, Ikonen T, Seppala EH, et al. Germline alterations of the RNASEL gene, a candidate HPC1 gene at 1q25, in patients and families with prostate cancer. Am J Hum Genet 2002;70:1299–1304.
24. Rennert H, Bercovich D, Hubert A, et al. A novel founder mutation in the RNASEL gene, 471delAAAG, is associated with prostate cancer in Ashkenazi Jews. Am J Hum Genet 2002;71:981–984.
25. Wang L, McDonnell SK, Elkins DA, et al. Analysis of the RNASEL gene in familial and sporadic prostate cancer. Am J Hum Genet 2002;71:116–123.

26. Silverman RH. Implications for RNase L in prostate cancer biology. Biochemistry 2003;42:1805–1812.

27. Bova GS, Partin AW, Isaacs SD, et al. Biological aggressiveness of hereditary prostate cancer: long-term evaluation following radical prostatectomy. J Urol 1998;160:660–663.

28. Sakr WA, Partin AW. Histological markers of risk and the role of high-grade prostatic intraepithelial neoplasia. Urology 2001;57:115–120.

29. Rubin MA, De Marzo AM. Molecular genetics of human prostate cancer. Mod Pathol 2004;17:380–388.

30. Nelson WG, DeMarzo AM, DeWeese TL. The molecular pathogenesis of prostate cancer: focus on the earliest steps. Eur Urol 2001;39:8–11.

31. DeMarzo AM, Nelson WG, Isaacs WB, Epstein JI. Pathological and molecular aspects of prostate cancer. Lancet 2003;361:955–964.

32. De Marzo AM, Meeker AK, Zha S, et al. Human prostate cancer precursors and pathobiology. Urology 2003;62:55–62.

33. Bostwick DG, Pacelli A, Lopez-Beltran A. Molecular biology of prostatic intraepithelial neoplasia. Prostate 1996;29:117–134.

34. Moore RA. The evolution and involution of the prostate gland. Am J Pathol 1936;12:599–624.

35. Rich AR. On the frequency of occurrence of occult carcinoma of the prostate. J Urol 1934;33:215–223.

36. Franks LM. Atrophy and hyperplasia in the prostate proper. J Pathol Bacteriol 1954;68:617–621.

37. Feneley MR, Young MP, Chinyama C, et al. Ki-67 expression in early prostate cancer and associated pathological lesions. J Clin Pathol 1996;49:741–748.

38. Weinstein RS, Gardner WA. Pathology and pathobiology of the urinary bladder and prostate. In: Monographs in pathology, no 34. Baltimore, Md: Williams & Wilkins, 1992, p xi, p 221.

39. McNeal JE. Normal histology of the prostate. Am J Surg Pathol 1988;12:619–633.

40. De Marzo AM, Marchi VL, Epstein JI, et al. Proliferative inflammatory atrophy of the prostate: implications for prostatic carcinogenesis. Am J Pathol 1999;155:1985–1992.

41. Ruska KM, Sauvageot J, Epstein JI. Histology and cellular kinetics of prostatic atrophy. Am J Surg Pathol 1998;22:1073–1077.

42. Putzi MJ, De Marzo AM. Morphologic transitions between proliferative inflammatory atrophy and high-grade prostatic intraepithelial neoplasia. Urology 2000;56:828–832.

43. Montironi R, Mazzucchelli R, Scarpelli M. Precancerous lesions and conditions of the prostate: from morphological and biological characterization to chemoprevention. Ann NY Acad Sci 2002;963:169–184.

44. Liavag I. Atrophy and regeneration in the pathogenesis of prostatic carcinoma. Acta Pathol Microbiol Scand 1968;73:338–350.

45. Shah R, Mucci NR, Amin A, et al. Postatrophic hyperplasia of the prostate gland: neoplastic precursor or innocent bystander? Am J Pathol 2001;158:1767–1773.

46. Macoska JA, Trybus TM, Wojno KJ. 8p22 loss concurrent with 8c gain is associated with poor outcome in prostate cancer. Urology 2000;55:776–782.

47. Tsujimoto Y, Takayama H, Nonomura N, et al. Postatrophic hyperplasia of the prostate in Japan: histologic and immunohistochemical features and p53 gene mutation analysis. Prostate 2002;52:279–287.

48. Nakayama M, Bennett CJ, Hicks JL, et al. Hypermethylation of the human glutathione S-transferase-pi gene (GSTP1) CpG island is present in a subset of proliferative inflammatory atrophy lesions but not in normal or hyperplastic epithelium of the prostate: a detailed study using laser-capture microdissection. Am J Pathol 2003;163:923–933.

49. Lee WH, Morton RA, Epstein JI, et al. Cytidine methylation of regulatory sequences near the pi-class glutathione S-transferase gene accompanies human prostatic carcinogenesis. Proc Natl Acad Sci USA 1994;91:11733–11737.

50. Lin X, Tascilar M, Lee WH, et al. GSTP1 CpG island hypermethylation is responsible for the absence of GSTP1 expression in human prostate cancer cells. Am J Pathol 2001;159:1815–1826.

51. Millar DS, Ow KK, Paul CL, et al. Detailed methylation analysis of the glutathione S-transferase pi (GSTP1) gene in prostate cancer. Oncogene 1999;18:1313–1324.

52. Zha S, Gage WR, Sauvageot J, et al. Cyclooxygenase-2 is up-regulated in proliferative inflammatory atrophy of the prostate, but not in prostate carcinoma. Cancer Res 2001;61:8617–8623.

53. Parsons JK, Nelson CP, Gage WR, et al. GSTA1 expression in normal, preneoplastic, and neoplastic human prostate tissue. Prostate 2001;49:30–37.

54. van Leenders GJ, Gage WR, Hicks JL, et al. Intermediate cells in human prostate epithelium are enriched in proliferative inflammatory atrophy. Am J Pathol 2003;162:1529–1537.

55. De Marzo AM, Nelson WG, Meeker AK, et al. Stem cell features of benign and malignant prostate epithelial cells. J Urol 1998;160:2381–2392.

56. De Marzo AM, Meeker AK, Epstein JI, et al. Prostate stem cell compartments: expression of the cell cycle inhibitor p27Kip1 in normal, hyperplastic, and neoplastic cells. Am J Pathol 1998;153:911–919.

57. van Leenders G, Dijkman H, Hulsbergen-van de Kaa C, et al. Demonstration of intermediate cells during human prostate epithelial differentiation in situ and in vitro using triple-staining confocal scanning microscopy. Lab Invest 2000;80:1251–1258.

58. Verhagen AP, Ramaekers FC, Aalders TW, et al. Colocalization of basal and luminal cell-type cytokeratins in human prostate cancer. Cancer Res 1992;52:6182–6187.

59. So A, Goldenberg L, Gleave ME. Prostate specific antigen: an updated review. Can J Urol 2003;10:2040–2050.

60. Weir EG, Partin AW, Epstein JI. Correlation of serum prostate specific antigen and quantitative immunohistochemistry. J Urol 2000;163:1739–1742.

61. Gregorakis AK, Holmes EH, Murphy GP. Prostate-specific membrane antigen: current and future utility. Semin Urol Oncol 1998;16:2–12.

62. Bander NH, Nanus DM, Milowsky MI, et al. Targeted systemic therapy of prostate cancer with a monoclonal antibody to prostate-specific membrane antigen. Semin Oncol 2003;30:667–676.

63. Fong L, Small EJ. Immunotherapy for prostate cancer. Semin Oncol 2003;30:649–658.

64. Slingerland J, Pagano M. Regulation of the cdk inhibitor p27 and its deregulation in cancer. J Cell Physiol 2000;183:10–17.

65. Yang RM, Naitoh J, Murphy M, et al. Low p27 expression predicts poor disease-free survival in patients with prostate cancer. J Urol 1998;159:941–945.

66. Bloom J, Pagano M. Deregulated degradation of the cdk inhibitor p27 and malignant transformation. Semin Cancer Biol 2003;13:41–47.

67. Thomas GV, Schrage MI, Rosenfelt L, et al. Preoperative prostate needle biopsy p27 correlates with subsequent radical prostatectomy p27, Gleason grade and pathological stage. J Urol 2000;164:1987–1991.

68. Gstaiger M, Jordan R, Lim M, et al. Skp2 is oncogenic and overexpressed in human cancers. Proceedings of the National Academy of Sciences of the United States of America 2001;98:5043–5048.

69. Latres E, Chiarle R, Schulman BA, et al. Role of the F-box protein Skp2 in lymphomagenesis. Proc Natl Acad Sci USA 2001;98:2515–2520.

70. Drobnjak M, Melamed J, Taneja S, et al. Altered expression of p27 and Skp2 proteins in prostate cancer of African-American patients. Clin Cancer Res 2003;9:2613–2619.

71. Yang G, Ayala G, Marzo AD, et al. Elevated Skp2 protein expression in human prostate cancer: association with loss of the cyclin-dependent kinase inhibitor p27 and PTEN and with reduced recurrence-free survival. Clin Cancer Res 2002;8:3419–34126.

72. Umbas R, Schalken JA, Aalders TW, et al. Expression of the cellular adhesion molecule E-cadherin is reduced or absent in high-grade prostate cancer. Cancer Res 1992;52:5104–5109.

73. Lieberfarb ME, Lin M, Lechpammer M, et al. Genome-wide loss of heterozygosity analysis from laser capture microdissected prostate cancer using single nucleotide polymorphic allele (SNP) arrays and a novel bioinformatics platform dChipSNP. Cancer Res 2003;63:4781–4785.

74. St Croix B, Sheehan C, Rak JW, et al. E-Cadherin-dependent growth suppression is mediated by the cyclin-dependent kinase inhibitor p27(KIP1). J Cell Biol 1998;142:557–571.

75. Thomas GV, Szigeti K, Murphy M, et al. Down-regulation of p27 is associated with development of colorectal adenocarcinoma metastases. Am J Pathol 1998;153:681–687.

76. Li J, Yen C, Liaw D, et al. PTEN, a putative protein tyrosine phosphatase gene mutated in human brain, breast, and prostate cancer. Science 1997;275:1943–1947.

77. Suzuki H, Freije D, Nusskern DR, et al. Interfocal heterogeneity of PTEN/MMAC1 gene alterations in multiple metastatic prostate cancer tissues. Cancer Res 1998;58:204–209.

78. Cairns P, Okami K, Halachmi S, et al. Frequent inactivation of PTEN/MMAC1 in primary prostate cancer. Cancer Res 1997;57:4997–5000.

79. Rubin MA, Gerstein A, Reid K, et al. 10q23.3 loss of heterozygosity is higher in lymph node-positive (pT2-3,N+) versus lymph node-negative (pT2-3,N0) prostate cancer. Hum Pathol 2000;31:504–508.

80. Maehama T, Dixon JE. The tumor suppressor, PTEN/MMAC1, dephosphorylates the lipid second messenger, phosphatidylinositol 3,4,5-trisphosphate. J Biol Chem 1998;273:13375–13378.

81. Vazquez F, Sellers WR. The PTEN tumor suppressor protein: an antagonist of phosphoinositide 3-kinase signaling. Biochim Biophys Acta 2000;1470:M21–35.

82. Di Cristofano A, De Acetis M, Koff A, et al. Pten and p27KIP1 cooperate in prostate cancer tumor suppression in the mouse. Nat Genet 2001;27:222–224.

83. Majumder PK, Yeh JJ, George DJ, et al. Prostate intraepithelial neoplasia induced by prostate restricted Akt activation: the MPAKT model. Proc Natl Acad Sci USA 2003;100:7841–7846.

84. Bernal-Mizrachi E, Wen W, Stahlhut S, et al. Islet beta cell expression of constitutively active Akt1/PKB alpha induces striking hypertrophy, hyperplasia, and hyperinsulinemia. J Clin Invest 2001;108:1631–1638.

85. Malstrom S, Tili E, Kappes D, et al. Tumor induction by an Lck-MyrAkt transgene is delayed by mechanisms controlling the size of the thymus. Proc Natl Acad Sci USA 2001;98:14967–14972.

86. Condorelli G, Drusco A, Stassi G, et al. Akt induces enhanced myocardial contractility and cell size in vivo in transgenic mice. Proc Natl Acad Sci USA 2002;99:12333–12338.

87. Shioi T, McMullen JR, Kang PM, et al. Akt/protein kinase B promotes organ growth in transgenic mice. Mol Cell Biol 2002;22:2799–2809.

88. Majumder PK, Febbo PG, Bikoff R, et al. mTOR inhibition reverses Akt-dependent prostate intraepithelial neoplasia via regulation of apoptotic and Hif1-dependent pathways. Nature Medicine 2004;10:594–601.

89. Sansal I, Sellers WR. The biology and clinical relevance of the PTEN tumor suppressor pathway. J Clin Oncol 2004;22:2954–2963.

90. Tolcher AW. Novel therapeutic molecular targets for prostate cancer: the mTOR signaling pathway and epidermal growth factor receptor. J Urol 2004;171:S41–43; [discussion S4].

91. Grunwald V, DeGraffenried L, Russel D, et al. Inhibitors of mTOR reverse doxorubicin resistance conferred by PTEN status in prostate cancer cells. Cancer Res 2002;62:6141–6145.

92. Yong EL, Lim J, Qi W, et al. Molecular basis of androgen receptor diseases. Ann Med 2000;32:15–22.

93. Huggins C, Hodges CV. Studies on prostatic cancer: 1. The effect of castration, of estrogen and androgen injection on serum phosphatases in metastatic carcinoma of the prostate. Cancer Res 1941;1:293–297.

94. Shah RB, Mehra R, Chinnaiyan AM, et al. Androgen-independent prostate cancer is a heterogeneous group of diseases: lessons from a rapid autopsy program. Cancer Res 2004;64:9209–9216.

95. Roudier MP, True LD, Higano CS, et al. Phenotypic heterogeneity of end-stage prostate carcinoma metastatic to bone. Hum Pathol 2003;34:646–653.

96. Hofer MD, Bismar TA, Kuefer R, et al. Determining pathologic risk factors for disease progression in high risk prostate cancer patients treated with radical prostatectomy. http://demarzolab.pathology.jhmi.edu.

97. Mucci NR, Akdas G, Manely S, et al. Neuroendocrine expression in metastatic prostate cancer: evaluation of high throughput tissue microarrays to detect heterogeneous protein expression. Hum Pathol 2000;31:406–414.

98. Visakorpi T, Hyytinen E, Koivisto P, et al. In vivo amplification of the androgen receptor gene and progression of human prostate cancer. Nat Genet 1995;9:401–406.

99. Gelmann EP. Molecular biology of the androgen receptor. J Clin Oncol 2002;20:3001–3015.

100. Giovannucci E, Stampfer MJ, Krithivas K, et al. The CAG repeat within the androgen receptor gene and its relationship to prostate cancer. Proc Natl Acad Sci USA 1997;94:3320–3323.

101. Schoenberg MP, Hakimi JM, Wang S, et al. Microsatellite mutation (CAG24→18) in the androgen receptor gene in human prostate cancer. Biochem Biophys Res Commun 1994;198:74–80.

102. Trapman J, Cleutjens KB. Androgen-regulated gene expression in prostate cancer. Semin Cancer Biol 1997;8:29–36.

103. Sadi MV, Barrack ER. Image analysis of androgen receptor immunostaining in metastatic prostate cancer. Heterogeneity as a predictor of response to hormonal therapy. Cancer 1993;71:2574–2580.

104. Sadi MV, Walsh PC, Barrack ER. Immunohistochemical study of androgen receptors in metastatic prostate cancer. Comparison of receptor content and response to hormonal therapy. Cancer 1991;67:3057–3064.

105. Magi-Galluzzi C, Xu X, Hlatky L, et al. Heterogeneity of androgen receptor content in advanced prostate cancer. Mod Pathol 1997;10:839–845.

106. Chen CD, Welsbie DS, Tran C, et al. Molecular determinants of resistance to antiandrogen therapy. Nat Med 2004;10:33–39.

107. Gil-Diez de Medina S, Salomon L, Colombel M, et al. Modulation of cytokeratin subtype, EGF receptor, and androgen receptor expression during progression of prostate cancer. Hum Pathol 1998;29:1005–1012.

108. Linja MJ, Savinainen KJ, Saramaki OR, et al. Amplification and overexpression of androgen receptor gene in hormone-refractory prostate cancer. Cancer Res 2001;61:3550–3555.

109. Debes JD, Tindall DJ. Mechanisms of androgen-refractory prostate cancer. N Engl J Med 2004;351:1488–1490.

110. Nupponen NN, Visakorpi T. Molecular cytogenetics of prostate cancer. Microsc Res Tech 2000;51:456–463.

111. Nupponen NN, Kakkola L, Koivisto P, et al. Genetic alterations in hormone-refractory recurrent prostate carcinomas. Am J Pathol 1998;153:141–148.

112. Jenkins RB, Qian J, Lieber MM, et al. Detection of c-myc oncogene amplification and chromosomal anomalies in metastatic prostatic carcinoma by fluorescence in situ hybridization. Cancer Res 1997;57:524–531.

113. Steiner MS, Anthony CT, Lu Y, et al. Antisense c-myc retroviral vector suppresses established human prostate cancer. Hum Gene Ther 1998;9:747–755.

114. Thompson TC, Southgate J, Kitchener G, et al. Multistage carcinogenesis induced by ras and myc oncogenes in a reconstituted organ. Cell 1989;56:917–930.

115. Bubendorf L, Kononen J, Koivisto P, et al. Survey of gene amplifications during prostate cancer progression by high-throughout fluorescence in situ hybridization on tissue microarrays. Cancer Res 1999;59:803–806.

116. Ellwood-Yen K, Graeber TG, Wongvipat J, et al. Myc-driven murine prostate cancer shares molecular features with human prostate tumors. Cancer Cell 2003;4:223–238.

117. Reiter RE, Gu Z, Watabe T, et al. Prostate stem cell antigen: a cell surface marker overexpressed in prostate cancer. Proc Natl Acad Sci USA 1998;95:1735–1740.

118. Gu Z, Thomas G, Yamashiro J, et al. Prostate stem cell antigen (PSCA) expression increases with high Gleason score, advanced stage and bone metastasis in prostate cancer. Oncogene 2000;19:1288–1296.

119. Reiter RE, Sato I, Thomas G, et al. Coamplification of prostate stem cell antigen (PSCA) and MYC in locally advanced prostate cancer. Genes Chromosomes Cancer 2000;27:95–103.

120. Ross S, Spencer SD, Holcomb I, et al. Prostate stem cell antigen as therapy target: tissue expression and in vivo efficacy of an immunoconjugate. Cancer Res 2002;62:2546–2553.

121. Ferdinandusse S, Denis S, van Berkel E, et al. Peroxisomal fatty acid oxidation disorders and 58 kDa sterol carrier protein X (SCPx). Activity measurements in liver and fibroblasts using a newly developed method. J Lipid Res 2000;41:336–342.

122. Kotti TJ, Savolainen K, Helander HM, et al. In mouse alpha-methylacyl-CoA racemase, the same gene product is simultaneously

located in mitochondria and peroxisomes. J Biol Chem 2000;275:20887–20895.

123. Ockner RK, Kaikaus RM, Bass NM. Fatty-acid metabolism and the pathogenesis of hepatocellular carcinoma: review and hypothesis. Hepatology 1993;18:669–676.

124. Tamatani T, Hattori K, Nakashiro K, et al. Neoplastic conversion of human urothelial cells in vitro by overexpression of H_2O_2-generating peroxisomal fatty acyl CoA oxidase. Int J Oncol 1999;15:743–749.

125. Luo J, Zha S, Gage WR, et al. alpha-Methylacyl-CoA racemase: a new molecular marker for prostate cancer. Cancer Res 2002;62:2220–2226.

126. Rubin MA, Zhou M, Dhanasekaran SM, et al. alpha-Methylacyl coenzyme A racemase as a tissue biomarker for prostate cancer. JAMA 2002;287:1662–1670.

127. Dhanasekaran SM, Barrette TR, Ghosh D, et al. Delineation of prognostic biomarkers in prostate cancer. Nature 2001;412:822–826.

128. Welsh JB, Sapinoso LM, Su AI, et al. Analysis of gene expression identifies candidate markers and pharmacological targets in prostate cancer. Cancer Res 2001;61:5974–5978.

129. Luo J, Duggan DJ, Chen Y, et al. Human prostate cancer and benign prostatic hyperplasia: molecular dissection by gene expression profiling. Cancer Res 2001;61:4683–4688.

130. Jiang Z, Woda BA, Rock KL, et al. P504S: a new molecular marker for the detection of prostate carcinoma. Am J Surg Pathol 2001;25:1397–1404.

131. Kuefer R, Varambally S, Zhou M, et al. alpha-Methylacyl-CoA racemase: expression levels of this novel cancer biomarker depend on tumor differentiation. Am J Pathol 2002;161:841–848.

132. Rubin MA, Bismar TA, Andrén O, et al. Decreased AMACR expression in localized prostate cancer is associated with biochemical recurrence and cancer specific death. 2005;14:1424–1432.

133. Rogers CG, Yan G, Zha S, et al. Prostate cancer detection on urinalysis for alpha methylacyl coenzyme a racemase protein. J Urol 2004;172:1501–1503.

134. Sreekumar A, Laxman B, Rhodes DR, et al. Humoral immune to alpha-methylacyl-CoA racemase and prostate cancer. J Natl Cancer Inst 2004;96:834–43.

135. Zielie PJ, Mobley JA, Ebb RG, et al. A novel diagnostic test for prostate cancer emerges from the determination of alpha-methylacyl-coenzyme a racemase in prostatic secretions. J Urol 2004;172:1130–1133.

136. Sreekumar A, Laxman B, Rhodes DR, et al. Humoral immune response to alpha-methylacyl-CoA racemase and prostate cancer. J Natl Cancer Inst 2004;96:834–843.

137. Jiang Z, Wu CL, Woda BA, et al. P504S/alpha-methylacyl-CoA racemase: a useful marker for diagnosis of small foci of prostatic carcinoma on needle biopsy. Am J Surg Pathol 2002;26:1169–1174.

138. Beach R, Gown AM, De Peralta-Venturina MN, et al. P504S immunohistochemical detection in 405 prostatic specimens including 376 18-gauge needle biopsies. Am J Surg Pathol 2002;26:1588–1596.

139. Sanderson SO, Sebo TJ, Murphy LM, et al. An analysis of the p63/alpha-methylacyl coenzyme A racemase immunohistochemical cocktail stain in prostate needle biopsy specimens and tissue microarrays. Am J Clin Pathol 2004;121:220–225.

140. Browne TJ, Hirsch MS, Brodsky G, et al. Prospective evaluation of AMACR (P504S) and basal cell markers in the assessment of routine prostate needle biopsy specimens. Hum Pathol 2004;35:1462–1468.

141. Medes G, Thomas A, Weinhouse S. Metabolism of neoplastic tissue. IV. A study of lipid synthesis in neoplastic tissue slices in vitro. Cancer Research 1953;13.

142. Sabine JR, Abraham S, Chaikoff IL. Control of lipid metabolism in hepatomas: insensitivity of rate of fatty acid and cholesterol synthesis by mouse hepatoma BW7756 to fasting and to feedback control. Cancer Res 1967;27:793–799.

143. Ookhtens M, Kannan R, Lyon I, et al. Liver and adipose tissue contributions to newly formed fatty acids in an ascites tumor. PG-R146-53. Am J Physiol 1984;247.

144. Weiss L, Hoffmann GE, Schreiber R, et al. Fatty-acid biosynthesis in man, a pathway of minor importance. Purification, optimal assay conditions, and organ distribution of fatty-acid synthase. Biol Chem Hoppe Seyler 1986;367:905–912.

145. Baron A, Migita T, Tang D, et al. Fatty acid synthase: a metabolic oncogene in prostate cancer? J Cell Biochem 2004;91:47–53.

146. Epstein JI, Carmichael M, Partin AW. OA-519 (fatty acid synthase) as an independent predictor of pathologic state in adenocarcinoma of the prostate. Urology 1995;45:81–86.

147. Rossi S, Graner E, Febbo P, et al. Fatty acid synthase expression defines distinct molecular signatures in prostate cancer. Mol Cancer Res 2003;1:707–715.

148. Swinnen JV, Van Veldhoven PP, Timmermans L, et al. Fatty acid synthase drives the synthesis of phospholipids partitioning into detergent-resistant membrane microdomains. Biochem Biophys Res Commun 2003;302:898–903.

149. McMenamin ME, Soung P, Perera S, et al. Loss of PTEN expression in paraffin-embedded primary prostate cancer correlates with high Gleason score and advanced stage. Cancer Res 1999;59:4291–4296.

150. Van de Sande T, De Schrijver E, Heyns W, et al. Role of the phosphatidylinositol 3'-kinase/PTEN/Akt kinase pathway in the overexpression of fatty acid synthase in LNCaP prostate cancer cells. Cancer Res 2002;62:642–646.

151. Kumar-Sinha C, Ignatoski KW, Lippman ME, et al. Transcriptome analysis of HER2 reveals a molecular connection to fatty acid synthesis. Cancer Res 2003;63:132–139.

152. Signoretti S, Montironi R, Manola J, et al. Her-2-neu expression and progression toward androgen independence in human prostate cancer. J Natl Cancer Inst 2000;92:1918–1925.

153. Hochachka PW, Rupert JL, Goldenberg L, et al. Going malignant: the hypoxia-cancer connection in the prostate. Bioessays 2002;24:749–757.

154. Kuhajda FP, Pizer ES, Li JN, Mani NS, Frehywot GL, Townsend CA. Synthesis and antitumor activity of an inhibitor of fatty acid synthase. Proc Natl Acad Sci USA 2000;97:3450–3454.

155. De Schrijver E, Brusselmans K, Heyns W, et al. RNA interference-mediated silencing of the fatty acid synthase gene attenuates growth and induces morphological changes and apoptosis of LNCaP prostate cancer cells. Cancer Res 2003;63:3799–3804.

156. Pizer ES, Pflug BR, Bova GS, et al. Increased fatty acid synthase as a therapeutic target in androgen-independent prostate cancer progression. Prostate 2001;47:102–110.

157. Graner E, Tang D, Rossi S, et al. The isopeptidase USP2a regulates the stability of fatty acid synthase in prostate cancer. Cancer Cell 2004;5:253–261.

158. Clegg DJ, Wortman MD, Benoit SC, McOsker CC, Seeley RJ. Comparison of central and peripheral administration of C75 on food intake, body weight, and conditioned taste aversion. Diabetes 2002;51:3196–3201.

159. Magee JA, Araki T, Patil S, et al. Expression profiling reveals hepsin overexpression in prostate cancer. Cancer Res 2001;61:5692–5696.

160. Stamey TA, Warrington JA, Caldwell MC, et al. Molecular genetic profiling of Gleason grade 4/5 prostate cancers compared to benign prostatic hyperplasia. J Urol 2001;166:2171–2177.

161. Vasioukhin V. Hepsin paradox reveals unexpected complexity of metastatic process. Cell Cycle 2004;3.

162. Klezovitch O, Chevillet J, Mirosevich J, et al. Hepsin promotes prostate cancer progression and metastasis. Cancer Cell 2004;6:185–195.

163. Rubin MA. Using molecular markers to predict outcome. J Urol 2004;172:S18–21 [discussion S2].

164. Voeller HJ, Augustus M, Madike V, et al. Coding region of NKX3.1, a prostate-specific homeobox gene on 8p21, is not mutated in human prostate cancers. Cancer Res 1997;57:4455–4459.

165. Bowen C, Bubendorf L, Voeller HJ, et al. Loss of NKX3.1 expression in human prostate cancers correlates with tumor progression. Cancer Res 2000;60:6111–6115.

166. Kim MJ, Bhatia-Gaur R, Banach-Petrosky WA, et al. Nkx3.1 mutant mice recapitulate early stages of prostate carcinogenesis. Cancer Res 2002;62:2999–3004.

167. He WW, Sciavolino PJ, Wing J, et al. A novel human prostate-specific, androgen-regulated homeobox gene (NKX3.1) that maps to 8p21, a region frequently deleted in prostate cancer. Genomics 1997;43:69–77.

168. Bieberich CJ, Fujita K, He WW, et al. Prostate-specific and androgen-dependent expression of a novel homeobox gene. J Biol Chem 1996;271:31779–31782.

169. Sciavolino PJ, Abrams EW, Yang L, et al. Tissue-specific expression of murine Nkx3.1 in the male urogenital system. Dev Dyn. 1997;209:127–138.

170. Korkmaz CG, Korkmaz KS, Monola J, et al. Analysis of androgen regulated homeobox gene NKX3.1 during prostate carcinogenesis. J Urol. 2004 Sep;172(3):1134–9.

171. Bhatia-Gaur R, Donjacour AA, Sciavolino PJ, et al. Roles for Nkx3.1 in prostate development and cancer. Genes Dev. 1999;13:966–977.

172. Magee JA, Abdulkadir SA, Milbrandt J. Haploinsufficiency at the Nkx3.1 locus. A paradigm for stochastic, dosage-sensitive gene regulation during tumor initiation. Cancer Cell 2003;3:273–283.

173. Francis NJ, Kingston RE. Mechanisms of transcriptional memory. Nat Rev Mol Cell Biol 2001;2:409–421.

174. Mahmoudi T, Verrijzer CP. Chromatin silencing and activation by Polycomb and trithorax group proteins. Oncogene 2001;20:3055–3066.

175. Varambally S, Dhanasekaran SM, Zhou M, et al. The polycomb group protein EZH2 is involved in progression of prostate cancer. Nature 2002;419:624–629.

176. Rhodes DR, Sanda MG, Otte AP, Chinnaiyan AM, Rubin MA. Multiplex biomarker approach for determining risk of prostate-specific antigen-defined recurrence of prostate cancer. J Natl Cancer Inst 2003;95:661–668.

177. Sellers WR, Loda M. The EZH2 polycomb transcriptional repressor—a marker or mover of metastatic prostate cancer? Cancer Cell 2002;2:349–350.

178. Rhodes DR, Barrette TR, Rubin MA, Ghosh D, Chinnaiyan AM. Meta-analysis of microarrays: interstudy validation of gene expression profiles reveals pathway dysregulation in prostate cancer. Cancer Res 2002;62:4427–4433.

179. Wang R, Xu J, Saramaki O, et al. PrLZ, a novel prostate-specific and androgen-responsive gene of the TPD52 family, amplified in chromosome 8q21.1 and overexpressed in human prostate cancer. Cancer Res 2004;64:1589–1594.

180. Rubin MA, Varambally S, Beroukhim R, et al. Overexpression, amplification, and androgen regulation of TPD52 in prostate cancer. Cancer Res 2004;64:3814–3822.

181. Sasaki H, Yukiue H, Kobayashi Y, et al. Expression of the MTA1 mRNA in thymoma patients. Cancer Lett 2001;174:159–163.

182. Toh Y, Kuwano H, Mori M, Nicolson GL, Sugimachi K. Overexpression of metastasis-associated MTA1 mRNA in invasive oesophageal carcinomas. Br J Cancer 1999;79:1723–1726.

183. Toh Y, Oki E, Oda S, et al. Overexpression of the MTA1 gene in gastrointestinal carcinomas: correlation with invasion and metastasis. Int J Cancer 1997;74:459–463.

184. Toh Y, Pencil SD, Nicolson GL. A novel candidate metastasis-associated gene, mta1, differentially expressed in highly metastatic mammary adenocarcinoma cell lines. cDNA cloning, expression, and protein analyses. J Biol Chem 1994;269:22958–22963.

185. Hofer MD, Kuefer R, Varambally S, et al. The role of metastasis-associated protein 1 in prostate cancer progression. Cancer Res 2004;64:825–829.

186. Martin DB, Gifford DR, Wright ME, et al. Quantitative proteomic analysis of proteins released by neoplastic prostate epithelium. Cancer Res 2004;64:347–355.

187. Santagata S, Demichelis F, Riva A, et al. JAGGED1 expression is associated with prostate cancer metastasis and recurrence. Cancer Res 2004;64:6854–6857.

188. Singh D, Febbo PG, Ross K, et al. Gene expression correlates of clinical prostate cancer behavior. Cancer Cell 2002;1:203–209.

189. Luo JH, Yu YP, Cieply K, et al. Gene expression analysis of prostate cancers. Mol Carcinog 2002;33:25–35.

190. Ramaswamy S, Ross KN, Lander ES, Golub TR. A molecular signature of metastasis in primary solid tumors. Nat Genet 2003;33:49–54.

191. Adam BL, Qu Y, Davis JW, et al. Serum protein fingerprinting coupled with a pattern-matching algorithm distinguishes prostate cancer from benign prostate hyperplasia and healthy men. Cancer Res 2002;62:3609–3614.

192. Petricoin EF, 3rd, Ornstein DK, Paweletz CP, et al. Serum proteomic patterns for detection of prostate cancer. J Natl Cancer Inst 2002;94:1576–1578.

193. Cher ML, MacGrogan D, Bookstein R, Brown JA, Jenkins RB, Jensen RH. Comparative genomic hybridization, allelic imbalance, and fluorescence in situ hybridization on chromosome 8 in prostate cancer. Genes Chromosomes Cancer 1994;11:153–162.

194. Visakorpi T, Kallioniemi AH, Syvanen AC, et al. Genetic changes in primary and recurrent prostate cancer by comparative genomic hybridization. Cancer Res 1995;55:342–347.

195. Joos S, Bergerheim US, Pan Y, et al. Mapping of chromosomal gains and losses in prostate cancer by comparative genomic hybridization. Genes Chromosomes Cancer 1995;14:267–276.

196. Abate-Shen C, Shen MM. Molecular genetics of prostate cancer. Genes Dev 2000;14:2410–2434.

197. Kononen J, Bubendorf L, Kallioniemi A, et al. Tissue microarrays for high-throughput molecular profiling of tumor specimens. Nat Med 1998;4:844–847.

198. Rubin MA. Tech.Sight. Understanding disease cell by cell. Science 2002;296:1329–1330.

199. Lindeman N, Waltregny D, Signoretti S, Loda M. Gene transcript quantitation by real-time RT-PCR in cells selected by immunohistochemistry-laser capture microdissection. Diagn Mol Pathol 2002;11:187–192.

200. Emmert-Buck MR, Bonner RF, Smith PD, et al. Laser capture microdissection. Science 1996;274:998–1001.

201. Strausberg RL. The Cancer Genome Anatomy Project: new resources for reading the molecular signatures of cancer. J Pathol 2001;195:31–40.

202. Strausberg RL, Greenhut SF, Grouse LH, Schaefer CF, Buetow KH. In silico analysis of cancer through the Cancer Genome Anatomy Project. Trends Cell Biol 2001;11:S66–71.

203. Rhodes DR, Yu J, Shanker K, et al. ONCOMINE: A Cancer Microarray Database and Integrated Data-Mining Platform. Neoplasia 2004;6:1–6.

204. Bova GS, Parmigiani G, Epstein JI, Wheeler T, Mucci NR, Rubin MA. Web-based tissue microarray image data analysis: initial validation testing through prostate cancer Gleason grading. Hum Pathol 2001;32:417–427.

205. Paez JG, Janne PA, Lee JC, et al. EGFR mutations in lung cancer: correlation with clinical response to gefitinib therapy. Science 2004;304:1497–500.

206. Smith JR, Freije D, Carpten JD, et al. Major susceptibility locus for prostate cancer on chromosome 1 suggested by a genome-wide search. Science 1996;274:1371–1374.

207. Berthon P, Valeri A, Cohen-Akenine A, et al. Predisposing gene for early-onset prostate cancer, localized on chromosome 1q42.2-43. Am J Hum Genet 1998;62:1416–1424.

208. Gibbs M, Stanford JL, McIndoe RA, et al. Evidence for a rare prostate cancer-susceptibility locus at chromosome 1p36. Am J Hum Genet 1999;64:776–787.

209. Xu J, Meyers D, Freije D, et al. Evidence for a prostate cancer susceptibility locus on the X chromosome. Nat Genet 1998;20:175–179.

210. Berry R, Schroeder JJ, French AJ, et al. Evidence for a prostate cancer-susceptibility locus on chromosome 20. Am J Hum Genet 2000;67:82–91.

Etiology of prostate cancer

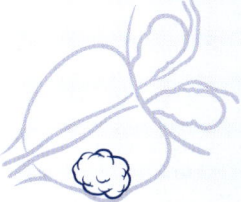

Concepts in the etiology of prostate cancer 17

Edith Canby-Hagino, Robin J Leach, Ian M Thompson

INTRODUCTION

Concepts in etiology of prostate cancer have evolved coincidentally with our deepening understanding of the complex interplay between the human genome and the environment. Given the heterogeneity of prostate cancers with regard to age of onset and aggressiveness, a unifying etiology for the majority of prostate cancers eludes discovery at this time and may not exist. In considering the etiology of prostate cancer, one can not remove suspect causes from the context of the interwoven domains of genetic determinants, endocrine milieu, and environmental exposure.

GENETIC DETERMINANTS

HEREDITARY PROSTATE CANCER

Based on twin studies, 42% of the risk for prostate cancer is the result of heritable factors.[1] However, only 10% of prostate cancers may be attributed to highly penetrant autosomal dominant genes and exhibit a mendelian pattern of inheritance.[2] While many candidate genes have been implicated in hereditary prostate cancer, their function and role in prostate carcinogenesis have not been clearly elucidated.

Numerous genome-wide linkage analyses of families with hereditary prostate cancer have suggested the presence of prostate cancer susceptibility genes on several chromosomes, and candidate genes at these loci have been identified; they are reviewed in more detail elsewhere in this text. The sheer number of candidate loci and genes for hereditary prostate cancer and the lack of consistent appearance of these candidates across ethnic, racial, and regional boundaries suggest, like sporadic prostate cancers, a complex interaction between genetic and environmental factors.

POLYMORPHISMS OF ANDROGEN AND OTHER METABOLIC LOCI

The majority of the hereditary loci have not been shown to play a major role in sporadic disease. This has led many investigators to propose that common variants in prostate-related genes may play a role in sporadic disease. These variants contribute slight-to-increased risk, but in combination could contribute to a genetic influence on sporadic disease. One such group of prostate-related genes is the androgen metabolic loci.

The androgen receptor (AR) gene has been the subject of substantial scrutiny with regard to both risk and progression of prostate cancer. Numerous studies have identified a shortened CAG trinucleotide repeat length in exon 1 to be associated with increased risk as well as associated with some cases of advanced, hormone-refractory disease.[3,4] The CAG repeat encodes a glutamine repeat in the N-terminal transactivation domain of the AR protein. In-vitro studies suggest that long CAG repeat lengths are associated with decreased transactivation of testosterone once it is bound to the AR.[5] Theoretically, this might exert a protective effect against the development of prostate cancer by decreasing prostatic epithelial proliferation in response to androgens.

More recently, several studies refute the association between shortened CAG repeat and prostate cancer risk.[6]

It is possible that earlier studies included a larger proportion of cases with clinically evident disease, reflecting the stage migration induced by widespread PSA screening. Perhaps CAG repeat length is more important in the etiology of clinically aggressive prostate cancer.[7]

The type II isozyme of steroid 5α-reductase, encoded by the *SRD5A2* gene, has also come under intense scrutiny, particularly in light of the recent completion of the Prostate Cancer Prevention Trial (PCPT).[8] Polymorphisms in SRD5A2 have functional consequences in vitro.[9] The functional significance of these polymorphisms and how they might affect risk for development of prostate cancer is currently the subject of intense study, and they may play a more important role in prognosis than carcinogenesis. Substitution for alanine by threonine at codon 49 (Ala49Thr) of SRD5A2 appears to confer five-fold greater enzymatic activity of 5α-reductase and has been associated with poor-prognosis prostate cancer, particularly in Hispanic and African-American men.[10,11] Finasteride, tested as a preventive agent in PCPT, has decreased affinity for isozyme produced by the Ala49Thr variant.[12] This may explain the relatively increased fraction of higher grade prostate cancers in the finasteride group, which was in fact similar to the rate of high-grade cancers in the placebo group.

Genes involved in biosynthesis of testosterone have also been implicated in prostate carcinogenesis. Cytochrome p450c17, encoded by the *CYP17* gene, catalyzes two important steps in the synthesis of testosterone in both the testis and adrenal gland. Some reports have linked a T to C polymorphism in the 5′ untranslated region (designated as A1 and A2 alleles) with an increased risk of prostate cancer in white males, others in hereditary cancer, while other have found no association with prostate cancer risk.[13–18]

Chromosome band 1p13 contains two homologous and closely linked genes, *HSD3B1* and *HSD3B2*, which code for 3β-hydroxysteroid dehydrogenase, an enzyme that catalyzes reductive reactions that inactivate dihydrotestosterone. The enzyme is thought to play an important role in regulating intraprostatic androgen levels.[19] Case-control studies of *HSD3B2* genetic polymorphisms have identified a complex series of $(TG)_n(TA)_n(CA)_n$ repeats to be substantially different among different populations at risk of prostate cancer.[20] A comprehensive screening of DNA from patients with and without prostate cancer identified 11 single nucleotide polymorphisms, 4 of which were informative.[21] Men with the variant genotypes at either B1-Asn367Thr or B2-C7519G were found to have a substantially increased risk of prostate cancer.

SOMATIC MUTATIONS

Genetic damage that leads to malignant transformation accumulates over a lifetime, a fact that may help explain why age is the single most important risk factor associated with the development of prostate cancer. Somatic mutations that accumulate with aging arise from both exogenous (e.g., environment, occupation, diet) and endogenous (e.g., inflammation) sources. The risk of prostate cancer associated with aging has been strongly linked to inherent ability to repair and respond to DNA damage, and the tendency of tumor suppressor genes to lose function with aging.[22,23]

Certain germline defects in DNA repair have been associated with specific cancer syndromes and extreme radiosensitivity, such as Nijmegen breakage syndrome and ataxia–telangiectasia. Given the lack of association of prostate cancer with such cancer-radiosensitivity syndromes, it is likely that more subtle, functional variations in DNA damage response and repair contribute to prostate cancer etiology. A number of polymorphisms in DNA repair genes have been linked to prostate cancer risk, including *BRCA1*, *BRCA2*, *CHEK2*, *XRCC1*, *ERCC1*, *OGG1* and *ATM*.[24–26] Given the relatively low prevalence of these genes, it is likely that these polymorphisms contribute to, but are not the sole causes of, accumulated DNA damage leading to initiation of prostate cancer.

When DNA damage is irreparable, the expected cellular response is initiation of apoptosis through a complex cascade of signals mediated by the ATM gene and affected by p53.[27] Many genes involved in the progressive signaling that culminates in apoptosis have been designated as tumor suppressor genes, given that their loss of function is associated with increased risk of malignancy.

Mutation, downregulation, or otherwise compromised function of tumor suppressor genes have been implicated in both the initiation and progression of prostate cancer. Function can be altered by mutation, methylation of the promoter, or modification of a gene's protein product; it is usually bi-allelic. One possible candidate tumor suppressor gene on 8p is *NKX3-1*. *NKX3-1* is expressed in normal prostate epithelial cells. Loss of either one or both *NKX3-1* alleles becomes increasingly common in prostate lesions as they progress from intraepithelial neoplasia to local, then metastatic and androgen independent tumors.[28]

Another tumor suppressor gene that may play a role in both initiation and progression of prostate cancer is *PTEN* on 10q23.[29] PTEN inactivates secondary messengers (including AKT, a serine/threonine kinase), which are phosphorylated in response to several growth factors, including insulin-like growth factor 1 (IGF1). Loss of PTEN results in increased phosphorylation of AKT, downregulation of the apoptotic mechanism, and increased proliferation of cells that might otherwise not be permitted to replicate. Loss of PTEN is associated with high Gleason score and advanced stage, and mutations of PTEN have been identified in up to a third of hormone-refractory prostate cancers.[30] Loss of PTEN has been identified both in high grade prostatic intraepithelial neoplasia and invasive carcinoma, suggesting that it is an early event in prostatic carcinogenesis. Complicating the evaluation of this marker has been the observation of substantial variation in PTEN defects at different metastatic sites.[31]

Genetic alterations in the classic tumor suppressor genes *RB1* and *p53* are less frequent in primary prostate cancer, but are commonly present in metastatic or hormone-refractory disease. Loss of their effects may be less important in initiation of prostate cancer, but may be critical to the development of aggressive, progressive disease. Loss of heterozygosity may be seen at the *RB1* locus (13q14.3); however, *RB1* does not appear to play a substantial role in the disease.[32] Using microcell hybrid techniques, introduction of chromosome 13 prevented development of metastases in a prostate cancer cell line; however, *RB1* specifically did not appear to play a role in suppressing metastases, thus implicating additional loci on chromosome 13 potentially related to the metastatic process.[33]

The oncogenes *MYC*, *ERBB2*, and *BCL2* have been observed in advanced and hormone refractory prostate cancer, but not commonly in low-stage and low-grade prostate cancers, suggesting that mutations of proto-oncogenes usually occur as secondary events after malignant degeneration.[34–36]

Somatic alterations in chromosomes associated with aging are also implicated in prostate cancer etiology. All eukaryotic chromosomes have telomeres on their ends, which consist of repeating units of 6 base pairs (TTAGGG) and binding proteins. Telomeres protect the chromosome ends from being misidentified as double-strand DNA breaks and help prevent inappropriate recombination.[37] Telomere length decreases successively with every cell replication. After 50 to 100 doublings, telomeres reach a critically short length, at which point cells undergo senescence and are arrested from further division. This process provides nonspecific protection against replication of cells that have accumulated unfavorable genetic alterations over time, but is not fail safe. Critical telomere shortening in animal models leads to chromosomal instability. This results in increased incidence of cancers, which are felt to be due to chromosomal fusions, breakage, and rearrangements.[38]

Telomerase, a ribonucleoprotein enzyme, acts as a reverse transcriptase to maintain or increase telomere length. The precise role of telomere length and telomerase expression in relation to prostatic carcinogenesis remains to be identified, but changes appear to occur early during prostate carcinogenesis.[39] Studies have identified both increased telomerase expression and (paradoxically) shortened telomere length in high-grade prostatic intraepithelial neoplasia and invasive cancers.[40]

Functional alteration in *GSTP1*, one of several genes coding for a glutathione-S-transferase (GST), is also likely to be an important early event in prostatic carcinogenesis. Glutathione transferases are a class of antioxidant enzymes designated as "caretakers" whose primary function is to catalyze the binding of electrophilic reactive oxygen species (both exogenous and endogenous) to glutathione, thereby detoxifying these DNA-damaging agents. Germline polymorphisms of the GST family of genes may have functional consequences that modify cancer risk, but prostate cancer case-control studies of GST polymorphisms fail to establish a clear association.[41–45]

A strong association has been found between somatic alteration of GST function and subsequent development of prostate cancer. Loss of *GSTP1* expression through hypermethylation of CpG islands in the *GSTP1* promoter region is suspected to be a very early event in carcinogenesis in the prostate.[46] Hypermethylation of the *GSTP1* promoter with subsequent loss of *GSTP1* expression has been found in 70% of high-grade prostatic intraepithelial neoplasias, and up to 100% of invasive prostate cancers.[40,46–56] Additionally, *GSTP1* hypermethylation has also been identified in prostate biopsies with histologic findings of proliferative inflammatory atrophy.[57] It is speculated that prostate epithelial proliferation in the setting of absent *GSTP1* "caretaker" function and an inflammatory environment rich in reactive oxygen species leads to replication of progressively more damaged DNA, culminating in neoplasia.[40]

ANDROGENS

There is little doubt that a lifetime of variable exposure of the prostate to androgens plays an important role in prostate carcinogenesis. The hormonal milieu in which prostate cancer develops has received the greatest attention in the study of prostate cancer etiology, yet remains ill defined. Long-term absence of androgen exposure to the prostate appears to protect against the development of prostate cancer, but a dose-response relationship between androgen levels and prostate cancer risk has not been established.

The primary androgen of the prostate is dihydrotestosterone (DHT), which is irreversibly catalyzed from testosterone by 5α-reductase. Dihydrotestosterone binds to intracytoplasmic ARs with much greater affinity than testosterone, and binding of DHT to the AR enhances translocation of the steroid–receptor complex into the nucleus and activation of androgen-response elements when compared with testosterone.[58] There are two isoenzymes of 5α-reductase, the product of two separate genes (type 1 on chromosome 5; type 2 on chromosome 2). Type-1 5α-reductase is expressed primarily in the skin and liver, while the type-2 enzyme is expressed predominantly in prostate epithelium and other genital tissues.[59]

Functional type-2 5α-reductase is a prerequisite for normal development of the prostate and external genitalia in males. The importance of 5α-reductase in genital development was first identified through studies of male pseudohermaphrodites in the 1960s.[60] An inherited deficiency in 5α-reductase activity in karyotypically normal males results in ambiguous genitalia, pseudovaginal perineoscrotal hypospadias, fully differentiated (although sometimes undescended) testes, normal Wolffian ductal systems, and an under-developed prostate. Although virilization occurs with the onset of puberty (presumably from hepatic conversion of testosterone to DHT by type-1 5α-reductase), the prostate remains underdeveloped.[61]

Insufficient exposure of the prostate to DHT appears to protect against the development of prostate cancer. Transrectal ultrasonography of males with inherited 5α-reductase deficiency demonstrates miniscule prostatic tissue, and biopsies demonstrate tissue consistent with prostatic stroma (fibrous connective tissue and smooth muscle), but no identifiable epithelial tissue.[62]

In addition to the lack of enzyme activity, a lack of substrate may also protect against the development of prostate cancer. The reader is referred to a review of long-term consequences of castration in Skoptzy, Chinese, and Ottoman eunuchs.[63] Medical studies described in this review were performed on men with mean duration of castration ranging from 18 to 54 years. Subjects were found to have atrophic and frequently impalpable prostates.

Additional evidence for the role of DHT in prostatic carcinogenesis comes from population-based studies that demonstrated an association between benign prostatic hyperplasia (BPH) and prostate cancer with levels of testosterone and DHT. Wu et al found that total and bioavailable testosterone are highest in Asian Americans, intermediate in African Americans, and lowest in whites.[64] These investigators also demonstrated that the DHT:testosterone ratio was highest in African Americans, intermediate in whites, and lowest in Asian Americans. This distribution of DHT:testosterone ratios parallels both incidence and mortality due to prostate cancer in these racial groups.[65]

The variations in DHT-testosterone and prostate cancer incidence have been associated with genetic polymorphisms of *SRD5A1* and *SRD5A2*, the genes that code for 5α-reductase, and are described in more detail above.

Although exposure of the prostate to androgens seems to be prerequisite for later development of prostate cancer, the duration and magnitude of androgen exposure needed to set the stage for carcinogenesis is not known. Both case-control and prospective epidemiologic studies have been employed to characterize the relationship between circulating levels of androgens and risk of prostate cancer, with mixed results. The strongest evidence in support of a positive relationship between circulating androgen levels and prostate cancer risk comes from the longitudinal Physician's Health Study, which identified a 2.6-fold increase in odds for prostate cancer for men with testosterone levels in the upper quartile, and a 54% reduction in odds for prostate cancer in men with sex hormone binding globulin (SHBG) in the upper quartile.[66] This is in contrast to the longitudinal Finnish Mobile Clinic Health Examination Survey, and a variety of case-control studies, which find no association between circulating androgens, SHBG, and prostate cancer risk.[67–71]

INFLAMMATION

Inflammation is a justifiable suspect in the causation of prostate cancer, given the frequent finding of inflammation on prostate biopsies, and the known deleterious effects of endogenous reactive oxygen species on DNA. Oxidant stresses from exogenous and endogenous sources are implicated in the accumulation of DNA damage that occurs with aging and subsequently leads to malignancy.[72] The oxidant stresses of chronic inflammation that lead to malignant degeneration are believed to be responsible for a number of human cancers, including colorectal, esophageal, gastric, bladder, and hepatocellular carcinomas.[72] The common finding of chronic inflammation in prostate biopsy specimens points to a possible association between prostatitis and subsequent development of prostate cancer.

Inflammatory cells in the prostate produce a variety of compounds designed to eradicate infectious microorganisms, many of which have potential to cause oxidative damage to DNA. These compounds include superoxide, hydrogen peroxide, oxygen free radicals, and peroxynitrite.[73] The inflammatory response stimulates the production of prostaglandins. Prostaglandins are part of a large family of regulatory molecules called eicosanoids, which include long-chain oxygenated polyunsaturated fatty acids derived from arachidonic acid. Cyclooxygenase (COX) enzymes catalyze the rate-limiting step of prostaglandin synthesis, converting arachidonic acid to the intermediate prostaglandin G2 via oxidative cyclization.[74]

Two isoforms of COX have been identified: *COX1* (on chromosome 9) and *COX2* (on chromosome 1).[75,76] COX1 and COX2 share identical catalytic mechanisms to generate the same products, but COX2 has a larger substrate-binding region, making it bind more efficiently to some substrates.

COX1 is expressed constitutively, with relatively constant levels and activity in most tissues, and is responsible for production of prostaglandins involved in normal physiologic functions, such as protection of gastric epithelium from an acidic environment, regulation of renal blood flow, and maintenance of normal platelet functions.

In contrast, COX2 expression is low or absent in most tissues at baseline, but expression can be rapidly induced and then return to basal levels in response to a number of inflammatory or mitogenic stimuli, including bacterial lipopolysaccharides, pro-inflammatory cytokines (interleukins 1β and 2 [IL1β, IL2] and tumor necrosis factor-α [TNF-α]), epidermal and platelet derived growth factors and androgens.[74,77] *COX2* expression is suppressed by corticosteroids and anti-inflammatory cytokines (IL4, IL10, and IL13).[74,78]

Prostaglandins resulting from *COX2* expression mediate a variety of responses to tissue injury and hypoxia, including apoptosis, cellular proliferation and angiogenesis. Induction of *COX2* appears to increase cellular resistance to apoptotic signaling. Proposed mechanisms for this include increased *BCL-2* expression (leading to inhibition of apoptosis), consumption of arachidonic acid substrate (leading to decreased production of proapoptotic ceramide), and decreased nitric oxide signaling.[74,77,79] *COX2* expression may also stimulate cellular proliferation through AKT phosphorylation.[80] Finally, *COX2* induction leads to increased expression of proangiogenic molecules, including vascular endothelial growth factor (VEGF), basic fibroblast growth factor (bFGF), thromboxane A2, prostaglandins E2 and I2 (PGE2 and PGI2).[74,81,82]

The potential for COX2 to inhibit apoptosis and promote proliferation and angiogenesis in an inflammatory, free-radical rich environment heightens the risk for replication of cells with genetic damage and is a proposed mechanism for inflammation-induced prostate cancers. Histopathologic evidence for this can be found in the diagnosis of proliferative inflammatory atrophy (PIA), in which epithelial proliferation arises in atrophic foci.[40] These foci are usually identified in the peripheral zone (the site of most prostate cancers), are usually accompanied by a chronic inflammatory infiltrate, and are frequently associated with high-grade prostatic intraepithelial neoplasia (PIN) or invasive prostate cancer.[83]

OBESITY

Multiple studies have correlated both a higher risk of prostate cancer and adverse outcomes after treatment with obesity. At this time, it is not clear whether obesity is an etiologic factor, affects treatment efficacy, or both. A number of changes are characteristic in the obese male that all may contribute to prostate cancer risk. Possible explanations for the apparent increased risk and worsened prognosis of prostate cancer in obese men include alterations in circulating estrogens and androgens, leptin, and oxidative stresses associated with dietary indiscretion.

OBESITY AND ANDROGENS

Population-based studies demonstrate an inverse relationship between circulating androgen levels and measures of obesity. The Tromso study, which included 1548 community-dwelling Norwegian men aged 25 to 84 years, demonstrated an inverse relationship between levels of testosterone and waist circumference, used as a surrogate measure of obesity.[84] Similarly, in a study of 1558 Danish military recruits, testosterone and SHBG decreased with increasing body mass index (BMI, another surrogate measure of obesity), while free testosterone as well as estradiol increased with increasing BMI.[85] Interestingly, in this study, though both testosterone and SHBG decreased, the fraction of free, bioavailable testosterone increased, perhaps providing more substrate for conversion to DHT.

A small, prospective, randomized controlled study of obese Finnish men suggests that treatment of obesity may modify risk for prostate cancer. After 10 weeks of a calorie-restricted diet, the men in the treatment group experienced a mean weight loss of 21 kilograms and experienced a rise in serum testosterone and SHBG levels, accompanied by a decrease in circulating levels of insulin and leptin.[86] These effects persist if men are able to maintain their weight loss.[87]

As noted above, the relationship between circulating levels of androgens and risk of prostate cancer is not clearly defined. There are no conclusive data that the reduction in circulating androgens seen in the obese state is linked to prostate cancer risk; and, as will be noted below, it may be that this reduction alters the presentation of prostate cancer, so that usual screening practices may be less effective in obese men.

Upon binding of DHT or other androgens to the AR, the steroid–receptor complex then binds to various androgen response elements (AREs) in the 5′ regulatory regions of various target genes, including the prostate-specific antigen (PSA) gene. Upon binding, various coactivators are recruited to the ARE site to regulate gene expression. Androgens are the most important activators of PSA expression.[88] Obesity or other factors which lower circulating androgen levels may decrease PSA production.

We have recently examined 2779 men who had no evidence of prostate cancer from a community-dwelling cohort. Using a linear contrast analysis to examine linear trend in mean PSA compared with rank-ordered covariates, we found that the level of PSA fell with each quintile of body mass index. Indeed, the least squares means for PSA for the lowest quintile of BMI was 1.01 ng/ml while the level for the highest quintile of BMI was 0.690 ng/ml.[89] These data would suggest that some of the current data suggesting worse prognostic features and adverse outcomes among obese men, when controlling for other prognostic factors, may be related to a delayed diagnosis of disease due to reduced levels of PSA, perhaps related to lower androgen levels.[90]

OBESITY AND LEPTIN

Leptin is an adiposity-related hormone, found at higher levels in obese individuals compared to lean individuals, and is reduced in the states of caloric restriction or starvation.[91] This 16 kDa peptide is secreted by adipocytes and acts systemically and in the central nervous system (CNS). In the CNS, leptin interacts with the arcuate nucleus of the hypothalamus to regulate feeding-related peptides such as neuropeptide Y, resulting in a decrease in feeding behavior and an increase in thermogenesis. Leptin is not released in response to meals, but instead regulates fats mass by helping to balance caloric consumption with energy expenditure.[92] In addition, normal levels of leptin are required for maintenance of gonadotropin secretion, an adaptive response that reduces the likelihood of reproduction in times of starvation.[93-95]

Outside of the CNS, leptin acts on a variety of peripheral cell types, which may serve to explain the association between obesity, prostate cancer, and prostate cancer with poor prognosis. The first report investigating leptin level and risk of prostate cancer by Lagiou et al showed no significant association.[96] In 2001, Chang et al reported a significant positive association between increased leptin levels and larger prostate cancer tumor volume.[91] Later that year, a nested case/control study derived from the Swedish arm of the World Health Organization Monitoring of Trends and Determinants in Cardiovascular Disease (WHO MONICA) study identified a 2.6-fold increased risk of prostate cancer in men with moderately increased leptin levels.[97] A subsequent study of Chinese men identified a positive association of waist-to-hip ratio (a measure of obesity) with prostate cancer risk, but a similar study of Norwegian men found no association between leptin levels and prostate cancer risk.[98,99]

In anticipation of results from these large studies, in vitro research is underway to elucidate possible mechanisms for leptin's role in prostate carcinogenesis. Leptin has been shown to stimulate proliferation of the androgen-independent prostate cancer cell lines DU145 and PC-3.[100,101] In addition, leptin appears to induce expression of VEGF and bFGF as well as cell migration, all of which are requisite for support of an invasive and growing malignancy.[102]

The argument for a role for leptin in prostate carcinogenesis is far from over. A recent case/control study from Portugal identified that prostate cancer patients were almost five times more likely to carry a genetic polymorphism that results in increased leptin expression, compared with controls.[103] It can be expected that future evaluations of the Prostate Cancer Prevention Trial and the San Antonio Center of Biomarkers of Risk for Prostate Cancer (SABOR) will provide more extensive evidence defining the relationship between leptin and prostate cancer risk in the near future.[3,8]

OBESITY AND OXIDATIVE STRESS

Oxidative stress induced by obesity creates a dangerous backdrop for mitogenic effects of leptin on prostate cells, increasing the potential for replication of cells with genetic damage. White fat in mammals serves not only as an important energy reservoir, but also as an endocrine organ, with secretion of cytokines and agents with cytokine-like activity, including tumor necrosis factor -α (TNFα), IL1β, IL6, IL8, IL10, transforming growth factor-β (TGFβ), as well as soluble receptors for these agents.[104] Obese individuals demonstrate significantly elevated markers of oxidative stress and lipid peroxidation, compared with normal-weight individuals. A number of studies, including the Framingham Study, have shown that BMI and waist circumference show significant positive correlation with plasma thiobarbituric acid reactive substance (TBARS) and urinary 8-epi-prostaglandin F2a, which are markers for lipid peroxidation and oxidative stress.[105,106] Treatment of obesity through reduction in fat intake and increased exercise has been shown to reduce oxidative stress as measured by urinary 8-epi-prostaglandin F2a, suggesting that lifestyle modification could be important in reducing the risk of prostate cancer.[107]

VITAMIN D, VITAMIN D RECEPTOR, AND CALCIUM

Since the observations of Hanchette and Schwartz that risk of prostate cancer death was geographically related to ultraviolet light exposure, a substantial amount of effort has examined the link of calcium and vitamin D with prostate cancer.[108] Vitamin D (1,25-dihydroxy-vitamin D3) is an essential vitamin that is a part of the steroid hormone superfamily. Human sources include both diet and sunlight-mediated conversion of pre-hormones in the skin.

A mechanism linking low levels of vitamin D to prostate carcinogenesis has not been elucidated, but a litany of findings from case-control studies suggest an association with prostate cancer risk, including the following:

1. Men with prostate cancer have lower levels of vitamin D compared with men without prostate cancer.[109]
2. Higher calcium intake (resulting in lower vitamin D levels) is associated with increased risk of prostate cancer.[110–112]
3. Higher fructose levels (fructose should reduce serum phosphate and, therefore, stimulate vitamin D production) are associated with a lower risk of prostate cancer.[110]

The antineoplastic effects of Vitamin D against prostate cancer can be supported by numerous in vitro and animal studies. Vitamin D exerts antiproliferative effects via cell cycle regulation in prostate cancer cell lines and xenografts.[113-118] At the present, both vitamin D (calcitriol) and newly developed vitamin D analogs are being explored as single agents and as adjuncts to chemotherapy in prostate cancer patients.[119]

The risk association between vitamin D level and prostate cancer risk is not clear cut. A recently published study of Nordic men consisting of 622 prostate cancer cases and 1451 matched controls shows that the distribution of risk for prostate cancer is U-shaped, relative to vitamin D levels, with increased risk at both low and high levels of vitamin D.[120] Possible explanations for increased risk with high levels of vitamin D include co-consumption of vitamin A from oily fish, other unknown dietary constituents that may be pro-neoplastic, or increased 24-hydroxylase activity, leading to increased degradation and decreased intraprostatic levels of 1, 25-dihydroxyvitamin D3.

Furthermore, a number of studies show either no or only weak associations of vitamin D levels with prostate cancer risk. A death-certificate based case-control study including 97,873 cases and 83,421 controls from 24 states showed no association between sunlight exposure and risk of death from prostate cancer.[121] The US Physicians' Health Study likewise showed no association between vitamin D levels and prostate cancer risk, although it did demonstrate an association between higher consumption of calcium and dairy products with increased risk for prostate cancer.[112,122] Likewise, the US Health Professionals Follow-up Study also failed to show a significant inverse relationship between vitamin D and prostate cancer.[123]

The conflicting findings regarding vitamin D and prostate cancer risk may be explained not by vitamin D levels, but by variants in the vitamin D receptor (VDR). Distribution of genetic polymorphisms of the VDR gene vary among ethnicities, which may provide a truer explanation for the geographic distribution of prostate cancer death; especially if populations used to study the link between ultraviolet exposure and prostate cancer risk are not ethnically diverse. Overall, these polymorphisms may not predict presence or prognosis of prostate cancer, but may be important determinants of risk and outcome in specific ethnic groups.[124] Polymorphisms resulting in VDR with lower activity have been associated with increased risk for prostate cancer, as well as with increased risk of biochemical recurrence following radical prostatectomy.[124-126]

CONCLUSIONS

It is clear that the process of carcinogenesis of prostate cancer is extremely complex. The interplay of constitutional, behavioral, and somatic factors, against the backdrop of various processes occurring during aging, interact to set into motion a series of events that ultimately are manifest through the diagnosis of prostate cancer. Complicating the understanding of this process are the various confounds associated with the diagnosis of the disease in clinical trials, in general populations, and in epidemiologic studies. Additionally, the blurred distinction of what constitutes biologically-consequential prostate cancer versus an indolent tumor with minimal-to-no risk over time, hampers the full understanding of the interaction of these factors. Future advances in the understanding of the etiology of prostate cancer will require prospective acquisition of these behavioral, constitutional, and somatic measures to understand which are essential elements and how these factors interact.

REFERENCES

1. Lichtenstein P, Holm NV, Verkasalo PK, et al. Environmental and heritable factors in the causation of cancer—analyses of cohorts of twins from Sweden, Denmark, and Finland [see comment]. N Engl J Med 2000;343:78–85.
2. Karan D, Lin MF, Johansson SL, Batra SK. Current status of the molecular genetics of human prostatic adenocarcinomas. Int J Cancer 2003;103:285–293.
3. Balic I, Graham ST, Troyer DA, et al. Androgen receptor length polymorphism associated with prostate cancer risk in Hispanic men. J Urol 2002;168:2245–2248.
4. Taplin ME, Rajeshkumar B, Halabi S, et al. Androgen receptor mutations in androgen-independent prostate cancer: Cancer and Leukemia Group B Study 9663. J Clin Oncol 2003;21:2673–2678.
5. Tut TG, Ghadessy FJ, Trifiro MA, Pinsky L, Yong EL. Long polyglutamine tracts in the androgen receptor are associated with reduced trans-activation, impaired sperm production, and male infertility. J Clin Endocrinol Metab 1997;82:3777–3782.
6. Freedman ML, Pearce CL, Penney KI, et al. Systematic evaluation of genetic variation at the androgen receptor locus and risk of prostate cancer in a multiethnic cohort study. Am J of Hum Genet 2005;76:82–90.
7. Giovannucci E. Is the androgen receptor CAG repeat length significant for prostate cancer? [comment]. Cancer Epidemiol Biomarkers Prev 2002;11:985–986.
8. Thompson IM, Goodman PJ, Tangen CM, et al. The influence of finasteride on the development of prostate cancer. [see comment]. N Engl J Med 2003;349:215–224.
9. Makridakis NM, Reichardt JK. Molecular epidemiology of androgen-metabolic loci in prostate cancer: predisposition and progression. J Urol 2004;171:S25–28; discussion S8–9.
10. Makridakis NM, Ross RK, Pike MC, et al. Association of mis-sense substitution in SRD5A2 gene with prostate cancer in African-American and Hispanic men in Los Angeles, USA. Lancet 1999;354:975–978.
11. Jaffe JM, Malkowicz SB, Walker AH, et al. Association of SRD5A2 genotype and pathological characteristics of prostate tumors. Cancer Res 2000;60:1626–1630.
12. Makridakis NM, di Salle E, Reichardt JK. Biochemical and pharmacogenetic dissection of human steroid 5 alpha-reductase type II. Pharmacogenetics 2000;10:407–413.
13. Loukola A, Chadha M, Penn SG, et al. Comprehensive evaluation of the association between prostate cancer and genotypes/haplotypes in CYP17A1, CYP3A4, and SRD5A2. Eur J Hum Genet 2004;12:321–332.
14. Cicek MS, Conti DV, Curran A, et al. Association of prostate cancer risk and aggressiveness to androgen pathway genes: SRD5A2, CYP17, and the AR. Prostate 2004;59:69–76.

15. Nam RK, Zhang WW, Trachtenberg J, et al. Comprehensive assessment of candidate genes and serological markers for the detection of prostate cancer. Cancer Epidemiol Biomarkers Prev 2003;12:1429–1437.

16. Gsur A, Bernhofer G, Hinteregger S, et al. A polymorphism in the CYP17 gene is associated with prostate cancer risk. Int J Cancer 2000;87:434–437.

17. Lunn RM, Bell DA, Mohler JL, Taylor JA. Prostate cancer risk and polymorphism in 17 hydroxylase (CYP17) and steroid reductase (SRD5A2). Carcinogenesis 1999;20:1727–1731.

18. Wadelius M, Andersson AO, Johansson JE, Wadelius C, Rane E. Prostate cancer associated with CYP17 genotype. Pharmacogenetics 1999;9:635–639.

19. Coffey DS. The molecular biology of the prostate. In Prostate Diseases, 1st ed. Philadelphia: WB Saunders; 1993.

20. Devgan SA, Henderson BE, Yu MC, et al. Genetic variation of 3 beta-hydroxysteroid dehydrogenase type II in three racial/ethnic groups: implications for prostate cancer risk. Prostate 1997;33:9–12.

21. Chang BL, Zheng SL, Hawkins GA, et al. Joint effect of HSD3B1 and HSD3B2 genes is associated with hereditary and sporadic prostate cancer susceptibility. Cancer Res 2002;62:1784–1789.

22. Goode EL, Ulrich CM, Potter JD. Polymorphisms in DNA repair genes and associations with cancer risk. [erratum appears in Cancer Epidemiol Biomarkers Prev. 2003;12:1119]. Cancer Epidemiol Biomarkers Prev 2002;11:1513–1530.

23. Li LC, Okino ST, Dahiya R. DNA methylation in prostate cancer. Biochim Biophys Acta 2004;1704:87–102.

24. Dong X, Wang L, Taniguchi K, et al. Mutations in CHEK2 associated with prostate cancer risk. Am J Hum Genet 2003;72:270–280.

25. Goode EL, Ulrich CM, Potter JD. Polymorphisms in DNA repair genes and associations with cancer risk. Cancer Epidemiol Biomarkers Prev 2002;11:1513–1530.

26. Hu JJ, Hall MC, Grossman L, et al. Deficient nucleotide excision repair capacity enhances human prostate cancer risk. Cancer Res 2004;64:1197–1201.

27. Zhou BB, Elledge SJ. The DNA damage response: putting checkpoints in perspective. Nature 2000;408:433–439.

28. Bowen C, Bubendorf L, Voeller HJ, et al. Loss of NKX3.1 expression in human prostate cancers correlates with tumor progression. Cancer Res 2000;60:6111–6115.

29. DeMarzo AM, Nelson WG, Isaacs WB, Epstein JI. Pathological and molecular aspects of prostate cancer. Lancet 2003;361:955–964.

30. Rubin MA, Gerstein A, Reid K, et al. 10q23.3 loss of heterozygosity is higher in lymph node-positive (pT2-3,N+) versus lymph node-negative (pT2-3,N0) prostate cancer. Hum Pathol 2000;31:504–508.

31. Suzuki H, Freije D, Nusskern DR, et al. Interfocal heterogeneity of PTEN/MMAC1 gene alterations in multiple metastatic prostate cancer tissues. Cancer Res 1998;58:204–209.

32. Latil A, Bieche I, Pesche S, et al. Loss of heterozygosity at chromosome arm 13q and RB1 status in human prostate cancer. Hum Pathol 1999;30:809–815.

33. Hosoki S, Ota S, Ichikawa Y, et al. Suppression of metastasis of rat prostate cancer by introduction of human chromosome 13. Asian J Androl 2002;4:131–136.

34. Qian J, Hirasawa K, Bostwick DG, et al. Loss of p53 and c-myc overrepresentation in stage T(2-3)N(1-3)M(0) prostate cancer are potential markers for cancer progression. Mod Pathol 2002;15:35–44.

35. Fossa A, Lilleby W, Fossa SD, Gaudernack G, Torlakovic G, Berner A. Independent prognostic significance of HER-2 oncoprotein expression in pN0 prostate cancer undergoing curative radiotherapy. Int J Cancer 2002;99:100–105.

36. Gurumurthy S, Vasudevan KM, Rangnekar VM. Regulation of apoptosis in prostate cancer. Cancer Metastasis Rev 2001;20:225–243.

37. Partin AW, Rodriguez R. Campbell's Urology, 8th ed. Saunders, 2002.

38. Blasco MA, Lee HW, Hande MP, et al. Telomere shortening and tumor formation by mouse cells lacking telomerase RNA.[see comment]. Cell 1997;91:25–34.

39. Sakr WA, Partin AW. Histological markers of risk and the role of high-grade prostatic intraepithelial neoplasia. Urology 2001;57:115–120.

40. De Marzo AM, Meeker AK, Zha S, et al. Human prostate cancer precursors and pathobiology. Urology 2003;62:55–62.

41. Aktas D, Hascicek M, Sozen S, Ozen H, Tuncbilek E. CYP1A1 and GSTM1 polymorphic genotypes in patients with prostate cancer in a Turkish population. Cancer Genet Cytogenet 2004;154:8185.

42. Ning B, Wang C, Morel F, et al. Human glutathione S-transferase A2 polymorphisms: variant expression, distribution in prostate cancer cases/controls and a novel form. Pharmacogenetics 2004;14:35–44.

43. Kidd LC, Woodson K, Taylor PR, Albanes D, Virtamo J, Tangrea JA. Polymorphisms in glutathione-S-transferase genes (GST-M1, GST-T1 and GST-P1) and susceptibility to prostate cancer among male smokers of the ATBC cancer prevention study. Eur J Cancer Prev 2003;12:317–320.

44. Medeiros R, Vasconcelos A, Costa S, et al. Metabolic susceptibility genes and prostate cancer risk in a southern European population: the role of glutathione S-transferases GSTM1, GSTM3, and GSTT1 genetic polymorphisms. Prostate 2004;58:414–420.

45. Nakazato H, Suzuki K, Matsui H, et al. Association of genetic polymorphisms of glutathione-S-transferase genes (GSTM1, GSTT1 and GSTP1) with familial prostate cancer risk in a Japanese population. Anticancer Res 2003;23:2897–2902.

46. Nakayama M, Bennett CJ, Hicks JL, et al. Hypermethylation of the human glutathione S-transferase-pi gene (GSTP1) CpG island is present in a subset of proliferative inflammatory atrophy lesions but not in normal or hyperplastic epithelium of the prostate: a detailed study using laser-capture microdissection. Am J Pathol 2003;163:923–933.

47. Harden SV, Sanderson H, Goodman SN, et al. Quantitative GSTP1 methylation and the detection of prostate adenocarcinoma in sextant biopsies. J Nat Cancer Inst 2003;95:1634–1637.

48. Harden SV, Guo Z, Epstein JI, Sidransky D. Quantitative GSTP1 methylation clearly distinguishes benign prostatic tissue and limited prostate adenocarcinoma. J Urol 2003;169:1138–1142.

49. Chu DC, Chuang CK, Fu JB, Huang HS, Tseng CP, Sun CF. The use of real-time quantitative polymerase chain reaction to detect hypermethylation of the CpG islands in the promoter region flanking the GSTP1 gene to diagnose prostate carcinoma. J Urol 2002;167:1854–1858.

50. Song JZ, Stirzaker C, Harrison J, Melki JR, Clark SJ. Hypermethylation trigger of the glutathione-S-transferase gene (GSTP1) in prostate cancer cells. Oncogene 2002;21:1048–1061.

51. Jeronimo C, Usadel H, Henrique R, et al. Quantitation of GSTP1 methylation in non-neoplastic prostatic tissue and organ-confined prostate adenocarcinoma. J Nat Cancer Inst 2001;93:1747–1752.

52. Lin X, Tascilar M, Lee WH, et al. GSTP1 CpG island hypermethylation is responsible for the absence of GSTP1 expression in human prostate cancer cells. Am J Pathol 2001;159:1815–1826.

53. Santourlidis S, Florl A, Ackermann R, Wirtz HC, Schulz WA. High frequency of alterations in DNA methylation in adenocarcinoma of the prostate. Prostate 1999;39:166–174.

54. Millar DS, Ow KK, Paul CL, Russell PJ, Molloy PL, Clark SJ. Detailed methylation analysis of the glutathione S-transferase pi (GSTP1) gene in prostate cancer. Oncogene 1999;18:1313–1324.

55. Brooks JD, Weinstein M, Lin X, et al. CG island methylation changes near the GSTP1 gene in prostatic intraepithelial neoplasia. Cancer Epidemiol Biomarkers Prev 1998;7:531–536.

56. Lee WH, Isaacs WB, Bova GS, Nelson WG. CG island methylation changes near the GSTP1 gene in prostatic carcinoma cells detected using the polymerase chain reaction: a new prostate cancer biomarker. Cancer Epidemiol Biomarkers Prev 1997;6:443–450.

57. Nakayama M, Gonzalgo ML, Yegnasubramanian S, Lin X, De Marzo AM, Nelson WG. GSTP1 CpG island hypermethylation as a molecular biomarker for prostate cancer. J Cell Biochem 2004;91:540–552.

58. Steers WD. 5alpha-reductase activity in the prostate. Urology 2001;58:17–24 [discussion].

59. Andriole G, Bruchovsky N, Chung LW, et al. Dihydrotestosterone and the prostate: the scientific rationale for 5alpha-reductase inhibitors in the treatment of benign prostatic hyperplasia. J Urol 2004;172:1399–1403.

60. Walsh PC, Madden JD, Harrod MJ, Goldstein JL, MacDonald PC, Wilson JD. Familial incomplete male pseudohermaphroditism, type 2. Decreased dihydrotestosterone formation in pseudovaginal perineoscrotal hypospadias. N Engl J Med 1974;291:944–949.

61. Imperato-McGinley J, Zhu YS. Androgens and male physiology: the syndrome of 5alpha-reductase-2 deficiency. Mol Cell Endocrinol 2002;198:51–59.

62. Imperato-McGinley J, Gautier T, Zirinsky K, et al. Prostate visualization studies in males homozygous and heterozygous for 5 alpha-reductase deficiency. J Clin Endocrinol Metab 1992;75:1022–1026.

63. Wilson JD, Roehrborn C. Long-term consequences of castration in men: lessons from the Skoptzy and the eunuchs of the Chinese and Ottoman courts.[see comment]. J Clin Endocrinol Metab 1999;84:4324–4331.

64. Wu AH, Whittemore AS, Kolonel LN, et al. Serum androgens and sex hormone-binding globulins in relation to lifestyle factors in older African-American, white, and Asian men in the United States and Canada. Cancer Epidemiol Biomarkers Prev 1995;4:735–741.

65. Hsing AW, Tsao L, Devesa SS. International trends and patterns of prostate cancer incidence and mortality. Int J Cancer 2000;85:60–67.

66. Gann PH, Hennekens CH, Ma J, Longcope C, Stampfer MJ. Prospective study of sex hormone levels and risk of prostate cancer.[see comment]. J Nat Cancer Inst 1996;88:1118–1126.

67. Stattin P, Lumme S, Tenkanen L, et al. High levels of circulating testosterone are not associated with increased prostate cancer risk: a pooled prospective study. Int J Cancer 2004;108:418–424.

68. Chen C, Weiss NS, Stanczyk FZ, et al. Endogenous sex hormones and prostate cancer risk: a case-control study nested within the Carotene and Retinol Efficacy Trial. Cancer Epidemiol Biomarkers Prev 2003;12:1410–1416.

69. Kaaks R, Lukanova A, Rinaldi S, et al. Interrelationships between plasma testosterone, SHBG, IGF-I, insulin and leptin in prostate cancer cases and controls. Eur J Cancer Prev 2003;12:309–315.

70. Heikkila R, Aho K, Heliovaara M, et al. Serum testosterone and sex hormone-binding globulin concentrations and the risk of prostate carcinoma: a longitudinal study. Cancer 1999;86:312–315.

71. Eaton NE, Reeves GK, Appleby PN, Key TJ. Endogenous sex hormones and prostate cancer: a quantitative review of prospective studies. Br J Cancer 1999;80:930–934.

72. Coussens LM, Werb Z. Inflammation and cancer.[see comment]. Nature 2002;420:860–867.

73. Potts JM, Pasqualotto FF. Seminal oxidative stress in patients with chronic prostatitis. Andrologia 2003;35:304–308.

74. Zha S, Yegnasubramanian V, Nelson WG, Isaacs WB, De Marzo AM. Cyclooxygenases in cancer: progress and perspective. Cancer Lett 2004;215:1–20.

75. DeWitt DL, Smith WL. Primary structure of prostaglandin G/H synthase from sheep vesicular gland determined from the complementary DNA sequence.[erratum appears in Proc Natl Acad Sci USA 1988 Jul;85:5056]. Proc Natl Acad Sci USA 1988;85:1412–1416.

76. Hla T, Neilson K. Human cyclooxygenase-2 cDNA. Proc Natl Acad Sci USA 1992;89:7384–7388.

77. Pruthi RS, Derksen E, Gaston K. Cyclooxygenase-2 as a potential target in the prevention and treatment of genitourinary tumors: a review. J Urol 2003;169:2352–2359.

78. Nagano S, Otsuka T, Niiro H, et al. Molecular mechanisms of lipopolysaccharide-induced cyclooxygenase-2 expression in human neutrophils: involvement of the mitogen-activated protein kinase pathway and regulation by anti-inflammatory cytokines. Int Immunol 2002;14:733–740.

79. Chan TA, Morin PJ, Vogelstein B, Kinzler KW. Mechanisms underlying nonsteroidal antiinflammatory drug-mediated apoptosis. Proc Natl Acad Sci USA 1998;95:681–686.

80. Leng J, Han C, Demetris AJ, Michalopoulos GK, Wu T. Cyclooxygenase-2 promotes hepatocellular carcinoma cell growth through Akt activation: evidence for Akt inhibition in celecoxib-induced apoptosis. Hepatology 2003;38:756–768.

81. Gately S. The contributions of cyclooxygenase-2 to tumor angiogenesis. Cancer Metastasis Rev 2000;19:19–27.

82. Yu HG, Li JY, Yang YN, et al. Increased abundance of cyclooxygenase-2 correlates with vascular endothelial growth factor-A abundance and tumor angiogenesis in gastric cancer. Cancer Lett 2003;195:43–51.

83. De Marzo AM, Marchi VL, Epstein JI, Nelson WG. Proliferative inflammatory atrophy of the prostate: implications for prostatic carcinogenesis. Am J Pathol 1999;155:1985–1992.

84. Svartberg J, von Muhlen D, Sundsfjord J, Jorde R. Waist circumference and testosterone levels in community dwelling men. The Tromso study. Eur J Epidemiol 2004;19:657–663.

85. Jensen TK, Andersson AM, Jorgensen N, et al. Body mass index in relation to semen quality and reproductive hormones among 1,558 Danish men. Fertility Sterility 2004;82:863–870.

86. Kaukua J, Pekkarinen T, Sane T, Mustajoki P. Sex hormones and sexual function in obese men losing weight. Obesity Res 2003;11:689–694.

87. Niskanen L, Laaksonen DE, Punnonen K, Mustajoki P, Kaukua J, Rissanen A. Changes in sex hormone-binding globulin and testosterone during weight loss and weight maintenance in abdominally obese men with the metabolic syndrome. Diabetes, Obesity Metab 2004;6:208–215.

88. Kim J, Coetzee GA. Prostate specific antigen gene regulation by androgen receptor. J Cell Biochem 2004;93:233–241.

89. Baillargeon J, Pollock BH, Kristal AR, et al. The association of body mass index and prostate-specific-antigen in a population-based study. Cancer 2005 (Epub ahead of print Jan 24).

90. Freedland SJ, Terris MK, Presti JC Jr, et al. Obesity and biochemical outcome following radical prostatectomy for organ confined disease with negative surgical margins. J Urol 2004;172:520–524.

91. Chang S, Hursting SD, Contois JH, et al. Leptin and prostate cancer. Prostate 2001;46:62–67.

92. Friedman JM, Halaas JL. Leptin and the regulation of body weight in mammals. Nature 1998;395:763–770.

93. Schurgin S, Canavan B, Koutkia P, Depaoli AM, Grinspoon S. Endocrine and metabolic effects of physiologic r-metHuLeptin administration during acute caloric deprivation in normal-weight women. J Clin Endocrinol Metab 2004;89:5402–5409.

94. Maciel MN, Zieba DA, Amstalden M, Keisler DH, Neves JP, Williams GL. Leptin prevents fasting-mediated reductions in pulsatile secretion of luteinizing hormone and enhances its gonadotropin-releasing hormone-mediated release in heifers. Biol Reprod 2004;70:229–235.

95. Wilson ME, Fisher J, Chikazawa K, et al. Leptin administration increases nocturnal concentrations of luteinizing hormone and growth hormone in juvenile female rhesus monkeys. J Clin Endocrinol Metab 2003;88:4874–4883.

96. Lagiou P, Signorello LB, Trichopoulos D, Tzonou A, Trichopoulou A, Mantzoros CS. Leptin in relation to prostate cancer and benign prostatic hyperplasia. Int J Cancer 1998;76:25–28.

97. Stattin P, Soderberg S, Hallmans G, et al. Leptin is associated with increased prostate cancer risk: a nested case-referent study. J Clin Endocrinol Metab 2001;86:1341–1345.

98. Hsing AW, Chua S Jr, Gao YT, et al. Prostate cancer risk and serum levels of insulin and leptin: a population-based study [see comment]. J Natl Cancer Inst 2001;93:783–789.

99. Stattin P, Kaaks R, Johansson R, et al. Plasma leptin is not associated with prostate cancer risk. Cancer Epidemiol Biomarkers Prev 2003;12:474–475.

100. Onuma M, Bub JD, Rummel TL, Iwamoto Y. Prostate cancer cell–adipocyte interaction: leptin mediates androgen-independent prostate cancer cell proliferation through c-Jun NH2-terminal kinase. J Biol Chem 2003;278:42660–42667.

101. Somasundar P, Frankenberry KA, Skinner H, et al. Prostate cancer cell proliferation is influenced by leptin. J Surg Res 2004;118:71–82.

102. Frankenberry KA, Somasundar P, McFadden DW, Vona-Davis LC. Leptin induces cell migration and the expression of growth factors in human prostate cancer cells. Am J Surg 2004;188:560–565.

103. Ribeiro R, Vasconcelos A, Costa S, et al. Overexpressing leptin genetic polymorphism (-2548 G/A) is associated with susceptibility to prostate cancer and risk of advanced disease. Prostate 2004;59:268–274.

104. Trayhurn P, Wood IS. Adipokines: inflammation and the pleiotropic role of white adipose tissue. Br J Nutr 2004;92:347–355.

105. Furukawa S, Fujita T, Shimabukuro M, et al. Increased oxidative stress in obesity and its impact on metabolic syndrome. J Clin Invest 2004;114:1752–1761.

106. Keaney JF, Jr., Larson MG, Vasan RS, et al. Obesity and systemic oxidative stress: clinical correlates of oxidative stress in the Framingham Study [see comment]. Arterioscler Thromb Vasc Biol 2003;23:434–439.

107. Roberts CK, Vaziri ND, Barnard RJ. Effect of diet and exercise intervention on blood pressure, insulin, oxidative stress, and nitric oxide availability. Circulation 2002;106:2530–2532.

108. Hanchette CL, Schwartz GG. Geographic patterns of prostate cancer mortality. Evidence for a protective effect of ultraviolet radiation. Cancer 1992;70:2861–2869.

109. Corder EH, Guess HA, Hulka BS, et al. Vitamin D and prostate cancer: a prediagnostic study with stored sera [see comment]. Cancer Epidemiol Biomarkers Prev 1993;2:467–472.

110. Giovannucci E, Rimm EB, Wolk A, et al. Calcium and fructose intake in relation to risk of prostate cancer. Cancer Res 1998;58:442–447.

111. Rodriguez C, McCullough ML, Mondul AM, et al. Calcium, dairy products, and risk of prostate cancer in a prospective cohort of United States men. Cancer Epidemiol Biomarkers Prev 2003;12:597–603.

112. Chan JM, Giovannucci EL. Dairy products, calcium, and vitamin D and risk of prostate cancer. Epidemiol Rev 2001;23:87–92.

113. Yang ES, Burnstein KL. Vitamin D inhibits G1 to S progression in LNCaP prostate cancer cells through p27Kip1 stabilization and Cdk2 mislocalization to the cytoplasm. J Biol Chem 2003;278:46862–46868.

114. Yang ES, Maiorino CA, Roos BA, Knight SR, Burnstein KL. Vitamin D-mediated growth inhibition of an androgen-ablated LNCaP cell line model of human prostate cancer. Mol Cell Endocrinol 2002;186:69–79.

115. Moffatt KA, Johannes WU, Hedlund TE, Miller GJ. Growth inhibitory effects of 1alpha, 25-dihydroxyvitamin D(3) are mediated by increased levels of p21 in the prostatic carcinoma cell line ALVA-31. Cancer Res 2001;61:7122–7129.

116. Vegesna V, O'Kelly J, Said J, Uskokovic M, Binderup L, Koeffle HP. Ability of potent vitamin D3 analogs to inhibit growth of prostate cancer cells in vivo. Anticancer Res 2003;23:283–289.

117. Guzey M, Kitada S, Reed JC. Apoptosis induction by 1alpha,25-dihydroxyvitamin D3 in prostate cancer. Mol Cancer Therapeutics 2002;1:667–677.

118. Getzenberg RH, Light BW, Lapco PE, et al. Vitamin D inhibition of prostate adenocarcinoma growth and metastasis in the Dunning rat prostate model system. Urology 1997;50:999–1006.

119. Crescioli C, Maggi M, Luconi M, et al. Vitamin D3 analogue inhibits keratinocyte growth factor signaling and induces apoptosis in human prostate cancer cells. Prostate 2002;50:15–26.

120. Tuohimaa P, Tenkanen L, Ahonen M, et al. Both high and low levels of blood vitamin D are associated with a higher prostate cancer risk: a longitudinal, nested case-control study in the Nordic countries [see comment]. Int J Cancer 2004;108:104–108.

121. Freedman DM, Dosemeci M, McGlynn K. Sunlight and mortality from breast, ovarian, colon, prostate, and non-melanoma skin cancer: a composite death certificate based case-control study. Occupat Environ Med 2002;59:257–262.

122. Gann PH, Ma J, Hennekens CH, Hollis BW, Haddad JG, Stampfer MJ. Circulating vitamin D metabolites in relation to subsequent development of prostate cancer. Cancer Epidemiol Biomarkers Prev 1996;5:121–126.

123. Platz EA, Leitzmann MF, Hollis BW, Willett WC, Giovannucci E. Plasma 1,25-dihydroxy- and 25-hydroxyvitamin D and subsequent risk of prostate cancer. Cancer Causes Control 2004;15:255–265.

124. Williams H, Powell IJ, Land SJ, et al. Vitamin D receptor gene polymorphisms and disease free survival after radical prostatectomy. Prostate 2004;61:267–275.

125. Oakley-Girvan I, Feldman D, Eccleshall TR, et al. Risk of early-onset prostate cancer in relation to germ line polymorphisms of the vitamin D receptor. Cancer Epidemiol Biomarkers Prev 2004;13:1325–1330.

126. Medeiros R, Morais A, Vasconcelos A, et al. The role of vitamin D receptor gene polymorphisms in the susceptibility to prostate cancer of a southern European population. J Hum Genet 2002;47:413–418.

Obesity and prostate cancer 18

Stephen J Freedland, William J Aronson

INTRODUCTION

Obesity is a rapidly growing epidemic. Today, over 30% of adults in the United States are obese compared with only 15% less than 20 years ago (Figures 18.1 and 18.2).[1] Obesity is associated with the development of multiple chronic diseases including coronary artery disease, hypertension, diabetes, asthma, and arthritis.[2] Obesity has also been linked to the development of several types of cancer including post-menopausal breast cancer and colon cancer.[3]

Prostate cancer is a major public health concern. It is the most commonly diagnosed non-skin cancer among men and the second leading cause of cancer death.[4] Despite the high prevalence of both prostate cancer and obesity, only recently have researchers begun to study the association between these two diseases in earnest. A PubMed literature search using the keywords "obesity" and "prostate cancer" in November 2004 demonstrated 134 papers of which 82 (61%) were published since January 1 2000, showing that the majority of the literature on obesity and prostate cancer has been written in the last 5 years.

There are several difficulties in trying to examine the association between obesity and prostate cancer. The first is the definition of obesity. Webster's dictionary defines obesity as "a condition characterized by excessive bodily fat."[5] However, how does one measure excessive bodily fat? One of the most common definitions of obesity is increased body mass index (BMI), which is calculated by dividing the weight in kilograms by the square of the height in meters. Both the World Health Organization and the National Institutes of Health define overweight as a BMI greater than 25

kg/m^2 (5'11" [1.8 m] man weighing 180 pounds [82 kg]) and obesity as a BMI greater than 30 kg/m^2 (5'11" [1.8 m] man weighing 215 pounds [98 kg]). While easy to calculate and, therefore, ideal for studies, BMI has its limitations. For example, body composition, such as whether someone is particularly muscular or thick-boned are not factored in to BMI calculations. Therefore, alternative measurements and definitions of obesity including waist-to-hip ratio (WHR), waist circumference, percentage body fat, skinfold thickness, crude weight, and lean body mass have all been used in various studies. Another difficulty encountered in studying obesity is that, due to the excess bodily fat, there are marked alterations in the serum concentrations of numerous hormones including testosterone, estrogen, insulin, insulin-like growth factor 1 (IGF1), and leptin, all of which have been linked to prostate cancer in some studies. In addition, obesity is highly correlated with dietary intake: on average, obese men consume more calories and greater amounts of dietary fat, both of which have been linked to cancer.[6]

A comprehensive review of all the various sequelae of obesity and their possible relationships to prostate cancer is beyond the scope of this chapter (Figure 18.3). Therefore, we will concentrate on recent studies examining the epidemiologic data relating obesity itself (predominantly, increased BMI) with risk of development, progression following therapy, and death from prostate cancer. We will also briefly touch on some new data suggesting that it may be harder to detect prostate cancers among obese men in the prostate-specific antigen (PSA) era leading to delayed diagnosis. For epidemiologic studies relating obesity to the risk of development of and death from prostate cancer, we will focus on results from large prospective

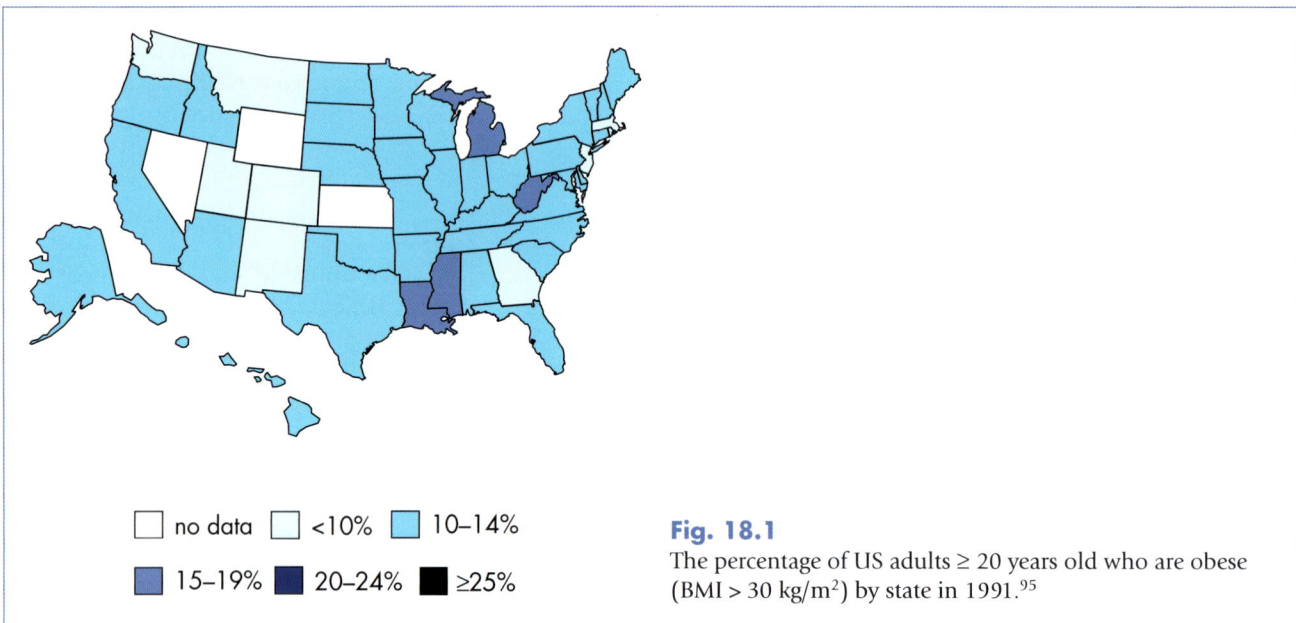

Fig. 18.1
The percentage of US adults ≥ 20 years old who are obese (BMI > 30 kg/m^2) by state in 1991.[95]

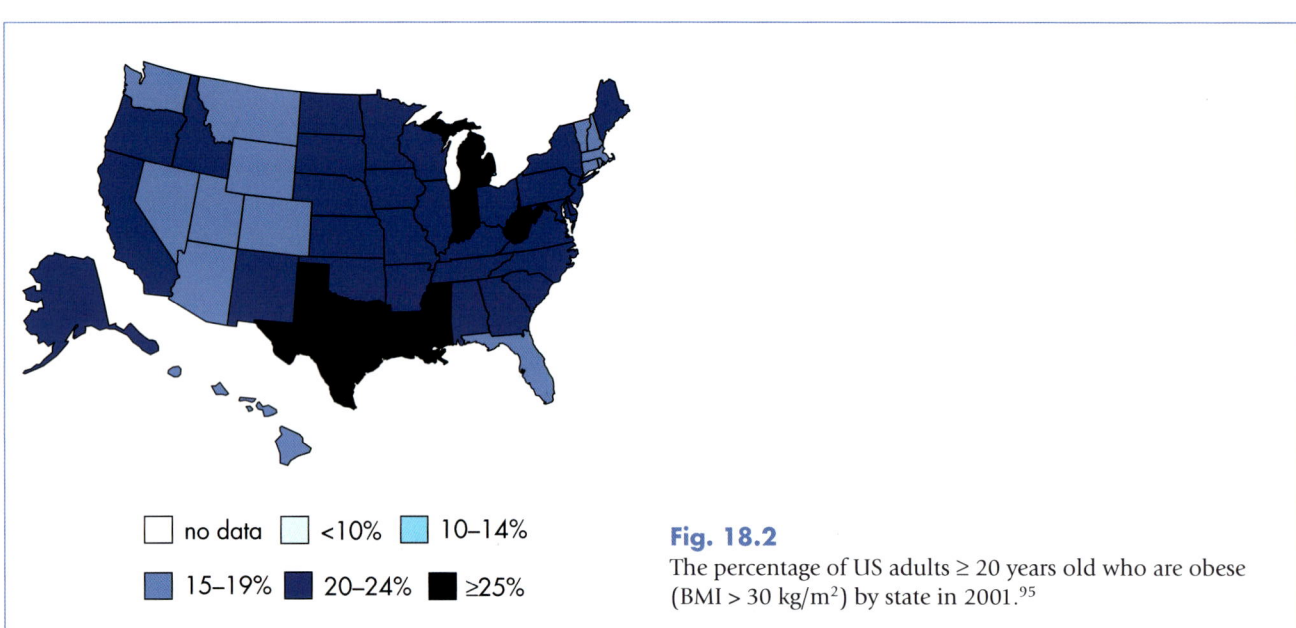

Fig. 18.2
The percentage of US adults ≥ 20 years old who are obese (BMI > 30 kg/m^2) by state in 2001.[95]

population-based studies. The reason for choosing these studies is they generally have larger sample sizes, thus allowing greater power to detect associations. In addition, exposure risk factors (e.g., body mass index) have been recorded prior to the event (i.e., diagnosis of prostate cancer), thus minimizing potential recall bias and any possible effects the tumor may have on the risk factor (i.e., advanced prostate cancer causing cachexia and thus lowering BMI, or hormone production by the tumor itself, etc.).

We will also briefly describe some of the hormonal sequelae of obesity and their relationship to prostate cancer with particular attention to insulin, the IGF-axis, and leptin. In addition, obesity is associated with decreased serum concentrations of testosterone and increased serum estradiol concentrations, both of which may play a key role in the development and progression

of prostate cancer in obese men. Though clearly important factors in understanding the association between obesity and prostate cancer, due to space limitations, we will only briefly mention the sex hormones. For detailed reviews regarding sex hormones or hormones in general and their relationship to prostate cancer, the reader is referred to Chapters 7, 9, and 10, and to reviews by Hsing et al, Kaaks et al, and Bosland.[7–9] In addition, the role of diet and physical activity is beyond the scope of this review, and the reader is referred to Chapter 17, and to reviews by Kolonel et al, Dagnelie et al, and Platz.[10–12] Finally, as we will outline below, results of the studies regarding obesity and prostate cancer often appear to conflict with one other, and so obtaining a unified "take-home" message is difficult. However, whenever possible we will try to point out differences between studies that may account for these discrepancies in findings, and attempt to summarize the literature into a bottom-line "take-home" message.

OBESITY AND RISK OF DEVELOPMENT OF PROSTATE CANCER

Prior studies examining the relationship between adult BMI and risk of developing prostate cancer have been mixed. Several large studies found that increased BMI in adulthood was associated with an increased risk of developing prostate cancer.[13-16] However, among these studies, some only showed increased risk for men in the highest BMI category,[14] and others found only a weak, albeit statistically significant, association with prostate cancer risk (RR 1.09 for highest versus lowest BMI category, 95% CI: 1.04–1.15).[15] On the other hand, numerous studies have found no association between adult BMI and prostate cancer risk.[17-21] More recently, several studies from the United States have found an inverse association between obesity and prostate cancer diagnosis. A prospective cohort study using data from the Health Professionals Follow-up Study found that increased BMI was associated with a decreased risk of developing prostate cancer, but only among men under 60 years old, or those with a family history.[22] Similarly, a population-based case-control study using data from the Surveillance, Epidemiology, and End Results (SEER) cancer registry also found an inverse association between increased BMI and prostate cancer risk.[23] Finally, a study of men undergoing prostate biopsy at a Veterans Affairs Medical Center (VAMC) found a lower prostate cancer detection rate among obese men.[24]

It is interesting to note that, historically, most studies found either a positive or null association between obesity and prostate cancer risk. However, several recent studies from the United States, largely during the PSA-era, suggest an inverse association. One possible explanation for this changing association is that PSA screening may be inherently biased against finding prostate cancer among obese men. Increasing evidence from several large population based studies suggest that obese men have lower PSA concentrations than normal weight men,[25-27] presumably the result of lower androgenicity among obese men resulting in less PSA production,[28] given that PSA production is under direct androgenic control.[29] Lower PSA concentrations would make obese men less likely to have an abnormal PSA test and undergo biopsy resulting in fewer cancers detected. In addition, obese men have larger prostates (Freedland et al, unpublished data).[30,31] Prostatic enlargement would make detection of an existent cancer less likely, given an equal sized tumor and an equal number of biopsy cores were obtained.[32,33] Combining lower PSA concentrations and prostatic enlargement would represent an inherent bias against detecting cancers among obese men. Consequently, if cancers are harder to detect among obese men this may lead to delayed diagnosis and subsequently later stage disease at the time of diagnosis. Indeed, in the biopsy-based study from men at the VAMC in which there was a lower prostate cancer detection rate among obese men,[24] when the data was reanalyzed adjusting for differences in PSA concentrations and prostate size, obese men actually had a higher rate of prostate cancer particularly high-grade cancer.[34] If this hypothesis of an inherent bias against the detectability of prostate cancer among obese men in the PSA-era were true, it would explain why an inverse association between obesity and prostate cancer has largely only been seen in the United States in recent years where PSA screening is commonplace. Moreover, delayed diagnosis among obese men would be expected to result in a higher percentage of obese men with advanced stage disease and worse outcomes after therapy.

Given the long protracted course of prostate cancer, it is felt that perhaps events that occur earlier in life may predispose to prostate cancer later in life. As such, examination of adulthood BMI may have missed the window when excess BMI and all its sequelae would have affected prostate cancer risk. To address this issue, several studies examined the relationship between prostate cancer risk and obesity earlier in life (age 10–30 years). Analogous to the findings when adulthood BMI was examined, these studies have demonstrated mixed results, with some studies finding a direct relationship

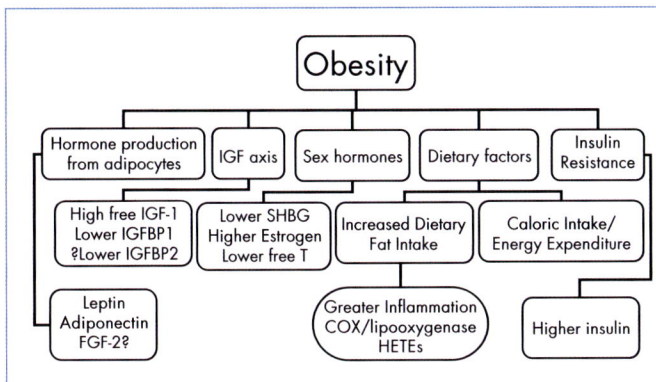

Fig. 18.3
Obesity and its related sequelae. Diagram is not intended to show all possible relationships between obesity and its sequelae, but merely to suggest that multiple factors associated with obesity may be important in prostate cancer biology.

between BMI early in life (age 20–30 years) and the risk for developing prostate cancer,[17,35] while others found obesity in early life (age 5 and 10 years) was protective for developing prostate cancer.[36]

OBESITY AND ONCOLOGIC OUTCOMES AFTER RADICAL PROSTATECTOMY

Several studies found that among men undergoing radical prostatectomy (RP), those with increased BMI had higher grade[37-39] and stage disease.[40] Two recent studies utilized large multi-institutional multiracial databases to address whether increased BMI was associated with higher biochemical failure rates following radical prostatectomy.[38,39] Both studies concluded that men with higher BMI (>30 kg/m^2 or >35 kg/m^2) were at increased risk of biochemical failure. Interestingly, both studies found that black men were more likely to be obese, which may explain, in part, the higher mortality from prostate cancer among black men. Further studies are needed to determine whether obese men are at increased risk for failure following other forms of primary therapy, including external beam radiation therapy and brachytherapy. Thus, though only two studies have examined this issue to date, both agreed that obesity was associated with greater risk of biochemical progression following radical prostatectomy.

OBESITY AND RISK OF DEATH FROM PROSTATE CANCER

While the relationship between obesity and prostate cancer risk is unclear, the relationship between obesity and mortality from prostate cancer is better established. Epidemiologic data has relatively consistently found a statistically significant positive association between increased BMI and risk of death from prostate cancer.[13,41,43] Several large prospective studies deserve particular attention. In 1959 and again in 1982, the American Cancer Society enrolled a cohort of participants for longitudinal studies on cancer, known as the Cancer Prevention Study (CPS) I and II, respectively. Men were then followed for 13 years in CPS-I and 14 years in CPS-II. Together these studies followed 816,268 men, during which time there were 5,212 prostate cancer deaths. Both CPS-I and CPS-II reported that obese men (BMI >30 kg/m^2) were significantly more likely to die from prostate cancer, with a 27% and 21% increased risk of prostate cancer death relative to normal weight men, respectively.[41] More details regarding CPS-II were recently published,

which showed that severely obese men (BMI >35 kg/m^2) were at even greater risk of death from prostate cancer (34% higher risk) relative to normal weight men.[42] The risk of death from prostate cancer appeared relatively linear in that as BMI increased above "normal," the risk of prostate cancer death steadily increased. A prospective study of 135,000 construction workers in Sweden found similar results in that men in the highest BMI category were 40% more likely to die from prostate cancer than men in the lowest BMI category.[13] Finally, a study from Scotland found that increased BMI among college students was associated with a 49% increased risk of prostate cancer death suggesting that events involved in prostate carcinogenesis and progression may occur years before actual tumor development.[44] Therefore, there appears to be near uniform consensus among multiple studies involving over a million men followed prospectively that obesity is associated with increased risk for prostate cancer death.

SEX STEROIDS (TESTOSTERONE AND ESTROGEN)

Androgens act in the prostate by binding and activating the androgen receptor resulting in enhanced transcription of genes involved in cellular proliferation, such as those encoding the mitogenic growth factors epidermal growth factor (EGF) and insulin-like growth factor 1 (IGF1).[45] Studies in animal models of prostate cancer further support the role for androgens in the development of prostate cancer.[46] Of interest, obese men are known to have decreased free testosterone levels.[28] This fact may, however, explain why obese men have more high-grade prostate cancers. In the Prostate Cancer Prevention Trial, men exposed to the 5α-reductase type II inhibitor finasteride developed more poorly differentiated tumors than the control group, possibly related to lower prostate dihydrotestosterone levels.[47] Recent data from retrospective studies suggest that testosterone may exert a differentiating effect on prostate cancer, and decreased serum testosterone levels have been associated with more advanced and poorly differentiated tumors at presentation.[48-51] In addition, a recent prospective cohort study found that men with lower serum testosterone were at higher risk for being diagnosed with high-grade prostate cancer.[52] Thus, the lower free testosterone levels found in obese men may predispose them to developing more poorly differentiated, advanced prostate cancers and partly explain the higher mortality of prostate cancer among obese men.

Obese men are known to have increased serum estradiol levels due to peripheral conversion of testosterone to estradiol by aromatase in adipocytes.[53] The exact role of estrogen in prostate cancer development and progression is unclear, but recent animal and experimental studies suggest that elevated estradiol levels may play an important role in testosterone induced carcinogenesis. Studies in mice with genetically altered aromatase or estrogen receptor expression found that estradiol combined with testosterone plays an important role in regulating proliferation and apoptosis of prostate cells.[45,54] In addition, Leav et al demonstrated that testosterone needed to be combined with estrogen to develop proliferative lesions in mouse prostate tissue.[55] Moreover, other investigators have found that chronic combined administration of testosterone with estrogens to the Noble rat model resulted in a high incidence of prostate tumors after 52 weeks of treatment, with precancerous lesions seen as early as 16 weeks.[56,57] Based on this experimental data, it is possible that elevated levels of estradiol in obese men may enhance the growth promoting effect of testosterone on prostate cancer.

Several more detailed review articles have been published regarding sex hormones and their relationship to prostate cancer.[7–9]

INSULIN

Obesity, in particular central adiposity, is associated with the metabolic syndrome that includes hyperinsulinemia and insulin resistance.[2] When coupled with inadequate beta-cell reserve, insulin resistance can result in diabetes. Moreover, in men with diabetes there is a progressive loss of beta-cell function such that over time men become hypoinsulinemic.[58] Therefore, though obesity itself is, in general, associated with increased serum insulin concentrations, diabetes, and particularly long-standing diabetes, is associated with decreased serum insulin concentrations. It has been suggested that elevated insulin concentrations among obese men may be one of the factors relating obesity to more aggressive prostate cancer.[52,59] This is based upon the fact that insulin binds to the insulin receptor (IR) which upregulates insulin response substrate-1 (IRS-1), resulting in activation of the mitogen-activated protein (MAP) kinase and phosphoinositol-3 kinase/Akt (PI3K-Akt) pathways ultimately leading to cell proliferation and improved survival.[60] These are the same pathways utilized by the related growth factor IGF1, which has been also associated with increased prostate cancer risk (see below).

If insulin is related to prostate cancer development, one would expect a reduced risk of prostate cancer among men with diabetes, particularly long-standing diabetes, who have low insulin concentrations. Indeed multiple epidemiologic studies have found a reduced

risk of prostate cancer among men with diabetes. Giovannucci et al, using data from the Health Professionals Follow-up Study, found that diabetes was associated with a decreased risk of developing prostate cancer and that the longer one had diabetes, the greater the risk reduction.[61] A similar inverse association between diabetes and prostate cancer risk was seen in the US Physicians' Health Study, a prospective study of nearly 15,000 male physicians in the United States during a 10-year follow-up,[62] as well as a prospective cohort study of 135,950 men with diabetes in Sweden.[63] However, not all prospective cohort studies have found similar results. For example, data from CPS-I suggested no relationship between diabetes and the risk of developing prostate cancer, except among men who had diabetes for more than 5 years who were at increased risk for prostate cancer.[64] Data from the National Health and Nutrition Survey I suggested that diabetic men were at increased risk of developing prostate cancer.[65]

Given the apparent conflicting results from some of these studies, a recent meta-analysis examined the association between prostate cancer risk and diabetes pulling data from 14 cohort and case-control studies.[66] The end conclusion of the meta-analysis was that diabetes appears to be protective for developing prostate cancer, though the risk reduction was slight (RR = 0.91; 95% CI, 0.86–0.96).

While diabetes is associated with lower serum insulin concentrations, the metabolic syndrome is associated with increased serum insulin concentrations and has been associated with increased risk of prostate cancer in a prospective cohort study in Finland.[67] Rather than relying on surrogates of insulin concentration (e.g., diabetes for low and metabolic syndrome for high), several studies have examined the association between directly measured insulin concentrations and prostate cancer risk. Using a case-control format of men from China, Hsing et al[68] found that higher serum insulin concentrations were associated with increased risk of prostate cancer. Moreover, among men with prostate cancer, high insulin concentrations are associated with higher-risk disease.[69] However, a recent nested case-control study using prediagnostic serum found no association between serum insulin and prostate cancer risk among men in the US, though it should be cautioned that the vast majority (95%) of men in this study had normal serum insulin concentrations, therefore, limiting the ability to comment about an association between insulin and prostate cancer in men with abnormal insulin concentrations.[21]

There are several difficulties in studying the association between insulin and prostate cancer. First, most studies do not directly measure insulin but rather use diabetes as a surrogate of low insulin. However, in the early and prediabetic phases, diabetes may be associated with increased insulin concentrations. Second, most studies have generally not discriminated between diabetes type I and type II. Third, given the overall prevalence of prostate cancer, any chronic disease that causes the patient to interact with their primary care provider more often would lead to greater opportunity for screening and potentially represent a bias for increased detection. When this is taken into account, the modest "protection" observed by diabetes may underestimate the strength of the true biological association between diabetes and prostate cancer development. Finally, insulin inhibits production of IGF-binding proteins 1 and 2 (IGFBP1 and IGFBP2), thereby increasing the free or bioactive IGF1 concentrations. Therefore, it is difficult to completely separate the actions of insulin from other prostate cancer growth factors. Though some conflicting data do exist, the majority of the data to date suggest that high-insulin states may be related to increased prostate cancer risk while low-insulin states may be protective. Collectively, these data suggest that insulin may be directly related to prostate cancer development and may underscore some of the association between obesity and prostate cancer.

INSULIN-LIKE GROWTH FACTOR AXIS

Insulin-like growth factor 1 is a polypeptide growth factor that circulates in the blood bound to one of several high-affinity IGFBPs (IGFBP1–6). In vitro, IGF1 stimulates growth of androgen-responsive and androgen-independent human prostate cancer cell lines.[70] In vivo, IGF1 is thought to be a growth factor for numerous different types of cancer, and elevated serum concentrations have been hypothesized as one of the main mechanisms associating obesity with mortality from multiple types of cancer, including prostate cancer.[42]

Increased IGF-1 concentrations are directly linked with dietary factors that have been associated with prostate cancer risk, including milk and other dairy products, calcium, and polyunsaturated fat intake, and are inversely correlated with protective dietary factors such as high vegetable consumption, particularly tomatoes.[71] This suggests that IGF1 may also underlie the relationship between various dietary components and prostate cancer risk. In addition, some studies,[8,72] but not all,[73] found that obesity is associated with increased free or bioactive IGF1 concentrations.

Additional indirect evidence supporting a link between IGF1 and prostate cancer comes from studies examining the association between adult height and prostate cancer risk. One of the main mechanisms through which growth hormone stimulates linear growth is through increased IGF1 expression. Therefore, the observation in some studies that taller men (who would have had higher circulating IGF1 levels during childhood and adolescence, though these were not directly measured in these studies) were at increased risk for development of and death from prostate cancer[15,41] further supports a possible link between IGF1 and prostate cancer.

Multiple epidemiologic studies, adjusting for BMI, found a direct positive correlation between serum IGF1 concentrations and the risk of prostate cancer development.[74–76] In addition, three separate meta-analyses all concluded that higher serum IGF1 levels were significantly associated with an increased risk for development of prostate cancer.[77–79] However, it should be noted that the majority of studies that found higher IGF1 levels were associated with prostate cancer were performed either prior to widespread PSA screening,[74] during periods of widespread PSA screening but using a high PSA cut-point for biopsy (>10 ng/mL),[76] or in countries where widespread PSA screening was not particularly common.[75,80] Thus, men in these studies were diagnosed with tumors at more advanced stages than commonly seen in the United States today. Indeed a follow-up study from the Physician's Health Study found that IGF1 correlated with advanced stage prostate cancer but not early clinically localized prostate cancer.[81] This raises the possibility that the majority of men in these studies who were later diagnosed with prostate cancer already had prostate cancer at the time of serum collection, and so higher IGF1 levels may also function as a tumor marker. Some authors have even examined whether IGF1 concentrations can be used, along with PSA, to help diagnose prostate cancer, with mixed results.[82,83] However, the fact that IGF1 concentrations increase after radical prostatectomy[84] argues against IGF1 as a useful tumor marker. Though much data supports that higher IGF1 concentrations may be involved in prostate cancer development, further studies are needed to determine whether elevated IGF1 concentrations can serve as a tumor marker.

Insulin-like growth factor 1 bioactivity is regulated by serum concentrations of the various IGFBPs, of which IGFBP3 is the predominate one. Thus, elevated IGFBP3 concentrations would result in lower free IGF1. While most studies found IGF1 concentrations were positively associated with prostate cancer risk, the results of studies examining serum IGFBP3 are less clear, with some studies finding a positive association and others finding a negative association. Using data from the Physician's Health Study, Chan et al found that increased IGFBP3, after adjusting for IGF1 levels, was associated with a decreased risk for developing prostate cancer.[74] However, several other studies found a weak positive association between IGFBP3 concentrations and prostate cancer risk, which were attenuated after adjustment for IGF1.[75,76] Two recent meta-analyses examining the association of IGFBP3 concentrations with prostate cancer risk came to different conclusions: one concluded no statistically significant association,[78] and one concluded increased IGFBP3 concentration was associated with increased prostate cancer risk.[79] However, recent concerns have been raised over the specificity of the assays used to measure IGFBP3 concentrations in some studies. Specifically, there is concern that various forms of IGFBP3 may be differentially detected by the assays and, therefore, serum from men with various stages of early prostate cancer may provide conflicting information due to the well-recognized prostatic protease cleavage of IGFBP3.[85] As a result, it is difficult to interpret many of the studies evaluating the association between IGFBP3 and prostate cancer risk.

In summary, IGF1 concentrations appear to be related to dietary factors associated with prostate cancer risk and have, in some studies, also been associated with obesity. The majority of studies, including multiple meta-analyses suggest elevated IGF1 concentrations are associated with increased prostate cancer risk. Given that many of these studies were done in unscreened populations, and IGF1 concentrations may be more strongly correlated with advanced disease, it is controversial whether IGF1 is etiologic in prostate cancer development or merely functions as a tumor marker. The studies examining the association between IGFBP3 and prostate cancer risk are mixed, with some showing a positive and others a negative association. Given concerns over the IGFBP3 assay used in some of these studies, further studies using a refined assay are needed to further explore any possible associations between IGFBP3 and prostate cancer development.

LEPTIN

Increasing evidence suggests that adipose tissue not only stores excess fat, but it can function as an endocrine organ. Adipocytes produce multiple polypeptide hormones, of which leptin is the best characterized. The normal physiologic role of leptin is to signal the brain that there are sufficient fat stores, which in turn results in curbing appetite.[86] However, most obese men have elevated leptin concentrations in line with their degree of adiposity.[87] Of unclear clinical significance, human prostate cancers have been shown to express leptin receptors.[88] In vitro, leptin stimulates growth of the androgen-independent cell lines DU145 and PC-3, but not the androgen-sensitive cell line, LNCaP.[89] Together, these data have given rise to the hypothesis that leptin may mediate some of the effects of obesity on prostate cancer.[90]

Given the possible relationship between leptin and prostate cancer, several studies examined the association between serum leptin concentrations and risk of developing prostate cancer. One nested case-control study found a positive correlation between prediagnostic serum leptin concentrations and prostate cancer risk (RR = 2.6; 95% CI, 1.3–5.2; comparing second and third quintiles versus first quintile serum leptin concentration, adjusted for multiple variables).[88] In addition, a recent study found that a particular polymorphism within the leptin gene that is associated with increased leptin production and secretion was associated with increased risk of prostate cancer, particularly advanced disease.[91] However, other studies using either a nested case-control design and prediagnostic serum[92] or a case-control design and serum obtained after prostate cancer diagnosis[68] found no association between serum leptin concentrations and prostate cancer risk. Among men with prostate cancer, two recent studies found that increased serum leptin concentrations were associated with larger, higher-grade, and more advanced tumors,[93,94] though a third study found no association between leptin concentrations and pathologic tumor stage.[95] The conflicting data regarding serum leptin concentrations and prostate cancer risk implies that it is unlikely that leptin concentration is a major risk factor for prostate cancer, though the number of studies that have addressed this issue is small. The fact that in-vitro leptin stimulates hormone-refractory but not hormone-sensitive prostate cancer cells suggests that leptin may play a role in late stage androgen-independent progression, though no studies have addressed this issue.

CONCLUSION

Obesity is clearly an epidemic in American society and elsewhere. Obesity is associated with multiple chronic medical problems. The relationship between obesity, its physiologic sequelae and the risk of developing prostate cancer is unclear. What is clear is that obese men are at significantly increased risk of death from prostate cancer. The exact reasons for this are unknown but likely multifactorial. It is probable that the hormonal sequelae of obesity, including alterations in serum concentrations of insulin, IGF1, and leptin, are involved to varying degrees. Attempts to reduce obesity in the general population are necessary. Whether lifestyle alterations after the diagnosis of prostate cancer can alter the natural history of the disease remains to be determined. Further studies are needed to determine the molecular basis for this increased risk of prostate cancer mortality among obese men. Moreover, additional studies are needed to examine the possible dual effect of obesity on risk of developing prostate cancer in general and on the risk of developing aggressive/fatal prostate cancer. Finally, further studies are warranted to assess to what degree there may be a bias in our ability to detect cancers among obese men leading to delayed diagnosis and worse outcomes.

ACKNOWLEDGMENTS

Supported by the National Institute of Health/National Cancer Institute SPORE Grant # P50 CA92131-01A1, CA100938, M01-RR00865 (WJA); the Department of Defense, Prostate Cancer Research Program, Grant #PC030666 (SJF), and the American Foundation for Urological Disease/American Urological Association Education and Research Scholarship Award (SJF). Views and opinions of, and endorsements by the authors do not reflect those of the US Army or the Department of Defense.

REFERENCES

1. Flegal KM, Carroll MD, Ogden CL, et al. Prevalence and trends in obesity among US adults, 1999–2000. JAMA 2002;288:1723–1727.

2. Mokdad AH, Ford ES, Bowman BA, et al. Prevalence of obesity, diabetes, and obesity-related health risk factors, 2001. JAMA 2003;289:76–79.

3. Bray GA. The underlying basis for obesity: relationship to cancer. J Nutr 2002;132:3451S–3455S.

4. Jemal A, Tiwari RC, Murray T, et al. Cancer statistics, 2004. CA Cancer J Clin 2004;54:8–29.

5. www.m-w.com, accessed 12-22-03.

6. Satia-Abouta J, Patterson RE, Schiller RN, et al. Energy from fat is associated with obesity in U.S. men: results from the Prostate Cancer Prevention Trial. Prev Med 2002;34:493–501.

7. Hsing AW, Reichardt JK, Stanczyk FZ. Hormones and prostate cancer: current perspectives and future directions. Prostate 2002;52:213–235.

8. Kaaks R, Lukanova A and Sommersberg B. Plasma androgens, IGF-1, body size, and prostate cancer risk: a synthetic review. Prostate Cancer Prostatic Dis 2000;3:157–172.

9. Bosland MC. The role of steroid hormones in prostate carcinogenesis. J Natl Cancer Inst Monogr 2000;27:39–66.

10. Kolonel LN, Nomura AM, Cooney RV. Dietary fat and prostate cancer: current status. J Natl Cancer Inst 1999;91:414–428.

11. Dagnelie PC, Schuurman AG, Goldbohm RA, et al. Diet, anthropometric measures and prostate cancer risk: a review of prospective cohort and intervention studies. BJU Int 2004;93:1139–1150.

12. Platz EA. Energy imbalance and prostate cancer. J Nutr 2002;132:3471S–3481S.

13. Andersson SO, Wolk A, Bergstrom R, et al. Englund A, Nyren O. Body size and prostate cancer: a 20-year follow-up study among 135006 Swedish construction workers. J Natl Cancer Inst 1997;89:385–389.

14. Veierod MB, Laake P, Thelle DS. Dietary fat intake and risk of prostate cancer: a prospective study of 25,708 Norwegian men. Int J Cancer 1997;73:634–638.

15. Engeland A, Tretli S, Bjorge T. Height, body mass index, and prostate cancer: a follow-up of 950000 Norwegian men. Br J Cancer 2003;89:1237–1242.

16. Putnam SD, Cerhan JR, Parker AS, et al. Lifestyle and anthropometric risk factors for prostate cancer in a cohort of Iowa men. Ann Epidemiol 2000;10:361–369.

17. Schuurman AG, Goldbohm RA, Dorant E, et al. Anthropometry in relation to prostate cancer risk in the Netherlands Cohort Study. Am J Epidemiol 2000;151:541–549.

18. Whittemore AS, Kolonel LN, Wu AH, et al. Prostate cancer in relation to diet, physical activity, and body size in blacks, whites, and Asians in the United States and Canada. J Natl Cancer Inst 1995;87:652–661.

19. Nilsen TI and Vatten LJ. Anthropometry and prostate cancer risk: a prospective study of 22,248 Norwegian men. Cancer Causes Control 1999;10:269–275.

20. Nomura A, Heilbrun LK, Stemmermann GN. Body mass index as a predictor of cancer in men. J Natl Cancer Inst 1985;74:319–323.

21. Hubbard JS, Rohrmann S, Landis PK, et al. Association of prostate cancer risk with insulin, glucose, and anthropometry in the Baltimore longitudinal study of aging. Urology 2004;63:253–258.

22. Giovannucci E, Rimm EB, Liu Y, et al. Body mass index and risk of prostate cancer in U.S. health professionals. J Natl Cancer Inst 2003;95:1240–1244.

23. Porter MP and Stanford JL. Obesity and the risk of prostate cancer. Prostate, 2004;62:316–321

24. Presti JC, Jr., Lee U, Brooks JD, et al. Lower body mass index is associated with a higher prostate cancer detection rate and less favorable pathological features in a biopsy population. J Urol 2004;171:2199–2202.

25. Gray MA, Delahunt B, Fowles JR, et al. Demographic and clinical factors as determinants of serum levels of prostate specific antigen and its derivatives. Anticancer Res 2004;24:2069–2072.

26. Baillargeon J, Pollock BH, Kristal AR, et al. The association of body mass index and prostate specific antigen in a population-based study. Cancer 2005;103:1092–1095.

27. Ku JH, Kim ME, Lee NK, et al. Influence of age, anthropometry, and hepatic and renal function on serum prostate-specific antigen levels in healthy middle-age men. Urology 2003;61:132–136.

28. Pasquali R, Casimirri F, Cantobelli S, et al. Effect of obesity and body fat distribution on sex hormones and insulin in men. Metabolism 1991;40:101–104.

29. Prins GS. Molecular biology of the androgen receptor. Mayo Clin Proc 2000;75: S32–35.

30. Dahle SE, Chokkalingam AP, Gao YT, et al. Body size and serum levels of insulin and leptin in relation to the risk of benign prostatic hyperplasia. J Urol 2002;168:599–604.

31. Hammarsten J, Hogstedt B. Hyperinsulinaemia as a risk factor for developing benign prostatic hyperplasia. Eur Urol 2001;39:151–158.

32. Kranse R, Beemsterboer P, Rietbergen J, et al. Predictors for biopsy outcome in the European Randomized Study of Screening for Prostate Cancer (Rotterdam region). Prostate 1999;39:316–322.

33. Finne P, Finne R, Auvinen A, et al. Predicting the outcome of prostate biopsy in screen-positive men by a multilayer perceptron network. Urology 2000;56:418–422.

34. Freedland SJ, Terris MK, Platz EA, et al. Body mass index as a predictor of possible cancer: development versus detection on biopsy. Urology 2005;66:108–113.

35. Dal Maso L, Zucchetto A, La Vecchia C, et al. Prostate cancer and body size at different ages: an Italian multicentre case-control study. Br J Cancer 2004;90:2176–2180.

36. Giovannucci E, Rimm EB, Stampfer MJ, et al. Height, body weight, and risk of prostate cancer. Cancer Epidemiol Biomarkers Prev 1997;6:557–563.

37. Rohrmann S, Roberts WW, Walsh PC, et al. Family history of prostate cancer and obesity in relation to high-grade disease and extraprostatic extension in young men with prostate cancer. Prostate 2003;55:140–146.

38. Freedland SJ, Aronson WJ, Kane CJ, et al. Impact of obesity on biochemical control after radical prostatectomy for clinically localized prostate cancer: a report by the Shared Equal Access Regional Cancer Hospital database study group. J Clin Oncol 2004;22:446–453.

39. Amling CL, Riffenburgh RH, Sun L, et al. Pathologic variables and recurrence rates as related to obesity and race in men with prostate cancer undergoing radical prostatectomy. J Clin Oncol 2004;22:439–445.

40. Amling CL, Kane CJ, Riffenburgh RH, et al. Relationship between obesity and race in predicting adverse pathologic variables in patients undergoing radical prostatectomy. Urology 2001;58:723–728.

41. Rodriguez C, Patel AV, Calle EE, et al. Body mass index, height, and prostate cancer mortality in two large cohorts of adult men in the United States. Cancer Epidemiol Biomarkers Prev 2001;10:345–353.

42. Calle EE, Rodriguez C, Walker-Thurmond K, et al. Overweight, obesity, and mortality from cancer in a prospectively studied cohort of U.S. adults. N Engl J Med 2003;348:1625–1638.

43. Snowdon DA, Phillips RL, Choi W. Diet, obesity, and risk of fatal prostate cancer. Am J Epidemiol 1984;120:244–250.

44. Okasha M, McCarron P, McEwen J, et al. Body mass index in young adulthood and cancer mortality: a retrospective cohort study. J Epidemiol Community Health 2002;56:780–784.

45. Ho E, Boileau TW, Bray TM. Dietary influences on endocrine-inflammatory interactions in prostate cancer development. Arch Biochem Biophys 2004;428:109–117.

46. McCormick DL, Rao KV, Dooley L, et al. Influence of N-methyl-N-nitrosourea, testosterone, and N-(4-hydroxyphenyl)-all-trans-retinamide on prostate cancer induction in Wistar-Unilever rats. Cancer Res 1998;58:3282–3288.

47. Thompson IM, Goodman PJ, Tangen CM, et al. The influence of finasteride on the development of prostate cancer. N Engl J Med 2003;349:215–224.

48. D'Amico AV, Chen MH, Malkowicz SB, et al. Lower prostate specific antigen outcome than expected following radical prostatectomy in patients with high grade prostate and a prostatic specific antigen level of 4 ng/ml or less. J Urol 2002;167:2025–2030.

49. Massengill JC, Sun L, Moul JW, et al. Pretreatment total testosterone level predicts pathological stage in patients with localized prostate cancer treated with radical prostatectomy. J Urol 2003;169:1670–1675.

50. Hoffman MA, DeWolf WC, Morgentaler A. Is low serum free testosterone a marker for high grade prostate cancer? J Urol 2000;163:824–827.

51. Schatzl G, Madersbacher S, Thurridl T, et al. High-grade prostate cancer is associated with low serum testosterone levels. Prostate 2001;47:52–58.

52. Platz EA, Leitzmann MF, Rifai N, et al. Sex steroid hormones and the androgen receptor gene CAG repeat and subsequent risk of prostate cancer in the PSA era. Cancer Epidemiol Biomarkers Prev 2005;14:1262–1269.

53. Calle EE, Kaaks R. Overweight, obesity and cancer: epidemiological evidence and proposed mechanisms. Nat Rev Cancer 2004;4:579–591.

54. Risbridger GP, Bianco JJ, Ellem SJ, et al. Oestrogens and prostate cancer. Endocr Relat Cancer 2003;10:187–191.

55. Leav I, Merk FB, Kwan PW, et al. Androgen-supported estrogen-enhanced epithelial proliferation in the prostates of intact Noble rats. Prostate 1989;15:23–40.

56. Bosland MC, Ford H, Horton L. Induction at high incidence of ductal prostate adenocarcinomas in NBL/Cr and Sprague-Dawley Hsd:SD rats treated with a combination of testosterone and estradiol-17 beta or diethylstilbestrol. Carcinogenesis 1995;16:1311–1317.

57. Drago JR. The induction of NB rat prostatic carcinomas. Anticancer Res 1984;4:255–256.

58. Scheen AJ. Pathophysiology of insulin secretion. Ann Endocrinol (Paris) 2004;65:29–36.

59. Barnard RJ, Aronson WJ, Tymchuk CN, et al. Prostate cancer: another aspect of the insulin-resistance syndrome? Obes Rev 2002;3:303–308.

60. Boyd DB. Insulin and cancer. Integr Cancer Ther 2003;2:315–329.

61. Giovannucci E, Rimm EB, Stampfer MJ, et al. Diabetes mellitus and risk of prostate cancer (United States). Cancer Causes Control 1998;9:3–9.

62. Zhu K, Lee IM, Sesso HD, et al. History of diabetes mellitus and risk of prostate cancer in physicians. Am J Epidemiol 2004;159:978–982.

63. Weiderpass E, Ye W, Vainio H, et al. Reduced risk of prostate cancer among patients with diabetes mellitus. Int J Cancer 2002;102:258–261.

64. Will JC, Vinicor F, Calle EE. Is diabetes mellitus associated with prostate cancer incidence and survival? Epidemiology 1999;10:313–318.

65. Steenland K, Nowlin S, Palu S. Cancer incidence in the National Health and Nutrition Survey I. Follow-up data: diabetes, cholesterol, pulse and physical activity. Cancer Epidemiol Biomarkers Prev 1995;4:807–811.

66. Bonovas S, Filioussi K, Tsantes A. Diabetes mellitus and risk of prostate cancer: a meta-analysis. Diabetologia 2004;47:1071–1078.

67. Laukkanen JA, Laaksonen DE, Niskanen L, et al. Metabolic syndrome and the risk of prostate cancer in Finnish men: a population-based study. Cancer Epidemiol Biomarkers Prev 2004;13:1646–1650.

68. Hsing AW, Chua S Jr, Gao YT, et al. Prostate cancer risk and serum levels of insulin and leptin: a population-based study. J Natl Cancer Inst 2001;93:783–789.

69. Lehrer S, Diamond EJ, Stagger S, et al. Increased serum insulin associated with increased risk of prostate cancer recurrence. Prostate 2002;50:1–3.

70. Iwamura M, Sluss PM, Casamento JB, et al. Insulin-like growth factor I: action and receptor characterization in human prostate cancer cell lines. Prostate 1993;22:243–252.

71. Gunnell D, Oliver SE, Peters TJ, et al. Are diet-prostate cancer associations mediated by the IGF axis? A cross-sectional analysis of diet, IGF-I and IGFBP-3 in healthy middle-aged men. Br J Cancer 2003;88:1682–1686.

72. Nam SY, Lee EJ, Kim KR, et al. Effect of obesity on total and free insulin-like growth factor (IGF)-1, and their relationship to IGF-binding protein (BP)-1, IGFBP-2, IGFBP-3, insulin, and growth hormone. Int J Obes Relat Metab Disord 1997;21:355–359.

73. Holmes MD, Pollak MN, Hankinson SE. Lifestyle correlates of plasma insulin-like growth factor I and insulin-like growth factor binding protein 3 concentrations. Cancer Epidemiol Biomarkers Prev 2002;11:862–867.

74. Chan JM, Stampfer MJ, Giovannucci E, et al. Plasma insulin-like growth factor-I and prostate cancer risk: a prospective study. Science 1998;279:563–566.

75. Stattin P, Bylund A, Rinaldi S, et al. Plasma insulin-like growth factor-I, insulin-like growth factor-binding proteins, and prostate cancer risk: a prospective study. J Natl Cancer Inst 2000;92:1910–1917.

76. Wolk A, Mantzoros CS, Andersson SO, et al. Insulin-like growth factor 1 and prostate cancer risk: a population-based, case-control study. J Natl Cancer Inst 1998;90:911–915.

77. Shaneyfelt T, Husein R, Bubley G, et al. Hormonal predictors of prostate cancer: a meta-analysis. J Clin Oncol 2000;18:847–853.

78. Renehan AG, Zwahlen M, Minder C, et al. Insulin-like growth factor (IGF)-I, IGF binding protein-3, and cancer risk: systematic review and meta-regression analysis. Lancet 2004;363:1346–1353.

79. Shi R, Berkel HJ, Yu H. Insulin-like growth factor-I and prostate cancer: a meta-analysis. Br J Cancer 2001;85:991–996.

80. Mantzoros CS, Tzonou A, Signorello LB, et al. Insulin-like growth factor 1 in relation to prostate cancer and benign prostatic hyperplasia. Br J Cancer 1997;76:1115–1118.

81. Chan JM, Stampfer MJ, Ma J, et al. Insulin-like growth factor-I (IGF-I) and IGF binding protein-3 as predictors of advanced-stage prostate cancer. J Natl Cancer Inst 2002;94:1099–1106.

82. Ismail HA, Pollak M, Behlouli H, et al. Serum insulin-like growth factor (IGF)-1 and IGF-binding protein-3 do not correlate with Gleason score or quantity of prostate cancer in biopsy samples. BJU Int 2003;92:699–702.

83. Scorilas A, Plebani M, Mazza S, et al. Serum human glandular kallikrein (hK2) and insulin-like growth factor 1 (IGF-1) improve the discrimination between prostate cancer and benign prostatic hyperplasia in combination with total and % free PSA. Prostate 2003;54:220–229.

84. Bubley GJ, Balk SP, Regan MM, et al. Serum levels of insulin-like growth factor-1 and insulin-like growth factor-1 binding proteins after radical prostatectomy. J Urol 2002;168:2249–2252.

85. Ali O, Cohen P, Lee KW. Epidemiology and biology of insulin-like growth factor binding protein-3 (IGFBP-3) as an anti-cancer molecule. Horm Metab Res 2003;35:726–733.

86. Yanovski JA, Yanovski SZ. Recent advances in basic obesity research. JAMA 1999;282:1504–1506.

87. Considine RV, Sinha MK, Heiman ML, et al. Serum immunoreactive-leptin concentrations in normal-weight and obese humans. N Engl J Med 1996;334:292–295.

88. Stattin P, Soderberg S, Hallmans G, et al. Leptin is associated with increased prostate cancer risk: a nested case-referent study. J Clin Endocrinol Metab 2001;86:1341–1345.

89. Onuma M, Bub JD, Rummel TL, et al. Prostate cancer cell-adipocyte interaction: leptin mediates androgen-independent prostate cancer cell proliferation through c-Jun NH2-terminal kinase. J Biol Chem 2003;278:42660–42667.

90. Ribeiro R, Lopes C, Medeiros R. Leptin and prostate: implications for cancer prevention—overview of genetics and molecular interactions. Eur J Cancer Prev 2004;13:359–368.

91. Ribeiro R, Vasconcelos A, Costa S, et al. Overexpressing leptin genetic polymorphism (-2548 G/A) is associated with susceptibility to prostate cancer and risk of advanced disease. Prostate 2004;59:268–274.

92. Stattin P, Kaaks R, Johansson R, et al. Plasma leptin is not associated with prostate cancer risk. Cancer Epidemiol Biomarkers Prev 2003;12:474–475.

93. Chang S, Hursting SD, Contois JH, et al. Leptin and prostate cancer. Prostate 2001;46:62–67.

94. Saglam K, Aydur E, Yilmaz M, et al. Leptin influences cellular differentiation and progression in prostate cancer. J Urol 2003;169:1308–1311.

95. Freedland SJ, Sokoll LJ, Mangold LA, et al. Serum leptin and pathological findings at the time of radical prostatectomy. J Urol 2005;173:773–776.

96. Ahluwalia IB, Mack KA, Murphy W, et al. State-specific prevalence of selected chronic disease-related characteristics—Behavioral Risk Factor Surveillance System, 2001. MMWR Surveill Summ 2003;52:1–80.

Chemoprevention of prostate cancer: concepts and evidence

19

Eric A Klein

INTRODUCTION

Carcinogenesis is a multistep molecular process induced by genetic and epigenetic changes that disrupt pathways controlling and the balance between cell proliferation, apoptosis, differentiation, and senescence. The presence of precursor lesions that represent intermediate stages between normal and malignant cells as long as 20 years before the appearance of cancer, coupled with the age-dependent incidence of most cancers, suggests that the carcinogenic process occurs slowly and during a protracted interval. In theory this provides the opportunity to intervene before a malignancy is established, using life-style changes such as dietary alterations, smoking cessation, or exercise, or by chemoprevention, defined as the use of natural or synthetic agents that reverse, inhibit, or prevent the development of cancer.[1] The goal of primary chemoprevention is to decrease the incidence of a given cancer, simultaneously reducing both treatment-related side effects and mortality. Effective chemoprevention requires the use of nontoxic (usually oral) agents that inhibit specific molecular steps in the carcinogenic pathway.

Prostate cancer is an attractive and appropriate target for primary prevention because of its incidence, prevalence, and disease-related mortality (Table 19.1). Although mortality from prostate cancer is decreasing, in the last 5 years alone more than 1 million men in the US have been newly diagnosed with this disease.[2] Despite prostate-specific antigen (PSA) induced stage migration, a high cure rate for localized disease, and improved understanding of prostate cancer biology, most men who develop metastatic disease are still destined to die of prostate cancer, with almost half a million deaths in the US between 1989 and 2001.[2] The burden of prostate cancer can also be measured in other terms. A recent study of complications after surgical therapy for localized disease in an unselected population-based cohort reported that at more than 18 months following radical prostatectomy, 8.4% of men were incontinent and 41.9% reported that their sexual performance was a moderate-to-large problem.[3] In a similarly designed study comparing outcomes after radiation to those after surgery, the radiation cohort reported an impotence rate of 61.5% and a significantly higher incidence of bowel problems.[4] Although many single-institution studies have reported better results in highly selected cohorts of treated patients, it is clear that the majority of men treated for localized disease in the

Table 19.1 The burden of prostate cancer in the United States

	Whites	African Americans	Total
Incidence*[†]	164.3	272.1	170.1
Mortality*[†]	30.2	73.0	32.9
New cases in 2004[†]	–	–	230,110
Mortality in 2004[†]	–	–	29,900
Lifetime risk of disease[‡]	16.6%	18.1%	–
Lifetime risk of death from disease[‡]	3.5%	4.3%	–

*Age-standardized per 100,000 population, 1996–2000.

[†]From Jemal A, Tiwari RC, Murray T, et al. Cancer Statistics 2004. CA Cancer J Clin 2004;54:8–29.

[‡]From Ries LAG, Kosary CL, Hankey BF, Miller BA, Edwards BK (eds). SEER Cancer Statistics Review, 1973-1995. Bethesda, MD: National Cancer Institute, 1998.

community pay a substantial price to be cured. Although most studies indicate that the vast majority of radiation or surgery patients would in retrospect choose to have the same therapy again, fear of cancer recurrence remains substantial for as long as 2 years after treatment.[5] It seems self-evident that an effective prevention strategy would spare many men this burden of diagnosis and cure.

The molecular pathogenesis of prostate cancer also lends itself to a primary prevention strategy. Several histologic lesions including atypical small acinar proliferation (ASAP), proliferative inflammatory atrophy (PIA), and prostatic intraepithelial neoplasia (PIN) that contain both genetic and epigenetic changes intermediate between normal prostatic epithelium and prostate cancer have been described. Clinically evident prostate cancer is rare in men under 50 years of age, while PIN is apparent at autopsy in men younger than 30 years. Furthermore, the prevalence of PIN is similar in populations at much different risks of developing clinically evident cancer, suggesting that external environmental influences are important and potentially modifiable.

TARGET POPULATIONS AND CLINICAL TRIAL DESIGN

Target populations appropriate for primary prevention studies can be subdivided into those with low, intermediate, and high risk of developing prostate cancer based on current epidemiologic evidence.[6–9] Each

group has its own clinical characteristics that lend advantages and disadvantages for trial design, endpoints, and statistical analysis (Table 19.2).[10] Based on the hypothesis that the specific molecular mechanisms underlying the development and/or progression of disease in each risk group and model may be unique and that different agents may be useful for each situation, it seems apparent that multiple potential chemopreventive agents should be tried in all risk groups and clinical models to best define which agents appear promising for large-scale studies. Testing of potentially active agents for secondary prevention in clinical models of patients with active disease is also appropriate (Table 19.3). The presurgical model allows for pre- and post-treatment tissue biopsies and is, therefore, useful for proof-of-principle demonstrations that a given agent is affecting its intended molecular target. The other models may yield useful strategies for the management of patients in specific clinical situations. The molecular mechanisms that underlie disease progression are likely to be different for each primary and secondary target population, and the results from a particular trial may not be generally applicable to other clinical scenarios.

There are numerous observations in the epidemiologic literature suggesting associations between various dietary, lifestyle, genetic and non-traditional factors and the risk of developing prostate cancer. In general is recognized that it will not be practicable to quantitate all of these factors in the conduct of a prevention trial, but if the trial is large enough these effects are likely to be equally and randomly distributed in all of the study arms. In

Table 19.2 Target populations for primary prevention

Risk group	Specific population	Advantages	Disadvantages
Low	General population	Easily definable Readily available Results widely applicable	Rate of progression slow Requires large study population and long follow-up interval Studies costly
Intermediate	African Americans	Higher risk than general population	Difficult to define Difficult to recruit because of perceived bias
	Genetic: Family history	Double or greater the risk of prostate cancer	Ascertainment bias Risk varies with number of affected family members, age of onset, and degree of relatedness Likely to be genetically heterogeneous
	HPC1 linked	Genetically homogeneous	Identification invasive and costly Affected subjects rare
	Other genes	Genetically homogeneous	Identification invasive and costly Affected subjects rare Risk of progression undefined
High	High-grade PIN	Highest known risk	Sampling error Diagnosis subjective Uncommon

HPC1, Hereditary Prostate Cancer 1 Gene; PIN, prostatic intraepithelial neoplasia.

Table 19.3 Models of secondary prevention

Model	Advantages	Disadvantages
Pre-surgical	Early-stage disease	Treatment period short
	Readily available study population	
	Pre- & post-treatment tissue available for biologic study	
Elevated PSA/negative biopsy	Well-defined histologic endpoint	Risk of progression undefined
		Sampling error
Adverse pathology after RP	High risk of progression	More advanced disease
		Clinical endpoint
Rising PSA after RP or RT	High risk of progression	Most advanced disease
		Clinical endpoint

PSA, prostate-specific antigen; RP, radical prostatectomy; RT, radiation therapy.

addition, most trials are designed to collect data relevant to these factors for secondary analysis and analysis of potential confounds for unexpected results.

FINASTERIDE AND THE PROSTATE CANCER PREVENTION TRIAL

The most significant event in chemoprevention of prostate cancer occurred with the publication of the results of the Prostate Cancer Prevention Trial (PCPT).[11] This landmark study, opened in 1993, was the first large-scale population based trial to test a chemopreventive strategy in men at risk for prostate cancer. The PCPT was based on two observations: 1) androgens are required for the development of prostate cancer; and 2) men with congenital deficiency of type 2 5α-reductase are unaffected by benign prostatic hyperplasia (BPH) and prostate cancer. The PCPT tested the hypothesis that treatment with finasteride, which induces an acquired deficiency of type 2 5α-reductase, would lower intraprostatic dihydrotestosterone (DHT) levels and thereby prevent prostate cancer. In PCPT, 18,882 men over 55 years with a normal digital rectal examination (DRE) and a PSA level of less than 3.0 ng/mL were randomly assigned to treatment with finasteride (5 mg/d) or placebo for 7 years. Prostate biopsy was recommended if the annual PSA level, adjusted for the effect of finasteride, exceeded 4.0 ng/mL or if the DRE was abnormal. The primary end point was the prevalence of prostate cancer during the 7 years of the study, as diagnosed by either for-cause biopsies (abnormal DRE or PSA) or by end-of-study biopsy. The trial was stopped approximately 15 months early by an independent Data Safety and Monitoring Committee because the primary endpoint of a 25% risk reduction on the finasteride arm was reached and sensitivity analyses suggested that additional follow-up would not change that outcome.

The main findings of the PCPT can be briefly summarized:

1. The prevalence of prostate cancer was reduced by 24.8% (HR = 0.75), from 24.4% to 18.4% in those randomized to finasteride compared with placebo.
2. The prevalence of Gleason grade 7–10 tumors was higher in the finasteride group than placebo (6.4% versus 5.1%, HR = 1.27).
3. The risk reduction associated with finasteride among risk groups defined by age, family history, race, and PSA were of the same general magnitude.
4. Sexual side effects were more common with finasteride, whereas urinary symptoms were more common with placebo.

Additional important observations include:

1. The risk reduction in the finasteride arm was seen in both clinically apparent tumors (those diagnosed "for cause" because of an elevated PSA or abnormal DRE) and end-of-study biopsies.
2. There were an equal number of deaths due to prostate cancer (5) in each study arm.
3. 98% of the tumors were clinically localized.
4. Finasteride-treated glands were 25% smaller than those in the placebo arm.

A number of relevant observations can be made about the results of the trial. Most surprising was the 24.4% prevalence of prostate cancer in the placebo arm, four times higher than the 6% assumed for the trial design. This discrepancy can be explained by the fact that the 6% assumption was based on SEER incidence estimates, which are derived from clinically evident cases and not on the prevalence in men undergoing biopsy for no reason other than being on the trial. Interestingly, the incidence of clinically evident cancers detected "for cause" by elevations in PSA or abnormal PSA was 7.2% at 7 years, roughly what was estimated by use of the SEER data. Another important observation is that a similar number of tissue cores were taken on end-of-study biopsy in both arms of the trial. Since the finasteride-treated glands were on average 25% smaller than those on the placebo arm, a relatively larger proportion of the gland was biopsied and evaluated histologically, leading to an increased chance of detecting cancer and suggesting the possibility that the risk reduction associated with finasteride may in fact be larger than observed. Finally, the data demonstrate a marked effect of finasteride on the prevalence of Gleason sum 6 tumors, no effect on the prevalence of Gleason sum 7 tumors, and a slight increase in the prevalence of Gleason sum 8 to 10 tumors.

There are two areas of continued debate over the results of the PCPT. The first is whether the Gleason sum 6 cancers that were "prevented" are biologically significant, which can be defined as destined to metastasize or kill the host. At present there are no biologic, clinical, pathologic, or radiographic markers that allow us to answer this question for an individual tumor. Either because of or in spite of this uncertainty, in the US 95% of patients with newly diagnosed Gleason sum 6 tumors choose some form of definitive therapy instead of watchful waiting.[12] This high treatment penetrance suggests that, even when lacking the ability to assign the biologic significance of a tumor, for affected men they are "clinically relevant" in that they lead to treatment and its attendant morbidity. The magnitude of their clinical relevance is illustrated by the large number of patients with biopsy Gleason sum 6 tumors who undergo surgery or brachytherapy by even the most selective academic practices.[13] Viewed in the context of "clinical relevance" as defined by current urologic practice, preventing grade 6 tumors by finasteride has the added advantage of preventing the anxiety, cost, and morbidity associated with their treatment. From a public health perspective, preventing the "burden of cure" in newly diagnosed patients should be added as a positive to the 25% reduction in risk of diagnosis and significant reduction in urinary symptoms associated with finasteride use.

The second question still under debate is whether the increased prevalence of higher grade tumors is real or artifactual. Finasteride is known to change the appearance of prostatic epithelium in a way that could bias interpretation, and the Gleason's grading system has never been validated on glands treated with antiandrogenic agents.[13,14] On the other hand, there are some plausible biologic hypotheses that suggest that the effect could be real,[13] and it is likely that until this issue is settled routine use of finasteride to prevent cancer will not be widely practiced. These and other biologic issues are currently being studied by a group of pathologists and scientists using the biologic repository (serum, white blood cells, and tissue) collected during the course of the study.

Deciding whether or not the advantages of taking finasteride (25% risk reduction for cancer, fewer urinary symptoms, and lower risk of intervention for urinary complaints, and avoiding the "burden of cure") outweigh the potential disadvantages of taking finasteride (potential excess mortality from extra cases of high-grade disease, the costs in both quality of life and dollars associated with excess sexual side effects, and the actual cost of finasteride itself) is complicated and will ultimately require detailed economic and quality-adjusted life-year analyses (Box 19.1). One recent mathematical model suggests a baseline 5:1 benefit-to-risk ratio as defined by the number of cancers prevented for each excess high-grade cancer in those taking finasteride.[15] This ratio increases to as much as 17:1 if half of the higher grade tumors are actually histologic artifact and if there was a 25% overdetection bias in the finasteride arm, and could be as low as 2:1 if only "for cause" biopsies are considered.

DUTASTERIDE

A second large scale industry-sponsored trial of another 5α-reductase inhibitor, dutasteride, has recently opened for accrual. This agent inhibits both type 1 and type 2 forms of 5α-reductase and has been shown to reduce the risk of prostate cancer in men treated for lower urinary tract symptoms related to benign prostatic enlargement compared with placebo. Eligibility for the REDUCE trial includes men with a PSA between 2 and 10 ng/mL and one prior negative prostate biopsy, representing a group at high risk for cancer on a subsequent biopsy. Target accrual is 8000 men in the United States and Europe.

SELENIUM

Selenium (Se) is an essential trace element occurring in both organic and inorganic forms. The organic form is

---

Box 19.1 Benefits and costs of finasteride as a preventative

Benefits

1. A 6.4% reduction in cancer prevalence
2. Fewer urinary symptoms & lower risk of acute urinary retention and need for surgical intervention for obstructive urinary symptoms
3. Avoidance of "burden of cure"

Costs

1. A 1.3% increase in high grade tumors
   - potential for more aggressive therapy
   - potential excess mortality
2. Sexual side effects and cost of treatment
3. Cost of finasteride

found predominantly in grains, fish, meat, poultry, eggs, and dairy products, and it enters the food chain via plant consumption. There is marked geographic variability of Se in food related to local soil content. Selenium is also widely available in over-the-counter supplements and multivitamins. It is widely distributed in body tissues and is an important constituent of many antioxidant enzymes.

Many epidemiologic observations support that Se acts to protect against the development of cancer. Both case-control and randomized placebo-controlled trials in humans also suggest that Se can decrease the risk of getting prostate cancer.[16] Vogt studied 445 men as part of a case-control study of cancers occurring disproportionately in African Americans.[17] In this study, serum Se levels were inversely proportional to the risk of prostate cancer (OR = 0.71, comparing highest and lowest quartiles), with no differences between whites and African Americans.

The strongest evidence for a protective effect of Se comes from the Nutritional Prevention of Cancer Trial, a randomized study of oral selenized yeast in patients with non-melanoma skin cancer. In that trial, 1312 participants took the equivalent of 200 mg/day of yeast versus placebo, and with a mean follow-up of 4.5 years the incidence of prostate cancer was reduced in the Se arm by two thirds compared with placebo. In an important update to this trial, Duffield-Lillico et al added an additional 25 months of follow-up to the study cohort to reach a mean of 7.45 years.[18] Reanalysis of the effect of Se supplementation continues to show a marked reduction on the incidence of prostate cancer (HR = 0.48). As in the initial analysis, the effect was strongest for those with a PSA less than 4 ng/mL and those with the lowest serum Se levels at study entry. The findings of this trial, where the incidence of prostate cancer was a secondary endpoint, serves as the basis for the use of Se in the large-scale Selenium and Vitamin E Cancer Prevention Trial (SELECT; vide infra). Support for the findings of this trial are lent by an analysis of the association between prostate cancer and baseline toenail Se level in the Netherlands Cohort Study.[19] After 6.3 years of follow-up, an inverse association between toenail Se level and prostate cancer risk was observed (OR = 0.69) in those with the highest levels. A less powerful but interesting autopsy study among Inuit, whose diet is rich in omega-3 polyunsaturated fatty acids and Se, found only one prostate cancer and no latent cancers in 61 males dying of other causes.[20]

Selenium inhibits tumorigenesis in a variety of experimental models, and a number of potential mechanisms have been proposed for its antitumorigenic effects.[16] Accumulating evidence suggests that Se works by inhibiting important early steps in carcinogenesis. Using methylselenic acid (MSA), a rapidly metabolized precursor of methylselenol (the form of Se active at the cellular level), Dong has demonstrated dose- and time-dependent growth inhibition and induction of apoptosis in the PC3 human prostate cancer cell line, and identified 12 clusters of Se-responsive genes by oligonucleotide array.[21] Cell cycle arrest induced by methylselenic acid was mediated in part by upregulation of p19^{INK4d} and p21^{WAF1} and down-regulation of CDK1, CDK2, and cyclin A. A confirmatory studying of LnCAP cells has demonstrated that MSA affects transcriptional levels of many cell cycle-regulated genes resulting in cell cycle arrest and decreased proliferation.[22] Methylselenic acid also modulated expression of many androgen-regulated genes, suppressed androgen receptor (AR) expression, and decreased levels of secreted PSA. Another important study has demonstrated that combining vitamin E succinate (VES, also known as α-tocopherol succinate) and MSA produced a synergistic effect on cell growth suppression, primarily mediated by augmenting apoptosis.[23] Along with previously published work, these studies suggest that Se in various forms works early in the carcinogenic pathway by blocking cell proliferation, promoting cell death, and inducing antioxidant enzymes, and that its effects are mediated by a variety of well-defined molecular pathways.

In-vivo studies also support the antitumorigenic role of Se in prostate cancer. In a dog model, Waters demonstrated that oral Se in various forms given over 7 months as a dietary supplement resulted in lower levels of DNA damage in prostatic epithelial cells and increased intraprostatic apoptosis compared with controls.[24] A study in men with normal pretreatment serum Se levels demonstrated that 200 μg/day oral Se resulted in statistically significant higher levels of Se in prostatic tissue compared with placebo in 51 men who underwent transurethral resection of the prostate for BPH.[25] Together these studies demonstrate that orally ingested Se reaches the prostate and modulates markers of oxidative stress relevant to the proposed molecular mechanisms of its protective effects.

Selenomethionine does not affect PSA secretion by LnCaP cells despite its antiproliferative effect.[26] This suggests that no PSA bias that could influence the decision to perform a prostate biopsy will be introduced in the many clinical trials of Se, including those at risk for prostate cancer (SELECT in North America, APPOSE in Australia, and PRECISE in Europe), those with a previous negative prostate biopsy, those with a biopsy demonstrating high-grade PIN, and in men choosing watchful waiting.[27,28]

VITAMIN E

Vitamin E is a family of naturally occurring, essential, fat-soluble vitamin compounds, which functions as the major lipid-soluble antioxidant in cell membranes. The most active form of vitamin E is α-tocopherol; it is also among the most abundant and is widely distributed in nature and the predominant form in human tissues. Alpha-tocopherol may influence the development of cancer through several mechanisms.

Alpha-tocopheryl succinate (VES), a derivative of vitamin E, is known to modulate prostate cancer cell growth. Recent work suggests that VES causes G1 cell cycle arrest by decreasing expression of the cell cycle regulatory proteins cyclin D1, D3, and E, and CDK2 and 4.[29] Thompson has demonstrated that the chromanol moiety (PMCol) of vitamin E has antiandrogen activity. In LNCap, PMCol produced a growth curve similar to that produced by the androgen receptor (AR) antagonist bicalutamide, inhibited PSA secretion and androgen-induced promoter activation, and did not affect AR protein expression levels.[30]

One large-scale randomized, placebo-controlled trial, the Alpha-Tocopherol, Beta-Carotene Cancer Prevention Trial (ATBC), supports the role of vitamin E in the prevention of prostate cancer. This was a randomized, double-blind, placebo-controlled trial of α-tocopherol (50 mg/day synthetic DL-α-tocopheryl acetate) and β-carotene (20 mg/day)—alone or in combination—among 29,133 male smokers aged 50 to 69 years at entry, designed with a primary endpoint of lung cancer incidence and mortality. In ATBC there was a statistically significant 32% reduction in prostate cancer incidence and a 41% lower mortality in those receiving α-tocopherol. An important postintervention follow-up assessment of cancer incidence and mortality in this study was recently reported, with an overall post-trial relative risk (RR) for prostate cancer of 0.88 for those receiving α-tocopherol.[31] The study concluded that the beneficial effects of supplemental α-tocopherol (and the deleterious effects on lung cancer incidence of β-carotene) disappeared during postintervention follow-up, suggesting that these agents affect the risk of cancer in real time, and that their effects wash out after discontinuation. This observation has important implications on the need for the long-term use of dietary supplements to prevent cancer, and presents interesting questions for public health policy on how best to make them available to populations at risk in the form of supplements or additions to the food supply.

Another randomized, double blind, placebo controlled lung cancer prevention trial, the β-Carotene and Retinol Efficacy Trial (CARET), lends support to the epidemiologic evidence that α-tocopherol may prevent prostate cancer. Analysis of serum micronutrients in CARET participants has demonstrated that low serum levels of α-tocopherol were associated with a higher risk of prostate cancer.[32]

SELECT—THE SELENIUM AND VITAMIN E CANCER PREVENTION TRIAL

The accumulated epidemiologic and biologic evidence that Se and vitamin E may prevent prostate cancer led to the design and launch of SELECT: the Selenium and Vitamin E Cancer Prevention Trial.[33] SELECT is an NCI-sponsored phase III, randomized, double-blind, placebo-controlled, population-based clinical trial designed to test the efficacy of selenium and vitamin E alone and in combination in the prevention of prostate cancer. The study has a 2 × 2 factorial design with a target accrual of 32,400. Eligibility criteria include age over 50 years for African Americans, over 55 years for whites, a DRE not suspicious for cancer, serum PSA less than 4 ng/mL, and normal blood pressure. Randomization will be equally distributed among four study arms (selenium + placebo, vitamin E + placebo, selenium + vitamin E, and placebo + placebo). Study duration is planned for 12 years, with a minimum of 7 and maximum of 12 years of intervention depending on the time of randomization. The study supplements consist of 200 μg L-selenomethionine, 400 mg of racemic α-tocopheryl, and an optional multivitamin containing no selenium or vitamin E.

The primary endpoint for SELECT is the clinical incidence of prostate cancer. Prostate biopsy will be performed at the discretion of study physicians according to local community standards based on abnormalities in DRE or elevations in serum PSA. Secondary endpoints will include prostate cancer-free survival, all-cause mortality, and the incidence and mortality of other cancers and diseases potentially impacted by the chronic use of Se and vitamin E. Other trial objectives include periodic quality of life assessments, assessment of serum micronutrient levels and prostate cancer risk, and studies of the evaluation of biologic and genetic markers with the risk of prostate cancer. The study design will permit detection of a 25% reduction in the incidence of prostate cancer for Se or vitamin E alone, with an additional 25% reduction for the combination of selenium and vitamin E compared with either agent alone. Since neither oral Se or vitamin E are known to affect serum PSA, no PSA adjustments are planned. SELECT reached full accrual of 32,400 men in April 2004. Initial data analysis is anticipated in 2006, and complete results in 2013.

VITAMIN D

Interest in vitamin D as a preventative agent for prostate cancer comes from several epidemiologic observations: 1) men living in Northern latitudes with less exposure to sunlight-derived UV (which converts inactive to active vitamin D in the skin) have a higher mortality rate from prostate cancer; 2) prostate cancer occurs more frequently in older men, in whom vitamin D deficiency is more common both because of less UV exposure and age-related declines in the hydroxylases responsible for synthesis of active vitamin D; 3) African Americans, whose skin melanin blocks UV radiation and inhibits activation of vitamin D, have the highest worldwide incidence and mortality rates for prostate cancer; 4) dietary intake of dairy products rich in calcium, which depresses serum levels of vitamin D, are associated with a higher risk of prostate cancer; and 5) native Japanese, whose diet is rich in vitamin D derived from fish, have a low incidence of prostate cancer. In addition, prostate cancer cells express vitamin D receptor, and several studies have demonstrated an antiproliferative effect of vitamin D on prostate cancer cell lines. A brief summation of the data supporting these observations has recently been published.[34] In support of the UV hypothesis, one case-control study has suggested a protective effect for individuals with more highly pigmented skin.[35] Additional data on the potential role of calcium and dairy intake is provided by analysis of the Cancer Prevention Study II Nutrition Cohort, a prospective cohort of 65,321 elderly men in the United States.[36] Participants in the study completed a detailed questionnaire on diet, medical history, and lifestyle at enrollment in 1992 to 1993. Multivariate-adjusted rate ratios demonstrated a modestly increased risk for prostate cancer for total calcium intake (dietary and via supplements; RR = 1.2) and high dietary calcium intake alone (>2000 versus <700 mg/day; RR = 1.6), but not for dairy intake. The results support the hypothesis that very high calcium intake above the daily recommendation may modestly increase risk. Microarray gene expression studies demonstrate that active vitamin D exerts its antiproliferative activity predominantly by inducing cell cycle arrest.[37] Use of vitamin D analogs in humans has been limited by their hypercalcemic effects, but newer analogs with more tolerable toxicity are currently being tested in phase I and II trials.

COX2 INHIBITORS

Nonsteroidal anti-inflammatory drugs (NSAIDs) function by nonselective inhibition of both COX1 and COX2, isoforms of cyclooxygenase that convert arachidonic acid to prostaglandins. COX1 is constitutively expressed and mediates preservation of renal blood flow and function, platelet aggregation and hemostasis, and cytoprotection of the gastrointestinal mucosa. COX2 is an inducible enzyme that mediates acute and chronic inflammation, pain, and cellular repair mechanisms. Inhibition of COX2 expression by NSAIDs, and by more selective drugs, blocks its proinflammatory effects and may underlie an important anticancer mechanism. Increased expression of COX2 is

known to correlate with increased angiogenesis, decreased apoptosis, increased tumor invasiveness, and immunosuppression in various tumors.[38] Prostate cancers express more COX2 than benign prostatic epithelium and several epidemiologic studies have noted an inverse association of prostate cancer and use of NSAIDs.[39] COX2 inhibition has been shown to induce apoptosis in several prostate cancer cell lines.[38] Recent work demonstrates that specific inhibition of COX2 by celecoxib and nimesulide reduced the expression of several androgen-inducible genes, repressed AR-mediated activation of PSA and hK2 promoter activity, and repressed AR protein expression.[40] Another study has demonstrated selective expression of COX2 in high-grade PIN in LPB-Tag transgenic mice, suggesting a role early in carcinogenesis.[41] These results support the hypothesis that inhibition of COX2 may be an effective preventive strategy.

SELECTIVE ESTROGEN RECEPTOR MODULATORS

Interest in selective estrogen receptor modulators (SERMs) as preventative agents is stimulated by an apparent role of estrogens in the pathogenesis of prostate cancer. Both prostate stroma and epithelial cells express estrogen receptor, and estrogens promote prostatic growth.[42] Epidemiologic evidence also supports a role for estrogen in prostate cancer, with age-related prostatic disease paralleling increases in serum estrogen levels and a low incidence of prostate cancer in cultures with diets rich in phytoestrogens.[43] Selective estrogen receptor modulators possess both agonistic and antagonistic estrogen-like activity and have been shown to repress prostate cancer growth in several transgenic mouse models. In the TRAMP model, toremifene reduces the incidence of high-grade PIN and cancer in an estrogen-dependent, androgen-independent mechanism.[44] This agent is currently under study in clinical trials in men with high-grade PIN on biopsy.

SOY

Legumes play an important role in the traditional diets of Eastern countries where prostate cancer incidence is low, but only a minor role in the West where the incidence is highest worldwide. Soybeans are unique among the legumes because they are a concentrated source of isoflavones, which have weak estrogenic activity. Several studies have demonstrated a consistent anticancer effect of soy-based diets compared with controls in a variety of prostate cancer animal models.[45] The major isoflavone components of soy, including genistein, daidzein, and their metabolites, inhibit benign and malignant prostatic epithelial cell growth, downregulate androgen-regulated genes, and reduce tumor growth in some animal models.[46,47,48] Recent work suggests these effects are mediated in part by inhibition of IGF1, resulting in cell-cycle arrest and induction of apoptosis, and by prostasome inhibition.[49,50] Genistein inhibits the growth of both androgen-dependent and androgen-independent prostate cancer cells in vitro.[51] Concentrations of these agents in seminal fluid are highest in men from soy-consuming countries.[45] These observations suggest that the effects of isoflavones are exerted locally within the prostate.

Epidemiologic evidence also supports the role of soy as an anticancer agent. Consumption of tofu is associated with a reduced risk of prostate cancer in those who consume tofu five times per week compared with once per week.[52] Japanese men excrete high levels of isoflavones in the urine, and urinary levels correlate with the intake of soybean-product.[53] In a follow-up study, the same investigators compared plasma levels of four isoflavenoids in 14 Japanese and 14 Finnish men. The mean plasma total isoflavenoid levels were 7 to 110 times higher in the Japanese men, and genistein occurred in the highest concentration.[54] These observations are of interest because Finnish men have one of the highest worldwide mortality rates for prostate cancer. A larger study of 59 countries demonstrated that prostate cancer mortality is inversely associated with estimated consumption of cereals, nuts and oilseed, and fish, and that soy products are protective with an effect size per kilocalorie at least four times as large as that of any other dietary factor.[55] A prospective study of 12,395 Seventh Day Adventists in California demonstrated that frequent consumption (> once/day) of soy milk was associated with a 70% reduction in the risk of developing prostate cancer.[56] Taken together, these epidemiologic observations support the hypothesis that soy and isoflavone consumption lowers the lifetime risk of developing or dying from prostate cancer.

No large-scale clinical trials using soy or soy-based products as preventative or therapeutic agents in prostate cancer have been reported. One study has demonstrated that healthy male subjects receiving 50 mg isoflavone mixture (Novasoy) twice daily for 3 weeks are protected from tumor necrosis factor-α (TNFα) induced NFκB activation.[57] In addition, a reduction of 5-hydroxymethyl-2'-deoxyuridine (5-OHmdU), a marker for oxidative DNA damage, was also observed following isoflavone supplementation. This preliminary study demonstrates that soy isoflavone supplementation may protect cells from oxidative stress-inducing agents by inhibiting NFκB activation and decreasing DNA adduct levels. Genestein, other isoflavones, and dietary intervention with soy are currently being studied in men at high risk of failure or with rising PSA after definitive treatment for localized prostate cancer,[58] and in men who have selected "watchful waiting" as primary therapy.[59]

LYCOPENE

Lycopene is a red–orange carotenoid found primarily in tomatoes and tomato-derived products including tomato sauce, tomato paste and ketchup, and other red fruits and vegetables. Lycopene is a highly unsaturated acyclic isomer of β-carotene, is the predominant carotenoid in human plasma, and possesses potent antioxidant activity. There is mixed epidemiologic evidence that lycopene consumption is associated with a lower risk of prostate cancer.[60] Lycopene inhibits the growth of benign and malignant prostatic epithelial cells in vitro.[61] In an in-vivo model where male rats were treated with N-methyl-N-nitrosourea and testosterone to induce prostate cancer, a protective effect was observed both for calorie restriction and tomato powder, but not for pure lycopene.[62] This observation suggests that tomato products contain compounds in addition to lycopene that modify prostate carcinogenesis, and that tomato phytochemicals and diet restriction may act by independent mechanisms. These observations also suggest that reduced caloric consumption and a diet rich in tomato-based foods may be more beneficial than taking oral lycopene supplements in reducing the risk of prostate cancer in humans.

Two non-placebo-controlled prospective clinical trials examining the effect of lycopene on known prostate cancer has been reported.[63,64] In the first trial, 26 men with clinically localized prostate cancer scheduled for radical prostatectomy were randomized to 15 mg lycopene p.o. b.i.d. for 3 weeks versus no lycopene preoperatively. Statistically significant reductions in serum PSA (18% drop vs. 14% increase) and in the rate of positive margins (from 72% to 17%) were observed in the lycopene group, with no differences seen in various biologic endpoints including serum IGF1, prevalence of high-grade PIN, and tumor expression of BCL2, bax, or connexin 43. The study is limited by a small sample size and significant differences in tumor burden between the intervention and control groups as assessed by pretreatment stage and tumor grade, which could account for the differences in pathologic findings. In the second trial, 32 patients with localized disease scheduled for radical prostatectomy ate tomato sauce-based pasta dishes for the 3 weeks (equivalent to 30 mg/day lycopene) before surgery. Serum and prostate lycopene concentrations were statistically significantly increased in the intervention group. Compared with preintervention levels, both leukocyte and prostate oxidative DNA damage were also reduced significantly after intervention. A small but statistically significant reduction in serum PSA was also observed (from 10.9

ng/mL to 8.7 ng/mL). Together these clinical trials support the hypothesis that lycopene is active against prostate caner and that additional larger studies with appropriate controls are indicated.

GREEN TEA

Green tea has been suggested as a prostate cancer preventative based on epidemiologic observations of a low incidence of prostate cancer among native Asians with a high dietary intake. Previous work has focused on the effects of polyphenols contained in green tea, but the molecular mechanism of their action has not been elucidated. Prostate cancer cell culture experiments have demonstrated that the major polyphenolic constituent of green tea (–)-epigallocatechin-3-gallate (EGCG) induces apoptosis, cell-growth inhibition, and cyclin kinase inhibitor WAF1/p21-mediated cell-cycle dysregulation.[65] Gene expression analysis found that EGCG treatment of LNCaP cells results in induction of growth-inhibitory genes that belong to the G-protein signaling network. In the TRAMP model, oral infusion of a polyphenolic fraction isolated from green tea (GTP) at a human achievable dose (equivalent to 6 cups of green tea/day) significantly inhibits tumor development and metastasis.[66] Additional work has shown that EGCG induces apoptosis by inhibiting fatty acid synthase (FAS).[67] Taken together, the data indicate that EGCG induces apoptosis in human prostate carcinoma cells by shifting the balance between pro- and antiapoptotic proteins in favor of apoptosis.

CONCLUSION

Prostate cancer is an attractive target for chemoprevention because of its ubiquity, treatment-related morbidity, long latency between premalignant lesions and clinically evident cancer, and defined molecular pathogenesis. The PCPT is the first firm evidence that this cancer can be prevented by a relatively nontoxic oral agent. New trials designed to test additional agents, many of which are antioxidants with antiandrogenic effects, are currently or are about to be tested in large scale human clinical trials. The current body of evidence is insufficient to make a routine recommendation of any dietary or nutritional supplement for the prevention of prostate cancer.

REFERENCES

1. Lieberman R, Kagan J, House MG, et al. Strategies for the chemoprevention of cancer. In Klein EA (ed): Management of Prostate Cancer, 2nd ed. Totowa, NJ: Humana Press, 2004, pp 71–106.

2. Jemal A, Tiwari RC, Murray T, et al. Cancer Statistics 2004. CA Cancer J Clin 2004;54:8–29.

3. Stanford JL, Feng Z, Hamilton AS, et al. Urinary and sexual function after radical prostatectomy for clinically localized prostate cancer: the Prostate Cancer Outcomes Study. JAMA 2000;283:354–360.

4. Potosky AL, Legler J, Albertsen PC, et al. Health outcomes after prostatectomy or radiotherapy for prostate cancer: results from the Prostate Cancer Outcomes Study. J Natl Cancer Inst 2000;92:1582–1592.

5. Mehta SS, Lubeck DP, Pasta DJ, et al. Fear of cancer recurrence in patients undergoing definitive treatment for prostate cancer: results from CaPSURE. J Urol 2003;170:1931–1933.

6. Landis SH, Murray T, Bolden S, et al. Cancer Statistics 1999. CA Cancer J Clin 1999;49:8–31.

7. Smith JR, Freije D, Carpten JD, et al. Major susceptibility locus for prostate cancer on chromosome 1 suggested by a genome-wide search. Science 1995;274:1371–1374.

8. Carter BS, Bova GS, Beaty T. Hereditary prostate cancer: Epidemiologic and clinical features. J Urol 1993;150:797–802.

9. Zlotta AR, Schulman CC. Clinical evolution of prostatic intraepithelial neoplasia. Eur Urol 1999;35:498–503.

10. Klein EA, Meyskens FL. Potential target populations and clinical models for testing chemopreventative agents. Urology 2001;57:171–173.

11. Thompson IM, Goodman PJ, Tangen CM, et al. The influence of finasteride on the development of prostate cancer. N Engl J Med 2003;349:215–224.

12. Harlan SR, Cooperberg MR, Elkin EP, et al. Time trends and characteristics of men choosing watchful waiting for initial treatment of localized prostate cancer: results from CaPSURE. J Urol 2003;170:1804–1807.

13. Thompson I, Klein EA, Lippman SM, et al. Prevention of Prostate Cancer with Finasteride: A U.S./European Perspective. Eur Urol 2003;44:650–655.

14. Civantos F, Soloway MS, Pinto JE. Histopathological effects of androgen deprivation in prostatic cancer. Semin Urol Oncol 1996;14:22–31.

15. Klein EA, Thompson IM, Tangen CM, et al. Assessing benefit and risk in prevention of prostate cancer: the Prostate Cancer Prevention Trial revisited. J Clin Oncol 2005;12 (Epub).

16. Klein EA. Selenium—epidemiology and basic science. J Urol 2004;171:S50–53.

17. Vogt TM, Ziegler RG, Graubard BI, et al. Serum Se and risk of prostate cancer in U.S. blacks and whites. Int J Cancer 2003;103:664–670.

18. Duffield-Lillico AJ, Dalkin BL, Reid ME, et al. Se supplementation, baseline plasma Se status, and incidence of prostate cancer: an analysis of the complete treatment period of the nutritional prevention of cancer study group. Br J Urol Intl 2003;91:608–612.

19. van den Brandt PA, Zeegers MP, Bode P, et al. Toenail selenium levels and the subsequent risk of prostate cancer: a prospective cohort study. Cancer Epidemiol Biomarkers Prev 2003;12:866–871.

20. Dewailly E, Mulvad G, Sloth Pedersen H, et al. Inuit are protected against prostate cancer. Cancer Epidemiol Biomarkers Prev 2003;12:926–927.

21. Dong Y, Zhang H, Hawthorne L, et al. Delineation of the molecular basis for Se-induced growth arrest in human prostate cancer cells by oligonucleotide array. Cancer Res 2003;63:52–59.

22. Zhao H, Whitfield ML, Xu T, et al. Diverse effects of methylseleninic acid on the transcriptional program of human prostate cancer cells. Mol Biol Cell 2003 Nov 14 [Epub ahead of print].

23. Zu K, Ip C. Synergy between selenium and vitamin E in apoptosis induction is associated with activation of distinctive initiator caspases in human prostate cancer cells. Cancer Res 2003; 63:6988–6995.

24. Waters DJ, Shen S, Cooley DM, et al. Effects of dietary Se supplementation on DNA damage and apoptosis in canine prostate. J Natl Cancer Inst 2003;95:237–241.

25. Gianduzzo TR, Holmes EG, Tinggi U, et al. Prostatic and peripheral blood selenium levels after oral supplementation. J Urol 2003;170:870–873.

26. Bhamre S, Whitin JC, Cohen HJ. Selenomethionine does not affect PSA secretion independent of its effect on LNCap growth. Prostate 2003;54:315–321.

27. Stratton MS, Reid ME, Schwartzberg G, et al. Selenium and prevention of prostate cancer in high-risk men: the Negative Biopsy Study. Anticancer Drugs 2003;14:589–594.

28. Stratton MS, Reid ME, Schwartzberg G, et al. Selenium and inhibition of disease progression in men diagnosed with prostate carcinoma: study design and baseline characteristics of the 'Watchful Waiting' Study. Anticancer Drugs 2003;14:595–600.

29. Ni J, Chen M, Zhang Y, et al. Vitamin E succinate inhibits human prostate cancer cell growth via modulating cell cycle regulatory machinery. Biochem Biophys Res Commun 2003;300:357–363.

30. Thompson TA, Wilding G. Androgen antagonist activity by the antioxidant moiety of vitamin E, 2,2,5,7,8-pentamethyl-6-chromanol in human prostate carcinoma cells. Mol Cancer Ther 2003;2:797–803.

31. Virtamo J, Pietinen P, Huttunen JK, et al. ATBC Study Group: Incidence of cancer and mortality following alpha-tocopherol and beta-carotene supplementation: a postintervention follow-up. JAMA 2003;290:476–485.

32. Goodman GE, Schaffer S, Omenn GS, et al. The association between lung and prostate cancer risk, and serum micronutrients: results and lessons learned from beta-carotene and retinol efficacy trial. Cancer Epidemiol Biomarkers Prev 2003;12:518–526.

33. Klein EA, Thompson IM, Lippman SM, et al. The Selenium and Vitamin E Cancer Prevention Trial. World J Urol 2003;21:21–27.

34. Peehl DM, Krishnan AV, Feldman D. Pathways mediating the growth-inhibitory actions of vitamin D in prostate cancer. J Nutr 2003;133:2461S–2469S.

35. Bodiwala D, Luscombe CJ, French ME, et al. Susceptibility to prostate cancer: studies on interactions between UVR exposure and skin type. Carcinogenesis 2003;24:711–717.

36. Rodriguez C, McCullough ML, Mondul AM, et al. Calcium, dairy products, and risk of prostate cancer in a prospective cohort of United States men. Cancer Epidemiol Biomarkers Prev 2003;12:597–603.

37. Krishnan AV, Peehl DM, Feldman D. Inhibition of prostate cancer growth by vitamin D: Regulation of target gene expression. J Cell Biochem 2003;88:363–371.

38. Pruthi RS, Derksen E, Gaston K. Cyclooxygenase-2 as a potential target in the prevention and treatment of genitourinary tumors: a review. J Urol 2003;169:2352–2359.

39. Hussain T, Gupta S, Mukhtar H. Cyclooxygenase-2 and prostate carcinogenesis. Cancer Lett 2003;191:125–135.

40. Pan Y, Zhang JS, Gazi MH, et al. The cyclooxygenase 2-specific nonsteroidal anti-inflammatory drugs celecoxib and nimesulide inhibit androgen receptor activity via induction of c-Jun in prostate cancer cells. Cancer Epidemiol Biomarkers Prev 2003;12:769–774.

41. Shappell SB, Olson SJ, Hannah SE, et al. Elevated expression of 12/15-lipoxygenase and cyclooxygenase-2 in a transgenic mouse model of prostate carcinoma. Cancer Res 2003;63:2256–2267.

42. Steiner MS, Raghow S. Antiestrogens and selective estrogen receptor modulators reduce prostate cancer risk. World J Urol 2003;21:31–36.

43. Denis L, Morton MS, Griffith K. Diet and its preventive role in prostatic disease. Eur Urol 1999; 35:377–387.

44. Raghow S, Hooshdaran MZ, Katiyar S. Toremifine prevents prostate cancer in the transgenic adenocarcinoma of mouse prostate model. Cancer Res 2002;62:1370–1376.

45. Klein EA, Prostate cancer. In Lang RS, Hansrud DD (eds): Clinical Preventive Medicine, 2nd ed. Chicago: AMA Press, 2004, pp 120–135.

46. Hedlund TE, Johannes WU, Miller GJ. Soy isoflavonoid equol modulates the growth of benign and malignant prostatic epithelial cells in vitro. Prostate 2003;54:68–78.

47. Cohen LA, Zhao Z, Pittman B, et al. Effect of soy protein isolate and conjugated linoleic acid on the growth of Dunning R-3327-AT-1 rat prostate tumors. Prostate 2003;54:169–168.

48. Yu L, Blackburn GL, Zhou JR. Genistein and daidzein downregulate prostate androgen-regulated transcript-1 (PART-1) gene expression induced by dihydrotestosterone in human prostate LNCaP cancer cells. J Nutr 2003;133:389–392.

49. Wang S, DeGroff VL, Clinton SK. Tomato and soy polyphenols reduce insulin-like growth factor-I-stimulated rat prostate cancer cell proliferation and apoptotic resistance in vitro via inhibition of intracellular signaling pathways involving tyrosine kinase. J Nutr 2003;133:2367–2376.

50. Kazi A, Daniel KG, Smith DM, et al. Inhibition of the proteasome activity, a novel mechanism associated with the tumor cell apoptosis-inducing ability of genistein. Biochem Pharmacol 2003;66:965–976.

51. Santibáñez JF, Navarro A, Martinez J. Genistein inhibits proliferation and in vitro invasive potential of human prostatic cancer cell lines. Anticancer Res 1997;17:1199–1204.

52. Severson KJ, Nomura AMY, Grove JS, et al. A prospective study of demographics, diet, and prostate cancer among men of Japanese ancestry in Hawaii. Cancer Res 1989;49:1857–1860.

53. Adlercreutz H, Honjo H, Higashi A, et al. Urinary excretion of lignans and isoflavonoid phytoestrogens in Japanese men and women consuming a traditional Japanese die. Am J Clin Nutr 1991 54:1093–1100.

54. Adlercreutz H, Markkanen H, Watanabe S. Plasma concentrations of phyto-oestrogens in Japanese men. Lancet 1993;342:1209–1210.

55. Hebert JR, Hurley TG, Olendzki BC, et al. Nutritional and socioeconomic factors in relation to prostate cancer mortality: a cross-national study. J Natl Cancer Inst 1998;90:1637–1647.

56. Jacobsen BK, Knutsen SF, Fraser GE. Does high soy milk reduce prostate cancer incidence? The Adventist Health Study (United States). Cancer Causes Control 1998;9:553–557.

57. Davis JN, Kucuk O, Djuric Z, et al. Soy isoflavone supplementation in healthy men prevents NF-kappaB activation by TNF-alpha in blood lymphocytes. Free Radic Biol Med 2001;30:1293–1302.

58. Bosland MC, Kato I, Melamed J, et al. Chemoprevention trials in men with prostate-specific antigen failure or at high risk for recurrence after radical prostatectomy: Application to efficacy assessment of soy protein. Urology 2001; 57:202–204.

59. Ornish DM, Lee KL, Fair WR, et al. Dietary trial in prostate cancer: Early experience and implications for clinical trial design. Urology 2001;57:200–201.

60. Giovannucci E, Clinton SK. Tomatoes, lycopene, and cancer: review of the epidemiologic literature. J Natl Cancer Inst 1999;91:317–331.

61. Obermuller-Jevic UC, Olano-Martin E, et al. Lycopene inhibits the growth of normal human prostate epithelial cells in vitro. J Nutr 2003;133:3356–3360.

62. Boileau TW, Liao Z, Kim S, et al. Prostate carcinogenesis in N-methyl-N-nitrosourea (NMU)-testosterone-treated rats fed tomato powder, lycopene, or energy-restricted diets. J Natl Cancer Inst 2003;95:1578–1586.

63. Kucuk O, Sarkar FH, Sakr W, et al. Phase II randomized clinical trial of lycopene supplementation before radical prostatectomy. Cancer Epidemiol Biomarkers Prev 2001;10:861–868.

64. Chen L, Stacewicz-Sapuntzakis M, Duncan C, et al. Oxidative DNA damage in prostate cancer patients consuming tomato sauce-based entrees as a whole-food intervention. J Natl Cancer Inst 2001;93:1872–1879.

65. Adhami VM, Ahmad N, Mukhtar H. Molecular targets for green tea in prostate cancer prevention. J Nutr 2003;133:2417S–2424S.

66. Hastak K, Gupta S, Ahmad N, et al. Role of p53 and NF-kappaB in epigallocatechin-3-gallate-induced apoptosis of LNCaP cells. Oncogene 2003;22:4851–4859.

67. Brusselmans K, De Schrijver E, Heyns W, et al. Epigallocatechin-3-gallate is a potent natural inhibitor of fatty acid synthase in intact cells and selectively induces apoptosis in prostate cancer cells. Int J Cancer 2003:106:856–862.

68. Ries LAG, Kosary CL, Hankey BF, et al. SEER Cancer Statistics Review, 1973–1995. Bethesda, MD: National Cancer Institute, 1998.

Molecular aspects of chemoprevention of prostate cancer

20

James D Brooks

INTRODUCTION

In many ways, prostate cancer lends itself to preventive approaches. Autopsy studies demonstrate that prostatic intraepithelial neoplasia (PIN—a putative prostate cancer precursor lesion) can be found in 29% to 46% of men in their fourth decade, and frank prostate cancer can be found in up to 34%.[1–3] However, prostate cancer usually does not become clinically manifest until most men are in their sixth decade and beyond, providing a large window for interventions designed to prevent the disease or slow its progression. The lifetime risk of prostate cancer diagnosis is approximately 18%, meaning that many men are at risk for the disease and, therefore, candidates for preventive intervention strategies.[4] Target populations at increased risk include African American men, men with a family history of prostate cancer and those carrying germline mutations in a handful of prostate cancer susceptibility genes.[5–8] The heightened awareness of prostate cancer motivates many men to take an interest in preventive interventions, evidenced by the high number of men who use nutritional supplements to either prevent prostate cancer or retard its progression.[9] The high prevalence, long latency, existence of high-risk populations, public awareness, and motivation of men to undertake preventive interventions provide an excellent foundation for developing effective prostate cancer prevention strategies.

Diverse evidence suggests that prostate cancer might be a preventable disease. Studies of Asian men demonstrate that their risk of prostate cancer increases dramatically as they emigrate from their native lands (where they have low incident rates) to the West.[10–18]

Three decades after their move, their risk of prostate cancer increases five-fold or more, and first generation Asian males born in the West assume incident rates approaching that of native whites.[15] The dramatic changes observed in incident rates following emigration implicate environmental factors as important in prostate carcinogenesis. However, unlike lung cancer in which smoking directly contributes to carcinogenesis, or liver cancer where hepatitis and aflatoxin have been strongly implicated, the features in the environment that contribute to prostate carcinogenesis remain a mystery. Given our rudimentary knowledge of the causes of prostate cancer, identification of effective preventive agents will prove challenging.

Epidemiologic studies have provided some clues to environmental factors that might contribute to prostate carcinogenesis and others that might protect against the disease. Although petroleum products and pesticides have been found to have a weak positive association with prostate cancer development,[19–22] most studies have implicated dietary factors as risk modifiers for prostate cancer.[11,23–31] Several studies have demonstrated an association between consumption of animal fats and an elevated prostate cancer risk.[31–33] Others studies have suggested that dietary micronutrients could exert a protective role and have noted an inverse association between prostate cancer risk and serum levels of or the intake of selenium, tomatoes and lycopene, vitamin E, green vegetables and cruciferous vegetables, soy, and vitamin D.[13,30,34–47] Two intervention trials have complemented these findings by suggesting that selenium or vitamin E could prevent prostate cancer compared with placebo.[48–51] The Prostate Cancer Prevention Trial (PCPT) demonstrated directly that finasteride results in a 25% decrease in prostate cancer compared with placebo in a large cohort of men.[52] While the epidemiologic studies provide some clues to potential prostate cancer prevention strategies, they also give some insight into biological features that contribute to prostate carcinogenesis.

BIOLOGICAL BASIS OF PROSTATE CANCER

Prostate carcinogenesis appears to be a multistep process wherein accumulated genetic damage and clonal selection results in dysplastic lesions, dysregulated cell growth, and, ultimately, carcinoma.[53,54] Prostate cancer shows many features of field carcinogenesis in that dysplastic lesions, or PIN, can be found diffusely starting at a young age and in association with carcinoma.[1,2] Like other malignancies, prostate cancer is often multifocal, and separate lesions can display distinct genetic alterations.[55,56] Yet, unlike other malignancies, few discrete genetic alterations have been found that are associated with progression from normal epithelium to dysplasia, low-grade carcinoma, high-grade carcinoma, metastasis, and ultimately to hormone refractory disease. In the absence of such knowledge, identification of the mechanisms underlying putative prostate cancer preventive agents has proved challenging. However, several important themes in prostate carcinogenesis are emerging and each is being investigated increasingly as potential targets of chemopreventive agents (Figure 20.1). Chemopreventive agents have been evaluated for their effects on androgen signaling, proliferation, oxidative stress, apoptosis, and several other important features of prostate carcinogenesis (Table 20.1).

Table 20.1 Selected targets and mechanisms of prostate cancer preventive agents		
Target mechanism	**Molecular targets**	**Representative agents**
Androgen signaling	5α-reductase	Finasteride, genistein
	AR binding	Casodex
	AR protein levels	Vitamin E, selenium, resveratrol
	Estrogen receptor	SERMs, genistein
Proliferation	Cyclins, cyclin-dependent kinases and many others	Vitamins E & D, selenium, retinoids, resveratrol, sulforaphane, lycopene
Inflammation	Free radicals	Vitamin E, lycopene, resveratrol, EGCG
	Carcinogen defenses	Sulforaphane, curcumin
Apoptosis	TGFβ, TRAIL others	Retinoids, resveratrol, selenium, EGCG
		Sulforaphane, COX2 inhibitors
Differentiation	TGFβ	Retinoids, vitamin D, phenyl-butyrate
Angiogenesis	FGF signaling	Genistein
	Thrombomodulin	Retinoids

AR, androgen receptor; COX2, cyclooxygenase 2; EGCG, epigallocatechin-3 gallate; FGF, fibroblast growth factor; SERMs, selective estrogen receptor modulators; TGFβ, transforming growth factor-β; TRAIL, tumor necrosis factor-related apoptosis-inducing ligand.

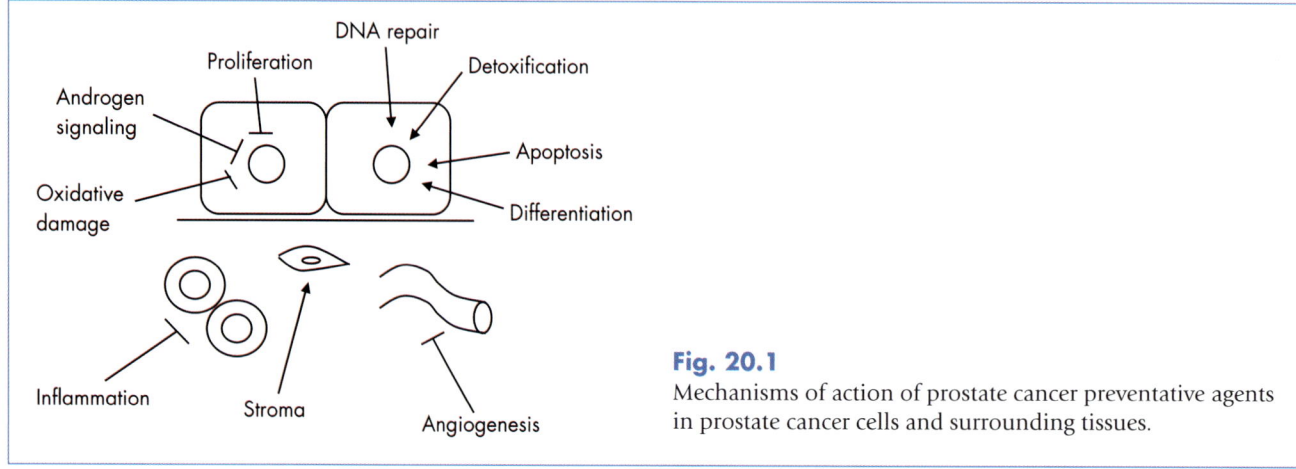

Fig. 20.1
Mechanisms of action of prostate cancer preventative agents in prostate cancer cells and surrounding tissues.

ANDROGENS AND STEROID HORMONE SIGNALING PATHWAYS

Since the 1940s, androgens have been known to be critical to prostate carcinogenesis and disease progression and this knowledge has served as the basis for androgen deprivation therapies for advanced prostate cancer.[57] Men castrated early in life have small rudimentary prostates and appear to be immune to prostatic diseases including prostate cancer. Although results are inconclusive, elevated prediagnostic serum testosterone levels have been associated with an increased risk of prostate cancer development.[58] Elevated serum androgen levels have been observed in African American men, a group at substantially higher risk for prostate cancer, compared with whites and Asian Americans.[59] Polymorphisms in the androgen receptor (AR) and androgen metabolizing genes that confer increased androgen signaling activity have been associated with increased risk for developing prostate cancer.[60–62] Thus the AR appears central to prostate carcinogenesis, and is critical to prostate biology.

In its unbound form, the AR is found largely in the cytoplasm; when it binds ligand, it is translocated to the nucleus of the prostate cell where it dimerizes and interacts with several coactivator proteins to form a complex that binds to transcriptional regulatory sequences known as androgen response elements (AREs).[63] Androgen receptor activation results in a transcriptional cascade of several hundred genes, some regulated directly through AREs and others indirectly either through pathways downstream of AR-regulated genes or through other mechanisms involving the AR protein complex.[64,65] These androgen responsive genes likely mediate the most important effects of androgen signaling in prostate cells: cell growth and differentiation into secretory epithelium.

The PCPT demonstrated unambiguously that disruption of androgen signaling prevents prostate cancer.[52] In PCPT, 18,882 asymptomatic men with low prostate-specific antigen (PSA) levels were randomly assigned to receive either placebo or finasteride, an inhibitor of 5α-reductase (type 2) that blocks conversion of testosterone to dihydrotestosterone (DHT), the primary androgen active in the prostate, which has a 10-fold higher affinity than testosterone for the AR. In the 9060 men who completed the full 7 years of therapy, cancer was detected in 18.4% of the men on finasteride and in 24.4% on placebo, for a risk reduction of 24.8%. Clouding these results was the finding of more cases of high grade cancer (Gleason 7–10) in the finasteride group compared with placebo (6.4% versus 5.1%). Regardless of the ultimate clinical application of the data from this trial, it demonstrates that modest inhibition of androgen signaling can reduce the incidence of prostate cancer and has promise of a prevention strategy. A second large randomized trial involving dutasteride (an inhibitor of both types 1 and 2 5α-reductase) that is underway will provide additional data on androgen blockage and prostate cancer prevention.[66]

Several candidate prostate cancer preventive agents appear to antagonize androgen signaling pathways (Figure 20.2). Both epidemiologic evidence and analysis of secondary endpoints of the Nutritional Prevention of Cancer (NPC) trial (in which selenized yeast was found to reduce prostate cancer diagnosis by 66% compared with placebo) have identified selenium as a promising prostate cancer preventive agent.[34,40,44,46,47,49,50] The means by which selenium might act to prevent cancer remain obscure, but are thought to involve incorporation of selenium into proteins as selenocysteine.[67] However, small organic selenium compounds such as methylselenic acid (MSA) will provide complete protection against carcinogenesis in animal models, and this effect is likely mediated through methylselenol.[68] Treatment of human prostate cancer cells in vitro with MSA produces profound changes in transcript levels of many androgen-regulated genes suggesting that it antagonizes androgen

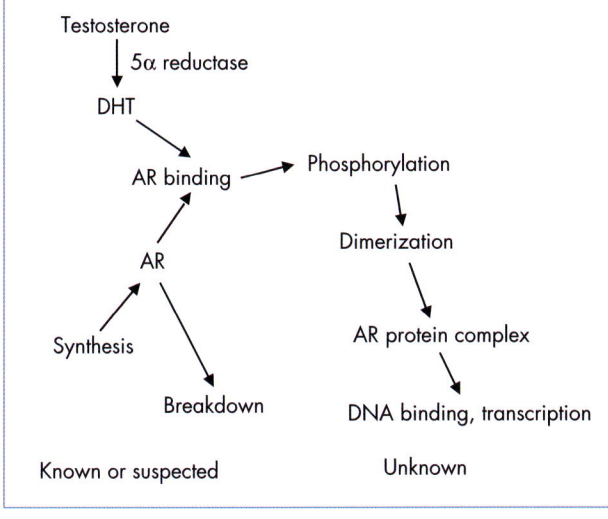

Fig. 20.2

Androgen signaling pathways that can be targeted by preventive compounds. On the left are portions of the androgen signaling pathway that are known or strongly suspected to be affected by preventive compounds. Portions of the signaling cascade on the right have not been found to be directly influenced by any preventive compounds.

signaling.[69] Furthermore, MSA reduces AR protein levels and levels of secreted PSA, and also significantly inhibits transcription of a PSA promoter–reporter construct. Somewhat surprisingly, selenomethionine, the form of selenium that is currently being used in the Selenium and vitamin E Cancer Prevention Trial (SELECT), does not appear to affect androgen signaling or PSA levels in vitro.[70] Therefore, it is possible that some selenium compounds act to prevent prostate cancer by antagonizing androgen signaling pathways; however, not all selenium compounds display this activity.

The α-tocopherol and β-carotene Cancer Prevention Study (TCCPS) led to the identification of vitamin E as a promising chemopreventive agent.[51] This trial was designed to test whether vitamin E (α-tocopherol), β-carotene, or the combination of the two could prevent lung cancer in 29,133 Finnish male smokers and is perhaps best known for the surprising and disappointing finding that β-carotene was associated with an increased incidence in lung cancer diagnosis compared with placebo. However, compared with placebo, α-tocopherol-treated men were found to have 30% lower chance of being diagnosed with prostate cancer and a 40% decrease in prostate cancer deaths.[48] Because serum α-tocopherol levels in the men receiving vitamin E was inversely related to serum testosterone and androstenedione levels, it was suggested that vitamin E reduces prostate cancer risk by reducing sex steroid levels.[71] Vitamin E might also directly antagonize androgen signaling. Vitamin E succinate (VES) will decrease intracellular and secreted PSA levels as well as AR transcript and protein levels in a ligand-independent fashion.[72] Intriguingly, VES appears to decrease AR levels largely by inhibiting translation by undefined mechanisms—a potentially novel means of interfering with androgen signaling.

Several foodstuff-derived polyphenols and isoflavones have been found to affect androgen signaling pathways. Recent epidemiologic evidence suggests that red wine (but not white wine, beer, or other alcoholic beverages) is associated with a decreased risk of prostate cancer diagnosis and progression.[73] Resveratrol, a trans-hydroxystilbene polyphenol, is found at high levels in red wine and has been implicated as a cancer preventive agent in several malignancies.[74] Resveratrol induces striking changes in gene expression in androgen responsive genes that strongly suggest that it antagonizes androgen signaling.[75–77] Furthermore, resveratrol decreases PSA secretion, and decreases AR protein levels, although the changes in AR protein levels occur long after changes in transcript levels of AR-responsive genes.[75] This suggests that resveratrol affects androgen signaling pathways at several steps. The soy-derived isoflavones genistein and daidzein also can modulate androgen-responsive genes globally, and have been found to influence steroid metabolism by inhibiting 5α-reductase and aromatase.[78–80] Several isoflavones, including genistein, will suppress DHT-induced PSA

production by human prostate cancer cells in vitro, again suggesting that these compounds can act by additional pathways to antagonize androgen signaling.[81]

Another mechanism by which candidate prostate cancer preventive agents might act is through modulation of other steroid signaling pathways. Estrogens were long used to treat advanced prostate cancer and were presumed to act by reducing testosterone levels to castrate levels. Recent evidence suggests that estrogens might have direct inhibitory effects on prostate cancer.[82] Several candidate preventive compounds have been found to act as weak antiestrogens or as selective estrogen receptor modulators (SERMs).[83–85] Soy is rich in phytoestrogens that can act as antiestrogens or SERMs, and licorice and the herbal preparation PC-SPES have been demonstrated to act as potent estrogens.[86,87] Toremifene, a SERM being evaluated as a breast cancer preventive agent, delays the onset and increases survival of transgenic adenocarcinoma of mouse prostate (TRAMP) animals.[85]

Therefore, inhibition of androgen signaling pathways and modulation of sex-steroid signaling pathways are emerging targets of many prostate cancer preventive agents. Understanding that agents might affect sex-steroid signaling pathways is critical, not simply because such knowledge could improve design of preventive strategies, but because it could influence design and interpretation of preventive intervention trials. For instance, agents that block androgen signaling could affect serum PSA levels, leading to fewer biopsies and fewer diagnoses in a treatment arm without a true reduction in prostate cancer rates. Furthermore, compounds that act as antiandrogens could affect interpretation of biopsies in individuals diagnosed with cancer by altering the histological appearance of tumors.

PROLIFERATION

Prostate cancer typically exhibits a low proliferative index, as would be expected given its long latency and protracted clinical course in most cases. Approximately 3% of prostate cancer cells stain positive for markers of proliferation by immunohistochemistry, which is far lower than many malignancies, although greater than the 0.2% of positively staining cells in normal prostate epithelium.[88] Proliferative index is higher in advanced-stage and high-grade prostate cancer, and increased proliferative index has been associated with adverse outcome in clinically localized prostate cancers.[89] Gene expression correlates of proliferation have been observed in biologically more aggressive forms of prostate cancer.[90,91] Thus, agents that target proliferation have potential to prolong the latency of subclinical prostate cancer and potentially slow progression of established disease.

Many candidate prostate cancer preventive compounds have been shown to affect prostate cancer cell growth or proliferation rates in some way. Investigators have demonstrated that a startling variety of candidate preventive compounds (selenomethionine, vitamin E, lycopene, methylselenic acid, resveratrol, sulindac sulfone, vitamin D, genistein, epigallocatechin gallate to name a few) will inhibit prostate cancer cell growth in vitro.[69,75,92–100] In many cases, compounds have been tested on both androgen-responsive and androgen-insensitive cells, thereby demonstrating that growth inhibition is not purely dependent upon androgen signaling blockade. The effects of many compounds have been refined to some extent by analysis of the cell cycle to identify the point at which the particular compound blocks cell growth. However, a single compound can often show different effects in different prostate cancer cell lines. Selenomethionine, for instance, produces G1 arrest in the LNCaP prostate cancer cell line and G2/M arrest in a PC-3 prostate cancer cell line that has been engineered to express the AR.[94] In addition, closely related compounds, such as selenomethionine and methylselenic acid, can produce growth arrest in different phases of the cell cycle within the same cell line.[69]

Candidate preventive compounds have also been tested for their ability to inhibit proliferation, tumor growth, and mortality in animal models of prostate cancer. Vitamin E, for instance will slow growth of LNCaP prostate cancer cell xenografts in nude mice that have been fed a high-fat diet.[101] Green tea polyphenols, genistein, flaxseed, toremifene, α-difluoromethylornithene, and flutamide have all been demonstrated to delay the onset of prostate cancer in the TRAMP model.[85,102–105] Tomato products and genistein have been shown to suppress sex accessory tissue cancers in Lobund-Wistar rats.[106,107] Thus in some in vivo model systems, candidate preventive agents have been demonstrated to suppress or slow growth. However, the exact mechanisms responsible for this growth suppression are poorly understood.

Attenuation of proliferation is a widely cited and tantalizing target for many prostate cancer preventive agents. Understanding how putative preventive compounds affect proliferation can be elusive and complex. Several studies have focused on the effects of preventive compounds on cell cycle regulatory proteins. Genistein, for example, induces expression of the cyclin-dependent kinase inhibitors p27 (KIP1) and p21 (WAF1) and induces G1 arrest in prostate cancer cells. However, it is unlikely that any of the preventive compounds decrease proliferation by directly modifying cell cycle regulatory proteins. Rather, these compounds likely act on upstream signaling pathways that influence cell cycle regulatory protein synthesis or turnover. Proliferation represents the integration of a host of positive and negative signals and involves a complex program of transcriptional and post-transcriptional changes in the cell. For instance, Whitfield et al have characterized 1134 transcripts that vary periodically as synchronized cells move through the cell cycle.[108] Resveratrol treatment of LNCaP cells in vitro leads to altered expression of 442 of these transcripts, and methylselenic acid affects 172.[69,75] Development of preventive compounds that target proliferation will depend upon defining the pathways altered in prostate cancer that are responsible for regulation of cell growth. While our current level of knowledge is meager at best, some signaling pathways, such as phosphoinositide 3 kinase (PI3K) appear to be important in prostate cancer and potentially targetable with biological therapies.[109]

INFLAMMATION

Several lines of evidence have recently converged that suggest that inflammation contributes to prostate carcinogenesis and might be a promising target for prostate cancer preventive interventions[110] (Figure 20.3). Inflammation has been implicated as a causative agent

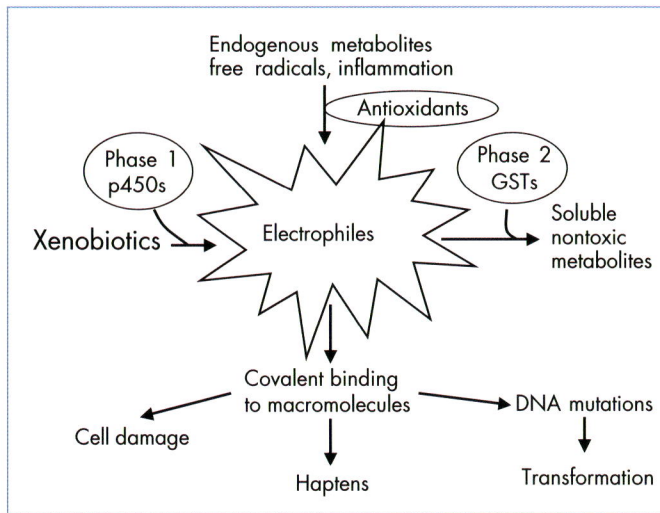

Fig. 20.3

Electrophilic compounds from endogenous sources (free radicals from cell signaling, metabolism, inflammation) and exogenous sources (dietary or environmental carcinogens) result in DNA damage and transformation. Many exogenous carcinogens are activated by oxidative phase 1 enzymes (p450s), while electrophiles are detoxified by phase 2 enzymes (e.g., glutathione transferases, glucuronosyl transferases, quinone oxidoreductases). Preventive compounds can act by quenching free radicals directly, decreasing phase 1 enzyme activation of carcinogens, or increasing electrophile metabolism by inducing phase 2 enzyme activity.

in several malignancies including liver, stomach, bladder, cervical, and colon cancers.[111] However establishment of a direct link between inflammation and prostate cancer poses several challenges. First, inflammation is extremely common in the prostate and can be found in over 95% of prostatectomy specimens.[112,113] Recently, careful pathologic assessment of inflammation in the prostate gland has led to identification of proliferative lesions associated with inflammatory cells called by various names such as simple atrophy, post-atrophic hyperplasia, and proliferative inflammatory atrophy (PIA).[114,115] Proliferative inflammatory atrophy lesions show many hallmarks of inflammation including overexpression of COX2, GSTP1, and GSTA1.[115] Coupled with this response is increased proliferation, increased expression of BCL2, and diminished apoptosis. This unholy alliance of proliferation and increased survival with apparent cellular stress due to inflammation has been proposed to set the stage for malignant transformation. Indeed, molecular genetic changes associated with prostate cancer such as gain of DNA sequences at the centromeric region of chromosome 8, p53 gene mutations and hypermethylation of GSTP1 promoter sequences,[114,116] have been identified in PIA lesions suggesting that they are a precursor to prostate cancer. Proliferative inflammatory atrophy lesions can be frequently found in association with PIN, a putative prostate cancer precursor lesion.

A second challenge in directly linking inflammation to prostate carcinogenesis is that the inflammatory response is complex and entails several biological processes. Usually, inflammation occurs in response to injury or invasive pathogens and is associated with eradication of the pathogen and damaged tissues, and wound healing, which involves tissue remodeling and regeneration so that normal function of the tissue can be re-established. Therefore, inflammation cannot be regarded in isolation, for it is associated with several processes that could contribute to prostate carcinogenesis including growth factor signaling, the secretion of cytokines (which have been shown to promote prostate cancer growth), stromal remodeling, angiogenesis, and epithelial growth.[117] In the mid-1980s, Dvorak noted many similarities between tumors and wound healing and suggested that tumors resemble wounds that do not heal.[118] Consistent with that observation, normal and malignant prostate tissues can be sorted based on a gene expression signature that captures the wound-healing phenotype.[119]

Despite these challenges, epidemiologic evidence has accumulated that links prostate cancer to inflammation. A meta-analysis of 23 case-control studies published between 1971 and 2000 reported statistically significant estimates of prostate cancer for a history of any sexually transmitted disease (RR = 1.4; 95% CI, 1.2–1.7), syphilis (RR = 2.3; 95% CI, 1.3–3.9), and gonorrhea (RR = 1.3; 95% CI, 1.1–1.6).[120] The finding that all sexually transmitted diseases (STDs) were associated with prostate cancer risk has led to the assertion that it is the inflammation in itself and not the particular pathogen that predisposes to prostate cancer. A second meta-analysis of 11 case-control studies found a 1.57-fold increased risk (OR 1.57, 95% CI, 1.01–2.45) of prostate cancer in men with a history of clinical symptoms of prostatitis, lending credence to the notion that the inflammation and not the pathogen contributes to prostate carcinogenesis.[121] The recent identification of the candidate prostate cancer susceptibility genes RNASEL and MSR1 has been proposed as further evidence that inflammation contributes significantly to prostate carcinogenesis. Germline inactivating mutations in the RNASEL gene have been identified in a subset of families with hereditary prostate cancer.[122] The protein RNASEL forms part of an endoribonuclease induced in response to viral infections and interferon signaling. RNASEL$^{-/-}$ mice show blunted interferon-α antiviral activity and decreased induction of apoptosis.[123] Similarly, MSR1 gene mutations have been identified in families with hereditary prostate cancer.[124] MSR1 is expressed in macrophages and MSR1$^{-/-}$ mice show increased susceptibility to some bacterial and viral infections and are prone to chronic infections and granuloma formation.[125] Since these susceptibility genes both influence host response to infection, it has been proposed that they set the stage for chronic inflammation that leads to prostate carcinogenesis.[110]

Use of anti-inflammatory agents such as aspirin or nonsteroidal anti-inflammatory drugs has been associated with a decreased risk of prostate cancer.[126,127] Although these agents might target inflammatory cells generally by decreasing cytokine production, a major target of these compounds are the cyclooxygenase (COX) enzymes. Cyclooxygenase 2 in particular has been associated with malignant transformation, enhanced tumor growth, and induction of angiogenesis.[128] Prostaglandin E$_2$ has been found at increased levels in prostate cancers compared to normal prostate tissue, although elevated levels of COX2 expression in prostate tissues have not been found consistently.[129,130] High levels of COX2 expression are seen in PIA lesions, raising the possibility that it plays a role in the early phases of prostate carcinogenesis. COX2 inhibitors will slow prostate cancer cell growth and enhance apoptosis in vitro, and will decrease tumor growth and prevent metastasis of prostate cancer in rat and mouse models of prostate cancer.[131–134] COX2 inhibitors are now being tested in a presurgical cohort for their ability to alter tissue prostaglandin levels and modulate biomarkers of proliferation, angiogenesis, oxidative damage and apoptosis.[135] However, concerns about the cardiovascular safety profile of selective COX2 inhibitors might temper enthusiasm for these agents in the future.

Epidemiologic evidence has also linked consumption of several foods and micronutrients to a decreased risk of prostate cancer. Consumption of tomatoes, green vegetables, α- and γ-tocopherol, soy, and red wine have all shown an inverse association with prostate cancer risk.[23,36,39–42,48,73] Critical components of each of these foods—lycopene in tomatoes, genistein in soy, chlorophyll in green vegetables and resveratrol in red wine—are antioxidants capable of directly quenching reactive oxygen and nitrogen species, much like α- and γ-tocopherol.[74,136–138] Again, these findings suggest a link between chronic inflammation and prostate cancer. As part of their bactericidal activity, inflammatory cells release reactive oxygen and nitrogen species that can cause collateral DNA damage resulting in mutations and ultimately malignant transformation. Both the NPC and TCCPT trials have added credence to the epidemiologic findings that antioxidants can prevent prostate carcinogenesis.[48,49] While tocopherols are known to be potent antioxidants, selenium has been assumed to act as an antioxidant since it is required for glutathione peroxidase (GPx) synthesis and activity. However, serum and erythrocyte GPx activities are unaffected by selenium supplementation, likely because these enzymes are synthesized at peak levels even in the face of dietary deficiencies of selenium.[49,139] It is possible that selenium supplementation could influence tissue GPx levels or modify detection of and response to free radicals.[140,141]

A molecular genetic finding common to most prostate cancers also suggests a link between inflammation, DNA damage, and prostate carcinogenesis. Regardless of grade or stage, more than 90% of prostate cancers lose expression of glutathione S-transferase-π due to extensive methylation of deoxycytidine residues in the 5′-regulatory regions of the *GSTP1* gene.[142–144] Loss of GSTP1 expression and promoter hypermethylation can be found in approximately 70% of PIN lesions and most cancers, and hypermethylation is never detected in normal tissues.[116,145] GSTP1 is one of the class of phase 2 enzymes that normally protect the cell against oxidants (such as lipid peroxides) and electrophiles that can act as mutagens.[146] Absent expression of GSTP1 in prostate cancer cells renders them more susceptible to DNA damage from PhIP (2-hydroxyamino-1-methyl-6-phenylimidazo(4,5-b)pyridine), a planar aromatic hydrocarbon found at high levels in charred meat.[147] *GSTP1*−/− mice show increased susceptibility to 7,12 dimethylbenz(a)anthracene-induced skin carcinogenesis.[148] *GSTP1* loss might, therefore, render prostate epithelial cells more vulnerable to reactive oxygen species or other endogenous or exogenous carcinogens.

Induction of expression of phase 2 enzymes has been long known to protect against a startling variety of carcinogen induced tumors.[149] Phase 2 enzyme inducing agents will decrease serum levels of alfatoxin in subjects living in hyperendemic areas of liver cancer and increase excretion of alfatoxin metabolites.[150,151] Foods associated with decreased prostate cancer risk contain several phase 2 enzyme-inducing agents, including selenium, resveratrol in red wine, genistein in soy, para-coumaric acid in tomatoes, and sulforaphane and other isothiocyanates in green vegetables, particularly cruciferous vegetables such as broccoli.[69,74,75,79,152–154] Sulforaphane, resveratrol, genistein, and methylselenic acid will induce phase 2 enzyme activity in prostate cancer cells in vitro.[69,75,79,152,153] Therefore, dietary agents associated with protection against prostate cancer might act both directly to quench reactive oxygen species, and indirectly by inducing cellular defenses.

APOPTOSIS

Prostate cancer growth depends on the balance between cell proliferation and apoptosis, or programmed cell death. Apoptotic rates in normal and malignant prostate epithelium are low, and loss of response to apoptotic signaling has been observed in early-stage prostate cancer as well as in hormone refractory disease, where antiapoptotic BCL2 protein levels can increase dramatically.[88,155] Enhancement of apoptosis has been investigated as a possible mechanism for many prostate cancer preventive agents. Increased apoptosis has been noted both in vitro and in vivo after treating prostate cancer cells with a number of candidate prostate cancer preventive compounds including genistein, resveratrol, EGCG, sulforaphane, selenium, vitamins D and E, and lycopene.[75,97,99,105,132,156] As seen in proliferation, the induction of apoptosis relies on integration of many signaling pathways, many of which are only beginning to be elucidated. Several compounds including COX2 inhibitors and resveratrol have been shown to block NFκB signaling, and NFκB activity will block programmed cell death.[111] NFκB has also been demonstrated to participate in tumor progression, to enhance tumor growth, and to increase metastases.[157] Intriguingly, NFκB is activated in response to inflammation, and might participate in the anticancer effects of anti-inflammatory, antiproliferative and proapoptotic preventive agents. Yet NFκB cannot explain the effects of all anti-inflammatory cancer preventive agents since activation of proapoptotic signaling pathways has also been demonstrated for several agents.

OTHER POSSIBLE MECHANISMS

Prostate tumor growth depends upon induction of blood vessel growth in the tumor (angiogenesis) to provide nutrients and oxygen. Several compounds inhibit angiogenesis, likely through their ability to suppress angiogenic protein expression (e.g. vascular endothelial growth factor [VEGF]) by the cancer cells.[131,158,159] Loss of PTEN activity has been implicated in prostate cancer, and agents that block the PI3/AKT/mTOR signaling pathway have been proposed as promising preventive agents.[109] Vitamin D and phenyl-butyrate appear to induce differentiation of cancer cells reflected in their inducing expression of genes associated with terminally differentiated prostate epithelium and inhibition of proliferation.[97,160] Similarly, prostate cancer development and progression has been linked to loss of the ability of prostate cancer cells to undergo senescence.[161] Induction of senescence pathways might represent a future avenue of prostate cancer preventive agent development.

SUMMARY

Progress in our understanding of prostate carcinogenesis and its prevention will come from the interplay of research into the molecular genetic events underlying prostate cancer and epidemiologic and basic studies in prostate cancer prevention. Increased understanding of the critical molecular genetic events in prostate carcinogenesis will lead to new approaches to prostate cancer prevention and, potentially, to the development of new compounds to target these pathways. On the other hand, identification and continued investigation of candidate preventive agents will contribute new insights in prostate cancer biology. For instance, the association of antioxidants with diminished risk of prostate cancer has fueled research into the role of inflammation in prostate carcinogenesis. Based on our current level of understanding, it is apparent that many candidate preventive agents are polyvalent—they work by many mechanisms. As we gain a more precise understanding of the mechanisms of action of prostate cancer preventive agents, it might be possible to design better agents or to combine agents that act synergistically. In the future, preventive interventions have great potential to contribute to decreasing death and suffering from prostate cancer.

REFERENCES

1. Sakr WA, Grignon DJ, Haas GP, et al. Epidemiology of high grade prostatic intraepithelial neoplasia. Pathol Res Pract 1995;191:838–841.

2. Sakr WA, Haas GP, Cassin BF, et al. The frequency of carcinoma and intraepithelial neoplasia of the prostate in young male patients. J Urol 1993;150:379–385.

3. Sakr WA, Partin AW. Histological markers of risk and the role of high-grade prostatic intraepithelial neoplasia. Urology 2001;57:115–120.

4. Stat bite: Lifetime risk of being diagnosed with cancer. J Natl Cancer Inst 2003;95:1745.

5. Gillanders EM, Xu J, Chang BL, et al. Combined genome-wide scan for prostate cancer susceptibility genes. J Natl Cancer Inst 2004;96:1240–1247.

6. Powell IJ. Prostate cancer and African-American men. Oncology (Huntingt) 1997;11:599–605; discussion 6–15 passim.

7. Steinberg GD, Carter BS, Beaty TH, et al. Family history and the risk of prostate cancer. Prostate 1990;17:337–347.

8. Carter BS, Beaty TH, Steinberg GD, et al. Mendelian inheritance of familial prostate cancer. Proc Natl Acad Sci USA 1992;89:3367–3371.

9. Boon H, Westlake K, Stewart M, et al. Use of complementary/alternative medicine by men diagnosed with prostate cancer: prevalence and characteristics. Urology 2003;62:849–853.

10. Breslow N, Chan CW, Dhom G, et al. Latent carcinoma of prostate of autopsy in seven areas. Int J Cancer 1977;20:680–688.

11. Brooks JD, Lee W-H, Nelson WG. Epidemiological and molecular features of prostatic carcinogenesis as clues for new prostate cancer prevention strategies. Canadian Journal of Urology (Suppl.) 1996;3:20–26.

12. Carter BS, Carter HB, Isaacs JT. Epidemiologic evidence regarding predisposing factors to prostate cancer. Prostate 1990;16:187–197.

13. DePrimo SE, Shinghal R, Vidanes G, et al. Prevention of prostate cancer. Hematol Oncol Clin North Am 2001;15:445–457.

14. Haenzel W, Kurihara M. Studies of Japanese migrants, I. Mortality from cancer and other diseases among Japanese men in the United States. J Natl Cancer Inst 1968;40:43–68.

15. Shimizu H, Ross RK, Bernstein L, et al. Cancers of the prostate and breast among Japanese and white immigrants in Los Angeles County. Br J Cancer 1991;63:963–966.

16. Whittemore AS, Wu AH, Kolonel LN, et al. Family history and prostate cancer risk in black, white, and Asian men in the United States and Canada. Am J Epidemiol 1995;141:732–740.

17. Wynder EL, Fujita Y, Harris RE, et al. Comparative epidemiology of cancer between the United States and Japan. A second look. Cancer 1991;67:746–763.

18. Yu H, Harris RE, Gao YT, et al. Comparative epidemiology of cancers of the colon, rectum, prostate and breast in Shanghai, China versus the United States. Int J Epidemiol 1991;20:76–81.

19. Van Maele-Fabry G, Willems JL. Prostate cancer among pesticide applicators: a meta-analysis. Int Arch Occup Environ Health 2004;77:559–570.

20. Van Maele-Fabry G, Willems JL. Occupation related pesticide exposure and cancer of the prostate: a meta-analysis. Occup Environ Med 2003;60:634–642.

21. Seidler A, Heiskel H, Bickeboller R, et al. Association between diesel exposure at work and prostate cancer. Scand J Work Environ Health 1998;24:486–494.

22. Nadon L, Siemiatycki J, Dewar R, et al. Cancer risk due to occupational exposure to polycyclic aromatic hydrocarbons. Am J Ind Med 1995;28:303–324.

23. Fair WR, Fleshner NE, Heston W. Cancer of the prostate: a nutritional disease? Urology 1997;50:840–848.

24. Hayes RB, Ziegler RG, Gridley G, et al. Dietary factors and risks for prostate cancer among blacks and whites in the United States. Cancer Epidemiol Biomarkers Prev 1999;8:25–34.

25. Kolonel LN, Yoshizawa CN, Hankin JH. Diet and prostatic cancer: a case-control study in Hawaii. Am J Epidemiol 1988;127:999–1012.

26. Kolonel LN. Nutrition and prostate cancer. Cancer Causes Control 1996;7:83–44.

27. Le Marchand L, Hankin JH, Kolonel LN, et al. Vegetable and fruit consumption in relation to prostate cancer risk in Hawaii: a reevaluation of the effect of dietary beta-carotene. Am J Epidemiol 1991;133:215–219.

28. Nomura AMY, Stemmermann GN, Lee J, et al. Serum micronutrients and prostate cancer in Japanese Americans in Hawaii. Cancer Epidemiol Biomarkers Prev 1997;6:487–491.

29. Ross RK, Shimizu H, Paganini-Hill A, et al. Case-control studies of prostate cancer in blacks and whites in southern California. J Natl Cancer Inst 1987;78:869–874.

30. West DW, Slattery ML, Robison LM, et al. Adult dietary intake and prostate cancer risk in Utah: a case-control study with special emphasis on aggressive tumors. Cancer Causes Control 1991;2:85–94.

31. Whittemore AS, Kolonel LN, Wu AH, et al. Prostate cancer in relation to diet, physical activity, and body size in blacks, whites, and Asians in the United States and Canada. J Natl Cancer Inst 1995;87:652–661.

32. Fleshner N, Bagnell PS, Klotz L, et al. Dietary fat and prostate cancer. J Urol 2004;171:S19–24.

33. Giovannucci E, Rimm EB, Colditz GA, et al. A prospective study of dietary fat and risk of prostate cancer. J Natl Cancer Inst 1993;85:1571–1579.

34. Brooks JD, Metter EJ, Chan DW, et al. Plasma selenium level before diagnosis and the risk of prostate cancer development. J Urol 2001;166:2034–2038.

35. Coates RJ, Weiss NS, Daling JR, et al. Serum levels of selenium and retinol and the subsequent risk of cancer. Am J Epidemiol 1988;128:515–523.

36. Cohen JH, Kristal AR, Stanford JL. Fruit and vegetable intakes and prostate cancer risk. J Natl Cancer Inst 2000;92:61–68.

37. Ghadirian P, Maisonneuve P, Perret C, et al. A case-control study of toenail selenium and cancer of the breast, colon, and prostate. Cancer Detect Prev 2000;24:305–313.

38. Giovannucci E, Ascherio A, Rimm EB, et al. Intake of carotenoids and retinol in relation to risk of prostate cancer. J Natl Cancer Inst 1995;87:1767–1776.

39. Giovannucci E. Tomatoes, tomato-based products, lycopene, and cancer: review of the epidemiologic literature. J Natl Cancer Inst 1999;91:317–331.

40. Helzlsouer KJ, Huang HY, Alberg AJ, et al. Association between alpha-tocopherol, gamma-tocopherol, selenium, and subsequent prostate cancer. J Natl Cancer Inst 2000;92:2018–2023.

41. Jacobsen BK, Knutsen SF, Fraser GE. Does high soy milk intake reduce prostate cancer incidence? The Adventist Health Study (United States). Cancer Causes Control 1998;9:553–557.

42. Kolonel LN, Hankin JH, Whittemore AS, et al. Vegetables, fruits, legumes and prostate cancer: a multiethnic case-control study. Cancer Epidemiol Biomarkers Prev 2000;9:795–804.

43. Kristal AR, Cohen JH, Qu P, Stanford JL. Associations of energy, fat, calcium, and vitamin D with prostate cancer risk. Cancer Epidemiol Biomarkers Prev 2002;11:719–725.

44. Nomura AM, Lee J, Stemmermann GN, et al. Serum selenium and subsequent risk of prostate cancer. Cancer Epidemiol Biomarkers Prev 2000;9:883–887.

45. Schwartz GG, Hulka BS. Is vitamin D deficiency a risk factor for prostate cancer? (Hypothesis). Anticancer Res 1990;10:1307–1311.

46. Willett WC, Polk BF, Morris JS, et al. Prediagnostic serum selenium and risk of cancer. Lancet 1983;2:130–134.

47. Yoshizawa K, Willett WC, Morris SJ, et al. Study of prediagnostic selenium level in toenails and the risk of advanced prostate cancer. J Natl Cancer Inst 1998;90:1219–1224.

48. Heinonen OP, Albanes D, Virtamo J, et al. Prostate cancer and supplementation with alpha-tocopherol and beta-carotene: incidence and mortality in a controlled trial. J Natl Cancer Inst 1998;90:440–446.

49. Clark LC, Combs GF, Jr., Turnbull BW, et al. Effects of selenium supplementation for cancer prevention in patients with carcinoma of the skin. A randomized controlled trial. Nutritional Prevention of Cancer Study Group. JAMA 1996;276:1957–1963.

50. Clark LC, Dalkin B, Krongrad A, et al. Decreased incidence of prostate cancer with selenium supplementation: results of a double-blind cancer prevention trial. Br J Urol 1998;81:730–734.

51. The effect of vitamin E and beta carotene on the incidence of lung cancer and other cancers in male smokers. The Alpha-Tocopherol, Beta Carotene Cancer Prevention Study Group [see comments]. N Engl J Med 1994;330:1029–1035.

52. Thompson IM, Goodman PJ, Tangen CM, et al. The influence of finasteride on the development of prostate cancer. N Engl J Med 2003;349:215–224.

53. Gonzalgo ML, Isaacs WB. Molecular pathways to prostate cancer. J Urol 2003;170:2444–2452.

54. Isaacs WB, Bova GS, Morton R, et al. Molecular and chromosomal alterations in prostate cancer. Cancer 1995:2004–2012.

55. Bastacky SI, Wojno KJ, Walsh PC, et al. Pathological features of hereditary prostate cancer. J Urol 1995;153:987–992.

56. Qian J, Bostwick DG, Takahashi S, et al. Chromosomal anomalies in prostatic intraepithelial neoplasia and carcinoma detected by fluorescence in situ hybridization. Cancer Res 1995;55:5408–5414.

57. Huggins C, Hodges CV. Studies on prostatic cancer: I. The effect of castration, of estrogen and of androgen injection on serum phosphatases in metastatic carcinoma of the prostate. 1941. J Urol 2002;168:9–12.

58. Barrett-Connor E, Garland C, McPhillips JB, et al. A prospective, population-based study of androstenedione, estrogens, and prostatic cancer. Cancer Res 1990;50:169–173.

59. Winters SJ, Brufsky A, Weissfeld J, et al. Testosterone, sex hormone-binding globulin, and body composition in young adult African American and Caucasian men. Metabolism 2001;50:1242–1247.

60. Makridakis NM, Reichardt JK. Molecular epidemiology of androgen-metabolic loci in prostate cancer: predisposition and progression. J Urol 2004;171:S25–28; discussion S8–9.

61. Giovannucci E, Stampfer MJ, Krithivas K, et al. The CAG repeat within the androgen receptor gene and its relationship to prostate cancer. Proc Natl Acad Sci USA 1997;94:3320–3323.

62. Ross RK, Bernstein L, Lobo RA, et al. 5-alpha-reductase activity and risk of prostate cancer among Japanese and US white and black males. Lancet 1992;339:887–889.

63. Sharma M, Li X, Wang Y, et al. hZimp10 is an androgen receptor co-activator and forms a complex with SUMO-1 at replication foci. Embo J 2003;22:6101–6114.

64. DePrimo SE, Diehn M, Nelson JB, et al. Transcriptional programs activated by exposure of human prostate cancer cells to androgen. Genome Biol 2002;3:RESEARCH0032.

65. Nelson PS, Clegg N, Arnold H, et al. The program of androgen-responsive genes in neoplastic prostate epithelium. Proc Natl Acad Sci USA 2002;99:11890–11895.

66. Andriole G, Bostwick D, Brawley O, et al. Chemoprevention of prostate cancer in men at high risk: rationale and design of the reduction by dutasteride of prostate cancer events (REDUCE) trial. J Urol 2004;172:1314–1317.

67. Ip C. The chemopreventive role of selenium in carcinogenesis. Adv Exp Med Biol 1986;206:431–447.

68. Ganther HE. Selenium metabolism, selenoproteins and mechanisms of cancer prevention: complexities with thioredoxin reductase. Carcinogenesis 1999;20:1657–1666.

69. Zhao H, Whitfield ML, Xu T, et al. Diverse effects of methylseleninic acid on the transcriptional program of human prostate cancer cells. Mol Biol Cell 2004;15:506–519.

70. Bhamre S, Whitin JC, Cohen HJ. Selenomethionine does not affect PSA secretion independent of its effect on LNCaP cell growth. Prostate 2003;54:315–321.

71. Hartman TJ, Dorgan JF, Woodson K, et al. Effects of long-term alpha-tocopherol supplementation on serum hormones in older men. Prostate 2001;46:33–38.

72. Zhang Y, Ni J, Messing EM, et al. Vitamin E succinate inhibits the function of androgen receptor and the expression of prostate-specific antigen in prostate cancer cells. Proc Natl Acad Sci USA 2002;99:7408–7413.

73. Schoonen WM, Salinas CA, Kiemeney LA, et al. Alcohol consumption and risk of prostate cancer in middle-aged men. Int J Cancer 2005;113:133–140.

74. Jang M, Cai L, Udeani GO, et al. Cancer chemopreventive activity of resveratrol, a natural product derived from grapes. Science 1997;275:218–220.

75. Jones S, DePrimo S, Whitfield M, Brooks JD. Resveratrol-induced gene expression profiles in human prostate cancer cells. Cancer Epidemiol Biomarkers Prev 2005;14:596–604.

76. Mitchell SH, Zhu W, Young CY. Resveratrol inhibits the expression and function of the androgen receptor in LNCaP prostate cancer cells. Cancer Res 1999;59:5892–5895.

77. Hsieh TC, Wu JM. Grape-derived chemopreventive agent resveratrol decreases prostate-specific antigen (PSA) expression in LNCaP cells by an androgen receptor (AR)-independent mechanism. Anticancer Res 2000;20:225–228.

78. Evans BA, Griffiths K, Morton MS. Inhibition of 5 alpha-reductase in genital skin fibroblasts and prostate tissue by dietary lignans and isoflavonoids. J Endocrinol 1995;147:295–302.

79. Takahashi Y, Lavigne JA, Hursting SD, et al. Using DNA microarray analyses to elucidate the effects of genistein in androgen-responsive prostate cancer cells: identification of novel targets. Mol Carcinog 2004;41:108–119.

80. Whitehead SA, Lacey M. Phytoestrogens inhibit aromatase but not 17beta-hydroxysteroid dehydrogenase (HSD) type 1 in human granulosa-luteal cells: evidence for FSH induction of 17beta-HSD. Hum Reprod 2003;18:487–494.

81. Rosenberg Zm Rosenberg RS, Jenkins DJ, Brown TJ, et al. Flavonoids can block PSA production by breast and prostate cancer cell lines. Clin Chim Acta 2002;317:17–26.

82. Oh WK. The evolving role of estrogen therapy in prostate cancer. Clin Prostate Cancer 2002;1:81–89.

83. Kim IY, Kim BC, Seong do H, et al. Raloxifene, a mixed estrogen agonist/antagonist, induces apoptosis in androgen-independent human prostate cancer cell lines. Cancer Res 2002;62:5365–5369.

84. Neubauer BL, McNulty AM, Chedid M, et al. The selective estrogen receptor modulator trioxifene (LY133314) inhibits metastasis and extends survival in the PAIII rat prostatic carcinoma model. Cancer Res 2003;63:6056–6062.

85. Raghow S, Hooshdaran MZ, Katiyar S, et al. Toremifene prevents prostate cancer in the transgenic adenocarcinoma of mouse prostate model. Cancer Res 2002;62:1370–1376.

86. Armanini D, Fiore C, Mattarello MJ, et al. History of the endocrine effects of licorice. Exp Clin Endocrinol Diabetes 2002;110:257–261.

87. DiPaola RS, Zhang H, Lambert GH, et al. Clinical and biologic activity of an estrogenic herbal combination (PC-SPES) in prostate cancer. N Engl J Med 1998;339:785–791.

88. Berges RR, Vukanovic J, Epstein JI, et al. Implication of cell kinetic changes during the progression of human prostatic cancer. Clin Cancer Res 1995;1:473–480.

89. Furuya Y, Kawauchi Y, Fuse H. Cell proliferation, apoptosis and prognosis in patients with metastatic prostate cancer. Anticancer Res 2003;23:577–581.

90. Lapointe J, Li C, Higgins JP, et al. Gene expression profiling identifies clinically relevant subtypes of prostate cancer. Proc Natl Acad Sci USA 2004;101:811–816.

91. Varambally S, Dhanasekaran SM, Zhou M, et al. The polycomb group protein EZH2 is involved in progression of prostate cancer. Nature 2002;419:624–629.

92. Liao S, Umekita Y, Guo J, et al. Growth inhibition and regression of human prostate and breast tumors in athymic mice by tea epigallocatechin gallate. Cancer Lett 1995;96:239–243.

93. Venkateswaran V, Fleshner NE, Klotz LH. Modulation of cell proliferation and cell cycle regulators by vitamin E in human prostate carcinoma cell lines. J Urol 2002;168:1578–1582.

94. Venkateswaran V, Klotz LH, Fleshner NE. Selenium modulation of cell proliferation and cell cycle biomarkers in human prostate carcinoma cell lines. Cancer Res 2002;62:2540–2545.

95. Venkateswaran V, Fleshner NE, Klotz LH. Synergistic effect of vitamin E and selenium in human prostate cancer cell lines. Prostate Cancer Prostatic Dis 2004;7:54–56.

96. Peehl DM, Skowronski RJ, Leung GK, et al. Antiproliferative effects of 1,25-dihydroxyvitamin D3 on primary cultures of human prostatic cells. Cancer Res 1994;54:805–810.

97. Peehl DM, Krishnan AV, Feldman D. Pathways mediating the growth-inhibitory actions of vitamin D in prostate cancer. J Nutr 2003;133:2461S–2469S.

98. Obermuller-Jevic UC, Olano-Martin E, Corbacho AM, et al. Lycopene inhibits the growth of normal human prostate epithelial cells in vitro. J Nutr 2003;133:3356–3360.

99. Knowles LM, Zigrossi DA, Tauber RA, et al. Flavonoids suppress androgen-independent human prostate tumor proliferation. Nutr Cancer 2000;38:116–122.

100. Goluboff ET, Shabsigh A, Saidi JA, et al. Exisulind (sulindac sulfone) suppresses growth of human prostate cancer in a nude mouse xenograft model by increasing apoptosis. Urology 1999;53:440–445.

101. Fleshner N, Fair WR, Huryk R, et al. Vitamin E inhibits the high-fat diet promoted growth of established human prostate LNCaP tumors in nude mice. J Urol 1999;161:1651–1654.

102. Raghow S, Kuliyev E, Steakley M, et al. Efficacious chemoprevention of primary prostate cancer by flutamide in an autochthonous transgenic model. Cancer Res 2000;60:4093–4097.

103. Gupta S, Ahmad N, Marengo SR, et al. Chemoprevention of prostate carcinogenesis by alpha-difluoromethylornithine in TRAMP mice. Cancer Res 2000;60:5125–5133.

104. Mentor-Marcel R, Lamartiniere CA, Eltoum IE, et al. Genistein in the diet reduces the incidence of poorly differentiated prostatic adenocarcinoma in transgenic mice (TRAMP). Cancer Res 2001;61:6777–6782.

105. Gupta S, Hastak K, Ahmad N, et al. Inhibition of prostate carcinogenesis in TRAMP mice by oral infusion of green tea polyphenols. Proc Natl Acad Sci USA 2001;98:10350–10355.

106. Boileau TW, Liao Z, Kim S, et al. Prostate carcinogenesis in N-methyl-N-nitrosourea (NMU)-testosterone-treated rats fed tomato powder, lycopene, or energy-restricted diets. J Natl Cancer Inst 2003;95:1578–1586.

107. Schleicher RL, Lamartiniere CA, Zheng M, et al. The inhibitory effect of genistein on the growth and metastasis of a transplantable rat accessory sex gland carcinoma. Cancer Lett 1999;136:195–201.

108. Whitfield ML, Sherlock G, Saldanha AJ, et al. Identification of genes periodically expressed in the human cell cycle and their expression in tumors. Mol Biol Cell 2002;13:1977–2000.

109. Tolcher AW. Novel therapeutic molecular targets for prostate cancer: the mTOR signaling pathway and epidermal growth factor receptor. J Urol 2004;171:S41–43; discussion S4.

110. Nelson WG, De Marzo AM, Isaacs WB. Prostate cancer. N Engl J Med 2003;349:366–381.

111. Marx J. Cancer research. Inflammation and cancer: the link grows stronger. Science 2004;306:966–968.

112. Gerstenbluth RE, Seftel AD, MacLennan GT, et al. Distribution of chronic prostatitis in radical prostatectomy specimens with up-regulation of bcl-2 in areas of inflammation. J Urol 2002;167:2267–2270.

113. Kohnen PW, Drach GW. Patterns of inflammation in prostatic hyperplasia: a histologic and bacteriologic study. J Urol 1979;121:755–760.

114. Shah R, Mucci NR, Amin A, et al. Postatrophic hyperplasia of the prostate gland: neoplastic precursor or innocent bystander? Am J Pathol 2001;158:1767–1773.

115. De Marzo AM, Marchi VL, Epstein JI, et al. Proliferative inflammatory atrophy of the prostate: implications for prostatic carcinogenesis. Am J Pathol 1999;155:1985–1992.

116. Nakayama M, Bennett CJ, Hicks JL, et al. Hypermethylation of the human glutathione S-transferase-pi gene (GSTP1) CpG island is present in a subset of proliferative inflammatory atrophy lesions but not in normal or hyperplastic epithelium of the prostate: a detailed study using laser-capture microdissection. Am J Pathol 2003;163:923–933.

117. Lucia MS, Torkko KC. Inflammation as a target for prostate cancer chemoprevention: pathological and laboratory rationale. J Urol 2004;171:S30–34; discussion S5.

118. Dvorak HF. Tumors: wounds that do not heal. Similarities between tumor stroma generation and wound healing. N Engl J Med 1986;315:1650–1659.

119. Chang HY, Sneddon JB, Alizadeh AA, et al. Gene expression signature of fibroblast serum response predicts human cancer progression: Similarities between tumors and wounds. PLoS Biology 2004;2:0001–0009.

120. Dennis LK, Dawson DV. Meta-analysis of measures of sexual activity and prostate cancer. Epidemiology 2002;13:72–79.

121. Dennis LK, Lynch CF, Torner JC. Epidemiologic association between prostatitis and prostate cancer. Urology 2002;60:78–83.

122. Carpten J, Nupponen N, Isaacs S, et al. Germline mutations in the ribonuclease L gene in families showing linkage with HPC1. Nat Genet 2002;30:181–184.

123. Zhou A, Paranjape J, Brown TL, et al. Interferon action and apoptosis are defective in mice devoid of 2′,5′-oligoadenylate-dependent RNase L. Embo J 1997;16:6355–6363.

124. Xu J, Zheng SL, Komiya A, et al. Germline mutations and sequence variants of the macrophage scavenger receptor 1 gene are associated with prostate cancer risk. Nat Genet 2002;32:321–325.

125. Thomas CA, Li Y, Kodama T, et al. Protection from lethal gram-positive infection by macrophage scavenger receptor-dependent phagocytosis. J Exp Med 2000;191:147–156.

126. Leitzmann MF, Stampfer MJ, Ma J, et al. Aspirin use in relation to risk of prostate cancer. Cancer Epidemiol Biomarkers Prev 2002;11:1108–1111.

127. Habel LA, Zhao W, Stanford JL. Daily aspirin use and prostate cancer risk in a large, multiracial cohort in the US. Cancer Causes Control 2002;13:427–434.

128. Basler JW, Piazza GA. Nonsteroidal anti-inflammatory drugs and cyclooxygenase-2 selective inhibitors for prostate cancer chemoprevention. J Urol 2004;171:S59–62; discussion S3.

129. Gupta S, Srivastava M, Ahmad N, et al. Over-expression of cyclooxygenase-2 in human prostate adenocarcinoma. Prostate 2000;42:73–78.

130. Zha S, Gage WR, Sauvageot J, et al. Cyclooxygenase-2 is up-regulated in proliferative inflammatory atrophy of the prostate, but not in prostate carcinoma. Cancer Res 2001;61:8617–8623.

131. Narayanan BA, Narayanan NK, Pittman B, et al. Regression of mouse prostatic intraepithelial neoplasia by nonsteroidal anti-inflammatory drugs in the transgenic adenocarcinoma mouse prostate model. Clin Cancer Res 2004;10:7727–7737.

132. Gupta S, Adhami VM, Subbarayan M, et al. Suppression of prostate carcinogenesis by dietary supplementation of celecoxib in transgenic adenocarcinoma of the mouse prostate model. Cancer Res 2004;64:3334–3343.

133. Srinath P, Rao PN, Knaus EE, Suresh MR. Effect of cyclooxygenase-2 (COX-2) inhibitors on prostate cancer cell proliferation. Anticancer Res 2003;23:3923–3928.

134. Narayanan BA, Condon MS, Bosland MC, et al. Suppression of N-methyl-N-nitrosourea/testosterone-induced rat prostate cancer growth by celecoxib: effects on cyclooxygenase-2, cell cycle regulation, and apoptosis mechanism(s). Clin Cancer Res 2003;9:3503–3513.

135. Heath EI, DeWeese TL, Partin AW, et al. The design of a randomized, placebo-controlled trial of celecoxib in preprostatectomy men with clinically localized adenocarcinoma of the prostate. Clin Prostate Cancer 2002;1:182–187.

136. Tikkanen MJ, Wahala K, Ojala S, et al. Effect of soybean phytoestrogen intake on low density lipoprotein oxidation resistance. Proc Natl Acad Sci USA 1998;95:3106–3110.

137. Di Mascio P, Kaiser S, Sies H. Lycopene as the most efficient biological carotenoid singlet oxygen quencher. Arch Biochem Biophys 1989;274:532–538.

138. Egner PA, Wang JB, Zhu YR, et al. Chlorophyllin intervention reduces aflatoxin-DNA adducts in individuals at high risk for liver cancer. Proc Natl Acad Sci USA 2001;98:14601–14606.

139. Hardell L, Degerman A, Tomic R, et al. Levels of selenium in plasma and glutathione peroxidase in erythrocytes in patients with prostate cancer or benign hyperplasia. Eur J Cancer Prev 1995;4:91–95.

140. Gladyshev VN, Factor VM, Housseau F, et al. Contrasting patterns of regulation of the antioxidant selenoproteins, thioredoxin reductase, and glutathione peroxidase, in cancer cells. Biochem Biophys Res Commun 1998;251:488–493.

141. Jacob C, Maret W, Vallee BL. Selenium redox biochemistry of zinc-sulfur coordination sites in proteins and enzymes. Proc Natl Acad Sci USA 1999;96:1910–1914.

142. Lee WH, Morton RA, Epstein JI, et al. Cytidine methylation of regulatory sequences near the pi-class glutathione S-transferase gene accompanies human prostatic carcinogenesis. Proc Natl Acad Sci USA 1994;91:11733–11737.

143. Lee W-H, Isaacs WB, Bova GS, et al. CG island methylation changes near the GSTP1 gene in prostatic carcinoma cells detected using the polymerase chain reaction: a new prostatic biomarker. Cancer Epidemiol Biomarkers Prev 1997;6:443–450.

144. Lin X, Tascilar M, Lee WH, et al. GSTP1 CpG island hypermethylation is responsible for the absence of GSTP1 expression in human prostate cancer cells. Am J Pathol 2001;159:1815–1826.

145. Brooks JD, Weinstein M, Lin X, et al. CG island methylation changes near the GSTP1 gene in prostatic intraepithelial neoplasia. Cancer Epidemiol Biomarkers Prev 1998;7:531–536.

146. Ketterer B, Meyer DJ. Glutathione transferases: a possible role in the detoxication and repair of DNA and lipid hydroperoxides. Mutat Res 1989;214:33–40.

147. Nelson CP, Kidd LC, Sauvageot J, et al. Protection against 2-hydroxyamino-1-methyl-6-phenylimidazo[4,5-b]pyridine cytotoxicity and DNA adduct formation in human prostate by glutathione S-transferase P1. Cancer Res 2001;61:103–109.

148. Henderson CJ, Smith AG, Ure J, et al. Increased skin tumorigenesis in mice lacking pi class glutathione S-transferases. Proc Natl Acad Sci USA 1998;95:5275–5280.

149. Talalay P, Fahey JW, Holtzclaw WD, et al. Chemoprotection against cancer by phase 2 enzyme induction. Toxicol Lett 1995;82–83:173–179.

150. Camoirano A, Bagnasco M, Bennicelli C, et al. Oltipraz chemoprevention trial in Qidong, People's Republic of China: results of urine genotoxicity assays as related to smoking habits. Cancer Epidemiol Biomarkers Prev 2001;10:775–783.

151. Jacobson LP, Zhang BC, Zhu YR, et al. Oltipraz chemoprevention trial in Qidong, People's Republic of China: study design and clinical outcomes. Cancer Epidemiol Biomarkers Prev 1997;6:257–265.

152. Brooks JD, Paton VG, Vidanes G. Potent induction of phase 2 enzymes in human prostate cells by sulforaphane. Cancer Epidemiol Biomarkers Prev 2001;10:949–954.

153. Brooks JD, Goldberg MF, Nelson LA, et al. Identification of potential prostate cancer preventive agents through induction of quinone reductase in vitro. Cancer Epidemiol Biomarkers Prev 2002;11:868–875.

154. Wattenberg LW. Inhibition of carcinogenesis by minor dietary constituents. Cancer Res 1992;52:2085s–2091s.

155. Colombel M, Symmans F, Gil S, et al. Detection of the apoptosis-suppressing oncoprotein bc1-2 in hormone-refractory human prostate cancers. Am J Pathol 1993;143:390–400.

156. Kucuk O, Sarkar FH, Sakr W, et al. Phase II randomized clinical trial of lycopene supplementation before radical prostatectomy. Cancer Epidemiol Biomarkers Prev 2001;10:861–868.

157. Greten FR, Eckmann L, Greten TF, et al. IKKbeta links inflammation and tumorigenesis in a mouse model of colitis-associated cancer. Cell 2004;118:285–296.

158. Dorai T, Cao YC, Dorai B, et al. Therapeutic potential of curcumin in human prostate cancer. III. Curcumin inhibits proliferation, induces apoptosis, and inhibits angiogenesis of LNCaP prostate cancer cells in vivo. Prostate 2001;47:293–303.

159. Fotsis T, Pepper M, Adlercreutz H, et al. Genistein, a dietary-derived inhibitor of in vitro angiogenesis. Proc Natl Acad Sci USA 1993;90:2690–2694.

160. Carducci MA, Nelson JB, Chan-Tack KM, et al. Phenylbutyrate induces apoptosis in human prostate cancer and is more potent than phenylacetate. Clin Cancer Res 1996;2:379–387.

161. Schwarze SR, DePrimo SE, Grabert LM, et al. Novel pathways associated with bypassing cellular senescence in human prostate epithelial cells. J Biol Chem 2002;277:14877–14883.

Testosterone and prostate safety

21

Alvaro Morales

FUNDAMENTAL CONCEPTS OF TESTOSTERONE ADMINISTRATION

The rapid increase in the aging population has brought new challenges and new solutions to the forefront of medical practice. It is a long and well-established fact that there are significant endocrinologic alterations (Table 21.1) associated with the aging process.[1,2] This has created a need for exploring issues related to hormonal supplementation in aging men. With the notable exception of thyroid replacement, the treatment of the remaining deficiencies is mired in controversy; which is particularly intense around androgen substitution. From the outset it should be established that there are four basic notions that require awareness when discussing the use of androgen replacement therapy (ART) in men. The first and most fundamental one is that the patient must have documented *and* symptomatic hypogonadism. In the same manner that a man with benign prostatic hyperplasia (BPH), another condition associated with aging, but without obstructive symptoms is, normally, not a candidate for treatment, a man with low or borderline-low serum level of testosterone and no manifestations of hypogonadism does not necessarily require treatment (Figure 21.1). Second, there should be no specific contraindications for ART. Third, the treating physician must be familiar and comfortable with his/her ability to diagnose and treat the condition. Finally, and perhaps most importantly, both the physician and the patient

Table 21.1 Hormonal alterations associated with aging in men

Decreased production
- Gonadotropin
- Testosterone
- Dehydroepiandrosterone
- Growth hormone
- Melatonin
- Thyroxin

Minimal changes
- Corticosteroids
- Estrogen

Increased production
- Sex hormone binding globulin
- Leptin

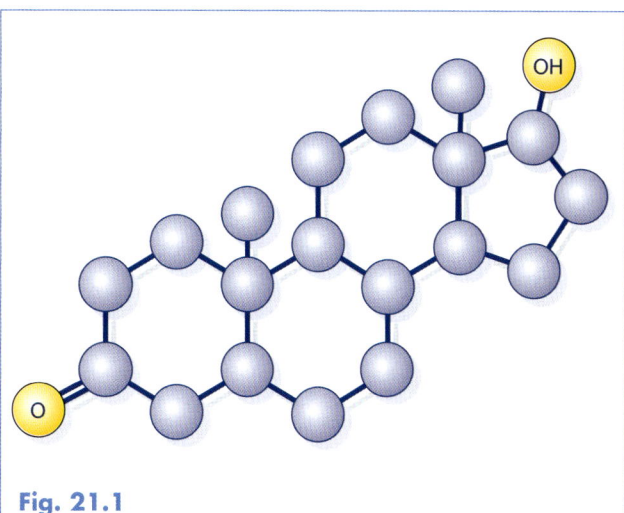

Fig. 21.1
The testerone steroid molecule.

Table 21.2 Most frequently used testosterone preparations

Type	Generic name	Trade name	Dose
Injectable	Testosterone cypionate	Depo-testosterone cypionate	200–400 mg every 3–4 weeks
	Testosterone enanthate	Delatestryl	200–400 mg every 4 weeks
	Testosterone undecanoate*	Nebido	1000 mg every 12 weeks
Oral/buccal	T buccal system	Striant	30 mg twice daily
	Methyltestosterone†	Metandren	10–30 mg/day
	Testosterone undecanoate‡	Andriol	120–160 mg/day
Transdermal	Testosterone patch	Androderm	6 mg/day
	Testosterone gel	Testoderm	10–15 mg/day
		Androgel/Testim	5–10 g/day

*Currently available only in countries of the European Union.

†As 17α alkylated testosterone products both fluoxymesterone and methyltestosterone are associated with serious liver toxicity.

‡Not available in the United States of America.

must commit to a regular follow-up schedule to assess the therapeutic response and potential adverse effects developing as a consequence of treatment. At present there is a wide and ever increasing choice of treatments for symptomatic late onset hypogonadism (SLOH).

TESTOSTERONE DELIVERY FORMULATIONS

Current, commercially available, testosterone preparations (Table 21.2) carry similar patterns of efficacy and safety, although each one exhibits some specific drawbacks, such as increased incidence of skin reactions or hematological alterations. At the end, the choice of one formulation over another largely depends on safety, availability, cost, convenience of use, and our familiarity with a specific product. Possible unwanted actions of ART are well recognized (Table 21.3). Most are rare, mild, easily detectable during follow-up, and readily correctable with dose modifications, switching to an alternative preparation, or discontinuation of treatment.

Table 21.3 Potential adverse effects of androgen replacement therapy

Organ/system	Potential adverse effects
Prostate/breast	BPH, gynecomastia, exacerbation of sub clinical carcinoma
Cardiovascular/lipids	Fluid retention, ↓HDL cholesterol
Liver	None except with methylated testosterone preparations (cholangitis, hepatomas)
Hematopoietic	Polycythemia
Mood	Irritability and hypersexuality with supraphysiological doses
Sleep	Exacerbation of sleep disorders (apnea)

BPH, benign prostatic hyperplasia; HDL, high-density lipoprotein.

SAFETY ISSUES RELATED TO ANDROGEN REPLACEMENT THERAPY

The two most prominent and worrisome potential adverse effects relate to prostate and cardiovascular safety. Regarding lipids and cardiovascular safety, it appears that hypogonadism is actually a promoter of atherosclerosis[3] in men. The efficacy of testosterone administration may go beyond a purely hormonal effect on lipid levels: Malkin et al[4] recently reported on a randomized, placebo controlled, crossover study of testosterone versus placebo in men with symptomatic hypogonadism. Those receiving testosterone showed a significant decrease in serum levels, not only of total cholesterol but of several proinflammatory cytokines (tumor necrosis factor-α [TNFα], interleukin 1β [IL1β]), which are risk factors for the development of complications from atheromatous plaques. Furthermore, the anti-inflammatory cytokine IL10 was increased following testosterone administration, confirming previous observations.[5] Despite these and many other encouraging results, the significance of lipid alterations, particularly lowering of high-density lipoprotein, although modest, remains to be established.

For the central theme of this chapter—prostate safety—many answers are not in and further research is clearly needed.[6] However, the extrapolation of the results of the Women's Health Initiative on hormonal replacement therapy (hormone replacement therapy [HRT]: estrogen ± progesterone) in postmenopausal women to the men's situation is uninformed and misleading: it does not take into consideration the large differences in the molecular structures and actions of the hormones themselves and the gender responses to them.[3,7] Although it is tempting to equate the possible effects of HRT in the development of breast cancer to ART in prostate cancer, the biological behavior and clinical management of the two tumors are markedly dissimilar. There is no controversy on the premise that the indiscriminate use (and particularly the abuse) of ART is completely inappropriate in clinical practice. But, the rational and well informed use of androgens is an important tool in the medical armamentarium. It must be recognized, however, that studies of the scope and magnitude of the Women's Health Initiative investigation are not available in men. In fact, studies of such magnitude are only at the planning stage. It has been estimated that, to have an adequate assessment in regards to risk of prostate cancer and ART alone, more than 5000 subjects and a 5-year follow-up will be needed.[8] Such a study will require these men to have a diagnosis of hypogonadism by history, physical examination, and biochemical confirmation, a task more complex than the simpler diagnosis of menopause. In addition, the men participating in the study should, ideally, be naive to ART. It is likely, however, that such a study will be underpowered and may not provide the definitive answers. A cohort of about 7000 participants may be more adequate. The Institute of Medicine (IOM)[6] has recently produced a series of recommendations suggesting the assessment of therapeutic response to testosterone in a limited number of subjects and, if a positive response is found, to proceed to large trials for safety. This implies that definitive answers will not be available for 10 to 15 years, at the earliest; and this is assuming that the limited studies currently available are considered sufficient to accept that there are benefits from testosterone supplementation therapy. The proposed large studies, beyond a doubt, are a necessary, worthwhile and urgent enterprise and one that demands careful planning and execution. But, as in many situations in clinical practice, when there are conditions for which definitive therapeutic evidence is incomplete the physician must be aware of the most credible information on hand regarding the advantages and drawbacks of ART, and follow guidelines and recommendations available from professional societies.

TESTOSTERONE AND PROSTATE SAFETY

A number of issues of immediate clinical importance in relation to prostate health need to be addressed for physicians who treat or are consulted about patients needing testosterone supplementation. The most relevant include: 1) the role of the androgen receptor; 2) the relationship between ART and benign prostatic hyperplasia (BPH); 3) the management of men with BPH and SLOH; 4) the role of testosterone in prostate cancer (CaP); 5) ART in men with SLOH successfully treated for CaP; 6) the basic, mandatory investigations prior to initiation of ART; and 7) the monitoring of men receiving ART.

A PRIMER ON THE PROSTATE AND ITS ANDROGEN RECEPTOR

The effects of androgens on the prostate gland are unquestionable and their effects have been documented to be dependent on the CAG repeat polymorphism of the androgen receptor;[9] however, although there has been a significant improvement in our understanding of the cellular and molecular mechanisms, they are not yet fully figured out.[10] They are described in detail in Chapter 9. Briefly, in the prostate, testosterone acts only as a prohormone. The effective androgen is the more potent dihydrotestosterone (DHT) which is converted from testosterone through the action of 5α-reductase. Different organs have variable amounts of 5α-reductase enzymes 1 and 2 (5αR1 and 2). The more prominent in the prostate, external genitalia, and skin is 5αR2, and its deficiency translates into minimal prostate growth and the presence of ambiguous external genitalia in boys who at puberty, however, exhibit the anticipated increase in muscle mass and male habitus. The glandular epithelium and a subset of endothelial cells are the primary androgen target tissues within the prostate. Dihydrotestosterone acts on these tissues' androgen receptors to generate a variety of androgen-induced stromal peptide growth factors or andromedins (e.g., prosurvival protein BCL2, vascular endothelial growth factor). Androgen deprivation, on the other hand, results in insufficient production of andromedins, which in turn upregulates the production of transforming growth factor-β1 (TGFβ1) that signals the apoptotic cascade in the secretory compartment of the prostatic epithelium.[11] The presence of 5αR1 in the prostate has also been documented,[12] but its function is less well understood. It appears that the enzyme regulates aromatase activity: high levels of 5αR1 are detected in normal glands, while the levels decrease as the prostate undergoes neoplastic transformation.[13] The elucidation of the mechanisms of androgen-dependent prostate cell growth, differentiation, and death is important because their manipulation has major consequences in the treatment of prostate neoplasms,[14] both benign and malignant.

THE ROLE OF ART IN BENIGN PROSTATIC HYPERPLASIA (BPH)

It is commonly accepted that the development of BPH is primarily mediated by intraprostatic events due to the action of 5α-DHT with active participation of estrogen (E_2).[15] Many studies have been conducted to determine the serum levels of sex steroids at the time of diagnosis of BPH[16]; this, of course, is an unreliable methodology since there is a recognized poor correlation between symptoms of lower urinary tract obstruction and the gland volume. A more convincing approach was the one used by the Physicians Health Study,[17] in which two groups of men were investigated with determination of serum sex steroid levels. Subjects had the biochemical assessment conducted before symptoms of BPH had developed. One group eventually required surgical treatment while the other one did not. Remarkably, the need for surgery did not correlate with androgen levels, but it did across quintiles of estrogen serum levels. Findings such as these, emphasize the importance of estrogen in the development of BPH and the interactions of sex steroids in benign prostate pathology.

Testosterone administration results not only in its conversion to 5α-DHT but, through the effect of aromatase, testosterone is also converted into estrogen. There are, therefore, two hormonal influences potentially promoting BPH in men receiving ART. Dihydrotestosterone, however, is non-aromatizable (in fact its administration suppresses the levels of estrogen) and for this reason it has been considered a "prostate-sparing androgen." There are, however, no studies with DHT replacement in hypogonadal men conclusively establishing a decrease in prostate volume, nor is there evidence for acute adverse effects of DHT on the prostate.[18–20] It is also recognized that prostate size increases with age in eugonadal men but not in their untreated hypogonadal counterparts. Similarly, when adult hypogonadal men are treated with androgens, they exhibit an increase in the gland volume but only to the size expected for normal men of the same age.[21] Some studies reported either no changes or a significant increase in prostate volume and prostate specific antigen (PSA) that, however, stayed within normal ranges.[22] More recent evidence from placebo-controlled, randomized trials of hypogonadal adult men receiving testosterone show that the difference between those men receiving androgens and those on placebo were insignificant with regard to prostate volume, prostate-specific antigen (PSA), or obstructive symptoms.[23] A report from the Baltimore Longitudinal Study of Aging[24] suggested that the risk of developing BPH might be predicted from the levels of PSA; however, this particular report did not include the levels of sex steroids in the subjects participating in the study. Whether this finding applies also to hypogonadal men before or during treatment (once a eugonadal state has been achieved) remains to be investigated. The availability of transdermal testosterone preparations has generated additional information in this regard. In a pivotal study by Wang et al[25] comparing two dosages of testosterone gel (50 and 100 mg) or testosterone patch single dose (5 mg), PSA elevations above 4 ng/dL occurred only in those receiving the gel (5/149). Decrease in urinary flow rate and deterioration of the International Prostate Symptom Score (I-PSS) were rare, and the changes were insignificant across doses and delivery forms. These findings

represented only the initial 3 months of monitoring but, with continuing observation, there were no significant changes at the 3-year follow-up.[26,27] A similar study, using a different transdermal testosterone gel, and for which only the short term results are available, reported essentially identical findings.[28] Although interesting and clinically reassuring, these and other studies were not specifically designed or powered to assess the impact of ART on the prostate and should be interpreted with caution.

MANAGEMENT OF MEN WITH BPH AND SLOH

As with most clinical situations where evidence-based guidelines do not exist, knowledge and good medical judgment play a crucial role. From the considerations on the effect of androgens on BPH, it is clear that some modest increase in the volume of the gland is to be expected after testosterone treatment in a hypogonadal man. Men with modest residual urine volumes and minimal symptoms of bladder outlet obstruction due to BPH (I-PSS < 8) can be safely treated with supplemental androgens. The situation is less well defined in the moderate category (I-PSS 8–15). Obviously, a man with severe symptoms and significant residual volumes can be tipped over into urinary retention by the administration of testosterone; therefore, ART is contraindicated. But the benefits of ART should not denied to a properly selected candidate because of the presence of mild, stable lower urinary obstructive symptoms. Treatment should only be postponed in those with moderate-to-severe obstructive symptoms until they have been successfully treated according to well established criteria.[29]

TESTOSTERONE AND CANCER OF THE PROSTATE

This issue needs to be discussed under two different situations: the natural endogenous androgen levels and those induced by the exogenous testosterone administration.

ENDOGENOUS LEVELS

Notwithstanding the lack of convincing evidence and the fact that the prevalence of prostate cancer increases as the levels of serum androgens decrease, there is a deep-rooted suspicion among physicians that androgen administration plays a fundamental causal role in the development of prostate cancer. This suspicion is based primarily on four facts: 1) experimental investigations in rodents have shown that artificially induced supranormal levels of testosterone result in the development of prostate cancer; 2) in the presence of profound hypogonadism, at puberty, the gland fails to develop; 3) most human prostate cancers respond promptly and dramatically to surgical or medical castration; and 4) the still controversial yet widely held impression that there is a positive relationship between androgen levels and prostate cancer in humans.[6] The picture is not clarified by the conflicting reports in the literature on the association of naturally occurring serum testosterone levels and the incidence of cancer of the prostate. The perplexing situation is appropriately illustrated by a sampling of the literature: a quantitative review and two meta-analyses addressing this issue together with two studies that investigated sex steroids in stored serum samples. The review of eight epidemiologic studies published by Eaton et al[30] found no significant differences in hormone levels between men developing CaP compared with those who did not. Shaneyfeld et al[31] concluded from their meta-analysis that men with either serum testosterone or insulin-like growth factor 1 (IGF1) in the upper quartiles of the population distribution have an approximately two-fold higher risk for developing prostate cancer. The second meta-analysis, by Slater and Oliver,[32] included 25 studies: 4 showed a positive association between high serum testosterone levels and CaP, in 6 high serum testosterone levels were associated with a reduced risk while in the remaining 15 there was no difference. Finally, the studies that assayed stored serum samples: the Massachusetts Male Aging Study (MMAS)[33] found that no evidence exists for a relationship between the levels of endogenous testosterone and the prevalence of CaP. More recently however, the Baltimore Longitudinal Study on Aging[34] using archival serum samples came to the opposite conclusion. These incongruous findings significantly muddle the field and help to fuel the controversy on the possibly detrimental effects of androgens in function of the prostate gland.

Support for the hypothesis that low testosterone levels prevents or delays the appearance of CaP has come from the recent results of a large finasteride trial: CaP was detected in 18% in the treatment group versus 24% in those receiving placebo.[35] The encouraging results, however, are tempered by the finding of a significantly higher proportion (37%) of poorly differentiated cancers in the finasteride group compared with the controls (22%). Despite the magnitude of the study in terms of numbers (n = 9060) and duration of follow-up (>7 years), only the statement that finasteride delays the appearance of CaP can be accepted with confidence from this study. It follows that some men with LOH may have sub-clinical CaP which manifests itself upon testosterone administration[36] and normalization of androgen levels; what could best be

described as sort of a testosterone provocative test for early detection of CaP.

Despite the large body of support for a positive relationship between male sex steroids and growth of prostate cells, there are a number of puzzling situations that are under active investigation. At the experimental level, a prostate cancer cell line (LNCaP) that requires initial stimulation by androgens to growth, is eventually suppressed by them.[37] At the clinical level, it is recognized that the incidence of CaP increases as the levels of testosterone decrease as part of the aging process.[15] Early studies showed that not all metastatic CaP is stimulated by androgen administration.[38] These and other observations led Prehn[39] to advance a well thought out but radical hypothesis, which he summarized with these words:

> "Contrary to prevalent opinion, declining rather than high levels of androgens probably contribute more to human prostate carcinogenesis and that androgen supplementation would probably lower the incidence of the disease. I will also consider the possibility that the growth of androgen-independent prostate cancers may be reduced by the administration of androgens."

Prehn's hypothesis is receiving renewed attention since evidence is now available indicating that among the various androgens, dehydroepiandrosterone (DHEA) inhibits development and proliferation of experimental prostate cancers.[40] Human research in this area would be important but fraught with ethical and clinical difficulties.

It is relevant to point out in this section, that strong epidemiologic evidence has been presented for a variety of factors influencing the development of CaP independently of sex hormones. They include nonsteroidal hormones (insulin, glucocorticoids),[41] genetic susceptibility, sexually transmitted agents, diet, and environmental carcinogens.[5,42,43] Whether any of these, alone or in combination, work synergistically with sex steroids has not been conclusively established. A significant body of experimental data indicating that prolactin plays an important role in the proliferation and survival of prostate epithelial cells, however, it has not been supported by observations in humans.[44] Similarly, it is well known that IGF1 and IGF2 are powerful regulators of cell proliferation, and the prostate is known to have IGF receptors.[45] It is also known that blocking the action of IGFs diminishes their proliferative effects in prostate cells[46] but this has not been documented in the clinical situation; in fact, it is claimed that there is no relation between IGF1 and prostate size, and that IGF2 may inhibit BPH and the development of prostate cancer.[47] Furthermore, middle-aged men with hypopituitarism receiving recombinant human growth hormone replacement for up to 2 years did not show any increases in PSA.[48] Finally, some growth factors, including IGF and epidermal growth factor (EGF) are capable of activating the androgen receptor and genes normally regulated by sex steroids.[49]

EXOGENOUS ANDROGEN ADMINISTRATION

Current standards of practice establish categorically that the administration of androgens is absolutely contraindicated in men suspected of or harboring prostate (and breast) cancer. This includes those with an abnormal digital rectal examination (DRE) and/or abnormal PSA in whom the diagnosis of carcinoma has not been excluded beyond doubt. However, a sub-clinical cancer can easily escape detection.[50] The presence of prostatic intraepithelial neoplasia (PIN) represents a major dilemma for the urologist. The experience of this is minimal and the information available limited to the extreme. Although Rhoden et al[51] concluded that ART "is not contraindicated in men with a history of PIN" their study included only 75 men followed for 12 months. These results must be viewed with much caution until further independent information is available.

The increasing use of testosterone preparations has made the issues involving ART and prostate cancer an important area of controversy with immediate clinical consequences. At present, there are no studies available to answer the question: "does testosterone administration induce prostate cancer?" This, beyond a doubt, constitutes the most important issue regarding safety in men receiving androgens. The IOM report[6] in its extensive review of the situation regarding ART recommended that prostate safety be considered a high priority in future clinical trials. Unfortunately the IOM also recommended that small studies be conducted initially to document the efficacy of testosterone treatment and only after efficacy has been confirmed should the matter of prostate safety—among other safety issues—be addressed. This puts the clinician in a precarious situation when dealing with a man with SLOH. Obviously, it is inappropriate to wait for 15 or more years until those important concerns are eventually settled. As mentioned above, limited studies have already clearly demonstrated efficacy of ART in the treatment of most of the manifestations of SLOH (for a recent and thorough review see Nieschlag & Behre[52]). In many of these studies, the changes induced in the prostate gland have been assessed directly (DRE, ultrasonography, biopsy) or by surrogate measures (urine flow, post-micturition residual volumes, PSA). All of those studies, however, are relatively small and lack sufficient power and follow-up for definitive answers. In short, these results although reassuring are far from definitive.

The increasing prevalence of localized CaP results in a large number of men undergoing curative procedures. Some of these men will present with SLOH. This presents a truly challenging situation. Should they receive androgen supplementation? If so when? Let us start admitting that today's physicians have an ingrained desire for deterrence of testosterone use in men with a history of prostate cancer. However, if one such man is considered cured and suffers from SLOH, should he be denied treatment? The facts are: 1) most men undergoing curative surgery for CaP do not undergo simultaneous castration; 2) most men undergoing radical surgery have normal serum testosterone levels; 3) although not fully recognized, serum testosterone levels increase after radical prostatectomy[53]; and 4) early evidence is being presented indicating that no detrimental effects have occurred in patients receiving testosterone after radical prostatectomy. With these facts and a commitment for close follow-up, the prudent treatment of SLOH with testosterone supplementation appears warranted. Once again, definitive evidence is simply not available.

BASELINE INVESTIGATIONS BEFORE ONSET OF ART

There are few areas in health care in which more medical and lay media controversy exists. The urologist dealing with SLOH needs to be aware of the salient points. As mentioned above, the extrapolation of the findings of the WHI regarding HRT in women to the situation in men is unwarranted. Although the results of large studies in men are not available (and there will not be for many years), a variety or organ systems have been studied during exogenous testosterone administration, and a number of facts allow the making of safe and rational clinical judgments

It is worth repeating that, ideally, a biochemical confirmation of hypogonadism should be present prior to onset of ART. A baseline DRE and PSA are mandatory. A lipid profile (total cholesterol, high and low density lipoproteins) and a complete blood count should be performed prior to administration of testosterone in order to establish if the treatment results in detrimental effects on lipids or hematological parameters. Liver and kidney function studies are also advisable to rule out preexisting hepatic or renal disease. Other investigations would depend on individual situations. For instance, if a man is to be treated for depression, osteoporosis, or sarcopenia, specific, condition-associated assessments are indicated.

THE FOLLOW-UP OF MEN ON ART

Periodic, competent monitoring of men receiving exogenous testosterone is mandatory. This is particularly important during the first year after onset of treatment, when potential adverse effects are most likely to occur. Quarterly visits are recommended for the first year. If no adverse effects are detected and the patient experiences an adequate response, annual visits are sufficient. At each visit, the response to ART should be assessed and dose modifications introduced if indicated. Digital rectal examination and PSA are mandatory as well as hemoglobin, hematocrit, and lipid profile. None of the current testosterone preparations is hepatotoxic but every manufacturer mentions in their inserts the possibility of liver damage; liver function studies are, therefore, left at the discretion of the physician. The possibility of fluid retention and gynecomastia should be explored, as well as any alterations in sleep patterns.

Prostate safety remains the paramount concern during testosterone replacement therapy. Any new finding on DRE (induration, nodularity) must be investigated. A great deal of importance is given to PSA velocity (PSAV) in these men. This is particularly useful if the patient has been watched for several years. For eugonadal men not receiving ART, the BLSA[54] found that an increase in PSAV of more than 0.1 ng/mL/year implies a greater risk of CaP. This criterion was not based, however, on hypogonadal men receiving ART. In the specific situation of men first starting ART, in whom sequential PSA readings over a long period are usually not available (but with PSA < 4 ng/mL), a rapid initial increase over the first few months of treatment, followed by stabilization of the levels would be expected. Under these circumstances, the recommendations of Bhasin et al[8] are practical and sensible: for follow-up periods less than 3 years, a PSAV greater than 0.4 ng/mL/year, while for periods more than 3 years a PSAV greater than 0.2 ng/mL/year indicate that there is a greater than average risk of CaP, and the patient should be dealt with accordingly. In patients starting testosterone treatment the crucial period is in the first 6 months, where increments in PSA are expected. However, increments of more than 0.5 ng/mL at 3 or 6 months are rare and concerning. Increases of this magnitude (even if the total level is <4 ng/mL) should trigger an assessment to rule out CaP.

RECOMMENDATIONS

A set of recommendations for men receiving ART were developed by an international panel of experts.[55] Those pertaining prostate safety are germane to this chapter and are reproduced below.

MONITORING THE PROSTATE

In men over the age of 40 years, digital rectal examination (DRE) and determination of serum prostatic specific antigen (PSA) are mandatory as baseline measurements of prostate health prior to therapy with androgens, every three (3) to six (6) months for the first 12 months, and yearly thereafter. Transrectal ultrasound guided biopsies of the prostate are indicated only if the DRE or the PSA are abnormal.

PROSTATE AND BREAST SAFETY—I

Androgen administration is absolutely contraindicated in men suspected of harboring carcinoma of the prostate or breast.

PROSTATE SAFETY—II

Men successfully treated for prostate cancer and suffering from symptomatic hypogonadism may become candidates for androgen therapy, after a prudent interval, if there is no evidence of residual cancer. The risk and benefits must be clearly understood by the patient and the follow-up must be particularly careful. No reliable evidence exists in favor of or against this recommendation. The clinician must exercise good clinical judgment together with adequate knowledge of the advantages and drawbacks of androgen therapy in this situation.

PROSTATE SAFETY—III

Androgen supplementation is contraindicated in men with severe bladder outlet obstruction due to an enlarged, clinically benign prostate. Moderate obstruction represents a partial contraindication to ART. After successful treatment of the obstruction, the contraindication can be lifted.

REFERENCES

1. Werner AA. The male climacteric: Report of two hundred and seventy three cases JAMA 1946;132:188–175.

2. Orrego JJ, Dimaraki E, Symons K, Barkan AL. Physiological testosterone replenishment in healthy elderly men does not normalize pituitary growth hormone output: Evidence against the connection between senile hypogonadism and somatopause. J Clin Endocrinol Metab 2004;87:3255–3260.

3. Hak AE, Witteman JCM, deJong FH, et al. Low levels of endogenous androgens increase the risk of atherosclerosis in elderly men: The Rotterdam Study. J Clin Endocrinol Metab 2002,87:3632–3639.

4. Malkin CJ, Pugh PJ, Jones RD, et al. The effect of testosterone replacement on endogenous inflammatory cytokines and lipid profiles in men. J Clin Endocrinol Metab 2004;89:3313–3318.

5. Liva SM, Voskhul RR. Testosterone acts directly on CD4+ lymphocytes to increase IL-10 production. J Immunol 2001;167:2060–2067.

6. Liverman CT, Blazer DG (eds). Institute of Medicine Report: Testosterone and Aging. Committee on Assessing the Need for Clinical Trials of Testosterone Replacement Therapy. National Academies Press, 2004.

7. Goderie-Plomp HM, van der Klift M, de Ronde W, et al. Endogenous sex hormones, sex hormone-binding globulin and the risk of incident vertebral fractures in elderly men and women: The Rotterdam Study. J Clin Endocrinol Metab 2004;89:3261–3269.

8. Bhasin S, Sing AB, Mac P, et al. Managing risk of prostate disease during testosterone replacement therapy of older men: Recommendations for a standard monitoring plan. J Androl 2003;24:299–306.

9. Zittzman M, Depenbusch M, Gromoll J, Nieschlag E. Prostate volume and growth in testosterone-substituted hypogonadal men are dependent on the CAG repeat polymorphism of the androgen receptor gene: a longitudinal pharmacogenetic study. J Clin Endocrinol Metab 2003;88:2049–2054.

10. Isaacs JT. Testosterone and the prostate. In Nieschlag E, Behre HM (eds): Testosterone, action deficiency, substitution, 3rd ed. Cambridge, UK: Cambridge University Press, 2004, pp 347–374.

11. Litvinov IV, De Marzo AM, Isaacs JT. Is the Achilles' heel for prostate cancer therapy a gain of function in androgen receptor signaling? J Clin Endocrinol Metab 2003;88:2972–2982.

12. Bonkhoff H, Stein U, Aumüller, Remberger K. Differential expression of 5-alpha reductase isoenzyme in the human prostate and prostatic carcinoma. Prostate 1996;29:261–267.

13. Bayne CW, Ross M, Miller WR, Habib F. A new role for 5α-reductase type 1 in prostate growth and disease. Elect J Oncol 2002; 152–57.

14. Nelson WG, De Marzo AM, Isaacs JT. Mechanisms of disease: Prostate cancer. N Engl J Med 2003;349:366–361.

15. Morales A. Androgen replacement therapy and prostate safety. Eur Urol 2002;41:113–120.

16. Marcelli M, Cunningham GR. Hormonal signaling in prostatic hyperplasia and neoplasia. J Clin Endocrinol Metab 1999;84:3463–3468.

17. Gann PH, Hennekens CH, Longcope C, et al. A prospective study of hormone plasma levels, non-hormonal factors and development of benign prostatic hyperplasia. Prostate 1995;26:40–49.

18. Kunelius P, Lukkarinen O, Anukksela ML, et al. The effect of transdermal dehydrotestosterone in the aging male: a prospective, randomized, double blind study. J Clin Endocrinol Metab 2002;87:1467–1472.

19. Wang C, Swerdloff RS. Editorial: Should the non-aromatizable androgen dehydrotestosterone be considered as an alternative to testosterone in the treatment of the andropause? J Clin Endocrinol Metab 2002;87:1462–1466.

20. Carson C III, Rittmaster R. The role of dehydrotestosterone in benign prostatic hyperplasia. Urology 2003;61:2–7.

21. Behre HM. Prostate volume in treated and untreated hypogonadal men in comparison to age-matched controls. Clin Endocrinol (Oxf) 1994;40:341–349.

22. Meikle AW, Arver S, Dobbs AS, et al. Prostate size in hypogonadal men treated with a nonscrotal permeation enhanced testosterone transdermal system. Urology 1997;49:191–196.

23. Tenover JL. Androgen deficiency in aging men. Aging Male 1998; (Suppl. 1):16–21.

24. Wright EJ, Fang J, Metter EJ, et al. Prostate specific antigen predicts the long-term risk of prostate enlargement: Results of the Baltimore Longitudinal Study of Aging. J Urol 2002;167:2484–2488.

25. Wang C, Swerdloff RS, Iranmanesh A, et al. Transdermal testosterone gel improves sexual function, mood, muscle strength and body composition parameters in hypogonadal men. J Clin Endocrinol Metab 2000;85:2839–2853.

26. Swerdloff RS, Wang C. Three year follow-up of androgen treatment in hypogonadal men: preliminary report with testosterone gel. Aging Male 2003;6:207–211.

27. Wang C, Cunningham G, Dobbs A, et al. Long-term testosterone gel (Androgel) treatment maintains beneficial effects on sexual function and mood, lean and fat mass and bone mineral density in hypogonadal men. J Clin Endocrinol Metab 2004;89:2085–2098.

28. McNicholas TA, Dean JD, Mulder H, et al. A novel testosterone gel formulation normalizes androgen levels in hypogonadal men, with improvements in body composition and sexual function. BJUI 2003;91:69–74.

29. AUA Practice Guidelines Committee. AUA Guideline on Management of Benign Prostatic Hyperplasia (2003). Chapter 1. Diagnosis and Treatment Recommendations. J Urol 2003;170:530–547.

30. Eaton NE, Reeves GK, Appleby PB, et al Endogenous sex hormones and prostate cancer: a quantitative review of prospective studies. Br J Cancer 199;80:930–934.

31. Shaneyfelt T, Husein R, Bubley G, et al. Hormonal predictors of prostate cancer: a meta-analysis. J Clin Oncol 2000;18:847–853.

32. Slater S, Oliver RTD. Testosterone: its role in the development of prostate cancer and potential risks for use as hormone replacement therapy. Drugs Aging 2000;17:431–439.

33. Mohr BA, Feldman HA, Kalih LA, et al. Are serum hormones associated with the risk of prostate cancer? Prospective results from the Massachusetts Male Aging Study. Urology 2001;57:930–935.

34. Parsons JK, Carter HB, Landis P, et al. High serum free testosterone is associated with an increased risk of prostate cancer: Results from the Baltimore Longitudinal Study on Aging. J Urol 2004;171:116[Abstract 439].

35. Thompson IM, Goodman PJ, Tangen CM, et al. The influence of finasteride in the development of prostate cancer. N Engl J Med 2003;349:215–224.

36. Morgentaler A, Bruning CO III, DeWolff WC. Occult prostate cancer in men with low serum testosterone levels. JAMA 1996;276:1904–1906

37. Knudsen KE, Arden KC, Cavanee WK. Multiple G1 regulatory elements control the androgen dependent proliferation of prostate carcinoma cells. J Biol Chem 1998;273:2013–2022.

38. Morales A, Connolly J, Burr R, Bruce AW. The use of radioactive phosphorus to treat bone pain in metastatica carcinoma of the prostate. Can Med Ass J 1970;103:372–375.

39. Prehn RT. On the prevention and therapy of prostate cancer by androgen administration. Cancer Res 1999;59:4161–4164.

40. Alagartè-Génin M, Cussenot O, Costa P. Prevention of prostate cancer by androgens: experimental paradox or clinical reality. Eur Urol 2004;46:285–295.

41. McKeehan WL, Adams PS, Rosser MP. Direct mitogenic effects of insulin, epidermal growth factor, glucocorticoid, cholera toxin, unknown pituitary factors and possibly prolactin, but not androgen on normal rat prostate epithelial cells in serum-free primary cell culture. Cancer Res 1984;44:1998–2010.

42. Stattin P, Soderberg S, Halmans G, et al. Leptin is associated with increased prostate cancer risk: A nested case-referent study. J Clin Endocrinol Metab 2001;86:1341–1345.

43. Plackson LA, Penson DF, Vaughn TL, et al. Cigarette smoking and risk of prostate cancer in middle age men. Cancer Epidemiol Biomarkers Prevention 2003;12:604–609.

44. Colao A, Vitale G, Di Sarno A, et al. Prolactin and prostate hypertrophy: A pilot observational, prospective, case control study in men with prolactinoma. J Clin Endocrinol Metab 2004;89:2770–2775.

45. Figueroa JA, De Raad S, Tadlock L, Speights VO, et al. Differential expression of insulin-like growth factor binding proteins in low versus high Gleason score prostate cancer. J Urol 1998;159:1379–1383.

46. Cohen P, Peehl DM, Graves HC, Rosenfeld RG. Biologic effects of prostate specific antigen as an insulin-like growth factor binding protein-3 protease. J Endocrinol 1994;142:407–415.

47. Harman SM, Metter EJ, Blackman MR, et al. Serum levels of insulin-like growth factor I (IGF-I), IGF-binding protein-3, and prostate specific antigen as predictors of clinical prostate cancer. J Clin Endocrinol Metab 2000;85:4258–4265.

48. Le Roux CW, Jenkins PJ, Chew SL, et al. Growth hormone replacement does not increase serum prostate-specific antigen in hypopituitary men over 50 years. Eur J Endocrinol 2002;147:59–63.

49. Feldman BJ, Feldman D. The development of androgen-independent prostate cancer. Nat Rev Cancer 2001;1:34–35.

50. Curran MJ, Bihrle W III. Dramatic rise in PSA after androgen replacement in a hypogonadal man with occult adenocarcinoma of the prostate. Urology 1999;53:423–424.

51. Rhoden EL, Morgentaler A. Testosterone replacement therapy in hypogonadal men at risk for prostate cancer: Results of 1 year of treatment in men with prostatic intraepithelial neoplasia. J Urol 2003;170:2348–2351.

52. Nieschlag E, Behre HM (eds). Testosterone: Action- Deficiency- Substitution. Cambridge, UK: Cambridge University Press, 2004.

53. Zhang PL, Rosen S, Veeramachaneni R, et al. Association between prostate cancer and serum testosterone levels. Prostate 2002;53:179–182.

54. Fang J, Metter EJ, Landis P, et al. PSA velocity for assessing prostate cancer risk in men with PSA levels between 2.0 and 4.0 ng/ml. Urology 2002;59:889–893.

55. Morales A, Buvat J, Gooren LJ, et al. Endocrine aspects of sexual dysfunction in men. J Sexual Med 2004;1:69–75.

Vitamin D, retinoids, and prostate cancer   22

Grenville M Oades

INTRODUCTION

Prostate cancer in men is the most commonly registered new malignant diagnosis and the second most commonly registered cause of cancer-related death in some countries. The specific causes of prostate cancer initiation and progression are not known, however, both genetics and the environment seem to play a significant role. It is accepted that prostate cancer develops and initially progresses slowly yet patients with metastatic, androgen-independent prostate cancer currently have few therapeutic options and their prognosis is bleak. The slow growth of prostate cancer and the discrepancy between the frequency of "latent" and clinically manifest disease suggest many factors may have a role in controlling the progression of this disease.

Vitamin D can be obtained from a few foods such as egg yolks and liver but the majority is produced as a result of normal sunlight exposure. Vitamin D_3 is produced by an ultraviolet light induced photolytic conversion of 7-dehydrocholesterol to previtamin D_3 followed by thermal isomerization in the skin. Vitamin D_3 then undergoes two hydroxylation steps. The first occurs primarily in the liver and the second in the kidney resulting in 1,25-dihydroxy vitamin D_3—1,25-$(OH)_2D_3$—the metabolically active compound[1] (Figure 22.1). Vitamin D and its hydroxylated metabolites are transported in the circulation bound to plasma proteins, their classical role being in calcium homeostasis. It is, however, now becoming clear that a host of other roles not directly related to calcium metabolism exist.

Retinoids are derivatives of vitamin A, a required nutrient, deficiency of which causes xerophthalmia. They are obtained from the diet in two forms, either from animal products as preformed fatty-acid retinyl esters (R-FA) or from fruit and vegetables as provitamin A carotenoids, such as β-carotene. These are converted in the gastrointestinal tract into retinol, the physiological

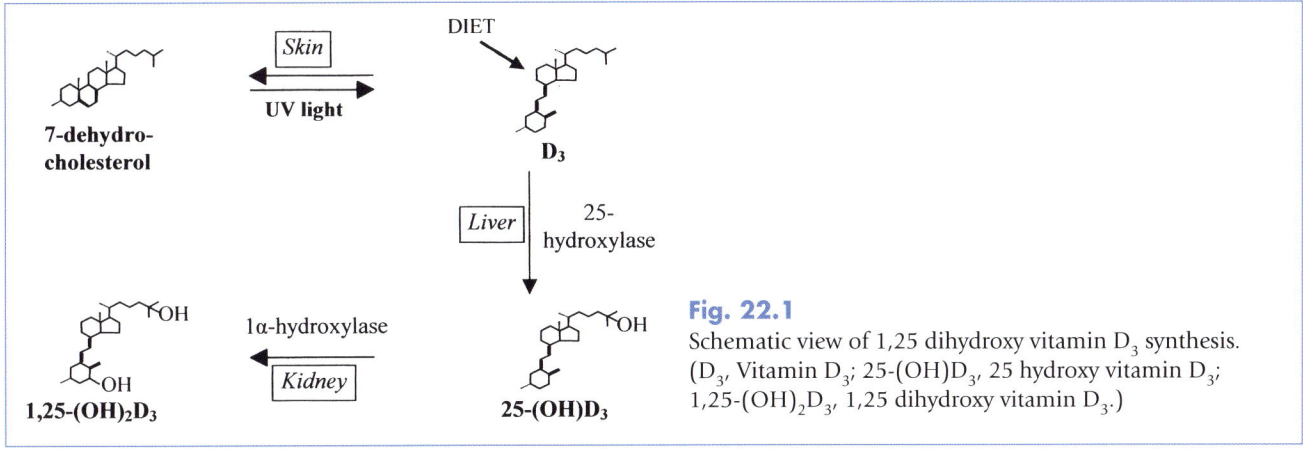

Fig. 22.1
Schematic view of 1,25 dihydroxy vitamin D_3 synthesis. (D_3, Vitamin D_3; 25-$(OH)D_3$, 25 hydroxy vitamin D_3; 1,25-$(OH)_2D_3$, 1,25 dihydroxy vitamin D_3.)

form of vitamin A. Fatty-acid retinyl esters are hydrolyzed in the enteric mucosa and by pancreatic enzymes, and β-carotene is cleaved into two retinol molecules. Retinol is absorbed by enterocytes and binds to cellular retinol-binding protein II. Here it is esterified to form R-FA and transported to the liver in chylomicrons through the lymph. Retinol is the major liver storage form of vitamin A and is transported to tissues bound to retinol-binding protein and transthyretin. There is an enterohepatic circulation of retinoids (Figure 22.2). In target cells retinol is oxidized to form the aldehyde retinal and all-*trans*-retinoic acid (ATRA) (Figure 22.3). All-*trans*-retinoic acid can in turn isomerize into 9-*cis*-retinoic acid (9cRA). Retinoids have well-characterized functions in vision and are recognized to have a role in growth, differentiation, and metastasis of normal and malignant cells.[2]

EPIDEMIOLOGY

In 1990, Schwartz and Hulka proposed that low levels of circulating $1,25\text{-}(OH)_2D_3$ were a risk factor for prostate cancer.[3] This hypothesis may offer at least a partial explanation of three known risk factors associated with prostate cancer: age, race, and residence in northern latitudes. Firstly, it is well recognized that the incidence of prostate cancer increases with increasing age. Vitamin D deficiency is extremely prevalent in the elderly due in part to a decreased environmental exposure to sunlight and a decreased capacity of older men to synthesize previtamin D_3.[4,5] Secondly, African-American men have almost twice the risk of prostate cancer as white men. They have also been shown to have an earlier onset of prostate cancer, a more advanced stage at diagnosis, and a higher mortality. These differences are not thought to be simply due to socio-economic variances between populations.[6] Racial pigmentation has been shown to significantly affect serum levels of $1,25\text{-}(OH)_2D_3$

following a standard dose of UVB radiation.[7] Thirdly, mortality rates from prostate cancer vary widely between countries. Some of these geographical variations may be attributable to differences in exposure to sunlight. Hanchette and Schwartz showed that mortality rates among white men in the USA were inversely correlated to geographic levels of UV radiation exposure.[8] Grant has recently estimated that approximately 1% of all deaths due to prostate cancer in the USA are related to insufficient exposure to UVB.[9]

Epidemiologic studies of the role of serum levels of $1,25\text{-}(OH)_2D_3$ in the etiology of prostate cancer have been controversial. Corder et al found that risk of prostate cancer decreased with higher serum levels of $1,25\text{-}(OH)_2D_3$ and that, in older men, low levels of $1,25\text{-}(OH)_2D_3$ were an important predictor of palpable tumors and high Gleason grade.[10] This correlation has, however, not been found in other studies.[11,12] It is possible that serum concentrations of $25\text{-}(OH)D_3$ are a better indicator of an individual's vitamin D status, as serum $1,25\text{-}(OH)_2D_3$ levels are under much tighter feedback control. In a recent study, a cohort of 19,000 men initially clinically free of prostate cancer was followed up for 14 years. In this group, 158 cases of prostate cancer were identified. Prostate cancer risk was inversely related to baseline serum levels of $25\text{-}(OH)D_3$ in men aged less than 52 years at entry.[13] A similar study of this metabolite in Japanese-American men has, however, failed to show a correlation.[14] Although there are animal models that suggest a chemopreventive

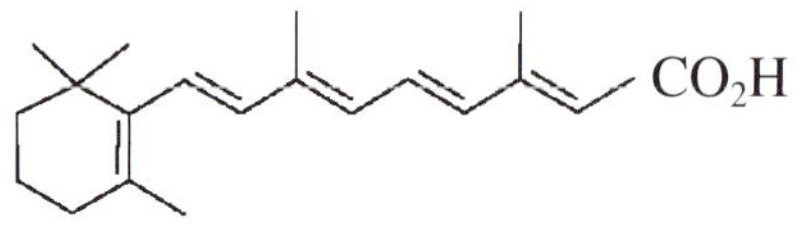

Fig. 22.3
All-*trans*-retinoic-acid.

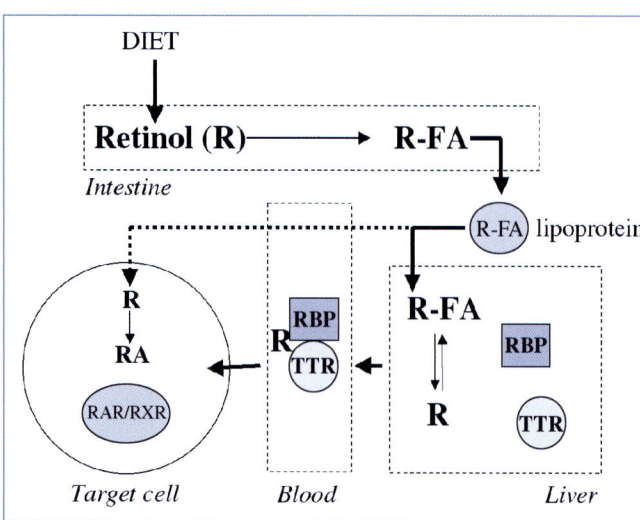

Fig. 22.2
Schematic overview of retinoid transport and metabolism. (RA, retinoic acid; RAR, retinoic acid receptor; RBP, retinol binding protein; R-FA, fatty acid retinyl esters; TTR, transthyretin; RXR, retinoid X receptor.)

action of vitamin D compounds against prostate cancer, there are no studies examining dietary vitamin D supplementation and subsequent risk of prostate cancer in a human population.

The role of retinoids in prostate cancer etiology is controversial. No consistent association has been found between dietary intake of preformed vitamin A or provitamin A carotenoids and risk of prostate cancer.[15] Several prospective studies based on serum retinol levels and prostate cancer risk have provided very inconsistent results. As with $1,25\text{-}(OH)_2D_3$, serum retinol levels are tightly homeostatically controlled, and only severe depletion of retinol stores in the liver will be reflected in decreased serum levels, limiting the usefulness of these studies. A chemopreventive activity of retinoids in animal models of prostate cancer has, however, been shown, but evidence of similar activity in human populations is lacking. The Carotene and Retinol Cancer Efficacy trial was a randomized, double-blind placebo controlled trial to assess the effect of 25,000 IU of retinyl palmitate plus 15 mg of β-carotene for the primary prevention of lung cancer but also looked at prostate cancer end points. There was no difference in prostate cancer incidence between the two arms of the study.[16] Indeed, a recent review of the cancer preventative potential of vitamin A concluded there was little evidence that vitamin A intake had any substantial protective effects.[15]

RECEPTORS

The actions of both retinoids and $1,25\text{-}(OH)_2D_3$ are mediated through high-affinity nuclear receptors that act as ligand activated transcription factors. These receptors belong to the steroid and thyroid hormone nuclear receptor superfamily. When activated by the relevant ligand, these receptors can directly regulate gene transcription by binding to response elements in the promoter regions of target genes.

Most of the biological actions of $1,25\text{-}(OH)_2D_3$ are mediated by the vitamin D receptor (VDR). In most cases, ligand-bound VDR heterodimerizes with the retinoid X receptor (RXR), an essential step for VDR function. The VDR is also capable of forming homodimers with itself, or heterodimers with the nuclear receptor for thyroid hormone. The VDR/RXR heterodimer has very low affinity for DNA in the absence of $1,25\text{-}(OH)_2D_3$. Binding of $1,25\text{-}(OH)_2D_3$ facilitates association with a vitamin D response element as well as inhibiting binding of 9cRA to RXR.[17] The VDR is universally expressed in the normal human prostate and localized primarily to secretory epithelial cells.[18] Expression is also more predominant in the peripheral as opposed to the central zone. It has been shown that $1,25(OH)_2D_3$ exerts both growth inhibitory and growth promoting effects on the prostate gland.[19–21]

Several common functional allelic variants of the VDR gene have been identified, and it has been postulated that these polymorphisms may be associated with an altered risk of prostate cancer. There have been a number of published reports that have examined these associations with mixed findings. A recent meta-analysis has, however, shown that four of the most commonly studied polymorphisms are unlikely to be major determinants of susceptibility to prostate cancer on a wide population basis.[22]

Many of the biological functions of retinoids are mediated through the actions of two families of nuclear receptors. These are the retinoic acid receptors (RARα, RARβ, and RARγ) and the retinoid X receptors (RXRα, RXRβ, and RXRγ). Both ATRA and 9cRA are ligands for the RARs while only 9cRA is a ligand for the RXRs. As with the VDR, many of the RARs also function as heterodimers with RXR, and binding of ligand promotes association with a retinoic acid response element.[2] Retinoid receptors are also widely expressed in the prostate and retinoids have been shown to be required for the normal development of the prostate gland in a mouse model.[23]

PRECLINICAL STUDIES

ANTIPROLIFERATIVE EFFECTS

Despite the inconsistent epidemiologic data linking Vitamin D and retinoids to prostate cancer, it seems likely that they do have a role in development of the normal human prostate. There is also strong experimental evidence that both vitamin D and retinoids play a part in prostate cancer, and may possibly provide future therapeutic strategies.

Vitamin D compounds inhibit the growth of primary cultures of prostate cancer and many established prostate cancer cell lines such as LNCaP, PC3 and DU145 (Figure 22.4).[24] The mechanism of inhibition appears to be by induction of cell cycle arrest and, in some instances, induction of apoptosis.

In agreement with findings in other tumor types, LNCaP cells have been shown to accumulate in the G1 phase of the cell cycle after treatment with $1,25\text{-}(OH)_2D_3$.[25] It appears that $1,25\text{-}(OH)_2D_3$ has a role in controlling the G1-S checkpoint in prostate cancer. Passage of the cell cycle checkpoints ultimately requires the activation of intracellular enzymes known as cyclin-dependent kinases (CDKs). The CDK inhibitor p21(CIP1) contains a functional vitamin D response element in its promoter region and can be transcriptionally regulated by $1,25\text{-}(OH)_2D_3$.[26] $1,25\text{-}(OH)_2D_3$ has been shown to induce cell cycle arrest and upregulation of p21(CIP1) in LNCaP, PC3 and DU145 cells, and the CDK inhibitor p27(KIP1) in LNCaP

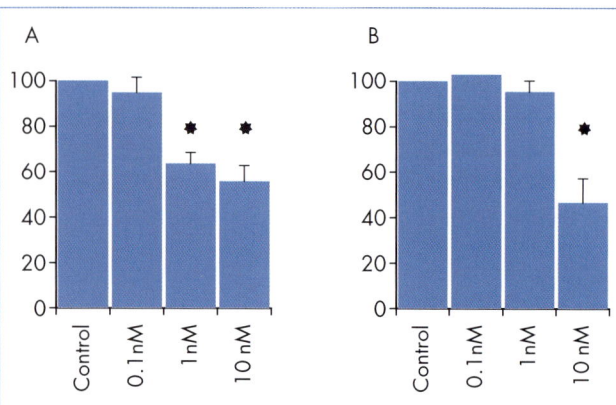

Fig. 22.4
Growth inhibition of LNCaP cells treated with 1,25-dihydroxy vitamin D_3 *(A)* or all-*trans*-retinoic-acid *(B)* for 6days. Cells were plated and treated with the indicated hormone concentration or with vehicle (0.1% ethanol). Growth inhibition assessed using sulforhodamine B (SRB) staining. Results expressed as a percentage of ethanol-treated control. Error bars represent means ±1 SD (n = 3). (*P < 0.05.)

cells.[27] Normally when retinoblastoma protein is phosphorylated, it looses its ability to complex with E2F transcription factors and restrain the cell cycle allowing cells to enter S phase. Decreased retinoblastoma protein phosphorylation, repressed E2F transcriptional activity, and decreased CDK2 activity, resulting in G1 arrest have also been shown.[28]

Apoptosis also seems to play a smaller role in the cellular response to 1,25-$(OH)_2D_3$ although this has not been consistently seen in all studies.[28–31] There is some evidence to suggest that the B_CL2 family of proteins plays a role in 1,25-$(OH)_2D_3$-induced apoptosis as 1,25-$(OH)_2D_3$ is capable of downregulating the antiapoptotic proteins B_CL2 and B_CLX_L in LN_CaP cells.[29]

Retinoids have also been shown to inhibit the growth of prostatic epithelial cells and established prostate cancer cell lines (see Figure 22.4). The exact mechanism by which retinoids regulate the growth of prostate cancer cells has not been completely elucidated. High concentrations of ATRA can certainly induce apoptosis in LNCaP cells, and several retinoids, like 1,25-$(OH)_2D_3$, appear to be associated with down regulation of B_CL2 expression.[32,33] Retinoids also have an effect on the G1 cell cycle regulatory proteins and can induce cell cycle arrest in a number of tumor types although studies in prostate cancer are limited.[34,35]

Effects exerted by retinoids on prostate cancer cell growth control and apoptosis are complex and often cell specific, mediated by specific RAR subtypes or even in a receptor-independent manner. Several studies have however suggested a crucial role for RARβ, which seems to be important in mediating the growth inhibitory effects of many retinoids. Loss of RARβ has been implicated in prostate carcinogenesis.[36]

ANTIMETASTATIC EFFECTS

Metastasis of tumor cells is a complex cascade involving a number of steps including angiogenesis, loss of tumor cell adhesion, invasion of the vasculature, evasion of host defense, arrest at a distant site, and establishment of new growth. There is evidence to suggest that 1,25-$(OH)_2D_3$ may interfere with this process in prostate cancer at a number of points; it has been shown to inhibit invasion, cell adhesion, and migration to the basement membrane matrix protein laminins in the DU145 and PC3 prostate cancer cell lines.[37] It has also been shown to inhibit DU145 invasiveness in a cell invasion assay and has antiangiogenic properties in a number of model systems.[38]

Retinoids have also been shown to reduce adhesion, motility, invasion, and expression of proteinases. In prostate cancer, retinoids have been shown to suppress exogenous endothelin 1 induced growth stimulation in LNCaP cells.[39] Retinoic acid can inhibit urokinase-mediated extracellular matrix degradation and invasion by DU145 human prostatic carcinoma cells.[40]

Retinoids have shown antiangiogenic effects in several systems. Both tumor and endothelial cells are directly affected by ATRA, which suppresses angiogenesis in vivo.[41,42] Both 9cRA and 13-*cis*-retinoic acid have also been shown to have antiangiogenic activity in a number of different tumor models in combination with interferons, however, data in prostate cancer is limited.

CLINICAL STUDIES

Based on the encouraging preclinical data, there have been a number of trials to evaluate the clinical role of 1,25-$(OH)_2D_3$ as a treatment for human prostate cancer. A small, non-randomized trial in 14 men with hormone-refractory metastatic disease treated with escalating doses of 1,25-$(OH)_2D_3$ up to 1.5 µg/day failed to show an objective response in any patient. In two patients there were declines in prostate-specific antigen (PSA) of 25% and 45%.[43] Eleven of the evaluated patients experienced grade I hypercalcemia.

In another study, seven patients with early recurrent prostate cancer following radical prostatectomy or radiotherapy were treated with escalating doses of 1,25-$(OH)_2D_3$ up to 2.5 µg/day.[44] Six of the seven patients showed a statistically significant decline in the rate of PSA rise and three patients maintained a stable serum

PSA for at least 1 year. Withdrawal of therapy resulted in the return of PSA velocity to pre-treatment levels. In this study, the dose of 1,25-$(OH)_2D_3$ was again limited by hypercalcemia and hypercalcuria, with one patient developing an asymptomatic renal calculus.

As the major toxicity of 1,25-$(OH)_2D_3$ is hypercalcemia, two studies addressed the question of the maximum tolerated dose of 1,25-$(OH)_2D_3$ that can be administered. Beer et al studied 15 patients with refractory malignancies including five with prostate cancer. They were given 1,25-$(OH)D_3$ at doses of up to 2.8 µg/kg in weekly pulses without dose limiting toxicity; however, only one patient had a stable PSA throughout the study period.[45] In a second study, 36 patients with advanced malignancy (including six with hormone-refractory prostate cancer) were administered 1,25-$(OH)_2D_3$ subcutaneously.[46] The maximum tolerated dose reached by any patient was 8 µg with dose-limiting toxicity being hypercalcemia as expected. Three patients developed renal calculi. No PSA response was seen in any of the prostate cancer patients, and three of these patients with diffuse bony metastasis experienced an increase in bone pain. This is in contrast to the observations of Van Veldhuizen et al.[47] In his phase II trial of 16 patients with hormone refractory prostate cancer, seven had baseline serum 25-$(OH)_2D_3$ below the normal range. Patients were given a daily dose of 2000 IU of ergocalciferol, a commercially available vitamin D analog, in combination with 500 mg oral calcium supplement. Four patients had an improvement in pain scores following treatment and twelve exhibited an increase in muscle strength. Five men had stable PSA levels, and one man showed a decrease in PSA during the study period. This study concluded that vitamin D deficiency develops in a significant percentage of patients with advanced hormone refractory prostate cancer. It is possible that vitamin D deficiency contributes to the osteoporosis and fractures in patients on long-term androgen ablation therapy for prostate cancer.[48,49] Vitamin D supplementation may be a useful adjunct for improving pain, muscle strength, and quality of life.

Clinical studies of retinoids are limited and have demonstrated only minimal efficacy. Shalev et al treated patients with PSA relapse following radical prostatectomy with 1 mg/kg/day of 13-*cis*-retinoic acid.[50] A modest PSA reduction was seen in 3 of 11 patients. Culnie et al undertook a phase II trial of intermittent ATRA in hormone-refractive prostate cancer. Patients received a single oral dose of 45 mg/m^2/day ATRA for 7 days followed by 7 days of no treatment, and then resumed treatment on day 15. This schedule was continued until progression or limiting toxicity occurred. Toxicity was mild but only 15% of patients achieved a biological response (>50% decrease in serum PSA).[51] Previously, a similar study had failed to show a response in any patient.[52] In a study by Kelly et al designed to look at pathologic endpoints, 14 patients with androgen-independent disease were treated with ATRA (50 mg/m^2 orally t.i.d). Clinical activity, assessed by radiographs and serum PSA, was minimal, and the majority of patients progressed within 3 months. The majority of cases (95%) showed no gross histologic changes and no difference in apoptotic or proliferative indices on pre- and post-treatment biopsies.[53]

CONCLUSION

It is likely that both Vitamin D and retinoids have some role to play in the development of the normal prostate. Their role in the development and progression of prostate cancer remains controversial. Epidemiologic evidence is patchy, and clinically apparent deficiency of both vitamin D and retinoids is rare in developed countries. It seems unlikely that dietary manipulation or lifestyle changes to alter the intake or synthesis of these compounds will have a significant impact on prostate cancer incidence.

Clinical studies have demonstrated only a modest efficacy of retinoids and vitamin D in the treatment of prostate cancer. Perhaps the most exciting prospect for the future lies in advances in medicinal chemistry. Analogs of vitamin D and retinoids are being developed with much greater potency and fewer side effects. It is possible that these compounds may have a role, alone or in combination with other agents, in the future treatment of this disease.

REFERENCES

1. Brown AJ, Dusso A, Slatopolsky E. Vitamin D. Am J Physiol 1999;277:F157–F175.
2. Sonneveld E, van der Saag PT. Metabolism of retinoic acid: implications for development and cancer. Int J Vitam Nutr Res 1998;68:404–410.
3. Schwartz GG, Hulka BS. Is vitamin D deficiency a risk factor for prostate cancer? (hypothesis). Anticancer Res 1990;10:1307–1312.
4. Baker MR, Peacock M, Nordin BE. The decline in vitamin D status with age. Age Ageing 1980;9:249–252.
5. MacLaughlin J, Holick MF. Aging decreases the capacity of human skin to produce vitamin D3. J Clin Invest 1985;76:1536–1538.
6. Thompson I, Tangen C, Tolcher A, et al. Association of African-American ethnic background with survival in men with metastatic prostate cancer. J Natl Cancer Inst 2001;93:219–225.
7. Matusoka LY, Wortsman J, Haddad JG, et al. Racial pigmentation and the cutaneous synthesis of vitamin D. Arch Dermatol 1991;127:536–538.
8. Hanchette CL, Schwartz GG. Geographic patterns of prostate cancer mortality. Evidence of a protective effect of ultraviolet radiation. Cancer 1992;70:2861–2869.
9. Grant WB. An estimate of premature cancer mortality in the U.S. due to inadequate doses of solar ultraviolet-B radiation. Cancer 2002;94:1867–1875.
10. Corder EH, Guess HA, Hulka BS, et al. Vitamin D and prostate cancer: a prediagnostic study with stored sera. Cancer Epidemiol Biomarkers Prev 1993;2:467–472.
11. Lerner EC, Qian Y, Blaskovich MA, et al. Ras CAAX peptidomimetic FTI-277 selectively blocks oncogenic Ras signaling by inducing cytoplasmic accumulation of inactive Ras-Raf complexes. J Biol Chem 1995;270:26802–26806.

12. Gann PH, Ma J, Hennekens CH, et al. Circulating vitamin D metabolites in relation to subsequent development of prostate cancer. Cancer Epidemiol Biomarkers Prev 1996;5:121–126.

13. Ahonen MH, Tenkanen L, Teppo L, et al. Prostate cancer risk and prediagnostic serum 25-hydroxyvitamin D levels (Finland). Cancer Causes Control 2000;11:847–852.

14. Nomura AM, Stemmermann GN, Lee J, et al. Serum vitamin D metabolite levels and the subsequent development of prostate cancer (Hawaii, United States). Cancer Causes Control 1998;9:425–432.

15. Vainio H, Rautalahti M. An international evaluation of the cancer preventive potential of vitamin A. Cancer Epidemiol Biomarkers Prev 1999;8:107–109.

16. Omenn GS, Goodman GE, Thornquist MD, et al. Risk factors for lung cancer and for intervention effects in CARET, the Beta-Carotene and Retinol Efficacy Trial. J Natl Cancer Inst 1996;88:1550–1559.

17. Thompson PD, Jurutka PW, Haussler CA, et al. Heterodimeric DNA binding by the vitamin D receptor and retinoid X receptors is enhanced by 1,25-dihydroxyvitamin D3 and inhibited by 9-cis-retinoic acid. Evidence for allosteric receptor interactions. J Biol Chem 1998;273:8483–8491.

18. Kivineva M, Blauer M, Syvala H, et al. Localization of 1,25-dihydroxyvitamin D3 receptor (VDR) expression in human prostate. J Steroid Biochem Mol Biol 1998;66:121–127.

19. Krill D, DeFlavia P, Dhir R, et al. Expression patterns of vitamin D receptor in human prostate. J Cell Biochem 2001;82:566–572.

20. Peehl DM, Skowronski RJ, Leung GK, et al. Antiproliferative effects of 1,25-dihydroxyvitamin D3 on primary cultures of human prostatic cells. Cancer Res 1994;54:805–810.

21. Krill D, Stoner J, Konety BR, et al. Differential effects of vitamin D on normal human prostate epithelial and stromal cells in primary culture. Urology 1999;54:171–177.

22. Ntais C, Polycarpou A, Ioannidis JP. Vitamin D receptor gene polymorphisms and risk of prostate cancer: a meta-analysis. Cancer Epidemiol Biomarkers Prev 2003;12:1395–1402.

23. Seo R, McGuire M, Chung M, et al. Inhibition of prostate ductal morphogenesis by retinoic acid. J Urol 1997;158:931–935.

24. Krishnan AV, Peehl DM, Feldman D. The role of vitamin D in prostate cancer. Recent Results Cancer Res 2003;164:205–221.

25. Blutt SE, Allegretto EA, Pike JW, et al. 1,25-dihydroxyvitamin D3 and 9-cis-retinoic acid act synergistically to inhibit the growth of LNCaP prostate cells and cause accumulation of cells in G1. Endocrinology 1997;138:1491–1497.

26. Liu M, Lee MH, Cohen M, et al. Transcriptional activation of the Cdk inhibitor p21 by vitamin D3 leads to the induced differentiation of the myelomonocytic cell line U937. Genes Dev 1996;10:142–153.

27. Campbell MJ, Elstner E, Holden S, et al. Inhibition of proliferation of prostate cancer cells by a 19-nor-hexafluoride vitamin D3 analogue involves the induction of p21waf1, p27kip1 and E-cadherin. J Mol Endocrinol 1997;19:15–27.

28. Zhuang SH, Burnstein KL. Antiproliferative effect of 1α, 25-dihydroxyvitamin D$_3$ in human prostate cancer cell line LNCaP involves reduction of cyclin-dependent kinase 2 activity and persistent G1 accumulation. Endocrinology 1998;139:1207.

29. Blutt SE, McDonnell TJ, Polek TC, et al. Calcitriol-induced apoptosis in LNCaP cells is blocked by overexpression of bcl-2. Endocrinology 2000;141:17.

30. Fife RS, Sledge GW, Jr., Proctor C. Effects of vitamin D3 on proliferation of cancer cells in vitro. Cancer Lett 1997;120:65–69.

31. Hsieh T, Wu JM. Induction of apoptosis and altered nuclear/cytoplasmic distribution of the androgen receptor and prostate-specific antigen by 1alpha,25-dihydroxyvitamin D3 in androgen-responsive LNCaP cells. Biochem Biophys Res Commun 1997;235:539–544.

32. Gao M, Ossowski L, Ferrari AC. Activation of Rb and decline in androgen receptor protein precede retinoic acid-induced apoptosis in androgen-dependent LNCaP cells and their androgen-independent derivative. J Cell Physiol 1999;179:336–346.

33. Zhang XK. Vitamin A and apoptosis in prostate cancer. Endocr Relat Cancer 2002;9:87–102.

34. Huss WJ, Lai L, Barrios RJ, et al. Retinoic acid slows progression and promotes apoptosis of spontaneous prostate cancer. Prostate 2004;61:142–152.

35. Niles RM. Signaling pathways in retinoid chemoprevention and treatment of cancer. Mutat Res 2004;555:97–105.

36. Lotan Y, Xu XC, Shalev M, et al. Differential expression of nuclear retinoid receptors in normal and malignant prostates. J Clin Oncol 2000;18:116–121.

37. Sung V, Feldman D. 1,25-Dihydroxyvitamin D3 decreases human prostate cancer cell adhesion and migration. Mol Cell Endocrinol 2000;164:133–143.

38. Schwartz GG, Wang MH, Zang M, et al. 1 alpha,25-Dihydroxyvitamin D (calcitriol) inhibits the invasiveness of human prostate cancer cells. Cancer Epidemiol Biomarkers Prev 1997;6:727–732.

39. Hsu JY, Pfahl M. ET-1 expression and growth inhibition of prostate cancer cells: a retinoid target with novel specificity. Cancer Res 1998;58:4817–4822.

40. Webber MM, Waghray A. Urokinase-mediated extracellular matrix degradation by human prostatic carcinoma cells and its inhibition by retinoic acid. Clin Cancer Res 1995;1:755–761.

41. Lingen MW, Polverini PJ, Bouck NP. Inhibition of squamous cell carcinoma angiogenesis by direct interaction of retinoic acid with endothelial cells. Lab Invest 1996;74:476–483.

42. Lingen MW, Polverini PJ, Bouck NP. Retinoic acid induces cells cultured from oral squamous cell carcinomas to become anti-angiogenic. Am J Pathol 1996;149:247–258.

43. Osborn JL, Schwartz GG, Smith DC, et al. Phase II trial of oral 1,25-dihydroxyvitamin D (calcitriol) in hormone refractory prostate cancer. Urologic Oncol 1995;1:195–198.

44. Gross C, Stamey T, Hancock S, et al. Treatment of early recurrent prostate cancer with 1,25-dihydroxyvitamin D$_3$ (calcitriol). J Urol 1998;159:2035–2040.

45. Beer TM, Munar M, Henner WD. A Phase I trial of pulse calcitriol in patients with refractory malignancies: pulse dosing permits substantial dose escalation. Cancer 2001;91:2431–2439.

46. Smith DC, Johnson CS, Freeman CC, et al. A Phase I trial of calcitriol (1,25-dihydroxycholecalciferol) in patients with advanced malignancy. Clin Cancer Res 1999;5:1339–1345.

47. Van Veldhuizen PJ, Taylor SA, Williamson S, et al. Treatment of vitamin D deficiency in patients with metastatic prostate cancer may improve bone pain and muscle strength. J Urol 2000;163:187–190.

48. Gallagher JC. The role of vitamin D in the pathogenesis and treatment of osteoporosis. J Rheumatol Suppl 1996;45:15–18.

49. Daniell HW, Dunn SR, Ferguson DW, et al. Progressive osteoporosis during androgen deprivation therapy for prostate cancer. J Urol JID - 0376374 2000;163:181–186.

50. Shalev M, Thompson TC, Frolov A, et al. Effect of 13-cis-retinoic acid on serum prostate-specific antigen levels in patients with recurrent prostate cancer after radical prostatectomy. Clin Cancer Res 2000;6:3845–3849.

51. Culine S, Kramar A, Droz JP, et al. Phase II study of all-trans retinoic acid administered intermittently for hormone refractory prostate cancer. J Urol 1999;161:173–175.

52. Trump DL, Smith DC, Stiff D, et al. A phase II trial of all-trans-retinoic acid in hormone-refractory prostate cancer: a clinical trial with detailed pharmacokinetic analysis. Cancer Chemother Pharmacol 1997;39:349–356.

53. Kelly WK, Osman I, Reuter VE, et al. The development of biologic end points in patients treated with differentiation agents: an experience of retinoids in prostate cancer. Clin Cancer Res 2000;6:838–846.

Molecular mechanisms of prostate carcinogenesis

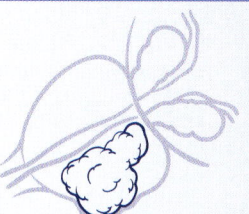

Mechanisms of prostate cancer progression 23

Kati P Porkka, Tapio Visakorpi

INTRODUCTION

Prostate cancer arises from glandular epithelium, most often in the peripheral zone of the prostate. Prostatic intraepithelial neoplasia (PIN) is also often found in the peripheral zone, and is believed to be a premalignant stage of, although not a prerequisite for, prostate carcinoma.[1] A special feature for prostate cancer is that a latent form of the disease is very common. Microscopic lesions of cancer have been found in autopsies from more than 50% of men between 70 and 80 years old.[2] A vast majority of these histologic cancers would most probably never develop into a clinical cancer. Whether these incidentally found small carcinomas represent the same disease entity as the clinically relevant, life-threatening tumors, is not really known.[3] Prostate cancer progression is a multistep process, in which an organ-confined tumor eventually invades through the capsule of the prostate into its surroundings and metastasizes to local lymph nodes and to distant organs, mainly bones (Figure 23.1). The growth and progression of prostate cancer is dependent on androgens. Therefore, the standard treatment for advanced prostate cancer has, for more than half a century, been hormonal therapy, such as castration or antiandrogens. However, during the treatment, an androgen-independent cancer cell population will eventually arise.[4] For such hormone-refractory tumors, no effective treatments are available.

Genetic alterations are believed to be the underlying causes of the above described clinical development and progression of prostate cancer. Such genetic mechanisms are, however, not fully understood. The novel tools of genetics have helped to identify some critical genetic aberrations, but many are still to be discovered. In this chapter, we describe chromosomal and gene aberrations that have been found in prostate cancer, especially those that are characteristic of the late progression of the disease.

CHROMOSOMAL ABERRATIONS

Several methods, such as traditional cytogenetics (G-banding), analysis of loss of heterozygosity (LOH), and comparative genomic hybridization (CGH), have been used to detect chromosomal aberrations in prostate cancer. Traditional cytogenetics has been very uninformative due to the fact that prostate cancer cells do not grow well in vitro. On the other hand, only a few whole genome-wide LOH analyses have so far been performed. Therefore, the most informative genome-wide analysis tool utilized has been CGH, which allows detection of both gains and losses of DNA sequence copy numbers. Studies using GCH have revealed two main features characteristic to prostate cancer. First, in early-stage prostate cancer losses of the genetic material are much more common than gains or amplifications,[5] indicating that tumor suppressor genes, which are believed to harbor the frequently deleted regions, probably play an important role in the early tumorigenesis of the prostate. Second, gains and amplifications are seen in metastatic and hormone-refractory tumors, suggesting that the late stage of the disease is characterized by oncogene activation.[5]

The most common chromosomal alterations in early prostate cancer detected by CGH are losses of 6q (~20%), 8p (~30%), 13q (~30%), 16q (~20%), and 18q (~20%). In the advanced disease, the frequency of

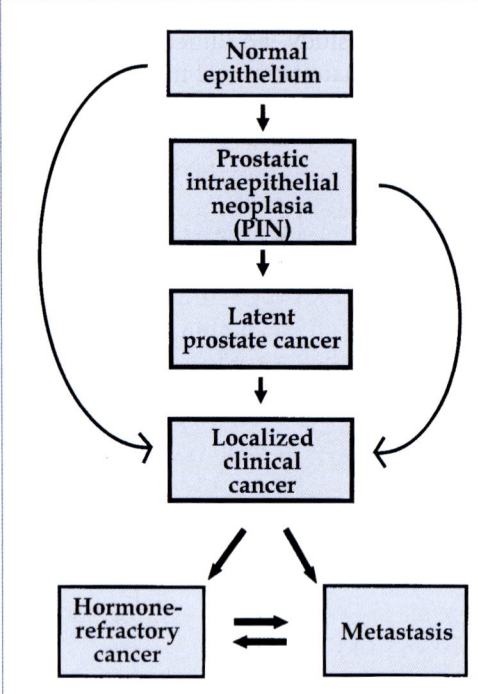

Fig. 23.1
Multi-step progression of prostate cancer. The cancer arises from normal epithelial cells, at least in some cases through a premalignant lesion called prostatic intraepithelial neoplasia (PIN). The common latent microscopic prostate cancer may also be a pre-stage of clinical cancer. However, the potential of the latent cancer to progress into a theoretically life-threatening clinical cancer is not really known. Prostate cancer metastasizes, in the first place, mainly to local lymph nodes and bone. The growth of the vast majority of prostate cancers is androgen-dependent. However, during androgen withdrawal, a hormone-refractory tumor clone eventually emerges.

alterations in these chromosome arms is higher, for example losses of 8p and 13q are found in up to 80% of cases. In addition, losses of 10q (~40%) and 17p (~40%) as well as gains of 7p/q (40%), 8q (~80%) and Xq (~40%) are common in the advanced stage of disease (Table 23.1).[6]

Table 23.1 The most common chromosomal alterations in untreated primary and hormone-refractory prostate carcinomas according to comparative genomic hybridization (CGH)

Chromosomal arm	Frequency of alteration in prostate carcinoma samples*	
	Untreated tumors (%)	Hormone-refractory tumors (%)
Losses:		
6q	~20	30–40
8p	~30	70–80
10q	~10	40–50
13q	~30	50–60
16q	~20	45–55
18q	~20	~20
Gains:		
8q	~5	70–90
7p/q	~10	40–60
Xq	~0	35–55

*Frequencies according to Visakorpi T, Kallioniemi AH, Syvänen AC et al. Genetic changes in primary and recurrent prostate cancer by comparative genomic hybridization. Cancer Res 1995;55:342–347 and Nupponen NN, Kakkola L, Koivisto P, Visakorpi T. Genetic alterations in hormone-refractory recurrent prostate carcinomas. Am J Pathol 1998;153:141–148.

CHROMOSOMAL ALTERATIONS IN THE EARLY DEVELOPMENT OF PROSTATE CANCER

The most commonly deleted chromosomal regions in prostate cancer are 8p and 13q. These alterations are the earliest chromosomal changes detected in prostate cancer, as they can be found already in high-grade PIN lesions.[7] From the 8p region, at least two minimally deleted regions, 8p21 and 8p22, have been identified, suggesting that several tumor suppressor genes may be located at 8p. The strongest candidate target gene for the loss of 8p is a homeobox gene *NKX3.1*, located at 8p21,[8] but no mutations in the remaining allele of the *NKX3.1* have been found.[9] However, the *NKX3.1* knock-out mouse models have demonstrated that even a loss of one allele can lead to hyperplasia and PIN-like lesions in the mouse prostate.[10,11] Thus, *NKX3.1* could be a target of haploinsufficiency. For the 13q loss, several target genes have been suggested, such as *RB1*, *BRCA2*, and *EDNRB*. However, no strong evidence in support of any of these genes exists.

Losses of 16q have been detected in 20% of early and 40% to 50% of metastatic and hormone-refractory prostate carcinomas in CGH analyses.[5,12,13] Perhaps the most intensively studied putative target gene for the 16q loss is E-cadherin (*CDH1*), located at 16q22. E-cadherin is a Ca^{2+}-dependent homotypic cell–cell adhesion molecule. Decreased expression of E-cadherin has been reported especially in poorly differentiated and aggressive tumors.[14,15] Surprisingly, prostate cancer metastases seem to express high levels of E-cadherin.[16] According to various LOH studies, the common minimally deleted region appears to be at 16q23-q24, excluding the E-cadherin locus at 16q22.[7] In addition, no mutations in the E-cadherin gene have been identified in prostate cancer.[17,18]

CHROMOSOMAL ALTERATIONS ASSOCIATED WITH THE PROGRESSION OF PROSTATE CANCER

Losses of 10q and 17p as well as gains of 7p/q, 8q, and Xq seem to be especially common in late-stage prostate cancer. Deletions at 10q have been found in up to 50% of hormone-refractory and metastatic prostate tumors.[5,12,13] According to CGH studies, the minimal regions of the 10q deletions are at 10cen-q21 and at 10q26,[13] whereas the highest rate of LOH has been reported at the region 10q23-q24.[19,20] As we will discuss later in the chapter, PTEN is likely to be one of the target genes for 10q loss.

Gain of 8q is the most common chromosomal alteration detected in hormone-refractory and metastatic prostate carcinomas by CGH, with a frequency of approximately 70% to 90% in advanced tumors.[5,12,13] Gain of 8q has been shown to be associated with an aggressive phenotype and poor prognosis of prostate cancer.[21,22] Although the gain usually covers the entire long arm of chromosome 8, two independently amplified subregions, 8q21 and 8q23-q24, have been identified (Figure 23.2).[12,13] Probably the most intensively studied putative target gene for the 8q gain is the well characterized oncogene MYC, located at 8q24. Recently, it was shown that transgenic mice expressing human MYC in prostate develop PIN lesions as well as invasive adenocarcinomas.[23] In humans, MYC has been shown to be amplified in prostate carcinomas,[24,25] and its increased copy number seems to be associated with poor prognosis in prostate cancer.[26] Even though overexpression of MYC, determined by

immunohistochemistry, has been reported in prostate cancer,[24] in our recent study no difference in MYC expression, detected by quantitative real-time polymerase chain reaction (RT-PCR), was found between benign prostatic hyperplasia (BPH) and prostate carcinoma samples (Figure 23.3).[27] In addition, MYC expression in prostate and breast cancer cell lines was not associated with the copy number of the MYC gene, suggesting that MYC is probably not a common target gene of the 8q gain.

By using suppression subtraction and cDNA microarray hybridization (and a combination of these), we have recently identified three putative target genes for the 8q23-24 gain: EIF3S3, KIAA0196, and RAD21.[25,28] These genes seem to be amplified in about 30% of hormone-refractory prostate carcinomas (see Figure 23.2). Amplification of EIF3S3 is also associated with high Gleason score and advanced clinical stage of the disease.[29] According to the quantitative RT-PCR analyses, EIF3S3, KIAA0196, and RAD21 are also overexpressed in prostate carcinomas compared with BPH tumors (see Figure 23.3).[27,28]

The EIF3S3 gene encodes for a p40 subunit of eukaryotic translation initiation factor 3 (eIF3), which plays a key role in the translation initiation pathway by binding to 40S ribosomal subunits in the absence of other translational components and helps to maintain the 40S and 60S subunits in a dissociated state.[30] However, the function of the p40 subunit itself is unknown. RAD21 (also known as hr21, Scc1, Mcd1, NXP1, or KIAA0078), on the other hand, is a human ortholog of the Schizosaccharomyces pombe RAD21. It is a component of the cohesin complex that holds sister chromatids together during mitosis.[31,32] It has also been reported that a caspase-mediated cleavage of the RAD21 protein occurs during apoptosis, causing amplification of the proapoptotic death signal.[33,34] The function of KIAA0196 is unknown, and it shows no homologies to known genes.

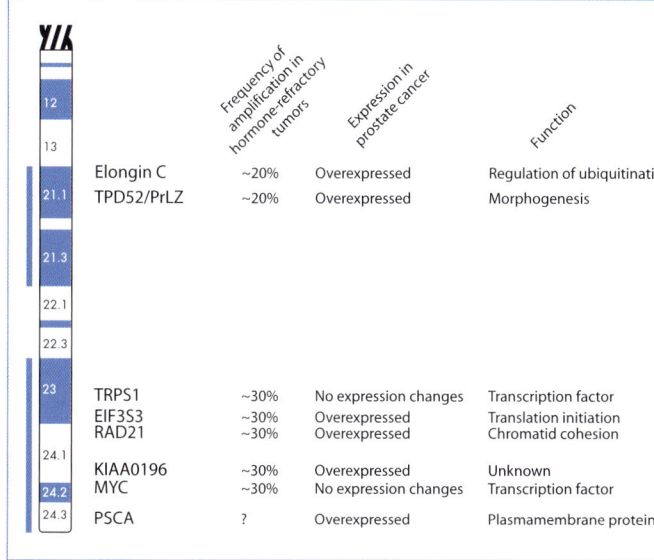

	Frequency of amplification in hormone-refractory tumors	Expression in prostate cancer	Function
Elongin C	~20%	Overexpressed	Regulation of ubiquitination
TPD52/PrLZ	~20%	Overexpressed	Morphogenesis
TRPS1	~30%	No expression changes	Transcription factor
EIF3S3	~30%	Overexpressed	Translation initiation
RAD21	~30%	Overexpressed	Chromatid cohesion
KIAA0196	~30%	Overexpressed	Unknown
MYC	~30%	No expression changes	Transcription factor
PSCA	?	Overexpressed	Plasmamembrane protein

Fig. 23.2
Gain of the long arm of chromosome 8 (8q) is one of the most common chromosomal aberrations in advanced-stage prostate cancer. According to comparative genomic hybridization (CGH) analyses, two minimal regions of gains can be identified: 8q21 and 8q23-q24. The suggested target genes for these gains are shown, as well as data on amplification frequency and expression.[25,27–29,40,41]

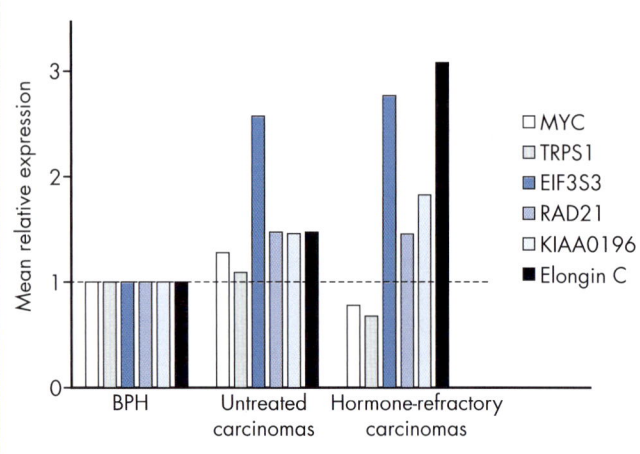

Fig. 23.3

Relative expression of putative target genes for 8q gain according to quantitative RT-PCR.[27,28] The values are normalized against the expression in benign prostate hyperplasia (BPH). *EIF3S3* and *RAD21* genes are overexpressed in both untreated and hormone-refractory tumors, whereas the gene coding for Elongin C and *KIAA0196* are overexpressed, especially in hormone-refractory tumors. *TRPS1* and *MYC* are not overexpressed in prostate cancer.

Other target genes suggested for the 8q23-24 amplification are, for example, the prostate stem cell antigen gene (*PSCA*) and *TRPS1/GC79*.[35,36] *PSCA* was identified, by using the representational difference analysis (RDA) method, in search for genes that are upregulated during prostate cancer progression.[35] Expression of the PSCA protein has been reported to correlate with prostate tumor stage and grade and androgen independence,[37] but studies on the mRNA level have not confirmed this correlation.[38] *TRPS1* was first discovered by differential display as a transcript showing higher expression in androgen-dependent than in androgen-independent prostate cell line.[39] We have found amplifications of the *TRPS1* gene in about one third of hormone-refractory prostate carcinomas, but we did not detect any differences in *TRPS1* expression between BPH and prostate carcinoma samples in quantitative RT-PCR analysis (see Figure 23.3).[27]

For the minimal amplification region at 8q21, only few candidate target genes have been suggested. Using the cDNA microarray technique, we and others have detected two overexpressed genes from this region: Elongin C (*TCEB1*) and *PrLZ/TPD52*.[40,41] Both genes have been found to be amplified in prostate carcinomas, especially in metastatic and hormone-refractory tumors.[40-42] In addition, the PrLZ protein has been shown to be overexpressed in clinical prostate carcinomas.[41,42] However, elevated expression of PrLZ has been detected also in PIN lesions,[41,42] suggesting that increased expression of PrLZ is an early event in the development of prostate cancer and may thus not be related to 8q gain.[41] *TCEB1*, on the other hand, is amplified in about 20% of hormone-refractory prostate carcinomas, but not in early cancer .[40] In addition, the expression of Elongin C is significantly higher in hormone-refractory than untreated carcinoma (see Figure 23.3). Elongin C seems to have at least two functions. First, it is a subunit of the Elongin complex (SIII), containing also subunits A and B, that activates transcription performed by RNA polymerase II. Binding of Elongin A to the subunits B and C reactivates the RNA polymerase, preventing pausing of the transcription.[43]

For tumorigenesis, the second function of Elongin C may be more important; this relates to the degradation of hypoxia-inducible factor 1α (HIF1α). A complex formed by Elongin B and C, Cul2, Rbx1, as well as von Hippel-Lindau (VHL) proteins targets other proteins, such as HIF1α for ubiquitinylation-mediated degradation. Mutations in VHL, which are often found in renal cancer, abrogate the binding of Elongin C to VHL,[44-47] preventing the ubiquitination and degradation of HIF1α. This in turn results in increased expression of their target-genes, such as the vascular endothelial growth factor (VEGF), platelet-derived growth factor β-chain (PDGFβ), and transforming growth factor-α (TGFα), thus promoting tumor growth.[47] The role of Elongin C in the interaction with VHL seems to be protective against tumorigenesis. Thus, the functional significance of the overexpression and amplification of the gene in prostate cancer remains unclear. Since it has been shown that the Elongin C protein is capable of forming complexes with several proteins,[48] it is possible that it has other, unidentified functions that could promote tumorigenesis.

Gain at both arms of the chromosome 7 has frequently been detected in prostate cancer in CGH analyses.[5,49] In FISH analysis, at least one extra copy of the entire chromosome 7 is often observed in prostate carcinoma samples,[50-54] and aneusomy of chromosome 7 has been shown to be associated with advanced tumor stage and poor prognosis of prostate cancer.[21,50,52,54] One of the target genes suggested is a receptor tyrosine kinase *MET*, a well-known oncogene. Overexpression of the MET protein and mRNA has been shown in high-grade tumors and metastases, but in some studies *MET* expression has been detected also in a high number of PIN lesions,[55-58] in which additional copies of chromosome 7 are infrequent.

Another candidate target gene for the gain of chromosome 7 has been the caveolin gene (*CAV1*). Positive immunostaining of the CAV1 protein has been shown to be associated with poor prognosis of prostate cancer, and functional studies have demonstrated the oncogenic potential of the *CAV1* gene in prostate cancer cells.[59-62] Paradoxically, other researchers have reported results indicating that *CAV1* displays tumor suppressive activities, and that the expression of *CAV1* is decreased in human malignancies.[63-67] Therefore, it is unclear whether *CAV1* is acting like an oncogene or like a tumor suppressor gene. It is also possible that the specific function of *CAV1* is highly cell- and context-dependent, which is why further studies with prostate cancer cells and samples are required to elucidate its role in the progression of prostate cancer. Of note, no high-level amplifications of *CAV1* have been found in prostate cancer.[13]

A third putative target gene for gain of chromosome 7 is the enhancer of zeste homolog 2 (*EZH2*). It is a component of the polycomb repressive complex 2 (PRC2), which is required for silencing of the *HOX* genes during embryogenesis. Recent studies have shown that *EZH2* is highly expressed in metastatic prostate cancer, and the increased expression of *EZH2* in primary prostate carcinomas is associated with poor prognosis and recurrence of the disease.[68-70] Inhibition of the *EZH2* expression has been shown to decrease the proliferation rate of prostate cancer as well as other cancer cells,[68,71] whereas its ectopic expression gives a growth advantage to cells,[71] demonstrating the oncogenic potential of *EZH2*. Amplifications of the *EZH2* locus at the chromosomal region 7q35 have been detected in various cancer types.[71] Also, one prostate cancer xenograft has been found to contain *EZH2* gene amplification (Saramäki OR and Visakorpi T, unpublished work), but the frequency of the *EZH2* amplification in prostate cancer is not known. Based on the CGH data it is probably low.

Gain of chromosome X has been detected by CGH in over 50% of hormone-refractory prostate cancers, whereas in primary tumors it is not commonly found.[5] At the region Xq12-q13, even high-level amplifications have been detected.[5] The gene for the androgen receptor (AR) is located at this region, and it is the most likely target gene for the Xq gain. The significance of AR and the AR signaling pathway in the progression of prostate cancer is discussed in more detail in the following chapters.

GENES INVOLVED IN THE PROGRESSION OF PROSTATE CANCER

TP53

The tumor suppressor gene *TP53* is the most commonly mutated gene in human cancers. It codes for the tumor protein p53, which is a key regulator of the cell cycle, controlling the transition from the G1 phase to the S phase. Under conditions conducive to DNA damage,

TP53 can either induce apoptosis or arrest the cell cycle for DNA repair.[72] Mutated p53 has a prolonged half-life, leading to nuclear accumulation of the abnormal protein. Because of the nuclear accumulation, the presence of the *TP53* mutation can be indirectly detected by immunohistochemistry. The frequency of *TP53* mutations in prostate cancer has been studied using both the immunohistochemical detection of the protein and sequencing of the gene. According to most studies, mutations in *TP53* are rare indeed in early, localized prostate cancer, whereas in advanced (metastatic and/or hormone-refractory) prostate carcinomas they are found in approximately 20% to 40% of cases.[73-75] Nuclear accumulation of the p53 has also been shown to be associated with poor prognosis.[74]

PTEN

Deletions and mutations of *PTEN* have been observed in a high proportion of advanced prostate carcinomas.[76-79] The *PTEN* gene encodes a dual specificity phosphatase that regulates crucial signal transduction pathways. It mainly functions as a lipid phosphatase and targets phosphatidylinositol 3,4,5-trisphosphate (PIP3).[78] By dephosphorylating PIP3, PTEN downregulates the AKT/PKB signaling pathway that promotes cell survival and inhibits apoptosis. Since the frequency of LOH at the *PTEN* locus has been reported to be higher than the rate of mutations,[80] it has been suggested that *PTEN* could be targeted by haploinsufficiency. Indeed, a heterozygous PTEN$^{+/-}$ TRAMP mouse model demonstrates that the loss of one allele of *PTEN* results in an increased rate of prostate cancer progression.[81] Mouse models also suggest a gene dosage dependent cooperation between *NKX3.1* and *PTEN*.[82] Interestingly, it was recently shown that the downstream effector of *PTEN*, AKT, is commonly phosphorylated in prostate cancer, and the phosphorylation is associated with poor prognosis.[83] One mechanism for the AKT phosphorylation is most likely the loss of *PTEN* function. *PTEN* is also involved in downregulation of the mTOR pathway, which can be inhibited also by a drug called rapamycin. It has been shown that prostate cancer xenografts with inactive *PTEN* are more sensitive to rapamycin than xenografts with wild-type *PTEN*.[84]

ANDROGEN RECEPTOR GENE

Due to the androgen-dependence of the growth of prostate cancer, it is natural that prostate carcinomas have been screened for AR mutations in many studies. The vast majority of the studies have indicated that AR mutations are rare in untreated prostate cancers.[85] In addition, mutations are infrequently found in tumors treated by castration alone.[86] However, AR mutations have been detected in approximately 10% to 20% of patients treated with antiandrogens, such as flutamide and bicalutamide.[87-88] It has also been demonstrated that at least some of these mutations alter the ligand specificity of the AR, and that the receptor may paradoxically be activated by the antiandrogens.[88-89]

We originally demonstrated that the AR gene is amplified in 30% of hormone-refractory prostate carcinomas from patients treated with androgen withdrawal.[90] This finding has subsequently been confirmed by several studies.[91] No amplifications have been found in untreated tumors suggesting that androgen withdrawal selected the gene amplification.[92] This suggests that tumors with AR gene amplification may be androgen hypersensitive instead of independent. Indeed, we have also shown that patients with AR gene amplification respond better to second-line maximal androgen blockade than patients without the amplification.[92] The AR gene amplification leads to the overexpression of the gene as expected. However, somewhat surprisingly, we and others have now shown that almost all hormone-refractory prostate carcinomas express high levels of AR.[93-94] Mechanisms for AR overexpression in tumors not containing the gene amplification remain unknown. However, in their recent work, Chen et al[95] showed that even a modest overexpression of AR is capable of converting androgen-dependent growth of prostate cancer cells into independent growth. Expression of AR also transformed an AR antagonist to an agonist. Thus, it seems that overexpression of AR is truly a common mechanism for androgen-independence of prostate cancer.

CONCLUSION

Studies of novel drugs, such as trastuzumab, imatinib, and gefitinib, have clearly demonstrated that tumors containing alterations in genes encoding the targets of these drugs are susceptible to these compounds.[96-99] Thus, it seems that genetic alterations may pinpoint potential therapeutic targets for antineoplastic agents. Therefore, the identification of genetic changes in prostate cancer is truly important. Androgen receptor signaling clearly is one pathway that should be considered as a potential therapeutic target. The currently available hormonal therapies, including antiandrogens, are just not efficient enough in inhibiting AR-transactivation. Clearly novel drugs targeting AR in prostate cancer tissue should be developed.

In addition, we still need to find other genes that are commonly altered in this disease. It is almost amazing how few recurrent mutations have been found in prostate cancer. It may be that it is not mutations but epigenetic changes, haploinsufficiency, or gene dosage (i.e., aneuploidy) that are the main forms of genetic aberrations in prostate cancer. The functional significance of these mechanisms compared with mutations are, however, more difficult to evaluate. Indeed, more studies are required.

REFERENCES

1. DeMarzo AM, Nelson WG, Isaacs WB, et al. Pathological and molecular aspects of prostate cancer. Lancet 2003;361:955–964.
2. Sheldon CA, Williams RD, Fraley EE. Incidental carcinoma of the prostate: a review of the literature and critical reappraisal of classification. J Urol 1980;124:626–631.
3. Selman SH. "Latent" carcinoma of the prostate: a medical misnomer? Urology 2000;56:708–711.
4. Arnold JT, Isaacs JT. Mechanisms involved in the progression of androgen-independent prostate cancers: it is not only the cancer cell's fault. Endocr Relat Cancer 2002;9:61–73.
5. Visakorpi T, Kallioniemi AH, Syvänen AC, et al. Genetic changes in primary and recurrent prostate cancer by comparative genomic hybridization. Cancer Res 1995;55:342–347.
6. Nupponen NN, Visakorpi T. Molecular cytogenetics of prostate cancer. Microsc Res Tech 2000;51:456–463.
7. Dong JT. Chromosomal deletions and tumor suppressor genes in prostate cancer. Cancer Metastasis Rev 2001;20:173–193.
8. He WW, Sciavolino PJ, Wing J, et al. A novel human prostate-specific, androgen-regulated homeobox gene (NKX3.1) that maps to 8p21, a region frequently deleted in prostate cancer. Genomics 1997;43:69–77.
9. Voeller HJ, Augustus M, Madike V, et al. Coding region of NKX3.1, a prostate-specific homeobox gene on 8p21, is not mutated in human prostate cancers. Cancer Res 1997;57:4455–4459.
10. Abdulkadir SA, Magee JA, Peters TJ, et al. Conditional loss of Nkx3.1 in adult mice induces prostatic intraepithelial neoplasia. Mol Cell Biol 2002;22:1495–1503.
11. Bhatia-Gaur R, Donjacour AA, Sciavolino PJ, et al. Roles for Nkx3.1 in prostate development and cancer. Genes Dev 1999;13:966–977.
12. Cher ML, Bova GS, Moore DH, et al. Genetic alterations in untreated metastases and androgen-independent prostate cancer detected by comparative genomic hybridization and allelotyping. Cancer Res 1996;56:3091–3102.
13. Nupponen NN, Kakkola L, Koivisto P, et al. Genetic alterations in hormone-refractory recurrent prostate carcinomas. Am J Pathol 1998;153:141–148.
14. Umbas R, Schalken JA, Aalders TW, et al. Expression of the cellular adhesion molecule E-cadherin is reduced or absent in high-grade prostate cancer. Cancer Res 1992;52:5104–5109.
15. Umbas R, Isaacs WB, Bringuier PP, et al. Decreased E-cadherin expression is associated with poor prognosis in patients with prostate cancer. Cancer Res 1994;54:3929–3933.
16. Rubin MA, Mucci NR, Figurski J, et al. E-cadherin expression in prostate cancer: a broad survey using high-density tissue microarray technology. Hum Pathol 2001;32:690–697.
17. Suzuki H, Komiya A, Emi M, et al. Three distinct commonly deleted regions of chromosome arm 16q in human primary and metastatic prostate cancers. Genes Chromosomes Cancer 1996;17:225–233.
18. Li C, Berx G, Larsson C, et al. Distinct deleted regions on chromosome segment 16q23-24 associated with metastases in prostate cancer. Genes Chromosomes Cancer 1999; 24:175–182.
19. Gray IC, Phillips SM, Lee SJ, et al. Loss of the chromosomal region 10q23-25 in prostate cancer. Cancer Res 1995;55:4800–4803.
20. Lacombe L, Orlow I, Reuter VE, et al. Microsatellite instability and deletion analysis of chromosome 10 in human prostate cancer. Int J Cancer 1996;69:110–113.
21. Alers JC, Rochat J, Krijtenburg PJ, et al. Identification of genetic markers for prostatic cancer progression. Lab Invest 2000;80:931–942.
22. van Dekken H, Alers JC, Damen IA, et al. Genetic evaluation of localized prostate cancer in a cohort of forty patients: gain of distal 8q discriminates between progressors and nonprogressors. Lab Invest 2003;83:789–796.
23. Ellwood-Yen K, Graeber TG, Wongvipat J, et al. Myc-driven murine prostate cancer shares molecular features with human prostate tumors. Cancer Cell 2003;4:223–238.

24. Jenkins RB, Qian J, Lieber MM, et al. Detection of c-myc oncogene amplification and chromosomal anomalies in metastatic prostatic carcinoma by fluorescence in situ hybridization. Cancer Res 1997;57:524–531.

25. Nupponen NN, Porkka K, Kakkola L, et al. Amplification and overexpression of p40 subunit of eukaryotic translation initiation factor 3 in breast and prostate cancer. Am J Pathol 1999;154:1777–1783.

26. Sato K, Qian J, Slezak JM, et al. Clinical significance of alterations of chromosome 8 in high-grade, advanced, nonmetastatic prostate carcinoma. J Natl Cancer Inst 1999;91:1574–1580.

27. Savinainen KJ, Linja MJ, Saramaki OR, et al. Expression and copy number analysis of TRPS1, EIF3S3 and MYC genes in breast and prostate cancer. Br J Cancer 2004;90:1041–1046.

28. Porkka KP, Tammela TL, Vessella RL, et al. RAD21 and KIAA0196 at 8q24 are amplified and overexpressed in prostate cancer. Genes Chromosomes Cancer 2004;39:1–10.

29. Saramäki O, Willi N, Bratt O, et al. Amplification of EIF3S3 gene is associated with advanced stage in prostate cancer. Am J Pathol 2001;159:2089–2094.

30. Asano K, Vornlocher HP, Richter-Cook NJ, et al. Structure of cDNAs encoding human eukaryotic initiation factor 3 subunits. Possible roles in RNA binding and macromolecular assembly. J Biol Chem 1997;272:27042–27052.

31. Nasmyth K, Peters JM, Uhlmann F. Splitting the chromosome: cutting the ties that bind sister chromatids. Science 2000;288:1379–1385.

32. Hirano T. Chromosome cohesion, condensation, and separation. Annu Rev Biochem 2000;69:115–144.

33. Chen F, Kamradt M, Mulcahy M, et al. Caspase proteolysis of the cohesin component RAD21 promotes apoptosis. J Biol Chem 2002;277:16775–16781.

34. Pati D, Zhang N, Plon SE. Linking sister chromatid cohesion and apoptosis: role of Rad21. Mol Cell Biol 2002;22:8267–8277.

35. Reiter RE, Gu Z, Watabe T, et al. Prostate stem cell antigen: a cell surface marker overexpressed in prostate cancer. Proc Natl Acad Sci USA 1998; 95:1735–1740.

36. Chang GT, Steenbeek M, Schippers E, et al. Characterization of a zinc-finger protein and its association with apoptosis in prostate cancer cells. J Natl Cancer Inst 2000;92:1414–1421.

37. Gu Z, Thomas G, Yamashiro J, et al. Prostate stem cell antigen (PSCA) expression increases with high gleason score, advanced stage and bone metastasis in prostate cancer. Oncogene 2000;19:1288–1296.

38. Ross S, Spencer SD, Holcomb I, et al. Prostate stem cell antigen as therapy target: tissue expression and in vivo efficacy of an immunoconjugate. Cancer Res 2002;62:2546–2553.

39. Chang GT, Blok LJ, Steenbeek M, et al. Differentially expressed genes in androgen-dependent and -independent prostate carcinomas. Cancer Res 1997;57:4075–4081.

40. Porkka K, Saramaki O, Tanner M, et al. Amplification and overexpression of Elongin C gene discovered in prostate cancer by cDNA microarrays. Lab Invest 2002;82:629–637.

41. Wang R, Xu J, Saramaki O, et al. PrLZ, a novel prostate-specific and androgen-responsive gene of the TPD52 family, amplified in chromosome 8q21.1 and overexpressed in human prostate cancer. Cancer Res 2004;64:1589–1594.

42. Rubin MA, Varambally S, Beroukhim R, et al. Overexpression, amplification, and androgen regulation of TPD52 in prostate cancer. Cancer Res 2004;64:3814–3822.

43. Aso T, Lane WS, Conaway JW, et al. Elongin (SIII): a multisubunit regulator of elongation by RNA polymerase II. Science 1995;269:1439–1443.

44. Duan DR, Pause A, Burgess WH, et al. Inhibition of transcription elongation by the VHL tumor suppressor protein. Science 1995;269:1402–1406.

45. Kibel A, Iliopoulos O, DeCaprio JA, et al. Binding of the von Hippel-Lindau tumor suppressor protein to Elongin B and C. Science 1995;269:1444–1446.

46. Stebbins CE, Kaelin WG Jr, Pavletich NP. Structure of the VHL-ElonginC-ElonginB complex: implications for VHL tumor suppressor function. Science 1999;284:455–461.

47. Kaelin WG Jr. Molecular basis of the VHL hereditary cancer syndrome. Nat Rev Cancer 2002;2:673–682.

48. Kamura T, Sato S, Haque D, et al. The Elongin BC complex interacts with the conserved SOCS-box motif present in members of the SOCS, ras, WD-40 repeat, and ankyrin repeat families. Genes Dev 1998;12:3872–3881.

49. Alers JC, Krijtenburg PJ, Vis AN, et al. Molecular cytogenetic analysis of prostatic adenocarcinomas from screening studies: early cancers may contain aggressive genetic features. Am J Pathol 2001;158:399–406.

50. Alcaraz A, Takahashi S, Brown JA, et al. Aneuploidy and aneusomy of chromosome 7 detected by fluorescence in situ hybridization are markers of poor prognosis in prostate cancer. Cancer Res 1994;54:3998–4002.

51. Visakorpi T, Hyytinen E, Kallioniemi A, et al. Sensitive detection of chromosome copy number aberrations in prostate cancer by fluorescence in situ hybridization. Am J Pathol 1994;145:624–630.

52. Bandyk MG, Zhao L, Troncoso P, et al. Trisomy 7: a potential cytogenetic marker of human prostate cancer progression. Genes Chromosomes Cancer 1994;9:19–27.

53. Wang RY, Troncoso P, Palmer JL, et al. Trisomy 7 by dual-color fluorescence in situ hybridization: a potential biological marker for prostate cancer progression. Clin Cancer Res 1996;2:1553–1558.

54. Cui J, Deubler DA, Rohr LR, et al. Chromosome 7 abnormalities in prostate cancer detected by dual-color fluorescence in situ hybridization. Cancer Genet Cytogenet 1998;107:51–60.

55. Pisters LL, Troncoso P, Zhau HE, et al. c-met proto-oncogene expression in benign and malignant human prostate tissues. J Urol 1995;154:293–298.

56. Humphrey PA, Zhu X, Zarnegar R, et al. Hepatocyte growth factor and its receptor (c-MET) in prostatic carcinoma. Am J Pathol 1995;147:386–396.

57. Watanabe M, Fukutome K, Kato H, et al. Progression-linked overexpression of c-Met in prostatic intraepithelial neoplasia and latent as well as clinical prostate cancers. Cancer Lett 1999;141:173–178.

58. Knudsen BS, Gmyrek GA, Inra J, et al. High expression of the Met receptor in prostate cancer metastasis to bone. Urology 2002;60:1113–1117.

59. Yang G, Truong LD, Wheeler TM, et al. Caveolin-1 expression in clinically confined human prostate cancer: a novel prognostic marker. Cancer Res 1999;59:5719–5723.

60. Nasu Y, Timme TL, Yang G, et al. Suppression of caveolin expression induces androgen sensitivity in metastatic androgen-insensitive mouse prostate cancer cells. Nat Med 1998;4:1062–1064.

61. Tahir SA, Yang G, Ebara S, et al. Secreted caveolin-1 stimulates cell survival/clonal growth and contributes to metastasis in androgen-insensitive prostate cancer. Cancer Res 2001;61:3882–3885.

62. Li L, Yang G, Ebara S, et al. Caveolin-1 mediates testosterone-stimulated survival/clonal growth and promotes metastatic activities in prostate cancer cells. Cancer Res 2001;61:4386–4392.

63. Galbiati F, Volonte D, Engelman JA, et al. Targeted downregulation of caveolin-1 is sufficient to drive cell transformation and hyperactivate the p42/44 MAP kinase cascade. EMBO J 1998;17:6633–6648.

64. Zhang W, Razani B, Altschuler Y, et al. Caveolin-1 inhibits epidermal growth factor-stimulated lamellipod extension and cell migration in metastatic mammary adenocarcinoma cells (MTLn3). Transformation suppressor effects of adenovirus-mediated gene delivery of caveolin-1. J Biol Chem 2000;275:20717–20725.

65. Bender FC, Reymond MA, Bron C, et al. Caveolin-1 levels are down-regulated in human colon tumors, and ectopic expression of caveolin-1 in colon carcinoma cell lines reduces cell tumorigenicity. Cancer Res 2000;60:5870–5878.

66. Wiechen K, Diatchenko L, Agoulnik A, et al. Caveolin-1 is down-regulated in human ovarian carcinoma and acts as a candidate tumor suppressor gene. Am J Pathol 2001;159:1635–1643.

67. Wiechen K, Sers C, Agoulnik A, et al. Down-regulation of caveolin-1, a candidate tumor suppressor gene, in sarcomas. Am J Pathol 2001;158:833–839.

68. Varambally S, Dhanasekaran SM, Zhou M, et al. The polycomb group protein EZH2 is involved in progression of prostate cancer. Nature 2002;419:624–629.

69. Rhodes DR, Sanda MG, Otte AP, et al. Multiplex biomarker approach for determining risk of prostate-specific antigen-defined recurrence of prostate cancer. J Natl Cancer Inst 2003;95:661–668.

70. Foster CS, Falconer A, Dodson AR, et al. Transcription factor E2F3 overexpressed in prostate cancer independently predicts clinical outcome. Oncogene 2004;23:5871–5879.

71. Bracken AP, Pasini D, Capra M, et al. EZH2 is downstream of the pRB-E2F pathway, essential for proliferation and amplified in cancer. EMBO J 2003;22:5323–5335.

72. Morris SM. A role for p53 in the frequency and mechanism of mutation. Mutat Res 2002;511:45–62.

73. Bookstein R, MacGrogan D, Hilsenbeck SG, et al. p53 is mutated in a subset of advanced-stage prostate cancers. Cancer Res 1993;53:3369–3373.

74. Visakorpi T, Kallioniemi OP, Heikkinen A, et al. Small subgroup of aggressive, highly proliferative prostatic carcinomas defined by p53 accumulation. J Natl Cancer Inst 1992;84:883–887.

75. Navone NM, Troncoso P, Pisters LL, et al. p53 protein accumulation and gene mutation in the progression of human prostate carcinoma. J Natl Cancer Inst 1993;85:1657–1669.

76. Cairns P, Okami K, Halachmi S, et al. Frequent inactivation of PTEN/MMAC1 in primary prostate cancer. Cancer Res 1997;57:4997–5000.

77. Gray IC, Stewart LM, Phillips SM, et al. Mutation and expression analysis of the putative prostate tumour-suppressor gene PTEN. Br J Cancer 1998;78:1296–1300.

78. McMenamin ME, Soung P, Perera S, et al. Loss of PTEN expression in paraffin-embedded primary prostate cancer correlates with high Gleason score and advanced stage. Cancer Res 1999;59:4291–4296.

79. Maehama T, Dixon JE. The tumor suppressor, PTEN/MMAC1, dephosphorylates the lipid second messenger, phosphatidylinositol 3,4,5-trisphosphate. J Biol Chem 1998;273:13375–13378.

80. Fernandez M, Eng C. The expanding role of PTEN in neoplasia: a molecule for all seasons? Clin Cancer Res 2002;8:1695–1698.

81. Kwabi-Addo B, Giri D, Schmidt K, et al. Haploinsufficiency of the Pten tumor suppressor gene promotes prostate cancer progression. Proc Natl Acad Sci USA 2001;98:11563–11568.

82. Kim MJ, Cardiff RD, Desai N, et al. Cooperativity of Nkx3.1 and Pten loss of function in a mouse model of prostate carcinogenesis. Proc Natl Acad Sci USA 2002;99:2884–2889.

83. Ayala G, Thompson T, Yang G, et al. High levels of phosphorylated form of Akt-1 in prostate cancer and non-neoplastic prostate tissues are strong predictors of biochemical recurrence. Clin Cancer Res 2004;10:6572–6578.

84. Neshat MS, Mellinghoff IK, Tran C, et al. Enhanced sensitivity of PTEN-deficient tumors to inhibition of FRAP/mTOR. Proc Natl Acad Sci USA 2001;98:10314–10319.

85. Culig Z, Klocker H, Bartsch G, et al. Androgen receptor mutations in carcinoma of the prostate: significance for endocrine therapy. Am J Pharmacogenomics 2001;1:241–249.

86. Wallen MJ, Linja M, Kaartinen K, et al. Androgen receptor gene mutations in hormone-refractory prostate cancer. J Pathol 1999;189:559–563.

87. Taplin ME, Bubley GJ, Shuster TD, et al. Mutation of the androgen-receptor gene in metastatic androgen-independent prostate cancer. N Engl J Med 1995;332:1393–1398.

88. Haapala K, Hyytinen ER, Roiha M, et al. Androgen receptor alterations in prostate cancer relapsed during a combined androgen blockade by orchiectomy and bicalutamide. Lab Invest 2001;81:1647–1651.

89. Hara T, Miyazaki J, Araki H, et al. Novel mutations of androgen receptor: a possible mechanism of bicalutamide withdrawal syndrome. Cancer Res 2003;63:149–153.

90. Visakorpi T, Hyytinen E, Koivisto P, et al. In vivo amplification of the androgen receptor gene and progression of human prostate cancer. Nat Genet 1995;9:401–406.

91. Elo JP, Visakorpi T. Molecular genetics of prostate cancer. Ann Med 2001;33:130–141.

92. Palmberg C, Koivisto P, Kakkola L, et al. Androgen receptor gene amplification at the time of primary progression predicts response to combined androgen blockade as a second-line therapy in advanced prostate cancer. J Urology 2000; 164:1992–1995.

93. Linja MJ, Savinainen KJ, Saramäki OR, et al. Amplification and overexpression of androgen receptor gene in hormone-refractory prostate cancer. Cancer Res 2001;61:3550–3555.

94. Latil A, Bieche I, Vidaud D, et al. Evaluation of androgen, estrogen (ER alpha and ER beta), and progesterone receptor expression in human prostate cancer by real-time quantitative reverse transcription-polymerase chain reaction assays. Cancer Res 2001;61:1919–1926.

95. Chen CD, Welsbie DS, Tran C, et al. Molecular determinants of resistance to antiandrogen therapy. Nat Med 2004;10:33–39.

96. Druker BJ, Talpaz M, Resta DJ, et al. Efficacy and safety of a specific inhibitor of the BCR-ABL tyrosine kinase in chronic myeloid leukemia. N Engl J Med 2001;344:1031–1037.

97. Slamon DJ, Leyland-Jones B, Shak S, et al. Use of chemotherapy plus a monoclonal antibody against HER2 for metastatic breast cancer that overexpresses HER2. N Engl J Med 2001;344:783–792.

98. Lynch TJ, Bell DW, Sordella R, et al. Activating mutations in the epidermal growth factor receptor underlying responsiveness of non-small-cell lung cancer to gefitinib. N Engl J Med 2004;350:2129–2139.

99. Paez JG, Janne PA, Lee JC, et al. EGFR mutations in lung cancer: correlation with clinical response to gefitinib therapy Science 2004;304:1497–1500.

Inherited susceptibility for prostate cancer—family and case-control studies

Jianfeng Xu, Sarah Linström, Henrik Grönberg, William B Isaacs

INTRODUCTION

The clustering of prostate cancer in families was noted by researchers as early as the mid 1950s.[1] Over 40 years ago, Woolf reported that deaths due to prostate cancer were three times higher among the fathers and brothers of men dying from prostate cancer than among deceased relatives of men dying from other causes.[2] Since then, numerous studies have consistently documented the increased risk of prostate cancer associated with family history. Indeed, along with age and race, family history is among the most consistent prostate cancer risk factors identified to date. This chapter will provide an overview of efforts to understand and characterize the genetic mechanisms underlying inherited susceptibility for prostate cancer.

CANCER GENETICS IN 2005

The late 20th century witnessed a revolution in our ability to understand mechanisms of carcinogenesis at the molecular level. The work of Vogelstein, Kinzler, and others firmly implanted the concept of cancer as a genetic disease—a process propelled by genetic instability and clonal selection—as a guiding principle.[3] Advances in technology, bioinformatics, and intellectual concepts provided the basis for classifying cancer genes as tumor suppressors acting to prevent cancer formation, and oncogenes, which provided positive forces for carcinogenesis. These genes could be inactivated or activated respectively, either by somatic alterations as is the case in sporadic disease, or at the germline level resulting in an inherited predisposition for cancer, which can manifest as familial clusters. This paradigm was evoked repeatedly as cancer genes such as *APC* and *VHL* were discovered and characterized through studies of specific cancer-prone families, providing an elegant foundation for both inherited and non-inheritited forms of colorectal and renal cell carcinoma, respectively.[3,4] While the identification of these "major" genes provided extensive insight into the genetic mechanisms underlying these two common cancers, the frequencies of deleterious, mutated forms of these genes are quite low in the general population, and they can not account for most of the cancer burden in the population; nor, for that matter, for the majority of familial clustering of these cancers. The underlying suspicion, based upon twin studies among others (see below), was that many common cancers still have an important genetic component, but rather than being caused by a single, major gene, some other more complex combination of genetic effects may be involved. With the sequencing of the human genome came a better appreciation of the variability that is common in the human population; that is, the human genome sequence contains many differences between individuals. While most of these differences are subtle—for example, single base substitutions, or SNPs (single nucleotide polymorphisms)—the possibility was proposed that these common variants in DNA sequence may play an important role in determining, or at least modifying, an individual's risk of developing common diseases such as cancer and diabetes. Testing this "common variant/common disease" hypothesis in many diseases has led to an avalanche of association studies where the frequency of genetic variants or alleles at a given locus are compared among individuals with and without a particular disease.[5] While these studies remain in an initial phase, at least a basic understanding of the specific genetic influences that determine or modify prostate cancer risk seems within our grasp. Below, we discuss both approaches to the study of prostate cancer genetics, that is: 1) family studies aimed at identifying major genes (genes that greatly increase risk); and 2) association studies, which are more efficient at identifying weaker but more common genetic influences.

FAMILY HISTORY, SEGREGATION ANALYSES, AND TWIN STUDIES— SUPPORT FOR A GENETIC ETIOLOGY

Positive family history is the most consistently identified risk factor for prostate cancer. Johns and Houlston recently reviewed over 22 reported studies and summarized these data by meta-analysis, concluding that having a first degree relative increases risk by over two-fold (RR = 2.5; 95% confidence interval [CI], 2.2–2.8).[6] This risk increased to higher levels when more than one first degree relative was affected. Furthermore, the meta-analysis emphasized a higher prostate cancer risk conferred by: 1) having an affected brother rather than an affected father; and 2) having a positive family history with disease diagnoses at younger than 65 years, compared with men that have a positive family history and diagnoses at 65 years. These findings are summarized in Figure 24.1.

By fitting patterns of familial aggregation of a disease in the general population with several alternative modes of inheritance (e.g., a major gene model, an environmental model, and/or polygene model), segregation analysis can provide inferences as to the specific model that best describes the transmission of the disease in families. Multiple segregation analyses have been performed for prostate cancer. Each has

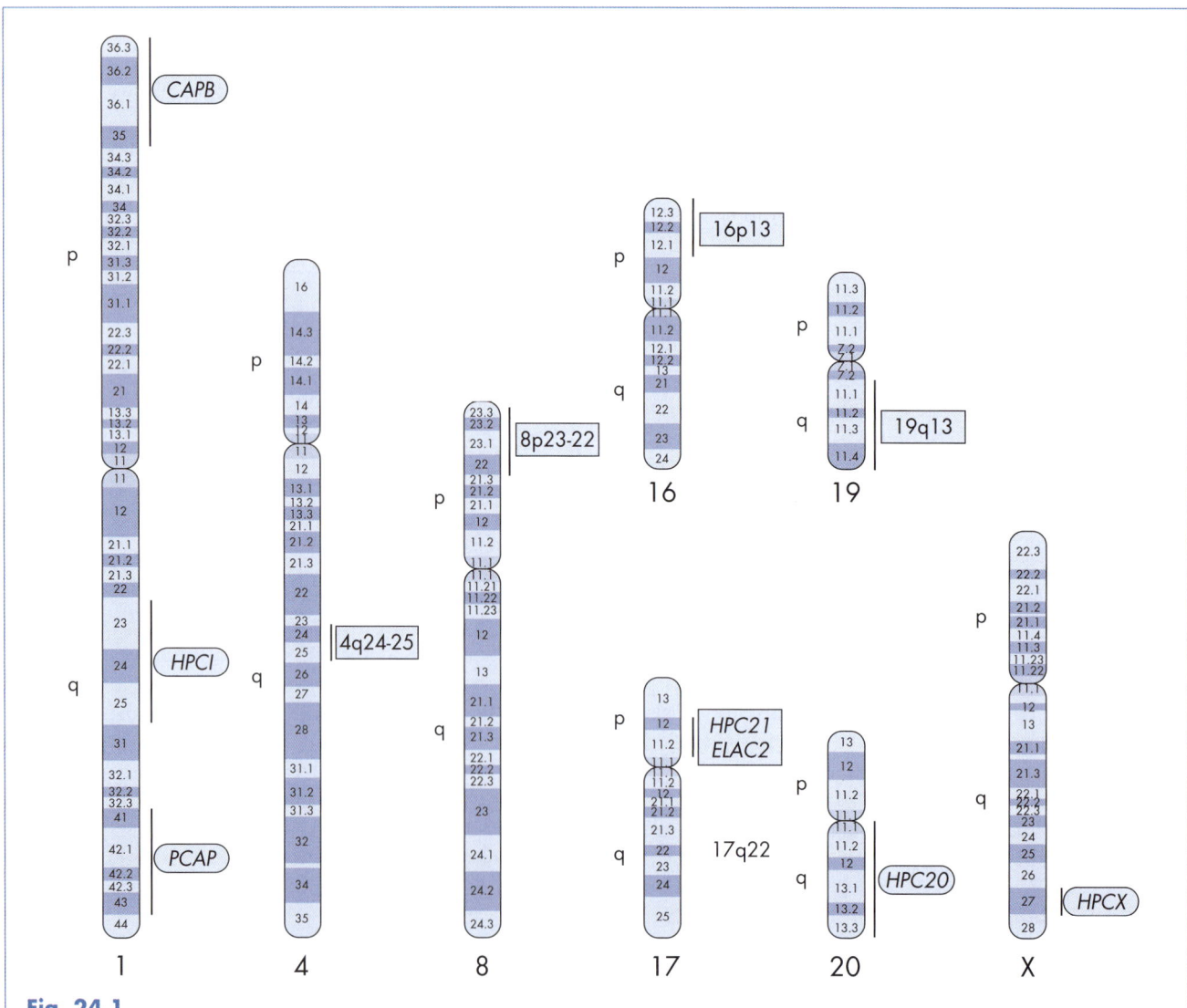

Fig. 24.1
Regions of prostate cancer susceptibility genes identified from linkage studies in hereditary and familial prostate cancer families (adapted from Simard et al 2003[89]).

indicated that familial clustering was consistent with the action of one or more "high risk" genes.[7] Briefly, these studies can be summarized as follows: 1) familial aggregation of prostate cancer is consistent with the autosomal dominant inheritance of a rare, high-risk allele; 2) an inherited form of prostate cancer is estimated to account for a significant proportion of early onset disease and as many as 9% of prostate cancer cases overall; 3) a dominant model is the best fit for younger age of onset families, while a recessive or X-linked model is the best fit for older age of onset in families; and 4) two-gene models fit the data better than single-gene models. So, while there is no consensus for which model is best in segregation analysis, in general this statistical approach supports a genetic etiology as being responsible for familial clustering of prostate cancer.

Twin studies comparing disease concordance rates for a given disease for identical (monozygotic) versus fraternal (dizygotic) twins is another method for testing for evidence of a genetic etiology. Of multiple twin studies performed in prostate cancer, the largest one, performed by Lichtenstein et al suggested that as much as 42% of prostate cancer can be attributable to heritable factors.[8] Interestingly, this fraction was higher than that estimated for either breast or colon cancer (Figure 24.2). On the basis of these types of studies, overwhelming evidence now exists to support a strong genetic influence in the etiology of at least some fraction of prostate cancer cases.

SO IT'S GENETIC: NOW WHAT?

In contrast to the strong evidence that supports this conclusion that prostate cancer is genetic, the definition and characterization of exactly what constitutes the genetic influence in prostate carcinogenesis is far more nebulous. Several major approaches have been taken to define the genes involved in inherited susceptibility for prostate cancer. As alluded to above, it is hypothesized that two types of genes are involved in prostate cancer susceptibility. One type are rare, high penetrance, major susceptibility genes in which germline mutations confer greatly increased risk for the disease and, therefore, can lead to familial clustering of prostate cancer. Genetic linkage and family-based association studies in hereditary prostate cancer families are commonly used to identify this type of gene. The other type of genes are more common, low penetrance, risk modifier genes, where germline sequence variants confer modest increases in risk and primarily contribute to sporadic prostate cancer. Genetic association studies in case-control study populations are commonly used to identify this type of gene.

LINKAGE STUDIES

The strong indication from segregation analyses that a subset of prostate cancer was likely due to the action of one or more major genes has led to large efforts worldwide to collect families with multiple men affected with prostate cancer for linkage studies. The linkage approach has been very successful in the identification of major susceptibility genes for other common cancers, such as those of the breast (*BRCA1* and *BRCA2*) and colon (*APC*, *hMSH2*). In 1993, Carter et al proposed criteria for families likely to carry major prostate cancer susceptibility genes. The operational definition of a family having three or more first degree relatives as a hereditary prostate cancer (HPC) family has been widely used in these efforts. Using linkage analysis, systematic searches in cancer families using genetic markers at intervals along each chromosome can provide powerful statistical evidence of the existence and location of disease predisposing genes. *HPC1* (hereditary prostate cancer 1) on chromosome 1 was the first locus implicated in prostate cancer using this approach.[9] Additional loci have been reported, including *HPCX* at *Xq27-28*,[10] *PCAP* at *1q43*,[11] *CAPB* at 1p36,[12] *HPC20* at 20q13,[13] 8p22-23.[14] In late 2003, the results of eight genome-wide screens were published simultaneously. A number of novel regions,

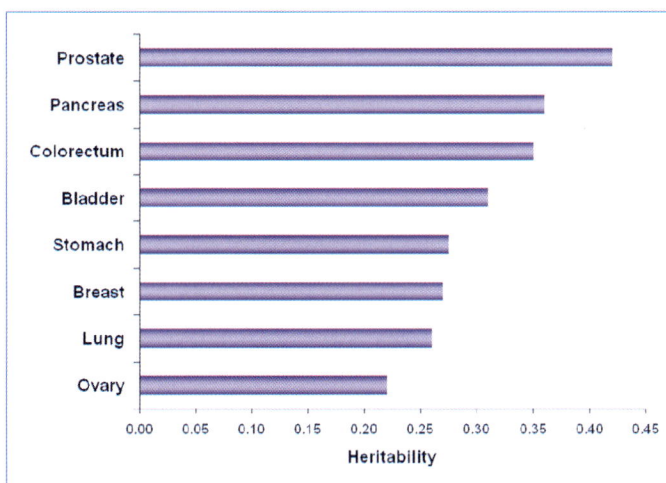

Fig. 24.2
Heritability from a large twin study in Sweden, Denmark, and Finland (Lichtenstein et al. 2000).[8]

as well as several previously described regions, were identified.[15-22] Most recently, the largest combined linkage analysis in 426 HPC families was reported, finding strong linkage at 17q22.[23] In general, few of the reported linkages have been convincingly replicated in independent study populations (see below for discussion).[24] Additional and larger studies are needed to confirm and narrow the linkage regions and ultimately identify the genes responsible for these linkages. An ongoing linkage analysis of over 1100 prostate cancer families collected by the members of the International Consortium for Prostate Cancer Genetics (ICPCG) should prove beneficial in this respect.

CANDIDATE MAJOR SUSCEPTIBILITY GENES IDENTIFIED BY POSITIONAL CLONING APPROACHES

The goal of linkage studies is to identify regions of the genome likely to contain prostate cancer susceptibility genes. In general, regions of linkage are large and may contain hundreds of genes, making the task of specific gene identification difficult. To date, as a result of positional information from linkage studies, three genes have been identified as candidates for major susceptibility genes for prostate cancer. The first one, *ELAC2/HPC2* at 17p11 was identified from extended high-risk HPC families collected in Utah.[25,26] The second reported prostate cancer gene, *RNASEL*, was identified among HPC families from the Johns Hopkins Hospital, after 6 years of intensive positional cloning aimed at the *HPC1* locus.[27] A gene at 8p22-23, *MSR1* (or *SR-A*), was the third reported prostate cancer gene. These latter two genes share related functions as they both play roles in the innate immune system (*RNASEL* in anti-viral defense and *MSR1* in antibacterial defense), suggesting that genetic variation in this system may modify risk for prostate cancer. Inactivating mutations that co-segregate with prostate cancer have been reported in each of these genes in at least one or more prostate cancer families. Overall, the confirmation of these genes across different study populations, however, has been inconsistent.[7] Thus, despite extensive efforts using linkage analysis, a gene which reproducibly accounts for more than a small percentage of familial prostate cancer cases has not been found. When one considers the heterogeneity of prostate cancer, this is perhaps not unexpected (see below), but suggests that new strategies are needed.

CASE-CONTROL ASSOCIATION STUDIES OF PROSTATE CANCER

With realization from linkage analyses that major genes may play a limited role in prostate cancer susceptibility, more interest has focused upon association studies to identify genes that may have more common, albeit weaker, risk alleles. These studies are typically performed in study populations of men with and without prostate cancer, often without regard to family history. As discussed above, these case-control studies have been greatly aided by the increased understanding of the variability of the human genome sequence among different individuals and the concept that common diseases may be due to common genetic variants in the population.[5] Thus, by simply examining the frequency of polymorphic alleles, typically SNPs, among cases and controls, associations between genes and disease risk can be rapidly assessed. A large number of genes involved in critical processes that occur in prostate cells—such as androgen action and metabolism, growth factor signaling, carcinogen detoxification, DNA repair, and inflammation—are being systematically evaluated in this fashion. Additionally, genome-wide association studies of prostate cancer involving thousands to millions of genetic markers are being contemplated and initiated; these are likely to implicate a large number of genes as affecting prostate cancer risk.

We have performed a review of the published literature regarding prostate cancer and genetic variation using PubMed. Only case-control association studies have been included in this search. The requirement for a significant association was either an association with a *P*-value below 0.05 or a confidence interval not including 1. An inclusion criterion of at least 100 cases and 100 controls left 59 SNPs and 8 microsatellites in 36 genes residing on 18 chromosomes (listed in Table 24.1), all associated with prostate cancer in at least one published study. The mean sizes of the studies were 199 cases and 247 controls.

GENES INVOLVED IN THE METABOLISM OF ANDROGENS

Genes involved in the metabolism of androgens have been hypothesized to play important roles in prostate cancer development because of the critical role androgens play in the growth of prostatic cells, and strong evidence from epidemiologic and clinical observations.[89] Currently, most association studies have evaluated only one or two functional sequence variants among a handful of candidate genes, such as *AR*, *SRD5A2*, *CYP17*, and *HSD3Bs*. Positive associations (with estimates of RR < 1.5 in most of the studies) have been reported for each of these genes, although results from confirmation studies have not been consistent. The inconsistent results may reflect small sample sizes in some studies and incomplete evaluation of other potentially important sequence variants in these genes. Considering that many other genes in this pathway are potentially important in the formation and inactivation of androgens, evaluations of association between genes in androgen pathways and prostate cancer risk are just beginning.

Table 24.1 Single nucleotide polymorphisms (SNPs) and microsatellites associated with prostate cancer

Reference	Gene	SNP/microsatellite	Location
Zheng et al[28]	AMACR	Met9Val Asp175Gly Ser201Leu Lys277Glu	5p13.2-q11.1
Balic et al[29] Chang et al[30] Giovannucci et al[31] Hsing et al[32] Ingles et al[33] Mononen et al[34] Mononen et al[35] Stanford et al[36] Xue et al[37]	AR	GGC repeat GGN repeat Arg726Leu	Xq11.2-q12
Wang et al[38]	CCND1	870A/G	11q13
Ikonen et al[39]	CDH1	S270A	16q22.1
Iughetti et al[40]	COL18A1	Asp104Asn	21q22.3
Panguluri et al[41]	COX2	−297C/G	1q25.2-q25.3
Habuchi et al[42] Wadelius et al[43] Yamada et al[44]	CYP17	5′ promoter region T/C	10q24.3
Latil et al[45] Suzuki et al[46]	CYP19	STRP in Intron 4 Arg264Cys	15q21.1
Acevedo et al[47] Chang et al[48] Murata et al[49] Murata et al[50]	CYP1A1	Msp1 3801T/C Ile462Val	15q22-q24
Chang et al[51] Tanaka et al[52]	CYP1B1	−263G/A −1001C/T −13C/T +142C/G Gly119Thr	2p21
Ferreira et al[53]	CYP2E1	Dral (Intron 6)	10q24.3-qter
Rybicki et al[54]	ERCC2	Asp312Asn	19q13.3
Cancel–Tassin[55] Suzuki et al[56] Tanaka et al[57]	ESR1	GGGA repeat codon 10 (T/C)	6q25.1
Acevedo et al[47] Kidd et al[58]	GSTM1	Homozygous deletion of gene	1p13.3
Medeiros et al[59]	GSTM3	3 bp deletion	1p13.3
Kote–Jarai et al[60]	GSTP1	Ile105Val	11q13
Nam et al[61]	GSTT1	Homozygous deletion of gene	22q11.23
Rökman et al[62] Suarez et al[63]	HPC2/ELAC2	Glu622Val Ala541Thr Ser217Leu	17p11.2
Margiotti et al[64]	HSD17B3	Gly289Ser	9q22
Chang et al[65]	HSD3B1	Asn367Thr	1p13.1
Nam et al[66]	IGF1	19–repeat allele	12q22-q23
McCarron et al[67]	Il10	1082A/G	1q31-q32
McCarron et al[67]	Il8	251A/T	4q13-q21
Nam et al[66]	KLK2	Arg226Trp	19q13.41
Hawkins et al[68]	LZTS1	2812G/A 2883T/C 3329C/T 4361C/T	8p22

Table 24.1 *continued*

Reference	Gene	SNP/microsatellite	Location
Miller et al[69]	MSR1	Pro3	8p22
Xu et al[70]		Indel1	
Xu et al[71]		IVS5–59	
		Pro275Ala	
		INDEL7	
		Arg293X	
Hamasaki et al[72]	NAT2	Slow acetylator	8p22
Hsing et al[73]	NCOA3	CAG/CAA repeat	20q12
Xu et al[74]	OGG1	11657A/G	3p26.2
		6803C/G	
		7143A/G	
Riley et al[75]	PGK1	STR	Xq13
Nakazato et al[76]	RNASEL	Arg462Gln	1q25
Rökman et al[77]		Asp541Glu	
Wang et al[78]		Glu265X	
Li et al[79]	SRD5A2	3001G/A	2p23
Loukola et al[80]		Val89Leu	
Makridakis et al[81]		Ala49Thr	
Nam et al[82]			
Nowell et al[83]	SULT1A1	Arg213His	16p12.1
Henner et al[84]	TP53	Arg72Pro	17p13.1
Correa–Cerro et al[85]	VDR	poly(A)–micros	12q12-q14
Habuchi et al[86]		Taq1 RFLP	
Ingles et al[33]		Bsml 825 bp	
Medeiros et al[87]			
Taylor et al[88]			
McCarron et al[67]	VEGF	1154G/A	6p12

Amino acids: Ala, alanine; Arg, arginine; Asn, asparagine; Asp aspartate; Glu, glutamate; Gly, glycine; His, histidine; Ile, isoleucine; Leu, leucine; Lys, lysine; Met, methionine; Pro, proline; Ser, serine; Thr, threonine; Val, valine. Bases: A, adenine; C, cytosine; Guanine; N, any base; T, thymine.

bp, base pairs; RFLP, restriction fragment length polymorphism.

GENES ENCODING PHASE I AND PHASE II ENZYMES

The genes encoding Cytochrome p450 (CYP) enzymes (phase I enzymes) make up a multiple-gene "superfamily" that plays an important role in steroidogenesis and in the activation or detoxification of environmental chemicals such as polycyclic aromatic hydrocarbons, benzo(a)pyrene, and heterocyclic amines. In contrast, phase II enzymes, such as the glutathione S-transferase (GST) family, facilitate excretion of carcinogenic compounds by conjugating metabolic intermediates to water-soluble forms. Genetic association studies between prostate cancer risk and genes in this pathway include *CYP1A1, CYP2D6, CYP17A2, CYP3A4, GST, NAT1,* and *NAT2,* although only a limited number of functional sequence variants have been evaluated in each gene. Positive association with prostate cancer has been reported for each of these genes (and most had an RR<1.5).[90] Many other genes that encode for Phase I and II enzymes still need to be evaluated.

DNA REPAIR GENES

Common polymorphisms in DNA repair genes may alter protein function and an individual's capacity to repair damaged DNA; deficits in repair capacity may lead to genetic instability and carcinogenesis. Associations between polymorphisms in DNA repair genes with cancer in the colon and breast have been intensively studied; however, association with prostate cancer has not been as commonly reported. Two sequence variants (11657A/G in the gene and Ser326Cys in the protein product) of the human oxoguanine glycosylase 1 (hOGG1),[74] have been reported to be associated with prostate cancer risk, and the association of hOGG1 confirmed in a subsequent study.[91] Results from such studies suggest that altered DNA repair capacity may also play an important role in prostate cancer development. Considering that there are 133 genes known to be involved in the DNA repair pathway thus far,[92] a systematic evaluation of the impact of DNA repair gene polymorphisms on prostate cancer risk is warranted.

INFLAMMATORY GENES

Chronic or recurrent inflammation has been implicated in the initiation and development of multiple human cancers, including those affecting the stomach, liver, colon, and bladder.[93,94] A role for chronic inflammation in the etiology of prostate cancer has been proposed.[95] Studies examining association between prostate cancer risk and factors related to chronic inflammation such as occurrence of prostatitis, sexually transmitted diseases (STDs), and intake of nonsteroidal anti-inflammatory drugs (NSAIDs) provide epidemiologic evidence that is consistent with chronic inflammation playing a role in prostate cancer development. The fact that two of three prostate cancer susceptibility genes (MSR1 and RNASEL) identified through positional cloning approaches are involved in innate immunity and inflammation suggests a further link between inflammation and prostate cancer.[27,70] In addition, recent findings of association between prostate cancer risk and sequence variants in MIC1,[96] TLR4,[97] and the TLR6-1-10 gene cluster,[98] as well as other cytokine genes,[67] provides a specific link between inflammatory genes and prostate cancer risk.

ASSOCIATION STUDIES OF OTHER GENES

Many other genes have been evaluated for their association with prostate cancer risk. Among these, the genes encoding insulin (INS),[99] vascular endothelial growth factor (VEGF),[67] vitamin D receptor (VDR),[100] and prostate-specific antigen (PSA)[37,101] have been evaluated in multiple studies. In addition, association studies have been reported at least once for the following genes: cyclin D1 gene (CCND1),[102] deleted in liver cancer 1 gene (DLC1),[103] cyclin dependent kinases N1A and N1B (CDKN1A and CDKN1B),[104,105] peroxisome proliferator-activated receptor-γ (PPARγ),[106] and alpha-methylacyl-CoA racemase (AMCAR).[107]

OTHER MAJOR CANCER GENES AS PROSTATE CANCER RISK FACTORS

In addition to linkage analyses and association studies, a third approach has been to study the possible roles of genes responsible for other cancer predisposing

syndromes as prostate cancer susceptibility genes. This approach has led to some interesting leads. The BRCA2 gene has been implicated in early onset prostate cancers,[108] and both CHEK2 and NBS1, genes involved in breast cancer susceptibility and the Nijmegen breakage syndrome, respectively, have been found to be mutated in prostate cancer families in different study populations.[109–112] That these three genes are all involved in DNA repair indicates that defects in the ability to repair damage to DNA and maintain genomic integrity predispose prostate epithelial cells, like many other cells in the body, to malignant transformation.

DISCUSSION AND CONCLUSIONS

Where is the study of familial prostate cancer, and prostate cancer susceptibility in general, taking us? It is hoped that by extensive study of prostate cancer pedigrees and an in-depth analysis and appreciation of other cancers, and other diseases co-occurring in prostate cancer families, we can optimize more effectively the predictive information of family history. It will most likely be important to provide more clinical detail regarding the prostate cancers that compose the family history, rather than considering all cases with a positive biopsy of equal significance (see below). In addition, defining genes that affect prostate cancer risk can potentially provide otherwise unattainable insight into the mechanisms of prostate carcinogenesis and lead towards the identification of novel therapeutic targets. That multiple genes involved in the inflammatory process (e.g., MSR1,[71] MIC1,[96] TRL4,[97] IL10[67]) are implicated through genetic studies provides a unique and compelling impetus for further study of this process in the development of prostate cancer.[94]

Whereas progress has been made in identifying genes associated with both sporadic and familial prostate cancer, there is much left to be learned, and many findings in this area have been difficult to replicate. Why is this so? There are a number of possibilities to consider. In general, prostate cancer is a very heterogeneous disease, with a complex etiology involving both genetic influences as well as strong, well-documented environmental influences, and, inevitably, interactions between the two. The fraction of prostate cancer that may be due to any single factor, such as a single gene, may be quite small and hard to detect, particularly in the midst of many competing etiologies. Another factor is the prevalence of this disease. Current estimates from the Prostate Cancer Prevention Trial suggest that as many as 1 in 4 American men over age 63 years, if biopsied, would be diagnosed as having prostate cancer.[113] At this frequency in the population, many familial clusters of prostate cancer are due simply to chance alone. Thus, in any collection of prostate cancer families, there will be families resulting from shared genetics, shared environmental factors, shared genetics interacting with shared environmental factors, as well as those due to chance alone, and some (perhaps most) due to some combination of these factors. Only when we restrict the phenotype under study can we reasonably hope to simplify this situation. For example, having large enough study populations so that well-defined subsets of prostate cancer can be emphasized is a possible solution. Unlike families where two or more relatives have positive biopsies, which is quite a common occurrence, families with multiple first degree relatives with prostate cancers having poor prognostic features are relatively rare. Will focusing on this type of prostate cancer simplify the picture? Only in a study population that is large enough and well enough characterized can such a question be addressed. The collaborative effort undertaken by the ICPCG and its 1800 HPC families has this capacity.[114] Will focusing on only a subset of prostate cancer decrease the relevance of any discoveries made as a consequence, with respect to prostate cancer in general? It is of note that it was through the study of families with a familial adenomatous polyposis (FAP), a syndrome that accounts for only a very small fraction of all colon cancers, or even familial colon cancer, which led to the identification of the *APC* gene, a gene which is inactivated in the majority of colon cancers, both familial and sporadic.[3]

In summary, despite extensive efforts and a number of promising leads, a major gene that can be used to identify individuals at high risk for prostate cancer has not been identified. However, a more focused analysis of clinically distinct subsets of prostate cancer (e.g., early onset, aggressive disease) could yield important insight into this question. Well-designed case-control studies that can identify alleles consistently associated with prostate cancer risk should be informative in this respect. As prostate cancer stands to become an even larger medical burden as the world's population ages, it is imperative that a better understanding of the molecular genetics of prostate cancer be acquired. Indeed, if the promise of the revolution in molecular medicine is to be realized with respect to prostate cancer, increased efforts utilizing better methodologies and technologies and large, well-characterized study populations are urgently needed to effectively confront this research problem.

REFERENCES

1. Morganti G, Gianferrari L, Cresseri A, et al. Recherches clinico-statistiques et genetiques sur les neoplasies de la prostate. Acta Genet 1956;6:304–305.

2. Woolf CM. An investigation of the familial aspects of carcinoma of the prostate. Cancer 1960;13:739–744.

3. Kinzler KW, Vogelstein B. Lessons from hereditary colorectal cancer. Cell 1996;87:159–170.

4. Linehan WM, Zbar B. Focus on kidney cancer. Cancer Cell 2004;6:223–228. Erratum in: Cancer Cell 2004;6:423.

5. Lohmueller KE, Pearce CL, Pike M, et al. Meta-analysis of genetic association studies supports a contribution of common variants to susceptibility to common disease. Nat Genet 2003;33:177–182.

6. Johns LE, Houlston RS. A systematic review and meta-analysis of familial prostate cancer risk. BJU Int 2003;91:789–794.

7. Schaid DJ. The complex genetic epidemiology of prostate cancer. Hum Mol Genet 2004; 13 Spec No 1:R103–R121.

8. Lichtenstein P, Holm NV, Verkasalo PK, et al. Environmental and heritable factors in the causation of cancer: analyses of cohorts of twins from Sweden, Denmark, and Finland. N Engl J Med 2000;343:78–85.

9. Smith JR, Freije D, Carpten JD, et al. Major susceptibility locus for prostate cancer on chromosome 1 suggested by a genome-wide search. Science 1996;274:1371–1374.

10. Xu J, Meyers D, Freije D, et al. Evidence for a prostate cancer susceptibility locus on the X chromosome. Nat Genet 1998;20:175–179.

11. Berthon P, Valeri A, Cohen-Akenine A, et al. Predisposing gene for early-onset prostate cancer, localized on chromosome 1q42.2-43. Am J Hum Genet 1998;62:1416–1424.

12. Gibbs M, Stanford JL, McIndoe RA, et al. Evidence for a rare prostate cancer-susceptibility locus at chromosome 1p36. Am J Hum Genet 1999;64:776–787.

13. Berry R, Schroeder JJ, French AJ, et al. Evidence for a prostate cancer-susceptibility locus on chromosome 20. Am J Hum Genet 2000;67:82–91.

14. Xu J, Zheng SL, Chang B, et al. Linkage and association studies of prostate cancer susceptibility gene on 8p22-23. Am J Hum Genet 2001;69341–350.

15. Edwards S, Meitz J, Eles R, et al. Results of a genome-wide linkage analysis in prostate cancer families ascertained through the ACTANE consortium. Prostate 2003;57:270–279.

16. Xu J, Gillanders EM, Isaacs SD, et al. Genome-wide scan for prostate cancer susceptibility genes in the Johns Hopkins hereditary prostate cancer families. Prostate 2003;57:320–325.

17. Cunningham JM, McDonnell SK, Marks A, et al. Genome linkage screen for prostate cancer susceptibility loci: results from the Mayo Clinic Familial Prostate Cancer Study. Prostate 2003;57:335–346.

18. Lange EM, Gillanders EM, Davis CC, et al. Genome-wide scan for prostate cancer susceptibility genes using families from the University of Michigan prostate cancer genetics project finds evidence for linkage on chromosome 17 near BRCA1. Prostate 2003;57:326–334.

19. Janer M, Friedrichsen DM, Stanford JL, et al. Genomic scan of 254 hereditary prostate cancer families. Prostate 2003;57:309–319.

20. Schleutker J, Baffoe-Bonnie AB, Gillanders E, et al. Genome-wide scan for linkage in Finnish hereditary prostate cancer (HPC) families identifies novel susceptibility loci at 11q14 and 3p25-26. Prostate 2003;57:280–289.

21. Witte JS, Suarez BK, Thiel B, et al. Genome-wide scan of brothers: replication and fine mapping of prostate cancer susceptibility and aggressiveness loci. Prostate 2003;57:298–308.

22. Wiklund F, Gillanders EM, Albertus JA, et al. Genome-wide scan of Swedish families with hereditary prostate cancer: suggestive evidence of linkage at 5q11.2 and 19p13.3. Prostate 2003;57:290–297.

23. Gillanders EM, Xu J, Chang BL, et al. Combined genome-wide scan for prostate cancer susceptibility genes: evidence of linkage at 17q22. JNCI 2004;96:1240–1247.

24. Easton DF, Schaid DJ, Whittemore AS, et al. International Consortium for Prostate Cancer Genetics. Where are the prostate cancer genes?—A summary of eight genome wide searches. Prostate 2003;57:261–269.

25. Tavtigian SV, Simard J, Teng DH, et al. A candidate prostate cancer susceptibility gene at chromosome 17p. Nat Genet 2001;27:172–180.

26. Rebbeck TR, Walker AH, Zeigler-Johnson C, et al. Association of HPC2/ELAC2 genotypes and prostate cancer. Am J Hum Genet 2000;67:1014–1019.

27. Carpten J, Nupponen N, Isaacs S, et al. Germline mutations in the ribonuclease L gene in families showing linkage with HPC1. Nat Genet 2002;30:181–184.

28. Zheng SL, Chang BL, Faith DA, et al. Sequence variants of alpha-methylacyl-CoA racemase are associated with prostate cancer risk. Cancer Res 2002;62:6485–6488.

29. Balic I, Graham ST, Troyer DA, et al. Androgen receptor length polymorphism associated with prostate cancer risk in Hispanic men. J Urol 2002;168:2245–2248.

30. Chang BL, Zheng SL, Hawkins GA, et al. Polymorphic GGC repeats in the androgen receptor gene are associated with hereditary and sporadic prostate cancer risk. Hum Genet 2002;110:122–129.

31. Giovannucci E, Stampfer MJ, Krithivas K, et al. The CAG repeat within the androgen receptor gene and its relationship to prostate cancer. Proc Natl Acad Sci USA 1997;94:3320–3323.

32. Hsing AW, Gao YT, Wu G, et al. Polymorphic CAG and GGN repeat lengths in the androgen receptor gene and prostate cancer risk: a population-based case-control study in China. Cancer Res 2000;60:5111–5116.

33. Ingles SA, Ross RK, Yu MC, et al. Association of prostate cancer risk with genetic polymorphisms in vitamin D receptor and androgen receptor. J Natl Cancer Inst 1997;89:166–170.

34. Mononen N, Ikonen T, Autio V, et al. Androgen receptor CAG polymorphism and prostate cancer risk. Hum Genet 2002;111:166–171.

35. Mononen N, Syrjäkoski K, Matikainen M, et al. Two percent of Finnish prostate cancer patients have a germ-line mutation in the hormone-binding domain of the androgen receptor gene. Cancer Res 2000;60:6479–6481.

36. Stanford JL, Just JJ, Gibbs M, et al. Polymorphic repeats in the androgen receptor gene: molecular markers of prostate cancer risk. Cancer Res 1997;57:1194–1198.

37. Xue W, Irvine RA, Yu MC, et al. Susceptibility to prostate cancer: interaction between genotypes at the androgen receptor and prostate-specific antigen loci. Cancer Res 2000;60:839–841.

38. Wang L, Habuchi T, Mitsumori K, et al. Increased risk of prostate cancer associated with AA genotype of cyclin D1 gene A870G polymorphism. Int J Cancer 2003;103:116–120.

39. Ikonen T, Matikainen M, Mononen N, et al. Association of E-cadherin germ-line alterations with prostate cancer. Clinical Cancer Research 2001;7:3465–3471.

40. Iughetti P, Suzuki O, Godoi PH, et al. A polymorphism in endostatin, an angiogenesis inhibitor, predisposes for the development of prostatic adenocarcinoma. Cancer Res 2001;61:7375–7378.

41. Panguluri RC, Long LO, Chen W, et al. COX-2 gene promoter haplotypes and prostate cancer risk. Carcinogenesis 2004;25:961–966.

42. Habuchi T, Liqing Z, Suzuki T, et al. Increased risk of prostate cancer and benign prostatic hyperplasia associated with a CYP17 gene polymorphism with a gene dosage effect. Cancer Res 2000; 60:5710–5713.

43. Wadelius M, Andersson AO, Johansson JE, et al. Prostate cancer associated with CYP17 genotype. Pharmacogenetics 1999;9:635–639.

44. Yamada Y, Watanabe M, Murata M, et al. Impact of genetic polymorphisms of 17-hydroxylase cytochrome P-450 (CYP17) and steroid 5alpha-reductase type II (SRD5A2) genes on prostate-cancer risk among the Japanese population. Int J Cancer 2001;92:683–686.

45. Latil AG, Azzouzi R, Cancel GS, et al. Prostate carcinoma risk and allelic variants of genes involved in androgen biosynthesis and metabolism pathways. Cancer 2001;92:1130–1137.

46. Suzuki K, Nakazato H, Matsui H, et al. Genetic polymorphisms of estrogen receptor alpha, CYP19, catechol-O-methyltransferase are associated with familial prostate carcinoma risk in a Japanese population. Cancer 2003;98:1411–1416.

47. Acevedo C, Opazo JL, Huidobro C, et al. Positive correlation between single or combined genotypes of CYP1A1 and GSTM1 in relation to prostate cancer in Chilean people. Prostate 2003;57:111–117.

48. Chang BL, Zheng SL, Isaacs SD, et al. Polymorphisms in the CYP1A1 gene are associated with prostate cancer risk. Int J Cancer 2003;106:375–378.

49. Murata M, Watanabe M, Yamanaka M, et al. Genetic polymorphisms in cytochrome P450 (CYP)1A1, CYP1A2, CYP2E1, glutathione S-transferase (GST) M1 and GSTT1 and susceptibility to prostate cancer in the Japanese population. Cancer Lett 2001;165:171–177.

50. Murata M, Shiraishi T, Fukutome K, et al. Cytochrome P4501A1 and glutathione S-transferase M1 genotypes as risk factors for prostate cancer in Japan. Jpn J Clin Oncol 1998;28:657–660.

51. Chang BL, Zheng SL, Isaacs SD, et al. Polymorphisms in the CYP1B1 gene are associated with increased risk of prostate cancer. Br J Cancer 2003;89:1524–1529.

52. Tanaka Y, Sasaki M, Kaneuchi M, et al. Polymorphisms of the CYP1B1 gene have higher risk for prostate cancer. Biochem Biophys Res Commun 2002;296:820–826.

53. Ferreira PM, Medeiros R, Vasconcelos A, et al. Association between CYP2E1 polymorphisms and susceptibility to prostate cancer. Eur J Cancer Prev 2003;12:205–211.

54. Rybicki BA, Conti DV, Moreira A, et al. DNA repair gene XRCC1 and XPD polymorphisms and risk of prostate cancer. Cancer Epidemiol Biomarkers Prev 2004;13:23–29.

55. Cancel-Tassin G, Latil A, Rousseau F, et al. Association study of polymorphisms in the human estrogen receptor alpha gene and prostate cancer risk. Eur Urol 2003;44:487 490.

56. Suzuki K, Nakazato H, Matsui H, et al. Association of the genetic polymorphism of the CYP19 intron 4[TTTA]n repeat with familial prostate cancer risk in a Japanese population. Anticancer Res 2003;23:4941–4946.

57. Tanaka Y, Sasaki M, Kaneuchi M, et al. Polymorphisms of estrogen receptor alpha in prostate cancer. Mol Carcinog 2003;37:202–208.

58. Kidd LC, Woodson K, Taylor PR, et al. Polymorphisms in glutathione-S-transferase genes (GST-M1, GST-T1 and GST-P1) and susceptibility to prostate cancer among male smokers of the ATBC cancer prevention study. Eur J Cancer Prev 2003;12:317–320.

59. Medeiros R, Vasconcelos A, Costa S, et al. Metabolic susceptibility genes and prostate cancer risk in a southern European population: the role of glutathione S-transferases GSTM1, GSTM3, and GSTT1 genetic polymorphisms. Prostate 2004;58:414–420.

60. Kote-Jarai Z, Easton D, Edwards SM, et al. Relationship between glutathione S-transferase M1, P1 and T1 polymorphisms and early onset prostate cancer. Pharmacogenetics 2001;11:325–330.

61. Nam RK, Zhang WW, Trachtenberg J, et al. Comprehensive assessment of candidate genes and serological markers for the detection of prostate cancer. Cancer Epidemiol Biomarkers Prev 2003;12:1429–1437.

62. Rökman A, Ikonen T, Mononen N, et al. ELAC2/HPC2 involvement in hereditary and sporadic prostate cancer. Cancer Res 2001;61:6038–6041.

63. Suarez BK, Gerhard DS, Lin J, et al. Polymorphisms in the prostate cancer susceptibility gene HPC2/ELAC2 in multiplex families and healthy controls. Cancer Res 2001;61:4982–4984.

64. Margiotti K, Kim E, Pearce CL, et al. Association of the G289S single nucleotide polymorphism in the HSD17B3 gene with prostate cancer in Italian men. Prostate 2002;53:65–68.

65. Chang BL, Zheng SL, Hawkins GA, et al. Joint effect of HSD3B1 and HSD3B2 genes is associated with hereditary and sporadic prostate cancer susceptibility. Cancer Res 2002;62:1784–1789.

66. Nam RK, Zhang WW, Trachtenberg J, et al. Single nucleotide polymorphism of the human kallikrein-2 gene highly correlates with serum human kallikrein-2 levels and in combination enhances prostate cancer detection. J Clin Oncol 2003;21:2312–2319.

67. McCarron SL, Edwards S, Evans PR, et al. Influence of cytokine gene polymorphisms on the development of prostate cancer. Cancer Res 2002;62:3369–3372.

68. Hawkins GA, Mychaleckyj JC, Zheng SL, et al. Germline sequence variants of the LZTS1 gene are associated with prostate cancer risk. Cancer Genet Cytogenet 2002;137:1–7.

69. Miller DC, Zheng SL, Dunn RL, et al. Germ-line mutations of the macrophage scavenger receptor 1 gene: association with prostate cancer risk in African-American men. Cancer Res 2003;63:3486–3489.

70. Xu J, Zheng SL, Komiya A, et al. Germline mutations and sequence variants of the macrophage scavenger receptor 1 gene are associated with prostate cancer risk. Nat Genet 2002;32:321–325.

71. Xu J, Zheng SL, Komiya A, et al. Common sequence variants of the macrophage scavenger receptor 1 gene are associated with prostate cancer risk. Am J Hum Genet 2003;72:208–212.

72. Hamasaki T, Inatomi H, Katoh T, et al. N-acetyltransferase-2 gene polymorphism as a possible biomarker for prostate cancer in Japanese men. Int J Urol 2003;10:167–173.

73. Hsing AW, Chokkalingam AP, Gao YT, et al. Polymorphic CAG/CAA repeat length in the AIB1/SRC-3 gene and prostate cancer risk: a population-based case-control study. Cancer Epidemiol Biomarkers Prev 2002;11:337–341.

74. Xu J, Zheng SL, Turner A, et al. Associations between hOGG1 sequence variants and prostate cancer susceptibility. Cancer Res 2002;62:2253–2257.

75. Riley DE, Krieger JN. Short tandem repeat polymorphism linkage to the androgen receptor gene in prostate carcinoma. Cancer 2001;92:2603–2608.

76. Nakazato H, Suzuki K, Matsui H, et al. Role of genetic polymorphisms of the RNASEL gene on familial prostate cancer risk in a Japanese population. Br J Cancer 2003;89:691–696.

77. Rökman A, Ikonen T, Seppälä EH, et al. Germline alterations of the RNASEL gene, a candidate HPC1 gene at 1q25, in patients and families with prostate cancer. Am J Hum Genet 2002;70:1299–1304.

78. Wang L, McDonnell SK, Elkins DA, et al. Analysis of the RNASEL gene in familial and sporadic prostate cancer. Am J Hum Genet 2002;71:116–123.

79. Li Z, Habuchi T, Mitsumori K, et al. Association of V89L SRD5A2 polymorphism with prostate cancer development in a Japanese population. J Urol 2003;169:2378–2381.

80. Loukola A, Chadha M, Penn SG, et al. Comprehensive evaluation of the association between prostate cancer and genotypes/haplotypes in CYP17A1, CYP3A4, and SRD5A2. Eur J Hum Genet 2004;12:321–332.

81. Makridakis NM, Ross RK, Pike MC, et al. Association of mis-sense substitution in SRD5A2 gene with prostate cancer in African-American and Hispanic men in Los Angeles, USA. Lancet 1999;354:975–978.

82. Nam RK, Toi A, Vesprini D, et al. V89L polymorphism of type-2, 5-alpha reductase enzyme gene predicts prostate cancer presence and progression. Urology 2001;57:199–204.

83. Nowell S, Ratnasinghe DL, Ambrosone CB, et al. Association of SULT1A1 phenotype and genotype with prostate cancer risk in African-Americans and Caucasians. Cancer Epidemiol Biomarkers Prev 2004;13:270–276.

84. Henner WD, Evans AJ, Hough KM, et al. Association of codon 72 polymorphism of p53 with lower prostate cancer risk. Prostate 2001;49:263–266.

85. Correa-Cerro L, Berthon P, Häussler J, et al. Vitamin D receptor polymorphisms as markers in prostate cancer. Hum Genet 1999;105:281–287.

86. Habuchi T, Suzuki T, Sasaki R, et al. Association of vitamin D receptor gene polymorphism with prostate cancer and benign prostatic hyperplasia in a Japanese population. Cancer Res 2000;60:305–308.

87. Medeiros R, Morais A, Vasconcelos A, et al. The role of vitamin D receptor gene polymorphisms in the susceptibility to prostate cancer of a southern European population. Journal of Human Genetics 2002;47:413–418.

88. Taylor JA, Hirvonen A, Watson M, et al. Association of prostate cancer with vitamin D receptor gene polymorphism. Cancer Res. 1996;56:4108–4110.

89. Simard J, Dumont M, Labuda D, et al. Prostate cancer susceptibility genes: lessons learned and challenges posed. Endocr Relat Cancer 2003;10:225–259.

90. Chen C. Risk of prostate cancer in relation to polymorphisms of metabolic genes. Epidemiol Rev 2001;23:30–35.

91. Chen L, Elahi A, Pow-Sang J, et al. Association between polymorphism of human oxoguanine glycosylase 1 and risk of prostate cancer. J Urol 2003;170:2471–2474.

92. http://www.cgal.icnet.uk/DNA_Repair_Genes.html.

93. Coussens LM, Werb Z. Inflammation and cancer. Nature 2002;420:860–867.

94. Nelson WG, De Marzo AM, Isaacs WB. Prostate cancer. N Engl J Med 2003;349:366–381.

95. De Marzo AM, Marchi VL, et al. Proliferative inflammatory atrophy of the prostate: implications for prostatic carcinogenesis. Am J Pathol 1999;155:1985–1992.

96. Lindmark F, Zheng SL, Wiklund F, et al. The H6D polymorphism in the Macrophage Inhibitory Cytokine Gene 1 (MIC-1) is associated with Prostate Cancer. J Natl Cancer Inst 2004;96:1248–1254.

97. Zheng SL, Augustsson-Balter K, Chang B, et al. Sequence variants of toll-like receptor 4 are associated with prostate cancer risk: results from the Cancer Prostate in Sweden Study. Cancer Res 2004;64:2918–2922.

98. Sun J, Wiklund F, Zheng SL, et al. Sequence variants in Toll-like receptor gene cluster (TLR6-TLR1-TLR10) are associated with prostate cancer risk. JNCI 2005;97:525–32.

99. Ho GY, Melman A, Liu SM, et al. Polymorphism of the insulin gene is associated with increased prostate cancer risk. Br J Cancer 2003;88:263–269.

100. Coughlin SS, Hall IJ. A review of genetic polymorphisms and prostate cancer risk. Ann Epidemiol 2002;12:182–196.

101. Xu J, Meyers DA, Sterling DA, et al. Association studies of serum prostate-specific antigen levels and the genetic polymorphisms at the androgen receptor and prostate-specific antigen genes. Cancer Epidemiol Biomarkers Prev 2002;11:664–669.

102. Koike H, Suzuki K, Satoh T, et al. Cyclin D1 gene polymorphism and familial prostate cancer: the AA genotype of A870G polymorphism is associated with prostate cancer risk in men aged 70 years or older and metastatic stage. Anticancer Res 2003;23:4947–4951.

103. Zheng SL, Mychaleckyj JC, Hawkins GA, et al. Evaluation of DLC1 as a prostate cancer susceptibility gene: mutation screen and association study. Mutat Res 2003;528:45–53.

104. Kibel AS, Suarez BK, Belani J, et al. CDKN1A and CDKN1B polymorphisms and risk of advanced prostate carcinoma. Cancer Res 2003;63:2033–2036.

105. Chang BL, Zheng SL, Isaacs SD, et al. A polymorphism in the CDKN1B gene is associated with increased risk of hereditary prostate cancer. Cancer Res 2004;64:1997–1999.

106. Paltoo D, Woodson K, Taylor P, Albanes D, et al. Pro12Ala polymorphism in the peroxisome proliferator-activated receptor-gamma (PPAR-gamma) gene and risk of prostate cancer among men in a large cancer prevention study. Cancer Lett 2003;191:67–74.

107. Zheng SL, Chang B, Isaacs SD, et al. Sequence variants of α-methylacyl-CoA racemase are associated with prostate cancer risk. Cancer Res 2002;62:6485–6488.

108. Edwards SM, Kote-Jarai Z, Meitz J et al., Two percent of men with early-onset prostate cancer harbor germline mutations in the BRCA2 gene. Am J Hum Genet 2003;72:1–12.

109. Seppala EH, Ikonen T, Mononen N, et al. CHEK2 variants associated with hereditary prostate cancer. Br J Cancer 2003;89:1966–1970.

110. Cybulski C, Gorski B, Debniak T, et al. NBS1 is a prostate cancer susceptibility gene. Cancer Res 2004;64:1215–1219.

111. Cybulski C, Huzarski T, Gorski B, et al. A novel founder CHEK2 mutation is associated with increased prostate cancer risk. Cancer Res 2004;64:2677–2679.

112. Dong X, Wang L, Taniguchi K, et al. Mutations in CHEK2 associated with prostate cancer risk. Am J Hum Genet 2003;72:270–280.

113. Thompson IM, Goodman PJ, Tangen CM, et al. The influence of finasteride on the development of prostate cancer. N Engl J Med 2003;349:215–224.

114. www.icpcg.org.

Prostate cancer stem cells 25

Aamir Ahmed, Isabelle Bisson, Charlotte Foley, John R Masters

STEM CELLS

How an organism maintains and replenishes specialized tissues over its lifetime is an intriguing question. For example, the hematopoietic system produces billions of cells of many different types every day. Yet the entire system can be produced and maintained by a tiny pool of hematopoietic stem cells.[1]

Stem cell concepts arose in part from studies of testicular teratoma,[2] which are capable of generating almost every possible cell type. Evidence for stem cells has been obtained in many tissues, including brain, liver, skin, and bone marrow, in which stem cell research was pioneered. Adult stem cells can be described as the small fraction of cells within a specialized tissue that are responsible for the regeneration, maintenance and replenishment of the cells within that tissue.[3,4] Stem cells are characterized by their capacity for self-renewal, pluripotency, and long lifespan.

The concept that normal tissues are maintained by stem cells may be equally valid for cancer. If prostate cancer contains stem cells that are responsible for the development and maintenance of the cancer, the implications for understanding and treatment are potentially profound. In this chapter, stem cell theory is considered first in relation to normal tissues and in particular the prostate. Then the information on normal stem cells informs and guides the subsequent discussion on stem cells in neoplasia and in prostate cancer in particular.

SELF-RENEWAL

If the adult stem cells regenerate, maintain, and repair a specific tissue over its lifetime, how can the stem cells achieve this without being depleted? The answer probably lies in traits considered to be specific to stem cells: self-renewal and long lifespan.

Self-renewal occurs during a cell division in which one or both of the daughter cells are stem cells that retain the same developmental potential as the parental stem cell.[5] Self-renewal could be symmetric or asymmetric, i.e., a parental stem cell giving rise to two daughter stem cells or one daughter stem cell and a progenitor cell (a cell programmed for differentiation[6]), respectively. Asymmetric self-renewal of stem cells gives rise to a hierarchy (Figure 25.1), in which one daughter cell retains identical genetic and functional properties of the parent cell rather than becoming a progenitor cell.[6]

The majority of the evidence substantiating the concept of adult stem cells comes from the bone marrow (see Dick[6] for review). In the hematopoietic system a model has been proposed in which hematopoietic stem cells (HSCs) sit at the apex of a hierarchy of lineage-committed, specialized cells, with four possible fates for HSCs: depletion, maintenance, expansion, and death.[6]

In the depletion mode, both the daughter cells become committed to specialization resulting in an initial reduction and subsequent extinction of the stem cell pool. So HSCs are thought to generate at least one daughter cell that retains the property of the parent stem cell via the maintenance or expansion mode in order to preserve the stem cell pool.[6] A further possible outcome is the death of both daughter cells.

LONGEVITY AND PREVENTION OF SENESCENCE IN STEM CELLS

As stem cells maintain tissues during the lifetime of an animal; it is thought that they have strict regulatory

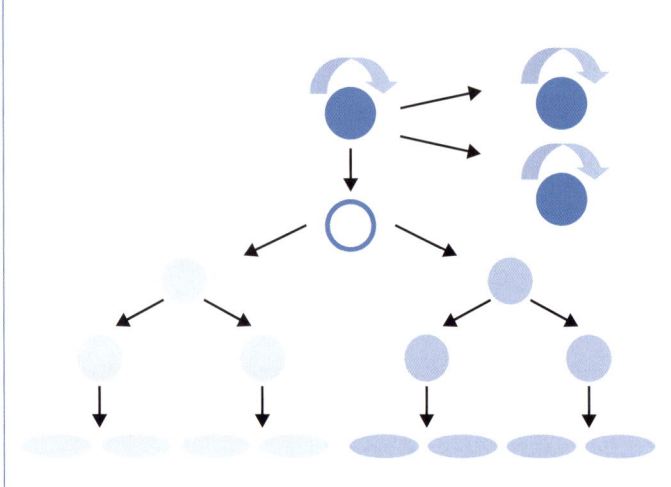

Figure 25.1
Models of stem cell hierarchy in normal tissue. In normal tissues, stem cells *(filled cells)* with high self-renewal capacity (depicted by *arrows*) produce, by asymmetrical division, a new stem cell and a progenitor cell (also known as transit amplifying cells; *hollow cell*) with higher proliferative potential. These progenitor cells upon further cell division become differentiated cells within the tissue *(flat cells)*. The progenitor cells can lead to different lineages *(round light and dark gray cells)*. Conversely, stem cells may undergo symmetrical division to generate two new stem cells. Local or distant signals and various signaling pathways might dictate the decision to undergo a symmetrical or an asymmetrical division.
Adapted from Dick JE. Stem cells: Self-renewal writ in blood. Nature 2003;423:231–233.

mechanisms to delay senescence.[5] Two mechanisms have been delineated: a telomere-dependent and a telomere-independent mechanism.[7–12]

Telomeres are repetitive, noncoding DNA sequences at the end of human chromosomes. Erosion of telomeres with successive cell divisions is considered to be one of the mechanisms regulating cell senescence.[13] Telomerase, a ribonucleoprotein, prevents telomere shortening by adding TTAGGG repeats to the 3' end of chromosomes.[14] In most somatic cells, telomerase activity is low or not detectable, leading to the progressive erosion of telomeres with each cell division.[13,15] Conversely, longer living or immortalized cells have been shown to have higher levels of telomerase.[16]

Hematopoietic stem cells express low-to-moderate levels of telomerase, but the expression levels only partially protect the telomere erosion in these cells.[9] These studies led to the understanding that telomere-independent pathways may also regulate prevention of cell senescence in HSCs, including epigenetic events such as histone modification and chromatin remodeling.

Proteins from the Polycomb family are epigenetic chromatin modifiers involved in cancer development and also in the maintenance of embryonic and adult stem cells.[17] It follows that genes involved in chromatin remodeling and gene expression, such as members of the Polycomb (and also Trithorax families, see Orlando[18] for a review) family, might be directly involved in decisions that affect stem cell fate, including self-renewal, senescence, and possibly aging.[5,17]

Bmi1 was initially identified as a human proto-oncogene that belongs to the Polycomb family of proteins.[17,19] Stem cells express high levels of *Bmi1* and investigations of the mechanism of *Bmi1* action suggest that this protein plays a crucial role in self-renewing cell divisions of adult HSCs as well as neural stem cells, but that it is less critical for the generation of differentiated progeny.[5,10,20–22]

PLURIPOTENCY

To give rise to and maintain complex tissues, the stem cell must be pluripotent, i.e., have the capability to give rise to one or more hierarchies of differentiated cells.[23] Pluripotency is well characterized in the hematopoietic system, where HSCs can reconstitute all cells of the blood (see Weissman[23] for a review). Stem cells from the central nervous system (CNS) can differentiate into neurons, astrocytes, and oligodendrocytes both in vitro and in vivo.[24–28]

Not only do adult stem cells give rise to cell lineages of the tissue of origin, but under certain conditions may differentiate into cell lineages other than the tissue of origin. Thus it has been demonstrated that neural stem cells can differentiate into a variety of hematopoietic cells, including the myeloid and the lymphoid cell lineages.[29] Conversely, under experimental cell culture conditions, mesenchymal stem cells from human and rodent bone marrow can differentiate into cells bearing neuronal markers.[30] Whether this process occurs in vivo due to migration or multipotency of adult stem cells from different tissue remains to be established.[32]

The dual properties of self-renewal and pluripotency are the two main criteria for the identification of stem cells. How should self-renewal and pluripotency be assessed? There are now established protocols to measure these features,[24,27,33] and these methods are briefly discussed in the next section.

ADULT STEM CELL ISOLATION FROM SOLID TISSUES

While characterization of HSCs has led the field and added greatly to our understanding, technical difficulties have meant that the isolation of stem cells from solid tissues has lagged. A major hurdle has been the lack of suitable culture systems that maintain stem cells in culture in an undifferentiated state.[34] A further difficulty is the lack of stem cell surface markers from these tissues[34] (see below). Nonetheless, fractions of cells displaying self-renewal and pluripotency have been isolated from various solid tissues, such as the brain, skin, breast, and eye.[34-38]

TECHNIQUES FOR THE ISOLATION, PROPAGATION AND CHARACTERIZATION OF STEM CELLS

The first hurdle is to extract the small population of stem cells within a solid tissue specimen. A frequently used approach is enzymatic (either collagenase or trypsin) digestion of the solid tissue, followed by mechanical dissociation to yield a single-cell suspension of a mixture of cell types.

Thereafter, a number of techniques have been employed to select stem cells, including fluorescence activated cell sorting (FACS; to select populations of cells with Hoechst 33342 dye exclusion capability or cell surface protein expression), differential collagen adhesion, in-vitro culture of dissociated cells at variable density to permit the formation of either: 1) colonies attached to tissue culture plates; or 2) sphere formation in suspension.[24]

Cell lines with stem cell properties have been established from human or rodent tissues by immortalization with viral genes.[31,39] A human mammary cell line was able to generate ductal-acinar structures in a basement-membrane gel.[31] However, the process of immortalization can itself introduce genetic changes that may alter cellular properties (e.g., self-renewal and prevention of senescence), and, therefore, their relevance to normal tissues and cancer is as yet unclear.

Few model systems using primary culture have been developed that allow the propagation of stem or progenitor cells.[34] Techniques have recently been developed for the cultivation of normal mammary epithelial cells so that they can be maintained in a relatively undifferentiated state. When primary cultures of mammalian mammary epithelium are grown on a solid support they undergo limited replication and differentiation in a highly regulated manner.[36,40,41]

Primary culture of neural stem cells has been advanced by growing the cells as neurospheres, thereby maintaining an undifferentiated, pluripotential population of cells in suspension.[40,42] The spheres float in the culture medium and contain between 4% and 20% stem cells, the remaining cells being at various stages of differentiation. This approach has been used for the isolation and purification of stem cells from various solid tissues.[22,24,33,36,37,43] Self-renewal using the sphere formation technique is assessed by dispersing the cells within the primary sphere and plating single cells to observe a new round of sphere formation (secondary spheres, considered to be self-renewed individual cells

from the primary sphere[24]). This procedure is repeated at least three times to validate self-renewal capability of individual cells.

Colony formation has been used in attempts to isolate stem cells from the prostate and other tissues.[44-46] The initial processing of tissue is identical in colony forming and sphere assays (i.e., mechanical and enzymatic digestion), but the assays differ according to whether the cells are adherent. This and the presence of serum are important factors as epithelial cells are anchorage-dependent for growth and differentiation.[36,47] Another concern is that attached colonies of different morphologies can be observed, and these are not robustly defined.[48,49] Finally, the number of cells within an attached colony can be up to tens of thousands,[48,49] making the identification of individual self-renewing cells more difficult.

Various methods have been utilized to study pluripotency, including facilitated cell attachment to ionically charged glass,[24] the use of solid matrices such as matrigel,[50] and inoculation of stem cell enriched cell fractions into animals.[29,32,33,35] To be considered as candidate stem cells, the cells must show pluripotency.[35,51] For example, the self-renewing spheres from adult brain have the potential to differentiate into three different neuronal lineages: neurons, astrocytes, and oligodendrocytes.[35] This is performed, for example, in the case of neural stem cells, by plating on poly-L-ornithine-coated glass coverslips and allowing the cells to grow for 1 to 8 days.[24,33]

STEM CELL MARKERS

Various proteins have been described as stem cell markers. Some of these proteins are expressed on the cell membranes and so are good candidates for isolating stem cells.

As stem cells form a very small fraction of the total cellular component of the tissues, most stem cell isolation techniques are essentially an enrichment process. Methods of enrichment rely upon the expression of selected membrane proteins using a variety of cell sorting techniques, maintaining the integrity of the cells if they are to be cultured.

Two classes of membrane proteins—cell surface molecules (cluster of differentiation [CD] antigens) and solute carrier proteins—have been used.[52,53] The side population is enriched for stem cells and is characterized by the increased ability of the cells to efflux the nuclear dye Hoechst 33342. Side population cells express high levels of a membrane transporter protein, called BCRP1 (or ABCG2), belonging to the family of multi-drug resistance proteins (ABC family), which facilitates the extrusion of Hoechst 33342 dye.[53-55] The side population cells are also identified by the absence of expression of another cell membrane protein called CD34. Transporter proteins such as the members of P-glycoprotein family of ABC transporters have thus been identified as markers for these cells.[53]

Other proteins (e.g., nestin, Oct4 and Bmi1) have also been identified as markers for stem cells in certain tissues.[12,22,24,53] It has been suggested that proteins such as Bmi1 are required for self-renewal of stem cells, but not for survival or differentiation (thus distinguishing stem cells from progenitors[5,56]). Therefore, some of these proteins markers may facilitate the distinction of stem and non-stem cells. Stem cell markers may not be identical in stem cells from different tissues.

ISOLATION OF ADULT STEM CELLS FROM THE PROSTATE

A recent search of the ISI Web of Science (Thomson, ISI) with the terms "prostate/prostatic epithelial/stem cells" yielded a handful of citations,[48,49,57–63] compared with the thousands of hits using the term "hematopoietic stem cells."

One of the first reports extending the concept of stem cells to the prostate was that of Isaacs and Coffey.[64] Following castration in rats, some basal epithelial cells persist in the prostate. On androgen replacement, the prostate regains its original size,[64] and the epithelial cell population expands. It was concluded that a stem cell population in the basal layer is capable of reconstituting the prostate epithelium.

Bonkhoff and Remberger[65] also proposed a stem cell model for the prostate, suggesting that a small population in the basal cell layer gives rise to all epithelial cell lineages encountered in the normal, hyperplastic, and neoplastic prostate. This population of cells was characterized mainly on the basis of staining with cytokeratins specific for the basal epithelial cells and proliferation associated antigens (such as Ki67, PCNA, and MiB1). These reports[64,65] provide no direct evidence of either self-renewal or pluripotency.

Some studies have tried to identify the subpopulation containing the stem cells. Liu et al[66] separated epithelial cells from the basal and luminal layers and studied these in isolation and with stromal cells. When the basal cells (CD44+), isolated using flow cytometry, were co-cultured with stromal cells, they produced prostate-specific antigen (PSA), suggesting differentiation into luminal cells. As the Bonkhoff and Remberger[65] model of prostate stem cells suggests that stem cells are likely to be present in the basal compartment, the authors reasoned that the CD44+ basal cells possess characteristics of stem cells and are the candidate progenitors of luminal cells. However, no direct evidence for either formation of epithelial like structures or more importantly demonstration of self-renewal was provided.

In two further studies, the ability of single cells to proliferate and form colonies was equated with stem and transit amplifying (progenitor or precursor) cells.[67,68] Peehl et al[69] first described the colony-forming ability of primary cultures of human prostate epithelial cells. Hudson et al[49] extended this work by identifying two distinct colony types on the basis of morphology, i.e., small irregular (approximately 90% of the total number of colonies formed on a plate) and large regular (approximately 10% of the total number of colonies formed on a plate). Evidence of a very high proliferative capacity of the large colonies, coupled with indications of pluripotency based on Matrigel assays of isolated colonies was provided.[49] However, no attempt was made to test whether the cells from the large colonies possess the ability to self-renew.

Also using colony-forming ability in vitro, Collins et al[48] suggested that putative prostate stem cells preselected on the basis of CD44 expression, express higher levels of $\alpha2$-integrin subunit than other cells within the basal layer. About 1% of basal cells were integrin "bright," and these cells could be selected directly from the tissue on the basis of rapid adhesion to type I collagen. Using a similar approach, these authors[70] have also suggested that the cell membrane protein CD133 may also be a marker for putative prostate stem cells.

The Collins study provides the strongest evidence of pluripotency of a cell population isolated from adult prostate. When a basal cell population (1×10^5 to 1×10^6 from the prostate was inoculated into mice, glandular structures developed that stained for PSA and prostatic acid phosphatase.[48] Although it is probable that self-renewing, pluripotent adult prostate stem cells were present in the cell fraction used in the xenografts, various other committed progenitor and differentiation cells present in this fraction might also have given rise to the glandular structures. Furthermore, like other previous attempts to isolate prostate stem cells, no direct evidence of self-renewal of individual cells within this heterogeneous cell fraction was provided.[48,49,70]

Bhatt et al[57] used a fluorescent dye (Hoechst 33342) exclusion approach to identify side populations of prostate cells.[71] Bhatt et al[57] suggested that a subpopulation that accounts for less than 2% of the total cell population could contain the prostate stem cells. Again, experiments to demonstrate either self-renewal or pluripotency have not yet been described.

Telomerase expression was used to identify a subpopulation of prostate cells assumed to contain stem cells.[15] The expression of telomerase was used as an indicator for regulation of senescence and longevity of cells. The telomerase activity was localized to the prostate epithelial basal cells and not to luminal cells.[15]

The authors did not isolate this population for further analysis of self-renewal or pluripotency, but by using the telomerase assay this study provides further evidence that the stem cell population is localized to the basal layer.

The reports on the isolation of putative human prostate stem cells are a step forward, but none of the cell populations were simultaneously shown to have the two essential properties of self renewal and pluripotency. Therefore, the definitive identification and characterization of adult human prostate stem cells has yet to be achieved.

In animals, it is possible to identify stem cells in situ on the basis of their slow turnover and consequent retention of labeled nucleotides. For example, when mice are treated with bromodeoxyuridine, the cells that retain the labeled DNA are long-lived and divide slowly—characteristics of stem cells. Using this technique,[103] it was found that cell fractions containing putative stem cells have greater proliferative activity in vitro and can reconstitute highly branched glandular ductal structures in collagen gels. Cells retaining the label were localized to the proximal region of the ducts.[103]

TUMOR INITIATING OR CANCER STEM CELLS

Cancers may have a stem cell hierarchy similar to that described in the previous section for normal tissues.[72] The concept that the growth and maintenance of a cancer is dependent on a tiny fraction of cells with distinct characteristics has profound implications for the understanding and treatment of cancer.[73]

CANCERS CONTAIN STEM CELLS

Most of the early evidence that cancers contain pluripotent stem cells was derived from studies on hematopoietic malignancies[74] (see Nowell[75] for a review). In many cancers, all the cells appear to have the same abnormal karyotype. The classic example is chronic myeloid leukemia (CML) characterized by the Philadelphia chromosome (Ph[1]). Ph[1] arises through reciprocal translocation between chromosomes 22 and 9. A second line of evidence is based on the inactivation of one of the two X chromosomes in females, and uses genes that are present on the X-chromosome and have a number of isozymes, such as glucose-6-phosphate dehydrogenase. In heterozygous females, typically only one isozyme is expressed, suggesting a monoclonal origin. A third line of evidence is based on the immunoglobulin class expressed by multiple myeloma, which is typically identical in all the tumor cells.

COLONY-FORMING ASSAYS

Various colony-forming assays were developed to study clonogenic cells from leukemias and solid cancers both in vivo and in vitro.[76] One of these methods was called the "human tumor stem cell assay." The tumor was disaggregated by mechanical or enzymatic procedures and the resulting suspension containing mainly single cells plated in a semi-solid medium (agar, agarose, or methylcellulose). A few cells (0.01–1%) gave rise to colonies. Only a small proportion of these showed "self-renewal," in that they had the ability to be disaggregated and replated.[67] The observation that only a small fraction of the cancer cells are able to develop into colonies was equated with the stem cell concept.

The relationship between clonogenic cells and stem cells is uncertain. As with normal cells, the majority of the colonies would be expected to arise from transit amplifying/progenitor cells. There is no means yet available to distinguish the colonies derived from putative stem cells from those derived from non-stem cells within the population, although large size is thought to be an indicator for stem cell colonies.

There were some attempts to use the "human tumor stem cell assay" to study the sensitivity of individual tumors to chemotherapeutic drugs in a variety of cancers.[77] However, the results regarding "individualized chemotherapy" were controversial, and there was considerable criticism of the methodology on theoretical and technical grounds.[78]

STEM CELL HIERARCHIES IN LEUKEMIAS

One of the problems associated with colony-forming assays is that they do not distinguish between stochastic and deterministic models of stem cells. In the stochastic model, all or a much larger proportion of the cells have the capacity to develop colonies. However, each potentially clonogenic cell has only a low probability of developing into a colony, perhaps depending on environmental cues such as growth factors and cell–cell interactions. In the deterministic model, potentially clonogenic cells have defined characteristics and a high probability of developing colonies.

A method of distinguishing between the stochastic and deterministic models was demonstrated for acute myeloid leukemia (AML).[79] Cells selected on the basis of expression of the cell surface proteins $CD34^+D38^-$ were engrafted in non-obese diabetic/severe combined immunodeficient (NOD/SCID) mice.[80-82] The $CD34^+D38^-$ cells formed a variable fraction of the AML cells, up to a maximum of 0.2%. Only these cells were capable of engrafting in NOD/SCID mice following the injection of as few as 5000 cells. Crucially, these cells could be serially transplanted to further mice. $CD34^+D38^+$ cells failed to engraft when up to 500,000 cells were injected. These data support the deterministic model, showing that only a small defined fraction of the cancer cells retain self-renewal capacity. Nevertheless, environmental cues such as growth factors and cell–cell interactions may control the rate of stem cell division.

Another question is whether the cancer stem cell hierarchy of differentiation recapitulates that in the normal tissue from which the cancer was derived. Evidence for this proposal has again been obtained in leukemia stem cells. The most primitive hematopoietic stem cells are the long-term HSC (LT-HSC). A single LT-HSC is sufficient to sustain the complete hematopoietic system of an individual. Long-term HSCs can give rise to short-term HSCs (ST-HSCs), and these in turn can produce lineage-committed progenitor cells (LCPs) responsible for one or a few hematopoietic cell lineages. In the mouse, LT-HSCs give rise to differentiated cells for the life of the mouse, whereas ST-HSCs and LCPs reconstitute lethally irradiated mice for less than 8 weeks.

In order to study leukemia stem cell hierarchy, AML cells were tagged with a gene expressing green fluorescent protein and transplanted into NOD/SCID mice. By tracking individual clones (according to the integration site of the gene) through serial transplants, it was found that both long-term (contributed throughout the serial transplantation) and short-term (occurred transiently) leukemia stem cells were present. Interestingly, a few clones only appeared in the secondary transplants, suggesting that some of the stem cells proliferate very slowly. The data from this study demonstrate that leukemia stem cells have a similar hierarchy to normal HSCs.[83]

The work on AML stem cells, if it can be translated to cancer in general, supports the view that cancers are caricatures of the normal tissue.[84] The cancer stem cells retain the ability to self-renew, and indeed may have a higher rate of self-renewal than normal stem cells. The cancer stem cells also have the capacity to follow normal developmental programs to a varying extent, producing cancers with greater or lesser degrees of differentiation.

STEM CELLS IN SOLID CANCERS

Studies on solid cancers have lagged behind those on hematopoietic malignancies. The delay has been due partly to the greater difficulties producing single suspensions and identifying cell surface markers that are specific for stem cells. Recently however, progress has been made in studies of breast and brain cancers.

Al-Hajj et al[79] established a protocol for the isolation of a subset of cells from breast tumors that have stem cell properties, using the cell membrane protein markers $CD44^+$ and $CD24^{-/low}$. Because breast cancer tissue contains a mixture of cell types, including hematopoietic, fibroblast, endothelial, and mesothelial cells, flow sorting of lineage markers was used to exclude these cells (Lin^+). Single-cell suspensions were separated

into fractions according to the expression of the cell surface markers and injected into the mammary fat pad of NOD/SCID mice.[79] Only a small proportion of the cells were able to develop tumors in mice, the $Lin^-ESA^+D44^+CD24^{low/-}$ fraction. As few as 200 of these cells developed cancers, and the calculations made suggested that this represents at least a 50-fold enrichment for tumor-initiating cells.

Importantly, the xenografts had similar characteristics to the cancers from which they were derived, and contained a similar proportion of cells with the same cell surface characteristics. These cells could be serially transplanted, demonstrating self-renewal.

Techniques used to grow normal neural stem cells were applied to brain tumors.[85] Tumor spheres were grown that could be disaggregated and replated to form secondary spheres. Cytogenetic studies on two of the samples grown in vitro indicated that the cells had genetic changes typical of the tumors of origin. The putative brain cancer stem cells that formed neurospheres were restricted to the fraction of the cells that expressed CD133. Cells derived from tumor spheres were shown to be pluripotent, although the cells preferentially differentiated down the lineage predominant in the tumor of origin (neuronal or glial).

Similar studies were performed on pediatric brain tumors, also showing the stem cell properties of pluripotency and serial recloning.[86] In contrast to normal neural stem cells, the tumor stem cells lived longer and were capable of differentiating into cells expressing a dual cell lineage phenotype, both neuronal and glial. Following grafting to neonatal rat brains, the neurosphere cells migrated, differentiated into neurons and glia, and continued to proliferate for 4 weeks.

IS CANCER A DISEASE OF STEM CELLS?

Cancer could be derived from almost any cell in any lineage. Nevertheless, the concept that cancer usually arises in normal stem cells fits best with the evidence available. There are two strong theoretical reasons for believing that cancer arises in normal stem cells. In most tissues, stem cells are the only cells with a sufficiently long lifespan to generate and pass on the initiating genetic change in cancer. Secondly, both normal and cancer stem are the only cells with the ability to self-renew.[87]

There is evidence that some AML and CML are derived from HSCs (see review by Passegue et al[88]). For most AML, the only cells capable of transmitting the disease in NOD/SCID mice are $CD34^+D38^-$, like normal HSCs.[81,83] This suggests that HSCs are the origin of the leukemia. The t(8,21) translocation is a frequent genetic change found in AML, generating an AML1-ETO fusion protein. This fusion protein can be detected in both normal and leukemic cells in remission, but these cells are not leukemic and can differentiate normally.[89,90] This finding suggests that the translocation occurred in normal HSCs, and that the leukemia developed as a result of further mutation in a subset of HSCs or their progeny. The recent demonstration by Dick's group that the leukemic stem cell compartment is structured as a hierarchy, similar to that of the normal hematopoietic stem cell, provides the strongest evidence yet obtained that, at least in many AML, the target for the initiating genetic change is a normal stem cell.[83]

There is also evidence that the leukemic stem cells express cell surface features characteristic of normal HSCs.[81,83] Similarly the cancer stem cells isolated from pediatric brain cancers also express, at least at the RNA level, genes expressed by neural stem cells, including CD133, *musashi-1*, *sox-2*, *melk*, *PSP*, and *Bmi1*.[86]

Cancer can also arise under certain circumstances from committed progenitor cells or differentiated cells.[88] However, much of this evidence comes from transgenic mice, where the expression of the genes is targeted to committed cells, and, therefore, may not be directly relevant to spontaneous cancer in man.

SIGNALING PATHWAYS CONTROLLING CANCER STEM CELLS

There is evidence of the involvement of various signaling pathways in the maintenance or promotion of stem cell self-renewal such as Notch, PTEN, Sonic hedgehog, and Wnt signaling pathways.[73,87] The transcriptional repressor Bmi1[20] is a factor controlling the proliferative capacity of both normal and leukemic stem cells. Because of the many similarities between normal and cancer stem cells, it seems reasonable to propose that similar pathways control the balance between stem cell self-renewal and commitment to differentiation.

PROGRESSION OF CANCER

The evidence discussed so far indicates that the initiating event or events in cancer development occur in normal stem cells. The theory suggests that cancer attempts to recapitulate normal development,[84] but, for reasons that are not yet clear, the differentiation is only partially successful, and only variably corresponds to the normal tissue-specific pattern. The model accommodates the probability that further genetic changes occur in downstream progenitors (which already carry the genetic changes in the stem cell), and that these cells may be responsible for cancer progression.

PROSTATE CANCER STEM CELLS

Although there is no direct evidence yet available for prostate cancer stem cells, it has been proposed that both benign prostatic hyperplasia[64] and prostate cancers contain stem cells.[61,91,92] Evidence for pluripotent stem cells has been obtained in a xenograft model.[93] For the definitive identification of prostate cancer stem cells, a number of technical advances are needed, including a methodology for reproducibly cloning single cells from cancer samples and the identification of cell surface markers for normal and prostate cancer stem cells.

Prostate cancer cells have proven difficult to grow in vitro. The number of authentic continuous cell lines is small, and many of the cell lines claimed to originate from prostate cancer are derived from other tissues or are cross-contaminated.[94] It is possible to grow primary cultures of human prostate cancer cells, and to confirm their origin from cancer using genetic analysis,[95] but in this study the primary cultures were not cloned.

The "human tumor stem cell assay" was applied to prostate cancer.[96-98] However, the technical and theoretical problems associated with the procedures[78] limited the extent to which the assay was applied.

IMPLICATIONS OF PROSTATE CANCER STEM CELLS

The stem cell concept has profound implications for the management of prostate cancer. The idea that the growth and maintenance of the cancer is dependent on a tiny fraction of cells that have distinct characteristics is the basis for a novel approach to treatment—cancer stem cell therapy. The theory suggests that eradicating this small fraction of cells has the potential to cure the cancer. However, the theory cannot be tested until treatments are developed that reliably eradicate cancer stem cells.

Androgen ablation for the treatment of prostate cancer may kill the more differentiated cells, but may spare the small fraction of slowly dividing stem cells. This theory implies that responses to chemotherapy or endocrine therapy are due to the response of the transit amplifying and differentiated cells. While remission is achieved temporarily in most patients, the stem cells survive to mutate further and bypass subsequent attempts to use the same therapy. This scenario may explain why hormone resistance almost inevitably develops follows endocrine treatment for advanced or metastatic prostate cancer.[99,100] Using a human prostate cancer xenograft, evidence was obtained for the clonal expansion of androgen-independent cells at a frequency of between one in one hundred thousand and one in a million.[101]

There is also the possibility that stem cells are inherently resistant to chemotherapy. One means of enriching for stem cells is to use the side population, based on their exclusion of a dye and sensitivity to verapamil. The cell fraction excludes this dye because it has a high concentration of a pump in its cell membrane that actively pumps drugs out of the cell, making the cells more resistant to cytotoxic agents that can be effluxed by this mechanism. There is evidence that human prostate tissue contains a side population.[57]

The importance of the transcriptional repressor and stem cell marker Bmi1 was discussed in relation to normal hematopoietic and leukemia stem cells.[20] Prostate cancer cells overexpress a protein of the same family called EZH2, whose level of expression is associated with prognosis.[102]

In conclusion, evidence is accumulating that the stem cell theory applies to both normal and neoplastic prostate. Selective targeting of stem cells in the prostate may eventually offer an alternative to surgery or radiotherapy for clinically localized disease. Effective cancer stem cell therapy may require targeting to the cancer stem cells due to differences between normal and cancer stem cells. Prostate cancer stem cell therapy also offers a distant possibility of an effective treatment for men with advanced prostate cancer, eradicating the cells that hormone therapy does not kill.

REFERENCES

1. Kondo M, Wagers AJ, Manz MG, et al. Biology of hematopoietic stem cells and progenitors: implications for clinical application. Annu Rev Immunol 2003;21:759–806.
2. Stevens LC. Studies on transplantable testicular teratomas of strain 129 mice. J Natl Cancer Inst 1958;20:1257–1275.
3. Till JE, McCulloch EA. A direct measurement of the radiation sensitivity of normal mouse bone marrow cells. Radiat Res 1961;14:213–222.
4. Blau HM, Brazelton TR, Weimann JM. The evolving concept of a stem cell: entity or function? Cell 2001;105:829–841.
5. Park IK, Morrison SJ, Clarke MF. Bmi1, stem cells, and senescence regulation. J Clin Invest 2004;113:175–179.
6. Dick JE. Stem cells: Self-renewal writ in blood. Nature 2003;423:231–233.
7. Morrison SJ, Prowse KR, Ho P, et al. Telomerase activity in hematopoietic cells is associated with self-renewal potential. Immunity 1996;5:207–216.
8. Pathak S. Organ- and tissue-specific stem cells and carcinogenesis. Anticancer Res 2002;22:1353–1356.
9. Yui J, Chiu CP, Lansdorp PM. Telomerase activity in candidate stem cells from fetal liver and adult bone marrow. Blood 1998;91:3255–3262.
10. Lessard J, Baban S, Sauvageau G. Stage-specific expression of polycomb group genes in human bone marrow cells. Blood 1998;91:1216–1224.
11. Molofsky AV, Pardal R, Iwashita T, et al. Bmi-1 dependence distinguishes neural stem cell self-renewal from progenitor proliferation. Nature 2003;425:962–967.
12. Park IK, Qian D, Kiel M, et al. Bmi-1 is required for maintenance of adult self-renewing haematopoietic stem cells. Nature 2003;423:302–305.
13. Levy MZ, Allsopp RC, Futcher AB, et al. Telomere end-replication problem and cell aging. J Mol Biol 1992;225:951–960.
14. Morin GB. The human telomere terminal transferase enzyme is a ribonucleoprotein that synthesizes TTAGGG repeats. Cell 1989;9:521–529.
15. Paradis V, Dargere D, Laurendeau I, et al. Expression of the RNA component of human telomerase (hTR) in prostate cancer, prostatic intraepithelial neoplasia, and normal prostate tissue. J Pathol 1999;189:213–218.
16. Kim NW, Piatyszek MA, Prowse KR, et al. Specific association of human telomerase activity with immortal cells and cancer. Science 1994;266:2011–2015.
17. Valk-Lingbeek ME, Bruggeman SW, van Lohuizen M. Stem cells and cancer; the polycomb connection. Cell 2004;118:409–418.
18. Orlando V. Polycomb, epigenomes, and control of cell identity. Cell 2003;112:599–606.
19. van Lohuizen M, Verbeek S, Scheijen B, et al. Identification of cooperating oncogenes in E mu-myc transgenic mice by provirus tagging. Cell 1991;65:737–752.
20. Lessard J, Sauvageau G. Bmi-1 determines the proliferative capacity of normal and leukaemic stem cells. Nature 2003;423:255–260.
21. Lessard J, Schumacher A, Thorsteinsdottir U, et al. Functional antagonism of the Polycomb-Group genes eed and Bmi1 in hemopoietic cell proliferation. Genes Dev 1999;13:2691–2703.
22. Molofsky AV, Pardal R, Iwashita T, et al. Bmi-1 dependence distinguishes neural stem cell self-renewal from progenitor proliferation. Nature 2003;425:962–967.
23. Weissman IL. Stem cells: units of development, units of regeneration, and units in evolution. Cell 2000;100:157–168.
24. Rietze RL, Valcanis H, Brooker GF, et al. Purification of a pluripotent neural stem cell from the adult mouse brain. Nature 2001;412:736–739.
25. Gage FH. Mammalian neural stem cells. Science 2000;287:1433–1438.
26. Reynolds BA, Weiss S. Generation of neurons and astrocytes from isolated cells of the adult mammalian central nervous system. Science 1992;255:1707–1710.
27. Qian X, Shen Q, Goderie SK, et al. Timing of CNS cell generation: a programmed sequence of neuron and glial cell production from isolated murine cortical stem cells. Neuron 2000;28:69–80.
28. Morshead CM, van der Kooy D. Disguising adult neural stem cells. Curr Opin Neurobiol 2004;14:125–131.
29. Bjornson CRR, Rietze RL, Reynolds BA, et al. Turning brain into blood: A hematopoietic fate adopted by adult neural stem cells in vivo. Science 1999;283:534–537.
30. Sanchez-Ramos J, Song S, Cardozo-Pelaez F, A et al. Adult bone marrow stromal cells differentiate into neural cells in vitro. Exp Neurol 2000;164:247–256.
31. Gudjonsson T, Villadsen R, Nielsen HL, et al. Isolation, immortalization, and characterization of a human breast epithelial cell line with stem cell properties. Genes Dev 2002;16:693–706.
32. Mezey E, Chandross KJ, Harta G, et al. Turning blood into brain: Cells bearing neuronal antigens generated in vivo from bone marrow. Science 2000;290:1779–1782.
33. Li H, Liu H, Heller S. Pluripotent stem cells from the adult mouse inner ear. Nat Med 2003;9:1293–1299.
34. Dontu G, Al Hajj M, Abdallah WM, et al. Stem cells in normal breast development and breast cancer. Cell Prolif 2003;36:59–72.
35. McKay R. Stem cells in the central nervous system. Science 1997;276:66–71.
36. Dontu G, Abdallah WM, Foley JM, et al. In vitro propagation and transcriptional profiling of human mammary stem/progenitor cells. Genes Dev 2003;17:1253–1270.
37. Tropepe V, Coles BL, Chiasson BJ, et al. Retinal stem cells in the adult mammalian eye. Science 2000;287:2032–2036.
38. Toma JG, Akhavan M, Fernandes KJ, et al. Isolation of multipotent adult stem cells from the dermis of mammalian skin. Nat Cell Biol 2001;3:778–784.
39. Kondo T, Setoguchi T, Taga T. Persistence of a small subpopulation of cancer stem-like cells in the C6 glioma cell line. Proc Natl Acad Sci USA 2004;101:781–786.
40. Reynolds BA, Weiss S. Clonal and population analyses demonstrate that an EGF-responsive mammalian embryonic CNS precursor is a stem cell. Dev Biol 1996;175:1–13.
41. Romanov SR, Kozakiewicz BK, Holst CR, et al. Normal human mammary epithelial cells spontaneously escape senescence and acquire genomic changes. Nature 2001;409:633–637.

42. Weiss S, Dunne C, Hewson J, et al. Multipotent CNS stem cells are present in the adult mammalian spinal cord and ventricular neuroaxis. J Neurosci 1996;16:7599–7609.

43. Carpenter MK, Cui X, Hu ZY, et al. In vitro expansion of a multipotent population of human neural progenitor cells. Exp Neurol 1999;158:265–278.

44. Verfaillie CM, Pera MF, Lansdorp PM. Stem cells: hype and reality. Hematology (Am Soc Hematol Educ Program) 2002;369–391.

45. Humphries RK, Eaves AC, Eaves CJ. Self-renewal of hemopoietic stem cells during mixed colony formation in vitro. Proc Natl Acad Sci USA 1981;78:3629–3633.

46. Johnson GR, Metcalf D. Pure and mixed erythroid colony formation in vitro stimulated by spleen conditioned medium with no detectable erythropoietin. Proc Natl Acad Sci USA 1977;74:3879–3882.

47. Streuli CH, Gilmore AP. Adhesion-mediated signaling in the regulation of mammary epithelial cell survival. J Mammary Gland Biol Neoplasia 1999;4:183–191.

48. Collins AT, Habib FK, Maitland NJ, et al. Identification and isolation of human prostate epithelial stem cells based on alpha(2)beta(1)-integrin expression. J Cell Sci 2001;114:3865–3872.

49. Hudson DL, O'Hare M, Watt FM, et al. Proliferative heterogeneity in the human prostate: evidence for epithelial stem cells. Lab Invest 2000;80:1243–1250.

50. Aarum J, Sandberg K, Haeberlein SL, et al. Migration and differentiation of neural precursor cells can be directed by microglia. Proc Natl Acad Sci USA 2003;100:15983–15988.

51. Jiang Y, Jahagirdar BN, Reinhardt RL, et al. Pluripotency of mesenchymal stem cells derived from adult marrow. Nature 2002;418:41–49.

52. Zhou S, Morris JJ, Barnes Y, Lan L, et al. Bcrp1 gene expression is required for normal numbers of side population stem cells in mice, and confers relative protection to mitoxantrone in hematopoietic cells in vivo. Proc Natl Acad Sci USA 2002;99:12339–12344.

53. Zhou S, Schuetz JD, Bunting KD, et al. The ABC transporter Bcrp1/ABCG2 is expressed in a wide variety of stem cells and is a molecular determinant of the side-population phenotype. Nat Med 2001;7:1028–1034.

54. Welm BE, Tepera SB, Venezia T, et al. Sca-1(pos) cells in the mouse mammary gland represent an enriched progenitor cell population. Dev Biol 2002;245:42–56.

55. Bunting KD. ABC transporters as phenotypic markers and functional regulators of stem cells. Stem Cells 2002;20:11–20.

56. Krishnamurthy P, Ross DD, Nakanishi T, et al. The stem cell marker Bcrp/ABCG2 enhances hypoxic cell survival through interactions with heme. J Biol Chem 2004;279:24218–24225.

57. Bhatt RI, Brown MD, Hart CA, et al. Novel method for the isolation and characterisation of the putative prostatic stem cell. Cytometry Part A 2003;54A:89–99.

58. Signoretti S, Waltregny D, Dilks J, et al. p63 is a prostate basal cell marker and is required for prostate development. Am J Pathol 2000;157:1769–1775.

59. Anderson KM, Bonomi P, Harris JE. Does an inability to eradicate normal stem cells preclude the cure of some cancers? Medical Hypotheses 1996;47:31–34.

60. Foster CS, Dodson A, Karavana V, et al. Prostatic stem cells. J Pathol 2002;197:551–565.

61. De Marzo AM, Nelson WG, Meeker AK, et al. Stem cell features of benign and malignant prostate epithelial cells. J Urol 1998;160:2381–2392.

62. De Marzo AM, Meeker AK, Epstein JI, et al. Prostate stem cell compartments—Expression of the cell cycle inhibitor p27(Kip1) in normal, hyperplastic, and neoplastic cells. Am J Pathol 1998;153:911–919.

63. Bonkhoff H, Remberger K. Morphogenesis of benign prostatic hyperplasia and prostate carcinoma. Pathologe 1998;19:12–20.

64. Isaacs JT, Coffey DS. Etiology and disease process of benign prostatic hyperplasia. Prostate Suppl 1989;2:33–50.

65. Bonkhoff H, Remberger K. Differentiation pathways and histogenetic aspects of normal and abnormal prostatic growth: a stem cell model. Prostate 1996;28:98–106.

66. Liu AY, True LD, LaTray L, et al. Cell-cell interaction in prostate gene regulation and cytodifferentiation. Proc Natl Acad Sci USA 1997;94:10705–10710.

67. Buick RN, Pollak MN. Perspectives on clonogenic tumor cells, stem cells, and oncogenes. Cancer Res 1984;44:4909–4918.

68. Popova NV, Teti KA, Wu KQ, et al. Identification of two keratinocyte stem cell regulatory loci implicated in skin carcinogenesis. Carcinogenesis 2003;24:417–425.

69. Peehl DM, Wong ST, Stamey TA. Clonal growth characteristics of adult human prostatic epithelial cells. In Vitro Cell Dev Biol 1988;24:530–536.

70. Richardson GD, Robson CN, Lang SH, et al. CD133, a novel marker for human prostatic epithelial stem cells. J Cell Sci 2004;117:3539–3545.

71. Goodell MA, Brose K, Paradis G, et al. Isolation and functional properties of murine hematopoietic stem cells that are replicating in vivo. J Exp Med 1996;183:1797–1806.

72. Mackillop WJ, Ciampi A, Till JE, et al. A stem cell model of human tumor growth: implications for tumor cell clonogenic assays. J Natl Cancer Inst 1983;70:9–16.

73. Reya T, Morrison SJ, Clarke MF, Weissman IL. Stem cells, cancer, and cancer stem cells. Nature 2001;414:105–111.

74. McCulloch EA. The stem cell origin of neoplasia. 1984. National Cancer Institute Monograph.

75. Nowell PC. The clonal evolution of tumor cell populations. Science 1976;194:23–28.

76. Steel GG, Stephens TC. Stem cells in tumours. In Potten CS (ed): Stem cells: their identification and characterisation. London: Churchill Livingstone, 1983, pp 271–293.

77. Salmon SE, Hamburger AW, Soehnlen B, et al. Quantitation of differential sensitivity of human-tumor stem cells to anticancer drugs. N Engl J Med 1978;298:1321–1327.

78. Selby P, Buick RN, Tannock I. A critical appraisal of the "human tumor stem-cell assay". N Engl J Med 1983;308:129–134.

79. Al Hajj M, Wicha MS, Benito-Hernandez A, et al. Prospective identification of tumorigenic breast cancer cells. Proc Natl Acad Sci USA 2003;100:3983–3988.

80. Lapidot T, Sirard C, Vormoor J, et al. A cell initiating human acute myeloid leukaemia after transplantation into SCID mice. Nature 1994;367:645–648.

81. Bonnet D, Dick JE. Human acute myeloid leukemia is organized as a hierarchy that originates from a primitive hematopoietic cell. Nat Med 1997;3:730–737.

82. Larochelle A, Vormoor J, Hanenberg H, et al. Identification of primitive human hematopoietic cells capable of repopulating NOD/SCID mouse bone marrow: implications for gene therapy. Nat Med 1996;2:1329–1337.

83. Hope KJ, Jin L, Dick JE. Acute myeloid leukemia originates from a hierarchy of leukemic stem cell classes that differ in self-renewal capacity. Nature Immunology 2004;5:738–743.

84. Pierce GB, Speers WC. Tumors as caricatures of the process of tissue renewal: prospects for therapy by directing differentiation. Cancer Res 1988;48:1996–2004.

85. Singh SK, Clarke ID, Terasaki M, et al. Identification of a cancer stem cell in human brain tumors. Cancer Res 2003;63:5821–5828.

86. Hemmati HD, Nakano I, Lazareff JA, et al. Cancerous stem cells can arise from pediatric brain tumors. Proc Natl Acad Sci USA 2003;100:15178–15183.

87. Pardal R, Clarke MF, Morrison SJ. Applying the principles of stem-cell biology to cancer. Nat Rev Cancer 2003;3:895–902.

88. Passegue E, Jamieson CH, Ailles LE, et al. Normal and leukemic hematopoiesis: are leukemias a stem cell disorder or a reacquisition of stem cell characteristics? Proc Natl Acad Sci USA 2003;100:11842–11849.

89. Miyamoto T, Nagafuji K, Akashi K, et al. Persistence of multipotent progenitors expressing AML1/ETO transcripts in long-term remission patients with t(8;21) acute myelogenous leukemia. Blood 1996;87:4789–4796.

90. Miyamoto T, Weissman IL, Akashi K. AML1/ETO-expressing nonleukemic stem cells in acute myelogenous leukemia with 8;21

chromosomal translocation. Proc Natl Acad Sci USA 2000;97:7521–7526.

91. Bonkhoff H. Role of the basal cells in premalignant changes of the human prostate: a stem cell concept for the development of prostate cancer. Eur Urol 1996;30:201–205.

92. van Leenders GJ, Schalken JA. Stem cell differentiation within the human prostate epithelium: implications for prostate carcinogenesis. BJU Int 2001;88 Suppl 2:35–42.

93. Huss WJ, Gray DR, Werdin ES, et al. Evidence of pluripotent human prostate stem cells in a human prostate primary xenograft model. Prostate 2004;60:77–90.

94. van Bokhoven A, Varella-Garcia M, Korch C, et al. Molecular characterization of human prostate carcinoma cell lines. Prostate 2003;57:205–225.

95. Bright RK, Vocke CD, Emmert-Buck MR, et al. Generation and genetic characterization of immortal human prostate epithelial cell lines derived from primary cancer specimens. Cancer Res 1997;57:995–1002.

96. Kirkels WJ, Pelgrim OE, Hoogenboom AM, et al. Patterns of tumor colony development over time in soft-agar culture. Int J Cancer 1983;32:399–406.

97. Dittrich C, Schmidbauer CP, Havelec L, et al. Assessment of the human tumor cloning assay for urologic malignancies with special emphasis on bladder cancer. Oncology 1986;43:40–45.

98. Sakuramoto T, Kubota Y, Kitajima N, et al. [Soft agar culture of human prostatic carcinoma—effect of testosterone on the clonal growth of the cells]. Hinyokika Kiyo 1985;31:1717–1721.

99. Bui M, Reiter RE. Stem cell genes in androgen-independent prostate cancer. Cancer Metastasis Rev 1998;17:391–399.

100. Feldman BJ, Feldman D. The development of androgen-independent prostate cancer. Nat Rev Cancer 2001;1:34–45.

101. Craft N, Chhor C, Tran C, et al. Evidence for clonal outgrowth of androgen-independent prostate cancer cells from androgen-dependent tumors through a two-step process. Cancer Res 1999;59:5030–5036.

102. Varambally S, Dhanasekaran SM, Zhou M, et al. The polycomb group protein EZH2 is involved in progression of prostate cancer. Nature 2002;419:624–629.

103. Tsujimura A, Koikawa Y, Salm S, et al. Proximal location of mouse prostate epithelial stem cells: a model of prostatic homeostasis. J Cell Biol 2002;157:1257–1265.

Rationale for molecular markers of prostate cancer 26

Lionel L Bañez, Shiv Srivastava, Judd W Moul

INTRODUCTION

What we presently know about the disease entity known as prostate cancer has grown tremendously since the first documented case by Langstaff in 1815.[1] Accumulation of knowledge since the mid-1980s has risen logarithmically, bolstered by the advancement of the molecular sciences. Experts in cancer biology and oncology recognize that molecular makers will play a major role not only in scientific investigations on prostate cancer but also in the clinical aspects of diagnosis, prognosis, therapeutics, and post-therapeutic monitoring.[2] The continuous growth and interest in the study of pertinent biomarkers of disease are reflected in the translational research initiatives emphasizing the need to "bridge the gap" between the basic science discoveries and clinical utility of the biomarkers ultimately benefiting the patients.[3] It is the purpose of this chapter to provide evidence that molecular markers have promising potential to impact upon the changing face of prostate cancer. Comprehensive details on the biology and current performance of these molecular markers are beyond the scope of this chapter and will be discussed elsewhere.

PROSTATE-SPECIFIC ANTIGEN—A MOLECULAR MARKER HISTORICAL PERSPECTIVE

To fully appreciate and comprehend the impact of molecular markers on present-day prostate oncology, one has to revisit the history of the archetypal significant molecular marker for prostate cancer (Figure 26.1). Prostate-specific antigen (PSA) was discovered almost half a century after prostatic acid phosphatase (PAP), the first key serum marker for monitoring of prostate cancer relapse.[4–5] In 1986, the United States Food and Drug Administration initially approved the use of serum PSA for post-therapeutic monitoring of prostate cancer relapse. Adapting the decision-making paradigm for ultrasound-guided prostate biopsy based on digital rectal examination (DRE) findings and serum PSA measurements in men suspected of having prostate malignancy led to its approval for use in early detection and prostate cancer screening.[6] Widely-used since the 1980s, PSA screening has led to a massive stage shift, wherein a decrease in prevalence of advanced stage disease at the time of diagnosis along with a decline in death rates due to prostate cancer[7] underscores the difference one significant biomarker makes to the epidemiology of this disease.

The clinical utility of PSA has extended beyond static serum measurements for early detection and post-treatment follow-up with the conception of PSA derivatives, and the discovery of its isoforms. PSA density, which factors in the size of the prostate gland with serum PSA,[8] PSA velocity (rate of increase of serum PSA over time),[9] PSA complexed with α1-antichymotrypsin (PSA-ACT)[10] and age-specific PSA cutoffs[11] are currently being used to improve prostate cancer specificity and minimize false positives due to benign prostate conditions, such as benign prostatic hyperplasia (BPH) and prostatitis, that also cause a modest elevation of serum PSA. The most frequently used method to increase cancer specificity involves measuring uncomplexed or free PSA (FPSA), which is usually higher in BPH, and computing the percentage

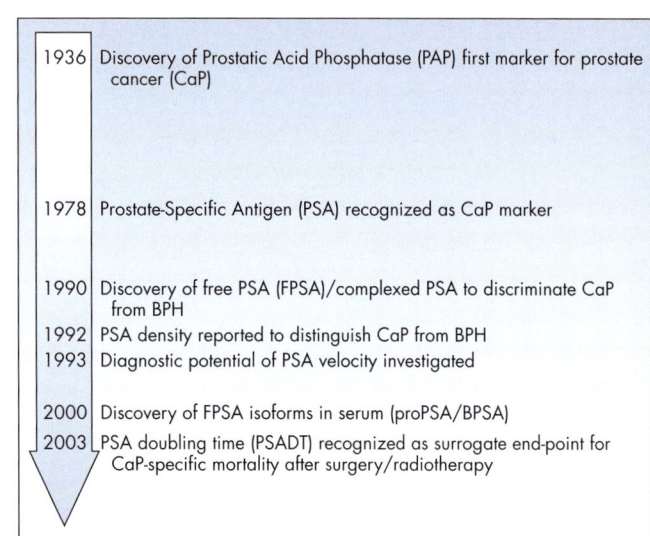

Fig. 26.1
Historic perspective of prostate-specific antigen and its utility in the management of prostate cancer. (BPH, benign prostatic hyperplasia; CaP, prostate cancer.)

ratio of free to total PSA (%FPSA).[12] As much as 20% of unnecessary biopsies may be avoided by using %FPSA missing only 5% of cancers that tend to be low-grade.[13] Ongoing studies on the diagnostic potential of the precursor form of PSA, proPSA have renewed scientific interest in investigating the various isoforms of this classical prostate cancer molecular marker.[14] Prognostic potential of PSA has evolved from traditional monitoring of post-treatment PSA to determine biochemical recurrence[15] to more definitive prognosticators such as PSA doubling time (PSA-DT), which serves as a surrogate end-point for cancer-specific mortality after primary treatment with radical prostatectomy or radiation therapy.[16] The effects of PSA as a molecular biomarker of prostate cancer are definitely far-reaching, as they are dynamic, galvanizing its place in the study of prostate cancer as the standard to which future markers will be measured.[17]

GENETIC BASIS FOR MOLECULAR MARKERS

The genetic basis for molecular markers is rooted in the mutations and other genetic alterations observed through intensive research investigations of the prostate cancer genome. Promising leads both in biology and translational research areas are beginning to emerge from recent genomics and proteomics technology, as well as some traditional approaches.[18] However, heterogeneity of prostate cancer has been one of the key factors that has impeded molecular characterization of prostate cancer.[19] Though much remains to be learned about specific molecular defects associated with prostate cancer onset and progression, the past decade has given us a host of candidate molecular markers that may be of value in the conduct of scientific research and clinical practice.

The genetic paradigm that carcinogenesis and neoplastic transformation is accompanied by progressive and cumulative changes in various genes has been influential to studies directed at searching for a genetic basis for prostate cancer.[20] Gene alterations that are thought to affect only the familial subset of prostate cancers are not entirely clear. Reports on familial prostate cancer susceptibility genes such as *RNASEL*[21] and *MSR1*[22] are provocative and are gradually lending to our understanding of underlying genetic mechanisms of disease. Deletions in certain chromosomal regions have also been identified in prostate cancer, and include 2q13-q33, 5q14-q23, 6q16-q22, 7q22-q32, 8p21-p22, 9p21-p22, 10q23-q24, 12p12-13, 13q14-q21, 16q22-24, and 18q21-q24.[23] Thorough evaluation of prostate cancer-related proto-oncogenes, tumor suppressor genes, and metastasis suppressor genes are currently underway to uncover useful biomarkers and targets for novel gene-based therapies.

Proto-oncogenes normally encode various proteins that function as growth factors, growth factor receptors, regulators of transcription and replication, as well as modifiers of protein function. Alterations in these critical processes of normal cell proliferation can cause neoplasia and aberrant cell growth. Therefore, it is plausible that therapeutic options may be directed at these genetic aberrations. The proto-oncogenes that have been implicated in prostate cancer are listed in Table 26.1. Among them, c-*MYC*[24] and c-*ERBB2*[25] have been extensively studied, however, results have been conflicting and no single oncogene has been conclusively linked with the initiation and early progression of prostate cancer. Recently, genes involved in signal transduction pathways coding for transcription factors which integrate signals that regulate cell growth and differentiation, stress responses and tumorigenesis such as *ERG1*[26] may provide possible oncogenic basis of disease.

Table 26.1 Genes implicated in primary prostate cancer*

Gene	Chromosome locus	Protein function
Oncogenes		
BCL2	18q21.3	Suppresses apoptosis
c-ERBB2	17p11.2	Receptor complex component
EZH2	7q35	Transcription repressor
c-MYC	8q24.12	Regulates gene transcription
n-MYC	2p24.1	Regulates gene transcription
H-RAS	11p15.5	Intrinsic GTPase activity
N-RAS	1p13.2	Intrinsic GTPase activity
K-RAS2	12p12.1	Intrinsic GTPase activity
RAF	3p25	Signal transduction
Tumor suppressor genes		
BRCA1	17q21	Central role in DNA repair
BRCA2	13q12.3	May participate in DNA repair associated pathway
CDH1 (E-cadherin)	16q22.1	Cell adhesion; invasion suppressor
GSTP1	11q13	Conjugation of reduced glutathione
KLF6	10p15	Transcription activator
MSR1	8p22–23	Mediates endocytosis of nutrient macromolecules
p53	17p13.1	Regulates cell division
PTEN	10q23.3	Regulates AKT1 signaling pathway
RB	13q14.1–14.2	Regulates other genes
RNASEL	1q25	Mediates interferon activity and resistance to viral infection
ST7	7q31.1	Unknown

*Information researched from GeneCards online database (http://bioinfo.weizmann.ac.il/cards/index.shtml).

Defects in tumor suppressor genes (TSGs) and the absence of their products may induce neoplasia. From a molecular standpoint, TSGs can be considered attractive targets for cancer chemoprevention.[27] Studies exploring the role of TSGs in prostate cancer involve examining prostate cancers for regions of consistent loss of heterozygosity (LOH), linkage analysis in familial prostate cancer pedigrees, and positional cloning. Tumor suppressor genes implicated in prostate cancer are listed in Table 26.1. Among these, *PTEN*, which acts as a negative regulator of the AKT pathway,[28] was found to be inactivated in primary prostate cancer.[29] Concurrent with proto-oncogenes, investigating these TSGs will provide better insight in prostate tumorigenesis and would potentially elucidate prognostic markers and accessible targets for therapy.

It is thought that products of metastasis suppressor genes function to prevent extraprostatic spread of prostate cancer and are involved in progression of prostate cancer from localized to disseminated disease.[30] The metastasis suppressor genes implicated in prostate cancer include *KAI1*, which codes for a TM4 protein that functions in cell-extracellular matrix binding,[31] *CD44* for which decreased expression was demonstrated to be an independent prognostic marker for surgically treated prostate cancer,[32] and maspin, which is regulated by the TSG encoding p53 and is associated with inhibition of tumor cell invasion and metastasis.[33]

Understanding the genetics and signaling pathways that impact treatable hormone-sensitive prostate cancer to its lethal hormone-refractory form is being addressed through studies on the androgen receptor (*AR*) gene. *AR* mutations, gene amplification, elevated expression of *AR*, and frequency of trinucleotide (CAG and GGC) repeats[34] have been extensively studied in human prostate cancer and in experimental models. In general, it appears that gain of *AR* function may associate with prostate cancer.

In addition to the analysis of chromosomal hot spots, current strategies for defining prostate cancer-specific genetic alterations include comparison of the global gene expression profiles in cancer cells and corresponding normal cells by differential display,[35] serial analysis of gene expression (SAGE),[36] and cDNA microarrays.[37] Innovative techniques of sample acquisition such as laser capture microdissection (LCM) under direct microscopic visualization permit rapid one-step procurement of pure malignant or benign cell populations from a heterogeneous section of prostate tissue.[38]

Earlier studies have shown that prostate-specific membrane antigen (PSMA),[39] human glandular kallikrein 2 (HK2)[40] and telomerase[41] show prostate cancer-associated elevated expression and have promising potential diagnostic or prognostic utility. Prostate cancer gene-discovery efforts identified genes showing prostate cancer associated overexpression such as prostate stem cell antigen (PSCA),[42] PCGEM1,[43] PSGR,[44] PMEPA1,[45] differential display 3 (DD3),[46] and STEAP,[47] which are not only prostate-specific/abundant but also show elevated expression in cancer and may have diagnostic or prognostic value. Studies evaluating prostate cancer-associated high-throughput gene expression profiling also revealed consistent overexpression of HEPSIN[48–49] and AMACR[50–51] in prostate cancer, and these genes represent attractive targets for biomarkers and novel therapy. However, decreased expression of HEPSIN as well as AMACR have been noted in tumors associated with advanced disease. Conversely, reduced or loss of expression of prostate cancer-associated genes such as that encoding pi-class glutathione S-transferase (GSTP1),[52] p27,[53] p63,[54] maspin,[55] annexin 7 (ANX7)[56] and NKX3.1[57] may also be potentially useful in defining prostate cancer onset or progression. Prostate cancer markers currently being studied for clinical use are listed in Table 26.2. Both mutational and gene-expression strategies are now providing prostate cancer-specific molecular signatures that need to be validated in prospective fashion and in the multicenter setting.

CANDIDATE MARKERS—MEETING THE CHALLENGES

As previously mentioned, scientific advancements in the molecular sciences within the last decades have intensified current investigations in biomarker research especially in the cancer field. This rapid evolution in cutting-edge molecular technology provides the infrastructure that has led to the current discovery and development of markers that exerts its influence in nearly every clinical aspect of prostate cancer today. Through meticulous evaluation and validation, the benefits gained from use of molecular markers are attempting to address the current unmet needs seen in clinical practice.

SCREENING AND EARLY DETECTION

Though the contribution of PSA to the early diagnosis of prostate cancer is seldom questioned, the limitation of the clinical assay in terms of poor specificity and low positive predictive value, especially in the "gray zone" (2.5–10 ng/mL),[58] cannot be ignored. Recent large-scale chemopreventive trials, such as the Prostate Cancer Prevention Trial (PCPT), have provided valuable insight on the natural history of prostate cancer and quantifiable limitations in both the specificity and

sensitivity of the presently accepted early detection strategies.[59] The alarming finding that 15.4% of the tumors that would have been otherwise missed, due to negative DRE findings and serum PSA of less than 4 ng/mL, were actually high-grade tumors has surpassed concerns of poor specificity in some respects.[60] These limitations in the classical molecular marker PSA necessitate the elucidation of novel molecular markers, which not only detect prostate malignancy with greater accuracy but distinguish between indolent low-grade cancer that may be treated with watchful waiting and lethal high-grade disease that requires more radical treatment options and closer post-treatment follow-up.

Succeeding studies on the nature of PSA has led to in-depth characterization of the various isoforms of PSA that may overcome specificity issues. The ratio of the zymogen proPSA, which constitutes a third of the total FPSA in serum of prostate cancer patients, was shown to improve specificity for cancer detection.[61] ProPSA can be further subdivided into its subforms: [–7] pPSA (its native form), [–5] pPSA and [–4] pPSA (truncated forms), and [–2] pPSA (also truncated), the subform most associated with prostate cancer.[62]

Limitations initially seen in single-marker assays are being addressed by multi-analyte proteomics approaches.[63] High-throughput techniques are being complemented by innovative bioinformatics analysis leading to the introduction of the protein profiling paradigm wherein patterns of low abundance proteins in serum as elucidated by surface enhanced laser desorption/ionization (SELDI) mass spectrometry are thought to contain diagnostic information.[64] Preliminary studies with promising high sensitivities and high specificities using optimized sample and ProteinChip processing protocols[65–66] or mass spectrometers with improved resolutions[67] have progressed to multi-institutional collaborative efforts to address issues of portability and reproducibility[68] with promising preliminary results.[69]

Other molecular-based techniques, such as detection of circulating epithelial cells in the peripheral blood of prostate cancer patients through reverse transcription polymerase chain reaction (RT-PCR) utilizing prostate markers such as PSA[70–71] and HK2,[71] have received renewed interest due to technical improvement and perceived additional value for prognosis and post-treatment monitoring. Unconventional but accessible biologic specimens, such as voided urine collected after prostatic massage, have been proven to be an alternative resource for clinical diagnostic and prognostic assays utilizing molecular markers such as DD3.[72]

TISSUE DIAGNOSIS

Molecular markers are providing pathologists with objective parameters that aid in accurate tissue

Table 26.2 Known and candidate molecular markers of prostate cancer by subcellular location*

Location	Marker	Function
Nucleus	Cyclin D1	Essential for the control of the cell cycle at the G1/S (start) transition
	Id-1	Transcription factor which regulates cellular differentiation
	EZH2	May be involved in the regulation of gene transcription and chromatin structure
	Ki67	Accelerates apoptosis by inducing the release of cytochrome c and activation of CASP3
	KLF6	Transcriptional activator with a possible role in B-cell growth and development
	MXI1	Regulator of growth-related genes
	NFκB	Involved in immune response and acute phase reactions
	NKX3.1	Transcription factor, which regulates proliferation of glandular epithelium in prostate
	p16	Cyclin-dependent kinase inhibitor which regulates proliferation of cells
	p21	Cyclin-dependent kinase inhibitor
	p27	Cyclin-dependent kinase inhibitor
	PC-1	Binds RNA and hydrolyzes nucleoside 5′ triphosphates
	PDEF	Interacts with the androgen receptor and activates PSA gene expression
	RB1	Acts as tumor suppressor
	TERT	Reverse transcriptase essential for the replication of chromosome termini
Nucleus/cytoplasm	AKT1	General protein kinase capable of phosphorylating several known proteins
	DD3	Noncoding gene of unknown function
	p53	Tumor suppressor which acts as a regulator of other genes
	PART1	Unknown
	PCGEM1	Noncoding gene of unknown function
	PSDR1	Exhibits an oxidoreductive catalytic activity towards retinoids
	UROC28	Choline/ethanolamine kinase with unknown biological function
Cytoplasm	BAX	Accelerates programmed cell death by antagonizing the apoptosis repressor BCL2
	Caspase 8	Responsible for TNFRSF6/FAS-mediated and TNFRSF1A-induced cell death
	DRG1	May play a role in cell proliferation, differentiation and death
	ETK/BMK	Activity is required for interleukin 6 (IL6)-induced differentiation and signal transduction
	GSTP1	Conjugation of reduced glutathione to hydrophobic electrophiles
	HSP27	Chaperone involved in stress resistance and actin organization
	HSP70	Chaperone involved in cell stress response
	HSP90	Molecular chaperone with ATPase activity
	PCTA1	Unknown
	PI3K	Lipid kinase involved in signaling
	PIM1	Involved in signal transduction in blood cells
	PTEN	Potential tumor suppressor involved in regulation of AKT1 signaling pathway
	RASSF1	Binds RAS and is involved in cell signaling
	RNASEL	Endoribonuclease which mediates interferon action and resistance to viral infection
Mitochondria	AMACR	Racemization and stereoisomerization of fatty acid CoA esters
	BCL2	Involved in membrane permeability and apoptosis
	COX2	Prostaglandin synthase which mediates inflammatory response
Other cellular organelles	Catenin	Cytoskeletal component which binds cadherin and is involved in cell adhesion
	CTSB	Lysosomal thiol protease which is believed to participate in turnover of proteins
	GRP78	Facilitating the assembly of multimeric protein complexes in microsomal membrane
Plasma membrane	Annexin 2	Calcium-regulated membrane-binding protein
	Cadherin-1	Calcium dependent cell adhesion proteins
	CAV1	Scaffolding protein involved in endocytosis and signaling
	CD34	Adhesion molecule with a role in early hematopoiesis
	CD44	Receptor for hyaluronic acid which mediates cell-cell and cell-matrix interactions
	EGFR	Receptor for EGF involved in the control of cell growth and differentiation

Table 26.2 *continued*

Location	Marker	Function
	EphA2	Tyrosine kinase involved in cell signaling
	Fas	Recruits caspases which mediate programmed cell death
	Hepsin	Plays an essential role in cell growth and maintenance of cell morphology
	HER2/NEU	Essential component of a neuregulin-receptor complex
	KAI1	Associates with CD4 or CD8 and delivers signals for the TCR/CD3 pathway
	MSR1	Membrane glycoproteins implicated in the deposition of cholesterol in arterial walls
	PATE	Unknown
	PMEPA1	Interacts with NEDD4 and regulates cell growth
	Prostasin	Serine protease which acts as a cell invasion suppressor
	Prostein	Unknown
	PSCA	Unknown
	PSGR	Putative odorant receptor
	PSMA	Folate hydrolase involved in cell stress response and prostate tumor progression
	RTVP1	Tumor suppressor inactivated by methylation in prostate cancer
	ST7	Unknown
	STEAP	Unknown
	TMPRSS2	Serine protease with uncertain biological function
	TRPM2	Calcium channel whose isoform inhibits calcium influx and susceptibility to cell death
	TRPP8	Calcium channel up-regulated in prostate cancer and other malignancies
Secreted	A2M	Inhibits proteases by a unique "trapping" mechanism
	IGF1	Growth factors functionally related to insulin but with higher growth-promoting activity
	IGF2	Promotes growth and is influenced by placental lactogen during fetal development
	IGFBP2	Prolongs the half-life of the IGFs and alter their interaction with their cell surface receptors
	IGFBP3	Prolongs the half-life of the IGFs and alter their interaction with their cell surface receptors
	IL6	Plays an essential role in the final differentiation of B-cells into Ig-secreting cells
	IL8	Chemotactic factor that attracts neutrophils, basophils, and T-cells
	KLK2	Glandular kallikreins cleave Met-Lys/Arg-Ser bonds to release Lys-bradykinin
	OPN	Binds tightly to hydroxyapatite, functions in integrin binding and cell-matrix interaction
	PAP	Might be a stress protein involved in the control of bacterial proliferation
	Prostase	Serine protease involved in extracellular matrix degradation
	PSA	Hydrolyzes seminal vesicle protein leading to the liquefaction of the seminal coagulum
	TIMP1	Inactivates metalloproteinases
	TIMP2	Inactivates metalloproteinases
	VEGF	Growth factor active in angiogenesis, vasculogenesis and endothelial cell growth
Extracellular	Maspin	Blocks the growth, invasion, and metastatic properties of mammary tumors

*Information researched from GeneCards online database (http://bioinfo.weizmann.ac.il/cards/index.shtml).

diagnosis. The gold standard for diagnosing prostate adenocarcinoma remains histopathologic confirmation of core biopsy samples. Though recommendations in increasing the number of core biopsies done from sextant to 10- or 12-cores are thought to decrease missed cancers,[73] interpretation of core biopsies can prove difficult since tissue diagnosis is often based on a limited amount of explicitly malignant glands amidst benign glands. Nonmalignant glands may be differentiated from their malignant counterparts through immunohistochemical (IHC) staining with keratin 903, a high-molecular-weight cytokeratin[74] or a basal cell cocktail containing 34βE12 (a cytokeratin) and p63 (a nuclear protein homologous to p53), both of which selectively stain for basal cells, which are absent in adenocarcinoma.[75] To further delineate tumor from benign tissue, protein markers that are highly overexpressed in prostate cancer such as α-methyl-CoA racemase (AMACR) are being investigated for their value in aiding accurate tissue diagnosis.[76] Epigenetic modification such as hypermethylation of CpG islands in the promoter region of the pi class of glutathione

S-transferase (GSTP1) occurs with very high frequency in prostate cancer.[52] Hypermethylation of GSTP1 demonstrated by quantitative methylation-specific polymerase chain reaction (QMSP) assay was shown to improve sensitivity of tissue diagnosis when combined with histopatholologic review.[77]

PRETREATMENT STAGING AND IMAGING

Although the value of modern axial imaging for preoperative staging is evident in other urologic malignancies, namely renal, bladder, and testicular cancer, the utility of computerized tomography[78] and endorectal coil magnetic resonance imaging (MRI) in prostate cancer remains unconvincing.[79] Alternative approaches to prostate imaging are made possible by taking advantage of appropriate cell surface membrane proteins. ProstaScint™ scan (111 In-CYT-356, Cytogen Corp., Princeton, NJ) which uses a radiolabeled monoclonal antibody to PSMA, an extensively studied type II integral membrane protein that is known to translocate from the cytosol in normal prostate epithelium to the plasma membrane in prostate cancer[80] was demonstrated to give a positive predictive value of 67% for detection of malignant extraprostatic extension in a prospective trial.[81]

PROGNOSIS AND RISK ASSESSMENT

Predicting which prostate cancer patient will suffer clinical metastasis, develop difficult end-stage hormone-insensitivity, and ultimately succumb to the disease is a palpable dilemma in which molecular markers may augment current strategies.[82] In clinical practice, risk assessment for progression of prostate cancer after primary therapy relies variably on clinical and pathologic features of the disease. Pretreatment serum PSA levels, along with clinical stage by DRE, and Gleason score of diagnostic needle biopsy specimens remain the mainstays used for clinical decision-making.[83] Serial measurements of PSA and computation of PSA-DT following surgery or radiation therapy for prostate cancer was shown to be a reliable surrogate end point for prostate cancer-specific mortality.[16] A short post-treatment PSA-DT heralds an ominous prognosis, and recommendations for initiating androgen suppression therapy may delay the imminent onset of metastatic disease.[84]

It is well accepted in clinical practice that clinical, demographic, and pathologic parameters may be used in various nomograms that have proven useful in predicting biochemical recurrence.[85] Recently, the addition of pretreatment plasma levels of interleukin 6 soluble receptor (IL6SR) and transforming growth factor-β (TGFβ1) was shown to improve the performance of a nomogram containing standard clinical parameters by a substantial margin.[86] Further confirmatory studies concluded that preoperative plasma TGFβ1 and IL6SR are associated with regional lymph node metastasis, occult metastasis at the time of surgery, and disease progression.[87] These compelling findings emphasize that molecular markers, which reflect the biologic behavior of the underlying prostatic malignancy, may be as valuable prognosticators as clinicopathologic parameters.

High-throughput molecular profiling has provided systematic interrogation of the prostate cancer genome for candidate prognostic biomarkers that can predict aggressiveness of disease. The polycomb group family protein EZH2 was observed to be overexpressed in hormone-refractory metastatic prostate cancer using microarray analysis[88] and, when multiplexed with E-cadherin (ECAD), a cell-adhesion molecule that correlates with adverse prognosis in prostate cancer,[89] may help define patients who are high-risk for recurrence.

PHARMACOGENOMICS AND TARGETED THERAPY

The treatment of patients with hormone-refractory metastatic prostate cancer continues to be plagued with morose morbidity and rising mortality while its mainstay modalities (hormone manipulation and chemotherapy) remain suboptimal and are accompanied by crippling side effects. Molecular markers, through pharmacogenomics, maximize efficacy and minimize unwanted ramifications by targeting specific molecular moieties using novel pharmacologic agents.[90] Success in in-vitro and animal model studies[91] have advanced to phase I and II clinical trials[92–93] which exploit cellular and molecular mechanisms of prostate cancer tumorigenesis, progression, and metastasis; including specific signaling pathways, cell cycle regulation, signal transduction, angiogenesis, apoptosis, and androgen regulation. Inhibition of platelet-derived growth factor receptor (PDGFR) with imatinib mesylate (formerly STI571, Gleevec, Novartis Pharmaceuticals Corp., East Hanover, NJ)[94] and epidermal growth factor receptor (EGFR) with gefitinib (Iressa, ZD1839, AstraZeneca, Macclesfield, UK)[95] continue to provide promising results for treatment of hormone-refractory prostate cancer. Whether used in combination with chemotherapeutic agents[92] or through dual-agent molecular targeting such as anti-EGFR monoclonal antibody,[96] as the knowledge base for the underlying biologic mechanisms of these molecules grows, innovative ways of enhancing the desired pharmacologic effect may be developed. Alternatively, prostate cancer cell-surface markers such as PSMA can also be exploited for targeted systemic therapy by focusing an immune response on or by delivery of highly cytotoxic agents to the cancer cells.[97]

IMMUNOTHERAPY

Exploitation of the immune system requires a comprehensive understanding of the mechanisms of immunity and the molecular markers that can be utilized in immunomodulatory manipulation. Advances in tumor immunology, molecular techniques, gene therapy, and increased understanding of the immune system has led to renewed interest in the development of prostate cancer vaccines.[98] Investigation of antigen-specific vaccines such as DNA-based vaccines,[99] protein-based vaccines,[100] recombinant viral or bacterial vaccines,[101] transfected autologous[102] or antigen-pulsed dendritic cell vaccines,[103] and tumor cell vaccines[104] constitute the bulk of the developing tumor immunotherapeutic armamentarium directed against prostate cancer.

CONCLUSIONS

The importance of molecular markers in prostate cancer is self-evident and cannot be overemphasized. Ubiquitously, the onset of the PSA era denotes the vast potential that biologic markers have and they can, indeed, transform modern medicine and disease epidemiology. Dissection of the prostate cancer genome and evaluation of molecular markers provides us with insight into the underlying biologic processes of the disease. Presently, resourceful utilization of molecular markers has been demonstrated to potentially augment every clinical aspect of prostate cancer: from early detection and tissue diagnosis; to risk assessment and prognosis; to treatment and post-treatment monitoring. New and improved molecular applications are being discovered and developed at such a rapid rate that scientific researchers are pushing technology to their very limits. This technological infrastructure combined with the wealth of knowledge on prostate cancer genomics, cytogenetics and molecular biology have translated into a plethora of promising candidate markers waiting to be validated and brought to the clinics.

REFERENCES

1. Langstaff RH, Polskey HJ. Prostatic malignancy. In Ballenger EG, Fontz WA, Hamer HG, Leis B (eds): History of Urology, vol. 2. Baltimore, MD: Wilkins & Wilkins Co., 1933, p 187.
2. Partin AW, Carter HB, Epstein JI, et al. The biology of prostate cancer: new and future directions in predicting tumor behavior. Monogr Pathol 1992:198–218.
3. Holtgrewe HL. The Economics of Prostate Cancer. In Murphy G, Khoury S, Partin AW, et al (eds): Prostate Cancer. Plymouth, UK: Health Publication Ltd, 2000, pp 497–514.
4. Sproul EE. Acid phosphatase and prostate cancer: historical overview. Prostate 1980;1:411–413.
5. Wang MC, Valenzuela LA, Murphy GP, et al. Purification of a human prostate specific antigen. Invest Urol 1979;17:159–163.
6. Catalona WJ, Smith DS, Ratliff TL, et al. Measurement of prostate-specific antigen in serum as a screening test for prostate cancer. N Engl J Med 1991;324:1156–1161. Erratum: N Engl J Med 1991;325:1324.
7. Sarma AV, Schottenfeld D. Prostate cancer incidence, mortality, and survival trends in the United States: 1981–2001. Semin Urol Oncol 2002;20:3–9.
8. Benson MC, Whang IS, Pantuck A, et al. Prostate specific antigen density: a means of distinguishing benign prostatic hypertrophy and prostate cancer. J Urol 1992;147:815–816.
9. Carter HB, Pearson JD. PSA velocity for the diagnosis of early prostate cancer. A new concept. Urol Clin North Am 1993;20:665–670.
10. Christensson A, Bjork T, Nilsson O, et al. Serum prostate specific antigen complexed to alpha 1-antichymotrypsin as an indicator of prostate cancer. J Urol 1993;150:100–105.
11. Oesterling JE, Jacobsen SJ, Chute CG, et al. Serum prostate-specific antigen in a community-based population of healthy men. Establishment of age-specific reference ranges. JAMA 1993;270:860–864.
12. Catalona WJ, Smith DS, Wolfert RL, et al. Evaluation of percentage of free serum prostate-specific antigen to improve specificity of prostate cancer screening. JAMA 1995;274:1214–1220.
13. Catalona WJ, Partin AW, Slawin KM, et al. Use of the percentage of free prostate-specific antigen to enhance differentiation of prostate cancer from benign prostatic disease: a prospective multicenter clinical trial. JAMA 1998;279:1542–1547.
14. Mikolajczyk SD, Grauer LS, Millar LS, et al. A precursor form of PSA (pPSA) is a component of the free PSA in prostate cancer serum. Urology 1997;50:710–714.
15. Oesterling JE, Chan DW, Epstein JI, et al. Prostate specific antigen in the preoperative and postoperative evaluation of localized prostatic cancer treated with radical prostatectomy. J Urol 1988;139:766–772.
16. D'Amico AV, Cote K, Loffredo M, et al. Determinants of prostate cancer specific survival following radiation therapy during the prostate specific antigen era. J Urol 2003;170:S42–46.
17. Han M, Gann PH, Catalona WJ. Prostate-specific antigen and screening for prostate cancer. Med Clin North Am 2004;88:245–265.
18. Hanash SM. Global profiling of gene expression in cancer using genomics and proteomics. Curr Opin Mol Ther 2001;3:538–545.
19. Aihara M, Wheeler TM, Ohori M, et al. Heterogeneity of prostate cancer in radical prostatectomy specimens. Urology 1994;43:60–66.
20. Verma RS, Manikal M, Conte RA, et al. Chromosomal basis of adenocarcinoma of the prostate. Cancer Invest 1999;17:441–447.
21. Carpten J, Nupponen N, Isaacs S, et al. Germline mutations in the ribonuclease L gene in families showing linkage with HPC1. Nat Genet 2002;30:181–184.
22. Xu J, Zheng SL, Komiya A, et al. Germline mutations and sequence variants of the macrophage scavenger receptor 1 gene are associated with prostate cancer risk. Nat Genet 2002; 32:321–325.
23. Dong JT. Chromosomal deletions and tumor suppressor genes in prostate cancer. Cancer Metastasis Rev 2001;20:173–193.
24. Buttyan R, Sawczuk IS, Benson MC, et al. Enhanced expression of the c-myc protooncogene in high-grade human prostate cancers. Prostate 1987;11:327–337.
25. Kuhn EJ, Kurnot RA, Sesterhenn IA, et al. Expression of the c-erbB-2 (HER-2/neu) oncoprotein in human prostatic carcinoma. J Urol 1993;150:1427–1433.
26. Petrovics G, Liu A, Shaheduzzaman S, et al. Frequent overexpression of ETS-related gene (ERG1) in prostate cancer transcriptome reveals its diagnostic and prognostic potential. Oncogene 2005;24:3847–3852.
27. Kopelovich L, Crowell JA, Fay JR. The epigenome as a target for cancer chemoprevention. J Natl Cancer Inst 20033;95:1747–1757.
28. Wu X, Senechal K, Neshat MS, et al. The PTEN/MMAC1 tumor suppressor phosphatase functions as a negative regulator of the phosphoinositide 3-kinase/Akt pathway. Proc Natl Acad Sci USA 1998;95:15587–15591.
29. Li J, Yen C, Liaw D, et al. PTEN, a putative protein tyrosine phosphatase gene mutated in human brain, breast, and prostate cancer. Science 1997;275:1943–1947.

30. Yoshida BA, Chekmareva MA, Wharam JF, et al. Prostate cancer metastasis-suppressor genes: a current perspective. In Vivo 1998;12:49–58.

31. Mashimo T, Watabe M, Hirota S, et al. The expression of the KAI1 gene, a tumor metastasis suppressor, is directly activated by p53. Proc Natl Acad Sci USA 1998;95:11307–11311.

32. Noordzij MA, van Steenbrugge GJ, Schroder FH, et al. Decreased expression of CD44 in metastatic prostate cancer. Int J Cancer 1999;84:478–483.

33. Zou Z, Zhang W, Young D, et al. Maspin expression profile in human prostate cancer (CaP) and in vitro induction of Maspin expression by androgen ablation. Clin Cancer Res 2002;8:1172–1177.

34. Giovannucci E, Stampfer MJ, Krithivas K, et al. The CAG repeat within the androgen receptor gene and its relationship to prostate cancer. Proc Natl Acad Sci USA. 1997;94:3320–3323. Erratum: Proc Natl Acad Sci USA 1997;94:8272.

35. Liang, P, Pardee AB. Differential display of eukaryotic messenger RNA by means of the polymerase chain reaction. Science 1992;257:967–971.

36. Velculescu VE, Zhang L, Vogelstein B, et al. Serial analysis of gene expression. Science 1995;70:484–487.

37. Chena M, Shalon DS, Davis RW, et al. Quantitative monitoring of gene expression patterns with a complementary DNA microarrays. Science 1995;270:467–470.

38. Emmert-Buck MR, Bonner RF, Smith PD, et al. Laser capture microdissection. Science 1996;274:998–1001.

39. Elgamal AA, Holmes EH, Su SL, et al. Prostate-specific membrane antigen (PSMA): current benefits and future value. Semin Surg Oncol 2000;18:10–16.

40. Becker C, Noldus J, Diamandis E, et al. The role of molecular forms of prostate-specific antigen (PSA or hK3) and of human glandular kallikrein 2 (hK2) in the diagnosis and monitoring of prostate cancer and in extra-prostatic disease. Crit Rev Clin Lab Sci 2001;38:357–399.

41. Sommerfeld HJ, Meeker AK, Piatyszek MA, et al. Telomerase activity: a prevalent marker of malignant human prostate tissue. Cancer Res 1996;56:218–222.

42. Reiter RE, Gu Z, Watabe T, et al. Prostate stem cell antigen: a cell surface marker overexpressed in prostate cancer. Proc Natl Acad Sci USA 1998;95:1735–1740.

43. Srikantan V, Zou Z, Petrovics G, et al. PCGEM1: a Novel Prostate Specific Gene is overexpressed in prostate cancer. Proc Natl Acad Sci USA 2000;97:12216–12221.

44. Xu L, Stackhouse BG, Florence K, et al. PSGR, A novel prostate-specific gene with homology to a G-protein coupled receptor, is overexpressed in prostate cancer. Cancer Res 2000;60:6568–6572.

45. Xu L, Shanmugam N, Segawa T, et al. A novel androgen-regulated gene, PMEPA1, located on chromosome 20q13 exhibits high level expression in prostate. Genomics 2000;66:257–263.

46. Bussemakers MJH, Van Bokhoven A, Verhaegh GW, et al. DD3: a new prostate-specific gene, highly overexpressed in prostate cancer. Cancer Res 1999;59:5975–5979.

47. Hubert RS, Vivanco I, Chen E, et al. STEAP: a prostate-specific cell-surface antigen highly expressed in human prostate tumors. Proc Natl Acad Sci USA 1999;96:14523–14528.

48. Magee JA, Araki T, Patil S, et al. Expression profiling reveals Hepsin overexpression in prostate cancer. Cancer Res 2001;61:5692–5696.

49. Srikantan V, Valladares M, Rhim JS, et al. HEPSIN inhibits cell growth/invasion in prostate cancer cells. Cancer Res. 2002;62:6812–6816.

50. Rubin MA, Zhou M, Dhanasekaran SM, et al. alpha-Methylacyl coenzyme A racemase as a tissue biomarker for prostate cancer. JAMA 2002;287:1662–1670.

51. Luo J, Zha S, Gage WR, et al. Alpha-methylacyl-CoA racemase: a new molecular marker for prostate cancer. Cancer Res 2002;62:2220–2226.

52. Lee WH, Morton RA, Epstein JI, et al. Cytidine methylation of regulatory sequences near the pi-class glutathione S-transferase gene accompanies human prostatic carcinogenesis. Proc Natl Acad Sci USA 1994;91:11733–11737.

53. Yang RM, Naitoh J, Murphy M, et al. Low p27 expression predicts poor disease-free survival in patients with prostate cancer. J Urol 1998;159:941–945.

54. Parsons JK, Gage WR, Nelson WG, et al. p63 protein expression is rare in prostate adenocarcinoma: implications for cancer diagnosis and carcinogenesis. Urology 2001;58:619–624.

55. Zou Z, Gao C, Nagaich AK, et al. p53 regulates the expression of the tumor suppressor gene maspin. J Biol Chem 2000;275:6051–6054.

56. Srivastava M, Bubendorf L, Srikantan V, et al. ANX7, a candidate tumor suppressor gene for prostate cancer. Proc Natl Acad Sci USA 2001;98:4575–4580.

57. He WW, Sciavolino PJ, Wing J, et al. A novel human prostate-specific, androgen-regulated homeobox gene (NKX3.1) that maps to 8p21, a region frequently deleted in prostate cancer. Genomics 1997;43:69–77.

58. Hernandez J, Thompson IM. Prostate-specific antigen: a review of the validation of the most commonly used cancer biomarker. Cancer 2004;101:894–904.

59. Thompson IM, Goodman PJ, Tangen CM, et al. The influence of finasteride on the development of prostate cancer. N Engl J Med 2003;349:215–224.

60. Thompson IM, Pauler DK, Goodman PJ, et al. Prevalence of prostate cancer among men with a prostate-specific antigen level < or =4.0 ng per milliliter. N Engl J Med 2004;350:2239–2246. Erratum: N Engl J Med 2004;351:1470.

61. Mikolajczyk SD, Catalona WJ, Evans CL, et al. Proenzyme forms of prostate-specific antigen in serum improve the detection of prostate cancer. Clin Chem 2004;50:1017–1025.

62. Mikolajczyk SD, Catalona WJ, Evans CL, et al. Proenzyme forms of prostate-specific antigen in serum improve the detection of prostate cancer. Clin Chem 2004;50:1017–1025.

63. Wulfkuhle JD, Liotta LA, Petricoin EF. Proteomic applications for the early detection of cancer. Nat Rev Cancer 2003;3:267–275.

64. Wright GL Jr. SELDI ProteinChip MS: a platform for biomarker discovery and cancer diagnosis. Expert Rev Mol Diagn 2002;2:549–563.

65. Adam BL, Qu Y, Davis JW, et al. Serum protein fingerprinting coupled with a pattern-matching algorithm distinguishes prostate cancer from benign prostate hyperplasia and healthy men. Cancer Res 2002;62:3609–3614.

66. Bañez LL, Prasanna P, Sun L, et al. Diagnostic potential of serum proteomic patterns in prostate cancer. J Urol 2003 Aug;170:442–446.

67. Ornstein DK, Rayford W, Fusaro VA, et al. Serum proteomic profiling can discriminate prostate cancer from benign prostates in men with total prostate specific antigen levels between 2.5 and 15.0 ng/ml. J Urol 2004;172:1302–1305.

68. Grizzle WE, Semmes OJ, Basler J, et al. The early detection research network surface-enhanced laser desorption and ionization prostate cancer detection study: A study in biomarker validation in genitourinary oncology. Urol Oncol 2004;22:337–343.

69. Semmes OJ, Feng Z, Adam BL, et al. Evaluation of serum protein profiling by surface-enhanced laser desorption/ionization time-of-flight mass spectrometry for the detection of prostate cancer: I. Assessment of platform reproducibility. Clin Chem 2005;51:102–112.

70. Gao CL, Rawal SK, Sun L, et al. Diagnostic potential of prostate-specific antigen expressing epithelial cells in blood of prostate cancer patients. Clin Cancer Res 2003;9:2545–2550.

71. Ylikoski A, Pettersson K, Nurmi J, et al. Simultaneous quantification of prostate-specific antigen and human glandular kallikrein 2 mRNA in blood samples from patients with prostate cancer and benign disease. Clin Chem 2002;48:1265–1271.

72. Hessels D, Klein Gunnewiek JM, van Oort I, et al. DD3 (PCA3)-based molecular urine analysis for the diagnosis of prostate cancer. Eur Urol 2003;44:8–15.

73. Ravery V, Goldblatt L, Royer B, et al. Extensive biopsy protocol improves the detection rate of prostate cancer. J Urol 2000;164:393–396.

74. Hedrick L, Epstein JI. Use of keratin 903 as an adjunct in the diagnosis of prostate carcinoma. Am J Surg Pathol 1989;13:389–396.

75. Shah RB, Kunju LP, Shen R, et al. Usefulness of basal cell cocktail (34betaE12 + p63) in the diagnosis of atypical prostate glandular proliferations.Am J Clin Pathol 2004;122:517–523.

76. Magi-Galluzzi C, Luo J, Isaacs WB, et al. Alpha-methylacyl-CoA racemase: a variably sensitive immunohistochemical marker for the diagnosis of small prostate cancer foci on needle biopsy. Am J Surg Pathol 2003;27:1128–1133.

77. Harden SV, Sanderson H, Goodman SN, et al. Quantitative GSTP1 methylation and the detection of prostate adenocarcinoma in sextant biopsies. J Natl Cancer Inst 20035;95:1634–1637.

78. Levran Z, Gonzalez JA, Diokno AC, et al. Are pelvic computed tomography, bone scan and pelvic lymphadenectomy necessary in the staging of prostatic cancer? Br J Urol 1995;75:778–781.

79. Perrotti M, Kaufman RP Jr, Jennings TA, et al. Endo-rectal coil magnetic resonance imaging in clinically localized prostate cancer: is it accurate? J Urol 1996;156:106–109.

80. Pinto JT, Suffoletto BP, Berzin TM, et al. Prostate-specific membrane antigen: a novel folate hydrolase in human prostatic carcinoma cells. Clin Cancer Res 1996;2:1445–1451.

81. Polascik TJ, Manyak MJ, Haseman MK, et al. Comparison of clinical staging algorithms and 111indium-capromab pendetide immunoscintigraphy in the prediction of lymph node involvement in high risk prostate carcinoma patients. Cancer 1999;85:1586–1592.

82. Kumar-Sinha C, Chinnaiyan AM. Molecular markers to identify patients at risk for recurrence after primary treatment for prostate cancer. Urology 2003;62 Suppl 1:19–35.

83. D'Amico AV, Moul J, Carroll PR, et al. Cancer-specific mortality after surgery or radiation for patients with clinically localized prostate cancer managed during the prostate-specific antigen era. J Clin Oncol 2003;21:2163–2172.

84. D'Amico AV, Moul JW, Carroll PR, et al. Surrogate end point for prostate cancer-specific mortality after radical prostatectomy or radiation therapy. J Natl Cancer Inst 2003;95:1376–1383.

85. Diblasio CJ, Kattan MW. Use of nomograms to predict the risk of disease recurrence after definitive local therapy for prostate cancer. Urology 2003;62 Suppl 1:9–18.

86. Kattan MW, Shariat SF, Andrews B, et al. The addition of interleukin-6 soluble receptor and transforming growth factor beta1 improves a preoperative nomogram for predicting biochemical progression in patients with clinically localized prostate cancer. J Clin Oncol 2003;21:3573–3579.

87. Shariat SF, Kattan MW, Traxel E, et al. Association of pre- and postoperative plasma levels of transforming growth factor beta(1) and interleukin 6 and its soluble receptor with prostate cancer progression. Clin Cancer Res 2004;10:1992–1999.

88. Varambally S, Dhanasekaran SM, Zhou M, et al. The polycomb group protein EZH2 is involved in progression of prostate cancer. Nature 2002;419:624–629.

89. Giroldi LA, Schalken JA. Decreased expression of the intercellular adhesion molecule E-cadherin in prostate cancer: biologic significance and clinical implications. Cancer Metastasis Rev 1993;12:29–37.

90. Barton J, Blackledge G, Wakeling A. Growth factors and their receptors: new targets for prostate cancer therapy. Urology 2001;58:114–122.

91. Kim SJ, Uehara H, Yazici S, et al. Simultaneous blockade of platelet-derived growth factor-receptor and epidermal growth factor-receptor signaling and systemic administration of paclitaxel as therapy for human prostate cancer metastasis in bone of nude mice. Cancer Res 2004;64:4201–4208.

92. Mathew P, Thall PF, Jones D, et al. Platelet-derived growth factor receptor inhibitor imatinib mesylate and docetaxel: a modular phase I trial in androgen-independent prostate cancer. J Clin Oncol 2004;22:3323–3329.

93. Rao K, Goodin S, Levitt MJ, et al. A phase II trial of imatinib mesylate in patients with prostate specific antigen progression after local therapy for prostate cancer. Prostate 2005;62:115–122.

94. Tiffany NM, Wersinger EM, Garzotto M, et al. Imatinib mesylate and zoledronic acid in androgen-independent prostate cancer. Urology 2004;63:934–939.

95. Bonaccorsi L, Marchiani S, Muratori M, et al. Gefitinib ('IRESSA', ZD1839) inhibits EGF-induced invasion in prostate cancer cells by suppressing PI3 K/AKT activation. J Cancer Res Clin Oncol 2004;130:604–614.

96. Huang S, Armstrong EA, Benavente S, et al. Dual-agent molecular targeting of the epidermal growth factor receptor (EGFR): combining anti-EGFR antibody with tyrosine kinase inhibitor. Cancer Res 2004;64:5355–5362.

97. Nanus DM, Milowsky MI, Kostakoglu L, et al. Clinical use of monoclonal antibody HuJ591 therapy: targeting prostate specific membrane antigen. J Urol 2003;170:S84–88.

98. Liu M, Acres B, Balloul JM, et al. Gene-based vaccines and immunotherapeutics. Proc Natl Acad Sci USA 2004;101 Suppl 2:14567–14571.

99. Wolchok JD, Gregor PD, Nordquist LT, et al. DNA vaccines: an active immunization strategy for prostate cancer. Semin Oncol 2003;30:659–666.

100. Meidenbauer N, Harris DT, Spitler LE, et al. Generation of PSA-reactive effector cells after vaccination with a PSA-based vaccine in patients with prostate cancer. Prostate 2000;43:88–100.

101. Eder JP, Kantoff PW, Roper K, et al. A phase I trial of a recombinant vaccinia virus expressing prostate-specific antigen in advanced prostate cancer. Clin Cancer Res 2000;6:1632–1638.

102. Heiser A, Coleman D, Dannull J, et al. Autologous dendritic cells transfected with prostate-specific antigen RNA stimulate CTL responses against metastatic prostate tumors. J Clin Invest 2002;109:409–417.

103. Lodge PA, Jones LA, Bader RA, et al. Dendritic cell-based immunotherapy of prostate cancer: immune monitoring of a phase II clinical trial. Cancer Res 2000;60:829–833.

104. Vieweg J, Rosenthal FM, Bannerji R, et al. Immunotherapy of prostate cancer in the Dunning rat model: use of cytokine gene modified tumor vaccines. Cancer Res 1994;54:1760–1765.

Molecular biology of serum biomarkers for prostate cancer

Robert W Veltri

INTRODUCTION AND BACKGROUND

Prostate-specific antigen (PSA) and its molecular derivatives have revolutionized the detection, diagnosis, and clinical management of prostate cancer (CaP), however, this tumor marker currently is positive in cases that are cancer-free in approximately 75% of the biopsy cases.[1,2] In spite of major advances in PSA technology, including assays for complex PSA, free PSA, proPSA (–2, –5, and –7 truncated forms), only limited improvements in the specificity for detection of prostate cancer have been demonstrated.[2–5]

A molecular assessment of biomarkers in oncology has been derived from the definition of clonal epigenetic and genetic alterations identified as DNA sequence alterations, changed RNA, and/or protein differential expression in preneoplasia and histologic progression in cancer.[6] Several studies have demonstrated that transformation of a normal cell into a malignant cell requires a series of genetic changes (or "hits")[7–11] such as point mutations, DNA methylation events in promoters or exons, chromosome deletions, insertions, amplifications, and translocations.[12–14] Additionally, several classes of well-characterized nuclear organelles (spliceosomes, centrosomes, telomeres, and nucleosomes), gene families (High Mobility Group Proteins (HMGA), ATPase chromatin remodeling complex (SWI/SNF), retinoid acid receptors (RARs), matrix associated receptors (MARs), etc.), and key structural and regulatory proteins (e.g., nuclear matrix proteins, HMGA proteins, nuclear histones H1, H2A, H2B, H3, and H4, and SWI/SNF complex) have been identified as being important to the maintenance of nuclear chromatin structure, transcription, and cell

function in cancer.[15–22] Given the general spectrum of molecular events that are known to occur during premalignant and malignant transformation and metastasis, numerous alterations in several pathways have been observed providing considerable opportunities to identify new biomarkers in prostate cancer using blood and urine markers.[23–25]

In the field of prostate cancer, the benefits of the advances in molecular biology of carcinogenesis have reaped major improvements in our current understanding of prostate cancer etiology and molecular pathogenesis and have identified the importance of hereditary (genetic susceptibility), epigenetics, and somatic gene defects that are responsible for the development and progression of this disease.[26–29] Human prostate cancer (HPC) susceptibility genes have been described on chromosome 1q24-25 (HPC1), 1q42-2-q43 Predisposing for Prostate Cancer (PCaP), 1q36 (CARB), 16q23.2, 17p11 (HPC2), 20q13 (HPC20) and chromosome Xq27-28 (HPCX).[29] The HPC1 gene has been cloned (*RNASEL*), and the HPC2 gene (*ELAC2*) has also been cloned. Key susceptibility genes that appear to be important in the host response to infections and inflammation are the macrophage scavenger receptor (*MSR*) on chromosome 8p22 and *RANSEL* on chromosome 1q24-25 (HPC1). Also, several polymorphic variants of three genes (androgen receptor (*AR*), cytochrome p450 (*CYP17*), and Steroid 5-Alpha-reductase 2 (*SRD5A2*), which have suggested a role for viral or bacterial infections as well as chronic inflammation in the development of prostate cancer.[26] In fact, the prostate cancer patient's diet, as well as demonstration of chronic inflammation possibly through infection and/or autoimmune mechanisms, has also been implicated in the cause and progression of prostate cancer.[28-32] Additionally, our knowledge of the molecular pathogenesis of prostate cancer development and progression, in terms of several somatic alterations (mutations, chromosome losses and gains, losses in key gene functions, amplifications, hypermethylation events) that have been identified and characterized, has uncovered novel biomarkers of value to detection and prognosis, as well as new therapeutic strategies for chemoprevention and chemotherapy of androgen-independent prostate cancer.[26-32] Several investigators have identified candidate diagnostic and prognostic biomarkers involved in neuroendocrine differentiation, cell proliferation, apoptosis, and androgen receptor (AR) biology, as well as tumor suppressor genes (Phosphatase and tensin homolog (*PTEN*) Homeobox 3A (*NKX3.1*), *p53*, etc.), oncogenes (*HER2/NEU*, *c-MYC*), hypermethylation Glutathione S-Transferase, P1 (*GSTP1*), and disease-associated polymorphisms.[28,29,31]

During the 1990s, urologists observed a rapid changing of the natural history of the biology of prostate cancer as a result of expanding PSA screening and public awareness, generated through support groups and widespread education including the internet, that have dramatically impacted clinical management of this disease. The widespread use of serum PSA and the growing acceptance of prostate cancer early detection have led to a profound stage migration of prostate cancer at diagnosis and a reduction in mortality.[33-36] Prostate cancer detected in the past using PSA testing and digital rectal examination (DRE) has transitioned from a disease in the 1980s and early 1990s that was often palpable with elevated PSAs to a disease today that presents as usually as clinically nonpalpable (clinical stage T1c) disease with a PSA between 2.5 and 8 ng/mL. Today, a majority of men (~75%) diagnosed have clinically significant stage T1c disease, detected by only an abnormal PSA test, with an associated increase in lead time of approximately 5 years for prostate cancer diagnosis.[36,37] The above changing demographics for prostate cancer, when they are diagnosed early with organ-confined (OC) tumors, are curable with radical prostatectomy (90–95%) or with radiation therapy (80–95%).[36-40]

As a result of increased screening of men for prostate cancer in this contemporary era of detection, men may be identified earlier resulting in a significant lead time bias (5–6 years) producing overdiagnosed cases that may influence survival outcomes due to tumors that may never become life threatening.[41] What is needed as a result of these changing demographics is a need to accurately predict aggressiveness of earlier diagnosed, smaller organ-confined tumors and to manage such patients with curative intent. Epstein et al[42] described a pretreatment expectant management criterion—based on PSA density and qualitative and quantitative pathologic findings on needle biopsy—for predicting small volume cancers in men with T1c disease, which was subsequently modified for a more extensive biopsy sampling procedure. Carter et al subsequently applied this approach successfully for expectant management to men with T1c disease having small organ-confined tumors with the expectation to treat for curative intent.[43,44] Also, the study of this patient sample was recently extended to assess additional new cases and also to perform multivariate analysis of criteria to predict biopsy pathologic progression and at least one variable, at a cut-off of 20% free PSA, contributed to prediction of progression.[45]

Additionally, also because of the rapidly changing demographics of prostate cancer, it is necessary to employ a comprehensive diagnostic systematic biopsy mapping strategy that thoroughly samples all lobes of the prostate bilaterally (apex, mid, and base) with special attention to the mid and lateral area of the peripheral zone; this is required to detect clinically significant prostate cancer.[46] As mentioned above, the changes represented in the patients surveyed since the early 1990s has also reflected a major shift in the biopsy and pathologic Gleason scores aggregating today in the range of 6 to 7, and the tumor volumes are usually smaller.[33-37] In spite of these changes, the critical importance of the biology of prostate cancer as it relates to accurate prediction of prognosis using novel biomarkers is uniformly based upon the accurate assessment of pathologic stage (organ-confined versus non-organ confined), Gleason score (primary, secondary, and even tertiary grading) and the molecular serum PSA profile at the time of diagnosis.[2-5,23,33-37] Subsequently, several investigators have assessed combinations of variables multivariately to produce computational algorithms or models to predict prostate cancer outcomes. Such models often necessitate key pathologic and clinical variables including PSA to evaluate pathologic stage and prognosis either preoperatively[47-53] or postoperatively.[54-58] Furthermore, repeated evaluation of long-term follow-up of prostate cancer patients has confirmed the importance of the several parameters such as pretreatment PSA level, PSA velocity, PSA doubling time, postoperative pathologic grade and stage, and age, in the likelihood of biochemical recurrence and ultimately distant metastases and death caused by prostate cancer.[37-39,59] Finally, the added contribution of novel biomarker(s) to the predictive accuracy of the best existing algorithms or models versus when the biomarker(s) are not included in the model results, also referred to as the concordance index, must be tested and clinically validated.[60] Given this background, let us evaluate the current molecular biology used to identify new biomarkers of the blood (Figure 27.1).

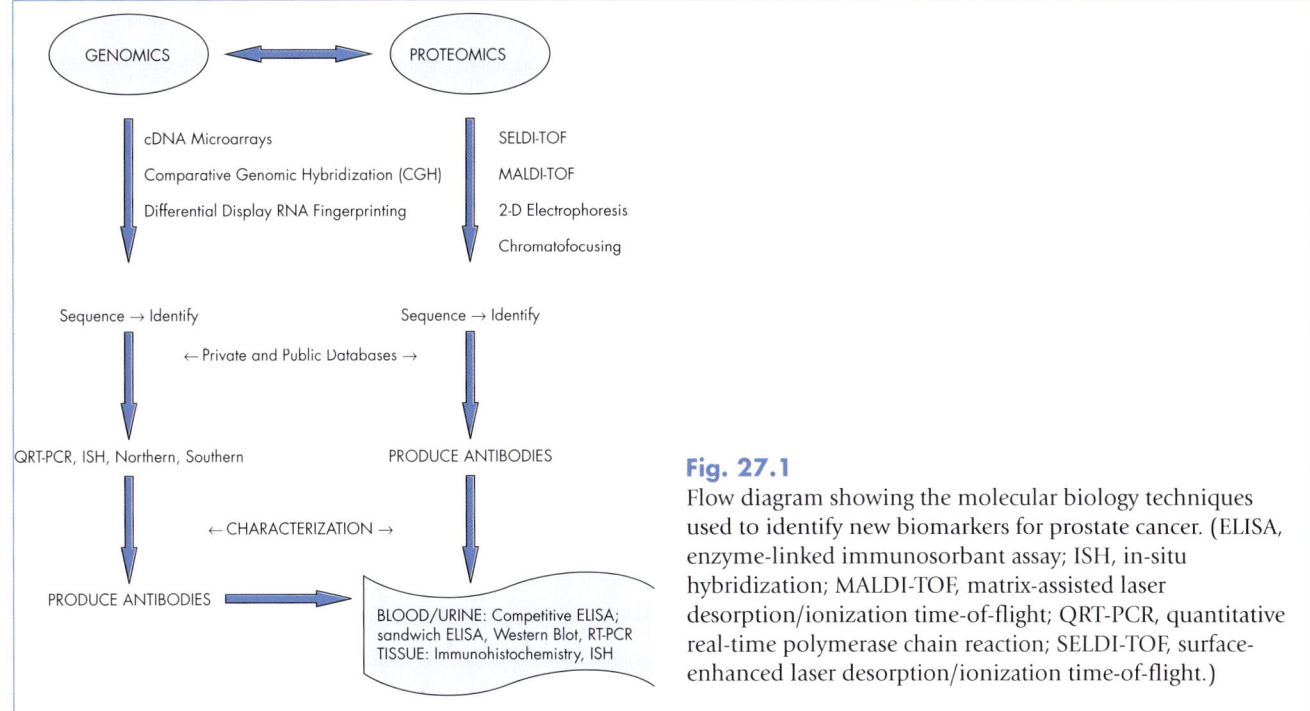

Fig. 27.1
Flow diagram showing the molecular biology techniques used to identify new biomarkers for prostate cancer. (ELISA, enzyme-linked immunosorbant assay; ISH, in-situ hybridization; MALDI-TOF, matrix-assisted laser desorption/ionization time-of-flight; QRT-PCR, quantitative real-time polymerase chain reaction; SELDI-TOF, surface-enhanced laser desorption/ionization time-of-flight.)

SINGLE MOLECULAR SERUM BIOMARKERS

PROSTATE-SPECIFIC MEMBRANE ANTIGEN

A recent review of the biochemistry and biology of the prostate-specific membrane antigen (PSMA) in human tissues and prostate cancer surveys the differential regulation of the molecule, its enzymatic functions, and its potential as a biomarker for in-vivo imaging and immunotherapy.[61] The gene encoding PSMA is located on chromosome 11p11-12; PMSA is a type-II membrane glycoprotein with a molecular weight of approximately 100 kDa, and three domains: an intracellular (amino acids: 1–18), a transmembrane (amino acids: 19–43), and a large extracellular (amino acids: 44–750) domain.[62] In the central nervous system, PSMA metabolizes the brain neurotransmitter, *N*-acetyl-aspartyl-glutamate (NAAG) and is called NAALADase. In the intestine, PSMA is found in the proximal small intestine where it removes γ-linked glutamates from poly-γ-glutamated folate (FOLH1) or as a carboxypeptidase, glutamate carboxypeptidase II (GCPII). Another interesting potential targeting feature of PSMA expression in the prostate is that it is overexpressed in the neovasculature of prostate and other tumors, but not in normal tissues of the prostate.[63,64] The PSMA gene is found on 11p11-12 and a gene encoding a PSMA-like molecule is located at 11q14.3, however only the PSMA molecule on chromosome 11p11-12 is overexpressed in prostate cancer.

In the prostate, there are three alternatively spliced variants of PSMA, one of which, PSM' located at the 5'end of PSMA cDNA, is known to be differentially expressed in normal prostate, benign prostatic hyperplasia (BPH), and prostate cancer. A study by Su et al[65] using RT-PCR demonstrated that the PSMA:PSM' ratio is between 3 and 6 in prostate cancer, upregulated compared with BPH (0.76–1.6) and normal prostate (0.075–0.45). However, given the extensive amount of information available about the biochemistry and biology of PSMA and its in-vivo imaging and therapeutic potential, there is only negligible data available to assess serum PSMA in clinical management of prostate cancer patients compared with the vast amount of data on PSA.[61,65]

Today, only a few studies have investigated PSMA protein levels in the blood of patients with prostate disease, in spite of numerous publications regarding the production of numerous new monoclonal antibodies made to PSMA.[64,66] The existing assays can only be characterized as research assays and the clinical data represent preliminary testing and not validation for a new clinical assay for assessment of diagnostic clinical performance. Reports to date utilized Western slot blot, a competitive enzyme-linked immunosorbent assay (ELISA), and more recently the use of Immuno-SELDI (surface-enhanced laser desorption/ionization). A competitive ELISA developed by Horoszewicz et al using 9h10-A4 and 7E11-C5 monoclonal antibodies found an increased PSMA level in 47% (20/43) of prostate cancer patients versus only 5% (3/66) of non-affected cases and negative in 30 normal blood donors.[67] Other investigators had employed a competitive ELISA and Western blotting and confirmed increasing expression with higher grade and stage, thus implicating PSMA in recurrence and progression.[68-70] A significant effort has been made to demonstrate tissue expression using quantitative immunoassays in the LNCaP cell line, human prostate cancer, and normal or BPH tissues, as well as in metastatic tissue, seminal fluid, and urine,[71-74] but none of these assays were developed into serum immunoassays.[65] However, Xiao et al[75] reported the use of an Immuno-SELDI assay for PSMA. The Immuno-SELDI assay utilized the 7E11-C5 IgG1 monoclonal antibody developed by Horoszewicz et al,[67] and the ProteinChip array was coated with 1 μg G-protein and then residual active sites were blocked with 1 M ethanolamine, washed and treated with 1.5 μg 7E11-C5 monoclonal antibody. The assay was formatted to create a 96-well array and the same exact clinical samples were processed that were run using Western blotting.[76] The results of the Immuno-SELDI assay clearly revealed that serum PSMA using the 7E11-C5 antibody differentiated prostate cancer (623.1 ng/mL; n = 17) from BPH (117.1 ng/mL; n = 10) significantly (p < 0.001). The authors showed considerable age-related overlap in serum activity in normal and BPH cases over 50 years of age.

In summary, the existing data clearly indicate that PSMA should be validated in a prospective clinical trial using a standardized immunoassay with several PSMA antibody epitopes.[64,66] The latter should select the best cocktail of monoclonal antibodies that might be ultimately developed into a new test for the detection and monitoring of prostate cancer patients.

PROSTATE-STEM CELL ANTIGEN

Prostate stem-cell antigen (PSCA) is a 123 amino-acid glycoprotein discovered in the LAPC-4 prostate cancer xenograft.[77] It is a glycosyl phosphatidylinositol anchored cell surface protein that bears homology to stem cell antigen 2. An immunohistochemistry analysis of PSCA using a 246-patient tissue microarray (TMA) revealed that it correlated with Gleason score, PSA level, and seminal vesicle invasion.[78] An analysis of PSCA expression at the protein level by immunohistochemistry and RNA level using in-situ hybridization (ISH) of PSC-mRNA of paraffin embedded BPH (n = 20), high-grade prostatic intraepithelial neoplasia (HGPIN; n = 20), prostate cancer (n = 48) and 9-androgen-independent prostate cancers.[79] The protein expression of the PSCA and PSC-mRNA was 8/11 (72.7%) in HGPIN, 40/48 (83.4%) in prostate cancer, 2/20 (20%) in BPH. The PSCA expression increased with higher Gleason score and prostate cancer stage, as well as with progression to metastasis. At this time there is no evidence in the literature for PSCA being detected in serum or plasma using the reagents available, including several antibodies. However, Hara et al[79] conducted a comparison of RT-PCR using a nested approach for PCSA,

PSMA, and PSA with only 1.0 mL of peripheral blood in a total of 58 prostate cancer cases and 71 nonmalignant cases. Among the 58 prostate cancer cases, the staging value was PCSA > PSA > PSMA, and, hence, PCSA may be a useful biomarker for staging based upon a higher incidence of extraprostatic disease. Therefore, these data would suggest that a serious attempt needs to be made to study PSCA as a serum/plasma biomarker in prostate cancer, given the existing bioreagents already available to develop immunoassays.

CAVEOLIN 1

Caveolin 1 (CAV1) is the major structural protein of caveolae and functions in signal transduction and lipid transport. It is preferentially secreted by prostate cancer epithelial cells and is subsequently captured by high density lipoprotein (HDL3) and transported into the serum. Immunohistochemical data demonstrated that CAV1 is overexpressed in metastatic prostate cancer and is an independent prognostic biomarker based upon its correlation to biochemical recurrence, higher Gleason scores, positive margins, seminal vesicle involvement, and lymph node metastasis.[80,81] Preliminary results for a serum test are based on results of using a modified Western slot blot and detected CAV1 in HDL3.[82] These investigators assessed 16 prostate cancer sera and 16 control sera using a Western slot blot and showed that 4/16 (25%) of controls and 15/16 (94%) patient's sera exhibited positive CAV1 activity. Subsequently, Tahir et al[82] developed a sensitive ELISA test (lower limit = 0.017 ng/mL) with an intra-assay coefficient of variation (COV) of 2.29% to 6.74% and an interassay COV of 2.81% to 6.43% that worked equally well in serum and plasma. In 102 men with clinically localized prostate cancer, the CAV1 median was 0.463 ng/mL, which was significantly higher than that of 81 normal healthy control men at a median of 0.324 ng/mL (p = 0.0446). The results for the ELISA in 107 men with BPH were a median of 0.172 ng/mL (p = 0.0317). Of note, unlike the immunohistochemistry reported above, the serum ELISA results did not correlate well with postoperative pathology variables such as Gleason grade, positive margins, lymph node status, extracapsular extension, and seminal vesicle invasion. The report by Tahir et al[82] provides solid evidence that their sandwich two-polyclonal antibody assay should be validated in another laboratory with different clinical specimens to confirm these clinical observations. Next, a prospective multi-institutional study should be conducted to validate the use of CAV1 as a biomarker for detection and recurrence clinical claims, and the trial would need to include men that are also taking statins for cholesterol control to assess any impact of this class of drugs on the diagnostic accuracy it might have for prostate cancer management.

INSULIN-LIKE GROWTH FACTORS AND THEIR BINDING PROTEINS

The insulin-like growth factor (IGF) system has both mitogenic and antiapoptotic effects on both normal and malignantly transformed epithelial cells. The majority of circulating IGF1 originates in the liver, but its bioactivity in tissues is dependent upon IGF binding protein 3 (IGFBP3) levels at the local and systemic level, limiting the availability of IGF1 to bind to its receptors. Serum protease activity (i.e., from PSA and others) may modulate the bioavailability of IGF1 to its receptors and its mitogenic effects in the prostate. It is important to note that both IGF1 and IGFBP3 are produced in substantial amounts (high ng/mL concentrations) in the circulation and, hence, are readily amenable for quantitation in patients; IGFBP3 is produced at 4 to 5 times the levels of IGF1. A nested case-controlled study utilized the Physicians' Health Study cohort to evaluate IGF1 as a risk factor for prostate cancer in 151 cases and controls, and it indicated a positive association between IGF1 and a risk for prostate cancer.[83] Chan et al used an ELISA to assay for IGF1, IGF2 and IGFBP3 using bioreagents from Diagnostics Systems Laboratory in Webster, Texas. Using age-standardized characteristics, the IGF1 levels within quartiles were established among the 151 control men, and IGF1 remained a significant independent variable to predict prostate cancer risk after inclusion of quartiles of weight, height, body mass index, lycopene, androgen receptor CAG repeats, and plasma hormone levels in logistic regression multivariate models ($p > 0.001$). The relative risk (RR) increased from 1.0 in the first quartile to 4.32 in the fourth quartile. There was no significant association between Gleason grade and stage between the first and fourth quartile groups. The risk for prostate cancer was greater in men older than 60 years of age. When IGF1 was evaluated multivariately by stratifying the patient sample according to PSA (≤ 4.0 and >4.0): when the prediagnostic PSA was above 4.0, the RR increased from 3.92 in the first quartile to 17.5 in the fourth quartile; in the group where PSA was less than or equal to 4.0, the RR went from 1.00 in the first quartile to 4.57 in the fourth quartile, after adjustment for age, smoking and IGFBP3 levels.

Another study by Chan et al[84] assessed 530 case patients and 534 controls in a nested case-control study in the Physicians' Health Study and concluded that IGF1 and IGFBP3 predict the risk of developing advanced prostate cancer. Subsequently, several prostate cancer screening studies were performed to evaluate IGF1 and IGFBP3 for predicting prostate cancer and the results were controversial, with some results being supportive while others proved unsupportive to the hypothesis.[85–91] Therefore, the potential use of IGF1 as a biomarker for prostate cancer detection does not appear, by itself, to replace PSA; nor does it appear that; if combined with PSA; it can improve sensitivity without compromising specificity. However, the disparity of results may due to the fact that PSA relates to tumor presence whereas IGF1 and IGFBP3 are circulating factors that may be risk factors for the development of prostate cancer as a result of the biologic activities of these molecules.

A follow-up study by Chan et al[84] studied the association between Gleason score and stage (A–D) in a case-control study of 530 case patients and 534 control subjects, matched for age and smoking status, in the prospective Physicians' Health Study. Conditional logistic regression models were used to estimate RRs for prostate cancer associated with IGF1 and IFGBP3, stratified by Gleason score (≥ 7 versus <7) and stage (early A + B versus late C + D). Plasma levels of IGF1 and IGFBP3 were predictive of advanced stage (C or D) but not early (A or B) prostate cancer. There was no association between IGF1 and IGFBP3 levels and Gleason score stratified using only Gleason 7. Combining PSA and IGF1 and IGFBP3 did not significantly improve the diagnostic performance of prostate cancer screening in this case-control study group. Unfortunately, repeated studies using IGF1 and IGFBP3 that were controlled for age, smoking, and other factors do not appear to be clinically useful for prostate cancer screening. However, for IGF1 and/or IGFBP3, the data appear to suggest some associations between tumor volume[92] and advanced tumor stage,[84,85,93] which may indicate that these two molecules may involve different aspects of the pathophysiology of prostate disease; however, PSA still appears to be more highly correlated with the presence of prostate cancer.

In summary, IGF1 and IFGBP3 require re-examination of their possible roles as biomarkers for detection and/or advanced staging of prostate cancer in a contemporary prospective study that addresses these and other parameters needed in the clinical management of prostate cancer.

INTERLEUKINS (CYTOKINES)

Diet, lifestyle factors, and chronic inflammation and oxidative damage of DNA through infection and/or autoimmune mechanisms have been implicated as having a key role in the development and progression of prostate cancer.[28,31,32] In fact, there is good evidence for chronic inflammation in the form of proliferative inflammatory atrophy (PIA), one of the earliest precursor lesions for prostate cancer.[32] Interleukin 6 (IL6) is a cytokine that is known to regulate immunity, differentiation, apoptosis, cell survival, and pro-liferation.[94,95] The IL6 molecule interacts with the plasma membrane receptor complex and signal transduction involves activation of the JAK (Janus kinase) tyrosine kinase family member, leading to activation of the STAT (signal transducers and activators of transcription) family.[96] Increased levels of IL6, its soluble receptor (IL6SR), tumor necrosis factor-α (TNFα) and transforming growth factor-β1 (TGFβ1) have all been reported in advanced stages of prostate cancer and metastasis-related morbidity.[97–99] Shariat et al[97] confirmed the prognostic value of circulating IL6 and IL6SR in a group of 120 men who underwent radical prostatectomy, 19 with prostate cancer metastatic to the lymph nodes, 10 with metastatic bone prostate cancer, and 44 healthy men without cancer. Kattan et al[98] combined pretreatment PSA, biopsy Gleason, clinical stage, and two cytokines (IL6SR and TGFβ1) to generate a nomogram biochemical (PSA) progression. In addition to IL6 and IL6SR (concentration, pg/mL) being useful as circulating biomarkers in prostate cancer, Veltri et al[100] reported that serum IL8 levels (pg/mL) increased in a patient cohort that included various stages of prostate cancer (A–D) and was able to clinically distinguish BPH from prostate cancer. Also in this study, when serum free/total PSA (f/tPSA) levels were combined with IL8 levels the area under the curve (AUC) (Figure 27.2) of the receiver operator curve (ROC) (AUC-ROC) was 0.8993 versus f/tPSA alone with and AUC-ROC of 0.7830 ($p < 0.0001$). Subsequently, others have confirmed not only the potential clinical significance of IL6 and IL8 in key pro-inflammatory events that occur in prostate cancer but also their importance to the progression of the disease to distant metastasis.[101–104] The importance of circulating cytokines to the biology and pathogenesis of this disease make measurement of these biomarkers extremely important for detection as well as assessment of progression of prostate cancer and monitoring of treatment. The major weakness of utilizing such biomarkers, alone or in combination, is the requirement for a good medical history in order to identify underlying nonmalignant inflammatory conditions (such as arthritis, asthma, infections, etc.) that may impact the diagnostic and prognostic accuracy of these variables. A panel of cytokines and receptors needs to be studied prospectively to assess their diagnostic and prognostic value to manage prostate cancer patients.

ANDROGEN LEVELS IN PROSTATE CANCER

Androgens mediate prostate growth, and prostate cancer can be treated by androgen ablation by surgery or chemical castration. Testosterone is primarily produced by the testes and circulates mostly bound to serum hormone-binding globulin (SHBG); it also binds to serum albumin. Testosterone is metabolized by type 2 5α-reductase to dihydrotestosterone (DHT) in the prostate, and DHT has a higher affinity (five-fold) for the intraprostatic AR.[105]

In a study of the Baltimore Longitudinal Study of Aging (BLSA), Carter et al[106] compared LH, total testosterone, and free testosterone in 16 men without prostatic disease, 20 men with BPH, 16 men with local/regional prostate cancer, and 4 men with metastatic prostate cancer. A comparison of the groups at 0 to 5, 5 to 10, and 10 to 15 years before diagnosis showed no differences in age-adjusted LH, testosterone, free testosterone, or SHBG levels. In the Physicians Health Study, Gann et al[107] in a nested-case control study identified 222 men who developed prostate cancer and 390 control subjects to study testosterone, DHT, 3α-androstanediol glucuronide (AAG), estradiol, SHBG, and prolactin. Employing conditional logistic regression modeling in this larger patient cohort, a strong correlation was observed between the levels of testosterone and SHBG (r = 0.55) and the risk for prostate cancer. In a study from Norway (Janus Serum Bank) of 59 men with prostate cancer, diagnosed between 1973 and 1994, and 180 controls (age-matched) there was no correlation for testosterone and SHBG levels and risk for prostate cancer.[108] Another pooled study from Norway and Sweden of 708 men who were diagnosed with prostate cancer versus 2242 control men who were not, there was no correlation between testosterone and SHBG levels and the risk for prostate cancer.[109]

The studies from Norway and Sweden contradict the results from the Physician Health Study with regard to the predictive value of testosterone and SHBG as risk

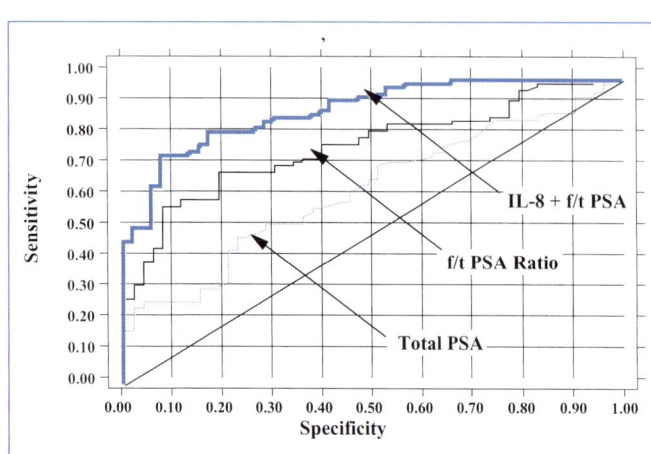

Fig. 27.2

Ability of total prostate-specific antigen (PSA; ng/mL), free-to-total (f/t) PSA ratio, and interleukin 8 (IL8; pg/mL) to distinguish benign prostatic hyperplasia and clinical stages A to D of prostate cancer (n = 146). Area under the curve: total PSA, 0.6269; f/t PSA ratio, 0.7830; IL8 + f/t PSA, 0.8993.

factors for prostate cancer and, hence, make it difficult to assess testosterone and SHBG as biomarkers for risk for prostate cancer. The inconsistencies for hormone levels as predictors for the risk for development of prostate cancer will require additional studies to fulfill the criteria needed to determine the potential of these biomarkers to assess risk and clinical value for management of prostate cancer patients.

VASCULAR ENDOTHELIAL GROWTH FACTOR

Angiogenesis is necessary for tumor growth and metastasis[110] and is important in prostate cancer progression as evidenced by immunohistochemical studies.[111,112] Based upon these earlier observations and subsequent development of several commercial-based ELISA-based assays, candidate biomarkers in the circulation became viable for clinical studies. A cohort of 215 men who underwent radical prostatectomies for clinically localized prostate cancer, and 9 cases with bone metastatic prostate cancer, and 40 controls were studied for vascular endothelial growth factor (VEGF) and serum vascular cell adhesion molecule 1 (sVCAM1).[113] Increased concentrations of VEGF were found with pathologic Gleason sum greater than or equal to 7.0, extraprostatic extension, and presence of lymph node metastasis. Vascular endothelial growth factor was independently associated with biochemical progression after adjustment for standard postoperative pathology.[113] Urinary VEGF was measured in men with prostate cancer undergoing radiation therapy, and it was found that there was an association with local, regional disease and metastasis.[114] In fact, stepwise logistic regression demonstrated that urinary VEGF was an independent predictor of progression-free survival following radiation therapy. These two studies clearly demonstrate the potential for VEGF as a candidate blood and/or urinary biomarker to predict progression in men with prostate cancer. Expanded validation studies need to be conducted for VEGF as a marker for

progression, and then VEGF needs to be utilized in clinical trials that apply the technology to assess new therapies for men with biochemical progression.

PROSTATE BREAST OVEREXPRESSED GENE 1

Prostate breast overexpressed gene 1 (*PBOV1* or UC28) was identified by differential display RNA finger-printing and found to be upregulated in prostate, breast, and bladder cancers; the protein can be found in patient's serum.[115] The PBOV1 gene maps to human chromosome 6q23-24 and is known to be overexpressed in prostate cancer with increasing Gleason grade and stage at both mRNA and protein levels. Using a first generation ELISA that employed mouse antibody demonstrated PBOV1 in the serum of normal, BPH, and prostate cancer cases, and compared results with total serum PSA (Figure 27.3). Subsequently, rabbit polyclonal antibodies were produced against two synthetic peptides (Peptide B, amino acids 4–21; Peptide C, amino acids 54–74), and their reactivity was assessed in TMAs from human prostate cancer blood and in the LNCaP cell line.[111]

At the 2004 AACR meeting,[116] we reported differential expression by immunohistochemistry (Figure 27.4) in a TMA with the AutoCyte Pathology Workstation Immuno-software on 174 cases of biochemical recurrence with metastasis, and illustrated that normal-appearing and prostate cancer epithelia differentially stained with PBOV1 significantly (p < 0.001). Recently, using the same rabbit anti-PBOV1 antibody, it has been determined in our laboratory that two proteins (~17 kDa and ~34 kDa) were found in the blood and in the LNCaP cell line by Western Blot using both Anti-A and Anti-C synthetic PBOV1 peptide antibodies (unpublished data). Also, using a Western blot approach, we can identify the blood protein when the human serum is preprocessed to remove immunoglobulins and albumin, or using molecular ultrafiltration with a 50 kDa protein filter. These preprocessing approaches improved the resolution

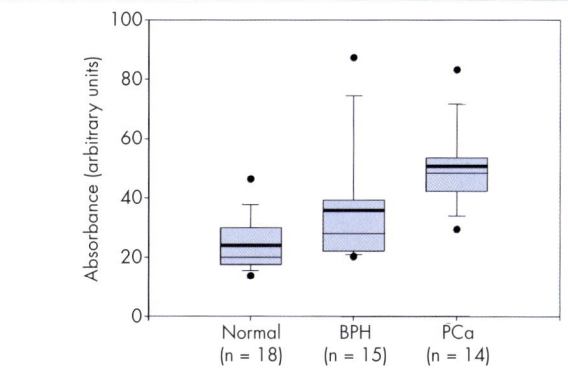

Logistics regression analysis	PBOV1	PSA	PBOV1 + PSA
Area under ROC (χ² p-value	0.8024 (0.0315)	0.7619 (0.0209)	0.8381 (0.0034)

Fig. 27.3
Detection of PBOV1 protein in human serum specimens. (BPH, benign prostatic cancer; PCa, prostate cancer; PSA, prostate-specific antigen.)

PBOV1 (UC28) IHC -MATCHED PZ ADJACENT NORMAL AREA

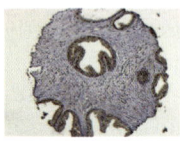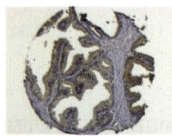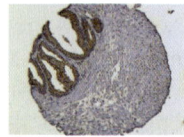

PBOV1 (UC28) - PZ CANCER AREA

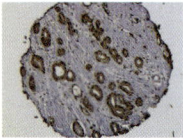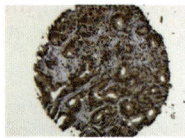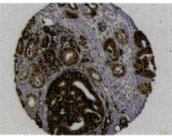

Fig. 27.4
Immunohistochemistry of histologic sections of a tissue microarray from prostate cancer patients with recurrence. (IHC, immunohistochemistry; PZ, periferal zone.)

of the 17 kDa and 34 kDa proteins in the serum without compromising their identification. Next, we used the Immuno-SELDI technique with a protein-G ProteinChip (Ciphergen) method to differentiate 10 normal, 10 BPH, and 10 prostate cancer cases. The anti-A PBOV1 rabbit antisera significantly separated the three groups of patient's sera (unpublished data). Additional molecular characterization of the PBOV1 (UC28) serum protein are in progress, as are expanded clinical studies regarding its utility for the management of prostate cancer. Monoclonal antibodies are being produced and a sandwich ELISA is currently being developed for large screening studies to validate our preliminary studies of PBOV1 in serum.

NMP48 (50.8 kDa) BIOMARKER

Recently, Hlavaty et al[117] discovered at unique 50.8 kDa prostate cancer-associated protein using mass spectroscopy with the Ciphergen system. Subsequently, Hlavaty et al[118] characterized the 50.8 kDa protein as a vitamin-D binding protein (VDP) using peptide mass fingerprinting by mass spectroscopy. A preliminary assessment of VDP used a mass spectroscopy assay with the Ciphergen Series PBS-1 ProteinChip system on WCX-2 chips. All prostate serum clinical specimens were preprocessed to remove lipids, IgG, and albumin and then fractionated using high-performance liquid chromatography (HPLC) on a Protein-Pak Q 8HR anion exchange column (Waters, Milford, MA). Specimens were scored as positive for the 50.8 kDa protein if a peak was found in the region of interest whose height was at least three times the baseline. The positive serum results were as follows: 50/52 prostate cancer cases (96%); 5/20 biopsy-confirmed benign conditions (25%); 3/10 BPH (30%), and 2/50 normals (4%). Currently, a prospective clinical trial for this biomarker using the mass spectroscopic assay is being conducted by Matritech, Inc.

DD3^PCA3 URINE MOLECULAR BIOMARKER

Using differential display to compare normal versus prostate cancer mRNA expression patterns, Bussemaker et al[119] identified *DD3* prostate-specific gene on chromosome 9q21-22. The gene was found to be alternatively spliced, alternative polyadenylation was observed, and no open reading frame was detected suggesting that DD3 may function as a noncoding RNA. Next, de Kok et al[120] developed a real-time quantitative RT-PCR (QRT-PCR) assay for DD3^PCA3 that could be used for tissue, ejaculate, urine, or prostatic massage fluid. Using the QRT-PCR of de Kok,[120] Hessels et al[121] developed a urine test and evaluated 108 men who underwent a biopsy with a serum PSA value of greater than 3.0 ng/mL: 24 of these men were found to have prostate cancer, and the QRT-PCR-DD3^PCA3 was positive in 16/24 (67%) with a negative predictive value of 90%. The QRT-PCR-DD3^PCA3 assay is currently being offered by one commercial urology pathology laboratory, and a molecular biology diagnostic company has been licensed to develop a clinical assay.

GLUTATHIONE *S*-TRANSFERASE-pi 1

Glutathione *S*-transferases (GSTs) represent a large family of detoxifying enzymes that catalyze conjugation with reactive chemical species using reduced glutathione. These enzymes function as dimers composed of subunit polypeptides from four main classes that include α, μ, π, and θ.

The π-class of GSTs (GSTP1) appears to be useful for detoxifying heterocyclic amines resulting from ingestion of well-done or charred meats.[122] The review lists key assays for CpG island hypermethylation, which include Southern blot, PCR of DNA treated with (5m)C-sensitive restriction endonucleases (RE-PCR), bisulfite genomic sequencing (BGS), and today the more commonly employed bisulfite modification of DNA followed by selective PCR amplification for specific target DNA sequences containing (5m)C (MS-PCR). Each of these assays, although sensitive for detection of methylated CpG islands, has technical limitations of either false positives or, in the case of MS-PCR, false negatives. Both the RE-PCR and MS-PCR assays can be performed using QRT-PCR.[122] This review demonstrates repeatedly the accurate detection of hypermethylated CpG islands in much higher levels in PIN, prostate cancer tissue (surgical specimens or biopsies), as well as in ejaculates, urine, plasma, and prostatic secretions from prostate cancer patients.[122]

Cairns et al[123] reported the detection of *GSTP1* with MS-PCR in 22/28 (79%) of prostate tumor tissues, while 6/22 (27%) urine sediments were positive. Goessl et al improved the detection of prostate cancer using urine obtained after prostatic massage.[124] They found, also using mass spectroscopy-polymerase chain reaction (MS-PCR), 1/45 (2%) positive in BPH, 2/7 (29%) for PIN cases, and 15/22 (68%) with organ-confined prostate cancer, versus 14/18 (78%) with locally advanced or metastatic prostate cancer. Using a fluorescent-modified genomic sequencing approach for MS-PCR, Goessl et al[125] were successful in the detection of *GSTP1* in 18/20 (90%) of prostate cancer tumors, 23/32 (72%) plasma or serum samples, 4/8 (50%) of ejaculates, and 22/29 (76%) urine samples tested. Gonzalgo et al[126] reported the detection of *GSTP1* in clean catch urine obtained immediately post-biopsy from 45 men who underwent TRUS biopsy, employing the MS-PCR method. Hypermethylation of the *GSTP1* gene was detected in only 18/36 (50%) of informative cases, and a total of 7/18 (39%) of prostate cancer cases were positive. A total of 7/21 (33%) patients biopsied had no evidence of prostate cancer while 4/6 (67%) of the biopsies with atypia or high-grade PIN were positive. This group demonstrated the clinical utility of a noninvasive approach for screening for prostate cancer in a high-risk population, however, with a compromised sensitivity and specificity that needs to be addressed in future studies. The use of MS-PCR to routinely measure *GSTP1* hypermethylation in tissue samples, plasma, serum, urine, and ejaculates is clearly and reproducibly feasible, and should be used in the clinical management of prostate cancer patients to improve the detection of specificity for the detection of prostate cancer. There are currently commercial ventures planning to use this molecular approach to detect prostate cancer.

ALPHA-METHYLACYL COENZYME A RACEMASE

The α-methylacyl coenzyme A racemase (AMACR) gene, found on chromosome 5, was identified by several groups as being up-regulated at the mRNA and protein level. The AMACR enzyme is responsible for the conversion of *R* to *S* stereoisomers of branched-chain fatty acids, a metabolic process necessary for their β-oxidation.[127] Using a Western blot analysis with voided urine specimens obtained from 26 men following their biopsy procedure, AMACR reactivity was detected in 18/26 (69%) patients and, of the 12 patients with positive biopsies, sensitivity was 100% with a specificity (5/12 false positives) of 58%. The feasibility of a urine test for AMACR was demonstrated, setting the stage for development of an ELISA-based assay and expanded studies for a noninvasive screening diagnostic test for prostate cancer that may be useful in conjunction with the PSA test.

To reaffirm the findings at the protein level, Zeilie et al[128] performed RT-PCR using prostatic excretions in 21 cases including 10 with prostate cancer, 2 men with HGPIN, and 9 cancer-free individuals. By combining AMACR RT-PCR and PSA RT-PCR (normalized) or the AMACR:PSA ratio, the combined assays correctly detected 100% of the 9 cancer-free individuals and 7/10 (70%) of the prostate cancer cases. These two studies demonstrated the diagnostic potential of AMACR for prostate cancer. Attention is required to develop appropriately standardized ELISA-type immunoassays and well-designed prospective clinical trials to validate the biomarker for prostate cancer diagnosis.

CELL-FREE CIRCULATING DNA

The accurate measurement of cell-free DNA in the blood is complicated in preclinical processing as it involves collection of the blood and sample preparation; DNA isolation protocols can impact DNA results.[129,130] A study conducted by Jung et al[131] in 32 organ-confined stage pN0M0, 30 stage pN1M0, and 29 stage M1 prostate cancer cases revealed that only in bone metastases (n = 29) did a significant increase in cell-free DNA occur (McNemar's test, P = 0.006) and this parameter predicted survival probability as reliably as PSA (31 ng/mL cut-off) or osteoprotegerin (3.7 pmol/L).

Another study by Allan et al[132] used QIAamp to isolate DNA and QRT-PCR to measure cell-free DNA in 37 patients prior to biopsy, within 1 hour of biopsy, and 2 weeks later. Employing a cut-off of 1000 GE/mL an ROC analysis had a diagnostic sensitivity of 85% and specificity of 73% for prostate cancer and HGPIN cases. Clearly, much more work would be required to standardize preclinical sample processing, DNA extraction, and DNA quantitation methods, and then a prospective clinical trial would need to be conducted to verify the diagnostic and prognostic potential of detection of cell-free DNA in serum and/or plasma.

ANTIBODY ARRAY PROFILING IN PROSTATE CANCER

The identification of biomarkers from human patient's serum has been assessed by a variety of proteomic technologies. The use of high throughput targeted-antibody arrays has afforded the opportunity to scan for tumor biomarkers using array technology that conserves precious clinical samples and also permits the scanning of numerous cancer tumor-associated proteins by several methods.[133] Several biomarker categories can be scanned using at least two formats for the assays being performed: 1) direct labeling, in which covalent labeling of all "tagged" proteins of interest provides a direct method of detecting conjugation of patient's antigens with targeted-antibody arrays; and 2) direct sandwich assays involve detection of patient's antigen bound to the specific targeted-antibody arrays via a specific cocktail of reagents that detect the antigen–antibody (Ag-Ab) immune complexes using radiometric, fluorescence, and/or chromogen-based technology. Miller et al[134] screened 184 unique antibodies and identified five known proteins of interest in 33 prostate cancer patients and 20 control sera (von Willebrand factor, immunoglobulin M, α1-chymotrypsin, villin, and immunoglobulin G) using two different substrates—polyacrylamide hydrogels and poly-1-lysine-coated glass slides—coated with the antibodies of interest. This reduction to practice by this group is a viable and practical alternative for identifying new candidates for blood biomarkers in prostate cancer. The counterpart to this approach is to use the molecular fractions of protein complexes separated by a variety of methods such as 2D liquid chromatography (chromatofocusing) from cell lines, such as LNCaP. Bouwman et al[135] coated over 1760 LNCaP molecular protein fractions on poly-L-lysine coated slides and evaluated 25 prostate cancer and 25 normal sera for antibodies that were specific to some of these fractionated proteins. Upon statistical analysis 38/1760 protein fractions of the LNCaP cell line adsorbed to prostate cancer sera rather than normal sera and, upon more detailed multivariate analysis of the 38 LNCaP variables, were assessed in a cross-validation study and yielded 84% accuracy. This approach offers another unique method for characterizing the humoral immune response to cancer proteins.[135,136]

The above technologies offer a dual proteomics approach to identifying both new candidate antibodies from a known characterized array of commercial and/or research-derived antibodies and detection of specific human patient-derived antibodies (various immunoglobulin classes), which can react to protein fractions obtained from several prostate cancer cell lines and other human resources. Encouragingly, one study of specific application of the latter approach by Seekumar et al[137] determined the response of 46 prostate cancer patients and 28 control subjects to AMACR and validated the results in 151 prostate cancer cases and 259 control subjects yielding a sensitivity of 77.8% and specificity of 80.6%.

Difficulties that must be resolved in such studies will be reproducibility of the assay technology as it relates to the bulk availability of bioreagents, and their quality assurance over time in a large single lot or multiple lots from various manufacturers in the former antibody array technology. In the latter approach, it will be even more difficult as the reagents needed to characterize the complex patterns must be generated reproducibly from large and complex patient cohorts, under good manufacturing practice (GMP), to test, for example, staging, progression, response to therapies, etc. These novel approaches in the future need to be more broadly tested and expanded to validate their potential routine clinical applications.

PROTEOMICS PATTERNS BASED UPON MASS SPECTROSCOPY

The development of powerful and sensitive new methods, such as matrix-assisted laser desorption/ionization time-of-flight (MALDI-TOF) mass spectrometry, have facilitated the characterization of proteins by mass spectrometry.[138,139] Hutchins and Yip[140] subsequently introduced the concept of surface-enhanced laser desorption/ionization (SELDI). This technology is a type of affinity-based mass spectrometry in which the protein sample is directly applied to a pretreated surface termed the "ProteinChip" (Ciphergen Biosystems ProteinChip, Fremont, CA). The versatility of this technology lies within the unique surface chemistry of the SELDI and begins by coating the samples with a light, absorbing material. Once in place, a pulsed ultraviolet laser (typically nitrogen) provides the desorption energy from each sample on the ProteinChip. These ions are accelerated through an electrical field to a detector; their peptide mass is derived from measurement of time-of-flight (TOF) of the ions through the electric field to the detector, and is related to the ion analyte mass-to-charge (m/z) ratio. A peptide mass map, referred to as a retentate map (retained proteins on the ProteinChip), is generated, which displays individual proteins as separate peaks on the basis of their mass and charge. This approach has recently been applied to cancer protein profiling to identify proteomic patterns in cancer.[138–142]

Several laboratories have become involved with characterizing proteomic patterns in the serum of prostate cancer patients. In fact, some rather remarkable statistics have evolved from several studies. Adam et al[143] required nine m/z ratio peaks and reported 83% sensitivity and 97% specificity for prostate cancer detection using an IMAC-Cu binding chip, and Petricoin et al[144] identified nine m/z peaks employing a C16 hydrophobic binding chip and achieved a 95% sensitivity and 78% to 83% specificity. Qu et al[145] used the IMAC-Cu protein-binding chip to identify 12 m/z peaks and reported 97% to 100% sensitivity and 97% to 100% specificity for detecting prostate cancer in patient sera. Of importance, however, is that from these three prostate cancer studies, all of the results were obtained using totally different m/z ratio peaks. Wagner et al[146] from the EVMS group studied 300 prostate cancer patients and employed 13 m/z peaks and a two-stage linear support vector machines (SVM)-based computational method to characterize a four-group classification system and obtained 87% accuracy. Banez et al[147] used an approach that combined two ProteinChips (weak cation exchange array and a copper affinity capture array) to identify 11 m/z ratios and trained a decision algorithm tree model on a set of 106 prostate cancer patients and 56 controls and then validated the study using separate set of 62 prostate cancer patients and 30 controls, generating a sensitivity of 85% and a specificity of 85% using this technique. Another approach was used by Li et al[148] of Johns Hopkins Medical Institutions group, who studied 345 men (246 prostate cancer cases, 99 men without cancer) to identify a proteomic pattern based upon data collected from two ProteinChips (IMAC3 and WCX2). They identified a group of three proteins (PC-1, PC-2, and PC-3) and trained a model using a subset of the 345 patients and then tested the linear regression model to generate a sensitivity of 76% and specificity of 45%, which was a significant improvement over PSA testing, which yielded a sensitivity of 57%.

One major concern in these studies is the biologic and biochemical reproducibility of these various serum profiling assays, because the results require different peptides having completely different m/z ratios, and then a variety of computational tools are utilize to provide a range of predictive accuracy measurements. Another critical factor is the historical literature reports known biomarker molecular assays that tend to be in the nanogram to picogram concentration range and even lower, whereas the Ciphergen ProteinChip detects low-molecular-weight biomarkers in prostate cancer sera that tend to be in the mg/L range (~1000-fold higher). The likelihood that the changes being identified in the sera of the prostate cancer patients by SELDI are from the prostate are unlikely, rather they are most likely from acute phase reactions, inflammation, cachexia, infection, and other metabolic changes manifested by the cancer patients. Although, such a clinical tool could be valuable in the future, until the instrumentation and clinical laboratory processing steps are standardized to generate valid clinical results, the technology remains developmental. However, the SELDI-TOF and other more sophisticated mass spectroscopy instrumentation technology remains extremely useful for discovery of new biomarkers.[142]

CIRCULATING PROSTATE AND PROSTATE CANCER CELLS

The concept of circulating tumor cells (CTCs) in the blood has a long history; Engell documented the phenomenon clinically in 1955.[150] Subsequently, the technical issue has become one of developing technology with sufficient sensitivity and specificity to reliably examine the clinical impact of these cells in cancer biology.[150–154] The emphasis has been on the ability to accurately detect, identify, and quantify these blood-borne cells, which are the keys to clarifying the role of whole-cell shedding into the blood. In addition, accurate enumeration of CTCs may provide insight into the processes of tumor growth and regression, metastasis, and disease progression, and it may allow definition of the linkage between CTC numbers and clinical status.

In the area of urologic oncology, Johns Hopkins Medical Institutions developed a method to isolate, identify, and monitor residual micrometastatic disease by detection of circulating prostate cancer cells, in the blood.[155,156] They were able to identify and characterize circulating prostate cancer cells in the blood of patients with metastatic disease. Other research laboratories have also used immunomagnetic technologies to isolate and characterize CTCs; Ellis et al[157] found PSA-positive cells prior to therapy initiation in 54% of the bone marrow and 24% of the peripheral blood samples they tested, while another group, Ady et al,[158] was able to detect circulating HER2NEU-positive epithelial cells in 6/11 (54%) metastatic prostate cancer patients and only in 3/31 patients with localized prostate cancer. Figure 27.5 illustrates a novel technology developed into a commercial system by Immunicon® (Huntingdon Valley, PA) that combines an automated sample preparation system for immunomagnetic epithelial cell selection in 7.5 mL whole blood samples with fluorescence-labeled monoclonal antibodies and a semi-automated fluorescence microscope system to count and characterize the captured cells.[159,160] The criteria for an object to be defined as a CTC includes round-to-oval morphology, a visible nucleus (DAPI positive), positive staining for cytokeratin and negative staining for CD45. The Immunicon® technology was recently utilized to verify a rise in CTC numbers and their correlation with both disease progression and overall survival in metastatic prostate cancer patients.[161,162] The results of a recent prospective, multi-center trial incorporating the Immunicon® technology also demonstrated that CTC levels were a strong predictor of rapid progression and death in metastatic breast cancer patients.[163] This technology is currently

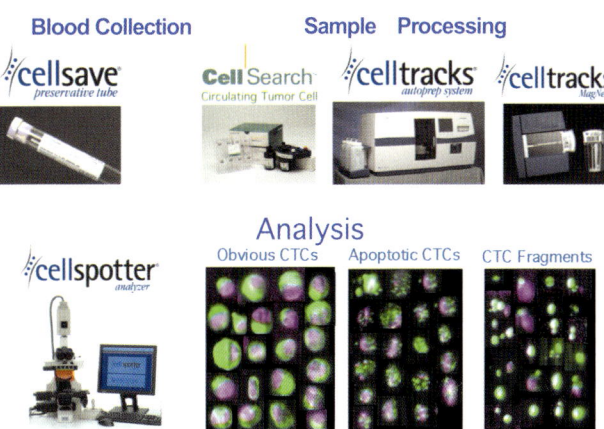

Fig. 27.5

Components of the Immunicon CellSearch™ assay. (CTCs, circulating tumor cells.)

Allard WJ, Matera J, Miller MC, et al. Tumor cells circulate in the peripheral blood of all major carcinomas but not in healthy subjects or patients with nonmalignant diseases. Clin Cancer Res 2004;10:6897–6904.

being commercialized for breast cancer under a license to Veridex LLC, a Johnson and Johnson Company (Raritan, NJ), and there are several hospital laboratories implementing the technology for this disease while research is continuing to develop the CTC method for other cancers. Hopefully, other image analysis companies will step forward to invent further changes to make the technology more cost-effective and routinely available for the clinical laboratory to better manage prostate cancer treatment.

Table 27.1 Single molecular biomarkers in the blood of prostate cancer

| Biomarkers | Correlation to | | | Assays | Tissue | Serum | Urine |
	Grade	Stage	Progression				
PSMA	+	+	+	IHC, Western blot	+	+	+
				Competitive ELISA	+	+	0
				Sandwich ELISA	+	0	+
				ImmunoSELDI	0	+	0
PSCA	+	+	+	IHC	+	0	0
				ISH	+	0	0
Caveolin 1	+	+	+	IHC	+	0	0
				Western blot	+	+	0
				Sandwich ELISA	0	+	0
Testosterone	0	0	0	RIA	?	+	+
VEGF	+	+	+	ELISA	?	+	+
UC28 (*PBOV1*)	+	+	+	ELISA	+	+	+ → 0
				ImmunoSELDI, ELISA	0	+	0
NMP48 (50.8 kDa)	?	?	?	Mass spectroscopy	0	+	?
DD3[PCA3]	+	+	?	QRT-PCR	+	+	0
GSTP1	+	+	+	SB, RE-PCR, MS-PCR	+	+	+

ELISA, enzyme-linked immunosorbant assay; IHC, immunohistochemistry; ISH, in-situ hybridization; MS-PCR, methylation specific polymerase chain reaction; PSCA, prostate stem-cell antigen; PSMA, prostate-specific membrane antigen; RE-PCR, restriction endonuclease polymerase chain reaction; RIA, radio-immunoassay; QRT-PCR, quantitative real-time polymerase chain reaction; SB, southern blot; SELDI, surface-enhanced laser desorption/ionization; VEGF, vascular endothelial growth factor.

Table 27.2 Multiple molecular biomarkers in the blood of prostate cancer

| Biomarkers | Correlation to | | | Assays | Tissue | Serum | Urine |
	Grade	Stage	Progression				
IGF1	+	+	+	ELISA	+	+	0
IGF2	?	?	?	ELISA	?	+	0
IGFBP3	+	+	+	ELISA	+	+	0
Interleukins:							
IL6	+	+	+	ELISA, IHC	+	+	0
IL6SR	+	+	+	ELISA	+	+	0
IL8	+	+	+	ELISA, IHC	+	+	0
TNFα	+	+	+	ELISA, IHC	+	+	0
TGFβ1	+	+	+	ELISA, IHC	+	+	0
Circulating DNAs	+	+	+	Electrophoresis, QRT-PCR	0	+	?
Proteomics	+	+	+	SELDI-TOF	+	+	+
Circulating cells	0	0	+	Immunomagnetic technology Image analysis	0	+	0

ELISA, enzyme-linked immunosorbant assay; IGF, insulin-like growth factor; IGFBP, insulin-like growth factor binding protein; IHC, immunohistochemistry; IL, interleukin; ISH, in-situ hybridization; QRT-PCR, quantitative real-time polymerase chain reaction; SELDI-TOF, surface-enhanced laser desorption/ionization time-of-flight; TGF, transforming growth factor; TNF, tumor necrosis factor.

Box 27.1 Process for development of a new biomarker

Phase I

Identification of "good biomarker candidates for early detection of prostate cancer." Assemble clinical specimens, evaluate biomarkers, and prioritize list of candidates as "good biomarkers for success" based on established criteria.

- Tissue specificity of markers using Northern analysis and reverse transcriptase polymerase chain reaction (RT-PCR)

- Test differential activity in normal, benign prostatic hyperplasia (BPH) and prostate cancer tissues by RT-PCR, ISH, and IHC. Include other normal and matched tumor types.

- Confirm bioactivity of new marker based upon using well documented Gleason grade (sum), pathologic stage, and tumor volume cases.

- Assess sensitivity and specificity of biomarker in tissue, serum or plasma and/or urine if reagents are available.

Phase II

- Testing biomarker on larger local sample sets. Preliminary evaluation of new biomarker in tissue and serum, plasma and/or urine.

- Quality assure all bioreagents and format and standardize bioassays.

- Conduct expanded testing using a statistically valid larger local retrospective sample size (e.g., prostate biopsies, broad sets of tissue microarrays and serum, plasma, and/or urine).

- Confirm sensitivity, specificity and predictive accuracy in tissue and serum, plasma and/or urine including ROC curves to assess known parameters with new biomarker.

Phase III

- Multicenter prospective clinical trials to validate clinical utilities for screening and monitoring.

- Identify a qualified industrial partner to commercialize the test.

- Cooperatively design a prospective clinical trial to validate the new biomarker with standardized bioassays.

- Validate the diagnostic utility for screening and/or monitoring.

Phase IV

- Commercialize the new biomarker with diagnostic clinical claims.

- If the biomarker is to be manufactured for sale and distribution, an FDA submission is required with claims.

- If the biomarker assay is going to be directly marketed to a clinical laboratory (hospital or central reference laboratory), the chemical, molecular or immunoassay-based technology must be established and validated for this operating environment using all appropriate certifications.

- Using good manufacturing practices (GMP) establish manufacturing production, quality control and packaging requirements.

SUMMARY

The field of the molecular serum biomarkers in prostate cancer as evidenced by the above survey offers numerous opportunities to advance the clinical management of prostate cancer from detection to monitoring through the response to current and new therapies (Tables 27.1 and 27.2). However, for this field to mature from an area of interesting research to one of clinical utility, the process needs to change from one of discovery and research to a phased development approach that includes partnering with industry to generate hospital and central reference clinical laboratory tests that are reimbursable (Box 27.1). Clearly, the range of possibilities of new candidate blood biomarkers is extensive, and the process of sorting out the winners needs to begin using a process that has worked in the past but must be followed to completion.

REFERENCES

1. Catalona WJ, Richie JP, Ahmenn FR, et al. Comparison of digital rectal examination and serum prostate specific antigen in the early detection of prostate cancer: results of a multicenter clinical trial of 6,630 men. J Urol 1994;151:1283–90.

2. Polascik TJ, Oesterling JE, Partin AW. Prostate specific antigen: a decade of discovery—What we have learned and where we are going. J Urol 1999;162:293–306.

3. Catalona WJ, Smith DS, Wolfert RL, et al. Evaluation of percentage of free prostate-specific antigen to improve specificity of prostate cancer screening. JAMA 1995;274:1214–1220.

4. Miller MC, O'Dowd GJ, Partin AW, et al. Contemporary use of complexed PSA and calculated free PSA for early detection of prostate cancer: impact of changing disease demographics. Urology 2001;57:1105–1111.

5. Khan MA, Partin AW, Rittenhouse HG, et al. Evaluation of pro-PSA for the early detection of prostate cancer in men with a total PSA range of 4.0–10 ng/ml. J Urology 2003;170:723–726.

6. Hanahan D, Weinberg RA. The hallmarks of cancer. Review. Cell 2000;100:57–70.

7. Rountree MR, Bachman KE, Herman JG, et al. DNA methylation, chromatin inheritance, and cancer. Oncogene 2001;20: 3156–3165.

8. Fearon ER. Molecular genetic studies of the adenoma-carcinoma sequence. Adv Intern Med 1994;39:123–147.

9. Knudson AG. Two genetic hits (more or less) to cancer. Nature Rev 2000;1:157–162.

10. Fearon ER. A genetic basis for multi-step pathway of colorectal tumorigenesis. Princess Takamatsu Symp 1991;22:37–48.

11. Vogelstein B, Kinzler KW. The multistep nature of cancer. Trends Genet 1993;9:138–141.

12. Jones PA, Takai D. The role of DNA methylation in mammalian epigenetics. Science 2001;293:1068–1070.

13. Robertson K. DNA methylation and chromatin—unraveling the tangled web. Oncogene 2002;21:5361–5379.

14. Ehrlich M. DNA methylation in cancer: too much, but also too little. Oncogene 2002;21: 5400–5413.

15. Stein GS, Montecino M, van Wijnen AJ, et al. Nuclear structure-gene—interrelationships: implications for aberrant gene expression in cancer. Cancer Res 2000;60:2067–2076.

16. Holth LT, Chadee DN, Spencer VA, et al. Chromatin, nuclear matrix and cytoskeleton: role of cell structure in neoplastic transformation (review). Int J Oncol 1998;13:827–837.

17. Konety BR, Getzenberg RH. Nuclear structural proteins as biomarkers of cancer. J Cell Biochem 1999;32:183–191.

18. Leman ES, Getzenberg RH. Nuclear matrix proteins as biomarkers in prostate cancer. J Cell Biochem 2002;86:213–223.

19. Reeves R, Beckerbauer L. HMGI/Y proteins: flexible regulators of transcription and chromatin structure. Biochim Biophys Acta 2001;1519:13–29.

20. Berger SL, Felsenfeld G. Chromatin goes global. Mol Cell, 2001;8:263–268.

21. Duensing S, Munger K. Centrosome abnormalities, genomic instability and carcinogenic progression. Biochim Biophys Acta 2001;1471:81–88.

22. Jenewein T, Allis CD. Translating the histone code. Science 2002;293:1074–1079.

23. Bok RA, Small EJ. Bloodborne biomolecular markers in prostate cancer development and progression. Nat Rev Cancer 2002;2:918–926.

24. Srivastava S, Gopal-Srivastava R. Biomarkers in cancer screening: A public health perspective. J Nutr 2002;132:2471S–2475S.

25. Pritzker KPH. Cancer biomarkers: Easier said than done. Clin Chem 2002;48:1147–1150.

26. De Marzo AM, Nelson WG, Isaacs WB, et al. Pathological and molecular aspects of prostate cancer. Lancet 2003;361:955–964.

27. Nelson WG, De Marzo AM, Isaacs WB. Mechanisms of disease: Prostate cancer. N Engl J Med 2003;349:366–381.

28. Foley R, Hollywood D, Lawler M. Molecular pathology of prostate cancer: the key to identifying new biomarkers of the disease. Endocr Rel Cancer 2004;11:477–488.

29. Montironi R, Scarpelli M, Beltran AL. Carcinoma of the prostate: inherited susceptibility, somatic gene defects and androgen receptors. Virchows Arch 2004;444:503–508.

30. Hsing AW, Devesa SS. Trends and patterns in prostate cancer incidence and mortality. What do they suggest? Epidemiol Rev 2001;23:3–13.

31. Nelson WG, DeWeese TL, De Marzo AM. The diet, prostate inflammation, and the development of prostate cancer. Cancer Metastasis Rev 2002;21:3–16.

32. Platz EA, DeMarzo AM. Epidemiology of inflammation and prostate cancer. J Urol 2004;171:36–40.

33. Soh S, Kattan MW, Berkman S, et al. Has there been a recent shift in the pathological features and prognosis of patients treated with radical prostatectomy. J Urol 1997;157:2212–2218.

34. Carter HB, Pearson JD. Prostate specific antigen (PSA) testing for early diagnosis of prostate cancer: Formulation of guidelines. Urology 1999;54:780–786.

35. Greenlee RT, Hill-Harmon MB, Murray T, et al. Cancer statistics, 2001. CA Cancer J Clin 2001;51:15.

36. Stamey TA, Donaldson AN, Yemoto CE, et al. Histological and clinical findings in 896 consecutive prostates treated only with radical retropubic prostatectomy: epidemiologic significance of annual changes. J Urol 1998;160:2412–2417.

37. Pound CR, Partin AW, Eisenberger MA, et al. Natural history of progression after PSA elevation following radical prostatectomy. JAMA 1999;281:1591–1597.

38. Han M, Partin AW, Pound CR, et al. Long-term biochemical disease-free and cancer-specific survival following anatomic radical retropubic prostatectomy. The 15-year Johns Hopkins experience. Urol Clin North Am 2001;28:555–565.

39. Millikan R, Logothetis C. Update of the NCCN guidelines for treatment of prostate cancer. Oncology 1997;11:180–193.

40. Shipley WU, Thames HD, Sandler HM, et al. Radiation therapy for clinically localized prostate cancer: a multi-institutional pooled analysis. JAMA 1999;281:1598–1604.

41. Etzioni R, Penson DF, Legler JM, et al. Overdiagnosis due to prostate-specific antigen screening: lessons from U.S. prostate cancer incidence trends. J Natl Cancer Inst 2002;94:981.

42. Epstein JI, Walsh PC, Carmichael M, et al. Pathologic and clinical findings to predict tumor extent of nonpalpable (stage T1c) prostate cancer. JAMA 1994;271:368.

43. Carter HB, Sauvageot J, Walsh PC, et al. Prospective evaluation of men with stage T1c adenocarcinoma of the prostate. J Urol 1997;157:2206–2209.

44. Carter HB, Walsh PC, Landis P, Epstein JI. Expectant management of nonpalpable prostate cancer with curative intent: preliminary results. J Urol 2002;167:1231–1234.

45. Khan MA, Carter HB, Epstein JI, et al. Can PSA derivatives and pathological parameters predict significant change in expectant management criteria for men with prostate cancer? J Urol 2003;170:2274–2278.

46. Presti JC, O'Dowd GJ, Miller MC, et al. Extended peripheral zone biopsy schemes increase cancer detection rates and minimize variance in PSA and age-related cancer rates – results of a community multipractice study. J Urol 2003;169:125–129.

47. Khan MA, Partin AW. Mini-reviews. Partin Tables: past and present. BJU Intl 2002;92:7–11.

48. Veltri RW, Miller MC, Partin AW, et al. Prediction of prostate carcinoma stage by quantitative biopsy pathology. Cancer 2001;91:2322–2328.

49. Graefen M, Haese A, Pichlmeier U, et al. A validated strategy for side specific prediction of organ confined prostate cancer: a tool to select for nerve sparing radical prostatectomy. J Urol 2001;165:857–863.

50. Veltri RW, Miller MC, Mangold LA, et al. Prediction of pathological stage in patients with clinical stage T1c prostate cancer: the new challenge. J Urol 2002;168:100–104.

51. Partin AW, Mangold LA, Lamm DM, et al. Contemporary update of prostate cancer staging nomograms (Partin Tables) for the new millennium. Urology 2001;58:843–848.

52. Kattan MW, Stapleton AM, Wheeler TM, et al. Evaluation of a nomogram used to predict the pathologic stage of clinically localized prostate carcinoma. Cancer 1997;79:528–537.

53. Narayan P, Gajendran V, Taylor SP, et al. The role of transrectal ultrasound-guided biopsy-based staging, preoperative serum prostate-specific antigen, and biopsy Gleason score in prediction of final pathologic diagnosis in prostate cancer. Urology 1995;46:205–212.

54. Pound CR, Partin AW, Epstein JI, et al. Prostate-specific antigen after anatomic radical retropubic prostatectomy. Patterns of recurrence and cancer control. Urol Clin North Am 1997;24:395–406.

55. Khan MA, Partin AW, Mangold LA, et al. Probability of biochemical recurrence by analysis of pathologic stage, Gleason score, and margin status for localized prostate cancer. Urology 2003;62:866–871.

56. Kattan MW, Scardino PT. Prediction of progression: nomograms of clinical utility. Clin Prostate Cancer. 2002;1:90–96.

57. Kattan MW, Eastham J. Algorithms for prostate-specific antigen recurrence after treatment of localized prostate cancer. Clin Prostate Cancer 2003;1:221–226.

58. Veltri RW, Khan MA, Miller MC, et al. Ability to predict metastasis based on pathology findings and alterations in nuclear structure of normal-appearing and cancer peripheral zone epithelium in the prostate. Clin Cancer Res 2004;10:3465–3473.

59. Khan MA, Partin AW. Management of high risk population with locally advanced prostate cancer. Oncologist 2003;8:259–269.

60. Kattan MW. Judging new markers by their ability to improve predictive accuracy. JNCI 2003;95:634–635.

61. Ghosh A, Heston DW. Tumor target prostate specific membrane antigen (PSMA) and its regulation of prostate cancer. J Cell Biochem 2004;91:528–539.

62. Israel RS, Powell CT, Fair WR, et al. Molecular cloning of a complimentary DNA encoding a prostate-specific membrane antigen. Cancer Res 1993;53:227–230.

63. Silver DA, Pellicer I, Fair WR, et al. Prostate-specific membrane antigen expression in normal and malignant human tissues. Clin Cancer Res 1997;3:81–85.

64. Chang SS, Reuter VE, Heston DW, et al. Five different anti-prostate-specific membrane antigen (PSMA) antidotes confirm PSMA expression in tumor-associated neovasculature. Cancer Res 1999;59:3192–3198.

65. Su SL, Huang IP, Fair WR, et al. Alternatively spliced variants of prostate-specific membrane antigen RNA: Ratio of expression as a potential measurement of progression. Cancer Res 1995;55:1441–1443.

66. Tino WT, Huber MJ, Lake TP, et al. Isolation and characterization of monoclonal antibodies specific for protein conformational epitopes present in prostate-specific membrane antigen. Hybridoma 2000;19:249–257.

67. Horoszewicz JS, Kawinski E, Murphy GP. Monoclonal antibodies to a new antigenic marker in epithelial prostatic cells and serum of prostatic cancer patients. Anticancer Res 1987;7:927–936.

68. Douglas TH, Morgan TO, McLeod DG, et al. Comparison of serum prostate specific membrane antigen, prostate specific antigen and free prostate specific antigen levels in radical prostatectomy patients. Cancer 1997;80:107–114.

69. Murphy GP, Maguire RT, Roger B, et al. Comparison of serum PSMA, PSA levels with results of Cytogen-356 ProstaScint scanning in prostate cancer patients. Prostate 1997;28:281–285.

70. Rochan YP, Horoszewicz JS, Boyton AL, et al. Western blot assay for prostate-specific membrane antigen in serum of prostate cancer patients. Prostate 1994;25:2119–223.

71. Troyer JK, Beckett ML, Wright GL. Location of prostate-specific membrane antigen in the LNCaP prostate carcinoma cell line. Prostate 1997;30:232–242.

72. Sweat SD, Pacelli A, Murphy GP, et al. Prostate-specific antigen expression is greatest in prostate adenocarcinoma and lymph node metastasis. Urology 1998;52:637–640.

73. Solokoff RL, Norton KC, Gasior CL, et al. A dual-monoclonal sandwich assay for prostate-specific membrane antigen: Levels in tissues, seminal fluid and urine. Prostate 2000;43:150–157.

74. Ross JS, Sheehan CE, Fisher HAG, et al. Correlation of prostate-specific membrane antigen expression with disease recurrence in prostate cancer. Clin Cancer Res 2003;9:6357–6362.

75. Xiao Z, Adam BL, Cazares LH, et al. Quantitation of prostate-specific membrane antigen by a novel protein biochip immunoassay discriminates benign and malignant prostate disease. Cancer Res 2001;61: 6029–6033.

76. Beckett ML, Cazares LH, Vihaou A, et al. Prostate-specific membrane antigen levels in sera from healthy men and patients with benign prostate hyperplasia or prostate cancer. Clin Cancer Res 1999;5:4034–4040.

77. Reiter RE, Gu Z, Watabe T, et al. Prostate stem cell antigen: a cell surface marker overexpressed in prostate cancer. Proc Natl Acad Sci USA. 1998;95: 1735–1740.

78. Han KR, Seligson DB, Liu X, et al. Prostate-stem cell antigen expression is associated with Gleason score, seminal vesicle invasion and capsular invasion in prostate. J Urol 2004;171:1117–1121.

79. Hara N, Kasahara T, Kawasaki T, et al. Reverse transcriptase-polymerase chain reaction of prostate specific membrane antigen and prostate stem cell antigen in one milliliter of peripheral blood: value for staging of staging of prostate cancer. Clin Cancer Res 2002;6:1794-1799.

80. Yang G, Truong LD, Timme TL, et al. Elevated expression of Caveolin is associated with prostate and breast cancer. Clin Cancer Res 1998;4: 1873–1880.

81. Yang G, Truong LD, Wheeler TM, et al. Caveolin-1 expression in clinically confined human prostate cancer: a novel prognostic marker. Cancer Res 1999;59:5719–5723.

82. Tahir SA, Ren C, Timme TL, et al. Development of an immunoassay for Caveolin-1: A novel biomarker for prostate cancer. Clin Cancer Res 2003;9:3653–3659.

83. Chan JM, Stampfer MJ, Giovannucci E, et al. Plasma insulin-like growth factor-1 and prostate cancer risk: a prospective study. Science 1998;279: 563–566.

84. Chan JM, Stampfer MJ, Ma J, et al. Insulin-like growth factor-1 (IGF-1) and IGF binding protein-3 as predictors of advanced-stage prostate cancer. J Natl Cancer Inst 2002;94:1099–1109.

85. Harman SM, Metter EJ, Blackman MR, et al. Serum levels of insulin-like growth factor 1 (IGF-1), IGF-II, IGB binding factor-3 and PSA as predictors of clinical prostate cancer. J Clin Endocrinol Metab 2000;85: 4258-4265.

86. Wolk A, Andersson SO, Mantzoros CS, et al. Can measurements of IGF-1 and IFGBP-3 improve the sensitivity of prostate cancer screening? Lancet 2000;356:1902–1903.

87. Djavan B, Bossa B, Seitz C, et al. Insulin-like growth factor 1 (IGF-1) and IGF-1 density, and IGF-1/PSA ratio for prostate cancer detection. Urology 1999;54:603–606.

88. Cutting CWM, Hunt C, Nisbet JA, et al. Serum insulin-like growth factor-1 is not a useful marker of prostate cancer. BJU Intl 1999;83:996–999.

89. Finne P, Auvinen A, Koisten H, et al. Insulin-like growth factor-1 is not a useful marker of prostate cancer in men with elevated levels of prostate specific antigen. J Clin Endocrinol Metab 2000;85:2744–2747.

90. Ismail H, Pollak M, Behlouli H, et al. Insulin-like growth factor-1 and insulin-like growth factor binding protein-3 for prostate cancer detection in patient undergoing prostate biopsy. J Urol 2002;168:2426–2430.

91. Baffa R, Reiss K, El-Gabry EA, et al. Low serum insulin-like growth factor-1 (IGF-1): a significant association with prostate cancer. Tech Urol 2000:6:236–239.

92. Sarma AV, Jaffe CA, Schottenfeld D, et al. Insulin-like growth factor-1, insulin-like growth factor binding protein-3, and body mass index; clinical correlates of prostate volume among black men. Urology 2002;59:362–367.

93. Miyata Y, Sakai H, Tamayoshi H, et al. Serum insulin-like growth factor binding protein-3/prostate-specific antigen ratio is a useful predictive marker in patients with advanced prostate cancer. Prostate 2003;54:125–132.

94. Hobisch A, Eder IE, Putz T, et al. Interleukin-6 regulates prostate-specific protein expression in prostate carcinoma cells by activation of androgen receptor. Cancer Res 1998;58:4640–4645.

95. Chung TD, Yu JJ, Spiotto MT. Characterization of the role of IL-6 in the progression of prostate cancer. Prostate 1999;38:199–207.

96. Heinrich PC, Behrmann I, Haan S, et al. Principles of interleukin-6 (IL-6) type cytokine signaling and its regulation. Biochem J 2003;374:1–20.

97. Shariat SH, Andrews B, Kattan M, et al. Plasma levels of ineterleukin-6 and its soluble receptor are associated with prostate cancer progression and metastasis. Urology 2003;58:1008–1015.

98. Kattan MW, Shariat SF, Andrews B, et al. The addition of interleukin-6 soluble receptor and transforming growth factor beta-1 improves a preoperative nomogram for predicting biochemical progression in patients with clinically localized prostate cancer. J Clin Oncol 2003;21:3573–3579.

99. Michalaki V, Syrigos K, Charles P, et al. Serum levels of IL-6 and TNF-α correlate with clinicopathological features and patient survival in patients with prostate cancer. Br J Cancer 2004;90:2312–2316.

100. Veltri RW, Miller MC, Zhao G, et al. Interleukin-8 serum levels in patients with benign prostatic hyperplasia and prostate cancer. Urology 1999;53:139–147.

101. Pfitzenmaier J, Vessella R, Higano CS, et al. Elevation of cytokine levels in cachectic patients with prostate carcinoma. Cancer 2003;97:1211–1216.

102. Steiner GE, Newman ME, Paikl D, et al. Expression and function of pro-inflammatory interleukin IL-17 and IL-17 receptor in normal, benign hyperplastic, and malignant prostate. Prostate 2003;56:171–182.

103. Lehrer S, Diamond EJ, Mamkine B, et al. Serum interleukin-8 is elevated in men with prostate cancer and bone metastasis. Tech Cancer Res Treatment 2004;5:411.

104. Konig JE, Senge T, Allhoff EP, et al. Analysis of the inflammatory network in benign hyperplasia and prostate cancer. Prostate 2004;58:121–129.

105. Coffey DS. The molecular biology of the prostate. In: Molecular Biology in Urology. Lepor H, Lawson RK (eds): Philadelphia: WB Saunders, 1993, pp 28–56.

106. Carter HB, Pearson JD, Metter EJ, et al. Longitudinal evaluation of serum androgen levels with and without prostate cancer. Prostate 1995;27:25–31.

107. Gann PH, Hennekens CH, Ma J, Longscope C, et al. Prospective study of sex hormone levels and risk of prostate cancer. J Natl Cancer Inst 1996;88:1118–1126.

108. Vatten LJ, Ursin G, Ross RK, et al. Androgens in serum and the risk of prostate cancer: A nested case-control study from the Janus serum bank in Norway. Cancer Epidemiol Biomarkers Prev 1997;6:967–969.

109. Stattin P, Lumme S, Tenkakanen L, et al. High levels of circulating testosterone are not associated with increased prostate cancer risk: A pooled prospective study. Int J Cancer 2004;108:418–424.

110. Folkman J. What is the evidence that tumors are angiogenesis dependent? J Natl Cancer Inst 1990;82:4–6.

111. Silberman MA, Partin AW, Veltri RW, et al. Tumor angiogenesis correlates with progression after radical prostatectomy but not with Gleason sum 5–7 adenocarcinoma of the prostate. Cancer 1997;79:772–779.

112. Huss WJ, Hanrahan CF, Barrios RJ, et al. Angiogenesis and prostate cancer: Identification of a molecular progression switch. Cancer Res 2001;61:2736–2743.

113. Shariat SF, Anwuri VA, Lamb DJ, et al. Association of preoperative levels of vascular endothelial growth factor and soluble vascular cell adhesion molecule-1 with lymph node status and biochemical progression after radical prostatectomy. J Clin Oncol 2004;22:1655–1663.

114. Chan LW, Moses MA, Goley E, et al. Urinary VEGF and MMP levels as predictive markers of 1-year progression-free survival in cancer patients treated with radiation therapy: A longitudinal study of protein kinetics throughout tumor progression and therapy. J Clin Oncology 2004;22:499–506.

115. An Gang, Ng AY, Reddy Meka CS, et al. Cloning and characterization of UROC28, a novel gene overexpressed in prostate, breast and bladder cancers. Cancer Res 2000;60:7014–7020.

116. Veltri RW, Van Rootselaar C, Bales W, et al. PBOV1 (UC28): A novel biomarker with potential utility in the management of prostate cancer. Proc AACR 2004;45:625 [Abstract #2707].

117. Hlavaty JJ, Partin AW, Kusinitz K. Mass spectroscopy as a discovery tool for identifying serum markers. Clin Chem 2001;47:1924–1926.

118. Hlavaty JJ, Partin AW, Shue MJ, et al. Identification and preliminary clinical evaluation of a 50.8 kDa serum marker for prostate cancer. Urology 2003;61:1261–1265.

119. Bussemakers MJ, van Bokhoven A, Verhaegh GW, et al. DD3: a new prostate-specific gene, highly overexpressed in prostate cancer. Cancer Res 1999;59:5975–5979.

120. de Kok JB, Verhaegh GW, Roelof RW, et al. DD3 (PCA3), a sensitive and specific marker to detect prostate tumors. Cancer Res 2002;62:2695–2698.

121. Hessels D, Jacqueline MT, Klein G, et al. DD3(PCA3)-based molecular urine analysis for diagnosis of prostate cancer. Eur Urol 2003;44:8–16.

122. Nakayama N, Gonzalgo ML, Yegnasubramanian S, Lin X, De Marzo AM, Nelson WG. GSTP1 CpG island hypermethylation as a molecular biomarker for prostate cancer. J Cell Biochem 2004;91:540–552.

123. Cairns P, Esteller M, Herman JG, et al. Molecular detection of prostate cancer in urine by GSTP1 hypermethylation. Clin Cancer Res 2001;7:2727–2730.

124. Goessl C, Muller M, Heicappell R, et al. DNA-based detection of prostate cancer in urine after prostatic massage. Urology 2001;58:335–338.

125. Goessl C, Muller M, Heicappell R, et al. DNA-based detection of prostate cancer in blood, urine, and ejaculates. Ann NY Acad Sci 2001;945:51–58.

126. Gonzalgo ML, Pavlovich CP, Lee SM, et al. Prostate cancer detection by GSTP1 methylation analysis of post-biopsy urine specimens. Clin Cancer Res 2003;9:2673–2677.

127. Rogers C, Yan G, Zha S, et al. Prostate cancer detection on urinalysis for α-methylacyl coenzyme A Racemase protein. J Urol 2004;172:1501–1503.

128. Zeilie PJ, Mobley JA, Ebb RG, et al. A novel diagnostic test for prostate cancer emerges from the determination of α-methylacyl coenzyme A racemase in prostatic secretions. J Urol 2004;172:1130–1133.

129. Swinkles DW, Weigerinck E, Steeger EAP, et al. Effects of blood processing protocols on cell-free DNA quantification in plasma. Clin Chem 2003;49:515–526.

130. Wu TS, Zhang D, Chia JH, et al. Cell-free DNA: measurement in various carcinomas and establishment of normal reference range. Clin Chim Acta 2002;321:77–87.

131. Jung K, Stephan C, Lewandowski M, et al. Increased cell-free DNA in plasma of patients with metastatic spread in prostate cancer. Cancer Letts 2004;205:173–180.

132. Allan D, Butt A, Cahill D, et al. Role of cell-free plasma DNA as a diagnostic marker for prostate cancer. Ann NY Acad Sci 2004;1022:76–80.

133. Haab BB. Methods and applications of antibody microarrays in cancer research. Proteomics 2003;3:2116–2122.

134. Miller JC, Zhou H, Kwekei J, et al. Antibody microarray profiling of human prostate cancer sera: Antibody screening and identification of potential markers. Proteomics 2003;3:56–63.

135. Bouwman K, Qiu J, Zhou H, et al. Microarray of tumor derived proteins uncover a distinct pattern of prostate cancer serum immunoreactivity. Proteomics 2003;3:2200–2207.

136. Seekumar A, Laxman B, Rhodes DR, et al. Humoral immune response to α-methylacyl-CoA racemase and prostate cancer. J Natl Cancer Inst 2004;96:834–843.

137. Yan F, Sreekumar A, Laxman B, et al. Protein microarrays using liquid phase fractionation of cell lysates. Proteomics 2003;3:1228–1235.

138. Banks RE, Dunn MJ, Hochstrasser DF, et al. Proteomics: new perspectives, new biomedical opportunities. Lancet, 2000;356:1749–1756.

139. Chambers G, Lawrie L, Cash P, et al. Proteomics: a new approach to the study of disease. J Pathol 2000;192:280–288.

140. Hutchens T, Yip T. New desorption strategies for the mass spectrometric analysis of macromolecules. Rapid Commun Mass Spectrom 1993;7:546–580.

141. Srinivas PR, Srivastava S, Hanash S, et al. Proteomics in early detection of cancer. Clin Chem 2001;47:1901–11.

142. Gretzer MB, Partin AW, Chan DW, et al. Modern tumor marker discovery in urology: surface enhanced laser desorption and ionization (SELDI). Rev Urol 2003;5:81–89.

143. Adam BL, Vlahou A, Semmes OJ, et al. Proteomic approaches to biomarker discovery in prostate and bladder cancers. Proteomics 2001;1:1264–1270.

144. Petricoin EF, Ardekani AM, Hit BA, et al. Use of proteomic patterns in serum to identify ovarian cancer. Lancet 2002;359:572–577.

145. Qu Y, Adam BL, Yasui Y, et al. Boosted decision tree analysis of surface-enhanced desorption/ionization mass spectral serum profiles discriminates prostate cancer from noncancer patients. Clin Chem 2001;48:1835–1843.

146. Wagner M, Naik DN, Pothen A, et al. Computational protein biomarker predictions: a case study for prostate cancer. BMC Bioinformatics 2004;5:26–35.

147. Banez LL, Prasanna P, Sun L, et al. Diagnostic potential of serum proteomic patterns in prostate cancer. J Urol 2003;170:442–446.

148. Li J, White N, Zhang Z, et al. Detection of prostate cancer using serum proteomics pattern in a histologically confirmed population. J Urol 2004;171:1782–1787.

149. Wang ZP, Eisenberger MA, Carducci MA, et al. Identification and characterization of circulating prostate carcinoma cells. Cancer 2000;88:2787–2795.

150. Engell HC. Cancer cells in the circulating blood. Acta Chir Scand 1955;210:10–70.

151. Goldblatt SA, Nadel EM. Cancer cells in the circulating blood: a critical review II. Acta Cytol 1965;9:6–20.

152. Kiseleva NS, Magamadov YC. Hematogenous dissemination of tumor cells and metastasis formation in Ehrlich ascites tumor. Neoplasma 1972;19:257–275.

153. Herbeuval R, Duheille J, Goerdert-Herbeuval C. Diagnosis of unusual blood cells by immunofluorescence. Acta Cytol 1965;9:73–82.

154. Stevenson JL, von Haam E. The application of immunofluorescence technique to the cytodiagnosis of cancer. Acta Cytol 1966;10:15–20.

155. Wang ZP, Eisenberger MA, Carducci MA, et al. Identification and characterization of circulating prostate carcinoma cells. Cancer 2000;88:2787–2795.

156. Ts'o PO, Pannek J, Wang ZP, et al. Detection of intact prostate cancer cells in the blood of men with prostate cancer. Urology 1997;49:881–885.

157. Ellis WJ, Pfitenmaier J, Colli J, et al. Detection and isolation of prostate cancer cells from peripheral blood and bone marrow. Urology 2003;61:277–281.

158. Ady N, Morat L, Fizazi K, et al. Detection of Her-2/neu- positive circulating epithelial cells in prostate cancer patients. Br J Cancer 2004;90:443–448.

159. Terstappen LW, Rao C, Gross S, et al. Flow cytometry—principles and feasibility in transfusion medicine. Enumeration of epithelial derived tumor cells in peripheral blood. Vox Sang 1998;74:269–274.

160. Terstappen LW, Rao C, Gross S, et al. Peripheral blood tumor cell load reflects the clinical activity of the disease in patients with carcinoma of the breast. Int J Oncol 2000;17:573–578.

161. Moreno JG, O'Hara SM, Gross S, et al. Changes in circulating carcinoma cells in patients with metastatic prostate cancer correlate with disease status. Urology 58:2001;386–392.

162. Miller MC, Gross S, Allard WJ, et al. Circulating tumor cells (CTC) predict survival in patients with metastatic prostate cancer. Proc Am Assoc Cancer Res 45:2004;A5270.

163. Cristofanilli M, Hayes DF, Budd GT, et al. Circulating tumor cells: A novel prognostic factor for newly diagnosed breast cancer. J Clin Onc, 2005; 23:1420–1430.

Molecular biology of tissue biomarkers for prostate cancer 28

John S Lam, Robert E Reiter

INTRODUCTION

Anatomic and clinical staging remains the mainstay by which clinical decisions are directed in patients diagnosed with prostate cancer. The tumor-node-metastasis (TNM) staging system is the most commonly used system, in which tumors are staged according to primary tumor size and presence or absence of either lymph node or distant metastasis. The widespread use of prostate-specific antigen (PSA) as a screening test for prostate cancer has led to an impressive stage migration with more patients presenting with organ-confined disease. Although current clinical and pathologic features provide useful information allowing clinicians to stratify patients into different risk categories and dictate treatment, differences remain in terms of accurately predicting outcome for any particular patient.[1] In the PSA era, more patients are presenting within a very narrow range of these parameters, thus limiting the predictive value of staging and prognosis. Furthermore, there are currently no means to assess which tumors are clinically significant. In addition, the identification of molecular targets involved in the tumorigenesis and progression of prostate cancer will provide opportunities for the development of new agents with greater therapeutic potential and better specificity. Therefore, additional diagnostic and prognostic biomarkers, as well as ones that will serve as therapeutic targets, are urgently needed for prostate cancer.

DETECTION AND ANALYSIS OF PROSTATE CANCER BIOMARKERS

Advances in molecular biology have led to the availability of a wide variety of biomarkers for prostate cancer (Table 28.1).[2] Immunohistochemical staining is typically used to detect tissue-based biomarkers. Specimens consist of either prostate needle biopsies or the entire surgical specimen obtained after radical prostatectomy. The predictive value of biopsy specimens is often hampered by the multifocal and heterogeneous nature of prostate cancer, thereby leading to sampling error. Although analysis of the entire prostate avoids this problem, in many cases one would like to scrutinize the prognostic marker prior to definitive treatment. Fluorescence in-situ hybridization (FISH) utilizes fluorescently labeled DNA probes to identify chromosomal abnormalities. Centromeric probes attach to the centromeres of chromosomes and allow for the number of copies of a given chromosome within a cell to be determined. Normal cells harbor two copies of a chromosome, whereas malignant cells will often have additional copies. Locus-specific probes provide information on whether a given gene (or an area on a chromosome) is amplified or deleted. Some biomarkers can be detected at the protein level by enzyme-linked immunosorbent assay (ELISA) or at the RNA level by reverse transcription-polymerase chain reaction (RT-PCR) (Figure 28.1). The field of proteomics allows for the protein "signature" of a given disease process to be analyzed. Surface-enhanced laser desorption/ionization time of flight (SELDI-TOF) mass spectrometry is an affinity-based mass spectrometry by which proteins are selectively adsorbed to a chemically modified substrate. Weakly bound proteins are washed away and the remaining samples are analyzed by mass spectrometry. This allows the identification of disease-associated proteins from specimens, such as tissue, urine, and serum. Finally, genetic markers may be useful in predicting outcome. Much work has been done in elucidating genetic mutations and/or polymorphisms that may play a role in prostate cancer.

Table 28.1 Prostate cancer tissue biomarkers

Biomarker	Function	Application
Promising		
Ki67	Nuclear cell proliferation antigen	D, P
P27	Cyclin-dependent kinase inhibitor (tumor suppressor)	D, P, T
Skp2	Tumor suppressor protein regulator	D, P
E-cadherin	Cell adhesion molecule	D, P
PTEN	Tumor suppressor protein	D, P, T
TGFβ1	Growth factor	D, P, T
TGFβ1 receptor type I	Tyrosine kinase receptor	D, P, T
Telomere length	Control of cellular senescence	D, P, T
Hepsin	Serine protease	D, P, T
AMACR	Fatty acid metabolism enzyme	D
Androgen receptor	Androgen receptor	D, P, T
Unclear/more studies needed		
P53	Tumor suppressor protein	D, P
BCL2	Apoptosis-related protein	D, P, T
C-CAM1	Cell adhesion molecule	D
CD44	Cell adhesion molecule	D, T
HYAL1-type HAase	Breaks down hyaluronic acid (hyaluronidase)	D, P
Integrin	Cell adhesion molecule	D
Selectin	Cell adhesion molecule	D
ERBB1/EGFR	Tyrosine kinase receptor	D, T
ERBB2/HER2/NEU	Tyrosine kinase receptor	D, T
ERBB3	Tyrosine kinase receptor	D
HRG	Tyrosine kinase receptor ligand	D, P
IGFR	Tyrosine kinase receptor	D, T
VEGF	Growth factor	D, T
VEGFR	Tyrosine kinase receptor	D, T
Microvessel density	Angiogenesis	D, P
FGF	Growth factor	D
FGFR	Tyrosine kinase receptor	D, T
NGF	Growth factor	D
trkA	Tyrosine kinase receptor	D, T
gp75NGFR	Tyrosine kinase receptor	D, T
NKX3.1	Transcription factor	D
Maspin	Tumor suppressor protein	D
On the horizon		
C-MYC	Transcription factor	D, P, T
PSCA	Stem cell antigen	D, T
N-cadherin	Cell adhesion molecule	D
EZH2	Transcriptional repressor	D, P
E2F3	Transcription factor	D, P
Thymosin β15	Actin binding protein	D, P

D, diagnosis; FGF, fibroblast growth factor; FGFR, FGF receptor; HAase, hyaluronidase; HRG, heregulin; IGFR, IGF receptor; NGF, nerve growth factor; P, prognosis; PSCA, prostate stem cell antigen; PTEN, phosphatase and tensin homolog deleted on chromosome 10; T, therapy; TGFβ1, Transforming growth factor β1; VEGF, vascular endothelial growth factor; VEGFR, VEGF receptor; AMACR, alpha-methylacyl Co A rasemase.

PROMISING BIOMARKERS FOR PROSTATE CANCER

Ki67

BIOLOGY

Ki67 is a nuclear antigen present throughout the cell cycle (G1, S, G2, and mitosis), but not at rest (G0), and its expression is associated with cellular proliferation.[3] During interphase, the antigen can be exclusively detected within the nucleus, whereas in mitosis most of the protein is relocated to the surface of the chromosomes. The Ki67 protein was originally defined by the prototype monoclonal antibody Ki-67, which was generated by immunizing mice with nuclei of the Hodgkin's lymphoma cell line L428. When the antigen was found to be a protein and the primary structure could be deduced from the corresponding cDNA, it revealed no homology to any known polypeptide.

CLINICAL CORRELATES

Multiple studies have demonstrated that elevated expression of Ki67 is associated with an adverse prognosis in prostate cancer. Ki67 has been shown to be an independent and significant prognostic factor for disease-specific survival in multivariate analysis.[4,5] In 106 patients with stage T1 to T3 prostate cancer treated with external beam radiation therapy (EBRT), elevated Ki67-staining of biopsy specimens correlated with poor progression-free survival (median follow-up: 62 months).[6] In a separate study involving 104 patients treated by radical prostatectomy, surgical specimens stained for Ki67 in the area of highest tumor grade.[7] Ki67 expression was significantly associated with time to biochemical failure, age, grade, stage, margin status, tumor size, and preoperative PSA. After multivariate analysis, only stage, PSA, and Ki67 expression were retained as significant independent predictors of time to biochemical recurrence. A similar study of 180 patients treated with radical prostatectomy also demonstrated an inverse correlation between Ki67 expression and disease-free survival.[8] Ki67 expression has also been shown to predict disease progression following initial hormonal therapy in patients with advanced prostate cancer.[9] Recently, a large multicenter study of 537 patients reported that Ki67 expression was the most significant determinant of distant metastasis and disease-specific survival in patients following androgen deprivation and radiation therapy.[10] In the future, the pretherapeutic assessment of Ki67 expression may become of increasing importance in the evaluation of tumor aggressiveness and the selection of adequate treatment. In a multiparametric analysis, which assessed p53, BCL2, and Ki67 expression in core needle biopsies

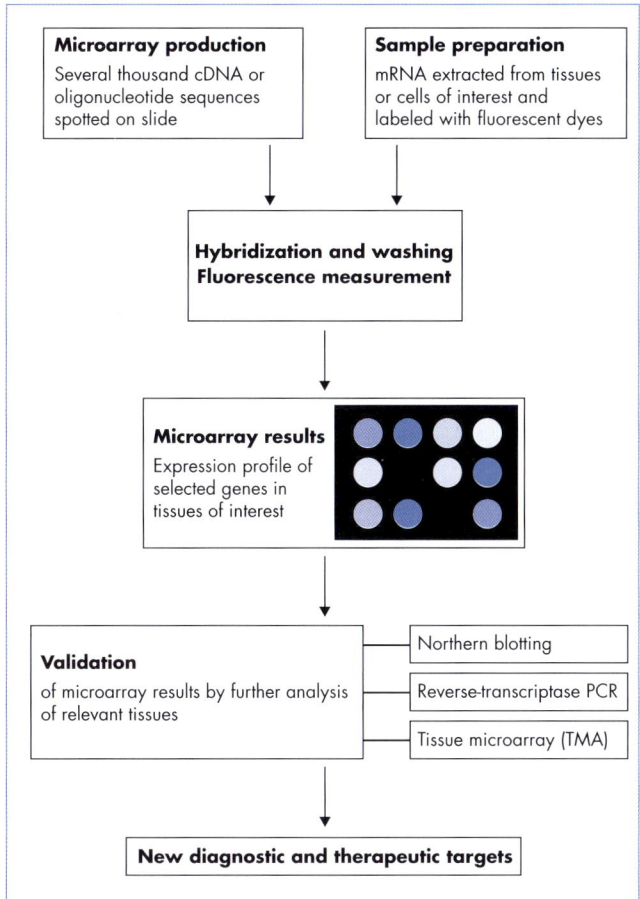

Fig. 28.1

Microarrays allow the analysis of patterns of expression of large numbers of genes in tissues of interest, such as localized prostate cancer. Visual representations of data show spots of different colors and intensities for genes expressed in either or both tissues at differing levels.

Rubin, et al. alpha-Methylacyl coenzyme A racemase as a tissue biomarker for prostate cancer. JAMA 2002;287:1662–1670.[75]

of prostate tumors, Ki67 was the only independent predictor of tumor-specific survival.[11]

OVERVIEW

Ongoing efforts to resolve the biological function of Ki67 will contribute to improving the understanding of the complex regulatory network that governs cell proliferation and support the acceptance of Ki67 as a general proliferation marker. Thus, Ki67 may serve as a significant diagnostic and prognostic biomarker for prostate cancer in patients managed with a variety of treatment modalities.

p27

BIOLOGY

p27 (Kip1) is a member of the universal cyclin-dependent kinase inhibitor family and is a putative tumor suppressor gene.[12] The p27 gene encodes for a cyclin-dependent kinase inhibitor that regulates progression of the cell cycle from G1 to S phase by binding to and inhibiting the cyclin E-CDK2 complex, thereby playing a role in cell cycle arrest and apoptosis.[13] Dysregulation of p27 expression may be a critical early event in the development of prostate cancer since reduced expression of p27 removes a cell-cycle block in human prostate epithelial cells. It has recently been shown that a ubiquitin E3 ligase, the SCF[SKP] complex (SKP1, CUL-1/CDC53 and the F-box protein SKP2), mediates the polyubiquitination of p27.[14] SKP2 is a positive regulator of G1 to S transition and promotes ubiquitin-mediated proteolysis of the cyclin-dependent kinase inhibitor p27. SKP2, the substrate-targeting subunit of the SCF complex, binds to the phosphorylated p27 and targets p27 for many cancers. Thus, upregulation of SKP2 ubiquitin ligase should result in decreased p27 and subsequent loss of cell cycle control.

CLINICAL CORRELATES

Several groups have observed that primary prostate cancers with lower levels of p27 protein were more biologically aggressive.[15–18] Expression of p27 has been shown to progressively decrease with higher tumor grade and stage in radical prostatectomy specimens.[16–20] Expression of p27 in needle biopsy specimens has also been shown to be inversely correlated with tumor stage and grade.[20] Moreover, in a multivariate analysis of a cohort of 52 Spanish patients treated with radical prostatectomy, low p27 expression by immuno-histochemical staining of the surgical specimen was the lone independent predictor of biochemical recurrence.[21] At 3 years, 59% of patients with low p27 expression had a PSA recurrence, whereas only 18% of patients with normal p27 expression relapsed. Similarly, in a separate study of 86 patients treated with radical prosta-tectomy, low p27 expression was a strong independent predictor of disease-free survival, second only to patho-logic stage.[18] Low p27 expression also correlated with seminal vesicle involvement and positive surgical mar-gins. The prognostic value of p27 is particularly impor-tant in organ-confined disease, which has up to a 20% PSA recurrence rate at 5 years. Furthermore, multivari-ate analysis demonstrated that loss of p27 confers a five-fold relative risk of biochemical recurrence inde-pendent of Gleason grade and preoperative PSA in patients with pathologic T2a to T3b disease. Therefore, absent or low levels of p27 protein expression appears to be an adverse prognostic factor in patients with clini-cally organ confined disease treated by radical prostate-ctomy. In addition, patients with positive surgical margins and low p27 expression have a relative risk of recurrence of 3.4 (p < 0.04).[2] Moreover, in patients with positive margins, low or absent p27 staining carries the

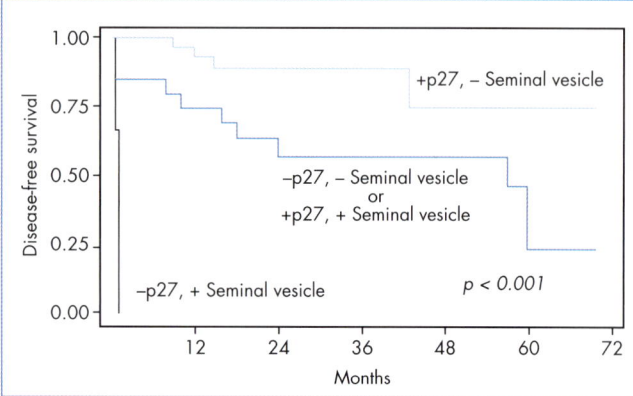

Fig. 28.2
Positive surgical margins: impact of p27 and stage on survival. Kaplan–Meier Disease-free survival curves for patients with organ-confined disease stratified by p27 expression.

same prognostic significance as seminal vesicle invasion (Figure 28.2). Thus, p27 status might help determine whether a patient with a positive margin would benefit from adjuvant radiation or other adjuvant therapies. Importantly, p27 status at the time of the initial prostate biopsy also appears to predict biochemical recurrence. In a study of 161 men with subsequent surgical management, p27 immunostaining in less than 45% of the cells resulted in significant preoperative risk stratification for time to PSA failure (HR 2.41, p = 0.010) (Figure 28.3).[23] This relationship retained significance in multivariate analysis. Furthermore, P27 expression in the prostate biopsy was a significant predictor of PSA failure for pathologically organ-confirmed disease, but not for those with non-organ-confirmed disease.[22] Therefore, p27 may be an important prognostic factor at the time of diagnosis.

SKP2 levels assessed by immunohistochemistry have been shown to be dramatically increased in both prostatic intraepithelial neoplasia (PIN) and radical prostatectomy specimens.[24] In addition, the level of SKP2 expression was positively correlated with preoperative PSA, Gleason score, and stage. A higher SKP2 labeling index also negatively impacted biochemical recurrence-free survival after radical prostatectomy. In another study, 51 samples from needle biopsies, transurethral resection and radical prostatectomy were analyzed for p27 and SKP2 expression.[25] SKP2 expression demonstrated a significant and direct correlation with malignancy.

Furthermore, SKP2 expression positively correlated with Gleason score and PSA. In addition, patients with metastases had significantly higher Skp2 and Ki67 expression than those with organ confined disease. SKP2 levels significantly correlated with Ki67, whereas an inverse correlation was found between p27 and SKP2.

OVERVIEW

The degradation of cyclin-dependent kinase inhibitors p21 and p27 by proteasome-dependent proteolysis may allow for the use of targeted therapies, such as bortezomib (PS-341, Millennium, Cambridge, MA), a proteasome inhibitor. Treatment with proteasome inhibitors results in cell-cycle arrest and a coordinated increase in p27 levels in advance of apoptosis. In addition, drugs that target its specific ubiquitin ligase may be useful. In summary, p27 is an excellent independent predictor of biologic behavior of prostate cancer, particularly in organ-confined disease, and may predict response to hormonal ablation therapy.

PTEN

BIOLOGY

Phosphatase and tensin homolog deleted on chromosome ten (PTEN)/mutated in multiple

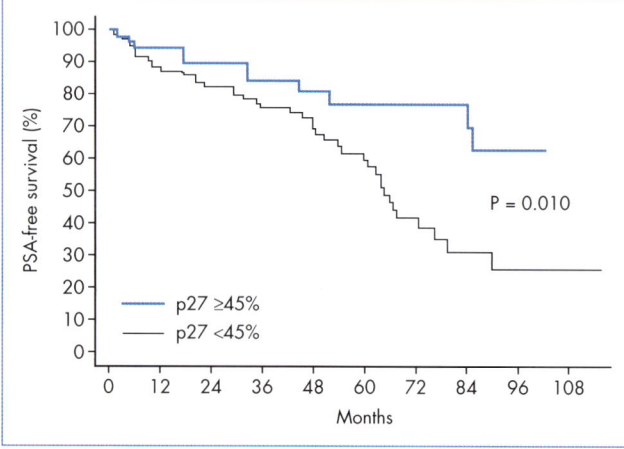

Fig. 28.3
Kaplan–Meier survival curves for PSA recurrence after radical prostatectomy stratified by greater than or less than 45% of tumor cells in prostate needle biopsy specimen staining positive for p27. (PSA, prostate-specific antigen.)

advanced cancers (MMAC)/transforming growth factor-β (TGFβ)-regulated and epithelial cell-enriched phosphatase (TEP1) is a candidate tumor suppressor gene located at 10q2.3.[26] PTEN is a phospholipid phosphatase that acts as a negative regulator in the phosphatidylinositol-3,4,5-triphosphate (PIP3)/Akt (also called protein kinase B) signaling pathway (Figure 28.4).[27] The end result of this pathway is to inhibit apoptosis and promote proliferation. PTEN dephosphorylates and thereby inactivates PIP3 and inhibits phosphatidylinositol 3-kinase (PI3K)-dependent activation of Akt, a serine-threonine kinase.[28] Thus, deletion or inactivating mutations of PTEN will lead to constitutive activation of PIP3 and Akt with subsequent uncontrolled cellular proliferation. Activation of PI3K and Akt has been shown to provide a survival signal in response to nerve growth factor (NGF), insulin-like growth factor 1 (IGF1), platelet-derived growth factor (PDGF), interleukin 3 (IL3), and the extracellular matrix.[29,30] Akt is likely to send survival signals by phosphorylating multiple targets, including the BCL2 family member Bad and the cell death pathway enzyme caspase 9.[31,32] Homozygous inactivation of PTEN/MMAC/TEP1 occurs in a large number of different types of tumors,[33–36] including advanced prostate cancer.[35,37] Interestingly, PTEN appears to suppress cell growth by distinct mechanisms in different types of tumors, producing G1 cell cycle arrest in glioblastoma cells, but inducing apoptosis in carcinomas. In addition, PTEN-deficient cell lines show an accelerated entry into S phase, which is accompanied by downregulation of p27.[38] These studies suggest that PTEN modulates both cell survival and cell-cycle progression. Furthermore, the role for PTEN in cellular signaling via the mitogen-activated protein kinase (MAPK) signaling pathways has been defined.[39] PTEN dephosphorylates Shc and focal adhesion kinase (FAK), which is subsequently followed by inhibition of Ras activation, followed by further downstream effects targeting the extracellular signal-regulated kinases (ERK) pathway of MAPK signaling.

CLINICAL CORRELATES

Loss of heterozygosity (LOH) at the PTEN locus has been observed in 29% to 42% of prostate tumors, and screening for homozygous deletions has identified a second mutational event in 43% of prostate tumors.[35,40] LOH at 10q was found in 11 of 60 tumors (18%) that were localized to the prostate, but also in 12 of 20 pelvic metastases (60%). This suggests that PTEN may be an important tumor suppressor in a subset of prostate cancers and inactivation of PTEN may be an important secondary genetic event that contributes to prostate cancer progression. In 109 primary prostate tumors, loss of PTEN expression, as assessed by immuno-histochemical staining, was found in 20% of primary prostate tumors and highly correlated with elevated

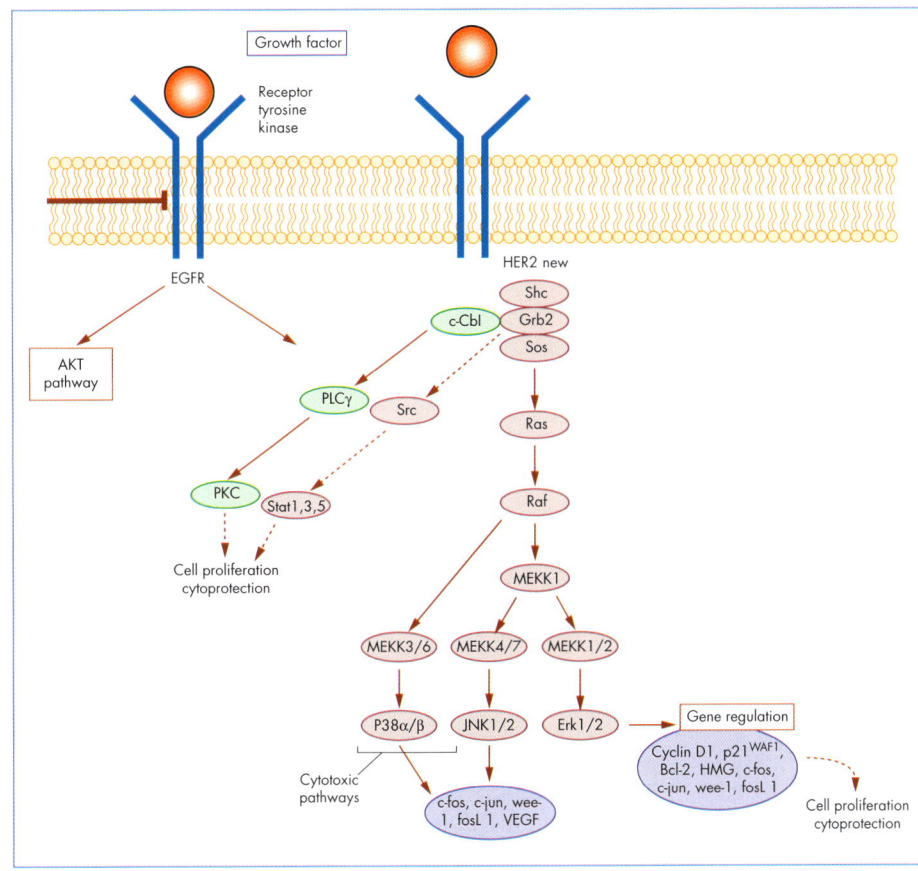

Fig. 28.4
The phosphatidylinositol 3-kinase (PI3K)/Akt/PTEN pathway. Secreted ligands such as insulin-like growth factor (IGF1) bind to and activate their transmembrane receptors (IGFR). Receptor activation results in the recruitment of PI3K to the receptor. Akt activation results in the phosphorylation of a number of downstream target substrates. PTEN is an enzyme that specifically dephosphorylates the phosphorylated lipids (PI-3,4,5-P3) produced by PI3K and dampens or blocks activation of the pathway. Tumor cells lacking PTEN contain elevated levels of PI-3,4,5-P3 and consequently have constitutively activated Akt and phosphorylation of down Akt targets. Substrates of Akt are involved in the regulation of both cell proliferation and cell death.

Gleason score and advanced stage.[41] Loss of PTEN expression has also been shown to be an independent predictor of biochemical failure in men treated by radical prostatectomy.[42]

OVERVIEW

Several studies have shown that loss of PTEN in cell lines and tumors results in elevated levels of Akt. Therefore, loss of PTEN might be useful as a factor predictive of success for therapies directed against this pathway. One of the downstream kinases activated in the PIP3/Akt pathway is mTOR (mammalian target of rapamycin). PTEN loss or inactivation leads to overactive mTOR and unchecked cellular proliferation.[43,44] Blocking mTOR should in essence take over the inhibitory role of the defective or deficient PTEN. Rapamycin and rapamycin analogs, such as CCI-779 (Wyeth, Madison, NJ) and RAD001 (Novartis, East Hanover, NJ), can target mTOR and inhibit its activation of substrates (S6 kinase and 4E-BP1) leading to tumor growth arrest. PTEN tumor suppressor gene mutations have also been shown to correlate with increased S6 kinase activity and phosphorylation of ribosomal S6 protein providing evidence for activation of the FRAP/mTOR pathway in these cells. In accordance, PTEN mutation makes tumors dramatically more responsive to treatment with CCI-779 than tumors with normal PTEN.[45] Thus, targeted therapy using an mTOR inhibitor is currently being studied in phase II clinical trials as neoadjuvant therapy in patients whose needle biopsies stain negative for PTEN by immunohistochemistry. Thus, PTEN may be a useful diagnostic and prognostic biomarker, as well as one that may help select patients for targeted therapies.

E-CADHERIN

BIOLOGY

E-cadherin is a cell adhesion molecule (CAM) associated with cell–cell and cell–matrix interaction, leukocyte function, and tumor invasion, and metastasis in a variety of tumors. E-cadherin or L-CAM belongs to the cadherin family, which is subdivided into at least three types: E-, P-, and N-cadherins.[46] E-cadherin is present in virtually all types of epithelial cells, although it is also found in glia and some types of neurons. The E-cadherin gene is located on chromosome 16q22.1 and encodes a cell membrane glycoprotein that is involved in intercellular adhesion.[46] The long arm of chromosome 16 (16q) is deleted in 30% of primary and more than 70% of metastatic prostate cancer by LOH analysis.[47] E-cadherin functions as a Ca^{2+}-dependent epithelial CAM. Its intracellular domain binds directly to β-catenin and, along with α-catenin, links E-cadherin to the underlying actin cytoskeleton.[46] In addition to its role in adhesion, β-catenin has been implicated in the Wnt signal transduction pathway and links the adenomatous polyposis coli (APC) tumor suppressor protein with transcription factors of the lymphoid enhancer factor/T-cell factor (LEF/TCF) family.[48] Loss of E-cadherin function may endow tumor cells with a relative growth advantage over normal contact-inhibited cells. E-cadherin expression, as assessed by immunohistochemistry, has been shown to be decreased or absent in prostate cancer.[47] E-cadherin has also been shown to mediate inhibition of invasion and proliferation via the induction of p27 in three-dimensional culture.[49] These findings link extracellular stimuli to the cell-cycle machinery and suggest a role for E-cadherin and p27 as suppressors of both invasion and growth.[50]

CLINICAL CORRELATES

Clinically, decreased or absent E-cadherin expression in prostate cancer is associated with tumor grade, advanced clinical stage, and poor survival.[47,51] An immuno-histochemical analysis evaluating 89 prostatectomy specimens demonstrated that E-cadherin expression was inversely correlated with Gleason grade, stage, presence of metastasis, and survival; and loss of E-cadherin staining was a powerful predictor of poor outcome and overall survival.[51] Decreased expression of E-cadherin in radical prostatectomy specimens has been shown to portend an elevated risk of PSA recurrence in patients with T2 tumors.[52] Furthermore, abnormal E-cadherin expression in radical prostatectomy specimens has strongly been associated with the detection of prostate cancer cells in the peripheral blood.[53] Hypermethylation of the E-cadherin promoter has also been shown to correlate with reduced or absent E-cadherin protein staining in prostate cancer specimens, and the severity of hypermethylation has been associated with higher tumor grade.[54] Demethylation restored E-cadherin mRNA transcription in prostate cancer lines.

OVERVIEW

It is unequivocal that mutations or reversible defects in cadherins and catenins are important in prostate cancer. These molecules act as both tumor suppressors and invasion suppressors. In addition, transcriptional regulation is achieved through β-catenin, and this signaling pathway may be an attractive target for therapy, since mutational changes of the many components affecting β-catenin functionality have been found in multiple human cancer types. Alternatively, upregulation of cadherin mediated cell–cell adhesion might be another therapeutic target by attempting to counteract signaling and simultaneously induce cell–cell adhesion. In summary, E-cadherin may be a useful diagnostic and prognostic biomarker, as well as a therapeutic target for prostate cancer.

TRANSFORMING GROWTH FACTOR-BETA 1

BIOLOGY

Transforming growth factor-β1 (TGFβ1) is one of more than 30 structurally related polypeptides that include activins, bone morphogenic proteins, and other TGFβs.[55] These proteins regulate diverse processes including cell proliferation, apoptosis, differentiation, migration, chemotaxis, immune response, and angiogenesis. The signaling cascade begins at the cell surface, where TGFβ ligand binding acts to bring together two receptors, type I and type II.[55] The type II receptor activates the type I receptor, which in turn phosphorylates and activates a group of transcription factors known as mothers against decapentaplegic-related (Smad) proteins.[56] The TGFβ superfamily of cytokines plays a role in the control of cellular proliferation, chemotaxis, angiogenesis, and cellular differentiation; however, TGFβ1 can also play opposing roles in tumor development. In the initial phase of tumorigenesis it may act as a tumor suppressor, but, during the later phases, it may function as a tumor promoter.[57] The TGFβ promoting activities for angiogenesis, immunosuppression, and synthesis of extracellular matrix provide an appropriate microenvironment for rapid tumor growth and metastasis,[58] and it plays an important role in the regulation of extracellular matrix synthesis, degradation, and remodelling.[58] These activities indirectly assist tumor progression in the invasion and metastasis phases. Transforming growth factor-β1 stimulates the synthesis of collagens, fibronectin, proteoglycans, tenascin, thrombospondin, plasminogen activator inhibitor 1 (PAI1), and tissue inhibitor of metalloproteases 1 (TIMP1), which are relevant in tumor invasion and metastasis.

CLINICAL CORRELATES

Loss of the inhibitory effects of TGFβ1 has been associated with cancer progression, and elevated local and circulating levels have correlated with prostate cancer invasion and metastasis.[59,60] Immuno-histochemical studies have demonstrated increased expression of TGFβ1 in prostate cancer epithelium compared to normal prostate.[61] Furthermore, increased TGFβ1 staining has been shown to be associated with higher tumor grade and presence of metastases.[62] Downstream alterations involving the expression of TGFβ1 receptors and Smads are also implicated in cancer and various other disorders in humans. In a study of 52 patients that underwent radical prostatectomy, loss of TGFβ1 receptor type I was significantly associated with poor prognosis.[63] In another study of 118 patients who underwent radical prostatectomy, TGFβ1 was significantly associated

with a loss of TGFβ1 receptor type I and type II expression.[64] Furthermore, loss of TGFβ1 receptor type I expression was an independent predictor of biochemical progression. Thus, in the absence of an intact signaling pathway, TGFβ1 may promote tumorigenesis.

OVERVIEW

The activated TGFβ1 signaling pathway is emerging as an attractive target in cancer and functionally relevant variants of this pathway may lead to the identification of individuals with a higher cancer risk. Therapies include blocking or neutralizing TGFβ1, which may restore or enhance immune recognition of tumor. In addition, inhibitors of the TGFβ1 signaling pathway may lead to delays in tumor progression and improvements in overall survival. In summary, TGFβ1 and its receptors may be useful diagnostic and prognostic markers for prostate cancer, as well as potential therapeutic targets.

HEPSIN

BIOLOGY

Hepsin is a type II membrane-associated serine protease originally found as a cDNA clone in a human liver cDNA library.[65] The hepsin gene encodes for a 417 amino acid single-chain protein with a molecular mass of 51 kDa.[66] The primary amino acid sequence of hepsin shows a high level of identity with trypsin and trypsin-like blood clotting factors.[67] The hepsin gene was found to be highly overexpressed in prostate cancer tissue compared with nonmalignant and benign prostatic hyperplasia (BPH) tissue.[68,69] It was recently demonstrated in a mouse model that hepsin overexpression in prostate epithelium caused disorganization of the basement membrane and promoted primary prostate cancer progression and metastasis to liver, lung, and bone.[70]

CLINICAL CORRELATES

Immunohistochemical studies revealed strongest expression of hepsin in high-grade PIN lesions, followed by primary prostate cancer, hormone refractory prostate cancer, and benign prostate tissue to the lowest degree.[67] In one study, lower hepsin expression was seen in patients with postoperative PSA failure, higher Gleason scores, and larger tumors, indicating an inverse correlation of hepsin expression with patient prognosis.[68] However, in a more recent and larger series, hepsin expression was associated with higher T stage and Gleason scores indicating a positive correlation between hepsin expression and probability of cancer progression.[71]

OVERVIEW

The structure and its homology with other serine proteases strongly imply a possible role for hepsin not only for promoting tumor growth, but also for cancer therapy. As a cell surface molecule that is overexpressed in prostate cancer, it may be a potential therapeutic target. Thus, hepsin may be a useful diagnostic and prognostic biomarker, in particular for distinguishing more aggressive (Gleason grade 4/5) tumors.

ALPHA-METHYLACYL CoA RACEMASE OR P504S

BIOLOGY

Alpha-methylacyl CoA racemase (AMACR) or P504S is a fatty acid metabolism enzyme overexpressed in prostate cancer and high-grade PIN.[72] It plays an important role in the β-oxidation of branched-chain fatty acids and fatty acid derivatives by catalyzing the conversion of several forms of (2R)-methyl-branched chain fatty acyl-coenzyme A to their (S)-stereoisomers. The gene for AMACR is located on chromosome 5p13 and encodes a 382 amino acid protein.

CLINICAL CORRELATES

The results of a number of studies from multiple institutions have demonstrated the AMACR is an important positive tissue marker for prostate cancer regardless of tumor grade, with a sensitivity ranging from 82% to 100% and a specificity ranging from 79% to 100% in prostate biopsies.[72–74] In one study, significant over expression of AMACR in prostate cancer was found in three of four independent DNA microarray analyses (n = 128 specimens) and tissue microarray specimens including 17 metastatic prostate cancers.[75] Another study found that over 95% of prostate cancers stained positively for AMACR, whereas less than 4% of histologically normal prostate epithelium was positive.[72] They also demonstrated 81% and 93% AMACR positivity in 32 metastatic prostate cancers from nonhormone refractory disease and 14 hormone refractory prostate cancers, respectively. Yet another study evaluated 405 clinical specimens including 376 prostate needle biopsies with P504S monoclonal antibody, and reported that a total of 153 of 186 biopsies (82%) with prostate cancer were positive for AMACR, while 21% of the foci of benign prostate epithelium showed focal, faint, and noncircumferential luminal staining.[76] The utility of this marker for prostate cancer has been extended by combining immunohistochemistry for AMACR with staining for the nuclear protein, p63, a basal cell marker in the prostate that is absent in prostate cancer.[72] Combined staining for p63 and AMACR resulted in a

pattern that greatly facilitated the identification of malignant prostate cells.[77,78] Current data show that treatment of prostate cancer with radiation and/or hormonal therapy has no overall effect on AMACR overexpression demonstrating that this immunostain is useful in the detection of cancer in post-treatment biopsies.[79] There have been no studies thus far that have demonstrated an association between AMACR and histoprognostic factors, such as Gleason score, pathologic stage, or margin status.[72,75] No association has also been found between AMACR expression and preoperative PSA levels, biochemical recurrence rates, and the Ki67 labeling index as a marker of tumor cell proliferation. Regardless, the consistency and magnitude of cancer cell-specific expression of AMACR may render it an important new marker of prostate cancer and its use in combination with basal specific 34βE12 and/or p63 staining may lead to a method for improved identification of prostate cancers.

OVERVIEW

AMACR is the first gene identified from prostate cancer by cDNA microarrays to be suitable for clinical practice and to improve the diagnosis of prostate cancer. Although it has limitations with respect to sensitivity and specificity, AMACR will no doubt become a standard adjunctive stain used by pathologists seeking to reach a definitive diagnosis in prostate biopsies considered to be atypical, but not diagnostic of malignancy on hematoxylin and eosin sections alone. This immunostain is currently in clinical use at multiple institutions, including the authors' own.

TELOMERE LENGTH AND TELOMERASE ACTIVITY

BIOLOGY

Mammalian aging occurs in part because of a decline in the restorative capacity of tissue stem cells. These self-renewing cells are rendered malignant by a small number of oncogenic mutations, and overlapping tumor suppressor mechanisms—such as $p16^{INK4a}$-RB, ARF-p53, and the telomere—have evolved to ward against this possibility. These beneficial antitumor pathways, however, appear also to limit stem cell lifespan, thereby contributing to aging. Telomeres are unique structures at the ends of all eukaryotic chromosomes and are composed of repeats of 6 base pairs as well as several different binding proteins that serve to protect chromosome ends from being recognized as double-strand breaks from illegitimate recombination.[80] Telomeres cannot be fully replicated during cell division and are subjected to progressive shortening, unless they are lengthened by the enzyme telomerase (a reverse transcriptase enzyme that catalyzes the synthesis of further telomeric DNA repeats) or by an alternative pathway referred to as alternative lengthening of telomeres. Telomerase activity allows for continued proliferation of cells by restoration and/or preservation of at least a minimal telomere length, which can be detected in 80% to 95% of tumor cells. The telomerase holoenzyme consists of the catalytic subunit reverse transcriptase protein (hTERT), the telomerase RNA template subunit (hTR), and other associated proteins. Moreover, the hTERT gene is regulated by different oncogenes including c-*MYC*, *BCL2*, *HER2*, and *RAS*, which seem to play an important role in prostate cancer progression.

CLINICAL CORRELATES

The importance of the telomere in prostate cancer as a diagnostic and prognostic marker has been investigated. In one study, telomere lengths in prostate cancer tissue were significantly and consistently shorter than those from adjacent normal tissue or BPH tissue.[81] In agreement with these results, hTERT immunoreactivity was found in high-grade prostate tumors (Gleason score >4).[82] A puzzling aspect of results on the relation between telomere length, telomerase activity, and prostate cancer is that telomerase activity has been shown to be increased in prostate cancers.[81,83] This may be due to activation of telomerase in tumor cells containing short telomeres in order to maintain telomere function. Another study demonstrated that death and disease recurrence in men with prostate cancer was significantly associated with reduced telomere DNA content, presumably reflecting shortened telomeres.[84] Telomerase activity has also been correlated with prostate tumor aggressiveness. In particular, compared with low-grade tumors, high-grade tumors have maximally activated telomerase, and a significant correlation between the telomerase activity and the Gleason score has been found.[85]

OVERVIEW

These findings suggest that telomerase might represent a very good candidate for targeted therapy in prostate tumors. In addition, considering the multigenic defects of prostate cancer, the combination of anti-telomerase strategies with conventional drugs and/or molecules capable of interfering with oncogenic pathways might efficiently improve the response of this tumor. In summary, results obtained from several different groups have shown that telomere shortening is a prevalent diagnostic and prognostic biomarker in prostate cancer and that it occurs early in the process of prostate carcinogenesis. Telomerase may also serve as a valuable diagnostic marker, as well as a potential target of therapy.

ANDROGEN RECEPTOR

BIOLOGY

Androgens are required for the development of the normal prostate and prostate cancer.[86] Androgens act through the androgen receptor (AR), which belongs to the steroid receptor superfamily of ligand-dependent transcription factors.[86] The AR gene is located on the long arm of the X chromosome at Xq11-12. The AR has a central role in mediating the biologic effects of androgens to different downstream genes. Proposed mechanisms of progression to androgen-independent growth include loss of AR expression; amplification of the AR gene; mutations of the AR gene, including shortened numbers of CAG nucleotide repeat sequences; activation of AR signaling pathway; recruitment of coactivators, such as ARA70; and presence of alternative signaling pathways, so that the AR is no longer relevant to disease progression.[87] It has also been suggested that other signaling pathways, such as HER2/NEU, could activate the AR pathway, especially when androgen levels are low.

CLINICAL CORRELATES

Immunohistochemistry studies have demonstrated AR expression in primary, advanced, and hormone-refractory prostate cancers, suggesting that disease progression is not necessarily associated with loss of AR expression.[88] In addition, considerable heterogeneity of AR expression in specimens and among patients has been reported.[89-91] Increased heterogeneity of AR expression has been shown to be associated with higher Gleason grade.[89] A recent immunohistochemical analysis of AR and Ki67 expression in 640 radical prostatectomy specimens demonstrated that a high level of AR expression was positively correlated with clinical stage, lymph node status, extracapsular extension, seminal vesicle invasion, and Gleason score.[92] High levels of AR correlated with high Ki67 index and also predicted a higher probability of recurrence. Multivariate analysis showed that a high level of AR expression was an independent prognostic indicator of biochemical recurrence-free survival.

OVERVIEW

A number of recent studies have suggested that most hormone-refractory prostate tumors may in fact be still androgen dependent.[87] Identification of these abnormalities (e.g., mutation, amplification, or overexpression) may identify androgen resistant tumors. The AR is likely to be a major therapeutic target in prostate cancer. Blockade of AR with intracellular antibodies or antisense RNA can abolish hormone-refractory prostate cancer in animal models, supporting this hypothesis. Much work is being performed to understand AR regulation and structure, with the goal of developing new AR antagonists. Thus, the AR may be a useful diagnostic and prognostic marker for prostate cancer, as well as an important therapeutic target.

OTHER BIOMARKERS FOR PROSTATE CANCER

BCL2

BIOLOGY

The BCL2 gene is the prototype of a newly described class of oncogenes that modulate apoptosis.[93] It was initially discovered through the translocation in follicular lymphomas (t14,18) and has subsequently been found to be involved in the carcinogenesis of various epithelial tumors.[94,95] Overexpression of BCL2 has also been found to play a role in a number of human malignancies.[95] An increase in intracellular Ca^{2+} concentration has been implicated as an important signaling event associated with cell death in prostatic epithelial cells.[96] BCL2 has been shown to inhibit the depletion of the endoplasmic reticulum Ca^{2+} pool and thereby inhibit capacitative influx of extracellular Ca^{2+}.[97]

BCL2 is normally expressed in the basal cells of the prostate glandular epithelium, which are resistant to the effects of androgen withdrawal.[98] In contrast, BCL2-negative secretory glandular epithelial cells undergo apoptotic cell death in response to androgen deprivation.[98] High levels of BCL2 expression are seen with greater frequency as prostate cancers progress from localized (7% of tumors overexpressing BCL2) to metastasizing androgen-dependent (17%) to androgen-independent (67%) tumors.[96] Several groups have also shown that androgen-independent prostate cancers are typically immunoreactive for BCL2 protein.[98,99] Thus, BCL2 may enable prostate cancer cells to remain viable despite castrate levels of androgen, and hormone ablation therapy may be selecting for BCL2 positive cells that fail to undergo apoptosis after hormone withdrawal.

Expression of BCL2 within prostate cancer cells has been associated with resistance to cell death induction by various chemotherapeutic agents. A mechanism by which BCL2 induces its antiapoptotic effect may be through the regulation of microtubule integrity.[100] Anticancer drugs that inhibit microtubule formation, such as paclitaxel and vinblastine, also induce BCL2 phosphorylation leading to its inactivation and apoptotic cell death. In contrast, drugs that damage DNA, such as doxorubicin and cisplatin, do not induce BCL2 phosphorylation or inhibit microtubule

formation. Phosphorylation of BCL2 involves the serine or threonine protein kinase c-RAF1.[101] In contrast, the antiapoptotic function of BCL2 may require phosphorylation of serine 70, one of several residues targeted by the c-JUN *N*-terminal kinase.[102,103] Furthermore, it has been suggested that BCL2 can target RAF1 to mitochondrial membranes, and the localization of RAF1 on the outer mitochondrial membrane protects cells from undergoing apoptosis, resulting in the phosphorylation of the proapoptotic protein, Bad. Growth factor activation of PI3K/Akt signaling pathway also results in the phosphorylation of BAD, thereby promoting cell survival.

CLINICAL CORRELATES

Evidence for the role of BCL2 as a biomarker in prostate cancer has been mixed. Expression of BCL2 in prostate needle biopsy specimens has been shown to predict biochemical failure in patients treated with radiation.[6,104] Similarly, several studies have confirmed that BCL2 expression in prostatectomy specimens correlates with higher rates of biochemical recurrence in patients who underwent radical prostatectomy for clinically localized prostate cancer.[52,105] However, in contrast to the radiotherapy studies, BCL2 staining in the preoperative biopsy specimen did not correlate with outcome.[105] In addition, BCL2 expression was significantly associated with poorer disease-specific and overall survival in a cohort of 221 elderly prostate cancer patients (median age, 75 years) followed expectantly.[106] However, this correlation failed to retain its significance after multivariate analysis. Expression of BCL2 has also been shown to be an adverse prognostic indicator in patients with locally advanced or metastatic prostate cancer receiving hormonal therapy.[99]

OVERVIEW

Induction of apoptotic cell death after androgen ablation or chemotherapy may be enhanced through functional inhibition of BCL2 with molecules such as antisense oligonucleotides (ASOs), which are short synthetic stretches of chemically modified DNA capable of specifically hybridizing to the mRNA of a target gene.[107] Based on the available data, BCL2 may be used as a diagnostic and prognostic marker, and may also be a promising therapeutic target.

p53

BIOLOGY

p53 is a tumor suppressor gene that encodes for a nuclear transcription factor that functions in cell cycle control, DNA repair, and apoptosis, and has been intensively studied in a wide range of human malignancies.[108] In response to DNA damage, wild-type p53 arrests cells in the G1 phase or induces apoptosis,[108] and is regulated by a number of inputs. The ataxia–telangiectasia gene product is thought to detect DNA damage, which in turn activates the cHK1 and cHK2 serine-threoine kinases that can phosphorylate and activate p53 in the damage response pathway. In response to DNA damage, p21 is induced by p53, which leads to p53-induced G1 arrest as a consequence of inhibition of cyclin-dependent kinase activity. p53 is in turn negatively regulated by MDM2, which targets p53 for protein degradation. Finally, the gene encoding the cell cycle regulator p16[INK4a] also encodes a second protein p14[ARF]. The alternative reading frame (ARF) protein is induced by a number of oncogenic signals and blocks the ability of MDM2 to degrade p53. The p53 gene is located on the short arm of chromosome 17 and LOH on chromosome 17p occurs in 16% of prostate cancers, with a range of 5% to 38%.[109–111] LOH for p53 in one allele, most often occurs in exons 5 through 8 and can either result in no protein being produced or production of a dysfunctional protein. Cells having such p53 mutations are genetically unstable, and they are prone to developing further mutations leading to tumor progression. Wild-type p53 has a short half-life and is normally expressed at low levels in G0 and G1 phases. In contrast, most p53 missense mutations result in a protein with a much longer half-life, facilitating detection by immunohistochemistry.[112,113] However, immunohistochemistry will not identify in-frame deletions, splicing errors, or nonsense mutations.[114]

CLINICAL CORRELATES

Studies have shown that p53 expression correlates with higher Gleason score, nuclear grade, pathologic stage, and proliferation in localized primary prostate cancer and that an increase in p53 mutations is present in advanced prostate cancer, with the highest incidence occurring in androgen-independent tumors.[115] A number of studies have suggested that p53 might have prognostic value in patients with prostate cancer. In a study evaluating archival paraffin-embedded radical prostatectomy specimens from 139 patients, immunohistochemical staining for p53 protein nuclear expression was positively associated with rising grade and stage, and was an independent predictor of disease-free survival.[116] In a study of 221 prostate cancer patients who underwent watchful waiting (median follow-up, 15 years), the degree of p53 nuclear accumulation in the biopsy specimen was significantly associated with disease-specific survival in both the overall study population as well as the subgroup of 125 patients with clinically localized disease.[117] Similarly, several studies have reported that nuclear accumulation of p53 in radical prostatectomy specimens correlates with increased risk of PSA recurrence and reduced disease-specific survival.[105,118,119] Of note, one study demonstrated that expression of p53 in radical prostatectomy specimens was significantly associated with biochemical recurrence, whereas p53 levels in preoperative biopsy specimens was not.[105] Positive p53 staining heralded PSA failure in patients with localized tumors treated with radiation.[104,120] Finally, in a study of patients with locally advanced prostate cancer treated with a combination of radiation and maximal androgen blockade versus radiation alone, abnormal p53 protein expression by immunohistochemistry of pretreatment prostate specimens (needle biopsy or transurethral resection) was significantly associated with an increased incidence of distant metastasis and decreased progression-free and overall survival.[121] Interestingly, time to metastasis was unrelated to p53 status in patients treated with radiation alone.

OVERVIEW

Unfortunately, the data for p53 have not been uniformly positive. Multiple studies have also failed to demonstrate a relationship between p53 and outcome, including disease-specific survival in advanced prostate cancers treated with hormone ablation,[122] PSA recurrence following radical prostatectomy,[52] and PSA recurrence in radical prostatectomy patients subsequently treated with neoadjuvant androgen ablation and salvage radiotherapy.[123] A major limitation of p53 in predicting behavior is that its inactivation occurs primarily in advanced disease.

EPIDERMAL GROWTH FACTOR RECEPTOR TYROSINE KINASE FAMILY

BIOLOGY

There are four members of the epidermal growth factor receptor (EGFR) tyrosine kinase family: ERBB1, ERBB2, ERBB3, and ERBB4.[124] The majority of prostate cancers express ERBB1, ERBB2, and ERBB3, but little or no ERBB4.[125] ERBB1 is the EGFR, and has frequently been found to be overexpressed in tumors of epithelial origin. Amplification of the ERBB1/EGFR gene has not been detected in prostate cancer, but overexpression of this receptor is common. In nearly all prostate cancer cell lines and tissues surveyed, an autocrine loop of TGFα/EGF and ERBB1/EGFR exists, replacing the requirement for the normal stromal-derived ligand.[124] Inhibition of ERBB1/EGFR autocrine loop or the kinase activity of the receptor prevents the growth of prostate cancer cells, indicating an essential role of ERBB1/EGFR signaling in their growth.

ERBB2, also called NEU (for the rat homology) or HER2 (human EGF receptor 2), is a member of the ERBB/EGFR family. Located on chromosome 17p, it is a transmembrane tyrosine kinase growth factor receptor.

HER2/NEU may also play a role in advanced prostate cancer and in the progression to androgen-independent growth. A study showed that HER2/NEU could modulate responses in the setting of low androgen levels by restoring AR function, resulting in ligand-independent growth and clinical progression of the cancer.[126] Other studies have shown that HER2/NEU can increase growth rate, PSA level, and AR transactivation in prostate cancer cells through the MAPK pathway (Figure 28.5).[127]

CLINICAL CORRELATES

The expression of EGFR has been associated with Gleason score, PSA level, and development of hormone-refractory disease.[128] A recent study has demonstrated that HER2/NEU protein expression increases progressively from untreated patients to those preoperatively treated with maximal androgen blockade (MAB) in androgen-independent tumors. A panel of prostate specimens obtained from patients treated with surgery alone, MAB followed by surgery, or MAB alone who subsequently progressed to metastatic, androgen-independent disease revealed that only 25% of the surgery alone group stained positive for HER2/NEU, whereas 59% of the MAB/surgery group and 78% of the androgen-independent group were positive.[129] Moreover, those patients treated with MAB demonstrated amplification of HER2/NEU mRNA by FISH analysis, while patients treated by surgery alone did not manifest gene amplification. These data suggest that HER2/NEU expression increases with progression to androgen independence. In contrast, in a study of 88 radical prostatectomy specimens (presumably androgen dependent), HER2/NEU gene amplification was found in 8 of 86 (9.3%) tumors and amplification was at low to moderate levels.[130] Several studies have also suggested that HER2/NEU carries a negative prognostic significance in prostate cancer. In a study of 112 patients undergoing curative radiotherapy for localized prostate cancer, HER2/NEU expression in the needle biopsy specimen was inversely correlated with both progression-free survival and disease-specific survival.[131] Similarly, in 70 Spanish patients diagnosed with metastatic prostate cancer and treated with MAB, HER2/NEU immunohistochemical overexpression led to decreased mean cancer-specific survival from 54 months to 33 months.[132] In contrast, a study of 113 patients treated by radical prostatectomy showed that HER2/NEU gene amplification by FISH correlated with shorter time to biochemical recurrence in univariate analysis, but did not reach significance in multivariate analysis with grade and DNA ploidy.[133] In addition, HER2/NEU protein expression by immunohistochemistry was not significantly associated with biochemical recurrence.

OVERVIEW

Several small-molecule inhibitors of the EGFR tyrosine kinase ATP binding site have been developed and have entered clinical testing. Phase I studies with ZD1839 (AstraZeneca, Walthem, MA) have shown activity in patients with advanced prostate cancer. The use of humanized monoclonal antibodies against the EGFR is another approach being explored. C225 (ImClone, New York, NY) is a chimeric antibody comprising a mouse anti-EGFR conjugated to a human IgG1 constant region. Phase I/II studies have established safety and feasibility in combination with cytotoxic agents in patients with hormone refractory prostate cancer.

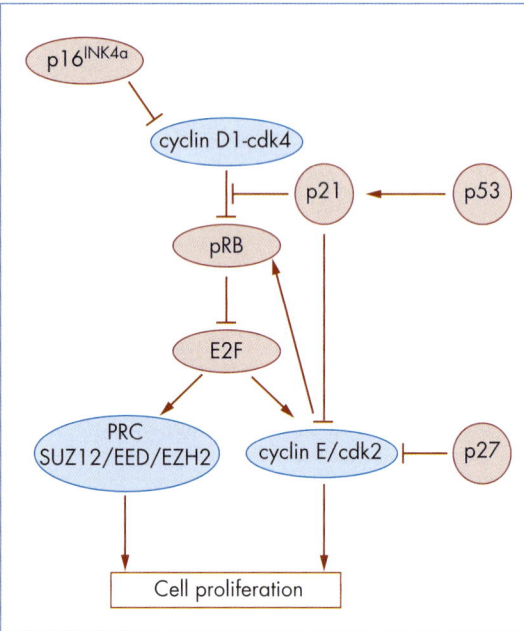

Fig. 28.5

The epidermal growth factor receptor (EGFR) and HER2/NEU signaling pathway. Secreted growth factor ligands, such as EGF or heregulin bind to and activate their respective transmembrane receptors (EGFR and HER2/NEU). Activation of the receptor triggers the conversion of RAS from the inactive guanosine nucleotide diphosphate (GDP)-bound state to the active guanine nucleotide triphosphate (GTP)-bound state. In the active state, RAS triggers the activation of the mitogen-activated protein kinase (MAPK) cascade, inducing RAF activation, which in turn activates MEK and then MAPK (Erk1 and Erk2).

ABX-EGF (Abgenix, Fremont, CA) is a fully human monoclonal antibody against the EGFR that has shown efficacy as a single agent. Small-molecule inhibitors of the EGFR tyrosine kinase may also be used to target HER2/NEU. Recombinant monoclonal antibodies targeting HER2/NEU, such as trastuzumab (Genentech, South San Francisco, CA), have been evaluated. Pertuzumab (2C4, Genentech) is another recombinant antibody against HER2/NEU being evaluated. In summary, EGFR and HER2/NEU may useful diagnostic markers, as well as important therapeutic targets for prostate cancer.

INSULIN-LIKE GROWTH FACTORS, THEIR BINDING PROTEINS, AND THEIR RECEPTORS

BIOLOGY

The local expression of IGF1, IGF binding proteins (IGFBPs), and IGF receptors (IGFRs) has been shown to be associated with tumor prognosis, progression, pathologic stage, and tumor grade in patients with colon, breast, lung, and prostate cancers.[134] Insulin-like growth factor 1 contributes to the development of prostate cancer by stimulating cell proliferation and by inhibiting apoptosis in prostate epithelium.[135] It is bound and inhibited by IGFBP3 in the blood,[134] and binds and activates both the IGF1 receptor (IGF1R) and the insulin receptor.[136] Activation of these receptors results in growth activation and metabolic change, respectively. The IGF1R signal transduction activates both the MAPK and PI3K/Akt pathways, which are essential for the growth stimulatory effects of IGF1.

CLINICAL CORRELATES

Several studies have reported that circulating levels of IGFs and IGFBPs have been associated with increased risk for prostate cancer. The main IGFBP produced by prostate epithelial cells is IGFBP2. Immunohistochemical studies have shown that IGFBP2 immunoreactivity is higher and IGFBP3 is lower in prostate cancer tissue.[137]

OVERVIEW

Antibodies to IGF1R have been shown to inhibit IGF1R phosphorylation and reduce anchorage-independent growth of several cell types.[138] OSI-774 (OSI, Melville, NY), a tyrosine kinase-binding quinazoline, inhibiting both ERBB1/HER1/EGFR and ERBB2/HER2/NEU has been shown to inhibit IGF1R activity.[139] In summary, the data is limited for IGF and IGFBP as tissue biomarkers, whereas IGFR may be a useful target for therapy in prostate cancer.

VASCULAR ENDOTHELIAL GROWTH FACTORS AND THEIR RECEPTORS

BIOLOGY

Blood vessel and lymphatic development depends on members of the vascular endothelial growth factor (VEGF) family of proteins and their receptors.[140] Vascular endothelial growth factors A, B, C, D, and E, and placental growth factor (PlGF) bind to tyrosine kinase receptors, inducing receptor dimerization and activation and the transduction of signals that direct cellular functions. The VEGF receptor (VEGFR) family includes VEGFR1 (also known as FLT1), VEGFR2 (also known as KDR), and VEGFR3 (also know as FLT4), which belong to a superfamily of receptor tyrosine kinases characterized by extracellular immunoglobulin homology domains and a split tyrosine kinase intracellular domain.

CLINICAL CORRELATES

The clinical relevance of tumor angiogenesis has been investigated in several human tumor types. Tumor angiogenesis, measured as microvessel density (MVD) and determined immunohistochemically using a polyclonal antibody against factor VIII, has been shown to be associated with higher tumor stage and grade in 98 prostate cancer specimens.[141] Multivariate survival analysis revealed that MVD and tumor grade were the only independent markers for prostate cancer progression. In another study, immunohistochemical analysis of VEGFA, basic fibroblast growth factor (bFGF), and C-MET expression in 98 radical prostatectomy specimens demonstrated that VEGFA and C-MET expression increased with tumor stage and grade, while bFGF expression increased only with tumor stage. In addition to VEGFA, C-MET seemed to be important and clinically relevant to the induction of angiogenesis in prostate cancer, mainly through its effect on MVD.[142] In another study, immunohistochemical analysis of VEGFC, VEGFD, and VEGFR3 expression was performed in 37 localized prostate cancer specimens.[143] The presence of VEGFR3-positive vessels was associated with lymph node metastasis, Gleason grade, extracapsular extension, and surgical margin status. In addition, VEGFR3 staining highlighted lymphatic invasion by VEGFC-positive/VEGFD-positive cancer cells. These results suggest that paracrine activation of lymphatic endothelial cell VEGFR3 by VEGFC and/or VEGFD may be involved in lymphatic metastasis.

OVERVIEW

Several strategies that target antiangiogenesis are being evaluated. These include bevacizumab (Genentech), a recombinant humanized antibody against VEGFA and small molecule inhibitors targeting VEGFR tyrosine kinase, such as ZD4190 (AstraZeneca), ZD6474 (AstraZeneca), and SU5416 (Pfizer, New York, NY). In summary, angiogenesis markers may be useful diagnostic biomarkers for prostate cancer, as well as potential therapeutic targets.

CD44

BIOLOGY

CD44 (85 kDa) is a transmembrane glycoprotein that belongs to the immunoglobulin (Ig) superfamily of cell adhesion molecules and participates in specific cell–cell and cell–extracellular matrix interactions.[144] Dozens of alternatively spliced CD44 isoforms have been reported that may differ in matrix binding capabilities. The expression of CD44 is considered to be a unique marker for the basal-cell population in the prostate gland.[145] Much attention regarding CD44-mediated metastasis regulation has been given to hyaluronate, which is the principle matrix ligand for CD44. However, recent studies show that the CD44-hyaluronate interaction is not necessary for CD44-mediated metastasis suppression.[146] More important to CD44-mediated suppression may be its cytoplasmic attachments to actin-associated proteins of the merlin/ezrin/radixin/moesin family, including merlin/NF2, a reported tumor suppressor of neurofibromatosis.

CLINICAL CORRELATES

The prognostic role of CD44 in prostate cancer has been studied, and it appears that CD44 can function as a metastatic suppressor.[147] Loss of CD44 protein expression has been associated with other adverse prognostic factors such as high grade tumor and aneuploid DNA content.[148] Hypermethylation of the CD44 gene is often detected in metastatic prostate cancer specimens.[149] Patients with lymph node metastases are much more likely to have decreased staining for CD44 in resected primary and metastatic lesions.[150] In addition, loss of CD44 in radical prostatectomy specimens has been shown to be an independent predictor of biochemical recurrence.[151]

OVERVIEW

The signaling pathways controlled by metastasis suppressor gene products are being defined, and strategies for reactivation of these genes in metastatic cancers are currently being investigated. An exciting possibility is that antimetastasis therapies currently under investigation, such as matrix metalloproteinase inhibitors and antiangiogenesis compounds, may be potentiated by the reactivation of metastasis suppressor expression and activity. In summary, CD44 expression

may be a useful diagnostic and prognostic marker, as well as a potential therapeutic target for prostate cancer.

BIOMARKERS ON THE HORIZON

c-MYC

BIOLOGY

c-MYC is one of the first members of the large helix-loop-helix leucine zipper family of transcription factors. These members share a common three-dimensional protein structure, and the ability to recognize a DNA-binding element known as an E-box. c-MYC binds to DNA in partnership with MAX, which results in transcriptional activation.[152] MAX also forms heterodimers with the MAD family of proteins, of which MXI1 is a member.[153] MAD–MAX complexes result in repression of transcription. MAD proteins act as an antagonist of c-MYC.[154] The c-MYC gene is mapped to chromosome 8q24 and is amplified in a significant number of advanced prostate cancers.[155]

CLINICAL CORRELATES

Fluorescence in-situ hybridization analysis has identified high-level amplification of c-MYC in more than 20% of recurrent and metastatic prostate cancers.[155,156] Amplification of c-MYC correlates with high levels of c-MYC protein expression.[155] In a study of tumor samples from 144 patients with high grade prostate cancer, c-MYC amplification assessed by FISH predicted systemic progression and cancer-specific death in patients with high-grade advanced tumors.[157] The use of FISH on tissue microarrays also showed high-level c-MYC amplification in 11% of metastases from patients with hormone-refractory disease.[158] On the other hand, FISH analysis of 195 organ-confined radical prostatectomy specimens demonstrated a correlation between c-MYC amplification and Gleason grade, but not between c-MYC amplification and biochemical recurrence.[159]

OVERVIEW

The universal deregulation of c-MYC gene expression in tumor cells suggests that this oncogene represents an attractive target for cancer therapeutics. Recent experimental evidence suggest that even a brief inhibition of c-MYC expression may be sufficient to permanently stop tumor growth and induce regression of tumors.[160] In addition, target genes downstream of c-MYC represent attractive targets for therapy. In summary, c-MYC may be a useful diagnostic and prognostic marker for prostate cancer, in particular for recurrent or advanced disease, as well as potential therapeutic target.

PROSTATE STEM CELL ANTIGEN

BIOLOGY

Prostate stem cell antigen (PSCA) is a 123 amino acid glycoprotein first identified in the LAPC-4 prostate xenograft mode of human prostate cancer.[161] It is a glycosyl phosphatidylinositol anchored cell surface protein related to the Ly6/Thy1 family of cell surface antigens that bears 30% identity to stem cell antigen type 2 (SCA2), a cell surface marker of immature thymic lymphocytes.[162,163] The gene encoding PSCA maps to chromosome 8q24.2, a region of genetic gain/amplification in a large percentage of advanced prostate cancers.[161,164] The expression of PSCA in normal tissues is largely prostate specific, but PSCA transcripts and protein have been found in the transitional epithelium of the bladder and neuroendocrine cells of the stomach.[165,166] Prostate stem cell antigen has also recently been shown to be expressed by a majority of both muscle-invasive and superficial bladder cancers.[167]

CLINICAL CORRELATES

In-situ hybridization and immunohistochemical analyses have demonstrated that PSCA expression is detected in 94% and overexpressed in about 40% of clinically localized and 100% of bone-metastatic prostate cancer specimens.[165] The genes for PSCA and c-MYC are co-amplified in locally advanced prostate tumors, suggesting a role for PSCA in the progression of this disease.[168] One immunohistochemical study demonstrated that PSCA expression was shown to increase with Gleason grade, tumor stage, and metastasis.[165] The expression of PSCA is maintained in androgen-independent prostate cancer, and PSCA is highly expressed in metastatic disease. A tissue microarray analysis constructed from 246 radical prostatectomy specimens demonstrated that high PSCA intensity was associated with adverse prognostic factors such as high Gleason score, seminal vesicle invasion, and capsular involvement (Figure 28.6).[169]

OVERVIEW

A strength of this marker is its potential as a therapeutic target. Monoclonal antibodies against PSCA have been shown to inhibit prostate cancer tumor growth and metastasis in animal models, offering hope that PSCA might be an excellent therapeutic target as well as a prognostic indicator in aggressive, c-MYC amplified tumors.[170] In summary, PSCA may a useful diagnostic and prognostic marker, as well as a therapeutic target for prostate cancer.

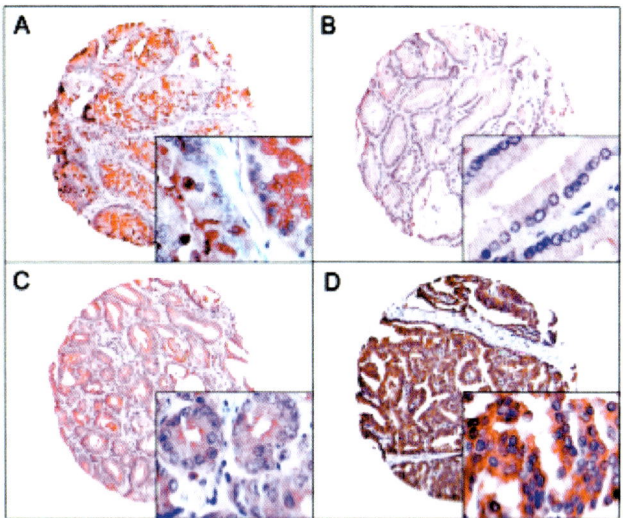

Fig. 28.6
A, A rare case of heterogeneous staining with PSCA antibody. B, Weak stain or PSCA intensity 1. C, Moderate stain or PSCA intensity 2. D, Strong stain or PSCA intensity 3. (Main images ×10; insets ×40.)

EZH2 AND E2F3

BIOLOGY

EZH2 (polycomb group protein enhancer of zeste homolog 2) is a transcriptional repressor, which is the catalytic subunit of the polycomb repressor complex 2, and can methylate lysines 9 and 27 on histone H3.[171] Its expression is controlled by the E2F transcription factors. Transcription factor E2F3 has a central role in linking cell cycle proteins, such as cyclins, cyclin-dependent kinases (CDKs), and the protein product of the retinoblastoma (RB) gene, pRB, to the expression of a variety of genes involved in cellular proliferation as part of the pRB-E2F pathway (Figure 28.7). The genes modulated by E2F3 have roles in a variety of cellular processes that are altered during cell transformation, such as apoptosis, cell cycle transition, DNA synthesis, transcription, and signal transduction.

CLINICAL CORRELATES

EZH2 has been shown to be overexpressed at the mRNA level in hormone-refractory metastatic prostate cancer relative to localized prostate cancer.[171] In a separate study, the same group assessed a panel of 14 candidate prognostic biomarkers identified utilizing tissue microarrays in a cohort of 259 patients who had undergone radical prostatectomy for localized prostate cancer. They determined that patients whose tumors exhibited moderate or strong immunostaining for EZH2 coupled with, at most, moderate expression of E-cadherin had a relative risk of approximately 3.0 for biochemical recurrence, even after adjusting for

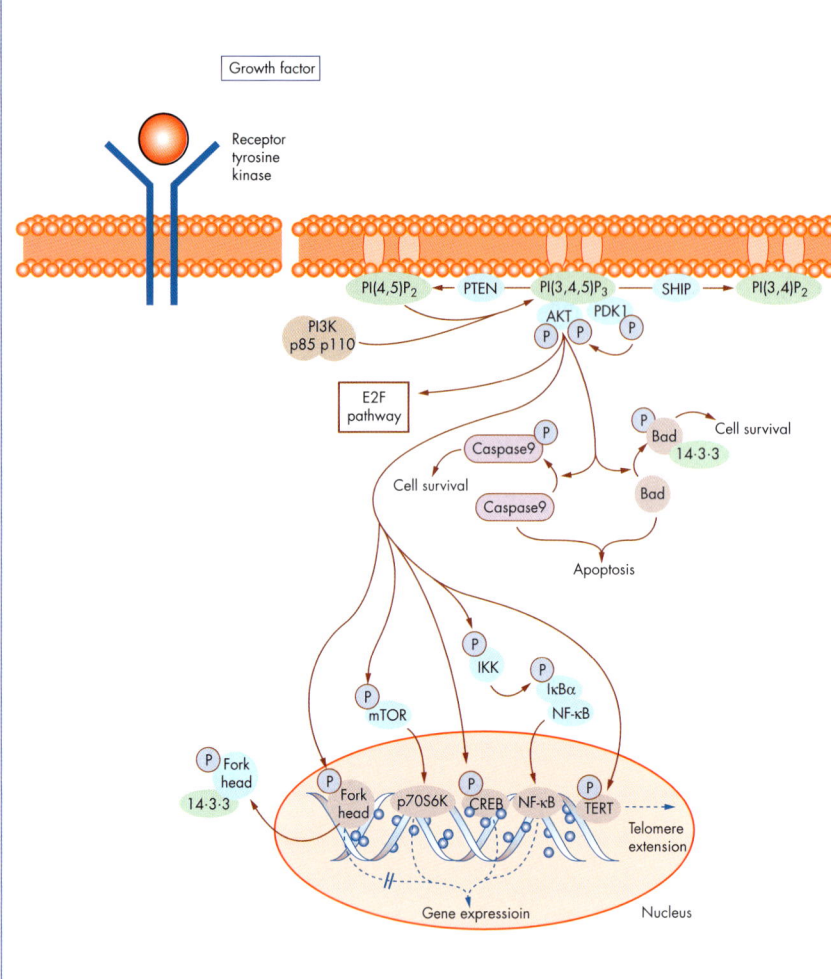

Fig. 28.7

The pRB-E2F pathway. This pathway is centered on the regulation of the protein product of the retinoblastoma (RB) gene, pRB, and the E2F transcription factor family. The E2F family is a critical regulator of the transcription of genes involved in cell proliferation and cell cycle progression. The RB protein can bind to E2F and the RB-E2F complex acts to repress or turn off transcription of the E2F target genes. This complex can be inactivated by phosphorylation of RB by the cyclin D1 and cyclin-dependent kinase (CDK4) complex leading to the activation of E2F transcription. Cyclin D1 and CDK4 are subjected to inhibitory regulation of the CDK inhibitor (CDKI) p16^{INK4a}. In addition to phosphorylating pRB, cyclin E is also an important transcriptional target of the RB/E2F complex. The CDKI p27 is a critical regulator of cyclin E/CDK2 activity and is a critical regulator of the G1 checkpoint downstream of pRB. EZH2 expression is controlled by the E2F transcription factors. EZH2 is part of the polycomb repressive complex (PRC). p53 is a transcription factor that can induce the production of p21 and result in cell-cycle arrest as a consequence of inhibition of CDK activity. In addition, p53 can induce programmed cell death.

stage, grade, and preoperative PSA.[171] Thus, EZH2/E-cadherin status might prove useful in identifying a high-risk cohort of patients following radical prostatectomy.

E2F transcription factors, including E2F3, directly modulate expression of EZH2. High levels of nuclear E2F3 expression occur in a high proportion of human prostate cancers. Patients with prostate cancer exhibiting immunohistochemically detectable nuclear E2F3 expression had poorer overall survival and disease-specific survival than patients without detectable E2F3 expression.[172] Multivariate analysis selected E2F3 expression as an independent factor predicting overall and disease-specific survival.

OVERVIEW

The published data on EZH2 and the E2F3 control protein pRB suggests that the pRB-E2F control axis may have a critical role in modulating aggressiveness in prostate cancer. In summary, EZH2 and E2F3 expression may serve as useful diagnostic and prognostic markers for prostate cancer.

THYMOSIN BETA 15

BIOLOGY

Thymosin-β15 is an actin-binding protein cloned by differential mRNA display as a result of overexpression in the Dunning prostate cancer cell line.[173] It binds monomeric actin and retards actin polymerization. Thymosin-β15 has been shown to directly regulate cell motility in prostate cancer cell lines.[174] Thymosin-β15 may prove to be a more useful marker than PSA for identifying patients at high risk of prostate cancer metastasis, since it is not expressed in prostate tissue from noncancerous prostate glands or in tissue obtained from patients without metastatic tumors.[174]

CLINICAL CORRELATES

In-situ hybridization studies showed that thymosin-β15 staining was most extensive and intense in high-grade (Gleason score, 8–10) cancers, followed by moderately differentiated prostate cancers with Gleason scores of 6 to 7.[173] In addition, strong staining was present in both lymph node and bone metastases. In contrast, all cases of BPH were negative. Staining intensity was demonstrated to strongly correlate with poor clinical outcome and may be a potentially important marker to identify high-risk patients with moderately differentiated, clinically localized prostate cancer.[175] In patients that stained 3+ (strongest staining), 62% developed bone failure compared with 13% of those patients whose specimens stained 1+ (weakest staining) (p = 0.01). The 5-year freedom from PSA failure was 25% for those patients with 3+ staining compared with 83% for those with 1+ staining (p = 0.02).

OVERVIEW

Thymosin-β15 may prove to be a more useful marker than PSA for identifying patients at high risk of prostate cancer metastasis. It represents a powerful predictor of subsequent development of metastases when expressed in localized prostate cancer.

CONCLUSIONS

One of the most important challenges in prostate cancer today is the inability to predict the behavior of an individual tumor in an individual patient. Improved diagnostic and prognostic biomarkers are needed for prostate cancer, and the use of these markers should ultimately translate into increased lifespan and quality of life. Proteomics and DNA methylation assays may soon be used in sensitive and specific diagnostic testing of serum and tissues for cancer. Expression arrays may be used to establish both a more specific diagnosis and prognosis for a particular tumor. The challenge ahead is to conclusively determine the role these genes play as prognostic and/or predictive markers, using large, retrospective, possibly multicenter databases with long-term follow-up. Potential therapeutic targets are also beginning to emerge, which will result in novel and more specific therapeutic modalities. The exponential growth of techniques in molecular biology and the progressive elucidation of the biological pathways of prostate cancer offer hope that this demand will soon be met.

REFERENCES

1. Hernandez J, Thompson IM. Prostate-specific antigen: A review of the validation of the most commonly used cancer biomarker. Cancer 2004;101:894–904.
2. Chin JL, Reiter RE. Genetic alterations in prostate cancer. Curr Urol Rep 2004;5:157–165.
3. Scholzen T, Gerdes J. The Ki-67 protein: from the known and the unknown. J Cell Physiol 2000;182:311–322.
4. Aaltomaa S, Lipponen P, Vesalainen S, et al. Value of Ki-67 immunolabelling as a prognostic factor in prostate cancer. Eur Urol 1997;32:410–415.
5. Borre M, Bentzen SM, Nerstrom B, et al. Tumor cell proliferation and survival in patients with prostate cancer followed expectantly. J Urol 1998;159:1609–1614.
6. Pollack A, Cowen D, Troncoso P, et al. Molecular markers of outcome after radiotherapy in patients with prostate carcinoma: Ki-67, bcl-2, bax, and bcl-x. Cancer 2003;97:1630–1638.
7. Halvorsen OJ, Haukaas S, Hoisaeter PA, et al. Maximum Ki-67 staining in prostate cancer provides independent prognostic information after radical prostatectomy. Anticancer Res 2001;21:4071–4076.
8. Bettencourt MC, Bauer JJ, Sesterhenn IA, et al. Ki-67 expression is a prognostic marker of prostate cancer recurrence after radical prostatectomy. J Urol 1996;156:1064–1068.
9. Matsuura H, Hayashi N, Kawamura J, et al. Prognostic significance of Ki-67 expression in advanced prostate cancers in relation to disease progression after androgen ablation. Eur Urol 2000;37:212–217.
10. Pollack A, DeSilvio M, Khor LY, et al. Ki-67 staining is a strong predictor of distant metastasis and mortality for men with prostate cancer treated with radiotherapy plus androgen deprivation: Radiation Therapy Oncology Group Trial 92-02. J Clin Oncol 2004;22:2133–2140.
11. Bubendorf L, Tapia C, Gasser TC, et al. Ki67 labeling index in core needle biopsies independently predicts tumor-specific survival in prostate cancer. Hum Pathol 1998;29:949–954.
12. Fero ML, Rivkin M, Tasch M, et al. A syndrome of multiorgan hyperplasia with features of gigantism, tumorigenesis, and female sterility in p27(Kip1)-deficient mice. Cell 1996;85:733–744.
13. Polyak K, Kato JY, Solomon MJ, et al. p27Kip1, a cyclin-Cdk inhibitor, links transforming growth factor-beta and contact inhibition to cell cycle arrest. Genes Dev 1994;8:9–22.
14. Pagano M, Tam SW, Theodoras AM, et al. Role of the ubiquitin-proteasome pathway in regulating abundance of the cyclin-dependent kinase inhibitor p27. Science 1995;269:682–685.
15. Cordon-Cardo C, Koff A, Drobnjak M, et al. Distinct altered patterns of p27KIP1 gene expression in benign prostatic hyperplasia and prostatic carcinoma. J Natl Cancer Inst 1998;90:1284–1291.
16. Cote RJ, Shi Y, Groshen S, et al. Association of p27Kip1 levels with recurrence and survival in patients with stage C prostate carcinoma. J Natl Cancer Inst 1998;90:916–920.
17. Tsihlias J, Kapusta LR, DeBoer G, et al. Loss of cyclin-dependent kinase inhibitor p27Kip1 is a novel prognostic factor in localized human prostate adenocarcinoma. Cancer Res 1998;58:542–548.
18. Yang RM, Naitoh J, Murphy M, et al. Low p27 expression predicts poor disease-free survival in patients with prostate cancer. J Urol 1998;159:941–945.
19. Cheville JC, Lloyd RV, Sebo TJ, et al. Expression of p27kip1 in prostatic adenocarcinoma. Mod Pathol 1998;11:324–328.
20. Thomas GV, Schrage MI, Rosenfelt L, et al. Preoperative prostate needle biopsy p27 correlates with subsequent radical prostatectomy p27, Gleason grade and pathological stage. J Urol 2000;164:1987–1991.
21. Ribal MJ, Fernandez PL, Lopez-Guillermo A, et al. Low p27 expression predicts biochemical relapse after radical prostatectomy in patients with clinically localised prostate cancer. Anticancer Res 2003;23:5101–5106.
22. Freedland SJ, de Gregorio F, Sacoolidge JC, et al. Predicting biochemical recurrence after radical prostatectomy for patients with organ-confined disease using p27 expression. Urology 2003;61:1187–1192.
23. Freedland SJ, deGregorio F, Sacoolidge JC, et al. Preoperative p27 status is an independent predictor of prostate specific antigen failure following radical prostatectomy. J Urol 2003;169:1325–1330.
24. Yang G, Ayala G, De Marzo A, et al. Elevated Skp2 protein expression in human prostate cancer: association with loss of the cyclin-dependent kinase inhibitor p27 and PTEN and with reduced recurrence-free survival. Clin Cancer Res 2002;8:3419–3426.
25. Ben-Izhak O, Lahav-Baratz S, Meretyk S, et al. Inverse relationship between Skp2 ubiquitin ligase and the cyclin dependent kinase inhibitor p27Kip1 in prostate cancer. J Urol 2003;170:241–245.

26. Li J, Yen C, Liaw D, et al. PTEN, a putative protein tyrosine phosphatase gene mutated in human brain, breast, and prostate cancer. Science 1997;275:1943–1947.

27. Vivanco I, Sawyers CL. The phosphatidylinositol 3-kinase AKT pathway in human cancer. Nat Rev Cancer 2002;2:489–501.

28. Maehama T, Dixon JE. The tumor suppressor, PTEN/MMAC1, dephosphorylates the lipid second messenger, phosphatidylinositol 3,4,5-trisphosphate. J Biol Chem 1998;273:13375–13378.

29. Downward J. PI 3-kinase, Akt and cell survival. Semin Cell Dev Biol 2004;15:177–182.

30. Franke TF, Kaplan DR, Cantley LC. PI3K: downstream AKTion blocks apoptosis. Cell 1997;88:435–437.

31. Datta SR, Dudek H, Tao X, et al. Akt phosphorylation of BAD couples survival signals to the cell-intrinsic death machinery. Cell 1997;91:231–241.

32. Cardone MH, Roy N, Stennicke HR, et al. Regulation of cell death protease caspase-9 by phosphorylation. Science 1998;282:1318–1321.

33. Bostrom J, Cobbers JM, Wolter M, et al. Mutation of the PTEN (MMAC1) tumor suppressor gene in a subset of glioblastomas but not in meningiomas with loss of chromosome arm 10q. Cancer Res 1998;58:29–33.

34. Liu W, James CD, Frederick L, et al. PTEN/MMAC1 mutations and EGFR amplification in glioblastomas. Cancer Res 1997;57:5254–5257.

35. Cairns P, Okami K, Halachmi S, et al. Frequent inactivation of PTEN/MMAC1 in primary prostate cancer. Cancer Res 1997;57:4997–5000.

36. Risinger JI, Hayes AK, Berchuck A, Barrett JC. PTEN/MMAC1 mutations in endometrial cancers. Cancer Res 1997;57:4736–4738.

37. Suzuki H, Freije D, Nusskern DR, et al. Interfocal heterogeneity of PTEN/MMAC1 gene alterations in multiple metastatic prostate cancer tissues. Cancer Res 1998;58:204–209.

38. Sun H, Lesche R, Li DM, et al. PTEN modulates cell cycle progression and cell survival by regulating phosphatidylinositol 3,4,5,-trisphosphate and Akt/protein kinase B signaling pathway. Proc Natl Acad Sci U S A 1999;96:6199–6204.

39. Gu J, Tamura M, Yamada KM. Tumor suppressor PTEN inhibits integrin- and growth factor-mediated mitogen-activated protein (MAP) kinase signaling pathways. J Cell Biol 1998;143:1375–1383.

40. Teng DH, Hu R, Lin H, et al. MMAC1/PTEN mutations in primary tumor specimens and tumor cell lines. Cancer Res 1997;57:5221–5225.

41. McMenamin ME, Soung P, Perera S, Kaplan I, Loda M, Sellers WR. Loss of PTEN expression in paraffin-embedded primary prostate cancer correlates with high Gleason score and advanced stage. Cancer Res 1999;59:4291–4296.

42. Halvorsen OJ, Haukaas SA, Akslen LA. Combined loss of PTEN and p27 expression is associated with tumor cell proliferation by Ki-67 and increased risk of recurrent disease in localized prostate cancer. Clin Cancer Res 2003;9:1474–1479.

43. Mita MM, Mita A, Rowinsky EK. The molecular target of rapamycin (mTOR) as a therapeutic target against cancer. Cancer Biol Ther 2003;2:S169–177.

44. Gao N, Zhang Z, Jiang BH, Shi X. Role of PI3K/AKT/mTOR signaling in the cell cycle progression of human prostate cancer. Biochem Biophys Res Commun 2003;310:1124–1132.

45. Neshat MS, Mellinghoff IK, Tran C, et al. Enhanced sensitivity of PTEN-deficient tumors to inhibition of FRAP/mTOR. Proc Natl Acad Sci USA 2001;98:10314–10319.

46. Cavallaro U, Christofori G. Cell adhesion and signalling by cadherins and Ig-CAMs in cancer. Nat Rev Cancer 2004;4:118–132.

47. Umbas R, Schalken JA, Aalders TW, et al. Expression of the cellular adhesion molecule E-cadherin is reduced or absent in high-grade prostate cancer. Cancer Res 1992;52:5104–5109.

48. Behrens J, von Kries JP, Kuhl M, et al. Functional interaction of beta-catenin with the transcription factor LEF-1. Nature 1996;382:638–642.

49. St Croix B, Sheehan C, Rak JW, Florenes VA, Slingerland JM, Kerbel RS. E-Cadherin-dependent growth suppression is mediated by the cyclin-dependent kinase inhibitor p27(KIP1). J Cell Biol 1998;142:557–571.

50. Thomas GV, Szigeti K, Murphy M, Draetta G, Pagano M, Loda M. Down-regulation of p27 is associated with development of colorectal adenocarcinoma metastases. Am J Pathol 1998;153:681–687.

51. Umbas R, Isaacs WB, Bringuier PP, et al. Decreased E-cadherin expression is associated with poor prognosis in patients with prostate cancer. Cancer Res 1994;54:3929–3933.

52. Wu TT, Hsu YS, Wang JS, Lee YH, Huang JK. The role of p53, bcl-2 and E-cadherin expression in predicting biochemical relapse for organ confined prostate cancer in Taiwan. J Urol 2003;170:78–81.

53. Loric S, Paradis V, Gala JL, et al. Abnormal E-cadherin expression and prostate cell blood dissemination as markers of biological recurrence in cancer. Eur J Cancer 2001;37:1475–1481.

54. Li LC, Zhao H, Nakajima K, et al. Methylation of the E-cadherin gene promoter correlates with progression of prostate cancer. J Urol 2001;166:705–709.

55. Massague J. TGF-beta signal transduction. Annu Rev Biochem 1998;67:753–791.

56. Ten Dijke P, Goumans MJ, Itoh F, Itoh S. Regulation of cell proliferation by Smad proteins. J Cell Physiol 2002;191:1–16.

57. Derynck R, Akhurst RJ, Balmain A. TGF-beta signaling in tumor suppression and cancer progression. Nat Genet 2001;29:117–129.

58. Massague J, Blain SW, Lo RS. TGFbeta signaling in growth control, cancer, and heritable disorders. Cell 2000;103:295–309.

59. Ivanovic V, Melman A, Davis-Joseph B, Valcic M, Geliebter J. Elevated plasma levels of TGF-beta 1 in patients with invasive prostate cancer. Nat Med 1995;1:282–284.

60. Shariat SF, Shalev M, Menesses-Diaz A, et al. Preoperative plasma levels of transforming growth factor beta(1) (TGF-beta(1)) strongly predict progression in patients undergoing radical prostatectomy. J Clin Oncol 2001;19:2856–2864.

61. Perry KT, Anthony CT, Steiner MS. Immunohistochemical localization of TGF beta 1, TGF beta 2, and TGF beta 3 in normal and malignant human prostate. Prostate 1997;33:133–140.

62. Wikstrom P, Stattin P, Franck-Lissbrant I, Damber JE, Bergh A. Transforming growth factor beta1 is associated with angiogenesis, metastasis, and poor clinical outcome in prostate cancer. Prostate 1998;37:19–29.

63. Kim IY, Ahn HJ, Lang S, et al. Loss of expression of transforming growth factor-beta receptors is associated with poor prognosis in prostate cancer patients. Clin Cancer Res 1998;4:1625–1630.

64. Shariat SF, Menesses-Diaz A, Kim IY, Muramoto M, Wheeler TM, Slawin KM. Tissue expression of transforming growth factor-beta1 and its receptors: correlation with pathologic features and biochemical progression in patients undergoing radical prostatectomy. Urology 2004;63:1191–1197.

65. Leytus SP, Loeb KR, Hagen FS, Kurachi K, Davie EW. A novel trypsin-like serine protease (hepsin) with a putative transmembrane domain expressed by human liver and hepatoma cells. Biochemistry 1988;27:1067–1074.

66. Tsuji A, Torres-Rosado A, Arai T, et al. Hepsin, a cell membrane-associated protease. Characterization, tissue distribution, and gene localization. J Biol Chem 1991;266:16948–16953.

67. Magee JA, Araki T, Patil S, et al. Expression profiling reveals hepsin overexpression in prostate cancer. Cancer Res 2001;61:5692–5696.

68. Dhanasekaran SM, Barrette TR, Ghosh D, et al. Delineation of prognostic biomarkers in prostate cancer. Nature 2001;412:822–826.

69. Welsh JB, Sapinoso LM, Su AI, et al. Analysis of gene expression identifies candidate markers and pharmacological targets in prostate cancer. Cancer Res 2001;61:5974–5978.

70. Klezovitch O, Chevillet J, Mirosevich J, Roberts RL, Matusik RJ, Vasioukhin V. Hepsin promotes prostate cancer progression and metastasis. Cancer Cell 2004;6:185–195.

71. Stephan C, Yousef GM, Scorilas A, et al. Hepsin is highly over expressed in and a new candidate for a prognostic indicator in prostate cancer. J Urol 2004;171:187–191.

72. Luo J, Zha S, Gage WR, et al. Alpha-methylacyl-CoA racemase: a new molecular marker for prostate cancer. Cancer Res 2002;62:2220–2226.

73. Jiang Z, Wu CL, Woda BA, et al. Alpha-methylacyl-CoA racemase: a multi-institutional study of a new prostate cancer marker. Histopathology 2004;45:218–225.

74. Jiang Z, Woda BA, Wu CL, Yang XJ. Discovery and clinical application of a novel prostate cancer marker: alpha-methylacyl CoA racemase (P504S). Am J Clin Pathol 2004;122:275–289.

75. Rubin MA, Zhou M, Dhanasekaran SM, et al. alpha-methylacyl coenzyme A racemase as a tissue biomarker for prostate cancer. JAMA 2002;287:1662–1670.

76. Beach R, Gown AM, De Peralta-Venturina MN, et al. P504S immunohistochemical detection in 405 prostatic specimens including 376 18-gauge needle biopsies. Am J Surg Pathol 2002;26:1588–1596.

77. Signoretti S, Waltregny D, Dilks J, et al. p63 is a prostate basal cell marker and is required for prostate development. Am J Pathol 2000;157:1769–1775.

78. Parsons JK, Gage WR, Nelson WG, De Marzo AM. p63 protein expression is rare in prostate adenocarcinoma: implications for cancer diagnosis and carcinogenesis. Urology 2001;58:619–624.

79. Yang XJ, Laven B, Tretiakova M, et al. Detection of alpha-methylacyl-coenzyme A racemase in postradiation prostatic adenocarcinoma. Urology 2003;62:282–286.

80. Neumann AA, Reddel RR. Telomere maintenance and cancer—look, no telomerase. Nat Rev Cancer 2002;2:879–884.

81. Sommerfeld HJ, Meeker AK, Piatyszek MA, Bova GS, Shay JW, Coffey DS. Telomerase activity: a prevalent marker of malignant human prostate tissue. Cancer Res 1996;56:218–222.

82. Iczkowski KA, Pantazis CG, McGregor DH, Wu Y, Tawfik OW. Telomerase reverse transcriptase subunit immunoreactivity: a marker for high-grade prostate carcinoma. Cancer 2002;95:2487–2493.

83. Wymenga LF, Wisman GB, Veenstra R, Ruiters MH, Mensink HJ. Telomerase activity in needle biopsies from prostate cancer and benign prostates. Eur J Clin Invest 2000;30:330–335.

84. Donaldson L, Fordyce C, Gilliland F, et al. Association between outcome and telomere DNA content in prostate cancer. J Urol 1999;162:1788–1792.

85. Kamradt J, Drosse C, Kalkbrenner S, et al. Telomerase activity and telomerase subunit gene expression levels are not related in prostate cancer: a real-time quantification and in situ hybridization study. Lab Invest 2003;83:623–633.

86. Debes JD, Tindall DJ. Mechanisms of androgen-refractory prostate cancer. N Engl J Med 2004;351:1488–1490.

87. Chen CD, Welsbie DS, Tran C, et al. Molecular determinants of resistance to antiandrogen therapy. Nat Med 2004;10:33–39.

88. van der Kwast TH, Tetu B. Androgen receptors in untreated and treated prostatic intraepithelial neoplasia. Eur Urol 1996;30:265–268.

89. Magi-Galluzzi C, Xu X, Hlatky L, et al. Heterogeneity of androgen receptor content in advanced prostate cancer. Mod Pathol 1997;10:839–845.

90. Miyamoto KK, McSherry SA, Dent GA, et al. Immunohistochemistry of the androgen receptor in human benign and malignant prostate tissue. J Urol 1993;149:1015–1019.

91. Sadi MV, Walsh PC, Barrack ER. Immunohistochemical study of androgen receptors in metastatic prostate cancer. Comparison of receptor content and response to hormonal therapy. Cancer 1991;67:3057–3064.

92. Li R, Wheeler T, Dai H, Frolov A, Thompson T, Ayala G. High level of androgen receptor is associated with aggressive clinicopathologic features and decreased biochemical recurrence-free survival in prostate: cancer patients treated with radical prostatectomy. Am J Surg Pathol 2004;28:928–934.

93. Hockenbery D, Nunez G, Milliman C, Schreiber RD, Korsmeyer SJ. Bcl-2 is an inner mitochondrial membrane protein that blocks programmed cell death. Nature 1990;348:334–336.

94. Cleary ML, Sklar J. Nucleotide sequence of a t(14;18) chromosomal breakpoint in follicular lymphoma and demonstration of a breakpoint-cluster region near a transcriptionally active locus on chromosome 18. Proc Natl Acad Sci USA 1985;82:7439–7443.

95. Cory S, Huang DC, Adams JM. The Bcl-2 family: roles in cell survival and oncogenesis. Oncogene 2003;22:8590–8607.

96. Furuya Y, Krajewski S, Epstein JI, Reed JC, Isaacs JT. Expression of bcl-2 and the progression of human and rodent prostatic cancers. Clin Cancer Res 1996;2:389–398.

97. Marin MC, Fernandez A, Bick RJ, et al. Apoptosis suppression by bcl-2 is correlated with the regulation of nuclear and cytosolic Ca^{2+}. Oncogene 1996;12:2259–2266.

98. Colombel M, Symmans F, Gil S, et al. Detection of the apoptosis-suppressing oncoprotein bc1-2 in hormone-refractory human prostate cancers. Am J Pathol 1993;143:390–400.

99. Apakama I, Robinson MC, Walter NM, et al. bcl-2 overexpression combined with p53 protein accumulation correlates with hormone-refractory prostate cancer. Br J Cancer 1996;74:1258–1262.

100. Haldar S, Basu A, Croce CM. Bcl2 is the guardian of microtubule integrity. Cancer Res 1997;57:229–233.

101. Blagosklonny MV, Schulte T, Nguyen P, Trepel J, Neckers LM. Taxol-induced apoptosis and phosphorylation of Bcl-2 protein involves c-Raf-1 and represents a novel c-Raf-1 signal transduction pathway. Cancer Res 1996;56:1851–1854.

102. Ito T, Deng X, Carr B, May WS. Bcl-2 phosphorylation required for anti-apoptosis function. J Biol Chem 1997;272:11671–11673.

103. Maundrell K, Antonsson B, Magnenat E, et al. Bcl-2 undergoes phosphorylation by c-Jun N-terminal kinase/stress-activated protein kinases in the presence of the constitutively active GTP-binding protein Rac1. J Biol Chem 1997;272:25238–25242.

104. Scherr DS, Vaughan ED, Jr., Wei J, et al. BCL-2 and p53 expression in clinically localized prostate cancer predicts response to external beam radiotherapy. J Urol 1999;162:12–16;discussion 16–17.

105. Stackhouse GB, Sesterhenn IA, Bauer JJ, et al. p53 and bcl-2 immunohistochemistry in pretreatment prostate needle biopsies to predict recurrence of prostate cancer after radical prostatectomy. J Urol 1999;162:2040–2045.

106. Borre M, Stausbol-Gron B, Nerstrom B, Overgaard J. Immunohistochemical BCL-2 and Ki-67 expression predict survival in prostate cancer patients followed expectantly. Prostate Cancer Prostatic Dis 1998;1:268–275.

107. Gleave ME, Miayake H, Goldie J, Nelson C, Tolcher A. Targeting bcl-2 gene to delay androgen-independent progression and enhance chemosensitivity in prostate cancer using antisense bcl-2 oligodeoxynucleotides. Urology 1999;54:36–46.

108. Levine AJ, Momand J, Finlay CA. The p53 tumour suppressor gene. Nature 1991;351:453–456.

109. Brewster SF, Browne S, Brown KW. Somatic allelic loss at the DCC, APC, nm23-H1 and p53 tumor suppressor gene loci in human prostatic carcinoma. J Urol 1994;151:1073–1077.

110. Cunningham JM, Shan A, Wick MJ, et al. Allelic imbalance and microsatellite instability in prostatic adenocarcinoma. Cancer Res 1996;56:4475–4482.

111. Uchida T, Wada C, Wang C, et al. Microsatellite instability in prostate cancer. Oncogene 1995;10:1019–1022.

112. McDonnell TJ, Navone NM, Troncoso P, et al. Expression of bcl-2 oncoprotein and p53 protein accumulation in bone marrow metastases of androgen independent prostate cancer. J Urol 1997;157:569–574.

113. Navone NM, Troncoso P, Pisters LL, et al. p53 protein accumulation and gene mutation in the progression of human prostate carcinoma. J Natl Cancer Inst 1993;85:1657–1669.

114. Bookstein R, MacGrogan D, Hilsenbeck SG, Sharkey F, Allred DC. p53 is mutated in a subset of advanced-stage prostate cancers. Cancer Res 1993;53:3369–3373.

115. Yang G, Stapleton AM, Wheeler TM, et al. Clustered p53 immunostaining: a novel pattern associated with prostate cancer progression. Clin Cancer Res 1996;2:399–401.

116. Bauer JJ, Sesterhenn IA, Mostofi KF, McLeod DG, Srivastava S, Moul JW. p53 nuclear protein expression is an independent prognostic marker in clinically localized prostate cancer patients undergoing radical prostatectomy. Clin Cancer Res 1995;1:1295–1300.

117. Borre M, Stausbol-Gron B, Overgaard J. p53 accumulation associated with bcl-2, the proliferation marker MIB-1 and survival in patients with prostate cancer subjected to watchful waiting. J Urol 2000;164:716–721.

118. Deliveliotis C, Skolarikos A, Karayannis A, et al. The prognostic value of p53 and DNA ploidy following radical prostatectomy. World J Urol 2003;21:171–176.

119. Quinn DI, Henshall SM, Head DR, et al. Prognostic significance of p53 nuclear accumulation in localized prostate cancer treated with radical prostatectomy. Cancer Res 2000;60:1585–1594.

120. Ritter MA, Gilchrist KW, Voytovich M, Chappell RJ, Verhoven BM. The role of p53 in radiation therapy outcomes for favorable-to-

intermediate-risk prostate cancer. Int J Radiat Oncol Biol Phys 2002;53:574–580.

121. Grignon DJ, Caplan R, Sarkar FH, et al. p53 status and prognosis of locally advanced prostatic adenocarcinoma: a study based on RTOG 8610. J Natl Cancer Inst 1997;89:158–165.

122. Omar EA, Behlouli H, Chevalier S, Aprikian AG. Relationship of p21(WAF-I) protein expression with prognosis in advanced prostate cancer treated by androgen ablation. Prostate 2001;49:191–199.

123. Rigaud J, Tiguert R, Decobert M, et al. Expression of p21 cell cycle protein is an independent predictor of response to salvage radiotherapy after radical prostatectomy. Prostate 2004;58:269–276.

124. Barnes CJ, Kumar R. Biology of the epidermal growth factor receptor family. Cancer Treat Res 2004;119:1–13.

125. Robinson D, He F, Pretlow T, Kung HJ. A tyrosine kinase profile of prostate carcinoma. Proc Natl Acad Sci USA 1996;93:5958–5962.

126. Craft N, Shostak Y, Carey M, Sawyers CL. A mechanism for hormone-independent prostate cancer through modulation of androgen receptor signaling by the HER-2/neu tyrosine kinase. Nat Med 1999;5:280–285.

127. Yeh S, Lin HK, Kang HY, Thin TH, Lin MF, Chang C. From HER2/Neu signal cascade to androgen receptor and its coactivators: a novel pathway by induction of androgen target genes through MAP kinase in prostate cancer cells. Proc Natl Acad Sci USA 1999;96:5458–5463.

128. Di Lorenzo G, Tortora G, D'Armiento FP, et al. Expression of epidermal growth factor receptor correlates with disease relapse and progression to androgen-independence in human prostate cancer. Clin Cancer Res 2002;8:3438–3444.

129. Signoretti S, Montironi R, Manola J, et al. Her-2-neu expression and progression toward androgen independence in human prostate cancer. J Natl Cancer Inst 2000;92:1918–1925.

130. Mark HF, Feldman D, Das S, et al. Fluorescence in situ hybridization study of HER-2/neu oncogene amplification in prostate cancer. Exp Mol Pathol 1999;66:170–178.

131. Fossa A, Lilleby W, Fossa SD, Gaudernack G, Torlakovic G, Berner A. Independent prognostic significance of HER-2 oncoprotein expression in pN0 prostate cancer undergoing curative radiotherapy. Int J Cancer 2002;99:100–105.

132. Morote J, de Torres I, Caceres C, Vallejo C, Schwartz S Jr, Reventos J. Prognostic value of immunohistochemical expression of the c-erbB-2 oncoprotein in metastasic prostate cancer. Int J Cancer 1999;84:421–425.

133. Ross JS, Sheehan CE, Hayner-Buchan AM, et al. Prognostic significance of HER-2/neu gene amplification status by fluorescence in situ hybridization of prostate carcinoma. Cancer 1997;79:2162–2170.

134. Yu H, Rohan T. Role of the insulin-like growth factor family in cancer development and progression. J Natl Cancer Inst 2000;92:1472–1489.

135. Cohen P, Peehl DM, Lamson G, Rosenfeld RG. Insulin-like growth factors (IGFs), IGF receptors, and IGF-binding proteins in primary cultures of prostate epithelial cells. J Clin Endocrinol Metab 1991;73:401–407.

136. Renehan AG, Zwahlen M, Minder C, O'Dwyer ST, Shalet SM, Egger M. Insulin-like growth factor (IGF)-I, IGF binding protein-3, and cancer risk: systematic review and meta-regression analysis. Lancet 2004;363:1346–1353.

137. Thrasher JB, Tennant MK, Twomey PA, Hansberry KL, Wettlaufer JN, Plymate SR. Immunohistochemical localization of insulin-like growth factor binding proteins 2 and 3 in prostate tissue: clinical correlations. J Urol 1996;155:999–1003.

138. Hailey J, Maxwell E, Koukouras K, Bishop WR, Pachter JA, Wang Y. Neutralizing anti-insulin-like growth factor receptor 1 antibodies inhibit receptor function and induce receptor degradation in tumor cells. Mol Cancer Ther 2002;1:1349–1353.

139. Moyer JD, Barbacci EG, Iwata KK, et al. Induction of apoptosis and cell cycle arrest by CP-358,774, an inhibitor of epidermal growth factor receptor tyrosine kinase. Cancer Res 1997;57:4838–4848.

140. Ferrara N, Gerber HP, LeCouter J. The biology of VEGF and its receptors. Nat Med 2003;9:669–676.

141. Strohmeyer D, Rossing C, Strauss F, Bauerfeind A, Kaufmann O, Loening S. Tumor angiogenesis is associated with progression after radical prostatectomy in pT2/pT3 prostate cancer. Prostate 2000;42:26–33.

142. Strohmeyer D, Strauss F, Rossing C, et al. Expression of bFGF, VEGF and c-met and their correlation with microvessel density and progression in prostate carcinoma. Anticancer Res 2004;24:1797–1804.

143. Zeng Y, Opeskin K, Baldwin ME, et al. Expression of vascular endothelial growth factor receptor-3 by lymphatic endothelial cells is associated with lymph node metastasis in prostate cancer. Clin Cancer Res 2004;10:5137–5144.

144. Weber GF, Ashkar S, Glimcher MJ, Cantor H. Receptor-ligand interaction between CD44 and osteopontin (Eta-1). Science 1996;271:509–512.

145. Liu AY, True LD, LaTray L, et al. Cell-cell interaction in prostate gene regulation and cytodifferentiation. Proc Natl Acad Sci USA 1997;94:10705–10710.

146. Gao AC, Lou W, Sleeman JP, Isaacs JT. Metastasis suppression by the standard CD44 isoform does not require the binding of prostate cancer cells to hyaluronate. Cancer Res 1998;58:2350–2352.

147. Gao AC, Lou W, Dong JT, Isaacs JT. CD44 is a metastasis suppressor gene for prostatic cancer located on human chromosome 11p13. Cancer Res 1997;57:846–849.

148. Kallakury BV, Yang F, Figge J, et al. Decreased levels of CD44 protein and mRNA in prostate carcinoma. Correlation with tumor grade and ploidy. Cancer 1996;78:1461–1469.

149. Lou W, Krill D, Dhir R, et al. Methylation of the CD44 metastasis suppressor gene in human prostate cancer. Cancer Res 1999;59:2329–2331.

150. Noordzij MA, van Steenbrugge GJ, Schroder FH, Van der Kwast TH. Decreased expression of CD44 in metastatic prostate cancer. Int J Cancer 1999;84:478–483.

151. Vis AN, Noordzij MA, Fitoz K, Wildhagen MF, Schroder FH, van der Kwast TH. Prognostic value of cell cycle proteins p27(kip1) and MIB-1, and the cell adhesion protein CD44s in surgically treated patients with prostate cancer. J Urol 2000;164:2156–2161.

152. Foley KP, Eisenman RN. Two MAD tails: what the recent knockouts of Mad1 and Mxi1 tell us about the MYC/MAX/MAD network. Biochim Biophys Acta 1999;1423:M37–47.

153. Lee TC, Ziff EB. Mxi1 is a repressor of the c-Myc promoter and reverses activation by USF. J Biol Chem 1999;274:595–606.

154. Queva C, Hurlin PJ, Foley KP, Eisenman RN. Sequential expression of the MAD family of transcriptional repressors during differentiation and development. Oncogene 1998;16:967–977.

155. Jenkins RB, Qian J, Lieber MM, Bostwick DG. Detection of c-myc oncogene amplification and chromosomal anomalies in metastatic prostatic carcinoma by fluorescence in situ hybridization. Cancer Res 1997;57:524–531.

156. Nupponen NN, Kakkola L, Koivisto P, Visakorpi T. Genetic alterations in hormone-refractory recurrent prostate carcinomas. Am J Pathol 1998;153:141–148.

157. Sato K, Qian J, Slezak JM, et al. Clinical significance of alterations of chromosome 8 in high-grade, advanced, nonmetastatic prostate carcinoma. J Natl Cancer Inst 1999;91:1574–1580.

158. Bubendorf L, Kononen J, Koivisto P, et al. Survey of gene amplifications during prostate cancer progression by high-throughout fluorescence in situ hybridization on tissue microarrays. Cancer Res 1999;59:803–806.

159. Tsuchiya N, Slezak JM, Lieber MM, Bergstralh EJ, Jenkins RB. Clinical significance of alterations of chromosome 8 detected by fluorescence in situ hybridization analysis in pathologic organ-confined prostate cancer. Genes Chromosomes Cancer 2002;34:363–371.

160. Prochownik EV. c-Myc as a therapeutic target in cancer. Expert Rev Anticancer Ther 2004;4:289–302.

161. Reiter RE, Gu Z, Watabe T, et al. Prostate stem cell antigen: a cell surface marker overexpressed in prostate cancer. Proc Natl Acad Sci USA 1998;95:1735–1740.

162. Antica M, Wu L, Scollay R. Stem cell antigen 2 expression in adult and developing mice. Immunol Lett 1997;55:47–51.

163. Classon BJ, Boyd RL. Thymic-shared antigen-1 (TSA-1). A lymphostromal cell membrane Ly-6 superfamily molecule with a putative role in cellular adhesion. Dev Immunol 1998;6:149–156.

164. Cher ML, MacGrogan D, Bookstein R, Brown JA, Jenkins RB, Jensen RH. Comparative genomic hybridization, allelic imbalance, and fluorescence in situ hybridization on chromosome 8 in prostate cancer. Genes Chromosomes Cancer 1994;11:153–162.

165. Gu Z, Thomas G, Yamashiro J, et al. Prostate stem cell antigen (PSCA) expression increases with high gleason score, advanced stage and bone metastasis in prostate cancer. Oncogene 2000;19:1288–1296.

166. Ross S, Spencer SD, Holcomb I, et al. Prostate stem cell antigen as therapy target: tissue expression and in vivo efficacy of an immunoconjugate. Cancer Res 2002;62:2546–2553.

167. Amara N, Palapattu GS, Schrage M, et al. Prostate stem cell antigen is overexpressed in human transitional cell carcinoma. Cancer Res 2001;61:4660–4665.

168. Reiter RE, Sato I, Thomas G, et al. Coamplification of prostate stem cell antigen (PSCA) and MYC in locally advanced prostate cancer. Genes Chromosomes Cancer 2000;27:95–103.

169. Han KR, Seligson DB, Liu X, et al. Prostate stem cell antigen expression is associated with gleason score, seminal vesicle invasion and capsular invasion in prostate cancer. J Urol 2004;171:1117–1121.

170. Saffran DC, Raitano AB, Hubert RS, Witte ON, Reiter RE, Jakobovits A. Anti-PSCA mAbs inhibit tumor growth and metastasis formation and prolong the survival of mice bearing human prostate cancer xenografts. Proc Natl Acad Sci USA 2001;98:2658–2663.

171. Varambally S, Dhanasekaran SM, Zhou M, et al. The polycomb group protein EZH2 is involved in progression of prostate cancer. Nature 2002;419:624–629.

172. Foster CS, Falconer A, Dodson AR, et al. Transcription factor E2F3 overexpressed in prostate cancer independently predicts clinical outcome. Oncogene 2004;23:5871–5879.

173. Bao L, Loda M, Janmey PA, Stewart R, Anand-Apte B, Zetter BR. Thymosin beta 15: a novel regulator of tumor cell motility upregulated in metastatic prostate cancer. Nat Med 1996;2:1322–1328.

174. Bao L, Loda M, Zetter BR. Thymosin beta15 expression in tumor cell lines with varying metastatic potential. Clin Exp Metastasis 1998;16:227–233.

175. Chakravatri A, Zehr EM, Zietman AL, et al. Thymosin beta-15 predicts for distant failure in patients with clinically localized prostate cancer-results from a pilot study. Urology 2000;55:635–638.

Biologic response modifiers and prostate cancer

29

Bob Djavan, Yan Kit Fong

INTRODUCTION

Prostate cancer is the most common malignancy in men in the Western world, affecting 1 in 6 American men at some time in their life. It was the cause of death in more than 28,000 American men in 2003 alone.[1] With the effective tumor marker, PSA, being used commonly as a screening tool, more cases of early, localized prostate cancer are being detected. Unfortunately, approximately 10% of patients are still diagnosed with metastatic disease[1] at initial presentation and 30% to 40% of patients with apparently localized disease who are treated with curative intent ultimately develop clinical or biochemical progression.[2–10] Though most patients will initially respond to androgen deprivation therapy, the vast majority will eventually develop androgen-independent disease, which usually leads to death. Thus, hormone–refractory prostate cancer (HRPC) poses a great challenge to both urologists and oncologists. The search for better drugs to treat HRPC patients continues, and it is hoped that understanding of the biologic response and underlying molecular mechanisms of metastatic prostate cancer will shed some light on this pursuit.

This chapter will first review the tumorigenesis and progression of prostate cancer, especially the entity of HRPC. Clinical trials of several molecular targets involved are discussed. Next, the important steps of metastasis such as invasion and angiogenesis are presented, together with a variety of potential biologic response modifiers.

TUMORIGENESIS AND PROGRESSION OF PROSTATE CANCER

Prostate cancer, like any cancer, is associated with an uncontrolled proliferation and loss of apoptotic potential leading to the development of tumor masses. Prostate epithelial cells are fundamentally dependent on the presence of androgens for growth and differentiation, eventually dying by the process of apoptosis.[11] Removal of androgens results in their death via apoptosis.[12] However, prostate cancer cells, specifically androgen-independent tumors, have developed mechanisms to overcome the loss of androgen. The culprits include amplification and overexpression of androgen receptors (AR),[13] and more importantly the postulated alternative growth signaling by several growth factors.

ANDROGEN GROWTH SIGNALING AND DIFFERENTIATION THERAPY (Figure 29.1)

Androgen growth signaling is activated through the androgen receptor, an important member of the nuclear hormone receptor superfamily that includes steroid receptors, retinoid receptors, thyroid hormone receptors, vitamin D_3 receptors and peroxisome proliferator–activator receptors (PPAR)[14]. In normal prostate development, AR signaling plays a key role in specifying the normal prostate architecture and the differentiation pathways. Promoting differentiation can lead to cell cycle arrest (terminal differentiation), restoration of normal homeostasis, and in some cases apoptosis. Thus androgen-related family members are potential targets for differentiation therapy for prostate cancer, including HRPC.

VITAMIN D

Low serum levels of vitamin D[15] and 1,25-dihydroxy vitamin D (calcitriol)[16] were found to be risk factors for

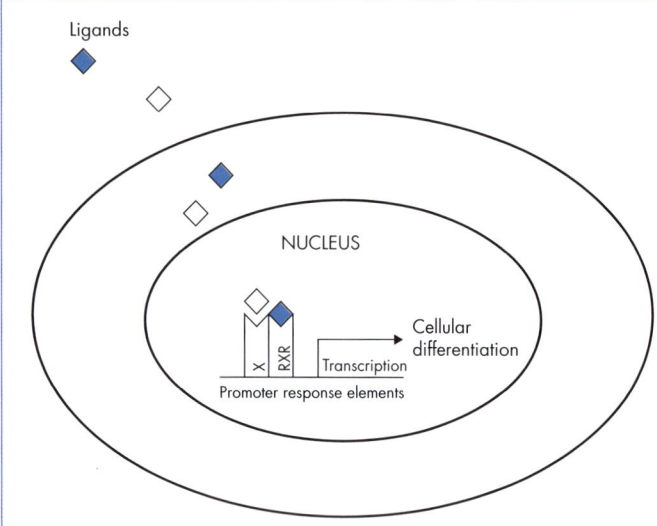

Ligands

NUCLEUS

Cellular differentiation

Transcription

Promoter response elements

Fig. 29.1
Differentiation therapy in prostate cancer. Ligands, such as vitamin D and prostaglandin, bind to their respective receptor X leading to heterodimerization of retinoid X receptor (RXR). This complex in turn binds to the promoter response element, such as vitamin D response element (VDRE) and peroxisome promoter response element (PPRE), and results in differentiation of malignant cells.

development of prostate cancer. Functional vitamin D3 receptors are expressed by prostate cancer, LNCaP, PC-3, and DU-145 cell lines, and primary prostate epithelial cells derived from patients with normal prostate and benign prostatic hyperplasia cells.[17–19] Binding of the receptor results in dimerization with retinoid X receptor (RXR) forming a heterodimer that regulates target gene transcription through the vitamin D response elements. This complex binds not only calcium metabolism regulatory genes but also genes such as those encoding c-FOS, c-MYC, p21, p27 and HOX A10, which are involved in cellular differentiation and proliferation.[20] Through these interactions, vitamin D controls differentiation and cell cycle arrest or apoptosis. Several in-vitro and animal experimental studies have demonstrated that calcitriol induces differentiation and reduces cellular proliferation,[18,19] enhances PSA secretion and AR expression,[17,18] and inhibits prostate adenocarcinoma growth alone as a monotherapy[21] and in combination with paclitaxel.[22] Gross et al treated early recurrent prostate cancer, defined by rising PSA in patients who had received definitive surgery or radiotherapy, with oral calcitriol and found that the agent decreased the rate of rising PSA in six of seven patients.[23] However, hypercalciuria was noted in each patient and two patients developed asymptomatic small nephrolithiasis. Though oral calcitriol alone was not effective in HRPC,[24] early results of combination of calcitriol and chemo-therapeutic agents were promising.[25–27]

PEROXISOME PROLIFERATOR-ACTIVATED RECEPTOR

The PPAR is another member of the nuclear receptor superfamily that functions as a regulator of numerous genes and induces differentiation in multiple tissues. It is known to be activated by several ligands that include prostaglandin,[28] arachidonic acid metabolites,[29] and an

important class of anti-diabetic drug, troglitazone.[30] Binding of the ligand results in a heterodimer with the RXR that affects the peroxisome proliferator response elements in the promoters of target genes. Transcription of these genes activates adipocyte differentiation and potential tumor suppressor-like functions in several cell types. The PPAR is highly expressed in prostate cancer cell lines[31–33] and prostatic intraepithelial neoplasia.[33] In-vitro and animal studies with two important ligands, 15-deoxy-δ-12,14-prostaglandin J_2 (15δ-PG J_2) and troglitazone have shown growth inhibition of prostate cancer cells.[31,32,34] In clinical trials, Hisatake et al reported PSA stabilization and notable decrease in PSA velocity after troglitazone (600–800 mg/day) in a patient with an androgen-dependent recurrence as defined by a rising PSA after radical prostatectomy.[35] Mueller and investigators treated 41 patients with either androgen-dependent (n = 12) or androgen-independent (n = 29) recurrences after definitive local therapy with troglitazone (800 mg/day) for at least 12 weeks.[31] An unexpectedly high incidence of prolonged stabilization of PSA, and the absence of new metastases and disease-related symptoms were noted. After 16 months of treatment, though one man had nearly undetectable level of PSA, no patients with androgen-independent cancer experienced more than 50% PSA decrease. Treatment was generally well tolerated with a single case of transient grade 3 transaminitis. Unfortunately, troglitazone was withdrawn from the market in the United States in 2000 due to reported idiosyncratic liver toxicity. Another similar drug, rosigliazone, is undergoing phase II trial in patients with PSA recurrence after local therapy.

GROWTH FACTOR RECEPTORS SIGNALING AND SIGNAL TRANSDUCTION (Figure 29.2)

Signal transduction refers to the way external stimuli by hormones and growth factors are transferred to the

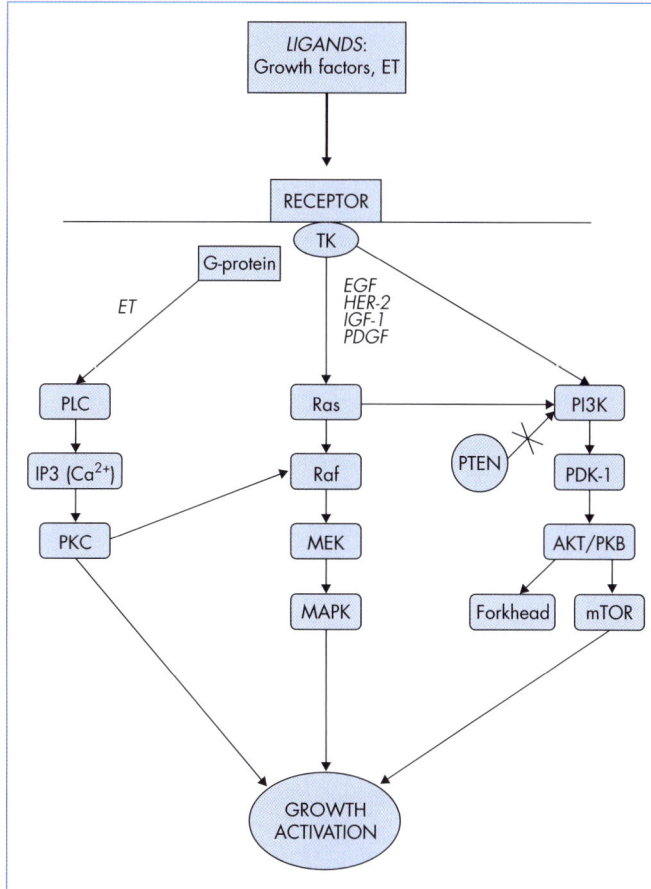

Fig. 29.2
Important signal transduction pathways in prostate cancer. Different ligands such as growth factors and endothelins bind to their respective receptors to elicit the different signal cascades. Important intercascade crosstalk is shown. (AKT/PKB, protein kinase B; IP3, inositol-triphosphate; MAPK, mitogen-activated protein kinase; MEK, mitogen-activated protein kinase; mTOR, mammalian target of rapamycin; PDK1, 3-phosphoinositide-dependent protein kinase; PI3K, phosphatidylinositol 3-kinase; PKC, protein kinase C; PLC, phospholipase C; PTEN, phosphatase and tensin homolog deleted from chromosome 10; TK, tyrosine kinase.)

nucleus after binding to the receptor. A different way of signal transduction is achieved by phosphorylation and activation of a chain of downstream enzymes after ligand binding, resulting in a wide variety of cellular responses on both DNA and protein level involved in cell proliferation, differentiation, and apoptosis. For signal transduction, tyrosine kinase, serine and threonine kinases, and G-coupled receptors play an important role in many signal transduction pathways. Important examples of such pathways, including phosphatidylinositol 3-kinase/AKT (PI3K-AKT), mitogen-activated protein kinase (MAPK), and transforming growth factor-β (TGFβ)-Smad pathways, show "crosstalk." Crosstalk indicates that activation of one pathway may alter the response to activation of other pathways by activation or mutual inhibition.

Small peptide growth factors, operating through autocrine and paracrine loops, are frequently the initiating agents for these signals. Numerous growth factors (Table 29.1) have been implicated in prostate cancer development, growth and metastasis. Although some of these processes are also regulated in part by androgens, dysregulation of these pathways also occurs independent of androgen control. Thus, the androgen-independent state may be driven by many of these growth factors and their downstream mediators.

ERBB RECEPTOR FAMILY SIGNALING

The ERBB receptor family consists of 4 members: ERBB1/epidermal growth factor receptor (EGFR), ERBB2/HER2/NEU, ERBB3, and ERBB4. The important ligands include epidermal growth factor (EGF) and transforming growth factor-α (TGFα) for ERBB1 and heregulin for ERBB3 and ERBB4. Epidermal growth factor is a mitogen required for normal prostate epithelial cells and is found in large quantities in normal human prostatic fluid and prostate cancer cells.[36] The EGFR has an extracellular binding domain and a cytoplasmic domain with tyrosine kinase activity. Both EGF and its receptor appear to signal mainly through the MAPK pathway, enhancing protein kinase A activity[37] and also induce AR signaling.[38] The EGFR was associated with Gleason score, PSA level, and development of androgen-independent disease.[39] In addition to its role in prostate cancer progression, EGFR also plays a role in prostate tumor cell invasion and metastasis. It is overexpressed in DU-145 cells with enhanced metastatic potential[40] and the invasiveness is reduced with EGFR-specific kinase inhibitor in the transgenic adenocarcinoma mouse prostate (TRAMP).[41]

The other important member of the ERBB receptor family is ERBB2/HER2, but there have been no identified agonistic ligands for the receptor. The possibility exists that

Table 29.1 Growth factor and receptors in prostate cancer and important inhibitors

Factor/ligands	Ligand expression levels	Receptors	Receptor expression levels	Important Inhibitors
Epidermal growth factor (EGF)	↑	ERBB1/EGFR	↑	Cetuximab, Gefitinib
–	–	HER2/NEU	↑	Trastuzumab, Gefitinib
Insulin-like growth factor 1 (IGF1)	↑	IGF1R	↑	OSI-774
Platelet-derived growth factor (PDGF)	↑	PDGFR	↑	Imatinib
Endothelin 1	↑	ETA	↑	Atrasentan
Vascular epithelial growth factor (VEGF)	↑/↓	FLT1 and FLK1	↑	Rhuα-VEGF
Basic fibroblast growth factor (bFGF)	↑	FGF2	↓	TNP-470

overexpression of HER2 may result in spontaneous homodimerization resulting in signal transduction like EGF, but without the need for an activating ligand. HER2 is overexpressed in prostate cancer patients[42,43] and amplification of the HER2 oncogene in prostate cancer was demonstrated in several series.[44-46] More importantly, increased HER2 mRNA and protein expression were seen in tumors that progressed from an androgen-dependent state to HRPC.[47] Moreover, Craft et al found that overexpression of HER2 in androgen-dependent prostate cancer could stimulate androgen-independent growth, and AR signaling could be activated in the absence of ligand.[47] All these findings make ERBB receptor signaling inhibition enticing, especially in HRPC.

ERBB2 receptor signaling can be inhibited at two levels: 1) recombinant antibodies against the receptor; and 2) inhibition of receptor-associated tyrosine kinase activity. In preclinical trials, inhibition of both EGFR using monoclonal antibodies C225 (ceftuximab) and HER2 with the monoclonal antibodies trastuzumab and 2C4 resulted in growth reduction in prostate cancer cells.[49-51,52] Surprisingly, trastuzumab had antitumor activity in xenografts of hormone-dependent prostate cancer but not in hormone-independent tumors.[53] Early clinical data of trastuzumab monotherapy in HRPC showed no objective response, but in combination with paclitaxel, the treatment regimen showed stable disease or partial response in 6 of 20 patients.[54] It is noteworthy that inhibition of HER2 results in PSA downregulation, rendering PSA serum levels less useful for monitoring of tumor response in these patients.[55] Finally, though HER2 overexpression was associated with advanced disease, response to trastuzumab was independent of the expression levels.[54]

Tyrosine kinase activation is an early event in the cellular signaling pathways that can lead to cell growth and/or division, cellular differentiation and cell activation (e.g., in immune responses). Conversely, tyrosine kinase inhibition

is expected to halt the downstream intracellular signaling and inhibit cell growth. The first oral EGFR inhibitor, gefitinib, was described in 1996. The antitumor activity of gefitinib has been demonstrated in a range of human tumor xenografts, including prostate cancer.[56-58] Similar to trastuzumab, gefitinib seems most effective in combination with chemotherapy[59] and inferior to paclitaxel monotherapy in xenograft models of androgen-independent prostate cancer.[60] Furthermore, preclinical studies of combination of gefitinib with antiandrogen bicalutamide showed greater efficacy than a higher dose of bicalutamide alone against a moderately androgen-independent tumor xenograft.[56] The efficacy and tolerability of gefitinib monotherapy have been investigated in four open label, multicenter, phase I dose escalation studies involving patients with a variety of solid malignant tumors.[61-64] Gefitinib was well tolerated in all four trials, with the most common adverse events being diarrhea, nausea, rash/acne, vomiting, and asthenia. In prostate cancer, phase I study data showed disease-related symptom improvement in 8 of 12 evaluable patients using gefitinib monotherapy with durations up to 6 months.[65] Early data from two pilot trials combining gefitinib with either mitoxantrone/prednisolone or docetaxel/estramustine regimens in prostate cancer showed PSA responses in up to 47% of patients, whereas pain responses in up to 43% and 41%, respectively.[66] However, another phase II study in 40 patients with metastatic hormone resistant prostate cancer with minimal clinical symptoms suggested little activity.[67] Moreover, it was found that regrowth of the human tumor xenograft rapidly followed the termination of treatment,[58,60] suggesting that the drug effect is cytostatic rather than cytotoxic and the agent needs dosing for long intervals.

INSULIN-LIKE GROWTH FACTOR SIGNALING

Insulin-like growth factor (IGF1) binds and activates both the IGF1 receptor (IGF1R) and insulin receptor.

Signal transduction via IGF1R activates both MAPK and PI3K/AKT pathways, which are essential for the growth stimulatory effects of IGF1.[68] IGF1 is also known to act downstream of the c-MYC oncogene and so block entry into the apoptotic pathway, especially after castration.[69] It binds to and is inhibited by IGF binding protein 3 (IGFBP3). In fact, an increased level of IGF1 is associated with increased risk of prostate cancer,[70,71] and a decreased level of IGFBP3 predictive of advanced prostate cancer.[72,73] Insulin-like growth factor 1 has also been found to stimulate the gene expression of BCL2, Bclx and MCL1 in prostate cell lines[74] and may be involved in the progression or development of prostate cancer, in particular androgen independence. Further evidence of the involvement of IGF1 was reported by Fiebig et al,[75] who found that prostate cancer cells overexpressed metalloproteinase 9 after being exposed to IGF1.

Therefore, antibodies to IGF1 appear as a promising treatment modality for inhibition of cell growth.[76] Unfortunately, no other clinical data is available to date about this treatment approach in prostate cancer. However, OSI-774 (tyrosine kinase inhibitor) has been shown to inhibit IGF1 activity besides inhibiting both ERBB1 and ERBB2.[77] There is crosstalk between EGFR and IGF1R, and it has been suggested that tyrosine kinase inhibitors may partially exert their growth inhibitory effects through IGF1R signal inhibition.[78] As such, IGF1 levels may be useful to predict treatment response and should be included as a marker in trials on tyrosine kinases known to inhibit IGF1R activity.

PLATELET-DERIVED GROWTH FACTOR SIGNALING

Platelet-derived growth factor (PDGF) family is another subset of the receptor tyrosine kinases (RTKs), and binding of the ligand causes receptor dimerization, kinase activation, cross phosphorylation, and signal transduction. This signaling occurs mainly through interactions with PI3K, and activation of the RAS/RAF/MAPK pathway.[79,80] Platelet-derived growth factor is also involved in activation of several oncogenes[81] and is a potent mitogen that inhibits apoptosis. In humans, PDGF receptors (PDGFRs) are not expressed in normal prostate epithelium and BPH, but are overexpressed in high-grade PIN[82] and adenocarcinomas of the prostate.[83] Moreover, PDGFR is also identified by reverse transcriptase polymerase chain reaction and immunohistochemisty in metastatic bone lesions.[84]

Imatinib mesylate (STI571) was initially found to inhibit BCR-ABL oncoprotein and has been FDA-approved for the treatment of chronic myeloid leukemia.[85] Besides, imatinib mesylate binds and inhibits tyrosine kinase activity of the PDGF. In nude mouse xenograft model, oral imatinib mesylate resulted in 50% reduction in the development of bone and lymph node metastasis.[86] Addition of paclitaxel further reduced the development of bone and lymph node metastases to 65% to 75%. Reduction of interstitial pressures by PDGF inhibition is the proposed mechanism of the synergistic effect.[87] An ongoing clinical trial involving 40 patients with advanced prostate cancer on imatinib mesylate would shed further light to the efficacy of this agent in prostate cancer.[88] Another PDGFR inhibitor is lefunomide (SU101). In a phase II clinical trial in heavily pretreated patients with HRPC, 3 of 39 patients showed more than 50% PSA decrease, 1 of 19 had an actual measurable partial response, and 9 of 35 had improvement of disease symptoms.[89] Interestingly, PDGFR expression was noted in 80% of bone marrow metastases, whereas 88% of primary prostate tumor archival specimens revealed significant expression. Thus, it is postulated that PDGFR is crucial early in prostate tumorigenesis, making it a feasible target for early prostate cancer treatment, and also PDGFR expression denotes a subset of prostate neoplasm that confer a poor prognosis that will more likely develop eventual metastatic disease.

PTEN AND AKT-MTOR SIGNALING

The PI3K pathway is regulated at least in part by the functional PTEN (phosphatase and tensin homolog deleted on chromosome 10). Inactivation of PTEN gene (10q23) has been documented with high frequency in a broad spectrum of malignancies, including prostate cancer, and results in unregulated stimulation of the AKT/PI3K pathway.[90–92] PTEN mutations occur in approximately 49% of prostate carcinomas.[93] A surge in phosphorylated AKT (activated) is found in PIN, compared with adjacent normal epithelium.[94] mTOR (mammalian target of rapamycin) is a serine-threonine kinase that is activated through PI3K/AKT pathway. Inhibition of mTOR affects the activity of two separate downstream pathways that control the translation of specific mRNAs required for cell cycle traverse from G1 to S phase, resulting in growth arrest in the G1 phase of the cell cycle.

Inhibition of mTOR by rapamycin (sirolimus) is particular effective in PTEN-negative tumors.[95–97] Among several mTOR inhibitors in clinical development for cancer therapy, CCI-779, a rapamycin derivative, has completed phase I trials as a single agent using intravenous formulation and oral formulalation.[98] It is currently in combination studies with other anticancer drugs and results are pending.

ENDOTHELIN SIGNALING

Endothelins (ETs)—which include three 21-amino-acid peptides ET1 (expressed in endothelial cells), ET2 (in kidney and testis) and ET3 (in brain)—are potent vasoconstricting peptides, involved in the pathophysiology of different malignancies.[99,100] Endothelins exert their effects by binding to two distinct cell surface ET receptors, ETA and ETB. ETB binds the three peptide isotypes with equal affinity, while ETA binds ET1 with higher affinity than the other isoforms. Ligand binding to the endothelin receptor results in activation of a pertussis toxin-insensitive G protein that stimulates phospholipase C activity and increases intracellular calcium levels, activation of protein kinase C and MAPK, and p125 focal adhesion kinase (FAK) phosphorylation. Endothelin 1 is also involved in the activation of EGF- and IGF-related kinases and MAPK.[101,102] Stimulation of these different signaling cascades by ET1 explains its diverse functions in vasoconstriction, mitogenesis, and inhibition of apoptosis. Moreover, ET1 is also involved in tumor neovascularization through upregulation of vascular endothelial growth factor (VEGF),[103,104] tumor invasion via enhancement of secretion of matrix-degrading proteinases such as matrix metalloproteinases (MMPs),[105] and osteogenesis by increasing synthesis of both collagenous and noncollagenous proteins that include osteopontin and osteocalcin.[106]

The ET axis has recently been identified as contributing to the pathophysiology of advanced prostate cancer.[107,108] The most extensively studied endothelin inhibitor is atrasentan (ABT-637), which binds to ETA receptors and antagonizes the effects of ET1. Phase I trial evaluation showed that the maximum-tolerated dose was 60 mg/day.[109] In this trial, stabilization and decline of PSA occurred in 66% of patients. In a randomized double-blinded phase II study, 288 patients with HRPC were enrolled and treated with atrasentan 2.5 mg and 10 mg administered orally once daily.[109] In the evaluable patients (n = 244), atrasentan 10 mg significantly delayed time to clinical and biochemical progression, maintained total and bone alkaline phosphatase concentrations compared with the placebo-treated group, and bone pain was less frequent in the atrasentan arm compared with the placebo arm. The most common side effects included rhinitis, peripheral edema, and headache. A phase III trial with atrasentan in non-metastasized prostate cancer and another phase II combination trial of a new ETA inhibitor (YM 598) and chemotherapy are ongoing.

ANGIOGENESIS AND METASTASIS

The steps in the progression to metastasis include angiogenesis, cell attachment, and invasion (basement membrane degradation). As tumors grow, they require new blood vessels from which they obtain oxygen and nutrients, and without which they are unable to grow beyond 2 mm.[111] Angiogenesis can be divided into several steps: proliferation of endothelial cells,

breakdown of extracellular matrix, migration of endothelial cells toward the chemotactic angiogenic stimulus (e.g., VEGF), and finally tube formation followed by circulation through the lumen. This complex process is regulated by a number of angiogenic factors such as VEGF and inhibitors, making it an attractive target for a biologic modifier.

VASCULAR ENDOTHELIAL GROWTH FACTOR SIGNALING

Vascular endothelial growth factor was the first selective angiogenic growth factor to be purified, and is still a preeminent molecule in this area. Tissue staining has demonstrated that human prostate cancer is positive for VEGF, while BPH and normal prostate cells displayed little VEGF staining and vascularity.[112] Other studies have demonstrated that castration inhibits prostate cancer VEGF production, but had no effect on other angiogenic factors.[113] Moreover, increased VEGF expression has been related to neuroendocrine differentiation in prostate cancer, a known poor prognostic factor for survival.[114,115] Taken together, these data suggest that prostate tumor growth advantage conferred by VEGF expression appears to be a consequence of stimulation of angiogenesis. The receptors for VEGF are fms-like tyrosine kinase 1 (FLT1) and fetal liver kinase 1 (FLK1), both expressed in prostate cancer.[116] The receptor tyrosine kinase FLK1 associates with VEGF as a high-affinity ligand and is suggested to have a crucial role in angiogenesis.[117]

In androgen-independent xenograft of prostate cancer, rhuα-VEGF, a humanized monoclonal antibody targeting VEGF, showed growth inhibition in prostate cancer cells.[118] After cessation of intraperitoneal antibody administration, xenograft tumor regrowth occurred. Additional growth inhibition was noted in mice treated with a combination of rhuα-VEGF and paclitaxel.[118] ZD6474, a tyrosine kinase inhibitor showed specific inhibition of VEGF signaling in addition to anti-EGF and anti-basic fibroblast growth factor (bFGF) activity.[119] This novel drug showed a dose-dependent regression of established PC3 xenografts in nude mice after oral administration. ZD4190 is another potent inhibitor of VEGF-stimulated human vascular endothelial cell proliferation in vitro. Chronic once daily oral dosing of ZD4190 to mice bearing established human tumor xenografts (breast, lung, prostate, and ovarian) elicited significant antitumor activity.[120]

Thalidomide was marketed in Europe as a sedative, but was withdrawn 30 years ago because it has potent teratogenic effects that cause stunted limb growth (dysmelia) in humans. It is now re-emerging in cancer and inflammation treatment for its immunomodulatory and angiogenesis blocking properties.[121] It blocks the activity of not only VEGF but also fibroblast growth factor (FGF) and interleukin 6 (IL6), and showed anticancer activity in several solid and hematologic malignancies. In a phase II study of thalidomide in patients with HRPC, a total of 27% of all patients (n = 63) had a decline in PSA of greater than or equal to 40%, often associated with improvement of clinical symptoms.[122] These data suggest that antiangiogenesis agents such as ZD6474 and thalidomide used as monotherapy showed moderate efficacy in prostate cancer and further evaluation of these agents in hormone naïve patients would be useful.

FIBROBLAST GROWTH FACTOR SIGNALING

The FGF family consists of a group of polypeptides associated with a wide variety of processes such as angiogenesis, hematopoiesis, and wound healing. Serum levels of FGFs are elevated in prostate cancer patients,[123] especially those with high-grade lesions.[123,124] Expression of the isoforms FGF receptors 1 and 2 (FGFR1 and FGFR2) was associated with PIN,[125] but FGFR expression was not changed in prostate cancer, and FGFR2 was even found to be downregulated in HRPC.[126]

TNP-470, a synthetic analog of fumagillin was shown to prevent binding of bFGF to low-affinity heparin sulfate proteoglycans[127] and inhibit endothelial cell growth in vitro.[128] In preclinical trials, PC-3 cell xenograft tumor growth was inhibited by TNP-470, which is also synergistic when used with cisplastin.[129] However, a phase I trial of TNP-470 in 33 patients with metastatic and androgen-independent prostate cancer showed no definite antitumor effect.[130] Recently, a CKD-731 analog has been developed and is reported to have 1000-fold more inhibition of endothelial cell growth than TNP-470.[131] In general, the fumagillin analog shows some promise and may provide the specificity needed to suppress endothelial mitogens without being prohibitively toxic.

OTHER ANGIOGENESIS INHIBITORS

Endostatin was discovered as an angiogenesis inhibitor produced by hemangioendothelioma, and was determined to be a 20 kDa *C*-terminal fragment of collagen XVIII. Endostatin was demonstrated to inhibit endothelial proliferation specifically and was found to be a potent inhibitor of angiogenesis and tumor growth.[132,133] In a transgenic mouse model with spontaneous prostate cancer tumorigenesis, endostatin prolonged survival time in mice for an additional 74 days.[134] Interestingly, angiostatin, an internal fragment of plasminogen, is another potent inhibitor of angiogenesis, which selectively inhibits endothelial cell proliferation.[135] When given systematically, angiostatin potently inhibits tumor growth and can maintain metastatic and primary tumors in a dormant state defined by a balance of cell proliferation and apoptosis

of tumor cells. Supplementing agents of endogenous origin, such as plasminogen, which is subsequently cleaved into angiostatin by the process of proteolysis by tumors, and endostatin may prove useful to reduce primary tumor growth and the establishment of metastasis that requires neovascularization.[133,136,137] This novel form of treatment for prostate cancer may prove to be effective when used in combination with other treatment modalities in the future.

INVASION AND METASTASIS

Proximity to blood vessels is paramount to a tumor's ability to reach the circulation, the step to metastasis is attachment and invasion of cells into the vasculature. Attachment of epithelial cells involves several junctional structures including desmosomes and tight junctions. These contacts are mediated by calcium-dependent interactions with the cadherin cell-adhesion molecule family (E-cadherin). Disruption of the cadherin–catenin complex decreases cell–cell adhesion, and low levels of E-cadherin have been associated with a more aggressive type of prostate cancer.[138] In contrast, CD44 is a protein involved in cell adhesion to the extracellular matrix protein hyaluronic acid and high cell expression correlates with poor outcome. Blocking of CD44 with antibodies has been shown to inhibit metastasis.[139] Protease inhibitors that inhibit basement membrane proteases are a class of molecules that may impede the tumor cell's ability to penetrate the vasculature as the basement membrane forms a barrier. Matrix metalloproteases are proteins that break down basement membranes, while tissue inhibitors of metalloproteases (TIMP) are regarded as invasion inhibitors. Increased tissue levels of MMP2 and MMP9, and absence of TIMP1 and TIMP2 correlated with higher Gleason score; while TIMP1 and TIMP2 overexpression were found in organ confined disease.[140]

MATRIX METALLOPROTEASE INHIBITORS

Several MMP inhibitors have been tested in preclinical and clinical trials for prostate cancer. Tetracycline derivative CMT-3 was found to inhibit both tumor growth and metastasis in rat model.[141] Stearns et al found that IL10 treatment of PC-3ML cell tumors in mouse models resulted in stimulation of TIMP1 and inhibition of MMP2 and MMP-9, thus reduced the number of spinal metastasis and increased the tumor-free survival rates.[142] Marimastat (BB-2516) was the first MMP inhibitor to have entered clinical trials in the field of oncology and completed phase I and phase II trials in prostate and colon cancer patients.[143] The drug was generally well tolerated and 58% response rate (complete response defined as no increase of PSA over the study period and partial response defined as less than 25% increase in PSA per 4 weeks) was reported using doses greater than 50 mg twice daily.[144]

UROKINASE-TYPE PLASMINOGEN ACTIVATOR

Urokinase-type plasminogen activator (uPA) plays a key role in tissue degradation in both normal and cancerous tissues. Overexpression of uPA has been reported in many cancers, including prostate, and particularly in a portion of HRPCs. Prostate cancer cell lines with gene amplification for high uPA expression are more sensitive to the urokinase inhibitor, amiloride compared with those without.[145] In a mouse model implanted with prostate cancer cell line Dunning R3227 that overexpresses uPA, a selective inhibitor of uPA enzymatic activity 4-iodobenzothiophene-2-caboxamide (B-428) resulted in a marked decrease in primary tumor volume as well as in the development of tumor metastasis when compared with controls.[146]

CONCLUSION

Understanding the biology of prostate cancer, including tumorigenesis, progression to HRPC, angiogenesis, and cancer cell invasion, is vital for the development of new drugs targeted at the different molecular levels. Since treatment for localized prostate cancer is probably optimal today, researches should be dedicated to the understanding and management of HRPC to improve the overall survival in prostate cancer patients. We have reviewed therapy targeted at the different levels such as androgen signaling (tumorigenesis), growth factors signaling (progression to HRPC), and angiogenesis and protease inhibition (metastasis). Among them, ERBB tyrosine kinase receptor inhibitor (gefitinib), endothelin 1 receptor inhibitor (atrasentan) and PDGF receptor inhibitor (imatinib) offer the most promise as they have completed both phase I and II trials. Combination with chemotherapy seems to improve the cytotoxicity of most of these drugs with minimal side effects and appears to be the best treatment strategy for HRPC and metastatic disease.

REFERENCES

1. Jemal A, Murray T, Samuels A, et al. Cancer statistics, 2003. CA Cancer J Clin 2003;53:5–26.
2. Amling CL, Blute ML, Bergstrah EJ, et al. Long-term hazard of progression after radical prostatectomy for clinically localized prostate cancer: continued risk of biochemical failure after 5 years. J Urol 200;164:101–105.
3. Pound CR, Partin AW, Epstein JI, et al. Prostate specific antigen after anatomic radical prostatectomy: patterns of recurrence and cancer control. Urol Clin North Am 1997;24:395–406.
4. Laufer M, Pound CR, Carducci MA, et al. Management of patients with rising prostate specific antigen after radical prostatectomy. Urology 2000;55:309–315.
5. Dilliioglugil O, Leibman BD, Kattan MW, et al. Hazard rates for progression after radical prostatectomy for clinically localized prostate cancer. Urology 1997;50:93–97.
6. Pound CR, Partin AW, Eisenberger MA, et al. Natural history of progression after PSA elevation following radical prostatectomy. JAMA 1999;281:1591–1597.
7. Lee WR, Hanks GE, Schultheiss TE, et al. Localized prostate cancer treated by external beam radiotherapy alone: serum PSA driven outcome analysis. J Clin Oncol 1995;13:464–469.
8. Sandler HM, McLaughlin PW, Kish KE, et al. Results of 3D conformal radiotherapy in the treatment of 707 patients with localized prostate cancer. Int J Radiat Oncol Biol Phys 1995;32:141–144.
9. Blasko JC, Wallner K, Grimm PD, et al. Prostate specific antigen based disease control following ultrasound guided ^{125}Iodine implantation for T1/T2 prostatic carcinoma. J Urol 1995;154:1096–1099.
10. Kupelian P, Elshaikh M, Reddy C, et al. Comparison of the efficacy of local therapies for localized prostate cancer in the prostate specific antigen era: a large single-institution experience with radical prostatectomy and external-beam radiotherapy. J Clin Oncol 2002;20:3376–3385.
11. Denmeade SR, Lin XS, Isaacs JT. Role of programmed (apoptotic) cell death during the progression and therapy for prostate cancer. Prostate 1996;28:251–265.
12. Berges RR, Vukanovic J, Epstein JI. Implication of the cell kinetic changes during the progression of human prostatic cancer. Clin Cancer Res 1995;1:473–480.
13. Linja MJ, Savinainen KJ, Saramaki OR. Amplification and overexpression of androgen receptor gene in hormone-refractory prostate cancer. Cancer Res 2001;61:3550–3555.
14. Hart SM. Modulation of nuclear receptor dependent transcription. Biol Res 2002;35:295–303.
15. Schwartz GG, Hulka BS. Is vitamin D deficiency a risk factor for prostate cancer? (Hypothesis). Anti-cancer Res 1990;1307–1311.
16. Corder EH, Guess HA, Hulka BS, et al. Vitamin D and prostate cancer: a prediagnostic study with stored sera. Cancer Epidemiol Biomarkers Prev 1993;2:467–472.
17. Miller GJ, Stapleton GE, Ferrara JA, et al. The human prostatic carcinoma cell line LNCaP expresses biologically active, specific receptors for 1,25-dihydroxyvitamin D3. Cancer Res 1992;52:515–520.
18. Skowronski RJ, Peehl DM, Feldman D. Vitamin D and prostate cancer:1,25-dihydroxyvitamin D3 receptors and actions in human prostate cancer cell lines. Endocrinology 1993;132:1952–1960.
19. Peehl DM, Skowronski RJ, Leung GK, et al. Antiproliferative effects of 1,25-dihydroxyvitamin D3 on primary cultures of human prostate cells. Cancer Res 1994;54:805–810.
20. Freedman LP. Transcriptional targets of the vitamin D3 receptor mediated cell cycle arrest and differentiation. J Nutr 1999;129:581S–586S.
21. Getzenberg RH, Light BW, Lapco PE, et al. Vitamin D inhibition of prostate adenocarcinoma growth and metastasis in the Dunning rat prostate model system. Urology 1997;50:999–1006.
22. Modzelewski RA, Hershberger PA, Johnson CS, et al. Apoptotic effects of paclitaxel and calcitriol in rat dunning MLL and human PC-3 prostate tumor cells in vitro. Proc Am Assoc Cancer Res 1999;40:580a.
23. Gross C, Stamey T, Hancock S, et al. Treatment of early recurrent prostate cancer with 1,25-dihydroxyvitamin D3 (calcitriol). J Urol 1998;159:2035–2040.
24. Osborn JL, Schwartz GG, Smith DC, et al. Phase II trial of oral 1,25-dihydroxyvitamin D3 (calcitriol) in hormone refractory prostate cancer. Urol Oncol 1995;1:195–198.
25. Beer TM, Eilers KM, Garzotto M, et al. Weekly high-dose calcitriol and docetaxel in metastatic androgen-independent prostate cancer. J Clin Oncol 2003;21:123–128.
26. Trump DL, Serafine S, Brufsky A, et al. High dose calcitriol (1,25-dihydroxyvitamin D3) + dexamethasone in androgen independent prostate cancer (AIPC). Proc Am Soc Clin Oncol 2000;19:337a.
27. Johnson CS, Egorin MJ, Zuhowski R, et al. Effects of high dose calcitriol (1,25-dihydroxyvitamin D3) on the pharmacokinetics of paclitaxel or carboplastin: results of two phase I studies. Proc Am Soc Clin Oncol 2000;19:210a.

28. Kliewer SA, Forman BM, Blumberg B, et al. Differential expression and activation of a family of murine peroxisome proliferator-activated receptors. Proc Natl Acad Sci USA 1994:91:7355–7359.

29. Yu K, Bayona W, Kallen W, et al. Differential activation of the peroxisome proliferator-activated receptors by eicosanoids. J Biol Chem 1995;270:975–983.

30. Smith MR, Kantoff PW. Peroxisome proliferator-activated receptor gamma (PPARgamma) as a novel target for prostate cancer. Invest New Drugs 2002;20:195–200.

31. Mueller E, Smith M, Sarraf P, et al. Effects of ligand activation of peroxisome proliferator-activated receptor gamma in human prostate cancer. Proc Natl Acad Sci USA 2000;97:990–995.

32. Butler R, Mitchell SH, Tindall DJ, et al. Nonapoptotic cell death associated with S-phase arrest of prostate cancer cells via the peroxisome proliferator-activated receptor gamma ligand, 15-deoxy-delta-12,14-prostaglandnin J2. Cell Growth Differ 2000;11:49–61.

33. Segawa Y, Yoshimura R, Hase T, et al. Expression of peroxisome proliferator-activated receptor (PPAR) in human prostate cancer. Prostate 2002;51:108–116.

34. Kubota T, Koshizuka K, Williamson EA, et al. Ligand for peroxisome proliferator-activated receptor gamma (troglitazone) has potent antitumor effect against human prostate cancer both in vitro and in vivo. Cancer Res 1998;58:3344–3352.

35. Hisatake J, Ikezoe T, Carey M, et al. Down regulation of prostate specific antigen expression by ligands for peroxisome proliferator-activated receptor gamma in human prostate cancer. Cancer Res 2000;60:5494–5498.

36. Fowler JE, Lau JLY, Ghosh L, et al. Epidermal growth factor receptors and prostate carcinoma: an immunohistochemical study. J Urol 1988;139:857–861.

37. Putz T, Culig Z, Eder IE, et al. Epidermal growth factor (EGF) receptor blockade inhibits the action of EGF, insulin-like growth factor 1, and a protein kinase A activator on the mitogen-activated protein kinase pathway in prostate cancer cell lines. Cancer Res 1999;59:227–233.

38. Culig Z, Hobisch A, Cronauer MV, et al. Androgen receptor activation in prostatic tumor cell lines by insulin-like growth factor-1, keratinocyte growth factor, and epidermal growth factor. Cancer Res 1994;54:5474–5478.

39. Di Lorenzo G, Tortora G, D'Armiento FP, et al. Expression of epidermal growth factor receptor correlates with disease relapse and progression to androgen-independence in human prostate cancer. Clin Cancer Res 2002;8:3438–3444.

40. Turner T, Chen P, Goodly LJ, et al. EGF receptor signaling enhances in vivo invasiveness of DU-145 human prostate carcinoma cells. Clin Exp Metastasis 1996;14:409–418.

41. Kassis J, Moellinger J, Lo H, et al. A role for phospholipase C-gamma-mediated signaling in tumor cell invasion. Clin Cancer Res 1999;5:2251–2260.

42. Mellon JK, Thompson S, Charlton RG, et al. p53, c-erbB-2 and the epidermal growth factor receptor in benign and malignant prostate. J Urol 1992;147:495–499.

43. Kuhn EJ, Kurnot RA, Sesterhenn IA. Expression of the c-erb-B-2 (HER-2/neu) oncoprotein in human prostatic carcinoma. J Urol 1993;150:1427–1433.

44. Ross JS, Sheehan CM, Hayner-Buchan AM, et al. HER-2/neu gene amplification status in prostate cancer by fluorescence in situ hybridization. Hum Pathol 1997;28:827–833.

45. Kallakury BV, Sheehan CE, Ambros RA, et al. Correlation of p34cdc2 cyclin-dependent kinase overexpression, CD44s downregulation, and HER-2/neu oncogene amplification with recurrence in prostatic adenocarcinomas. J Clin Oncol 1998;16:1302–1309.

46. Mark HF, Feldman D, Das S, et al. Fluorescence in situ hybridization study of HER-2/neu oncogene amplification in prostate cancer. Exp Mol Pathol 1999;66:170–178.

47. Signoretti S, Montironi R, Manola J, et al. Her-2-neu expression and progression toward androgen independence in human prostate cancer. J Natl Cancer Inst 2000;92:1918–1925.

48. Craft NA, Shostak Y, Carey M, et al. A mechanism for hormone-independent prostate cancer through modulation of androgen receptor signaling by the Her-2/neu tyrosine kinase. Nature Med 1999;5:280–285.

49. Karashima T, Sweeney P, Slaton JW, et al. Inhibition of angiogenesis by the antiepidermal growth factor receptor antibody ImClone C225 in androgen-independent prostate cancer growing orthotopically in nude mice. Clin Cancer Res 2002;8:1253–1264.

50. Mendoza N, Phillips GL, Silva J, et al. Inhibition of ligand-mediated HER-2 activation in androgen-independent prostate cancer. Cancer Res 2002;62:5485–5488.

51. Ye D, Mendelsohn J, Fan Z. Augmentation of a humanized anti-HER-2 mAb 4D5 induced growth inhibition by a human-mouse chimeric anti-EGF receptor mAb C225. Oncogene 1999;18:731–738.

52. Agus DB, Akita RW, Fox WD, et al. A potential role for activated HER-2 in prostate cancer. Semin Oncol 2000;27:76–83.

53. Agus DB, Scher HI, Higgins B, et al. Response of prostate cancer to anti-Her-2/neu antibody in androgen-dependent and -independent human xenograft models. Cancer Res 1999;59:4761–4764.

54. Morris MJ, Reuter VE, Kelly WK, et al. HER-2 profiling and targeting in prostate carcinoma. Cancer 2002;94:980–986.

55. Lee MS, Igawa T, Yuan TC, et al. ErbB-2 signaling is involved in regulating PSA secretion in androgen-independent human prostate cancer LNCaP C-81 cells. Oncogene 2003;22:781–796.

56. Sirotnak FM, She Y, Lee F, et al. Studies with CWR 22 xenografts in nude mice suggest that ZD 1839 may have a role in the treatment of both androgen-dependent and androgen-independent human prostate cancer. Clin Cancer Res 2002;8:3870–3876.

57. Vincenti C, Festuccia C, Gravina GL, et al. Prostate cancer cell proliferation is strongly reduced by the epidermal growth factor receptor tyrosine kinase inhibitor ZD 1839 in vitro on human cell lines and primary cultures. J Cancer Res Clin Oncol 2003;129:165–174.

58. Wakeling AE, Guy SP, Woodburn JR, et al. ZD1830 (Iressa): an orally active inhibitor of epidermal growth factor signaling with potential for cancer therapy. Cancer Res 2002;62:5749–5754.

59. Ciardiello F, Caputo R, Bianco R, et al. Antitumor effect and potentiation of cytotoxic drugs activity in human cancer cells by ZD-1839 (Iressa), an epidermal growth factor receptor-selective tyrosine kinase inhibitor. Clin Cancer Res 2000;6:2053–2063.

60. Sirotnak FM, Zakowski MF, Miller VA, et al. Efficacy of cytotoxic agents against human tumor xenografts is markedly enhanced by coadministration of ZD 1839 (Iressa), an inhibitor of EGFR tyrosine kinase. Clin Cancer Res 2000;6:4885–4892.

61. Baselga J, Rischin D, Ranson M, et al. Phase I safety, pharmacokinetic, and pharmacodynamic trial of ZD1839, a selective oral epidermal growth factor receptor tyrosine kinase inhibitor, in patients with five selected solid tumor types. J Clin Oncol 2002;20:4292–4302.

62. Herbst RS, Madox AM, Rothenberg ML, et al. Selective oral epidermal growth factor receptor tyrosine kinase inhibitor ZD 1839 is generally well-tolerated and has activity in non-small-cell lung cancer and other solid tumors: results of a phase I trial. J Clin Oncol 2002;20:3815–3825.

63. Negoro S, Nakagawa K, Fukuoka M, et al. Final results of a phase I intermittent dose-escalation trial of ZD 1839 (Iressa) in Japanese patients with various solid tumors. Proc Am Soc Clin Oncol 2001;20:324a.

64. Ranson M, Hammond LA, Ferry D, et al. ZD 1839, a selective oral epidermal growth factor receptor-tyrosine kinase inhibitor, is well tolerated and active in patients with solid, malignant tumors: results of a phase I trial. J Clin Oncol 2002;20:2240–2250.

65. Barton J, Blackledge G, Wakeling A. Growth factors and their receptors: new targets for prostate cancer therapy. Urology 2001;58:114–122.

66. Trump D, Wilding G, Small E, et al. A pilot trials of ZD 1839 (Iressa), an orally active, selective epidermal growth factor receptor tyrosine kinase inhibitor (EGFR-TKI), in combination with docetaxel and estramustine in patients with hormone-refractory prostate cancer (HRPC). J Urol 2003;169:244.

67. Moore M, Winquist E, Pollak M, et al. A randomized phase II study of two doses of ZD 1839 in patients with hormone refractory prostate cancer (HRPC): a NCI Canada Clinical Trials Group Study. Ann Oncol 2002;13:90–97.

68. Burroughs KD, Oh J, Barrett JC, et al. Phosphatidyinositol 3-kinase and mek 1/2 are necessary for insulin-like growth factor-1-induced vascular endothelial growth factor synthesis in prostate epithelial cells: a role for hypoxia-inducible factor-1? Mol Cancer Res 2003;1:312–22.

69. Cross TG, Scheel-Toellner D, Henriquez NV, et al. Serine/threonine protein kinases and apoptosis. Exp Cell Res 2001;256:34–41.

70. Djavan B, Bursa B, Seitz C, et al. Insulin-like growth factor-1 (IGF-1), IGF-1 density, and IGF-1/PSA ratio for prostate cancer detection. Urology 1999;54:603–606.

71. Shi R, Berkel HJ, Yu H. Insulin-like growth factor-1 and prostate cancer: a meta-analysis, Br J Cancer 2001;85:991–996.

72. Chan JM, Stampfer MJ, Ma J, et al. Insulin-like growth factor-1 (IGF-1) and IGF binding protein-3 as predictors of advanced-stage prostate cancer. J Natl Cancer Inst 2002;94:1099–1106.

73. Shariat SF, Lamb DJ, Kattan MW, et al. Association of preoperative plasma levels of insulin-like growth factor I and insulin-like growth factor binding proteins-2 and -3 with prostate cancer invasion, progression, and metastasis. J Clin Oncol 2002;20:833–841.

74. Datta SR, Dudek H, Tao X. Akt phosphorylation of BAD couples survival signals to the cell intrinsic death machinery. Cell 1997;91:234–241.

75. Fiebig AA, Persad S. The role of IGF-1 signaling via PI-3 kinase pathway in prostate cancer invasion. Proc Am Assoc Cancer Res 2003;44:3265.

76. Hailey J, Maxwell E, Koukouras K, et al. Neutralizing anti-insulin-like growth factor receptor 1 antibodies inhibit receptor function and induce receptor degradation in tumor cells. Mol Cancer Ther 2002;1:1349–1353.

77. Moyer JD, Barbacci EG, Iwata KK, et al. Induction of apoptosis and cell cycle arrest by CP-358,774, an inhibitor of epidermal growth factor receptor tyrosine kinase. Cancer Res 1997;57:4838–4848.

78. van der Poel HG. Smart drugs in prostate cancer. Eur Urol 2004;45:1–17.

79. Wennstrom S, Hawkins P, Cooke F, et al. Activation of phosphoinositide-3-kinase is required for PDGF-stimulated membrane ruffling. Curr Biol 1994;5:385–393.

80. Wennstrom S, Siegbahn A, Yokote K, et al. Membrane ruffling and chemotaxis transduced by the PDGF beta-receptor require the binding site for phosphoinositol 3-kinase. Oncogene 1994;9:651–660.

81. Heldin CH, Westermark B. Mechanism of action and in vivo role of platelet-derived growth factor. Physiol Rev 1999;79:12283–12316.

82. Fudge K, Bostwick DG, Stearns ME. Platelet-derived growth factor A and B chains and the alpha and beta-receptors in prostatic intraepithelial neoplasia. Prostate 1996;29:282–286.

83. Fudge K, Wang CY, Stearns ME. Immunohistochemistry analysis of platelet-derived growth factor A and B chains and platelet-derived growth factor alpha and beta-receptor expression in benign prostatic hyperplasias and Gleason-graded human prostate adenocarcinomas. Mod Pathol 1994;7:549–554.

84. Chott A, Zijie S, Morganstern D, et al. Tyrosine kinases expressed in vivo by human prostate cancer bone marrow metastases and loss of the type I insulin-like growth factor receptor. Am J Pathol 1999;155:1271–1279.

85. Druker BJ, Talpaz M, Resta DJ, et al. Efficacy and safety of a specific inhibitor of the BCR-ABL tyrosine kinase in chronic myeloid leukemia. N Engl J Med 2001;344:1031–1037.

86. Uehara H, Kim SJ, Karashima T, et al. Effects of blocking platelet-derived growth factor-receptor signaling in a mouse model of experimental prostate cancer bone metastases. J Natl Cancer Inst 2003;95:458–470.

87. Pietras K, Ostman A, Sjoquist M, et al. Inhibition of platelet-derived growth factor receptors reduces interstitial hypertension and increases transcapillary transport in tumors. Cancer Res 2001;61:2929–2934.

88. George D. Platelet-derived growth factor receptors: a therapeutic target in solid tumors. Semin Oncol 2001;28:27–33.

89. Ko YJ, Small EJ, Kabbinavar T, et al. A multi-institutional phase II study of SU101, a platelet-derived growth factor receptor inhibitor, for patients with hormone-refractory prostate cancer. Clin Cancer Res 2001;7:800–805.

90. Whang YE, Wu X, Suzuki H, et al. Inactivation of the tumor suppressor PTEN/MMAC1 in advanced human prostate cancer through loss of expression. Proc Natl Acad Sci USA 1998;95:5246–5250.

91. Li J, Yen C, Liaw D, et al. PTEN, a putative protein tyrosine phosphatase gene mutation in human brain, breast, and prostate cancer. Science 1997;275:1943–1947.

92. McMenamin ME, Soung P, Perera S, et al. Loss of PTEN expression in paraffin-embedded primary prostate cancer correlates with high Gleason score and advanced stage. Cancer Res 1999;59:4291–4296.

93. Feilotter HE, Nagai MA, Boag AH, et al. Analysis of PTEN and the 10q23 region in primary prostate carcinomas. Oncogene 1998;16:1743–1748.

94. Paweletz CP, Charboneau L, Bischel VE, et al. Reverse phase protein microarrays which capture disease progression show activation of pro-survival pathways at the cancer invasion front. Oncogene 2001;20:1981–1989.

95. van der Poel H, Hanrahan C, Zhong H, et al. Rapamycin induces Smad activity in prostate cancer cell lines. Urol Res 2003;30:380–386.

96. Grunwald V, DeGraffenried L, Rissel D, et al. Inhibitors of mTOR reverse doxorubicin resistance conferred by PTEN status in prostate cancer cells. Cancer Res 2002;62:6141–6145.

97. Mousses S, Wagner U, Chen Y, et al. Failure of hormone therapy in prostate cancer involves systematic restoration of androgen responsive genes and activation of rapamycin sensitive signaling. Oncogene 2001;20:6718–6723.

98. Dancey JE. Clinical development of mammalian target of rapamycin inhibitors. Hematol Oncol Clin North Am 2002;16:1101–1114.

99. Levin ER. Endothelins. N Eng J Med 1995;333:356–363.

100. Masaki T. The endothelin family: an overview. J Cardiovasc Pharmacol 2000;35:S3-S5.

101. Daub H, Weiss FU, Wallasch C, et al. Role of transactivation of the EGF receptor in signaling by G-protein-coupled receptors. Nature 1996;379:557–560.

102. Battistini B, Chailler P, D'Orleans-Juste P, et al. Growth regulatory properties of endothelins. Peptides 1993;14:385–399.

103. Salani D, Taraboletti G, Rosano L, et al. Endothelin-1 induces an angiogenic phenotype in cultured endothelial cells and stimulates neovascularisation in vivo. Am J Pathol 2000;157:1703–1711.

104. Spinella F, Rosano L, Di Castro V, et al. Endothelin-1 induces vascular endothelial growth factor by increasing hypoxia-inducible factor 1α in ovarian carcinoma cells. J Biol Chem 2002;277:27850–27855.

105. Salani D, Di Castro V, Nicotra MR, et al. Role of endothelin-1 in neovascularization of ovarian carcinoma. Am J Pathol 2000;157:1537–1547.

106. Shioide M, Noda M. Endothelin modulates osteopointin and osteocalcin messenger ribonucleic acid expression in rat osteoblastic osteosarcoma cells. J Cell Biochem 1993;53:176–180.

107. Nelson JB, Hedican SP, George DJ, et al. Identification of endothelin-1 in the pathophysiology of metastatic adenocarcinoma of the prostate. Nat Med 1995;1:944–949.

108. Nelson JB, Chan-Tack K, Hedican SP, et al. Endothelin-1 production and decreased endothelin B receptor expression in advanced prostate cancer. Cancer Res 1996;56:663–668.

109. Carducci MA, Nelson JB, Bowling MK, et al. Atrasentan, an endothelin-receptor antagonist for refractory adenocarcinomas: safety and pharmacokinetics. J Clin Oncol 2002;20:2171–2281.

110. Carducci MA, Padley RJ, Breul J, et al. Effect of endothelin-A receptor blockade with atrasentan on tumor progression in men with hormone-refractory prostate cancer: a randomized, phase II, placebo-controlled trial. J Clin Oncol 2003;21:679–689.

111. Folkman J, Klagbrun M. Angiogenic factors. Science 1987;235:442–447.

112. Ferrer FA, Miller LJ, Adrwis I, et al. Angiogenesis and prostate cancer: in vivo and in vitro expression of angiogenesis factors by prostate cancer cells. Urology 1998;51:161–167.

113. Joseph IB, Isaacs JT. Potentiation of the angiogenic ability of linomide by androgen ablation involves down-regulation of vascular endothelial growth factor in human androgen-responsive prostatic cancers. Cancer Res 1997;57:1054–1057.

114. Harper ME, Glynne-Jones E, Goddard L, et al. Vascular endothelial growth factor (VEGF) expression in prostatic tumors and its relationship to neuroendocrine cells. Br J Cancer 1996;74:910–916.

115. Theodorescu D, Broder SR, Boyd JC, et al. Cathepsin D and chromogranin A as predictors of long-term disease specific survival after radical prostatectomy for localized carcinoma of the prostate. Cancer 1997;80:2109–2119.

116. Ferrer FA, Miller LJ, Lindquist R, et al. Expression of vascular endothelial growth factor receptors in human prostate cancer. Urology 1999;54:567–572.

117. Millauer B, Wizigmann-Voss S, Schnurch H, et al. High affinity VEGF binding and development expression suggest Flk-1 as a major regulator of vasculogenesis and angiogenesis. Cell 1993;72:835–846.

118. Fox WD, Higgins B, Maise KM, et al. Antibody to vascular endothelial growth factor slows growth of an androgen-independent xenograft model of prostate cancer. Clin Cancer Res 2002;8:3226-3321.

119. Wedge SR, Ogilvie DJ, Dukes M, et al. ZD 6474 inhibits vascular endothelial growth factor signaling, angiogenesis, and tumor growth following oral administration. Cancer Res 2002;62:4645–4655.

120. Wedge SR, Ogilvie DJ, Dukes M, et al. ZD 4190: an orally active inhibitor of vascular endothelial growth factor signaling with broad-spectrum antitumor efficacy. Cancer Res 2000;60:970–975.

121. Macpherson GR, Franks M, Tomoaia-Cotisel A, et al. Current status of thalidomide and its role in the treatment of metastatic prostate cancer. Crit Rev Oncol Hematol 2003;46:49–57.

122. Figg WD, Dahut W, Duray P, et al. A randomized phase II trial of thalidomide, an angiogenesis inhibitor, in patients with androgen-independent prostate cancer. Clin Cancer Res 2001;7:1888–1893.

123. Kohli M, Kaushal V, Spencer HJ, et al. Prospective study of circulating angiogenic markers in prostate specific antigen (PSA)- stable and PSA-progressive hormone-sensitive advanced prostate cancer. Urology 2003;61:765–769.

124. Dorkin TJ, Robinson MC, Marsh C, et al. aFGF immunoreactivity in prostate cancer and its co-localisation with bFGF and FGF8. J Pathol 1999;189:564–569.

125. Huss WJ, Barrios RJ, Foster BA, et al. Differential expression of specific FGF ligand and its receptor isoforms during angiogenesis associated with prostate cancer progression. Prostate 2003;54:8–16.

126. Naimi B, Latil A, Fournier G, et al. Down-regulation of (IIIb) and (IIIc) isoforms of fibroblast growth factor receptor 2 (FGFR2) is associated with malignant progression in human prostate. Prostate 2002;52:245–252.

127. Bond SJ, Klein SA, Anderson GL, et al. Interaction of angiogenesis inhibitor TNP-470 with basic fibroblast growth factor receptors. J Surg Res 2002;92:18–22.

128. Ingeber D, Fujita T, Kishimoto S, et al. Synthetic analogues of fumagillin that inhibits angiogenesis and suppress tumor growth. Nature 1990;348:555–557.

129. Yamaoka M, Yamamoto T, Ikeyama S, et al. Angiogenesis inhibitor TNP-470 (AGM-1470) potently inhibits the tumor growth of hormone-independent human breast and prostate carcinoma cell lines. Cancer Res 1993;53:5233–5236.

130. Logothetis CJ, Wu KK, Finn LD, et al. Phase I trial of the angiogenesis inhibitor TNP-470 for progressive androgen-independent prostate cancer. Clin Cancer Res 2001;7:1198–1203.

131. Han CK, Ahn SK, Choi NS, et al. Design and synthesis of highly potent fumagillin analogues from homology modeling for a human MetAP-2. Biog Med Chem Lett 2000;10:39–43.

132. O'Reilly MS, Holmgren L, Chen C, et al. Angiostatin induces and sustains dormancy of human primary tumors in mice. Nature Med 1996;2:689–692.

133. O'Reilly MS, Boehm T, Shing Y, et al. Endostatin: an endogenous inhibitor of angiogenesis and tumor growth. Cell 1997;88:277–285.

134. Yokoyama Y, Green JE, Sukhatme VP, et al. Effect of endostatin on spontaneous tumorigenesis of mammary adenocarcinoma in a transgenic mouse model. Cancer Res 2000;60:4362–4365.

135. O'Reilly MS. Angiostatin: an endogenous inhibitor of angiogenesis and tumor growth. Exs 1997;79:273–294.

136. Gately S, Twardowski P, Stack MS, et al. Human prostate carcinoma cells express enzymatic activity that converts human plasminogen to the angiogenesis inhibitor, angiostatin. Cancer Res 1996;56:4887–4890.

137. Gately S, Twardowski P, Stack MS, et al. The mechanism of cancer-mediated conversion of plasminogen to the angiogenesis inhibitor angiostatin. Proc Natl Acad Sci USA 1997;94:10868–10672.

138. Luo J, Lubaroff DM, Hendrix MJ. Suppression of prostate cancer invasive potential and matrix metalloproteinase activity by E-cadherin transfection. Cancer Res 1999;59:3552–3556.

139. Seiter S, Arch R, Reber S, et al. Prevention of tumor metastasis formation by ant-variant CD44. J Exp Med 1993;177:443–455.

140. Wood M, Fudge K, Mohler JL, et al. In situ hybridization studies of metalloproteniases 2 and 9 and TIMP-1 and TIMP-2 expression in human prostate cancer. Ann N York Acad Sci 1999;15:246–258.

141. Lokeshwar BL. MMP inhibition in prostate cancer. Ann NY Acad Sci 1999;878:271–289.

142. Stearns ME, Fudge K, Garcia F, et al. IL-10 inhibition of human prostate PC-3 ML cell metastases in SCID mice: IL-10 stimulation of TIMP-1 and inhibition of MMP-2/MMP-9 expression. Invasion Metast 1997;17:62–74.

143. Nemunaitis J, Poole C, Primrose J, et al. Combined analysis of studies of the effects of the matrix metalloproteinase inhibitor marimastat on serum tumor markers in advanced cancer: selection of a biologically active and tolerable dose for longer-term studies. Clin Cancer Res 1998;4:1101–1109.

144. Steward WP. Marimastat (BB2516): Current status of development. Cancer Chemother Pharmacol 1999;43:S56–S60.

145. Helenius MA, Saramaki OR, Linja MJ, et al. Amplification of urokinase gene in prostate cancer. Cancer Res 2001;61:5340–5344.

146. Rabbani SA, Harakidas P, Davidson DJ, et al. Prevention of prostate cancer metastasis in vivo by a novel synthetic inhibitor of urokinase-type plasminogen activator (uPA). Int J Cancer 1995;63:840–845.

Cell adhesion molecules in prostate cancer

30

Jack A Schalken

INTRODUCTION

The role of cell adhesion molecules in the development of prostate cancer has gained true interest since 1992.[1] The combination of molecular genetic studies, differential gene expression analyses, and the, at that time, recent insight that E-cadherin can act as an invasion suppressor protein led the author of this chapter, together with Dr William B Isaacs (Johns Hopkins Hospital, Baltimore) to the hypothesis that in fact E-cadherin could contribute to prostate cancer progression as an invasion/metastasis suppressor gene. Since then, more than 100 peer reviewed papers have been published on the role of cadherins in prostate cancer, and the cadherin family is, therefore, the most intensely studied group of adhesion molecules in prostate cancer.

The cadherins mediate the physical interaction between two neighboring cells in a calcium dependent and predominantly homotypic/homophilic way, by establishing a link with the actin cytoskeleton. The integrins are linked to the microfilament network as well and, with cancer progression, the integrin expression pattern and their counter-receptors change (Figure 30.1). The cell adhesion molecules are grouped according to conserved structural motifs, and their importance as progression markers became apparent in the second half of the 1980s. The adhesion molecules mediate very specific cell–cell and cell–matrix interactions, and in fact "… what a cell touches, determines what a cell does…" became a common quote in cancer biology, for example, polarization and differentiation are all dependent on cell–cell and cell–matrix interactions. The finding that β-catenin, one of the anchor/catenating molecules linking E-cadherin with the cytoskeleton is also directly involved in a nuclear localized transcription initiation complex with T-cell factors[2] established the first firm link between adhesion and gene regulation. Current textbooks can not, therefore, deal with adhesion molecules as an isolated entity, but these proteins should be considered in the integral context of the "outside-in and inside-out" signaling machinery. I will review the insight on cell adhesion molecules in prostate cancer, per subfamily and give a perspective on the developing field in relation to the wnt/wingless pathway (wnt/Wg) and epithelial–mesenchymal transitions (EMTs).

CELL ADHESION MOLECULES AS SERUM MARKERS

The first cell adhesion molecule that was studied as a marker in prostate cancer was carcinoembryonic antigen (CEA),[3] although it should be noted that at that time CEA was not described as a cell adhesion molecule. The use of CEA, in the context of all available tumor makers was reported on quite extensively, and CEA is not considered as a useful marker for prostate cancer, despite the more recent insight that other members from the CEA family might be more promising.[4] More recently, the potential of soluble intercellular adhesion molecule 1 (ICAM1)/CD56 and CD44 was studied in cell lines[5] that appeared to secrete detectable levels of these. The level of circulating adhesion molecules was tested in a cohort of patients in which ICAM1, vascular cell adhesion molecule (VCAM) and E-selectin were measured; the authors concluded that there is limited utility of these circulating adhesion molecules as markers.[6]

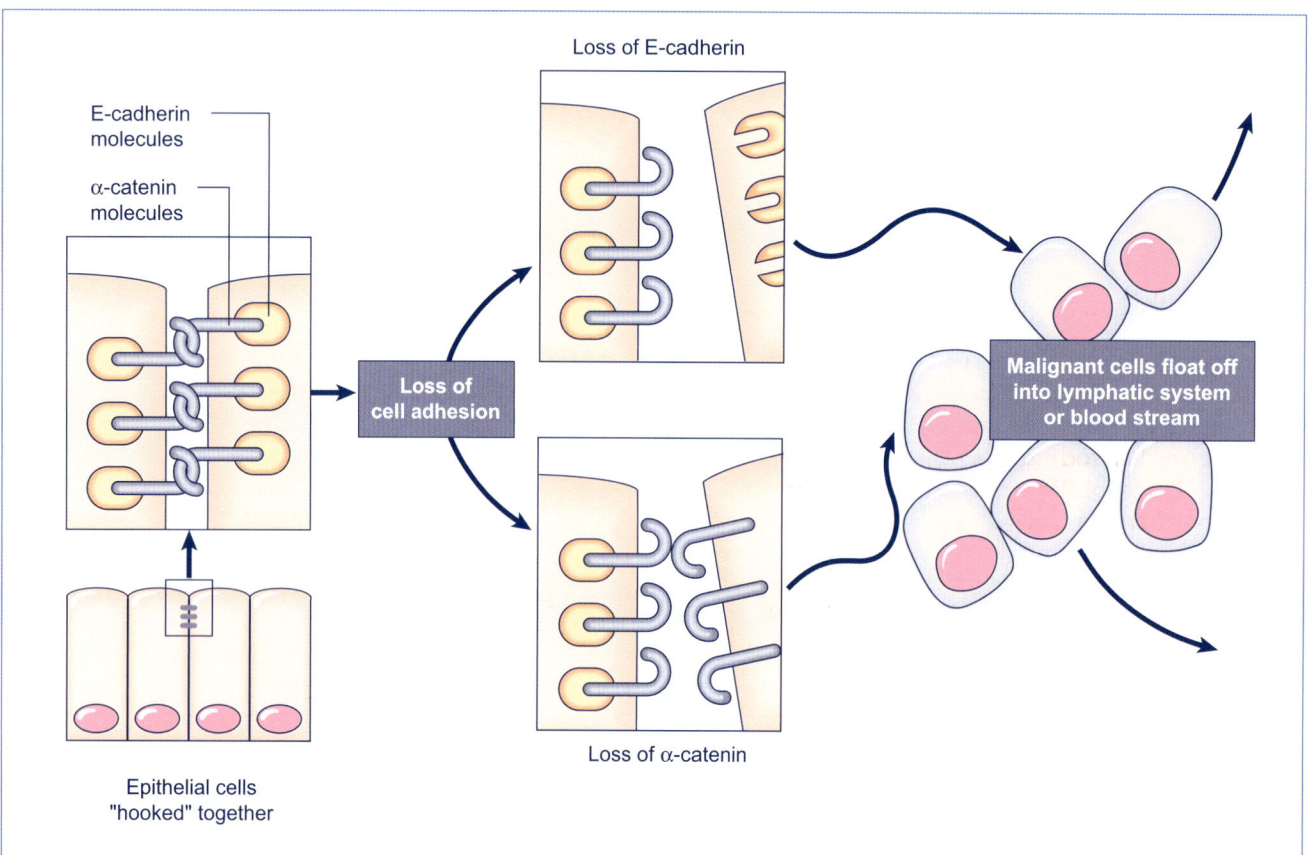

Fig. 30.1

Diagram to illustrate the role of E-cadherin and α-catenin in linking cells together. Loss of either E-Cadherin or α-catenin may allow malignant cells to float off into the circulation and metastasize.

CADHERINS

At the time that the cadherins gained research interest among cancer biologists, including myself, they were thought to represent a small set of structurally related proteins. The epithelial cadherin (E-cadherin) was a challenging member for tumor biology studies, since the teams of Birchmeier and Mareel had convincingly shown that there was a biologic functional relation between loss of E-cadherin and acquisition of invasive potential.[7] The role of cadherins in development and cancer progression as reviewed by Takeichi posed challenging questions.[8] The hypothetical relationship between loss of E-cadherin expression and cancer progression, assessed by immunohistochemistry was established by Umbas et al.[9,10] A number of studies confirmed the initial findings.[11–13] The translation of these findings into a useful clinical setting (i.e., the prognosis of extracapsular prostatic disease using biopsy specimens) is cumbersome due to the multifocality and heterogeneity so characteristic to prostate cancer.[14,15] The more recent studies on the expression of E-cadherin in metastatic lesions led to the hypothesis that E-cadherin is transiently down regulated and re-expressed at the secondary site.[13,16,17] This is, in fact, in agreement with an EMT during cancer progression.

The first implicit evidence of an EMT was provided by Tomita et al,[18] who observed and described a "cadherin switch" in prostate cancer progression—that is, the loss of E-cadherin was associated with de-novo expression of N- and OB-cadherin, two mesenchymal cadherin subtypes.

The mechanisms leading to defective E-cadherin function seem to be quite diverse; somatic mutations in the E-cadherin gene have been reported, whereas in a subset of prostate cancers β-catenin is mutated.[19,20] The E-cadherin gene in prostate cancer seems to be predominantly transcriptionally silenced. This can be by methylation of the promotor,[21–23] even though evidence for this mechanism is only obtained for a subset of aggressive cancers. Direct modulation of E-cadherin through a specific set of transcription factors appears to be more common. The transcription factors snail and slug that can interact with the essential E-boxes in the promoter of E-cadherin[24,25] deserve particular interest, since these are known to be essential for EMTs.[26] Recently, a number of reports appeared on the role of snail and slug, as well as their expression in human carcinomas, indicating that this may be a pivotal step in the EMT. Snail and slug expression is reported to increase with cancer progression and can serve as a switch to downregulate E-cadherin and upregulate matrix metalloproteinases

(MMPs) and induce angiogenesis.[26–31] Moreover, snail can be a direct target of wnt signaling.[32–35] These findings define a potential mechanism whereby wnt signaling stabilizes snail and β-catenin proteins in a tandem fashion so as to cooperate in transcriptional programs that control an EMT.

INTEGRINS

Integrins are the major metazoan receptors for extracellular matrix proteins and, in vertebrates, also play important roles in certain cell–cell adhesions. Integrins are heterodimeric cell surface receptors that mediate heterophilic cell–cell interactions and interactions between cells and the extracellular matrix. As such, they are involved in morphogenic processes during development, as well as in the maintenance of normal tissue architecture in fully developed organs. The interaction with the extracellular matrix via transmembrane connections to the cytoskeleton results in the activation of many intracellular signaling pathways. Since the recognition of the integrin receptor family in the late 1980s,[36] they have become the best-understood cell adhesion receptors. Eight β-subunits can assort with 18 α-subunits to form 24 distinct integrins. These can be considered in several subfamilies based on evolutionary relationships. Integrins and their ligands play key roles in development and immune responses (for a review see Hynes et al[37]).

Despite the tremendous advances in this field including an array of integrin knockout mice (~27), relatively little is known on the role of integrins in prostate development and cancer. One of the most remarkable changes in integrin expression in prostate cancer is the loss of α4β6, the receptor for LN5, marking the hemidesmosomal contact of epithelial cells with the basement membrane.[38] Considering that prostate cancer is characterized by the absence of true basal cells, the loss of α4β6 can be interpreted as a loss of this cell population, similarly to P-cadherin[39] and keratin 14. The progressive loss of α4β6 from non-malignant prostate epithelium, to PIN,[40] to cancer supports this interpretation. Human prostate cancer is devoid of expression of α6, β2, and β3 integrins.[41] The integrin matrix receptors that are most consistently reported to be expressed in prostate cancer are the "RGD" receptors (having the arginine-glycine-aspartate recognition sequence) α5β1 and α3β1[42] associated with fibronectin-dependent migration. Whereas rather little is known on changes in integrin expression in prostate cancer, the lack of attachment with the basement membrane (loss of α4β6) and increased propensity to migrate over fibronectin-based matrices seem to emerge as a common pathway. Initial evidence for the activation of integrin based signaling through focal adhesion kinase (FAK) is in agreement with such a model.[43]

IMMUNOGLOBULIN SUPERFAMILY

The common characteristic of the immunoglobulin superfamily proteins is the subdomains resembling immunoglobulin repeats. The neural cell adhesion molecule (NCAM) is found to be upregulated in prostate cancer and may be associated with neural invasion.[44] The cell adhesion molecule C-CAM was identified as an androgen-regulated suppressor of prostate growth.[45,46] The downregulation of C-CAM has been confirmed in a number of studies most recently by Busch et al,[47] and is even pursued as therapeutic target.[45,48,49]

OTHER ADHESION MOLECULES

Some adhesion molecules can not, as yet, be classified into one of the large families and will discussed separately.

CD44

As mentioned in the introduction, cell adhesion molecules were once believed to function primarily in tethering cells to extracellular ligands. Cadherins and integrins now have well-recognized functions in cell signaling. The CD44 transmembrane glycoprotein family adds new aspects to these roles by participating in signal-transduction processes—not only by establishing specific transmembrane complexes, but also by organizing signaling cascades through association with the actin cytoskeleton.[50] CD44 and its associated partner proteins monitor changes in the extracellular matrix that influence cell growth, survival, and differentiation. The designation CD44 describes a group of type I transmembrane proteins which share *N*-terminal and *C*-terminal sequences. These molecules differ in the central extracellular domain, which consists of sequences encoded by ten variant exons that may be included in various combinations or be completely absent; they also differ by cell-type specific addition of glycosaminoglycan and carbohydrate moieties.[51] CD44 was thought to contribute to the metastatic phenotype by acquiring certain properties through alternative splicing.[52] Certain splice variants (CD44v) can promote the metastatic behavior of cancer cells. In human colon and breast cancer, the presence of epitopes encoded by exon v6 on primary resected tumor material indicates poor prognosis. Metastasis-promoting splice variants differ from those that seem not to have a role in the induction of metastasis by the formation of homomultimeric complexes in the plasma membrane of cells. This may increase their affinity to ligands such as hyaluronate. The affinity can be further regulated over a range from low to very high by cell-specific modification. The fact that CD44v epitopes are found on normal epithelial cells such as skin, cervical epithelium, and bladder enforces cautious evaluation of the significance of CD44v expression in human cancer. Nevertheless, certain epitopes can serve as tools in early diagnosis of certain cancers and will facilitate the development of specific targeted therapy.

It is now recognized that cancer cells can recruit characteristics of CD44 through variable mechanisms.[53,54] CD44 is intensely studied in prostate cancer. One of the first indications that CD44 can have pleiotropic effects in cancer progression came from studies on human prostate cancer specimens. Initial studies using prostate cancer cell lines suggested a relation between increased CD44 expression and prostate cancer progression.[55,56] However, the first report analyzing human prostate cancer tissue showed a paradoxical downregulation of CD44 in cancer and expression of variant CD44 isoforms (v3 and v6) in prostate basal cells.[57] Also in prostate cancer metastases, CD44 expression was reduced or absent.[58] Gao et al even suggested that CD44 could act as a tumor suppressor gene in prostate cancer.[59,60] The reduced expression of CD44 appeared to be associated with a poor prognosis.[61,62] The only relationship between a CD44 isoform and cancer progression is the report of Aaltoma et al,[63] who conclude that CD44v3 expression is associated with prostate cancer progression. Surprisingly, in a more recent study, they do not support this conclusion.[64] Thus, the literature to date is quite consistent that in prostate cancer and its metastasis CD44 expression is lost.

EPITHELIAL AND ACTIVATED LEUKOCYTE CELL ADHESION MOLECULES

Epithelial cell adhesion molecule (EpCAM) is a 40 kDa antigen recognized by antibody 19A1, and is overexpressed in a number of carcinomas including prostate cancer.[65] The new generation antibody against EpCAM, ING1, is now being pursued for therapeutic purposes.[66] In the future the combination with taxol or navelbine might be considered since this upregulates EpCAM expression.[67]

Activated leukocyte cell adhesion molecule (ALCAM/CD166) is involved with homophilic and heterophilic cell adhesion through as yet unknown mechanisms. It can be recruited to the cell membrane coordinately with E-cadherin by a catenin,[68] and it is upregulated in low-grade prostate cancer,[69] but expression is lost in high-grade cancer. Like cadherins and integrins, ALCAM function is dependent on an intact actin filament network.[70] Although many questions remain to be resolved, a common picture in which coordinated interactions in the subcortical cytoskeleton are triggered emerges.[71]

SUMMARY AND PERSPECTIVES

Since the late 1980s, cell adhesion molecules have been studied extensively in prostate carcinogenesis. A summary of changes in expression of adhesion molecules is presented in Table 30.1. Whereas the clinical implications so far seem to be rather limited, the most intriguing insight obtained is that cell adhesion molecules are integral part of "outside-in and inside-out" signaling. The wnt signal seems to initiate a coordinate switch towards proliferation via the canonical wnt/Wg pathway, activating proliferation associated genes such as c-MYC and p21 via β-catenin/T-cell factors and EMT by regulating snail, a transcription factor controlling repression of E-cadherin and MMPs. Consequently, this pathway is in the limelight as target for therapy. Considering that both APC and β-catenin mutations are frequently found in human cancers, leading to constitutive activation of β-catenin/T-cell factor-induced transcription, this suggests that to affect this pathway the target need to be chosen downstream of APC/β-catenin/GSK3β. Significant advances have already been made. The exact molecular interaction between wnt signaling, GSK3β, and snail/slug is not yet know, but again intervention with the EMT switch provides a challenge for drug development.

Table 30.1 Changes in expression of adhesion molecules in prostate cancer

Adhesion molecule	Upregulated	Downregulated	Mutated	SNP
Cadherins	Cadherin 11-OB	E-cadherin/α-catenin	β-catenin	−160C/A
	Cadherin 2-N			E-cadherin promoter
	Protocadherin[72]			
Integrins	α5β1	α6β4		
	α5β3	β3, β3, β4		
IgG-like	NCAM	C-CAM		
Miscellaneous	EpCAM	CD44		

C-CAM, belongs to a class of androgen-repressed genes associated with enriched stem/amplifying cell population after prolonged castration; EpCAM, epithelial cell adhesion molecule; NCAM, neural cell adhesion molecule; SNP, single nucleotide polymorphism.

REFERENCES

1. Bussemakers MJ, van Moorselaar RJ, Giroldi LA, et al. Decreased expression of E-cadherin in the progression of rat prostatic cancer. Cancer Res 1992;52:2916–2922.

2. Behrens J, von Kries JP, Kuhl M, et al. Functional interaction of beta-catenin with the transcription factor LEF-1. Nature 1996;382:638–642.

3. Guinan P, Dubin A, Bush I, et al. The CEA test in urologic cancer: an evaluation and a review. Oncology 1975;32:158–168.

4. Scorilas A, Chiang PM, Katsaros D, et al. Molecular characterization of a new gene, CEAL1, encoding for a carcinoembryonic antigen-like protein with a highly conserved domain of eukaryotic translation initiation factors. Gene 2003;310:79–89.

5. Rokhlin OW, Cohen MB. Soluble forms of CD44 and CD54 (ICAM-1) cellular adhesion molecules are released by human prostatic cancer cell lines. Cancer Lett 1996;107:29–35.

6. Perabo F, Sharma S, Gierer R, et al. Circulating intercellular adhesion molecule-1 (ICAM-1), vascular cell adhesion molecule-1 (VCAM-1) and E-selectin in urological malignancies. Indian J Cancer 2001;38:1–7.

7. Behrens J, Mareel MM, Van Roy FM, et al. Dissecting tumor cell invasion: epithelial cells acquire invasive properties after the loss of uvomorulin-mediated cell-cell adhesion. J Cell Biol 1989;108:2435–2447.

8. Takeichi M. Cadherin cell adhesion receptors as a morphogenetic regulator. Science 1991;251:1451–1455.

9. Umbas R, Isaacs WB, Bringuier PP, et al. Decreased E-cadherin expression is associated with poor prognosis in patients with prostate cancer. Cancer Res 1994;54:3929–3933.

10. Umbas R, Schalken JA, Aalders TW, et al. Expression of the cellular adhesion molecule E-cadherin is reduced or absent in high-grade prostate cancer. Cancer Res 1992;52:5104–5109.

11. Kuniyasu H, Troncoso P, Johnston D, et al. Relative expression of type IV collagenase, E-cadherin, and vascular endothelial growth factor/vascular permeability factor in prostatectomy specimens distinguishes organ-confined from pathologically advanced prostate cancers. Clin Cancer Res 2000;6:2295–2308.

12. Kallakury BV, Sheehan CE, Winn-Deen E, et al. Decreased expression of catenins (alpha and beta), p120 CTN, and E-cadherin cell adhesion proteins and E-cadherin gene promoter methylation in prostatic adenocarcinomas. Cancer 2001;92:2786–2795.

13. Rubin MA, Mucci NR, Figurski J, et al. E-cadherin expression in prostate cancer: a broad survey using high-density tissue microarray technology. Hum Pathol 2001;32:690–697.

14. Ruijter E, van de KC, Aalders T, et al. Heterogeneous expression of E-cadherin and p53 in prostate cancer: clinical implications. BIOMED-II Markers for Prostate Cancer Study Group. Mod Pathol 1998;11:276–281.

15. Ruijter ET, Werahera PN, van de Kaa CA, et al. Detection of abnormal E-cadherin expression by simulated prostate biopsy. J Urol 1998;160:1368–1371.

16. Bryden AA, Freemont AJ, Clarke NW, et al. Paradoxical expression of E-cadherin in prostatic bone metastases. BJU Int 1999;84:1032–1034.

17. Bryden AA, Hoyland JA, Freemont AJ, et al. E-cadherin and beta-catenin are down-regulated in prostatic bone metastases. BJU Int 2002;89:400–403.

18. Tomita K, van Bokhoven A, van Leenders GJ, et al. Cadherin switching in human prostate cancer progression. Cancer Res 2000;60:3650–3654.

19. Chesire DR, Isaacs WB. Beta-catenin signaling in prostate cancer: an early perspective. Endocr Relat Cancer 2003;10:537–560.

20. Chesire DR, Ewing CM, Sauvageot J, et al. Detection and analysis of beta-catenin mutations in prostate cancer. Prostate 2000;45:323–334.

21. Chung WB, Hong SH, Kim JA, et al. Hypermethylation of tumor-related genes in genitourinary cancer cell lines. J Korean Med Sci 2001;16:756–761.

22. Li LC, Zhao H, Nakajima K, et al. Methylation of the E-cadherin gene promoter correlates with progression of prostate cancer. J Urol 2001;166:705–709.

23. Woodson K, Hayes R, Wideroff L, et al. Hypermethylation of GSTP1, CD44, and E-cadherin genes in prostate cancer among US Blacks and Whites. Prostate 2003;55:199–205.

24. Bussemakers MJ, Giroldi LA, van Bokhoven A, et al. Transcriptional regulation of the human E-cadherin gene in human prostate cancer cell lines: characterization of the human E-cadherin gene promoter. Biochem Biophys Res Commun 1994;203:1284–1290.

25. Giroldi LA, Bringuier PP, de Weijert M, et al. Role of E boxes in the repression of E-cadherin expression. Biochem Biophys Res Commun 1997;241:453–458.

26. Bolos V, Peinado H, Perez-Moreno MA, et al. The transcription factor Slug represses E-cadherin expression and induces epithelial to mesenchymal transitions: a comparison with Snail and E47 repressors. J Cell Sci 2003;116:499–511.

27. Miyoshi A, Kitajima Y, Kido S, et al. Snail accelerates cancer invasion by upregulating MMP expression and is associated with poor prognosis of hepatocellular carcinoma. Br J Cancer 2005;92:252–258.

28. Miyoshi A, Kitajima Y, Sumi K, et al. Snail and SIP1 increase cancer invasion by upregulating MMP family in hepatocellular carcinoma cells. Br J Cancer 2004;90:1265–1273.

29. Ohkubo T, Ozawa M. The transcription factor Snail downregulates the tight junction components independently of E-cadherin downregulation. J Cell Sci 2004;117:1675–1685.

30. Peinado H, Marin F, Cubillo E, et al. Snail and E47 repressors of E-cadherin induce distinct invasive and angiogenic properties in vivo. J Cell Sci 2004;117:2827–2839.

31. Yokoyama K, Kamata N, Fujimoto R, et al. Increased invasion and matrix metalloproteinase-2 expression by Snail-induced mesenchymal transition in squamous cell carcinomas. Int J Oncol 2003;22:891–898.

32. Bachelder RE, Yoon SO, Franci C, et al. Glycogen synthase kinase-3 is an endogenous inhibitor of Snail transcription: implications for the epithelial-mesenchymal transition. J Cell Biol 2005;168:29–33.

33. Schlessinger K, Hall A. GSK-3beta sets Snail's pace. Nat Cell Biol 2004;6:913–915.

34. Yook JI, Li XY, Ota I, et al. Wnt-dependent regulation of the E-cadherin repressor snail. J Biol Chem 2005;280:11740–11748.

35. Zhou BP, Deng J, Xia W, et al. Dual regulation of Snail by GSK-3beta-mediated phosphorylation in control of epithelial-mesenchymal transition. Nat Cell Biol 2004;6:931–940.

36. Hynes RO. Integrins: a family of cell surface receptors. Cell 1987;48:549–554.

37. Hynes RO, Lively JC, McCarty JH, et al. The diverse roles of integrins and their ligands in angiogenesis. Cold Spring Harb Symp Quant Biol 2002;67:143–153.

38. Nagle RB, Knox JD, Wolf C, et al. Adhesion molecules, extracellular matrix, and proteases in prostate carcinoma. J Cell Biochem Suppl 1994;19:232–237.

39. Jarrard DF, Paul R, van Bokhoven A, et al. P-Cadherin is a basal cell-specific epithelial marker that is not expressed in prostate cancer. Clin Cancer Res 1997;3:2121–2128.

40. Davis TL, Cress AE, Dalkin BL, et al. Unique expression pattern of the alpha6beta4 integrin and laminin-5 in human prostate carcinoma. Prostate 2001;46:240–248.

41. Murant SJ, Handley J, Stower M, et al. Co-ordinated changes in expression of cell adhesion molecules in prostate cancer. Eur J Cancer 1997;33:263–271.

42. MacCalman CD, Brodt P, Doublet JD, et al. The loss of E-cadherin mRNA transcripts in rat prostatic tumors is accompanied by increased expression of mRNA transcripts encoding fibronectin and its receptor. Clin Exp Metastasis 1994;12:101–107.

43. Tremblay L, Hauck W, Aprikian AG, et al. Focal adhesion kinase (pp125FAK) expression, activation and association with paxillin and p50CSK in human metastatic prostate carcinoma. Int J Cancer 1996;68:164–171.

44. Li R, Wheeler T, Dai H, et al. Neural cell adhesion molecule is upregulated in nerves with prostate cancer invasion. Hum Pathol 2003;34:457–461.

45. Hsieh JT, Earley K, Pong RC, et al. Structural analysis of the C-CAM1 molecule for its tumor suppression function in human prostate cancer. Prostate 1999;41:31–38.

46. Hsieh JT, Luo W, Song W, et al. Tumor suppressive role of an androgen-regulated epithelial cell adhesion molecule (C-CAM) in prostate carcinoma cell revealed by sense and antisense approaches. Cancer Res 1995;55:190–197.

47. Busch C, Hanssen TA, Wagener C, et al. Down-regulation of CEACAM1 in human prostate cancer: correlation with loss of cell polarity, increased proliferation rate, and Gleason grade 3 to 4 transition. Hum Pathol 2002;33:290–298.

48. Estrera VT, Luo W, Phan D, et al. The cytoplasmic domain of C-CAM1 tumor suppressor is necessary and sufficient for suppressing the tumorigenicity of prostate cancer cells. Biochem Biophys Res Commun 1999;263:797–803.

49. Kleinerman DI, Zhang WW, Lin SH, et al. Application of a tumor suppressor (C-CAM1)-expressing recombinant adenovirus in androgen-independent human prostate cancer therapy: a preclinical study. Cancer Res 1995;55:2831–2836.

50. Ponta H, Sherman L, Herrlich PA. CD44: from adhesion molecules to signalling regulators. Nat Rev Mol Cell Biol 2003;4:33–45.

51. Ponta H, Wainwright D, Herrlich P. The CD44 protein family. Int J Biochem Cell Biol 1998;30:299–305.

52. Ponta H, Sleeman J, Dall P, et al. CD44 isoforms in metastatic cancer. Invasion Metastasis 1994;14:82–86.

53. Herrlich P, Morrison H, Sleeman J, et al. CD44 acts both as a growth- and invasiveness-promoting molecule and as a tumor-suppressing cofactor. Ann NY Acad Sci 2000;910:106–118; discussion 118–120.

54. Herrlich P, Sleeman J, Wainwright D, et al. How tumor cells make use of CD44. Cell Adhes Commun 1998;6:141–147.

55. Lokeshwar BL, Lokeshwar VB, Block NL. Expression of CD44 in prostate cancer cells: association with cell proliferation and invasive potential. Anticancer Res 1995;15:1191–1198.

56. Welsh CF, Zhu D, Bourguignon LY. Interaction of CD44 variant isoforms with hyaluronic acid and the cytoskeleton in human prostate cancer cells. J Cell Physiol 1995;164:605–612.

57. Kallakury BV, Yang F, Figge J, et al. Decreased levels of CD44 protein and mRNA in prostate carcinoma. Correlation with tumor grade and ploidy. Cancer 1996;78:1461–1469.

58. Nagabhushan M, Pretlow TG, Guo YJ, et al. Altered expression of CD44 in human prostate cancer during progression. Am J Clin Pathol 1996;106:647–651.

59. Gao AC, Lou W, Ichikawa T, et al. Suppression of the tumorigenicity of prostatic cancer cells by gene(s) located on human chromosome 19p13.1-13.2. Prostate 1999;38:46–54.

60. Gao AC, Lou W, Dong JT, et al. CD44 is a metastasis suppressor gene for prostatic cancer located on human chromosome 11p13. Cancer Res 1997;57:846–849.

61. Noordzij MA, van Steenbrugge GJ, Schroder FH, et al. Decreased expression of CD44 in metastatic prostate cancer. Int J Cancer 1999;84:478–483.

62. Noordzij MA, van Steenbrugge GJ, Verkaik NS, et al. The prognostic value of CD44 isoforms in prostate cancer patients treated by radical prostatectomy. Clin Cancer Res 1997;3:805–815.

63. Aaltomaa S, Lipponen P, Viitanen J, et al. Prognostic value of CD44 standard, variant isoforms 3 and 6 and -catenin expression in local prostate cancer treated by radical prostatectomy. Eur Urol 2000;38:555–562.

64. Aaltomaa S, Lipponen P, Ala-Opas M, et al. Expression and prognostic value of CD44 standard and variant v3 and v6 isoforms in prostate cancer. Eur Urol 2001;39:138–144.

65. Poczatek RB, Myers RB, Manne U, et al. Ep-Cam levels in prostatic adenocarcinoma and prostatic intraepithelial neoplasia. J Urol 1999;162:1462–1466.

66. de Bono JS, Tolcher AW, Forero A, et al. ING-1, a monoclonal antibody targeting Ep-CAM in patients with advanced adenocarcinomas. Clin Cancer Res 2004;10:7555–7565.

67. Thurmond LM, Stimmel JB, Ingram AC, et al. Adenocarcinoma cells exposed in vitro to Navelbine or Taxol increase Ep-CAM expression through a novel mechanism. Cancer Immunol Immunother 2003;52:429–437.

68. Tomita K, van Bokhoven A, Jansen CF, et al. Coordinate recruitment of E-cadherin and ALCAM to cell-cell contacts by alpha-catenin. Biochem Biophys Res Commun 2000;267:870–874.

69. Kristiansen G, Pilarsky C, Wissmann C, et al. ALCAM/CD166 is up-regulated in low-grade prostate cancer and progressively lost in high-grade lesions. Prostate 2003;54:34–43.

70. Nelissen JM, Peters IM, de Grooth BG, et al. Dynamic regulation of activated leukocyte cell adhesion molecule-mediated homotypic cell adhesion through the actin cytoskeleton. Mol Biol Cell 2000;11:2057–2068.

71. Zimmerman AW, Nelissen JM, van Emst-de Vries SE, et al. Cytoskeletal restraints regulate homotypic ALCAM-mediated adhesion through PKCalpha independently of Rho-like GTPases. J Cell Sci 2004;117:2841–2852.

72. Chen MW, Vacherot F, De La TA, et al. The emergence of protocadherin-PC expression during the acquisition of apoptosis-resistance by prostate cancer cells. Oncogene 2002;21:7861–7871.

Apoptosis and prostate cancer 31

Sinead E Walsh, John M Fitzpatrick, R William G Watson

INTRODUCTION

Cell death, in a dynamic balance with cell proliferation, is necessary to maintain homeostatic control of cell numbers,[1] with 10 billion cells dying in an average adult every day, simply to keep balance with the numbers of new cells arising from the body's stem cell populations. Cell death occurs principally as a result of damage, but it also occurs under controlled conditions, such as in the sculpturing of organs in an embryo and the elimination of T cells once they have fought an infection.

The two main ways in which cells die are by necrosis and apoptosis (programmed cell death).[2,3] However, there are emerging intermediary forms of cell death, such as "aponecrosis," which shares certain features with both necrosis and apoptosis.[4,5] Necrotic death is a chaotic, uncontrolled process, and occurs as a result of severe injury to the cell. It is characterized by the swelling and rupture of the cell, due to uncontrolled regulation of fluids and ions. In contrast, apoptosis, which was discovered in 1972,[1] is a controlled, energy-dependent process resulting in the death of a cell and its efficient removal by surrounding phagocytes.

Though apoptosis is a necessary process, the disruption of apoptosis is associated with two major disease processes. Inappropriate activation is associated with pathologic loss of cells such as in neurodegenerative diseases, whereas inadequate apoptosis leads to accumulation of cells as in cancer.[6,7] In the early stages, prostate cancer is a relatively slow-growing malignancy, and studies have shown that inhibition of apoptosis rather than enhanced cellular proliferation is more critical for its development.[8] For this reason, chemotherapeutic drugs that target rapidly proliferating cells are ineffective in treating prostate cancer. Instead, treatments such as androgen ablation, which induces apoptosis by removing survival factors, are the mainstay of prostate cancer therapy. Unfortunately, this inevitably fails, causing progression to androgen-independent disease, and, therefore, new mechanisms of inducing apoptosis must be sought.

DEFINITIONS AND CHARACTERISTICS OF APOPTOSIS

Cells undergoing apoptosis all demonstrate similar characteristics, but individual cell types may differ in the extent to which they express these changes. These changes include both cytoplasmic and nuclear deconstruction. Within the cytoplasm, structural proteins such as actin microtubules are cleaved to break down the cellular scaffold, and enzymatic proteins whose functions are no longer required by the dying cell are inactivated. Nuclear changes include compaction of chromatin and internucleosomal double-stranded cutting of DNA by endonucleases, producing fragments ranging from 700 bp to 50 kbp in size.[9] The nucleus is then broken down to form multiple fragments. Fragmentation, or blebbing of the plasma membrane begins by the flipping of phosphatidylserine from the inner plasma membrane to the cell surface. Finally, these cell surface protuberances separate to produce membrane-enclosed apoptotic bodies of varying size, within which the closely packed cytoplasmic organelles remain well preserved. The entire process of apoptosis can be completed in under 30 minutes, and the fragmented cell is quickly and efficiently removed by phagocytes. For this reason, few apoptotic cells are visible in tissue specimens, but apoptosis can readily be measured in cultured cells. Morphologic assessment is the classical method of identifying cells demonstrating distinct characteristics of apoptosis, such as membrane blebbing. Also, the exposure of phosphatidylserine can be detected by the antibody Annexin V. The nuclear collapse that is the hallmark of apoptosis has as its biochemical correlate the "DNA ladder" on agarose gel electrophoresis. DNA fragmentation can also be detected by terminal transferase mediated dUTP-biotin nick end labeling (TUNEL), or staining with propidium iodide, a DNA-intercalating agent.

The systematic cleavage of proteins to bring about the demise of the dying cell is centrally dependent on a number of proteins, especially the proteolytic enzymes called the caspases. Apoptosis can be induced by extrinsic (death receptor) and intrinsic (mitochondrial) pathways. Though the apoptosis-inducing agents differ, they ultimately converge on a central pathway involving activation of "executioner" caspases. Also, there is a great deal of communication or "crosstalk" between the cell surface receptors, the mitochondria, and another stress-sensing organelle, the endoplasmic reticulum (ER). The series of events in the apoptotic process, as described here, may seem straightforward; however, the important decision of the cell—to live or die—is regulated by competing and conflicting signals from the cell surface and numerous organelles within the cell, which control a vast myriad of proteins. Though there has been an explosion of knowledge in the area of programmed cell death since the term "apoptosis" was coined in 1972, many gaps in our understanding remain. A major goal in apoptosis research in prostate cancer is to understand the molecular changes causing apoptosis in androgen-independent disease. When this question is addressed, it will allow identification of new therapies to effectively treat androgen-independent prostate cancer, an urgent issue for clinicians. This chapter will specifically focus on the death receptor, mitochondria, and ER triggers of the apoptotic pathway and their role in prostate cancer (for a review of prostate cell apoptosis see Coffey et al[10]).

RECEPTOR-MEDIATED CELL DEATH PATHWAYS

Numerous transmembrane receptors exist on the plasma membrane of each cell that function in transferring extracellular signals into the cell. Among these, "death receptors" such as members of the tumor necrosis factor (TNF) family have been identified. These include TNF receptor 1 (TNFR1) and Fas, which, on interaction with the corresponding antigens, TNFα and Fas ligand (FasL) can initiate death signals through "death domains" in their receptors.[11–13] FasL can function in either autocrine (self-activation) or paracrine (activated by neighboring cells) mechanisms, leading to cell death.[14] Apo2 ligand or tumor necrosis

factor-related apoptosis-inducing ligand (TRAIL) is another of the several members of the tumor necrosis factor gene superfamily that induce apoptosis through engagement of death receptors. TRAIL was discovered in 1995,[15] and is considered a promising cancer therapeutic agent due to its ability to selectively kill tumor cells. There are two receptors that TRAIL binds to that contain a death domain motif; death receptor 4 (TRAILR1)[16] and death receptor 5 (TRAILR2).[17] However, there are two other receptors; TRAILR3 and R4 which have a normal extracellular domain but a truncated, nonfunctional death domain, which are described as decoy receptors.[18] In addition, a soluble decoy receptor, osteoprotegerin (OPG), has recently been identified, which may function as a paracrine survival factor.[19]

The signaling mechanism by which Fas, TNFR1, and TRAIL receptors induce cell death still remains somewhat unclear. However, from our knowledge we surmise that their ligation results in the formation of the death-inducing signaling complex (DISC).[18] This then results in the binding of the adaptor protein Fas-associated death domain (FADD).[20] The TNFR1-associated proteins (TRADD)[21] also bind but only on activation of the Fas and TNFR1 receptors and are not involved in TRAIL-induced activation. These adapter proteins and the formation of the DISC then results in the activation of caspase 8.[22] The activation of caspase 8 by death receptors can directly activate caspase 3, which in turn causes a "caspase cascade." Alternatively, caspase 8 can amplify the apoptotic signal by eliciting the help of the mitochondria. This is mediated by cleaving the proapoptotic protein Bid, producing truncated Bid (tBid), which integrates into the mitochondrial membrane,[23] releasing a host of other proapoptotic proteins (see below). Either pathway of caspase activation results in a common end-point—the induction of apoptosis. It is important to identify which mechanism of caspase activation occurs in each cell type, and under what conditions, as this will help to locate the points of apoptotic resistance in these cells.

RECEPTOR CELL DEATH PATHWAYS AND PROSTATE CANCER

Prostate cancer cell lines have been shown to express the receptors for FasL,[24] TNFα[25] and TRAIL[26] but only certain cells undergo apoptosis in response to these ligands.

FAS

Despite increased expression of Fas and FasL[24] on the surface of prostatic intraepithelial neoplasia (PIN) and prostate cancer cells, they are resistant to apoptotic induction, indicating that the resistance to apoptosis must occur downstream of the receptor. Both cFLIP (cellular Flice-like inhibitory protein) and the formation

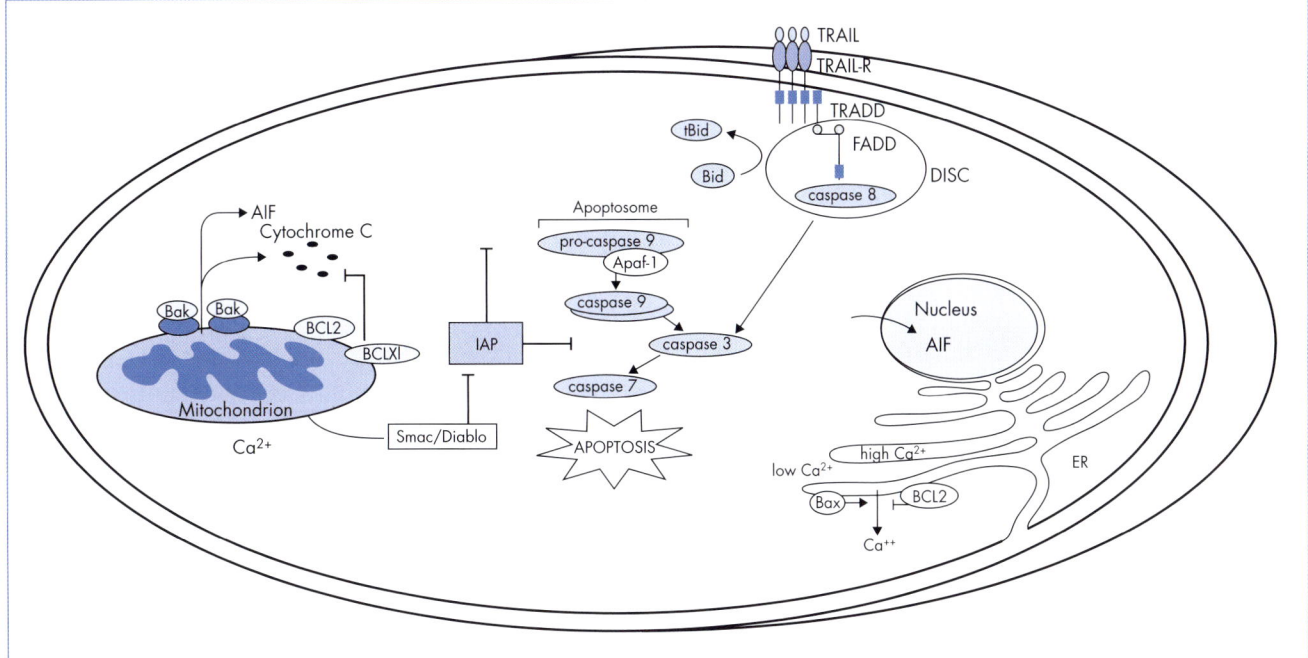

Fig. 31.1

Cross talk between the death receptor, mitochondria and endoplasmic reticulum pathways of apoptosis in prostate cancer cells.

of the DISC are important regulators of the downstream activation of the caspase cascade from death receptor induced apoptosis. Resistance to Fas-mediated apoptosis has been associated with increased expression of cFLIP. Inhibitors of the pro-survival protein, Akt not only reduce the expression of cFLIP but also enhance the recruitment of FADD and formation of the DISC.[27] Antisense oligonucleotides to cFLIP has been shown to downregulate its protein expression and sensitizes DU-145 cells to CH-11 (Fas antibody)-induced apoptosis, indicating a central role for cFLIP in apoptotic resistance.[28] Radiation has also been shown to increase the sensitivity of LNCaP cells to Fas-mediated apoptosis through increased Fas expression.[29] JNK activation has also been shown to play a central role in resistance to Fas-induced apoptosis in prostate cancer cells, with specific ability to decrease the expression of the Fas/FADD-interacting kinase HIPK3.[30] In addition, the interaction between FADD and caspase 8 is defective in DU-145 cells, but strategies that inhibit JNK signaling restore the affinity of FADD for caspase-8 and their ability to undergo Fas receptor mediated apoptosis.[30]

TRAIL

The sensitivity of prostate cancer cells to TRAIL may be influenced by the levels of the decoy receptor, OPG. Hormone independent PC3 and DU-145 cells produce 10- to 20-fold more OPG than LNCaP cells, which is negatively correlated with the capacity of TRAIL to induce apoptosis in these cells.[31] Sensitizing for TRAIL-induced apoptosis can be mediated by radiation, which upregulates DR5 as well as downstream regulators of the apoptotic pathway.[32] A number of specific and non-specific approaches have also been shown to regulate both Fas- and TRAIL-induced apoptosis downstream of the receptor, either at the level of the mitochondria or caspase activation. Thiol[33] and pH[34] alter Fas- and TRAIL-induced apoptosis via caspase and mitochondrial pathways. Oxidants, including nitric oxide sensitize prostate cancer cells to TRAIL via inactivation of NFκB, mediated through the inhibition of the antiapoptotic protein, BCLXL.[35] Chemotherapeutic agents including cisplatin, etoposide, and doxorubicin also sensitize prostate cancer cell lines to TRAIL-induced apoptosis.[36] The X-linked inhibitor of apoptosis protein (XIAP), a potent inhibitor of caspase activity has been shown to be central in TRAIL resistance.[37] Specific inhibition of XIAP using antisense oligonucleotides increases the sensitivity of prostate cancer cells to TRAIL induced apoptosis.[38]

To summarise, though prostate cancer cells express death receptors, the death receptor pathways in these cells seem to depend on down-stream effectors, such as the mitochondria to fully execute apoptosis. Focused research into receptor-mitochondrial signaling should help unravel why these tumor cells become resistant to receptor-induced apoptosis. Also, the mitochondria represent targets for manipulation, which could be targeted in conjunction with death ligand treatments such as TRAIL to overcome apoptotic resistance in prostate cancer.

MITOCHONDRIAL-MEDIATED APOPTOSIS

The primary function of mitochondria is to produce energy, in the form of ATP, which is necessary for the cell to live. However, a paradoxical function was discovered in the 1990s, when research showed that mitochondria are in fact central players in apoptosis. It was noticed that, shortly before the onset of apoptosis, the carefully-sustained mitochondrial membrane potential (MMP) is lost.[39] Furthermore, it emerged that cytochrome c, a "simple" electron-shuttling protein in the electron transport chain, becomes a potent proapoptotic molecule when released from the mitochondria.[40] For these reasons, mitochondria have been given the title of "both the giver and taker of life." There is a delicate balance within the cell of pro- and antiapoptotic molecules, which is often perturbed in cancer cells.

Mitochondria have the ability to sense the induction of apoptosis within the cell, and also to interpret extrinsic cell death signals from death receptors. Though the signaling mechanisms involved are not fully understood, one hypothesis is that the changing ratio of BCL2 family proteins on the outer mitochondrial membrane predict apoptosis occurrence or resistance.[41] The BCL2 family of proteins contains proapoptotic members such as Bax, Bak, and BCL2 homology domain 3 (BH3)-only proteins; antiapoptotic members include BCL2, and BCLXL.[42] A crucial step in mitochondrial-mediated apoptosis is the loss of MMP, but, despite intensive efforts, the mechanism responsible for membrane depolarization has not been conclusively described, and so remains a controversial issue. At present, two mechanisms have been described and each may function under different physiological circumstances. Briefly, the first mechanism involves opening of the permeability transition (PT) pore on the inner membrane, allowing small molecules such as water to pass through. This leads to loss of MMP as ions equilibrate across the membrane, and the swelling of the matrix due to the influx of water can be sufficient to burst the outer membrane, releasing lethal proteins from the intermembrane space. The second mechanism involves BCL2 family members acting directly on the outer mitochondrial membrane to release proapoptotic proteins from the mitochondrial intermembrane space (reviewed in detail by Green and Kroemer[43])

If cell damage exceeds a certain threshold, the proapoptotic BCL2 family members Bax or Bak have been proposed to form high molecular weight oligomeric pores in the mitochondrial membrane through which cytochrome c can pass. Pore formation might be stimulated by changes in the pH or by BH3-only proteins such as truncated BID (tBID). Truncated BID is formed by caspase 8 cleavage, which primarily occurs at activated TNFα or Fas receptors.[23] The translocation of tBID from the cell surface to the mitochondria links receptor-mediated and mitochondrial-mediated apoptosis. How tBid interacts with Bak/Bax to make the mitochondrial membrane permeable is still under dispute. To counteract spurious initiation of apoptosis, antiapoptotic BCL2 and BCLXL appear to inhibit formation of pores in the mitochondrial membrane, thus preventing cytochrome c release. Once released, cytochrome c in association with apoptosis associated factor 1 (APAF1), leads to formation of the apoptosome, activating pro-caspase 9, which then activates caspases 3 and 7 in a caspase cascade. These caspases lead to cleavage of cellular substrates resulting in apoptosis.[44] Even at the point of cytochrome c release, there are safety mechanisms in place, including the "inhibitor of apoptosis" proteins, specifically, XIAP, which can bind to and inhibit the activity of caspase 9, preventing it from activating caspases 3 and 7.[45] A counter measure, ensuring the completion of apoptosis is the release of SMAC/DIABLO from the mitochondria, which promotes caspase activation by binding to and inhibiting XIAP.[46,47] Another protein released from the mitochondria during apoptosis is apoptosis inducing factor (AIF), which translocates from the mitochondria to the nucleus, and plays a role in DNA condensation and fragmentation.[48] This complex balancing act between pro- and antiapoptotic proteins ensures the survival of healthy cells, while eliminating damaged ones. However, slight perturbations in these pathways, such as elevated levels of XIAP could lead to cancer progression.[49]

MITOCHONDRIAL-MEDIATED APOPTOSIS AND PROSTATE CANCER

Strong evidence suggests that the mitochondrial pathway of apoptosis is activated in prostate cancer cell death.[41] These studies showed the importance of the Bax/BCL2 ratio as a determinant of apoptosis—cells with relatively high Bax expression underwent apoptosis in response to androgen ablation. Also, many investigators have reported increased BCL2 expression in androgen-independent prostate cancer.[50,51] This is corroborated by the fact that numerous experiments employing death ligands in prostate cancer cells, require concomitant mitochondrial instability in order to induce apoptosis.[34,52] The importance of the Bax/BCL2 ratio in prostate cancer cells has been exploited by causing adenoviral-mediated Bax overexpression both in vitro and in vivo, inducing the mitochondrial pathway of apoptosis.[53] In a separate study, it was revealed that protein kinase C epsilon (PKCε), an oncoprotein expressed in prostatic epithelial cells, can interact with the Bax protein, thus interrupting signaling via the mitochondrial death pathway. Induction of PKCε alone in LNCaP cells caused a significant resistance to phorbol ester-induced apoptosis. This resistance was associated with the inhibition of phorbol ester-induced Bax conformational rearrangements, which are necessary for Bax oligomerization, integration into the mitochondrial membrane, and cytochrome c release.[54] In an in-vivo model of PC3 cell tumors grown in nude mice, injections of a Bax overexpression system caused 25% regression in tumor size.[55] This data convincingly shows that the apoptotic pathway can be manipulated both in vitro and in vivo by Bax overexpression; however, the apoptotic-inducing effect is not specific to prostate cancer cells, and so can cause death in many other cell types, which could lead to adverse side effects in treated patients.[56,57] This has led to the development of a prostate-specific promoter, to direct Bax overexpression to prostate cancer cells.[58] Whereas the Bax/BCL2 ratio may favor increased BCL2 in certain prostate cancer patients, a variety of other mutations/protein alterations may be present in other cases.

Another link between mitochondria and prostate cancer was discovered by Hermann et al in 2003,[59] who analyzed the protein cytochrome c oxidase in human prostate tissue specimens. Cytochrome c oxidase is made up of subunits, and those that make up the catalytic core are synthesized from mitochondrial DNA, while the remaining subunits are synthesized from nuclear DNA. A significant shift in the amount of nuclear-encoded subunits relative to mitochondrial-encoded subunits was noticed during the progression of prostate cancer, and this shift begins even in the premalignant stage. This research highlights the importance of nuclear DNA-encoded mitochondrial proteins, and also the need to fully characterize the often forgotten mitochondrial proteome.[59]

Another determinant of apoptotic susceptibility in prostate cancer cells may be the overexpression of antiapoptotic proteins, which act immediately downstream of the mitochondria. Tissue microarray experiments have shown that XIAP, survivin, cIAP1 and cIAP2 proteins are all overexpressed in prostate carcinoma compared with benign prostate tissue. These proteins, which are the only known endogenous inhibitors of caspases, have frequent elevated expression in PIN lesions, suggesting that expression changes in these proteins may be an initiating event in prostate carcinogenesis.[60]

ENDOPLASMIC RETICULUM-MEDIATED APOPTOSIS

A third mechanism of apoptosis induction is that involving the ER. The ER is a subcellular organelle connected to the plasma membrane, the nucleus, and mitochondria. The luminal volume of the ER takes up one-tenth the volume of the entire cell, and functions in folding, sorting, and modifying newly synthesized proteins. Other functions include maintaining intracellular Ca^{2+} homeostasis and synthesizing lipids and sterols. A variety of conditions, such as loss of the oxidizing environment in the ER lumen, Ca^{2+} imbalance, hypoxia/ischemia, or an overload of proteins can lead to the accumulation of unfolded proteins in the ER, activating ER-stress-induced pathways.[61,62] The ER stress response is an evolutionary conserved cellular response where ER-localized chaperones are induced, protein synthesis is slowed down, and a protein degrading system is initiated, which enables the cell to deal with accumulated proteins.[63–65] This complex response is coordinated by three ER membrane proteins; Ire1 (α and β), ATF6 and PERK which can sense protein aggregation and trigger the stress response.[66,67] Ire1 and PERK are normally maintained in an inactive state by being bound to a molecular chaperone called Bip. When proteins accumulate in the ER, Bip dissociates allowing Ire1α and PERK to become active.[68] PERK then phosphorylates the translation initiation factor eIF2α, thereby blocking protein synthesis.[67] ATF6 and Ire1 act in concert to initiate a transcriptional response in the nucleus. They induce the expression of ER-directed chaperones, which bind to ER proteins, preventing them from aggregating and denaturing.

Ultimately, this protective response gives the cell time to recover from a stress; however, prolonged ER-stress leads to apoptosis through mechanisms that are not fully understood. It is known that a transcription factor pathway and a caspase-dependent pathway can be activated. In the first pathway, Ire1 is thought to switch to act as a proapoptotic protein, by upregulating the transcription factor, GADD153/CHOP, which may amplify the proapoptotic signal by altering the balance between BCL2 and Bax.[69,70] The anti-apoptotic protein, Bcl2 not only localizes at the mitochondria, but also at the ER/cytoplasm interface. Its importance in preventing apoptosis was shown by directing BCL2 to the ER through linking it to cytochrome c, which blocked most types of apoptosis.[71] The survival mechanism by which BCL2 at the ER blocks apoptosis is enigmatic, though three or four possibilities exist.[72] ER stress or other apoptotic stimuli might also activate caspases at the ER surface and induce apoptosis independent of the mitochondria. Murine caspase 12 (with high homology to human caspases 1 and 4) resides predominantly on the outer ER membrane.[73] Caspase 12 is activated by chemicals such as thapsigargin, which induces ER stress by interfering with the SERCA Ca^{2+} pump (which pumps Ca^{2+} into the ER). The existence of a human caspase 12 remains a controversial issue. Functional caspase 12 has been cloned from the mouse and the rat, but not from humans, although a sequence has been identified in the human genome that shows identity to murine caspase 12. This sequence, however, contains nine premature stop codons that produce various truncated forms of the protein.[74] Questions remain whether mutations could override these stop codons to produce a fully functional caspase 12, and also whether a caspase 12 sequence exists at a different location in the human genome, or if other human caspases carry out its functions.

Research into ER-mediated apoptosis via calcium signaling has been developed to a greater extent. Endoplasmic reticulum stress can lead to the release of Ca^{2+} from the ER and subsequent production of reactive oxygen species (ROS) from the highly oxidizing environment of the lumen of the ER.[75] A substantial release of Ca^{2+} from the ER could lead to altered mitochondrial functions, as high cytosolic Ca^{2+} can induce a loss in mitochondrial transmembrane potential, which results in the release of cytochrome c and formation of the apoptosome.[76]

ENDOPLASMIC RETICULUM-MEDIATED APOPTOSIS AND PROSTATE CANCER

A role for Ca^{2+} released from the ER has been shown in some models of apoptosis, but the mechanisms involved and the functional significance of this in prostate cancer is unclear. A study by Nutt in 2002 showed that some apoptotic stimuli were associated with emptying of the ER Ca^{2+} pool in human PC3 prostate cancer cells. This mobilization of ER Ca^{2+} was associated with an increase in mitochondrial Ca^{2+} levels, causing release of cytochrome c, DNA fragmentation, and cell death. This did not occur in Bax-null DU145 cells, which demonstrates that Bax-mediated alterations in ER, as well as mitochondria, regulate the Ca^{2+} signals upstream of cytochrome c release in some examples of apoptosis. Work by Isaacs et al[77] has investigated the role of thapsigargin (TG) in ER-mediated apoptosis in prostate cancer cells. As androgen-independent prostate cancer exhibits a low rate of proliferation, TG was chosen as it is a proliferation-independent cytotoxic agent, which induces apoptosis by perturbing intracellular free Ca^{2+}. It was shown that TG induces two waves of Ca^{2+} signaling in prostate cancer cells: the first is a transient, reversible nanomolar rise in Ca^{2+}, which induces new gene transcription and translation; this is followed by a secondary micromolar rise in Ca^{2+} which irreversibly commits the cell to apoptosis via a calmodulin/calcineurin cascade.[77] Other extracellular factors have shown to influence ER calcium concentrations (ER $[Ca^{2+}]$). Insulin-like growth factor (IGF), which increases cell growth, induces an increase in ER $[Ca^{2+}]$, whereas TNFα, which induces apoptosis, reduces ER $[Ca^{2+}]$ in LNCaP prostate cancer cells. The ER $[Ca^{2+}]$ is directly correlated with the expression of the Ca^{2+} pump subunit, SERCA2b. Thus, both ER $[Ca^{2+}]$ and ER calcium pump expression are central targets for determining LNCaP cell life or death induced by growth modulators.[78] Caspase 12 has reportedly been implicated in genistein-induced Ca^{2+}-mediated apoptosis in MCF-7 human breast cancer cells.[79] However, the presence of a functional caspase 12 in prostate cancer has not yet been investigated.

DISCUSSION

From the published literature exploring apoptosis in prostate cancer cells, an emerging theme of crosstalk between pathways is clearly evident. The death receptor pathways in some prostate cancer cells utilise the mitochondria to amplify the apoptotic signal. Signaling between the two is often perturbed in prostate cancer cells, such as LNCaP, thus preventing apoptosis. The ratio of BCL2/Bax is not only important in regulating mitochondrial integrity, but also influences the permeability of the endoplasmic reticulum to Ca^{2+} ions, and possibly ROS. Also, elevated levels of antiapoptotic proteins such as the "inhibitor of apoptosis proteins" may influence apoptotic susceptibility arising from all three apoptotic triggers.

A new theme for both scientists and clinicians is that of "targeted therapies." However, this may prove difficult in the treatment of prostate cancer due to the heterogeneity of the disease, as almost every gene mentioned in this chapter has been shown to be involved in some cancers. This chapter has demonstrated the complexity of the apoptotic pathway and the number of sites by which cancer can interfere with its manipulation. It is important to understand the normal biology of prostate epithelial cells before we determine and treat the abnormalities that occur in prostate cancer. This underlies the importance of basic science research running in parallel with research using clinically-relevant samples.

REFERENCES

1. Kerr JFR, Wyllie AH, Currie AR. Apoptosis: a basic biological phenomenon with wide-ranging implications in tissue kinetics. Br J Cancer 1972;26:239–257.
2. Gerschenson L, Rotello, RJ. Apoptosis: a different type of cell death. FASEB J 1992;6:2450–2455.
3. Cohen JJ. Apoptosis. Immunol Today 1993;14:126–130.
4. Formigli L, Papucci L, Tani A, et al. Aponecrosis: morphological and biochemical exploration of a syncretic process of cell death sharing apoptosis and necrosis. J Cell Physiol 2000;182:41–49.
5. Papucci L, Formigli L, Schiavone N, et al. Apoptosis shifts to necrosis via intermediate types of cell death by a mechanism depending on c-myc and bcl-2 expression. Cell Tissue Res 2004;316:197–209.
6. Carson DA, Ribeiro JM. Apoptosis and disease. Lancet 1993;341:1251–1254.
7. Kerr JFR, Winterford CM, Harmon BV. Apoptosis: Its significance in cancer and cancer therapy. Cancer 1994;73:2013–2026.
8. Tu H, Jacobs SC, Borkowski A, et al. Incidence of apoptosis and cell proliferation in prostate cancer: relationship with TGF-beta1 and bcl-2 expression. Int J Cancer 1996;69:357–363.
9. Sun XM, Cohen GM. Mg^{2+} dependent cleavage of DNA into kilobase pair fragments is responsible for the initial degradation of DNA in apoptosis. J Biol Chem 1994;269:14857–14860.

10. Coffey RN, Watson RWG, Fitzpatrick JM. Signalling for the caspases: their role in prostate cell apoptosis. J Urol 2001;165:5–14.

11. Nagata S, Golstein P. The Fas Death factor. Science 1995;267:1449–1456.

12. Suda T, Nagata S. Purification and characterisation of the Fas-ligand that induces apoptosis. J Exp Med 1993;179:873–879.

13. Nagata S, Takashi S. Fas and Fas ligand: 1pr and gld mutations. Immunol Today 1994;16:39–43.

14. Dhein J, Walczak H, Baumler C, et al. Autocrine T-cell suicide mediated by APO-1(Fas/CD95). Nature 1995;373:438–441.

15. Pitti RM, Marsters SA, Rupert S, et al. Induction of apoptosis by Apo-2 ligand, a new member of the tumor necrosis factor cytokine family. J Biol Chem 1996;31:12687–12690.

16. Pan G, O'Rourke K, Chinnaiyan AM, et al. The receptor for the cytotoxic ligand TRAIL. Science 1997;276:111–113.

17. Sheridan JP, Marsters SA, Pitti RM, et al. Control of TRAIL-induced apoptosis by a family of signalling and decoy receptors. Science 1997;277:818–821.

18. Le Blanc HN, Ashkenazi A. Apo2L/TRAIL and its death and decoy receptors. Cell Death Diff 2003;10:66–75.

19. Shipman CM, Croucher PI. Osteoprotegerin is a soluble decoy receptor for tumor necrosis factor-related apoptosis-inducing ligand/Apo2 ligand and can function as a paracrine survival factor for human myeloma cells. Cancer Res 2003;63:912–6.

20. Chinnaiyan AM, O'Rourke K, Tewari M, et al. FADD, a novel death domain-containing protein, interacts with the death domain of Fas and initiates apoptosis. Cell 1995;81:505–512.

21. Hsu H, Xiong J, Goeddel DV. The TNF receptor 1-associated protein TRADD signals cell death and NF-κB activation. Cell 1995;81:495–504.

22. Alnemri ES, Livingston DJ, Nicholson DW, et al. Human ICE/CED-3 protease nomenclature. Cell 1996;87:171.

23. Li H, Zhu H, Xu CJ, et al. Cleavage of Bid by caspase 8 mediates the mitochondrial damage in the Fas pathway of apoptosis. Cell 1998;94:491–501.

24. Jiang J, Ulbright TM, Zhang S, et al. Fas and Fas ligand expression is elevated in prostatic intraepithelial neoplasia and prostatic carcinoma. Cancer 2002;95:296–300.

25. Jaruga-Killeen E, Rayford W. TNF receptor 1 is involved in the induction of apoptosis by the cyclin dependent kinase inhibitor p27Kip1 in the prostate cancer cell line PC3. FASEB J 2005;19:139–141.

26. Voelkel-Johnson C. An antibody against DR4 (TRAIL-R1) in combination with doxorubicin selectively kills malignant but not normal prostate cells. Cancer Biol Ther 2003;2:289–290.

27. Shimada K, Nakamura M, Ishida E, et al. The molecular mechanism of sensitization to Fas-mediated apoptosis by 2-methoxyestradiol in PC3 prostate cancer cells. Mol Carcinogen 2004;39:1–9.

28. Hyer ML, Sudarshan S, Kim Y, et al. Downregulation of c-FLIP sensitises DU145 prostate cancer cells to Fas-mediated apoptosis. Cancer Biol Ther 2002;1:401–406.

29. Shimada K, Nakamura M, Ishida E, et al. Androgen and the blocking of radiation-induced sensitisation to Fas-mediated apoptosis through c-jun induction in prostate cancer cells. Int J Radiat Biol 2003;79:451–462.

30. Curtin JF, Cotter TG. JNK regulates HIPK3 expression and promotes resistance to Fas-mediated apoptosis in DU-145 prostate carcinoma cells. J Biol Chem 2004;279:17090–17100.

31. Holen I, Croucher PI, Hamdy FC, et al. Osteoprotegerin (OPG) is a survival factor for human prostate cancer cells. Cancer Res 2002;62:1619–1623.

32. Shankar S, Singh TR, Srivastava RK. Ionising radiation enhances the therapeutic potential of TRAIL in prostate cancer in vitro and in vivo: Intracellular mechanisms. Prostate 2004;61:35–49.

33. Coffey RN, Watson RW, Hegarty PK, et al. Priming prostate carcinoma cells for increased apoptosis is associated with up-regulation of the caspases. Cancer 2001;92:2297–2308.

34. Lee YJ, Song JJ, Kim JH, et al. Low extracellular pH augments TRAIL-induced apoptotic death through the mitochondria-mediated caspase signal transduction pathway. Exp Cell Res 2004;293:129–143.

35. Huerta-Yepz S, Vega M, Jazirehi A, et al. Nitric oxide sensitises prostate carcinoma cell lines to TRAIL-mediated apoptosis via inactivation of NF-kappa B and inhibition of Bcl-xl expression. Oncogene 2004;23:4993–5003.

36. Munshi A, McDonnell TJ, Meyn RE. Chemotherapeutic agents enhance TRAIL-induced apoptosis in prostate cancer cells. Cancer Chemother Pharmacol 2002;50:46–52.

37. Ng CO, Bonavida B. X-linked inhibitor of apoptosis (XIAP) blocks Apo2 ligand/tumour necrosis factor-related apoptosis-inducing ligand-mediated apoptosis of prostate cancer cells in the presence of mitochondrial activation: sensitization by overexpression of second mitochondrial-derived activator of caspase/direct IAP-binding protein with low pH (Smac/DIABLO). Mol Cancer Ther 2002;1:1051–1058.

38. Amantana A, London CA, Iversen PL, et al. X-linked inhibitor of apoptosis protein inhibition induces apoptosis and enhances chemotherapy sensitivity in human prostate cancer cells. Mol Cancer Ther 2004;3:699–707.

39. Zamzami NEA. Reduction in mitochondrial potential constitutes an early irreversible step of programmed lymphocyte death in vivo. J Exp Med 1995;181:1661–1672.

40. Liu X, Kin CN, Yang J, et al. Induction of apoptotic program in cell-free extracts: Requirement for dATP and cytochrome c. Cell 1996;86:147–157.

41. Perlman H, Zhang X, Chen MW, et al. An elevated bax/bcl-2 ratio corresponds with the onset of prostate epithelial cell apoptosis. Cell Death Differ 1999;6:48–54.

42. Cory S, Adams JM. The Bcl2 family: regulators of the cellular life-or-death switch. Nature Reviews Cancer 2002;2:647–656.

43. Green DR, Kroemer G. The pathophysiology of mitochondrial cell death. Science 2004;305:626–629.

44. Slee EA, Harte MT, Kluck RM, et al. Ordering the cytochrome c-initated caspase cascade: hierarchial activation of caspases-2, -3, -6, -7, -8 and -10 in a caspase-dependent manner. J Cell Biol 1999;144:281–292.

45. Deveraux QL, Takahashi R, Salvesen GS, et al. X-linked IAP is a direct inhibitor of cell-death proteases. Nature 1997;388:300–304.

46. Orrenius S. Mitochondrial regulation of apoptotic cell death. Toxicol Lett 2004;149:19–23.

47. Green DR, Kroemer G. The pathophysiology of mitochondrial cell death. Science 2004;275:626–629.

48. Susin SA, Lorenzo HK, Zamzami N, et al. Molecular characterization of mitochondrial apoptosis-inducing factor. Nature 1999;305:441–446.

49. Krajewska M, Krajewski S, Banares S, et al. Elevated expression of Inhibitor of apoptosis proteins in prostate cancer. Clin Can Res 2003;9:4914–4925.

50. McDonnell TJ, Troncoso P, Brisbay SM, et al. Expression of the protooncogene bcl-2 in the prostate and its association with emergence of androgen-independent prostate cancer. Cancer Res 1992;52:6940–6944.

51. Colombel M, Symmans F, Gil S, et al. Detection of the apoptosis supressing oncoprotein Bcl-2 in hormone refractory human prostate cancers. Am J Pathol 1993;143:390–400.

52. Liang Y, Eid MA, Lewis RL, et al. Mitochondria from TRAIL-resistant prostate cancer cells are capable of responding to apoptotic stimuli. Cellular Signalling 2005;17:243–251.

53. Xiaoying L, Marani M, Yu J, et al. Adenovirus-mediated Bax overexpression for the induction of therapeutic apoptosis in prostate cancer. Cancer Res 2001;61:186–191.

54. McJilton M, Van Sikes C, Wescott GC, et al. Protein kinase C epsilon interacts with Bax and promotes survival of human prostate cancer cells. Oncogene 2003;22:7958–7968.

55. Li H, Zhu H, Xu CJ, et al. Adenoviral-mediated Bax overexpression for the induction of therapeutic apoptosis in prostate cancer. Cancer Res 2001;61:186–191.

56. Kagawa S, Pearson SA, Ji L. A binary adenoviral vector system for expressing high levels of the proapoptotic gene bax. Gene Ther 2000;7:75–79.

57. Kagawa S, Gu J, Swisher SG, et al. Antitumor effect of adenovirus-mediated Bax gene transfer on p53-sensitive and p53-resistant cancer lines. Cancer Res 2000;60:1157–1161.

58. Zhang J, Thomas TZ, Kasper S, et al. A small composite probasin promoter confers high levels of prostate-specific gene expression through regulation by androgens and glucocorticoids in vitro and in vivo. Endocrinology 2000;141:4698–4710.

59. Hermann PC, Gillespie JW, Charboneau L, et al. Mitochondrial proteome: altered cytochrome c oxidase subunit levels in prostate cancer. Proteomics 2003;3:1801–1810.

60. Krajewska M, Krajewski S, Steven Banares, et al. Elevated expression of inhibitor of apoptosis proteins in prostate cancer. Clin Can Res 2003;9:4914–4925.

61. Pahl HL, Baeleurle PA. A novel signal transduction pathway from the endoplasmic reticulum to the nucleus is mediated by transcription factor NF-kappaB. EMBO 1995;14:2580–2588.

62. Price BD, Calderwood SK. Gadd45 and Gadd153 messenger RNA levels are increased during hypoxia and after exposure of cells to agents which elevate the levels of the glucose-regulated proteins. Cancer Res 1992;52:3814–3817.

63. Brewer JW, Diehl JA. PERK mediates cell-cycle exit during the mammalian unfolded protein response. Proc Natl Acad Sci USA 2000;97:12396–12397.

64. Prostko CR, Brostrom MA, Malara EM, et al. Phosphorylation of eukaryotic initation factor (eIF) 2 alpha and inhibition of eIF2B in Gh3 pituitary cells by perturbants of early protein processing that induce GRP78. J Biol Chem 1992;267:16751–16754.

65. Kozutsumi Y, Segal M, Normington K, et al. The presence of malfolded proteins in the endoplasmic reticulum signals the induction of glucose-regulated proteins. Nature 1988;332:462–464.

66. Tirasophon W, Welhinda AA, Kaufman RJ. A stress response pathway from the endoplasmic reticulum to the nucleus requires a novel bifunctional protein kinase/endoribonuclease (Ire1p) in mammalian cells. Genes Dev 1998;12:1812–1824.

67. Shi Y, Vattem KM, Sood R, et al. Identification and characterisation of pancreatic eukaryotic initiation factor 2 alpha-subunit kinase, PEK, involved in translation control. Mol Cell Biol 1998;18:7499–7509.

68. Bertolotti A, Zhang Y, Hendershot LM, et al. Dynamic interaction of BiP and ER stress transducers in the unfolded-protein response. Nat Cell Biol 2000;2:326–332.

69. Wang XZ, Harding HP, Zhang Y, et al. Cloning of mammalian Ire1 reveals diversity in the ER stress responses. EMBO 1998;17:5708–5717.

70. Ghribi O, Herman MM, DeWitt DA, et al. Abeta (1-42) and aluminum induce stress in the endoplasmic reticulum in rabbit hippocampus, involving nuclear translocation of gadd 153 and NF-kappaB. Brain Res Mol Brain Res 2001;96:30–38.

71. Lee ST, Hoeflich KP, Wasfy GW, et al. Bcl-2 targeted to the endoplasmic reticulum can inhibit apoptosis induced by Myc but not etoposide in Rat-1 fibroblasts. Oncogene 1999;18:3520–3528.

72. Hacki J, Egger L, Monney L, et al. Apoptotic crosstalk between the endoplasmic reticulum and mitochondria controlled by Bcl2. Oncogene 2000;19:2286–2295.

73. Nakagawa T, Zhu H, Morishima N, et al. Caspase-12 mediates endoplasmic-reticulum-specific apoptosis and cytotoxicity by amyloid-beta. Nature 2000;403:98–103.

74. Fischer H, Koenig U, Eckhart L, et al. Human caspase 12 has acquired deleterious mutations. Biochem Biophys Res Commun 2002;293:722–726.

75. McCullough KD, Martindale JL, Klotz LO, et al. Gadd153 sensitizes cells to endoplasmic reticulum stress by down-regulating Bcl2 and perturbing the cellular redox state. Mol Cell Biol 2001;21:1249–1259.

76. Scorrano L, Oakes SA, Opferman JT, et al. BAX and BAK regulation of endoplasmic reticulum Ca++: A control point for apoptosis. Science 2003;300:135–139.

77. Tombal B, Weeraratna AT, Denmeade SR, et al. Thapsigargin induces a calmodulin/calcineurin-dependent apoptotic cascade responsible for the death of prostate cancer cells. Prostate 2000;43:303–317.

78. Humez S, Legrand G, Vanden-Abeele F, et al. Role of endoplasmic reticulum calcium content in prostate cancer cell growth regulation by IGF and TNFalpha. J Cell Physiol 2004;201:201–213.

79. Sergeev IN. Genistein induces Ca++-mediated, calpain/caspase-12 dependent apoptosis in breast cancer cells. Biochem Biophys Res Commun 2004;321:462–467.

Cellular proliferation and senescence in prostate cancer

32

Alan K Meeker, Donald S Coffey

INTRODUCTION

With aging, the human prostate gland exhibits a startling propensity for both benign and malignant neoplasia. Estimates for 2004 predicted 230,110 new cases of prostate cancer in the United States, representing the majority (33%) of new cancer cases in men (excluding skin cancer). Currently, US males have a 1 in 6 lifetime risk of developing clinical prostate cancer, and prostate cancer is the second leading cause of cancer deaths in US men (29,900 deaths estimated for 2004).[1]

Both benign prostatic hyperplasia (BPH) and prostate cancer display striking increases in incidence with advancing age. It is estimated that up to 80% of men 80 years or older possess clinically undetected foci of prostate cancer.[2] The populations of several industrialized nations are aging at an increasingly rapid pace. Currently in the United States approximately 1 in 5 of the population is aged 60 years or over, and persons 85 years or older comprise the fastest growing segment of the population. According to the US Census Bureau, the rate of growth of those 60+ is projected to be three-and-a-half times as high as that of the total population by 2010. This demographic transition towards the aged means that, despite the welcome advances in early detection and treatment that are believed to have led to declining mortality rates over roughly the past decade, prostate cancer will likely remain a significant clinical burden for the foreseeable future.

Cancer is primarily a disease of aberrant cell growth in which the rate of proliferation is no longer counterbalanced by the rate of cell death. In normal cells, multiple mechanisms act to stringently control cell growth, thus helping to prevent the development of cancer. How is it that these mechanisms are bypassed during tumorigenesis, and what makes increasing age such a potent risk factor for prostate cancer? This chapter focuses on these questions and their potential clinical impact in the realms of prostate cancer prognosis, treatment, and prevention.

CONTROL OF CELLULAR PROLIFERATION

For primitive single-celled organisms the rate (and extent) of cellular proliferation typically proceeds at a maximum; limited only by external environmental factors such as nutrient availability and space constraints. The development of multicellular organisms allowed for a division of labor between germline cells, the physical genomes of which are passed directly on to the next generation, and somatic cells that serve to protect and maintain the germline.[3] This represents a remarkable degree of cooperation in that the somatic cells have essentially surrendered their individual proliferative potential (their so-called "immortality") for the common goal of ensuring transfer of their shared genome into the next generation. Extreme examples of such cellular altruism are terminally differentiated, post-mitotic cells such as neurons and muscle myocytes, which can last a lifetime without ever dividing. Interestingly, these types of cells rarely become cancerous. On the other hand, certain cell populations, notably those in many epithelial tissues, undergo continuous turnover throughout life, and several of these same epithelial tissues comprise the most common sites of cancer development in adults; with marked increases in cancer incidence with age.

In the normal state, multiple growth control pathways maintain the precise balance between cell birth and cell death required for the striking homeostasis observed in renewal tissues. These systems include a broad array of paracrine and endocrine effectors, such as positive and negative growth factors, cytokines, and hormones; as well as specific physical cell–cell and cell–extracellular matrix (ECM) contacts that act to limit cell proliferation to only that strictly necessary for repair and maintenance of the tissue. Proliferating cells harboring activating mutations in genes involved in such growth regulatory networks are at risk of malignant transformation. Indeed, many oncogenes and tumor suppressor genes are members of growth factor signaling pathways that positively or negatively, respectively, affect cell division.[4–6] Increased proliferation, as assessed by Ki67 immunohistochemical staining, has been shown to be a prognostic marker for prostate cancer recurrence following surgery, for metastases, and poor survival following radiotherapy.[7–10] Likewise, several recent studies examining the cell cycle inhibitor p27 in prostate cancer have found decreased p27 expression to correlate with proliferation status and to be an independent predictor of relapse and decreased survival time (reviewed in Tsihlias et al[11]).

Unlike several other cancers in which one or a small number of genes are frequently found to be mutated, analyses of prostate cancer has revealed a plethora of changes, many of which have strong links to cell proliferation.[12,13] Many such positive and negative regulators have been studied in the laboratory mouse where their respective overexpression or deletion results in prostatic hyperplasia, prostatic intraepithelial neoplasia (PIN), or cancer to varying degrees. Examples include the androgen receptor (AR), members of the fibroblast growth factor (FGF)/FGF receptor family, keratinocyte growth factor (KGF), Insulin-like growth factor 1 (IGF1), transforming growth factor-β receptor (TGFβR), retinoic acid receptors (RAR, RXR), the PTEN tumor suppressor, homeobox gene Nkx3.1, Akt kinase, and the MYC and RAS oncogene products.[14]

In order to limit the development and accrual of potentially carcinogenic mutations, organisms employ several safeguards; protection that is especially important in large long-lived species where there is ample time for mutations to accumulate. These safeguards can be classified into four general categories:

- Damage recognition and repair.
- Cellular hierarchies that reduce the need for proliferation of long-lived tissue stem cells.
- Protective systems that act to prevent genomic damage.
- Elimination of damaged cells from the proliferative pool.

Each of these systems and their potential importance with respect to prostate cancer are described below.

DNA DAMAGE REPAIR

Many different agents are genotoxic and can directly damage DNA. For example, reactive oxygen species generated either as byproducts of aerobic metabolism within the cell, or from external sources such as inflammation, the diet, or environmental exposures, can chemically attack DNA. Likewise, radiation and errors in the process of DNA replication itself can lead to DNA damage such as single- and double-strand DNA breaks. The types of lesions generated are diverse, and, therefore, cells possess several different systems that can specifically recognize and repair them. Notably, inherited genetic defects in such repair systems often result in an elevated susceptibility to cancer, although this increased risk is typically evident only in specific organs or tissues.[15] Well-known examples include defects in mismatch repair genes leading to hereditary colon cancer and the involvement of the BRCA1 and BRCA2 genes in hereditary breast and ovarian cancers. These same genes have also been found altered in subsets of sporadic cancer cases.[15] To date however, defective DNA damage repair genes do not appear to be major contributors to the development of prostate cancer.

CELLULAR HIERARCHIES AND TISSUE STEM CELLS

Terminally differentiated cells lost due to injury, death, or physical removal must be replaced in order to maintain tissue integrity and function. The ultimate source for replenishment of these cells are long-lived progenitor stem cells. These relatively undifferentiated cells are capable of giving rise to the multiple types of fully differentiated cells within a given tissue.

As mentioned previously, DNA replication itself can cause damage to the genetic material. Should this damage (or damage from other sources) go unrepaired before replication ensues then an incorrect nucleotide base or bases may be inserted into the newly synthesized DNA strand, thus becoming locked in as a permanent mutation in one of the daughter cells following cell division. Subsequent divisions of the mutated DNA template propagates the error to subsequent daughter cells. Therefore, the risk of mutation accumulation is higher in dividing versus nondividing cells, and the longer the division history of a given cell in a proliferating population, the greater the chance for accruing carcinogenic mutations in critical growth control genes. This problem is compounded by the possibility that such a mutation may endow the cell with a growth advantage, in which case that cell's descendants will be over-represented in subsequent generations leading to an expanding target population at risk for further mutagenic "hits"—a process referred to as clonal expansion.[16,17]

Given the above, it would seem then that, due to their persistence and proliferative competence, stem cells would be in particular danger of malignant transformation. One solution to this problem is to keep the proliferation rate of reserved tissue stem cells (which may last a lifetime) to a minimum. This may be accomplished by shifting the proliferative burden away from these long-lived cells to their shorter-lived proximal descendants. In this scenario, a stem cell divides asymmetrically, giving rise to two different daughter cells, one of which replaces the original stem cell, while the other becomes a so-called transient amplifying (TA) or transient proliferating (TP) cell. These TA/TP cells then divide for a limited period of time, giving rise to the nondividing terminally differentiated cells that make up the bulk of the tissue.[18,19] In certain tissues, this hierarchical model appears to be reflected in an ordered spatial arrangement of cells. For instance, in the crypts of the intestinal mucosa, terminally differentiated cells lie at the surface and in the upper regions of the crypt structure. These cells, which are continuously being lost, arise from an area of intense proliferation (TA/TP cells) further down the crypt, which, in turn, is thought to be descended from a limited number of infrequently dividing stem cells residing at the base of the crypt. A key concept here is the idea that stem cells are located in a specialized compartment (microenvironment) called the stem-cell niche. It is here that stem cells are thought to receive signals via specific cell–cell contacts and signaling molecules that instruct the stem cells to maintain their comparatively undifferentiated state and may impact on the timing of their division[18,20]

Although they may be spared extensive division, stem cells are long-lived and do not undergo terminal differentiation; therefore, it has been proposed that they may be the primary targets for carcinogenesis.[21–24] Unfortunately, unlike the well-stratified multilayered architecture of the rapidly dividing skin or intestinal epithelia, stem cells have not been definitively localized within the prostate, although their existence has been inferred from tissue and cell transplantation studies, plus the fact that the residual cells remaining within the involuted prostate following castration can fully regenerate the gland upon restoration of testosterone.[25,26] Similarly, while well characterized cell surface markers allow the ex-vivo isolation of stem cells of the hematopoietic system, no such unequivocal markers of prostatic stem cells have yet been identified.

The prostatic epithelium primarily consists of two phenotypically distinct cell types—basal cells and luminal cells. One or two layers of basal epithelial cells lie atop the basement membrane, above the fibromuscular stroma. Basal cells appear fairly undifferentiated, strongly express high-molecular-weight cytokeratins such as CK5, CK14, and CK15, and also express p63 protein, the antiapoptotic protein BCL2, and the protective enzyme glutathione-S-transferase-pi (GSTP1). Directly above the basal cell layer are the highly differentiated tall columnar secretory epithelial cells, which communicate with the lumens of the prostatic ducts and acini. These luminal epithelial cells strongly express cytokeratins CK8 and CK18 and are CK5-negative.[27] Prostatic luminal cells are highly dependent on androgens for their survival and are the sites of production of androgen-regulated prostatic secretions such as prostate-specific antigen (PSA).[28] Since the majority of proliferative activity occurs in the basal cell layer, and at least a subset of basal cells are competent to renew the prostate, it is presumed that the prostatic epithelial stem cells reside here. However, arguing against the idea that these stem cells are the targets for prostate carcinogenesis is the fact that the phenotypes of both prostate adenocarcinoma and PIN (the presumed precursor to prostate cancer) most closely resemble that of *luminal* secretory cells (e.g., CK5⁻, GSTP1⁻, PSA⁺, PSAP⁺).[29,30] An alternative hypothesis proposes that partially differentiated TA/TP cells rather than undifferentiated stem cells are the actual targets for malignant transformation in the prostate.[27,31] These TA/TP cells are thought to lie on the path between the basal stem cells and the highly differentiated luminal secretory cells. Indeed, through multiple-label immunofluorescence, cells with intermediate phenotypes between these two extremes have been observed in the human prostate, and a variably present third cell layer that is negative for the proliferation inhibitory protein p27 has been noted between the basal and luminal layers.[32–34] Thus, TA/TP cells manifest some of the differentiated phenotypic markers of luminal secretory cells but also carry with them features from the stem cell compartment, such as protection from apoptosis and proliferative competence—features also found in cancer cells. In contrast, cell division in the benign proliferative disorder BPH occurs in the basal cells, which maintain their genome protective mechanisms thus preventing genetic instability and clonal expansion.[27]

Recent studies on the hedgehog signaling pathway in the prostate may have important implications both for prostate cancer and prostate stem cell biology. This pathway is one of several highly conserved developmental signaling pathways first identified in Drosophila that contribute to various human cancers when they become dysregulated. The hedgehog pathway consists of a family of secreted protein signaling molecules, cell surface receptors, and downstream intracellular effector molecules, required for normal prostate development as well as androgen-induced regeneration of the residual gland following castration.[35] In the adult prostate, this pathway may act to regulate stem-cell renewal and the proliferative response during repair of tissue damage. It has been proposed that inappropriate and prolonged pathway activation, perhaps in response to chronic inflammation or injury, may contribute to tumor development.[36] Prostate cancer cells express and positively respond to hedgehog pathway ligands, and the pathway is active in prostate cancer cell lines.[35,37] Notably, forced pathway activation in normal prostate epithelial cells in culture is sufficient to immortalize and transform them.[35] In the prostate, the hedgehog pathway induces expression of the oncogene *Bmi1* which may underlie the immortalization as it has been shown to activate the telomere maintenance enzyme telomerase, inhibit both p14 and p16 growth inhibitory proteins, and is able to immortalize human breast epithelial cells.[38-40] The hedgehog pathway inhibitor cyclopamine inhibits the growth of prostate cancer cells in vitro and, strikingly, has produced durable tumor regressions in a human prostate cancer xenograft model.[35]

Clearly, more work needs to be done in order to understand prostate stem-cell biology and its relationship to prostate cancer, and this is currently an active area of investigation.

PROTECTION AGAINST GENOME DAMAGE

As previously described, cells encounter a host of intrinsic and extrinsic chemical compounds capable of damaging DNA. To counter these threats, cells employ an array of protective molecules and enzymes. For example, oxidative species such as oxy-radicals can be neutralized with antioxidants such as β-carotene, lycopene, and vitamin E, or by enzymes such as superoxide dismutase, catalase, or one of several peroxidases. In the prostate, the enzyme GSTP1 functions to detoxify oxidants, free radicals, and electrophilic carcinogens and is normally expressed in basal cells. This makes sense as the basal layer is the primary site of proliferating cells in the prostate, and the prostatic epithelial stem cells are thought to reside here. Interestingly, GSTP1 is not expressed in prostate cancer due to repressive hypermethylation of cytosines in so-called CpG islands within the regulatory region of the GSTP1 gene.[41,42] Methylation of the GSTP1 gene is also apparent in a significant fraction of PIN lesions, therefore, it occurs early during prostate carcinogenesis and, thus, may be playing a causal role.[43]

Cell proliferation in a setting of genotoxic stress and inadequate genome protection has recently been proposed to play a key role in the earliest stages of prostate cancer development.[12] Focal microscopic regions of atrophic epithelia associated with inflammation have been found to be highly proliferative compared with normal prostatic epithelia and have, therefore, been given the name proliferative inflammatory atrophy (PIA; reviewed in De Marzo et al[44]). Proliferative inflammatory atrophy is an attractive candidate prostate cancer precursor for several reasons: 1) it is common in the peripheral zone of the prostate, where the majority of adenocarcinomas arise; 2) like PIN, there is decreased p27 expression in PIA and increased proliferation in luminal epithelial cells; 3) PIA lesions are enriched for cells of intermediate phenotype, often express BCL2 and, perhaps as a result of this, display low levels of apoptosis; 4) GSTP1, GSTA1, and COX2 are broadly expressed, likely induced by oxidative stress from local inflammation; and 5) PIA lesions display small but significant frequencies of abnormal GSTP1 promoter methylation.[43]

The current model put forward for involvement of PIA in prostate carcinogenesis proposes that PIA represents regenerative lesions responding to damage from inflammation or other, as yet uncharacterized, sources. An overall increase in proliferation is accompanied by expansion of the intermediate cell pool, and an increased ratio of proliferating luminal cells to proliferating basal cells. It is thought that cells dividing in this genotoxic environment, perhaps those rare cells that have lost GSTP1 expression, may accrue carcinogenic mutations and thus progress onward towards PIN or cancer.[44]

NEUTRALIZATION OF DAMAGED CELLS

As discussed above, cells have several ways of avoiding and repairing DNA damage. However, damage is inevitable as no maintenance or repair process is perfect. For this reason, organisms have developed failsafe mechanisms to prevent damaged or partially transformed cells from proliferating extensively, which, if allowed, could give rise to a malignant tumor. The most well known and well understood of such mechanism is the process of programmed cell death, otherwise known as apoptosis, in which cells are induced to commit suicide.[45] There is evidence that, at least in fibroblasts and lymphocytes, the ability to undergo apoptosis decreases with increasing age, and this has also been proposed as a potential factor in prostate pathology.[46] Damaged cells can also be eliminated by other means including autophagy (self-digestion), necrosis, or mitotic catastrophe due to lethal defects in the machinery of mitosis. However, our understanding of these alternatives to apoptosis is still in its infancy.[47] Apart from cell death, another way to constrain cells at risk for malignant transformation is the non-lethal process called senescence.

CELLULAR SENESCENCE

The phenomenon of cellular senescence was first described in a series of classic studies in the early 1960s by Hayflick and Moorhead in which they showed, contrary to the reigning paradigm, that normal cultured human cells had a finite in-vitro lifespan.[48] These researchers found that following an initial period of robust proliferation the growth rate of normal cells in culture slows, ultimately halting altogether. This cessation of growth, subsequently termed the "Hayflick limit," is accompanied by distinctive morphologic changes, particularly a greatly enlarged and flattened cell shape. There is also a marked increase in the number of cells that stain positively for so-called senescence-associated β-galactosidase (SAβgal) that is active at low pH. In initial studies, it was proposed that this represented a highly specific marker for senescent cells.[49] However, subsequent studies have since shown that, while staining does correlate positively with senescence, it does not appear to be highly specific; rather it seems also to mark cells experiencing various forms of stress.[50,51]

Senescent cells do not die but rather remain metabolically active in an arrested state, resistant to apoptosis, and distinct from quiescent cells that can be driven back into the cell cycle with mitogenic stimuli.[52,53] At the molecular level, senescent cells primarily arrest in the G1 phase of the cell cycle due to the simultaneous downregulation of growth promoting genes and upregulation of growth inhibitory genes.[54,55]

There has been great interest regarding in-vitro senescence as a possible cellular model for the study of ageing. Over the past four decades much work has been done trying to understand the biology of the senescent cell. Although much of this work has made use of fibroblast cell lines, other cell types, including prostatic stromal and epithelial cells, have also been shown to undergo senescence.[56,57]

As described previously, proliferating cells are at risk of developing procarcinogenic mutations, and the more divisions a cell undergoes the greater the risk. Since senescence places strict limits on division potential, it has been proposed to have evolved as a tumor suppressive mechanism acting to prevent the outgrowth of transformed clones should they arise.[58,59] However, senescence may be a double-edged sword as studies on senescent human fibroblasts in vitro have revealed intriguing changes in gene expression that could act to provide a permissive environment for the growth of transformed epithelial cells, even as the fibroblasts themselves become irreversibly growth arrested. Such changes include the expression of matrix remodeling proteases, soluble growth factors, and proinflammatory cytokines and chemokines, such as MCP1, Groα, and interleukins 15 and 1β (IL15 and IL1β) involved in the recruitment and activation of neutrophils and macrophages. It has been pointed out that the overall phenotype of senescent fibroblasts appears in many ways similar to that of activated fibroblasts found in the setting of wound healing.[60,61] Furthermore, co-culture studies have shown that senescent fibroblasts selectively stimulate premalignant and malignant cells, and promote tumor formation in vivo. Therefore, should senescent fibroblasts accumulate with age (expected, given their resistance to apoptosis), it is conceivable that they may change the normal reciprocal stromal–epithelial communication in such a way as to foster the survival and growth of nearby transformed epithelial cells.[61] Furthermore, through their expression of soluble proinflammatory factors they may also help instigate and/or sustain chronic inflammation, which is commonly seen in the prostate and also increases with age.[62–64] The accumulation of senescent fibroblasts with age is a prerequisite for such hypotheses, however, such accumulation has been challenged, at least in the case of dermal fibroblasts.[65] Unfortunately, there are no reliable markers for unequivocally identifying senescent cells in situ. The putative senescence marker SAβgal has been assessed in prostate BPH tissues in two independent studies, but positive staining was only seen in a proportion of *epithelial* cells while no staining was evident in the prostatic stroma in either study and, as discussed previously, this marker is not senescence-specific.[49,66,67] Functionally, prostatic stroma from older donors was seen to have less growth potential than stroma from younger donors, possibly reflecting senescent cells in the older donors' stroma.[67] However, the older donors in this study were all BPH patients while the younger samples were obtained from organ donation or cystoprostatectomy, and so differences in the study groups may have contributed to the observed growth rate differences.

Finally, what relationship, if any, senescent fibroblasts may have to the abnormal, so-called "reactive stroma" associated with many cancers (including prostate cancer) that also displays a wound healing-type behavior remains to be determined.[68,69]

For human cells, progressive telomere shortening determines the Hayflick limit.[70] Telomeres are essential structures composed of specialized terminal DNA sequence repeats complexed with telomere-binding proteins and are located at the ends of every human chromosome.[71] Telomeric DNA tracts are composed of 1000 to 2000 tandem repeats of the noncoding hexanucleotide sequence TTAGGG and are dynamic entities. Telomeres are subject to shortening during cell division because of their incomplete replication during DNA synthesis—the "end replication problem—thus telomere length serves as a proxy for the number of times a cell has divided.[72] In addition, telomere shortening may also result from unrepaired single-strand breaks caused by oxidative damage.[73,74] Conversely, telomere length may be increased by the telomere synthetic enzyme telomerase or, in rare instances, via telomerase-independent genetic recombination.[75,76] The classic observations of Hayflick on fibroblasts appear to be explained by the progressive shortening of telomeres acting as a "mitotic clock" counting down cell divisions and signaling the onset of cellular senescence once one or more telomeres reaches a critical threshold length.[70] In normal cells, telomeres keep track of the cell's division history and, therefore, senescence due to progressive telomere shortening is referred to as "replicative senescence." Importantly, forced expression of telomerase can prevent telomere shortening and thus prevent replicative senescence and endow cells with unlimited replicative potential—i.e. "immortalization."[77,78]

Precisely how short telomeres trigger the onset of senescence is still being worked out. Evidence to date implicates the tumor suppressor protein p53 in the response to shortened telomeres, perhaps functioning in the recognition of short telomeres as a form of DNA damage; however, there is also evidence for a p53-independent response to dysfunctional telomeres involving the cell cycle inhibitory protein p16.[79]

At least 85% of prostate cancers and all established prostate cancer cell lines tested possess active telomerase, while normal prostate tissue is telomerase-negative; further reinforcing the concept that senescence represents a strong barrier against tumorigenesis. Indeed, careful study has revealed that telomere length maintenance is a required step for human cells to become malignant; confirming the long-held belief that cellular immortalization is a prerequisite for carcinogenesis.[80]

Telomerase activity in the prostate is androgen regulated. Both normal prostate and BPH tissues free of cancer are typically telomerase-negative, while activity is strong in the stem cell-enriched residual tissue remaining following castration. Upon restoration of androgen, this activity subsides as the gland regrows.[81–83] In androgen-responsive prostate cancer cells, this normal regulation of telomerase is inverted—telomerase is active in the presence of androgen but decreases dramatically upon either androgen-withdrawal, bicalutamide administration, or, in a human prostate cancer xenograft model, castration.[84–87] While the precise details of this aberrant regulation remain to be elucidated, potential positive regulators of telomerase in the prostate have been identified and include the oncogene product c-MYC and the polycomb protein CBX7, which was recently identified in a screen for genes upregulated in human prostate epithelial cells that had bypassed senescence.[88]

In the prostate, the senescence barrier may be crucial in limiting cancer formation. Telomere lengths have recently been found to be abnormally short in the vast majority of high-grade PIN lesions. Therefore, in order for these lesions to progress further to invasive carcinoma, they must presumably overcome replicative senescence.[89,90] Since the majority of PIN lesions are not thought to progress, telomere-based replicative senescence may represent a critical bottleneck responsible for restraining the outgrowth of most PIN lesions. This idea fits with the fact that most primary prostate cancers possess telomerase activity, since only those PIN lesions able to activate telomerase would be competent to fully progress to become invasive cancer. Of note, BPH cells display the opposite phenotype—approximately normal telomere lengths and no telomerase activity—arguing against any extensive proliferation of individual cells or cell lineages during the genesis of BPH.[81] This implies that BPH is a more global proliferative disorder affecting many cells at once, while prostate cancer appears to be a clonal disease in which, during the process of tumorigenesis, extensive cell division has occurred in the absence of telomerase. In addition, very short telomeres can initiate chromosomal instability, and so these observations may also help explain the severe genetic abnormalities that typify prostate cancers but are lacking in BPH.

Over the past several years, it has become clear that the senescent phenotype is a common endpoint initiated by several disparate triggers including: DNA damage, oxidative stress, radiation, inappropriate activity of growth factor pathways, activated oncogenes, and other forms of acute and chronic stress, all of which are potentially procarcinogenic.[91] Thus, telomere-based replicative senescence is but one type of cellular senescence, and these other stimuli may induce senescence long before telomeres shorten to the threshold level required for initiating the Hayflick limit. As expected, in such cases forced telomerase expression does not bypass senescence.[92]

Two major growth regulatory pathways participate in the initiation and maintenance of senescent growth arrest, namely the p53 and pRB pathways. Abrogation of these pathways, for instance by certain viral oncoproteins, bypasses replicative senescence, and, not surprisingly, these proteins are prominent tumor suppressors, frequently altered in human cancers. Usually, progression through the cell cycle requires the action of specific cyclin-dependent kinases (CDKs) that become activated by association with specific protein partners known as cyclins.[93] For example, progression from the G1 to S (DNA synthetic) phase of the cell cycle requires cyclin D1 binding to and activating CDK4 and CDK6 which, in turn, act to phosphorylate pRb thus removing pRb's repressive influence on cell division (Figure 32.1). A critical level of growth control is effected by CDK inhibitor proteins (CDKIs), of which there are two families, which act in part to counterbalance the growth promoting action of the CDKs.[94] The first family of CDKIs, the INK4 family, includes p15^{INK4B}, p16^{INK4A}, p18^{INK4C}, and p19^{INK4D} (also known as p19^{ARF} or p14^{ARF}). These proteins bind to

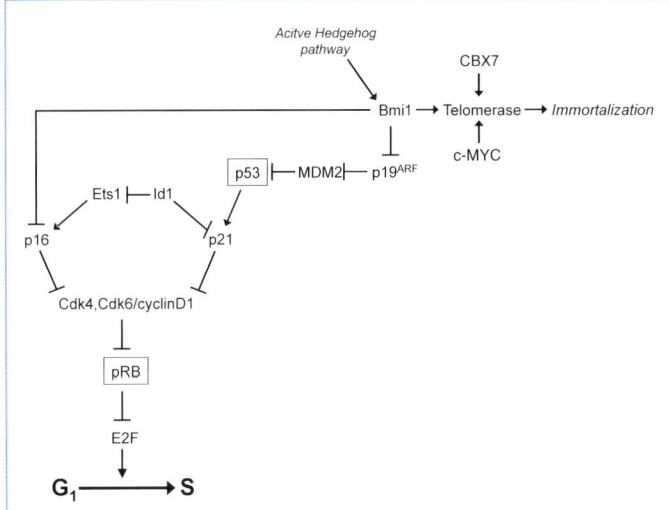

Fig. 32.1

Partial map of the regulatory network governing progression from the G1 to S phase of the cell cycle. Arrows represent positive regulation while T-junctions represent suppression. Regulatory mechanisms may include changes in gene transcription, protein modification, protein function, or protein stability.

CDK4 and CDK6 preventing their association with, and activation by, cyclin D1, thus acting to prevent pRB phosphorylation with the effect that progression from G1 to S is blocked. Members of the second CDKI family, the CIP/KIP family, include p21[CIP1], p27[KIP1], and p57[KIP2]. These CDKIs act broadly to inhibit CDK–cyclin complexes and also block pRB phosphorylation. It is not surprising to find that CDKIs also act as tumor suppressors and that many are lost or inactivated in various cancers.[11]

Some CDKIs have also been found to function in the initiation or maintenance of senescence. In particular, levels of p16 and p21 (in addition to p53) are often seen to increase as fibroblasts approach replicative senescence. While p53 and p21 levels may decline once senescence has been reached, p16 typically remains elevated and, therefore, may play a role in maintaining the senescent state. This is supported by recent work indicating that p16 seems to facilitate pRB-dependent formation of stable repressive chromatin foci at growth promoting genes in senescent cells.[95] These foci may explain the irreversibility of the growth arrest observed for p16-induced senescence.[96]

Several studies have been performed aimed at identifying the molecular changes that occur during the senescence of normal prostate epithelial cells in culture. Like fibroblasts, senescent prostate epithelial cells predominately accumulate in the G1 phase of the cell cycle, exhibit low levels of hyperphosphorylated pRb and other markers of cell proliferation such as PCNA, and low CDK2 activity.[66,67,97–99] As discussed above, the p53 tumor suppressor and its target gene p21 play a pivotal role in initiating senescence in fibroblasts. Similarly, Jarrard et al observed increases in p53 and p21 (and p15) in prostate epithelial cells approaching senescence, with these levels returning back to baseline in terminal senescence.[57] Focusing on the subset of genes that were both upregulated at senescence and downregulated during immortalization, three genes stood out: *BRAR*, a chemokine located on chromosome

5q; *DOC1*, a gene of unknown function downregulated in ovarian cancer; and *IGFBP3* a member of the IGF growth signaling pathway.

Several genes upregulated in senescent fibroblasts, such as ECM-degrading proteases, growth factors, and cytokines are also upregulated in senescing prostatic epithelial cells including IGF1, TGFβ, IL1, and IL6.[57,98] These results imply that, like fibroblasts, senescing epithelial cells may also display a phenotype that promotes the growth of neighboring nonsenescent cells and may contribute to induction or exacerbation of localized inflammation. The repeated findings of alterations of members of the IGF signaling pathway is especially intriguing, as this axis appears important in age-related pathologies including prostate cancer.[100–103]

Increased expression of p16 appears to be a universal finding among studies of prostate epithelial cell senescence, likely accounting for their low level of phosphorylated pRb and consequent G1 cell cycle arrest.[67,97–99] The increased levels of p16 may result from decreased levels of Id1 that normally functions to inhibit p16 transcription via Ets transcription factors.[98] p16 is often inactivated in human tumors either through mutation, deletion, or promoter hypermethylation.[15] However, p16 is infrequently mutated or methylated in prostate cancer.[104–106] On the other hand, loss of heterozygosisty (LOH) of the chromosomal vicinity of the p16 gene is observed in approximately 1 in 5 primary prostate cancers and 1 in 2 metastases, while LOH for pRB has been observed in approximately 30% of cases.[104]

Paradoxically, p16 *protein* expression is upregulated in high-grade PIN and in more than 80% of prostate cancer cases.[107–109] Given the fact that these lesions are proliferative, it would seem that despite its elevated expression p16 is ineffective in halting cell cycle progression in these settings. This may be due to inactivation of the p16/pRB pathway downstream of p16. For instance, as alluded to, LOH has been observed in a significant fraction (~30%) of prostate cancer cases and immunostaining for pRB is lacking in a significant number of prostate cancer tissues.[109,110] Alternatively, it is possible that p16-expressing cells are actually senescent but are stimulating the proliferation of neighboring cancer cells.

IMPLICATIONS OF CELLULAR SENESCENCE FOR THERAPY

As previously discussed, the majority of prostate tumors have abnormally short telomeres and are apparently immortal due to activation of the enzyme telomerase. This is a common phenotype shared by most epithelial cancers that appear to have succeeded in bypassing the senescence tumor-suppressor checkpoint at some point during their development through combinations of p53 and pRB pathway inactivation and telomere length maintenance, typically via telomerase activation. Given these observations, it would be natural to assume that tumor cells are incapable of senescing, however, this appears not to be the case. For example, various chemotherapeutic agents, differentiating agents (e.g., sodium butyrate), and radiation can induce a senescent-like arrest in tumor cells (reviewed in Shay and Roninson[92]). The prostate cancer cell line LNCaP displays approximately 10% to 15% of cells staining positively for SAβgal under normal culture conditions, possibly representing the continual generation of senescent cells.[111] It may be that cancer cells have selectively overcome *replicative* senescence (for instance, via telomerase) but that they remain able to senesce in response to other initiating factors. Along these lines, Shay and Roninson have proposed that senescence may be at work in some prostate cancers treated with radiation therapy.[92] This stems from results in which complete tumor regressions took a year or more after radiation treatment in some patients.[112] There are also indications that some growth inhibitory factors associated with senescent prostate epithelial cells such as IGFBP3, IGFBPRP1, and maspin, are markers of good prognosis.[99,113,114]

In a provocative study, by Schmitt et al, the ability of tumor cells to senesce was shown to have a profound impact on treatment outcome.[115] In this study, which involved a transgenic B-cell lymphoma mouse model, mice bearing tumors capable of undergoing drug-induced senescence had a significantly more favorable outcome following chemotherapy. When apoptosis was inhibited in the tumor cells (by forced expression of BCL2), senescence became the dominant response to treatment with cyclophosphamide. A key finding by these authors was: "The initial response to chemotherapy did not necessarily predict treatment outcome." Thus tumors may fail to regress (tumor cell death) following treatment but still produce a favorable outcome due to the induction of a cytostatic senescence response.[115] If true, then this will have important implications for the assessment of treatment efficacy.

Finally, as with senescent fibroblasts, some senescent prostate epithelial cells also secrete soluble paracrine growth stimulatory or inhibitory factors that may act to either promote or retard the growth of neighboring nonsenescent epithelial cells, and thus may be potentially procarcinogenic in some cases. Early evidence suggests that the difference between the growth promoting versus growth inhibitory phenotype may be related to the particular repertoire of CDKIs expressed in the senescent epithelial cells. This could help to explain the paradoxical unfavorable prognoses for prostate cancers expressing p16 or p21.[92]

The p16 gene is infrequently mutated in prostate cancer, and the protein is typically at low or undetectable levels in the normal prostate. However, it is expressed in PIN and in more than one half of prostate cancers, where it has been found to be an independent predictor of relapse following radical prostatectomy.[107,116,117] Then again, these findings were for organ-confined disease, and a recent study involving locally advanced disease treated with radiation therapy or radiation therapy plus androgen ablation found a *loss* of p16 protein to be correlated with adverse clinical outcome.[118]

As with p16, several studies have also found the CDKI protein p21 to be an unfavorable prognostic marker for prostate cancer. It has been positively correlated with high tumor grade, tumor proliferation (Ki67 labeling index), and also found to be an independent marker of biochemical recurrence (reviewed in Knillova et al[119]). On the other hand, not all studies support this correlation for p21. Interestingly, Sarkar et al found p21 to be a marker of disease-free survival only in whites, not in African Americans, indicating the potential for significant dependence on patient ethnicity.[120]

CONCLUSIONS

Given the altered phenotypes observed for both senescent fibroblasts and senescent prostatic epithelial cells described above, we may speculate on their potential impact on the development of prostate cancer as men age. Although senescent cells do not proliferate, they may accumulate over time, and their altered functions may act to promote the transformation and growth of nearby transformed cells by:

1. Attracting and stimulating immune effector cells leading to chronic inflammation, which in turn causes local cell turnover in a genotoxic environment. A vicious cycle may then become established as inflammation could lead to increased numbers of proinflammatory senescent cells.

2. Stimulation of epithelial cell growth due to paracrine growth factors secreted by senescent cells and the release of growth factors from the ECM due to ECM degradation activity.
3. Creation of a permissive environment for tumor cell invasion via senescent cells' ECM-remodeling activities.

Thus, it appears that aging may foster the development of prostate cancer in two ways. First, by the simple accrual over time of pro-oncogenic mutations in long-lived tissue stem cells—an inevitable occurrence since no maintenance process is 100% efficient. Second, as cells become senescent, their phenotype can alter in ways that promote the growth of surrounding cells, particularly transformed cells, and also promote inflammation via proinflammatory cytokines.[60,61] Again, this could initiate a viscous cycle, in which inflammation drives further proliferation locally, producing more senescent cells that then feedback and sustain the inflammatory response (Figure 32.2). Such a process could help to explain the existence of focal inflammation in the prostate; a common histologic finding that increases with age but the etiology of which is poorly understood at present.[62–64]

Senescent stroma resembles the activated stroma seen in wound healing.[60,61] The altered stromal–epithelial signaling in such an activated state may lead to continuous tissue regeneration in an environment of chronic inflammation, perhaps resulting in PIA. Over time, epithelial stem cells or intermediate cells with stem-like properties proliferating in this genotoxic environment

may suffer mutations in key growth regulatory pathways, such as the hedgehog signaling pathway, leading to clonal expansion of the abnormal cells, and culminating in the emergence of PIN. During this process, telomeres will shorten due to proliferation and/or oxidative stress. Telomere-based replicative senescence may then act to limit the majority of PIN lesions from progressing further, but it may also lead to the appearance of senescent stromal and epithelial cells with growth-promoting phenotypes. Despite the stringent barrier to tumorigenesis posed by cellular senescence, rare mutant cells may bypass senescence and continue to divide, eventually experiencing critical telomere shortening and concomitant chromosomal instability, and leading to further oncogenic mutations resulting in invasive cancer. Finally, immortalization by telomere length stabilization, most commonly through telomerase activation, is required to allow for unlimited tumor expansion.

A full understanding of the details of senescence-related processes potentially involved in prostate tumorigenesis will hopefully lead to new targets for therapy. For instance, the findings of hedgehog pathway activation and the reliance on telomerase in most prostate cancers gives hope that inhibitors of these pathways may be efficacious in treating this disease. Likewise, it appears that even without apoptosis the induction of senescence in tumor cells may be a valid therapeutic goal, albeit one requiring a broader definition of what constitutes a positive clinical response. However, there are indications that not all senescent cells behave equally—in some cases, senescing cancer cells may act to stimulate the growth and survival

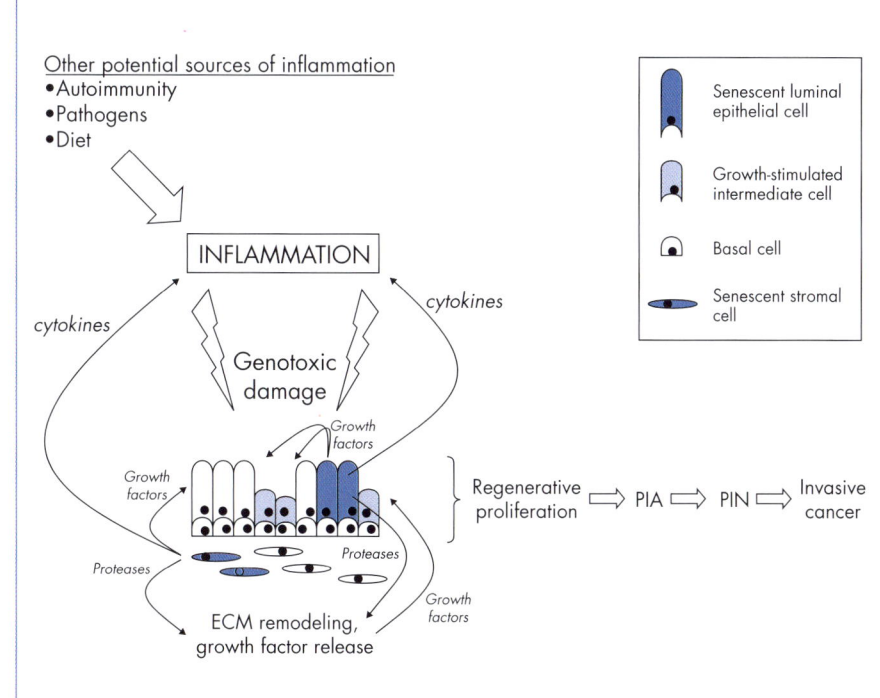

Fig. 32.2
Model for role of senescent cells in promoting prostate cancer. Senescent stromal and epithelial cells may stimulate neighboring cells by expressing positive growth factors or releasing bound growth factors from the extracellular membrane (ECM). Senescent cells may also stimulate inflammation via secreted cytokines. Inflammation can cause genotoxic damage and incite regenerative proliferation causing mutations and the production of more senescent cells that positively feedback on the inflammation promoting a viscous cycle. Chronic stimulation and damage eventually leads to the production of mutated stem cells/transient amplifying intermediate cells, prostatic inflammatory atrophy (PIA), prostatic intraepithelial neoplasia (PIN), and cancer.

of the surrounding non-senescing tumor cells. Effective senescence-based therapies then would be those that guide senescent cells into either growth-neutral or growth-inhibitory modes.

Finally, one can envision contributions from this field of study to the area of chemoprevention. Should it be shown that senescent cells actually do accumulate and contribute to prostate tumorigenesis then strategies aimed at either preventing their accumulation or eliminating them from the prostate may help to reduce the incidence of prostate cancer as men age.

REFERENCES

1. Jemal A, Tiwari RC, Murray T, et al. Cancer statistics, 2004. CA Cancer J Clin 2004;54:8–29.

2. Ruijter E, van de Kaa C, Miller G, et al. Molecular genetics and epidemiology of prostate carcinoma. Endocr Rev 1999;20:22–45.

3. Kirkwood TB. Immortality of the germ-line versus disposability of the soma. Basic Life Sci 1987;42:209–218.

4. Hartwell L. Defects in a cell cycle checkpoint may be responsible for the genomic instability of cancer cells. Cell 1992;71:543–546.

5. Vogelstein B, Kinzler KW. Cancer genes and the pathways they control. Nat Med 2004;10:789–799.

6. Weinberg RA. Oncogenes, antioncogenes, and the molecular bases of multistep carcinogenesis. Cancer Res 1989;49:3713–3721.

7. Cowen D, Troncoso P, Khoo VS, et al. Ki-67 staining is an independent correlate of biochemical failure in prostate cancer treated with radiotherapy. Clin Cancer Res 2002;8:1148–1154.

8. Li R, Heydon K, Hammond ME, et al. Ki-67 staining index predicts distant metastasis and survival in locally advanced prostate cancer treated with radiotherapy: an analysis of patients in radiation therapy oncology group protocol 86-10. Clin Cancer Res 2004;10:4118–4124.

9. Stapleton AM, Zbell P, Kattan MW, et al. Assessment of the biologic markers p53, Ki-67, and apoptotic index as predictive indicators of prostate carcinoma recurrence after surgery. Cancer 1998;82:168–175.

10. Pollack A, DeSilvio M, Khor LY, et al. Ki-67 staining is a strong predictor of distant metastasis and mortality for men with prostate cancer treated with radiotherapy plus androgen deprivation: Radiation Therapy Oncology Group Trial 92-02. J Clin Oncol 2004;22:2133–2140.

11. Tsihlias J, Kapusta L, Slingerland J. The prognostic significance of altered cyclin-dependent kinase inhibitors in human cancer. Annu Rev Med 1999;50:401–423.

12. Nelson WG, De Marzo AM, Isaacs WB. Prostate cancer. N Engl J Med 2003;349:366–381.

13. Visakorpi T. The molecular genetics of prostate cancer. Urology 2003;62:3–10.

14. Roy-Burman P, Wu H, Powell WC, et al. Genetically defined mouse models that mimic natural aspects of human prostate cancer development. Endocr Relat Cancer 2004;11:225–254.

15. Sherr CJ. Principles of tumor suppression. Cell 2004;116:235–246.

16. Cairns J. Mutation selection and the natural history of cancer. Nature 1975;255:197–200.

17. Nowell PC. The clonal evolution of tumor cell populations. Science 1976;194:23–28.

18. Potten CS. Stem Cells. Cambridge: Academic Press, 1997.

19. Isaacs JT, Coffey DS. Etiology and disease process of benign prostatic hyperplasia. Prostate Suppl 1989;2:33–50.

20. Foster CS, Dodson A, Karavana V, et al. Prostatic stem cells. J Pathol 2002;197:551–565.

21. Potten CS, Loeffler M. Stem cells: attributes, cycles, spirals, pitfalls and uncertainties. Lessons for and from the crypt. Development 1990;110:1001–1020.

22. Pierce GB. Neoplasms, differentiations and mutations. Am J Pathol 1974;77:103–118.

23. Bonkhoff H, Remberger K. Differentiation pathways and histogenetic aspects of normal and abnormal prostatic growth: a stem cell model. Prostate 1996;28:98–106.

24. Kinbara H, Cunha GR, Boutin E, et al. Evidence of stem cells in the adult prostatic epithelium based upon responsiveness to mesenchymal inductors. Prostate 1996;29:107–116.

25. Sugimura Y, Cunha GR, Donjacour AA. Morphological and histological study of castration-induced degeneration and androgen-induced regeneration in the mouse prostate. Biol Reprod 1986;34:973–983.

26. Huss WJ, Gray DR, Werdin ES, et al. Evidence of pluripotent human prostate stem cells in a human prostate primary xenograft model. Prostate 2004;60:77–90.

27. De Marzo AM, Nelson WG, Meeker AK, et al. Stem cell features of benign and malignant prostate epithelial cells. J Urol 1998;160:2381–2392.

28. Isaacs JT, Lundmo PI, Berges R, et al. Androgen regulation of programmed death of normal and malignant prostatic cells. J Androl 1992;13:457–464.

29. Bostwick DG, Pacelli A, Lopez-Beltran A. Molecular biology of prostatic intraepithelial neoplasia. Prostate 1996;29:117–134.

30. Sakr WA, Grignon DJ. Prostatic intraepithelial neoplasia and atypical adenomatous hyperplasia. Relationship to pathologic parameters, volume and spatial distribution of carcinoma of the prostate. Anal Quant Cytol Histol 1998;20:417–423.

31. Verhagen AP, Ramaekers FC, Aalders TW, et al. Colocalization of basal and luminal cell-type cytokeratins in human prostate cancer. Cancer Res 1992;52:6182–6187.

32. Schalken JA, van Leenders G. Cellular and molecular biology of the prostate: stem cell biology. Urology 2003;62:11–20.

33. Wang Y, Hayward S, Cao M, et al. Cell differentiation lineage in the prostate. Differentiation 2001;68:270–279.

34. De Marzo AM, Meeker AK, Epstein JI, et al. Prostate stem cell compartments: expression of the cell cycle inhibitor p27Kip1 in normal, hyperplastic, and neoplastic cells. Am J Pathol 1998;153:911–919.

35. Karhadkar SS, Bova GS, Abdallah N, et al. Hedgehog signalling in prostate regeneration, neoplasia and metastasis. Nature 2004;431:707–712.

36. Beachy PA, Karhadkar SS, Berman DM. Tissue repair and stem cell renewal in carcinogenesis. Nature 2004;432:324–331.

37. Sanchez P, Hernandez AM, Stecca B, et al. Inhibition of prostate cancer proliferation by interference with SONIC HEDGEHOG-GLI1 signaling. Proc Natl Acad Sci USA 2004;101:12561–12566.

38. Dimri GP, Martinez JL, Jacobs JJ, et al. The Bmi-1 oncogene induces telomerase activity and immortalizes human mammary epithelial cells. Cancer Res 2002;62:4736–4745.

39. Jacobs JJ, Kieboom K, Marino S, et al. The oncogene and Polycomb-group gene bmi-1 regulates cell proliferation and senescence through the ink4a locus. Nature 1999;397:164–168.

40. Kiyono T, Foster SA, Koop JI, et al. Both Rb/p16INK4a inactivation and telomerase activity are required to immortalize human epithelial cells. Nature 1998;396:84–88.

41. Lee WH, Morton RA, Epstein JI, et al. Cytidine methylation of regulatory sequences near the pi-class glutathione S-transferase gene accompanies human prostatic carcinogenesis. Proc Natl Acad Sci USA 1994;91:11733–11737.

42. Nakayama M, Gonzalgo ML, Yegnasubramanian S, et al. GSTP1 CpG island hypermethylation as a molecular biomarker for prostate cancer. J Cell Biochem 2004;91:540–552.

43. Nakayama M, Bennett CJ, Hicks JL, et al. Hypermethylation of the human glutathione S-transferase-pi gene (GSTP1) CpG island is present in a subset of proliferative inflammatory atrophy lesions but not in normal or hyperplastic epithelium of the prostate: a detailed study using laser-capture microdissection. Am J Pathol 2003;163:923–933.

44. De Marzo AM, Putzi MJ, Nelson WG. New concepts in the pathology of prostatic epithelial carcinogenesis. Urology 2001;57:103–114.

45. Hartwell LH, Kastan MB. Cell cycle control and cancer. Science 1994;266:1821–1828.

46. Warner HR. Aging and regulation of apoptosis. Curr Top Cell Regul 1997;35:107–121.

47. Okada H, Mak TW. Pathways of apoptotic and non-apoptotic death in tumour cells. Nat Rev Cancer 2004;4:592–603.

48. Hayflick L, Moorhead PS. The serial cultivation of human diploid cell strains. Exp Cell Res 1961;25:585–621.

49. Dimri GP, Lee X, Basile G, et al. A biomarker that identifies senescent human cells in culture and in aging skin in vivo. Proc Natl Acad Sci USA 1995;92:9363–9367.

50. Severino J, Allen RG, Balin S, et al. Is beta-galactosidase staining a marker of senescence in vitro and in vivo? Exp Cell Res 2000;257:162–171.

51. Untergasser G, Gander R, Rumpold H, et al. TGF-beta cytokines increase senescence-associated beta-galactosidase activity in human prostate basal cells by supporting differentiation processes, but not cellular senescence. Exp Gerontol 2003;38:1179–1188.

52. Wang E. Senescent human fibroblasts resist programmed cell death, and failure to suppress bcl2 is involved. Cancer Res 1995;55:2284–2292.

53. Chen QM. Replicative senescence and oxidant-induced premature senescence. Beyond the control of cell cycle checkpoints. Ann NY Acad Sci 2000;908:111–125.

54. Goldstein S. Replicative senescence: the human fibroblast comes of age. Science 1990;249:1129–1133.

55. Dimri GP, Campisi J. Molecular and cell biology of replicative senescence. Cold Spring Harb Symp Quant Biol 1994;59:67–73.

56. Cristofalo VJ. Cellular senescence: cell proliferation and its control. Adv Pathobiol 1980;7:100–114.

57. Schwarze SR, Shi Y, Fu VX, et al. Role of cyclin-dependent kinase inhibitors in the growth arrest at senescence in human prostate epithelial and uroepithelial cells. Oncogene 2001;20:8184–8192.

58. Sager R. Senescence as a mode of tumor suppression. Environ Health Perspect 1991;93:59–62.

59. Shay JW. Aging and cancer: are telomeres and telomerase the connection? Mol Med Today 1995;1:378–384.

60. Shelton DN, Chang E, Whittier PS, et al. Microarray analysis of replicative senescence. Curr Biol 1999;9:939–945.

61. Krtolica A, Parrinello S, Lockett S, et al. Senescent fibroblasts promote epithelial cell growth and tumorigenesis: a link between cancer and aging. Proc Natl Acad Sci USA 2001;98:12072–12077.

62. Platz EA, De Marzo AM. Epidemiology of inflammation and prostate cancer. J Urol 2004;171:S36–40.

63. Robinette CL. Sex-hormone-induced inflammation and fibromuscular proliferation in the rat lateral prostate. Prostate 1988;12:271–286.

64. Kohnen PW, Drach GW. Patterns of inflammation in prostatic hyperplasia: a histologic and bacteriologic study. J Urol 1979;121:755–760.

65. Cristofalo VJ, Allen RG, Pignolo RJ, et al. Relationship between donor age and the replicative lifespan of human cells in culture: a reevaluation. Proc Natl Acad Sci USA 1998;95:10614–10619.

66. Castro P, Giri D, Lamb D, et al. Cellular senescence in the pathogenesis of benign prostatic hyperplasia. Prostate 2003;55:30–38.

67. Choi J, Shendrik I, Peacocke M, et al. Expression of senescence-associated beta-galactosidase in enlarged prostates from men with benign prostatic hyperplasia. Urology 2000;56:160–166.

68. Tuxhorn JA, Ayala GE, Smith MJ, et al. Reactive stroma in human prostate cancer: induction of myofibroblast phenotype and extracellular matrix remodeling. Clin Cancer Res 2002;8:2912–2923.

69. Cunha GR, Hayward SW, Wang YZ. Role of stroma in carcinogenesis of the prostate. Differentiation 2002;70:473–485.

70. Harley CB, Futcher AB, Greider CW. Telomeres shorten during ageing of human fibroblasts. Nature 1990;345:458–460.

71. Blackburn EH. Structure and function of telomeres. Nature 1991;350:569–567

72. Levy MZ, Allsopp RC, Futcher AB, et al. Telomere end-replication problem and cell aging. J Mol Biol 1992;225:951–960.

73. Kruk PA, Rampino NJ, Bohr VA. DNA damage and repair in telomeres: relation to aging. Proc Natl Acad Sci USA 1995;92:258–262.

74. von Zglinicki T, Pilger R, Sitte N. Accumulation of single-strand breaks is the major cause of telomere shortening in human fibroblasts. Free Radic Biol Med 2000;28:64–74.

75. Greider CW, Blackburn EH. Identification of a specific telomere terminal transferase activity in Tetrahymena extracts. Cell 1985;43:405–413.

76. Reddel RR, Bryan TM, Colgin LM, et al. Alternative lengthening of telomeres in human cells. Radiat Res 2001;155:194–200.

77. Bodnar AG, Ouellette M, Frolkis M, et al. Extension of life-span by introduction of telomerase into normal human cells. Science 1998;279:349–352.

78. Vaziri H, Benchimol S. Reconstitution of telomerase activity in normal human cells leads to elongation of telomeres and extended replicative life span. Curr Biol 1998;8:279–282.

79. Jacobs JJ, de Lange T. Significant role for p16(INK4a) in p53-independent telomere-directed senescence. Curr Biol 2004;14:2302–2308.

80. Hahn WC, Counter CM, Lundberg AS, et al. Creation of human tumour cells with defined genetic elements. Nature 1999;400:464–468.

81. Sommerfeld HJ, Meeker AK, Piatyszek MA, et al. Telomerase activity: a prevalent marker of malignant human prostate tissue. Cancer Res 1996;56:218–222.

82. Meeker AK, Sommerfeld HJ, Coffey DS. Telomerase is activated in the prostate and seminal vesicles of the castrated rat. Endocrinology 1996;137:5743–5746.

83. Ravindranath N, Ioffe SL, Marshall GR, et al. Androgen depletion activates telomerase in the prostate of the nonhuman primate, *Macaca mulatta*. Prostate 2001;49:79–89.

84. Meeker AK. Telomere Dynamics and Androgen Regulation of Telomerase Enzymatic Activity in Normal and Pathological States of the Prostate. Baltimore: Johns Hopkins University School of Medicine, 2001.

85. Guo C, Armbruster BN, Price DT, et al. In vivo regulation of hTERT expression and telomerase activity by androgen. J Urol 2003;170:615–618.

86. Iczkowski KA, Bostwick DG. Prostate biopsy interpretation. Current concepts, 1999. Urol Clin North Am 1999;26:435–452.

87. Bouchal J, Kolar Z, Mad'arova J, et al. The effects of natural ligands of hormone receptors and their antagonists on telomerase activity in the androgen sensitive prostatic cancer cell line LNCaP. Biochem Pharmacol 2002;63:1177–1181.

88. Gil J, Bernard D, Martinez D, et al. Polycomb CBX7 has a unifying role in cellular lifespan. Nat Cell Biol 2004;6:67–72.

89. Meeker AK, Hicks JL, Platz EA, et al. Telomere shortening is an early somatic DNA alteration in human prostate tumorigenesis. Cancer Res 2002;62:6405–6409.

90. Vukovic B, Park PC, Al-Maghrabi J, et al. Evidence of multifocality of telomere erosion in high-grade prostatic intraepithelial neoplasia (HPIN) and concurrent carcinoma. Oncogene 2003;22:1978–1987.

91. Itahana K, Campisi J, Dimri GP. Mechanisms of cellular senescence in human and mouse cells. Biogerontology 2004;5:1–10.

92. Shay JW, Roninson IB. Hallmarks of senescence in carcinogenesis and cancer therapy. Oncogene 2004;23:2919–2933.

93. Miele L. The biology of cyclins and cyclin-dependent protein kinases: an introduction. Methods Mol Biol 2004;285:3–21.

94. Sherr CJ, Roberts JM. CDK inhibitors: positive and negative regulators of G1-phase progression. Genes Dev 1999;13:1501–1512.

95. Narita M, Nunez S, Heard E, et al. Rb-mediated heterochromatin formation and silencing of E2F target genes during cellular senescence. Cell 2003;113:703–716.

96. Beausejour CM, Krtolica A, Galimi F, et al. Reversal of human cellular senescence: roles of the p53 and p16 pathways. Embo J 2003;22:4212–4222.

97. Sandhu C, Peehl DM, Slingerland J. p16INK4A mediates cyclin dependent kinase 4 and 6 inhibition in senescent prostatic epithelial cells. Cancer Res 2000;60:2616–2622.

98. Untergasser G, Koch HB, Menssen A, et al. Characterization of epithelial senescence by serial analysis of gene expression: identification of genes potentially involved in prostate cancer. Cancer Res 2002;62:6255–6262.

99. Schwarze SR, DePrimo SE, Grabert LM, et al. Novel pathways associated with bypassing cellular senescence in human prostate epithelial cells. J Biol Chem 2002;277:14877–14883.

100. Lopez-Bermejo A, Buckway CK, Devi GR, et al. Characterization of insulin-like growth factor-binding protein-related proteins (IGFBP-rPs) 1, 2, and 3 in human prostate epithelial cells: potential roles for IGFBP-rP1 and 2 in senescence of the prostatic epithelium. Endocrinology 2000;141:4072–4080.

101. Sonntag WE, Lynch CD, Cefalu WT, et al. Pleiotropic effects of growth hormone and insulin-like growth factor (IGF)-1 on biological aging: inferences from moderate caloric-restricted animals. J Gerontol A Biol Sci Med Sci 1999;54:B521–538.

102. Slater M, Barden JA, Murphy CR. Changes in growth factor expression in the ageing prostate may disrupt epithelial-stromal homeostasis. Histochem J 2000;32:357–364.

103. Harman SM, Metter EJ, Blackman MR, et al. Serum levels of insulin-like growth factor I (IGF-I), IGF-II, IGF-binding protein-3, and prostate-specific antigen as predictors of clinical prostate cancer. J Clin Endocrinol Metab 2000;85:4258–4265.

104. Jarrard DF, Bova GS, Ewing CM, et al. Deletional, mutational, and methylation analyses of CDKN2 (p16/MTS1) in primary and metastatic prostate cancer. Genes Chromosomes Cancer 1997;19:90–96.

105. Nguyen TT, Nguyen CT, Gonzales FA, et al. Analysis of cyclin-dependent kinase inhibitor expression and methylation patterns in human prostate cancers. Prostate 2000;43:233–242.

106. Yegnasubramanian S, Kowalski J, Gonzalgo ML, et al. Hypermethylation of CpG islands in primary and metastatic human prostate cancer. Cancer Res 2004;64:1975–1986.

107. Lee CT, Capodieci P, Osman I, et al. Overexpression of the cyclin-dependent kinase inhibitor p16 is associated with tumor recurrence in human prostate cancer. Clin Cancer Res 1999;5:977–983.

108. Henshall SM, Quinn DI, Lee CS, et al. Overexpression of the cell cycle inhibitor p16INK4A in high-grade prostatic intraepithelial neoplasia predicts early relapse in prostate cancer patients. Clin Cancer Res 2001;7:544–550.

109. Jarrard DF, Modder J, Fadden P, et al. Alterations in the p16/pRb cell cycle checkpoint occur commonly in primary and metastatic human prostate cancer. Cancer Lett 2002;185:191–199.

110. Brooks JD, Bova GS, Isaacs WB. Allelic loss of the retinoblastoma gene in primary human prostatic adenocarcinomas. Prostate 1995;26:35–39.

111. Chang BD, Broude EV, Dokmanovic M, et al. A senescence-like phenotype distinguishes tumor cells that undergo terminal proliferation arrest after exposure to anticancer agents. Cancer Res 1999;59:3761–3767.

112. Cox JD, Kline RW. Do prostatic biopsies 12 months or more after external irradiation for adenocarcinoma, Stage III, predict long-term survival? Int J Radiat Oncol Biol Phys 1983;9:299–303.

113. Shariat SF, Lamb DJ, Kattan MW, et al. Association of preoperative plasma levels of insulin-like growth factor I and insulin-like growth factor binding proteins-2 and -3 with prostate cancer invasion, progression, and metastasis. J Clin Oncol 2002;20:833–841.

114. Machtens S, Serth J, Bokemeyer C, et al. Expression of the p53 and Maspin protein in primary prostate cancer: correlation with clinical features. Int J Cancer 2001;95:337–342.

115. Schmitt CA, Fridman JS, Yang M, et al. A senescence program controlled by p53 and p16INK4a contributes to the outcome of cancer therapy. Cell 2002;109:335–346.

116. Gu K, Mes-Masson AM, Gauthier J, et al. Analysis of the p16 tumor suppressor gene in early-stage prostate cancer. Mol Carcinog 1998;21:164–170.

117. Halvorsen OJ, Hostmark J, Haukaas S, et al. Prognostic significance of p16 and CDK4 proteins in localized prostate carcinoma. Cancer 2000;88:416–424.

118. Chakravarti A, Heydon K, Wu CL, et al. Loss of p16 expression is of prognostic significance in locally advanced prostate cancer: an analysis from the Radiation Therapy Oncology Group protocol 86-10. J Clin Oncol 2003;21:3328–3334.

119. Knillova J, Kolar Z, Hlobilkova A. The significance of key regulators of apoptosis in the development and prognosis of prostate carcinoma. II. Products of suppressor genes Rb and PTEN, CDKI, Fas. Biomed Pap Med Fac Univ Palacky Olomouc Czech Repub 2003;147:11–17.

120. Sarkar FH, Li Y, Sakr WA, et al. Relationship of p21(WAF1) expression with disease-free survival and biochemical recurrence in prostate adenocarcinomas (PCa). Prostate 1999;40:256–260.

Angiogenesis and prostate cancer

33

Mark Rochester, Jeremy Crew

INTRODUCTION

Angiogenesis is the growth of new blood vessels from existing ones. It is characterized by increased endothelial cell proliferation, migration, and new blood vessel formation, and it is crucial for physiologic processes, such as embryogenesis, and wound healing. It is also involved in pathologic conditions including psoriasis, endometriosis, ischemic heart disease, and rheumatoid arthritis. Much interest followed the discovery of its role in tumor biology.

Diffusion is adequate for oxygen and nutrient delivery to tumors up to 3 mm.[3] In order to grow, invade, and metastasize tumors need to develop a blood supply, as low oxygen tension occurs 100 to 200 μm from capillaries, at the limit for oxygen diffusion within extracellular fluid. In the 1970s Folkman demonstrated that tumor cells interact with their environment to stimulate new vessel growth and that growth and metastasis occurs rapidly once neovascularization has occurred.[1,2] Tumors are more vascular than normal tissue, and their new vessels differ from surrounding mature vessels.[3] Vascular architecture within areas of angiogenesis is disorganized and irregular with permeable endothelium as a result of incompetent intercellular junctions and incomplete basement membranes. This makes vessels "leaky"[4] and may increase tumor cell invasion and metastasis.

QUANTIFICATION OF ANGIOGENESIS

In the 1990s, the development of specific endothelial markers (CD31, CD34, and factor VIII related antigen) allowed accurate identification of endothelial cells using immunohistochemistry. This allowed microvessel density (MVD) within a tumor to be quantified as a marker of angiogenesis.[5] Many studies reported that quantification of angiogenesis within tumors yielded information regarding the response to radiotherapy,[6] chemotherapy,[7] and hormonal therapy, as well as prognosis.[8] Inconsistencies between results from different studies led to criticism of the lack of standardization of methodology. Various endothelial antibodies, vascular parameters (i.e., vessel numbers, surface area, or perimeter), quantification sites (i.e., hot spots, average over whole field, average over 3 representative areas), counting techniques, and statistical analyses have been employed. In 2002, the publication of the second international consensus on the methodology and evaluation of angiogenesis quantification attempted to address these issues.[9]

Factors involved in tumor angiogenesis have been investigated as possible surrogate markers for angiogenesis. Individual factors have been measured in most body compartments including tumor tissue, blood, serum, and urine. This approach has provided prognostic information as well as information regarding the interaction and expression of these factors within tumors.

The association between tumor grade and angiogenesis in prostate cancer was first shown by Wakui,[10] who showed that MVD predicted bone metastases. High MVD has also been shown to predict extraprostatic extension and lymph node metastases in prostate cancer,[11–13] and it is suggested that MVD can predict disease-free survival in radical prostatectomy[14] and overall survival in biopsies from patients managed by watchful waiting.[15]

THE ANGIOGENIC SWITCH

Normal endothelial cells are non-angiogenic, reflecting the balance between angiogenesis stimulators and inhibitors. In hypovascular tissues, such as cornea or cartilage, high levels of natural inhibitors prevent blood vessel development.[16] Altering the balance of competing factors can result in new blood vessel growth.

Similarly, in tumors, the generation of a blood supply is achieved through a shift in balance of these factors. The shift in favor of stimulators is known as the "angiogenic switch" (Figure 33.1), and occurs at an early stage. It may result from changes in the local environment, such as hypoxia, acidosis, and hypoglycemia, as well as mechanical strain due to tissue growth. Genetic mutation, causing dysregulation of angiogenic factors, may also affect the balance.

ANGIOGENESIS FACTORS

Most solid tumors produce a number of different angiogenic growth factors. These impact upon the angiogenic pathway at different points and vary in importance between tumor types. A large number of molecules with angiogenic capability have been described and are reviewed elsewhere.[17] The principle factors involved in the process are discussed in more detail, with particular reference to prostate cancer.

VASCULAR ENDOTHELIAL GROWTH FACTOR

Vascular endothelial growth factor A (VEGFA) is the most studied factor of a family of related proteins (VEGFA, -B, -C, -D, and placental growth factor). mRNA splice variants coding for different proteins produce further diversity. All the factors within the family are potent chemoattractants and mitogens for endothelial cells and are central to angiogenesis.

Vascular endothelial growth factor is produced by tumor cells, platelets, lymphocytes, and macrophages.

Its effects are mediated through receptors expressed mainly on endothelial cells. The most extensively investigated receptors are the flt1 and Flk1/KDR receptors. Once stimulated, the endothelial cells produce proteins that degrade the extracellular matrix (ECM) allowing migration and invasion. In addition, endothelial cell adhesion becomes incompetent, leading to increased permeability and further increase in interstitial plasminogen and plasmin.

Expression of VEGF within many tumors has been shown to be associated with a poor prognosis[18,19] and resistance to anticancer therapies. In prostate cancer studies have shown that cancer cells stain for VEGF, and that this correlates with MVD.[20] Normal and benign prostatic hyperplasia (BPH) tissue had little VEGF staining and vascularity.[21] The expression of VEGF has been linked to neuroendocrine differentiation in prostate cancer, a poor prognostic indicator.[22,23]

In-vivo studies of modified metastatic prostate cancer cell lines have suggested enhanced VEGF production and tumor vascularity compared with prostate cancer cells of lower metastatic potential.[24] When PC-3M (highly metastatic) and DU145 (poorly metastatic) are injected orthotopically into nude mice, angiogenesis is more evident in PC-3M tumors compared with DU145 tumours.[25]

MATRIX METALLOPROTEINASES

Matrix metalloproteinases (MMPs) are enzymes that cleave ECM components through their proteolytic action. The effect is to induce other angiogenic factors rather than directly stimulate endothelial cells. MMP2 (gelatinase A) and MMP9 (gelatinase B) are the most studied. Increased MMP2 expression by malignant prostatic epithelia has been shown to be an independent predictor of decreased survival.[26] Endogenous inhibitors of MMPs are seen, known as tissue inhibitors of MMP (TIMPs), perhaps producing a controlled environment of proteolysis. An imbalance of MMPs and TIMPs has been shown in malignant prostatic epithelium.[27]

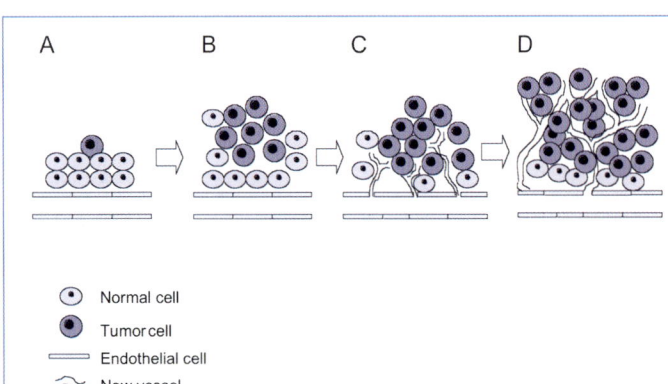

A B C D

⊙ Normal cell
◉ Tumor cell
═ Endothelial cell
∿ New vessel

Fig. 33.1
The angiogenic switch. Tumor begins as dormant nodule (A). Cells survive by diffusion until the tumor is 2–3 mm³ (B). A change in the balance of stimulating inhibiting factors, the "angiogenic switch" leads to new vessel sprouting (C), and the continually growing tumor develops its own blood supply (D).

THYMIDINE PHOSPHORYLASE

Thymidine phosphorylase (platelet-derived endothelial growth factor) is an enzyme involved in pyrimidine metabolism. It catalyses phosphorylation of thymidine to 2-deoxy-D-ribose-1-phosphate, and its angiogenic action appears to be mediated through extracellular 2-deoxy-D-ribose. Thymidine phosphorylase may have a role in allowing solid tumors to withstand hypoxia and enhance invasion and metastasis through induction of VEGF, interleukins, and MMP1. Thymidine phosphorylase mRNA expression correlated with the protein expression level, MVD, and Gleason score in one prostate cancer study. It also correlated with VEGF expression and blood flow, but not with stage or prostate-specific antigen (PSA),[28] supporting previous work that suggested stromal cell expression might play an important role in tumor angiogenesis in prostate cancer.[29]

BASIC FIBROBLAST GROWTH FACTOR

The fibroblast growth factors (FGFs) are a family of nine structurally related peptides expressed by the prostate in varying levels.[30] They regulate ECM production and contribute to angiogenesis in tumours.[12] Basic fibroblast growth factor (bFGF) exerts its action through binding to the tyrosine kinase FGF receptor 1. Angiogenesis induction has been demonstrated in response to bFGF in the rabbit corneal model.[31] It has been shown that VEGF and bFGF are synergistic for angiogenesis induction.[32] Elevated levels of bFGF have been demonstrated in the urine of some prostate cancer patients,[33] and high serum levels have also been found.[34] In vitro, androgen-independent, moderately metastatic DU145 and highly metastatic PC3- cells produce active bFGF, and express large amounts of FGF receptor mRNA, in contrast to nonmetastatic LNCaP.[35] The more aggressive PC-3M cell line is more angiogenic and displays greater bFGF staining than the less aggressive DU145 cell line.[25] No correlation of urinary and serum VEGF and bFGF with prognosis has been found.[36,37]

TRANSFORMING GROWTH FACTOR-β

The role of transforming growth factor-β (TGFβ) in prostate cancer is unclear. It inhibits epithelial cell growth and stimulates the growth of stromal cells. Prostate cancer cell growth in vitro is inhibited by TGFβ but this can be overcome by growth factors or ECM components.[38] Prostate cancer cells in vivo acquire resistance to inhibition by TGFβ as they become more aggressive. Overexpression of TGFβ and loss of the TGFβ receptor are associated with poor prognosis in prostate cancer.[39] The expression of TGFβ correlates with tumor vascularity, grade, and metastasis,[40] and resistance to TGFβ growth inhibition and TGFβ stimulated angiogenesis and metastasis may explain this variable role. Epithelial cell TGFβ staining is more extensive in prostate cancer than in BPH,[41] and increased intracellular staining is found in patients with lymph node involvement compared with patients with localized disease.[42] This supports the concept of TGFβ enhancing tumorigenicity in contrast to its inhibitory role in benign tissue.

ANDROGENS/MACROPHAGES

Androgens are involved in blood flow regulation in the prostate in vivo.[43,44] Castration inhibits VEGF expression and induces apoptosis of endothelial cells that precedes the apoptosis of tumor cells in vivo.[45] Chemical castration 7 to 28 days prior to radical prostatectomy results in tremendous recruitment of inflammatory cells in resected histologic specimens.[46] Tumor-associated macrophages (TAMs) play an important role in tumor angiogenesis.[47] Reduced infiltration of TAMs has been associated with prostate cancer progression,[48] and they can influence alterations of the local ECM, induce endothelial cells to migration or proliferation, and inhibit vascular growth.[49]

CYCLOOXYGENASE 2

Cyclooxygenase 2 (COX2) plays a role in hypoxia-induced angiogenesis through its interaction with VEGF. In BPH, membranous expression of COX2 in luminal glandular cells occurs without stromal expression. In cancer, epithelial COX2 expression was four-fold greater in one study, with a change in the staining pattern from membranous to cytoplasmic, and COX2 levels were higher in more poorly differentiated tumours.[50]

ANGIOGENESIS INHIBITORS

The discovery of endogenous inhibitors of angiogenesis attracted widespread interest due to the potential as anticancer therapy. It may appear a paradox that tumors produce inhibitors of angiogenesis until it is appreciated that temporal and spatial coordination of expression of these factors is essential for successful neovascularization. Their presence may explain why tumor cells may remain dormant for many years as tumor cell apoptosis (due to hypoxia) balances proliferation. Net loss of inhibitors resulting in an angiogenic switch would favor increased tumor cell survival with tumor "awakening."

- Angiostatin was the first endogenous inhibitor to be characterized. It is a 38 kDa protein originally isolated from the urine from the Lewis Lung carcinoma mouse model,[51] and led to the discovery of other inhibitors. These include angiostatin (cleaved from plasminogen), serpin antithrombin,[52] PEX,[53] 14 kDa prolactin fragment,[54] laminin,[55] and endostatin, among others. PC3 tumors in nude mice maintain quiescence on systemic administration of angiostatin.[56]

- Endostatin is related to angiostatin and is the best-studied endogenous inhibitor.[57,58] Disappointingly, the significant preclinical success with this peptide has not been translated in successful human trials.[59–61,62]

- Prostate-specific antigen is a serine protease. It has been shown that PSA can convert plasminogen to biologically active angiostatin-like fragments[63] and reduce the proliferation, migration, and invasion of endothelial cell lines after stimulation by FGF2 and VEGF.[64] Recombinant PSAs have been developed that inhibit angiogenesis in vitro and in vivo.[65] In contrast, PSA does not directly affect the proliferation of PC3 cells.[64,66] These effects may contribute to the slow progression of prostate cancer as PSA elevations may be part of a physiological response to combat tumor progression.

- Thrombospondin 1 (TSP1) is a 430 kDa antiangiogenic glycoprotein. It inhibits the activity of VEGF and bFGF in a range of cell types.[67,68,69] This effect appears in part to be controlled through the p53 tumor suppressor gene.[67] Transfection of DU145 cells with the TSP1 gene does not exert any growth inhibitory activity in vitro, but overexpression inhibits growth in vivo and lowers MVD.[70] Decreased expression of TSP1 in prostate cancer when compared with that in BPH or PIN has suggested a role in tumor progression.[71]

- Overexpression of IL-10 in primary prostate cancer cell cultures followed by orthotopic implantation in SCID mice induces TIMP1 expression and inhibits MMP2 expression.[72] The relationship between interleukin 10 (IL10) signaling and TIMP has also been demonstrated in primary cultures.[73] Decreased metastatic ability and enhanced survival followed. Conversely, expression of TGFβ in the same tumor model induces MMP2 expression, with increased metastases and reduced survival.[72]

HYPOXIC REGULATION OF ANGIOGENESIS

As a tumor outgrows its blood supply, inner cells become hypoxic. Maintenance of tumor growth at times of cellular stress, including hypoxia, is required for invasion and metastasis. Tumor hypoxia is associated with increased aggression and poor survival.[74] An appreciation of the pathways involved in hypoxic signaling and their link with angiogenesis is essential for understanding tumor biology.

Several transcription factors are involved in the pathway with most attention focused on hypoxia-inducible factor 1 (HIF1). In a normoxic environment HIF1α is highly unstable and is rapidly degraded, mediated through the ubiquitinE3 ligase complex. The von Hippel Lindau (VHL) protein forms part of this complex and is responsible for binding HIF1α prior to proteolysis. Proteolysis is blocked if the VHL gene is mutated. In hypoxic environments HIF1β is stabilized and translocates to the nucleus to bind with HIF1β. This leads to the transcription and upregulation of a complex array of gene pathways including VEGF, the glycolytic pathway, endothelial adhesion, cell proliferation, and

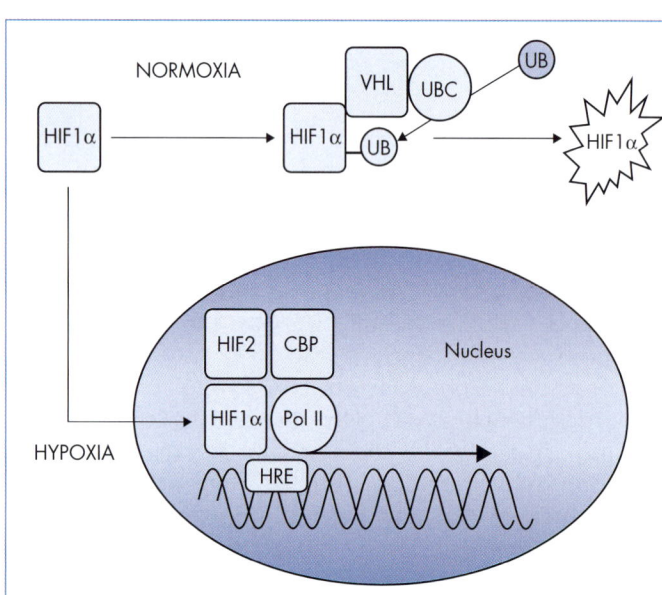

Fig. 33.2
The role of hypoxia-inducible factor 1α (HIF1α). At normal oxygen tension (normoxia), prolyl hydroxylase acts on its substrate HIF1α to allow formation of an association with von-Hippel-Lindau protein (VHL) and ubiquitinylation complex (UBC). Ubiquitinylation of HIF1α leads to its degradation. In contrast, under hypoxic conditions, prolyl hydroxylase cannot act on HIF1α. This allows its passage to the nucleus, where it binds with HIF2 and CReb binding protein (CBP) to sequences of DNA known as hypoxic response elements (HRE) to stimulate target gene expression by DNA polymerase II (Pol II).

urokinase, as well as others (Figure 33.2).[75] It has also been shown to downregulate angiogenesis inhibitors[76]

Tumor cell lines with mutant HIF1α grow more slowly and with reduced angiogenesis; HIF1α increases growth rate and metastatic ability in prostate cancer cells independent of the oxygen tension in the cellular environment.[77] The HIF1α protein levels are higher in prostate cancer than benign glands.[78] Hypoxia upregulates VEGF expression in prostate cancer in vitro,[79] and it has been shown that this occurs through phosphoinositol 3 (PI3) kinase signaling.[80] Inhibition of HIF1α signaling may of therapeutic value.

ANTIANGIOGENIC THERAPY

Traditional approaches to treating solid tumors are inadequate as tumor resistance and relapse is common. Targeting the neovasculature offers a new treatment modality, and angiogenic vessels can be selectively targeted through differences in surface markers between angiogenic and quiescent endothelial cells.[81,82] Antiangiogenic cancer strategies are attractive options as they may be less susceptible to resistance than conventional anticancer treatment, since endothelial cells are non-neoplastic and, therefore, genetically stable in contrast to the labile tumor cells.

Several synthetic inhibitors of MMPs have been developed. In vivo studies with intraperitoneal injections of A-177430 showed dose-dependent reduction in tumor volumes, with the maximum dose showing almost complete arrest of tumor growth.[83] Marimastat is another MMP currently being tested in phase III trials.[84] Side effects such as arthralgia and myalgia may reduce patient tolerance of Marimastat treatment.[85]

TNP-470 directly inhibits the growth of endothelial cells and is a synthetic analog of fumagillin, an antibiotic secreted by *Aspergillus fumigatus*.[86] In-vitro studies have also shown growth inhibiting effects on LNCaP cells. In contrast, PSA secretion per cell was induced 1.1- to 1.5-fold following TNP-470 exposure.[86] A phase I trial showed no definite efficacy in prostate cancer and further clinical trials have been cancelled until further notice. Antiangiogenic activity has also been identified in an extract of *Rabdosia rubescens*, a component of the dietary supplement PC SPES, proposed as a treatment for advanced prostate cancer.[87]

Thalidomide is best known as an antiemetic with devastating teratogenic side effects. The limb defects are a result of inhibition of blood vessel growth in the fetus, and it has been subsequently shown that the drug inhibits FGF2 and VEGF-induced angiogenesis.[88,89] In a phase II study in patients with androgen-independent prostate cancer, a PSA decline of more than 50% was noted in 14% of the patients; 28% had more than 40% decline of PSA.[90] A series of thalidomide analogs have

been developed with activity against both endothelial and prostate cancer cells in vitro.[91]

Drugs are also under investigation that inhibit endothelial-specific integrin signaling. Angiogenesis depends on the adhesive interactions between vascular cells and the ECM mediated through integrins. Integrin avβ3 has been identified as the most important integrin and is 4-fold increased during angiogenesis. A monoclonal antibody to avβ3 (Vitaxin) blocks angiogenesis induced by FGF2[92] and has entered phase I trials.[93]

SU5416, a selective inhibitor of VEGFR2, has been in clinical trials for the treatment of advanced malignancies.[94] Unfortunately, in prostate cancer, no effect of SU5416 on PSA secretion or time to progression was detectable in patients, and further evaluation of SU5416 in prostate cancer has been halted.[95]

SU6668 blocks VEGF, FGF, and PDGF receptor signaling and induced regressions of a diverse panel of large established human tumor xenografts.[96] Investigations are ongoing in phase I clinical trials.

Curcumin is a plant extract, which is a dietary factor in the Asian diet apart from the soy-based products. It has pleiotropic inhibitory effects on receptor tyrosine kinases such as the signaling mediated by the VEGF and EGF receptors. In LNCaP cells curcumin caused a decrease in cell proliferation and a significant decrease in MVD,[97,98] and it has been shown to cause radiosensitization in PC3 cells.[99]

Suramin is a polysulfonated naphthylurea previously used for the treatment of patients with trypanosomiasis and acquired immunodeficiency syndrome (AIDS). It has the ability to bind several growth factors, antagonizing their growth-promoting effects, and has demonstrated direct antiproliferative effects against prostatic tumor cell lines.[100] Suramin has a narrow therapeutic window with common dose-limiting effects including adrenal insufficiency, coagulation abnormalities, peripheral neuropathy, and death, but with close monitoring of serum levels the drug can be safely administered with limited, but significant efficacy.[101] The combination of suramin and the chemotherapeutic agent epirubicin did not suggest major improvements compared with suramin alone in a phase II trial.[102] Another phase II trial has recently been published with a PSA response rate of 37% in hormone resistant cancer.[103]

Takei et al have developed small interfering RNAs (siRNAs) targeting human VEGF. This approach dramatically inhibited the secretion of VEGF in PC3 cells and suppressed tumor angiogenesis and tumor growth in a xenograft model.[104] Delivery of molecular therapeutics such as siRNAs or antisense oligonucleotides can be difficult as a result of instability. The authors used atelocollagen to give a profound increase in stability of their duplexes with associated functional effect.

ZD1839 (Iressa) is a selective EGFR-tyrosine kinase inhibitor in clinical trials in cancer patients. Experimental evidence has been provided for a link between EGFR signaling and angiogenic mechanisms. Both EGF and TGFα can upregulate the production of VEGF in human cancer cells.[105] The antitumor effect of ZD1839 has been shown to be accompanied by inhibition in the production of autocrine and paracrine growth factors that both sustain autonomous local growth and facilitate angiogenesis.[106] Hence, although this agent primarily targets a growth factor receptor, part of its action may be attributed to its antiangiogenic properties.

ADJUVANT ANTIANGIOGENIC THERAPY

Recent preclinical studies have suggested that radiotherapy in combination with antiangiogenic agents enhances the therapeutic effect of ionizing radiation. The hypoxic tumor microenvironment also contributes to the interaction between these agents and ionizing radiation. Hypoxia stimulates upregulation of angiogenic and tumor-cell survival factors, giving rise to tumor proliferation, radioresistance, and angiogenesis. Preclinical evidence suggests that antiangiogenic agents reduce tumor hypoxia and provides a rationale for combining these agents with ionizing radiation. Angiogenesis inhibitors have been shown to attenuate the angiogenic effects of radiation-induced prostate cancer cell growth factor production and amplify the direct anti-endothelial action of radiation in vitro.[107]

Despite the success of preclinical studies, effects in clinical trials have been disappointing. This failure of molecular biology to be translated to the bedside may be a consequence of the complexity of the molecular pathways involved. Further possible limitations of antiangiogenic therapy have been suggested by recent studies demonstrating that some tumors have vessel density similar to normal tissue and thus exhibit non-angiogenic phenotypes.[108,109]

The exploration of the pathways involved in angiogenesis continues to gain momentum. The importance of angiogenesis in determining tumor prognosis is no longer a matter for debate, although there is no clinical application in human cancer management as yet. Antiangiogenesis therapy continues to attract considerable attention, and a number of targets have been identified, although in-vivo results have not transferred effectively to clinical trials. However, there remains concern that randomly targeting one factor or one particular pathway may have only limited clinical success. Different angiogenic pathways may predominate within different tumors and within the same tumor at different stages of development. Identification of the crucial pathways in prostate cancer remains the challenge to allow accurate and therapeutic targeting of tumor blood supply.

REFERENCES

1. Folkman J. Tumor angiogenesis: therapeutic implications. N Engl J Med 1971;285:1182–1186.
2. Folkman J. What is the evidence that tumors are angiogenesis dependent? J Natl Cancer Inst 1990;82:4–6.
3. Carmeliet P, Jain RK. Angiogenesis in cancer and other diseases. Nature 2000;407:249–257.
4. Dvorak HF, Nagy JA, Feng D, et al. Vascular permeability factor/vascular endothelial growth factor and the significance of microvascular hyperpermeability in angiogenesis. Curr Top Microbiol Immunol 1999;237:97–132.
5. Weidner N, Folkman J, Pozza F, et al. Tumor angiogenesis: a new significant and independent prognostic indicator in early-stage breast carcinoma. J Natl Cancer Inst 1992;84:1875–1887.
6. Hall MC, Troncoso P, Pollack A, et al. Significance of tumor angiogenesis in clinically localized prostate carcinoma treated with external beam radiotherapy. Urology 1994;44:869–875.
7. Inoue K, Slaton JW, Karashima T, et al. The prognostic value of angiogenesis factor expression for predicting recurrence and metastasis of bladder cancer after neoadjuvant chemotherapy and radical cystectomy. Clin Cancer Res 2000;6:4866–4873.
8. Dickinson AJ, Fox SB, Persad RA, et al. Quantification of angiogenesis as an independent predictor of prognosis in invasive bladder carcinomas. Br J Urol 1994;74:762–766.
9. Vermeulen PB, Gasparini G, Fox SB, et al. Second international consensus on the methodology and criteria of evaluation of angiogenesis quantification in solid human tumours. Eur J Cancer 2002;8:1564–1579.
10. Wakui S, Furusato M, Itoh T, et al. Tumour angiogenesis in prostatic carcinoma with and without bone marrow metastasis: a morphometric study. J Pathol 1992;168:257–262.
11. Fregene TA, Khanuja PS, Noto AD, et al. Tumor-associated angiogenesis in prostate cancer. Anticancer Res 1993;13:2377–2381.
12. Weidner N, Carroll PR, Flax J, et al. Tumor angiogenesis correlates with metastasis in invasive prostate carcinoma. Am J Pathol 1993;143:401–409.
13. Brawer MK, Deering RE, Brown M, et al. Predictors of pathologic stage in prostatic carcinoma. The role of neovascularity. Cancer 1994;73:678–687.
14. Silberman MA, Partin AW, Veltri RW, et al. Tumor angiogenesis correlates with progression after radical prostatectomy but not with pathologic stage in Gleason sum 5 to 7 adenocarcinoma of the prostate. Cancer 1997;79:772–779.
15. Borre M, Offersen BV, Nerstrom B, et al. Microvessel density predicts survival in prostate cancer patients subjected to watchful waiting. Br J Cancer 1998;78:940–944.
16. Gonzales M, Weksler B, Tsuruta D, et al. Structure and function of a vimentin-associated matrix adhesion in endothelial cells. Mol Biol Cell 2001;12:85–100.
17. Nicholson B, Theodorescu D. Angiogenesis and prostate cancer tumor growth. J Cell Biochem 2004;91:125–150.
18. Crew JP, O'Brien T, Bradburn M, et al. Vascular endothelial growth factor is a predictor of relapse and stage progression in superficial bladder cancer. Cancer Res 1997;57:5281–5285.
19. Edgren M, Lennernas B, Larsson A, et al. Serum concentrations of VEGF and b-FGF in renal cell, prostate and urinary bladder carcinomas. Anticancer Res 1999;19:869–873.
20. Ferrer FA, Miller LJ, Andrawis RI, et al. Vascular endothelial growth factor (VEGF) expression in human prostate cancer: in situ and in vitro expression of VEGF by human prostate cancer cells. J Urol 1997;157:2329–2333.
21. Ferrer FA, Miller LJ, Andrawis RI, et al. Angiogenesis and prostate cancer: in vivo and in vitro expression of angiogenesis factors by prostate cancer cells. Urology 1998;51:161–167.
22. Harper ME, Glynne-Jones E, Goddard L, et al. Vascular endothelial growth factor (VEGF) expression in prostatic tumours and its relationship to neuroendocrine cells. Br J Cancer 1996;74:910–916.
23. Noordzij MA, van der Kwast TH, van Steenbrugge GJ, et al. The prognostic influence of neuroendocrine cells in prostate cancer: results of a long-term follow-up study with patients treated by radical prostatectomy. Int J Cancer 1995;62:252–258.

24. Balbay MD, Pettaway CA, Kuniyasu H, et al. Highly metastatic human prostate cancer growing within the prostate of athymic mice overexpresses vascular endothelial growth factor. Clin Cancer Res 1999;5:783–789.

25. Connolly JM, Rose DP. Angiogenesis in two human prostate cancer cell lines with differing metastatic potential when growing as solid tumors in nude mice. J Urol 1998;160:932–936.

26. Trudel D, Fradet Y, Meyer F, et al. Significance of MMP-2 expression in prostate cancer: an immunohistochemical study. Cancer Res 2003;63:8511–8515.

27. Brehmer B, Biesterfeld S, Jakse G. Expression of matrix metalloproteinases (MMP-2 and -9) and their inhibitors (TIMP-1 and -2) in prostate cancer tissue. Prostate Cancer Prostatic Dis 2003;6:217–222.

28. Kikuno N, Yoshino T, Urakami S, et al. The role of thymidine phosphorylase (TP) mRNA expression in angiogenesis of prostate cancer. Anticancer Res 2003;23:1305–1312.

29. Okada K, Yokoyama K, Okiharak K, et al. Immunohistochemical localization of platelet-derived endothelial cell growth factor expression and its relation to angiogenesis in prostate. Urology 2001;57:376–381.

30. Benharroch D, Birnbaum D. Biology of the fibroblast growth factor gene family. Isr J Med Sci 1990;26:212–219.

31. Gaudric A, N'Guyen T, Moenner M, et al. Quantification of angiogenesis due to basic fibroblast growth factor in a modified rabbit corneal model. Ophthalmic Res 1992;24:181–188.

32. Pepper MS, Ferrara N, Orci L, et al. Potent synergism between vascular endothelial growth factor and basic fibroblast growth factor in the induction of angiogenesis in vitro. Biochem Biophys Res Commun 1992;189:824–831.

33. Nguyen M, Watanabe H, Budson AE, et al. Elevated levels of an angiogenic peptide, basic fibroblast growth factor, in the urine of patients with a wide spectrum of cancers. J Natl Cancer Inst 1994;86:356–361.

34. Meyer GE, Yu E, Siegal JA, et al. Serum basic fibroblast growth factor in men with and without prostate carcinoma. Cancer 1995;76:2304–2311.

35. Nakamoto T, Chang CS, Li AK, et al. Basic fibroblast growth factor in human prostate cancer cells. Cancer Res 1992;52:571–577.

36. Walsh K, Sherwood RA, Dew TK, et al. Angiogenic peptides in prostatic disease. BJU Int 1999;84:1081–1083.

37. Bok RA, Halabi S, Fei DT, et al. Vascular endothelial growth factor and basic fibroblast growth factor urine levels as predictors of outcome in hormone-refractory prostate cancer patients: a cancer and leukemia group B study. Cancer Res 2001;61:2533–2536.

38. Morton DM, Barrack ER. Modulation of transforming growth factor beta 1 effects on prostate cancer cell proliferation by growth factors and extracellular matrix. Cancer Res 1995;55:2596–2602.

39. Shariat SF, Mensesses-Diaz A, Kim IY, et al. Tissue expression of transforming growth factor-beta1 and its receptors: correlation with pathologic features and biochemical progression in patients undergoing radical prostatectomy. Urology 2004;63:1191–1197.

40. Wikstrom P, Stattin P, Franck-Lissbrant I, et al. Transforming growth factor beta1 is associated with angiogenesis, metastasis, and poor clinical outcome in prostate cancer. Prostate 1998;37:19–29.

41. Truong LD, Kadmon D, McCune BK, et al. Association of transforming growth factor-beta 1 with prostate cancer: an immunohistochemical study. Hum Pathol 1993;24:4–9.

42. Eastham JA, Truong LD, Rogers E, et al. Transforming growth factor-beta 1: comparative immunohistochemical localization in human primary and metastatic prostate cancer. Lab Invest 1995;73:628–635.

43. Hartley-Asp B, Vukanovic J, Joseph IB, et al. Anti-angiogenic treatment with linomide as adjuvant to surgical castration in experimental prostate cancer. J Urol 1997;158:902–907.

44. Lekas E, Johansson M, Widmark A, et al. Decrement of blood flow precedes the involution of the ventral prostate in the rat after castration. Urol Res 1997;25:309–314.

45. Jain RK, Safabakhsh N, Sckell A, et al. Endothelial cell death, angiogenesis, and microvascular function after castration in an androgen-dependent tumor: role of vascular endothelial growth factor. Proc Natl Acad Sci USA 1998;95:10820–10825.

46. Mercader M, Bodner BK, Moser MT, et al. T cell infiltration of the prostate induced by androgen withdrawal in patients with prostate cancer. Proc Natl Acad Sci USA 2001;98:14565–14570.

47. Lissbrant IF, Stattin P, Wikstrom P, et al. Tumor associated macrophages in human prostate cancer: relation to clinicopathological variables and survival. Int J Oncol 2000;17:445–451.

48. Shimura S, Yang G, Ebara S, et al. Reduced infiltration of tumor-associated macrophages in human prostate cancer: association with cancer progression. Cancer Res 2000;60:5857–5861.

49. Sunderkotter C, Steinbrink K, Goebeler M, et al. Macrophages and angiogenesis. J Leukoc Biol 1994;55:410–422.

50. Madaan S, Abel PD, Chaudhary KS, et al. Cytoplasmic induction and over-expression of cyclooxygenase-2 in human prostate cancer: implications for prevention and treatment. BJU Int 2000;86:736–741.

51. O'Reilly MS, O' Reilly MS, Holmgren L, et al. Angiostatin: a novel angiogenesis inhibitor that mediates the suppression of metastases by a Lewis lung carcinoma. Cell 1994;79:315–328.

52. O'Reilly MS, Pirie-Shepherd S, Lane WS, et al. Antiangiogenic activity of the cleaved conformation of the serpin antithrombin. Science 1999;285:1926–1928.

53. Brooks PC, Silletti S, von Schalscha TL, et al. Disruption of angiogenesis by PEX, a noncatalytic metalloproteinase fragment with integrin binding activity. Cell 1998;92:391–400.

54. Ferrara N, Clapp C, Weiner R. The 16K fragment of prolactin specifically inhibits basal or fibroblast growth factor stimulated growth of capillary endothelial cells. Endocrinology 1991;129:896–900.

55. Yao L, Pike SE, Tosato G. Laminin binding to the calreticulin fragment vasostatin regulates endothelial cell function. J Leukoc Biol 2002;71:47–53.

56. O'Reilly MS, Holmgren L, Chen C, et al. Angiostatin induces and sustains dormancy of human primary tumors in mice. Nat Med 1996;2:689–692.

57. O'Reilly MS, Boehm T, Shing Y, et al. Endostatin: an endogenous inhibitor of angiogenesis and tumor growth. Cell 1997;88:277–285.

58. Dixelius J, Dixelius J, Sasaki T, et al. Endostatin-induced tyrosine kinase signaling through the Shb adaptor protein regulates endothelial cell apoptosis. Blood 2000;95:3403–3411.

59. Yoon SS, Eto H, Lin CM, et al. Mouse endostatin inhibits the formation of lung and liver metastases. Cancer Res 1999;59:6251–6256.

60. Perletti G, Concari P, Giardini R, et al. Antitumor activity of endostatin against carcinogen-induced rat primary mammary tumors. Cancer Res 2000;60:1793–1796.

61. Yokoyama Y, Green JE, Sukhatme VP, et al. Effect of endostatin on spontaneous tumorigenesis of mammary adenocarcinoma in a transgenic mouse model. Cancer Res 2000;60:4362–4365.

62. Chen CT, Lin J, Li Q, et al. Antiangiogenic gene therapy for cancer via systemic administration of adenoviral vectors expressing secretable endostatin. Hum Gene Ther 2000;11:1983–1996.

63. Heidtmann HH, Nettelbeck DM, Mingels A, et al. Generation of angiostatin-like fragments from plasminogen by prostate-specific antigen. Br J Cancer 1999;81:1269–1273.

64. Fortier AH, Nelson BJ, Grella DK, et al. Antiangiogenic activity of prostate-specific antigen. J Natl Cancer Inst 1999;91:1635–1640.

65. Fortier AH, Leiby DA, Narayanan RB, et al. Recombinant prostate specific antigen inhibits angiogenesis in vitro and in vivo. Prostate 2003;56:212–219.

66. Denmeade SR, Litvinov I, Sokoll LJ, et al. Prostate-specific antigen (PSA) protein does not affect growth of prostate cancer cells in vitro or prostate cancer xenografts in vivo. Prostate 2003;56:45–53.

67. Grossfeld GD, Ginsberg DA, Stein JP, et al. Thrombospondin-1 expression in bladder cancer: association with p53 alterations, tumor angiogenesis, and tumor progression. J Natl Cancer Inst 1997;89:219–227.

68. Grossfeld GD, Carroll PR, Lindeman N, et al. Thrombospondin-1 expression in patients with pathologic stage T3 prostate cancer undergoing radical prostatectomy: association with p53 alterations, tumor angiogenesis, and tumor progression. Urology 2002;59:97–102.

69. Doll JA, Reiher FK, Crawford SE, et al. Thrombospondin-1, vascular endothelial growth factor and fibroblast growth factor-2 are key functional regulators of angiogenesis in the prostate. Prostate 2001;49:293–305.

70. Jin RJ, Kwak C, Lee SG, et al. The application of an anti-angiogenic gene (thrombospondin-1) in the treatment of human prostate cancer xenografts. Cancer Gene Ther 2000;7:1537–1542.

71. Vallbo C, Wang W, Damber JE. The expression of thrombospondin-1 in benign prostatic hyperplasia and prostatic intraepithelial neoplasia is decreased in prostate cancer. BJU Int 2004;93:1339–1343.

72. Stearns ME, Rhim J, Wang M. Interleukin 10 (IL-10) inhibition of primary human prostate cell-induced angiogenesis: IL-10 stimulation of tissue inhibitor of metalloproteinase-1 and inhibition of matrix metalloproteinase (MMP)-2/MMP-9 secretion. Clin Cancer Res 1999;5:189–196.

73. Wang M, Hu Y, Shima I, et al. IL-10/IL-10 receptor signaling regulates TIMP-1 expression in primary human prostate tumor lines. Cancer Biol Ther 2002;1:556–563.

74. Vaupel P, Kelleher DK, Hockel M. Oxygen status of malignant tumors: pathogenesis of hypoxia and significance for tumor therapy. Semin Oncol 2001;28:29–35.

75. Maxwell PH, Ratcliffe PJ. Oxygen sensors and angiogenesis. Semin Cell Dev Biol 2002;13:29–37.

76. Laderoute KR, Alarcon RM, Brody MD, et al. Opposing effects of hypoxia on expression of the angiogenic inhibitor thrombospondin 1 and the angiogenic inducer vascular endothelial growth factor. Clin Cancer Res 2000;6:2941–2950.

77. Zhong H, Agani F, Baccala AA, et al. Increased expression of hypoxia inducible factor-1alpha in rat and human prostate cancer. Cancer Res 1998;58:5280–5284.

78. Zhong H, De Marzo AM, Laughner E, et al. Overexpression of hypoxia-inducible factor 1alpha in common human cancers and their metastases. Cancer Res 1999;59:5830–5835.

79. Cvetkovic D, Movsas B, Dicker AP, et al. Increased hypoxia correlates with increased expression of the angiogenesis marker vascular endothelial growth factor in human prostate cancer. Urology 2001;57:821–825.

80. Zhong H, Chiles K, Feldser D, et al. Modulation of hypoxia-inducible factor 1alpha expression by the epidermal growth factor/phosphatidylinositol 3-kinase/PTEN/AKT/FRAP pathway in human prostate cancer cells: implications for tumor angiogenesis and therapeutics. Cancer Res 2000;60:1541–1545.

81. Pasqualini R, Ruoslahti E. Organ targeting in vivo using phage display peptide libraries. Nature 1996;380:364–366.

82. Arap W, Pasqualini R, Ruoslahti E. Cancer treatment by targeted drug delivery to tumor vasculature in a mouse model. Science 1998;279:377–380.

83. Rabbani SA, Harakidas P, Guo Y, et al. Synthetic inhibitor of matrix metalloproteases decreases tumor growth and metastases in a syngeneic model of rat prostate cancer in vivo. Int J Cancer 2000;87:276–282.

84. Steward WP. Marimastat (BB2516): current status of development. Cancer Chemother Pharmacol 1999;43 Suppl:S56–60.

85. Steward WP, Thomas AL. Marimastat: the clinical development of a matrix metalloproteinase inhibitor. Expert Opin Investig Drugs 2000;9:2913–2922.

86. Horti J, Dixon SC, Logothetis CJ, et al. Increased transcriptional activity of prostate-specific antigen in the presence of TNP-470, an angiogenesis inhibitor. Br J Cancer 1999;79:1588–1593.

87. Meade-Tollin LC, Wijeratne EM, Cooper D. Ponicidin and oridonin are responsible for the antiangiogenic activity of *Rabdosia rubescens*, a constituent of the herbal supplement PC SPES. J Nat Prod 2004;67:2–4.

88. D'Amato RJ, Loughnan MS, Flynn E, et al. Thalidomide is an inhibitor of angiogenesis. Proc Natl Acad Sci USA 1994;91:4082–4085.

89. Kenyon BM, Browne F, D'Amato RJ. Effects of thalidomide and related metabolites in a mouse corneal model of neovascularization. Exp Eye Res 1997;64:971–978.

90. Figg WD, Arlen P, Gulley J, et al. A randomized phase II trial of thalidomide, an angiogenesis inhibitor, in patients with androgen-independent prostate cancer. Clin Cancer Res 2001;7:1888–1893.

91. Capitosti SM, Hansen TP, Brown ML. Thalidomide analogues demonstrate dual inhibition of both angiogenesis and prostate cancer. Bioorg Med Chem 2004;12:327–336.

92. Brooks PC, Montogomery AM, Rosenfeld M, et al. Integrin alpha v beta 3 antagonists promote tumor regression by inducing apoptosis of angiogenic blood vessels. Cell 1994;79:1157–1164.

93. Gutheil JC, Campbell TN, Pierce PR, et al. Targeted antiangiogenic therapy for cancer using Vitaxin: a humanized monoclonal antibody to the integrin alphavbeta3. Clin Cancer Res 2000;6:3056–3061.

94. Mendel DB, Laird AD, Smolich BD, et al. Development of SU5416, a selective small molecule inhibitor of VEGF receptor tyrosine kinase activity, as an anti-angiogenesis agent. Anticancer Drug Des 2000;15:29–41.

95. Stadler WM, Cao D, Vogelzang NJ, et al. A randomized Phase II trial of the antiangiogenic agent SU5416 in hormone-refractory prostate cancer. Clin Cancer Res 2004;10:3365–3370.

96. Laird AD, Vajkoczy P, Shawver LK, et al. SU6668 is a potent antiangiogenic and antitumor agent that induces regression of established tumors. Cancer Res 2000;60:4152–4160.

97. Dorai T, Gehani N, Katz A. Therapeutic potential of curcumin in human prostate cancer-I. Curcumin induces apoptosis in both androgen-dependent and androgen-independent prostate cancer cells. Prostate Cancer Prostatic Dis 2000;3:84–93.

98. Dorai T, Gehani N, Katz A. Therapeutic potential of curcumin in human prostate cancer. II. Curcumin inhibits tyrosine kinase activity of epidermal growth factor receptor and depletes the protein. Mol Urol 2000;4:1–6.

99. Chendil D, Ranga RS, Meigooni D, et al. Curcumin confers radiosensitizing effect in prostate cancer cell line PC-3. Oncogene 2004;23:1599–1607.

100. Church D, Zhang Y, Rago R, et al. Efficacy of suramin against human prostate carcinoma DU145 xenografts in nude mice. Cancer Chemother Pharmacol 1999;43:198–204.

101. Garcia-Schurmann JM, Schulze H, Haupt G, et al. Suramin treatment in hormone- and chemotherapy-refractory prostate cancer. Urology 1999;53:535–541.

102. Falcone A, Antonuzzo A, Danesi R, et al. Suramin in combination with weekly epirubicin for patients with advanced hormone-refractory prostate carcinoma. Cancer 1999;86:470–476.

103. Vogelzang NJ, Karrison T, Stadler WM, et al. A Phase II trial of suramin monthly × 3 for hormone-refractory prostate carcinoma. Cancer 2004;100:65–71.

104. Takei Y, Kadomatsu K, Yuzawa Y, et al. A small interfering RNA targeting vascular endothelial growth factor as cancer therapeutics. Cancer Res 2004;64:3365–3370.

105. Goldman CK, Kim J, Wong WL, et al. Epidermal growth factor stimulates vascular endothelial growth factor production by human malignant glioma cells: a model of glioblastoma multiforme pathophysiology. Mol Biol Cell 1993;4:121–133.

106. Ciardiello F, Caputo R, Bianco R, et al. Inhibition of growth factor production and angiogenesis in human cancer cells by ZD1839 (Iressa), a selective epidermal growth factor receptor tyrosine kinase inhibitor. Clin Cancer Res 2001;7:1459–1465.

107. Abdollahi A, Lipson KE, Han X, et al. SU5416 and SU6668 attenuate the angiogenic effects of radiation-induced tumor cell growth factor production and amplify the direct anti-endothelial action of radiation in vitro. Cancer Res 2003;63:3755–3763.

108. Pezzella F, Di Bacco A, Andreola S, et al. Angiogenesis in primary lung cancer and lung secondaries. Eur J Cancer 1996;32A:2494–2500.

109. Pandey J, Bannout A, Wendell DL. The Edpm5 locus prevents the "angiogenic switch" in an estrogen-induced rat pituitary tumor. Carcinogenesis 2004;25(10):1829–1838.

Endothelin and prostate cancer 34

Joel B Nelson

INTRODUCTION

Hormone-refractory prostate cancer remains true to its middle name: it is largely refractory to attempts to delay its progression. New targets and new therapies are demanded. Through a review of the available literature on endothelin and several preclinical observations, the endothelin axis has emerged as one such target. In phase II and III clinical trials of atrasentan, a potent and selective endothelin receptor A subtype (ETA) antagonist, disease progression was delayed in some men. This well-tolerated, oral agent may help convert advanced prostate cancer to a more chronic disease. This review will discuss the endothelin axis, preclinical rationale, and some of the available clinical trial data on this promising new approach.

ENDOTHELIN AXIS

In 1988, a graduate student in Japan published a stunning paper in the journal *Nature* about the isolation

and characterization of a new, 21-residue peptide produced by porcine aortic endothelial cells as the most potent vasoconstrictor, called endothelin.[1] The vasoconstrictor activity of endothelin was at least 10 times more potent than that reported for angiotensin II, and 100 times more potent, on a molar basis, than norepinephrine. Since then, over 16,000 publications listing endothelin as a key word have appeared in the scientific literature. This peptide, now termed endothelin 1 (ET1; Figure 34.1), was subsequently found to be part of a family of endothelins, which includes ET2, ET3 and the sarafotoxins (isolated from the venom of the Israeli burrowing asp).[2] The active form of ET1 is derived from a 39-amino acid precursor peptide, "big ET1," following proteolytic cleavage of the *C*-terminal portion of the molecule by an endothelin-converting enzyme.[3]

Two receptors have been identified for members of the endothelin family: endothelin receptor A (ETA) and endothelin receptor B (ETB) are members of the seven-transmembrane-segment G-protein-coupled superfamily. ETA has a higher affinity for ET1 and ET2, and lower for ET3. ETB binds all three endothelin ligands identically, and may play an important role in ligand clearance. Collectively, the ET family of ligands and the ET receptors are termed the "ET axis."[4]

As a biologic mediator, ET1 is ubiquitous: ET1 is produced by a large variety of cells from a wide range of mammalian species.[5] It has been identified in plasma, cerebrospinal fluid, urine, breast milk, and amniotic fluid.[6–10] Of particular interest to the topic at hand, an immunoreactive form of ET1 was found in large quantity in human seminal fluid from both intact and vasectomized men, where the testicular contribution to the ejaculate has been eliminated, indicating a prostatic and/or seminal vesicle source.[11]

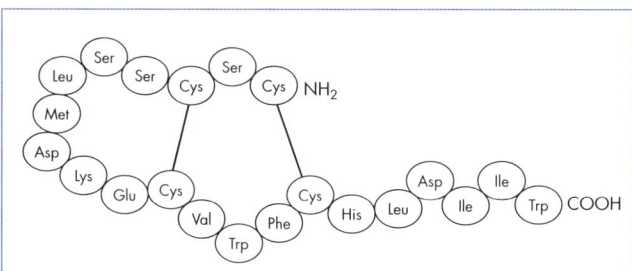

Fig. 34.1
Amino acid structure of endothelin 1 (ET1).

Indeed, the concentrations of endothelin 1 in the ejaculate are amongst the highest reported in any body fluid.

Production of ET1 in the prostate is by luminal epithelial cells and may contribute to the contractility of the prostate stroma.[12,13] In-vitro studies also showed a mitogenic effect on cultured smooth muscle cells from a human prostate.[14] The action of ET1 on the prostate may be paracrine, since both ETA and ETB have been identified in the normal human prostate.[12]

ENDOTHELIN 1 IN PROSTATE CANCER

The magnitude difference between concentrations of ET1 in seminal fluid compared with those in plasma are reminiscent of those seen with prostate-specific antigen (PSA), where concentrations are measured in the mg/dl range in the semen compared with ng/dl quantities in circulation. Indeed, ET1 levels in plasma samples from men with hormone-refractory prostate cancer were compared with those from men with clinically localized disease and those without prostate cancer, and, as a group, were found to be significantly increased.[15] Local concentrations of ET1 are believed to be several fold higher than levels in circulation (where ET1 half-life is 3.5 minutes), as man has exquisite homeostatic mechanisms to control the concentrations of this most potent peptide.[16] These increases in ET1 in prostate cancer may be associated with the loss of the expression and activity of the enzyme responsible for its cleavage, neutral endopeptidase 24.11, seen in androgen-independent prostate cancer cell lines and prostate cancer samples from androgen ablated men.[17] Every prostate cancer cell line studied produced ET1 mRNA and protein.[15] Endothelin 1 specific immunohistochemistry of primary prostate cancers and of tissues obtained from men dying from prostate cancers was present almost without exception.[18]

ENDOTHELIN RECEPTORS IN PROSTATE CANCER

Both ETA and ETB receptors are found in the normal prostate: ETA receptor binding has been found predominantly in the stromal component of the prostate, whereas ETB binding is predominantly in epithelial luminal cells.[19] It was surprising, therefore, when no ETB binding sites could be detected in human prostate cancer cell lines.[18] Among the possible mechanisms for downregulation of receptor expression was frequent somatic methylation of the ETB receptor gene, EDNRB, observed in prostate cancer and, now, in a variety of malignancies. Embedded in the gene for the

receptor in the 5′ regulatory region is a CpG-rich sequence, referred as a CpG island. Somatic methylation of CpG islands in regulatory regions of genes has been associated with decreased transcriptional activity; this hypermethylation was found in 5/5 human prostate cancer cell lines, 15/21 primary prostate cancer tissues, and 8/14 prostate cancer metastases, or about 70% of the total number of samples examined.[20] Others have shown EDNRB methylation to be associated with increased tumor stage and grade.[21,22] Although no hypermethylation was observed in normal tissues using Southern-blot analysis,[20] others have observed EDNRB methylation in benign prostatic hyperplasia (BPH) tissues using a more sensitive polymerase chain reaction approach.[23] Hypermethylation of EDNRB has also been observed in colon and bladder cancers, nasopharyngeal carcinoma, and lung cancer, suggesting ETB silencing may have more global role in carcinogenesis.[24–26]

Unlike the loss of ETB in prostate cancer, increased ETA expression has been associated with progression of prostate cancer. In an immunohistochemical evaluation of 51 specimens, 71% were positive for ETA expression, which increased to 100% in patients with bone metastasis. Gleason scores of between 8 and 10 had particularly high rates of ETA staining, as did those cancer cells penetrating the prostatic capsule.[27] Unpublished data from our group, examining 140 primary prostate cancers, shows high ETA expression in 73% and low expression in 27%. These findings suggest the expression of the endothelin receptors may be useful prognosticators in prostate cancer and, potentially more importantly, selection of those who may benefit from receptor blockade.

EFFECTS OF ENDOTHELIN 1 ON CANCER CELLS IN VITRO

Shortly after the discovery of ET1 and the generation of ET1-specific antibodies, it was shown that many epithelial carcinomas, and, in particular, those associated with a local desmoplastic stromal response secrete ET-1 (pancreatic, colon, breast, etc.).[28,29] In addition to production of ET1, some cells proliferated in a dose-dependent manner when stimulated by ET1, most notably ovarian carcinoma, suggesting autocrine activity.[30,31] Although a mitogenic effect was also observed in prostate cancer cell lines, the response was weak.[15]

Unlike the effects of ET1 alone on cell growth, the combination ET1 and polypeptide growth factors, such as epidermal growth factor, greatly increased proliferation compared with either factor alone.[32] This synergistic growth effect, observed in only one prostate cancer cell line, where most of the effects were simply additive,[18] may be the result of transactivation of the peptide growth factor signaling pathway by ET1.[33] Secretion of ET1 was also increased by cytokines and growth factors active in prostate stroma–epithelium interactions. Both ET1 and its precursor big ET1 were produced in greater quantities by the human PC3 and DU145 human prostate cancer cell line in response to stimulation with interleukin 1β, interleukin 1α, tumor necrosis factor-α, transforming growth factor-β1, or epidermal growth factor.[34,35]

Defects in apoptosis are believed to underlie hormone-refractory prostate cancer progression.[36] Endothelin 1 can inhibit apoptosis in prostate cancer cell lines, following exposure to an apoptotic agent, such as paclitaxel. For example, apoptosis is readily induced in rat prostate cancer cell line MLL treated with paclitaxel, but the addition of ET1 significantly reduced the amount of cell death, an effect mediated through the ETA receptor. Similar results were seen with the PPC-1 cell line treated with the apoptosis-inducing FAS ligand. Endothelin 1 induces the expression of AKT, leading to the phosphorylation and inactivation of the proapoptotic protein, Bad.[37] It was also found that ET1 exposure led to a reduction in the expression of the proapoptotic proteins Bad, Bak, or Bax. Interestingly, re-expression of ETB in prostate cancer induces apoptosis, increases expression of the same pro-apoptotic proteins, and increases sensitivity to paclitaxel.[38]

ENDOTHELIN AXIS AND BONE METASTASES

Many investigators have found ET1 to be a potent stimulator of osteoblasts, the bone cell responsible for the osteoblastic response. Osteoblasts have high affinity ETA receptors, at a density (approximately 10[5] per cell) greatly exceeding the density on prostate cancer cells.[39] A significant part of the original hypothesis that ET1 had a role in prostate cancer progression was based on its effects on osteoblasts, as shown in a new-bone-forming model.[15] To study the effects of the ET axis in established bone, the WISH (a transformed human amnion cell line inducing a robust osteoblastic response) tumor model was used. The WISH cell line produces ET1, and stable transfection with an ET1-overexpression cDNA construct generated clones producing 18-fold more bioactive ET1. In this model, these ET1-overexpressing clones produced significantly more new bone when implanted in the lower leg of nu/nu mice.[40] These areas of new bone formation were significantly decreased in animals treated with a selective ETA receptor antagonist A127722, the racemic version of atrasentan. These findings have been supported by the recent report by Yin et al, indicating the causal role of ET1 in the pathogenesis of osteoblastic bone metastases in a breast carcinoma model.[41]

ENDOTHELIN AXIS AND PAIN

Among the complaints voiced by men with advanced prostate cancer, none is a frequent or as loud as pain, particularly associated with bone metastases. It has been found that ET1 induced hyperalgesia and pain in a variety of model systems, including a dramatic pain response in a man undergoing infusion of ET1 into a brachial artery.[42-44] The mechanistic pattern of ET1-induced pain appeared to be novel, unresponsive at usual doses to cyclooxygenase inhibitors such as indomethicin or ibuprofen, suggesting that agents specifically targeting ET1 activity, like ETA antagonists, could be useful in alleviating pain.[45] As a mediator of pain, ET1, acting through the ETA receptor, had both direct effects on nerve, and as a potentiator of other noxious stimuli.[46-50] In a new murine model of cancer pain, ET1-producing tumors created within bone were significantly more painful than other tumors not producing ET1: local administration of an ETA antagonist and atrasentan (ABT-627) significantly blocked this effect.[51,52]

ATRASENTAN (ABT-627)

The discovery of ET1 as the preeminent vasoconstrictor galvanized the biomedical world—and, in particular, the pharmaceutical industry—with the promise of a new mechanism for cardiovascular disease and its treatment. Like many companies, Abbott Laboratories developed an agent, ABT-627, which, at the time of disclosure, was the most potent and selective ETA receptor antagonist (Figure 34.2). ABT-627, or atrasentan, is a highly potent (Ki = 0.034 nM) and selective (1800-fold) ETA receptor antagonist, blocking the biologic effects of ET1 in a host of in-vitro and in-vivo model systems.[53,54] With a

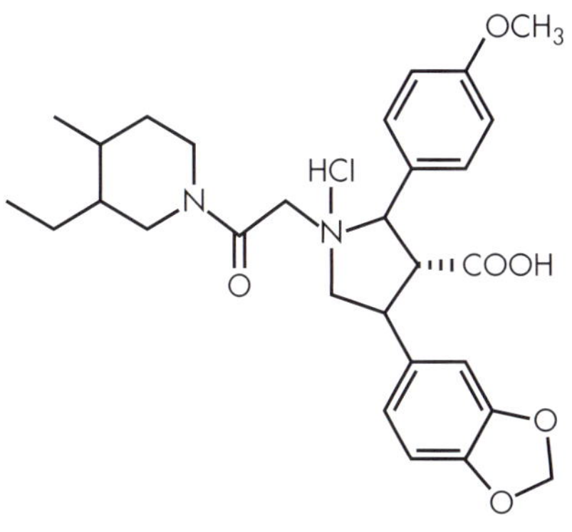

Fig. 34.2
Chemical structure of atrasentan (ABT-627). The brand name of atrasentan is Xinlay.

possible indication of hypertension in mind, atrasentan was developed as an orally bioavailable agent with a half-life of 25 hours, favoring once-per-day dosing. Single-dose pharmacokinetic studies with atrasentan in normal male volunteers demonstrated a terminal half-life range of 20 to 25 hours with extensive tissue distribution. Consistent with its vasoactive nature, the most frequent adverse events were transient headache, rhinitis, and nausea. As seen throughout the subsequent trials in cancer, atrasentan did not induce hepatic or hematologic toxicity.[55] With the promise of the clinical trials in men with prostate cancer, atrasentan has been given the brand name Xinlay.

PHASE 1 TRIALS

Based on the preclinical findings described above and the availability of potent and selective ETA receptor antagonists, like atrasentan, it was both reasonable and strategic to target ET-1 in men with prostate cancer. Therefore, two phase 1 clinical trials were performed to assess the safety and pharmacokinetics of atrasentan in men with hormone-refractory prostate cancer and other patients with refractory adenocarcinomas.[56,57] In both studies, patients were treated for 28 days with escalating oral atrasentan doses (2.5 to 95 mg) and then were eligible for an extension study. Like phase 1 in normal males, the most common side-effects were headache, rhinitis, and peripheral edema. In one trial, dose-limiting toxicity (headache) was seen at 75 mg; in the other study no maximum tolerated dose was found in the dose range studied (up to 95 mg).

In men with hormone-refractory prostate cancer, the PSA level was unchanged or decreased in 68% (15/22), with declines ranging from 5% to 95% (Figure 34.3). There was no obvious correlation between dose and PSA declines. In 7 of 10 patients (70%) with narcotic requiring pain, atrasentan reduced pain, as measured by the visual analog scale (VAS). These results, although not placebo controlled and from short, open-label trials were, nevertheless, compelling, driving the clinical trial effort forward.

PHASE 2 TRIALS

M96-500

Based on the preclinical findings implicating ET1 in pain described above, the hypothesis that ectopic secretion of ET1 by metastatic prostate cancer cells could directly induce pain,[15] and the reduction in pain observed in some patients in the phase 1 clinical trials, a phase 2 trial was designed to address the benefit of atrasentan in relieving prostate-cancer induced pain. In this first, double-blind, placebo-controlled human study of the modulation of pain using an endothelin receptor antagonist, 131 men with hormone-refractory metastatic prostate cancer with disease-related pain requiring opioid analgesics were enrolled in three study groups: 43 were randomized to the placebo arm; 40 were randomized to the 2.5 mg atrasentan arm; and 48 were randomized to the 10 mg atrasentan arm.

Not unexpectedly, in men with symptomatic, hormone-refractory disease, progression was common: 81 subjects (62%) discontinued study drug before the planned 84 days of treatment. There was no statistically significant differences in response rates for the primary endpoint (pain relief at week 12). In the 10 mg atrasentan group, however, a trend toward improvement in pain without increased analgesic consumption was seen: the average VAS pain score for subjects receiving 10 mg atrasentan decreased 8% from baseline, while the average VAS pain score for placebo subjects increased 8% from baseline. Statistically significant improvement was seen for the 10 mg atrasentan group versus placebo ($P \leq 0.05$) at week 12 for two pain domains in the brief pain inventory (BPI): pain interference with relations with other people ($P = 0.031$), and worst pain in the last 24 hours ($P = 0.030$).

M96-594

Based on the PSA responses observed in the phase 1 trials, efficacy of atrasentan in delaying disease progression was studied in a double-blind placebo-controlled phase 2 trial in men with asymptomatic, hormone-refractory, metastatic prostate cancer.[58] At 72 sites in the United

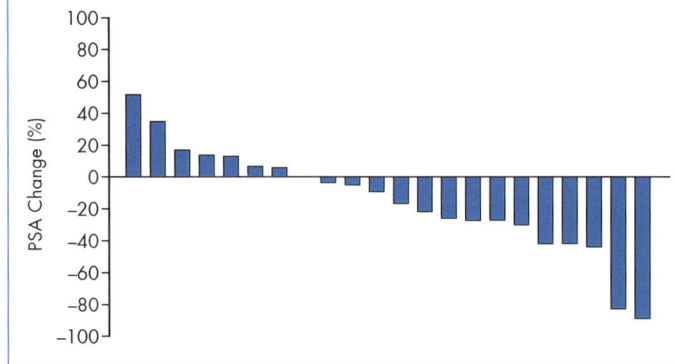

Fig. 34.3
Percentage changes in serum prostate-specific antigen (PSA) in men with hormone-refractory prostate cancer after 28 days of atrasentan (ABT-627) in the phase 1, dose escalation clinical trials. Each bar represents an individual patient.

States and Europe, 288 men were randomized to receive daily oral doses of placebo or 2.5 mg or 10 mg atrasentan. The primary endpoint was time to disease progression, as defined by new lesions, pain requiring opioids, and disease-related symptoms requiring intervention. Secondary endpoints included time to PSA progression, changes in bone markers, and quality of life.

In the intent-to-treat analysis, median time to disease progression was 183 days in the 10 mg atrasentan-treated patients compared with 137 days for the placebo group (P = 0.13). In the evaluable subset (n = 244), there was a significant (P = 0.021) delay in disease progression from 129 days (placebo) to 196 days (10 mg atrasentan) (Figure 34.4). In both the intent-to-treat and in the evaluable subset there was a significant (P = 0.002) delay in PSA progression in the 10 mg atrasentan group; median time to PSA progression was more than twice (155 days) that of placebo (71 days). As observed in the previous trials, atrasentan was well tolerated, with headache, edema, and rhinitis being the most common side effects. Like phase 1, men reaching an endpoint were permitted to enter an open-label atrasentan study: this design, with significant placebo crossover confounds any survival analysis. Nevertheless, when one combines atrasentan treatment into a single arm, there was a significant (P = 0.03) survival advantage compared with placebo in the evaluable subset (HR = 0.69).[59]

Due to preclinical data implicating the ET axis in the osteoblastic response of bone to cancer, markers of bone deposition (alkaline phosphatase, bone alkaline phosphatase) and bone resorption (N-telopeptides, C-telopeptides, and deoxypyridinoline) were also studied in this trial.[60] At baseline, not surprisingly, there were significant elevations in markers of both bone deposition and bone resorption, ranging from 1.4 to 2.7 fold above normal. Also not surprisingly, men on placebo had significant (P < 0.001) increases in both sets of markers, consistent with disease progression. It was startling, however, that men on atrasentan, in a dose-dependent fashion, had a stabilization of these markers, suggesting a disruption in the expected progression in bony sites (Figure 34.5). Bone scan index, a semi-quantitative measure of changes in bone scan, was studied, in a blinded fashion, in a subset of these men. Although not significant, there was a strong trend favoring the 10 mg atrasentan arm (P = 0.066). Collectively, these finding were the first strong indication that atrasentan may be most active in men with bone-metastatic prostate cancer, a theme repeated in phase 3.

PHASE 3 TRIALS

M00-211

The results in phase 2, showing a significant delay in disease progression in the evaluable subset, lead to the design and implementation of two phase 3 clinical trials. One study, referred to as M00-211, was designed to essentially duplicate the time to disease progression

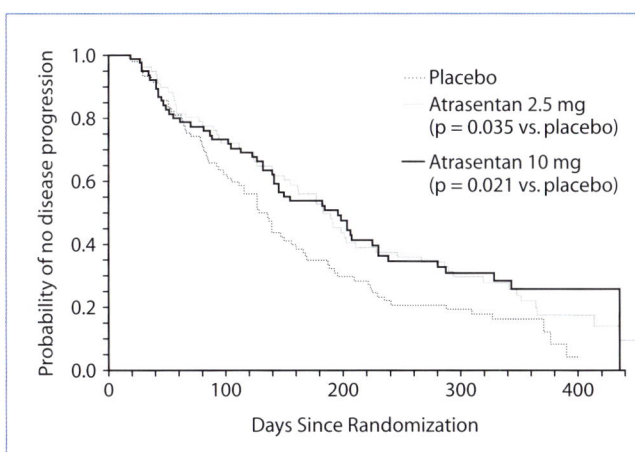

Fig. 34.4

Evaluable subset from a phase 2 clinical trial (M96-594) of atrasentan (2.5 mg and 10 mg) compared with placebo in men with metastatic, hormone-refractory prostate cancer. There was a significant delay in disease progression with atrasentan.

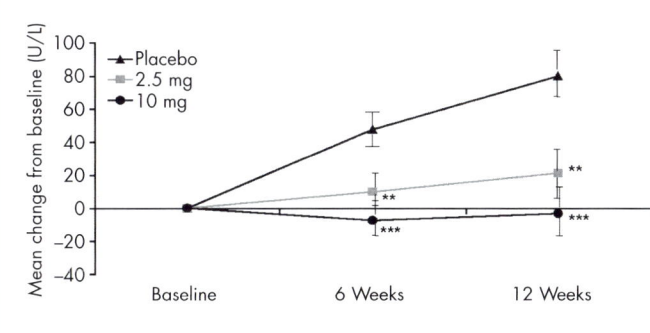

Fig. 34.5

In phase 2 clinical trials (M96-500 and M96-594) atrasentan significantly limited the rise in bone alkaline phosphatase, as a marker of bone deposition, compared with placebo over 12 weeks (**P < 0.01; ***P <0.001).

phase 2 trial (M96-594), with a few notable differences. Given the increased response rate in the 10 mg atrasentan without an increase in side effects, the phase 3 trial had only placebo and 10 mg arms. The second difference was a mandated objective evaluation of disease progression to reduce, as much as possible, PSA bias. Therefore, unlike the phase 2 study, where radiographic imaging was performed for clinical indications, in the phase 3 M00-211 study, bone scans and axial imaging were performed every 3 months. The primary endpoint (disease progression), secondary endpoints (PSA progression, markers of bone metabolism, quality of life), and enrollment criteria (asymptomatic, metastatic hormone-refractory prostate cancer) were otherwise the same.

A total of 809 men were enrolled (401 placebo, 408 atrasentan 10 mg) in the phase 3 study.[61] In the intent-to-treat population, atrasentan exhibited a nonsignificant trend in delayed TTP (log-rank, $P = 0.091$; HR, 1.14; 95% confidence intervals, 0.98–1.34). As in phase 2, the evaluable, per-protocol analysis (329 placebo, 342 atrasentan 10 mg) was significant in favor of atrasentan 10 mg (log-rank, p = 0.007; HR, 1.26; 95% CI, 1.06–1.50). Secondary endpoints (PSA progression, bone marker progression and certain quality of life tools) all significantly favored atrasentan 10 mg.

In a hypothesis-generating exercise, patients were stratified based on the characteristics of their metastatic disease at enrollment (bone only, bone and soft tissue, soft tissue only) to determine if a particular disease presentation favored better response to atrasentan. Consistent with the preclinical, and earlier clinical trials, those men with bone metastases (with or without soft tissue metastases) enjoyed the most significant delays in disease progression compared with placebo-treated patients with the same characteristics. Since 85% of the men enrolled into this trial had bone metastases, this finding is pertinent to the large majority of hormone refractory prostate cancer patients, to the design of subsequent trials, and to the possible use of atrasentan clinically.

Despite a series of trials all showing consistency in the response to atrasentan, the absence of a significant delay in time to disease progression in the intent-to-treat analysis in a pivotal trial is disappointing. When small but real effects are detected, one can perform a meta-analysis to strengthen the power of an observation. When one analyzes the phase 2 (M96-594) and phase 3 (M00-211) studies of atrasentan (n = 1097) with nearly identical patient populations, very similar trial designs and endpoints, there is a significant ($P = 0.013$) delay in disease progression in the intent-to-treat analysis, favoring atrasentan. There are several issues to consider when performing a robust meta-analysis: 1) Are the individual study protocols followed? In this analysis, yes; 2) Is there data selection bias? In this analysis, no. Every study performed in this population with this agent

is included; 3) Is there patient group heterogeneity? In this analysis, no. The patient populations are almost identical in the two studies; 4) there is no study-by-study treatment interaction. Based on this robust meta-analysis and its findings, Abbott Laboratories, the sponsors of these trials, has announced an intention to file a New Drug Application (NDA) for atrasentan (Xinlay) with the Food and Drug Administration (FDA).

ONGOING CLINICAL TRIALS

M00-244

A second phase 3 clinical trial (M00-244) is ongoing. This is another double-blind placebo-controlled trial, designed to determine if atrasentan 10 mg can delay disease progression in men with rising PSA on hormonal therapy, but who do not yet have radiographic or clinical evidence of metastatic disease. Obviously, this is a population earlier in their disease progression. When closed to new accrual in May 2003, a total of 942 men had been enrolled. Results are expected from the trial in 2005.

M00-366

A phase 2 clinical trial (M00-366) is also ongoing. This is double-blind, placebo-controlled in men who have undergone a radical prostatectomy, have evidence of biochemical failure by rising PSA, with a PSA doubling time of less than 12 months. Several studies have shown a short PSA doubling time is associated with more rapid progression. To enrich the study with men with progressive and threatening disease, the trial is designed to examine differences in the rate of rise of PSA these men, as defined by two doublings. Given an enrollment requiring PSA doubling more rapid than every 12 months, the study should be evaluable in 2005.

Finally, given the recent approval of taxotere for the treatment of hormone-refractory prostate cancer and preclinical data supporting a combination of atrasentan and the taxanes, a phase 1 trial of atrasentan and taxotere is underway. Likewise, the activity of the bisphosphonates in preventing skeletal-related events in advanced prostate cancer coupled with the activity of atrasentan in this compartment has led to a phase 1 study of the combination of zometa and atrasentan.

SUMMARY

The endothelin axis has emerged as a unique target for the treatment of metastatic prostate cancer—particularly in the skeleton. The consistency of findings in preclinical models and in phase 1, phase 2, and phase 3 clinical trials all support an ongoing investigation of agents designed to disrupt this axis. Although many questions remain unanswered in this area, translational researchers can be encouraged that the development of an idea into mature clinical trials need not be complacent. It has been less than 10 years since the publication of the original hypothesis to a commitment to seek approval for atrasentan as new drug for hormone-refractory prostate cancer.

REFERENCES

1. Yanagisawa M, Kurihara H, Kimura S, et al. A novel potent vasoconstrictor peptide produced by vascular endothelial cells. Nature 1988;332:411–415.

2. Inoue A, Yanagisawa M, Kimura S, et al. The human endothelin family: Three structurally and pharmacologically distinct isopeptides predicted by three separate genes. Proc Natl Acad Sci USA 1989;86:2863–2867.

3. Kimura S, Kasuya Y, Sawamura T, et al. Conversion of big endothelin-1 to 21-residue endothelin-1 is essential for expression of full vasoconstrictor activity: structure-activity relationships of big endothelin-1. J Cardiovasc Pharmacol 1989;13:S5–7.

4. Nelson JB, Carducci MA. The role of the endothelin axis in prostate cancer. Prostate J 1999;1:126–130.

5. Battistini B, D'Orleans-Juste P, Sirois P. Biology of disease. Endothelins: Circulating plasma levels and presence in other biologic fluids. Lab Invest 1993;68:600–628.

6. Ando K, Hirata Y, Shichiri M, et al. Presence of immunoreactive endothelin in human plasma. FEBS Lett 1989;245:164–166.

7. Yamaji T, Johshita H, Ishibashi M, et al. Endothelin family in human plasma and cerebrospinal fluid. J Clin Endocrinol Metab 1990;71:1611–1615.

8. Berbinschi A, Ketelslegers JM. Endothelin in urine. Lancet 1989;2:46.

9. Lam H-C, Takahashi K, Ghatei MA, et al. Presence of immunoreactive endothelin in human milk. FEBS Lett 1990;261:184–186.

10. Casey ML, Word RA, MacDonald PC. Endothelin-1 gene expression and regulation of endothelin mRNA and protein biosynthesis in avascular human amnion: Potential source of amniotic fluid endothelin. J Biol Chem 1991;266:5762–5768.

11. Casey ML, Byrd W, MacDonald PC. Massive amounts of immunoreactive endothelin in human seminal fluid. J Clin Endocrinol Metabol 1992;74:223–225.

12. Prayer-Galetti T, Rossi GP, Belloni AS, et al. Gene expression and autoradiographic localization of endothelin-1 and its receptors A and B in the different zones of the normal human prostate. J Urol 1997;157:2334–2339.

13. Lagenstroer P, Tang R, Shapiro E, et al. Endothelin-1 in the human prostate: tissue levels, source of production and isometric tension studies. J Urol 1993;150:495–499.

14. Saita Y, Yazawa H, Koizumi T, et al. Mitogenic activity of endothelin on human cultured prostatic smooth muscle cells. Eur J Pharmacol 1998;349:123–128.

15. Nelson JB, Hedican SP, George DJ, et al. Identification of endothelin-1 in the pathophysiology of metastatic adenocarcinoma of the prostate. Nature Med 1995;1:944–949.

16. Nelson JB, Opgenorth TJ, Fleisher LA, et al. Perioperative plasma endothelin-1 and big endothelin-1 concentrations in elderly patients undergoing major surgical procedures. Anesth Analg 1999;88:898–903.

17. Papandreou CN, Usmani B, Geng Y, et al. Neutral endopeptidase 24.11 loss in metastatic human prostate cancer contributes to androgen-independent progression. Nature Med 1998;4:50–57.

18. Nelson JB, Chan-Tack K, Hedican SP, et al. Endothelin-1 production and decreased endothelin B receptor expression in advanced prostate cancer. Cancer Res 1996;56:663–668.

19. Kobayashi S, Tang R, Wand B, et al. Localization of endothelin receptors in the human prostate. J Urol 1994;151:763–766.

20. Nelson JB, Lee W-H, Nguyen SH, et al. Methylation of the 5' CpG island of the endothelin B receptor gene is common in human prostate cancer. Cancer Res 1997;57:35–37.

21. Woodson K, Hanson J, Tangrea J. A survey of gene-specific methylation in human prostate cancer among black and white men. Cancer Lett 2004;205:181–188.

22. Yegnasubramanian S, Kowalski J, Gonzalgo ML, et al. Hypermethylation of CpG islands in primary and metastatic human prostate cancer. Cancer Res 2004;64:1975–1986.

23. Jeronimo C, Henrique R, Campos PF, et al. Endothelin B receptor gene hypermethylation in prostate adenocarcinoma. J Clin Pathol 2003;56:52–55.

24. Pao MM, Tsutsumi M, Liang G, et al. The endothelin receptor B (EDNRB) promoter displays heterogeneous, site specific methylation patterns in normal and tumor cells. Human Mol Genet 2001;10:903–910.

25. Lo K-W, Tsang Y-S, Kwong J, et al. Promoter hypermethylation of the EDNRB gene in nasopharyngeal carcinoma. Int J Cancer 2002;95:651–655.

26. Cohen AJ, Belinsky S, Franklin W, et al. Molecular and physiologic evidence for 5' CpG island methylation of the endothelin B receptor gene in lung cancer. Chest 2002;121:27S–28S.

27. Gohji K, Kitazawa S, Tamada H, et al. Expression of endothelin receptor A associated with prostate cancer progression. J Urol 2001;165:1033–1036.

28. Suzuki N, Matsumoto H, Kitada C, et al. Production of endothelin-1 and big-endothelin-1 by tumor cells with epithelial-like morphology. J Biochem 1989;106:736–741.

29. Kusuhara M, Yamaguchi K, Nagasaki K, et al. Production of endothelin in human cancer cell lines. Cancer Res 1990;50:3257–3261.

30. Schichiri M, Hirata Y, Nakajima T, et al. Endothelin-1 is an autocrine/paracrine growth factor for human cancer cell lines. J Clin Invest 1991;87:1867–1871.

31. Nelson JB, Bagnato A, Battistini B, et al. The endothelin axis: emerging role in cancer. Nature Reviews Cancer 2003;3:110–116.

32. Brown KD, Littlewood CJ. Endothelin stimulates DNA synthesis in Swiss 3T3 cells. Synergy with polypeptide growth factors. Biochem J 1989;263:977–980.

33. Daub H, Weiss FU, Wallasch C, et al. Role of transactivation of the EGF receptor in signalling by G-protein-coupled receptors. Nature 1996;379:557–560.

34. Le Brun G, Aubin P, Soliman H, et al. Upregulation of endothelin 1 and its precursor by IL-1β, TNF-α, and TGF-β in the PC3 human prostate cancer cell line. Cytokine 1999;11:157–162.

35. Granchi S, Brocchi S, Bonaccorsi L, et al. Endothelin-1 production by prostate cancer cell lines is up-regulated by factors involved in cancer progression and down-regulated by androgens. Prostate 2001;49:267–277.

36. Berges RR, Furuya Y, Remington L, et al. Cell proliferation, DNA repair, and p53 function are not required for programmed death of prostatic glandular cells induced by androgen ablation. Proc Natl Acad Sci 1993;90:8910–8914.

37. Udan MS, Pflug BR, Nelson JB. Endothelin-1 promotes survival of prostate cancer cells through activation of AKT. J Urol 2000;163:31.

38. Pflug BR, Nelson JB, Udan MS. Endothelin-B receptor mediates apoptosis in prostate cancer cells. J Urol 2001;165:50.

39. Takuwa Y, Ohue Y, Takuwa N, et al. Endothelin-1 activates phospholipase C and mobilizes Ca++ from extra- and intracellular pools in osteoblastic cells. Am J Physiol 1989;257:E797–803.

40. Nelson JB, Nguyen SH, Wu-Wong JR, et al. New bone formation in an osteoblastic tumor model is increased by endothelin-1 overexpression and decreased by endothelin A receptor blockade. Urology 1999;53:1063–1069.

41. Yin JJ, Mohammad KS, KaKonen SM, et al. A causal role of endothelin-1 in the pathogenesis of osteoblastic bone metastases. Proc Natl Acad Sci 2003;100:10954–10959.

42. Ferreira SH, Romitelli M, de Nucci G. Endothelin-1 participation in overt and inflammatory pain. J Cardiovascular Pharmacol 1989;13:S220–222.

43. Raffa RB, Schupsky JJ, Martinez RP, et al. Endothelin-1 induced nociception. Life Sci 1991;49:PL61–65.

44. Dahlof B, Gustafsson D, Hedner T, et al. Regional haemodynamic effects of endothelin-1 in rat and man: unexpected adverse reaction. J Hypertens 1990;8:811–817.

45. Raffa RB, Schupsky JJ, Lee DK, et al. Characterization of endothelin-induced nociception in mice: evidence for a mechanistically distinct analgesic model. J Pharmacol Exp Ther 1996;278:1–7.

46. Davar G, Hans G, Fareed MU, et al. Behavioral signs of acute pain produced by application of endothelin-1 to rat sciatic nerve. Neuroreport 1998;9:2279–2283.

47. Gokin AP, Fareed MU, Pan HL, et al. Local injection of endothelin-1 produces pain-like behavior and excitation of nociceptors in rats. J Neurosci 2001;21:5358–5366.

48. Zhou Z, Davar G, Strichartz G. Endothelin-1 (ET-1) selectively enhances the activation gating of slowly inactivating tetrodotoxin-resistant sodium currents in rat sensory neurons: a mechanism for pain-inducing actions of ET-1. J Neurosci 2002;22:6325–6330.

49. Piovezan AP, D'Orleans-Juste P, Souze GE, et al. Endothelin-1-induced ET(A) receptor-mediated nociception, hyperalgesia and oedema in the mouse hind-paw: modulation by simultaneous ET(B) receptor activation. Br J Pharmacol 2000;129:961–968.

50. De-Melo JD, Tonussi CR, D'Orleans-Juste P, et al. Articular nociception induced by endothelin-1, carrageenan and LPS in native and previously inflamed knee-joints in the rat: inhibition by endothelin receptor antagonists. Pain 1998;77:261–269.

51. Wacnik PW, Eikmeier LJ, Ruggles TR, et al. Functional interactions between tumor and peripheral nerve: morphology, algogen identification, and behavioral characterization of a new murine model of cancer pain. J Neurosci 2001;21:9355–9366.

52. Peters CM, Lindsay TH, Pomonis JD, et al. Endothelin and the tumorigenic component of bone cancer pain. Neurosci 2004;126:1043–1052.

53. Opgenorth TJ, Adler AL, Calzadilla SV, et al. Pharmacological characterization of A-127722: An orally active and highly potent ETα-selective receptor antagonist. J Pharmacol Exp Ther 1996;276:473–481.

54. Verhaar MC, Grahn AY, van Weerdt AWM, et al. Pharmacokinetics and pharmacodynamic effects of ABT-627, an oral ETA selective endothelin antagonist, in humans. Br J Clin Pharmacol 2000;49:562–573.

55. Samara E, Dutta S, Cao G, et al. Single-dose pharmacokinetics of atrasentan, and endothelin-A receptor antagonist. J Clin Pharmacol 2001;41:397–403.

56. Carducci MA, Nelson JB, Bowling MK, et al. Atrasentan, an endothelin-receptor antagonist for refractory adenocarcinomas: safety and pharmacokinetics. J Clin Oncol 2002;20:2171–2180.

57. Zonnenberg BA, Groenewegen G, Janus TJ, et al. Phase I dose-escalation study of the safety and pharmacokinetics of atrasentan: an endothelin receptor antagonist for refractory prostate cancer. Clin Cancer Res 2003;9:2965–2972.

58. Carducci MA, Padley RJ, Breul J, et al. The effect of endothelin-A receptor blockade with atrasentan on tumor progression in men with hormone refractory prostate cancer: a randomized, placebo controlled trial. J Clin Oncol 2003;21:679–689.

59. Carducci MA, Nelson JB, Humerickhouse R, et al. Effects of atrasentan on progression and survival in men with hormone refractory prostate cancer: follow-up study M96-594. J Clin Oncol 2002;21:178a.

60. Nelson JB, Nabulsi AA, Vogelzang NJ, et al. Suppression of prostate cancer induced bone remodeling by the endothelin receptor A antagonist atrasentan. J Urol 2003;169:1143–1149.

61. Carducci M, Nelson JB, Saad F, et al. Effects of atrasentan on disease progression and biological markers in men with metastatic hormone-refractory prostate cancer: Phase 3 study. J Clin Oncol 2004;22:384s.

Mechanisms of androgen independence

35

Glenn J Bubley, Steven P Balk

INTRODUCTION

Approximately 80% to 90% of patients with bone metastasis from prostate cancer (CaP) will respond to androgen deprivation therapy.[1,2] However, the duration of response is finite, averaging 12 to 18 months.[3] Combining androgen receptor (AR) antagonists with androgen deprivation therapy has not resulted in a meaningful improvement in survival compared with androgen ablative monotherapy.[4,5] Androgen deprivation administered earlier in the course of the disease, for instance prior to the onset of bone disease, has a longer duration of response, but the overwhelming majority of men will still eventually become resistant to this form of therapy.

Prostate cancer that recurs, either biochemically or clinically, after androgen ablative therapy has been termed hormone-refractory or androgen-independent (AI) CaP. As will be discussed below, the term hormone-refractory is something of a misnomer, as a number of hormonal therapies have some effectiveness after androgen ablation. However, the response rates to these therapies are generally modest and responses are of short duration.[6–8] Although there are an increasing number of treatments available for men with AI disease, the median survival is less than 2 years.[9] What has perplexed physicians for over 50 years is the mechanism of resistance to androgen ablative therapy. If it were possible to understand how CaP cells are able to adapt and thrive in the relative absence of androgens, then insights into therapeutic strategies might follow.

ANDROGEN RECEPTOR AND PROSTATE CANCER BIOLOGY

Most hormone-naive tumors express the AR and are dependent on signaling through androgens for cell growth or survival. Interestingly, the majority of CaPs that recur following androgen deprivation continue to secrete prostate-specific antigen (PSA). The expression of PSA is induced by androgens. In fact, the pattern of genes expressed by AI CaP is very similar to the pattern observed for hormone-naive tumors prior to androgen ablation.[10] Therefore, it appears as if androgen-independent tumors remain dependent on AR signaling, and multiple studies have focused on the role of the AR signaling in disease progression.

The androgen receptor is a sex hormone receptor and a member of nuclear receptor superfamily.[11–13] It has a structure similar to other steroid hormone receptors. The AR amino-terminal, encoded by exon 1, comprises about half of the protein and can independently strongly stimulate transcription. DNA binding is mediated by a central DNA binding domain (exons 2 and 3) that binds to specific DNA sequences (androgen responsive elements, AREs) located in androgen-regulated genes. Androgen binding is mediated by the carboxy-terminal ligand binding domain, comprising exons 4 to 8. In the absence of androgen, the AR associates with a heat shock protein 90 complex that functions as a chaperone to maintain the AR in a ligand binding conformation. Upon androgen binding, the AR undergoes a conformational change that results in formation of a homodimer, DNA binding, and recruitment of multiple transcription factors that activate the transcription of androgen dependent genes.

ANDROGEN RECEPTOR IN ANDROGEN-INDEPENDENT PROSTATE CANCER

EXPRESSION

The AR is expressed in the majority of androgen-independent CaP, importantly often at increased levels relative to the primary tumors.[14–17] Our cDNA microarray expression studies of metastatic AI versus primary CaP averages approximately 5-fold higher levels of AR message in the AI tumors (manuscript in preparation). Increased AR expression is a consistent finding in cDNA studies in AI cell lines.[18] Moreover, AR immunostaining reveals a strong nuclear pattern of expression in AI CaP, even in patients treated with a luteinizing hormone-releasing hormone (LHRH) agonist and bicalutamide.[19] In contrast, AR expression is not increased in primary androgen-dependent CaP relative to normal prostate epithelium.[20–23] These observations suggest that there is selective pressure to increase AR expression in response to androgen deprivation therapy.

One mechanism for increased AR expression is gene amplification. Importantly the AR gene is amplified in up to 30% of patients with AI disease.[24,25] The AR expressed in AI CaP also appears to be transcriptionally active as these tumors express high levels of multiple genes that are normally AR regulated, including PSA and prostate-specific membrane antigen (PSMA). Finally, in experimental models of AI disease, disruption of AR function by either a hammerhead ribozyme[26] or by RNA interference (manuscript submitted) inhibits tumor growth. Taken together, these observations indicate that the AR remains active in AI CaP through mechanisms that are refractory to the usual androgen deprivation therapies.

MUTATIONS

One mechanism proposed to account for AR activity in AI CaP is mutations of the receptor. In-vitro studies have shown that AR deletion mutants with the entire carboxy-terminal ligand-binding domain removed are constitutively active in the absence of androgens,[27,28] but such mutations have not been identified in patients. However, several groups have found AR missense mutations in AI CaP patients.[16,22,29–33] For example, our group used reverse transcriptase polymerase chain reaction (PCR) amplification and DNA sequencing to

analyze the AR expressed in bone marrow metastases from patients with advanced AI disease. In these studies any candidate mutations were confirmed by repeat amplification and sequencing, while polymorphisms were ruled out by sequencing the AR gene from peripheral blood mononuclear cells.[16,32] Results from these studies and additional samples are summarized in Table 35.1. Sequencing of the AR ligand-binding domain has revealed AR mutations in 12 of 44 patients. Significantly, the majority of the mutations were in patients treated with an AR antagonist (flutamide) in conjunction with androgen ablation (combined androgen blockade). In this group mutations were found in 9 of 21 samples, versus 3 of 23 samples from monotherapy-treated patients. This finding suggested that flutamide treatment was selecting for tumor cells with AR mutations.

Table 35.1 Summary of androgen receptor (AR) mutations in bone marrow metastases from androgen-independent prostate cancer patients treated initially with androgen ablation monotherapy versus combined androgen blockade with flutamide

Monotherapy	AR	Combined	AR
Orchiectomy	Gln902Arg	Orchiectomy + F	WT
Orchiectomy	Multiple*	Orchiectomy + F	Und
Orchiectomy	WT	LHRH + F	Thr877Ser
Orchiectomy	WT	LHRH + F	His874Tyr
Orchiectomy	WT	LHRH + F	Ala721Thr
Orchiectomy	WT	LHRH + F	WT
Orchiectomy	WT	LHRH + F	Val715Met
Orchiectomy	Und	LHRH + F	Thr877Ala
Orchiectomy	Und	LHRH + F	WT
Orchiectomy	WT	LHRH + F	Thr877Ala
Orchiectomy	WT	LHRH + F	Thr877Ala
Orchiectomy	WT	LHRH + F	WT
Orchiectomy	WT	LHRH + F	Thr877Ala, Thr877Ser†
LHRH	WT	LHRH + F	WT
LHRH	WT	LHRH + F	WT
LHRH	Und	LHRH + F	Thr877Ala
LHRH	WT	LHRH + F	WT
LHRH	WT	LHRH + F	WT
LHRH	Und	LHRH + F	WT
LHRH	Asp890Asn	LHRH + F	WT
LHRH	WT	LHRH + F	WT
LHRH	WT		
DES	Und		

DES, diethylstilbesterol (an estrogen) LHRH, leutinizing hormone-releasing hormone; F, flutamide; WT, wildtype; Und, undetectable AR by PCR amplification.

*A single AR with 4 mutations was detected.

†Two mutant ARs detected in biopsy.

The mutation found most frequently in the flutamide-treated patients (Thr877Ala, codon 877 threonine to alanine) was identical to the mutation identified initially in the LNCaP cell line.[34] Importantly, this mutant AR is strongly stimulated by 4-hydroxyflutamide (the active metabolite of flutamide), as well as by estradiol and progesterone. The functional consequences of the other mutants were similarly assessed by transfecting each mutant AR into an AR-negative cell line, in conjunction with an androgen-regulated luciferase reporter gene. These experiments demonstrated that 4-hydroxyflutamide also stimulated the Val715Met, His874Tyr, and Thr877Ser mutations identified in the flutamide-treated patients.[32,35] In contrast, the Asp890Asn and Gln902Arg mutants from the monotherapy patients were not stimulated by 4-hydroxyflutamide. Significantly, bicalutamide was still an antagonist of these mutant ARs in-vitro, and clinical responses to bicalutamide were observed in patients bearing these mutations.[7]

The detection of gain-of-function AR mutations indicates that there is strong selective pressure to maintain AR activity after androgen ablation therapy. This conclusion is also supported by the report of a cortisol-stimulated mutant AR from an AI CaP bone marrow metastasis.[36] Nonetheless, mutation of the AR gene is not likely to be a frequent mechanism for AR activity in AI disease, as mutations have been detected in only a minority of patients. The variable rate for the detection of AR mutations may reflect in part different patient populations, tumor from primary versus metastatic sites, methods used to detect mutations, and whether the patients were treated with flutamide.[16,22,29–33]

COACTIVATORS AND CO-REPRESSORS

The transcriptional activity of the AR and other steroid hormone receptors is mediated through a large and growing number of interacting proteins that function as coactivators, co-repressors, or otherwise modulate transcriptional activity (Figure 35.1).[37] The best characterized of these coactivators are the steroid receptor coactivator (SRC) proteins (SRC1, –2, and –3).[38–43] These coactivators bind to agonist-liganded nuclear receptors, with binding to the AR mediated by independent sites in the AR amino-terminus and the carboxy-terminal ligand binding domain.[44–48] The SRC proteins enhance transcriptional activity through intrinsic histone acetyltransferase activity and binding of additional factors, such as CREB binding protein (CBP) and p300. However, although the SRC proteins can clearly augment AR transcriptional activity in the presence of androgens, their possible role in AI CaP has not been clear.

Importantly, recent studies have found increased expression of SRC1 and SRC2 (TIF2, murine GRIP1) in clinical samples from AI CaP.[49,50] Studies in vitro further indicate that SRC1 can augment AR transcriptional activity in the presence of therapeutic levels of bicalutamide.[19] Taken together with high levels of AR, these findings indicate that increased coactivator expression could be a mechanism contributing to AR activity in androgen-independent CaP.

Co-repressor proteins make important contributions to the biology of multiple nuclear receptors, such as the thyroid hormone receptor and retinoid receptors. The best characterized of these co-repressors are NCoR and

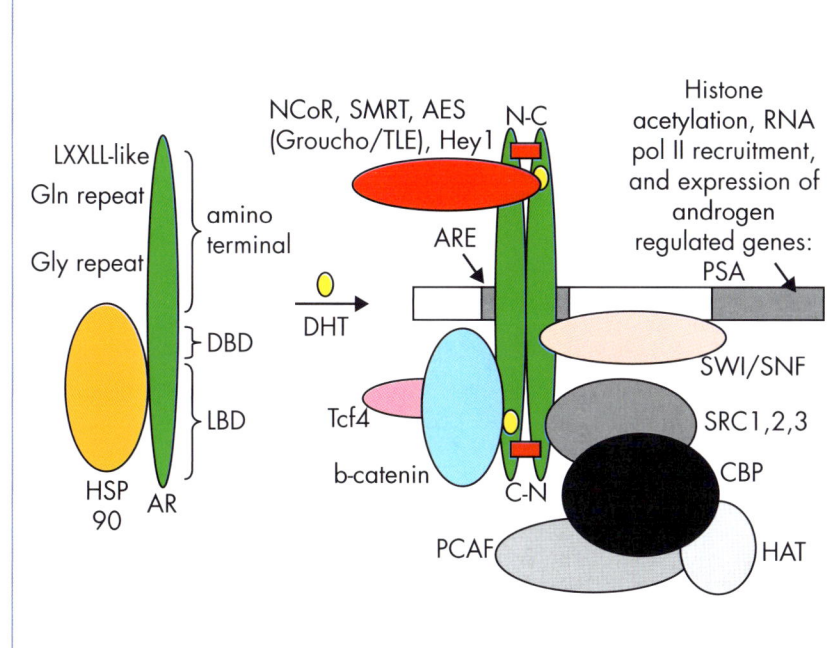

Fig. 35.1
Androgen receptor structure and function: AR, Androgen receptor; Gln, glutamine repeats within the AR; Gly, glycine repeats within the AR; LXXLL, amino acid binding site within the amino terminal of the AR; Hsp90, Heat shock protein 90; DBD, DNA binding domain of the AR; LBD, ligand binding domain of the AR; DHT, dihydrotestosterone; N-C, N-terminal-C-terminal interaction of the AR; Tcf4, T cell factor 4, along with beta catenin a AR co-activator; N-COR, SMRT, AES, Groucho/TLE, Hey, potential co:repressors or part of the co:repressor complex for the AR; SRC1,2,3, steroid receptor co:activator proteins. The following are part of the transcriptional complex. CBP, creb-binding protein; HAT, histone acetyltransferase; PCAF, P 300 associated factor; SWI/SNF, chromatin helicases.

SMRT, which bind to unliganded nuclear receptors and repress transcription through recruitment of histone deacetylases.[51,52] Importantly, the activities of tamoxifen and raloxifene in breast cancer reflect their ability to induce alternative conformations of the estrogen receptor that favor NCoR binding.[53–55] Nonetheless, a physiological role for co-repressors in regulating the AR and other steroid hormone receptors has been uncertain, as unliganded steroid hormone receptors appear to be sequestered away from DNA. However, recent reports indicate that the AR can be regulated by co-repressors,[56,57] including NCoR.[58] These findings suggest the development of selective agonists that favor AR-co-repressor binding as an alternative approach to block AR function.

Finally, it should be emphasized that there is a large and rapidly growing list of additional proteins that appear to interact with and modulate the AR. While some of these proteins may function as general coactivators or co-repressors of AR transcriptional activity, others may modulate AR activity selectively on subsets of promoters.

ACTIVATION BY GROWTH FACTOR AND SIGNAL TRANSDUCTION PATHWAYS

Androgen-independent disease may be mediated by AR activation though signaling and growth factor receptor pathways. At least in vitro, AR activation in the apparent absence of androgens has been reported in response to stimulation by several growth factors and signal transduction pathways including protein kinase A and protein kinase C.[59–64] The reason for great interest in these observations is that it connects pathways that may be important in AI disease, and for which there is evidence from some experimental models. For instance, it has been demonstrated that stimulation of LNCaP cells with growth factors such as epidermal growth factor (EGF), keratinocyte growth factor (KGF), or insulin like growth factor 1 (IGF1) results in enhanced cell growth and PSA secretion, independent of androgen.[59,65] In an animal model of AI disease, Sawyers et al demonstrated that increased expression the HER2/NEU growth factor receptor, a member of the EGF-receptor family, resulted in enhanced activity of the AR, even in the absence of androgen stimulation.[66]

Activation of phosphoinositol 3 (PI3) kinase pathway may also enhance the transition to AI cell growth. The PTEN gene product encodes a phosphatidylinositol phosphatase that antagonizes the activity of PI3 kinase.[67] Loss of PTEN function, therefore, leads to maintenance of PI3 kinase signaling in a chronically activated state and further downstream activation of the AKT/mTOR pathway, which is associated with proliferation and resistance to apoptosis. Importantly, the PTEN gene seems to be lost more frequently in AI disease.[68] However, even in PTEN-positive cells, the AKT/mTOR pathway can be activated further by growth factor stimulation.

Interleukin 6 (IL6) can also stimulate ligand-independent AR activation, which may be mediated by signal transducer and activator of transcription 3 (a signal transduction protein, STAT3).[69,70] However, in cases where AR antagonists were examined, AR activation could be inhibited by bicalutamide at concentrations well within those achieved in vivo in patients.[71] It is important to underscore that, in many experimental models of AI disease, antiandrogen treatment at concentrations easily achievable in vivo blocks the effects of growth factor and signal transduction stimulation. Therefore, these models are not fully consistent with the clinical behavior of AI CaP, which as above does not often respond to therapy with AR antagonists

Other signal transduction pathways that may modulate the AR are Erks, β-catenin, and caveolin. One report has shown ligand-independent AR activity on the complex PSA promoter/enhancer in cells transfected with a constitutively activated MAP kinase kinase (MEKK1) and this activity was only partially blocked by bicalutamide.[72] Also, it has been shown that the AR can interact directly with β-catenin and caveolin.[73–77] There have also been interactions observed between the AR and cyclins, cyclin dependent kinases, and cyclin dependent kinase inhibitors.[78–81] Therefore, interactions between the AR and these modulating proteins may be another promising target for novel AR antagonists

It is not known with certainty how stimulation by growth factors and signal transduction pathways would result in activation of the AR. Some of the effects of growth factor and signaling pathways may be mediated by AR phosphorylation, but the role of phosphorylation in regulating AR activity remains uncertain.[12] There is also an emerging literature demonstrating that AR (and many other transcription factors) can be regulated by acetylation, and by conjugation to ubiquitin and the related protein small ubiquitin-like modifier (SUMO).[82] These alterations in AR protein structure may alter AR stability or other of its functional properties. Finally, AR can effect cell signaling systems by nongenomic mechanisms as evidenced by the fact that these reactions occur within a time frame too short to implicate regulation of AR-expressed genes.[83]

ALTERATION OF CELL CYCLE PROTEINS AND ANDROGEN-INDEPENDENT DISEASE

A fruitful avenue of research into potential molecular mechanisms of AI disease is to interrogate clinical samples from patients at this stage of disease. The *MYC* oncogene has been shown to be amplified in almost approximately 10% of cases refractory stages, but only rarely in hormone-sensitive disease.[84] In experimental models of AI disease, disruption of *MYC* by RNA interference alters the cell phenotype.[85] This is of interest as this gene product is involved in cell cycle regulation and cell division.

Progression to AI disease may also involve alterations in other critical cell-cycle regulatory proteins such as the cyclin-dependent kinase inhibitor p27 (kip1).[86] Loss of p27 is observed more frequently in metastatic CaP[87] and seems to be an independent marker of poor disease outcome in primary disease.[88] Interestingly in an animal model of CaP, the combination of loss of p27 and heterozygous loss of PTEN results in the development of CaP.[89]

There may be other alterations involving the evolution of CaP to the hormone refractory state that are related to loss of the normal control for cell death. Very interestingly, increased expression of the antiapoptotic gene, *BCL2*, leads to androgen independence in LNCaP cells.[90] In experimental systems, inhibition of ras signaling can restore hormonal sensitivity to a CaP cell line in vivo.[91]

WHAT IS LEARNED REGARDING ANDROGEN-INDEPENDENT DISEASE FROM SECONDARY HORMONAL MANIPULATIONS

Although second line or salvage hormonal therapies are less effective than primary hormonal therapy, the responses observed in some patients to these therapies provide genuine insight into potential mechanisms of androgen independence.

Some patients treated with antiandrogens in combination with LHRH agonists have been shown to experience a clinical response following discontinuation of the antiandrogen.[92] Molecular analysis of the AR from patients treated with long term flutamide and who have a withdrawal response reveal that at least some of these patients have a point mutation in the AR that alters the function of the protein such that it is stimulated, rather than inhibited, by flutamide.[92] Some of these patients will respond to bicalutamide, albeit for a relatively brief period.[6,7]

Insight into AI disease can also be gleaned from an evaluation of the effects of ketoconazole.[93] Although ketoconazole may have non-hormonal antitumor properties, it is likely that as a salvage therapy it is effective by reducing adrenal hormonal synthesis. In fact, at the doses prescribed, ketoconazole so effectively inhibits the synthesis of adrenal cortical hormones that it is necessary to co-administer replacement doses of glucocorticoids. It is thought that androstenedione and other adrenal androgens may either directly stimulate

the androgen receptor, or be converted to testosterone at the tissue level. In fact, in one study, patients who had become refractory to ketoconazole were shown to have higher levels of adrenal hormonal synthesis than those achieved at the beginning of treatment.[8] These data suggest that AI disease may result in part from residual levels of androgens present in tumor tissues. There may increased synthesis of androgens within tumor tissues during the progression to AI disease.[94]

Estrogens such as DES have been shown to be effective in the treatment of CaP. DES has an approximately 25% response rate.[95] The mechanism of response to DES in AI disease is not known. However, it is known that AI cells express other steroid receptors in addition to the androgen receptor. For example prostate cells and perhaps CaP cells express the beta form of the estrogen receptor (ERβ). It is also possible that circulating androgens or even the metabolism of androgens at the tissue level could be effected by DES. Besides ERβ, other nuclear receptors have been targeted for therapy in AI disease. Responses to vitamin D analogs such as calcitrol,[96] and to retinoids,[97] suggest that these nuclear receptors might play a role in AI disease.

CONCLUSIONS

Obviously one of the more important and vexing problems facing CaP patients is the progression of the disease to the hormone-refractory state. It is generally accepted that the eventual failure of androgen ablation therapy is due to the outgrowth of tumors cells present at the initiation of therapy that are either fully or partially AI, with cells in the latter case evolving over time into more fully AI cells. The consistent expression of the AR and of androgen-regulated genes by AI CaP, and the selection for tumor cells with AR gene amplification and activating AR mutations, indicate that continued AR activity is necessary for the outgrowth of these tumor cells.

How might AR activity be maintained despite the decrement in androgen levels? One hypothesis is that the AR is "hyper-responsive" to androgen signaling, even by minute quantities of androgen. This hyper-responsiveness might be the result of altered structure or expression of the AR, or altered interaction with coactivating or co-repressing proteins, or as the result of crosstalk with other signal transduction pathways, such as those involved from growth factor receptors. Another hypothesis is that, despite multiple hormonal measures, during the evolution of AI disease androgen metabolism is enhanced within CaP cells in such a manner that concentrations of ligand sufficient for AR activation are maintained. It is also quite possible that there are other pathways involved with progression to the hormone-refractory state that are totally independent of the androgen receptor.

REFERENCES

1. Catalona WJ. Management of cancer of the prostate. N Engl J Med 1994;331:996–1004.

2. Denmeade SR, Isaacs JT. A history of prostate cancer treatment. Nat Rev Cancer 2002;2:389–396.

3. Isaacs W, De Marzo A, Nelson W. Focus on prostate cancer. Cancer Cell 2002;2:113–116.

4. Eisenberger MA, Blumenstein BA, Crawford ED, et al. Bilateral orchiectomy with or without flutamide for metastatic prostate cancer. N Engl J Med 1998;339:1036–1042.

5. Caubet JF, Tosteson TD, Dong EW, et al. Maximum androgen blockade in advanced prostate cancer: a meta-analysis of published randomized controlled trials using nonsteroidal antiandrogens. Urology 1997;49:71–78.

6. Scher HI, Liebertz C, Kelly WK, et al. Bicalutamide for advanced prostate cancer: the natural versus treated history of disease. J Clin Oncol 1997;15:2928–2938.

7. Joyce R, Fenton MA, Rode P, et al. High dose bicalutamide for androgen independent prostate cancer: effect of prior hormonal therapy. J Urol 1998;159:149–153.

8. Small EJ, Halabi S, Dawson NA, et al. Antiandrogen withdrawal alone or in combination with ketoconazole in androgen independent prostate cancer: a phase III trial. J Clin Oncol 2004;22:1025–1033.

9. Oefelein MG, Agarwal PK, Resnick MI. Survival of patients with hormone refractory prostate cancer in the prostate specific antigen era. J Urol 2004;171:1525–1528.

10. Mousses S, Wagoner U, Chen Y, et al. Failure of hormone therapy in prostate cancer involves systematic restoration of androgen responsive genes and activation of rapamycin sensitive signaling. Oncogene 2001;20:6718–6713.

11. Mangelsdorf DJ, Thummel C, Beato M, et al. The nuclear receptor superfamily: the second decade. Cell 1995;83:835–839.

12. Quigley CA, De Bellis A, Marschke KB, et al. Androgen receptor defects: historical, clinical, and molecular perspectives. Endocr Rev 1995;16:271–321.

13. Brinkmann AO, Blok LJ, de Ruiter PE, et al. Mechanisms of androgen receptor activation and function. J Steroid Biochem Mol Biol 1999;69:307–313.

14. van der Kwast TH, Schalken J, Ruizeveld de Winter JA, et al. Androgen receptors in endocrine-therapy-resistant human prostate cancer. Int J Cancer 1991;48:189–193.

15. Ruizeveld de Winter JA, Janssen PJ, Sleddens HM, et al. Androgen receptor status in localized and locally progressive hormone refractory human prostate cancer. Am J Pathol 1994;144:735–746.

16. Taplin ME, Bubley GJ, Shuster TD, et al. Mutation of the androgen-receptor gene in metastatic androgen-independent prostate cancer. N Engl J Med 1995;332:1393–1398.

17. Hobisch A, Culig Z, Radmayr C, et al. Distant metastases from prostatic carcinoma express androgen receptor protein. Cancer Res 1995;55:3068–3072.

18. Chen CD, Welsbie DS, Tran C, et al. Molecular determinants of resistance to antiandrogen therapy. Nat Med 2004;10:33–39

19. Masiello D, Cheng S, Bubley GJ, et al. Bicalutimide functions as an androgen receptor antagonist by assembly of a transcriptionally inactive receptor. J Biol Chem 2002;277:26321–26326.

20. Leav I, McNeal JE, Kwan PW, et al: Androgen receptor expression in prostatic dysplasia (prostatic intraepithelial neoplasia) in the human prostate: an immunohistochemical and in situ hybridization study. Prostate 1996;29:137–145.

21. Tsuji M, Kanda K, Murakami Y, et al. Biologic markers in prostatic intraepithelial neoplasia: immunohistochemical and cytogenetic analyses. J Med Invest 1999;46:35–41.

22. Harper ME, Glynne-Jones E, Goddard L, et al. Expression of androgen receptor and growth factors in premalignant lesions of the prostate. J Pathol 1998;186:169–177.

23. Sweat SD, Pacelli A, Bergstralh EJ, et al. Androgen receptor expression in prostatic intraepithelial neoplasia and cancer. J Urol 1999;161:1229–1232.

24. Visakorpi T, Hyytinen E, Koivisto P, et al. In vivo amplification of the androgen receptor gene and progression of human prostate cancer. Nat Genet 1995;9:401–406.

25. Koivisto P, Kononen J, Palmberg C, et al. Androgen receptor gene amplification: a possible molecular mechanism for androgen deprivation therapy failure in prostate cancer. Cancer Res 1997;57:314–319.

26. Zegarra-Moro OL, Schmidt LJ, Huang H, et al. Disruption of androgen receptor function inhibits proliferation of androgen-refractory prostate cancer cells. Cancer Res 2002;62:5632–5636.

27. Jenster G, van der Korput HA, van Vroonhoven C, et al. Domains of the human androgen receptor involved in steroid binding, transcriptional activation, and subcellular localization. Mol Endocrinol 1991;5:1396–1404.

28. Simental JA, Sar M, Lane MV, et al. Transcriptional activation and nuclear targeting signals of the human androgen receptor. J Biol Chem 1991;266:510–518.

29. Culig Z, Hobisch A, Cronauer MV, et al. Mutant androgen receptor detected in an advanced-stage prostatic carcinoma is activated by adrenal androgens and progesterone. Mol Endocrinol 1993;7:1541–1550.

30. Suzuki H, Sato N, Watabe Y, et al. Androgen receptor gene mutations in human prostate cancer. J Steroid Biochem Mol Biol 1993;46:759–765.

31. Suzuki H, Akakura K, Komiya A, et al. Codon 877 mutation in the androgen receptor gene in advanced prostate cancer: relation to antiandrogen withdrawal syndrome. Prostate 1996;29:153–158.

32. Taplin ME, Bubley GJ, Ko YJ, et al. Selection for androgen receptor mutations in prostate cancers treated with androgen antagonist. Cancer Res 1999;59:2511–2515.

33. Zhao XY, Boyle B, Krishnan AV, et al. Two mutations identified in the androgen receptor of the new human prostate cancer cell line MDA PCa 2a. J Urol 1999;162:2192–2199.

34. Veldscholte J, Ris-Stalpers C, Kuiper GG, et al. A mutation in the ligand binding domain of the androgen receptor of human LNCaP cells affects steroid binding characteristics and response to anti-androgens. Biochem Biophys Res Commun 1990;173:534–540.

35. Fenton MA, Shuster TD, Fertig AM, et al. Functional characterization of mutant androgen receptors from androgen-independent prostate cancer. Clin Cancer Res 1997;3:1383–1388.

36. Zhao XY, Malloy PJ, Krishnan AV, et al. Glucocorticoids can promote androgen-independent growth of prostate cancer cells through a mutated androgen receptor. Nat Med 2000;6:703–706.

37. McKenna NJ, Lanz RB, O'Malley BW. Nuclear receptor coregulators: cellular and molecular biology. Endocr Rev 1999;20:321–344.

38. Onate SA, Tsai SY, Tsai MJ, et al. Sequence and characterization of a coactivator for the steroid hormone receptor superfamily. Science 1995;270:1354–1357.

39. Voegel JJ, Heine MJ, Zechel C, et al. TIF2, a 160 kDa transcriptional mediator for the ligand-dependent activation function AF-2 of nuclear receptors. EMBO J 1996;15:3667–3675.

40. Torchia J, Rose DW, Inostroza J, et al. The transcriptional co-activator p/CIP binds CBP and mediates nuclear-receptor function. Nature 1997;387:677–684.

41. Hong H, Kohli K, Garabedian MJ, et al. GRIP1, a transcriptional coactivator for the AF-2 transactivation domain of steroid, thyroid, retinoid, and vitamin D receptors. Mol Cell Biol 1997;17:2735–2744.

42. Anzick SL, Kononen J, Walker RL, et al. AIB1, a steroid receptor coactivator amplified in breast and ovarian cancer. Science 1997;277:965–968.

43. Takeshita A, Cardona GR, Koibuchi N, et al. TRAM-1, A novel 160-kDa thyroid hormone receptor activator molecule, exhibits distinct properties from steroid receptor coactivator-1. J Biol Chem 1997;272:27629–27634.

44. Ding XF, Anderson CM, Ma H, et al. Nuclear receptor-binding sites of coactivators glucocorticoid receptor interacting protein 1 (GRIP1) and steroid receptor coactivator 1 (SRC-1): multiple motifs with different binding specificities. Mol Endocrinol 1998;12:302–313.

45. Berrevoets CA, Doesburg P, Steketee K, et al. Functional interactions of the AF-2 activation domain core region of the human androgen receptor with the amino-terminal domain and with the transcriptional coactivator TIF2 (transcriptional intermediary factor2). Mol Endocrinol 1998;12:1172–1183.

46. Webb P, Nguyen P, Shinsako J, et al. Estrogen receptor activation function 1 works by binding p160 coactivator proteins. Mol Endocrinol 1998;12:1605–1618.

47. Alen P, Claessens F, Verhoeven G, et al. The androgen receptor amino-terminal domain plays a key role in p160 coactivator-stimulated gene transcription. Mol Cell Biol 1999;19:6085–6097.

48. Bevan CL, Hoare S, Claessens F, et al. The AF1 and AF2 domains of the androgen receptor interact with distinct regions of SRC1. Mol Cell Biol 1999;19:8383–8392.

49. Gregory CW, He B, Johnson RT, et al. A mechanism for androgen receptor-mediated prostate cancer recurrence after androgen deprivation therapy. Cancer Res 2001;61:4315–4319.

50. Fujimoto N, Mizokami A, Harada S, et al. Different expression of androgen receptor coactivators in human prostate. Urology 2001;58:289–294.

51. Horlein AJ, Naar AM, Heinzel T, et al. Ligand-independent repression by the thyroid hormone receptor mediated by a nuclear receptor co-repressor. Nature 1995;377:397–404.

52. Chen JD, Evans RM. A transcriptional co-repressor that interacts with nuclear hormone receptors. Nature 1995;377:454–457.

53. Smith CL, Nawaz Z, O'Malley BW. Coactivator and corepressor regulation of the agonist/antagonist activity of the mixed antiestrogen, 4-hydroxytamoxifen. Mol Endocrinol 1997;11:657–666.

54. Brzozowski AM, Pike AC, Dauter Z, et al Molecular basis of agonism and antagonism in the oestrogen receptor. Nature 1997;389:753–758.

55. Shiau AK, Barstad D, Loria PM, et al. The structural basis of estrogen receptor/coactivator recognition and the antagonism of this interaction by tamoxifen. Cell 1998;95:927–937.

56. Yu X, Li P, Roeder RG, et al. Inhibition of androgen receptor-mediated transcription by amino-terminal enhancer of split. Mol Cell Biol 2001;21:4614–4625.

57. Yuan X, Lu ML, Li T, et al. SRY interacts with and negatively regulates androgen receptor transcriptional activity. J Biol Chem ;276:46647–46654.

58. Cheng S, Brzostek S, Lee SR, et al. Inhibition of the dihydrotestosterone activated androgen receptor by the corepressor NCoR. Mol Endocrinol, in press.

59. Culig Z, Hobisch A, Cronauer MV, et al. Androgen receptor activation in prostatic tumor cell lines by insulin-like growth factor-I, keratinocyte growth factor and epidermal growth factor. Eur Urol 1995;27:45–47.

60. Ikonen T, Palvimo JJ, Kallio PJ, et al. Stimulation of androgen-regulated transactivation by modulators of protein phosphorylation. Endocrinology 1994;135:1359–1366.

61. de Ruiter PE, Teuwen R, Trapman J, et al. Synergism between androgens and protein kinase-C on androgen-regulated gene expression. Mol Cell Endocrinol 1995;110:1–6.

62. Nazareth LV, Weigel NL. Activation of the human androgen receptor through a protein kinase A signaling pathway. J Biol Chem 1996;271:19900–19907.

63. Blok LJ, de Ruiter PE, Brinkmann AO. Forskolin-induced dephosphorylation of the androgen receptor impairs ligand binding. Biochemistry 1998;37:3850–3857.

64. Sadar MD. Androgen-independent induction of prostate-specific antigen gene expression via cross-talk between the androgen receptor and protein kinase A signal transduction pathways. J Biol Chem 1999;274:7777–7783

65. Putz T, Culig Z, Eder IE, et al. Epidermal growth factor receptor blockade inhibits the action of EGF, insulin like growth factor I, and a protein kinase activator in prostate cancer cell lines. Cancer Res 1999;59:227–233.

66. Craft N, Shostak Y, Carey M, et al. A mechanism for hormone-independent prostate cancer through modulation of androgen receptor signaling by the HER-2/neu tyrosine kinase. Nat Med 1999;5:280–285.

67. Whang Y, Xu X, Suzuki H, et al. Inactivation of the tumor suppressor PTEN/MMAC1 advanced prostate cancer through loss of expression. Proc Natl Acad Sci 1998;95:5246–5250.

68. McMenamin ME, Soung P, Perera S, et al. Loss of PTEN expression in paraffin-embedded primary prostate cancer correlates with high Gleason score and advanced stage. Cancer Res 1999;59:4291–4296.

69. Hobisch A, Eder IE, Putz T, et al. Interleukin-6 regulates prostate-specific protein expression in prostate carcinoma cells by activation of the androgen receptor. Cancer Res 1998;58:4640–4645.

70. Chen T, Wang LH, Farrar WL. Interleukin 6 activates androgen receptor-mediated gene expression through a signal transducer and activator of transcription 3-dependent pathway in LNCaP prostate cancer cells. Cancer Res 2000;60:2132–2135.

71. Cockshott ID, Cooper KJ, Sweetmore DS, et al. The pharmacokinetics of Casodex in prostate cancer patients after single and during multiple dosing. Eur Urol 1990;18:10–17.

72. Abreu-Martin MT, Chari A, Palladino AA, et al. Mitogen-activated protein kinase kinase kinase 1 activates androgen receptor-dependent transcription and apoptosis in prostate cancer. Mol Cell Biol 1999;19:5143–5154.

73. Truica CI, Byers S, Gelmann EP. Beta-catenin affects androgen receptor transcriptional activity and ligand specificity. Cancer Res 2000;60:4709–4713.

74. Yang G, Truong LD, Timme TL, et al. Elevated expression of caveolin is associated with prostate and breast cancer. Clin Cancer Res 1998;4:1873–1880.

75. Lu ML, Schneider MC, Zheng Y, et al. Caveolin-1 interacts with androgen receptor. A positive modulator of androgen receptor mediated transactivation. J Biol Chem 2001;276:13442–13451.

76. Yeh S, Lin HK, Kang HY, et al. From HER2/Neu signal cascade to androgen receptor and its coactivators: a novel pathway by induction of androgen target genes through MAP kinase in prostate cancer cells. Proc Natl Acad Sci USA 1999;96:5458–5463.

77. Lin HK, Yeh S, Kang HY, et al. Akt suppresses androgen-induced apoptosis by phosphorylating and inhibiting androgen receptor. Proc Natl Acad Sci USA 2001;98:7200–7205.

78. Knudsen KE, Cavenee WK, Arden KC. D-type cyclins complex with the androgen receptor and inhibit its transcriptional transactivation ability. Cancer Res 1999;59:2297–2301.

79. Yamamoto A, Hashimoto Y, Kohri K, et al. Cyclin E as a coactivator of the androgen receptor. J Cell Biol 2000;150:873–880.

80. Gregory CW, Hamil KG, Kim D, et al. Androgen receptor expression in androgen-independent prostate cancer is associated with increased expression of androgen-regulated genes. Cancer Res 1998;58:5718–5724.

81. Reutens AT, Fu M, Wang C, et al Cyclin D1 binds the androgen receptor and regulates hormone-dependent signaling in a p300/CBP-associated factor (P/CAF)-dependent manner. Mol Endocrinol 2001;15:797–811.

82. Poukka H, Karvonen U, Janne OA, et al. Covalent modification of the androgen receptor by small ubiquitin-like modifier 1 (SUMO-1). Proc Natl Acad Sci USA 2000;97:12145–14150.

83. Baron S, Manin M, Beaudoin C, et al. Androgen receptor mediates non-genomic activation of phosphatidylinositol 3-OH kinase in androgen sensitive epithelial cells. J Biol Chem 2004;279:14579–14586.

84. Bubendorf L, Kononen J, Kiovisto P, et al. Survey of gene amplifications during prostate cancer progression by high throughput fluorescence in situ hybridization on tissue microarrays. Cancer Res 1999;59:803–806.

85. Bernard D, Pourtier-Manzanedo A, Gil J, et al. Myc confers androgen-independent prostate cancer cell growth. J Clin Invest 2003;112:1724–1731.

86. Waltregny D, Leav I, Signoretti S, et al. Androgen-driven prostate epithelial cell proliferation and differentiation in vivo involve the regulation of p27. Mol Endocrinol 2001;15:765–782.

87. Fernandez PL, Arce Y, Farre X, et al. Expression of p27/Kip1 is down regulated in human prostate carcinoma progression J Pathol 1999;187:563–566.

88. Freedland SJ, deGregorio F. Scoolidge JC, et al. Pre operative p27 status is an independent predictor of prostate specific antigen failure following radical prostatectomy J Urol 2003;169:1325–1330.

89. Di Cristofana A, De Acetis M, Koff A, et al. Pten and p27kip1 cooperate in prostate cancer tumor progression in the mouse. Nat Genet 2001;27:222–224.

90. McDonnell TJ, Troncoso P, Brisbay SM, et al. Expression of the protooncogene bcl-2 in the prostate and its assocaition with emergence of androgen-independent prostate cancer. Cancer Res 1992;52:6940–6944.

91. Bakin RE, Goeli D, Bissonette EA, et al. Attenuation of Ras signaling restores androgen sensitivity to hormone-refractory C4-2 prostate cancer cells. Cancer Res 2003;63:1975–1980.

92. Scher HI, Kelly WK. Flutamide withdrawal syndrome: its impact on clinical trials in hormone-refractory prostate cancer. J Clin Oncol 1993;11:1566–1572

93. Buchanen G, Yang M, Harris JM, et al. Mutations at the boundary of the hinge and ligand binding domain of the androgen receptor confer increased transactivation function. Mol Endocrinol 2001;15:46–56.

94. Small EJ, Baron AD, Fippin L, et al. Ketoconazole retains activity in advanced prostate cancer patients with progression depsite flutamide withdrawal. J Urol 1007;157:1204–1207.

94. Mohler JL, Gregory CW, Ford OH, et al. The androgen axis on recurrent prostate cancer. Clin Cancer Res 2004;10:440–448.

95. Oh WK, Kantoff PW, Weinberg V, et al. Prospective, multicenter, randomized phase II trial of the herbal supplement PC-SPES and diethylstilbesterol in patients with androgen-independent prostate cancer. J Clin Oncol 2004;22:3705–3712.

96. Beer TM, Lemmon D, Lowe BA, et al. High-dose weekly oral calcitrol in patients with a rising PSA after prostatectomy or radiation for prostate cancer Cancer 2003;97:1217–1224.

97. Hammond LA, Brown G, Keedwell RG, et al. The prospects of retinoids in the treatment of prostate cancer. Anticancer Drugs 2002;13:781–790.

Knockout models of prostate carcinogenesis

36

Brent W Sutherland, Norman M Greenberg

INTRODUCTION

It is estimated that prostate cancer will be the most diagnosed of all human cancers in 2005 and will continue to remain the second leading yearly cause of cancer related deaths amongst men in the United States (American Cancer Society, Facts and Figures; www.cancer.org). Despite considerable research effort, the underlying causes of prostate cancer remain elusive, and, therefore, we have yet to appreciably influence the efficacy of current therapeutic intervention strategies aimed towards preventing or treating advanced disease.[1–3]

Prostate cancer is a disease mostly unique to aging men, and our understanding of the natural history of prostate cancer remains uncertain, in part, because of the heterogeneous nature of both the disease and the patient population. It is generally accepted, however, that prostate cancer progresses slowly, originating from focal hyperplasias or atrophic inflammatory regions representing early-stage disease through low- and high-grade prostatic epithelial neoplasia (PIN) lesions to become adenocarcinomas that can metastasize to distant sites, most notably to bone. Similar to most if not all cancer, genetic alterations are likely requisite for initiation and progression to advanced disease.[4] Interestingly, many of the well-known and characterized tumor susceptibility genes are not mutated with high frequency in prostate tumors. Rather, prostate tumors appear to exhibit tremendous diversity in identifiable genetic lesions both between and within individual tumors[5] (recently reviewed by several authors[6–8]). It has, therefore, been challenging to identify and isolate clinically relevant prostate cancer tumor susceptibility genes and to develop appropriate and valid models that accurately mimic the uncertain natural history of the human disease. Indeed, significant technical advances have now allowed many groups to develop genetically engineered mouse (GEM) models of spontaneous autochthonous prostate cancer that should help us to understand the mechanisms underlying the initiation, progression and metastatic spread of prostate cancer at the molecular level. Several classes of transgenic mouse models of prostate cancer have been developed in which expression of heterologous genes of interest (GOI) have been enforced in prostate-specific fashion, and these have been recently reviewed.[9–14] The purpose of this discourse will, therefore, be to focus on the development and characterization of "knock-out" and related conditional GEM models that are especially promising in their ability to dissect the role of gene function through ablation in somatic cells, and to discuss recent advances in prostate cancer biology afforded through the application of such strategies. Finally, important considerations for the development of next generation prostate cancer model systems will be examined.

PROSTATE CANCER: FROM THE MOUSE PERSPECTIVE

Rodents rarely develop spontaneous prostate cancer, so the background incidence is fortuitously low. Even though the Lobund–Wistar (L-W) rat will develop tumors in the dorsolateral and anterior prostatic lobes that exhibit progression to androgen independent and metastatic disease,[15] only one in four L-W rats develop such cancers, and only after a long latency period. So investigators have turned to strategies that, for the most part, modulate the expressivity of specific genes implicated by analyses of clinical tissue to generate autochthonous models that hopefully mimic the natural history of prostate cancer with a high degree of penetrance and reproducibility. Indeed, a number of models have been generated that carry lesions in regions exhibiting high frequencies of chromosomal instability during prostate cancer progression including 8p, 10q, 13q, and 17p,[16-24] that encode genes predicted to possess tumor suppression functions such as Nkx3.1 (8p), PTEN (10q), Mxi1 (10q), and Rb (13q).[22-29] Current knockout model strategies can be roughly grouped into three categories (Table 14.1). These are 1) the germline knockouts that allow for detailed investigation of the consequence of defined genetic lesions, loss of heterozygosity (LOH) and/or haploinsufficiency; 2) the bigenic/complex knockouts that help us to characterize how combinations of specific genetic lesions can influence initiation and/or progression; and 3) the conditional knockout models that allow us to control and study the temporal and spatial pattern of a given genetic lesion in a restricted number of cells.

GERMLINE KNOCKOUTS: IS IT HAPLOINSUFFICIENCY OR HAPLOSUFFICIENCY?

Nkx3.1

Clinical data supports a tumor suppressor role for Nkx3.1. It is highly expressed in the prostate gland, maps to a genomic region (8p21) associated with a high frequency of LOH in prostate tumors, and loss of Nkx3.1 protein expression correlates with prostate cancer progression.[23,30-33] Germline knockouts were first generated by Bhatia-Gaur et al to more thoroughly investigate the association between Nkx3.1 and prostate disease.[34] These targeted deletions were in regions in exon 2 that included the homeodomain. While other groups used slightly different targeting strategies,[35-37] all of the resulting models demonstrated that homozygous loss of Nkx3.1 could influence cellular proliferation prior to terminal differentiation, culminating in prostatic epithelial hyperplasia with focal dysplasia that could increase in severity with age. Even though Nkx3.1$^{-/-}$ mice exhibited progression from non-neoplastic hyperplasias to neoplastic mouse PIN lesions with focal atypia (mPIN as defined in ref. 38), additional genetic events appear to be required for progression to advanced metastatic disease, as overt invasive carcinoma or metastasis has not been observed in any of theses models.[34-37] This generally supports the

notion that multiple genetic mutations likely cooperate with Nkx3.1 loss to drive prostate cancer progression.

An interesting observation from these studies was the lobe-specific severity of epithelial hyperplasia and dysplasia in the mice. The most prominent phenotype was in the anterior prostate (AP), followed by the dorsolateral prostates (DLP) and low to absent in the ventral prostate (VP) except for the description of hyperplasia in the ventral lobe by Tanaka et al.[37] This may have been influenced, in part, by the strains used in these studies, especially given the recent report of how strain-related variations in gene expression can modulate cancer development and progression in transgenic models.[39] Interestingly, in a subsequent study, Kim et al[40] examined the effects of Nkx3.1 null mutations in multiple strains, including C57Bl/6J as used by Tanaka et al,[37] and subtle differences in the occurrence of mPIN were also observed between strains.

All groups discussed the possibility that haplo-insufficiency at Nkx3.1 explains the preneoplastic and mPIN phenotypes. One group demonstrated that loss of Nkx3.1 protein (but not mRNA expression) is likely associated with, or at least a prerequisite for, progression of non-neoplastic hyperplasias to neoplastic mPIN lesions,[40,41] while another demonstrated that complete loss of Nkx3.1 activity might not be an absolute prerequisite for progression to mPIN.[42] However, both stochastic loss and dose dependent reduction of key downstream targets such as intelectin, and angiopoietin 2 have been reported.[42] As well, all the germline knockout models demonstrated that loss of Nkx3.1 profoundly effects prostate development, in that all lobes exhibited developmental hypoplasia culminating in loss of prostatic duct complexity with significantly reduced ductal branch morphogenesis, and that titration of Nkx3.1 expression in the C57Bl/6J background was related to a significant reduction in ventral prostate wet weight.[37]

PTEN/Mmac1

Extensive clinical and experimental data supports a tumor suppressor role for the PTEN gene, encoding "phosphatase and tension homolog deleted from chromosome 10",[43] in multiple, if not most, somatic cell malignancies (recently reviewed by Sansall and Sellers[44]). In particular, many groups have reported that LOH and/or reduced PTEN protein expression is commonly associated with primary and advanced prostate cancers.[24,26,43,45-49] Germline knockouts, such as those described by Di Cristofano et al,[50] were generated to investigate the putative association between PTEN and tumorigenesis by deleting exons 4 and 5 (encoding for the entire PTEN-phosphatase domain and part of the two α-helix motifs flanking the catalytic core). Other groups subsequently generated models by targeted deletion of

Table 36.1 Genetically engineered mouse (GEM) gene knockout models

	Strain background	Normal prostate	Abnormal development with or without agenesis, hypoplasia or atrophy	Non-neoplastic proliferation epithelium or stroma, focal or diffuse with or without atypia	mPIN with or without atypia	Neoplastic proliferation with documented progression to invasive carcinoma	with documented metastasis	Reference
Single germline								
Estrogen receptor	C57Bl/6J	+						127
RAR-gamma2		+						128
RAR-gamma			+					128
p53	C57Bl/6J		+					129
p63	C57Bl/6J		+					130
Hoxd-13	129/SvImJ;C57Bl/6J		+					131
prolactin	NI		+					132
p27KIP1;Cdkn1b	C57Bl/6J			+				69
aromatase (cyp19)	C57Bl/6J			+				86
Mix1	NI			+				78
Nkx3.1	129/SvImJ;C57Bl/6J		+	+				37
Nkx3.1	C57Bl/6J		+	+				38
Nkx3.1	C57Bl/6J		+	+				36
Nkx3.1	129/SvImJ and 129/SvImJ;C57Bl/6J		+	+	+			35
PTEN;Mmac1	C57Bl/6J		a+	a+				51
PTEN;Mmac1	129/SvImJ;C57Bl/6J		NI	a+	a+			52
PTEN;Mmac1	129/SvImJ;C57Bl/6J		NI	a+	a+	a+		54
Bigenic/Complex								
Nkx3.1 × p27KIP1	129/SvImJ × C57Bl/6J			b+	b+			89
PTEN × p27KIP1	C57Bl/6J × C57Bl/6J			b+	b+	b+		92
Nkx3.1 × PTEN	129/SvImJ × C57Bl/6J			+	b+	b+	b+	42
PTEN × TRAMP	129/SvImJ × C57Bl/6J			b+	b+	b+	b+	96
Erg1 × TRAMP or CR2-T-Ag	C57Bl/6J × C57Bl/6J or FVB/N			+	+	c+	+	133
PTEN+/– PTEN-Hy	C57Bl/6J × NI			+	+	+		55
Conditional								
RXR-alpha-LoxP × PB-Cre4	NI		+	+	+			121
Rb-LoxP x × PB-Cre	C57Bl/6J × 129/SvImJ			+	+			128
Nkx3.1-LoxP × PSA-Cre	C57Bl/6J × C57Bl/6J			+	+	+		36
PTEN-LoxPx × MMTV-LTR-Cre	NI			+	+	+		109
PTEN-LoxP× × FB-Cre4 or PB-Cre	C57Bl/6J × C57Bl/6J/6xDBA2 or FVB			+	+	+	+	55
PTEN-LoxP × P3-Cre4	129/Balb/c × C57Bl/6J/6xDBA2			+	+	+	+	110

a+, homozygous null mutant mice are embryonic lethal, heterozygous mice for one null allele and one wild type allele examined in these studies; b+, acceleration or synergistic effect in cancer progression as compared to individual mutant mice alone; c+, delayed progression from mPIN to invasive carcinoma as compared to individual mutant mice alone; NI, not indicated.

part of exon 5 or targeted deletion of exons 3, 4, and 5.[51,52] Although homozygous loss of both PTEN alleles proved to be early-embryonic lethal in these models, they all demonstrate how loss of just one PTEN allele could dramatically influence cellular proliferation and malignant transformation, culminating in epithelial cell hyperplasia and overt neoplasia in multiple organ types, including the prostate gland. Indeed, these groups described that PTEN haploinsufficiency could result in moderate focal prostate epithelial cell hyperplasia and dysplasia. Furthermore, progression to mPIN (with or without documented progression to invasive adenocarcinoma) has been reported in these models, albeit at low penetrance and with advanced age (40–65 weeks).[51–53] One group reported that LOH at PTEN rather than haploinsufficiency was associated with advanced prostate tumors (3/3 tumors analyzed),[53] a finding consistent with some but not all clinical data.[47] However, the influence of LOH and/or haploinsufficiency in early disease states (hyperplasia and/or mPIN) was not addressed in that study. Indeed, a subsequent study (as discussed in the bigenic/complex mouse models section) using a complex breeding strategy and multiple GEM transgenic mice—including the PTEN[+/-] mice generated by Di Cristofano et al[50]—eloquently demonstrated how subtle dose-dependent stochastic titration of protein expression was associated with the early stages of prostate cancer progression.[54]

p27KIP1

Both clinical and experimental data suggest that p27KIP1, a negative regulator of cell cycle progression, plays a tumor suppressor role in multiple cancer types including prostate (reviewed by several authors[55,56]). Although mutation of this gene has rarely been identified in somatic cell tumors,[57,58] a genetic polymorphism is associated with increased risk of hereditary prostate cancer,[59] and genomic instability in the region containing the p27KIP gene is associated with prostate cancer progression.[60] Moreover, loss or mis-localization of p27KIP1 protein expression is associated with prostate cancer progression and/or poor disease-free survival.[61–64] Three independent research groups generated germline p27KIP1 knockouts to investigate an association with cell growth and differentiation.[65–67] One group targeted exon 1 (cyclin-CDK inhibition domain), while the other two groups deleted both exon 1 and 2.[65–67] All models demonstrated how homozygous loss of the p27KIP1 gene could profoundly influence the regulation of cellular proliferation processes culminating in increased total body size and organ size (multiple organs including the prostate). Of the organs examined, increased total size was largely attributed to hyperplastic proliferation rather than increased cellular size, however, prostate glands were

not examined to this detail. Interestingly, although multiple organs exhibited hyperplastic lesions, the only evidence of progression to overt tumor formation was in the pituitary gland.[67] In subsequent studies, loss of p27KIP1 in the prostate gland profoundly influenced the regulation of cellular proliferation culminating in global prostatic hyperplasia.[68] Prostate glands from mice at 14 months of age demonstrated increased rates of prostatic cell proliferation both in the epithelial and stromal compartments, and the total number of acini per gland was significantly increased. However, progression of hyperplastic lesions to mPIN or invasive adenocarcinoma has not yet been documented. Again, and similar to the conclusions of the Nkx3.1 knockout studies, multiple genetic mutations likely cooperate with p27KIP1 loss to drive prostate cancer progression. In contrast to Knudson's "two-mutation" criterion for a tumor suppressor gene,[69] Fero et al[70] conclusively demonstrated that both mice that were nullizygous and those that were heterozygous for the p27KIP1 gene were predisposed to tumorigenesis in multiple tissues, albeit to different degrees of penetrance, when challenged with irradiation or chemical carcinogens that can induce genetic lesions with stochastic variability.

Mxi1

Clinical and experimental data implicate a tumor suppressor role for Mxi1, a MAD family protein[71] in multiple tumor types, including that of the prostate. Mxi1 resides on chromosomal region 10q, which exhibits high frequency of genomic instability in multiple cancers, including prostate cancer.[27–29] Mxi1 is involved in the regulation of cellular proliferation and differentiation though the negative regulation of the MYC oncoprotein, a finding consistent with presumed tumor suppression activity.[72–76] To further investigate the association between Mxi1 and tumorigenesis, a germline knockout model was generated through the deletion of an exon required for the production of both mouse Mxi1 isoforms.[77] This model demonstrated that homozygous loss of Mxi1 could profoundly influence cell homeostatic processes, culminating in both increased proliferation responses and/or in cellular atrophy in multiple organ types, including the prostate. Mice lacking Mxi1 developed modest regions of focal prostatic epithelial cell hyperplasia with evidence of dysplasia and nuclear atypia that became progressively more severe with age, albeit with moderate penetrance (6/11 mice examined). Consistent with a role for Mxi1 in cell cycle regulation, increased cellular proliferation was readily demonstrated by Ki67 expression in lesions of hyperplasia in Mxi1[-/-] mice. However, as neither mPIN nor invasive adenocarcinoma was apparent in these mice, additional genetic mutations are likely prerequisite for advanced prostate disease. Of note, the phenotypic consequence of Mxi1 loss appeared to be very age dependent (onset >7 months). These observations might support the notion that intrinsic age-dependent factors could significantly influence or modify tumor suppressor activities attributed to Mxi1.

Cyr19 (aromatase)

Experimental evidence indicates that early estrogen exposure (imprinting) can influence homeostasis in the fully developed prostate gland, as alterations in growth, androgen receptor expression and predisposition to non-neoplastic transformation are associated with abnormal estrogen exposure in rodent models.[78–84] To further explore this association, prostate glands were obtained and characterized[85] from a knockout model generated through the targeted disruption of cyr19 exon IX.[86] Cyr19 encodes the aromatase enzyme required to convert androgens to estrogen, thus Cyr19$^{-/-}$ mice are, in effect, estrogen deficient. This model demonstrated that estrogen deficiency could profoundly influence normal prostate gland physiology. Mice deficient in estrogen displayed significantly increased levels of serum testosterone (T), 5α-dihydrotestosterone (DHT) and prolactin (PRL). Interestingly, tissues samples of the anterior prostate exhibited significantly increased levels of DHT while levels in other lobes of the prostate were indistinguishable from those of nontransgenic mice. Cyr19 mutant mice also exhibited significantly increased levels of the androgen receptor (AR) in epithelial but not stromal cells in all lobes. Furthermore, prostate lobes appeared significantly larger in mutant mice with a balanced increase in the volumes of the epithelial, interstitial and luminal compartments. However, the severity of abnormal prostatic growth in response to loss of estrogens appeared to be lobe and age dependent. The VP and DLP of estrogen-deficient mice exhibited, on average, a size increase of more than 50%, while the AP exhibited on average a 29% increase in size (all age groups combined). Moreover, significant age-dependent differences in growth advantage of the AP were reported. The 8- to 14-week-old mice exhibited a 40% increase in wet weight, while 16- to 26-week-old mice exhibited a corresponding 21% increase, and 48- to 56-week-old mice exhibited a 25% increase. It was interesting to note that, although all lobes of estrogen deficient mice were clearly enlarged based on wet weight, only the VP exhibited evidence of abnormal histology with increased in-folding of epithelial luminal cells that could become progressively more severe with age. However, progression to mPIN or invasive adenocarcinoma has not been reported in any lobe in mutant mice as old as 56 weeks of age. Thus, as for most other single germline knockouts described, additional and possibly multiple genetic hits would be required to ultimately drive progression to advanced prostate disease.

BIGENIC/COMPLEX KNOCKOUT MODELS: HOW MANY HITS DOES IT TAKE?

Single lesion germline knockout models demonstrate a "proof of principle" that complete or partial loss of tumor suppressor activity can be causally related to the initiation of early prostate cancer events. However, these models also demonstrate that additional genetic mutations are likely required for progression to invasive carcinoma and/or metastasis. To further elucidate which combinations of genetic lesions can result in prostate tumorigenesis, many groups have combined germline knockout and transgenic models to generate bigenic and higher order complex models systems.

Nkx3.1 × PTEN

Germline knockout models have clearly established that Nkx3.1 or PTEN deficiency can influence the initiation and sometimes the progression of prostate disease. To determine whether loss of both Nkx3.1 and PTEN tumor suppressors would cooperate in prostate cancer progression, a germline Nkx3.1;PTEN knockout model was generated by crossing Nkx3.1$^{+/-}$ and PTEN$^{+/-}$ virgin males.[34,41,51] Compound heterozygous Nkx3.1$^{+/-}$;PTEN$^{+/-}$ mutant mice (mixed C57Bl/6J;129/SvJ strain background) were then intercrossed to produce cohorts of mice containing all 6 viable genotypes (embryos with the PTEN$^{-/-}$ genotype are embryonic lethal, as previously described). In general, this complex model eloquently demonstrated a causal synergy in prostate cancer initiation and progression to advanced disease.[41,87] Indeed, the loss or reduction in level of both the Nkx3.1 and PTEN tumor suppressor gene products resulted in a significantly reduced time to tumor formation (latency) and an increase in penetrance with respect to mPIN, and, significantly, an increase in invasive adenocarcinoma and, in some instances, metastatic disease. Unlike the vast majority of the control Nkx3.1$^{+/+}$;PTEN$^{+/-}$ mice, 6-month-old Nkx3.1$^{-/-}$;PTEN$^{+/-}$ mice—and to a lesser but significant extent Nkx3.1$^{+/-}$;PTEN$^{+/-}$ mice—routinely exhibited severe mPIN with multifocal lesions of poorly differentiated cells containing areas of focal nuclear atypia. By 12 months of age, mPIN was evident in all Nkx3.1$^{-/-}$;PTEN$^{+/-}$ and Nkx3.1$^{+/-}$;PTEN$^{+/-}$ mutant mice, whereas 66% of control Nkx3.1$^{+/+}$;PTEN$^{+/-}$ mice exhibited mPIN by this age. In young mice (<1 year of age), the cooperation between Nkx3.1 and PTEN in prostate tumorigenesis appears limited to influencing the rate of progression to severe mPIN as mice did not frequently develop invasive carcinoma or metastasis. However, using a complex combined knockout/xenograft model, Abate-Shen et al[87] demonstrated that prostate tissue obtained from young (8 months of age) Nkx3.1$^{+/-}$;PTEN$^{+/-}$ mice could develop invasive carcinoma after multiple rounds of serial transplantation into nude mice, suggesting that additional stochastic events could facilitate progression under selective pressure of transplantation. Furthermore, aged intact Nkx3.1[+/-];PTEN[+/-] mutant mice (12 to 15 months of age) could develop invasive carcinoma (22/26 mice) and lymph node metastasis (4/16) at a higher frequency than control Nkx3.1[+/+];PTEN[+/-] mice, even though 7/13 mice exhibited invasive carcinoma with no indication of metastasis. Interestingly, a much higher frequency of invasive carcinoma was observed in the DLP than the AP and VP, in agreement with other observations that sensitivities to neoplastic transformation may be lobe-specific.

This model eloquently demonstrated that while loss of the PTEN wild-type allele was associated with mPIN lesions, loss or mutational inactivation of the remaining wild-type Nkx3.1 locus was not. However, Nkx3.1 protein loss, through a currently unknown mechanism, might precede or be requisite for prostate cancer progression. Androgen independence for the onset of mPIN in mice deficient in both Nkx3.1 and PTEN has been reported,[87] but evidence of androgen-independent progression to advanced disease states was not routinely observed in mice as old as 9 months of age.

Nkx3.1 × p27KIP1

Loss of the tumor suppressors Nkx3.1 or p27KIP1 are each causally linked to the initiation of early non-neoplastic prostate lesions. To investigate whether loss of both Nkx3.1 and p27KIP1 tumor suppressors could cooperate in prostate cancer progression, a germline Nkx3.1;p27KIP1 bigenic knockout model was generated by crossing Nkx3.1[+/-] and p27KIP1 mutant mice.[35,65,88] Heterozygous Nkx3.1[+/-];p27KIP1[+/-] mice (on a mixed C57Bl/6J;129SvImJ strain background) were then intercrossed to generate cohort mice containing all 9 viable genotypes. In general, this model system demonstrated that loss or titration of both Nkx3.1 and p27KIP could lead to an increased incidence of severe hyperplasia in the AP, unfortunately the only lobe examined in this study.[88] Most dramatically, by 24 weeks of age all Nkx3.1[-/-];p27KIP1[-/-] mice developed severe prostatic epithelial cell hyperplasia with significant nuclear atypia. Furthermore, and consistent with haploinsufficiency, mice completely lacking one tumor suppressor that were heterozygous for the other gene (in either combination) developed hyperplasia at higher frequency than control mice. These mice did not develop hyperplasia at the same frequency or as rapidly as the double nullizygous mice that exhibited a significantly increased rate of proliferation compared with all other genotypes in the study. Interestingly, p27KIP1[-/-] mice concurrently showed a modest but significant increase in the rate of apoptosis that was by

itself influenced by Nkx3.1. However, unlike the Nx3.1;PTEN compound bigenic knockout model, cooperation between Nkx3.1 and p27KIP1 loss appeared to be limited to initiation and/or early stage events, as progression to advanced disease was not evident in mice as old as 9 months of age. These findings show that not all combinations of tumor susceptibility loss are sufficient to drive progression toward more advanced disease. Consistent with other models,[40-42] haploinsufficiency of Nkx3.1 was documented with respect to hyperplasia and/or mPIN in this model.[88] That focal areas of Nkx3.1 protein loss were observed in both Nkx3.1[+/-];p27KIP1[-/-] and Nkx3.1[+/+];p27KIP1 mutant mice (or conversely, loss of p27KIP protein expression in Nkx3.1[-/-];p27KIP1[+/-] and Nkx3.1[-/-];p27KIP1[+/+] mice in some lesions), supports a synergy between Nkx3.1 and p27KIP1 protein loss and prostate cancer progression.

PTEN × p27KIP1

As previously discussed, PTEN and p27KIP1 knockout models validate the important role of these tumor suppressors in the initiation and progression of multiple organ tumor types, including that of the prostate gland. Interestingly, experimental evidence indicates a functional, albeit indirect, association between PTEN and p27KIP1 tumor suppressor activity through Akt kinase that is downstream of PTEN and upstream of p27KIP1.[89,90] To further investigate whether PTEN and p27KIP1 tumor could cooperate in tumorigenesis, a germline PTEN;p27KIP1 bigenic knockout model was generated by crossing PTEN[+/-] and p27KIP1[-/-] mutant mice in a C57Bl/6J strain background.[50,66,91] This model clearly demonstrated a profound cooperation between loss of these tumor suppressor genes with respect to tumor initiation, progression and aggressiveness given the significantly reduced animal survival (mean survival of 15.06 ± 0.18 weeks for PTEN[+/-];p27KIP1[-/-] mutant mice and 35.9 ± 2.05 weeks for PTEN[+/-];p27KIP1[+/-] mice versus 51.01 ± 1.48 weeks for control PTEN[+/-] mice). Of note, this synergistic effect was particularly prominent in the prostate gland where all PTEN[+/-];p27KIP1[-/-] mutant mice (13/13 mice) developed adenocarcinoma by 3 to 5 months of age, while only 9/18 PTEN[+/-] mice exhibit similar pathology, and only after 9 months of age. Moreover, evidence of progression to invasive carcinoma was often associated with prostate tumor lesions in the PTEN[+/-];p27KIP1[-/-] mice with 25% of lesions showing ruptures in nascent basement membranes. Interestingly, this model also demonstrated significant lobe-specific differences with respect to tumor penetrance. While 100% of animals developed tumors in the DLP and 85% in the AP, there was no evidence of invasive carcinoma in the VP. This is certainly similar to the phenotype of the VP in the

Nkx3.1 knockout models.[34–36] Of significant note, recent clinical data demonstrate that the combined loss of both PTEN and p27KIP1 protein expression is associated with advanced tumor grade and increased risk of recurrence.[92,93]

PTEN × TRAMP

Substantial clinical and experimental data links LOH at PTEN with many cancers. However, contrary to the two hit criteria for a tumor suppressor gene,[69] discordance between LOH and mutational inactivation of the remaining wild-type allele has been reported by many groups.[46,48,49] To further investigate the association between PTEN loss and prostate cancer initiation and progression, PTEN deficiency was examined in the context of spontaneous prostate cancer using the transgenic adenocarcinoma of the mouse prostate (TRAMP) model.[94] TRAMP is a well-characterized model of spontaneous prostate cancer, generated by the directed expression of the simian virus 40 (SV40) early genes (T and t) to terminally differentiated prostate epithelial cells. TRAMP mice display spontaneous prostate disease that closely mimics the natural history of the clinical disease including androgen independence and metastatic disease.[12,38,94] To generate the PTEN[+/−];TRAMP complex model,[95] germline PTEN[+/−] knockout mice in a 129/SvImJ strain background were crossed with TRAMP mice in a C57Bl/6J strain background.[51,94] TRAMP[+] male progeny were then placed into a large cohort study (70 animals) such that one half of the mice were expected to be PTEN[+/−] and the other half PTEN[+/+]. (PTEN genotypes were assessed at necropsy to prevent potential experimental bias). As enforced expression of the SV40 oncogenes is driven by the rat probasin promoter (active in terminally differentiated prostate epithelial cells), PTEN deficiency would be expected to precede oncogenic induced malignant transformation in this model. Similar to other PTEN-based knockout models, this model demonstrated that deficiency in PTEN tumor suppressor activity was causally linked to and could cooperate with oncogene gain-of-function events to drive prostate cancer progression cumulating in an increased rate of prostate cancer progression. The PTEN[+/−];TRAMP compound mice exhibited significantly decreased survival (185 ± 9 days) compared with PTEN[+/+];TRAMP mice (226 ± 10 days). At necropsy, similar pathologic features were observed in prostates procured from PTEN[+/−];TRAMP and PTEN[+/+];TRAMP mice. Moreover, equal proportions (approximately 30%) of mice died of local rather than metastatic disease, indicating that PTEN loss likely influenced the aggressiveness of primary tumor growth more than metastatic spread. Interestingly, in 13 of 19 (68%) mice examined, LOH demonstrated in primary tumors corresponded to loss of the wild-type PTEN allele. The 6 mice not exhibiting LOH showed no evidence of mutational inactivation in the remaining wild-type PTEN allele and Western blot analyses confirms the protein expression was still retained in the primary tumors. Of significant note, spontaneous LOH at the PTEN locus was demonstrated in a large proportion of primary tumors in control PTEN[+/+];TRAMP mice (9 of 19 tumors examined). Furthermore, on the basis of Kaplin–Meier survival analyses, either complete PTEN inactivation (mice that exhibited LOH of the remaining wild-type allele) or partial inactivation (mice that contained one wild-type PTEN allele: PTEN[+/−];TRAMP, or PTEN[+/+];TRAMP mice that exhibited spontaneous LOH) was significantly correlated with reduced survival when compared to TRAMP mice that retained both wild-type copies of the PTEN, findings entirely consistent with a causal relationship between PTEN haploinsufficiency and prostate cancer progression.

PTEN TITRATION DEFICIENCY MODEL

To further investigate this association between PTEN dose and prostate cancer progression, Trotman et al generated an eloquent but rather complex PTEN titration deficiency model.[54] This model required a series of complex breeding strategies that included crossing germline PTEN[+/−] mice[50] with germline PTEN[hy/+] mice,[54] where the hypomorph (hy) PTEN allele generated by transcriptional interference exhibited reduced expression of wild-type PTEN. In this mouse series, progeny containing the genotypes PTEN,[+/+] PTEN[hy/+], PTEN[+/−] and PTEN[hy/−] in sequential order exhibited progressively lower PTEN protein doses (titration). This model also employed breeding strategies that involved crossing mice containing LoxP-targeted PTEN alleles (PTEN[LoxP/LoxP] mice) with one of two Cre recombinase activator mouse strains to generate prostate-specific PTEN conditional mutant mice. In this mouse series, PTEN(LoxP/LoxP) mice crossed with the PB-Cre4 mouse strain[96] exhibited homozygous loss of PTEN at a higher penetrance (all lobes) and in a higher percentage of prostate epithelial cells than PTEN[LoxP/LoxP] mice crossed with the PB-Cre mouse strain.[97] In general, this complex titration model eloquently demonstrated that discrete dose-dependent reductions in PTEN expression could be causally linked to different stages of prostate cancer progression, culminating in a PTEN dose-dependent reduction in latency of early prostate cancer events and progression to invasive adenocarcinoma and metastasis. Importantly, subtle differences in PTEN dose profoundly influenced the prostate cancer phenotype. PTEN[hy/−] mice exhibited severe hyperplasia with reduced latency and complete penetrance, abnormal cellular differentiation and an increased rate of progression from mPIN to invasive carcinoma when compared with PTEN[+/−] mice. When compared with PB-Cre[+];PTEN[LoxP/LoxP] mice, the PB-Cre4[+];PTEN[LoxP/LoxP] mice exhibited more rapid (reduced latency) and robust (higher penetrance) prostate enlargement and more advanced pathology displaying diffuse (all lobes), severe prostate epithelial cell hyperplasia with cellular dysplasia by 2 to 3 months of age. Most strikingly, this model also demonstrated that prostate-specific deletion of PTEN could significantly influence prostate cancer progression compared with germline PTEN deficiency. All PB-Cre4;PTEN[LoxP/LoxP] and PB-Cre;PTEN[LoxP/LoxP] mice exhibited invasive carcinomas by 6 months of age, but only 25% of 6 month old PTEN[hy/−] mice displayed a similar phenotype. Of significant note and consistent with the well documented indirect role of PTEN in the regulation of Akt kinase activity (for recent review refer to Sansal and Sellers[44]), this model further demonstrated a causal association between PTEN status and Akt activation as the dose-dependent loss of PTEN correlated with increased P-Akt protein levels and activation or downregulation of Akt kinase targets p27KIP1, FOXO3, and mTOR. These findings support PTEN dose as a molecular switch that can determine the natural history of early lesions and tumor progression.

PTEN × P53

Substantial clincial data indicates that LOH of PTEN and mutation of the p53 tumor suppressor genes are frequent in many human cancers, and Chen et al[133] recently investigated whether an association between PTEN loss and prostate cancer initiation and progression is influenced by p53 inactivation.

A PTEN × P53 conditional knockout model was generated whereby LoxP modified PTEN[54] and p53[98] alleles were conditionally ablated in prostate epithelial cells using the PB-Cre4+ mouse line[96]. This model demonstrated a synergistic for somatic loss of PTEN and p53 in prostate cancer progression. PB-Cre4+;PTEN[LoxP/LoxP]/p53[LoxP/LoxP] mice exhibited invasive prostate cancer by 10 weeks of age and mice invariably died by 7 months of age (1/16 mice containing somatic loss of PTEN alone died within this age). These mice did not develop metastatic lesions and hormone dependence was not investigated. In a wild-type p53 background, complete (but not partial) loss PTEN lead to cellular senescence, while sustained proliferation was observed in a p53 deficient background. Consistent with a previous report[95], these finding help to explain the discordance between LOH at the PTEN locus and mutational inactivation of both PTEN alleles predicated be Knudson's two-hit hypothesis[69]. Thus human cancers might maintain cells with one functional PTEN allele as loss of both alleles likely promotes cellular senescence rather than tumor growth.

CONDITIONAL KNOCKOUTS: MORE SIMILAR TO THAT OF THE HUMAN DISEASE?

Although family history is associated with increased risk, no hereditary prostate cancer gene has yet been conclusively identified (recently reviewed by Isaacs and Kainu[99]). Rather, most prostate cancers are thought to arise from sporadic mutations in terminally differentiated prostatic epithelial cells. In this respect, germline knockout models might not be predicted to accurately mimic the natural history of most prostate cancers. Furthermore, in general, tumor suppressor genes representing the major targets of knockout strategies tend to regulate cellular processes that are typically required for generalized cellular homeostasis processes. Therefore, and not surprisingly, many germline knockout strategies have indeed proven to be either nonviable or, if viable, with systemic and/or organ-confined defects. For example, homozygous loss of Rb or PTEN will cause embryonic lethality, while severe prostate developmental hypoplasia is associated with homozygous loss of Nkx3.1. Therefore, many groups have chosen to develop models that mimic somatic loss of tumor suppressor gene function in order to characterize causal relationships with prostate disease.

RETINOBLASTOMA

Retinoblastoma (Rb), the prototype tumor suppressor gene, plays a pivotal role in cell cycle control, largely though interactions with the E2F family of transcription factors.[100] Consistent with the role of suppressing prostate cancer, Rb maps to a genomic region (13q) that exhibits loss at a high frequency in prostate tumors.[18–22] As well, LOH at Rb occurs with high frequency in both early- and late-stage prostate cancer, and significantly reduced mRNA expression levels are observed in many tumors.[101–104] The embryonic lethality of Rb nullizygous mice precluded their use to investigate the association between the Rb tumor suppressor and prostate disease.[105–107] Therefore, to circumvent germline lethality, a prostate-specific conditional Rb knockout model was recently generated using the Cre/LoxP strategy.[108] A mouse expressing Cre recombinase (PB-Cre) exclusively in terminally differentiated epithelial cells of the VP[97] was crossed with mice carrying a LoxP-modified Rb allele.[108] Mice heterozygous for Rb[LoxP/+] were then intercrossed, and mice containing all possible genotypes were generated. This approach demonstrated that both complete and partial loss of the Rb tumor suppressor was causally linked to prostate cancer initiation. Early-onset focal mPIN (without documented progression to invasive carcinoma) was recognized in ventral prostates of both PB-Cre$^+$;Rb$^{LoxP/LoxP}$ and PB-Cre$^+$;Rb$^{LoxP/+}$ mutant mice as young as 12 weeks of age. By 18 weeks, mice exhibited a significant increase in abnormal ductal lesions (Cre$^+$;Rb$^{LoxP/LoxP}$, 24.6% abnormal; PB-Cre$^+$;Rb$^{LoxP/+}$, 30% abnormal; control age-matched littermates, 16% abnormal). The percentage of abnormal epithelium per duct was determined to range from 0% to 50%, thus highlighting how remarkably similar these lesions were to clinical disease with respect to their sporadic and focal nature.

A desmoplastic response and thickening of the smooth muscle layer was concomitant with an increase in cyclin E levels in the Cre$^+$;Rb$^{LoxP/LoxP}$ mice, and the increase in proliferation index helped establish a causal relationship between somatic Rb loss and mPIN. Interestingly, loss of somatic Rb expression was often spatially correlated with pronounced epithelial herniations and compromised basement membrane and smooth muscle layers, consistent with pre- or minimally invasive carcinoma. However, since the mice did not exhibit evidence of progression to metastatic carcinoma by 52 weeks of age, additional genetic lesions, such as loss of p53 function in TRAMP mice, are likely prerequisite for progression to advanced disease states.

PTEN

Germline PTEN$^{+/-}$ deficiency models (PTEN null mice were embryonic lethal) demonstrated a causal relationship between partial PTEN loss and multiorgan malignant transformation. Unfortunately, such mice display a tendency to die at a relatively young age, precluding thorough examination of associations between PTEN loss and prostate cancer progression. To this end, two independent PTEN conditional knockout models have been described.[109,110] For the most part, both models were generated using similar strategies whereby LoxP-modified PTEN alleles[111,112] were used to conditionally ablate expression in a Cre recombinase dependent fashion specifically in terminally differentiated prostate epithelial cells. One group used a highly prostate-specific Cre recombinase expression mouse line (PB-Cre4$^+$) where Cre expression is driven by the probasin promoter,[96,110] and another group used a more generalized Cre recombinase expression system (MTTV-Cre$^+$) driven by the mouse mammary tumor virus promoter.[109–113] With general agreement, these conditional models demonstrated a significant role for somatic loss of PTEN, not only in prostate cancer initiation, but one group eloquently demonstrated that somatic loss of PTEN could also drive prostate cancer progression through to advanced androgen-independent disease.[110] In a large cohort investigation, PB-Cre4$^+$;PTEN$^{LoxP/LoxP}$ mice demonstrated focal areas of epithelial hyperplasia by 4 weeks of age. Indeed, the model generated by Wang et al[110] demonstrated that somatic cell loss of PTEN could drive

progression to mPIN by 6 weeks of age, invasive carcinoma by 9 to 29 weeks of age, and metastatic disease, most notability to lymph nodes or lung, by 29 weeks of age. Of note, gene expression microarray analyses of tumor tissue from these mice generated expression "signature profiles" that were somewhat similar to that of clinical prostate tumor tissue specimens, findings that strongly support a role for PTEN loss in the natural history of clinical prostate cancer disease.

Nkx3.1

Germline Nkx3.1 knockout models demonstrated that Nkx3.1 loss is linked to early prostate disease (hyperplasia), however, all prostate lobes exhibited severe developmental hypoplasia. To further investigate the association between loss of Nkx3.1 and prostate disease independent of early developmental associated defects, a prostate-specific conditional Nkx3.1 knockout model was generated by multiple rounds of subsequent mating involving PSA-Cre$^+$, Nkx3.1$^{LoxP/LoxP}$ and Nkx3.1$^{LoxP/-}$ mice.[35] Mice containing the PSA-Cre$^+$;Nkx3.1$^{LoxP/LoxP}$, PSA-Cre$^+$;Nkx3.1$^{LoxP/+}$, PSA-Cre$^+$;Nkx3.1$^{LoxP/-}$, Nkx3.1$^{LoxP/LoxP}$, or Nkx3.1$^{LoxP/+}$ genotypes were examined. This model demonstrated that targeted disruption of Nkx3.1 alleles in somatic prostate epithelia could profoundly influence cellular proliferation and neoplastic progression culminating in areas of focal hyperplasia that increase in severity with age. Furthermore progression to mPIN, with evidence of nuclear atypia but not invasive carcinoma, was demonstrated by increased proliferation index, persistence of E-cadherin expression and partial loss of high-molecular-weight cytokeratin in the basal cell compartment. Of significant note, progression to mPIN in mice containing prostate-specific Nkx3.1 gene deletions occurs with shortened latency and increased penetrance compared with germline Nkx3.1 knockout counterparts (89% of Cre$^+$;Nkx3.1$^{LoxP/LoxP}$ mice exhibit mPIN by 21 to 25 weeks of age but few germline Nkx3.1$^{-/-}$ knockout models progress to mPIN, as previously discussed). This model demonstrated haploinsufficiency of Nkx3.1 in tumor suppressor activity, as expression was readily apparent in areas of hyperplasia. Consistent with previous findings[40–42] a virtual loss of Nkx3.1 protein expression but not mRNA expression was reported in mPIN lesions.

RETINOID X RECEPTOR-ALPHA

Extensive clinical and experimental data links retinoid action with the inhibition of cancer development, including prostate cancer. Retinoids significantly inhibit prostate tumor growth in animal models such as the Lobund–Wister Rat model,[114,115] and exogenous addition of retinoids can significantly inhibit growth-related processes in prostate cancer cell culture models.[116–118] Germline loss of retinoid X receptor-α (RXRα), a nuclear retinoid receptor, was found to be embryonic lethal.[119,120] However a prostate-specific conditional RXRα knockout model[121] was generated using the PB-Cre4+ activator mice[96] and mice homozygous for LoxP-modified RXRα4, where the LoxP sites flank exon 4.[122] This model demonstrated a causal role for the loss of retinoid signaling pathways in unregulated cellular proliferation culminating in multifocal prostate epithelial cell hyperplasia by 4 months of age. Progression to mPIN was evident at 5 months. These lesions rapidly progressed in severity with age, exhibiting significantly increased proliferation, cell stratification, and cytological atypia. Notably, progression to invasive carcinoma was not evident in the mice up to 15 months of age, supporting the notion that additional genetic insults are likely required to cooperate with loss of retinoid-mediated signaling events to drive progression to advanced prostate disease. Interestingly, this model demonstrated how loss of retinoid receptor signaling could influence ductal tip morphogenesis in a lobe-specific manner as increased ductal tip branching was observed in lateral and anterior lobes. Furthermore, haploinsufficiency for RXR activity was inferred since PB-Cre4+;RXRα^LoxP/+ mice could exhibit similar pathologic lesions to those of PB-Cre4+;RXRα^LoxP/LoxP, albeit with a longer latency period (hyperplasia by 11 months of age and mPIN by 14 months of age).

WHERE DO WE GO FROM HERE?

Towards the goal to understand and effectively treat prostate disease, the long-term goals of GEM model development will be: 1) to identify predictive diagnostic markers; 2) to identify and validate therapeutic targets; and 3) to facilitate preclinical studies to determine the efficacy of therapeutic intervention strategies in a cost-effective manner.

Still early in the development cycle, GEM prostate adenocarcinoma conditional knockout (PACK) models have and will continue to provide revealing insights into our understanding of prostate cancer biology. Indeed, two key observations from the aforementioned knockout models underscore the necessity to continue development of experimental GEM PACK systems: 1) most simple and complex models display pathology consistent with early stage hyperplasia and PIN *without documented progression* to invasive adenocarcinoma; and 2) in current models that do exhibit documented progression to invasive adenocarcinoma, *penetrance is modest at best*, while metastatic spread and androgen-independent disease states are not clearly evident. In general, multiple mutational hits are likely requisite for clinical prostate cancer progression and next generation bigenic/complex knockout models that target genes involved in multiple and distinct "tumorigenic pathways" might more faithfully mimic the natural history of the clinical disease. For instance, as genes involved in signaling pathways regulating proliferation (Nkx3.1, p27KIP1), survival (PTEN, Akt) and genome stability (p53) at the very least are independently linked to prostate disease (recently reviewed by several authors[7,8,123]), the combined perturbations of multiple pathway types might be predicted to create an ideal tumorigenic environment. Certainly, the recent finding that combined loss of PTEN and p27KIP1 is associated with advanced tumor grade and increased risk of recurrence supports this notion.[92,93] Since temporal and spatial patterns of mutational events likely influence the incidence and nature of prostate cancer, the use of various combinations of conditional gene ablation/expression strategies will greatly facilitate GEM PACK development for prostate cancer research.

SPECIFICITY, TIMING, AND PENETRANCE

Conditional knockout strategies often represent a multicomponent system. For the most part responder mice are engineered to carry a recombinase specific (i.e., LoxP) recognition sequence flanking all or part of the gene of interest. Only when these mice are crossed with activator strains harboring tissue-specific recombinase (i.e., Cre) will the conditional knockout occur in bigenic offspring carrying activator and responder alleles. Unlike temporally regulated systems that operate more like a "door bell button" to maintain or suppress target gene expression only so long as the inducer is present, somatic targeted DNA recombination in the bigenic mouse should behave more like a "light switch" and remain stable and irreversible. Hence, the expression of the recombinase is extremely important in determining the temporal and spatial pattern of somatic recombination. Thus, it is really "all about Cre." Although beyond the scope of this review, multiple prostate specific lines of Cre-expressing mice have now been described, each exhibiting unique patterns of expression.[35,96,97,110,113,124–126] Highlighting the potential power of Cre/LoxP technology, Trotman et al[54] demonstrated how the phenotype of a PACK GEM was dependent on the Cre activator, and how this influenced lobe specificity, focality, latency, and grade of prostate cancer. This underscores the need to employ multiple Cre activator lines to fully explore the range of phenotypes for each conditional PACK GEM model.

We anticipate that the next generation of activator mouse strains should allow us to independently target each of the four unique mouse prostate lobes given that the dorsal and anterior mouse prostate lobes might be more predisposed to tumor initiation and progression.

The next generation systems will also facilitate identification, isolation, and characterization of genetic modifier or predisposition loci that control how a phenotype might vary with strain background and as a consequence of a defined engineered genotype. For example, when Nkx3.1$^{-/-}$ germline knockout mice were characterized in different genetic backgrounds profound and subtle phenotypic differences were observed in both developmental and prostate cancer phenotypes. In a pure C57BL/6 background, Nkx3.1$^{-/-}$ mice exhibited significantly reduced ventral prostate sizes compared to control littermates.[37] In contrast, when transmitted in 129/SvImJ or 129/SvImJ × C57BL/6, Nkx3.1$^{-/-}$ prostate lobes were indistinguishable based on wet weights.[34] With that said, in an independent investigation of strain contribution to phenotypic outcome, Kim et al have now demonstrated subtle effects in the occurrence and timing of mPIN formation.[40]

LASTLY…

We hope this review has demonstrated the utility of knockout based GEM strategies and the potential of this technology towards a common goal of understanding prostate disease. Certainly, as current and future technical advances permit, model systems of prostate disease that accurately mimic the full natural history of prostate cancer initiation and progression to advanced androgen-independent disease will undoubtedly be generated, characterized, and shared throughout the research community.

REFERENCES

1. Garnick MB. Hormonal therapy in the management of prostate cancer: from Huggins to the present. Urology 1997;49:5–15.
2. Laufer M, Denmeade SR, Sinibaldi VJ, et al. Complete androgen blockade for prostate cancer: what went wrong? J Urol 2000;164:3–9.
3. Smith PH. Carcinoma of prostate: case against immediate hormonal therapy. Prostate 1996;28:205–208.
4. Vogelstein B, Kinzler KW. Cancer genes and the pathways they control. Nat Med 2004;10:789–799.
5. Saric T, Brkanac Z, Troyer DA, et al. Genetic pattern of prostate cancer progression. Int J Cancer 1999;81:219–224.
6. De Marzo AM, DeWeese TL, Platz EA, et al. Pathological and molecular mechanisms of prostate carcinogenesis: implications for diagnosis, detection, prevention, and treatment. J Cell Biochem 2004;91:459–477.
7. DeMarzo AM, Nelson WG, Isaacs WB, et al. Pathological and molecular aspects of prostate cancer. Lancet 2003;361:955–964.
8. Mazzucchelli R, Barbisan F, Tarquini LM, et al. Molecular mechanisms in prostate cancer. A review. Anal Quant Cytol Histol 2004;26:127–133.
9. Kasper S, Smith JA Jr. Genetically modified mice and their use in developing therapeutic strategies for prostate cancer. J Urol 2004;172:12–19.
10. Park JH, Walls JE, Galvez JJ, et al. Prostatic intraepithelial neoplasia in genetically engineered mice. Am J Pathol 2002;161:727–735.
11. Ostrand-Rosenberg S. Animal models of tumor immunity, immunotherapy and cancer vaccines. Curr Opin Immunol 2004;16:143–150.
12. Winter SF, Cooper AB, Greenberg NM. Models of metastatic prostate cancer: a transgenic perspective. Prostate Cancer Prostatic Dis 2003;6:204–211.
13. Huss WJ, Maddison LA, Greenberg NM. Autochthonous mouse models for prostate cancer: past, present and future. Semin Cancer Biol 2001;11:245–260.
14. Roy-Burman P, Wu H, Powell WC, et al. Genetically defined mouse models that mimic natural aspects of human prostate cancer development. Endocr Relat Cancer 2004;11:225–254.
15. Pollard M. Lobund-Wistar rat model of prostate cancer in man. Prostate 1998;37:1–4.
16. Massenkeil G, Oberhuber H, Hailemariam S, et al. P53 mutations and loss of heterozygosity on chromosomes 8p, 16q, 17p, and 18q are confined to advanced prostate cancer. Anticancer Res 1994;14:2785–2790.
17. Alers JC, Krijtenburg PJ, Vis AN, et al. Molecular cytogenetic analysis of prostatic adenocarcinomas from screening studies: early cancers may contain aggressive genetic features. Am J Pathol 2001;158:399–406.
18. Alers JC, Rochat J, Krijtenburg PJ, et al. Identification of genetic markers for prostatic cancer progression. Lab Invest 2000;80:931–942.
19. Dong JT, Boyd JC, Frierson HF Jr. Loss of heterozygosity at 13q14 and 13q21 in high grade, high stage prostate cancer. Prostate 2001;49:166–171.
20. Dong JT, Chen C, Stultz BG, et al. Deletion at 13q21 is associated with aggressive prostate cancers. Cancer Res 2000;60:3880–3883.
21. Li C, Larsson C, Futreal A, et al. Identification of two distinct deleted regions on chromosome 13 in prostate cancer. Oncogene 1998;16:481–487.
22. Melamed J, Einhorn JM, Ittmann MM. Allelic loss on chromosome 13q in human prostate carcinoma. Clin Cancer Res 1997;3:1867–1872.
23. He WW, Sciavolino PJ, Wing J, et al. A novel human prostate-specific, androgen-regulated homeobox gene (NKX3.1) that maps to 8p21, a region frequently deleted in prostate cancer. Genomics 1997;43:69–77.
24. Feilotter HE, Nagai MA, Boag AH, et al. Analysis of PTEN and the 10q23 region in primary prostate carcinomas. Oncogene 1998;16:1743–1748.
25. Voeller HJ, Augustus M, Madike V, et al. Coding region of NKX3.1, a prostate-specific homeobox gene on 8p21, is not mutated in human prostate cancers. Cancer Res 1997;57:4455–4459.
26. Steck PA, Pershouse MA, Jasser SA, et al. Identification of a candidate tumour suppressor gene, MMAC1, at chromosome 10q23.3 that is mutated in multiple advanced cancers. Nat Genet 1997;15:356–362.
27. Edelhoff S, Ayer DE, Zervos AS, et al. Mapping of two genes encoding members of a distinct subfamily of MAX interacting proteins: MAD to human chromosome 2 and mouse chromosome 6, and MXI1 to human chromosome 10 and mouse chromosome 19. Oncogene 1994;9:665–668.
28. Shapiro DN, Valentine V, Eagle L, et al. Assignment of the human MAD and MXI1 genes to chromosomes 2p12-p13 and 10q24-q25. Genomics 1994;23:282–285.
29. Wechsler DS, Hawkins AL, Li X, et al. Localization of the human Mxi1 transcription factor gene (MXI1) to chromosome 10q24-q25. Genomics 1994;21:669–672.
30. Bova GS, Carter BS, Bussemakers MJ, et al. Homozygous deletion and frequent allelic loss of chromosome 8p22 loci in human prostate cancer. Cancer Res 1993;53:3869–3873.
31. Bergerheim US, Kunimi K, Collins VP, et al. Deletion mapping of chromosomes 8, 10, and 16 in human prostatic carcinoma. Genes Chromosomes Cancer 1991;3:215–220.
32. Bergerheim US, Collins VP, Ekman P, et al. Recessive genetic mechanisms in the oncogenesis of prostatic carcinoma. Scand J Urol Nephrol Suppl 1991;138:93–96.
33. Bowen C, Bubendorf L, Voeller HJ, et al. Loss of NKX3.1 expression in human prostate cancers correlates with tumor progression. Cancer Res 2000;60:6111–6115.
34. Bhatia-Gaur R, Donjacour AA, Sciavolino PJ, et al. Roles for Nkx3.1 in prostate development and cancer. Genes Dev 1999;13:966–977.

35. Abdulkadir SA, Magee JA, Peters TJ, et al. Conditional loss of Nkx3.1 in adult mice induces prostatic intraepithelial neoplasia. Mol Cell Biol 2002;22:1495–1503.

36. Schneider A, Brand T, Zweigerdt R, et al. Targeted disruption of the Nkx3.1 gene in mice results in morphogenetic defects of minor salivary glands: parallels to glandular duct morphogenesis in prostate. Mech Dev 2000;95:163–174.

37. Tanaka M, Komuro I, Inagaki H, et al. Nkx3.1, a murine homolog of Drosophila bagpipe, regulates epithelial ductal branching and proliferation of the prostate and palatine glands. Dev Dyn 2000;219:248–260.

38. Shappell SB, Thomas GV, Roberts RL, et al. Prostate pathology of genetically engineered mice: definitions and classification. The consensus report from the Bar Harbor meeting of the Mouse Models of Human Cancer Consortium Prostate Pathology Committee. Cancer Res 2004;64:2270–2305.

39. Qiu TH, Chandramouli GV, Hunter KW, et al. Global expression profiling identifies signatures of tumor virulence in MMTV-PyMT-transgenic mice: correlation to human disease. Cancer Res 2004;64:5973–5981.

40. Kim MJ, Bhatia-Gaur R, Banach-Petrosky WA, et al. Nkx3.1 mutant mice recapitulate early stages of prostate carcinogenesis. Cancer Res 2002;62:2999–3004.

41. Kim MJ, Cardiff RD, Desai N, et al. Cooperativity of Nkx3.1 and Pten loss of function in a mouse model of prostate carcinogenesis. Proc Natl Acad Sci USA 2002;99:2884–2889.

42. Magee JA, Abdulkadir SA, Milbrandt J. Haploinsufficiency at the Nkx3.1 locus. A paradigm for stochastic, dosage-sensitive gene regulation during tumor initiation. Cancer Cell 2003;3:273–283.

43. Li J, Yen C, Liaw D, et al. PTEN, a putative protein tyrosine phosphatase gene mutated in human brain, breast, and prostate cancer. Science 1997;275:1943–1947.

44. Sansal I, Sellers WR. The biology and clinical relevance of the PTEN tumor suppressor pathway. J Clin Oncol 2004;22:2954–2963.

45. Gray IC, Stewart LM, Phillips SM, et al. Mutation and expression analysis of the putative prostate tumour-suppressor gene PTEN. Br J Cancer 1998;78:1296–1300.

46. Pesche S, Latil A, Muzeau F, et al. PTEN/MMAC1/TEP1 involvement in primary prostate cancers. Oncogene 1998;16:2879–2883.

47. McMenamin ME, Soung P, Perera S, et al. Loss of PTEN expression in paraffin-embedded primary prostate cancer correlates with high Gleason score and advanced stage. Cancer Res 1999;59:4291–4296.

48. Wang SI, Parsons R, Ittmann M. Homozygous deletion of the PTEN tumor suppressor gene in a subset of prostate adenocarcinomas. Clin Cancer Res 1998;4:811–815.

49. Cairns P, Okami K, Halachmi S, et al. Frequent inactivation of PTEN/MMAC1 in primary prostate cancer. Cancer Res 1997;57:4997–5000.

50. Di Cristofano A, Pesce B, Cordon-Cardo C, et al. Pten is essential for embryonic development and tumour suppression. Nat Genet 1998;19:348–355.

51. Podsypanina K, Ellenson LH, Nemes A, et al. Mutation of Pten/Mmac1 in mice causes neoplasia in multiple organ systems. Proc Natl Acad Sci USA 1999;96:1563–1568.

52. Suzuki A, de la Pompa JL, Stambolic V, et al. High cancer susceptibility and embryonic lethality associated with mutation of the PTEN tumor suppressor gene in mice. Curr Biol 1998;8:1169–1178.

53. Stambolic V, Tsao MS, Macpherson D, et al. High incidence of breast and endometrial neoplasia resembling human Cowden syndrome in pten+/− mice. Cancer Res 2000;60:3605–3611.

54. Trotman LC, Niki M, Dotan ZA, et al. Pten dose dictates cancer progression in the prostate. PLoS Biol 2003;1:E59.

55. Lloyd RV, Erickson LA, Jin L, et al. p27kip1: a multifunctional cyclin-dependent kinase inhibitor with prognostic significance in human cancers. Am J Pathol 1999;154:313–323.

56. Macri E, Loda M. Role of p27 in prostate carcinogenesis. Cancer Metastasis Rev 1998;17:337–344.

57. Pietenpol JA, Bohlander SK, Sato Y, et al. Assignment of the human p27Kip1 gene to 12p13 and its analysis in leukemias. Cancer Res 1995;55:1206–1210.

58. Ponce-Castaneda MV, Lee MH, Latres E, et al. p27Kip1: chromosomal mapping to 12p12-12p13.1 and absence of mutations in human tumors. Cancer Res 1995;55:1211–1214.

59. Chang BL, Zheng SL, Isaacs SD, et al. A polymorphism in the CDKN1B gene is associated with increased risk of hereditary prostate cancer. Cancer Res 2004;64:1997–1999.

60. Kibel AS, Faith DA, Bova GS, et al. Loss of heterozygosity at 12P12-13 in primary and metastatic prostate adenocarcinoma. J Urol 2000;164:192–196.

61. Cheville JC, Lloyd RV, Sebo TJ, et al. Expression of p27kip1 in prostatic adenocarcinoma. Mod Pathol 1998;11:324–328.

62. Fernandez PL, Arce Y, Farre X, et al. Expression of p27/Kip1 is down-regulated in human prostate carcinoma progression. J Pathol 1999;187:563–566.

63. Yang RM, Naitoh J, Murphy M, et al. Low p27 expression predicts poor disease-free survival in patients with prostate cancer. J Urol 1998;159:941–945.

64. Cote RJ, Shi Y, Groshen S, et al. Association of p27Kip1 levels with recurrence and survival in patients with stage C prostate carcinoma. J Natl Cancer Inst 1998;90:916–920.

65. Fero ML, Rivkin M, Tasch M, et al. A syndrome of multiorgan hyperplasia with features of gigantism, tumorigenesis, and female sterility in p27(Kip1)-deficient mice. Cell 1996;85:733–744.

66. Kiyokawa H, Kineman RD, Manova-Todorova KO, et al. Enhanced growth of mice lacking the cyclin-dependent kinase inhibitor function of p27(Kip1). Cell 1996;85:721–732.

67. Nakayama K, Ishida N, Shirane M, et al. Mice lacking p27(Kip1) display increased body size, multiple organ hyperplasia, retinal dysplasia, and pituitary tumors. Cell 1996;85:707–720.

68. Cordon-Cardo C, Koff A, Drobnjak M, et al. Distinct altered patterns of p27KIP1 gene expression in benign prostatic hyperplasia and prostatic carcinoma. J Natl Cancer Inst 1998;90:1284–1291.

69. Knudson AG, Jr. Mutation and cancer: statistical study of retinoblastoma. Proc Natl Acad Sci USA 1971;68:820–823.

70. Fero ML, Randel E, Gurley KE, et al. The murine gene p27Kip1 is haplo-insufficient for tumour suppression. Nature 1998;396:177–180.

71. Zervos AS, Gyuris J, Brent R. Mxi1, a protein that specifically interacts with Max to bind Myc-Max recognition sites. Cell 1993;72:223–232.

72. Austen M, Cerni C, Henriksson M, et al. Regulation of cell growth by the Myc-Max-Mad network: role of Mad proteins and YY1. Curr Top Microbiol Immunol 1997;224:123–130.

73. McArthur GA, Laherty CD, Queva C, et al. The Mad protein family links transcriptional repression to cell differentiation. Cold Spring Harb Symp Quant Biol 1998;63:423–433.

74. Schreiber-Agus N, DePinho RA. Repression by the Mad(Mxi1)-Sin3 complex. Bioessays 1998;20:808–818.

75. Lee TC, Ziff EB. Mxi1 is a repressor of the c-Myc promoter and reverses activation by USF. J Biol Chem 1999;274:595–606.

76. Taj MM, Tawil RJ, Engstrom LD, et al. Mxi1, a Myc antagonist, suppresses proliferation of DU145 human prostate cells. Prostate 2001;47:194–204.

77. Schreiber-Agus N, Meng Y, Hoang T, et al. Role of Mxi1 in ageing organ systems and the regulation of normal and neoplastic growth. Nature 1998;393:483–487.

78. Jarred RA, Cancilla B, Prins GS, et al. Evidence that estrogens directly alter androgen-regulated prostate development. Endocrinology 2000;141:3471–3477.

79. Naslund MJ, Coffey DS. The differential effects of neonatal androgen, estrogen and progesterone on adult rat prostate growth. J Urol 1986;136:1136–1140.

80. Prins GS. Neonatal estrogen exposure induces lobe-specific alterations in adult rat prostate androgen receptor expression. Endocrinology 1992;130:2401–2412.

81. Prins GS, Birch L. The developmental pattern of androgen receptor expression in rat prostate lobes is altered after neonatal exposure to estrogen. Endocrinology 1995;136:1303–1314.

82. Pylkkanen L, Santti R, Newbold R, et al. Regional differences in the prostate of the neonatally estrogenized mouse. Prostate 1991;18:117–129.

83. Pylkkanen L, Makela S, Valve E, et al. Prostatic dysplasia associated with increased expression of c-myc in neonatally estrogenized mice. J Urol 1993;149:1593–1601.

84. vom Saal FS, Timms BG, Montano MM, et al. Prostate enlargement in mice due to fetal exposure to low doses of estradiol or diethylstilbestrol and opposite effects at high doses. Proc Natl Acad Sci USA 1997;94:2056–2061.

85. McPherson SJ, Wang H, Jones ME, et al. Elevated androgens and prolactin in aromatase-deficient mice cause enlargement, but not malignancy, of the prostate gland. Endocrinology 2001;142:2458–2467.

86. Fisher CR, Graves KH, Parlow AF, et al. Characterization of mice deficient in aromatase (ArKO) because of targeted disruption of the cyp19 gene. Proc Natl Acad Sci USA 1998;95:6965–6970.

87. Abate-Shen C, Banach-Petrosky WA, Sun X, et al. Nkx3.1;Pten mutant mice develop invasive prostate adenocarcinoma and lymph node metastases. Cancer Res 2003;63:3886–3890.

88. Gary B, Azuero R, Mohanty GS, et al. Interaction of Nkx3.1 and p27kip1 in prostate tumor initiation. Am J Pathol 2004;164:1607–1614.

89. Graff JR, Konicek BW, McNulty AM, et al. Increased AKT activity contributes to prostate cancer progression by dramatically accelerating prostate tumor growth and diminishing p27Kip1 expression. J Biol Chem 2000;275:24500–24505.

90. Nakamura N, Ramaswamy S, Vazquez F, et al. Forkhead transcription factors are critical effectors of cell death and cell cycle arrest downstream of PTEN. Mol Cell Biol 2000;20:8969–8982.

91. Di Cristofano A, De Acetis M, Koff A, et al. Pten and p27KIP1 cooperate in prostate cancer tumor suppression in the mouse. Nat Genet 2001;27:222–224.

92. Dreher T, Zentgraf H, Abel U, et al. Reduction of PTEN and p27kip1 expression correlates with tumor grade in prostate cancer. Analysis in radical prostatectomy specimens and needle biopsies. Virchows Arch 2004;444:509–517.

93. Halvorsen OJ, Haukaas SA, Akslen LA. Combined loss of PTEN and p27 expression is associated with tumor cell proliferation by Ki-67 and increased risk of recurrent disease in localized prostate cancer. Clin Cancer Res 2003;9:1474–1479.

94. Kaplan-Lefko PJ, Chen TM, Ittmann MM, et al. Pathobiology of autochthonous prostate cancer in a pre-clinical transgenic mouse model. Prostate 2003;55:219–237.

95. Kwabi-Addo B, Giri D, Schmidt K, et al. Haploinsufficiency of the Pten tumor suppressor gene promotes prostate cancer progression. Proc Natl Acad Sci USA 2001;98:11563–11568.

96. Wu X, Wu J, Huang J, et al. Generation of a prostate epithelial cell-specific Cre transgenic mouse model for tissue-specific gene ablation. Mech Dev 2001;101:61–69.

97. Maddison LA, Nahm H, DeMayo F, et al. Prostate specific expression of Cre recombinase in transgenic mice. Genesis 2000;26:154–156.

98. Chen Z, Trotman LC, Shaffer D, et al. Crucial role of p53-dependent cellular senescence in suppression of Pten-deficient tumorigenesis. Nature 2005;436:725–30.

99. Isaacs W, Kainu T. Oncogenes and tumor suppressor genes in prostate cancer. Epidemiol Rev 2001;23:36–41.

100. Dyson N. The regulation of E2F by pRB-family proteins. Genes Dev 1998;12:2245–2262.

101. Ittmann MM, Wieczorek R. Alterations of the retinoblastoma gene in clinically localized, stage B prostate adenocarcinomas. Hum Pathol 1996;27:28–34.

102. Phillips SM, Barton CM, Lee SJ, et al. Loss of the retinoblastoma susceptibility gene (RB1) is a frequent and early event in prostatic tumorigenesis. Br J Cancer 1994;70:1252–1257.

103. Phillips SM, Morton DG, Lee SJ, et al. Loss of heterozygosity of the retinoblastoma and adenomatous polyposis susceptibility gene loci and in chromosomes 10p, 10q and 16q in human prostate cancer. Br J Urol 1994;73:390–395.

104. Tricoli JV, Gumerlock PH, Yao JL, et al. Alterations of the retinoblastoma gene in human prostate adenocarcinoma. Genes Chromosomes Cancer 1996;15:108–114.

105. Clarke AR, Maandag ER, van Roon M, et al. Requirement for a functional Rb-1 gene in murine development. Nature 1992;359:328–330.

106. Jacks T, Fazeli A, Schmitt EM, et al. Effects of an Rb mutation in the mouse. Nature 1992;359:295–300.

107. Lee EY, Chang CY, Hu N, et al. Mice deficient for Rb are nonviable and show defects in neurogenesis and haematopoiesis. Nature 1992;359:288–294.

108. Maddison LA, Sutherland BW, Barrios RJ, et al. Conditional deletion of rb causes early stage prostate cancer. Cancer Res 2004;64:6018–6025.

109. Backman SA, Ghazarian D, So K, et al. Early onset of neoplasia in the prostate and skin of mice with tissue-specific deletion of Pten. Proc Natl Acad Sci USA 2004;101:1725–1730.

110. Wang S, Gao J, Lei Q, et al. Prostate-specific deletion of the murine Pten tumor suppressor gene leads to metastatic prostate cancer. Cancer Cell 2003;4:209–221.

111. Lesche R, Groszer M, Gao J, et al. Cre/loxP-mediated inactivation of the murine Pten tumor suppressor gene. Genesis 2002;32:148–149.

112. Suzuki A, Yamaguchi MT, Ohteki T, et al. T cell-specific loss of Pten leads to defects in central and peripheral tolerance. Immunity 2001;14:523–534.

113. Wagner KU, McAllister K, Ward T, et al. Spatial and temporal expression of the Cre gene under the control of the MMTV-LTR in different lines of transgenic mice. Transgenic Res 2001;10:545–553.

114. Pollard M, Luckert PH. The inhibitory effect of 4-hydroxyphenyl retinamide (4-HPR) on metastasis of prostate adenocarcinoma-III cells in Lobund-Wistar rats. Cancer Lett 1991;59:159–163.

115. Pollard M, Luckert PH, Sporn MB. Prevention of primary prostate cancer in Lobund-Wistar rats by N-(4-hydroxyphenyl)retinamide. Cancer Res 1991;51:3610–3611.

116. Esquenet M, Swinnen JV, Heyns W, et al. Control of LNCaP proliferation and differentiation: actions and interactions of androgens, 1alpha,25-dihydroxycholecalciferol, all-trans retinoic acid, 9-cis retinoic acid, and phenylacetate. Prostate 1996;28:182–194.

117. Esquenet M, Swinnen JV, Heyns W, et al. Triiodothyronine modulates growth, secretory function and androgen receptor concentration in the prostatic carcinoma cell line LNCaP. Mol Cell Endocrinol 1995;109:105–111.

118. de Vos S, Dawson MI, Holden S, et al. Effects of retinoid X receptor-selective ligands on proliferation of prostate cancer cells. Prostate 1997;32:115–121.

119. Kastner P, Grondona JM, Mark M, et al. Genetic analysis of RXR alpha developmental function: convergence of RXR and RAR signaling pathways in heart and eye morphogenesis. Cell 1994;78:987–1003.

120. Sucov HM, Dyson E, Gumeringer CL, et al. RXR alpha mutant mice establish a genetic basis for vitamin A signaling in heart morphogenesis. Genes Dev 1994;8:1007–1018.

121. Huang J, Powell WC, Khodavirdi AC, et al. Prostatic intraepithelial neoplasia in mice with conditional disruption of the retinoid X receptor alpha allele in the prostate epithelium. Cancer Res 2002;62:4812–4819.

122. Chen J, Kubalak SW, Chien KR. Ventricular muscle-restricted targeting of the RXRalpha gene reveals a non-cell-autonomous requirement in cardiac chamber morphogenesis. Development 1998;125:1943–1949.

123. Wang G, Reed E, Li QQ. Apoptosis in prostate cancer: progressive and therapeutic implications (Review). Int J Mol Med 2004;14:23–34.

124. Jin C, McKeehan K, Wang F. Transgenic mouse with high Cre recombinase activity in all prostate lobes, seminal vesicle, and ductus deferens. Prostate 2003;57:160–164.

125. Lu QY, Hung JC, Heber D, et al. Inverse associations between plasma lycopene and other carotenoids and prostate cancer. Cancer Epidemiol Biomarkers Prev 2001;10:749–756.

126. Cleutjens KB, van der Korput HA, Ehren-van Eekelen CC, et al. A 6-kb promoter fragment mimics in transgenic mice the prostate-specific and androgen-regulated expression of the endogenous prostate-specific antigen gene in humans. Mol Endocrinol 1997;11:1256–1265.

127. Eddy EM, Washburn TF, Bunch DO, et al. Targeted disruption of the estrogen receptor gene in male mice causes alteration of spermatogenesis and infertility. Endocrinology 1996;137:4796–4805.

128. Lohnes D, Kastner P, Dierich A, et al. Function of retinoic acid receptor gamma in the mouse. Cell 1993;73:643–658.

129. Colombel M, Radvanyi F, Blanche M, et al. Androgen suppressed apoptosis is modified in p53 deficient mice. Oncogene 1995;10:1269–1274.

130. Signoretti S, Waltregny D, Dilks J, et al. p63 is a prostate basal cell marker and is required for prostate development. Am J Pathol 2000;157:1769–1775.

131. Podlasek CA, Duboule D, Bushman W. Male accessory sex organ morphogenesis is altered by loss of function of Hoxd-13. Dev Dyn 1997;208:454–465.

132. Steger RW, Chandrashekar V, Zhao W, et al. Neuroendocrine and reproductive functions in male mice with targeted disruption of the prolactin gene. Endocrinology 1998;139:3691–3695.

133. Abdulkadir SA, Qu Z, Garabedian E, et al. Impaired prostate tumorigenesis in Egr1-deficient mice. Nat Med 2001;7:101–107.

Molecular mechanisms of metastasis in prostate cancer

37

Noel W Clarke, Mick D Brown

METASTATIC MECHANISMS IN THE PRIMARY TUMOR

One of the fundamental problems arising as a consequence of prostate cancer is the propensity of the disease to metastasize. Without this, the disease would cease to be the major public health problem that it is acknowledged to be. This metastatic tendency is predicated on specific molecular mechanisms and interactions that result in the coordinated and inexorable process of local invasion, extravasation, and distal migration from the primary site, and endothelial attachment, transmigration, and site-specific establishment of metastases at secondary sites. Basic knowledge relating to this structured mechanism has improved in recent years, but considerable deficiencies remain in our understanding of how and why this process occurs. Improving our understanding of the molecular mechanisms underpinning metastases is essential and will open the way for the application of novel therapies to treat this incurable condition.

LOCAL INVASION

Local invasion is a critical characteristic of all malignant tumors. It is one of the fundamental early steps in the metastatic process and without it, tumor spread cannot occur. To develop invasive potential, the malignant cell must downregulate its cell–cell and cell–matrix adhesive characteristics it must become motile and it must acquire the ability to break down the extracellular matrix using degradative enzymes. The means by which cells transformed by the malignant process invade and

migrate once they have become detached has been described as the three step invasion and metastasis theory.[1] It comprises the following steps:

1. Attachment to underlying extracellular matrix.
2. Digestion of basement membrane.
3. Migration to the interstitium.

Once the malignant cell has reached the interstitium, it must enter the vascular or lymphatic circulation by breaching the vascular or lymphatic endothelial barrier, a process which is described in detail below. From there, the cell migrates in the blood or lymphatic circulation and becomes arrested at a secondary endothelial site. It must then go through the process of endothelial binding, extravasation, and endothelial transmigration at that site before reaching the interstitium, where it can proliferate and/or coalesce with other metastasizing cells to form a micrometastasis. It will only do this if the environment at the secondary site is favorable (Figure 37.1).

PRIMARY SITE CELL–CELL AND CELL–MATRIX ADHESION

The maintenance of the architectural integrity of an organ depends fundamentally on cell–cell and cell–matrix binding. In the prostate, as in other structures, one of the main regulators of cell–cell binding function is the cadherin–catenin complex, whilst the cell matrix binding is largely a function of integrins, dimeric binding proteins which consist of α- and β-chain subunits.

Cadherins are transmembrane glycoproteins, of which E-cadherin is the best characterized in prostate cancer. It plays a critical role in embryogenesis and

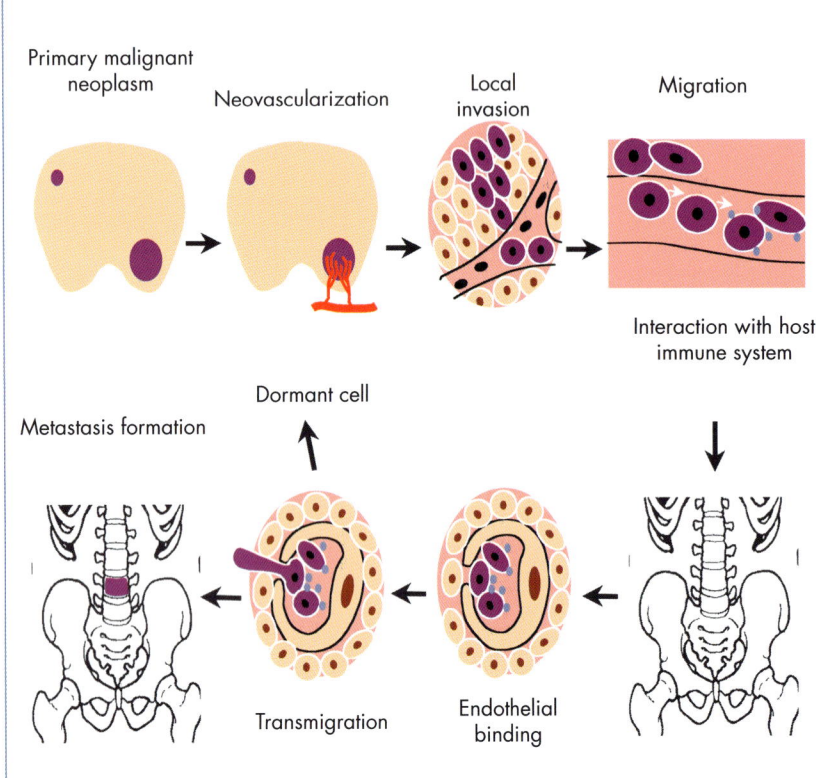

Primary malignant neoplasm

Neovascularization

Local invasion

Migration

Interaction with host immune system

Dormant cell

Metastasis formation

Transmigration

Endothelial binding

Fig. 37.1

The process of metastasis is characterized by proliferation, neovascularization, and extravasation at the primary site. In the circulation, malignant cells interact with the cellular and immune molecular mechanisms resulting in destruction in most instances. The surviving cells arrest at the secondary endothelial site by a process of lectin binding consolidated by integrin-based stabilization of the epithelial/endothelial binding. The cell then undergoes a process of active transmigration. The binding process is complete within 30 to 60 minutes, and the endothelial transmigration is complete by 24 hours. Once the cell gains the interstitium, it may remain dormant for an undefined period or it may coalesce with other cells and proliferate to form a metastatic cellular colony. When it does this, it will disturb the local physiological function at the secondary site leading to physiological dysfunction and anatomical disruption. The metastasis may also serve as a site from which further metastatic migration can occur.

organogenesis through intercellular adhesion and signalling.[2] The locus coding for E-cadherin (16q22.1) can be considered as a tumor-suppressor gene, as loss of function of this molecule facilitates cell detachment and has been shown to induce an invasive phenotype,[3] while transfection of E-cadherin cDNA into invasive adenocarcinoma cells can render them noninvasive.[4]

E-cadherin is attached intracellularly to structural proteins, the actin cytoskeleton, by interactive binding with intracellular catenin. The catenin complex comprises three protein molecules, α, β, and γ catenin, which interact to form binding sites for the intracellular domain of E-cadherin and the actin fibers of the cytoskeleton. Once bound to the internal cellular structure, the transmembrane cadherins then bind externally to other cadherin binding sites on the surface of adjacent cells. This cadherin–catenin complex plays an essential role in both morphogenesis[5] and subsequent structural and functional organization of epithelial cells.[6] Disruption of either component of this interaction has been shown to produce significant alterations in cellular behavior. Early in-vitro studies demonstrated the emergence of an invasive cellular phenotype following inhibition of cadherin mediated cell adhesion[3] and subsequent studies of tumor cell lines have shown that lack of cadherin expression is associated with invasive biopotential.[7] Indeed, loss of E-cadherin expression has been suggested as one of the key events in the transformation from adenoma to carcinoma.[8]

E-cadherin has been extensively studied in human cancers in recent years, resulting in it being proposed as a marker for metastatic biopotential in many tumours, and in particular E-cadherin expression is one of the more strongly supported molecular biological markers of prostate cancer behavior.

In primary prostatic carcinoma, aberrant expression of E-cadherin has been correlated to tumor grade and stage and, in particular, to the presence of bone metastases.[9–11] However, contrasting data have been published in relation to this. While confirming the correlation with tumor grade, one study found no relationship with tumor progression or with cancer-related death.[12] Conversely, in animal models of prostate cancer, absent E-cadherin expression has been described in metastasizing and nonmetastasizing tumor sublines.[7]

In an archival study to address this issue,[13] the loss of E-cadherin expression was studied in matching prostate primary tissue and prostatic bone metastases from the same patient. The results showed that strong E-cadherin protein expression was maintained in 4 of 10 specimens with untreated metastatic prostatic carcinoma, and in only one case was immunohistochemical staining entirely negative. A similar pattern was confirmed in 14 prospectively collected untreated metastatic specimens. In 11 of these, mRNA for E-cadherin was also detected using in-situ hybridization techniques. When the phenotype of the primary was compared with the metastasis, 13 of 14 had positive expression of mRNA for E-cadherin, and this was uniformly seen in the primary tumor cells of 10 cases. Comparing primary and metastatic tissue, decreased expression of E-cadherin mRNA was found in the metastasis in 9 cases, similar levels in 2 cases, and 3 metastatic specimens had higher levels of E-cadherin mRNA than their corresponding primary tumor.

These results suggest that the downregulation of E-cadherin expression is not, of itself, an essential step in the metastatic cascade. However, in the metastatic specimens in this study, reported E-cadherin levels were normal in only 3, and in 9 of 14 cases, the metastatic phenotype was associated with reduced E-cadherin expression when compared with the primary. Consequently, if E-cadherin is a clinically important invasion/metastasis suppressor, then transient functional downregulation may be a more likely mechanism in the metastatic process.

A number of hypotheses have been proposed to explain this phenomenon. Transient downregulation of E-cadherin has been attributed to changes in the local microenvironment. In cell lines, it has been shown that E-cadherin is re-expressed during in-vitro passages having been lost *in vivo*.[14] It is also postulated that E-cadherin expression in the metastatic phenotype may just be a continuation of the fluctuating unstable expression of E-cadherin exhibited by malignant cells.[7] Another potential mechanism is the disruption of homotypic binding by the local overproduction of products such as episialin by the tumor cells, which may mask the E-cadherin binding site.[15] However, the answer to this question in prostate and other cancers may lie in the inter-relationship between E-cadherin and catenin, and their functional intracellular binding.

The integrity of the cadherin–catenin complex and its anchorage to the actin cytoskeleton are required for effective E-cadherin mediated intercellular adhesion. Absence or dysfunction of the catenin component of this complex may lead to impaired cellular adhesion with apparently normal levels of E-cadherin.[13,16] In transitional cell bladder tumors, the immunohistochemical expression of E-cadherin and α-, β-, and γ-catenins are all associated with tumor grade,[17] which, in turn, correlates with metastasis. There is a 20% discrepancy between cadherin and catenin expression, but their independent prognostic values are similar, although only that for E-cadherin is statistically significant for survival. A similar pattern is found in colorectal neoplasms, where E-cadherin and α-catenin expression are correlated: decreased expression is associated with the presence of metastases. Similarly, in nasopharyngeal tumors the expression of both β-catenin and E-cadherin are markers of poor prognosis.[18] The expression of β-catenin is strongly associated with that of E-cadherin, and its prognostic significance is equivalent. There are slightly different patterns seen in melanocytic neoplasms. In these, decreased E-cadherin expression is a feature in early melanomas. However, in metastasizing primary tumors, E-cadherin is identified and localized to the membrane, while expression of α- and β-catenins is restricted to the cytoplasm.[19] This may suggest that differential cadherin and catenin expression may reflect differing stages in tumor metastasis.

Clinical studies of prostate cancer have confirmed the correlation between catenin subtype expression with tumor dedifferentiation and local stage.[20] Aberrant expression of α-catenin is rare in the presence of normal E-cadherin expression. In a study of 28 prostatic tumors, Murant et al found consistent abnormalities of E-cadherin expression, but there was also downregulation of α-catenin.[21] Umbas found this in only 4 of 52 cases,[22] but the combination occurred in patients with advanced disease, of whom 2 of 4 went on to die of prostate cancer, compared with just 2 of 9 patients with advanced disease exhibiting normal E-cadherin and α-catenin. The β-catenin molecule has dual functions in prostatic and other tissues. In addition to its role in the cadherin–catenin complex, it is also a regulator of signal transduction, acting by binding to DNA and activating gene transcription. Nuclear accumulation of β-catenin is mediated by mutation of the adenomatous polyposis coli (APC) tumor-suppressor gene in colorectal carcinoma, which is thought to contribute to neoplastic transformation.[23] There are few reports detailing abnormalities of β-catenin signaling acting as a sole regulator in prostate cancer: less than 4% of primary prostate tumors have been shown to have β-catenin mutations[24] and mutations of the APC gene have not been detected.[25] Therefore, the aberrant b-catenin expression would seem to relate predominantly to the function of the cadherin-catenin complex. This notion is supported by the study of matched primary and bone metastasis specimens.[13] In 13 of 14 primary tumors high expression of β-catenin was found (and was uniform in 11). By contrast, 12 of 14 metastases showed downgrading of β-catenin mRNA levels compared with their primary tumor, such that 5 of 14 metastases were entirely negative for β-catenin, and the remaining 9 had heterogeneous staining. There is, therefore, a striking contrast between the levels of β-catenin mRNA in the primary and in the metastasis in a manner that is consistent with downregulation of β-catenin and consequent dysfunction of the cadherin–catenin complex. This factor may, therefore, be an important early step in the metastatic process. There are, however, unexplained observations that run counter to this hypothesis. For example, β-catenin expression in the primary tumor does not appear to reflect the metastatic potential of tumors in some patients. Unfortunately, there are no comparable studies of β-catenin levels in prostatic bone metastases. Previous work, apart from the studies by Bryden et al, has only considered the level of expression in primary tumors, where expression mirrors tumor grade.[20]

This information and the lack of a defined role or mechanism for impaired E-cadherin function would suggest that relying on simple immunohistochemical expression of E-cadherin as a marker for metastatic potential may be an oversimplification.

These studies have demonstrated that the expression of E-cadherin protein and mRNA in prostatic bone metastases, and its intensity, is highly variable, although E-cadherin is usually present in prostatic metastases to bone. However, there is commonly a disruption of the E-cadherin/β-catenin axis, suggesting that, while E-cadherin is not lost from metastatic cells (or is re-expressed in the secondary site once it has been lost in the primary site), its functionality in association with β-catenin is impaired.

CELL–MATRIX ADHESION, MATRIX DEGRADATION, AND CELL MIGRATION/MOTILITY

Cell–matrix attachment is mediated by the integrin group of cell adhesion molecules in association with the cMet/HGF/SF axis (see below). Although there is significant variation in integrin expression between tumors, overexpression of the α6- and β3-integrins has been associated with increased invasion.[26,27] This suggests that they may function to anchor the malignant cell to the basement membrane to allow digestion, or that they are involved with initiation of transduction signals relating to the initiation of cell motility. Whatever the true mechanism, integrins are fundamentally important in the binding and migration process at metastatic sites.

Integrins work in conjunction with enzymes that degrade the extracellular matrix and the basement membrane. The extracellular matrix and basement membrane are composed mainly of type IV collagen, laminin, fibronectin, entactin, and tenascin.[28] Leukocytes and malignant cells are normally the only cells able to breach the basement membrane, and they do so by production of proteolytic enzymes, the matrix metalloproteinases (MMPs). There are currently 24 described MMPs,[29] and they are named according to their substrate. They include collagenases, matrilysin, stromelysins, and gelatinases, and their normal function is in the turnover and degradation of extracellular matrix. The MMPs are usually present in an inactivated form, and their activity is regulated by the tissue inhibitors of metalloproteinases (TIMPs). Imbalance in the MMP:TIMP system either by downregulation of TIMPs or by increased production of MMPs by tumor cells can lead to an invasive phenotype at the primary site.[30] Within the metastasis, this balance is also vitally important both in the degradation of the endothelial barrier[31] and in the establishment of metastases in bone marrow stroma *in vitro*[32,33] (see below).

At the apex of the proteolytic enzyme cascade is urokinase-type plasminogen activator (uPA). This is a serine protease most commonly associated with thrombolysis. However, it also has direct lytic activity on fibronectin, and through plasmin activates procollagenases. It is important in initiating MMP action, a phenomenon which has been shown to be particularly important in the development of prostate cancer metastases.[32]

Increased motility is mediated by loss of intercellular adhesion and a concomitant activation of the ability of cells to move independently. In time-lapse video microscopic studies, Lang et al[34,35] showed that invasive prostate cancer cells displayed a fibroblast-like morphology (Figure 37.2) and that they were very motile. The mechanisms of this motility are probably under the control of a number of factors but two important ones are the Rho/Ras axis and the mitogenic growth factor c-MET (hepatocyte growth factor).

THE RHO/RAS AXIS

Cell motility and migration in prostate and other cancer cells is linked integrally to Ras and the GTP-binding proteins Rho, Rac, and Rab. These are important for many cellular functions including cytoskeletal assembly, intracellular signaling, and the physical movement of cell membrane areas and of whole cells.[36]

Ras is a small (21 kDa) transmembranous glycosylated protein responsible for regulating downstream cellular functions such as cell proliferation, nuclear transcription, apoptosis, and invasion[37] (Figure 37.3). It acts as a membrane transducer whereby extracellular signals bind

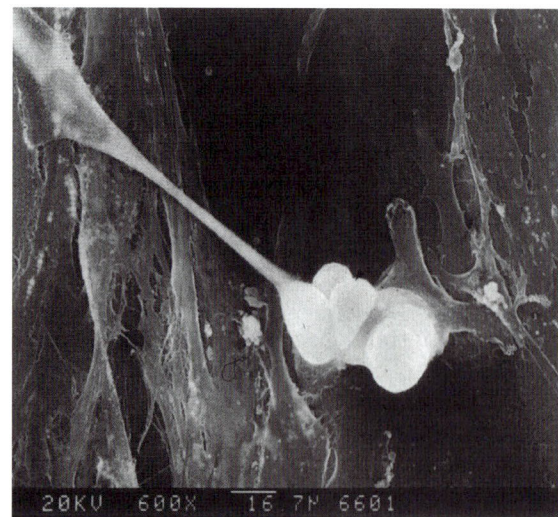

Fig. 37.2
An isolated human prostate epithelial cell *(white)* grown in co-culture with human bone marrow stroma. The cell has long filamentous processes that enable it to bind to the stromal surface. Time-lapse video-microscopy of these cells shows them to be highly motile, changing binding sites regularly, and gradually undermining the bone marrow structure.
Courtesy of S Lang et al. The Prostate 1998[35]

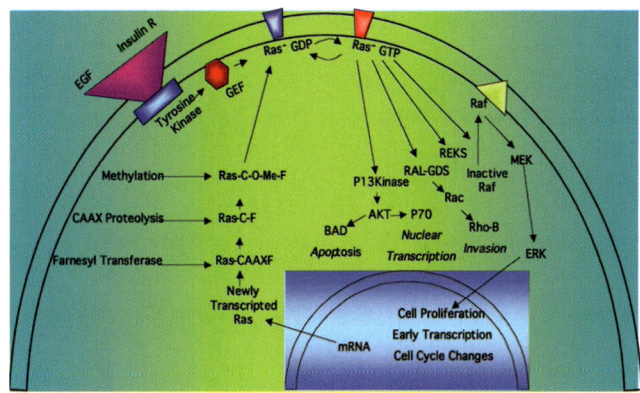

Fig. 37.3
Schematic diagram demonstrating the Ras signaling pathway and its linkage to the Rho/RAC cellular motility axis.

to receptor tyrosine kinases resulting in the activation of Ras and subsequent downstream events.[38,39] It is part of a larger "superfamily" including proteins such as Ral, Rho, Rac, and Raf.[40] The Ras subfamily, which takes part in the majority of cell signaling, consists of h-, k-, n-, r-, and m-Ras. Ras mutations are common in human cancers and are responsible for about 30% of solid tumors, but only 3% of prostate cancers.[38] Therefore, the vast majority of prostate cancer epithelial cells should have normal Ras function.

The Ras-linked kinase cascade is dependent on several events following receptor tyrosine kinase (RTK) stimulation; RTK activates ERB and SRC to recruit FAK and thus Raf (Ras activating factor) to the inner cell membrane.[41] This in turn directs the Ras-GDP and Ras-

GTP equilibrium towards the phosphorylated GTP product.[40] Following a fixed GTP-Ras signal, there are a number of effector pathways that control a wide variety of cellular functions[42] including cell morphology, gene transcription,[39] cell motility, invasiveness,[43] cell survival, apoptosis,[44] cell–cell binding, and proliferation.

The Rho family of GTPases are similar in structure and synthesis to the Ras family: their activation is downstream of Ras and hence Ras-dependent. The Rho family currently comprises Rho A, B, C, E, G, RAC1, Rac2, CDC42H5, and TC10—all proteins involved in cell movement. It has also been suggested[45] that the role of Rho GTPase is in the actin dynamics that guide cell axon growth and movement. Cell movement in this case could occur by means of a "molecular clutch," which involves the extension of filopodia bound to the cortical actin network and a fixed extracellular ligand. This results in movement of the whole body of the cell towards the attractant (Figure 37.4).

Prevention of Rho synthesis or activity should result in reduced cell motility with a corresponding reduction in invasion of cells across endothelial barriers. This Ras/Rho mechanism is thought to be important in cellular migration and the development of metastases from prostate and other cancers. This has been shown *in vitro* by studies that have utilized compounds known to inhibit the prenylation pathway. In studies using the mevalonate pathway (and thus RhoA) inhibiting bisphosphonate zoledronic acid, it has been shown in breast cancer *in vitro* that cancer cell motility is reduced and that this effect is ultimately a consequence of inhibition of RHOA.[46] In similar studies in prostate

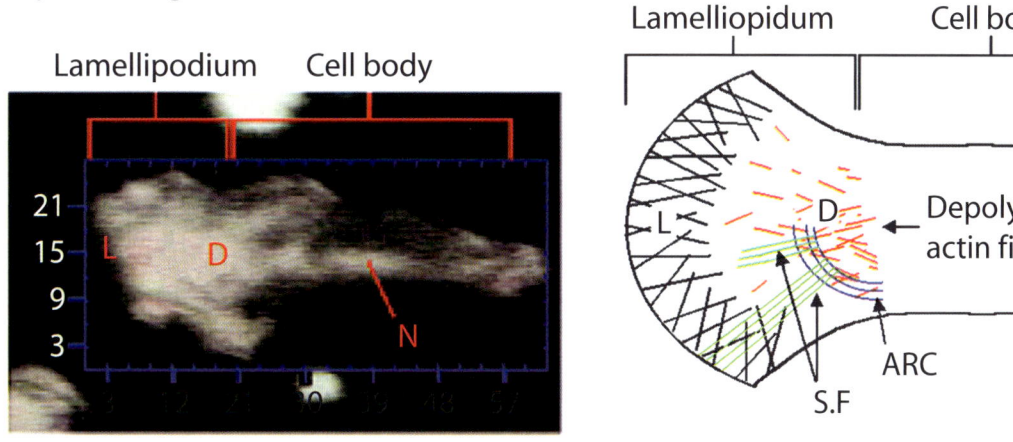

Fig. 37.4
Optical image of a motile prostate cancer cell with a lamellipodial extension *(N)* projecting out in the direction of cellular travel. The schematic diagram shows the internal architecture of the lamellipodium, with actin filaments linking the internal cellular structure to the external lipid cellular membrane. These filaments undergo a constant process of polymerization and destruction resulting in movement of the lamellipodium and forward movement of the cell.
Courtesy of E Gazi, ProMPT GU Research Group Manchester.

cancer, Montague et al[31] also demonstrated that cell motility and the cellular transmigration of primary prostate cancer and prostate cancer cell lines across human bone marrow endothelial barriers and in human bone marrow stromal co-culture was inhibited using the same compound. In a further series of experiments, in which both the farnesyl and geranyl-geranyl prenylation pathways were inhibited using a potent prenylation inhibitor,[47] the migration and motility of prostate cancer epithelial cells was reduced dramatically after the inhibition of Ras prenylation (and therefore Rho inhibition). It is therefore likely that the Ras/Rho axis is activated in the process of prostate cancer metastasis, and that this underpins the important acquisition of cell motility in cancer metastasis. The reasons for this are not currently understood, but the phenomenon is unlikely to be due to Ras mutation per se. As mentioned previously, Ras mutations are only found in approximately 3% of prostate cancers.[38]

THE c-MET/HEPATOCYTE GROWTH FACTOR AXIS

"Scatter factor" (SF) or "hepatocyte growth factor" (HGF) is so named because of its ability to cause cohesive epithelial colonies to scatter, and because of its mitogenic properties originally described in hepatocytes.[48] The HGF/SF axis represents a classical ligand/receptor transduction signaling system, the receptor being c-MET. This is membrane bound and was first described in 1984.[49] The HGF/SF is secreted by stromal cells, and it mediates stromal/epithelial signaling (reviewed by Knudsun and Edlund[50]). The c-MET/HGF/SF system is known to be important in the development of cancers *in vitro* and in animal systems, where it has been shown to influence carcinogenesis, tumor cell invasion[51-53] and metastasis.[54,55,56]

In the prostate, c-MET/HGF/SF regulates branching morphogenesis during development. This requires the invasion of prostate epithelial cells in to the prostatic stroma, and it is this process that may be dysregulated during the process of malignant transformation.[51] In normal prostate, the expression of c-MET is confined to the basal and intermediate layers of the prostate glandular epithelium,[50,57] while in malignancy, the c-MET expression is more generalized.[57] It localizes to keratin 5 and keratin 18 expressing cells, i.e., those known to arise from the putative stem cell compartment.[58,59] In studies of men presenting with prostate cancer c-MET has been shown to be expressed in 43 to 85% of primary tumours.[60-62] This level of expression is increased in metastases, particularly in bone. In a study of 86 patients, the expression of c-MET in the 41 bone metastases studied was high (approximately 100%) in all evaluable specimens. The rate of expression was lower in lymph nodes, with only 54%, but

this level was significantly higher than that seen in the primary tissue.[63] The c-MET/HGF/SF axis, therefore, seems to be of relevance in the sequence of events leading to the development of prostatic metastases and in particular, to the establishment of prostatic metastases in bone marrow.

c-MET is multifunctional and the mechanisms underpinning its influence remain to be determined fully. However, there are a number of known effects that lend weight to the understanding of the process by which this receptor ligand axis produces its effects. The c-MET/HGF/SF receptor/ligand activation influences the binding of prostatic epithelial cells to each other and to the underlying stroma by its influence on cadherins, catenins, and integrins, thus liberating the cells from their surrounding structural attachments (the importance of cadherin/catenin binding in relation to this has been discussed above). c-MET expression is known to have a direct effect on E-cadherin expression and β-catenin binding[64] by a process of β-catenin binding and phosphorylation.[65] This has the effect of downregulating epithelial cell–cell binding, a phenomenon which is known to be associated with metastatic behavior, as observed by Umbas[22] and Bryden et al.[13]

In addition, c-MET affects epithelial/stromal binding by inducing changes in integrin expression and signaling in prostatic and other tumors. It is likely that the differential changes in integrin signaling, affecting basal cells expressing integrins-α2, 3, and 6 and -β1 and 4, have a significant effect on triggering growth and motility/migration.[51] The α2/β1 intergrin has been shown to be particularly influential in the metastatic process in bone marrow stroma *in vitro*,[34,35] but this is unlikely to be the only factor. An additional influence may be the inhibition of motility arising as a consequence of met blockade. It is known that inhibition of c-MET activation will decrease primary prostate colony formation in human bone marrow co-culture,[66] and that inhibition of c-MET by viral transfection will prevent tumor cell migration and invasion.[67] The true reasons for these observations are incompletely understood, but it is possible that they may be related to the known relationship between MET and the Rho GTPases[69] and the documented activation of MMP secretion by MET. The Rho pathway in relation to prostatic and other cellular motility (described above) is fundamentally important to metastasis formation. In addition, it has been shown that c-MET induction causes MMP production.[69] MMPs are also essential to prostate cancer cell migration and to the establishment of prostatic metastases *in vitro*[32,33] and there is a demonstrable link between the MMP/TIMP axis in prostate cancer migration across endothelial and barriers *in vitro* (Figure 37.5).[31]

In summary, it is likely that the c-MET/HGF/SF axis is a key component of prostate cancer epithelial cell detachment, migration, and metastasis, and that this process arises as a consequence of multiple effects on the process by which the epithelial cell detaches from its primary anatomical site, and the way in which the motile processes in that cell are activated. Because of this influential role, the c-MET/HGF/SF axis is an attractive target for novel therapeutic modulation in the prevention of and treatment of prostatic bone metastases

the bone marrow. Cells isolated from the bone marrow were often clumped together[81] in a manner consistent with work reported in other solid tumors (e.g., breast cancer) and with all other prostate studies to date.[82] On the basis of this it could be argued that the correct term for these isolated cells is the plural "micrometastases" and not the singular "micrometastasis."[83]

PROSTATE CANCER CELLS IN CIRCULATION

In all primary tumors, malignant cells enter the circulation, particularly as the local tumor load increases. This may be a function of the size of the tumor, although it is more likely that it relates to dedifferentiation and the acquisition of the metastatic phenotype. It is certainly true that the more aggressive tumors metastasize early at a point when the primary component may still be small.

The presence of circulating cells at an early stage in the clinical natural history has been demonstrated in various cancers, where they are detectable in both blood and bone marrow. In 1980, Sloane et al were successful in detecting disseminated tumor cells in the bone marrow of breast cancer patients[70] and, since then, other workers have shown the presence of occult tumor cells in bone marrow. These have potential prognostic value as has been demonstrated in breast, colorectal and non-small cell lung cancer.[71-73] This phenomenon has been also been confirmed recently in larger studies of malignant cellular isolation from the peripheral blood of women with breast cancer.[74] Many studies addressing this subject refer to breast cancer, in which the prevalence of micrometastases in bone marrow has been noted to be between 2% and 48%, and in which a mostly positive correlation has been reported in relation to the presence of positive axillary lymph nodes.[75-77] Studies of gastrointestinal, lung, head, neck, and pancreatic tumors have documented a micrometastatic rate of approximately 38.5%.[78] Studies on prostate cancer are restricted to local or early disease and are hampered by relatively small numbers. However, the micrometastatic rates observed are consistent with those reported in other solid tumours.[76,79,80] The presence of these cells may therefore represent an early stage of dissemination. However, there is currently no firm evidence that the detection of prostate epithelial cells in the peripheral circulation or the bone marrow necessarily leads to the subsequent development of a metastasis in the skeleton.

In investigations in our laboratory, the number of prostate cells isolated from bone marrow was relatively low but extraction was more consistently reliable from the bone marrow than from peripheral blood, suggesting that there is a process by which cells are concentrated in

PROSTATE TUMOR CELL CLEARANCE FROM PERIPHERAL BLOOD

Whilst it is now clear that there is a background of circulating cells from the primary tumor in the blood and bone marrow of patients with prostate and other cancers, the fate of the individual cell once it escapes from the primary site is poorly understood. This gap in knowledge has been assisted recently by studies of humans and in *in-vitro* studies using human tissue.

Iatrogenic shedding of cells in to the peripheral circulation is known to occur in clinical situations such as prostate manipulation during transurethral resection of the prostate (TURP),[84,85] radical prostatectomy,[86] prostate biopsy[87] and brachytherapy.[88] These reports have all shown that prostate epithelial cells are disseminated but notwithstanding this observed effect, there is no perceptible increase in the clinical rate of metastasis development in patients where this phenomenon has been reported. This may relate to an individual cell's ability to propagate (see below) or to other unknown factors. Whatever the truth of this, there is a process by which cells are "cleared" from the circulation at a steady state. Price et al demonstrated circulating cell clearance within 4 weeks in 91% of patients who had detectable prostate epithiel cells (PECs) in prostate biopsy samples following.[87] This time scale, however, is probably far too long and the speed of cell clearance from the circulation is almost certainly much more rapid than this. Chambers et al[33] have proposed that this process is mainly a function of arrest of relatively large epithelial cells (or clumps of cells) in the first capillary bed that they encounter. However, this cannot be the sole explanation: if it were, the incidence of pulmonary and hepatic metastases would be much higher than it actually is in prostate, breast, and a number of other cancers. There is likely to be an additional component predicated on differential binding properties of prostate cancer cells and the influence of chemo-attraction and activated cellular motility. In an in-vitro model of prostate epithelial cell binding to human bone marrow endothelium, it has been shown that the process of epithelial/endothelial binding is virtually complete within 1 hour[89] and that once that process has occurred, the epithelial cell migrates through the endothelial barrier within 24 hours.[88] This series of laboratory findings is supported by the results of reverse transciptase polymerase chain reaction (RT-PCR) measurements in men undergoing TURP. A series of measurements using RT-PCR based techniques on peripheral blood taken in and around the operative period during prostatic resection showed that prostatic epithelial cells appeared in the circulation at the commencement of surgery, but they were undetectable within 2 hours of the cessation of the surgical procedure.[90] It is clear, therefore, that a cell, once it enters the circulation, is rapidly taken out, almost certainly by binding to an endothelial surface at a secondary site.

Whilst the tumor cells remain in the circulation they may circulate freely but they may also interact with platelets to form a tumor–platelet thrombus. This "clumping" phenomenon has been mentioned above[81] and is a phenomenon that possibly aids the formation of metastases by: 1) stabilizing tumor cell arrest in the vasculature; 2) stimulating tumor cell proliferation; 3) promoting tumor cells extravasation by potentiating tumor cell-induced endothelial cell retraction; and 4) enhancing tumor cell interaction with the extracellular matrix.[26] However, this cell platelet interaction is not an absolute prerequisite to binding, migration, and metastasis formation. It has been shown clearly that the process of endothelial binding and retraction *in vitro* does occur without the presence of platelets or cellular clumping/coalescence.[88]

There are other reasons why epithelial cells from prostate and other cancers might be eliminated from the peripheral circulation. One is the antitumor efficiency of the immune system. This is mediated primarily by the action of NK/LAK cells, macrophages and cytolytic T lymphocytes.[91] Immune recognition of neoplastic cells, as demonstrated by a lymphoplasmacytic response, is generally considered a favorable prognostic sign in human malignancies.[92] However, this necessitates the expression of class I and class II major histocompatibility (MHC) antigens during the presentation of cellular tumor antigens to the immune system. Loss of class I antigens has been associated with poorer prognosis in small cell lung cancer, breast cancer and laryngeal carcinoma,[93,94] while decreased expression of HLA-A, B, and C are found in locoregional metastases of malignant melanoma.[95] Avoidance of immune surveillance appears to be associated with tumor progression and, indeed, it has been demonstrated that metastatic prostate cancer cells lose HLA expression,[96] thereby facilitating avoidance of immune recognition and cell epithelial cell elimination.

Another factor that may influence prostate cell survival in the circulation is that many tumor cells are unable to survive the deformation required to pass through the microvasculature.[97] This deformation process has been demonstrated elegantly in a series of time lapse confocal microscopic studies showing the changes in cellular shape and size during cellular transmigration through the endothelial barrier[88] (Figure 37.6).

METASTATIC INEFFICIENCY AND THE STEM CELL CONCEPT

Another factor that accounts for the absence of metastatic development in the presence of significant numbers of cancer cells in circulation is the differing potential of cellular subtypes to propagate. It has been shown experimentally that many tumor cells arrest but fail to initiate growth, and that many micrometastases fail to progress to macroscopic tumours.[98] This may be a manifestation of the terminally differentiated state of the individual cells. In prostate cancer, particularly when it is advanced, large numbers of cells are shed in to the circulation at a constant rate. However, only a tiny fraction go on to form active metastases. It is also known from in-vitro studies (e.g. Lang et al[34]) that cells must be present in critical number before a metastatic colony will begin to grow. Estimates of "metastatic inefficiency," i.e., the number of tumor cells entering the vascular or lymphatic system, varies. Fidler,[99] in an in-vivo animal model, suggested that a threshold level of 10^5 tumor cells was needed in the circulation at any one time in order for a metastasis to develop. In a tumor injection model of highly metastatic melanoma cells, only 1% went on to form macrometastases, while in one report in renal cell carcinoma only 4 of 10 patients developed metastases, despite shedding a median of 3.7×10^7 cancer cells per day into the circulation for at least 180 days.[100] These gross cell numbers do not, however, take in to account the fact that not all of the cells entering the circulation have the capacity to continue dividing. A large proportion will be terminally differentiated and will have lost the capacity for continued regeneration. The regenerative component is likely to arise in the stem cell compartment of the prostate. In studies of the prostate stem cell phenotype, it is known that there is a "stem component" from which accelerated and continued growth occurs from a very small number of cells.[58,59,101–103] This prostate "stem compartment" arises in the basal layers of the prostate, and when it is isolated by cell separation and fax analysis it has been shown to constitute a maximum of 1% of all the epithelial cells.[104] It may, therefore, be the case that the number of prostate stem cells or transient amplifying cells (TAP cells) appearing in the circulation is the most critical determinant of metastatic development. At present there is no reliable way to mark these cells *in vivo* in a manner that would enable differentiation from the rest of the prostate cell population.

DISTAL ATTACHMENT AND TUMOR CELL TRANSMIGRATION THROUGH ENDOTHELIUM

Tumor cell arrest on endothelial surfaces in the circulation and the subsequent transendothelial

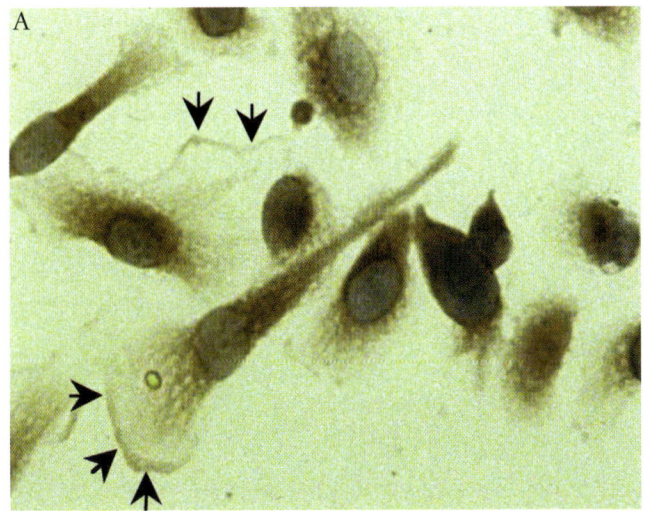

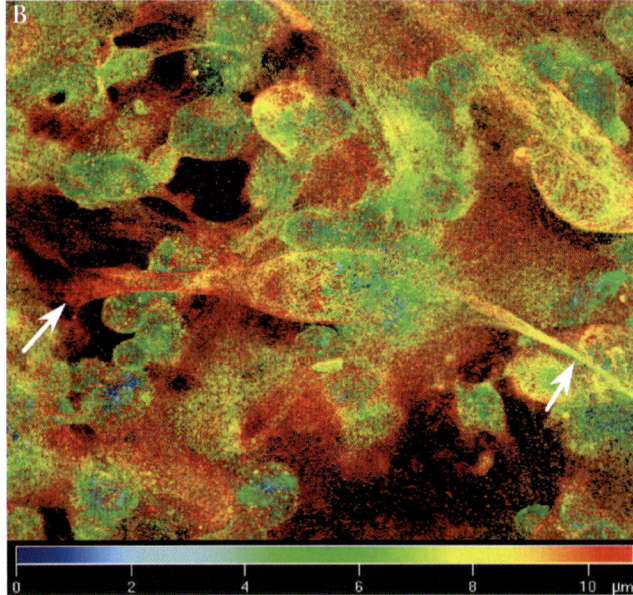

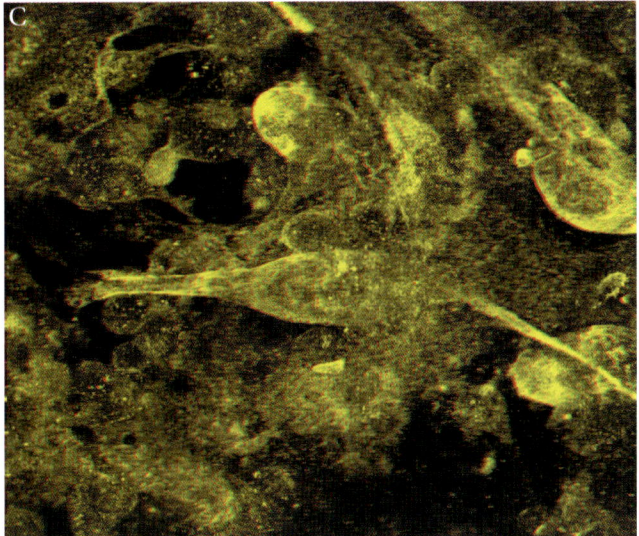

Fig. 37.5

A, Photomicrograph showing matrix metalloproteinase 7 (MMP7) immunocytochemical staining of prostate cancer cells in culture. High levels of MMP7 staining are seen at the leading edge of the cell in relation to the ruffling border at the margin of the pseudopodial extension *(arrows)* (magnification ×400). *B & C,* Confocal 3D-imaging of prostate cancer cells in bone marrow co-culture showing prostate cellular invasion of bone marrow stroma. *B,* False color image of a PC3 cell within the BMS: Blue being 0 μm, closest to the viewer (top of bone marrow stroma [BMS]) through to red 10 μm, furthest away from the viewer (bottom of the BMS layer). Using morphology for identification, *left arrow* shows the leading pseudopodia of a PC-3 cell with *right arrow* showing the trailing end. *C,* 3D-image of the same picture showing the PC3 cell underneath the BMS. MMP concentrations are seen to be highest at the leading edge of the cell. The cells also have the extended "fibroblastic" morphology typical of motile cells.

Courtesy of C Hart, ProMPT GU Research Group Manchester.

migration of tumor cells are key events in cancer metastasis in prostate and other cancers. Tumor cell–endothelial interactions are thought to involve multiple adhesive interactions, akin to the "docking and locking" hypothesis at the molecular level.[26] The initial step is thought to involve selectins; this interaction is then stabilized by integrin binding.[105] These are not the only binding steps, since antibodies to CD11a, CD18, LFA-1, and CD31 have also been shown to interfere with the binding process.[106]

Site-specific adhesion determinants may play a role in the preferential metastasis of tumors to certain organs. Some of the molecules postulated to be involved in tumor–endothelial adhesion include platelet-endothelial cell adhesion molecule 1 (PECAM1 or CD31), a member of the immunoglobulin superfamily,[107] and α4β1-integrin and sialyl Lewis X, which bind to the endothelial cells through E-selectin and VCAM1.[108]

After adhering to the surface of endothelial cells, tumor cells must penetrate the endothelial junction (Figure 37.6). The endothelial cell appears to be actively involved in permitting transmigration, as there are dynamic changes in the expression and localization of adhesion molecules including N-cadherin, VE-cadherin and PECAM1.[109]

Following endothelial cell retraction, the tumor cells once more adhere to the underlying extracellular matrix. Binding to laminin and type IV and type V collagens is mediated by β1- and β4-integrins, whilst binding to hyaluronan, fibronectin, type I collagen, and cellular migration is mediated through β1-integrin (amongst other integrins) and CD44.[108,110–113] The process of cellular migration is also influenced significantly by chemoattractants such as chemokines specific to the secondary site (see below). The understanding of this process of secondary site binding and extravasation in prostate cancer has been

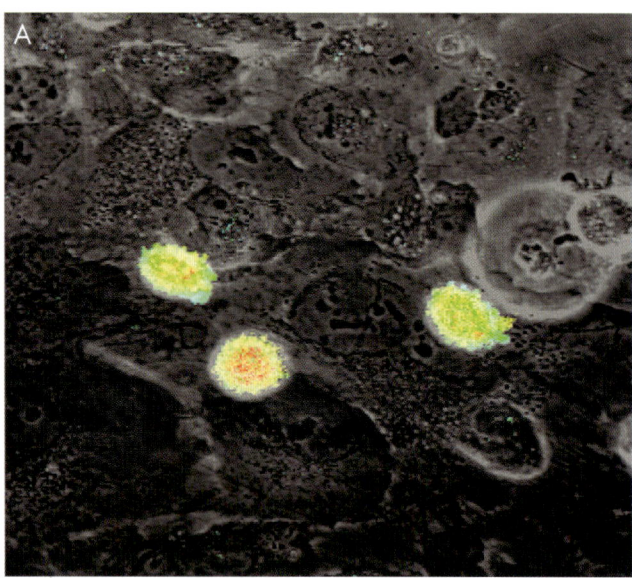

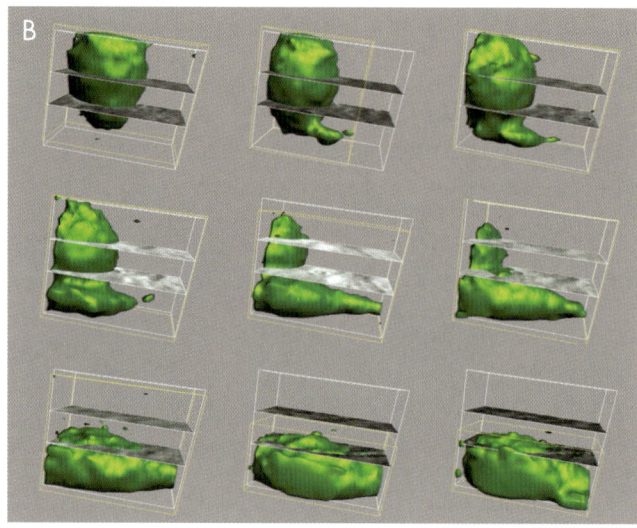

Fig. 37.6

Green fluorescent protein (GFP)-transfected cells: binding and movement through endothelium. Photomicrograph of a bone marrow endothelial monolayer *(gray)* seeded with prostate cancer PC3 cells transfected with green fluorescent protein *(bright green) (A)*. The cells bind to the junctional areas of the endothelium within 30–60 minutes. Thereafter they induce retraction of the bone marrow endothelial layer and migrate through in to the interstitium (see Figure 37.7). This process involves active cellular movement and cellular expansion *(B)* as shown by the time-lapse volumetric reconstructions of one of these GFP-marked cells as it extravasates through the endothelial monolayer.

Courtesy of Hart, Brown et al. Br J Cancer 2005.

facilitated and augmented by the development of co-culture models using human bone marrow and both primary prostate cells and cell lines to study the early mechanisms of epithelial binding, migration through endothelial barriers,[32,88,89] and the establishment of prostate epithelial colonies in human bone marrow.[34,35]

In studies using isolated human bone marrow endothelial cells and specific binding assays, the binding characteristics and the duration of the binding process have been measured.[88] These experiments have shown that the process of epithelial/endothelial cell binding is complete within 90 minutes (confirming the clinical findings of McIntyre et al[89]). They have also demonstrated that the binding depends fundamentally on the β1-integrin component of the cell matrix integrin binding mechanism. Furthermore, using different endothelial types and benign and malignant prostate epithelial cells, it has been shown that prostate epithelial cells bind more avidly to bone marrow endothelial surfaces than to other endothelia, and that benign and malignant cells have the same binding capacity for those endothelial surfaces. Why then, do metastases not develop from the proliferative prostate epithelial cells known to be present in the circulation during prostatic resection for benign prostatic hyperplasia (BPH)? The answer to this question lies in the differential ability of the prostate epithelial cell to migrate across the endothelial barrier. This has been demonstrated by in-vitro studies using green fluorescent protein (GFP)-transfected prostate cancer cells in

conjunction with time-lapse confocal microscopy. This has enabled cellular tracking measurements of benign and malignant prostate epithelial cells in epithelial/endothelial co-cutlure.[88] This series of experiments has demonstrated that the prostate cancer cells bind to the junctional areas of the endothelial barrier (figure 37.6), where they precipitate retraction of the endothelial layer, followed by migration of the epithelial cell through the ensuing endothelial defect in a process that involves the active movement of motile prostate cells (figure 37.6 and 37.7). The observed cellular migration across the endothelial barrier is complete within 24 hours of cellular binding and, importantly, *only* malignant cells will transmigrate through the endothelial layer. Benign cells will bind in the same way as malignant ones, but they will not pass across the endothelial barrier in to the interstitium.[88]

Study of this mechanism is critical to the understanding and potential treatment of metastases in prostate cancer. Once bound, prostate epithelial cells induce rapid endothelial cell retraction, but the precise mechanism inducing that retraction, an essential component of cellular transmigration, is at present unclear. A major component of the signaling cascade modulating endothelial permeability is the intracellular level of Ca^{2+}.[114] Studies by Lewalle et al[115] demonstrated that the binding of breast epithelial cells to Human Umbilical Vein Endothelial Cells (HUVECs) induced a transitory rise in HUVEC intracellular concentration of Ca^{2+}, resulting in endothelial retraction and epithelial migration. This rise in Ca^{2+} levels and retraction of the endothelial layer is entirely dependent on cell–cell contact, and inhibition of this rise in intracellular Ca^{2+} concentration inhibited breast epithelial transendothelial migration. Binding of prostate epithelial cells and melanoma cells also induces raised intracellular Ca^{2+} levels,[116] correlating with increased binding of the epithelial cells. Previous studies by our group have shown that treatment of a bone marrow endothelial cell line with the bisphosphonate zoledronic acid, a potent calcium chelating agent and blocker of the mevalonate transduction pathway, tightens the endothelial to endothelial cell binding in the absence of prostate epithelial cells. However, the tightening of this binding has not been observed with high doses (100 μM) of the weaker bisphosphonate pamidronate, or with EDTA, both of which are potent Ca^{2+}-chelating agents.[31] Therefore, it is unlikely that endothelial retraction relates to increased levels of extracellular Ca^{2+}, although the effects on intracellular Ca^{2+} levels at the higher concentrations observed in relation to endothelial binding experiments are unknown.[31] The effect is more likely to be related to Ras/Rho mechanisms and the release of specific degradative enzymes such as MMPs. This inhibitory effect has been demonstrated using specific inhibitors of the prenylation step[47] and by measurement of local TIMP/MMP concentrations.[31]

The effect of Ras/Rho inhibition in reducing the ability of prostate cancer cells to invade across endothelial barriers towards bone marrow suggests that a major component affecting cancer cell migration is inhibition of the transduction pathways related to the Rho axis. This inhibitory effect in prostate cancer has been demonstrated *in vitro* using both zoledronic acid[31] and the prenylation inhibitor AZD3409.[47,48] The inhibitory effect of both of these compounds is known to be related to the Rho pathway through

Ras linkage.[117] Inhibition of this pathway affects downstream prenylation of small GTPases such as Rho, which is known to be involved integrally in cell motility. Therefore, an early event following β1-integrin binding in prostate cancer cells may be the induction of a specific pathway or pathways relating to Ras and subsequently Rho. Whether or not this is a consequence of flux in intracellular calcium levels within endothelial cells remains to be determined. The role of the β1-integrin component and the interaction between the prostate epithelial cell with the endothelial tight cell junction in relation to induced rises in intracellular Ca^{2+} concentrations is certainly worthy of further study.

Malignant prostate cells migrate across the endothelial barrier in similar manner to melanoma cells.[109] After binding rapidly to the endothelial junctions, the prostate epithelial cells show marked membrane blebbing and lamellipodia formation at the point of contact between the two cell surfaces. The prostate epithelial cell then generates a pseudopodal extension which penetrates the endothelial cell layer, the endothelial cells retract and the prostate cell then moves through the endothelial barrier (Figures 37.6 and 37.7). As with the migration across endothelia observed in melanoma cells, prostate epithelial transmigration is considerably slower than leukocyte transmigration, with 29% of cells completing the transit within 4 hours.[88] This extravasation time is comparable to that observed for melanoma cells,[109] rat ascites hepatoma cells[118] and other tumor cells.[119] However, it has been shown that over 50% of monocytes can cross an endothelium within the first hour of contact[120,121.] without inducing endothelial cell retraction. This difference may be due to the fact that epithelial cells are larger then monocytes and therefore require greater retraction of the endothelium, thus resulting in the significantly increased time of invasion.

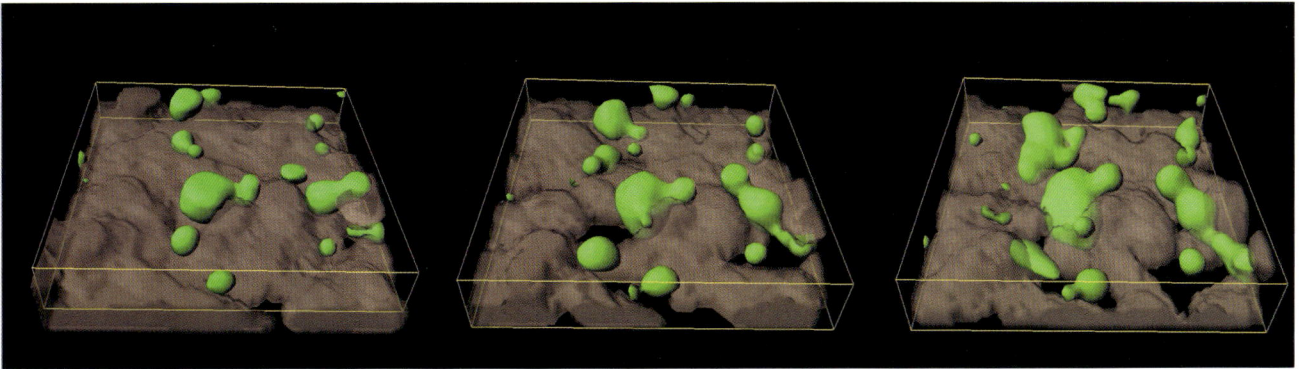

Fig. 37.7

Reconstructed confocal microscopic image of prostate cancer cells transfected with green fluorescent protein *(green)* seeded on to a bone marrow endothelial monolayer *(gray)* and photographed sequentially with time-lapse confocal microscopy. *A,* The cells binding to the junctional areas of the endothelium. *B,* The endothelial cells have started to retract, leaving gaps in the endothelial barrier. *C,* The epithelial cells then migrate through in to the underlying interstitium.

Courtesy of Dr M Brown and Dr S Bagley, ProMPT GU Research Group, Manchester.

BONE MARROW STROMAL INVASION

Once through the endothelial barrier the cells require several key elements to be present to develop into an overt metastasis. There are a number of uncertainties in this area, and it has been shown by RT-PCR-based and whole cell extraction studies that malignant epithelial cells can remain dormant in the bone marrow for considerable periods of time. There are certain key elements that are required for propagation to enable development in to a metastasis including a critical cell number, cell–cell crosstalk via specific integrins,[34,35] cellular motility,[34,66] and the presence of active degradative enzymes[32,33] particularly MMPs such as MMP2 and MMP7,[32,122,123] and their activator, uPA.[32,124–126] The balance of MMPs and TIMPs is also critical.[31] In these co-culture experiments, the establishment of metastatic colonies and the motility of primary and prostate cancer cell lines was inhibited by escalating doses of the zoledronic acid. One of the main reasons for this was the effect on TIMP2 levels, which were elevated 800-fold following treatment. This resulted in a reduction of MMP activation, a factor known to be important in the establishment of prostatic metastatic development *in vitro*.[32]

CHEMOATTRACTION AT THE SECONDARY SITE: CHEMOKINES AND LIPIDS

The "seed/soil" hypothesis of Paget is exemplified by prostate cancer, which has an obvious predilection for the red bone marrow of the axial skeleton.[127] Once there, it disturbs the integrated and balanced function of the skeleton, and it displaces the red bone marrow leading to marrow dysfunction, ultimately precipitating bone marrow failure. This is not a characteristic that is unique to prostate cancer; indeed, a number of studies, many of them recent, have shown the preference that many epithelial cancers have to metastasize in a similar manner. These include cancers of the kidney,[128] lung[129] breast,[130] and skin.[131,132] Two characteristics that may contribute to this homing phenomenon are the presence of chemokines and the affinity for energy-rich sources, such as specific lipids, which are freely available within adipocytes in the red bone marrow.

The chemokine axis is one of the main mechanisms responsible for the "homing" of hematologic and immunologic cells to specific targets in the body. Cells from a number of epithelial tumor types share many of the trafficking characteristics of this hematopoietic stem cell (HSC) homing system.[130] The homing of the HSC to the bone marrow during fetal life and after bone marrow transplantation has been well characterized, the key

molecular axis being the CXC chemokine stromal derived factor 1 (SDF1 or CXCL12) and its receptor CXCR4 (CD186). This model is supported by the knowledge that both bone marrow endothelial cells and osteoblasts express SDF1,[133–135] CXCR4 knockouts do not show hematopoietic engraftment of the bone marrow,[136] and that the level of expression of CXCR4 expression by HSC determines their ability to engraft the bone marrow.[137] It is now known that the CXCR4/SDF1 axis also plays an important role in the targeting of solid tumor metastases to the bone marrow. It has been shown to be important in various primary tumors including those from the breast,[131] kidney,[138] lung,[129] pancreas,[139] and prostate.[127,140] It has also been shown *in-vitro* that CXCR4 and SDF1 are involved in the motility process: interactions alongside CCR7/CCL21 trigger pseudopodal invasion by malignant breast epithelial cells by a process of actin polymerization.[130] This has led to the hypothesis that CXCR4 is the key component of metastatic implantation in bone marrow, and that it represents an important therapeutic target for metastatic bone disease, such as that arising from prostate cancer. Blockade of the CXCR4 signaling pathway in malignant breast epithelial cells either by neutralizing antibodies[130] or by peptide antagonists such as T140,[141] has been shown to inhibit metastasis *in vivo*.

In a series of experiments using migration chambers in prostate cancer co-cultures to measure the influence of SDF1 signaling via CXCR4, the results of Sun et al,[140] have shown that the level of CXCR4 expression increased with increasing malignancy, with the greatest expression being observed in the aggressively metastatic cell line PC3 and in human bone metastasis sections. This increasing expression also suggests that CXCR4/SDF1 signaling may be one of the key signaling pathways for metastatic spread to the bone. Furthermore, the importance of this pathway has been demonstrated by Taichman et al[127] utilizing a matrigel basement membrane invasion assay to show that SDF1 signaling induced both DU145 and PC3 cells to invade. However, Hart et al,[88] using recombinant SDF1 and T140 inhibitors have shown that the CXCR4/SDF1signaling pathway is not the sole chemoattractant in the spread of prostate epithelial cells to the bone. This study has confirmed that whilst SDF1 is a potent stimulus for invasion, the level of invasion it induces is significantly less than that seen by using either bone marrow endothelial (BME) cells and/or bone marrow stroma (BMS) alone. This measured phenomenon was reinforced in these experiments by the observation that use of T140 (a specific CXCR4 antagonist peptide), at a concentration which blocked prostate epithelial cell invasion in response to maximum levels of SDF1 signaling, did not completely block invasion towards either BME or BMS completely. Thus, the CXCR4/SDF1 signaling pathway is important in prostate cancer metastasis, but it is not the only signaling pathway involved.[88]

Another potentially important stimulus is the requirement for the metastasizing prostate cancer cell to seek out a lipid source. It is well known that cancer cells are metabolizing rapidly and, as a consequence, they have a fundamental requirement for lipid, either for utilization as an energy source, or for utilization in the cellular processes involved in tumor cell maintenance, proliferation, and migration. In an *in-vitro* study,[142] it was shown that PC3 cells grew rapidly in the vicinity of lipid cells in bone marrow. Further studies[143] have shown that prostate cancer cells take up lipid rapidly as soon as they are seeded on to human bone marrow (Figure 37.8). Furthermore, specific lipids act as a strong chemoattractant for prostate cancer cells. Arachidonic acid, an omega-6 lipid, results in rapid migration of PC3 cells towards bone marrow stroma, and this effect is blocked by competitive inhibition using omega-3 lipids. Additional evidence for the importance of this effect is provided by experiments of lipid depletion in bone marrow. The attractant property of human bone marrow for prostate cancer cells is abolished if the bone marrow stroma is depleted of lipid cells prior to epithelial cellular seeding.[143] Thus, it is confirmed that specific lipids are involved in the metastatic process, and they may, therefore, be an important determinant of the site of early prostate cancer cell implantation and metastatic growth.

MOLECULAR MECHANISMS OF METASTATIC PROSTATE CANCER IN BONE/BONE MARROW

Once established at the secondary site in bone marrow, the prostatic micrometastasis develops in the bone marrow space, often in close association with the bone surface, where the osteoblast/fibroblast microenvironment is disturbed locally. It has been postulated that the first event in this metastatic developmental process is osteoblast-mediated bone resorption leading to release of stimulatory cytokines from the bone surface and a cycle of resorption/tumor stimulation. However, in personal observation by the author of serial micrometastases from human metastatic bone biopsies taken from men with prostate cancer, this phenomenon has not been observed. The first event in the process is always a stimulation of fibroblastic elements in the bone marrow and local stimulation of osteoblasts (Figure 37.9). As the metastasis develops, it induces an imbalance of the carefully regulated skeletal cycle, uncoupling bone resorption from bone formation, with the result that there is accelerated bone formation and resorption occurring synchronously. This is caused by changes in local cytokine production and interaction.

A number of stimulating factors have been identified in relation to "osteoblastic" metastases in prostate cancer. These mechanisms have become much clearer in recent years. One important discovery is that of the influence of the endothelin axis. Endothelins are 21-amino-acid peptides with multiple functions. There are three types (endothelin 1, 2, and 3), and they act via the endothelin receptors ET_a and ET_b. They are synthesized in vascular endothelial cells and their functions include vasoconstriction, nociception, and the physiological regulation of bone function. It is this latter effect that is important in relation to prostate cancer, particularly through the actions of ET_1 and its receptor ET_a. The work by Nelson and Carducci (reviewed by Nelson[144]) has shown that exogenous ET_1 induces prostate cancer proliferation and enhances the mitogenic effects of insulin-like growth factor (IGF) and epidermal growth factor (EGF). More importantly in relation to prostate cancer metastasis in bone, ET_1 production is one of the major factors responsible for

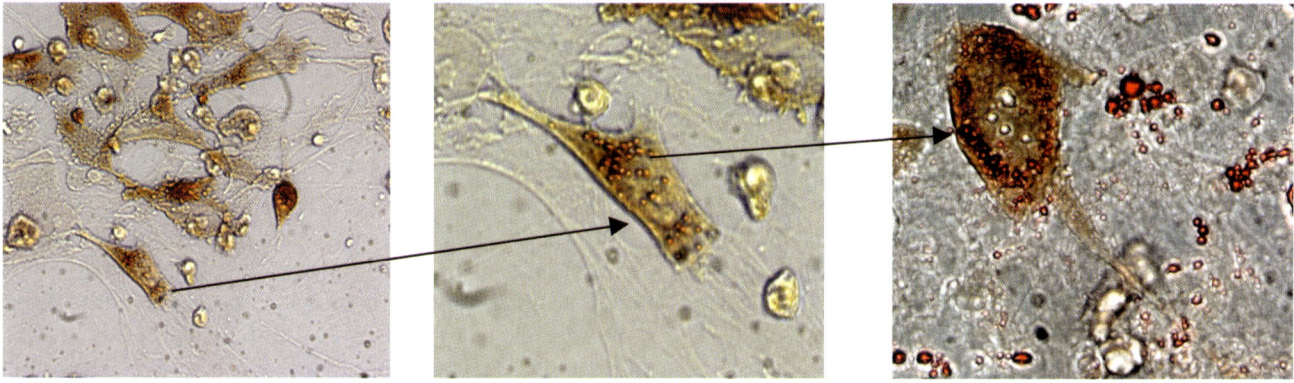

Fig. 37.8

A, Micrograph showing lipid uptake by a prostate cancer cell in co-culture. *B,* The lipid droplets (Nile red staining globules) are taken up rapidly by the prostate cancer cell and have been shown to be intracellular using sectional confocal microscopy. *C,* The lipid droplets are more clearly demonstrated in the prostate cancer cells in co-culture at higher magnification in human bone marrow stroma. The prostate cancer cells have an affinity for the adipocytes and co-localize with these in the bone marrow. Courtesy of Brown M et al. 2005. PromPT GU Research Group, Paterson Insitute Manchester).

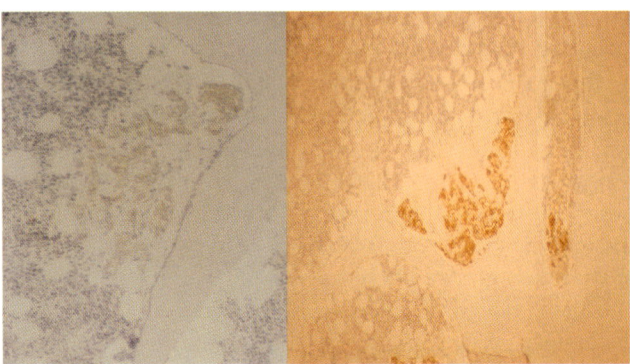

Fig. 37.9
Photomicrographs of two bone biopsies taken by the author from different prostate cancer patients. These show the typical appearance of early "micrometastases" from prostate cancer. The epithelial cells are stained for prostate-specific antigen (PSA) and show as brown. The cell colonies lie close to the bone surface (uniformly pale) where they are stimulating early osteoblastic activity. In the surrounding bone marrow, the fibroblasts are stimulated to induce a desmoplastic reaction. There is no evidence of bone resorption at this stage of the disease process.

osteoblast overstimulation.[145] Prostate epithelial cells produce ET_1, and its receptor ET_a is present throughout the prostate gland.[146–148] Endothelin 1 is also produced by prostate cancer cells in a bone environment.[149] In a series of experiments using an osteoblast mouse model,[145] it has been shown that tumors producing ET_1 (such as prostate cancer) act via the ET_a receptors on the osteoblast to stimulate accelerated bone formation. This abnormal activity can be blocked by the effects of the ET_1 inhibitor, ABT-627 (Atrasentan).[144]

Although it is important in this process, ET1 is not the only osteoblast stimulator in prostate cancer metastases. Other factors include upregulation of the Wnt pathway (known to be upregulated in prostate cancer), and the production of cytokines such as bone morphogenetic protein (BMG), transforming growth factor-β (TGFβ), IGF, vascular epithelial growth factor (VEGF), platelet-derived growth factor (PDGF), and MD Anderson bone factor (MDABF).[150] One interesting aspect of the cytokine balance and its effect in prostate cancer metastases relates to the IGF axis and PTHrP, which is known to be produced in prostate cancer bone metastases.[151,152] Prostate-specific antigen (PSA), a known protease, can cleave PTHrP (a fact that might explain why PTHrP is measurable in the peripheral circulation patients with breast cancer but not in those with prostate cancer) and, therefore, shift the balance within the immediate milieu of the prostate metastasis from bone resorption to formation.[153,154] Furthermore, PSA can also cleave IGF binding protein 3 (IGFBP3), which in turn increases the levels of IGF1. This too would have the effect of shifting the axis of stimulation by the metastatic

prostate cancer cells towards increasing osteoblast activity.[155]

This osteoblast overactivity is responsible for the measurable increase in bone volume in prostate cancer bone metastases[156,157] and for the accelerated bone mineralization rate as measured by double tetracycline labeling in human prostate cancer bone biopsy specimens.[158] The prostate tumor-generated bone in these deposits is formed as abnormal "woven" bone. This is characteristic of bone produced in high turnover states, and it is responsible for the well-described sclerotic appearance measured histomorphometrically[157] and seen radiologically in over 90% of patients with metastatic prostate cancer.[159]

The traditional view of prostate cancer as an "osteoblastic" disease obscured the fact that the disease is responsible for major bone destruction for many years. The resorptive effects of prostate cancer were suggested initially on the basis of preliminary histologic studies in bone[160] and the phenomenon was subsequently proven unequivocally on the basis of histomorphometric measurement of human metastatic bone biopsies[156,157] and biochemical measurement of bone resorption products in humans.[161,162] The paradox of increasing bone volume in the presence of bone resorption is explained by histomorphometric studies showing that the resorption of the existing skeleton is accompanied by synchronous replacement of abnormal woven bone, which, itself, undergoes further resorption.[157] This produces a measurable increase in bone volume in the presence of wholesale destruction of the normal skeleton.

The molecular mechanisms responsible for the lytic process arise, like the formative "blastic" process, as a consequence of abnormal levels of soluble growth factors produced by the invading prostatic tumor. This in turn stimulates abnormal osteoclast activity, which is responsible for the bone resorption. Osteoclast recruitment, differentiation, and activation by tumors is incompletely understood, but it is thought to be related to osteoblast stimulation, probably as a consequence of over expression of NFKB (RANK ligand) by osteoblasts and the production of osteoprotogerin, known to be increased in prostate cancer metastasis.[163] This effect may be occurring by stimulation by macrophage colony stimulating factor (MCSF), the receptor activator of the NFKB ligand (RANK ligand) and osteoprotegerin.[164,165] Osteoblasts secrete the RANK ligand, which then induces osteoclast differentiation by binding the RANK surface receptor on the osteoclast precursor. This in turn stimulates osteoclastogenesis.[164] The protein, osteoprotegerin plays a key regulatory role in this process by competing for the RANK binding site on osteoclast precursors. A cofactor in this process may be PTH-rP. Cancer cells are unable to express RANK ligand and cannot, therefore, stimulate osteoclastogenesis by this route. However, when PTH-rP is present (as shown in murine osteoblasts and hematopoietic progenitors in culture[166]) osteoclasts differentiate in the absence of other stimulatory agents, thus suggesting that PTHrP has a facilitatory role. PTH-rP is a major factor in bone resorption in breast cancer[167] and is expressed in both primary and bone metastases in prostate cancer.[151,152]

CONCLUSION

The molecular mechanisms of metastasis in prostate cancer are complex and involve a number of specific steps and inter-related mechanisms. The primary epithelial cells must have the ability to detach, migrate, and avoid the host defences to reach a secondary site where they bind to the local endothelium in a site-specific manner. If the cell has the capacity to propagate, it will migrate in to the interstitium, attracted by a number of chemoattractive factors. Once there, provided the environment is favorable, it will form a metastatic colony of cells which, because of its ability to produce active cytokines that disrupt the normal controlled milieu, will disrupt the balanced local homeostatic mechanisms, leading to architectural disruption and a continued cycle of tumor proliferation and migration. Continued improvements in the understanding of the molecular mechanisms controlling this process will help to develop novel therapies with the prospect of controlling this progressively fatal condition.

REFERENCES

1. Liotta L. Tumour invasion and metastases—role of the extracellular matrix. Rhodes Memorial Lecture. Cancer Res 1986;46:1–7.
2. Birchmeier W, Behrens J. Cadherin expression in carcinomas: the role in the formation of cell junctions and prevention of invasiveness. Biochem Biophys Acta 1994;1198:11–26.
3. Frixen U, Behrens J, Sachs M, et al. E-cadherin mediated cell-cell adhesion prevents invasiveness of human carcinoma cells. J Cell Biol 1991;113:173–185.
4. Vleminckx K, Vakaet L Jr, Mareel M, et al. Genetic manipulation of E-cadherin expression by epithelial tumor cells reveals an invasion suppressor role. Cell 1991;66:107–119.
5. Takeichi M. Cadherin cell adhesion receptors as a morphogenetic regulator. Science 1991;251:1451–1455.
6. Näthke I, Hinck L, Swedlow JR, et al. Defining interactions and distributions of cadherin and catenin complexes in polarized epithelial cells. J Cell Biol 1994;125:1341–1352.
7. Bussemakers M, van Moorselaar RJA, Giroldi LA, et al. Decreased expression of E-cadherin in the progression of rat prostatic cancer. Cancer Res 1992;52:2916–2922.
8. Perl A, Wilgenbus P, Dahl U, et al. A causal role for E-cadherin in the transition from adenoma to carcinoma. Nature 1998;392:190–193.
9. Umbas R, Schalken JA, Aalders TW, et al. Expression of the cellular adhesion molecule E-caherin is reduced or absent in high grade prostate cancer. Cancer Res 1992;52:5104–5109.
10. Umbas R, Isaacs WB, Bringuier PP, et al. Decreased E-cadherin expression is associated with poor prognosis in patients with prostate cancer. Cancer Res 1994;54:3929–3933.
11. Cheng L, Nagabhushan M, Pretlow TP, et al. Expression of E-cadherin in primary and metastatic prostate cancer. Am J Path 1996;148:1375–1380.
12. McWilliam L, Knox WF, Hills C, et al. E-cadherin expression fails to predict progression and survival in prostate cancer [Abstract]. J Urol 1996;155:516–526.
13. Bryden AAG, Freemont AJ, Clarke NW, et al. Paradoxical expression of E-cadherin in prostate bone metastases. Br J Urol 1999:84:1032–1034.
14. Mareel M, Behrens J, Birchmeier W, et al. Down regulation of E-cadherin expression in Madin Darby canine kidney (MDCK) cells inside tumors of nude mice. Int J Cancer 1991;47:922–928.
15. Ligtenberg M, Buijs F, Vos HL, et al. Suppression of cellular aggregation by high levels of episialin. Cancer Res 1992;52:2318–2324.
16. Shimoyama Y, Nagafuchi A, Fujita S, et al. Cadherin dysfunction in a human cancer cell line: possible involvement of loss of -catenin expression in reduced cell-cell adhesiveness. Cancer Res 1992;52:5770–5774.
17. Shimazu T, Schalken JA, Giroldi LA, et al. Prognostic value of cadherin associated molecules (alpha, beta, gamma catenins and p120cas) in bladder tumours. Cancer Res 1996;56:4154–4158.
18. Zheng Z, Pan J, Chu B, et al. Downregulation and abnormal expression of E-cadherin and beta-catenin in nasopharyngeal carcinoma: close association with advanced disease stage and lymph node metastasis. Hum Pathol 1999;30:458–466.
19. Silye R, Karayiannakis AJ, Syrigos KN, et al. E-cadherin/catenin complex in benign and malignant melanocytic lesions. J Pathol 1998;186:350–355.
20. Morita N, Uemura H, Tsumatani K, et al. E-cadherin and alpha-, beta- and gamma-catenin expression in prostate cancers: correlation with tumour invasion. Br J Cancer 1999;79:1879–1883.
21. Murant S, Handley J, Stower M, et al. Co-ordinated changes in expression of cell adhesion molecules in prostate cancer. Eur J Cancer 1997;33:263–271.
22. Umbas R, Isaacs WB, Bringuier PP, et al. Relation between aberrant alpha catenin expression and loss of cadherin function in prostate cancer. Int J Cancer 1997;74:374–377.
23. Tetsu O, McCormick F. Beta-catenin regulates expression of cyclin D1 in colon carcinoma cells. Nature 1999;398:422–426.
24. Voeller H, Truica CI, Gelmann EP. Beta-catenin mutations in prostate cancer. Cancer Res 1998;58:2520–2523.
25. Suzuki H, Aida S, Akimoto S, et al. State of adenomatous polyposis coli gene and ras oncogenes in Japanese prostate cancer. Jap J Cancer Res 1994;85:847–852.
26. Honn K, Tang DG. Adhesion molecules and tumor cell interaction with endothelium and subendothelial matrix. Cancer Metastasis Rev 1992;11:353–375.
27. Cress A, Rabinovitz I, Zhu W, et al. The alpha 6 beta 1 and alpha 6 beta 4 integrins in human prostate cancer progression. Cancer Metastasis Rev 1995;14:219–228.
28. Nagle R, Knox JD, Wolf C, et al. Adhesion molecules, extracellular matrix, and proteases in prostate carcinoma. J Cell Biochem 1994;19:232–237.
29. Overall CM, Lopez-Otin C. Strategies for MMP inhibition in cancer: innovations for the post-trial era. Nat Rev Cancer 2002;2:657–672.
30. Lokeshwar B, Selzer MG, Block NL, et al. Secretion of matrix metalloproteinases and their inhibitors (tissue inhibitor of metalloproteinases) by human prostate in explant cultures: reduced tissue inhibitor of metalloproteinase secretion by malignant tissues. Cancer Res 1993;53:4493–4498.
31. Montague R, Hart CA, George NJ, et al. Differential inhibition of invasion and proliferation by bisphosphonates: anti metastatic potential of zoledronic acid in prostate cancer. Eur Urol 2004;46,389–402.
32. Hart CA, Scott LJ, Bagley S, et al. Role of proteolytic enzymes in prostate bone metastasis formation: *in vitro* and *in vivo* studies. Br J Canc 2002;86:1136–1142.
33. Chambers AF, Groom AC, MacDonald IC. Dissemination and growth of cancer cells in metastatic sites. Nat Rev Cancer 2002:2:563–572.
34. Lang S, Clarke NW, George NJ, et al. Primary prostatic epithelial cell binding to human bone marrow stroma and the role of alpha2beta1 integrin. Clin Exp Metast 1997;15:218–227.
35. Lang S, Clarke NW, George NJR, et al. Interaction of prostate epithelial cells from benign and malignant tumor tissue with bone-marrow stroma. Prostate 1998;34:203–213.

36. Oxford G, Theodorescu D. Ras superfamily monomeric G proteins in carcinoma cell motility. Cancer Lett 2003;189:117–28.

37. Johnston SR. Farnesyl transferase inhibitors: a novel targeted therapy for cancer. Lancet Oncol 2001;2, 18–26.

38. Adjei A. Blocking oncogenic Ras signaling for cancer therapy. J Natl Cancer Inst 2001:93:1062–1074.

39. Hu L, Shi Y, Hsu JH, et al. Downstream effectors of oncogenic ras in multiple myeloma cells. Blood 2003;101:3126–3135.

40. Cohen LH, Pieterman E, van Leeuwen RE, et al. Inhibitors of prenylation of Ras and other G-proteins and their application as therapeutics. Biochem Pharmacol 2000;60:1061–1068.

41. Graham TE, Pfeiffer JR, Lee RJ, et al. MEK and ERK activation in ras-disabled RBL-2H3 mast cells and novel roles for geranylgeranylated and farnesylated proteins in Fc epsilonRI-mediated signaling. J Immunol 1998;161:6733–6744.

42. Kelloff GJ, Lubet RA, Fay JR, et al. Farnesyl protein transferase inhibitors as potential cancer chemopreventives. Cancer Epidemiol Biomarkers Prev 1997;6:267–282.

43. van Golen KL, Bao L, DiVito MM, et al. Reversion of RhoC GTPase-induced inflammatory breast cancer phenotype by treatment with a farnesyl transferase inhibitor. Mol Cancer Ther 2002;1:575–583.

44. Peters DG, Hoover RR, Gerlach MJ, et al. Activity of the farnesyl protein transferase inhibitor SCH66336 against BCR/ABL-induced murine leukemia and primary cells from patients with chronic myeloid leukemia. Blood 2001;97:1404–1412.

45. Giniger E. How do Rho family GTPases direct axon growth and guidance? A proposal relating signaling pathways to growth cone mechanics. Differentiation 2002;70:385–396.

46. Denoyelle C, Hong L, Vannier JP, et al. New insights into the actions of bisphosphonate zoledronic acid in breast cancer cells by dual RhoA-dependent and -independent effects. Br J Cancer 2003;88:1631–1633.

47. Khafagy R, Hart C, Stephens T, et al. In vitro effects of the prenyl transferase inhibitor AZD3409 on prostate cancer epithelial cells. Proc Asco 2004.

48. Rosen EM, Nigam SK, Goldberg ID. Scatter factor and the cMet receptor: a paradigm for mesenchymal-epithelial interaction. J Cell Biol 1994;127:1783–1787.

49. Cooper CS, Park M, Blair DG, et al Molecular cloning of a new transforming gene from a chemically transformed human cell line. Nature 1984;311:29–33.

50. Knudsen BS, Edlund E. Prostate cancer and the cMet hepatocyte growth factor. Adv Cancer Res 2004;91:31–67.

51. Behrens J, Weidner K, Frixen UH, et al. The role of E cadherin and scatter factor in tumour invasion and cell motility. EXS 1991;59:109–126.

52. Rong S, Bodescot M, Blair DG, et al. Tumorigenicity of the met proto-oncogene and the gene for hepatocyte growth factor. Mol Cell Biol 1992;12:5152–5158.

53. Rong S, Segal S, Anver M, et al Invasiveness and metastasis of NIH-3T3 cells induced by met-hepatocyte growth factor / scatter factor autocrine stimulation. Proc Natl Acad Sci USA 1994;91:4731–4735.

54. Jeffers M, Rong S, Woude GE. Hepatocyte growth factor / scatter factor-Met signaling in tumorigenicity and invasion/metastasis. J Mol Med 1996;74:505–513.

55. Jeffers M, Fiscella M, Webb CP et al. The mutationally activated met receptor mediates motility and metastasis. Proc Natl Acad Sci 1998;95:14417–14422.

56. Kurimoto S, Moriyama N, Horie S, et al. Co-expression of hepatocyte growth factor and its receptor in human prostate cancer. Histochem J 1998;30.

57. Van Leenders G, van Balken B, Aalders T, et al. Intermediate cells in normal and malignant prostate epithelium express cMet: Implications for prostate cancer invasion. Prostate 2002;51:98–107.

58. Bonkhoff H, Stein U, Remberger K. The proliferative function of basal cells in the normal and hyperplastic human prostate. Prostate 1994;24:114–118.

59. Bonkhoff H. Analytical molecular pathology of epithelial-stromal interactions in the normal and neoplastic prostate. Anal Quant Cytol Histol 1998;20:437–432.

60. Humphrey P, Zhu X, Zarnegar R, et al. Hepatocyte growth factor and its receptor (c-MET) in prostatic carcinoma. Am J Pathol 1995;147:386–396.

61. Pisters L, Troncoso P, Zhau HE, et al. c-met proto-oncogene expression in benign and malignant human prostate tissues. J Urol 1995;154:293–298.

62. Watanabe M, Fukutome K, Kato H, et al. Progression linked over-expression of cMet in prostatic intraepithelial neoplasia and latent as well as clinical prostate cancers. Cancer Lett 1999;141:173–178.

63. Knudsen BS, Gmyrek GA, Inra J, et al. High expression of cMet receptor in prostate cancer metastasis to bone. Urology 2002;60:1113–1117.

64. Birchmeier W, Brinkmann V, Niemann C, et al. Role of HGF/SF and c-Met in morphogenesis and metastasis of epithelial cells. Ciba Found Symp 1997;212:230–240.

65. Monga SP, Mars WM, Pediaditakis P, et al. Hepatocyte growth factor induces wnt independent translocation of beta catenin after met-beta catenin dissociation in hepatocytes. Cancer Res 2002;62:2064–2071.

66. Lang SH, Clarke NW, George NJR, et al. Scatter factor influences the formation of prostate epithelial colonies in bone marrow stroma *in vitro*. Clin Exp Metastasis 1999;17:333–340.

67. Kim SJ, Johnson M, Koterba K, et al. Reduced cMet expression by an adenovirus expressing a cMet ribozyme inhibits tumorigenic growth and lymph node metastases of PC3-LN4 prostate tumour cells in an orthotopic nude mouse. Clin Canc Res 2003:9:5161–5170.

68. Miao H, Nickel CH, Cantley LG, et al. EphA kinase activation regulates HGF-induced epithelial branching morphogenesis. J Cell Biol 2003;162:1281–1292.

69. Fujiuchi Y, Nagakawa O, Murukami K, et al. Effect of hepatocyte growth factor on invasion of prostate cancer cell lines. Oncol Reports 2003;10:1001–1006.

70. Sloane JP, Ormerod MG, Neville AM. Potential pathological application of immunocytochemical methods to the detection of micrometastases. Cancer Res 1980;40:3079–3082.

71. Diel IJ, Kaufmann M, Goerner R, et al. Detection of tumor cells in bone marrow of patients with primary breast cancer: a prognostic factor for distant metastasis. J Clin Oncol 1992;10:1534–1539.

72. Lindemann F, Schlimok G, Dirschedl P, et al. Prognostic significance of micrometastatic tumour cells in bone marrow of colorectal cancer patients. Lancet 1992;340:685–689.

73. Pantel K, Riethmuller G. Micrometastasis detection and treatment with monoclonal antibodies. Curr Top Microbiol Immunol 1996;213:1–18.

74. Cristofanilli M, Budd GT, Ellis M, et al. Circulating tumour cells, disease progression and survival in metastatic breast cancer. N Engl J Med 2004:351:824–826.

75. Berger U, Bettelheim R, Mansi JL, et al. The relationship between micrometastases in the bone marrow, histopathologic features of the primary tumor in breast cancer and prognosis. Am J Clin Pathol 1988;90:1–6.

76. Mansi JL, Easton D, Berger U, et al. Bone marrow micrometastases in primary breast cancer: prognostic significance after 6 years' follow-up. Eur J Cancer 1991;27:1552–1555.

77. Diel IJ, Kaufmann M, Costa SD, et al. Micrometastatic breast cancer cells in bone marrow at primary surgery: prognostic value in comparison with nodal status. J Natl Cancer Inst 1996;88:1652–1658.

78. Funke I, Schraut W. Meta-analyses of studies on bone marrow micrometastases: an independent prognostic impact remains to be substantiated. J Clin Oncol 1998;16:557–566.

79. Pantel K, Schlimok G, Angstwurm M, et al. Methodological analysis of immunocytochemical screening for disseminated epithelial tumor cells in bone marrow. J Hematother 1994;3:165–173.

80. Slovin S F, Scher HI. Detectable tumor cells in the blood and bone marrow: smoke or fire? Cancer 1998;83:394–398.

81. Bhatt RI. Identification and Characterisation of the Putative Prostatic Stem Cell. Manchester University MD Thesis, 2005.

82. Pantel K, Cote RJ, Fodstad O. Detection and clinical importance of micrometastatic disease. J Natl Cancer Inst 1999;91:1113–1124.

83. Pikarsky E, Peretz T. Bone marrow metastases in breast cancer. N Engl J Med 2000;343:577–578.

84. Straub B, Muller M, Krause H, et al. Detection of prostate-specific antigen RNA before and after radical retropubic prostatectomy and transurethral resection of the prostate using "Light-Cycler"-based quantitative real-time polymerase chain reaction. Urology 2001;58:815–820.

85. Heung YM, Walsh K, Sriprasad S, et al. The detection of prostate cells by the reverse transcription-polymerase chain reaction in the circulation of patients undergoing transurethral resection of the prostate. BJU Int 2000;85:65–69.

86. Eschwege P, Dumas F, Blanchet P, et al. Haematogenous dissemination of prostatic epithelial cells during radical prostatectomy. Lancet 1995;346:1528–1530.

87. Price DK, Clontz DR, Woodard WL 3rd, et al. Detection and clearance of prostate cells subsequent to ultrasound-guided needle biopsy as determined by multiplex nested reverse transcription polymerase chain reaction assay. Urology 1998;52:261–266; discussion 266–267.

88. Hart C, Brown M, Bagley S, et al. Invasive characteristics of human prostatic epithelial cells: understanding the metastatic process. Br J Cancer 2005;1–10.

89. Scott LJ, Hart C, Clarke NW, et al. Interactions of human prostate epithelial cells with bone marrow endothelium: binding and invasion. Br J Cancer 2001;84:1417–1423.

90. McIntyre IG, Bhatt RI, Clarke NW. Isolation of epithelial cells from blood and bone marrow of prostate cancer patients. Pros Cancer Pros Dis 2002;5:S21.

91. Alonso-Varona A, Palomares T, Bilbao P, et al. Tumor-host interaction in non-random metastatic pattern distribution. Bull Cancer 1996;83:27–38.

92. Brightmore T, Greening WP, Hamlin I. An analysis of clinical and histopathological features in 101 cases of carcinoma of breast in women under 35 years of age. Br J Cancer 1970;24:644–669.

93. Doyle A, Martin WJ, Funa K, et al. Markedly decreased expression of class I histocompatibility antigens, protein, and mRNA in human small-cell lung cancer. J Exp Med 1985;161:1135–1151.

94. Concha A, Esteban F, Cabrera T, et al. Tumor aggressiveness and MHC class I and II antigens in laryngeal and breast cancer. Semin Cancer Biol 1991;2:47–54.

95. Ruiter D, Mattijssen V, Broeker E-B, et al. MHC antigens in human melanomas. Semin Cancer Biol 1991;2:35–45.

96. Blades R, Keating PJ, McWilliam LJ, et al. Loss of HLA class I expression in prostate cancer: implications for immunotherapy. Urology 1995;46:681–686.

97. Weiss L. Deformation driven lethal damage to cancer cells. Its contribution to metastatic inefficiency. Cell Biophys 1991;18:73–79.

98. Luzzi K, MacDonald IC, Schmidt EE, et al. Multistep nature of metastatic inefficiency: dormancy of solitary cells after successful extravasation and limited survival of early micrometastases. Am J Pathol 1998;153:865–873.

99. Fidler IJ. Metastasis: quantitative analysis of distribution and fate of tumor emboli labeled with 125 I-5-iodo-2′-deoxyuridine. J Natl Cancer Inst 1970;45:773–782.

100. Glaves D, Huben RP, Weiss L. Haematogenous dissemination of cells from human renal adenocarcinomas. Br J Cancer 1988;57:32–35.

101. Collins AT, Habib FK, Maitland NJ, et al. Identification and isolation of human prostate epithelial stem cells based on alpha(2)beta(1)-integrin expression. J Cell Sci 2001;114:3865–3872.

102. Hudson DL, O'Hare M, Watt FM, et al. Proliferative heterogeneity in the human prostate: evidence for epithelial stem cells. Lab Invest 2000;80:1243–1250.

103. Brown M, Samuel J, Gilmore P, et al. Characterisation and phenotype of the recently defined prostate SP population: the quest for the prostate cancer stem cell. Proc ASCO 2005.

104. Bhatt RI, Brown M, Hart C, et al. A novel method for the isolation and characterization of the putative prostatic stem cell. Cytometry 2003;54A:89–99.

105. Orr F, Sanchez-Sweatman OH, Kostenuik P, et al. Tumour-bone interactions in skeletal metastases. Clin Orthopaedics Related Res 1995;312:19–33.

106. Lehr J, Pienta KJ. Preferential adhesion of prostate cancer cells to a human bone marrow endothelial cell line. J Natl Cancer Inst 1998;90:118–123.

107. Tang D, Chen YQ, Newman PJ, et al. Identification of PECAM-1 in solid tumor cells and its potential involvement in tumor cell adhesion to endothelium. J Biol Chem 1993;268:22883–22894.

108. Zetter B. Adhesion molecules in tumor metastasis. Semin Cancer Biol 1993;4:219–229.

109. Voura E, Sandig M, Siu CH. Cell-cell interactions during transendothelial migration of tumor cells. Microsc Res Tech 1998;43:265–275.

110. Sneath R, Mangham DC. The normal structure and function of CD44 and its role in neoplasia. Mol Pathol 1998;51:191–200.

111. Rabinovitz I, Nagle RB, Cress AE. Integrin alpha 6 expression in human prostate carcinoma cells is associated with a migratory and invasive phenotype *in vitro* and *in vivo*. Clin Exper Metast 1995;13:481–491.

112. Harsten M, Grove AS Jr, Woog JJ. The role of the integrin family of adhesion molecules in the development of tumors metastatic to the orbit. Ophthalmol Plas Recostruct Surg 1997;13:227–238.

113. Trikha M, Raso E, Cai Y, et al. Role of alphaII(b)beta3 integrin in prostate cancer metastasis. Prostate 1998;35:185–192.

114. Curry FE. Modulation of venular microvessel permeability by calcium influx into endothelial cells. Faseb J 1992;6:2456–2466.

115. Lewalle J, Calaldo D, Baiou K, et al. Endothelial cell intra cellular Ca^{2+} concentration is increased upon breast tumor cell contract and mediates tumour cell trans-endothelial cel migration. Clin Exp Metast 1998;16(1):21–29.

116. Pili R, Corda S, Passaniti A, et al. Endothelial cell Ca^{2+} increases upon tumor cell contact and modulates cell-cell adhesion. J Clin Invest 1993;92:3017–3022.

117. Virtanen SS, Vaananen HK, Harkonen PL, et al. Alendronate inhibits invasion of PC-3 prostate cancer cells by affecting the mevalonate pathway. Cancer Res 2002;62:2708–2714.

118. Ohigashi H, Shinkai K, Mukai M, et al. *In vitro* invasion of endothelial cell monolayer by rat ascites hepatoma cells. Jpn J Cancer Res 1989;80:818–821.

119. Kramer RH, Nicolson GL. Interactions of tumor cells with vascular endothelial cell monolayers: a model for metastatic invasion. Proc Natl Acad Sci USA 1979;76:5704–5708.

120. Sandig M, Negrou E, Rogers KA. Changes in the distribution of LFA-1, catenins, and F-actin during transendothelial migration of monocytes in culture. J Cell Sci 1997;110, 2807–2818.

121. To C, Tsao MS. The roles of hepatocyte growth factor/scatter factor and met receptor in human cancers [Review]. Oncol Reports 1998;5:1013–1024.

122. Gohji K, Fujimoto N, Hara I, et al. Serum matrix metalloproteinase-2 and its density in men with prostate cancer as a new predictor of disease extension. Intl J Cancer 1998;79:96–101.

123. Hashimoto K, Kihira Y, Matuo Y, et al. Expression of matrix metalloproteinase-7 and tissue inhibitor of metalloproteinase-1 in human prostate. J Urol 1998;160:1872–1876.

124. Rabbani S, Harakidas P, Davidson DJ, et al. Prevention of prostate-cancer metastasis *in vivo* by a novel synthetic inhibitor of urokinase-type plasminogen activator (uPA). Intl J Cancer 1995;63:840–845.

125. Van Veldhuizen PJ, Sadasivan R, Cherian R, et al. Urokinase-type plasminogen activator expression in human prostate carcinomas. Am Jf Med Sci 1996;312:8–11.

126. Kirchheimer J, Pfluger H, Ritschl P, et al. Plasminogen activator activity in bone metastases of prostatic carcinomas as compared to primary tumors. Inv Metast 1985;5:344–355.

127. Taichman RS, Cooper C, Keller ET, et al. Use of the stromal cell-derived factor-1/CXCR4 pathway in prostate cancer metastasis to bone. Cancer Res 2002;62:1832–1837.

128. Schrader AJ, Lechner O, Templin M, et al. CXCR4/CXCL12 expression and signalling in kidney cancer. Br J Cancer 2002;86:1250–1256.

129. Burger M, Glodek A, Hartmann T, et al. Functional expression of CXCR4 (CD184) on small-cell lung cancer cells mediates migration, integrin activation, and adhesion to stromal cells. Oncogene 2003;22:8093–8101.

130. Muller A, Homey B, Soto H, et al. Involvement of chemokine receptors in breast cancer metastasis. Nature 2001;410:50–56.

131. Murakami T, Maki W, Cardones AR, et al. Expression of CXC chemokine receptor-4 enhances the pulmonary metastatic potential of murine B16 melanoma cells. Cancer Res 2002;62:7328–7334.

132. Robledo MM, Bartolome RA, Longo N, et al. Expression of functional chemokine receptors CXCR3 and CXCR4 on human melanoma cells. J Biol Chem 2001;276:45098–45105.

133. Aiuti A, Webb IJ, Bleul C, et al. The chemokine SDF-1 is a chemoattractant for human CD34+ hematopoietic progenitor cells and provides a new mechanism to explain the mobilization of CD34+ progenitors to peripheral blood. J Exp Med 1997;185:111–120.

134. Hamada T, Mohle R, Hesselgesser J, et al. Transendothelial migration of megakaryocytes in response to stromal cell-derived factor 1 (SDF-1) enhances platelet formation. J Exp Med 1998;188:539–548.

135. Ponomaryov T, Peled A, Petit I, et al. Induction of the chemokine stromal-derived factor-1 following DNA damage improves human stem cell function. J Clin Invest 2000;106:1331–1339.

136. Aiuti A, Tavian M, Cipponi A, et al. Expression of CXCR4, the receptor for stromal cell-derived factor-1 on fetal and adult human lympho-hematopoietic progenitors. Eur J Immunol 1999;29:1823–1831.

137. Peled A, Petit I, Kollet O, et al. Dependence of human stem cell engraftment and repopulation of NOD/SCID mice on CXCR4. Science 1999;283:845–848.

138. Staller P, Sulitkova J, Lisztwan J, et al. Chemokine receptor CXCR4 downregulated by von Hippel-Lindau tumour suppressor pVHL. Nature 2003;425:307–311.

139. Koshiba T, Hosotani R, Miyamoto Y, et al. Expression of stromal cell-derived factor 1 and CXCR4 ligand receptor system in pancreatic cancer: a possible role for tumor progression. Clin Cancer Res 2000;6:3530–3535.

140. Sun YX, Wang J, Shelburne CE, et al. Expression of CXCR4 and CXCL12 (SDF-1) in human prostate cancers (PCa) *in vivo*. J Cell Biochem 2003;89:462–473.

141. Tamamura H, Hori A, Kanzaki N, et al. T140 analogs as CXCR4 antagonists identified as anti-metastatic agents in the treatment of breast cancer. FEBS Lett, 2003;550:79–83.

142. Tokuda Y, Satoh Y, Fujiyama C, et al. Prostate cancer cell growth is mediated by adipocyte—cancer cell interaction. Br J Urol Int 2003;91:716–720.

143. Hart C, Brown M, Bagley S, et al. Influence of Omega 3 and Omega 6 lipids on prostate cancer cell migration and proliferation in human bone marrow stroma. 2005 In Submission

144. Nelson J, Bagnato A, Battistini B, et al. The endothelin axis: emerging role in cancer. Nat Cancer Rev 2003;3:110–116.

145. Guise TA, Yin JJ, Mohammad KS. Role of endothelin-1 in osteoblastic metastases. Cancer 2003;97:3:779–784.

146. Nelson J, Hedican SP, George DJ, et al. Identification of endothelin-1 in the pathophysiology of metastatic adenocarcinoma of the prostate. Nat Med 1995;1:944–949.

147. Nelson J, Lee WH, Nguyen SH, et al. Endothelin-1 production and decreased endothelin B receptor expression in advanced prostate cancer. Cancer Res 1996;56:663–668.

148. Nelson J, Nguyen SH, Wu-Wong JR, et al. New bone formation in an osteoblastic tumour model is increased by ET-1 overexpression and decreased by ET-A receptor blockade. Urology 1999;53:2063–2069.

149. Chiao JW, Moonga BS, Yang YM, et al. Endothelin-1 from prostate cancer cells is enhanced by bone contact which blocks osteoclastic bone resorption Br J Cancer 2000;83:360–365.

150. Logothetis CJ, Lin SH. Osteoblasts in prostate cancer metastasis to bone. Nat Rev Cancer 2005;5:21–28.

151. Bryden AAG, Islam SH, Shanks JH, et al. Expression of PTH rP in bone metastases from prostate cancer. Prostate Cancer Prostate Dis 2002;40:673–676.

152. Bryden AAG, Hoyland J, Freemont AJ, et al. Parathyroid hormone related peptide and receptor expression in primary prostate cancer and bone metastases. Br J Cancer 2002;86:322–325.

153. Cramer SD, Chen Z, Peehl DM. Prostate specific antigen cleaves parathyroid hormone related protein in the PTH like domain: inactivation of PTHrP stimulated camp accumulation in mouse osteoclasts. J Urol 1996;156:526–531.

154. Iwamura M, Hellman J, Cockett AT, et al. Alteration of the hormonal bioactivity of parathyroid hormone related peptide (PTHrP) as a result of limited proteolysis by prostate specific antigen. Urology 1996;48:317–325.

155. Cohen P, Peehl DM, Graves H, et al. Biological effects of prostate specific antigen as an insulin like growth factor binding protein 3 protease. J Endocrinol 1994;142:407–415.

156. Charhon SA, Chapoy MC, Devlin EE, et al. Histomorphometric analysis of sclerotic bone metastasis from prostatic carcinoma from prostate cancer with special reference to osteomalacia. Cancer 1983;51:918–924.

157. Clarke NW, McLure J, George NJR. Morphometric evidence for bone destruction and replacement in metastatic prostate cancer. Br J Urol 1991;68:74–80.

158. Clarke NW, McClure J, George NJR. Osteoblast function and osteomalacia in metastatic prostate cancer. Eur Urol 1993;24:286–290.

159. Cook GB, Watson FR. Events in the natural history of prostate cancer: rising salvage, mean age distribution and contingency co-efficient. J Urol 1968;99:87–96.

160. Galasko CSB. Mechanisms of bone destruction in the development of skeletal metastases. Nature 1976;263:507–510.

161. Urwin GH, Percival RC, Harvey WJ, et al. Generalised increase in bone resorption in carcinoma of the prostate. Br J Urol 1985;57:721–72.

162. Clarke NW, McClure J, George NJR. Disodium pamidronate identifies differential osteoclastic bone resorption in metastatic prostate cancer. Br J Urol 1992;69:74.

163. Jung K, Lein M, Stephan C, et al. Comparison of 10 different bone turnover markers in prostatic carcinoma patients with bone metastatic spread: diagnostic and prognostic implications. Int J Cancer 2004;111:783–791.

164. Suda T, Takahasi N, Udagawa N, et al. Modulation of osteoclast differentiation and function modulation by new members of the tumour factor receptor by new members of the tumour necrosis factor receptor and ligand families. Endocr Rev 1999;20:345–357.

165. Tietelbaum SL. Bone resorption by osteoclasts. Science 2000;289;1504–1508.

166. Thomas RJ, Guise TA, Yin JJ, et al. Breast cancer cells interact with osteoblasts to support osteoclast formation. Endocrinology 1999;140:4451–4458.

167. Guise TA, Mundy GR. Cancer and Bone. Endocr Rev 1998;19:18–54.

Novel targets for prostate cancer immunotherapy 38

Johannes Vieweg, Andrew Jackson

INTRODUCTION

The treatment of recurrent or advanced prostate cancer has been evolving since the discovery that prostate tumors are hormone-dependent malignancies which respond to drugs reducing circulating testosterone levels or preventing binding of this ligand to the androgen receptor (AR). These insights initiated comprehensive searches to uncover the molecular mechanisms promoting prostate cancer development and progression. Despite our increased understanding of this disease, prostate cancer remains a leading cause of death in men. It is estimated that in the United States and Western Europe close to 185,000 men present with prostate cancer every year; almost one third of these newly diagnosed patients have locally advanced or metastatic disease.[1] Recurrent or metastatic prostate cancer is initially treated with androgen ablative therapy, but, despite primary or secondary hormonal manipulations, all patients eventually progress with androgen-independent disease, which is ultimately fatal. There are only limited treatment options for men who develop hormone-refractory prostate cancer, and the only systemic treatment modality that has shown impact on overall survival, albeit modestly, entails docetaxel and prednisone.[2] Therefore, the development of more effective and less toxic therapies will be pivotal in ultimately improving the outcome of prostate cancer patients.

A new class of highly targeted approaches, which seek to inhibit the cellular pathways that mediate tumor progression or differentiation to a hormone-independent state, or that render tumor cells resistant to apoptosis, are currently under preclinical and clinical development. Immunotherapy is one form of targeted therapy currently being explored for cancer therapy, demonstrating promise in animal models and in human clinical trials. Immunotherapy holds the promise of a new treatment modality that is tumor-specific, bears little toxicity, and, once fully developed, could have a long-lasting effect. The purpose of this chapter is to provide an overview of the molecular mechanisms and the clinical potential of emerging immunotherapeutic strategies that employ approaches based on either monoclonal antibodies (mAbs) or cancer vaccines in patients with recurrent or metastatic prostate cancer.

PROSTATE CANCER IMMUNOTHERAPY

Treatment strategies that specifically target the unique biologic aberrations associated with malignancy represent a significant and fundamental therapeutic paradigm shift in medical oncology since the advent of systemic therapies. Cancer immunotherapy is one form of targeted therapy exacting tumor cell death in a highly specific manner by taking advantage of the biologic differences between normal and cancerous cells. Although prostate cancer represents a heterogeneous disease, comprised of tumor cells with varying degrees of aggressiveness and response to therapy, primary prostate cancers share a relatively restricted set of characteristics crucial to facilitate the onset and propagation of malignant disease. Scientific advances in the molecular characterization of human tumors have now provided unprecedented opportunities to develop novel therapeutic strategies that not only target tumor-associated antigens (TAA), but also cellular proteins with critical roles in oncogenesis. Mechanisms that regulate tumor cell proliferation, control resistance to apoptotic signals, enable escape from the immune response, promote new blood vessel formation, and facilitate stromal–epithelial interactions are increasingly well understood, and approaches that specifically target these individual pathways have been developed and are currently undergoing preclinical and clinical evaluation.

The immune system is equipped with two different effector arms against tumors, each of which involves different effector cells and mechanisms of attack. Antibody-based approaches were the first form of immunotherapy to receive FDA approval for treating patients with solid or hematopoietic malignances. Antibodies such as rituximab (anti-CD20) and trastuzumab (anti-ErbB2)[3] represent a fast-growing class of cancer therapeutics in the rapidly expanding market for oncologic drugs. The recent success of mAb technology can be attributed to the development of standardized technologies that produce fully "human" or "humanized" antibodies through hybridoma technology in conjunction with protein engineering. Secondly, the discovery and characterization of highly relevant antigens that can serve as targets for mAb therapy has paved the way for effective antibody-based drugs that are currently being introduced into clinical practice.

The other major form of cancer immunotherapy, termed active immunotherapy, aims to activate T cells that kill tumor cells in an antigen-specific fashion. Therapeutic vaccines, one form of active immunotherapy, stimulate antitumor immune responses by priming T cells, which bind to TAA in context with molecules of the major histocompatibility complex (MHC). Tumor-associated antigen epitopes, recognized by cytotoxic T cells, are sequences of 8 to 11 amino acids attached to proteins or carbohydrates that reside on tumor cells, but that are absent or diminished on normal cells. Each T-cell receptor binds only to its cognate MHC–antigen complex. This strict recognition ensures that T cells are able to recognize subtle changes in the repertoire of antigens expressed by somatic cells, thus yielding the exquisite specificity typical of cellular immunity. T cells kill tumors not only through receptor-mediated pathways, but also by attracting other cellular components of the innate immune system (granulocytes, macrophages, natural killer T cells) to tumor sites, thereby exerting antitumor activity through production of reactive oxygen species, death receptor ligands, or granzymes. In contrast to mAbs, cancer vaccines have not yet met the criteria for effective cancer therapies by demonstrating therapeutic efficacy in clinical trials. However, limited clinical responses have been observed in numerous studies that have studied increasingly potent cancer vaccines over the past 20 years. As we have gained a clearer understanding of the molecular pathways that modulate the onset and propagation of human malignancy, even more potent cancer vaccine strategies have emerged that now allow effective modulation of immune responses in cancer patients, thereby optimizing the potential for clinical success.

PREVENTING IMMUNE EVASION

Since the mid-1990s, many prostate or prostate cancer-associated antigens have been cloned and much effort has been devoted in academic and biotechnology settings to identify clinically effective targets for either prostate cancer immunotherapy (reviewed by Vieweg and Dannull[4]). Prostate cancer cells express both tumor- and tissue-specific antigens that can be recognized by mAbs or by the T-cell arm of the immune system. Prostate-specific antigen (PSA), prostate membrane-associated antigen, and prostatic acid phosphatase represent prototypic TAAs that have been targeted in many experimental studies and also in immunotherapy clinical trials.[5] Although the expression of these antigens is highly restricted to either prostate-specific or prostate cancer-specific epithelia, their recognition by mAbs, their efficacy to elicit T-cell responses, and their expression in later stages of disease are highly variable. Moreover, the genetic instability of prostate tumors cells is well documented, as is the propensity of tumor cells to evade the immune system through a variety of genetic and epigenetic means.[6] Genetic changes affecting tumor antigens, such as point mutations, make the tumor less susceptible to immune attack, and, to further complicate matters, prostate malignancies often escape immune recognition and destruction through downregulation of MHC antigens,[7] as well as through disturbances involving antigen presentation pathways.[8] Recent clinical evidence suggests that these obstacles do not necessarily represent a major barrier for the development of effective immunotherapeutics. First, mAb-based therapies are not compromised by defects in MHC class I expression, or by disturbances of pathways affecting the antigen processing machinery. Secondly, the discovery and thorough delineation of molecular events involved in tumor progression and metastatic behavior has led to new therapeutic targets that may reduce the potential for immune escape. Since downregulation of genes required for tumor progression or survival is not an option for growing tumors, targeting these pathways may have high relevance to the development of novel immune-based cancer drugs. Given the complexity of the signaling pathway abnormalities present in most cancers, targeting these mechanisms has been shown to disrupt multiple aberrant signaling molecules instead of just one or two, which may eventually prove of unique therapeutic benefit. The difficult issue is which of the many approaches should be developed and how best to assess the response using standard and surrogate endpoints. Certainly, the future of prostate cancer therapy will undergo a dramatic evolution as a result of the continued interaction between the laboratory and the clinic.

TARGETING PATHWAYS THAT REGULATE TUMOR GROWTH AND SURVIVAL (Table 38.1)

The process of oncogenesis involves many incremental changes, allowing cells to proliferate, differentiate, metastasize, and resist immune control. Some of these changes involve the dysregulation of genes or proteins involved in the oncogenic process or in the maintenance of the oncogenic phenotype. The best explored mechanism to date by which prostate tumors differentiate into an androgen-independent phenotype is the amplification of the AR gene, causing continued signaling through a functional, but altered AR.[9] Amplified levels of the AR are accompanied by increased sensitivity to androgenic stimuli, thereby driving uninhibited proliferation.[10] Aside from androgen-mediated pathways, recent research has identified a number of alternative, highly relevant mechanisms that also impact tumor cell proliferation and metastatic behavior in prostate tumors. These pathways that can either involve or bypass the AR, have resulted in the identification of an increasing number of molecules that can be targeted by mAbs, T cells, or small molecule-based inhibitors.

GROWTH FACTOR RECEPTORS

Human tumors overexpress many growth factors and their receptors, providing a survival advantage over surrounding non-neoplastic tissues. In prostate cancer, many autocrine and paracrine pathways have been identified that stimulate cell proliferation due to the interplay between growth factor ligands and their cognate receptors in target tissues. Aside from cellular proliferation, growth factor pathways also regulate numerous other functions such as acquisition of apoptotic resistance, cell motility, invasive potential, and neo-angiogenesis. Several molecules and their receptors involved in phenotypic or oncogenic transformations have now been identified, including epidermal growth factor (EGF, ErbB1), platelet-derived growth factor (PDGF), insulin-like growth factor (IGF), vascular endothelial growth factor (VEGF), and transforming growth factor-β (TGFβ). Although the specific molecular components of each of these circuits may differ, there are commonalities in the activation of each pathway. In general, when one or more ligands of a growth factor family bind to specific cell surface receptors, they form a signaling complex that activates protein kinases, induces trans-autophosphorylation, and activates intracellular signaling pathways, resulting in gene transcription (Figure 38.1).

Monoclonal antibodies or vaccines targeting ligand-receptor binding or recognizing epitopes expressed by proteins or enzymes involved in cell signaling, provide a selective strategy to interfere with receptor/ligand interactions or downstream events, and, hence, may inhibit tumor growth. The rationale for targeting growth factor receptors rather than growth factors themselves is compelling because of the multiplicity of ligands for a given receptor and the lack of defined ligands for some of the family members.[11,12]

EPIDERMAL GROWTH FACTOR RECEPTOR (HER-2) SIGNALING PATHWAY

Two major malignancy-associated growth factor pathways that have been successfully exploited for cancer immunotherapy are those involving components of the tyrosine kinase receptor EGFR/HER-2 (Erb) signaling pathway. Fully humanized monoclonal antibodies have recently been developed that specifically bind to EGFR1 (ErbB1) or to HER-2/neu (ErbB2) receptors and prevent growth factor interaction with binding sites. Improved clinical response rates have been achieved using the anti-HER-2 mAb (trastuzumab [Herceptin]) in advanced breast cancer,[3] or using the anti-EGFR mAb (cetuximab [Erbitux]) in metastatic colon carcinoma.[13] Although considerable efforts are currently underway to translate these experiences to the field of prostate cancer, clinical results, thus far, have not been as promising as for other malignancies. Nevertheless, there are several lines of evidence that blockade of these common oncogenic pathways in a prostate cancer setting will eventually yield new reagents with demonstrable clinical activity. Several studies have shown that EGFR expression increases with prostate cancer progression.[14] Furthermore, concomitant upregulation of EGF and EGFR in advanced prostate cancers suggest the presence of an autocrine growth factor circuit between the membrane receptor and the corresponding ligand. Finally, EGFR is not only overexpressed but also mutated or deleted in 80% of prostate cancers, resulting in dedifferentiation, acquisition of androgen-independent disease, and resistance to apoptosis-inducing ligands.[15] Physiologically, at least six different ligands with unique roles activate EGFR1. These ligands include EGF, transforming growth factor-α (TGFα), amphiregulin, betacellulin, heparin-binding EGF, and epiregulin. Most recently mutations in the EGFR have been identified, in particular a ligand-independent mutant, EGFRvIII receptor, which has constitutive kinase activity in a large fraction of prostate cancers.[16]

The ErbB2/HER-2 (HER-2/neu) proto-oncogene encodes a 185-kDa transmembrane tyrosine kinase with a marked degree of identity with the EGFR. Despite this structural similarity, a ligand for HER-2 has, thus far, not yet been identified. In contrast to the other ErbB family members, HER-2 has a pair of inactive ligand-binding domains, which may account for the lack of defined ligands. Since the mid-1980s, many studies have shown

Table 38.1 Targeting of pathways involved in the regulation of tumor growth and survival

Pathway	Function	Therapy	Mechanism of action
Tumor growth and survival			
ErbB1	Prostate cancer mitosis	Cetuximab (ErbITUX, IMC-C225)	RA. Chimeric anti-EGFR mAb
			RA. Fully human anti-EGFR mAb
		ABX-EGF	RA/AA. Anti-EGFR mAb
		EMD72000	
ErbB2	Prostate cancer mitosis	Trastuzumab (Herceptin)	RA/CC/ADCC. Humanized mAb
		ErbB2 + GM-CSF	
		ErbB2 peptide +	T-cell vaccine
		Flt3 ligand	T-cell vaccine
TGFα1	Cell-cycle arrest & differentiation	*Anti-TGFα mAb	Cytokine inhibitor
		↓ immune functions	
Endoglin (CD105)	Endothelial TGFα receptor	*xenogenic CD105 vaccine	T-cell vaccine
Oncogenic phenotype			
TERT	Maintenance of telomere length	TERT mRNA-transfected DC	T-cell vaccine
		TERT peptide-loaded DC	T-cell vaccine
MUC1 (CD227)	Mucin modulating signal transduction	rVaccinia-MUC1 + IL2	T-cell vaccine
Gangliosides GM1b, GM2, GM3, GD1a, GD2	↑ cell growth—synergize with ErbB pathway ↓ immune functions		
Survivin	↓ apoptosis	*Survivin mRNA loaded DC	T-cell vaccine
Stromal/epithelial interactions			
VEGFR2	Endothelial cell mitosis, differentiation, migration & vessel stability	Endostatin	Endogenous angiogenesis inhibitor
		Bevacizumab (anti-VEGF mAb)	Cytokine inhibitor
	↑ capillary permeability & metastasis	Thalidomide	ΛΛ/T-cell stimulatory
MMP	Dissolution of interceding cellular matrix	*xenogenic MMP2	T-cell vaccine
	↑ invasion & metastasis		
ET-1	↑ mitosis, apoptosis, vasoconstricton	Atrasentan (ABT-627)	RA
	Tissue remodeling— ↑ MMP, ↓ TIMP		
TGFβ	Pro-angiogenic, ↑ VEGF, ↑ FGF-2	*LAP (TGFβ latency-associated peptide)	Cytokine-inhibitor
	Recruits stromal cells to form pericytes		
Antigen-processing			
HSP	Molecular chaperone for antigenic peptides	Oncophage (HSPPC96)	T-cell vaccine

*Preclinical stage only.

AA, antiangiogenic; ADCC, antibody-dependent cellular cytotoxicity; CC, cell cycle inhibition; DC, dendritic cell; ET-1, endothelin 1; FGF, fibroblast growth factor; HSP, heat-shock protein; IL2, interleukin-2; mAb, monoclonal antibody; MMP, matrix metalloproteinase; RA, receptor antagonist; TIMP, tissue inhibitor of matrix metalloproteinase; VEGF, vascular endothelial growth factor.

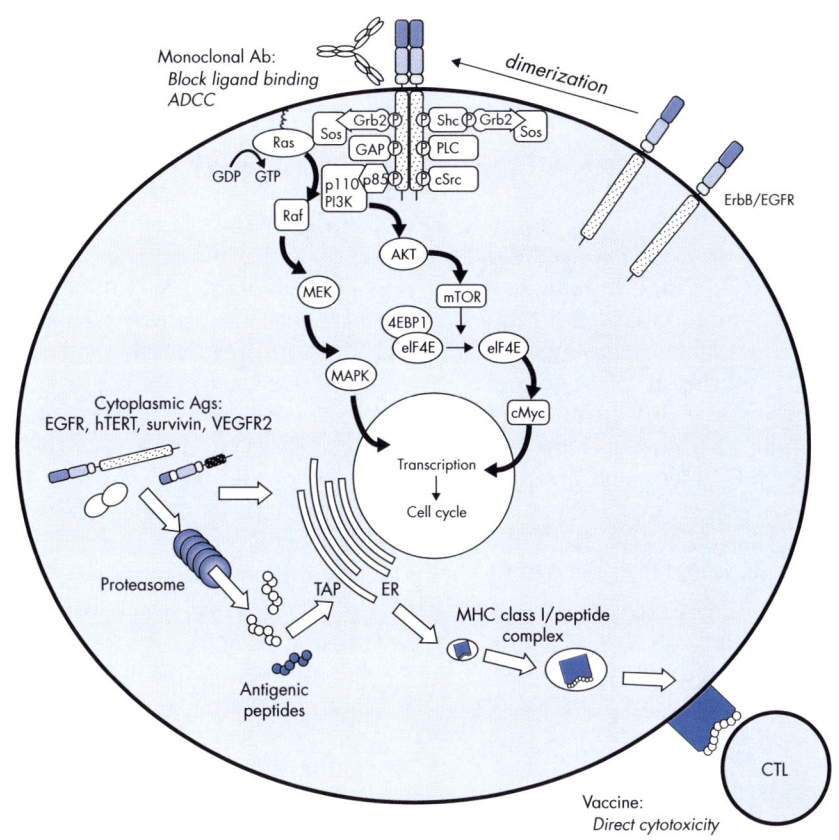

Fig. 38.1

Diagram depicting the signaling pathway of the epidermal growth factor receptor family (EGFR/ErbB1). Following receptor dimerization, a series of tyrosine-kinase mediated phosphorylation events leads to the recruitment of signaling components of the mitogen-activated protein kinase (MAPK) or the cMyc pathway. Triggering of these signals results in the assembly and gene transcription of factors controlling cell-cycle progression, proliferation, differentiation and apoptosis. In prostate cancer cells, pathways such as the EGFR signaling pathway play a key role in tumor growth and progression. Cell-surface EGFR serves as a target for monoclonal antibody (Ab) therapies (e.g., trastuzumab) that interfere with ligand binding and also trigger antibody-dependent cellular cytotoxicity (ADCC). Also shown is the antigen-processing pathway for cytosolic antigens including EGFR, human telomerase (hTERT), survivin, and vascular endothelial growth factor receptor 2 (VEGFR2). The principal proteolytic machinery allowing processing of cytosolic proteins is the proteasome, yielding antigenic peptides. Such peptides are then transported to the endoplasmic reticulum (ER) by TAP1 and TAP2 transporter molecules. After assembly with MHC class I molecules, peptide/MHC complexes are exported for display on the cell surface. Here, they can be targeted by cytotoxic T lymphocytes (CTL). When CTL recognize their specific targets on prostate cancer cells they induce cell death by a variety of means including release of perforin, granzyme B, and triggering apoptosis via the CD95/CD95L pathway. Considerable efforts are currently ongoing to identify novel antigenic proteins or glycoproteins present on prostate cancer cells or on stromal cells, such as blood vessels and tumor fibroblasts.

that HER-2/neu is a marker of poor prognosis, shorter overall survival, and biologic aggressiveness in breast cancer and in several other epithelial-origin carcinomas. Human HER-2 is overexpressed in approximately 63% of primary breast cancers and in 40% to 60% of metastatic prostate cancers, dependent on the clinical stage of the disease.[15] High levels of HER-2 receptors have been shown to promote spontaneous dimerization or transactivation by EGF-like ligands, resulting in the formation of EGFR/HER-2 heterodimers that trigger receptor activation and signaling, in part due to enhanced ligand affinity and decelerated dissociation. However, unlike in breast cancer, the usefulness of tar-

geting HER-2/neu in prostate cancer has been widely debated, since its expression in prostate cancer tissues is usually weak in intensity and focal in distribution. However, it is important to note that the activating mechanisms of HER-2 in prostate cancer are quite distinct from those identified in breast carcinomas. Most studies reported to date support the notion that HER-2 gene amplification occurs only infrequently in prostate cancer,[17] while HER-2 protein appears to be overexpressed, even in the absence of gene amplification, in a fraction of early-stage prostate cancers.[18,19] Therefore, the activation-state of HER-2 may play a more significant role than the absolute number of receptors that can be identified in target tissues. Other components involved in the Erb expression pathway can also be dysregulated in prostate cancer. For example EGFR1 and TGFα ligands are coexpressed, most pronounced in androgen independent prostate cancers,[19] suggesting the presence of an autocrine stimulation circuit in the majority of metastatic androgen-independent tumors.

Promising new cancer treatments include monoclonal antibodies directed against the extracellular domain of EGFR and/or HER-2. Fully humanized, EGFR-specific antibodies, including cetuximab, ABX-EGF, and EMD72000 are now available and are undergoing clinical investigation in metastatic prostate and other malignancies. Trastuzumab, the first monoclonal antibody to be approved by the FDA for the treatment of a solid tumor, targets the HER-2/neu gene product. Studies have shown that a major mechanism of trastuzumab-induced cell-cycle arrest results from the activation of the cyclin-dependent kinase (CDK) inhibitor p27(KIP1).[20] Alternatively, several studies have suggested that antibody-dependent cellular cytotoxicity (ADCC) is an important mechanism by which cellular killing can be induced even in the absence of HER-2/neu downmodulation.[21] In prostate cancer, expression of p27(KIP1) inversely correlates with tumor grade, suggesting potential mechanisms of resistance. However p27(KIP1) expression can be stimulated by vitamin D_3, the receptor of which is expressed in prostate cancer.[22] Therefore, it may be possible to modulate trastuzumab resistance by supplementing diet with $1\alpha,25$-dihydroxyvitamin D_3.

An alternative immune-based approach allowing the specific targeting of HER-2-expressing prostate cancer bone lesions was recently introduced by using redirected effector lymphocytes.[23] In this experimental study, adoptive transfer of engineered lymphocytes bearing ErbB2-specific chimeric receptors resulted in decreased tumor growth, reduced PSA secretion, and extended survival of tumor-bearing mice. Studies are currently ongoing to translate these experiences into more clinically relevant settings.

In summary, expanding knowledge of Erb-mediated signaling pathways suggests that dysregulation of these circuits play a critical role in prostate cancer progression and that strategies aimed at blocking this growth factor pathway may be of therapeutic importance, particularly in the setting of hormone-refractory disease.

OTHER PROTEIN TYROSINE KINASE RECEPTOR-MEDIATED PATHWAYS

Although considerable efforts have been devoted to the exploitation of aberrant Erb signaling pathways, other tyrosine kinases and their corresponding receptors may also represent appealing targets for intervention because of their more consistent overexpression and activation in prostate cancer tissues. Much interest has recently focused on one particular tyrosine kinase, termed EphA2, which physiologically appears to be a key regulator of many aspects of adult epithelial cell behavior.[24] Moreover, the Eph kinases appear to play crucial roles in vascular development and tumor formation. Several studies have shown that EphA2 is overexpressed or dysregulated in high-grade prostate intraepithelial neoplasia (PIN) and prostate neoplasms, consistent with its role as a powerful oncogene conferring malignant transformation and tumorigenic potential when overexpressed.[25] Several features render EphA2 a promising candidate target for mAb-based or T cell-based prostate cancer therapy. First, its transmembrane receptor is found at very high levels on malignant cells, but not on surrounding epithelium. Secondly, despite its overexpression, EphA2 fails to bind to its cognate ligand, termed ephrin A1, in malignant cells. Unlike with other receptor tyrosine kinases, ligand binding is not necessary to trigger EphA2 enzymatic activity in malignant disease. These receptor ligand interactions, however, are essential to downregulate tumor cell growth and proliferation. Therefore, any mAb or molecule designed to mimic actions of ephrin A1 may have the potential to reverse metastatic behavior by activating high levels of EphA2 on the tumor cell surface. This concept has been investigated in several experimental studies using either agonistic antibodies,[26] or EphA2 peptide-pulsed dendritic cell (DC) vaccines,[27] demonstrating inhibition of malignant cell behavior or inducing potent antitumor immunity against EphA2-expressing murine tumors. Upon further preclinical validation, it is reasonable to expect the initiation of human trials in prostate cancer and other EphA2 overexpressing malignancies.

TRANSFORMING GROWTH FACTOR-BETA PATHWAY

Transforming growth factor-β, a pleiotropic cytokine, is recognized as a key regulator of cell proliferation and differentiation, angiogenesis, and immune function in many cancer types. In nonmalignant prostate tissues, TGFβ provides inhibitory signals to epithelial cells by counterbalancing the mitogenic effects of various growth factors. Conversely, in malignancy components of the TGFβ signaling pathway are dysregulated, thereby rendering cancer cells insusceptible to the inhibitory effects of TGFβ. In an attempt to compensate for the loss of sensitivity to TGFβ, prostate cancers and surrounding stromal cells increase TGFβ production establishing a positive feedback circuit. The overexpression of TGFβ alters the host–tumor interactions that facilitate tumor progression, stimulate metastasis and angiogenesis, and induce profound immune suppression. It also has been shown that TGFβ modulates extracellular matrix metalloproteinase production and can stimulate adhesion of prostate cancer cells to bone cells, suggesting a potential involvement in the promotion of metastatic disease. Accordingly, loss of TGFβ receptor expression has been shown to represent a negative prognostic marker for prostate cancer patients,[28] and for subjects with other epithelial malignancies.[29]

Recent research has further demonstrated that tumor-derived TGFβ exerts profound immunosuppressive activity in cancer patients. Although the exact mechanisms by which TGFβ inhibits immune function are not fully understood, it appears that it mediates stimulation of immunoregulatory T cells and directly impairs the function and migration of antigen-presenting cells in the tumor-bearing host.[30,31] Therefore, any reagent that interferes with TGFβ signaling may not only impact on tumor progression, but also may reverse tumor-mediated immunosuppression in the cancer patient. Several studies have shown that TGFβ-neutralizing mAbs are capable of inhibiting the growth of tumors in mice,[31] and of correcting dendritic cell defects in patients with multiple myeloma.[32] Transforming growth factor-β signaling has also been shown to promote neo-angiogenesis in growing tumors. Particularly, CD105/endoglin, a vascular-specific TGFβ receptor, is markedly upregulated, but not mutated, in prostate cancer-induced blood vessels[33] and may, therefore, serve as an attractive target for immune-based strategies. Accordingly, a recent study demonstrated that it is possible to break tolerance against this self-antigen by vaccinating against epitopes expressed by xenogeneic CD105.[34] In this study, significant antitumor activity was induced by inhibition of angiogenesis in tumor tissues, while no apparent toxicity, including autoimmunity, was identified in immunized mice.

In summary, a number of strategies are currently being developed aiming to disrupt TGFβ signaling pathways in human prostate cancer and other malignancies. However, unlike strategies targeting Erb receptors, the exploration of TGFβ-targeting strategies remains, at this point, in an early stage of development.

TARGETING MOLECULES ESSENTIAL TO MAINTAIN THE ONCOGENIC PHENOTYPE

The recent identification of tumor antigens that are broadly expressed among many tumors has provided new opportunities for the development of effective immune-based cancer strategies. Antigenic targets such as human telomerase reverse transcriptase (TERT),[35] survivin,[36] or oncofetal antigen (immature laminin receptor)[37] are commonly overexpressed in many malignancies including prostate cancers and are, therefore, being investigated as potential therapeutic targets. Since these molecules are essential to facilitate tumor cell survival or for maintaining the oncogenic

phenotype, targeting of these molecules would make it more difficult for tumors to evade immune recognition by downregulating antigen expression.

TELOMERASE REVERSE TRANSCRIPTASE

Telomerase is a ribonucleoprotein in which the catalytic reverse transcriptase protein subunit uses its RNA as a template for the addition of telomeric repeat sequences to the ends of chromosomes.[38] Most somatic tissues and primary cultured cells possess low-to-undetectable telomerase activity, leading to a steady decline in telomere length with continued cell proliferation *in vivo* or with passage in culture.[39] However, human telomerase activity is transiently expressed in proliferating tissues such as activated T and B cells, hematopoietic progenitors, germ cells, and cells within intestinal and liver tissue. Also, TERT is dramatically overexpressed or reactivated in more than 80% of human cancers, raising the expectation that TERT could function as a "universal" tumor antigen.[35] In normal prostate or in benign prostate hypertrophy tissues, TERT enzymatic activity was found to be absent, while primary prostate cancer exhibited high levels of TERT activity.[40] Moreover, a positive correlation between TERT enzymatic activity and Gleason score has been reported.[41]

Vaccination strategies using TERT peptide-loaded DC[42] or with TERT mRNA-transfected DC[43] have been recently investigated in two independent clinical trials, suggesting the safety and immunologic efficacy of immunization against TERT, and providing a rationale for targeting TERT in a metastatic prostate cancer setting. In both studies, no significant toxicity was observed and vaccine-mediated stimulation of TERT-reactive T cells was reported in the majority of the treated subjects. Subsequent clinical trials are currently ongoing to further improve the immunologic and clinical responses observed with this type of investigational treatment.

SURVIVIN

One important, AR-independent event driving the oncogenic process involves the dysregulation of apoptotic (programmed cell death) mechanisms. Prostate cancers resist apoptosis due to defects in apoptotic pathways, bypassing internal surveillance and acquiring an invasive phenotype.[36] Several pro- or antiapoptotic mechanisms have been identified that play important roles in the differentiation to androgen-refractory disease. Protagonists of an expanding family of genes that regulate apoptosis comprise the tumor suppressor genes p53 and PTEN (phosphatase and tensin homolog),[44] and the antiapoptotic gene Bcl-2.[45] Interest has recently focused on survivin, a novel member of the inhibitor of apoptosis (IAP) gene family that counteracts cell death and controls mitotic progression.[46] Survivin is overexpressed in about 80% of prostate tumors and overexpression correlated positively with lymph-node positive disease, vascular invasion, and high Gleason grade.[47,48] Similar to TERT, downregulation of survivin inhibited tumor growth and metastatic progression in in-vitro and in-vivo models. Survivin is essential for ensuring normal cell division in the G2/M phase of the cell cycle. It is highly expressed in a cell cycle-regulated manner and localizes together with caspase 3 on microtubules within centrosomes.[49] Several studies have shown that inhibition of survivin function results both in a failure of cell division and induction of cell death.[49,50]

Several studies have now shown that targeting survivin by active immunization with HLA-A201-restricted peptides or survivin mRNA-loaded DC[51] is capable of protecting mice against tumor challenges and stimulating potent cytotoxic T lymphocyte (CTL) responses from the Peripheral Blood Mononuclear Cells (PBMC) of cancer patients. Although there have been no reports on the clinical utility of survivin in prostate cancer patients, a clinical phase I study using a survivin-derived peptide vaccine has demonstrated immunologic and objective clinical responses in patients with advanced colorectal carcinoma.[52]

TARGETS MISREGULATED DURING ONCOGENESIS

Epithelial mucins are cell-surface glycoproteins that line and protect the epithelial and glandular cell surfaces, where they are involved in cell–cell interactions and signaling.[53] Several human mucins (MUC1 to MUC8) have been identified, at least one of which (MUC1) is overexpressed and shows aberrant cell-surface expression on prostate cancer epithelial cells. MUC1 consists of a large, highly glycosylated core region that is comprised of 30 to 100 tandem repeats and a 20-amino acid sequence, all of which have been linked to the activity of the molecule. The protein is cleaved in the endoplasmic reticulum and the amino and carboxyl groups form a heterodimer on the cell surface. Oligosaccharides make up about 50% to 90% of mucin molecules. In the prostate, MUC1 is normally expressed on apical cell surfaces. When overexpressed or hyperglycosylated in tumor cells, the protein loses its polarized distribution. Altered expression disrupts the protein's physiologic role in cell signaling and cell adhesion and also exacts immunosuppressive properties. Hyperglycosylation of MUC1 changes the protein conformation to expose the tandem repeats on the cell surface. Studies have shown that this region can trigger both cytotoxic and humoral immune responses. Several studies have shown that MUC1 peptides can be processed and presented in con-

junction with MHC to the immune system for recognition, highlighting the potential relevance of MUC antigens in the development of immunotherapeutics.[54]

Active immunization with cell surface-based carbohydrate tumor antigens is also being explored as a possible therapeutic modality for prostate cancer, since the appearance of unusual, glycolipid- or glycoprotein-derived oligosaccharide motifs on the cell surface has been shown to correlate with more advanced cancer or hormone-refractory disease. A number of carbohydrate-based cancer vaccines that target the gangliosides GM2, GD2, GD3, and FucM1,[55] mucin-core structures such as TF, Tn, and S-Tn,[56] and blood group-related antigens, including globoH and LeY,[57] have been investigated in prostate cancer clinical trials. While measurable antibody responses were achieved, clinical efficacy remains to be demonstrated. Newer strategies seek to enhance the immunogenicity of glycoprotein or carbohydrate vaccines by conjugation with keyhole limpet hemocyanin (KLH) and by coadministration of classic immunological adjuvants such as the saponin derivatives QS-21 or GP-0100.[58]

TARGETING THE TUMOR STROMA

The well-documented genetic instability of tumor cells is responsible for their propensity to evade the immune system via a host of genetic and epigenetic mechanisms. Emergence of treatment-resistant variants will manifest itself in the face of increasingly effective therapeutic protocols, and, not unlike what is seen with chemotherapy, could defeat much of the promise of emerging therapeutics targeting defined TAAs. Immunologic targeting of the tumor stroma could significantly reduce the ability of tumor to evade immune destruction.[59] Tumor progression is critically dependent on the adjacent stroma consisting of blood vessels, smooth muscle cells, fibroblasts, and other cell types, collectively referred to as "tumor stroma." Immunizing against stromal products that are preferentially, though not necessarily exclusively, expressed by the tumor stroma could also impact on tumor growth, either by affecting stromal functions essential for tumor growth and/or by collateral damage caused by a local inflammatory reaction. For example, stimulating immune responses against angiogenesis-associated products expressed in the tumor vasculature could interfere with the vascularization process and inhibit tumor growth. Since stromal cells, unlike tumor cells, are diploid, genetically stable, and exhibit limited proliferative capacity, targeting the stroma could substantially reduce the incidence of immune evasion. Therefore, targeting of genetically stable stromal components or disrupting or stromal-epithelial interactions may offer new opportunities to impact on tumor progression.

ANTIANGIOGENIC STRATEGIES FOR PROSTATE CANCER

As prostate cancer growth and progression depends on vascular supply, angiogenic products are currently being explored to serve as targets for anticancer therapy. Microvessels supplying tumors are strikingly different than vessels elsewhere in the body by undergoing constant remodeling driven by tumor-secreted VEGF, angiopoietins and ephrin family members.[60] Recent studies have shown that the tumor stroma offers a broad range of potential molecular therapeutic targets. Vascular epithelial growth factor and its receptor VEGFR2, basic fibroblast growth factor (bFGF), and the angiotensin receptor Tie2 are among the molecules that have been targeted by monoclonal antibodies, small-molecule-based inhibitors, or vaccine-based strategies eliciting T-cell responses. Moreover, genes encoding highly specific targets for tumor endothelium have been identified. These include the tumor endothelial markers (TEM1, TEM5, and TEM8), which are abundantly expressed on tumor endothelium but absent from normal adult vessels[61] and the Robo4 gene, which is expressed during development.[62] Several studies have examined the antitumor efficacy mediated by immunization with paraformaldehyde-fixed xenogeneic endothelial cells,[63] xenogeneic CD105/endoglin,[34] VEGFR2 protein-loaded DC,[64] VEGFR2 cDNA-encoding salmonella-based vectors,[65] or DC transfected with VEGFR2, Tie2, or VEGF mRNA.[66] In all studies, tumor growth was significantly inhibited without induction of significant autoimmune pathology.

Recent studies have identified the critical role of the endothelin (ET) axis—including the vascular peptides ET-1, ET-2, ET-3 and the ET cell surface receptors ETA and ETB—in promoting mitogenesis, invasion, escape from programmed cell death, new vessel formation, abnormal osteogenesis, and the alteration of nociceptive stimuli.[67] Data suggest that ET-1/ETA signaling promotes the growth and progression of many tumors including prostate, breast, brain, melanoma, and bony metastases. In prostate cancer, ET-1 concentrations produced by epithelial cells are significantly elevated due to defective ET-1 clearance. Increasing ETA expression is also seen with advancing grade and stage. Multiple pathways exists by which the ET-1/ETA axis may promote prostate cancer progression.[68] In prostate cancer cell lines, ET-1 acts synergistically with other peptide growth factors as a mitogen, thereby modulating apoptosis and cell survival. Selective antagonists such as atrasentan have been shown to block the proliferative effects of exogenous ET-1 in both prostate cancer cells and osteoblasts.[69] Moreover, clinical studies suggested the role of atrasentan as a therapeutic target in patients with hormone-refractory prostate cancer. In a randomized phase II study enrolling 288 subjects with metastatic prostate cancer, atrasentan exhibited favorable toxicity profiles and significantly delayed time to clinical and biochemical tumor progression.[70] Comprehensive searches are underway to identify other, more effective or complementary means to target the endothelin axis in prostate and other malignancies.

TARGETING TUMOR-RESIDENT FIBROBLASTS

Fibroblasts represent a major component of the tumor stroma and the extracellular matrix. Matrix metalloproteinases (MMPs) or fibroblast activation protein-α (FAPα) are fibroblast-derived gene products involved in stromal–epithelial interactions, tumor invasion, metastasis, and the promotion of neo-angiogenesis.[71] Support for the concept of immunologically targeting fibroblast-derived factors was provided by a study in which a vaccine based on chicken MMP2 as a model antigen induced both protective and therapeutic antitumor immunity in tumor-bearing mice. In this study, angiogenesis was effectively inhibited within the tumor following vaccine treatment.[72]

Fibroblast activation protein-α, a serine protease expressed by activated fibroblasts, received recently increased attention as a potential antitumor target. Human FAPα is selectively expressed by fibroblasts surrounding epithelial carcinomas, but not by tumor epithelial cells, normal fibroblasts, or other normal tissues. It has been argued that FAPα exemplifies a pathway by which the tumor microenvironment is "conditioned" to provide a fertile "soil" for tumor invasion and metastasis.[60] Fibroblast activation protein-α has been shown to have both in-vitro dipeptidyl peptidase and collagenase activity, but its biologic function in the tumor microenvironment remains largely unknown. In one study, overexpression of murine FAPα in transfected cell lines was capable of promoting tumor growth in experimental animals.[73] Furthermore, animals immunized with recombinant FAPα developed polyclonal anti-FAPα antibodies that significantly inhibited FAPα enzymatic activity in vitro, and attenuated tumor growth in vivo. Recently, radiolabeled humanized mAbs directed against FAPα have been clinically tested, however, questions regarding the clinical efficacy of this strategy is yet to be determined in upcoming clinical trials.[74]

REGULATION OF ANTIGEN PROCESSING PATHWAYS

Antigens expressed by tumor cells must be processed in order to be recognized by activated T cells. Key regulators involved in this process are the heat shock proteins (HSPs), which aid in protein folding and protein trafficking between cellular compartments. During natural protein degradation, HSPs chaperone peptide antigens via the endoplasmatic reticulum (gp96 and calreticulin) or the cytoplasm (via HSP70, HSP90, and HSP110) as part of the normal antigen presentation pathway.[75] Heat shock proteins themselves are not immunogenic, but they activate an immune response to peptide antigens through binding toll-like receptors and the endocytic receptor protein CD91[76] expressed by DC and macrophages.

These complexes are efficiently taken up by DC via specific receptors such as CD91 and processed for antigen presentation. This presentation triggers an immune response to the antigenic peptide and activates maturation of the DC with subsequent release of pro-inflammatory cytokines and upregulation of co-stimulatory molecules. Active immunotherapy using autologous tumor-derived HSP/peptide complexes has been a major focus of investigation over the past years.[77] Studies have shown that tumor tissue is enriched with HSP/antigenic peptide complexes, which can be isolated, purified, and administered to patients. In clinical settings, HSPs have to be isolated from the patient's tumor, resulting in the generation of patient-specific, customized vaccines. However, and in direct relevance to the development of prostate cancer vaccines, allogeneic cell lines are also currently being explored as a source for HSP isolation. At present, HSPPC-96 (Oncophage) is in phase III development, enrolling subjects with metastatic renal cell carcinoma accessible by surgical resection.

Aside from their involvement in antigen presentation, HSPs have also shown to play a significant role in promoting prostate cancer progression and the development of hormone-refractory disease. Prior to ligand binding, the AR is complexed with HSP90 and other co-chaperones. AR-HSP90 interaction maintains AR in a high-affinity ligand-binding conformation that is required for efficient response to androgens. 17-Allylamino-17-demethoxygeldanamycin (17-AAG) is an inhibitor of the HSP90 chaperone protein. Inhibition of HSP90 function results in the proteasomal degradation of proteins that require this chaperone for maturation or stability. Clients of HSP90 include several proteins of potential importance in mediating prostate cancer progression, including wild-type and mutated AR, HER-2, and Akt.[78] In murine models of prostate cancer, 17-AAG causes the degradation of these client proteins at nontoxic doses and inhibits the growth of hormone-naive and castration-resistant tumors.[79] Cumulatively, these data suggest that inhibitors of HSP90 may represent a novel strategy for the treatment of patients with prostate cancer and clinical trials to test this hypothesis are currently ongoing.

CONCLUSIONS

Metastatic prostate remains a major health problem with marked impact upon our society. Continued need for clinically effective and less toxic therapies has prompted the development of novel antibody drugs or vaccine-based strategies targeting molecules or disrupting signaling circuits with critical roles in oncogenesis. Clinical responses to these therapies are predicated by the requirements that tumors appropriately express and present the antigenic target for immune recognition and that tumor cells depend on its function. However, the redundancy of many signaling pathways and the ability of tumors to use alternative mechanisms to maintain the oncogenic phenotype represent major obstacles for the successful development of targeted immunotherapies. One approach to overcome this obstacle is to inhibit either multiple stations along a given pathway or to concomitantly target multiple individual pathways. Clearly, successful cancer therapy will require a combination approach that includes multiple therapeutic steps and combinations.[80] Regarding the development of more effective cancer vaccines, mAb-mediated CTLA-4 blockade,[81] elimination of immunosuppressive regulatory T cells,[82] provision of potent co-stimulatory signals,[83] or silencing genes with immunosuppressive roles through small inhibitory RNA (siRNA)[84] or aptamer technologies[85] have been shown to improve the effectiveness of cancer immunotherapy in preclinical settings. Finally, conventional approaches such as radiation therapy or chemotherapy appear to have synergistic effects in context with passive and active immunotherapy by either potentiating mAb-mediated inhibition or by rendering tumor cells more susceptible to CTL lysis.[86] Without question, successful development of more effective prostate cancer therapies will rely on a thorough understanding of the molecular events modulating the oncogenic process and will require cooperative efforts that facilitate continued clinical translation.

REFERENCES

1. Ries LAG, Eisner MP, Kosary CL. SEER Cancer Statistics Review. Bethesda, MD: National Cancer Institute, 2002.

2. Petrylak DP, Tangen CM, Hussain MH, et al. Docetaxel and estramustine compared with mitoxantrone and prednisone for advanced refractory prostate cancer. N Engl J Med 2004;351:1513–1520.

3. Toi M, Takada M, Bando H, et al. Current status of antibody therapy for breast cancer. Breast Cancer 2004;11:10–14.

4. Vieweg J, Dannull J. Future Perspective: Immunotherapy and Vaccines in Prostate Cancer. In: Cummings KB (ed): Prostate Cancer. New York: Elsevier Science, 2004, pp 367–392.

5. Vieweg J, Dannull J. Technology insight: vaccine therapy for prostate cancer. Nat Clin Pract Urol 2005;2:1–8.

6. Karan D, Lin MF, Johansson SL, et al. Current status of the molecular genetics of human prostatic adenocarcinomas. Int J Cancer 2003;103:285–293.

7. Sanda MG, Restifo NP, Walsh JC, et al. Molecular characterization of defective antigen processing human prostate cancer. Nat Cancer Inst 1995;87:280–285.

8. Seliger B, Hohne A, Knuth A, et al. Analysis of the major histocompatibility complex class I antigen presentation machinery in normal and malignant renal cells: evidence for deficiencies associated with transformation and progression. Cancer Res 1996;56:1756–1760.

9. Linja MJ, Savinainen KJ, Saramaki OR, et al. Amplification and overexpression of androgen receptor gene in hormone-refractory prostate cancer. Cancer Res 2001;61:3550–3555.

10. Culig Z, Hoffmann J, Erdel M, et al. Switch from antagonist to agonist of the androgen receptor bicalutamide is associated with prostate tumour progression in a new model system. Br J Cancer 1999;81:242–251.

11. Ward CW, Garrett TP. Structural relationships between the insulin receptor and epidermal growth factor receptor families and other proteins. Curr Opin Drug Discov Devel 2004;7:630–638.

12. Xian CJ, Zhou XF. EGF family of growth factors: essential roles and functional redundancy in the nerve system. Front Biosci 2004;9:85–92.

13. Cunningham D, Humblet Y, Siena S, et al. Cetuximab monotherapy and cetuximab plus irinotecan in irinotecan-refractory metastatic colorectal cancer. N Engl J Med 2004;351:337–345.

14. Russell PJ, Bennett S, Stricker P. Growth factor involvement in progression of prostate cancer. Clin Chem 1998;44:705–723.

15. Di Lorenzo G, Tortora G, D'Armiento FP, et al. Expression of epidermal growth factor receptor correlates with disease relapse and progression to androgen-independence in human prostate cancer. Clin Cancer Res 2002;8:3438–3444.

16. Olapade-Olaopa EO, Moscatello DK, MacKay EH, et al. Evidence for the differential expression of a variant EGF receptor protein in human prostate cancer. Br J Cancer 2000;82:186–194.

17. Bubendorf L, Kononen J, Koivisto P, et al. Survey of gene amplifications during prostate cancer progression by high-throughout fluorescence in situ hybridization on tissue microarrays. Cancer Res 1999;59:803–806.

18. Arai Y, Yoshiki T, Yoshida O. c-erbB-2 oncoprotein: a potential biomarker of advanced prostate cancer. Prostate 1997;30:195–201.

19. Scher HI, Sarkis A, Reuter V, et al. Changing pattern of expression of the epidermal growth factor receptor and transforming growth factor alpha in the progression of prostatic neoplasms. Clin Cancer Res 1995;1:545–550.

20. Le XF, Claret FX, Lammayot A, et al. The role of cyclin-dependent kinase inhibitor p27Kip1 in anti-HER2 antibody-induced G1 cell cycle arrest and tumor growth inhibition. J Biol Chem 2003;278:23441–23450.

21. Gennari R, Menard S, Fagnoni F, et al. Pilot study of the mechanism of action of preoperative trastuzumab in patients with primary operable breast tumors overexpressing HER2. Clin Cancer Res 2004;10:5650–5655.

22. Huang YC, Chen JY, Hung WC. Vitamin D3 receptor/Sp1 complex is required for the induction of p27Kip1 expression by vitamin D3. Oncogene 2004;23:4856–4861.

23. Pinthus JH, Waks T, Malina V, et al. Adoptive immunotherapy of prostate cancer bone lesions using redirected effector lymphocytes. J Clin Invest 2004;114:1774–1781.

24. Walker-Daniels J, Coffman K, Azimi M, et al. Overexpression of the EphA2 tyrosine kinase in prostate cancer. Prostate 1999;41:275–280.

25. Zeng G, Hu Z, Kinch MS, et al. High-level expression of EphA2 receptor tyrosine kinase in prostatic intraepithelial neoplasia. Am J Pathol 2003;163:2271–2276.

26. Carles-Kinch K, Kilpatrick KE, Stewart JC, et al. Antibody targeting of the EphA2 tyrosine kinase inhibits malignant cell behavior. Cancer Res 2002;62:2840–2847.

27. Hatano M, Kuwashima N, Tatsumi T, et al. Vaccination with EphA2-derived T cell-epitopes promotes immunity against both EphA2-expressing and EphA2-negative tumors. J Transl Med 2004;2:40.

28. Kim IY, Ahn HJ, Lang S, et al. Loss of expression of transforming growth factor-beta receptors is associated with poor prognosis in prostate cancer patients. Clin Cancer Res 1998;4:1625–1630.

29. Bennett WP, el-Deiry WS, Rush WL, et al. p21waf1/cip1 and transforming growth factor beta 1 protein expression correlate with survival in non-small cell lung cancer. Clin Cancer Res 1998;4:1499–1506.

30. Nakamura K, Kitani A, Strober W. Cell contact-dependent immunosuppression by CD4+25+ regulatory T cells is mediated by cell surface-bound transforming growth factor beta. J Exp Med 2001;194:629–644.

31. Kobie JJ, Wu RS, Kurt RA, et al. Transforming growth factor beta inhibits the antigen-presenting functions and antitumor activity of dendritic cell vaccines. Cancer Res 2003;63:1860–1864.

32. Brown R, Murray A, Pope B, et al. Either interleukin-12 or interferon-gamma can correct the dendritic cell defect induced by transforming growth factor beta in patients with myeloma. Br J Haematol 2004;125:743–748.

33. Wikstrom P, Lissbrant IF, Stattin P, et al. Endoglin (CD105) is expressed on immature blood vessels and is a marker for survival in prostate cancer. Prostate 2002;51:268–275.

34. Tan GH, Wei YQ, Tian L, et al. Active immunotherapy of tumors with a recombinant xenogeneic endoglin as a model antigen. Eur J Immunol 2004;34:2012–2021.

35. Shay JW, Bacchetti S. A survey of telomerase activity in human cancer. Eur J Cancer 1997;33:787–791

36. Li F. Survivin study: what is the next wave? J Cell Physiol 2003;197:8–29.

37. Coggin JH Jr, Barsoum AL, Rohrer JW. Tumors express both unique TSTA and crossprotective 44 kDa oncofetal antigen. Immunol Today 1998;19:405–408.

38. Blackburn EH. Structure and function of telomeres. Nature 1991;350:569–573.

39. Hodes RJ. Telomere length, aging, and somatic cell turnover. J Exp Med 1999;190:153–156.

40. Sommerfeld HJ, Meeker AK, Piatyszek MA, et al. Telomerase activity: a prevalent marker of malignant human prostate tissue. Cancer Res 1996;56:218–222.

41. Kamradt J, Drosse C, Kalkbrenner S, et al. Telomerase activity and telomerase subunit gene expression levels are not related in prostate cancer: a real-time quantification and in situ hybridization study. Lab Invest 2003;83:623–633.

42. Vonderheide RH, Domchek SM, Schultze JL, et al. Vaccination of cancer patients against telomerase induces functional antitumor CD8+ T lymphocytes. Clin Cancer Res 2004;10:828–839.

43. Dannull J, Su Z, Boczkowski D, et al. Enhanced antigen presenting function of terminally matured dendritic cells after co-transfection with OX40 Ligand mRNA. Blood 2005; 105: 3206–3213.

44. Debes JD, Tindall DJ. Mechanisms of androgen-refractory prostate cancer. N Engl J Med 2004;351:1488–1490.

45. Zellweger T, Ninck C, Bloch M, et al. Expression patterns of potential therapeutic targets in prostate cancer. Int J Cancer 2005;113:619–628.

46. Andersen MH, Thor SP. Survivin—a universal tumor antigen. Histol Histopathol 2002;17:669–675.

47. Shariat SF, Lotan Y, Saboorian H, et al. Survivin expression is associated with features of biologically aggressive prostate carcinoma. Cancer 2004;100:751–757.

48. Kishi H, Igawa M, Kikuno N, et al. Expression of the survivin gene in prostate cancer: correlation with clinicopathological characteristics, proliferative activity and apoptosis. J Urol 2004;171:1855–1860.

49. Shin S, Sung BJ, Cho YS, et al. An anti-apoptotic protein human survivin is a direct inhibitor of caspase-3 and -7. Biochemistry 2001;40:1117–1123.

50. Reed JC, Reed SI. Survivin' cell-separation anxiety. Nature Cell Biology 1999;1:E199–E200.

51. Zeis M, Siegel S, Wagner A, et al. Generation of cytotoxic responses in mice and human individuals against hematological malignancies using survivin-RNA-transfected dendritic cells. J Immunol 2003;170:5391–5397.

52. Tsuruma T, Hata F, Torigoe T, et al. Phase I clinical study of anti-apoptosis protein, survivin-derived peptide vaccine therapy for patients with advanced or recurrent colorectal cancer. J Transl Med 2004;2:19.

53. Parry S, Silverman HS, McDermott K, et al. Identification of MUC1 proteolytic cleavage sites in vivo. Biochem Biophys Res Commun 2001;283:715–720.

54. Agrawal B, Reddish MA, Longenecker BM. In vitro induction of MUC-1 peptide-specific type 1 T lymphocyte and cytotoxic T lymphocyte responses from healthy multiparous donors. J Immunol 1996;157:2089–2095.

55. Livingston PO, Natoli EJ, Calves MJ, et al. Vaccines containing purified GM2 ganglioside elicit GM2 antibodies in melanoma patients. Proc Natl Acad Sci USA 1987;84:2911–2915.

56. Ragupathi G, Howard L, Cappello S, et al. Vaccines prepared with sialyl-Tn and sialyl-Tn trimers using the 4-(4-maleimidomethyl)cyclohexane-1-carboxyl hydrazide linker group result in optimal antibody titers against ovine submaxillary mucin and sialyl-Tn-positive tumor cells. Cancer Immunol Immunother 1999;48:1–8.

57. Wang ZG, Williams LJ, Zhang XF, et al. Polyclonal antibodies from patients immunized with a globo H-keyhole limpet hemocyanin vaccine: isolation, quantification, and characterization of immune responses by using totally synthetic immobilized tumor antigens. Proc Natl Acad Sci USA 2000;97:2719–2724.

58. Slovin SF, Ragupathi G, Musselli C, et al. Fully synthetic carbohydrate-based vaccines in biochemically relapsed prostate cancer: clinical trial results with alpha-N-acetylgalactosamine-O-serine/threonine conjugate vaccine. J Clin Oncol 2003;21:4292–4298.

59. Cheng JD, Weiner LM. Tumors and their microenvironments: tilling the soil. Commentary re: Scott AM et al. A Phase I dose-escalation study of sibrotuzumab in patients with advanced or metastatic fibroblast activation protein-positive cancer. Clin Cancer Res 2003;9:1590–1595.

60. Yancopoulos GD, Davis S, Gale NW, et al. Vascular-specific growth factors and blood vessel formation. Nature 2000;407:242–248.

61. Carson-Walter EB, Watkins DN, Nanda A, et al. Cell surface tumor endothelial markers are conserved in mice and humans. Cancer Res 2001;61:6649–6655.

62. Bicknell R, Harris AL. Novel angiogenic signaling pathways and vascular targets. Annu Rev Pharmacol Toxicol 2004;44:219–238.

63. Wei YQ, Wang QR, Zhao X, et al. Immunotherapy of tumors with xenogeneic endothelial cells as a vaccine. Nat Med 2000;6:1160–1166.

64. Li Y, Wang MN, Li H, et al. Active immunization against the vascular endothelial growth factor receptor flk1 inhibits tumor angiogenesis and metastasis. J Exp Med 2002;195:1575–1584.

65. Niethammer AG, Xiang R, Becker JC, et al. A DNA vaccine against VEGF receptor 2 prevents effective angiogenesis and inhibits tumor growth. Nat Med 2002;8:1369–1375.

66. Nair S, Boczkowski D, Moeller B, et al. Synergy between tumor immunotherapy and antiangiogenic therapy. Blood 2003;102:964–971.

67. Nelson J, Bagnato A, Battistini B, et al. The endothelin axis: emerging role in cancer. Nat Rev Cancer 2003;3:110–116.

68. Nelson JB, Hedican SP, George DJ, et al. Identification of endothelin-1 in the pathophysiology of metastatic adenocarcinoma of the prostate. Nat Med 1995;1:944–949.

69. Jimeno A, Carducci M. Atrasentan: targeting the endothelin axis in prostate cancer. Expert Opin Investig Drugs 2004;13:1631–1640.

70. Carducci MA, Padley RJ, Breul J, et al. Effect of endothelin-A receptor blockade with atrasentan on tumor progression in men with hormone-refractory prostate cancer: a randomized, phase II, placebo-controlled trial. J Clin Oncol 2003;21:679–689.

71. Nelson WG, Simons JW, Mikhak B, et al. Cancer cells engineered to secrete granulocyte-macrophage colony-stimulating factor using ex vivo gene transfer as vaccines for the treatment of genitourinary malignancies. Cancer Chemother Pharmacol 2000;46:S67–72.

72. Su JM, Wei YQ, Tian L, et al. Active immunogene therapy of cancer with vaccine on the basis of chicken homologous matrix metalloproteinase-2. Cancer Res 2003;63:600–607.

73. Cheng JD, Dunbrack RL, Jr., Valianou M, et al. Promotion of tumor growth by murine fibroblast activation protein, a serine protease, in an animal model. Cancer Res 2002;62:4767–4772.

74. Scott AM, Wiseman G, Welt S, et al. A Phase I dose-escalation study of sibrotuzumab in patients with advanced or metastatic fibroblast activation protein-positive cancer. Clin Cancer Res 2003;9:1639–1647.

75. Srivastava PK. Peptide-binding heat shock proteins in the endoplasmic reticulum: role in immune response to cancer and in antigen presentation. Adv Cancer Res 1993;62:153–177.

76. Li Z, Dai J, Zheng H, et al. An integrated view of the roles and mechanisms of heat shock protein gp96-peptide complex in eliciting immune response. Front Biosci 2002;7:731–751.

77. Tamura Y, Peng P, Liu K, et al. Immunotherapy of tumors with autologous tumor-derived heat shock protein preparations. Science 1997;278:117–120.

78. Solit DB, Basso AD, Olshen AB, et al. Inhibition of heat shock protein 90 function down-regulates Akt kinase and sensitizes tumors to Taxol. Cancer Res 2003;63:2139–2144.

79. Solit DB, Zheng FF, Drobnjak M, et al. 17-Allylamino-17-demethoxygeldanamycin induces the degradation of androgen receptor and HER-2/neu and inhibits the growth of prostate cancer xenografts. Clin Cancer Res 2002;8:986–993.

80. Pardoll D, Allison J. Cancer immunotherapy: breaking the barriers to harvest the crop. Nat Med 2004;10:887–892.

81. Hurwitz AA, Foster BA, Kwon ED, et al. Combination immunotherapy of primary prostate cancer in a transgenic mouse model using CTLA-4 blockade. Cancer Res 2000;60:2444–2448.

82. Shevach EM, McHugh RS, Piccirillo CA, et al. Control of T-cell activation by CD4+ CD25+ suppressor T cells. Immunol Rev 2001;182:58–67.

83. Su Z, Dannull J, Yang B, et al. Telomerase mRNA transfected dendritic cells stimulate antigen-specific CD8+ and CD4+ T-cell responses in patients with metastatic prostate cancer. J Immunol 2005; 174: 3798–3807.

84. Laderach D, Compagno D, Danos O, et al. RNA interference shows critical requirement for NF-kappa B p50 in the production of IL-12 by human dendritic cells. J Immunol 2003;171:1750–1757.

85. Santulli-Marotto S, Nair SK, Rusconi C, et al. Multivalent RNA aptamers that inhibit CTLA-4 and enhance tumor immunity. Cancer Res 2003;63:7483–7489.

86. Chakraborty M, Abrams SI, Coleman CN, et al. External beam radiation of tumors alters phenotype of tumor cells to render them susceptible to vaccine-mediated T-cell killing. Cancer Res 2004;64:4328–4337.

Clinical diagnosis and staging of prostate cancer

SECTION 5

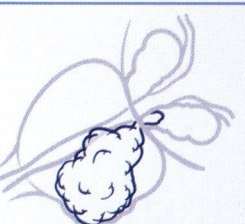

New concepts in the early detection of prostate cancer

39

Misop Han, William J Catalona

INTRODUCTION

The strategy for detecting prostate cancer has undergone drastic changes in the past two decades. Serum prostate-specific antigen (PSA) test has became widely available for screening of prostate cancer. Transrectal ultrasonography is now routinely used in guiding systemic prostate biopsies. Along with excellent surgical outcomes from an improved understanding of pelvic anatomy and modified surgical techniques,[1] early detection of prostate cancer has contributed to the improved outcomes of men with prostate cancer. In this chapter, we review a brief history of the current detection strategy for prostate cancer; then we review potential new markers for prostate cancer screening and detection. Finally, we discuss the rationale and results of early detection of prostate cancer.

PROSTATE SPECIFIC-ANTIGEN TESTING

HISTORY

Early detection of prostate cancer would not have been possible without PSA testing. Prostate-specific antigen is a serine protease that is produced by prostatic epithelium and periurethral glands. In seminal fluid, PSA plays a role in liquefaction of seminal coagulum.[2] Although it was initially discovered in the 1970s, early studies did not support the use of PSA testing for screening and early detection of prostate cancer.[3–5] Instead, they indicated that PSA was useful for monitoring patients with known prostate cancer.

Subsequently in 1986, the US Food and Drug Administration (FDA) approved PSA for monitoring early recurrence following surgery.[6] In 1987, Stamey et al described PSA elevations that occur with age, prostatitis, or benign prostatic hyperplasia (BPH), as well as with prostate cancer.[7] In 1990, Cooner et al reported that higher PSA levels were associated with the diagnosis of prostate cancer in a private urology practice-based screening program.[8] However, they performed prostate biopsies only for suspicious findings on digital rectal examination (DRE) or ultrasonography and not for elevated PSA levels alone.[8]

In 1991, Catalona et al reported in a community-based screening study that PSA could be used as a first-line screening test for prostate cancer and that PSA was more accurate in this regard than the DRE.[9] They also suggested that changes in PSA levels over time might be another means of detecting prostate cancer.[9] In 1991, Lilja, Stenman, and coworkers characterized the two forms of PSA, a free and complexed PSA, and showed a possible increase in specificity using free PSA.[10,11] In 1992, Carter et al reported that the rate of change of PSA ("PSA velocity") in archived serum samples was strongly associated with prostate cancer.[12] In the same year, Benson et al popularized the concept that the serum PSA divided by the prostate volume ("PSA density") was higher in men with cancer than those with BPH and recommended using PSA density measurements to select patients for biopsy,[13] and Oesterling proposed the use of age-specific PSA reference ranges for prompting biopsy.[14] In 1992, the American Cancer Society recommended PSA as a part of the annual physical examination, and, 2 years later, PSA was approved by the FDA as an aid to early prostate cancer detection.[15] In 1995, Moul et al reported upon race-specific PSA reference ranges for African-American men.[16] In the same year, Gann et al demonstrated that PSA levels in plasma samples were associated with the subsequent risk of developing prostate cancer in a study cohort that was not screened for prostate cancer.[17] In 1997, Catalona et al suggested lowering the PSA cutoff for recommending prostate biopsy to greater than 2.5 ng/mL, reporting a 22% positive biopsy rate in the 2.6 to 4.0 ng/mL PSA range.[18]

In 1995, in a retrospective study of archived serum samples, and in 1998 in a multi-institutional prospective screening study, Catalona et al demonstrated that measurements of the percentage of free PSA (%fPSA = (free PSA/total PSA) × 100) could help discriminate between BPH and prostate cancer in men whose PSA levels were between 4 and 10 ng/mL.[19,20] In 1988, based upon these studies, the FDA approved the free PSA test as an aid to early prostate cancer detection. In 1998, the FDA also approved the first complex PSA assay.

In 1997 and 2000, Mikolajczyk et al reported on the existence of other free PSA isoforms, including "B" (associated with BPH) PSA, "i" (a molecularly intact and inactive) PSA and "pro-" (proenzyme) PSA.[21,22] In 2003, Sokoll et al reported that the percentage of proPSA ((proPSA/fPSA) × 100) could discriminate between BPH and cancer better than %fPSA in men with a total PSA in the 2.5 to 4 ng/mL range.[23] In 2003, Catalona et al confirmed this and reported that proPSA measurements also preferentially identified more aggressive prostate cancers.[24,25]

CLINICAL USES

At present, the measurement of serum PSA level is widely used in the US for the screening and early detection of prostate cancer. It is also frequently used in determining the need for a repeat biopsy in men with previously negative prostate biopsy. Increasing serum PSA values are significantly associated with an increased risk of prostate cancer.[17] Traditionally, it was believed that if the serum PSA concentration was between 4 and 10 ng/mL approximately 25% of patients would have cancer detected with a needle biopsy of the prostate.[15] Subsequently, it has been shown from more extensive and repeat biopsies that 35% to 45% of men with PSA levels in this range have detectable prostate cancer, and the great majority of these tumors have the histopathologic features of clinically relevant tumors.[26–28] It also has been shown that more than 20% of men with PSA levels of 2.6 to 4 ng/mL have readily detectable prostate cancer.[18,29,30]

It is impossible to determine the actual sensitivity and specificity of PSA testing in a typical study where biopsies cannot be performed in all subjects, primarily for ethical reasons. In a recent study, Punglia et al used mathematical models to predict biopsy outcome among men with low PSA levels and estimated that the percentage of cancers missed using a 4 ng/mL cutoff as the threshold to recommend a biopsy is as high as 82% in men younger than 60 years of age and 65% in men aged 60 years or older.[31] It appears logical that reducing the PSA screening cutoff for recommending biopsy to below 4.0 ng/mL will detect more cancers at an early, potentially curable stage. There is evidence that this can be done without materially "over-detecting" possibly harmless cancers.[31]

IMPROVING THE ACCURACY

The measurement of PSA lacks a high degree of clinical specificity, since serum PSA levels can also be elevated with benign conditions such as BPH, prostatitis, recent ejaculation, and minor trauma to the prostate by DRE, catheterization, and urinary retention. Substantial efforts have been made to optimize PSA-based screening. The methods most extensively studied include: PSA "velocity," PSA "density," age-specific PSA reference ranges, percent free PSA, human kallikrein 2 (hK2), and measuring the levels of isoforms of PSA.

PROSTATE-SPECIFIC ANTIGEN VELOCITY

Prostate-specific antigen velocity measures the rate of change of PSA as a function of time.[12] An increase in the serum PSA level of 0.75 ng/mL per year has been reported to be suspicious for prostate cancer.[12] An important limitation of PSA velocity is that it takes time and multiple measurements to determine whether a biopsy is necessary. Because of "noise"—fluctuations of 10% to 15% that frequently occur in serial PSA measurements—experience has shown that PSA velocity is best used in a "common sense" manner. With prostate cancer and BPH, PSA levels rise persistently (the slope is usually steeper with cancer than with BPH); whereas, with prostatitis or trauma to the prostate gland, PSA levels may increase transiently and later decrease with resolution of the inflammation. In some men with prostatitis, antibiotic therapy can lower PSA levels, but in others antibiotics are ineffective at promptly restoring PSA levels to normal.[32] Frequently, PSA levels gradually return to normal with spontaneous resolution of the inflammation. However, a man might have cancer, BPH, and prostatitis simultaneously, which could produce confounded PSA patterns that are difficult to interpret.

PROSTATE-SPECIFIC ANTIGEN DENSITY

Benson et al popularized the concept that the serum PSA divided by the prostate volume ("PSA density") was higher in men with cancer than those with BPH and recommended using PSA density measurements to select patients for biopsy.[13] Since then, it has been reported that PSA density values higher than 0.15 are strongly associated with prostate cancer.[33,34] Other studies suggested that the commonly used cutoff of 0.15 is too high and misses cancer in many patients.[35] A PSA density cutoff in the range of 0.10 would provide more acceptable sensitivity for cancer detection, but specificity at that cutoff would be inadequate. Another major disadvantage of using PSA density measurements is that they require transrectal ultrasonography to accurately determine the prostate volume, which adds cost and patient discomfort to the screening process. The limited reproducibility of prostate volume measurements is another source of variability.[36]

AGE-SPECIFIC REFERENCE RANGES FOR PROSTATE-SPECIFIC ANTIGEN

Age-specific PSA reference ranges refers to using different PSA prompts or cutoffs for recommending prostate biopsy for patients in different age groups. The most commonly used age-specific PSA reference ranges are those suggested by Oesterling et al: 2.5 ng/mL for men in their 40s, 3.5 ng/mL in their 50s, 4.5 ng/mL in their 60s, and 6.5 ng/mL for men in their 70s or older.[14] These cutoffs would substantially reduce the number of negative biopsies performed. However, the use of age-specific reference ranges would miss or delay the detection of prostate cancer in 20% of men in their 60s and in 60% of men in their 70s.[37]

FREE/TOTAL PROSTATE-SPECIFIC ANTIGEN RATIO

Prostate-specific antigen forms that can be measured in serum or plasma by immunoassay include the noncomplexed, ~33 kDa form called "free" PSA (fPSA) and complexed forms (cPSA) bound to serum protease inhibitors, primarily α1-antichymotrypsin.[10,11,38] The total clinically measurable PSA concentration is equal to the concentration of fPSA plus the concentration of cPSA (Figure 39.1). Typically, between 70% and 90%

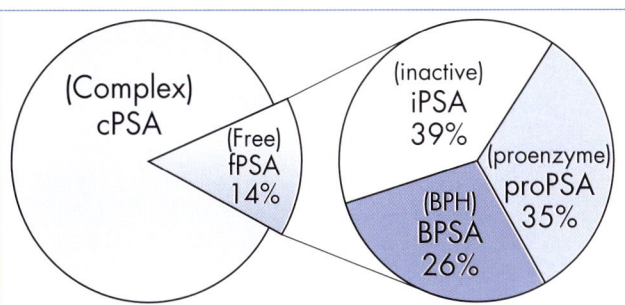

Fig. 39.1
Example proportions of prostate-specific antigen (PSA) isoforms in cancer serum with total PSA ranges 4 to 10 ng/mL. (BPH, benign prostatic hyperplasia.)

of the PSA in serum is in the cPSA form, with the remainder being fPSA.[10,11] The %fPSA in serum is increased in men with BPH because the inner portion ("transition zone") of the prostate gland, where BPH predominantly occurs, contains elevated levels of fPSA isoforms (iPSA and BPSA) that leak into the bloodstream.

Measurement of PSA isoforms, such as fPSA and cPSA, improves the discrimination between cancer and benign prostatic disease. In men with prostate cancer, the percentage of fPSA is lower, and more PSA is complexed in serum. For example, for men whose total PSA is in the 4 to 10 ng/mL range, a %fPSA higher than 25% is associated with only an 8% chance of finding cancer with a needle biopsy, while a %fPSA less than 10% is associated with a 56% chance of finding cancer.[20] Using a 25% cutoff for %fPSA for recommending biopsy detects 95% of cancers while avoiding 20% of unnecessary biopsies in the PSA range of 4 to 10 ng/mL.[20] Some investigators have suggested using a %fPSA to determine the need for repeat prostate biopsy.[39]

The %fPSA measurement is less robust in discriminating between cancer and benign prostate disease in the 2.6 to 4 ng/mL total PSA range. In one study of men with PSA of 2.6 to 4 ng/mL and benign DRE who underwent biopsy, a 25% fPSA cutoff would have detected 85% of cancers and avoided 19% of negative biopsies, while a 30% fPSA cutoff would have detected 93% of cancers and avoided only 9% of negative biopsies.[40]

Percent fPSA measurements can also be combined with lower PSA thresholds to reduce both false-positive and false-negative PSA testing results. For instance, Gann et al compared the traditional PSA cutoff of 4 ng/mL for recommending biopsy with a strategy that used a PSA cutoff of 3 to 10 ng/mL with a %fPSA cutoff of 20% or less.[41] The latter strategy would have detected 10% more cancers with 13% fewer biopsies.

FREE/TOTAL PROSTATE-SPECIFIC ANTIGEN SLOPE

The value of %fPSA slope in predicting the subsequent diagnosis of prostate cancer was first reported by Pearson et al from the Baltimore Longitudinal Study on Aging.[42] They reported that a falling %fPSA slope was the earliest sign of cancer, occurring approximately 10 years before the diagnosis of cancer and even before the total PSA level began to rise.[42] Subsequently, Ellis et al reported on longitudinal changes in the free/total PSA ratio from the β-Carotene/Retinol Efficacy Study.[43] Serial changes in free/total PSA ratio over 5 years in their study were so minimal as to render them clinically insignificant.[43] The increase in the total PSA level was more predictive of cancer. The results of Ellis et al were confirmed by Zhu et al.[44]

COMPLEXED PROSTATE-SPECIFIC ANTIGEN

Conflicting studies have been reported concerning the clinical value of cPSA. Some studies have reported that cPSA measurements provide more predictive information about the presence or absence of cancer than total PSA and predictive information equivalent to that provided by %fPSA.[45,46] In addition, some studies have reported that cPSA measurements are more accurate than %fPSA in total PSA ranges below 6 ng/mL.[47] These authors who are enthusiastic about the cPSA test maintain that, in the total PSA range of 2 to 6 ng/mL, cPSA should be the preferred first-line screening test for prostate cancer.[48]

In contrast, other studies have reported that %fPSA and percent cPSA both provide more information than total PSA, but the measurement of neither cPSA or fPSA alone provides more information than the ratio of either to total PSA.[49] Bartsch et al suggested using a percent cPSA in selecting men indicated for repeat biopsy procedure.[50]

Since total PSA equals the sum of fPSA and cPSA, the knowledge of any two of these measurements allows the calculation of the value of the third, and no one measurement should provide more predictive information than the other two. The reason for conflicting results is unknown, but the patient populations studied by different research groups might be an important factor.

A limitation of screening with cPSA measurements alone is that one does not necessarily know the total PSA level because it can vary considerably for any value of cPSA. For example, an individual with a cPSA of 6 ng/mL could have a total PSA as high as 10 ng/mL or as low as 6.5 ng/mL. In clinical practice, the results of using cPSA can be interpreted that the total PSA is higher than the cPSA, but how much higher is unknown.

HUMAN KALLIKREIN 2

Human kallikrein 2 is a member of the human kallikrein family that catalyzes the conversion of proPSA

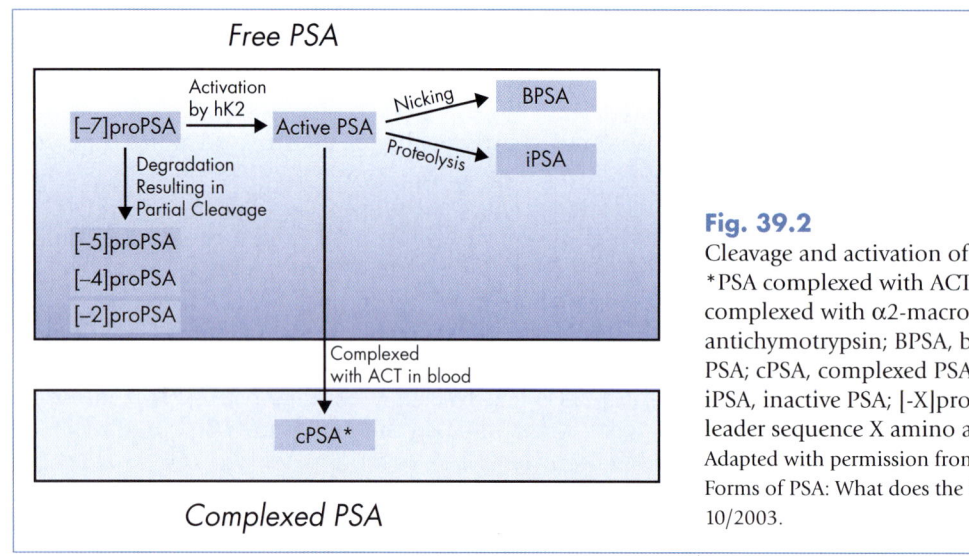

Fig. 39.2
Cleavage and activation of prostate-specific antigen (PSA). *PSA complexed with ACT is immunoreactive, but PSA complexed with α2-macroglobulin is not. (ACT, α1-antichymotrypsin; BPSA, benign prostatic hyperplasia PSA; cPSA, complexed PSA; hk2, human kallikrein 2; iPSA, inactive PSA; [-X]proPSA, proenzyme PSA with a leader sequence X amino acids long.)
Adapted with permission from Partin AW, Gretzer MB. Molecular Forms of PSA: What does the future hold? Urology Times 10/2003.

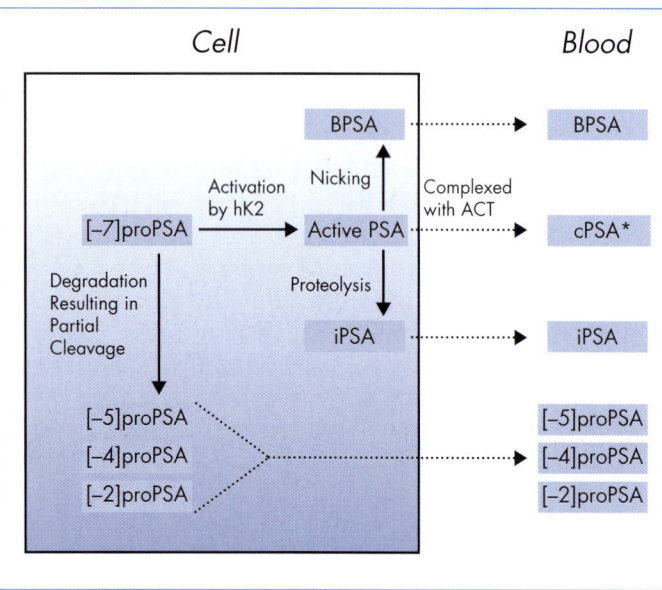

Fig. 39.3
Prostate-specific antigen (PSA) isoforms in cell and blood. *PSA-ACT is immunoreactive, but not PSA-α2-macroglobulin. (ACT, α1-antichymotrypsin; BPSA, benign prostatic hyperplasia PSA; cPSA, complexed PSA; hk2, human kallikrein 2; iPSA, inactive PSA; [-X]proPSA, proenzyme PSA with a leader sequence X amino acids long.)
Adapted with permission from Partin AW, Gretzer MB. Molecular Forms of PSA: What does the future hold? Urology Times 10/2003.

to active PSA by cleaving the 7-amino-acid peptide leader from the proPSA molecule[51-54] (Figures 39.2 and 39.3). It is present in very low concentrations (pg/mL) in the blood.[55] The levels of hK2 are higher in prostate cancer tissue than in BPH tissue. Also, the serum hK2 levels are higher in patients with prostate cancer. Studies have reported that the ratio of hK2 to percent free PSA in serum provides discriminatory information about the presence or absence of prostate cancer, especially in men with total PSA levels in the 2 to 4 ng/mL range.[56-58] With hK2 in the numerator (higher with cancer) and percent free PSA in the denominator (lower with cancer), the ratio magnifies the discrimination between cancer and BPH. Human kallikrein 2 also has been reported to be useful in predicting tumor stage and the proportion of Gleason patterns 4/5 in the tumor. However, the use of hK2 is limited by the difficulty in measuring its low concentrations in the blood. Future testing with multiple markers including hK2 (multiplex) testing with an appropriate algorithm may provide significantly greater clinical diagnostic information.

PROSTATE-SPECIFIC ANTIGEN ISOFORMS

Prostate cancer develops predominantly within the peripheral zone of the prostate gland. Studies of transition and peripheral zone tissues from the same prostate revealed other forms of fPSA, called proPSA (proenzyme PSA) and BPSA.[22,59] The proPSA is elevated in cancerous prostate tissue, while BPSA is elevated in nodular BPH transition zone tissue[22,59] (Figure 39.4). Both BPSA and proPSA are more disease-associated than the other forms of PSA that are measured in clinical practice, such as total PSA, fPSA, and cPSA. Virtually all of the PSA in prostate tissue is in the uncomplexed forms. Recently, research immunoassays have been developed to measure BPSA and proPSA forms in serum.[60]

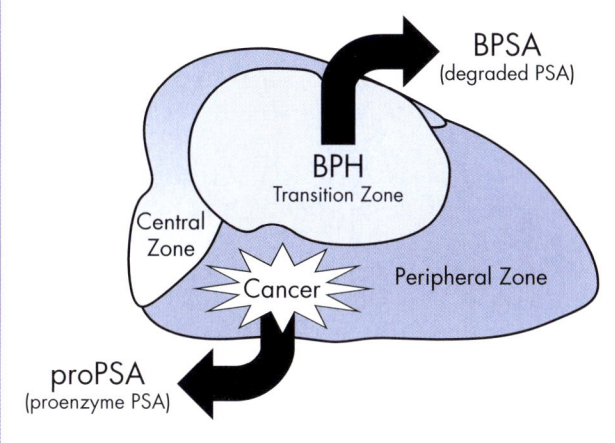

Fig. 39.4
Disease-associated forms of free prostate-specific antigen (PSA). (BPH, benign prostatic hyperplasia.)

Proenzyme PSA is the natural precursor form of PSA, but usually it is very rapidly converted to PSA.[21] For yet unknown reasons, proPSA accumulates in prostate cancer tissue. In addition to the native form of proPSA with a 7-amino-acid leader peptide fragment ([-7] proPSA), there are other degradation (not naturally occurring) forms of proPSA with truncated pro leader peptides. These consist primarily of proPSA with "pro" leader peptides of 5 ([-5]proPSA), 4 ([-4]proPSA), or 2 ([-2]proPSA) amino acids. The [-2]proPSA has received the most clinical attention, since it was the primary form found in tumor extracts and shows higher immuno-staining in cancerous prostate tissue.[61]

Proenzyme PSA can also significantly enhance the detection of prostate cancer in blood samples with either high or low percentages of fPSA.[24,25] The ratio of proPSA to free PSA has been shown in preliminary studies to be most predictive of cancer in patients with total PSA levels in the 2.6 to 4 ng/mL range, and as good or slightly better in the 4 to 10 ng/mL total PSA range.[24,62] If these studies are verified, it is possible that proPSA measurements might be preferable to free or complexed PSA as a marker for cancer in clinical use. With greater acceptance and use of lower PSA cutoffs, more men will be advised to undergo biopsy, and there will be a greater need to eliminate unnecessary biopsies.

CONTROVERSIES IN PROSTATE CANCER SCREENING

Screening for prostate cancer has been controversial since it was introduced in the early 1990s, and the controversy continues. Current controversies include the age at which to begin screening, the screening intervals to be used, the PSA threshold to be used for recommending a prostate biopsy, the need for repeat prostate biopsies, and biopsy protocols to be used for repeat biopsies.

AGE AT WHICH TO BEGIN SCREENING

The American Cancer Society and the American Urological Association recommend that screening with PSA measurement and DRE be offered to men with a life expectancy of at least 10 years, beginning at age 50 years in the general population, at age 45 in high-risk men (African Americans or men with a positive family history), and at age 40 in men with strong family history of early-onset disease. Other organizations, such as the American College of Physicians (ACP) and the U.S. Preventive Services Task Force, do not believe that, in the absence of randomized trials, there is sufficient evidence to support routine prostate cancer screening. However, ACP does encourage primary physicians to decide about screening on an individual basis, following discussion of the pros and cons with the patient. Recently, the 2004 National Comprehensive Cancer Network (NCCN) guidelines recommended that a DRE be done yearly and a PSA blood test be offered, beginning at age 50 years, to men who have at least a 10-year life expectancy, and to younger men who are at high risk.[63]

SCREENING HIGH-RISK MEN

There are limited data on screening results in high-risk men with a family history of early age onset prostate cancer. In a study of screening high-risk men aged 40 to 49 years, 8% overall had PSA greater than 2.5 ng/mL or suspicious findings on DRE.[64] These men were advised to undergo prostate biopsy. Approximately 50% of those biopsied had cancer detected and about 80% of cancers were organ-confined with favorable prognostic features. Only 7% of men had "possibly harmless" cancers, using the criteria reported by Epstein et al.[65]

PROSTATE-SPECIFIC ANTIGEN LEVELS IN YOUNGER MEN: AGED 40–60 YEARS OLD

In a study by Fang et al, the median PSA level for men aged 40 to 49 years was 0.6 ng/mL, and the median value for men aged 50 to 59 years was 0.7 ng/mL.[66] Men whose PSA level was higher than the median for their age group had a three-fold higher risk of prostate cancer within 10 to 25 years.[66] Antenor et al reported a similar trend from a prostate cancer screening study, except that the risks for being diagnosed with prostate cancer were even higher (12- to 22-fold higher relative risk of prostate cancer for men whose initial PSA level was higher than the median for their age group).[67] These results in a screened population are also consistent with those previously reported with Gann et al who related the baseline PSA with the subsequent risk of being diagnosed with prostate cancer using archived serum samples in a non-screened patient population.[17]

PROSTATE-SPECIFIC ANTIGEN THRESHOLD FOR A BIOPSY RECOMMENDATION

Presently, most physicians use the 4.0 ng/mL PSA threshold for recommending a prostate biopsy; however, there is accumulating evidence that using lower PSA cutoffs detect clinically relevant prostate cancer earlier. The positive biopsy rate is 22% to 25% it the 2.6 to 4 ng/mL PSA range.[18,30] Lower cutoffs increase the immediate biopsy rate; however, in about half of the patients, it merely moves up the time of biopsy by a few years. Approximately 81% to 85% of cancers are pathologically organ-confined when detected at a PSA level of 2.5 to 4 ng/mL, while about 17% may be clinically insignificant.

Results from several studies have shown that a higher proportion of patients are diagnosed with organ-confined cancer when lower PSA cutoffs are used, and the progression-free survival rates correlate with the PSA level at the time of diagnosis.[67,68] These studies also suggest that cancer can be detected earlier without materially over-detecting potentially harmless prostate cancer.

Krumholtz et al evaluated completely embedded radical prostatectomy specimens in men whose PSA was 2.6 to 4 ng/mL at the time of diagnosis versus those whose PSA was 4 to 10 ng/mL.[68] The cancer detected for the 2.6 to 4.0 ng/mL PSA had smaller cancer volumes, but there was no difference in the proportion of tumors that met published criteria of "clinically insignificant" or "clinically unimportant" cancer. Similar results were reported from the European Screening Trial.

Using lower PSA cutoffs raises the concern that more harmless cancers will be detected. For cancers that are high grade or high volume, it is not difficult to determine that they are potentially dangerous. It is more difficult—in fact, impossible—to state which cancers are truly harmless. However, an optimal screening strategy would not necessarily be designed to detect only high-volume, high-grade cancer. If this were the case, treatment outcomes would be compromised, since intervention might be applied too late. The goal of screening should be to detect cancers with favorable prognostic features, i.e., low PSA, low-volume, intermediate Gleason grade cancers that are organ-confined. This will lead to improved outcomes.

SCREENING INTERVALS

The American Urological Association and American Cancer Society recommend that annual screening should be offered to men who have a life expectancy of at least 10 years. Other screening interval models have been suggested, including screening at 2- or 4-year intervals.[69,70] One proposed model suggests beginning screening at age 40 years; then, if the PSA is less than 1 ng/mL and the DRE examination is not suspicious for cancer, re-screen at age 45 years; if the PSA is still below 1 ng/mL, re-screen again at age 50 years; then re-screen at 2-year intervals after age 50 as long as the PSA level remains below 1 ng/mL; if the PSA rises above 1 ng/mL, annual screening should be initiated.[70] Alternatively, Crawford et al suggested that if PSA was below 1 ng/mL, the patient would not need to be re-screened for 5 years; however, he recommended if the PSA level were 1 to 2 ng/mL, re-screening should be recommended every 2 years.[71]

The impetus for less frequent screening is that it potentially reduces costs and morbidity of screening and follow-up testing. Only a small percentage (1–2%) of men with very low PSA levels have rapid PSA rises. However, these men have the most aggressive cancers and the most to lose from delayed detection. The extent to which delays would compromise the outcomes of those who do have rapid rises is undetermined. Our results have shown that infrequent screening protocols could delay the detection of cancer in a significant proportion of patients.[72]

OVERDETECTION

There are also concerns about possible overdetection of prostate cancer. Etzioni et al reported on a computer model simulation of screening 2 million men enrolled in Medicare aged 60 to 84 years over 10 years.[73] Overdiagnosis of prostate cancer—defined as cancer that would not have been diagnosed during the man's lifetime due to death from competing causes—was reported to occur in 29% of whites and 44% of blacks diagnosed with cancer. However, the authors claimed that the majority of cancers would have presented clinically and only a minority of so-called "autopsy" cases would have been detected.[73] In this study, 4% of whites and 7% of blacks screened would have prostate cancer. The population screened in this computer simulation was much older than would be preferred for screening protocols (60 to 84 years old), largely because lower life expectancy reduces the benefits of screening and increases the likelihood of overdiagnosis. In actual clinical prostate cancer screening studies involving younger populations, most screen-detected prostate cancers have the features of clinically relevant tumors.[73–75]

ROLE OF DIGITAL RECTAL EXAMINATION IN PROSTATE CANCER SCREENING: IS IT NECESSARY IF THE PROSTATE-SPECIFIC ANTIGEN IS LOW?

In large prostate cancer screening programs, it is logistically difficult to provide a screening DRE to all men. Accordingly, in some screening studies, routine screening DRE is not included unless the PSA level is elevated.[76] In a large community-based prostate cancer screening study, there was a significant association between the PSA level and the likelihood of finding prostate cancer on a biopsy in men with findings suspicious for cancer on DRE.[77] However, it appeared that the only group of men who had very low rate of cancer was those with PSA values less than 1 ng/mL. In this study, among men who had PSA below 1 ng/mL and suspicious findings on DRE, 5% had prostate cancer diagnosed on needle biopsy.[77] If the PSA was 1 to 2.5 ng/mL and the DRE was suspicious, 14% had cancer detected, and, if the PSA was 2.6 to 4 ng/mL and

the DRE was suspicious, 30% had prostate cancer diagnosed.[77] Of the cancers detected, 80% were pathologically organ confined with clear surgical margins. Similar results were reported from the European Randomized Study of Screening for Prostate Cancer.[78,79] Recently, Thompson et al investigated the prevalence of prostate cancer among men who had a PSA level of 4.0 ng/mL or less and a benign DRE.[80] They found prostate cancer in 15% overall in men with a PSA level below 4.0 ng/mL, but 7% among men with a PSA level up to 0.5 ng/mL and as high as 27% among those with a PSA level between 3 and 4 ng/mL.[80]

HAS EARLY DETECTION OF PROSTATE CANCER MADE A DIFFERENCE?

If there were no effective treatment for prostate cancer, early detection would not be relevant. In 2002, Holmberg et al reported the first prospective, randomized trial to show that radical prostatectomy reduces metastases and mortality from prostate cancer.[81] In the intent-to-treat analysis of 695 men, these authors demonstrated that men in a radical prostatectomy arm have lower cancer-specific mortality, distant metastasis, local progression, and overall mortality compared with those in a watchful waiting arm.[81]

If treatment of early cancer is effective, then the goals for early detection should be: 1) to detect potentially harmful cancers while they are still curable to reduce cancer-related morbidity and mortality; 2) to avoid excessive morbidity and mortality from the screening and/or treatment; and 3) to have reasonable economic costs.

What trends would one see if early diagnosis were effective? Initially, there would be an increase in incidence rates, as previously undetectable cancers are detected. Subsequently, there would be a decline in incidence rates, as previously occult cancers are culled from the population. There would also be a higher new baseline incidence rate, because more of the prevalent cases would be detected. Earlier stage disease would be detected, and there would be a reduction in advanced-stage disease. One of the last trends to be observed would be a decrease in the morbidity and mortality rates from advanced cancer. Other expected trends would be: detecting more moderate-grade tumors and fewer low- and high-grade tumors; increasing the "relative" survival rate (survival relative to other causes of death); increasing detection of cancer at a younger age and at lower PSA levels. *All of these trends have occurred.*

These favorable trends do not prove that early detection improves outcomes. To prove that early detection is effective would require convincing results from a prospective, randomized trial or a sustained reduction in cancer-specific morbidity rates (difficult to measure accurately) or mortality rates in national cancer registries.

If it were proven that early detection does improve outcomes, it would remain necessary to determine: which patients benefit; how many cancers must be detected to save one life; the risk-benefit ratio in relation to side effects; and the economic costs in relation to the benefits.

What are the data currently available? Prostate cancer incidence and mortality rates for US men from 1973 to 2000 show striking changes in stage at diagnosis.[82] Between 1991 and 2000, the number of localized prostate cancer cases increased sharply and the numbers of regional and advanced cases decreased in return.[82] Since 1991, the number of well-differentiated and poorly-differentiated tumors decreased while the number of moderately-differentiated tumors increased.[82] Virtually all studies have shown that the great majority of PSA-detected tumors have the features of clinically important cancers (i.e., tumor volume and grade) and most are still confined to the gland.[73-75] It has been estimated that PSA screening advances the date of diagnosis by 5 to 13 years.[17,83]

Figure 39.5 illustrates the change in prostate cancer incidence rates from the National Cancer Institute's Surveillance, Epidemiology, and End Results (SEER) program. There was a sharp increase in prostate cancer incidence from 1988 to 1992, followed by a sharp decrease from 1992 to 1995, and a mild increase from 1995 to 1999, with a slope similar to the gradual increase observed before 1988. Figure 39.6 illustrates the change in prostate cancer mortality rates from 1973 to 1997. There was a peak of prostate cancer mortality in 1991, followed by a gradual decrease.

Relative survival rates are survival from cancer in relation to other typical causes of death. They can be increased by both lead-time bias (detecting cancers earlier) and length-time bias (preferentially detecting indolent cancers); however, they also are increased by early detection and effective treatment. The SEER data demonstrates that 5-year relative survival rates in whites

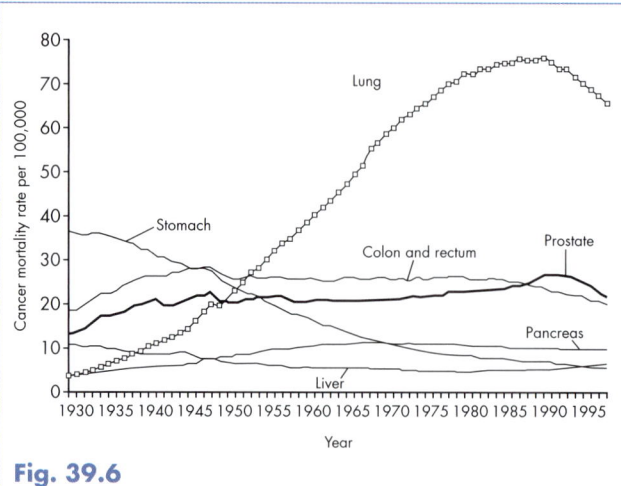

Fig. 39.6

Cancer mortality rates* for men in the US, 1930–1998. (*Age-adjusted to the 1970 US standard population.) Source: US Mortality Public Use Data Tapes 1960–1998, US Mortality Volumes 1930–1959, National Center for Health Statistics, Centers for Disease Control and Prevention, 2001.

have increased by 18% between 1986 and 1988, while the same rates have increased by 37% in blacks. To illustrate the potential importance of increasing relative survival rates, between 1992 and 1998, 5-year relative survival rates were 100% for men with local/regional disease versus 33.6% with distant disease.

How have these trends been interpreted by the cancer epidemiology community? The percentage of men receiving a PSA test has increased dramatically from 1.2% in 1988 to nearly 50% in 1999.[84] The percentage of prostate cancer treated for cure has also increased from 7% in 1983 to much higher in 1999. These data strongly suggest that PSA screening is playing some role in observed trends. Hankey et al from the National Cancer Institute stated, "...there is little uncertainty that PSA testing has left its mark on the vital statistics for prostate cancer. Several factors, especially the decline in the incidence of and mortality from distant stage disease, hold out the promise that PSA testing may lead to a sustained decline in prostate cancer mortality."[84] Some of the decline in mortality is probably attributable to more effective treatment, including improved surgical and radiation techniques as well as more widespread use of hormonal therapy. However, separating the contributions of screening and treatment is impossible, since there is an essential interaction between the success of therapy and the diagnosis of disease at an earlier stage.

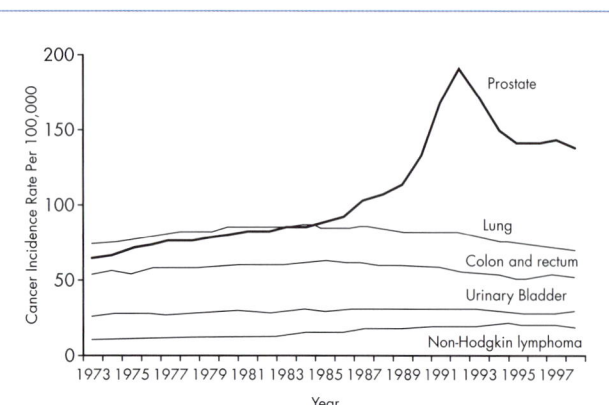

Fig. 39.5

Cancer incidence rates* for men in the US, 1973–1998, from the SEER data.[82] (*Age-adjusted to the 1970 US standard population.)

RANDOMIZED CLINICAL TRIALS

The Laval University/Quebec Screening Trial conducted from 1988 to 1998 studied 8137 screened and 46,193 non-screened men.[85,86] They reported a 69% reduction in prostate cancer mortality in screened men.[85] This trial was criticized for: 1) low statistical power; 2) possible selection bias, since only 23% of those invited participated in screening; 3) failure to use intention-to-treat analysis; and 4) a short observation period of 4 to 7 years.

There are two ongoing large-scale, randomized prostate cancer screening trials. The European Randomized Study of Screening for Prostate Cancer (ERSPC) is being conducted in seven countries (see Chapter 40).[87,88] In the US, the Prostate, Lung, Colorectal, Ovary (PLCO) Cancer Screening Trial is being conducted at 10 sites (see Chapter 42).[89–91] These two important randomized studies will address the effect of population screening with regard to reduction of prostate cancer specific mortality and quality of life issues.

The Tyrol screening trial, initiated in 1993, provided a PSA screening to two thirds of eligible men in the Tyrol region of Austria aged 45 to 75 years old (see Chapter 41).[92–94] Nearly all patients were treated for cure and there was virtually no watchful waiting. This study demonstrated a decrease in advanced-stage disease and a reduction in the prostate cancer mortality rate that was significantly greater in Tyrol than in other parts of Austria where prostate cancer screening was less widespread.

If the current cancer incidence and mortality trends are not caused by beneficial early detection and effective treatment, there are several possible alternative explanations. The early appearance of a survival benefit after the introduction of PSA screening suggests that earlier use of hormonal therapy also could be a factor (i.e., treatment of early recurrences may delay disease progression, and patients may die of unrelated causes before they die of prostate cancer). Another possible explanation could be the misclassification of the mortality cause. If a fixed percentage of deaths from other causes is misclassified as prostate cancer deaths, then, as the incidence rates of prostate cancer rise and fall, the prostate cancer mortality rates would also automatically rise and fall with them.[95] Other explanations to be considered are changes in diet and other environmental exposures; however, no exposures seem likely to explain the recent mortality trends.

The demonstration in a prospective, randomized clinical trial that radical prostatectomy is effective in preventing prostate cancer progression and mortality—coupled with the sustained decline in the incidence of and mortality from advanced-stage prostate cancer observed in the national SEER tumor registry and the downward trends of the clinical and pathologic features of the cancers detected—strongly suggests that PSA testing and subsequent effective treatment are *at least partially* responsible for the favorable prostate cancer mortality trends. We believe that with time the beneficial effects of early detection and effective treatment of prostate cancer will become even more apparent.

REFERENCES

1. Walsh PC, Donker PJ. Impotence following radical prostatectomy: insight into etiology and prevention. J Urol 1982;128:492–497.

2. Lilja H. A kallikrein-like serine protease in prostatic fluid cleaves the predominant seminal vesicle protein. J Clin Invest 1985;76:1899–1903.

3. Ablin RJ, Soanes WA, Bronson P, et al. Precipitating antigens of the normal human prostate. J Reprod Fertil 1970;22:573–574.

4. Ablin RJ, Bronson P, Soanes WA, et al. Tissue- and species-specific antigens of normal human prostatic tissue. J Immunol 1970;104:1329–1339.

5. Wang MC, Valenzuela LA, Murphy GP, et al. Purification of a human prostate specific antigen. Invest Urol 1979;17:159–163.

6. Ercole CJ, Lange PH, Mathisen M, et al. Prostatic specific antigen and prostatic acid phosphatase in the monitoring and staging of patients with prostatic cancer. J Urol 1987;138:1181–1184.

7. Stamey TA, Yang N, Hay AR, et al. Prostate-specific antigen as a serum marker for adenocarcinoma of the prostate. N Engl J Med 1987;317:909–916.

8. Cooner WH, Mosley BR, Rutherford CL Jr, et al. Prostate cancer detection in a clinical urological practice by ultrasonography, digital rectal examination and prostate specific antigen. J Urol 1990;143:1146–1152; discussion 1152–1154.

9. Catalona WJ, Smith DS, Ratliff TL, et al. Measurement of prostate-specific antigen in serum as a screening test for prostate cancer. N Engl J Med 1991;324:1156–1161.

10. Lilja H, Christensson A, Dahlen U, et al. Prostate-specific antigen in serum occurs predominantly in complex with alpha 1-antichymotrypsin. Clin Chem 1991;37:1618–1625.

11. Stenman UH, Leinonen J, Alfthan H, et al. A complex between prostate-specific antigen and alpha 1-antichymotrypsin is the major form of prostate-specific antigen in serum of patients with prostatic cancer: assay of the complex improves clinical sensitivity for cancer. Cancer Res 1991;51:222–226.

12. Carter HB, Pearson JD, Metter EJ, et al. Longitudinal evaluation of prostate-specific antigen levels in men with and without prostate disease. JAMA 1992;267:2215–2220.

13. Benson MC, Whang IS, Olsson CA, et al. The use of prostate specific antigen density to enhance the predictive value of intermediate levels of serum prostate specific antigen. J Urol 1992;147:817–821.

14. Oesterling JE, Jacobsen SJ, Cooner WH. The use of age-specific reference ranges for serum prostate specific antigen in men 60 years old or older. J Urol 1995;153:1160–1163.

15. Catalona WJ, Richie JP, Ahmann FR, et al. Comparison of digital rectal examination and serum prostate specific antigen in the early detection of prostate cancer: results of a multicenter clinical trial of 6,630 men. J Urol 1994;151:1283–1290.

16. Moul JW, Sesterhenn IA, Connelly RR, et al. Prostate-specific antigen values at the time of prostate cancer diagnosis in African-American men. JAMA 1995;274:1277–1281.

17. Gann PH, Hennekens CH, Stampfer MJ. A prospective evaluation of plasma prostate-specific antigen for detection of prostatic cancer. JAMA 1995;273:289–294.

18. Catalona WJ, Smith DS, Ornstein DK. Prostate cancer detection in men with serum PSA concentrations of 2.6 to 4.0 ng/mL and benign prostate examination. Enhancement of specificity with free PSA measurements. JAMA 1997;277:1452–1455.

19. Catalona WJ, Smith DS, Wolfert RL, et al. Evaluation of percentage of free serum prostate-specific antigen to improve specificity of prostate cancer screening. JAMA 1995;274:1214–1220.

20. Catalona WJ, Partin AW, Slawin KM, et al. Use of the percentage of free prostate-specific antigen to enhance differentiation of prostate cancer from benign prostatic disease: a prospective multicenter clinical trial. JAMA 1998;279:1542–1547.

21. Mikolajczyk SD, Grauer LS, Millar LS, et al. A precursor form of PSA (pPSA) is a component of the free PSA in prostate cancer serum. Urology 1997;50:710–714.

22. Mikolajczyk SD, Millar LS, Wang TJ, et al. "BPSA," a specific molecular form of free prostate-specific antigen, is found predominantly in the transition zone of patients with nodular benign prostatic hyperplasia. Urology 2000;55:41–45.

23. Sokoll LJ, Chan DW, Mikolajczyk SD, et al. Proenzyme psa for the early detection of prostate cancer in the 2.5-4.0 ng/ml total psa range: preliminary analysis. Urology 2003;61:274–276.

24. Bartsch G, Harninger W, Klocker H, et al. ProPSA Improves The Detection Of Prostate Cancer Compared To % Free PSA Or Complexed PSA In The 4-10 ng/mL Range and Especially In The 2-4 ng/mL PSA Range. In: Gillenwater JY(ed), American Urological Association Meeting; 2003. Chicago: 2003, p 1595.

25. Catalona W, Mikolajczyk SD, Linton HJ, et al. ProPSA Helps To Detect More Aggressive Prostate Cancer In The 2-4 ng/mL PSA Range. In: In: Gillenwater JY(ed), American Urological Association Meeting; 2003. Chicago: 2003, p 1128.

26. Durkan GC, Sheikh N, Johnson P, et al. Improving prostate cancer detection with an extended-core transrectal ultrasonography-guided prostate biopsy protocol. BJU Int 2002;89:33–39.

27. Chon CH, Lai FC, McNeal JE, et al. Use of extended systematic sampling in patients with a prior negative prostate needle biopsy. J Urol 2002;167:2457–2460.

28. Babaian RJ, Toi A, Kamoi K, et al. A comparative analysis of sextant and an extended 11-core multisite directed biopsy strategy. J Urol 2000;163:152–157.

29. Catalona WJ, Ramos CG, Carvalhal GF, et al. Lowering PSA cutoffs to enhance detection of curable prostate cancer. Urology 2000;55:791–795.

30. Babaian RJ, Johnston DA, Naccarato W, et al. The incidence of prostate cancer in a screening population with a serum prostate specific antigen between 2.5 and 4.0 ng/ml: relation to biopsy strategy. J Urol 2001;165:757–760.

31. Punglia RS, D'Amico AV, Catalona WJ, et al. Effect of verification bias on screening for prostate cancer by measurement of prostate-specific antigen. N Engl J Med 2003;349:335–342.

32. Bozeman CB, Carver BS, Eastham JA, et al. Treatment of chronic prostatitis lowers serum prostate specific antigen. J Urol 2002;167:1723–176.

33. Seaman E, Whang M, Olsson CA, et al. PSA density (PSAD). Role in patient evaluation and management. Urol Clin North Am 1993;20:653–663.

34. Bazinet M, Meshref AW, Trudel C, et al. Prospective evaluation of prostate-specific antigen density and systematic biopsies for early detection of prostatic carcinoma. Urology 1994;43(1):44–51; discussion 51–52.

35. Catalona WJ, Richie JP, deKernion JB, et al. Comparison of prostate specific antigen concentration versus prostate specific antigen density in the early detection of prostate cancer: receiver operating characteristic curves. J Urol 1994;152:2031–2036.

36. Terris MK, Stamey TA. Determination of prostate volume by transrectal ultrasound. J Urol 1991;145:984–987.

37. Catalona WJ, Southwick PC, Slawin KM, et al. Comparison of percent free PSA, PSA density, and age-specific PSA cutoffs for prostate cancer detection and staging. Urology 2000;56:255–260.

38. Christensson A, Laurell CB, Lilja H. Enzymatic activity of prostate-specific antigen and its reactions with extracellular serine proteinase inhibitors. Eur J Biochem 1990;194:755–763.

39. Djavan B, Zlotta A, Remzi M, et al. Optimal predictors of prostate cancer on repeat prostate biopsy: a prospective study of 1,051 men. J Urol 2000;163:1144–1148; discussion 1148–1149.

40. Roehl KA, Antenor JA, Catalona WJ. Robustness of free prostate specific antigen measurements to reduce unnecessary biopsies in the 2.6 to 4.0 ng/ml range. J Urol 2002;168:922–925.

41. Gann PH, Ma J, Catalona WJ, et al. Strategies combining total and percent free prostate specific antigen for detecting prostate cancer: a prospective evaluation. J Urol 2002;167:2427–2434.

42. Pearson JD, Luderer AA, Metter EJ, et al. Longitudinal analysis of serial measurements of free and total PSA among men with and without prostatic cancer. Urology 1996;48:4–9.

43. Ellis WJ, Etzioni R, Vessella RL, et al. Serial prostate specific antigen, free-to-total prostate specific antigen ratio and complexed prostate specific antigen for the diagnosis of prostate cancer. J Urol 2001;166:93–98; discussion 98–99.

44. Zhu H, Roehl KA, Antenor JA, et al. Clinical Value of Longitudinal Free-To-Total PSA Ratio Slope to Diagnosis of Prostate Cancer. In:

Gillenwater JY(ed), American Urological Association Meeting; 2002. Orlando, FL: 2002, p 840.

45. Brawer MK, Meyer GE, Letran JL, et al. Measurement of complexed PSA improves specificity for early detection of prostate cancer. Urology 1998;52:372–378.

46. Brawer MK, Cheli CD, Neaman IE, et al. Complexed prostate specific antigen provides significant enhancement of specificity compared with total prostate specific antigen for detecting prostate cancer. J Urol 2000;163:1476–1480.

47. Horninger W, Cheli CD, Babaian RJ, et al. Complexed prostate-specific antigen for early detection of prostate cancer in men with serum prostate-specific antigen levels of 2 to 4 nanograms per milliliter. Urology 2002;60:31–35.

48. Partin AW, Gretzer MB. Molecular forms of PSA: what does the future hold? Urology Times 2003; October: 1–2.

49. Okihara K, Cheli CD, Partin AW, et al. Comparative analysis of complexed prostate specific antigen, free prostate specific antigen and their ratio in detecting prostate cancer. J Urol 2002;167:2017–2023; discussion 2023–2024.

50. Bartsch G, Brawer MK, Cheli CD, et al. Predicting Cancer on Repeat Biopsy: Results Of A Multicenter Prospective Evaluation Of Complex PSA. In: Gillenwater JY(ed), American Urological Association Meeting; 2003. Chicago, IL: 2003, p 460.

51. Lovgren J, Rajakoski K, Karp M, et al. Activation of the zymogen form of prostate-specific antigen by human glandular kallikrein 2. Biochem Biophys Res Commun 1997;238:549–555.

52. Takayama TK, Fujikawa K, Davie EW. Characterization of the precursor of prostate-specific antigen. Activation by trypsin and by human glandular kallikrein. J Biol Chem 1997;272:21582–1588.

53. Young CY, Andrews PE, Montgomery BT, et al. Tissue-specific and hormonal regulation of human prostate-specific glandular kallikrein. Biochemistry (Mosc) 1992;31:818–824.

54. Murtha P, Tindall DJ, Young CY. Androgen induction of a human prostate-specific kallikrein, hKLK2: characterization of an androgen response element in the 5′ promoter region of the gene. Biochemistry (Mosc) 1993;32:6459–6464.

55. Black MH, Magklara A, Obiezu CV, et al. Development of an ultrasensitive immunoassay for human glandular kallikrein with no cross-reactivity from prostate-specific antigen. Clin Chem 1999;45:790–799.

56. Magklara A, Scorilas A, Catalona WJ, et al. The combination of human glandular kallikrein and free prostate-specific antigen (PSA) enhances discrimination between prostate cancer and benign prostatic hyperplasia in patients with moderately increased total PSA. Clin Chem 1999;45:1960–1966.

57. Partin AW, Catalona WJ, Finlay JA, et al. Use of human glandular kallikrein 2 for the detection of prostate cancer: preliminary analysis. Urology 1999;54:839–845.

58. Kwiatkowski MK, Recker F, Piironen T, et al. In prostatism patients the ratio of human glandular kallikrein to free PSA improves the discrimination between prostate cancer and benign hyperplasia within the diagnostic "gray zone" of total PSA 4 to 10 ng/mL. Urology 1998;52:360–365.

59. Chan TY, Mikolajczyk SD, Lecksell K, et al. Immunohistochemical staining of prostate cancer with monoclonal antibodies to the precursor of prostate-specific antigen. Urology 2003;62:177–181.

60. Linton HJ, Marks LS, Millar LS, et al. Benign prostate-specific antigen (BPSA) in serum is increased in benign prostate disease. Clin Chem 2003;49:253–259.

61. Mikolajczyk SD, Marker KM, Millar LS, et al. A truncated precursor form of prostate-specific antigen is a more specific serum marker of prostate cancer. Cancer Res 2001;61:6958–6963.

62. Niemela PM, Stueber T, Huland H, et al. A Novel Assay For Nicked, Multi-Chain Free PSA Enhances Discrimination Of Prostate Cancer Cases From Men With No Cancer and PSA-Levels of 2-10 ng/mL. In: Gillenwater JY(ed), American Urological Association Meeting; 2003. Chicago, IL: 2003.

63. Prostate Cancer: Treatment guidelines for Patients, Version IV; National Comprehensive Cancer Network, Practice Guidelines in Oncology; 2004, p 1–27.

64. Catalona WJ, Antenor JA, Roehl KA, et al. Screening for prostate cancer in high risk populations. J Urol 2002;168:1980–1983; discussion 1983–1984.

65. Epstein JI, Chan DW, Sokoll LJ, et al. Nonpalpable stage T1c prostate cancer: prediction of insignificant disease using free/total prostate specific antigen levels and needle biopsy findings. J Urol 1998;160:2407–2411.

66. Fang J, Metter EJ, Landis P, et al. Low levels of prostate-specific antigen predict long-term risk of prostate cancer: results from the Baltimore Longitudinal Study of Aging. Urology 2001;58:411–416.

67. Antenor JA, Roehl KA, Catalona W. Relation between PSA level at initial screening and subsequent cancer detection in a prostate cancer screening study. Supplement to the J Urol 2002;167:396.

68. Krumholtz JS, Carvalhal GF, Ramos CG, et al. Prostate-specific antigen cutoff of 2.6 ng/mL for prostate cancer screening is associated with favorable pathologic tumor features. Urology 2002;60:469–473; discussion 473–474.

69. Carter HB, Epstein JI, Chan DW, et al. Recommended prostate-specific antigen testing intervals for the detection of curable prostate cancer. JAMA 1997;277:1456–1460.

70. Ross KS, Carter HB, Pearson JD, et al. Comparative efficiency of prostate-specific antigen screening strategies for prostate cancer detection. JAMA 2000;284:1399–1405.

71. Crawford ED, Chia D, Andriole GL, et al. PSA Testing Interval, Reduction In Screening Intervals: Data From The Prostate, Lung, Colorectal and Ovarian Cancer (PLCO) Screening Trial. In: Gillenwater JY (ed), American Urological Association Meeting; 2002. Orlando, FL: 2002, p 397.

72. Grubb RL, Roehl KA, Antenor JA, et al. Delays In Cancer Detection Using 2 and 4 Year Screening Intervals For Prostate Cancer Screening In Men With Initial PSA < 2 ng/mL. In: Gillenwater JY(ed), American Urological Association Meeting; 2002. Orlando, FL: 2002, p 400.

73. Etzioni R, Penson DF, Legler JM, et al. Overdiagnosis due to prostate-specific antigen screening: lessons from U.S. prostate cancer incidence trends. J Natl Cancer Inst 2002;94:981–990.

74. Smith DS, Catalona WJ. The nature of prostate cancer detected through prostate specific antigen based screening. J Urol 1994;152:1732–1736.

75. Humphrey PA, Keetch DW, Smith DS, et al. Prospective characterization of pathological features of prostatic carcinomas detected via serum prostate specific antigen based screening. J Urol 1996;155:816–820.

76. Schroder FH, Roobol-Bouts M, Vis AN, et al. Prostate-specific antigen-based early detection of prostate cancer—validation of screening without rectal examination. Urology 2001;57:83–90.

77. Carvalhal GF, Smith DS, Mager DE, et al. Digital rectal examination for detecting prostate cancer at prostate specific antigen levels of 4 ng/ml or less. J Urol 1999;161:835–839.

78. Hoedemaeker RF, Rietbergen JB, Kranse R, et al. Comparison of pathologic characteristics of T1c and non-T1c cancers detected in a population-based screening study, the European Randomized Study of Screening for Prostate Cancer. World J Urol 1997;15:339–345.

79. Schroder FH, van der Maas P, Beemsterboer P, et al. Evaluation of the digital rectal examination as a screening test for prostate cancer. Rotterdam section of the European Randomized Study of Screening for Prostate Cancer. J Natl Cancer Inst 1998;90:1817–1823.

80. Thompson IM, Pauler DK, Goodman PJ, et al. Prevalence of prostate cancer among men with a prostate-specific antigen level < or =4.0 ng per milliliter. N Engl J Med 2004;350:2239–2246.

81. Holmberg L, Bill-Axelson A, Helgesen F, et al. A randomized trial comparing radical prostatectomy with watchful waiting in early prostate cancer. N Engl J Med 2002;347:781–789.

82. Stanford JL, Stephenson RA, Coyle LM, et al. Prostate Cancer Trends 1973-1995, SEER Program. Bethesda: National Cancer Institute, NIH; 1999. Report No.: 99-4543.

83. Draisma G, Boer R, Otto SJ, et al. Lead times and overdetection due to prostate-specific antigen screening: estimates from the European Randomized Study of Screening for Prostate Cancer. J Natl Cancer Inst 2003;95:868–878.

84. Hankey BF, Feuer EJ, Clegg LX, et al. Cancer surveillance series: interpreting trends in prostate cancer—part I: Evidence of the effects of screening in recent prostate cancer incidence, mortality, and survival rates. J Natl Cancer Inst 1999;91:1017–1024.

85. Labrie F, Candas B, Dupont A, et al. Screening decreases prostate cancer death: first analysis of the 1988 Quebec prospective randomized controlled trial. Prostate 1999;38:83–91.

86. Candas B, Cusan L, Gomez JL, et al. Evaluation of prostatic specific antigen and digital rectal examination as screening tests for prostate cancer. Prostate 2000;45:19–35.

87. Schroder FH, Bangma CH. The European Randomized Study of Screening for Prostate Cancer (ERSPC). Br J Urol 1997;79:68–71.

88. Schroder FH, Kranse R, Rietbergen J, et al. The European Randomized Study of Screening for Prostate Cancer (ERSPC): an update. Members of the ERSPC, Section Rotterdam. Eur Urol 1999;35:539–543.

89. Simpson NK, Johnson CC, Ogden SL, et al. Recruitment strategies in the Prostate, Lung, Colorectal and Ovarian (PLCO) Cancer Screening Trial: the first six years. Control Clin Trials 2000;21:356S–378S.

90. Hasson MA, Fagerstrom RM, Kahane DC, et al. Design and evolution of the data management systems in the Prostate, Lung, Colorectal and Ovarian (PLCO) Cancer Screening Trial. Control Clin Trials 2000;21:329S–348S.

91. Hayes RB, Reding D, Kopp W, et al. Etiologic and early marker studies in the prostate, lung, colorectal and ovarian (PLCO) cancer screening trial. Control Clin Trials 2000;21:349S–355S.

92. Bartsch G, Horninger W, Klocker H, et al. Prostate cancer mortality after introduction of prostate-specific antigen mass screening in the Federal State of Tyrol, Austria. Urology 2001;58:417–424.

93. Horninger W, Reissigl A, Rogatsch H, et al. Prostate cancer screening in the Tyrol, Austria: experience and results. Eur J Cancer 2000;36:1322–1335.

94. Horninger W, Reissigl A, Rogatsch H, et al. Prostate cancer screening in Tyrol, Austria: experience and results. Eur Urol 1999;35:523–538.

95. Feuer EJ, Merrill RM, Hankey BF. Cancer surveillance series: interpreting trends in prostate cancer—part II: Cause of death misclassification and the recent rise and fall in prostate cancer mortality. J Natl Cancer Inst 1999;91:1025–1032.

Screening for prostate cancer: the ERSPC study

40

Fritz H Schröder

INTRODUCTION

Screening for prostate cancer (PC) remains a controversial issue. While the value of early detection and the application of screening tests to individuals has been shown to lead to the diagnosis of usually confined and curable prostate cancer, the value of screening on a population basis has not been proven. In most healthcare systems, screening for prostate cancer will only become acceptable and financed once a significant prostate cancer mortality reduction has been shown in a randomized controlled study comparing a screening with a control arm. Other prerequisites relate to knowledge of the natural history, the effectiveness and acceptability of screening tests, the availability of effective treatment, and the lack of negative effects on quality of life, which might not be in balance with a potential advantage in terms of preventing prostate cancer related deaths.

The European Randomized Study of Screening for Prostate Cancer (ERSPC) was initiated in July 1994 after the initial participants, Belgium and The Netherlands, had completed their pilot studies. The pilot studies were mainly feasibility studies including randomization. The results were encouraging and led to the design of the protocol of ERSPC as a potential European study.

The main goal of ERSPC is to show or exclude in a randomized controlled screening study a positive effect of screening in the screening arm on prostate cancer mortality of at least 20%. Initial sample size calculations were based on a power of 80% to achieve this goal and were later corrected for participation rates and contamination rates by opportunistic screening. The most recent estimates of power and sample size are reported by de Koning et al.[1] The ERSPC considers the age group 55 to 69 years as the core age group. However,

the age segments of 50 to 54 years and 70 to 74 years, which are included in several of the local studies, will also be considered in the final evaluation. The screening interval is 4 years. From the very beginning, the study group realized that quality-of-life studies of all aspects of screening, treatment, and natural history of prostate cancer are an essential adjunct to the study of prostate cancer mortality. Such studies have been established in several centers. A third goal of ERSPC already established in 1993 was the evaluation of the screening tests, a task which was taken on by several centers, but mainly by Rotterdam.

Several recent reviews are available of all aspects of ERSPC.[2-4] The 2003 *British Journal of Urology International* supplement gives an update of the contributions of each individual center, the work of all the Committees, on quality control aspects and on the mechanism of functioning of the independent Data Monitoring Committee. Also, the supplement includes a complete list of the 169 publications related to ERSPC that have appeared up to the year 2003.

THE STRUCTURE OF ERSPC

From the very beginning, as the result of the pilot studies in Belgium and The Netherlands, it became evident that a randomized controlled trial of the anticipated size could for logistic and financial reasons not be conducted in *one* European country. Cooperation of other countries was, therefore, solicited. The precondition was that financing for the screening study in each individual country would be obtained by a local study group. At the same time, the international coordinator, author of this review, took on the challenge to obtain financing for the international coordination of the ERSPC, which included the running of a central database, financing of a semi-annual group meeting, and financing of all the Committees that were necessary to make this decentralized organization functional.

THE COMMITTEES

The **Scientific Committee** (SC) is the decision-taking body of the ERSPC. Each country assigns as many active participants as seems necessary; voting is, however, restricted to two members per country. The Scientific Committee meets two times per year and hears updates per country, a report of the central database, reports of the individual committees, and reports on scientific work that is conducted in individual countries and that is relevant to the progress of the study.

The independent **Data Monitoring Committee** (DMC) is an interdisciplinary committee of scientists that are not directly involved in running a local study group. The DMC is the ethical watchdog of the study. It has established flagging and stopping rules and follows the study along according to the semi-annual reports of the data center. The DMC is the only structure within ERSPC that receives endpoint-related information. The DMC has the right to discontinue the study in line with previously agreed criteria.

Causes of Death Committees are established nationally and internationally. The national Causes of Death Committee evaluates the cause of death in every individual case of prostate cancer within the screening and control group. The committee makes use of a previously agreed computerized algorithm.[5] The international Causes of Death Committee reviews doubtful cases. All Causes of Death Committees report directly to the central database.

The **Epidemiology Committee** (EC) has throughout the years given valuable advice about the set-up and the conduct of the study. It is chaired by the head of the independent data center. The EC shares responsibility on the data collection and presentation and supervises, together with the Scientific Committee, the performance of each individual country.

The **Quality Control Committee** (QCC) watches the conduct of each center, has taken responsibility for collecting information on contamination by opportunistic screening, and has the right to conduct site visits, which are also regularly conducted by the DMC.

The **PSA Committee** conducts a quality control program on the prostate-specific antigen (PSA) test and advises on all related matters.

The **Pathology Committee** has fulfilled a very important role in standardization of pathology reporting, quality control with relation to the Gleason system, and also in relation to the inevitable occurrence of false positive and false negative diagnosis.[6,7]

The decentralized structure of the ERSPC is very different from the Prostate, Lung, Colon, and Ovary (PLCO) screening trial conducted by the National Cancer Institute USA. Both trials have established a close affiliation and plans for common evaluation.[8] Further discussion and updating for the plans for a common evaluation of the ERSPC and the PLCO are at present ongoing.

CONDITIONS FOR PARTICIPATION AND CONTINUED PARTICIPATION IN ERSPC

Obviously, a very large trial with a decentralized structure will require very distinct rules and regulations for participation, and an agreement on procedures and a dataset that is identical for all participants. The ERSPC established these common rules for participation early on during the course of the study.

The minimal dataset is established with input from all centers. Latecomers had little input due to the fact that the study was ongoing. The minimal dataset includes baseline information on participants, the date and result of randomization per participant, information on comorbidity, the prostate cancer screening history, follow-up of all cancer cases in the screening and control arm, results of linkage to the regional cancer registries, the date and cause of death, identification of exclusions after randomization, and a number of other features specific to the screening arm. Detailed information is also required on all cancer cases in both arms concerning the screening history, the mechanism of diagnosis, the TNM staging, treatment, and follow-up information allowing the study of morbidity and causes of death. The central database is located by agreement in an institution that is not a study center. The central database and the datasheets that are used for semi-annual reporting of the individual countries to the central database reflect the minimal dataset on which plans for common analysis of all centers are based.

Obviously, the protocols of the individual countries, which are all reported in detail[4] have to take account of local cultural needs and ethical requirements, which are different in different European countries. Ethical rules allow randomization into a control group without knowledge of the participant. In other countries this type of population-based study is impossible. The ERSPC had to decide to allow two different schemes for randomization which are reproduced in Figure 40.1. Each randomization scheme has potential advantages and pitfalls. Randomization after obtaining an informed consent as it is required in Belgium, The Netherlands, Spain, and Switzerland obviously excludes men from the study who do not wish to be randomized. Participation rate is likely to be high in

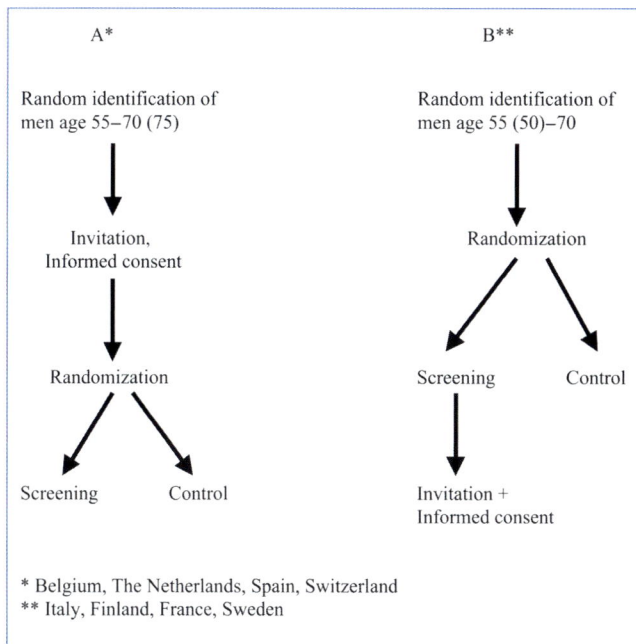

A*

Random identification of
men age 55–70 (75)

↓

Invitation,
Informed consent

↓

Randomization

↙   ↘

Screening   Control

B**

Random identification of
men age 55 (50)–70

↓

Randomization

↙   ↘

Screening   Control

↓

Invitation +
Informed consent

* Belgium, The Netherlands, Spain, Switzerland
** Italy, Finland, France, Sweden

Fig. 40.1
Randomization procedures in the ERSPC. Two different
schemes (A and B) for randomization are used by different
countries.

this setting because of the upfront commitment of men
to participate in the screening. In scheme B, which is
used in Finland, France, Italy, and Sweden participation
rate in the control arm is by definition 100%.
Participation in the screening arm is likely to be lower
because it requires consent to undergo screening after
randomization has taken place. Randomization
according to one of these two algorithms, however, is
a prerequisite for each of the European centers.
Furthermore, all centers are required to live up to the
minimal dataset; no center was permitted in without
having conducted a pilot study showing that
randomization in the local setting was feasible. Local
ethical approval was required; discipline was assured
by making decisions of the Scientific Committee
obligatory. Centers agreed to provide data to the central
database and the DMC on a semi-annual basis, and
there was agreement that all protocol changes would
have to be approved by the Scientific Committee. Other
more practical features relate to the inclusion of the
core age group of 55 to 69 years in every local study,
and repeat screening after an interval of 4 years
(exception Sweden where 2 years was accepted); an
identical screening procedure using PSA as the key
test was agreed. Slight differences per country were
accepted. The centers obliged themselves to guarantee a
follow-up of at least 10 years and preferably longer. Side
studies and publications per center are encouraged but
are to be presented and approved by the Scientific
Committee.

As the years went on, these regulations proved to be
practical and similar sets of criteria were established for

the right of continuous participation and for access to
the central database for common publications of several
centers on a given subject. This system has worked well.
Many aspects of screening for prostate cancer have been
addressed by local and group publications testified by
the complete list of references produced by the ERSPC
up to 2003.[9] Adherence by the individual centers to the
rules of participation and continued participation is
assured by the activities of the Quality Control
Committee, which has effectively interfered on several
occasions.

THE SCREENING PROCEDURES

At the time that the ERSPC was set up it was clear that
PSA made a major contribution to the early detection
of prostate cancer. The pioneering work by Catalona[10]
had shown that with the use of PSA prostate cancer
could be diagnosed more frequently and at earlier
stages. The role of rectal examination and transrectal
ultrasonography were even more uncertain than they
are at this time. The group decided in 1993 that
screening should include a determination of the PSA
levels in serum, and that, subsequently, if possible by
investigators blinded to the result of the PSA test, rectal
examination and transrectal ultrasonography should
be carried out as additional screening tests. This
procedure was followed until April 1997. In November
1995, because of an extremely low positive predictive
value (PPV) of rectal examination in men with PSA
values of between 0 and 0.9 ng/mL, it was
recommended to the group to discontinue rectal
examination in these men. From the beginning, the
Swedish group had utilized a PSA cutoff of 3.0 ng/mL
as a biopsy indication without using rectal
examination and ultrasonography as a screening test.
The group initially did not adopt this policy because of
uncertainties about the aggressiveness of cancer that
were missed by omitting rectal examination in the
PSA range below 4. Data from the ERSPC Rotterdam,
however, suggested that parameters of aggressiveness
were directly related to PSA levels.[11,12] In addition,
modeling of the results of biopsy if every participant in
the lower PSA range were biopsied showed that large
numbers of cancer were missed, specifically in the PSA
range 3.0 to 3.9 ng/mL.[13] On the basis of such data, it
was decided in 1997 to use PSA 3.0 ng/mL or higher
as a biopsy indication and to omit transrectal
ultrasonography and rectal examination as screening
tests. A validation of this new policy was subsequently
carried out in 7943 men.[14] The results are compared
with those from 8612 men screened with the original
regimen. The data are reproduced in Table 40.1.
Logistic regression analysis had estimated that half of
the cancers in the PSA range 3 to 4 ng/mL were missed.
The validation study showed that rectal examination

Table 40.1 Biopsy indications and cancer detection

		PSA 4.0 ng/mL + DRE or TRUS (1994–1996)	PSA >= 3.0 ng/mL; no DRE or TRUS (1996–1997)	p-value
A	Total number screened	8612	7943	–
B	Number of DRE and TRUS done [%]	8612 [100]	1302 [16.4]	<0.001
C	Number of biopsies for PSA 3.0–3.9 ng/mL	642	534	0.07
D	Total number of biopsies [%]	2365 [27.4]	1552 [19.5]	<0.001
E	Number with PC for PSA 3.0–3.9 ng/mL [%]	41 [6.4]	96 [18.0]	0.32
F	Total number with PC [detection rate, %]	430 [5.0]	377 [4.7]	0.47
G	Overall PPV* (F/D 100, %)	18.2	24.3	<0.001
H	PPV* for PSA 3.0–3.9 ng/mL (E/C 100, %)	6.4	18.0	<0.001

*PPV is calculated for intension to biopsy.

DRE, digital rectal examination; PC, prostate cancer; PSA, prostate-specific antigen; PPV, positive predictive value; TRUS, transrectal ultrasound.

Modified after Schröder FH, Roobol-Bouts M, Vis AN, Kwast TH van der, Kranse R. PSA based early detection of prostate cancer – Validation of screening without rectal examination. Urology 2001;57:83–90.

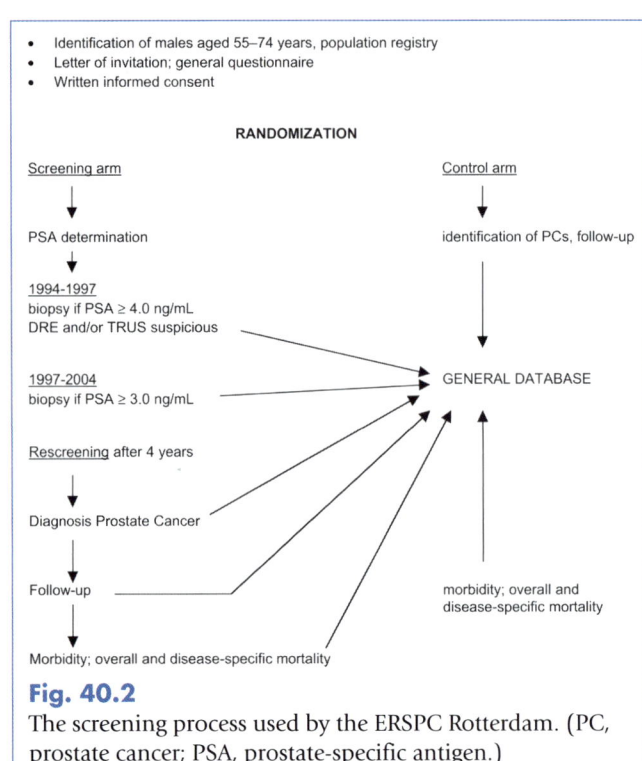

Fig. 40.2
The screening process used by the ERSPC Rotterdam. (PC, prostate cancer; PSA, prostate-specific antigen.)

missed two of three cancers in that PSA range. The detection rate in both sets of the Rotterdam study were almost identical and amounted to 5.0% and 4.7% respectively. The group realized at the time the change was applied that some aggressive cancers that occurred in the low PSA ranges might be missed by omitting rectal examination. The assumption, however, was that most of the cancers would be found at the subsequent screening round, still in a curable stage. Only the final outcome of the study can show whether these assumptions were correct. A flow diagram of the screening procedures of the Rotterdam study is given as an example in Figure 40.2.

BIOPSY TECHNIQUE

Up to the appearance of a paper by Eskew et al 1997,[15] a classical sextant prostatic biopsy was used. After this date, a recommendation was accepted to liberalize sextant biopsies, which according to the data of Eskew would only lead to missing 5% of cancers that would be detectable with 13 biopsies on average. In order to keep the ERSPC dataset consistent, most centers have not changed biopsy indications over time. However, in some centers where clinical practice changed uniformly toward the use of more biopsies, in order to stay in line

with the control group, a switch to screening with more than six biopsies was made. This is specifically the case in Finland.

SECOND ROUND TESTING

Second round testing in the ERSPC takes place after 4 years, with the exception of the Swedish study which re-screens after 2 years. The biopsy indication is unchanged: biopsies are recommended if a serum PSA level of 3.0 ng/mL or higher is found. This means that, as well as a smaller group of men who already had a biopsy indication during the first round but in whom no cancer was found, those men were biopsied who showed PSA progression from lower levels to levels above 3.0 ng/mL. Within the ERSPC, the risk of PSA progression to values above 4 ng/mL and values above 3 ng/mL were studied separately. Four-year PSA progression to above 3 ng/mL varied between 10% and 25% for PSA values in first round screening of 1 to 2.9 ng/mL.[16] In the combined Spanish and Rotterdam evaluation, the risk of PSA progression was shown to be strongly dependent on initial PSA values, age, and interval.[17] Probably the key observation, however, was made by comparing the PPV of PSA between round 1 and round 2.[18] In round 2 the correlation between PPV and PSA values above 3 ng/mL was lost. This means that the PPV of a PSA of 10 ng/mL was identical to that of a PSA of 3.0 ng/mL found in round 2. The data are illustrated in Figure 40.3. In the same study, it was shown that PSA doubling time and PSA velocity on a population basis added only very little to a PSA value of 3 ng/mL as a biopsy indication in round 2. This was confirmed in another study, which showed that only prostatic volume determined by ultrasound was a significant negative predictor. The relationship of prostatic volume to PPV is inverse. Prostatic cancer volume was compared for 185 radical prostatectomy cases of first round and 147 radical prostatectomy cases for second round cancers. 4-mm step sections were used to evaluate total tumor volume. While tumor volumes were significantly smaller in round 2, the correlation between PSA and tumor volumes remained significant in both rounds.[20] The available data are compatible with the view that even a 4-year interval is not sufficient to allow regrowth of cancers to a level that would restore the relationship between PSA and PPV seen in the first round. This is in line with recent observations on lead-time, which will be referred to later in this chapter.

RECTAL EXAMINATION

While our studies have clearly shown that rectal examination has an unacceptably low PPV in the low PSA ranges, its value with respect to selecting for cases that represent a risk to their carrier and can still be cured is unclear at this moment. It is likely that the overdiagnosis that is inherent to screening mainly occurs in those cases that are not palpable, and which are diagnosed exclusively by PSA-driven biopsies—the T1c cases. Studies that allow evaluation of rectal examination as a test to make screening more selective for aggressive and curable cases are urgently needed and, fortunately, ongoing.

PRESENT STATUS OF PROGRESS OF THE ERSPC

The ERSPC is far advanced. In all but one center, recruitment and second round screening has been completed. In the centers that joined ERSPC early on in

1994 and 1995, follow-up ranges between 6 and 7 years. The database was updated in May 2004 and contains 5534 prostate cancer cases detected in 205,897 men randomized either to the screening or control group. The data are given in Table 40.2. France only joined the ERSPC in 2003, and its input into the final analysis of ERSPC will be limited by the short follow-up period.

Data collection in all the ERSPC centers depends on linkage to regional cancer registries. All causes of deaths in prostate cancer cases are verified by local or international Causes of Death Committees. The process requires, on average, 1 year, which has to be added to the follow-up period of 10 years determined by the protocol based on power estimates (see below).

POWER AND OUTCOME

The power calculation of ERSPC as a whole was recently updated.[1] The diagram showing the development of power in relation to time and hypothetical differences in prostate cancer mortality, which may be discovered in the ERSPC, is reproduced as Figure 40.4. The calculations consider the so-called "core age group" of age 55 to 69 years, which is common to all participating centres; men of age 50 to 55 and 70 to 74 years will, however, be included in the final analysis. The calculations also take account of two major factors that influence the power of a randomized screening trial: participation rates and contamination. From Figure 40.4 it is obvious that power is very strongly dependent on the difference that eventually will occur between prostate cancer mortality in the screening and in the control arm. If the difference amounts to 20%, the study would only have a power of 70% by 2008. If, however, a difference of 30% were seen, a power of 80% would already be reached in 2005. It is on this background that the Scientific Committee has decided to initiate endpoint evaluations without statistical testing in 2004. Obviously, the results of such evaluations will only be made known at the level of the independent Data Monitoring Committee.

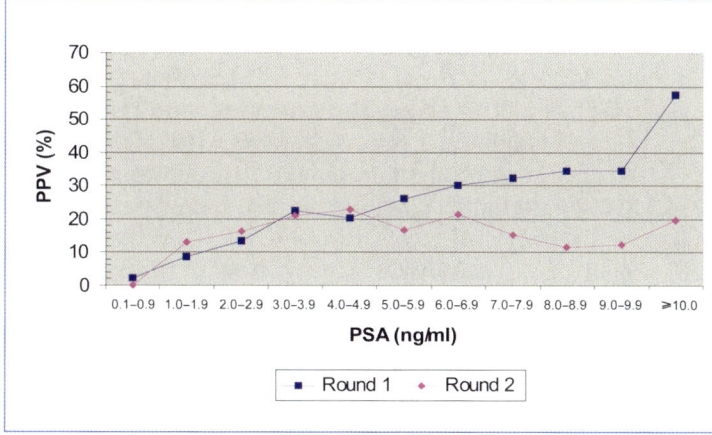

Fig. 40.3

Differences in the positive predictive value (PPV) of prostate-specific antigen (PSA) between the initial (first) and second screening rounds, stratified by PSA range.
Reprinted from Urology, 98, Raaijmakers R, Wildhagen MF, Ito K, et al. Prostate-specific antigen change in the European Randomized Study of Screening for Prostate Cancer, section Rotterdam, 316–320, 2004, with permission from Elsevier.

Table 40.2 European Randomized Study of Screening for Prostate Cancer (ERSPC) — recruitment and diagnosis of prostate cancer in eight participating countries, 1994–2004 (May)

Country	Randomization			Screened (C) [% of A]	Cancer in A [% of C]	Cancer in B [period]
	Screen (A)	Control [B]	Total			
Belgium	5055	5035	10,090	4483 [88.7]	189 [4.2]	127 [1991–2004]
Finland	32,000	48,458	80,458	20,792 [65.0]	1212 [5.8]	747 [1996–2004]
France [start 2003]	12,128	11,703	23,831	2031 [16.7]	25 [1.2]	12 [2003–2004]
Italy	7518	7495	15,013	5107 [67.9]	134 [2.6]	42 [1996–2004]
Netherlands	21,210	21,166	42,376	19,970 [94.1]	1580 [7.9]	574 [1994–2004]
Spain	2416	1862	4287	2416 [100]	76 [3.2]	15 [1996–2004]
Sweden	9972	9973	19,945	5855 [58.7]	431 [7.4]	292 [1994–2004]
Switzerland	4948	4958	9906	4938 [99.8]	160 [3.2]	2 [1998–2004]
Total	92,247	110,650	205,897	111,093*	3723* [4.04]	1811

*Data relate to all screening rounds, ongoing.

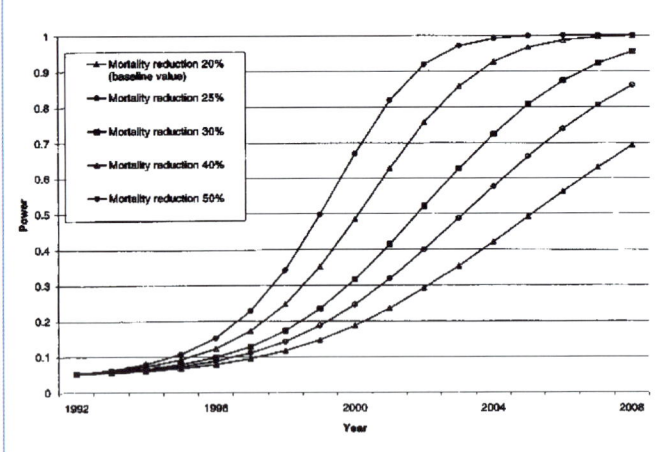

Fig. 40.4
Expected prostate cancer mortality in men entering the ERSPC trial after exclusion of prevalent prostate cancer cases at the start of the trial (as a percentage of national prostate cancer mortality rates).
From de Koning HJ, Liem MK, Baan CA, Boer R, Schroder FH, Alexander FE. ERSPC. Prostate cancer mortality reduction by screening: power and time frame with complete enrollment in the European Randomised Screening for Prostate Cancer (ERSPC) trial. Int J Cancer 2002;98:268–273.

CONTAMINATION

Contamination, the use of screening tests outside the screening protocol influences the power calculation adversely in an exponential fashion. The Scientific Committee of the ERSPC has agreed that contamination is to be studied in all centers. A recent summary of results per center is given by Ciatto et al.[21] The data are inhomogeneous and difficult to interpret. A clear definition of contamination is lacking. Prostate-specific antigen tests can be done for different reasons, and represent contamination only if the resulting biopsy indications in fact lead to biopsies. It is difficult to evaluate contamination at this level. In the Rotterdam center "effective contamination" in this sense was found in 3% of control group participants per year amounting potentially to a 30% contamination rate during the 10 year follow-up period.[22] However, contamination during the first years and during the last years of a follow-up period of 10 years cannot have the same impact on outcome, considering the protracted national history of prostate cancer. The sample size calculations

and the power calculations of the ERSPC take account of 20% of contamination overall. If this correction turns out to be insufficient, the only way to correct for this is by prolongation of follow-up, a measure that may have to be taken if this situation occurs.

LEAD-TIME AND OVERDIAGNOSIS

By definition, effective screening advances the point in time at which prostate cancer is diagnosed. The added time is called lead-time. Prostate cancer occurs in men in their 60s and 70s, a period of life in which other causes of death are prevalent. Population-based statistics show that, prior to the PSA era, which started in the early 1990s, one in two men diagnosed with prostate cancer would die of this disease (intercurrent death occurred in about 50%). McGregor estimated that with PSA-driven screening one in seven carriers of screen-detected prostate cancers might be at risk of dying of prostate cancer and could be saved by active treatment.[23] Overdiagnosis—defined as the diagnosis of cases that would otherwise not be diagnosed during a lifetime—varies according to different estimates between about 40% and 90%.[24] In relation to the Rotterdam section of the ERSPC, lead-times and overdiagnosis rates were estimated by MISCAN modelling.[25] The MISCAN data on lead-time and overdiagnosis are summarized in Table 40.3. The mean lead-time for the ERSPC study is estimated to be in the range of 11 to 12 years, overdiagnosis is in the range of 48% to 53%, and, with a 4-year screening interval, lifetime risk is raised by 65%. These numbers are worrisome and show that in the future it will be necessary to make screening for prostate cancer more selective for those cases that pose a threat to their carriers and are still curable. This issue may represent the main research task for our profession for years to come. The proper selection and follow-up of cases for watchful waiting may be the easiest approach.

FOLLOW-UP

Follow-up of all cancer cases and the determination of the causes of death of all noncancer cases are part of the dataset that has been agreed between all centers. Follow-up is achieved by yearly linkage to cancer registries and the statistical databases of the individual countries for non-cancer-related deaths. Several centers, in addition, follow all cancer cases by yearly chart review. All resulting data are reported on a semi-annual basis to the study group independent data center.

The period of follow-up of 10 years, which was used in the original sample size calculation of the ERSPC, was based on natural history data of clinical cases, obviously not on screen-detected cases. The natural history of screen-detected cases is still, to a large extent, unknown. The long lead-times calculated by different groups and different techniques,[24] which may be in the range or excess of 10 years, suggest that longer follow-up periods are necessary. The progress of the ERSPC will allow a better estimate of the needed follow-up period. Work on this issue is in progress. As shown above, the required follow-up period strongly depends on the potential

difference in prostate cancer mortality that may be shown between screening and control.

CONCLUSIONS

The ERSPC is far advanced and seems set to resolve the issue of whether mortality reduction from prostate cancer can be achieved by screening. Depending on the difference in mortality that may be seen between the two arms of the study, and taking account of the delay occurring through linkage to cancer registries, the endpoint of the ERSPC will probably be sometime between 2006 and 2010. If larger differences occur, obviously, such differences could be detected earlier. A more detailed summary of the ERSPC was recently published.[26]

The ERSPC has produced a wealth of information on various aspects of early detection of prostate cancer, as well as standardization of evaluation techniques used in the study. A regularly updated list of references is found on the website of the ERSPC (www.erspc.org). If the ERSPC, possibly in conjunction with PLCO, shows a significant difference in prostate cancer mortality at an acceptable price in terms of quality of life, this will lead to the acceptance of population-based screening of prostate cancer in most countries around the world. Healthcare providers may, however, find the amount of inherent overdiagnosis and overtreatment unacceptable. Here lies a major task for clinical research in years to come.

If the ongoing randomized studies do not show a significant reduction of prostate cancer mortality by screening, however, it is likely that opportunistic screening will still go on. The notion that prostate cancer can be detected early and treated early will remain convincing to some men, together with the clinical finding that prostate cancer with aggressive features can be treated effectively if diagnosed early.

ACKNOWLEDGMENTS

The author is grateful to Mrs Ellen van den Berg for managing this manuscript. The ERSPC has been supported by multiple national and international grants. The coordination has been continuously supported by the European Union programs "Europe against Cancer" and the "Framework Programmes 5 and 6." National support has recently been indicated in detail in Schröder et al.[26]

Table 40.3 Lead-time and overdetection

Single screen at age (years)	Mean lead-time (years)	Screening program	Mean lead-time (years)	Overdiagnosis %
55	12.3	yearly, 55–67	12.3	27
60	11.0	4-yearly, 55–67	11.2	38
65	9.5	4-yearly, 55–75	10.3	47
70	7.7			53
75	6.0			56

From Draisma et al. 2002

REFERENCES

1. de Koning HJ, Liem MK, Baan CA, et al. Prostate cancer mortality reduction by screening: power and time frame with complete enrollment in the European Randomised Screening for Prostate Cancer (ERSPC) trial. Int J Cancer. 2002;98:268–273.

2.   de Koning HJ, Auvinen A, Berenguer Sanchez A, et al; European Randomized Screening for Prostate Cancer (ERSPC) Trial; International Prostate Cancer Screening Trials Evaluation Group. Large-scale randomized prostate cancer screening trials: program performances in the European Randomized Screening for Prostate Cancer trial and the Prostate, Lung, Colorectal and Ovary cancer trial. Int J Cancer 2002;97:237–244.

3.   Schröder FH. Screening for Prostate Cancer. Urol Clin North Am 2003;30:239–251.

4.   Roobol MJ, Schröder FH (eds). BJUI supplement 2003:92 Suppl. 2.

5.   de Koning HJ, Blom J, Merkelbach JW, et al. Determining the cause of death in randomized screening trial(s) for prostate cancer. BJU Int 2003;Vol 92 (Suppl. 2):71–78.

6.   van der Kwast TH, Lopes C, Martikainen PM, et al. Report of the Pathology Committee: false-positive and false-negative diagnoses of prostate cancer. BJU Int 2003;92 (Suppl. 2):62–65.

7.   van der Kwast TH, Roobol MJ, Wildhagen MF, et al. Consistency of prostate cancer grading results in screened populations across Europe. BJU Int 2003;92 (Suppl. 2):88–91.

8.   Auvinen A, Rietbergen JBW, Denis LJ, et al. Prospective evaluation plan for randomised trials of prostate cancer screening. J Med Screening 1996;3:97–104.

9.   Roobol MJ and Schröder FH. European Randomized Study of Screening for Prostate Cancer: achievements and presentation. BJU Int 2003;92 (Suppl. 2):117–122.

10.   Catalona WJ, Smith DS, Ratliff TL, et al. Measurement of prostate-specific antigen in serum as a screening test for prostate cancer. N Engl J Med 1991;324:1156–1161.

11.   Schröder FH, Van der Maas PJ, Beemsterboer PMM, et al. Evaluation of the digital rectal examination (DRE) as a screening test for prostate cancer. J Natl Cancer Inst 1998;90:1817–1823.

12.   Schröder FH, van der Cruijsen-Koeter I, de Koning HJ, et al. Prostate cancer detection at low prostate specific antigen. J Urol 2000;163:806–812.

13.   Kranse R, Beemsterboer PMM, Rietbergen JBW, et al. Predictors for Biopsy Outcome in the European Randomized Study of Screening for Prostate Cancer (Rotterdam region). Prostate 1999;39:316–322.

14.   Schröder FH, Roobol-Bouts M, Vis AN, et al. PSA based early detection of prostate cancer—Validation of screening without rectal examination. Urology 2001;57:83–90.

15.   Eskew LA, Bare RL, McCullough DL. Systematic 5 region prostate biopsy is superior to sextant method for diagnosing carcinoma of the prostate. J Urol 1997;157:199–203.

16.   Schröder FH, Raaijmakers R, Postma R, et al. Four year PSA progression and diagnosis of prostate cancer in the European Randomized Study of Screening for Prostate Cancer (ERSPC), section Rotterdam. 2005;174:489–494.

17.   Paez A, Lujan M, Raaijmakers R, Berenguer A and members of ERSPC. Four-year prostate-specific antigen progression in the non-cancer population of the European Randomized Study of Screening for Prostate Cancer. BJU Int 2003;92 (Suppl. 2):84–87.

18.   Raaijmakers R, Wildhagen MF, Ito K, et al. Prostate-specific antigen change in the European Randomized Study of Screening for Prostate Cancer, section Rotterdam. Urology 2004;63:316–320.

19.   Roobol MJ, Kranse R, De Koning, HJ, et al. Prostate-specific antigen velocity at low prostate-specific antigen levels as screening tool for prostate cancer: Results of second screening round of ERSPC (Rotterdam). Urology 2004;63:309–315.

20.   Postma R. Personal communication 2004.

21.   Ciatto S, Zappa M, Villers A, et al. Contamination by opportunistic screening in the European Randomized Study of Prostate Cancer Screening. BJU Int 2003;92 (Suppl. 2):97–100.

22.   Otto SJ, van der Cruijsen IW, Liem MK, et al. Effective PSA contamination in the Rotterdam section of the European Randomized Study of Screening for Prostate Cancer. Int J Cancer 2003;105:394–399.

23.   McGregor M, Hanley JA, Boivin JF, et al. Screening for prostate cancer: estimating the magnitude of overdetection. CMAJ 1998;159:1368–1372.

24.   Draisma G, de Koning HJ. MISCAN: estimating lead-time and over-detection by simulation. BJU Int 2003;92 (Suppl. 2):106–111.

25.   Draisma G, Boer R, Otto SJ, et al. Lead times and overdetection due to prostate-specific antigen screening: estimates from the European Randomized Study of Screening for Prostate Cancer. J Natl Cancer Inst 2003;95:868–878.

26.   Schröder FH, Denis LJ, Roobol M and all participants of ERSPC. The story of the European Randomized Study of Screening for Prostate Cancer. BJU Int 2003;92 (Suppl. 2):1–13.

Screening for prostate cancer and its effect on mortality: the Tyrol study

41

Wolfgang Horninger, Andreas Berger, Alexandre Pelzer, Helmut Klocker,
Wilhelm Oberaigner, Dieter Schönitzer, Gianluca Severi,
Chris Robertson, Peter Boyle, Georg Bartsch

INTRODUCTION

In the early 90s, a remarkable increase in the incidence of prostate cancer in many countries, particularly in the United States,[1] was observed. This observation can be attributed to the widespread use of prostate-specific antigen (PSA), which was first approved for the detection of recurrent disease in patients with established prostate cancer in 1986. Thereafter, the potential of this test for early diagnosis of prostate cancer was soon recognized. From 1984 until 1994, PSA was increasingly used for diagnostic purposes. In 1984, PSA testing was used in 5.1% and in 1994 in 60.6% of all newly diagnosed prostate carcinomas.[2] It has been shown that a great number of cancers detected by PSA testing are clinically significant and potentially curable.[3-6]

However, the introduction of PSA testing in prostate cancer screening programs has also led to controversy surrounding several distinct issues, including the sensitivity and specificity of the screening test; treatment of early prostate cancer and, indeed, whether some cancers will do equally well if left untreated; and the side effects of therapy, particularly radical prostatectomy. The two most common cancer screening programs—Papanicolaou smears for cervical cancer and mammographic examination for breast cancer—came into common use and acceptance through widely different mechanisms: the results of randomized trials of mammographic screening for breast cancer, and the observation of the decrease in incidence and mortality from cervical cancer after the policy to introduce cervical cancer screening to populations. The present study reports the incidence and mortality rates of prostate cancer in the Federal State of Tyrol, Austria, where regular PSA testing has been made freely available to the population since 1993, and where use of the test has been high. This population is also characterized by being particularly stable. Prostate-specific antigen testing was not freely available in the rest of Austria, although it will have been used, probably evolving in a similar manner to the use in many Western countries. A comparison of the mortality rates between Tyrol and the rest of Austria allowed evaluation of the outcome of this natural experiment.

MATERIAL AND METHODS

In 1993, a mass screening project using PSA as the only screening test was launched in the Federal State of Tyrol (one of nine federal states of the Republic of Austria). Previously (1988 to 1992), both PSA and digital rectal examination (DRE) were available and used in the diagnostic workup of symptomatic patients and, in a limited way, for asymptomatic men. Since 1989, urologists at the Innsbruck University Hospital have promoted the concept of early prostate cancer detection using PSA and DRE. From 1989 to 1992, the number of PSA tests performed in this hospital rose from 2360 to 5878.

Tyrol is an alpine region in Western Austria with, at the 1991 census, 631,410 inhabitants (324,161 women and 307,249 men) in an area of 12,647 square kilometers. The region is dominated by the mountains of the Central Alps, and the distances to Innsbruck, the capital, where the central healthcare unit is located, are not too far (infrequently more than 100 kilometers). This geographic situation, as well as the willingness of the general population to participate in preventative medical programs, caused us to launch a statewide mass screening program with PSA as the only screening test for the early detection of prostate cancer. PSA testing was made freely available by the Social Insurance Company of the Federal State of Tyrol and the University Hospital of Innsbruck to all men aged 45 to 75 years. All men in this age range were advised and encouraged to undergo PSA testing, and information to this effect was distributed to all Tyrolean men by press, radio, and television.

The screening project was performed in collaboration with general practitioners, medical examiners, urologists, medical laboratories, and the Tyrol Blood Bank of the Red Cross. Informed consent was obtained from all volunteers participating in the program. All coworkers were fully informed of the guidelines for withdrawal, storage, and shipping of the blood samples. Prostate-specific antigen was assessed immediately on arrival of the blood or serum sample. All volunteers and/or referring physicians were informed about the results. In the case of elevated PSA levels, the volunteers were invited to undergo additional urologic evaluations, and the men with normal PSA levels were invited to have a repeated PSA test 12 months later. More than 80% of all volunteers found to have an elevated PSA level consented to an additional evaluation, which included DRE, transrectal ultrasonography (TRUS), and prostate biopsy. At the time of drawing blood for PSA measurement, no DRE was performed. Several scientific projects[7-11] have been published describing this screening program.

This mass screening program was provided free of charge to men between 45 and 75 years old and to younger men with a family history of prostate cancer. Age-referenced PSA levels[12] in combination with percent free PSA of less than 22%, were initially used as the biopsy criteria. Since October 1995, so called "bisected" PSA levels[13] (one half the age-specific reference ranges; Table 41.1) together with percent free PSA levels of less than 18% were used. Since 2001, complexed PSA was also included in our diagnostic workup. Screened volunteers with a PSA level greater than 10 ng/mL were recommended to undergo biopsy irrespective of their percent free PSA. Since March 1996, PSA transition zone density[11] has been introduced as an additional diagnostic parameter in selecting patients for biopsy to decrease the number of unnecessary biopsies. All men

who, according to bisected age-referenced levels and free PSA concentrations, had an elevated PSA concentration were invited to undergo additional urologic evaluation, including DRE and ultrasound-guided biopsies. Urologists performed the DREs and TRUS examinations.

Sextant biopsies were initially made using ultrasound guidance with an automatic biopsy gun and an 18-gauge needle; since 1995, 10 systematic biopsies were carried out, and since 2000, additional contrast enhanced color Doppler-targeted biopsies have been performed.

Patients presenting with organ-confined lesions (T1 and T2) underwent radical prostatectomy or external beam radiotherapy if surgery was not acceptable to them (70.2 Gy, single fraction 1.8 Gy, four-box technique); those with stage T3 lesions underwent external beam radiotherapy (70.2 Gy, single fraction 1.8 Gy, four-box technique); and those with metastatic disease underwent androgen deprivation therapy. Every patient with N1 or M1 disease received hormonal therapy. The policy was such that no patient was treated primarily by surveillance ("watchful waiting").

Data on cancer incidence have been available from the population-based Tyrol Cancer Registry since 1988. Cancer mortality data have been available, independently, from the Austrian Central Statistics Office since 1970. The underlying cause of death was attributed from the death certificates of all deaths in Austria by the Central Statistical Office in Vienna, where they were unaware of the study being performed in Tyrol. The numbers of cases and population estimates are available, annually, in 5-year classes of age. Prostate-specific antigen tests were available at no charge for men aged 45 to 75 years, although use among men on either side of these age limits also occurred.

All incidence and mortality rates were calculated for the truncated age range (40 to 79 years) using the World standard population as the reference.[14]

The principal hypotheses tested were:

1. Whether the prostate cancer mortality rates in Tyrol decreased from 1993.
2. Whether the trends in the prostate cancer mortality rates in Tyrol differed from those in the rest of Austria from 1993.

The trends in the mortality rates in Tyrol and the rest of Austria were compared within a Poisson regression model:

$$\log(\text{rate}) = \beta0 + \beta1(\text{year} - 1993) + \beta2(\text{year} - 1993)I(\text{year} \geq 1993) + \beta3\text{Tyrol} + \beta4\text{Tyrol} \times (\text{year} - 1993) + \beta5\text{Tyrol} \times (\text{year} - 1993)I(\text{year} \geq 1993)$$

This is a "change-point" model in which the term "I(year ≥ 1993)" is an indicator that permits a different slope from 1993 onward compared with before 1993. The parameter β0 gives the estimated log mortality rate in the rest of Austria in 1993; β3 represents the difference from this value in Tyrol. A priori, no

Table 41.1 Bisected age-specific reference ranges for total PSA	
Age (years)	**Normal range (ng/mL)**
45–49	0–1.25
50–59	0–1.75
60–69	0–2.25
70–75	0–3.25

difference was anticipated. The slope of the relationship between the log mortality rates and time was given by β1 in the rest of Austria and β1 + β4 in Tyrol; thus β4 represented the difference in slopes before 1993. The parameter β2 gave an estimate of any change in slope from 1993 onward compared with 1992 and before in the rest of Austria. If no change occurred, the estimated value would be about 0; if treatment advances have occurred, a negative estimate would be expected. In Tyrol, the change in the slope from 1993 onward was given by β2 + β5. Thus β5 was the crucial parameter in the analysis, as it measured the different slope in Tyrol compared with the rest of Austria from 1993 onward. The goodness of fit of the model was established on the basis of residual plots, and the hypothesis tests were based on changes in the deviance.[15] All statistical analysis was carried out using Splus 2000.[16]

In this analysis we used 1993 as the reference year. This was the beginning of the period at which the practice was different with regard to PSA testing in Tyrol compared with the rest of Austria and so represents the earliest time at which any changes in the trend associated with the mass screening program might theoretically begin. Any other choice of reference year, such as 1995, could be open to criticism on the basis of a post hoc choice, even though one might argue that the earliest time one might begin to see a real benefit from screening would be about 2 years after the introduction. This is because the median survival time for metastatic prostate cancer is about 18 months. If the mass screening program had an effect on the mortality rates, using the earlier date would tend to give conservative results, since no difference in the rates in the two regions should occur for a certain period after the introduction of the mass screening program. The estimated benefit of the mass screening program was calculated by comparing the observed and expected numbers of deaths in Tyrol and by examining the prostate cancer mortality trends in the two regions. The expected numbers of cases and deaths for each year in Tyrol were calculated using the average of the rates from 1986 to 1990 as the reference. The effect of using the data for 1988 to 1990 in the calculation of the expected values should be conservative for incidence and have no influence on mortality.

RESULTS

During 1993, when PSA testing became freely available, 32.3% of all Tyrolean men between 45 and 75 years old underwent PSA screening, and at least 70% of this population were tested at least once during the first 10 years of the study. At the laboratory of the Department of Urology, Innsbruck University, more than 96,000 men were screened at least once. Of these, 10,100 were aged 45 to 49 years and 4900 were aged 40 to 44 years. Thus, a substantial number of men aged 40 to 44 were screened, justifying the inclusion of this age group in the analysis of the incidence and mortality rates.

From 1993 to 2001, 6024 transrectal prostate needle biopsies—as described above—were performed. The overall prostate cancer detection rate was 30.2%. Table 41.2 shows the major and minor complications of the 6024 transrectal biopsies.

The incidence of prostate cancer in men aged 40 to 79 years in Tyrol increased from 1988 to 1994 and has remained constant since (Figure 41.1). The incidence of organ-confined disease (Stages I and II) continued to increase from 1988 until 1998, although the incidence of extraprostatic disease (Stage III) declined following a peak in 1994. The incidence of metastatic disease (Stage IV) has been declining since 1993 (Figure 41.2). The stage reported to the Cancer Registry is a mixture of clinical and pathologic stages.

Since the beginning of the screening project, a significant migration to lower total PSA levels in patients undergoing radical prostatectomy has been

Table 41.2 Complications of 6024 transrectal needle prostate biopsies (n = 6024)

Complications	%
Gross hematuria >1 day	12.5
Haemospermia	29.8
Significant pain	4.0
Rectal bleeding	0.6
Nausea	0.8
Fever >38.5°C	0.8
Epididymitis	0.7
Sepsis	0.3

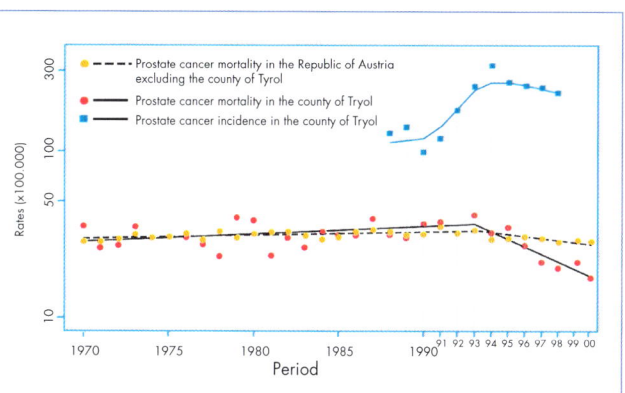

Fig. 41.1

Prostate cancer incidence rates in Tyrol and prostate cancer mortality rates in Tyrol and in the rest of Austria.

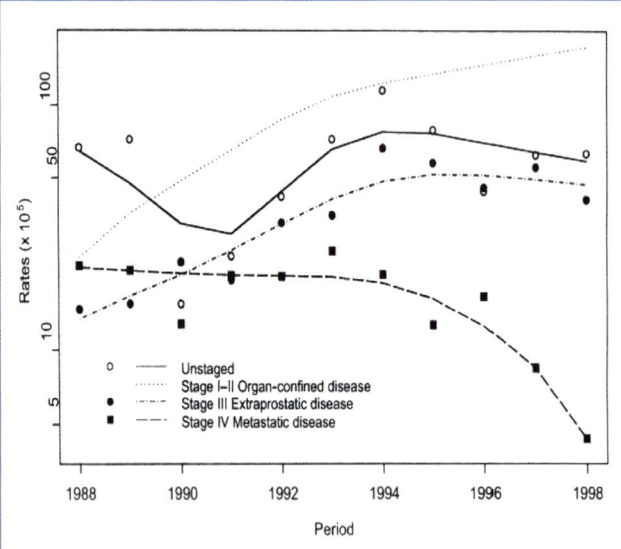

Fig. 41.2

Prostate cancer incidence rates in Tyrol by stage in men aged 40 to 79 years.

Table 41.4 Expected and observed numbers of prostate cancer deaths in the Federal State of Tyrol

Year	Deaths expected	Deaths observed [SMR % change]	SMR, % [95% CI]
1991	44	50	114 [84–150]
1992	43	44	101 [74–136]
1993*	43	52	121 [90–159]
1994	43	42	97 [70–132]
1995	45	45	101 [74–135]
1996	47	21	79 [56–109]
1997	49	33 [–32]	67 [46–94]
1998	52	30 [–42]	58 [39–82]
1999	55	37 [–33]	68 [48–93]
2000	57	32 [–44]	59 [39–80]

*Year when mass screening for prostate-specific antigen was introduced.

SMR, standardized mortality ratio.

observed. Subsequently, the rate of organ confined disease in radical prostatectomy increased from 28.7% in 1993 to over 80% in 2002 (Table 41.3).

The mortality from prostate cancer in Tyrol decreased significantly between 1993 and 2000, in contrast to the modest downward trend in prostate cancer death rates observed in the rest of Austria (see Figure 41.1). On the basis of the age-specific prostate cancer mortality rates in Tyrol between 1986 and 1990, 22 fewer prostate cancer deaths in the age range 40 to 79 occurred in 1998 than were expected, 18 fewer deaths than expected occurred in 1999 and 25 fewer deaths than expected occurred in the year 2000 (Table 41.4).

The fitted values of the model, described above, are shown in Figure 41.1. No significant difference was found between the trends in Tyrol and the rest of Austria

Table 41.3 Total prostate-specific antigen and stage migration in radical prostatectomies since 1993

Year	Mean PSA (ng/mL)	Stage (% of organ-confined prostate cancer)
1993	14.9	28.7
1994	14.2	27.6
1995	12.7	25.1
1996	9.7	55.8
1997	8.6	65.7
1998	6.3	67.2
1999	6.2	79.1
2000	5.8	82.1
2001	5.3	82.0
2002	4.8	81.0

before 1993 (χ^2 = 1.12, 1 degree of freedom, P = 0.29). The log mortality rates increased at a rate of 0.0113 (standard error [SE] 0.005) per year in Tyrol and 0.0057 (SE 0.0014) in the rest of Austria from 1970 up to and including 1992. No significant difference was found between the estimated rates in 1993 in the two regions of Austria (P = 0.13). A decrease in mortality occurred in Tyrol after 1993 (χ^2 = 12.74, 1 degree of freedom, P = 0.0004), where the log mortality rates decreased at a rate of 0.092 (SE 0.024) per year from 1993 onward. In the rest of Austria, the decrease was 0.0229 (SE 0.0064) per year. From 1993 onward, the trends in the rates show a significant difference between Tyrol and the rest of Austria (χ^2 = 7.55, 1 degree of freedom, P = 0.006). In the analysis, we assumed linear trends between the log mortality rates and year, permitting changes in slopes from 1993 onward in Tyrol and in the rest of Austria. We tested whether the change in the slope from 1993 onward was the same in Tyrol as in the rest of Austria. This hypothesis was rejected. Although no statistically significant differences were observed between Tyrol and the rest of Austria before 1993, the fitted value in Tyrol in 1993 was slightly higher than in the rest of Austria (see Figure 41.1), and this may have some implications for the change in the slope. To investigate the effect of this, we constrained the line before 1993 to be exactly the same in Tyrol as in the rest of Austria. This was achieved by setting $\beta3$ and $\beta4$ both equal to 0 in the model. The rate of increase in the log mortality rate was 0.0061 (SE 0.0013) per year, which was very similar to that for the rest of Austria, as Tyrol is a small part of Austria. In the rest of Austria, the rate of decrease from 1993 onward was 0.0246 (SE 0.0063) per year, and in Tyrol, it was 0.0709 (SE 0.0197) per year. The test statistic for the comparison of the slopes from 1993 onward was χ^2 = 5.38, P = 0.02. Thus, our conclusions were only slightly tempered.

Taking 1995 as the year at which the first change can be reasonably expected yielded a rate of decrease in the rest of Austria from 1995 onward of 0.0309 (SE 0.0104) per year; in Tyrol, it was 0.1505 (SE 0.0410) per year. The latter figure was almost double the corresponding decrease from 1993, and the rate of decrease in the rest of Austria was one-third greater. These rates of decrease are significantly different (χ^2 = 7.99, P = 0.0047). Constraining the lines to be identical in Tyrol and the rest of Austria before 1995 yielded very similar results. In the rest of Austria, the rate of decrease was 0.0328 (SE 0.0103) per year, and in Tyrol, it was significantly greater at 0.1259 (SE 0.0355) per year (P = 0.0098).

DISCUSSION

Three possibilities could lead to a reduction in the mortality rate from prostate cancer: 1) prevention of the disease; 2) detection of the disease at a stage when it is more likely to be curable; and 3) improvement in the outcome of therapy for metastatic disease. A fourth possibility, that screening would bring forward the time of death in some individuals, is very unlikely to explain the differences observed. Currently, screening for prostate cancer is in a phase of rapid development, with several different approaches used. The general acceptance of prostate cancer screening as a part of public healthcare programs can only be expected if the benefits in terms of mortality can be demonstrated.

The intermediate endpoints of cancer screening include migration to lower cancer stages at the time of diagnosis, a lower progression rate, and a higher survival rate. The endpoint of screening programs and the ultimate goal of all cancer research and treatment has to be a reduction in disease-related mortality and improvement in the quality of life. The latter is of particular concern when a screening program could result in more men living longer with cancer and the side effects of the disease and its treatment.[17] Screening programs may help control prostate cancer. The term "screening" should only be used if tests suitable for early detection are applied in a clearly defined program (e.g., in the form of population screening). In terms of the costs associated with this type of screening, only primary PSA screening would be acceptable. However, the sensitivity, specificity, and positive predictive value of PSA must be known and must be superior to other diagnostic tools suitable for screening.[18,19]

With screening procedures, there is usually a discrepancy between the sensitivity and specificity. In the case of prostate cancer, the cutoff for PSA as a biopsy criterion has to be lowered to improve sensitivity; however, that entails a great number of negative biopsies. Because of its low cost and complete standardization and automation, it would be very attractive to use total PSA as the only biopsy criterion.

However, to reduce the number of negative biopsies, additional diagnostic tests such as the assessment of percent free PSA and PSA transition zone density should be performed.[11] With the help of these two diagnostic tests, approximately 54% of negative biopsies could be avoided.[11] In evaluating this program, one should bear in mind that an "aggressive" screening policy has been combined with a complex decision algorithm to maximize prostate cancer detection without unacceptable biopsy rates. Agreement is general that a number of prerequisites have to be fulfilled before a screening program can be introduced as a health policy. These requirements have been described by Wilson and Jungner[20] in a classic paper.

No evidence is yet available from randomized trials that PSA-based screening can decrease prostate cancer mortality rates.[21] Nevertheless, the results obtained from the population-based Surveillance, Epidemiology, and End Results Program[22-25] show that the incidence of prostate cancer and the mortality rates have declined in recent years. The results of another study[26] suggest that screening for prostate cancer by DRE may be beneficial; screening by DRE was found to be much less common among men who died of histologically confirmed prostate cancer than among age-matched population controls. Currently two large, prospective studies are underway to examine the impact of PSA-based screening on prostate cancer mortality, but, to date, neither has a sufficiently long follow-up to document a reduction in mortality as a direct result of PSA-based screening.[27] The results reported here are from a unique natural experiment. The increase in incidence of prostate cancer after the introduction of a uniformly available and free testing program is precisely what is expected if a large proportion of men are screened. The continued increase in local disease incidence, indicating that PSA testing picks up early disease, and the constant decline in the incidence of prostate cancer that has distant spread at diagnosis in the population are encouraging. The fall in prostate cancer mortality rates in Tyrolean men contrasts with the more modest change taking place among all men of the same age in the rest of Austria (see Figure 41.1) and coincides from the temporal point of view with the introduction of PSA testing. The differences we report between the mortality rates in Tyrol and the rest of Austria bear strong similarities to two other phenomena. Mortality rates from cervical cancer in Nordic countries fell after screening became widely available, but not in Norway where it was not available.[28] In addition, the mortality rates from breast cancer in The Netherlands and the United Kingdom have both fallen since the introduction of mammographic screening programs,[29] in both cases too quickly to be due to the diagnosis and treatment of clinically undetectable cancers. The absence of a watchful waiting strategy in Tyrol has meant that some patients with Stage T3/4 disease will have been treated with hormonal therapy earlier than is usual in the disease course. Recent evidence suggests that earlier hormonal therapy may have a beneficial effect on survival.[30] The decline in mortality from prostate cancer seen in the men in the age range for which PSA testing was made available, and where acceptance of testing was high, is the first evidence from a geographically defined population, for which screening was available to all its members, that the policy of making PSA testing universally available and at no cost may have led to a reduction in death from prostate cancer in that population.

Many aspects of prostate cancer screening require better definition by randomized trials, including screening interval, issues relating to lead time, cutoff limits for a PSA test to be considered positive, and estimation of the benefits. Our study was not designed to investigate the important issues relating to economics and psychological impact. Although these necessary data are becoming available, the current demonstration of a decline in mortality from prostate cancer supports, but does not prove, the hypothesis that the policy of making PSA testing available to the population of Tyrol has led to a reduction in prostate cancer death rates. Also, the gap between the absolute numbers of deaths observed and those expected by the pre-PSA testing age-specific mortality rates has been growing in the age range liable to have been screened.

REFERENCES

1. Stanford JL, Stephenson RA, Coyle M, et al. Prostate Cancer Trends 1973–1995, SEER Program. NIH Publication No. 99-4543. Bethesda: National Cancer Institute, 1999, pp 7–15.
2. Jones GW, Mettlin C, Murphy GP, et al. Patterns of care for carcinoma of the prostate gland: results of a national survey of 1984 and 1990. J Am Coll Surg 1995;180:545-554.
3. Catalona WJ, Richie JP, Ahmann FR, et al. Comparison of digital rectal examination and serum prostate specific antigen in the early detection of prostate cancer: results of a multicenter clinical trial of 6,630 men. J Urol 1994;151:1283–1290.
4. Ohori M, Wheeler TM, Dunn JK, et al. The pathological features and prognosis of prostate cancer detectable with current diagnostic tests. J Urol 1994;152:1714–1720.
5. Smith DS, Catalona WJ. The nature of prostate cancer detected through prostate specific antigen based screening. J Urol 1994;152:1732–1736.
6. Slawin KM, Ohori M, Dillioglugil O, et al. Screening for prostate cancer: an analysis of the early experience. CA Cancer J Clin 1995;45:134–147.
7. Reissigl A, Pointner J, Horninger W, et al. Comparison of different PSA cutpoints for early detection of prostate cancer: results of a large screening study. Urology 1995;46:662–665.
8. Reissigl A, Pointner J, Horninger W, et al. PSA based screening for prostate cancer in asymptomatic younger males: pilot study in blood donors. Prostate 1997;30:20–25.
9. Reissigl A, Ennemoser O, Klocker H, et al. Frequency and clinical significance of transition zone cancer in prostate cancer screening. Prostate 1997;30:130–135.
10. Reissigl A, Klocker H, Horninger W, et al. Usefulness of the ratio free/total PSA in addition to total PSA levels in prostate cancer screening. Urology 1996;48:62–66.

11. Horninger W, Reissigl A, Klocker H, et al. Improvement of specificity in PSA based screening by using PSA transition zone density and percent free PSA in addition to total PSA levels. Prostate 1998;37:133–137.
12. Oesterling JE, Jacobsen SJ, Chute CG, et al. Serum prostate specific antigen in a community-based population of healthy men: establishment of age specific reference ranges. JAMA 1993;270:860–864.
13. Horninger W, Reissigl A, Rogatsch H, et al. Prostate cancer screening in the federal state of Tyrol, Austria. European Journal of Cancer 2000;36:1322–1335.
14. Boyle P, Parkin DM. Statistical methods for registries. In Jensen OM, Parkin DM, McLennan R, et al (eds): UROLOGY 58 (3), 2001 Cancer Registration: Principles and Methods, No. 95. Lyon: IARC Scientific Publication, 1995, pp 126–158.
15. McCullagh P, Nelder JA: Generalized Linear Models, 2nd ed. London: Chapman and Hall, 1989.
16. Splus 2000. User's Guide. Seattle: Data Analysis Products Division, Mathsoft, 1999.
17. Boyle P, Severi G: Epidemiology of chemoprevention of prostate cancer. Eur Urol 1999;35:370–376.
18. Catalona WJ, Smith DS, Ratliff TL, et al. Measurement of prostate specific antigen in serum as a screening test for prostate cancer. N Engl J Med 1991;324:1156–1161.
19. Mettlin C, Murphy GP, Babaian RJ, et al, for the Investigators of the American Cancer Society National Prostate Cancer Detection Project. The results of a five year early prostate cancer detection intervention. Cancer 1996;77:150–159.
20. Wilson JMG, Jungner G. Principles and Practice of Screening for Disease, Public Health Paper No. 34. Geneva: World Health Organization, 1969.
21. Von Eschenbach A, Ho R, Murphy GP, et al, for the American Cancer Society. Guidelines for the early detection of prostate cancer. Cancer 1997;80:1805–1807.
22. Smart CR. The results of prostate carcinoma screening in the U.S. as reflected in the Surveillance, Epidemiology, and End Results Program. Cancer 1997;80:1835–1844.
23. Hankey BF, Feuer EJ, Clegg LX, et al. Cancer surveillance series: interpreting trends in prostate cancer-part I: evidence of the effects of screening in recent prostate cancer incidence, mortality and survival rates. J Natl Cancer Inst 1999;91:1017–1024.
24. Feuer J, Merrill RM, Hankey BF. Cancer surveillance series: interpreting trends in prostate cancer—part II: cause of death misclassification and the recent rise and fall in prostate cancer mortality. J Natl Cancer Inst 1999;91:1025–1032.
25. Etzioni R, Legler JM, Feuer EJ, et al. Cancer surveillance series: interpreting trends in prostate cancer—part III: quantifying link between population prostate specific antigen testing and recent declines in prostate cancer mortality. J Natl Cancer Inst 1999;91:1033–1039.
26. Jacobsen SJ, Bergstralh EJ, Katusic SK, et al. Screening digital rectal examination and prostate cancer mortality: a population-based case-control study. Urology 1998;52:173–179.
27. Boyle P. Prostate specific antigen (PSA) testing as screening for prostate cancer: the current controversy. Ann Oncol 1998;9:1263–1264.
28. Laara E, Day NE, Hakama M. Trends in mortality from cervical cancer in the Nordic countries: association with organised screening programs. Lancet 1987;1:1247–1249.
29. van den Akker-van Marle E, de Konig H, Boer R, et al. Reduction in breast cancer mortality due to the introduction of mass screening in The Netherlands: comparison with the United Kingdom. J Med Screen 1999;6:30–34.
30. Messing EM, Manola J, Sarosdy M, et al. Immediate hormonal therapy compared with observation after radical prostatectomy and pelvic lymphadenectomy in men with node-positive prostate cancer. N Engl J Med 1999;341:1781–1788.

Lessons from the prostate cancer awareness week program and PLCO study

42

Paul D Maroni, E David Crawford

INTRODUCTION

Prostate Cancer Awareness Week (PCAW) and the Prostate, Lung, Colorectal, Ovarian (PLCO) Cancer Screening Trial are two ongoing projects attempting through different means to develop PSA demographics and determine the utility of screening for prostate cancer. While patient education is the primary goal of PCAW, a massive database containing demographic information, survey instruments, and blood/urine laboratory values/samples has accumulated over the last 15 years. In the early 1990s, the NIH began funding the PLCO trial designed to determine if screening for various malignancies reduces cause-specific and overall mortality. While we eagerly await end-point information from this trial, several studies have capitalized on the wealth of clinical data currently available. This chapter will describe the history of the two projects and review published data.

PROSTATE CANCER AWARENESS WEEK

The discovery and development of tools enabling the measurement of serum prostate-specific antigen (PSA) provided a unique opportunity not readily available for other solid organ malignancies. Screening techniques such as mammograms for breast cancer and endoscopy for colon cancer were well established in the conversations primary care physicians had with patients. While newly diagnosed prostate cancer cases and deaths rose through the 1980s, public understanding of the disease remained unmonitored and likely underemphasized. Prostate Cancer Awareness Week began as an instrument for educating the community about prostate cancer and has become a nationally recognized program that annually screens thousands of men in September.

In 1988, the senior author sought interest in sponsorship for a public awareness campaign from several organizations to participate in an endeavor of unspecified length using multiple community-based centers. Schering-Plough Corporation agreed to provide the funds to form the Prostate Cancer Education Council (PCEC), a multispecialty group of physicians and representatives from patient advocacy/minority groups with a common goal of promoting prostate cancer screening and awareness. As a first task, the PCEC created a survey measuring public knowledge, attitudes, and health practices. This study confirmed a tremendous lack of public awareness about general prostate cancer facts. For example, only half of men over 40 years had annual physical examinations and half again had a digital rectal exam (DRE) as cancer screening.[1] With the success of programs such as Breast Cancer Awareness Month and the Great American Smoke Out, an advertising campaign and media announcement officially designated the third week of September as Prostate Cancer Awareness Week to garner public attention. The screening exam consisted of a DRE and serum PSA test. Abnormal exams and PSA values greater than 4.0 ng/mL were reported to the patients, and they were encouraged to seek follow-up from their primary care physician. The first year of PCAW included over 90 participating centers and screened roughly 15,000 men. Celebrity participation has attracted public interest with well-known prostate cancer survivors, including retired U.S. Army General Norman Schwarzkopf, former Mayor of New York City Rudolph

Giuliani, and numerous actors. More recently, the National Football League in the U.S. has sponsored PCAW with a "Tackle Prostate Cancer" campaign allowing professional athletes to support local efforts.

Over the following 2 years, over a half-million men were screened at hundreds of screening sites, creating an incredible opportunity for data collection and investigation regarding screening for prostate cancer and demographic differences in the PSA test. The program was considered a resounding success, and the PCEC decided to continue its efforts indefinitely entirely under its own auspices. Participation waned in the mid 1990s as many previously participating sites developed their own awareness weeks conforming to local calendars, but the PCEC continued to provide technical assistance and educational and advertisement materials to designated PCAW sites. Initially, the screening was offered at no cost to patients, but ultimately sites were allowed to collect a nominal fee to offset the costs incurred from blood testing. Through the remainder of the 1990s and early 2000s, millions of men have been screened with tens of thousands diagnosed with and treated for prostate cancer as a result.

The PCAW population is largely white, tends towards higher education levels, and has a higher incidence of symptoms related to urinary function/prostatic disease. Ninety-one percent of screened men are white, with African-American, Latino, and Asian numbers less than half of those expected for a representative cross section of the US population (Figure 42.1).[1,2] Numerous efforts

have been made to increase minority recruitment, including the participation of African-American entertainers Danny Glover and Harry Belafonte as spokespeople for PCAW. Happily, 2003 saw a dramatic rise, with 16% of participants being African American. While minority rates of participation appear to be improving, patients with functional urinary issues may be over-represented in the PCAW population. In 2001 to 2002, 36% of men participating had moderate or severe symptoms, reaffirming the high prevalence of urinary symptoms in a voluntarily screened population.[3] While correlations between urinary symptoms and PSA are accepted but weak, the potential bias in the development of PSA metrics in a misrepresentative population is real but modest.[4] Despite the "awareness week" format, the assumption that symptomatic individuals preferentially seek care from free/inexpensive screening programs may not be accurate, since the proportion of symptomatic men in PCAW generally matches that observed in other community studies.[4]

The development of screening parameters for PSA were initially developed from a group of 860 men and women.[5] A concentration of 4 ng/mL represented 2 standard deviations above the mean and thus determined the threshold for further diagnostic testing, i.e., prostate biopsy. While nonscientific in its initial assignment, a large cohort study (6630 men) by Catalona et al confirmed the utility of this value.[6] Crawford et al examined the population from the 1993 PCAW, which included over 31,000 tested men with 6139 men (19.2%) with an elevated PSA (>4 ng/ml), a suspicious DRE, or both. Prostate needle biopsy was carried out in 1307 men, with cancer present in 322 (24.6% positive biopsy rate).[7] The positive predictive values for PSA greater than 4 ng/mL alone were 31.6%, abnormal DRE alone 25.5%, and abnormal DRE with elevated PSA was predictive 46.6% (Figure 42.2). Nearly 90% of cancers detected were clinically localized at the time of diagnosis reconfirming the efficiency and efficacy of PSA and DRE screening. Parenthetically, only 21.3% of men with an indication for biopsy actually followed-up with a biopsy, which highlights the problems of community/volunteer based studies.

With the attendant increase in PSA variation with aging, pegged threshold values for PSA by nature will designate older men for biopsy. While carcinoma of the prostate increases with age in autopsy studies, many of these cancers may have little clinical significance in the elderly. Oesterling et al addressed age-related increases in PSA by sampling 471 Minnesota men to develop age-specific reference ranges (ASRRs).[8] With PCAW, the availability of a large multiracial national section of men allowed for more specific investigation regarding standardized PSA values. Reference ranges based on age and race were a specific target of the 1993 and 1994 PCAW campaigns.[9] Data was published in 1996 using the records of over 77,000 screened individuals deemed

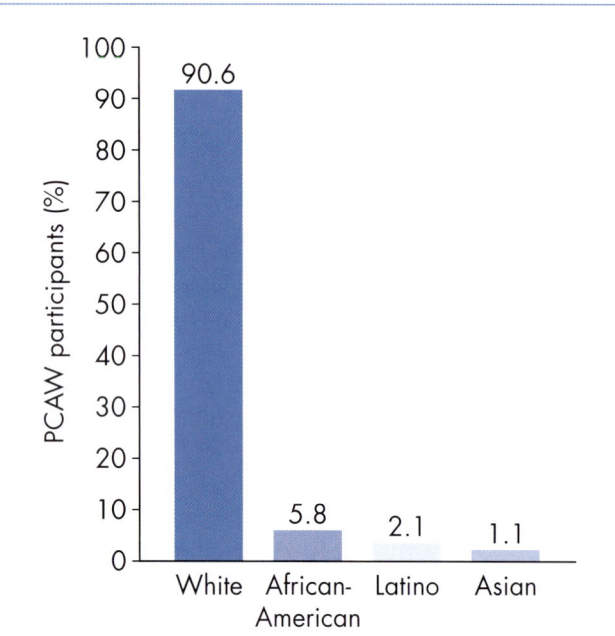

Fig. 42.1
Racial distribution of patients in Prostate Cancer Awareness Week.
Reprinted from Crawford ED. Prostate Cancer Awareness Week: September 22 to 28, 1997. CA Cancer J Clin 1997; 47:288–296.

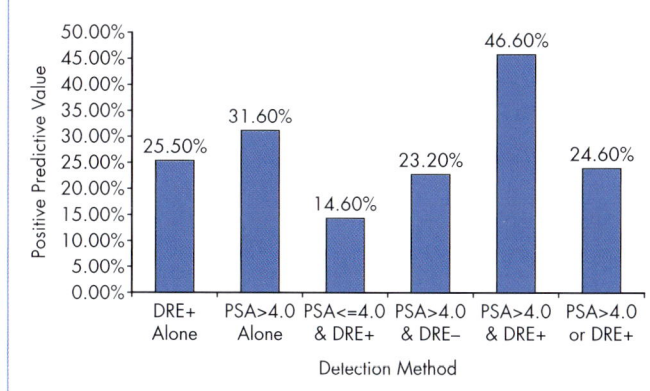

Fig. 42.2

Positive predictive value for prostate cancer detection. (DRE, digital rectal exam, PSA, prostate-specific antigen.) Reprinted with permission from Crawford ED, DeAntoni EP, Etzioni R, et al. Serum prostate-specific antigen and digital rectal examination for early detection of prostate cancer in a national community-based program, Urology 1996;47:863-869. Copyright©Elsevier, 1996.

free of prostate cancer and/or having a PSA of less than 20 ng/mL. The upper limits of the ASRRs represented the 95th percentile and were categorized by age alone and age/race combined. Significant differences in PSA were noted between age and most race groups. Of note, African Americans had higher PSA values with a higher variance relative to whites, an interesting phenomenon considering African Americans seem to have different prostate cancer physiology. As a result of this study, new ASRRs were developed for the IMx‰ assay. The University of Colorado group addressed the efficiency of these reference ranges several years later using a larger sample of men.[10] Of more than 116,000 screened men, 22,014 (19%) had an abnormal screening evaluation using a PSA of 4 ng/mL as the cutoff whereas 17,561 (15.1%) had an indication for biopsy if ASRRs (see above) were used. A dismal rate of men following up with prostate biopsies was again noted (18.9%). Positive predictive values were again calculated using similar models and assumptions (Table 42.1). While specificities were improved in ASRR models, sensitivities were slightly worse, thus missing men with prostate cancer, and recommendations were to continue using a PSA of 4 ng/mL as the cutoff. The clinical importance of early diagnosis in certain age groups will hopefully be answered by the PLCO study (see next section).

The screened population has also been used to examine myths surrounding the measurement of PSA. The impact of DRE on PSA was evaluated in a clinical trial involving 2,754 men.[11] Blood tests were taken before and after examinations. There was no statistical difference in pre- and post-DRE PSA levels, except that men with an already elevated PSA tended to have a further increase. These results were mirrored by a study pre- and post-ejaculation PSA test conducted in 750 men, where orgasm did not increase PSA except in men with previously abnormal levels.[12] Therefore, DRE and recent ejaculation should not interfere with PSA measurement in men with acceptable PSA levels. With the surging interest in complementary medicine, patients were surveyed regarding vitamin/herbal prostate medication use and relationship to urinary symptoms.[3] Use of alternative medical therapies were as common as the use of prescription medications in

patients with AUA SS (American Urologic Association Symptom Score) greater than 15, but the majority of men (64%) coped with symptoms without medications. Data from PCAW has also investigated risk factors for the development of prostate cancer.[13] No correlation was found between history of vasectomy and African-American race and small trends were noted with respect to body-mass index (BMI). Large populations of obese men have also been examined for serum parameters such as testosterone and cholesterol and the relationship to BMI. Men with BMIs greater than 30 were at 2.4 times the risk of having a serum testosterone below 300 ng/dL. These results suggest that serum testosterone and obesity should both be considered in risk stratification to minimize potential confounding.[14]

Cost-effective patient education and appropriate informed consent are two dilemmas of PCAW. One cannot easily explain the complex process of diagnosing, treating, and understanding prostate cancer to individuals from diverse socioeconomic backgrounds. DeAntoni et al followed a cohort of PCAW participants over a several year period and numerous frustrating facts highlight difficulties in mass education.[15] Briefly, participants generally have a poor understanding of the risks and benefits associated with screening that does not improve with longitudinal follow-up. This can flippantly be explained by a general interest in the male to "do" things to monitor general health, but more ominously, 84% of men believe prostate screening has been shown to save lives with virtually no understanding of the risks of screening.[16] These studies drove massive revisions to the educational material presented to patients, including the development of an informative website providing educational materials and newsletters year-round (www.pcaw.com). Also, barriers to medical care (e.g., lack of health insurance) might prevent men who would benefit from therapy from obtaining it. As an annual examiner in PCAW, one cannot relate the exasperation the senior author has seen in patients with very concerning rectal exams and a lack of resources to obtain appropriate follow-up.

Prostate Cancer Awareness Week continues to provide support for community screening programs while

Table 42.1 Distribution of efficiencies of abnormal prostate-specific antigen (PSA) alone, abnormal digital rectal examination (DRE) alone, and combined abnormal PSA and DRE. A, Using 4.0-ng/mL cutoff PSA in all 22,014 men. B, Using age-specific reference range cut-off PSA in all 17,561 men

	Abnormal PSA; normal DRE	Normal PSA; abnormal DRE	Abnormal PSA; abnormal DRE
A			
Number of men	7786	11,779	2449
Number of biopsies	1511	1835	814
Biopsy rate (%)	19.4	15.6	33.2
Number of positive biopsies	419	325	456
PPV (%)	27.7	17.7	56.0
SE (%)	34.9	27.1	38.0
SP (%)	63.1	49.0	87.9
FPR (%)	36.9	51.0	12.1
B			
Number of men	3333	12,718	1510
Number of biopsies	915	2114	535
Biopsy rate (%)	27.5	16.6	35.4
Number of positive biopsies	291	440	314
PPV (%)	31.8	20.8	63.7
SE (%)	27.1	41.0	31.8
SP (%)	75.0	32.8	92.2
FPR (%)	25.0	67.1	7.8

FPR, false positive rate; PPV, Positive predictive value; SE, sensitivity; SP, specificity.

Reprinted with permission from Crawford ED, Leewansangtong S, Goktas S, Holthaus K, Baier M. Efficiency of prostate-specific antigen and digital rectal examination in screening, using 4.0 ng/ml and age-specific reference range as a cutoff for abnormal values. Prostate 1999;38:296–302. Copyright ©1999.

attempting to answer difficult questions in urology. Targets for ongoing and future research projects involve verifying relationships of the sample population and the diseased prostate; for instance, the role of obesity in PSA and its various subtypes.

PROSTATE, LUNG, COLORECTAL, AND OVARIAN CANCER SCREENING TRIAL

The PLCO trial is an enormous NCI-funded randomized trial started in late 1992 designed to determine the effect of screening on cause-specific and overall mortality.[17] More than 154,000 men and women aged 55 to 74 enrolled in the study between 1992 and 2001 at 10 national centers. Subjects were randomized to receive routine care from their primary physician or screening for the above-mentioned cancers for a total of six years (Table 42.2). Participants are then followed for an additional 10 years and receive an annual questionnaire. Prostate cancer screening consists of six annual PSA tests and four annual DREs. Nearly 38,000 men were randomized to the screening arm, with the majority of patients in the 55 to 64 age groups. Again, minority groups are somewhat

underrepresented, but large numbers will hopefully allow reasonable deductions (Figure 42.3).[18]

Several interesting observations regarding PSA screening have come from this trial. Gelmann et al examined relationships between patient characteristics and free and total PSA values.[19] This study confirmed racial variability in PSA with higher levels in African Americans and lower in Asians. Free PSA also followed these trends, but the ratio appeared to remain stable over time. Smoking and weight appeared to have

Table 42.2 Screening schedule for Prostate, Lung, Colorectal, Ovarian (PLCO) study.

Test	Frequency
Prostate serum antigen (PSA)	Initial visit, annually for 5 years
Digital rectal exam (DRE)	Upon entry, annually for 3 years
Chest X-ray	Smokers upon entry, annually for 3 years
	Never smokers upon entry, annually for 2 years
Sigmoidoscopy	Upon entry, one after 5 years in study
Transvaginal ultrasound (TVU)	Upon entry, annually for 3 years
CA125	Initial visit, annually for 5 years

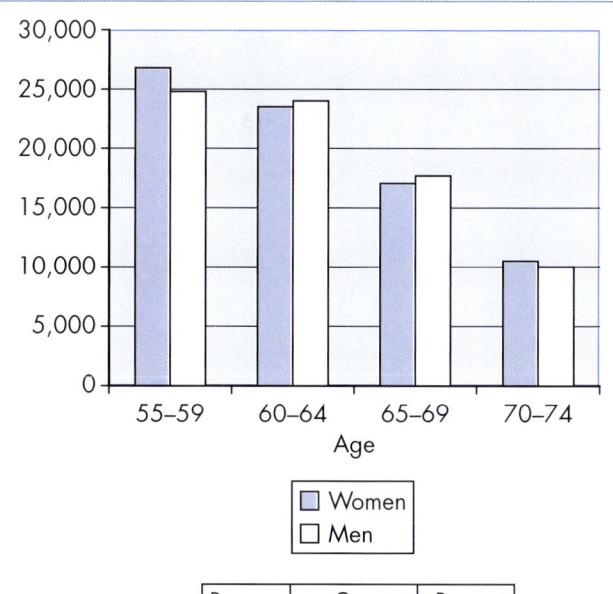

Race	Count	Percent
White	135,258	87.2
Black	7,829	5.1
Asian	5,579	3.6
Other	1,224	0.9

Fig. 42.3

PLCO baseline characteristics of enrolled participants.
Reprinted from Andriole GL, Reding D, Hayes RB, Prorok PC, Gohagan JK. The Prostate, Lung, Colon, and Ovarian (PLCO) cancer screening trial: status and promise. Urol Oncol 2004;22:358–361. Copyright©Elsevier, 2004.

negative effects on PSA and free PSA levels likely secondary to hormone metabolism. Investigators also suggested increasing the screening interval in certain individuals undergoing screening.[20] They found that of patients with PSA values less than 1 ng/mL, nearly 99% would have a PSA value less than 4 ng/mL after 4 additional years of screening. Likewise, in patients with PSA values between 1 and 2 ng/mL, 99% would have a PSA less than 4 ng/mL the following year. Patients in the 3 to 4 ng/mL range had a higher likelihood of reaching biopsy indications with 24% having a PSA greater than 4 ng/mL on follow-up blood test and 83% progressing to this endpoint by 4 years of screening. Recently, Kang et al used questionnaire data from the PLCO database to determine risk factors for nocturia and benign prostatic hyperplasia (BPH).[21] Whites and African Americans had relatively constant rates of BPH while Asian Americans appeared to be protected. Alcohol and possibly smoking are related to lower risks of BPH and nocturia.

The informative potential of the PLCO trial excites all physicians participating in the care of cancer patients in terms of diagnosis, treatment, and possibly prevention. This study will hopefully definitively confirm that screening for prostate cancer does save lives as well as develop efficient and effective screening protocols and

risk stratification. Quality-of-life analyses should help direct us toward practices and therapies that provide the most satisfaction for our patients. The NCI and investigators should be lauded for support of such a monumental and important project.

ACKNOWLEDGMENT

Acknowledgment to Albaha Barqawi, MD, for assistance with PCAW data.

REFERENCES

1. Crawford ED. Prostate Cancer Awareness Week: September 22 to 28, 1997. CA Cancer J Clin 1997;47:288–296.

2. US Census Bureau. Overview of race and Hispanic origin: Census 2000 brief. Issued March 2001:3.

3. Barqawi A, Gamito E, O'Donnell C, et al. Herbal and vitamin supplement use in a prostate screening population. Urology 2004;63:288–292.

4. Roehrborn CG, McConnell JD. Etiology, pathophysiology, epidemiology, and natural history of benign prostatic hyperplasia. In Walsh PC, Retik AB, Vaughan ED, et al, (eds): Campbell's Urology, 8th edn. Philadelphia: Saunders, 2002, pp1297–1336.

5. Myrtle JF, Klimley PG, Ivor LP, et al. Clinical utility of prostate-specific antigen (PSA) in the management of prostate cancer. Advance in Cancer Diagnostics. San Diego: Hybritech Inc., 1986.

6. Catalona WJ, Hudson MA, Scardino PT, et al. Selection of optimal prostate specific antigen cutoffs for early detection of prostate cancer: Receiver operating characteristic curves. J Urol 1994;152:2037–2042.

7. Crawford ED, DeAntoni EP, Etzioni R, et al. Serum prostate-specific antigen and digital rectal examination for early detection of prostate cancer in a national community-based program. Urology 1996;47:863–869.

8. Oesterling JE, Jacobsen SJ, Chute CG, et al, Serum prostate-specific antigen in a community-based population of healthy men: Establishment of age-specific reference ranges. JAMA 1993;270:860–864.

9. DeAntoni EP, Crawford ED, Oesterling JE, et al. Age- and race-specific reference ranges for prostate-specific antigen from a large community-based study. Urology 1996;48:234–239.

10. Crawford ED, Leewansangtong S, Goktas S, et al. Efficiency of prostate-specific antigen and digital rectal examination in screening, using 4.0 ng/ml and age-specific reference range as a cutoff for abnormal values. Prostate 1999;38:296–302.

11. Crawford ED, Schultz MJ, Clejan S, et al. The effect of digital rectal examination on prostate-specific antigen levels. JAMA 1992;267:2227–2228.

12. Simak R, Madersbacher S, Zhang ZF, et al. The impact of ejaculation on serum prostate-specific antigen. J Urol 1993;150:895–897.

13. Stone NN, Blum DS, DeAntoni EP, et al. Prostate cancer risk factor analysis among >50,000 men in a national study of prostate-specific antigen [abstract]. J Urol 1994;151:278A.

14. Barqawi A, O'Donnell C, Crawford ED. The relationship between testosterone, BMI, and cholesterol: data from the Prostate Cancer Awareness Week. Presented at 83rd Annual Meeting of the South Central Section of the AUA. Dublin, 2004 [abstract p272]

15. DeAntoni EP, Glode LM, Ross CA, et al. Knowledge, attitudes and health behaviours in a prostate cancer screening program: exhibiting the need for informed consent [abstract]. Pscho-Oncology 1996;5:154.

16. DeAntoni EP. Eight years of "Prostate Cancer Awareness Week." Cancer 1997;80:1845–1851.

17. Prorok PC, Andriole GL, Bresalier RS, et al. Design of the prostate, lung, colorectal and ovarian (PLCO) cancer screening trial. Control Clin Trials 2000;21:273S–309S.

18. Andriole GL, Reding D, Hayes RB, et al. The Prostate, Lung, Colon, and Ovarian (PLCO) cancer screening trial: status and promise. Urol Oncol 2004;22:358–361.

19. Gelmann EP, Chia D, Pinsky PF, et al. Relationship of demographic and clinical factors to free and total prostate-specific antigen. Urology 2001;58:561–566.

20. Crawford ED, Chia D, Andriole GL, et al. PSA changes as related to initial PSA: data from the Prostate, Lung, Colorectal and Ovarian cancer (PLCO) screening trial. Presented at American Society for Clinical Oncology Annual Meeting, Orlando, FL, May 2002.

21. Kang D, Andriole GL, Van De Vooren RC, et al. Risk behaviours and benign prostatic hyperplasia, BJU Intl 2004;93:1241–1245.

Clinical staging of prostate cancer: an overview

43

Mohamad E Allaf, H Ballentine Carter

INTRODUCTION

Clinical staging of prostate cancer aims to utilize pretreatment parameters to predict the true extent of disease. The goals of cancer staging are to allow the assessment of prognosis and facilitate educated decision-making regarding available treatment options. An accurate assessment of disease extent is critical for men with newly diagnosed prostate cancer, since pathologic stage is the most reliable means of predicting the outcome of definitive treatment in men with clinically localized cancer.[1] Available pretreatment modalities that can help predict the true disease extent in men with prostate cancer include: digital rectal examination (DRE), serum prostate-specific antigen (PSA), tumor grade, radiologic imaging, and pelvic lymphadenectomy. The local extent of disease can be predicted by a combination of DRE (Figure 43.1), serum tumor markers such as PSA, and tumor grade.

Although in unique circumstances imaging modalities may assist in the detection of extraprostatic spread of cancer, in the vast majority of cases these tests are not yet reliable. Pelvic lymphadenectomy remains the gold standard for the detection of lymph node spread in men at high risk for harboring occult lymph node metastases. Ultimately, clinical staging may provide the patient and urologist with valuable information regarding whether newly diagnosed prostate cancer is localized, locally advanced, or metastatic. This information helps guide management decisions.

STAGING: CLINICAL VERSUS PATHOLOGIC

Clinical staging is an assessment of the extent of disease using pretreatment parameters such as DRE, PSA, needle

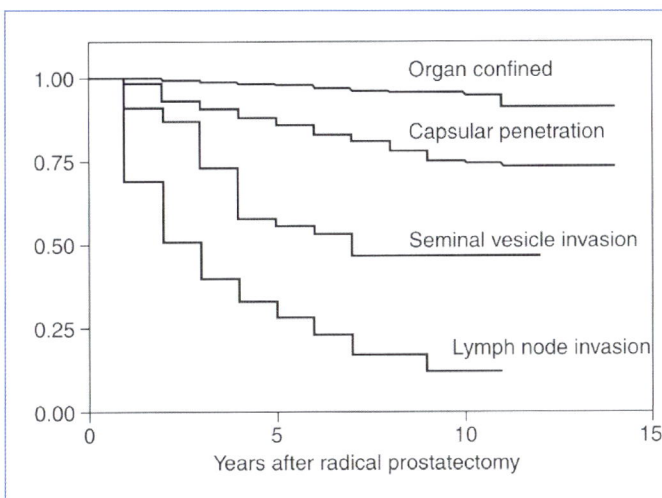

Fig. 43.1
Actuarial prostate-specific antigen (PSA) recurrence-free survival after radical prostatectomy stratified by pathologic stage. Curves represent organ confined disease, isolated capsular penetration, isolated seminal vesicle involvement, and lymph node involvement. Data adapted from the series of Patrick C. Walsh, The Johns Hopkins Hospital, 1982–1999.

biopsy findings, and radiologic imaging. Pathologic stage, on the other hand, is determined after prostate removal and involves careful histologic analysis of the prostate, seminal vesicles, and pelvic lymph nodes if a lymphadenectomy is performed. Thus, pathologic staging represents a more accurate estimate of the true disease burden and is more useful in the prediction of prognosis. Tumor volume and grade, extracapsular extension, and surgical margins are all accurately determined by pathologic staging. The importance of pathologic stage is underscored by the fact that biochemical recurrence-free survival and cancer-specific survival are both inversely related to the pathologic stage of disease (Figure 43.2). The most important pathologic criteria that predict prognosis after radical prostatectomy are tumor grade, surgical margin status, presence of extracapsular disease, seminal vesicle invasion, and pelvic lymph node involvement.[1-7]

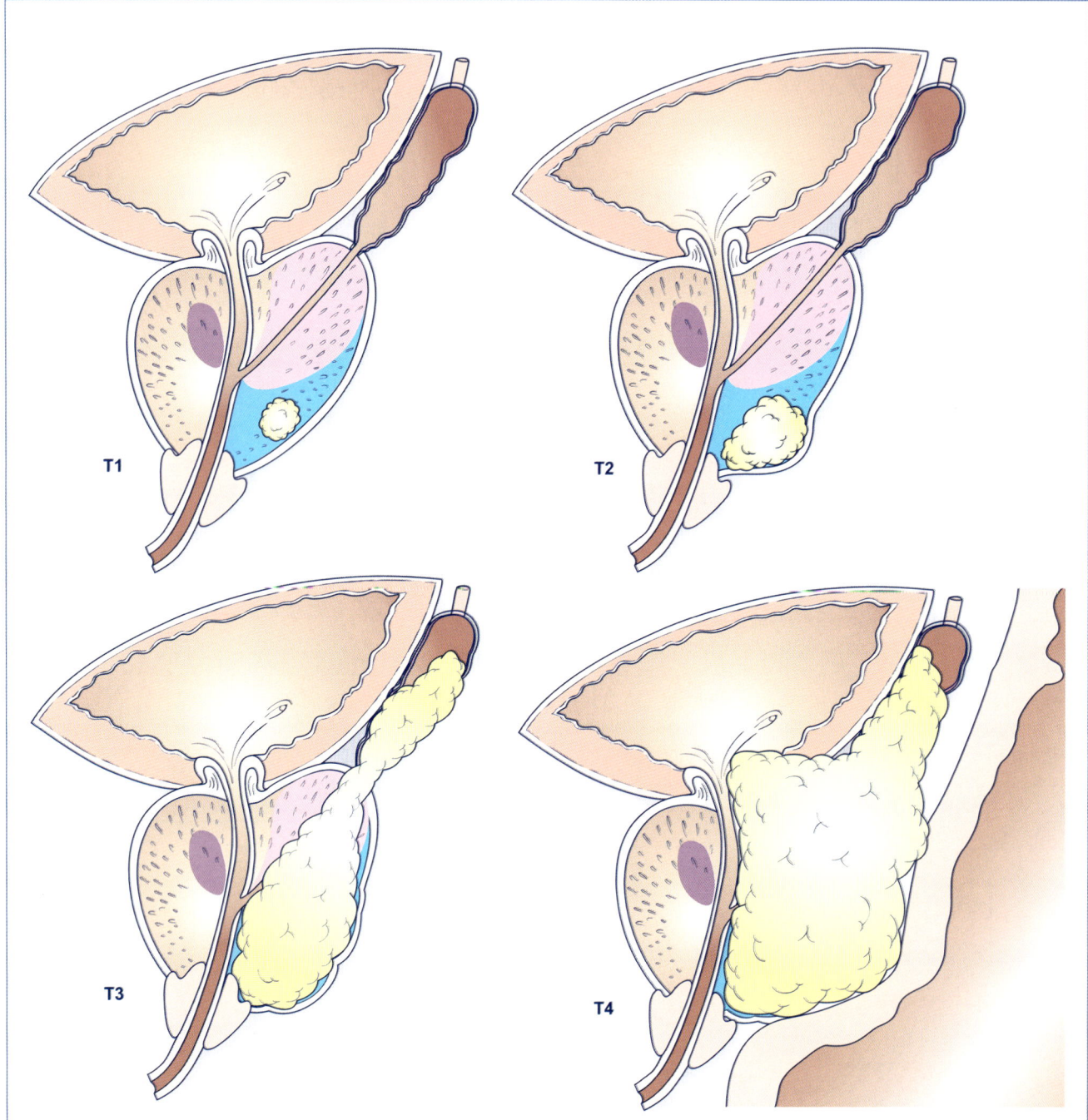

Fig. 43.2

Clinical staging of prostate cancer. Digital rectal examination and other modalities help to distinguish T1 from T2, T3 and T4 prostatic cancers.

CLINICAL STAGING CLASSIFICATION SYSTEMS

Two main classification systems for clinical staging exist today: the Whitmore–Jewett and tumor, node, metastasis (TNM) classification systems. Whitmore introduced the first clinical staging classification system for prostate cancer in 1956, and Jewett modified this in 1975.[8,9] The TNM system was first adopted in 1975 by the American Joint Committee for Cancer Staging and End Results Reporting (AJCC).[10] A new TNM classification system was adopted in 1992 by the AJCC and International Union Against Cancer (UICC) and this system was then modified in 1997 to reduce the subdivision of T2 disease from three categories (T2a, T2b and T2c) to two substages by combining single lobe disease (T2a and T2b) into a single stage (T2).[11,12] Several authors have questioned the 1997 modification arguing that the prior distinction between stages T2a and T2b is clinically important.[13,14] Table 43.1 summarizes and compares the Whitmore–Jewett and TNM staging schemes.

Interestingly, a nonpalpable lesion identified by imaging in the prostate is considered a T2 lesion by the current TNM clinical staging system. This is controversial in light of several studies documenting that transrectal ultrasound (TRUS) findings do not predict tumor extent in PSA-detected nonpalpable lesions.[15,16] In fact, most TRUS findings do not represent cancer, and the majority of cancer is not visualized by ultrasonography. Furthermore, Ohori et al reported no difference in cancer-specific survival between men with nonpalpable disease, regardless of whether their cancer was visible on TRUS.[17] Another recent study, however, contradicted these findings by concluding that men with nonpalpable prostate cancer and visible lesions on TRUS had a disease-free survival comparable to a group of men with palpable disease (T2); whereas men with nonpalpable disease and no suspicious findings on TRUS had better disease-free outcomes when compared with those with stage T2.[18] Therefore, this issue remains unresolved, and it is not unusual for urologists to classify all men with nonpalpable disease as T1c regardless of TRUS findings.

PREDICTION OF TUMOR EXTENT

COMBINED USE OF PRETREATMENT PARAMETERS

Although numerous pretreatment parameters correlate with the true extent of disease, on an individual basis no single parameter can accurately predict pathologic stage. Clinicians typically integrate the data available to determine the likelihood of disease extent. Nomograms and algorithms have been constructed to aid in the precise prediction of pathologic stage by using multiple clinical parameters. Taking into consideration the primary T stage based on DRE findings, serum PSA level, and Gleason grade, these algorithms have been shown to be accurate predictors of both cancer extent and long-term outcomes after treatment of the primary tumor.[19-24] One example of these nomograms, the Partin tables (Table 43.2), shows the percent probability of having a final pathologic stage based on logistic regression analyses for all three variables combined.[19,23,25] Such nomograms are constructed based on large numbers of patients who have undergone radical prostatectomy. D'Amico has suggested stratification of men into low risk (stages T1c to 2a disease, PSA 10 ng/mL or less and Gleason score 6 or less), intermediate risk (stage T2b disease or PSA greater than 10–20 ng/mL or less, or Gleason score 7), and high risk (stage T2c disease, or PSA greater than 20 ng/mL or Gleason score 8 or greater) disease, and has shown that freedom from disease at 10 years after radical prostatectomy is statistically significantly different for the risk categories: 83% for low risk, 46% for intermediate risk, and 29% for high risk disease.[26] Stratification of disease using these algorithms prior to treatment is useful for counseling men regarding the optimal treatment regimen.

PROSTATE NEEDLE BIOPSY

Histologic grade is the most important piece of information obtained from the needle biopsy. The Gleason grading system is the most commonly used classification scheme for the histologic grading of prostate cancer.[27] This system is based on a low magnification microscopic description of the architecture of the cancer. The predominant pattern (occupying the largest area of the specimen) is given a grade between 1 and 5. This number is then added to the grade assigned to the second most dominant pattern—thus a Gleason sum can be as low as 2 and as high as 10. Gleason grade has been shown to correlate with the pathologic extent of disease but, as stated above, is not sufficiently accurate when considered on its own.[3-5,28,29] The presence of a Gleason pattern 4 or greater or a Gleason sum of 7 or greater is particularly predictive of a poor prognosis. Due to the numerous multivariate analyses supporting the assertion that Gleason sum is a strong predictor of disease extent, some investigators have advocated that all new predictive indicators be compared with Gleason grade.[3,4,15,16,30] Only those parameters that prove to provide statistically independent predictive information should then be considered clinically useful.

Clinical staging algorithms may also incorporate other parameters from needle biopsy in making decisions such as the extent of disease (e.g., number of

Table 43.1 Prostate cancer staging systems

TNM 2002	TNM 1997	TNM 1992	Description	Whitmore–Jewett	Description
TX	TX	TX	Primary tumor cannot be assessed	None*	None
T0	T0	T0	No evidence of primary tumor	None	None
T1	T1	T1	Nonpalpable tumor—not evident by imaging	A	Same as TNM
T1a	T1a	T1a	Tumor found in tissue removed at TUR; 5% or less is cancerous and histologic grade ≤7	A1	Same as TNM
T1b	T1b	T1b	Tumor found in tissue removed at TUR; >5% is cancerous or histologic grade >7	A2	Same as TNM
T1c	T1c	T1c	Tumor identified by prostate needle biopsy due to elevation in PSA	None	None
T2	T2	T2	Palpable tumor confined to the prostate	B	Same as TNM
T2a		T2a	Tumor involves less than half of one lobe	B1	Tumor involves {1/2} lobe; surrounded by normal tissue on all sides
	T2a		Tumor involves one lobe or less	B1	Same as TNM
T2b		T2b	Tumor involves more than half of a lobe, but not both lobes	B1	Same as TNM
	T2b		Tumor involves more than one lobe (Bilateral)	B2	Same as TNM
T2c	None	T2c	Tumor involves more than one lobe (Bilateral)	B2	Same as TNM
T3	T3	T3	Palpable tumor beyond prostate	C1	Tumor <6 cm in diameter
	T3a	T3a	Unilateral extracapsular extension	C1	Same as TNM
T3a			Unilateral or bilateral extracapsular extension		
	T3b	T3b	Bilateral extracapsular extension	C1	Same as TNM
None	T3c	T3c	Tumor invades seminal vesicle(s)	C1	Same as TNM
T3b			Tumor invades seminal vesicle(s)		
T4	T4	T4	Tumor is fixed or invades adjacent structures—not seminal vesicle(s)	C2	Same as TNM
None	None	T4a	Tumor invades bladder neck, external sphincter, and/or rectum	C2	Same as TNM
None	None	T4b	Tumor invades levator muscle and/or fixed to pelvic wall	C2	Same as TNM
None	None	None	None	D0	Elevated prostatic acid phosphatase
NX	NX	NX	Regional lymph nodes cannot be assessed	None	None
N0	N0	N0	No lymph node metastases	None	None
N1	N1	N+	Involvement of regional lymph nodes	D1	Same as TNM
		N1	Metastases in single regional lymph node, ≤2 cm in dimension	D1	Same as TNM
None	None	N2	Metastases in single (>2 but ≤5 cm) or multiple with none >5 cm	D1	Same as TNM
None	None	N3	Metastases in regional lymph node >5 cm in dimension	D1	Same as TNM
M+	M+	M+	Distant metastatic spread	D2	Same as TNM
MX	MX	MX	Distant metastases cannot be assessed	None	None
M0	M0	M0	No evidence of distant metastases	None	None
M1	M1	M1	Distant metastases	D2	Same as TNM
M1a	M1a	M1a	Involvement of nonregional lymph nodes	D2	Same as TNM
M1b	M1b	M1b	Involvement of bones	D2	Same as TNM
M1c	M1c	M1c	Involvement of other distant sites	D2	Same as TNM
None	None	None	None	D3	Hormonal refractory disease

PSA, prostate-specific antigen; TNM, tumor, node, metastasis; TUR, transurethral resection.

Table 43.2 Updated Partin tables* showing the percent probability of having a final pathologic stage based on logistic regression analyses for all three variables combined (prostate-specific antigen [PSA] level, pathologic stage, and Gleason score).

PSA range ng/mL	Pathologic stage	Gleason score				
		2–4	5–6	3 + 4 = 7	4 + 3 = 7	8–10
Clinical stage T1c (nonpalpable; PSA elevated)						
0–2.5	Organ confined	95 (89–99)	90 (88–93)	79 (74–85)	71 (62–79)	66 (54–76)
	Capsular penetration	5 (1–11)	9 (7–12)	17 (13–23)	25 (18–34)	28 (20–38)
	Seminal vesicle (+)	–	0 (0–1)	2 (1–5)	2 (1–5)	4 (1–10)
	Lymph node (+)	–	–	1 (0–2)	1 (0–4)	1 (0–4)
2.6–4.0	Organ confined	92 (82–98)	84 (81–86)	68 (62–74)	58 (48–67)	52 (41–63)
	Capsular penetration	8 (2–18)	15 (13–18)	27 (22–33)	37 (29–46)	40 (31–50)
	Seminal vesicle (+)	–	1 (0–1)	4 (2–7)	4 (1–7)	6 (3–12)
	Lymph node (+)	–	–	1 (0–2)	1 (0–3)	1 (0–4)
4.1–6.0	Organ confined	90 (78–98)	80 (78–83)	63 (58–68)	52 (43–60)	46 (36–56)
	Capsular penetration	10 (2–22)	19 (16–21)	32 (27–36)	42 (35–50)	45 (36–54)
	Seminal vesicle (+)	–	1 (0–1)	3 (2–5)	3 (1–6)	5 (3–9)
	Lymph Node (+)	–	0 (0–1)	2 (1–3)	3 (1–5)	3 (1–6)
6.1–10.0	Organ confined	87 (73–97)	75 (72–77)	54 (49–59)	43 (35–51)	37 (28–46)
	Capsular penetration	13 (3–27)	23 (21–25)	36 (32–40)	47 (40–54)	48 (39–57)
	Seminal vesicle (+)	–	2 (2–3)	8 (6–11)	8 (4–12)	13 (8–19)
	Lymph node (+)	–	0 (0–1)	2 (1–3)	2 (1–4)	3 (1–5)
>10.0	Organ confined	80 (61–95)	62 (58–64)	37 (32–42)	27 (21–34)	22 (16–30)
	Capsular penetration	20 (5–39)	33 (30–36)	43 (38–48)	51 (44–59)	50 (42–59)
	Seminal vesicle (+)	–	4 (3–5)	12 (9–17)	11 (6–17)	17 (10–25)
	Lymph node (+)	–	2 (1–3)	8 (5–11)	10 (5–17)	11 (5–18)
Clinical stage T2a (palpable <half of one lobe)						
0–2.5	Organ confined	91 (79–98)	81 (77–85)	64 (56–71)	53 (43–63)	47 (35–59)
	Capsular penetration	9 (2–21)	17 (13–21)	29 (23–36)	40 (30–49)	42 (32–53)
	Seminal vesicle (+)	–	1 (0–2)	5 (1–9)	4 (1–9)	7 (2–16)
	Lymph node (+)	–	0 (0–1)	2 (0–5)	3 (0–8)	3 (0–9)
2.6–4.0	Organ confined	85 (69–96)	71 (66–75)	50 (43–57)	39 (30–48)	33 (24–44)
	Capsular penetration	15 (4–31)	27 (23–31)	41 (35–48)	52 (43–61)	53 (44–63)
	Seminal vesicle (+)	–	2 (1–3)	7 (3–12)	6 (2–12)	10 (4–18)
	Lymph node (+)	–	0 (0–1)	2 (0–4)	2 (0–6)	3 (0–8)
4.1–6.0	Organ confined	81 (63–95)	66 (62–70)	44 (39–50)	33 (25–41)	28 (20–37)
	Capsular penetration	19 (5–37)	32 (28–36)	46 (40–52)	56 (48–64)	58 (49–66)
	Seminal vesicle (+)	–	1 (1–2)	5 (3–8)	5 (2–8)	8 (4–13)
	Lymph node (+)	–	1 (0–2)	4 (2–7)	6 (3–11)	6 (2–12)
6.1–10.0	Organ confined	76 (56-94)	58 (54–61)	35 (30–40)	25 (19–32)	21 (15–28)
	Capsular penetration	24 (6–44)	37 (34–41)	49 (43–54)	58 (51–66)	57 (48–65)
	Seminal vesicle (+)	–	4 (3–5)	13 (9–18)	11 (6–17)	17 (11–26)
	Lymph node (+)	–	1 (0–2)	3 (2–6)	5 (2–8)	5 (2–10)
>10.0	Organ confined	65 (43–89)	42 (38–46)	20 (17–24)	14 (10–18)	11 (7–15)
	Capsular penetration	35 (11–57)	47 (43–52)	49 (43–55)	55 (46–64)	52 (41–62)
	Seminal vesicle (+)	–	6 (4–8)	16 (11–22)	13 (7–20)	19 (12–29)
	Lymph node (+)	–	4 (3–7)	14 (9–21)	18 (10–27)	17 (9–29)
Clinical stage T2b (palpable >half of one lobe, not on both lobes)						
0–2.5	Organ confined	88 (73–97)	75 (69–81)	54 (46–63)	43 (33–54)	37 (26–49)
	Capsular penetration	12 (3–27)	22 (17–28)	35 (28–43)	45 (35–56)	46 (35–58)

Continued...

Table 43.2 Updated Partin tables* showing the percent probability of having a final pathologic stage based on logistic regression analyses for all three variables combined (prostate-specific antigen [PSA] level, pathologic stage, and Gleason score). Continued

PSA range ng/mL	Pathologic stage	Gleason score				
		2–4	5–6	3 + 4 = 7	4 + 3 = 7	8–10
	Seminal vesicle (+)	–	2 (0–3)	6 (2–12)	5 (1–11)	9 (2–20)
	Lymph node (+)	–	1 (0–2)	4 (0–10)	6 (0–14)	6 (0–16)
2.6–4.0	Organ confined	80 (61–95)	63 (57–59)	41 (33–48)	30 (22–39)	25 (17–34)
	Capsular penetration	20 (5–39)	34 (28–40)	47 (40–55)	57 (47–67)	57 (46–68)
	Seminal vesicle (+)	–	2 (1–4)	9 (4–15)	7 (3–14)	12 (5–22)
	Lymph node (+)	–	1 (0–2)	3 (0–8)	4 (0–12)	5 (0–14)
4.1–6.0	Organ confined	75 (55–93)	57 (52–63)	35 (29–40)	25 (18–32)	21 (14–29)
	Capsular penetration	25 (7–5)	39 (33–44)	51 (44–57)	60 (50–68)	59 (49–69)
	Seminal vesicle (+)	–	2 (1–3)	7 (4–11)	5 (3–9)	9 (4–16)
	Lymph node (+)	–	2 (1–3)	7 (4–13)	10 (5–18)	10 (4–20)
6.1–10.0	Organ confined	69 (47–91)	49 (43–54)	26 (22–31)	19 (14–25)	15 (10–21)
	Capsular penetration	31 (9–53)	44 (39–49)	52 (46–58)	60 (52–68)	57 (48–67)
	Seminal vesicle (+)	–	5 (3–8)	16 (10–22)	13 (7–20)	19 (11–29)
	Lymph node (+)	–	2 (1–3)	6 (4–10)	8 (5–14)	8 (4–16)
>10.0	Organ confined	57 (35–86)	33 (28–38)	14 (11-17)	9 (6-13)	7 (4-10)
	Capsular penetration	43 (14–65)	52 (46–56)	47 (40–53)	50 (40–60)	46 (36–59)
	Seminal vesicle (+)	–	8 (5–11)	17 (12–24)	13 (8–21)	19 (12–29)
	Lymph node (+)	–	8 (5–12)	22 (15–30)	27 (16–39)	27 (14–40)
Clinical stage T2c (palpable on both lobes)						
0–2.5	Organ confined	86 (71–97)	73 (63–81)	51 (38–63)	39 (26–54)	34 (21–48)
	Capsular penetration	14 (3–29)	24 (17–33)	36 (26–48)	45 (32–59)	47 (33–61)
	Seminal vesicle (+)	–	1 (0–4)	5 (1–13)	5 (1–12)	8 (2–19)
	Lymph node (+)	–	1 (0–4)	6 (0–18)	9 (0–26)	10 (0–27)
2.6–4.0	Organ confined	78 (58–94)	61 (50–70)	38 (27–50)	27 (18–40)	23 (14–34)
	Capsular penetration	22 (6–42)	36 (27–45)	48 (37–59)	57 (44–70)	57 (44–70)
	Seminal vesicle (+)	–	2 (1–5)	8 (2–17)	6 (2–16)	10 (3–22)
	Lymph node (+)	–	1 (0–4)	5 (0–15)	7 (0–21)	8 (0–22)
4.1–6.0	Organ confined	73 (52–93)	55 (44–64)	31 (23–41)	21 (14–31)	18 (11–28)
	Capsular penetration	27 (7–48)	40 (32–50)	50 (40–60)	57 (43–68)	57 (43–70)
	Seminal vesicle (+)	–	2 (1–4)	6 (2–11)	4 (1–10)	7 (2–15)
	Lymph node (+)	–	3 (1–7)	12 (5–23)	16 (6–32)	16 (6–33)
6.1–10.0	Organ confined	67 (45–91)	46 (36–56)	24 (17–32)	16 (10–24)	13 (8–20)
	Capsular penetration	33 (9–55)	46 (37–55)	52 (42–61)	58 (46–69)	56 (43–69)
	Seminal vesicle (+)	–	5 (2–9)	13 (6–23)	11 (4–21)	16 (6–29)
	Lymph node (+)	–	3 (1–6)	10 (5–18)	13 (6–25)	13 (5–26)
>10.0	Organ confined	54 (32–85)	30 (21–38)	11 (7–17)	7 (4–12)	6 (3–10)
	Capsular penetration	46 (15–68)	51 (42–60)	42 (30–55)	43 (29–59)	41 (27–57)
	Seminal vesicle (+)	–	6 (2–12)	13 (6–24)	10 (3–20)	15 (5–28)
	Lymph node (+)	–	13 (6–22)	33 (18–49)	38 (20–58)	38 (20–59)

*Adapted from Partin AW, Mangold LA, Lamm DM, Walsh PC, Epstein JI, Pearson JD. Contemporary update of prostate cancer staging nomograms (Partin Tables) for the new millennium. Urology 2001;58: 843–848.

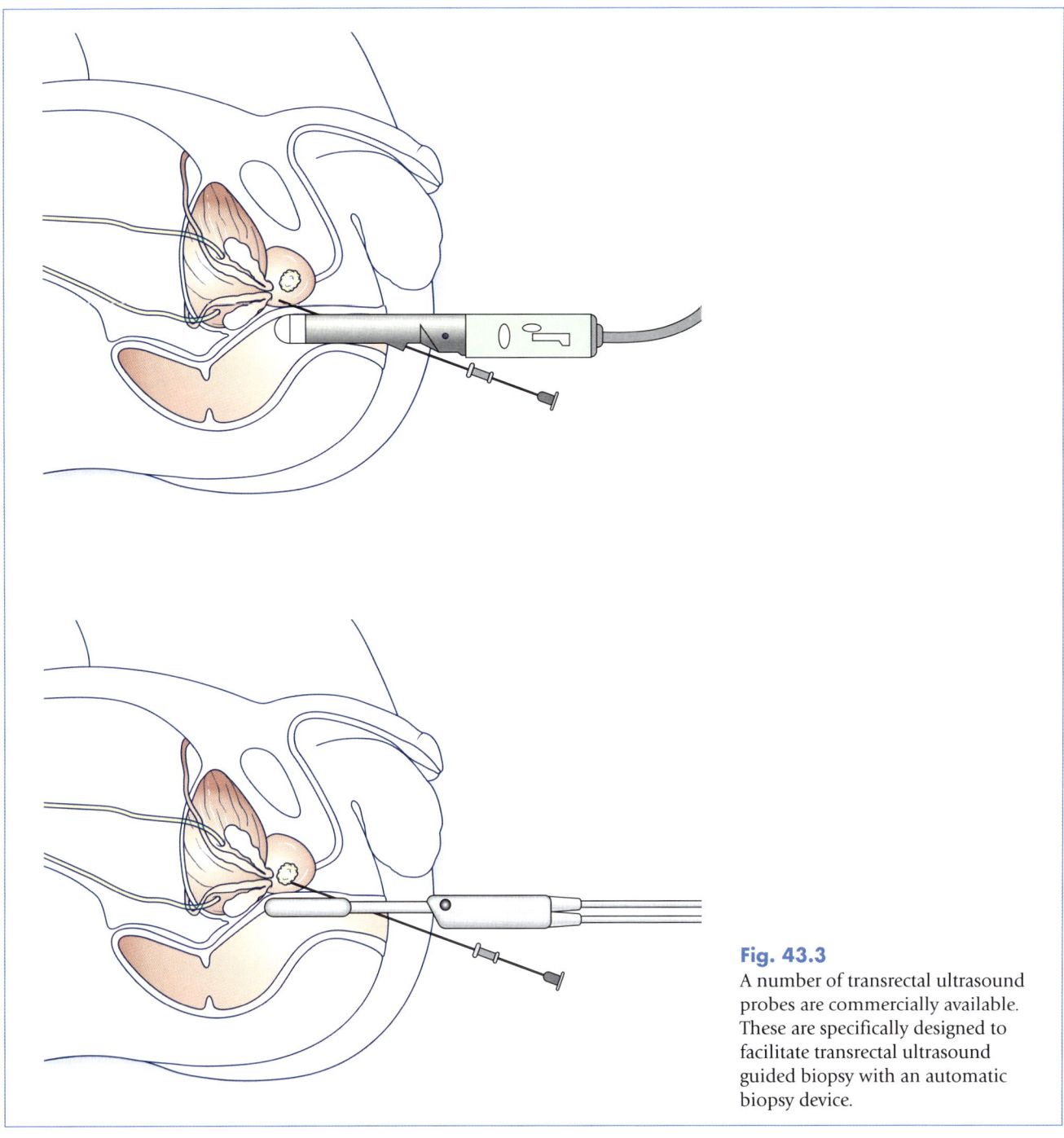

Fig. 43.3
A number of transrectal ultrasound probes are commercially available. These are specifically designed to facilitate transrectal ultrasound guided biopsy with an automatic biopsy device.

positive cores, percentage of positive cores), seminal vesicle involvement, invasion of periprostatic tissue, and perineural invasion (PNI). Prostate needle biopsy tumor extent is related to several pathologic endpoints in radical prostatectomy, such as tumor volume, margin status, and pathologic stage[31] (Figure 43.3). In addition, needle biopsy disease extent can be clinically useful in selecting candidates for expectant management programs and in predicting response to radiation therapy and radical prostatectomy.[32] Seminal vesicle invasion is associated with a poor prognosis, and, therefore, some authors have recommended biopsy of the seminal vesicles to improve staging.[33–36]

Other investigators noted that tumor in the periprostatic fat is associated with capsular penetration and, as a result, advocate biopsies of the prostatic capsule and seminal vesicles.[37] Recent reports have suggested, however, that routine biopsy of the seminal vesicles should only be reserved for cases with large palpable tumors located at the base of the prostate.[38,39] Although controversial, several studies have shown that PNI on a biopsy is associated with extracapsular extension of disease in the radical prostatectomy specimen.[40,41] Up to 75% of men with PNI on a biopsy will have capsular penetration on examination of the prostatectomy specimen. But it would appear that PNI is not an independent predictor of long-term outcome after radical prostatectomy.[42]

PROSTATE-SPECIFIC ANTIGEN

Prostate-specific antigen is a member of the human kallikrein gene family of serine proteases located on chromosome 19. It is the most important tumor marker available today for the diagnosis, staging, and monitoring of prostate cancer.[43] Serum PSA has been shown to correlate directly with pathologic stage and tumor volume.[44–46] Since PSA can be influenced by benign prostate hyperplasia (BPH) and tumor grade, and PSA levels overlap between stages, it cannot be used alone to accurately predict the extent of disease for an individual patient. Men with more advanced prostate cancer have higher grade and higher volume tumors that produce less PSA per gram of tumor.[47] Additionally, the contribution of BPH to overall serum PSA has been estimated to be 0.15 ng/mL of PSA per gram of BPH tissue.[48,49] Despite these confounding factors, 80% of men with PSA less than 4.0 ng/mL have pathologically organ-confined disease, 66% of men with PSA levels between 4.0 and 10.0 ng/mL have organ-confined disease, and more than 50% of men with PSA greater than 10.0 ng/mL have extraprostatic disease.[50,51] Additionally, 20% of men with PSA greater than 20 ng/mL and 75% of those with PSA greater than 50 ng/mL are found to have pelvic lymph node involvement.[19,47]

Pro-PSA is released from cells with a 7-amino-acid leader sequence that is cleaved by human kallikrein 2 (hK2) to produce active PSA. In addition to its potential role in cancer detection, some studies suggest that hK2 may be a useful predictor of pathologically organ-confined disease.[52] The role of pro-PSA, and other PSA isoforms, in prostate cancer staging remains unclear.[53] Multiple studies have found an association between percentage of free PSA and more extensive pathologic disease.[54,55] Most recently, a study found that men whose PSA level increases by more than 2.0 ng/mL/year before the diagnosis of prostate cancer have an increased risk of death from prostate cancer, despite undergoing radical prostatectomy.[56] The role of molecular forms of PSA and PSA kinetics in staging require further clarification before wide clinical use.

While prostatic acid phosphatase (PAP) elevations are directly related to the pathologic stage of prostate cancer, the closer relationship between PSA and disease extent has virtually eliminated the use of this parameter in clinical practice.[57] Prostatic acid phosphatase rarely adds additional information in those men who are considered to have clinically localized prostate cancer based on the results of DRE, PSA, and Gleason grade.[58] Nevertheless, two recent studies demonstrated that preoperative PAP levels may provide independent prognostic information with respect to predicting progression following radical prostatectomy.[59,60]

DIGITAL RECTAL EXAMINATION

Digital rectal examination determines whether a lesion is palpable and thus is a surrogate for the local extent of disease (clinical T stage). Because of its poor sensitivity and lack of reproducibility, DRE can both overestimate and underestimate the extent of disease. Studies from the 1970s demonstrated that, of men predicted to have extracapsular disease by DRE, only 25% were confirmed to have that finding on pathologic examination.[61,62] More recent studies in presumed organ-confined cases reveal a pattern of understaging or false-negative prediction of organ-confined status by DRE.[7] The sensitivity and specificity of DRE in determining organ-confined status was evaluated in a large series in which all DREs and radical prostatectomies were performed by one urologist with pathologic evaluations by a single pathologist.[19] In this series of 565 men in whom the DRE suggested organ confined disease (T2), 52% actually had organ-confined disease, 31% capsular penetration, and the remaining 17% exhibited either seminal vesicle or lymph node involvement. In this same series, of 36 men in whom extraprostatic disease was suspected on DRE (T3a), 19% were organ confined, 36% had capsular penetration, and 45% had either involvement of the seminal vesicles or lymph nodes. This represents a sensitivity of 52% and a specificity of 81% for prediction of organ-confined disease by DRE alone. When combined with other parameters, as mentioned earlier, DRE can assist in the precise prediction of overall tumor extent.

IMAGING

A variety of imaging modalities have been evaluated for staging prostate cancer. None of these techniques are sensitive enough to reliably detect the extraprostatic spread of prostate cancer. The inability to image microscopic disease limits the accuracy of current imaging modalities.

Radionuclide bone scan (bone scintigraphy) is the most sensitive modality for the detection of skeletal metastases.[63–65] This is in contrast to bone survey films (skeletal radiography), which require more than 50% of the bone density to be replaced with tumor before they can identify distant spread.[66,67] Today, skeletal radiography is only obtained to confirm a positive bone scan in men at low risk for bone metastases. Radionuclide bone scan can also screen for upper urinary tract obstruction and thus can obviate the need for further evaluation of the urinary tract in men with prostate cancer.[68] Since bone metastases at diagnosis are rare in men without bone pain in the PSA screening era, the routine use of bone scans in this population may not be useful and can create needless stress by detecting benign conditions that require further tests to rule out occult malignant disease. In addition, a strategy of using bone scintigraphy in the staging evaluation of all PSA screened men may not be cost effective.[69] Bone scans are not routinely obtained in patients with PSA levels less than 10 ng/mL and no bone pain. When a bone scan is performed, however, it provides a baseline evaluation for comparison in men who later may complain of bone pain.

The use of computed tomography (CT) and magnetic resonance imaging (MRI) to evaluate the local extent of disease and the possibility of nodal involvement is not routinely recommended due to the low sensitivity of these modalities.[70-72] Such tests may be appropriately reserved for high-risk patients such as those with locally advanced disease by DRE, a PSA greater than 20 ng/mL, or men with poorly differentiated cancer on needle biopsy. Furthermore, the cost effectiveness of these tests in populations with probabilities of lymph node involvement less than 30% has been questioned.[70-72] Given the rarity of lymph node involvement in screened populations, it appears that these imaging modalities are being overused in the staging of prostate cancer.[73]

Combined MRI and MR spectroscopy (MRS) are being evaluated for staging prostate cancer, but there is no evidence that these methods will overcome the current limitation of the inability to image microscopic disease.[74,75] Specialized techniques such as high-resolution MRI used in tandem with the intravenous administration of lymphotropic superparamagnetic nanoparticles may allow the detection of small and otherwise undetectable lymph-node metastases in patients with prostate cancer.[76] These techniques, however, require further clinical evaluation before widespread use.

Transrectal ultrasound is an insensitive method for detecting local extension of tumor, but some experts still believe that TRUS can add staging information over that gained with DRE.[70] Intravenous urography is rarely obtained to stage prostate cancer but can evaluate the upper urinary tract in cases of hematuria or suspected obstruction. A chest X-ray is generally a low-yield examination in the staging of prostate cancer, since lung metastases are exceedingly rare in the absence of widespread metastatic disease.

RADIOIMMUNOSCINTIGRAPHY

Monoclonal antibody radioimmunoscintigraphy (radiolabeled monoclonal antibody scan) is an approach used for the identification of microscopic cancer deposits in regional and distant sites. The ProstaScint scan (Cytogen Corp, Princeton NJ) utilizes this technology but has had limited accuracy in the detection of lymph node metastases due to the fact that

the antibody targets an intracellular epitope, which is exposed in dying or dead cells only.[77,78] Future generations of this technology that circumvent this limitation are currently being developed.

MOLECULAR STAGING

Molecular staging has focused on the detection of circulating prostate cancer cells either directly through centrifugation/immunostaining methods or indirectly by identifying the genetic message (mRNA) for prostate-specific biomarkers like PSA or prostate surface membrane antigen (PSMA) from circulating prostate cells.[79,80] The latter technique, referred to as reverse transcription polymerase chain reaction (RT-PCR), involves reverse transcription of circulating mRNA to complementary DNA (cDNA), and amplification of the DNA coding for the biomarker by polymerase chain reaction. Although studies have shown that these PCR assays are strong predictors of pathologic stage, their sensitivity for detecting circulating cancer cells has been variable among different investigators.[41,81,82] In addition, 25% of 65 men found to have organ confined disease at prostatectomy in one study had a positive PCR-PSA assay.[83] These men would have been denied surgery if one equated the PCR test results with incurable disease. Thus, until the significance of a positive PCR assay is known with long-term follow-up, men with clinically localized disease should not be denied curative treatment based on these tests.

PELVIC LYMPHADENECTOMY

The presence of lymph node metastasis in men diagnosed with clinically localized prostate cancer portends a poor prognosis. Accurate identification of these men allows more precise prognostication and may have important implications on the initiation of adjuvant therapy. While the prevalence of pelvic lymph node metastases correlates directly with T stage, serum PSA level, and biopsy grade, pelvic lymphadenectomy remains the most accurate staging modality for the detection of occult nodal involvement.[84] The advent of PSA screening has resulted in a steady decline in the incidence of lymph node metastasis from rates of 20% to 40% in the 1970s and 1980s to less than 6% today.[23,84] As a result of this stage shift, lymphadenectomy is often omitted preceding various curative treatment approaches (radical retropubic prostatectomy, perineal prostatectomy, and radiation therapy).[85] The criteria for laparoscopic pelvic lymphadenectomy prior to treatment are controversial and this procedure is often reserved for patients with Gleason score greater than 8, extraprostatic extension on DRE, PSA greater than 20 ng/mL, or when there is suspicion of enlarged lymph nodes on radiological evaluation.

Given the individual variation in prostatic lymphatic drainage patterns, some investigators have favored an extended pelvic lymphadenectomy in lieu of a limited dissection. A recent retrospective study demonstrated that an extended pelvic lymphadenectomy may maximize the detection rate of lymph node positive disease compared with a limited lymph node dissection in a contemporary series of PSA-screened men with clinically localized prostate cancer undergoing radical prostatectomy.[86] Information regarding the therapeutic value of such a strategy is confounded by the issue of stage migration and is difficult to evaluate in the absence of prospective trials.

REFERENCES

1. Pound CR, Partin AW, Epstein JI, et al. Prostate-specific antigen after anatomic radical retropubic prostatectomy. Patterns of recurrence and cancer control. Urol Clin North Am 1997;24:395–406.

2. Epstein J. Evaluation of radical prostatectomy capsular margins of resection: The significance of margins designated as negative, closely approaching and positive. Am J Surg Pathol 1990;14:626–632.

3. Epstein J, Pizov G, Walsh P. Correlation of pathologic findings with progression after radical retropubic prostatectomy. Cancer 1993;71:3582–3593.

4. Epstein J, Carmichael M, Pizov G, et al. Influence of capsular penetration on progression following radical prostatectomy: A study of 196 cases with long-term follow-up. J Urol 1993;150:135–141.

5. Partin AW, Pound CR, Clemens JQ, et al. Serum PSA after anatomic radical prostatectomy. The Johns Hopkins experience after 10 years. Urol Clin North Am 1993;20:713–725.

6. Jewett H. The present status of radical prostatectomy for stages A and B prostatic cancer. Urol Clin N Am 1975:105–124.

7. Walsh PC, Jewett HJ. Radical surgery for prostatic cancer. Cancer 1980;45:1906–1911.

8. Jewett H. Significance of the palpable prostatic nodule. JAMA 1956;160:838.

9. Whitmore WF Jr. Hormone therapy in prostatic cancer. Am J Med 1956;21:697–713.

10. Wallace D, Chisolm G, Hendry W. TNM classification for urological tumors (UICC)—1974. Br J Urol 1975;47:1–12.

11. Schroder F, Hermanek P, Denis L, et al. The TNM classification of prostate cancer. Prostate Suppl 1992;4:129–138.

12. Flemming I, Cooper J, Hemson D, et al. In: American Joint Committee on Cancer Staging Manual, 5th ed. Philadelphia: Lipincott, 1997, pp 219–222.

13. Iyer R, Hanlon A, Pinover W, et al. Outcome evaluation of the 1997 American Joint Committee on cancer staging system for prostate carcinoma treated by radiation therapy. Cancer 1999;85:1816–1821.

14. Han M, Walsh P, Partin A, et al. Ability of the 1992 and 1997 American Joint Committee on cancer staging systems for prostate cancer to predict progression-free survival after radical prostatectomy for stage T2 disease. J Urol 2000;164:89–92.

15. Ferguson J, Bostwick D, Suman V, et al. Prostate-specific antigen detected prostate cancer: Pathological characteristics of ultrasound visible versus ultrasound invisible tumors. Eur Urol 1995;27:8–12.

16. Epstein J, Walsh P, Carmichael M, et al. Pathologic and clinical findings to predict tumor extent of non-palpable (stage T1c) prostate cancer. JAMA 1994;271:368–374.

17. Ohori M, Utsunomiya T, Suyama K, et al. Is the definition of stage T1c prostate cancer correct: Do impalpable cancers visible on ultrasound differ from those not visible? J Urol 2000;63:182 [abstract #808].

18. Tiguert R, Gheiler E, Grignon D, et al. Patients with abnormal ultrasound of the prostate but normal digital rectal examination should be classified as having clinical stage T2 tumors. J Urol 2000;163:1486–1490.

19. Partin AW, Yoo J, Carter HB, et al. The use of prostate specific antigen, clinical stage and Gleason score to predict pathological stage in men with localized prostate cancer. J Urol 1993;150:110–4.

20. Kleer E, Oesterling JE. PSA and staging of localized prostate cancer. Urol Clin North Am 1993;20:695–704.

21. Kleer E, Larson-Keller JJ, Zincke H, et al. Ability of preoperative serum prostate-specific antigen value to predict pathologic stage and DNA ploidy. Influence of clinical stage and tumor grade. Urology 1993;41:207–216.

22. Humphrey PA, Walther PJ, Currin SM, et al. Histologic grade, DNA ploidy, and intraglandular tumor extent as indicators of tumor progression of clinical stage B prostatic carcinoma. A direct comparison. Am J Surg Pathol 1991;15:1165–1170.

23. Partin AW, Kattan MW, Subong EN, et al. Combination of prostate-specific antigen, clinical stage, and Gleason score to predict pathological stage of localized prostate cancer. A multi-institutional update. JAMA 1997;277:1445–1451.

24. Bluestein DL, Bostwick DG, Bergstralh EJ, et al. Eliminating the need for bilateral pelvic lymphadenectomy in select patients with prostate cancer. J Urol 1994;151:1315–1320.

25. Partin AW, Mangold LA, Lamm DM, et al. Contemporary update of prostate cancer staging nomograms (Partin Tables) for the new millennium. Urology 2001;58:843–848.

26. D'Amico AV, Whittington R, Malkowicz SB, et al. Predicting prostate specific antigen outcome preoperatively in the prostate specific antigen era. J Urol 2001;166:2185–2188.

27. Gleason D. Classification of prostatic carcinoma. Cancer Chemotherapy Report 1966;50:125–128.

28. Zincke H, Oesterling JE, Blute ML, et al. Long-term (15 years) results after radical prostatectomy for clinically localized (stage T2c or lower) prostate cancer. J Urol 1994;152:1850–1857.

29. Stein A, deKernion JB, Dorey F. Prostatic specific antigen related to clinical status 1 to 14 years after radical retropubic prostatectomy. Br J Urol 1991;67:626–631.

30. Epstein J, Walsh P, Brendler C. Radical prostatectomy for impalpable prostate cancer: The Johns Hopkins experience with tumors found on transurethral resection (Stages T1a and T1b) and on needle biopsy (Stage T1c). J Urol 1994;152:1721–1729.

31. Bismar TA, Lewis JS Jr, Vollmer RT, et al. Multiple measures of carcinoma extent versus perineural invasion in prostate needle biopsy tissue in prediction of pathologic stage in a screening population. Am J Surg Pathol 2003;27:432–440.

32. Carter HB, Walsh PC, Landis P, et al. Expectant management of nonpalpable prostate cancer with curative intent: preliminary results. J Urol 2002;167:1231–1234.

33. Stone N, Stock R, Parikh D, et al. Perineural invasion and seminal vesicle involvement predict pelvic lymph node metastasis in men with localized carcinoma of the prostate. J Urol 1998;160:1722–1726.

34. Stone N, Stock R, Unger P. Indications for seminal vesicle biopsy and laparoscopic pelvic lymph node dissection in men with localized carcinoma of the prostate. J Urol 1995;154:1392–1396.

35. Vallancien G, Bochereau G, Wetzel O, et al. Influence of preoperative positive seminal vesicle biopsy on the staging of prostatic cancer. J Urol 1994:1152–1156.

36. Terris M, McNeal J, Freiha F, et al. Efficacy of transrectal ultrasound-guided seminal vesicle biopsies in the detection of seminal vesicle invasion by prostate cancer. J Urol 1993;149:1035–1039.

37. Ravery V, Boccon-Gibod L, Dauge-Geffroy M, et al. Systematic biopsies accurately predict extracapsular extension of prostate cancer and persistent/recurrent detectable PSA after radical prostatectomy. Urology 1994;44:371–376.

38. Guillonneau B, Debras B, Veillon B, et al. Indications for preoperative seminal vesicle biopsies in staging of clinically localized prostatic cancer. Eur Urol 1997;32:160–165.

39. Terris M, Pham T, Issa M, et al. Routine transition zone and seminal vesicle biopsies in all patients undergoing transrectal ultrasound guided prostate biopsies are not indicated. J Urol 1997;157:204–206.

40. Egan AJ, Bostwick DG, Belt E, et al. Prediction of extraprostatic extension of prostate cancer based on needle biopsy findings: perineural invasion lacks significance on multivariate analysis. A

study of 229 consecutive cases of total perineal prostatectomy for cancer of the prostate. Am J Surg Pathol 1997;21:1496–1500.

41. de la Taille A, Katz A, Bagiella E, et al. Perineural invasion on prostate needle biopsy: an independent predictor of final pathologic stage. Urology 1999;54:1039–1043.

42. O'Malley KJ, Pound CR, Walsh PC, et al. Influence of biopsy perineural invasion on long-term biochemical disease-free survival after radical prostatectomy. Urology 2002;59:85–90.

43. Polascik TJ, Oesterling JE, Partin AW. Prostate specific antigen: a decade of discovery—what we have learned and where we are going. J Urol 1999;162:293–306.

44. Stamey TA, Yang N, Hay AR, et al. Prostate-specific antigen as a serum marker for adenocarcinoma of the prostate. N Engl J Med 1987;317:909–16.

45. Stamey TA, Kabalin JN, McNeal JE, et al. Prostate specific antigen in the diagnosis and treatment of adenocarcinoma of the prostate. II. Radical prostatectomy treated patients. J Urol 1989;141:1076–1083.

46. Noldus J, Graefen M, Huland E, et al. The value of the ratio of free-to-total prostate specific antigen for staging purposes in previously untreated prostate cancer. J Urol 1998;159:2004–2007; discussion 2007–2008.

47. Partin AW, Carter HB, Chan DW, et al. Prostate specific antigen in the staging of localized prostate cancer: influence of tumor differentiation, tumor volume and benign hyperplasia. J Urol 1990;143:747–752.

48. Benson MC, Whang IS, Pantuck A, et al. Prostate specific antigen density: a means of distinguishing benign prostatic hypertrophy and prostate cancer. J Urol 1992;147:815–816.

49. Benson MC, Whang IS, Olsson CA, et al. The use of prostate specific antigen density to enhance the predictive value of intermediate levels of serum prostate specific antigen. J Urol 1992;147:817–821.

50. Rietbergen JB, Hoedemaeker RF, Kruger AE, et al. The changing pattern of prostate cancer at the time of diagnosis: characteristics of screen detected prostate cancer in a population based screening study. J Urol 1999;161:1192–1198.

51. Catalona WJ, Smith DS, Ornstein DK. Prostate cancer detection in men with serum PSA concentrations of 2.6 to 4.0 ng/mL and benign prostate examination. Enhancement of specificity with free PSA measurements. JAMA 1997;277:1452–1455.

52. Haese A, Graefen M, Becker C, et al. The role of human glandular kallikrein 2 for prediction of pathologically organ confined prostate cancer. Prostate 2003;54:181–186.

53. Gretzer MB, Partin AW. PSA markers in prostate cancer detection. Urol Clin North Am 2003;30:677–686.

54. Southwick PC, Catalona WJ, Partin AW, et al. Prediction of post-radical prostatectomy pathological outcome for stage T1c prostate cancer with percent free prostate specific antigen: a prospective multicenter clinical trial. J Urol 1999;162:1346–1351.

55. Carter HB, Partin AW, Luderer AA, et al. Percentage of free prostate-specific antigen in sera predicts aggressiveness of prostate cancer a decade before diagnosis. Urology 1997;49:379–384.

56. D'Amico AV, Chen MH, Roehl KA, et al. Preoperative PSA velocity and the risk of death from prostate cancer after radical prostatectomy. N Engl J Med 2004;351:125–135.

57. Heller JE. Prostatic acid phosphatase: its current clinical status. J Urol 1987;137:1091–1103.

58. Burnett AL, Chan DW, Brendler CB, et al. The value of serum enzymatic acid phosphatase in the staging of localized prostate cancer. J Urol 1992;148:1832–1834.

59. Moul JW, Connelly RR, Perahia B, et al. The contemporary value of pretreatment prostatic acid phosphatase to predict pathological stage and recurrence in radical prostatectomy cases. J Urol 1998;159:935–940.

60. Han M, Piantadosi S, Zahurak ML, et al. Serum acid phosphatase level and biochemical recurrence following radical prostatectomy for men with clinically localized prostate cancer. Urology 2001;57:707–711.

61. Turner RD, Belt E. The results of 1,694 consecutive simple perineal prostatectomies. J Urol 1957;77:853–863.

62. Byar DP, Mostofi FK. Carcinoma of the prostate: prognostic evaluation of certain pathologic features in 208 radical prostatectomies. Examined by the step-section technique. Cancer 1972;30:5–13.

63. Schaffer DL, Pendergrass HP. Comparison of enzyme, clinical, radiographic, and radionuclide methods of detecting bone metastases from carcinoma of the prostate. Radiology 1976;121:431–434.

64. Gerber G, Chodak GW. Assessment of value of routine bone scans in patients with newly diagnosed prostate cancer. Urology 1991;37:418–422.

65. Terris MK, Klonecke AS, McDougall IR, et al. Utilization of bone scans in conjunction with prostate-specific antigen levels in the surveillance for recurrence of adenocarcinoma after radical prostatectomy. J Nucl Med 1991;32:1713–1717.

66. Lachman E. Osteoporosis — The potentialities and limitations of its roentgenologic diagnosis. Am J Roentgenol Radium Ther Nucl Med 1955;74:712–725.

67. Lentle BC, McGowan DG, Dierich H. Technetium-99M polyphosphate bone scanning in carcinoma of the prostate. Br J Urol 1974;46:543–548.

68. Narayan P, Lillian D, Hellstrom W, et al. The benefits of combining early radionuclide renal scintigraphy with routine bone scans in patients with prostate cancer. J Urol 1988;140:1448–1451.

69. Chybowski FM, Keller JJ, Bergstralh EJ, et al. Predicting radionuclide bone scan findings in patients with newly diagnosed, untreated prostate cancer: prostate specific antigen is superior to all other clinical parameters. J Urol 1991;145:313–318.

70. Rifkin MD, Zerhouni EA, Gatsonis CA, et al. Comparison of magnetic resonance imaging and ultrasonography in staging early prostate cancer. Results of a multi-institutional cooperative trial. N Engl J Med 1990;323:621–626.

71. Tempany CM, Zhou X, Zerhouni EA, et al. Staging of prostate cancer: results of Radiology Diagnostic Oncology Group project comparison of three MR imaging techniques. Radiology 1994;192:47–54.

72. Wolf JS, Jr., Cher M, Dall'era M, et al. The use and accuracy of cross-sectional imaging and fine needle aspiration cytology for detection of pelvic lymph node metastases before radical prostatectomy. J Urol 1995;153:993–999.

73. Kindrick AV, Grossfeld GD, Stier DM, et al. Use of imaging tests for staging newly diagnosed prostate cancer: trends from the CaPSURE database. J Urol 1998;160:2102–2106.

74. Kurhanewicz J, Vigneron DB, Males RG, et al. The prostate: MR imaging and spectroscopy. Present and future. Radiol Clin North Am 2000;38:115–138, viii–ix.

75. Yu KK, Scheidler J, Hricak H, et al. Prostate cancer: prediction of extracapsular extension with endorectal MR imaging and three-dimensional proton MR spectroscopic imaging. Radiology 1999;213:481–488.

76. Harisinghani MG, Barentsz J, Hahn PF, et al. Noninvasive detection of clinically occult lymph-node metastases in prostate cancer. N Engl J Med 2003;348:2491–2499.

77. Chang SS, Reuter VE, Heston WD, et al. Five different anti-prostate-specific membrane antigen (PSMA) antibodies confirm PSMA expression in tumor-associated neovasculature. Cancer Res 1999;59:3192–3198.

78. Troyer JK, Beckett ML, Wright GL, Jr. Location of prostate-specific membrane antigen in the LNCaP prostate carcinoma cell line. Prostate 1997;30:232–242.

79. Ts'o PO, Pannek J, Wang ZP, et al. Detection of intact prostate cancer cells in the blood of men with prostate cancer. Urology 1997;49:881–885.

80. Moreno JG, Croce CM, Fischer R, et al. Detection of hematogenous micrometastasis in patients with prostate cancer. Cancer Res 1992;52:6110–6112.

81. Cama C, Olsson CA, Raffo AJ, et al. Molecular staging of prostate cancer. II. A comparison of the application of an enhanced reverse transcriptase polymerase chain reaction assay for prostate specific antigen versus prostate specific membrane antigen. J Urol 1995;153:1373–1378.

82. Israeli RS, Miller WH Jr, Su SL, et al. Sensitive detection of prostatic hematogenous tumor cell dissemination using prostate specific antigen and prostate specific membrane-derived primers in the polymerase chain reaction. J Urol 1995;153:573–577.

83. Katz AE, Olsson CA, Raffo AJ, et al. Molecular staging of prostate cancer with the use of an enhanced reverse transcriptase-PCR assay. Urology 1994;43:765–775.

84. Parker CC, Husband J, Dearnaley DP. Lymph node staging in clinically localized prostate cancer. Prostate Cancer Prostatic Dis 1999;2:191–199.

85. Bishoff JT, Reyes A, Thompson IM, et al. Pelvic lymphadenectomy can be omitted in selected patients with carcinoma of the prostate: development of a system of patient selection. Urology 1995;45:270–274.

86. Allaf ME, Palapattu GS, Trock BJ, et al. Anatomical extent of lymph node dissection: impact on men with clinically localized prostate cancer. Journal of Urology 2004;172:1840–1844.

TNM and IUCC staging of prostate cancer

44

Lincol Olsen, J Brantley Thrasher, Jeffrey M Holzbeierlein

PHILOSOPHY OF THE TNM SYSTEM

The American Joint Committee on Cancer (AJCC) classification system (TNM staging) is based on the fact that cancers of an anatomic site act in similar ways. In general, as the primary tumor (T) grows it begins to invade locally and eventually spreads to regional lymph nodes that drain the area of the tumor (N). In addition to nodal disease the tumor may spread either by lymph drainage or by hematogenous spread and involve distant sites of the body or nonregional lymph nodes (i.e., metastasis, M). Evaluation by clinical means allows for the assignment of a clinical stage. In some instances, evaluation of the primary tumor and nodal disease may or may not be assessed accurately by clinical means and, if surgical intervention is pursued, a pathologic stage is assigned based on findings at the time of operation as well as histologic analysis of the primary tumor and regional lymph nodes.[1] This classification system is known as the TNM staging system and is identical to that of the International Union Against Cancer (IUCC).

TNM STAGING OF PROSTATE CANCER

The Whitmore–Jewett staging model was the first widely used staging system for prostate cancer (CaP), but was supplanted by the TNM staging system initially proposed in 1975. In 1992 a new TNM classification system was adopted, which was revised in 1997 by including T2b lesions in the T2a category and changing T2c lesions to T2b. This change was reversed in 2002 (Table 44.1). Once the tumor, nodes, and metastasis evaluations are made a stage (I to IV) is then assigned to the patient with CaP (Table 44.2).

The TNM staging system utilizes both clinical staging techniques as well as pathologic staging. Clinical staging is based on physical examination and imaging studies. Clinical understaging is common when compared to pathological staging.[3-5] Pathologic staging, including surgical margin status, presence of extracapsular extension, seminal vesicle invasion, and nodal status are the factors that are most predictive of disease outcome.[6-9]

CLINICAL STAGING

ASSESSMENT OF THE PRIMARY TUMOR (T STAGE)

The extent of the primary tumor (T stage) is primarily assessed by digital rectal examination (DRE). Occasionally radiographic images (transrectal ultra-sonography [TRUS]) may also be used to assess the primary tumor, however, it is controversial as to whether this should change the clinical T stage. A nodule or suspicious area of induration on prostate examination are the physical exam findings that are used to determine the T stage. A T1 lesion (the most common T stage seen in the United States) is one identified by abnormal prostate-specific antigen (PSA) or findings of adenocarcinoma on transurethral resection of the prostate with a normal DRE. A T2 lesion is a palpable lesion and is the second most common in the United States. Extracapsular spread, a nodule that is palpable beyond the prostate or a lesion that, on palpation, appears to invade the seminal vesicle, represents a T3 stage. A T4 lesion is one that is fixed to the pelvic side wall or invades adjacent structures other than the

Table 44.1 TNM staging of prostate cancer 2002

TNM		Description
Primary tumor clinical staging (T)		
Tx		Primary tumor unable to be assessed
T0		No evidence of primary tumor
T1		Tumor not apparent on palpation or imaging
	T1a	Incidental finding at TUR (<5%)
	T1b	Incidental finding at TUR (>5%)
	T1c	Tumor identified at time of biopsy (PSA elevation)
T2		Tumor confined within the prostate
	T2a	Tumor involves less than half a single lobe
	T2b	Tumor involves more than one half of a single lobe
	T2c	Tumor involves more than one lobe (Bilateral)
T3		Tumor not confined to the prostate
	T3a	Extension through the capsule
	T3b	Extension into the seminal vesicle(s)
T4		Tumor fixed or invades adjacent structures excluding seminal vesicles (bladder neck, external sphincter, rectum, levator muscles, and pelvic wall)
Pimary tumor pathologic staging (T)		
pT2		Organ confined
	pT2a/b	Unilateral involvement
	pT2c	Bilateral involvement
pT3		Extraprostatic extension
	pT3a	Capsular invasion
	pT3b	Seminal vesicle invasion
pT4		Invasion of contiguous structures
Regional lymph nodes (N)		
Nx		Regional lymph nodes not assessed
N0		No involvement of regional nodes
N1		Regional lymph node involvement
Distant metastasis (M)		
Mx		Distant metastasis not assessed
M0		No distant metastasis
M1		Distant metastasis
	M1a	Nonregional lymph node involvement
	M1b	Bone involvement
	M1c	Involvement of other distant sites

Table 44.2 Stage grouping in prostate cancer

	T	N	M
Stage I	T1a	N0	M0
Stage II	T1a–T2	N0	M0
Stage III	T3	N0	M0
Stage IV	T4	N0	M0
	Any T	N1	M0
	Any T	Any N	M1

seminal vesicles (i.e., bladder neck, external sphincter, rectum, levator muscle, or pelvic wall).[1]

DIGITAL RECTAL EXAMINATION

Traditionally, DRE has been the primary method of screening for CaP and assessment of clinical T stage for CaP. Gustafsson et al screened 1782 men and found that the positive predictive value (PPV) of an abnormal DRE when used alone in screening is 22%.[10] Digital rectal examination failed to identify 20 patients who were found to have CaP at biopsy (of 143 identified by TRUS). In addition, DRE is not sensitive or specific for evaluation of extracapsular extension. Multiple studies have assessed the usefulness of DRE in the staging of the primary tumor. O'Dowd et al compiled data from multiple radical prostatectomy series and found that the false-negative rate for DRE was 48%.[11] In addition the authors found that the specificity of DRE was less than 10% and that overall accuracy was only 57% when the examination was performed by one urologist and the pathologic slides were examined by one pathologist. Furthermore, DRE is subject to interobserver variability making the DRE subjective and poorly reproducible.[12–13] Other studies have found that lesions confined to the prostate on digital palpation actually extend through the capsule or into the seminal vesicles more than 55% of the time on pathologic examination[2–5] underscoring the problem of understaging associated with clinical staging. Although DRE lacks both specificity and sensitivity, it is currently the major modality to assess the clinical T stage and does provide a measure of probable recurrence. It becomes more useful when combined with Gleason score and PSA in predictive models such as the Kattan nomogram (Figure 44.1)

PROSTATE-SPECIFIC ANTIGEN

Although not currently included in the TNM staging system, PSA has been demonstrated to correlate with pathologic stage and tumor volume even though its value in predicting extracapsular extension at levels of 4 to 10 ng/mL has been reported to be only 33% to 47%.[14,15] At levels of 1 to 4 ng/mL, Partin et al found a positive predictive value of 64% for organ-confined disease.[14] Recent data from Catalona et al have recommended lowering the PSA cutoff to 2.5 ng/mL, which has resulted in organ confined rates of 88%.[16] High PSA values (>50 ng/mL) are predictive of extraprostatic disease with over 90% demonstrating pathologic T3 or T4 disease.[14] In addition, PSA is one of the most heavily weighted factors in the Kattan nomogram predictive model.

PROSTATE BIOPSY AND GLEASON SCORE

Currently, information gained from the prostate biopsy is not used in the evaluation of the clinical T stage. The

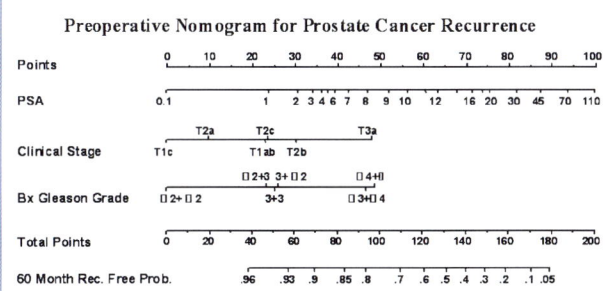

Fig. 44.1

Kattan nomogram for preoperative evaluation using prostate-specific antigen (PSA), clinical stage, and Gleason score as a predictor for prostate cancer recurrence.

Instruction for physician: Locate the patient's PSA on the PSA axis. Draw a line straight upwards to the Points axis to determine how many points towards recurrence the patient receives for his PSA. Repeat this process for the Clinical Stage and Biopsy Gleason Sum axes, each time drawing straight upward to the Points axis. Sum the points achieved for each predictor and locate this sum on the Total Points axis. Draw a line straight down to find the patient's probability of remaining recurrence free for 60 months, assuming he does not die of another cause first.

Note: This nomogram is not applicable to a man who is not otherwise a candidate for radical prostatectomy. You can use this only on a man who has already selected radical prostatectomy as treatment for his prostate cancer.

Instruction to patient: "Mr X, if we had 100 men exactly like you, we would expect between <predicted percentage from nomogram – 10%> and <predicted percentage from nomogram + 10%> to remain free of their disease at 5 years following radical prostatectomy, and recurrence after 5 years is very rare."

Kattan MW et al. JNCI 1998;90:766–771.

Gleason score is the most used method for histologic grading of CaP. Multiple studies have attempted to correlate the Gleason score with the risk of extracapsular extension.[14,15,17] For Gleason scores of 2 to 6, the rate of organ-confined disease is 68%, while those with Gleason scores of 7 and 10 had extracapsular extension and seminal vesicle invasion in 46% and 23% of cases, respectively. The Gleason score is not incorporated into clinical staging.

Goto et al examined the significance of the number of positive cores, the total length of cancer in the cores, and the percentage of poorly differentiated cancer in each core.[18] They found that 93% of patients with a PSA greater than 6 ng/mL had advanced pathologic stage if at least four biopsy cores had cancer, total length of cancer in all cores was at least 20 mm, and at least 10% of the cancer was poorly differentiated. Patients who did not meet these criteria had organ-confined disease in nearly 90% of cases. Although this data is not taken into account in clinical staging, many argue that it should be incorporated into future staging protocols.

TRANSRECTAL ULTRASOUND

Transrectal ultrasound is the most commonly used imaging modality for evaluation of the prostate. Prostate cancer classically appears as a hypoechoic lesion on ultrasound. Multiple studies have evaluated TRUS as a screening modality for CaP.[19,20] These studies have found that TRUS is unable to localize early prostate cancer and that it has a low PPV when used for screening (15–18%). In addition, TRUS only detects 64% of CaP in patients undergoing radical prostatectomy.[21]

Transrectal ultrasound has also been evaluated for staging of pathologically confirmed prostate cancer. Results from a large study by Rifkin et al found that in evaluating the prostate for extracapsular extension TRUS had an overall accuracy of 46% with sensitivity and specificity of 66% and 46% respectively.[22] The sensitivity of ultrasound imaging tends to improve with increasing stage whereas the specificity is inversely related to the stage of disease.[2]

More recently color Doppler has been used to evaluate CaP.[23] Areas of hypervascularity found in the peripheral zone of the prostate often represent CaP, and if isoechoic areas of hypervasularity have "chaotic flow" then they are also likely to be cancerous. Most important is the fact that areas without evidence of neovascularization are not neoplastic in more than 90% of cases. Many urologists feel that TRUS is not particularly useful in clinical staging, and do not currently incorporate findings either positive or negative into their T staging.

ENDORECTAL MAGNETIC RESONANCE IMAGING

Technological advancements have allowed for the use of endorectal coil magnetic resonance imaging (MRI) as another method of imaging the prostate. The images have increased resolutional capacity of the prostate with the ability to distinguish zonal anatomy and periprostatic tissue in a well-defined manner when compared with TRUS and computed tomography (CT)[24] (Figure 44.2). Results have varied significantly with this type of imaging as a preoperative evaluation. Some studies have failed to find an increased advantage of endorectal MRI over TRUS.[25] Others have found that it has good sensitivity for extracapsular extension (84–97%) and seminal vesicle invasion (84–93%) but lacks sensitivity for the same criteria (13–22% and 23–59%, respectively).[26,27] Unfortunately, because of the high false-positive rate of extracapsular extension of this study, many feel it may exclude some patients who should be referred for possible curative radical prostatectomy, or may incorrectly exclude patients from nerve sparing procedures. Additionally, there is a significant amount of inter-reader variability associated with endorectal MRI, with most of this variability attributed to reader experience.[28] This imaging modality is not currently incorporated into the clinical TNM staging system.

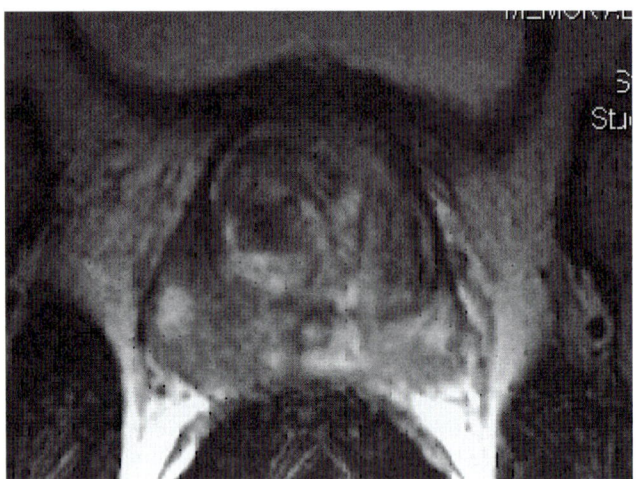

Fig. 44.2
Endorectal coil magnetic resonance imaging (MRI) of the prostate showing characteristic lesion of prostate cancer.

ASSESSMENT OF LYMPH NODE METASTASIS (N STAGE)

Clinical lymph node involvement is evaluated by imaging modalities when indicated. Relative indications include PSA greater than 20 ng/mL, Gleason greater than 8, or stage greater than T3. The regional lymph nodes that are most frequently involved are those of the true pelvis including the hypogastric, obturator, internal, and external iliac nodes. N0 represents no nodal involvement while N1 to N3 represent involvement of regional lymph nodes of varying size and number (see Table 44.1)[1]

COMPUTED TOMOGRAPHY

Computed tomography evidence of lymph node involvement is based on the measurements of a individual lymph nodes, with those over 1 cm considered suspicious. Two recent studies have shown high specificity (95–98%) for CT imaging of lymph nodes, however, the sensitivity was variable, with one of the studies finding a sensitivity of 25% while the other 78%.[29,30] In addition to low sensitivity, CT has a very low positive yield (1.5–12%) especially for patients with a PSA of less than 20 ng/mL.[31,32] Therefore, CT should usually be reserved for patients with a high likelihood of having nodal metastasis (T3 or greater disease, Gleason >8, PSA >20) or for those who are not likely to undergo traditional surgical staging (i.e., radical perineal prostatectomy).

POSITRON EMISSION TOPOGRAPHY

Positron emission topography (PET) scanning allows for visualization of increased metabolic activity after intravenous administration of a radiotracer. The radiotracer is concentrated in neoplastic cells and allows the clinician to evaluate nodal status. Prostate cancer has a relatively low metabolic rate and this contributes to the limitations of PET in its assessment. However, recent studies have shown PET scanning to be 72% to 93% accurate in detecting nodal metastasis.[33,34] This is an imaging modality that has shown promise and may help to stage nodal disease in patients with CaP in the future.

RADIO-IMMUNOSCINTIGRAPHY

Monoclonal antibodies directed at a glycoprotein of the prostate-specific membrane antigen (PSMA) have been developed and these may be useful in identifying nodal metastasis. The ProstaScint™ (Cytogen, Princeton, NJ) scan is the most commonly used of these scans. Rosenthal et al reported a PPV and negative PV (NPV) of 72% and 62%, respectively, with ProstaScint™ in patients with newly diagnosed CaP who had high risk of nodal metastases.[35] Another recent prospective study revealed a sensitivity and specificity of 62% and 72% compared with a sensitivity of 4% for CT and 15% for MRI.[36] It is currently FDA approved for those patients at high risk for nodal involvement and for those with a PSA recurrence after primary therapy. However, its usefulness has been questioned because the antibody targets an intracellular portion of the PSMA leading to decreased sensitivity. Newer antibodies, which may be directed at both the intracellular and extracelluar portion of PSMA or against other antigens specific for CaP, may improve the usefulness of this test for staging.

EVALUATION FOR METASTATIC DISEASE (M STAGE)

Any distant metastasis including bone and nonregional lymph nodes are characterized as M1 disease. Nonregional lymph nodes that may be secondarily involved are the common iliac, deep or superficial inguinal, aortic, and retroperitoneal nodes; if involved, this represents M1a disease. Bone involvement is classified as M1b, and all other metastasis are M1c disease.

Bone is the organ most often involved in CaP metastasis and bone scanning is the most common method used to detect metastasis to the bone. In patients with a PSA of less than 20 ng/mL, less than 0.5% of individuals will have a positive bone scan, and the mean PSA value of patients with a positive bone scan is greater then 150 ng/mL.[37] The majority of patients with positive bone scan have a PSA of more than 40 ng/mL.[38] This would suggest that staging bone scan can be omitted in patients with PSA values of less than 20 ng/mL in the absence of other factors such as high Gleason scores or advanced T-stage disease.

PATHOLOGIC STAGING

ASSESSMENT OF THE PRIMARY TUMOR (T STAGE)

Histopathologic analysis at the time of radical prostatectomy assesses the laterality of cancer as well as extracapsular extension, surgical margin status, and seminal vesicle involvement. As noted earlier, two key prognostic indicators at the time of radical prostatectomy are surgical margins and extraprostatic spread of the cancer. The probability of positive surgical margins is increased by increasing cancer stage and volume and by the experience of the surgeon.[39] It has been suggested that T2 tumors with positive surgical margins be considered pT2+ tumors due to the increased risk of recurrence with positive surgical margins. The T stage determined by pathologic analysis is shown in Table 44.1. Again, it should be noted that there was a change from the 1992 pathologic staging in the T2 category with the 1997 staging system.

ASSESSMENT OF THE NODAL STATUS

PELVIC LYMPHADENECTOMY

Pelvic lymphadenectomy is the gold standard for determining the presence of gross or microscopic metastasis to regional lymph nodes. It can be undertaken as a separate procedure before perineal prostatectomy or radiation treatment or at the time of radical retropubic prostatectomy. Multiple procedures for pelvic lymphadenectomy have been described, including laparoscopy[40] and mini laparotomy.[41] Bluestein et al evaluated the need for pelvic lymph node dissection (PLND) in 1632 men with CaP and found that only 39% of patients with clinical stages T1a to T2b would need staging PLND based on evaluation of PSA, Gleason score, and clinical stage.[42]

Some have suggested that extended PLND is more accurate in determining nodal involvement than a limited lymph node dissection. One study found that 24% of patients undergoing extended PLND at the time of radical prostatectomy were found to have nodal involvement.[43] These patients had an average PSA of 11 ng/mL, and there was no control group. Another study compared the incidence of nodal involvement in patients with clinically localized CaP when extended versus limited lymph node dissection was performed.[44] They found that only 8 of 123 patients with a mean PSA of 7.4 ng/mL had lymph node metastasis, and only 4 of these would not have been found on limited node dissection. Additionally, complications were three times as common when extended PLND was performed. It is currently unclear if extended lymphadenectomy has

advantages over limited PLND, and it is not performed routinely. Furthermore, some have advocated more extensive pathologic analysis of the lymph nodes, which include fat-clearing techniques, immunohistochemistry, or reverse transcriptase polymerase chain reaction (RT-PCR) for PSA to indicate lymph node involvement. However, currently this is not the standard pathologic assessment.

Because of the overall small percentages of positive lymph nodes in the United States attributed to aggressive screening and early detection, many have advocated omitting the pelvic lymph node dissection. However, most agree that those patients who have findings suggestive of pelvic lymphadenopathy during clinical staging, PSA greater than 20, Gleason 8 or higher, or palpable extraprostatic extension should undergo PLND.[45] This may be of particular importance in men who have elected not to undergo surgical intervention or in those who wish to have a perineal prostatectomy.

ON THE HORIZON

ARTIFICIAL INTELLIGENCE NETWORKS

Recently, the development of artificial intelligence networks or artificial neural networks (ANNs) has been applied to the staging of CaP. Artificial neural networks are information processing units that attempt to simulate the characteristics of biological systems.[46] In a study of 1200 men with clinically localized CaP, serum PSA, systematic biopsy results, and Gleason score results were analyzed by the ANN, the network had a sensitivity of 81% to 100% and a specificity of 72% to 75% for predicting surgical margins, seminal vesicle involvement, and lymph node involvement when compared with histologic examination. Only 2% of patients with lymph node involvement were misdiagnosed by the ANN, and none were found to have seminal vesicle involvement if the ANN did not predict it.[47]

REVERSE TRANSCRIPTASE POLYMERASE CHAIN REACTION

The RT-PCR reaction is a molecular biology technique that allows detection of cells circulating in the blood that produce PSA. Initial reports suggest that this technique is useful in identifying patients who would have treatment failures after radical prostatectomy.[48] Other reports by different groups have suggested that RT-PCR does not assist in clinical staging of CaP.[49] This tool is experimental and has no role in clinical staging at this time.

SUPERPARAMAGNETIC PARTICLES

A new method of localizing nodal metastasis is through the use of superparamagnetic particles that are highly lymphotrophic. This technique has recently been reported to be useful in clinical staging of CaP.[50] This study utilized lymphotrophic particles in combination with MRI to identify nodal disease. The results of MRI were compared with histopathologic sections of lymph nodes. All patients with nodal metastasis were identified with the combination MRI and lymphotrophic superparamagnetic particles. This technique is not widely used currently.

SUMMARY

TNM staging is the most widely used staging system for CaP. The most important factors in patient survival are surgical margins, extraprostatic extension, seminal vesicle involvement, and nodal metastasis, all of which are more accurately assessed by pathologic staging. The current modality for staging the primary tumor in CaP is DRE, however, some imaging modalities may provide useful information. Relative indications for assessing the nodal status of a patient include PSA of more than 20 ng/mL, Gleason 8 or higher, and T3 or greater disease. The reference standard for nodal involvement is pelvic lymphadenectomy; however, other modalities have shown promise in the clinical assessment of nodal disease. Assessment of metastatic disease is usually not indicated in patients with PSA greater than 20 ng/mL (unless high Gleason score or advanced T stage). In addition to the more common modalities of staging of CaP, there are several new techniques that have shown promise and may be incorporated into the staging system in the future.

REFERENCES

1. Flemming E, Cooper J, Hemson D, et al. American Joint Committee on Cancer Staging Manual 5th ed. Philadelphia: JP Lippincott, 1997, p 219.
2. Ohori M, Egawa S, Shinohara K, et al. Detection of microscopic extracapsular extension prior to radical prostatectomy for clinically localized prostate cancer. Br J Urol 1994;74:72–79.
3. Hamper U, Sheth S, Walsh P, et al. Capsular transgression of prostatic carcinoma: evaluation with transrectal US with pathologic correlation. Radiology 1991;178:791–795.
4. Tempany C, Zhou Z, Zerhouni E, et al. Staging of prostate cancer: results of Radiology Diagnostic Oncology Group project comparison of three MR imaging techniques. Radiology 1994;192:47–54.
5. Vapnek J, Hricak H, Shinohara K, et al. Staging accuracy of magnetic resonance imaging versus transrectal ultrasound in stages A and B prostatic cancer. Urol Int 1994;53:191–195.
6. Epstein J, Pizov G, Walsh P. Correlation of pathologic findings with progression after radical retropubic prostatectomy. Cancer 1993;71:3582–3593.
7. Catalona W, Smith D. 5-year tumor recurrence rates after anatomical radical retropubic prostatectomy for prostate cancer. J Urol 1994;152:1837–1842.
8. Partin A, Pound C, Clemens J, et al. Serum PSA after anatomic radical prostatectomy. The Johns Hopkins experience after 10 years. Urol Clin N Am 1993;20:713–725.
9. McNeal J, Villers A, Redwine E, et al. Capsular penetration in prostate cancer. Significance for natural history and treatment. Am J Surg Path 1990;14:240–247.
10. Gustafsson O, Norming U, Almgard L, et al. Diagnostic methods in the detection of prostate cancer: a study of a randomly selected population of 2,400 men. J Urol 1992;148:1827–1831.
11. O'Dowd G, Veltri R, Orozco R, et al. Update on the appropriate staging evaluation for newly diagnosed prostate cancer. J Urol 1997;158:687–698.
12. Smith D, Catalona W. Interexaminer variability of digital rectal examination in detecting prostate cancer. Urology 1995;45:70–74.
13. Varenhorst E, Berglund K, Lofman O, et al. Inter-observer variation in assessment of the prostate by digital rectal examination. Br J Urol 1993;72:173–176.
14. Partin A, Kattan M, Subong E, et al. Combination of prostate-specific antigen, clinical stage, and Gleason score to predict pathological state of localized prostate cancer. A multi-institutional update. JAMA 1997;277:1445–1451.
15. Narayan P, Gajendran V, Taylor S, et al. The role of transrectal ultrasound-guided biopsy-based staging, preoperative serum prostate-specific antigen, and biopsy Gleason score in prediction of final pathologic diagnosis in prostate cancer. Urology 1995;46:205–212.
16. Krumholtz J, Carvalhal G, Ramos C, et al. Prostate-specific antigen cutoff of 2.6 ng/mL for prostate cancer screening is associated with favorable pathologic tumor features. Urology 2002;60:469–473.
17. Oesterling J, Brendler C, Epstein J, et al. Correlation of clinical stage, serum prostatic acid phosphatase and preoperative Gleason grade with final pathological stage in 275 patients with clinically localized adenocarcinoma of the prostate. J Urol 1987;138:92–98.
18. Goto Y, Ohori M, Scardino P. Use of systematic biopsy results to predict pathologic stage in patients with clinically localized prostate cancer: a preliminary report. Int J Urol 1998;5:337–342.
19. Mettlin C, Lee F, Drago J, et al. The American Cancer Society National Prostate Cancer Detection Project. Findings on the detection of early prostate cancer in 2425 men. Cancer 1991;67:2949–2958.
20. Flanigan R, Catalona W, Richie J, et al. Accuracy of digital rectal examination and transrectal ultrasonography in localizing prostate cancer. J Urol 1994;152:1506–1509.
21. Ellis J, Tempany C, Sarin M, et al. MR imaging and sonography of early prostatic cancer: pathologic and imaging features that influence identification and diagnosis. AJR Amer J Roentgenol 1994;162:865–872.
22. Rifkin M, Zerhouni E, Gatsonis C, et al. Comparison of magnetic resonance imaging and ultrasonography in staging early prostate cancer. Results of a multi-institutional cooperative trial. N Engl J Med 1990;323:621–626.
23. Bree R. The role of color Doppler and staging biopsies in prostate cancer detection. Urology 1997;49:31–34.
24. Schnall M, Lenkinski R, Pollack H, et al. Prostate: MR imaging with an endorectal surface coil. Radiology 1989;172:570–574.
25. Ekici S, Ozen H, Agildere M, et al. A comparison of transrectal ultrasonography and endorectal magnetic resonance imaging in the local staging of prostatic carcinoma. BJU Int 1999;83:796–800.
26. Ikonen S, Karkkainen P, Kivisaari L, et al. Magnetic resonance imaging of clinically localized prostatic cancer. J Urol 1998;159:915–919.
27. Perrotti M, Kaufman R, Jennings T, et al. Endo-rectal coil magnetic resonance imaging in clinically localized prostate cancer: is it accurate? J Urol 1996;156:106–109.
28. Yu K, Hricak H, Alagappan R, et al. Detection of extracapsular extension of prostate carcinoma with endorectal and phased-array coil MR imaging: multivariate feature analysis. Radiology 1997;202:697–702.
29. Oyen R, Van Poppel H, Ameye F, et al. Lymph node staging of localized prostatic carcinoma with CT and CT-guided fine-needle aspiration biopsy: prospective study of 285 patients. Radiology 1994;190:315–322.
30. Rorvik J, Halvorsen O, Albrektsen G, et al. Lymphangiography combined with biopsy and computer tomography to detect lymph node metastases in localized prostate cancer. Scand J Urol Nephrol 1998;32:116–119.

31. Levran Z, Gonzalez J, Diokno A, et al. Are pelvic computed tomography, bone scan, and pelvic lymphadenectomy necessary in the staging of prostate cancer? Br. J Urol 1995;75:778–781.

32. Albertson P, Hanley J, Harlan L, et al. The positive yield of imaging studies in the evaluation of men with newly diagnosed prostate cancer: a population based analysis. J Urol 2000;163:1138–1143.

33. de Jong I, Pruim J, Elsinga P, et al. Preoperative staging of pelvic lymph nodes in prostate cancer by 11C-Choline PET. J Nucl Med 2003;44:331–335.

34. Salminen E, Hogg A, Binns D, et al. Investigations with FDG-PET scanning in prostate cancer show limited value for clinical practice. Acta Oncol 2002;41:425–429.

35. Rosenthal S, Haseman M, Polascik T. Utility of capromab pendetide (ProstaScint) imaging in the management of prostate cancer. Tech Urol 2001;7:27–37.

36. Manyak M, Hinkle G, Olsen J, et al. Immunoscintigraphy with indium-111-capromab pendetide: evaluation before definitive therapy in patients with prostate cancer. Urology 1999;54:1058–1063.

37. Chybowski F, Keller J, Bergstralh E, et al. Predicting radionuclide bone scan findings in patients with newly diagnosed, untreated prostate cancer: prostate specific antigen is superior to all other clinical parameters. J Urol 1991;145:313–318.

38. Kemp P, Maguire G, Bird N. Which patients with prostatic carcinoma require a staging bone scan? Br J Urol 1997;79:611–614.

39. Eastham J, Kattan M, Riedel E, et al. Variations among individual surgeons in the rate of positive surgical margins in radical prostatectomy specimens. J Urol 2003;170:2292–2295.

40. Schuessler W, Vancaillie T, Reich H, et al. Transperitoneal endosurgical lymphadenctomy in patients with localized prostate cancer. J Urol 1991;145:988–991.

41. Perrotti M, Gentle D, Barada J, et al. Mini-laparotomy pelvic lymph node dissection minimizes morbidity, hospitalization and cost of pelvic lymph node dissection. J Urol 1996;155:986–988.

42. Bluestein D, Bostwick D, Bergstralh E, et al. Eliminating the need for bilateral pelvic lymphadenectomy in select patients with prostate cancer. J Urol 1994;151:1315–1320.

43. Burkhard F, Bader P, Schneider E, et al. Reliability of preoperative values to determine the need for lymphadenectomy in patients with prostate cancer and meticulous lymph node dissection. Eur Urol 2002;42:84–90.

44. Clark T, Parekh D, Cookson M, et al. Randomized prospective evaluation of extended versus limited lymph node dissection in patients with clinically localized prostate cancer. J Urol 2003;169:145–147.

45. Sgrignoli A, Walsh P, Steinberg G, et al. Prognostic factors in men with stage D1 prostate cancer: identification of patients less likely to have prolonged survival after radical prostatectomy. J Urol 1994;152:1077–1081.

46. Cross S, Harrison R, Kennedy R. Introduction to neural networks. Lancet 1995;346:1075–1139.

47. Tewari A, Narayan P. Novel staging tool for localized prostate cancer: a pilot study using genetic adaptive neural networks. J Urol 1998;160:430–436.

48. Olsson C, de Vries G, Raffo A, et al. Preoperative reverse transcriptase polymerase chain reaction for prostate specific antigen predicts treatment failure following radical prostatectomy. J Urol 1996;155:1557–1562.

49. Sokoloff M, Tso C, Kaboo R, et al. Quantitative polymerase chain reaction does not improve preoperative prostate cancer staging: a clinicopathological molecular analysis of 121 patients. J Urol 1996;156:1560–1566.

50. Harisinghani M, Barentsz J, Hahn P, et al. Noninvasive detection of clinically occult lymph-node metastases in prostate cancer. N Engl J Med 2003;348:2491–2499.

Prostate-specific antigen: practical applications and future prospects

45

Daniel W Lin, Michael K Brawer

INTRODUCTION

Since the late 1980s, prostate-specific antigen (PSA) has established itself as the most important tumor marker in all solid tumor oncology and has become indispensable in the management of prostate cancer. Since the introduction of PSA-based screening, there has been a marked increase in the incidence of clinically, and pathologically, organ-confined disease, and the majority of prostate cancers diagnosed today are nonpalpable PSA-detected tumors (T1c).[1] Still, controversy surrounds the use of PSA as a routine screening tool, and, for this reason, great efforts have been devoted to understanding the relationship between PSA and tumor biology before, at the time of, and after prostate cancer diagnosis and treatment.

A central issue in this controversy is the fact that PSA is organ-specific, not cancer-specific, such that changes in serum PSA are not always a manifestation of cancer, but rather may be due to inflammation, trauma, or, most commonly, benign prostatic hyperplasia (BPH).[1,2] Furthermore, considerable overlap exists in PSA levels among men with prostate cancer and BPH, most evident in the so-called "diagnostic gray zone" of PSA: 4.0 to 10.0 ng/mL. Due to questions surrounding the specificity of PSA, a number of modalities have been proposed to increase the performance of this analyte, namely PSA-derivatives such as age-specific PSA, PSA density, PSA velocity, and PSA isoforms. Here, we will first present the practical applications of PSA and PSA derivatives in the diagnosis and management of prostate cancer and then introduce more recent developments in the burgeoning field of prostate cancer tumor markers.

PROSTATE-SPECIFIC ANTIGEN

First described in 1979, PSA is a single-chain 33-kDa serine protease belonging to the kallikrein family.[3] It is synthesized and secreted from prostate epithelial cells, encoded by an androgen responsive gene located on chromosome 19q13.3-13.4,[4] and serves to liquefy the seminal coagulum, releasing the spermatozoa.[5] While PSA was initially thought to be prostate-specific, it is found to small degrees in other non-prostatic tissues, although its presence in these non-prostatic sites amounts to little clinical significance.[6]

Once PSA enters the bloodstream, approximately 70% to 90% of the PSA is complexed, primarily to α1-antichymotrypsin (ACT) or α2-macroglobulin (AMG),[7,8] although there exist other minor complexed forms. The PSA bound to AMG is not detectable by immunoassays due to lack of exposed antigens; however, the PSA-ACT complex has sufficient antigenic epitopes for detection as complexed PSA (cPSA).[9] Complexed PSA is the major molecular form in serum, and the remainder is considered free PSA (fPSA). The half-life of PSA in serum has been reported to be between 2.2 and 3.2 days, with fPSA being cleared at a higher rate than complexed forms.[10,11] A brief discussion of PSA isoforms is included below, and a detailed discussion is presented elsewhere in this textbook.

CAUSES OF PROSTATE-SPECIFIC ANTIGEN ELEVATION

The prostatic lumen contains the highest concentrations of PSA, but it is closely guarded by barriers to the systemic circulation such as the basement membrane, the intervening stroma, the capillary basement membrane, and the capillary endothelial cell layer. Any forces that compromise or disrupt these layers may cause elevations in serum PSA.

The major causes of increased serum PSA include BPH, prostate cancer, prostate inflammation or infection, and prostate or perineal trauma.[12–14] The overlap in serum PSA levels between BPH and prostate cancer are well-established. Although the PSA per gram of tissue is higher in malignant versus benign prostate tissue, BPH is still the most common cause of elevated serum PSA. In addition to producing more PSA per gram of tissue, invasive prostate cancer disrupts the prostate–blood barrier, further increasing serum PSA. In men with prior negative prostate biopsies, prostate acute and chronic inflammation has been found to be more prevalent in patients with a serum PSA greater than 4 ng/mL compared with those with lower levels.[15] Furthermore, although some have reported that the %fPSA (fPSA/tPSA × 100) is not affected by the presence of inflammation,[16] others have shown that it is unable to distinguish chronic prostatitis from prostate cancer, as both may significantly decrease %fPSA.[17]

Lastly, from a practical standpoint, prostate "trauma" from cystoscopy, prostate biopsy, transurethral resection (TURP), vigorous digital rectal examination (DRE), or ejaculation may cause transient increases in PSA. Clearly, mechanical manipulations such as biopsy and TURP can significantly alter the serum PSA. In one study,[18] men undergoing biopsy experienced a median 7.9 ng/mL increase and those undergoing TURP a median elevation of 5.9 ng/mL. The median time for PSA to return to baseline following biopsy was 15 to 17 days and following TURP was 18 days. The changes in PSA following rigid and flexible cystoscopy were less pronounced at 0.1 and 0.5 ng/mL, respectively. Of note, fPSA reportedly is cleared more rapidly from circulation than complexed forms, thus the %fPSA may be altered more significantly after prostate manipulations.[19,20] While DRE has been shown to cause a transient and minimal increase in PSA, the PSA changes have been reported in multiple setting to have little clinical significance.[21] Likewise, ejaculation can minimally elevate the serum PSA for approximately 48 to 72 hours.[22] Taken as a whole, the current recommendations are that serum PSA levels after cystoscopy and DRE are accurate and reliable, a serum PSA level should not be obtained 48 to 72 hours post-ejaculation, and a period of at least 4 to 6 weeks should occur after a biopsy or TURP before PSA levels are measured.

PROSTATE-SPECIFIC ANTIGEN DERIVATIVES

Although the sensitivity of PSA is quite impressive, the positive predictive value (PPV) of PSA has still been

questioned. When PSA is 4.0 to 10.0 ng/mL, the PPV is 18% to 25% (mean 21%), and when PSA is greater than 10 ng/mL, the PPV is 58% to 64% (mean 61%).[23–25] As a result, methods to enhance the performance of PSA have evolved.

PROSTATE-SPECIFIC ANTIGEN DENSITY

PSA density (PSAD), the serum PSA divided by gland volume, has been suggested to improve PSA specificity. A PSA density of greater than 0.15 ng/mL has been shown to increase specificity of detection of prostate cancer when compared with total serum PSA,[26–29] however, the optimal cutoff is controversial. Early studies by Benson et al evaluated the efficacy of PSAD for prostate cancer detection.[26] The mean PSAD in those with prostate cancer and BPH was 0.581 and 0.044, respectively. No patient with BPH had a PSA density greater than 0.117, and only one had a density of 0.1 or greater. Of patients with a PSA density of 0.1 or greater, 97% had prostate cancer. Despite these promising results, this PSA modification involves multiple sources of potential error, such as ultrasound operator variability, assay variability, interindividual heterogeneous stromal/epithelial ratios, and sampling bias.[30] One large multicenter study[31] that compared PSA and PSAD for early detection of prostate cancer found that, in men with PSA of 4 to 10 ng/mL, if a PSAD cutoff of 0.15 was used, then 47% of the cancers would be missed, findings that have been supported by others. Others have promoted the use of transition zone PSAD (TZ-PSAD),[32] defined as the serum PSA divided by the volume of the transition zone. Although initial reports were encouraging, this parameter is subject to all the same sources of error of PSAD.[33] In summary, while PSAD and TZ-PSAD may boast an increased specificity and avoidance of up to 37% of biopsies, they risk missing an unacceptable number of clinically significant cancers.

PROSTATE-SPECIFIC ANTIGEN VELOCITY

The rate of change of PSA over time (PSA velocity) has been proposed to improve the PPV of PSA. Carter et al and others[34,35] first reported that an annual increase of 0.75 ng/mL per year in serum PSA indicated men who would develop or have developed prostate carcinoma. Using this cutoff, specificity reportedly increased to over 90% with 72% sensitivity in predicting prostate cancer in men with PSA less than 10.0 ng/mL. Importantly, the recommended interval between PSA measurements is 1.7 to 2.0 years, and at least three PSA measurements are recommended to obtain maximal benefit from using PSA velocity measurements.[36,37] Other studies debate the utility of PSA velocity owing to the significant intra-individual (biologic) variability and interassay (analytic) variability particularly in the setting of relatively short time intervals between PSA tests and PSA in the low ranges.[38-41] Additionally, PSA velocity requires longitudinal samples over many years, during which disease progression may occur. Furthermore, men harboring prostate cancer often have a PSA velocity of less than 0.75 ng/mL per year, especially those with PSA levels less than 4.0 ng/mL.[42] Still, the rate of change of PSA over time may prove to be a significant indicator of a malignant or premalignant change in prostate histology for patients with borderline elevations in serum PSA. A corollary to PSA velocity is the rate at which PSA doubles, or PSA doubling time (PSADT). This has been the subject of numerous recent investigations and will be discussed later in this chapter as it relates to prognostic predictions in newly diagnosed and recurrent prostate cancer.

AGE-SPECIFIC PROSTATE-SPECIFIC ANTIGEN

As it is well recognized that PSA increases with age, age-adjusted PSA ranges have been proposed to decrease the PSA threshold for biopsy in younger men while increasing the threshold in older men.[43,44] The rationale for these modifications in PSA cutoff points is to improve the test specificity in men 60 years or older while improving the test sensitivity in men younger than 60 years. One study compared the use of age-specific reference ranges (as defined by Oesterling et al[44]) versus a serum PSA cutoff of 4.0 ng/mL (regardless of age) in men over the age of 50.[45] The use of age-specific ranges minimally increased the PPV from 37% to 42%, but reduced the cancer detection rate from 5.7% to 3.8%; the authors determined that using a standard serum PSA cutoff of 4.0 ng/mL would have saved significantly more life-years compared with using age-specific ranges. One other very large study of 6600 men over the age of 50 years found that increasing the PSA thresholds in older men may result in 44% less biopsies, but at the expense of missing up to 47% of organ-confined cancer.[46] Furthermore, when reviewing the published reports of age-specific PSA, the standard deviation of PSA age-adjusted cutoffs increases with age such that the standard deviation is 0.44 ng for men 40 to 49 years old, however, the standard deviation is 1.27 ng for men 70 to 79 years old.[47] Taken as a whole, while this modification may increase the test sensitivity in younger men, it will also decrease the sensitivity in the older population with subsequent decreased detection rates in older men.

PROSTATE-SPECIFIC ANTIGEN ISOFORMS

As previously mentioned, PSA exists in multiple molecular forms in the serum, and the ability of these molecular forms to discriminate between prostate cancer and benign conditions has been well documented. A brief presentation of PSA isoforms will be presented here, as the issues surrounding PSA isoforms are dealt with in more detail in Chapter 46. Stenman[7] and Lilja[8] were pioneers in elucidating the relationship between different circulating molecular forms of PSA and risk of prostate cancer. For example, using a 25% free PSA cutoff yields a 95% sensitivity, 20% less biopsies, and only 5% missed cancers. Using free-to-total PSA ratio, the areas under the receiver operating characteristic curve (ROC-AUC) have been increased on average by 22% over PSA alone (Table 45.1). The performance of free-to-total PSA ratios improves in the diagnostic gray zone, in men with previous negative biopsies, and in men with prostate volumes less than 40 mL^3—three important and prevalent clinical situations.[48-52] More recently, advancement in immunoassay technology has yielded a serum assay for cPSA, which has been the subject of numerous reports investigating the performance of measuring this one analyte in the early detection of prostate cancer, rather than measuring two analytes to calculate the %fPSA, namely fPSA and tPSA.[53-55] Brawer et al first demonstrated improved specificity for cPSA over tPSA, 26.7% over 21.8%, respectively, at cutoffs that provided 95% sensitivity[56] (Table 45.2). Other studies have shown similar diagnostic performance, reporting that cPSA significantly improves the ROC-AUC over tPSA alone, Figure 45.1 shows these findings from a multicenter investigation,[57-59] however, other studies have shown minimal benefit of a single measurement of cPSA over total PSA (tPSA), particularly in studies composed of populations comprised of serum samples with equal tPSA distributions between the benign and cancer samples.[60-62] Others have evaluated the performance of cPSA in combination with tPSA (c:t PSA ratio), PSAD (cPSAD) and fPSA (f:c PSA ratio). For example, one study cited better performance using c/t PSA ratio specifically in the PSA 4 to 10 ng/mL range compared with cPSA alone; however, cPSA outperformed this c/tPSA ratio in the PSA 2 to 6 ng/mL range.[57] For example, within the tPSA range of 2.0 to 6.0 ng/mL, a cut-point of 2.2 ng/mL for cPSA and 2.5 ng/mL for PSA demonstrated specificities of 35% and 21.2%

Table 45.1 Percentage of free prostate-specific antigen (PSA) cutoffs, sensitivity, and specificity

Free PSA Cut-off (%)	Sensitivity, % (no.) of cancers detected [95% CI]	Specificity, % (no.) of unnecessary biopsies avoided [95% CI]
≤22	90 (341/379) [86–93]	29 (115/394) [25–34]
≤25	95 (358/379) [92–97]	20 (80/394) [16–24]

From Catalona WJ, Partin, AW, Slawin KM, et al. Use of the percentage of free prostate-specific antigen to enhance differentiation of prostate cancer from benign prostatic disease: A prospective multicenter clinical trial. JAMA 1998;279:1542–1547.

Table 45.2 Specificity of the different prostate-specific antigen (PSA) assays at selected sensitivities over the entire PSA range

Sensitivity (%)	Total PSA		cPSA		free/total PSA	
	Cutoff	Specificity	Cutoff	Specificity	Cutoff	Specificity
	(ng/mL)	(%)	(ng/mL)	(%)	(ng/mL)	(%)
100	1.0	3.1	0.89	6.2	67	0
97.5	2.28	12.9	1.67	14.7	32	8.9
95	3.06	21.8	2.52	26.7	28	15.6
90	3.4	25.3	2.94	33.8	24	26.2
85	3.86	31.1	3.34	38.7	22	32.4
80	4.11	35.6	3.98	51.6	19	46.2

From Brawer MK, Meyer GE, Letran JL, et al. Measurement of complexed PSA improves specificity for early detection of prostate cancer. Urology 1998;52:372–378.

respectively.[57] Lastly, one study reported that the intra-individual variability of cPSA was the greatest (25.4%) compared with other PSA tests, stating that the amount of change required for a significant difference between two cPSA readings (with 95% confidence) was 70.4%.[63]

In summary, the application of PSA isoforms has greatly improved the discrimination between benign disease and prostate cancer and will continue to change PSA screening efforts, particularly with the newly characterized PSA isoforms such as proPSA and BPSA (see below). These revelations in PSA isoforms must be guarded by the fact that varying the cutoff values of these ratios yields significantly different detection rates, and the reported utility of these modification include reports using various PSA assays subject to significant variability.

PROSTATE-SPECIFIC ANTIGEN IN LOW RANGE (2–4 ng/mL)

The incidence of prostate cancer in men with a serum PSA 2.0 to 4.0 ng/mL has been the subject of numerous reports.[64–66] The recent results from the Prostate Cancer Prevention Trial (PCPT)[67] reported that there was a significant prostate cancer detection rate in control arm participants who underwent biopsy at the end of study with PSA less than 4 ng/ml and normal DRE.[64] In this study, 15% of these control participants were found to have occult prostate cancer, and, of that group, 14% were high grade. More importantly the breakdown of PSA level versus incidence in this group was as followed: less than 0.5 ng/mL, 10%; 0.5 to 1.0 ng/mL, 10%; 1.1 to 2.0 ng/mL, 17%; 2.1 to 3 ng/mL, 24%;

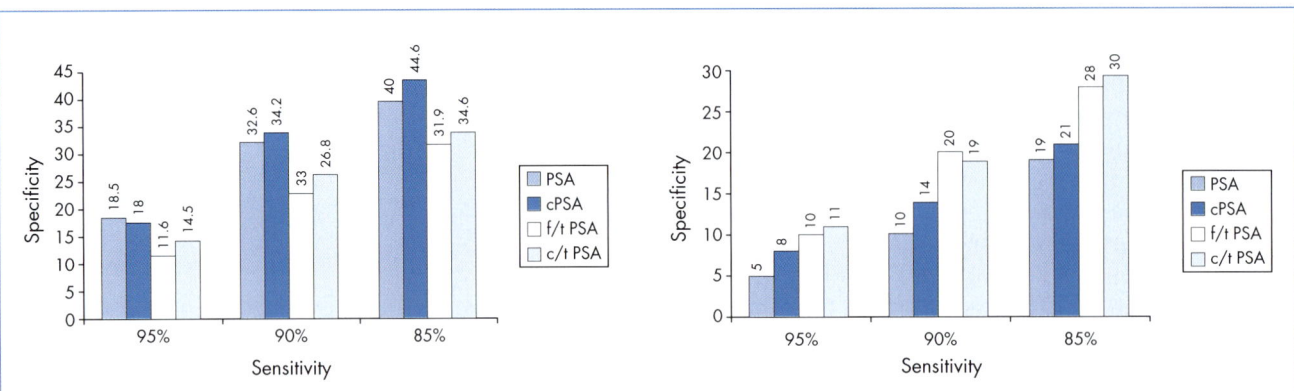

Fig. 45.1

Charts showing the prostate-specific antigen (PSA), complexed PSA (cPSA), ratio of free-to-total PSA (f/t PSA) and ratio of complexed-to-total PSA (c/t PSA) for all samples (n = 831) *(A)* and those within the range of 4 to 10 ng/mL PSA (n = 389) *(B)*. From Partin AW, Brawer MK, Bartsch G, et al. Complexed prostate specific antigen improves specificity for prostate cancer detection: results of a prospective multicenter clinical trial. J Urol 2003;170:1787.

and 3.1 to 4 ng/mL, 27%. The controversial issues surrounding the recommendation for prostate biopsy in this population include: 1) whether cancers found at a PSA 2 to 4 ng/mL are clinically "significant"; 2) whether a man with a PSA 2 to 4 ng/mL will progress to "abnormal" levels (above 4 ng/mL); and 3) whether detection and treatment of cancers at this lower PSA range result in improved disease control over treatment at PSA greater than 4 ng/mL.

Addressing one of these issues, Catalona et al[66] evaluated 914 men found to have a PSA 2.5 to 4.0 and a normal DRE on screening examination. Of these, 332 (36%) underwent biopsy of the prostate, and the overall positive biopsy rate was 22%. All prostate cancer cases were clinically localized. Of the patients undergoing radical prostatectomy, 81% were pathologically organ-confined, and only 17% were low volume and low grade, thus deemed possibly clinically insignificant. In Europe, Schroder et al[65] performed analysis of radical prostatectomy specimens from men with pre-radical prostatectomy PSA of 0 to 3.9 ng/mL, finding that at least 50% were clinically significant as defined by Gleason grade 7 or greater or any Gleason 4/5 components. Furthermore, 84% were organ confined. To address the issue of whether men with low PSA levels may eventually progress to abnormal levels or be diagnosed with prostate cancer, Gann et al[68] reported that comparing men with PSA levels less than 1.0 ng/mL with those with PSA levels of 2.0 to 3.0 ng/mL, the relative risk of being diagnosed with prostate cancer on follow-up was 5.5 (95% CI, 3.7–9.2); these findings suggest that men with a PSA starting in this relatively low range represent a population that is clearly at risk for occult prostate cancer or developing prostate cancer. These findings further imply that a substantial proportion of men with low PSA levels are eventually diagnosed with prostate cancer, supporting the lowered cut-point for prostate biopsy. Most recently, Punglia et al[46] evaluated cancer detection rates in a cohort of 6691 men who underwent routine screening of PSA. They reported that lowering the threshold for biopsy from 4.1 to 2.6 ng/mL in men younger than 60 years would double the cancer detection rate from 18% to 36% with a corresponding decrease in specificity only falling from 98% to 94%, further stating that if biopsies are performed in men younger than 60 when PSA was greater than 4.0 ng/mL, then 82% of the cancers would have been missed. To answer the question of whether finding prostate cancer at levels of PSA below 4 ng/mL results in improved cancer control is more difficult and poorly addressed to date. One study compared men undergoing radical prostatectomy with a PSA of 2 to 4 ng/mL with men undergoing surgery with PSA greater than 4 ng/mL, evaluating the probability of curable cancer as defined by organ-confined tumor or tumor with capsular penetration of low grade (Gleason <7), negative margins, and no seminal vesicle invasion or lymph node metastasis. The probability of finding curable cancer was not statistically different between these two groups of patients, suggesting that overall cure rates are not different if PSA is allowed to increase to levels above 4 ng/mL.[69]

One final consideration in men with low PSA is the utility of PSA modifications. There are now multiple single- and multi-institutional studies supporting the use of %fPSA in men with low total PSA.[32,66,70,71] For example, Catalona et al[72] retrospectively studied 368 archived serum samples from men who underwent prostate biopsy with a PSA of 2.5 to 4.0 ng/mL and a normal DRE. Using various free PSA cut-points between 10% and 15%, the PPV increased to as high as 46%, while only 10% to 36% of the men underwent biopsy. More cancers were detected per biopsy by using %fPSA to identify those men at highest risk rather than by simply lowering the total PSA cutpoint. Despite these promising results, the performance of fPSA in discriminating between cancer and benign disease at PSA values less than 4 ng/mL was less robust than its performance in the established diagnostic gray zone of PSA of 4 to 10 ng/mL.[72] Perhaps the more recently characterized precursor form of PSA, proPSA, will become most useful in this low PSA range (see later discussion). In summary, lowering the PSA threshold to 2.0 or 2.5 ng/mL, particularly in younger men, appears not only to increase the detection of clinically significant, yet organ-confined, prostate cancer but also identifies a cohort of men at high risk for the eventual diagnosis of prostate cancer, although the impact on disease-specific survival and utility of PSA isoforms in this low range remain to be characterized.

PROSTATE-SPECIFIC ANTIGEN KINETICS BEFORE AND AFTER PRIMARY TREATMENT

The rate at which PSA changes, or PSA doubling time (PSADT), both before primary treatment for prostate cancer and at time of disease recurrence after primary therapy, has been shown to independently predict disease outcome as reported by multiple investigators, most notably D'Amico et al.[73–79] After radical prostatectomy or radiotherapy, various cut-points for PSADT have been examined for their ability to predict disease progression and survival. For example, Pound et al[79] examined 315 men with biochemical recurrence after radical prostatectomy and followed them for clinical evidence of progression. They found that men with a PSADT of less than 10 months experienced significantly lower metastasis-free survival than men with PSADT more than 10 months. Other well-established clinicopathologic parameters such as

Gleason score and time from prostatectomy to biochemical failure also contributed to the nomogram for post-radical prostatectomy metastasis-free survival; however, importantly, PSADT was an independent factor in multivariate analysis. Other investigators have reported similar findings, although the cut-points for PSADT have been variable. Similarly, D'Amico et al studied 2751 men who underwent external beam radiotherapy as primary treatment for prostate cancer finding that a PSADT of less than 3 months was statistically significantly associated with prostate cancer-specific mortality (HR, 19.6; 95% CI 12.5–30.9).[77]

A more recent report that examines PSA velocity in the year preceding prostate cancer diagnosis significantly adds to the efforts to improve our abilities to predict disease aggression and to better counsel our patients about primary therapies.[80] These investigators examined 1095 patients with newly diagnosed prostate cancer who underwent prostatectomy and retrospectively examined the PSA velocity in the year preceding the diagnosis, showing that the rate of PSA rise in the year preceding prostate cancer diagnosis not only predicted adverse pathologic parameters and disease-free survival, but also, more importantly and uniquely, cancer-specific and overall survival following prostatectomy. A man with a PSA velocity of greater than 2 ng/mL/year was nearly 10 times more likely to die of prostate cancer than a man with a PSA velocity of less than 2 ng/mL/year. Still, the analysis of the subset of patients with PSA velocity greater than 2 ng/mL/year showed that grade, stage, and PSA remained important stratifying factors of both cancer-specific and overall survival, suggesting that although PSA velocity is an independent variable on multivariate analysis, the impact of these other well-established factors cannot be overlooked. A significant consideration in evaluating this study is that PSA velocity was only calculated by using the PSA measurement closest in time to diagnosis and all PSA values "within one year before diagnosis." At this time, most men who are diagnosed by PSA in the US have only a yearly PSA before a PSA is obtained that precipitates biopsy and a cancer diagnosis. If these findings correlate with the PSA velocities calculated over several years before a diagnosis of prostate cancer, and if these findings are confirmed by other large trials, then it certainly may affect the way we stratify for clinical trials, counsel patients for primary treatments, or screen with PSA.

The PSA level necessary to prove disease-free states after radiation therapy and the definition of PSA failure after radiation therapy or surgery have been controversial subjects that are beyond the scope of this chapter and will be addressed in other sections of this textbook.[81–84] Likewise, the rate of and relative decline in PSA after androgen ablation, chemotherapy, or other investigational agents has also been the subject of numerous reports.[85–87] To date, PSA has not been accepted as a surrogate marker for efficacy of various treatments in advanced prostate cancer.[88] However, the kinetics of PSA, whether by PSADT or PSA velocity, are gaining greater momentum as data emerges and likely will be used in the future for entry into clinical trials, risk stratification, and prediction modeling.

PROSTATE-SPECIFIC ANTIGEN ASSAY CONSIDERATIONS

In 1986, the US Food and Drug Administration (FDA) approved the first commercial immunoassay (Hybritech) for PSA; since then, assay standardization, assay variability, and ultrasensitive assays have been addressed in multiple reports. Much of the work in assay standardization is attributed to Stamey et al who were instrumental in convening scientific forums to discuss approaches and solutions to assay standards between different commercial and research assays.[89–91] The biological and analytical variation of the PSA assay has been addressed in numerous reports.[38–41,66] Ornstein et al[38] reported that there is a mean variation of approximately 15% in measurements of total PSA based on three PSA measurements drawn from subjects 2 weeks apart. Nixon et al[40] reported that the combined degree of biological and analytical variation could be as high as 20% to 46%. Prestigiacomo and Stamey[39] reported a mean coefficient of variation of 10.5% for between assay (analytical) and 23.5% for physiologic (biological) variation, concluding that the intra-individual physiologic variation is 2 to 3 times the inter-assay variation. While these studies were not entirely composed of prostate cancer patients and were highly populated with men having PSA less than 10 ng/dL, they define the substantial PSA variability due to assay and intra-individual variation. Lastly, several commercial assays are now available with substantially lower limits of PSA detection, or so-called, ultrasensitive assays.[92] There are several reports that examine the utility of these ultrasensitive assays in monitoring post-radical prostatectomy patients, reporting 1 to 3 years of lead time in predicting ultimate clinical recurrence.[93–96] For example, Haese et al[94] used an ultrasensitive assay in a cohort of 442 patients being followed for recurrence after radical prostatectomy. They found that 57% of biochemical failures were detected by ultrasensitive assay before the standard assay was positive, and the ultrasensitive assay results closely correlated with pathologic stage, Gleason grade, and margin status. Importantly, with the standard assay, only 25% of relapses were detected in the first year; however, this detection rate increased to 85.7% with the ultrasensitive assay. Other investigators believe that the role of ultrasensitive assays is limited due to the substantial false-positive tests (e.g., detectable PSA).[92] At this time, the significance of a positive ultrasensitive assay and resulting lead time gains are tempered by the lack of evidence to support early versus late treatments, of any type (e.g., hormonal manipulation, chemotherapy, or investigational) for recurrent prostate cancer.

FUTURE PROSPECTS

OTHER PSA ISOFORMS

The discovery and characterization of other PSA isoforms and related serine proteases represents perhaps the most promising improvements in the screening and detection of prostate carcinoma. As previously stated, PSA circulates in the serum in free (unbound) and complexed (bound to protease inhibitors) forms.[7,8] Free PSA is known to be composed of at least three distinct forms of inactive PSA: 1) proPSA, a proenzyme, or precursor form of PSA, associated with cancer[97,98]; 2) BPSA, an internally cleaved or degraded form more associated with BPH and the transition zone[99]; and 3) other minor variant inactive free PSA forms. Prostate-specific antigen bound to α1-antichymotrypsin (ACT) and α1-protease inhibitor (API) together comprise the measurable complexed PSA (cPSA).

The precursor form of PSA, proPSA, is cleaved to form several different measurable proteins. proPSA contains a 7-amino-acid leader sequence to the constituent amino acid sequence of mature active PSA and is termed [−7]proPSA. This 7-amino-acid sequence can be completely cleaved by human kallikrein 2 (hK2) to release active PSA[100,101]; however, incomplete removal of the 7-amino-acid leader sequence can yield other "clipped" or truncated forms with varying length leader sequence lengths, such as 2-, 4-, and 5-amino acid leaders, termed [−2]proPSA, [−4]proPSA, and [−5]proPSA, respectively.[102–104] There is substantial evidence that proPSA, particularly the truncated forms, is present in the serum of men with prostate cancer.[97,98,102,104] A recent report measured proPSA, fPSA, and cPSA in 1091 samples from multiple institutions to assess the comparative ability in early detection of prostate cancer.[105] In the range of tPSA 2.0 to 4.0 ng/mL, the [−2]proPSA assay had the highest specificity for cancer detection and was significantly greater than %fPSA or cPSA. Within the tPSA range of 2.0 to 10.0 ng/mL, the ratio of pPSA to fPSA (percent proPSA) yielded the highest ROC-AUC and was significantly increased compared to %fPSA and cPSA (p = 0.040 and <0.001, respectively). Percent proPSA spared 21% of unnecessary biopsies compared with 13% for %fPSA and 9% for cPSA.[105] Another recent report evaluated archived serum samples from 93 men with tPSA 4.0 to 10.0 ng/mL who underwent 12-core biopsies. When proPSA was added to tPSA and %fPSA, the overall test specificity increased from 23% for tPSA, to 33% for

%fPSA, to the maximal value of 44% for the three values in combination.[106]

Active PSA can be further metabolized to BPSA by internal cleavage or intact PSA (iPSA) by proteolysis. BPSA has been identified in BPH transition zone tissue and recently has been investigated for its ability to discriminate prostate cancer from benign disease. Khan et al[107] studied 161 men with a serum %fPSA value of less than 15%. The ROC-AUC was significantly better using the ratio of pPSA to BPSA than using %fPSA alone or tPSA: the AUC was 0.72, yielding a sensitivity and specificity of 90% and 46%, respectively. iPSA has also been examined for early detection of prostate cancer, with preliminary studies reporting that the ratios of iPSA to fPSA increase the sensitivity and specificity over the various established combinations of tPSA and fPSA.[108,109]

HUMAN KALLIKREIN 2

Human kallikrein 2 belongs to the same family of serine proteases as PSA and shares approximately 80% sequence identity with PSA.[110] Unlike PSA, hK2 expression incrementally increases from BPH to primary cancer and lymph node metastasis[111]; similarly, hK2 expression is increased in poorly differentiated cancer compared to well-differentiated disease.[112] Furthermore, hK2 expression has been reported to correlate with the pathologic stage of prostate cancer.[113–115] In multiple studies of men who underwent radical prostatectomy, hK2 and hK2-related parameters, such as hK2 density and hK2 to %fPSA ratio, independently predicted pathologic stage of clinically localized prostate cancer, particularly in the tPSA range below 10 ng/mL.[113,114]

Several investigators have evaluated the utility of hK2 in combination with serum PSA and/or fPSA for early detection of prostate cancer. While some reports specifically examine the value of total hK2,[116,117] the majority measure hK2 to fPSA ratio or hK2 multiplied by the f/t PSA ratio.[118–121] For instance, Becker et al[117] reported on 604 men undergoing prostate cancer screening with PSA greater than 3.0 ng/mL. In this study, hK2 multiplied by t/f PSA ratio provided improved sensitivity and specificity when compared to tPSA or %fPSA. Likewise, Nam et al[122] reported that mean hK2 and hK2 to fPSA ratio were significantly higher in men with prostate cancer compared with those who had benign disease. These studies suggest that hK2 may be used as an adjunct to PSA, however, no prospective multi-institutional studies have confirmed these assertions. Interestingly, others have examined the C/T hK2 polymorphism in 1287 men undergoing prostate biopsy.[123] The odds ratios for prostate cancer were significantly higher in men with one or more T allele than in those with no T allele (wild-type CC). Furthermore, when combined with serum hK2 levels, the combined adjusted odds ratio for having prostate cancer was 13.92 (95% CI, 6.6–29.2) for patients with high hK2 levels and at least one T allele, although another more recent report was unable to confirm this finding.[124]

SUMMARY

Novel isoforms of PSA and other serine proteases offer great promise in improving the diagnostic capabilities involved in prostate cancer screening, although these parameters will not be established or embraced until further multi-institutional and prospective trials are completed. Until this time, the use of PSA as detailed in the preceding sections should guide clinicians in their decision-making regarding prostate biopsy. The field of serum proteomics and high-throughput multiplex analyses has yielded encouraging data and may prove to be the new frontier for more sensitive and specific markers in prostate cancer.[125,126] As novel, evolving biomarkers of prostate cancer continue to emerge, the indications for biopsy will expand beyond the traditional PSA and DRE and promise to provide improved predictive capabilities and prognostic value.

REFERENCES

1. Cooperberg MR, Lubeck DP, Meng MV, et al. The changing face of low-risk prostate cancer: trends in clinical presentation and primary management. J Clin Oncol 2004;22:2141–2149.

2. Gelmann EP, Chia D, Pinsky PF, et al. Relationship of demographic and clinical factors to free and total prostate-specific antigen. Urology 2001;58:561–566.

3. Wang MC, Valenzuela LA, Murphy GP, et al. Purification of a human prostate specific antigen. Invest Urol 1979;17:159–163.

4. Riegman PH, Vlietstra RJ, Klaassen P, et al. The prostate-specific antigen gene and the human glandular kallikrein-1 gene are tandemly located on chromosome 19. FEBS Lett 1989;247:123–126.

5. Lilja H. A kallikrein-like serine protease in prostatic fluid cleaves the predominant seminal vesicle protein. J Clin Invest 1985;76:1899–1903.

6. Partin AW, Hanks GE, Klein EA, et al. Prostate-specific antigen as a marker of disease activity in prostate cancer. Oncology (Huntingt) 2002;16:1024–1038.

7. Stenman UH, Leinonen J, Alfthan H, et al. A complex between prostate-specific antigen and alpha 1-antichymotrypsin is the major form of prostate-specific antigen in serum of patients with prostatic cancer: assay of the complex improves clinical sensitivity for cancer. Cancer Res 1991;51:222–226.

8. Lilja H, Christensson A, Dahlen U, et al. Prostate-specific antigen in serum occurs predominantly in complex with alpha 1-antichymotrypsin. Clin Chem 1991;37:1618–1625.

9. Espana F, Sanchez-Cuenca J, Estelles A, et al. Quantitative immunoassay for complexes of prostate-specific antigen with alpha2-macroglobulin. Clin Chem 1996;42:545–550.

10. Stamey TA, Yang N, Hay AR, et al. Prostate-specific antigen as a serum marker for adenocarcinoma of the prostate. N Engl J Med 1987;317:909–916.

11. Oesterling JE, Chan DW, Epstein JI, et al. Prostate specific antigen in the preoperative and postoperative evaluation of localized prostatic cancer treated with radical prostatectomy. J Urol 1988;139:766–772.

12. Ruckle HC, Klee GG, Oesterling JE. Prostate-specific antigen: critical issues for the practicing physician. Mayo Clin Proc 1994;69:59–68.

13. Neal DE Jr, Clejan S, Sarma D, et al. Prostate specific antigen and prostatitis. I. Effect of prostatitis on serum PSA in the human and nonhuman primate. Prostate 1992;20:105–111.

14. Irani J, Levillain P, Goujon JM, et al. Inflammation in benign prostatic hyperplasia: correlation with prostate specific antigen value. J Urol 1997;157:1301–1303.

15. Nadler RB, Humphrey PA, Smith DS, et al. Effect of inflammation and benign prostatic hyperplasia on elevated serum prostate specific antigen levels. J Urol 1995;154:407–413.

16. Ornstein DK, Smith DS, Humphrey PA, et al. The effect of prostate volume, age, total prostate specific antigen level and acute inflammation on the percentage of free serum prostate specific antigen levels in men without clinically detectable prostate cancer. J Urol 1998;159:1234–1237.

17. Jung K, Meyer A, Lein M, et al. Ratio of free-to-total prostate specific antigen in serum cannot distinguish patients with prostate cancer from those with chronic inflammation of the prostate. J Urol 1998;159:1595–1598.

18. Oesterling JE, Rice DC, Glenski WJ, et al. Effect of cystoscopy, prostate biopsy, and transurethral resection of prostate on serum prostate-specific antigen concentration. Urology 1993;42:276–282.

19. Bjork T, Ljungberg B, Piironen T, et al. Rapid exponential elimination of free prostate-specific antigen contrasts the slow, capacity-limited elimination of PSA complexed to alpha 1-antichymotrypsin from serum. Urology 1998;51:57–62.

20. Partin AW, Piantadosi S, Subong EN, et al. Clearance rate of serum-free and total PSA following radical retropubic prostatectomy. Prostate Suppl 1996;7:35–39.

21. Crawford ED, Schutz MJ, Clejan S, et al. The effect of digital rectal examination on prostate-specific antigen levels. JAMA 1992;267:2227–2228.

22. Tchetgen MB, Song JT, Strawderman M, et al. Ejaculation increases the serum prostate-specific antigen concentration. Urology 1996;47:511–516.

23. Catalona WJ, Smith DS, Ratliff TL, et al. Measurement of prostate-specific antigen in serum as a screening test for prostate cancer. N Engl J Med 1991;324:1156–1161.

24. Catalona WJ, Smith DS, Ratliff TL, et al. Detection of organ-confined prostate cancer is increased through prostate-specific antigen-based screening. JAMA 1993;270:948–954.

25. Bretton PR. Prostate-specific antigen and digital rectal examination in screening for prostate cancer: a community-based study. South Med J 1994;87:720–723.

26. Benson MC, Whang IS, Pantuck A, et al. Prostate specific antigen density: a means of distinguishing benign prostatic hypertrophy and prostate cancer. J Urol 1992;147:815–816.

27. Bazinet M, Meshref AW, Trudel C, et al. Prospective evaluation of prostate-specific antigen density and systematic biopsies for early detection of prostatic carcinoma. Urology 1994;43:44–51.

28. Ohori M, Dunn JK, Scardino PT. Is prostate-specific antigen density more useful than prostate-specific antigen levels in the diagnosis of prostate cancer? Urology 1995;46:666–671.

29. Benson MC, Whang IS, Olsson CA, et al. The use of prostate specific antigen density to enhance the predictive value of intermediate levels of serum prostate specific antigen. J Urol 1992;147:817–821.

30. Brawer MK, Aramburu EA, Chen GL, et al. The inability of prostate specific antigen index to enhance the predictive the value of prostate specific antigen in the diagnosis of prostatic carcinoma. J Urol 1993;150:369–373.

31. Catalona WJ, Richie JP, deKernion JB, et al. Comparison of prostate specific antigen concentration versus prostate specific antigen density in the early detection of prostate cancer:receiver operating characteristic curves. J Urol 1994;152:2031–2036.

32. Djavan B, Zlotta A, Kratzik C, et al. PSA, PSA density, PSA density of transition zone, free/total PSA ratio, and PSA velocity for early detection of prostate cancer in men with serum PSA 2.5 to 4.0 ng/mL. Urology 1999;54:517–522.

33. Lin DW, Gold MH, Ransom S, et al. Transition zone prostate specific antigen density: lack of use in prediction of prostatic carcinoma. J Urol 1998;160:77–81.

34. Schmid HP, McNeal JE, Stamey TA. Observations on the doubling time of prostate cancer. The use of serial prostate-specific antigen in

patients with untreated disease as a measure of increasing cancer volume. Cancer 1993;71:2031–2040.

35. Carter HB, Morrell CH, Pearson JD, et al. Estimation of prostatic growth using serial prostate-specific antigen measurements in men with and without prostate disease. Cancer Res 1992;52:3323–3328.

36. Carter HB, Pearson JD, Waclawiw Z, et al. Prostate-specific antigen variability in men without prostate cancer: effect of sampling interval on prostate-specific antigen velocity. Urology 1995;45:591–596.

37. Carter HB, Pearson JD. Prostate-specific antigen velocity and repeated measures of prostate-specific antigen. Urol Clin North Am 1997;24:333–338.

38. Ornstein DK, Smith DS, Rao GS, et al. Biological variation of total, free and percent free serum prostate specific antigen levels in screening volunteers. J Urol 1997;157:2179–2182.

39 Prestigiacomo AF, Stamey TA. Physiological variation of serum prostate specific antigen in the 4.0 to 10.0 ng/ml range in male volunteers. J Urol 1996;155:1977–1980.

40. Nixon RG, Wener MH, Smith KM, et al. Biological variation of prostate specific antigen levels in serum: an evaluation of day-to-day physiological fluctuations in a well-defined cohort of 24 patients. J Urol 1997;157:2183–2190.

41. Nixon RG, Wener MH, Smith KM, et al. Day to day changes in free and total PSA: significance of biological variation. Prostate Cancer Prostatic Dis 1997;1:90–96.

42. Fang J, Metter EJ, Landis P, et al. PSA velocity for assessing prostate cancer risk in men with PSA levels between 2.0 and 4.0 ng/ml. Urology 2002;59:889–893.

43. Dalkin BL, Ahmann FR, Kopp JB. Prostate specific antigen levels in men older than 50 years without clinical evidence of prostatic carcinoma. J Urol 1993;150:1837–1839.

44. Oesterling JE, Jacobsen SJ, Chute CG, et al. Serum prostate-specific antigen in a community-based population of healthy men. Establishment of age-specific reference ranges. JAMA 1993;270:860–864.

45. Etzioni R, Shen Y, Petteway JC, et al. Age-specific prostate-specific antigen: a reassessment. Prostate Suppl 1996;7:70–77.

46. Punglia RS, D'Amico AV, Catalona WJ, et al. Effect of verification bias on screening for prostate cancer by measurement of prostate-specific antigen. N Engl J Med 2003;349:335–342.

47. Karazanashvili G, Abrahamsson PA. Prostate specific antigen and human glandular kallikrein 2 in early detection of prostate cancer. J Urol 2003;169:445–457.

48. Catalona WJ, Partin AW, Slawin KM, et al. Use of the percentage of free prostate-specific antigen to enhance differentiation of prostate cancer from benign prostatic disease: a prospective multicenter clinical trial. JAMA 1998;279:1542–1547.

49. Djavan B, Zlotta A, Remzi M, et al. Optimal predictors of prostate cancer on repeat prostate biopsy: a prospective study of 1,051 men. J Urol 2000;163:1144–1148.

50. Haese A, Graefen M, Noldus J, et al. Prostatic volume and ratio of free-to-total prostate specific antigen in patients with prostatic cancer or benign prostatic hyperplasia. J Urol 1997;158:2188–2192.

51. Stephan C, Lein M, Jung K, et al. The influence of prostate volume on the ratio of free to total prostate specific antigen in serum of patients with prostate carcinoma and benign prostate hyperplasia. Cancer 1997;79:104–109.

52. Partin AW, Catalona WJ, Southwick PC, et al. Analysis of percent free prostate-specific antigen (PSA) for prostate cancer detection: influence of total PSA, prostate volume, and age. Urology 1996;48:55–61.

53. Allard WJ, Zhou Z, Yeung KK. Novel immunoassay for the measurement of complexed prostate-specific antigen in serum. Clin Chem 1998;44:1216–1223.

54. Morris DL, Dillon PW, Very DL, et al. Bayer Immuno 1 PSA Assay: an automated, ultrasensitive method to quantitate total PSA in serum. J Clin Lab Anal 1998;12:65–74.

55. Wu JT, Zhang P, Liu GH, et al. Development of an immunoassay specific for the PSA-ACT complex without the problem of high background. J Clin Lab Anal 1998;12:14–19.

56. Brawer MK, Cheli CD, Neaman IE, et al. Complexed prostate specific antigen provides significant enhancement of specificity compared with total prostate specific antigen for detecting prostate cancer. J Urol 2000;163:1476–1480.

57. Partin AW, Brawer MK, Bartsch G, et al. Complexed prostate specific antigen improves specificity for prostate cancer detection: results of a prospective multicenter clinical trial. J Urol 2003;170:1787–1791.

58. Maeda H, Arai Y, Aoki Y, et al. Complexed prostate-specific antigen and its volume indexes in the detection of prostate cancer. Urology 1999;54:225–228.

59. Okegawa T, Noda H, Nutahara K, et al. Comparison of two investigative assays for the complexed prostate-specific antigen in total prostate-specific antigen between 4.1 and 10.0 ng/mL. Urology 2000;55:700–704.

60. Stamey TA, Yemoto CE. Examination of the 3 molecular forms of serum prostate specific antigen for distinguishing negative from positive biopsy: relationship to transition zone volume. J Urol 2000;163:119–126.

61. Lein M, Jung K, Elgeti U, et al. Comparison of the clinical validity of free prostate-specific antigen, alpha-1 antichymotrypsin-bound prostate-specific antigen and complexed prostate-specific antigen in prostate cancer diagnosis. Eur Urol 2001;39:57–64.

62. Jung K, Elgeti U, Lein M, et al. Ratio of free or complexed prostate-specific antigen (PSA) to total PSA: which ratio improves differentiation between benign prostatic hyperplasia and prostate cancer? Clin Chem 2000;46:55–62.

63. Bunting PS, DeBoer G, Choo R, et al. Intraindividual variation of PSA, free PSA and complexed PSA in a cohort of patients with prostate cancer managed with watchful observation. Clin Biochem 2002;35:471–475.

64. Thompson IM, Pauler DK, Goodman PJ, et al. Prevalence of prostate cancer among men with a prostate-specific antigen level < or =4.0 ng per milliliter. N Engl J Med 2004;350:2239–2246.

65. Schroder FH, van der Cruijsen-Koeter I, de Koning HJ, et al. Prostate cancer detection at low prostate specific antigen. J Urol 2000;163:806–812.

66. Catalona WJ, Smith DS, Ornstein DK. Prostate cancer detection in men with serum PSA concentrations of 2.6 to 4.0 ng/mL and benign prostate examination. Enhancement of specificity with free PSA measurements. JAMA 1997;277:1452–1455.

67. Thompson IM, Goodman PJ, Tangen CM, et al. The influence of finasteride on the development of prostate cancer. N Engl J Med 2003;349:215–224.

68. Gann PH, Hennekens CH, Stampfer MJ. A prospective evaluation of plasma prostate-specific antigen for detection of prostatic cancer. JAMA 1995;273:289–294.

69. Carter HB. A PSA threshold of 4.0 ng/mL for early detection of prostate cancer: the only rational approach for men 50 years old and older. Urology 2000;55:796–799.

70. Haese A, Dworschack RT, Partin AW. Percent free prostate specific antigen in the total prostate specific antigen 2 to 4 ng/ml range does not substantially increase the number of biopsies needed to detect clinically significant prostate cancer compared to the 4 to 10 ng/ml range. J Urol 2002;168:504–508.

71. Makinen T, Tammela TL, Hakama M, et al. Prostate cancer screening within a prostate specific antigen range of 3 to 3.9 ng/ml a comparison of digital rectal examination and free prostate specific antigen as supplemental screening tests. J Urol 2001;166:1339–1342.

72. Catalona WJ, Partin AW, Finlay JA, et al. Use of percentage of free prostate-specific antigen to identify men at high risk of prostate cancer when PSA levels are 2.51 to 4 ng/mL and digital rectal examination is not suspicious for prostate cancer: an alternative model. Urology 1999;54:220–224.

73. Roberts SG, Blute ML, Bergstralh EJ, et al. PSA doubling time as a predictor of clinical progression after biochemical failure following radical prostatectomy for prostate cancer. Mayo Clin Proc 2001;76:576–581.

74. Patel A, Dorey F, Franklin J, et al. Recurrence patterns after radical retropubic prostatectomy: clinical usefulness of prostate specific antigen doubling times and log slope prostate specific antigen. J Urol 1997;158:1441–1445.

75. D'Amico AV, Cote K, Loffredo M, et al. Determinants of prostate cancer specific survival following radiation therapy during the prostate specific antigen era. J Urol 2003;170:S42–S46.

76. D'Amico AV, Cote K, Loffredo M, et al. Determinants of prostate cancer-specific survival after radiation therapy for patients with clinically localized prostate cancer. J Clin Oncol 2002;20:4567–4573.

77. D'Amico AV, Moul J, Carroll PR, et al. Prostate specific antigen doubling time as a surrogate end point for prostate cancer specific mortality following radical prostatectomy or radiation therapy. J Urol 2004;172:S42–S46.

78. D'Amico AV, Moul JW, Carroll PR, et al. Surrogate end point for prostate cancer-specific mortality after radical prostatectomy or radiation therapy. J Natl Cancer Inst 2003;95:1376–1383.

79. Pound CR, Partin AW, Eisenberger MA, et al. Natural history of progression after PSA elevation following radical prostatectomy. JAMA 1999;281:1591–1597.

80. D'Amico AV, Chen MH, Roehl KA, et al. Preoperative PSA velocity and the risk of death from prostate cancer after radical prostatectomy. N Engl J Med 2004;351:125–135.

81. Critz FA, Levinson AK, Williams WH, et al. Prostate specific antigen nadir achieved by men apparently cured of prostate cancer by radiotherapy. J Urol 1999;161:1199–1203.

82. Zietman AL, Tibbs MK, Dallow KC, et al. Use of PSA nadir to predict subsequent biochemical outcome following external beam radiation therapy for T1-2 adenocarcinoma of the prostate. Radiother Oncol 1996;40:159–162.

83. Consensus statement: guidelines for PSA following radiation therapy. American Society for Therapeutic Radiology and Oncology Consensus Panel. Int J Radiat Oncol Biol Phys 1997;37:1035–1041.

84. Amling CL, Bergstralh EJ, Blute ML, et al. Defining prostate specific antigen progression after radical prostatectomy: what is the most appropriate cut point? J Urol 2001;165:1146–1151.

85. Smith DC, Pienta KJ. The use of prostate-specific antigen as a surrogate end point in the treatment of patients with hormone refractory prostate cancer. Urol Clin North Am 1997;24:433–437.

86. Matzkin H, Eber P, Todd B, et al. Prognostic significance of changes in prostate-specific markers after endocrine treatment of stage D2 prostatic cancer. Cancer 1992;70:2302–2309.

87. Miller JI, Ahmann FR, Drach GW, et al. The clinical usefulness of serum prostate specific antigen after hormonal therapy of metastatic prostate cancer. J Urol 1992;147:956–961.

88. Committee FA. Prostate Cancer Trials Could Use Composite PSA/Bone Scan Endpoint, 2004

89. Stamey TA, Prestigiacomo AF, Chen Z. Standardization of immunoassays for prostate specific antigen. A different view based on experimental observations. Cancer 1994;74:1662–1666.

90. Stamey TA. Second Stanford Conference on International Standardization of Prostate-Specific Antigen Immunoassays: September 1 and 2, 1994. Urology 1995;45:173–184.

91. Graves HC, Wehner N, Stamey TA. Comparison of a polyclonal and monoclonal immunoassay for PSA: need for an international antigen standard. J Urol 1990;144:1516–1522.

92. Junker R, Brandt B, Semjonow A, et al. The biologic lower detection limit of six ultrasensitive PSA assays. Anticancer Res 1999;19:2625–2628.

93. van Iersel MP, Thomas CM, Segers MF, et al. The use of 'ultrasensitive' prostate-specific antigen assays in the detection of biochemical recurrence after radical prostatectomy. Br J Urol 1996;77:418–422.

94. Haese A, Huland E, Graefen M, et al. Ultrasensitive detection of prostate specific antigen in the followup of 422 patients after radical prostatectomy. J Urol 1999;161:1206–1211.

95. Arai Y, Okubo K, Aoki Y, et al. Ultrasensitive assay of prostate-specific antigen for early detection of residual cancer after radical prostatectomy. Int J Urol 1998;5:550–555.

96. Ellis WJ, Vessella RL, Noteboom JL, et al. Early detection of recurrent prostate cancer with an ultrasensitive chemiluminescent prostate-specific antigen assay. Urology 1997;50:573–579.

97. Mikolajczyk SD, Grauer LS, Millar LS, et al. A precursor form of PSA (pPSA) is a component of the free PSA in prostate cancer serum. Urology 1997;50:710–714.

98. Mikolajczyk SD, Millar LS, Wang TJ, et al. A precursor form of prostate-specific antigen is more highly elevated in prostate cancer compared with benign transition zone prostate tissue. Cancer Res 2000;60:756–759.

99. Mikolajczyk SD, Millar LS, Wang TJ, et al. "BPSA," a specific molecular form of free prostate-specific antigen, is found predominantly in the transition zone of patients with nodular benign prostatic hyperplasia. Urology 2000;55:41–45.

100. Takayama TK, Fujikawa K, Davie EW. Characterization of the precursor of prostate-specific antigen. Activation by trypsin and by human glandular kallikrein. J Biol Chem 1997;272:21582–21588.

101. Rittenhouse HG, Finlay JA, Mikolajczyk SD, et al. Human Kallikrein 2 (hK2) and prostate-specific antigen (PSA): two closely related, but distinct, kallikreins in the prostate. Crit Rev Clin Lab Sci 1998;35:275–368.

102. Mikolajczyk SD, Marker KM, Millar LS, et al. A truncated precursor form of prostate-specific antigen is a more specific serum marker of prostate cancer. Cancer Res 2001;61:6958–6963.

103. Zhang WM, Leinonen J, Kalkkinen N, et al. Purification and characterization of different molecular forms of prostate-specific antigen in human seminal fluid. Clin Chem 1995;41:1567–1573.

104. Peter J, Unverzagt C, Krogh TN, et al. Identification of precursor forms of free prostate-specific antigen in serum of prostate cancer patients by immunosorption and mass spectrometry. Cancer Res 2001;61:957–962.

105. Catalona WJ, Bartsch G, Rittenhouse HG, et al. Serum pro prostate specific antigen improves cancer detection compared to free and complexed prostate specific antigen in men with prostate specific antigen 2 to 4 ng/ml. J Urol 2003;170:2181–2185.

106. Khan MA, Partin AW, Rittenhouse HG, et al. Evaluation of proprostate specific antigen for early detection of prostate cancer in men with a total prostate specific antigen range of 4.0 to 10.0 ng/ml. J Urol 2003;170:723–726.

107. Khan MA, Sokoll LJ, Chan DW, et al. Clinical utility of proPSA and "benign" PSA when percent free PSA is less than 15%. Urology 2004;64:1160–1164.

108. Steuber T, Nurmikko P, Haese A, et al. Discrimination of benign from malignant prostatic disease by selective measurements of single chain, intact free prostate specific antigen. J Urol 2002;168:1917–1922.

109. Nurmikko P, Pettersson K, Piironen T, et al. Discrimination of prostate cancer from benign disease by plasma measurement of intact, free prostate-specific antigen lacking an internal cleavage site at Lys145-Lys146. Clin Chem 2001;47:1415–1423.

110. Young CY, Andrews PE, Montgomery BT, et al. Tissue-specific and hormonal regulation of human prostate-specific glandular kallikrein. Biochemistry 1992;31:818–824.

111. Darson MF, Pacelli A, Roche P, et al. Human glandular kallikrein 2 expression in prostate adenocarcinoma and lymph node metastases. Urology 1999;53:939–944.

112. Tremblay RR, Deperthes D, Tetu B, et al. Immunohistochemical study suggesting a complementary role of kallikreins hK2 and hK3 (prostate-specific antigen) in the functional analysis of human prostate tumors. Am J Pathol 1997;150:455–459.

113. Haese A, Graefen M, Becker C, et al. The role of human glandular kallikrein 2 for prediction of pathologically organ confined prostate cancer. Prostate 2003;54:181–186.

114. Haese A, Graefen M, Steuber T, et al. Human glandular kallikrein 2 levels in serum for discrimination of pathologically organ-confined from locally-advanced prostate cancer in total PSA-levels below 10 ng/ml. Prostate 2001;49:101–109.

115. Haese A, Becker C, Noldus J, et al. Human glandular kallikrein 2: a potential serum marker for predicting the organ confined versus non-organ confined growth of prostate cancer. J Urol 2000;163:1491–1497.

116. Becker C, Piironen T, Pettersson K, et al. Discrimination of men with prostate cancer from those with benign disease by measurements of human glandular kallikrein 2 (HK2) in serum. J Urol 2000;163:311–316.

117. Becker C, Piironen T, Pettersson K, et al. Clinical value of human glandular kallikrein 2 and free and total prostate-specific antigen in serum from a population of men with prostate-specific antigen levels 3.0 ng/mL or greater. Urology 2000;55:694–699.

118. Magklara A, Scorilas A, Catalona WJ, et al. The combination of human glandular kallikrein and free prostate-specific antigen (PSA) enhances discrimination between prostate cancer and benign prostatic hyperplasia in patients with moderately increased total PSA. Clin Chem 1999;45:1960–1966.

119. Kwiatkowski MK, Recker F, Piironen T, et al. In prostatism patients the ratio of human glandular kallikrein to free PSA improves the discrimination between prostate cancer and benign hyperplasia

within the diagnostic "gray zone" of total PSA 4 to 10 ng/mL. Urology 1998;52:360–365.

120. Recker F, Kwiatkowski MK, Piironen T, et al. The importance of human glandular kallikrein and its correlation with different prostate specific antigen serum forms in the detection of prostate carcinoma. Cancer 1998;83:2540–2547.

121. Partin AW, Catalona WJ, Finlay JA, et al. Use of human glandular kallikrein 2 for the detection of prostate cancer: preliminary analysis. Urology 1999;54:839–845.

122. Nam RK, Diamandis EP, Toi A, et al. Serum human glandular kallikrein-2 protease levels predict the presence of prostate cancer among men with elevated prostate-specific antigen. J Clin Oncol 2000;18:1036–1042.

123. Nam RK, Zhang WW, Trachtenberg J, et al. Single nucleotide polymorphism of the human kallikrein-2 gene highly correlates with serum human kallikrein-2 levels and in combination enhances prostate cancer detection. J Clin Oncol 2003;21:2312–2319.

124. Chiang CH, Chen KK, Chang LS, et al. The impact of polymorphism on prostate specific antigen gene on the risk, tumor volume and pathological stage of prostate cancer. J Urol 2004;171:1529–1532.

125. Petricoin EF 3rd, Ornstein DK, Paweletz CP, et al. Serum proteomic patterns for detection of prostate cancer. J Natl Cancer Inst 2002;94:1576–1578.

126. Adam BL, Qu Y, Davis JW, et al. Serum protein fingerprinting coupled with a pattern-matching algorithm distinguishes prostate cancer from benign prostate hyperplasia and healthy men. Cancer Res 2002;62:3609–3614.

127. Mikolajczyk SD, Marks LS, Partin AW, et al. Free prostate-specific antigen in serum is becoming more complex. Urology 2002;59:797–802.

128. Catalona WJ, Partin AW, Slawin KM, et al. Use of the percentage of free prostate-specific antigen to enhance differentiation of prostate cancer from benign prostatic disease. A prospective multicenter clinical trial. JAMA 1998;279:1542–1547.

129. Brawer MK, Meyer GE, Letran JL, et al. Measurement of complexed PSA improves specificity for early detection of prostate cancer. Urology 1998;52:372–378.

Clinical applications of prostate-specific antigen isoforms

46

Eduardo I Canto, Kevin M Slawin

IS THE TOTAL PROSTATE-SPECIFIC ANTIGEN ERA COMING TO AN END?

The introduction of prostate-specific antigen (PSA) in the late 1980s revolutionized the diagnosis, staging, and management of prostate cancer. No other technology has had such a profound effect on the diagnosis and management of prostate cancer. Only the development of the grading system devised by Donald Gleason, M.D. Ph.D. in the early 1970s has had a comparable impact on prostate cancer staging.[1] The widespread use of PSA as a screening tool has resulted in a marked stage migration over the last two decades.[2,3] Because there have been no major breakthroughs in the treatment of prostate cancer since the late 1980s, most authors attribute the recent decline in prostate cancer-specific mortality to the use of PSA, both as a screening and as a management tool for prostate cancer. Over the last two decades, an increasing amount of data has accumulated to support this hypothesis.[2-4]

Although far from perfect, serum PSA testing in conjunction with digital rectal examination of the prostate (DRE) compares favorably with other cancer screening modalities. The positive predictive value (PPV) of a PSA above 4 ng/mL is 30% to 40%.[5] An abnormal mammogram for example, has a PPV of 10% to 20% and is an order of magnitude more expensive than PSA.[6] Nevertheless, the widespread acceptance of PSA, paradoxically, has led to a marked decrease in its utility for both prostate cancer screening and staging. The average yearly rise in serum PSA concentration in men with either prostate cancer or benign prostatic hyperplasia (BPH) is low (i.e., 0.75 ng/mL/year for cancer and 0.1–0.5 ng/mL/year for BPH). Therefore, as a larger percentage of the population enters the pool of men being screened on a yearly basis, the average PSA of men above the commonly used cutoff of 4 ng/mL moves ever closer to that cut-off point.[7,8] Unfortunately, because of the complex relationship between PSA, prostate cancer, and BPH, the clinical utility of PSA in this range for both staging and screening is modest at best. Therefore, the unprecedented impact of PSA and its widespread adoption for the screening of prostate cancer has severely taxed its performance for both screening and staging. Nevertheless, the PSA era will not come to an end until a more specific screening marker and a more sensitive staging and management tool become commercially available.

FREE PROSTATE-SPECIFIC ANTIGEN—A COMPLEX MIXTURE OF MOLECULES

Prostate-specific antigen, also known as seminogelase, seminin, P-30, human kallikrein 3, and γ-semino-protein, is a 33-kDa serine protease of the kallikrein family. It was first isolated from human serum in 1971, from human semen in 1978, and from prostate tissue in 1979.[9-11] It is produced in clinically significant quantities by prostate luminal epithelial cells only. These cells secrete PSA into the seminal fluid, where it degrades semenogelin I and II and fibronectin, the major gel-forming proteins of the human ejaculate, to allow the release of spermatozoa.[12,13] Prostate-specific antigen enters the circulation through an unknown mechanism reaching ng/mL concentrations, 10^6 times less than its concentration in the seminal fluid.[13] Because it is produced by normal, hyperplastic, and neoplastic prostate epithelial cells, it is an organ-specific rather than a tumor-specific marker. Moreover, the presence or absence of prostate cancer is only one of the biologic variables that influence the release of PSA into the circulation.[14] Because of these and other inherent, biologically determined drawbacks, PSA loses its specificity as a screening marker and its sensitivity as a staging tool when its serum concentration falls within 4 to10ng/mL range.

The quest for a better prostate cancer marker and the improvements in the technologies available for the study of proteins resulted in the identification of a growing number of distinct molecular forms of PSA. Shortly after the complementary DNA (cDNA) for PSA was cloned in 1987, it was observed that PSA isolated from human serum exists in either a bound (i.e., to α1-antichymotrypsin) or unbound form.[15,16] Serum concentrations of protease inhibitor-bound PSA, also known as complexed PSA (cPSA), were found to have a positive correlation with the presence of prostate cancer.[16] Conversely, serum concentrations of unbound, or free PSA (fPSA), as a fraction of total PSA, were found to have a negative correlation with the presence of prostate cancer.[17] Although the biologic explanation for this phenomenon eludes researchers, it was theorized that the loss of tissue architecture that results from disorganized cancer growth facilitates the binding of inhibitors delivered by the circulatory system or produced locally within prostate tissue. The result is that the amount of cPSA released into the bloodstream is greater than that released by benign prostate tissue. In contrast, PSA produced by BPH is secreted into the seminal plasma and must leak back through the intercellular space, where it is exposed to proteases, before reaching the circulation. Because cleaved, inactive forms for PSA are unable to bind protease inhibitors,

they remain unbound in the blood, comprising the fPSA fraction. Nevertheless, we now have evidence to prove that this hypothesis is not completely true because fPSA forms have been isolated that are released preferentially by prostate cancer.[18]

Approximately 75% of measurable serum PSA is irreversibly bound to the protease inhibitor α1-antichymotrypsin (PSA-ACT). A lesser fraction binds to α2-macroglobulin (AMG) forming PSA-AMG or to α1-protease inhibitor (PSA-API). The complexed PSA-AMG may retain part of its enzymatic activity, but neither PSA-ACT nor fPSA is enzymatically active.[16] α1-Antitrypsin has been shown to bind the active site of PSA and form a stable acyl-enzyme bond.[19]

Like many other secreted proteases, PSA is produced in an inactive form as a "pre-pro" peptide. The amino-terminal 17-amino-acids target the protein upon translation into the endoplasmic reticulum for secretion into the seminal spaces. These 17 amino acids define the "pre" peptide. The following 7 amino acids of the amino-terminus define the "pro" peptide and maintain the enzyme in inactive form until it reaches the seminal spaces. Here, one or more enzyme, cleaves the pro-peptide sequence off, activating the now mature PSA.[15] (Figure 46.1) Surprisingly, studies examining the actual amino-terminal sequences of the various inactive forms of fPSA in the seminal plasma, serum, and normal, hyperplastic, and cancerous prostate tissue have found that various alternatively processed forms of fPSA have retained some or all of the "pro" sequence of amino acids. In addition, mature inactive forms of PSA with and without internal cleavages have also been identified. (Figure 46.2)

The following fPSA molecular forms have been identified in human serum: mature but inactive non-

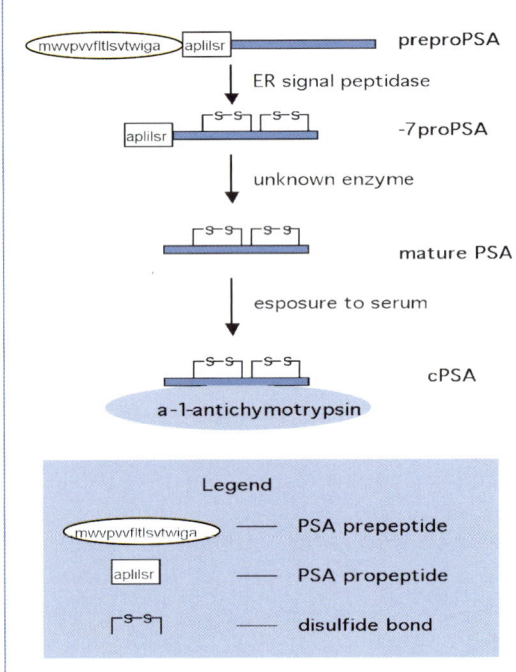

Fig. 46.1

Production of complex prostate-specific antigen (cPSA). PSA is produced as a pepropeptide. The leader "pre" sequence directs the nascent protein into the endoplasmic reticulum (ER), where a signal peptidase cleaves off the pre amino acids to give –7proPSA. An unknown enzyme cleaves off the pro amino acids to give mature PSA. Once it reaches the circulation, mature active PSA will bind α1-antichymotrypsin, forming cPSA.

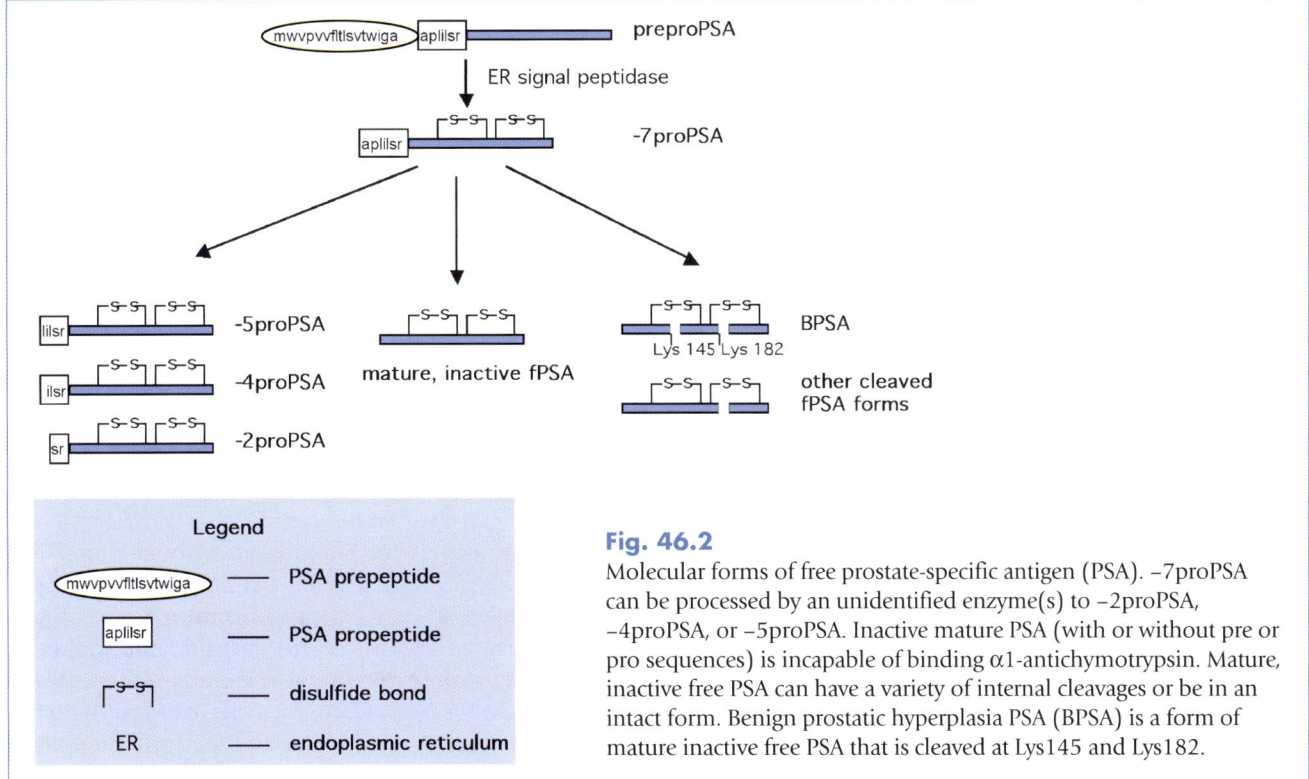

Legend

mwvpvvfltlsvtwiga ——— PSA prepeptide

aplilsr ——— PSA propeptide

S-S ——— disulfide bond

ER ——— endoplasmic reticulum

Fig. 46.2

Molecular forms of free prostate-specific antigen (PSA). –7proPSA can be processed by an unidentified enzyme(s) to –2proPSA, –4proPSA, or –5proPSA. Inactive mature PSA (with or without pre or pro sequences) is incapable of binding α1-antichymotrypsin. Mature, inactive free PSA can have a variety of internal cleavages or be in an intact form. Benign prostatic hyperplasia PSA (BPSA) is a form of mature inactive free PSA that is cleaved at Lys145 and Lys182.

cleaved PSA, inactive zymogen forms, including –2, –4, –5, and –7 proPSA, and cleaved, also inactive, forms of otherwise mature PSA, including cleavages at Ile1, His54, Phe157, Lys145, and Lys182 (see Figure 46.2). Zymogen forms of PSA were first noted when PSA was expressed using recombinant DNA in otherwise non-PSA-expressing mammalian and insect cells.[20–22] The first two studies that examined human serum reported conflicting results. Noldus et al, who were the first to purify PSA from pooled human serum in search of PSA isoforms, found both inactive mature PSA and cleaved forms, but not zymogen forms.[23] In contrast, using immunoabsorption rather than gel filtration, Mikolajczyk et al did find various zymogen forms of PSA, also known as proPSA, molecular forms[24] (see Figure 46.2). The absence of proPSA in the Noldus study probably was caused by contamination with

enzymatically active hK2, which has been shown to cleave proPSA forms to generate mature PSA. The purified PSA fraction of fPSA in the Noldus study displayed both trypsin and chymotrypsin-like activity. Prostate-specific antigen has only chymotrypsin-like activity, whereas hK2 has trypsin-like activity. Subsequent studies have confirmed the presence of proPSA molecular forms containing 2, 4, 5, or all 7 of the zymogen amino acids in the serum of patients with prostate cancer.[18,25] Recently, Mikolajczyk et al showed that zymogen forms of PSA are more abundant in peripheral than in transition zone tissue, and in prostate cancer than in normal peripheral zone.[18] (Table 46.1)

Inactive fPSA isolated from BPH tissue and seminal plasma has only a limited amount of the proPSA molecular forms. Conversely, inactive fPSA isolated from normal peripheral or normal transition zone tissue has

Table 46.1 Zone and pathology—specific markers as a fraction of total tissue prostate-specific antigen (PSA)[18]

Marker	TZ-N (PV < 25 mL) (mean %) n = 8	TZ-BPH (PV > 50 mL) (mean %) n = 10	PZ-N (mean %) n = 18	PZ-C (mean %) n = 18
BPSA	4.1	11.4	3.7	4.3
–2,–4proPSA	0.4	1.7	3.9	5.6
Inactive PSA	40.1	38.0	36.6	36.2

PV, prostate volume; PZ-C, peripheral zone with cancer; PZ-N, normal peripheral zone; TZ-BPH, transition zone with BPH; TZ-N, normal transition zone tissue.

only a limited amount of the internally cleaved, mature fPSA (median of 0.17 µg BPSA per mg total protein in normal transition zone tissue [n = 8]; median of 2.0 mg BPSA per µg total protein in transition zone tissue with BPH [n = 10]).[26] Inactivation of the fPSA in BPH tissue and seminal plasma is primarily the result of internal cleavages.[18,26–28] Although a variety of internal cleavage sites have been noted, the most abundant cleaved form of fPSA from BPH tissue is cleaved at Lys145 and Lys182.[26] This mature, enzymatically inactive form of fPSA has been dubbed BPSA, and it comprises about one third of the absolute fPSA in serum.[29]

CLINICAL APPLICATION OF FREE AND COMPLEXED PROSTATE-SPECIFIC ANTIGEN

Prostate-specific antigen has at least five epitopes. Binding to all five epitopes is hindered by the interaction of PSA with AMG. Conventional total PSA assays, therefore, detect both fPSA and cPSA (i.e., PSA-ACT) but not PSA-AMG. Two of the five epitopes of PSA are inaccessible to antibodies when the molecule is bound to ACT. Commercial fPSA assays are based on antibodies that specifically bind to the epitopes that are hidden when PSA is bound to ACT. The only cPSA assay approved by the U.S. Food and Drug Administration is based on antibody-mediated elimination of all fPSA followed by measurement of the remaining ACT-bound PSA (Bayer Immunol cPSA Assay, Bayer Diagnostics, Tarrytown, NY). There are at least three assays approved for %fPSA prostate cancer screening. Because the performance of these assays varies, the established cutoffs for each specific assay should be used.

SCREENING

The use of fPSA, expressed as a percent of total PSA, %fPSA (i.e., 100 × fPSA/total PSA), as an adjunct to PSA and DRE-based prostate cancer screening has gained significant acceptance since its FDA approval. It is approved for the risk stratification of patients with a normal DRE and PSA in the diagnostic gray zone of 4 to 10 ng/mL. The pivotal study that led to FDA approval was published in 2000 by a multicenter group. Using the Tandem-E fPSA assay, Catalona et al found that a fPSA cutoff of 25% could reduce the number of unnecessary biopsies by 20% while still detecting 95% of the cancers that would have been diagnosed had all patients with a PSA between 4 and 10 ng/mL been biopsied. This study showed conclusively that the risk of prostate cancer decreases as the %fPSA rises and that the use of %fPSA could improve the specificity of a PSA-based prostate cancer-screening program.[30]

With the recognition that up to 25% of men with a negative DRE and a PSA between 2.6 and 4 ng/mL may have prostate cancer, studies were carried out to evaluate %fPSA for its ability to improve the specificity of PSA-based prostate cancer screening in this setting. Using the Tandem-E fPSA assay, Catalona et al reported an 18% reduction in the number of unnecessary biopsies while maintaining a sensitivity of 90% when patients with a %fPSA below 27% and a total PSA between 2.6 and 4 ng/mL were biopsied.[31] In this study, 83% of the cancers diagnosed met criteria for clinical significance. Another large study using the Abbott AxSYM free PSA assay also found that %fPSA can improve the performance of PSA-based screening in men with PSA between 3 and 4 ng/mL. When a %fPSA cutoff of 19% was applied, 90% of cancers were detected and 44% of the biopsies performed were positive for cancer.[32]

The cPSA assay was developed with the goal of replacing both PSA and %fPSA. Even though early data suggested that cPSA by itself (not in a ratio to total PSA) could perform as well as %fPSA, large studies failed to confirm this finding. The largest multicenter study of cPSA showed that only when the range of total PSA was restricted to below 6 ng/mL did cPSA perform as well as %fPSA. For the 2 to 10 ng/mL range, only in a ratio to total PSA did cPSA perform as well as %fPSA.[33] Because it offers no significant improvement over %fPSA, even when in a ratio to total PSA, cPSA has failed to gain widespread use.

STAGING

The data available on the use of %fPSA for prostate cancer staging, unlike that on its use for prostate cancer screening, is inconclusive. Three large studies have evaluated the potential of %fPSA in prostate cancer staging. Only one of the three studies found %fPSA to be a stronger predictor than commonly used parameters such as Gleason grade and PSA. This large multicenter study evaluated 268 men with no palpable tumors and total PSA between 4 and 10 ng/mL who underwent radical prostatectomy. A value of 15% or less was found to correlate with unfavorable final pathology.[34] Nevertheless, two later studies found that %fPSA had a predictive value comparable to that of serum PSA and biopsy Gleason score in univariate analyses, although it failed to provide additional staging or prognostic information in multivariate analyses that included clinical stage, Gleason score, and PSA.[35,36]

Analysis of three recent studies evaluating cPSA as a staging tool for prostate cancer shows that in none of the studies did cPSA remain an independent predictor of final pathologic stage when Gleason score and PSA were included as predictors. In all three studies, cPSA provided the same staging information as did PSA.

When evaluated in a ratio to total PSA, the performance of cPSA actually declined.[37–39]

Although the use of %fPSA is far more common than the use of cPSA, %fPSA is not without drawbacks. The performance of %fPSA decreases when prostate size exceeds 40 mL. In these larger prostates, %fPSA has been shown to increase even in the presence of cancer.[40] Free PSA is less stable than cPSA under the commonly used storage conditions of 4 °C to –20 °C. For this reason, it is recommended that specimens that will not be processed within 8 hours for fPSA be stored at –70 °C. In contrast, loss of immunoreactivity of cPSA can be prevented by storage at –20 °C.[41] Finally, compared with fPSA, cPSA concentration has been shown to be less susceptible to changes associated with manipulation of the prostate such as DRE and cystoscopy.[42]

Although the molecular mechanisms behind the production of free and bound forms of PSA still are not completely understood, it has been observed that, at least in practical terms, the utility of %fPSA depends on the correlation between fPSA and prostate volume. Large studies have clearly shown that, in patients without prostate cancer, serum PSA concentration correlates with prostate volume. This correlation has been shown to be age dependent.[43] In the presence of prostate cancer, however, this correlation no longer holds true, presumably because of the significant impact that prostate cancer has on serum PSA levels. In contrast, recent studies demonstrate that serum fPSA (the absolute fPSA value, not in a ratio to PSA) concentration is proportional to prostate size, independent of age, and is maintained even in patients with prostate cancer.[29] In light of these observations, a simplistic, yet probably accurate, understanding of %fPSA is that it represents a serologic equivalent of PSA density (PSA/prostate volume), albeit inverted. In the absence of a serum marker known to be expressed only by prostate cancer, it is likely that the next generation of PSA-based screening strategies will continue to depend on ratios of markers that correlate with prostate volume and markers that correlate with the presence of prostate cancer. Indeed, as we review recent discoveries relating to the various molecular forms of fPSA, the concept of serologic equivalent of PSA density will take center stage.

CLINICAL APPLICATION OF MOLECULAR FORMS OF FREE PROSTATE-SPECIFIC ANTIGEN

Although the introduction of %fPSA has only modestly improved our effectiveness in screening prostate cancer, the clinical success of this assay renewed the urologic community's interest in the study of molecular forms of PSA. Recently, fluorogenic immunoassays have been developed that specifically recognize the various proPSA forms as well as the major cleaved fPSA form, known as BPSA. Using recombinant fusion protein products containing the various amino-terminal sequences of the known proPSA forms fused to hK2, Mikolajczyk et al developed four proPSA assays currently available for research use only. These include a –2proPSA assay, a –4proPSA assay, a combined –5 and –7proPSA assay, and a pan-proPSA assay. The combined –5 and –7proPSA assay detects both –5 and –7 zymogen forms. The pan-proPSA assay recognizes all proPSA forms.[24]

The isoform BPSA consists of mature PSA that has been inactivated by cleavages at Lys145 and Lys182. The cleavage at Lys182 generates a conformational change in this form of fPSA allowing for the selection of antibodies specific for fPSA forms with this internal cleavage. Unfortunately, the antibodies generated against BPSA detect fPSA molecular forms with a cleavage at Lys182 only, as well as those with cleavages at both Lys182 and Lys145. Nevertheless, tissue studies have demonstrated that the ratio of true BPSA (cleaved at both Lys182 and Lys145) to fPSA cleaved only at Lys182 is relatively fixed. Therefore, it is expected that the available assay for BPSA (which measures both fPSA cleaved at Lys182 only and fPSA cleaved at Lys182 and Lys145) overestimates by a fixed proportion the true concentration of BPSA.[44]

Understanding the ratios of fPSA molecular forms currently under study requires that the relationship between these various forms and both prostate cancer and BPH be made very clear. As noted above, the absolute concentration of fPSA correlates with prostate volume in both biopsy-negative and biopsy-positive patients. Nevertheless, we now know that fPSA is composed of both relatively cancer-specific and BPH-specific molecular forms (Figure 46.3; see also Figure

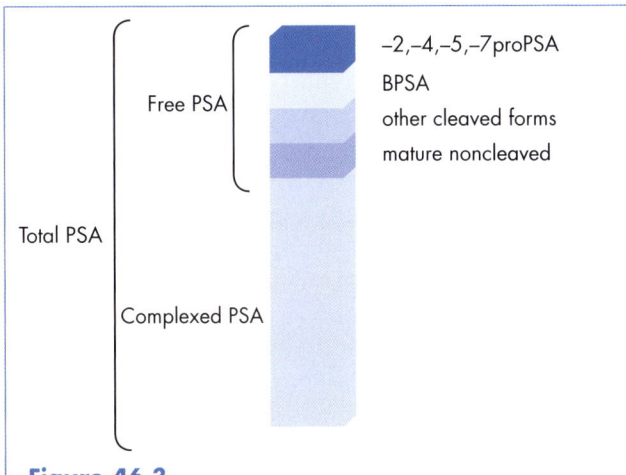

Figure 46.3

Heterogeneity of prostate-specific antigen (PSA). Total PSA is composed of complexed PSA and free PSA. Free PSA is comprised of proPSA molecular forms, a mature noncleaved form, and mature cleaved forms including BPSA.

39.4). The cancer-specific forms are zymogen forms of PSA: –2, –4, –5 and –7proPSA. The BPH-specific fPSA forms are exemplified by BPSA. If fPSA is composed of both cancer-specific and BPH-specific molecular forms and %fPSA is, indeed, a serologic equivalent of PSA density, then subtraction of the cancer-specific molecular forms from fPSA should improve the performance of %fPSA. On the other hand, subtraction of the BPH-specific form from fPSA should negatively affect its performance. Both of these hypotheses have been proven correct.[45]

Early data showed that absolute values of the zymogen forms of PSA could not discriminate between patients with and without cancer, probably because proPSA forms are made by both normal and neoplastic peripheral zone tissue (see Table 46.1). Given the success of %fPSA, it would be reasonable to evaluate ratios of relatively cancer-specific markers such as proPSA, PSA, and cPSA to markers that correlate with prostate volume, such as fPSA and BPSA, in order to generate new serologic PSA density equivalents. Both our data and that of others support –2proPSA/fPSA as the best marker for prostate cancer in men with PSA below 10 ng/mL.[45]

SCREENING

The clinical evaluation of these recently discovered molecular forms of fPSA has been facilitated by the availability of stored banks of serum generated for studies evaluating both PSA and %fPSA. It has been shown, using these stored serum samples, that proPSA forms, particularly –2proPSA/fPSA, modestly, yet consistently, outperform %fPSA in the diagnostic gray zone of 4 to 10 ng/mL PSA. In a study involving just over 1000 archived specimens, Catalona et al found that either –2proPSA or pan-proPSA in a ratio to fPSA outperformed both %fPSA and cPSA in the 4 to 10 ng/mL total PSA range. In this range of PSA, while maintaining a 90% sensitivity, pan-proPSA/fPSA spared 21% of unnecessary biopsies while %fPSA spared only 13% and cPSA spared 9% (P < 0.0001), a modest, yet statistically significant improvement.[46] Mikolajczyk et al studied 380 serum samples and also found that –2proPSA/fPSA modestly outperformed both %PSA and cfPSA. At a 90% sensitivity, –2proPSA/fPSA maintained a specificity of 21% compared with 20% and 19%, respectively, for %fPSA and cPSA.[47]

Studies focusing on the 2 to 4 ng/mL total PSA range have found a more robust improvement in the performance of PSA-based screening when including proPSA molecular forms of fPSA in the screening strategy. A small, initial study, including only 119 men with PSA between 2.5 and 4 ng/mL, found that the area under the curve (AUC) for proPSA/fPSA was larger than that of %fPSA (0.688 versus 0.567).[48] This trend was confirmed in the previously mentioned, much larger study by Catalona et al. In the 2 to 4 ng/mL PSA range, –2proPSA/fPSA had a specificity of 19% at 90% sensitivity compared with 10% and 11%, respectively, for %fPSA and cPSA.[46]

With the goal of further improving the specificity of PSA- and fPSA-based prostate cancer screening, attention has been extended from the diagnostic gray zone of total PSA between 4 and 10 ng/mL to the low-specificity range defined by %fPSA of less than 15%. Patients with a %fPSA of less than 15% have a probability of a positive biopsy of between 30% and 50%. Khan et al showed that the use of proPSA/BPSA can further reduce, by about half, the number of unnecessary biopsies in patients with %fPSA below 15% and PSA between 4 and 10 ng/mL, while maintaining a 90% sensitivity.[49] Comparable results were noted by Mikolajczyk et al using pan-proPSA/fPSA in patients with %fPSA below 15%. A 90% sensitivity was maintained and about one third of the unnecessary biopsies could have been avoided.[47]

STAGING

Data on prostate cancer staging using the various molecular forms of fPSA are less abundant than those for screening. This is due primarily to the need for surgery in order to obtain a pathologic stage. Nevertheless, an initial exploratory study involving a cohort of 62 consecutive prostatectomies from Baylor showed that the absolute preoperative levels of proPSA forms correlated with tumor volume and percent positive biopsy, and predicted extracapsular extension as well as risk of recurrence based on the stratification method defined by D'Amico et al. These associations remained significant after adjustment for the effects of total PSA, clinical stage, and biopsy Gleason score.[50]

In a larger study, Catalona et al confirmed these findings. They showed that –2proPSA/fPSA outperformed both cPSA and %fPSA in the prediction of final pathologic Gleason score greater or equal to 7 and/or extracapsular extension or a cancerous surgical margin. This finding held true for preoperative PSA values between 2 and 4 ng/mL and between 4 and 10 ng/mL. In the group with total PSA of 2 to 4 ng/mL, –2proPSA/fPSA had a specificity of 19% for detection of aggressive tumors at 90% sensitivity, while cPSA and %fPSA had 11% and 10% specificity, respectively. In the group with total PSA of 4 to 10 ng/mL, –2proPSA/fPSA had a specificity of 31% for detection of aggressive tumors at 90% sensitivity while cPSA and %fPSA had 19% and 20% specificity, respectively.[51]

MOLECULAR FORMS OF FREE PROSTATE-SPECIFIC ANTIGEN IN THE MANAGEMENT OF PROSTATE CANCER

In addition to screening and staging, molecular forms of fPSA may be useful in management and detection of recurrence after definitive therapy for prostate cancer. Both radiation and radical prostatectomy are associated with a low, yet significant, risk of recurrence over the 10 to 15 year period after primary therapy, even in the best of circumstances. Recurrence after either radiation or prostatectomy raises a number of important clinical questions. With either therapy, it may be important to determine if the recurrence is local or due to metastatic disease. From the patient's point of view, prognosis at the time of recurrence is of paramount importance. Although the clinical situation may vary greatly, a number of clinical and pathologic parameters may be used to direct further care and determine prognosis. However, there is still a need for serum markers capable of distinguishing between aggressive, likely metastatic, recurrence and indolent, likely local, recurrence.

The study of serum markers for evaluation of prostate cancer recurring after primary therapy is hindered by the need for long periods of follow-up and the involvement of additional practitioners other than the primary urologist in the patient's care. Nevertheless, although data are not yet available, studies are ongoing at Baylor to evaluate the use of molecular forms of fPSA and their ratios in the setting of post-prostatectomy PSA recurrence.

CONCLUSION

Serum PSA has become the most commonly used cancer test. Its success has fueled intense research in the field of molecular forms of PSA in both academia and industry. As a result, our understanding of the various molecular forms of PSA, particularly fPSA, has grown exponentially over the last two decades. The specific role in the screening, staging, and management of prostate cancer that one or more of the fPSA molecular forms will play in the near future is yet to be defined. Nevertheless, it is very likely that one or more of these new molecular forms of fPSA will improve our ability to screen, stage, and/or manage prostate cancer and thereby prolong the PSA era.

ACKNOWLEDGMENT

Special thanks to Carolyn Schum for her excellent editorial assistance.

REFERENCES

1. Gleason DF, Mellinger GT. Prediction of prognosis for prostatic adenocarcinoma by combined histological grading and clinical staging. J Urol 1974;111:58–64.
2. Roberts RO, Bergstralh EJ, Katusic SK, et al. Decline in prostate cancer mortality from 1980 to 1997, and an update on incidence trends in Olmsted County, Minnesota. J Urol 1999;161:529–533.
3. Ries LAG, Eisner MP, Kosary CL, et al (eds). 2000. SEER Cancer Statistics Review, 1973–1998. Bethesda: National Cancer Institute.
4. Bartsch G, Horninger W, Klocker H, et al. Decrease in prostate cancer mortality following introduction of prostate specific antigen (PSA) screening in the federal state of Tyrol, Austria. Annual meeting of the American Urological Association. Atlanta, 2000. [Abstract].
5. Gore JL, Shariat SF, Miles BJ, et al. Optimal combinations of systematic sextant and laterally directed biopsies for the detection of prostate cancer. J Urol 2001;165:1554–1559.
6. Kerlikowske K, Grady D, Barclay J, et al. Positive predictive value of screening mammography by age and family history of breast cancer. JAMA 1993;270:2444–2450.
7. Bonilla J, Roehrborn CG, McConnel JD. Patterns of prostate growth observed in placebo treated patients in the PLESS trial over four years. J Urol 1995;159:301A.
8. Carter HB, Pearson JD, Metter EJ, et al. Longitudinal evaluation of prostate-specific antigen levels in men with and without prostate disease. JAMA 1992;267:2215–2220.
9. Hara M, Inorre T, Fukuama T. Some physico-chemical characteristics of gamma-seminoprotein, an antigenic component specific for human seminal plasma. Jap J Legal Med 1971;25:322.
10. Sensabaugh GF. Isolation and characterization of a semen-specific protein from human seminal plasma: a potential new marker for semen identification. J Forensic Sci 1978;23:106–115.
11. Wang MC, Valenzuela LA, Murphy GP, et al. Purification of a human prostate specific antigen. Invest Urol 1979;17:159–163.
12. Lilja H. A kallikrein-like serine protease in prostatic fluid cleaves the predominant seminal vesicle protein. J Clin Invest 1985;76:1899–903.
13. Robert M, Gibbs BF, Jacobson E, et al. Characterization of prostate-specific antigen proteolytic activity on its major physiological substrate, the sperm motility inhibitor precursor/semenogelin I. Biochemistry 1997;36:3811–3819.
14. Henttu P, Liao SS, Vihko P. Androgens up-regulate the human prostate-specific antigen messenger ribonucleic acid (mRNA), but down-regulate the prostatic acid phosphatase mRNA in the LNCaP cell line. Endocrinology 1992;130:766–772.
15. Lundwall A, Lilja H. Molecular cloning of human prostate specific antigen cDNA. FEBS Lett 1987;214:317–322.
16. Stenman UH, Leinonen J, Alfthan H, et al. A complex between prostate-specific antigen and alpha 1- antichymotrypsin is the major form of prostate-specific antigen in serum of patients with prostatic cancer: assay of the complex improves clinical sensitivity for cancer. Cancer Res 1991;51:222–226.
17. Catalona WJ, Smith DS, Wolfert RL, et al. Evaluation of percentage of free serum prostate-specific antigen to improve specificity of prostate cancer screening. JAMA 1995;274:1214–1220.
18. Mikolajczyk SD, Millar LS, Wang TJ, et al. A precursor form of prostate-specific antigen is more highly elevated in prostate cancer compared with benign transition zone prostate tissue. Cancer Res 2000;60:756–759.
19. Peter J, Unverzagt C, Hoesel W. Analysis of free prostate-specific antigen (PSA) after chemical release from the complex with alpha(1)antichymotrypsin (PSA-ACT). Clin Chem 2000;46:474–482.
20. Kurkela R, Herrala A, Henttu P, et al. Expression of active, secreted human prostate-specific antigen by recombinant baculovirus-infected insect cells on a pilot-scale. Biotechnology (NY) 1995;13:1230–1234.
21. Kumar A, Mikolajczyk SD, Goel AS, et al. Expression of pro form of prostate-specific antigen by mammalian cells and its conversion to mature, active form by human kallikrein 2. Cancer Res 1997;57:3111–3114.
22. Kumar A, Mikolajczyk SD, Hill TM, et al. Different proportions of various prostate-specific antigen (PSA) and human kallikrein 2 (hK2)

forms are present in noninduced and androgen-induced LNCaP cells. Prostate 2000;44:248–254.

23. Noldus J, Chen Z, Stamey TA. Isolation and characterization of free form prostate specific antigen (f-PSA) in sera of men with prostate cancer. J Urol 1997;158:1606–1609.

24. Mikolajczyk SD, Grauer LS, Millar LS, et al. A precursor form of PSA (pPSA) is a component of the free PSA in prostate cancer serum. Urology 1997;50:710–714.

25. Mikolajczyk SD, Marker KM, Millar LS, et al. A truncated precursor form of prostate-specific antigen is a more specific serum marker of prostate cancer. Cancer Res 2001;61:6958–6963.

26. Mikolajczyk SD, Millar LS, Wang TJ, et al. "BPSA," a specific molecular form of free prostate-specific antigen, is found predominantly in the transition zone of patients with nodular benign prostatic hyperplasia. Urology 2000;55:41–45.

27. Chen Z, Chen H, Stamey TA. Prostate specific antigen in benign prostatic hyperplasia: purification and characterization. J Urol 1997;157:2166–2170.

28. Zhang WM, Leinonen J, Kalkkinen N, et al. Purification and characterization of different molecular forms of prostate-specific antigen in human seminal fluid. Clin Chem 1995;41:1567–1573.

29. Canto EI, Singh H, Shariat SF, et al. Serum BPSA outperforms both total PSA and free PSA as a predictor of prostatic enlargement in men without prostate cancer. Urology 2004;63:905–910; discussion 910–911.

30. Catalona WJ, Southwick PC, Slawin KM, et al. Comparison of percent free PSA, PSA density, and age-specific PSA cutoffs for prostate cancer detection and staging. Urology 2000;56:255–260.

31. Catalona WJ, Smith DS, Ornstein DK. Prostate cancer detection in men with serum PSA concentrations of 2.6 to 4.0 ng/mL and benign prostate examination. Enhancement of specificity with free PSA measurements. JAMA 1997;277:1452–1455.

32. Vashi AR, Wojno KJ, Henricks W, et al. Determination of the "reflex range" and appropriate cutpoints for percent free prostate-specific antigen in 413 men referred for prostatic evaluation using the AxSYM system. Urology 1997;49:19–27.

33. Partin AW, Brawer MK, Bartsch G, et al. Complexed prostate specific antigen improves specificity for prostate cancer detection: results of a prospective multicenter clinical trial. J Urol 2003;170:1787–1791.

34. Southwick PC, Catalona WJ, Partin AW, et al. Prediction of post-radical prostatectomy pathological outcome for stage T1c prostate cancer with percent free prostate specific antigen: a prospective multicenter clinical trial. J Urol 1999;162:1346–1351.

35. Tombal B, Querton M, de Nayer P, et al. Free/total PSA ratio does not improve prediction of pathologic stage and biochemical recurrence after radical prostatectomy. Urology 2002;59:256–260.

36. Graefen M, Karakiewicz PI, Cagiannos I, et al. Percent free prostate specific antigen is not an independent predictor of organ confinement or prostate specific antigen recurrence in unscreened patients with localized prostate cancer treated with radical prostatectomy. J Urol 2002;167:1306–1309.

37. Martinez M, Navarro S, Medina P, et al. The role of the complexed-to-total prostate-specific antigen ratio in predicting the final pathological stage of clinically localized prostate cancer. Eur Urol 2003;43:609–614.

38. Sokoll LJ, Mangold LA, Partin AW, et al. Complexed prostate-specific antigen as a staging tool for prostate cancer: a prospective study in 420 men. Urology 2002;60:18–23.

39. Taneja SS, Hsu EI, Cheli CD, et al. Complexed prostate-specific antigen as a staging tool: results based on a multicenter prospective evaluation of complexed prostate-specific antigen in cancer diagnosis. Urology 2002;60:10–17.

40. Meyer A, Jung K, Lein M, et al. Factors influencing the ratio of free to total prostate-specific antigen in serum. Int J Cancer 1997;74:630–636.

41. Arcangeli CG, Smith DS, Ratliff TL, et al. Stability of serum total and free prostate specific antigen under varying storage intervals and temperatures. J Urol 1997;158:2182–2187.

42. Lynn NN, Collins GN, O'Reilly PH. Prostatic manipulation has a minimal effect on complexed prostate-specific antigen levels. BJU Int 2000;86:65–67.

43. Roehrborn CG, Boyle P, Gould AL, et al. Serum prostate-specific antigen as a predictor of prostate volume in men with benign prostatic hyperplasia. Urology 1999;53:581–589.

44. Linton HJ, Marks LS, Millar LS, et al. Benign prostate-specific antigen (BPSA) in serum is increased in benign prostate disease. Clin Chem 2003;49:253–259.

45. Canto EI, Singh H, Shariat SF, et al. Comparison of %fPSA, %BPSA, [-2]pPSA/fPSA, and [-2]pPSA/BPSA for prostate cancer detection in men with total serum PSA concentrations between 4 and 10 ng/nl. 99th Annual Meeting of the American Urological Association, San Francisco, CA, 2004.

46. Catalona WJ, Bartsch G, Rittenhouse HG, et al. Serum pro prostate specific antigen improves cancer detection compared to free and complexed prostate specific antigen in men with prostate specific antigen 2 to 4 ng/ml. J Urol 2003;170:2181–2185.

47. Mikolajczyk SD, Catalona WJ, Evans CL, et al. Proenzyme forms of prostate-specific antigen in serum improve the detection of prostate cancer. Clin Chem 2004;50:1017–1025.

48. Sokoll LJ, Chan DW, Mikolajczyk SD, et al. Proenzyme PSA for the early detection of prostate cancer in the 2.5–4.0 ng/ml total psa range: preliminary analysis. Urology 2003;61:274–276.

49. Khan MA, Sokoll LJ, Chan DW, et al. Clinical utility of proPSA and "benign" PSA when percent free PSA is less than 15%. Urology 2004;64:1160–1164.

50. Shariat SF, Mikolajczyk SD, Singh H, et al. Preoperative serum levels of pro-PSA isoforms are associated with biologically aggressive prostate cancer. 98th Annual Meeting of the American Urological Association, San Francisco, CA, 2003.

51. Catalona WJ, Bartsch G, Rittenhouse HG, et al. Serum pro-prostate specific antigen preferentially detects aggressive prostate cancers in men with 2 to 4 ng/ml prostate specific antigen. J Urol 2004;171:2239–2244.

Radiographic anatomy of the prostate 47

Uday Patel, Hywel Evans

INTRODUCTION

Knowledge of the anatomy of the gland is essential for the understanding of the various pathologies of the gland, and aids understanding of the surgical approaches to prostate surgery. This chapter explores the gross and radiological anatomy of the gland, how it can be evaluated using the various currently available imaging modalities, and how this knowledge may assist surgical understanding and planning.

GROSS ANATOMY OF THE PROSTATE

The prostate is a gland situated between the bladder base and the pelvic floor. In shape it approximates to an inverted cone, with the base situated superiorly. The apex of the gland is paradoxically its most inferior portion adjacent to the external urethral sphincter. Dimensions of the unenlarged gland are 3 cm in height, 2.5 cm in depth, and 4 cm in width; and its volume is less than 25 ml or the size of a walnut. Beyond the age of 40 years, the gland tends to enlarge with the onset of benign prostatic hyperplasia.

SURFACE RELATIONS OF THE PROSTATE

The gland is described as having anterior, posterior, and inferolateral surfaces. Anteriorly lies the symphysis pubis, particularly over the lower portion of the gland. The posterior relations are the rectum with the seminal vesicles situated superiorly, behind the bladder neck. The reminder of the superior relation is the bladder neck.

Along its lateral surface lie the pelvic sidewalls and levator ani muscles. Of all these relations, the key structures are the neurovascular bundles, which contain the arteries and neural supply of the gland (Figure 47.1). Some of these neural fibers also supply the corpora cavernosa of the penis. They are located posterolaterally and are vulnerable during surgical dissection. Further surgical, and radiological, landmarks are the bladder neck, the external sphincter and the dorsal vein complex that overlies the apex of the gland. The urinary sphincters (i.e., the bladder neck and the external sphincter) fuse with the prostate gland and, during surgical dissection, damage to either or both may lead to incontinence. However, all these areas are also points of "prostate weakness" and pathways for local infiltration by prostate cancer. The surgeon needs added vigilance when the fasciae in these regions are being dissected during prostatectomy.

PERIPROSTATIC FASCIA

The prostate is surrounded by three layers of fascia. Denonvilliers' fascia is a fused layer of connective tissue situated posterior to the prostate, separating it from the rectum. It is formed from the fusion of the inferior elements of the rectovesical pouch. At the apex of the gland, this layer thins before terminating at the urethral sphincter. At its cranial extreme, posterior to the base of the prostate and the seminal vesicles, it is more substantial. Over the anterior surface, the prostatic fascia lies superficial to the prostatic venous plexus (of Santorini), with the dorsal vein of the penis anterior to the fascia. As it passes posterolaterally, it fuses with the third fascial layer, the levator fascia, to form the lateral pelvic fascia. The levator fascia lies against the pelvic

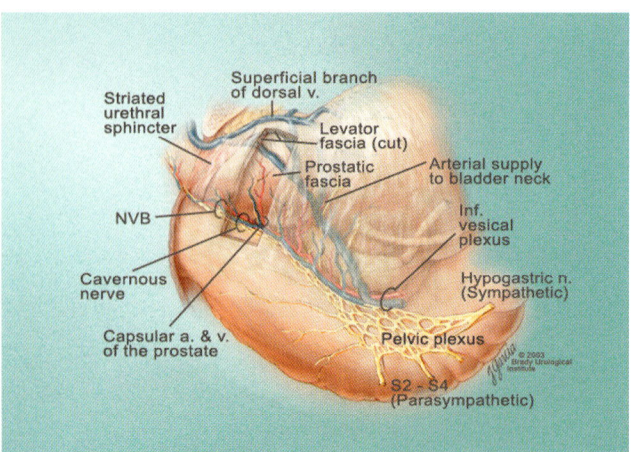

Fig. 47.1

This diagram illustrates the surface relations of the prostate. Of particular importance to the surgeon are the neurovascular bundles and prostatic venous plexus, and their relationship to the periprostatic fascial layers. The neurovascular bundles lie between the levator fascia and prostatic fascia. (NVB, neurovascular bundle.) (By courtesy of Patrick Walsh.)

floor, covering the levator ani muscles. The neurovascular bundles lie between the prostatic and levator fascia (see Figure 47.1).

PROSTATIC CAPSULE

The prostate does not have a true fibro-elastic capsule, but the surrounding 2 to 3 mm of stromal tissue is seen as a distinct boundary on imaging, it can be identified pathologically and is termed the prostatic capsule.[1] This capsule thins towards the apex, where it ceases to exist, making extracapsular spread more likely at the apex.[2] Further areas of capsular weakness are around the base of the gland, where the ejaculatory ducts pierce it, and those points along the posterolateral margins perforated by the neural and vascular supplies.

LOBAR AND ZONAL ANATOMY OF THE GLAND

In the early part of the twentieth century, the lobar anatomy of the gland was described, based on dissections along natural planes.[3] Five lobes were described—the anterior, middle, posterior, and two lateral lobes. The anterior lobe is a small area of the gland anterior to the urethra. The middle lobe refers to the region of the prostate between the ejaculatory ducts and the proximal urethra. The remaining gland at the back and to the sides represents the posterior and lateral lobes. In reality, clear anatomic distinction between zones is rarely demonstrated, and the lobar model has now fallen into disuse. Currently, the widely accepted description is the model of zonal anatomy, as described

by McNeal.[4,5] This description has useful correlates in imaging and in distribution of pathology in the gland. Under the zonal model, the prostate is described as having three glandular zones. These are the peripheral, central, transition (fibromuscular stroma) zones (Figure 47.2).

The peripheral zone (PZ) accounts for most of the glandular tissue in the young adult (about 70%). It lies behind the urethra and is bulkier around the base. Its lateral margins project substantially in an anterior direction, such that this zone is seen to "cup" the gland on imaging or gross pathology. These "cups" are termed the posterolateral margins or the anterior horns; tumor is more common in these horns. It is also a site of frequent extracapsular spread and positive surgical margins, as it lies adjacent to the neurovascular bundles. The prostatic ducts drain into the distal urethra, either side of the verumontanum of the urethra. The second largest glandular portion is the central zone (CZ), representing about 25% of the gland and lying anterior to the PZ. The ejaculatory ducts lie in the CZ. The transition zones (TZ) are two glandular areas adjacent to the urethra. The TZ accounts for less than 5% of the gland in the absence of benign prostatic hyperplasia (BPH). Histologically, the zones demonstrate subtle microscopic differences and McNeal proposed that the CZ may be of Woolfian duct origin as it displays similarity to the seminal vesicle epithelium; and that the rest of the gland originates from the urogenital sinus. A final histologic component of the gland is fibromuscular stroma that lies anterior to the urethra below the level of the verumontanum.

As well as being histologically distinct, the value of the zonal model is that it correlates with the common prostate pathologies. For as yet unknown reasons, cancer most commonly originates in the PZ, while BPH is principally a disease of the TZ and the periurethral glands. Furthermore, all these zones are readily demonstrated on imaging, most clearly by transrectal ultrasound (TRUS) and magnetic resonance imaging (MRI) as further explained below.

PROSTATIC BLOOD SUPPLY

The main arterial supply to the prostate arises from the inferior vesical artery, a branch of the anterior division of the internal iliac artery. The seminal vesicle is also supplied by branches of the inferior vesical artery. The supply is grouped into capsular and urethral branches.[6] The capsular branches are located in the lateral pelvic fascia posterolateral to the bladder. The capsular branches provide the blood supply to the outer prostatic tissue. The urethral branches of the inferior vesical artery enter the prostate posterolaterally at the junction of the bladder and prostate. The central portion of the gland receives the majority of its blood via this route.

A

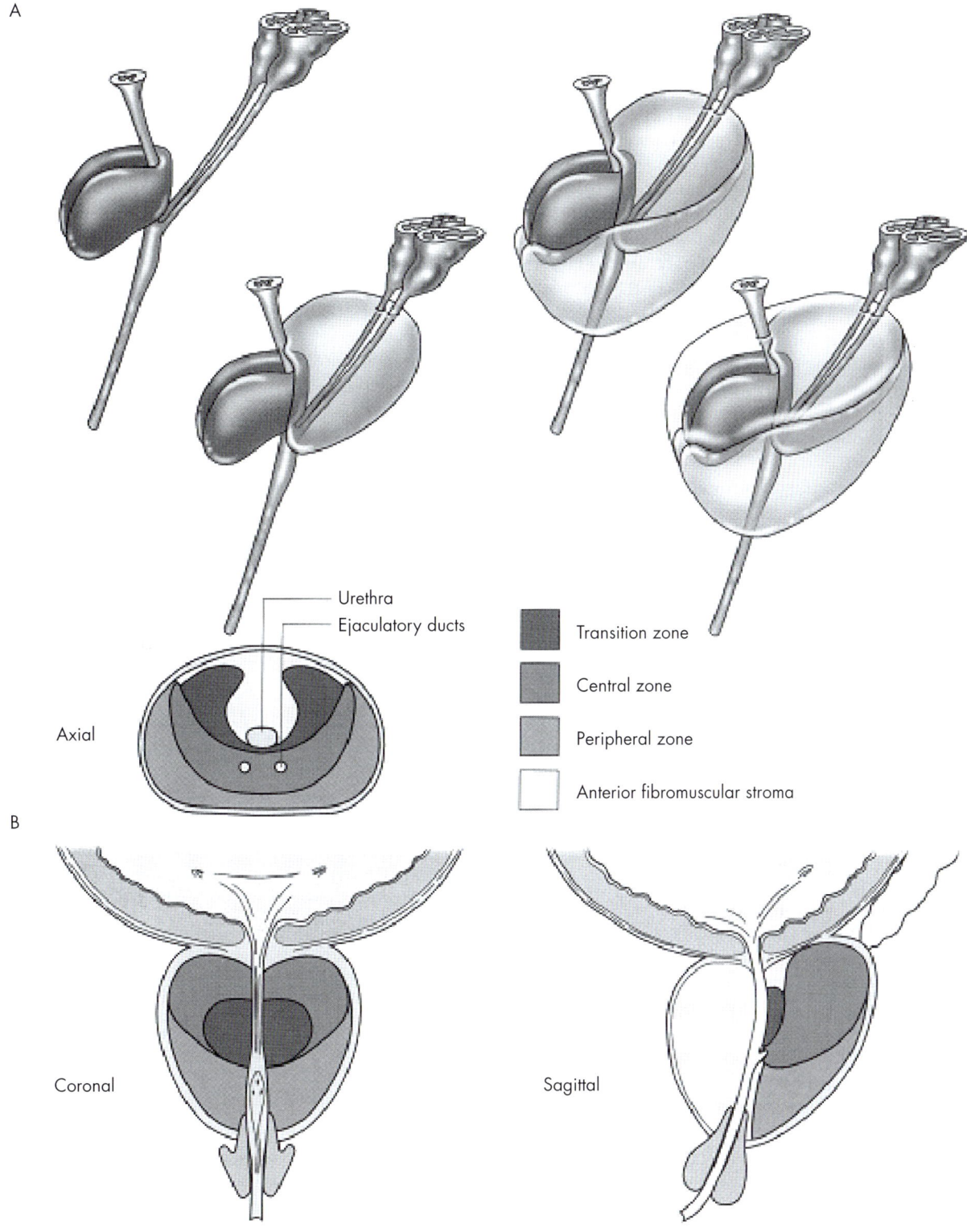

Urethra
Ejaculatory ducts

Transition zone

Central zone

Peripheral zone

Anterior fibromuscular stroma

Axial

B

Coronal

Sagittal

Fig. 47.2
The zonal model for prostate anatomy is now used in preference to the lobar descriptions often still encountered in anatomy texts. As the common pathologies largely tend to follow zonal patterns of distribution, the advantage of this model is clear. Prostate carcinoma is most frequently seen in the peripheral zone, which is seen to cup the remainder of the gland. The transition zone accounts for approximately 5% of gland volume in the normal gland. It is the principle site affected by benign prostatic hyperplasia and is, therefore, often far larger than this.

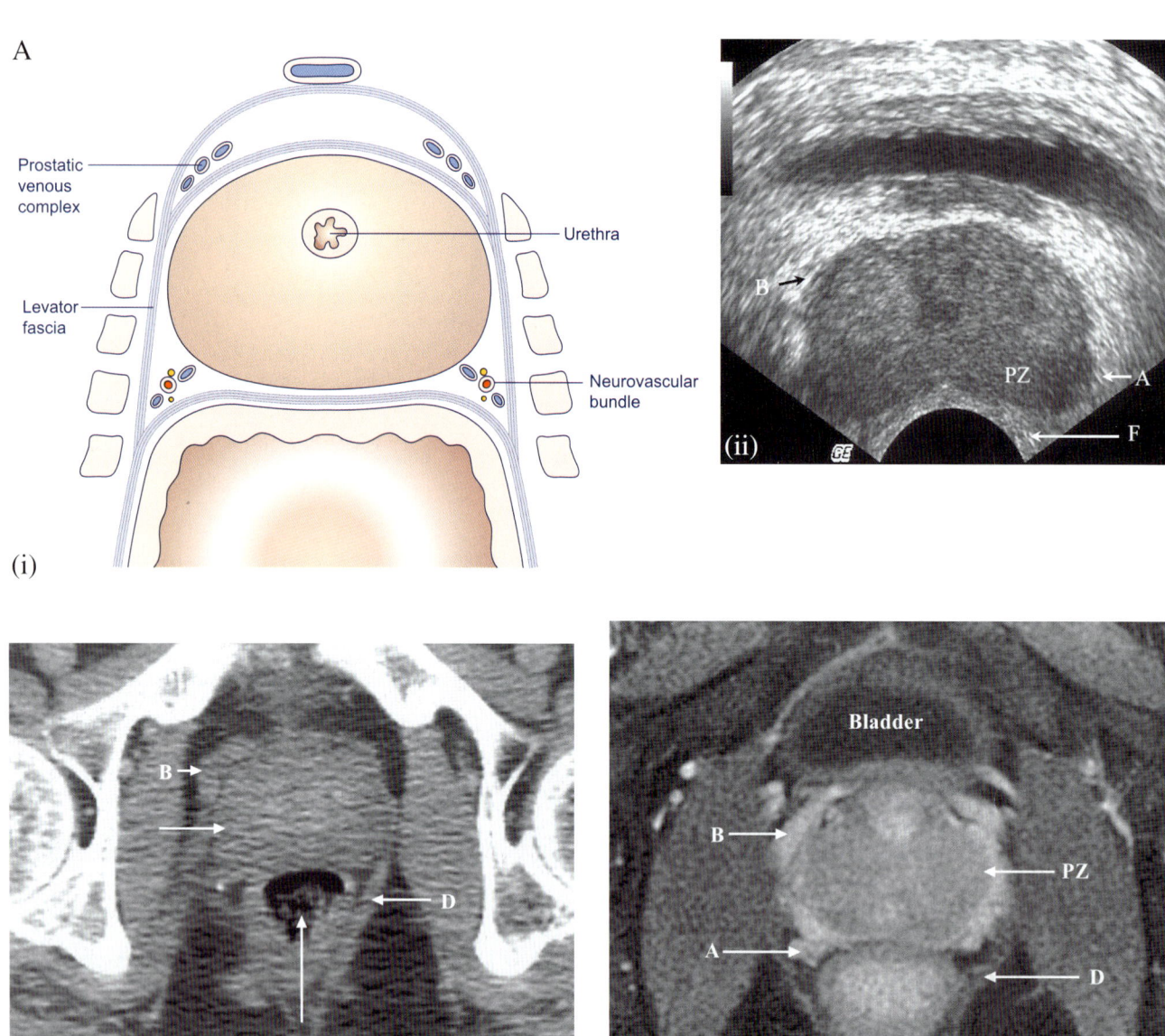

Fig. 47.3a–c

The above images are comparisons of the images obtained in the axial plane using transrectal ultrasound (TRUS) *(ii)*, computed tomography (CT) *(iii)*, and magnetic resonance imaging (MRI) *(iv)*, alongside a schematic diagram *(i)* of the axial plane at the base (A), midzone (B), and apex (C) of the prostate. The peripheral zone is well demonstrated with both TRUS and MRI, but is less easily appreciated with CT. For either open or laparoscopic prostatectomy, two of the key surgical landmarks are the neurovascular bundles and the deep and superficial venous plexi, and these structures are both well demonstrated using MRI, with TRUS also useful in this regard. CT poorly demonstrates the local periprostatic anatomy. (A, neurovascular bundles; B, prostatic venous plexus; C, prostatic fascia; D, levator ani; E, seminal vesicles; F, rectum; G, obturator internus; PZ, peripheral zone.) (Figure 47.3b(i) and 47.3c(i) by courtesy of Patrick Walsh.)

Venous drainage occurs via the venous plexus of Santorini. The surgical relevance of the venous plexus and the venous drainage of the penis is elegantly described by Walsh et al,[6,7] and their surgical control is an important step during prostatectomy, reducing the perioperative blood loss. The venous drainage of the penis, via the dorsal vein, comes into close contact with the prostate as it penetrates the urogenital diaphragm and divides into three main branches. The superficial branch lies anterior to the prostate and bladder neck. Here it sits between the puboprostatic ligaments (condensations of the visceral pelvic fascia) and is superficial to the prostatic fascia. The right and left lateral branches (or the deep veins) pass in a posterolateral direction, deep to the prostatic fascia. All of the major branches interconnect with adjacent venous complexes, particularly the lateral plexuses (with the internal pudendal vein, obturator and pelvic

B

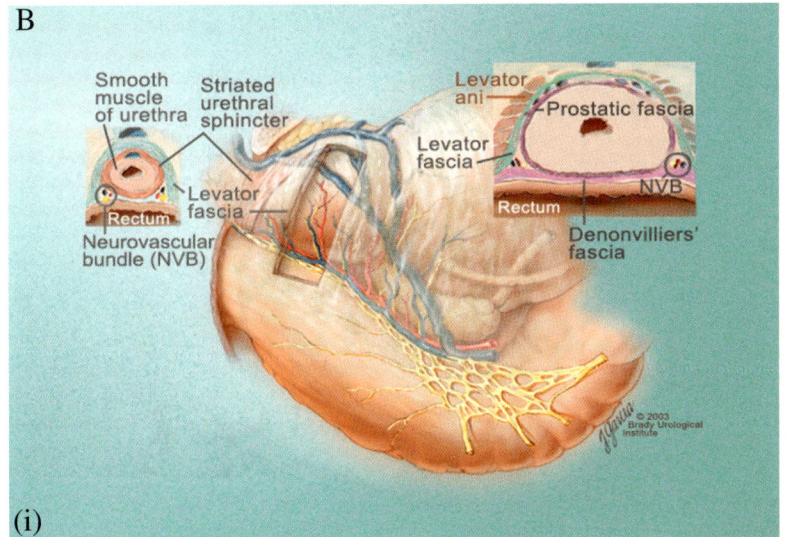

(i)

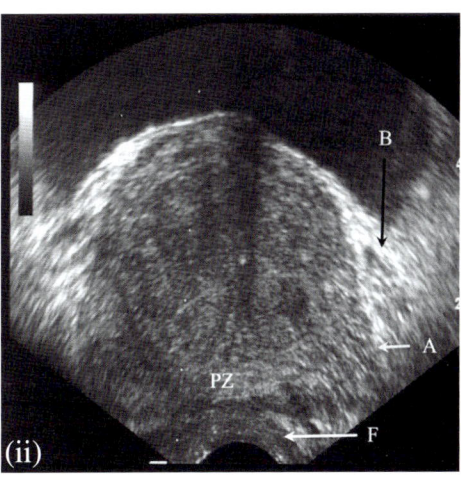

(ii)

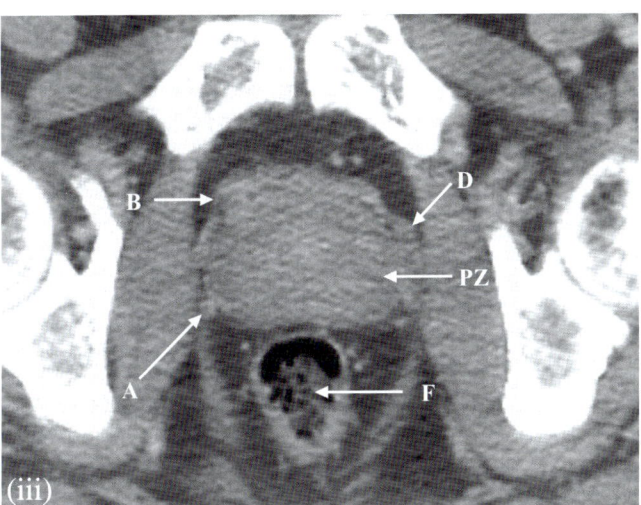

(iii)

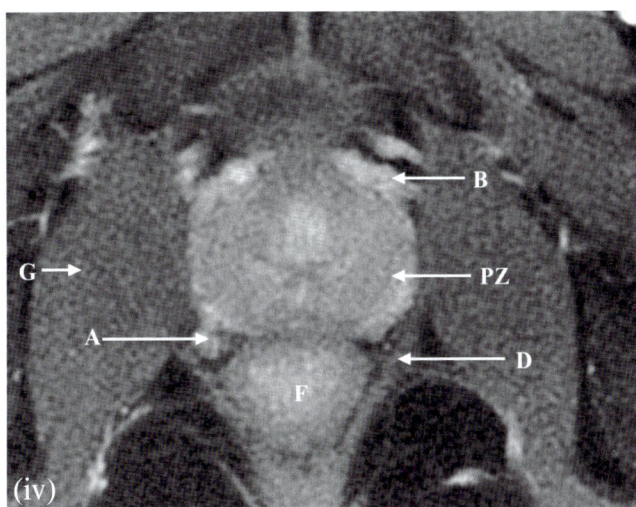

(iv)

Fig. 47.3b
(See caption 47.3a)

plexuses). Ultimately, drainage is via the inferior vesical vein and the iliac system.

PROSTATIC NERVE SUPPLY

From an imaging perspective as well as a surgical one, the vascular bundles act as a landmark for identifying the plexus of nerves running in the neurovascular bundle, as the nerve fibers are not large enough for macroscopic resolution. The nerves originate from the pelvic plexus and contain fibers from the inferior hypogastric plexus and parasympathetic fibers from the pelvic splanchnic nerves (S2, 3, and 4). The sympathetic fibers arise from the sacral sympathetic trunks after the latter have passed over the pelvic brim to lie medial to the sacral exit foramina. The visceral branches from these sacral ganglia mix with the parasympathetic fibers of the hypogastric plexus, which arise from the second, third, and fourth sacral

roots. The resulting plexus runs along the pelvic sidewall, and at the level of the prostate is situated within the lateral pelvic fascia, superficial to the prostatic fascia, and intimately related to the vascular bundles.

The branches of the plexus supplying the prostate only pierce the fascia of Denonvilliers and prostatic fascia at the site of entry into the gland. The branches of the pelvic plexus supplying the corpora cavernosa, and responsible for penile erection, also lie in the lateral pelvic fascia. They enter the penis by piercing the urogenital diaphragm.[7,8]

PROSTATIC LYMPHATIC DRAINAGE

Prostatic lymphatics drain into the periprostatic subcapsular network. From this network, the lymphatics drain to the internal iliac, external iliac and obturator chains.

C

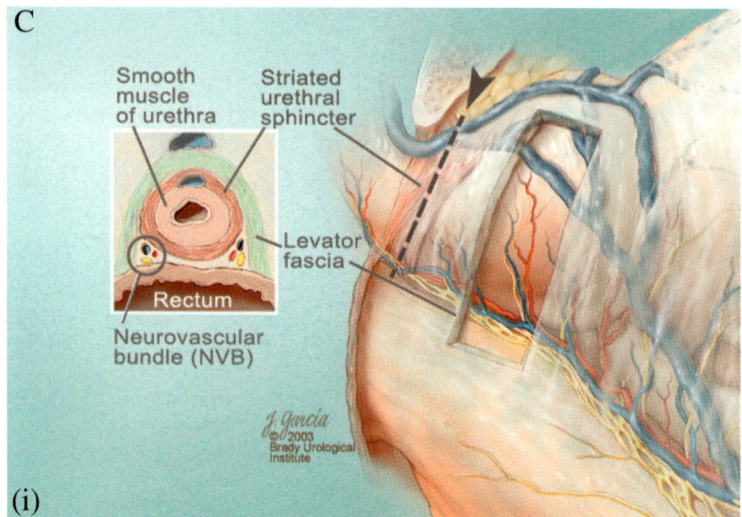

(i)

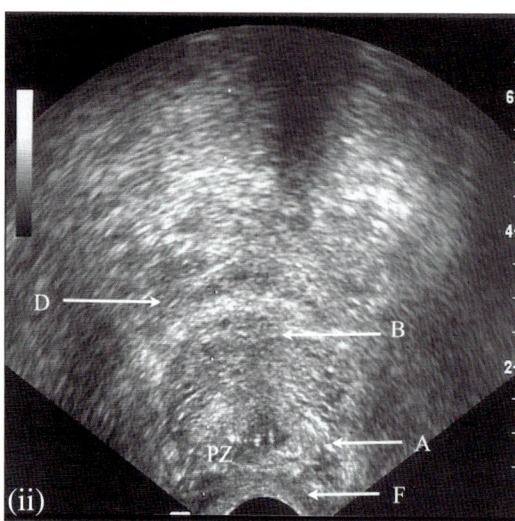

(ii)

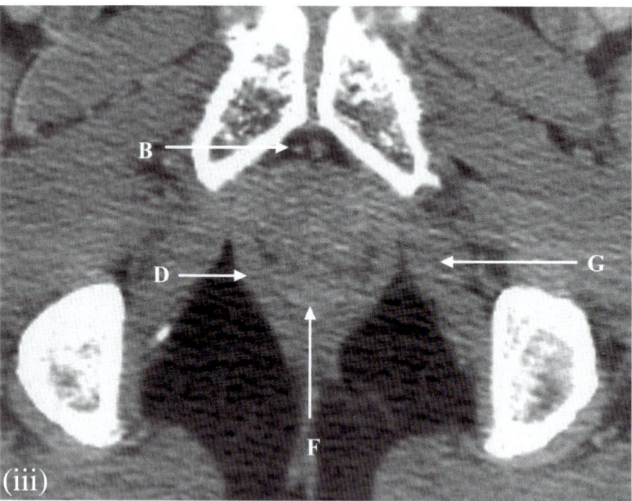

(iii)

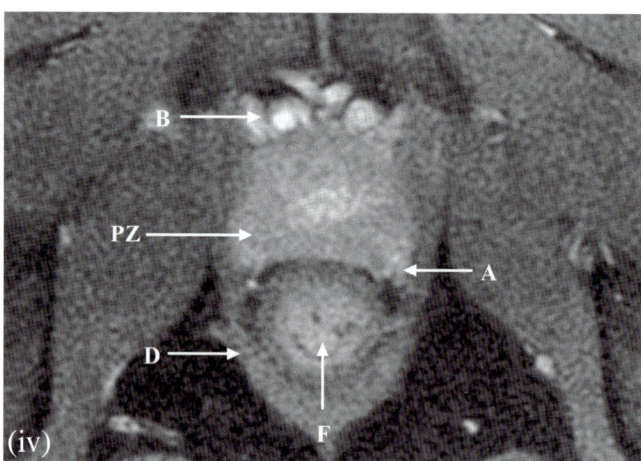

(iv)

Fig. 47.3c
(See caption 47.3a)

ACCESSORY OR PARAPROSTATIC STRUCTURES

The seminal vesicles, ejaculatory ducts and the urethral sphincters are important paraprostatic structures as all have a bearing on local cancer staging and surgery. The seminal vesicles are positioned against the posterior wall of the bladder, above the prostate. The thicker upper portion of Denonvilliers' fascia is a direct posterior relation, the ureter passing superomedial to the seminal vesicles and the neurovascular bundles lie in the groove between the prostate and vesicle. Blood supply to the vesicles is from branches of the middle rectal and vesical arteries. Medial to each vesicle lies the ampulla of the ductus deferens (or vas deferens). It approaches the prostate from the obturator fascia, after crossing the obturator vessels and nerve. The ampullae of the seminal vesicles fuse with the ampullae of the vasa to form the ejaculatory ducts that puncture the base of the gland, traverse through the central zone and empty into the verumontanum. This point is a pathway for local tumor extension into the seminal vesicles.

Urinary continence is dependent on the bladder neck sphincter and external urethral sphincter. The bladder neck has smooth muscle fibers contiguous with those of the prostate and seminal vesicles (the bladder neck is sometimes termed the internal sphincter), and the external sphincter is composed of striated muscle. This muscle is of slow twitch type, to enable tonic contraction and hence the striated external sphincter provides voluntary control of continence. Its preservation is of prime concern during prostatic surgery. It has a thin upper end that extends above the urogenital diaphragm, surrounding the distal prostatic urethra. The lower portion of the sphincter sits within the deep perineal pouch and is more bulbous in shape. A proportion of these fibers arise from the pubic rami and behave as a sling, passing posterior to the membranous urethra and inserting back onto the pubic rami. Some fibers insert posteriorly on the perineal body and a proportion encircle the urethra. Careful dissection of the external sphincter allows a continent bladder neck–urethral anastomosis.

RADIOLOGICAL ANATOMY OF THE PROSTATE GLAND

An unexpected bonus of the detailed imaging now possible of the prostate gland is that the zonal divisions described by McNeal are clearly resolvable. In particular the peripheral zone is seen as hyperechoic structure on TRUS and is of high signal on T2-weighted MRI. On computed tomography (CT), it is also often identifiable after contrast enhancement. Unfortunately, the remainder of the zones are not seen as clearly separate structures with current imaging; and on imaging the non-PZ glandular portions are sometimes collectively termed the inner gland, with the PZ being the outer gland. However, the reminder of the prostatic anatomy is better visualized on imaging with the urethra, neurovascular bundles, and seminal vesicles seen as separate and distinct (Figure 47.3).

All these modalities are useful for presurgical staging of prostate cancer, though with limitations. These items are covered more thoroughly elsewhere, but, briefly, the key points are asymmetry of anatomy and imaging "signal." The specificity of both TRUS and MRI is limited by the similar imaging characteristics of several benign disorders and post-biopsy appearances when compared with prostatic tumors, but on TRUS, tumors are seen as hypoechoic areas, although most tumors in contemporary practice are sonographically invisible. When seen, local extension may be identified as irregularity of the prostate capsule or periprostatic fat planes, neurovascular or seminal vesicle enlargement or hypoechogenicity. Ultrasound (TRUS) features suggestive of extracapsular disease in addition to obvious tumor spread include distortion of normal contour and capsular irregularity. Figures of up to 86% sensitivity and 94% specificity have been attributed to TRUS evaluation of local spread.[9] Reported sensitivity for seminal vesicle involvement ranges from 20% to 92%, and specificity 65% to 100%.[10]

On MRI, tumor is more consistently visualized. Appearance can vary depending on the magnet, but the majority of tumors will return lower signal on T2-weighted sequences compared with the surrounding normal, intermediate signal peripheral zone (Figure 47.4). Magnetic resonance imaging has been reported to have 92% sensitivity for tumor detection in the PZ. Sensitivity in the TZ is less due to the normally heterogeneous signal returned from benign prostatic hyperplasia.[11-13] Capsular involvement most commonly occurs adjacent to the neurovascular bundles at the site of neural perforation of the capsule, at the posterolateral aspect of the prostate.[14] Smooth or irregular bulging of the prostate, focal capsular thickening or retraction, asymmetry or direct involvement of the neurovascular bundles, and loss of definition of the rectoprostatic angle are all taken to represent signs of extracapsular

extension.[15] Magnetic resonance imaging is reported to have sensitivity and specificity of 21% to 63% and 85% to 97%, respectively for involvement of the seminal vesicles.[16-18] Involvement of the seminal vesicles is suggested by inability to visualize the ejaculatory duct, and low signal in the seminal vesicles on T2-weighted sequences (Figure 47.5). Tumors involving the whole peripheral zone will be less obvious, as they do not have the intrinsic contrast of adjacent normal tissue. In comparison, CT has poor sensitivity and specificity for assessment of local disease staging and extracapsular spread.[19]

SURGICAL LANDMARKS ON IMAGING

The central goal of curative surgical treatment for prostate cancer is total removal of the prostate gland (usually with the seminal vesicles), with preservation of urinary continence and erectile function. To achieve this, the gland should be removed with generous margins, as far as possible, around the expected pathways of local

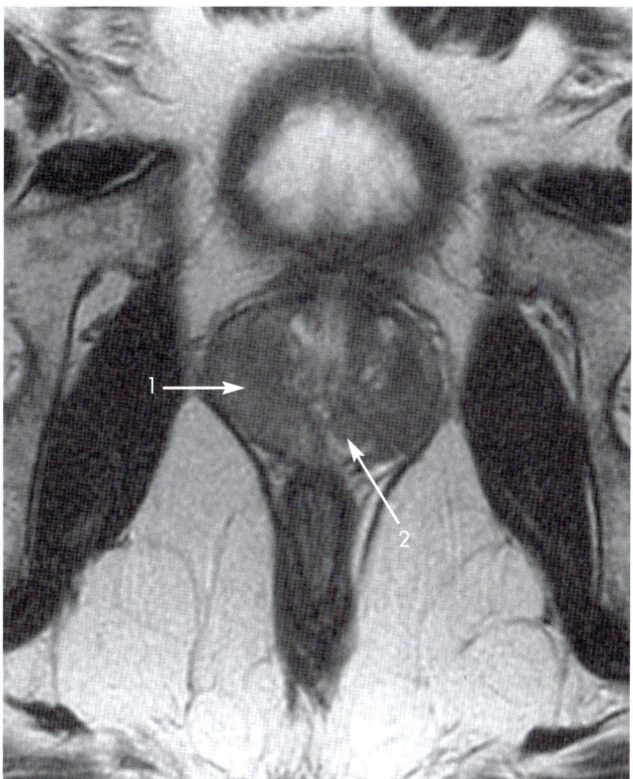

Fig. 47.4

This is a T2-weighted axial magnetic resonance image through the prostate showing extensive infiltration of the peripheral zone with low signal tumour *(1)*, leaving only a small region of normal relatively high-signal peripheral zone *(2)* posteriorly. The identification of pathology in the peripheral zone relies largely on the contrast between normal and abnormal tissue. This image illustrates the potential difficulty in identifying tumour if the gland is diffusely involved.

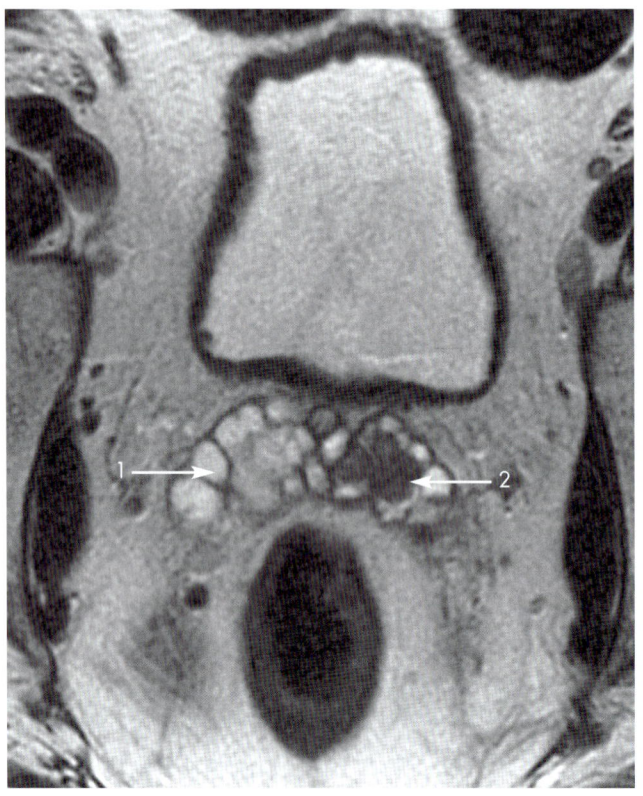

Fig. 47.5
This T2-weighted axial magnetic resonance imaging (MRI) scan through the seminal vesicles shows the contrast between normal high-signal *(1)* and infiltrated low-signal *(2)* seminal vesicle. MRI demonstrates involvement of the seminal vesicles more clearly than the other imaging modalities, although transrectal ultrasonography (TRUS) also has an important role.

cancer spread and with conservation of the neurovascular bundles and the external urethral sphincter. The areas where positive surgical margins are more likely are the apex, the posterolateral aspects, and the base of the gland. Surgical technique is associated with location of positive margins: with retropubic prostatectomy positive apical margins are more frequent, with laparoscopic surgery positive posterolateral margins, and with perineal prostatectomy positive basilar margins.

The figures illustrate correlations between the radiological anatomy and surgical landmarks that are crucial to these various operative approaches to the prostate gland.

REFERENCES

1. Jager G, Barentsz J. Prostate Cancer. In: Husband JES, Reznek RH (eds): Imaging in Oncology. London: ISIS Medical Media. 1998. pp 239–257.
2. Ayala GA, Ro JY, Babaian R, et al. The prostatic capsule: does it exist? Am J Surg Pathol 1989;13:21–27.
3. Lowsley OS. The development of the human prostate gland with reference to the development other structures at eh neck of the urinary bladder. Am J Anat 1912;13:299–349.
4. McNeal JE. Normal and pathologic anatomy of the prostate. Suppl Urol 1981;XVII:11–16.
5. McNeal JE. The prostate and prostatic urethra: a morphologic synthesis. J Urol 1972;107:1008–1016.
6. Walsh PC, Retic AB, Vaughan ED, et al. Anatomic radical retropubic prostatectomy. In: Campbell's Urology, 8th ed. Philidelphia: W B Saunders, 2002, pp 3109–3129.
7. Walsh PC. Anatomic radical retropubic prostatectomy: evolution of the surgical technique. J Urol 1990;160:2418–2424.
8. Lepor H, Gregerman M, Crosby R, et al. Precise localization of the autonomic nerves from the pelvic plexus to the corpora cavernosa: A detailed anatomical study of the adult male pelvis. J Urol 1985;133:207–212.
9. Salo JO, Kivisaari L, Ranniko S, et al. CT and transrectal ultrasound in the assessment of local extension of prostate cancer before radical retropubic prostatectomy. J Urol 1987;137:435–438.
10. Melchior SW, Brawer MK. Role of transrectal ultrasound and prostate biopsy. J Clin Ultrasound 1996;24:463–471.
11. Biondetti PR, Lee JKT, Ling D, et al. Clinical stage B prostate carcinoma: staging with MR imaging. Radiology 1987;162:325–329.
12. Bezzi M, Kressel HY, Allen KS, et al. Prostate carcinoma staging with MR imaging at 1.5 T. Radiology 1988;169:339–346.
13. Ling D, Lee JK, Heiken JP, et al. Prostatic carcinoma and benign prostatic hyperplasia: Inability of MR to distinguish between the two diseases. Radiology 1986;158:103–107.
14. McNeal JE, Viller AA, Redwine EA, et al. Capsular penetration in prostate carcinoma. Significance for natural history and treatment. Am J Surg Radiol 1990;14:240–247.
15. Chang SD, Hricak H. Radiological evaluation of the urinary bladder, prostate and urethra. In: Grainger RG, Allison DJ, Adam A, et al (eds) Diagnostic radiology, 4th ed. London: Churchill Livingstone, 2001, pp 1637–1643.
16. Tempany CMC, Zhou X, Zerhouni EA, et al. Prostate cancer: Results of radiology diagnostic oncology group project comparison of three MR imaging techniques. Radiology 1994;192:47–54.
17. Chelsky MJ, Schnall MD, Pollack HM, et al. Use of endorectal surface coil magnetic resonance imaging for local staging of prostate cancer. J Urol 1993;150:391–395.
18. Quinn SF, Franzini DA, Demlow TA, et al. MR imaging of prostate cancer with an endorectal surface coil technique: correlation with whole mount specimens. Radiology 1994;190:323–327.
19. Engeler CE, Wasserman NF, Zhang G. Preoperative assessment of prostatic carcinoma by computed tomography: weaknesses and new perspectives. Urology 1990;40:346–350.

Transrectal and transperineal ultrasound-guided biopsy of the prostate

48

J Robert Ramey, Leonard G Gomella

INTRODUCTION

Historically, prostatic biopsies were performed under digital guidance for the evaluation of a palpable abnormality found on digital rectal examination (DRE). First described by Wantanabe, et al in 1968,[1] transrectal ultrasonography (TRUS) did not gain widespread clinical implementation until the mid-1980s.[2] Subsequently, the development of serum prostate-specific antigen (PSA) assays and the TRUS-guided sextant biopsy technique[3] have led to a dramatic increase in the number of prostate biopsy procedures performed annually. The American Cancer Society estimates 230,110 new cases of prostate cancer will be diagnosed in the US in 2004.[4] With most published biopsy series quoting TRUS cancer detection rates of 25% to 33%, approximately 800,000 men undergo prostate biopsy in the US annually.

INDICATIONS FOR PROSTATE BIOPSY

Prior to the implementation of serum PSA testing, DRE served as the main screening tool for prostate cancer detection. Normal prostatic tissue has a moderately firm texture and the normal gland should have a symmetrical, smooth contour on DRE. The presence of any focal nodules or contour abnormalities should prompt a biopsy as they may represent an underlying area of adenocarcinoma regardless of the PSA level.

The ability to detect prostate cancer in its earliest stages is dramatically improved by PSA-based prostate cancer screening. Catalona et al have shown that using PSA for prostate cancer screening improves the detection rate of organ-confined disease[5] with prostate biopsy most commonly performed with a PSA greater than 4.0 ng/mL. Using this cutoff, several studies show a positive predictive value (PPV) of 17% to 28%.[6–9] On the other hand, recently published data from the Prostate Cancer Prevention Trial (PCPT) suggests that the PSA cutoff for biopsy may instead need to be altered downward.[10] In the PCPT, 2950 men in the placebo arm had PSA concentrations that remained below 4.0 ng/mL, yet 15.2% of them were found to have prostate cancer at their mandated end of study biopsy. Roughly 15% of the cancers were Gleason grade 7 or higher tumors, suggesting many of them developed clinically significant disease. Based on this data and a study by Catalona's group that indicated higher rates or organ confined disease at radical prostatectomy in screened men in the 2.6 to 4 ng/mL PSA range, many urologists now offer biopsy to patients with PSA levels greater than 2.5 ng/mL.[11]

Age, symptom status, and varying PSA thresholds based on age and race are included in some recommendations for prostate biopsy.[12,13] While the entire area of screening for prostate cancer through the use of PSA remains controversial, Box 48.1 includes some of the currently utilized indications for prostate biopsy. It should be noted that controversy with respect to the absolute PSA value to consider biopsy remains problematic. The trend at present is to consider lowering the threshold for an "abnormal" PSA in men under 60 years to 2.5 to 3.0 ng/mL[5,13] While the "normal" PSA level in older men is set slightly higher (i.e., in a 70 year old 5.5 to 6.5 ng/mL); this recommendation is not universally accepted.[12,13]

Refinements in PSA testing may be useful to guide prostate biopsy. Several studies have shown that in the presence of prostate cancer, the serum ratio of free PSA (fPSA) to total PSA (tPSA) becomes reduced compared with men without prostate cancer.[13–16] In patients with a PSA between 4.0 and 10.0 ng/mL a %fPSA cutoff of 25% has been shown to detect 95% of cancers while eliminating 20% of unnecessary biopsies. Further, the risk of prostate cancer increases as the %fPSA declines.[17] In most settings, free to total PSA is most commonly used to guide repeat prostate biopsy decisions. Prostate-specific antigen velocity changes (an increase of more than 0.75 to 1.0 ng/mL/year, regardless of initial PSA) are often associated with prostate cancer and may prompt biopsy.[13]

Repeat biopsy is indicated in the subset of patients found to have high-grade prostatic intraepithelial neoplasia (HGPIN) or atypical small acinar proliferation (ASAP) on their initial biopsy specimens. High-grade prostatic intraepithelial neoplasia represents a premalignant lesion and carries a 23% to 35% risk of detecting prostate cancer on subsequent biopsy.[18–20] The natural history of ASAP is less certain than that of HGPIN, but if present on initial biopsy it too carries an increased risk of discovering cancer on subsequent biopsy.[21,22] Thus, current recommendations are to re-biopsy patients in 3 to 6 months, or possibly sooner, if either of these findings are present on initial biopsy regardless of subsequent PSA values.

Contraindications to prostate biopsy include recent or active acute prostatitis or other conditions that would result in significant morbidity for the procedure, such as uncorrected coagulopathy or colorectal diseases.

ULTRASONOGRAPHIC IMAGING MODALITIES

Transrectal ultrasonography of the prostate is most commonly performed using gray-scale mode. A transducer capable of transmitting in the frequency range of 6 to 10 MHz should be employed for optimal imaging of the prostate. Both side and end fire endorectal probes may be used. The scanning angle of the probe should approach 180° to allow simultaneous visualization of the entire prostate in both the transverse and sagittal plane.

The gray-scale evaluation of the prostate begins with measurement of the gland in both the transverse and sagittal plane. This allows the gland volume to be calculated using the formula for a prolate ellipse (volume = length × width × height × 0.52).[23] Following these measurements, the prostate should be systematically imaged from base to apex in the transverse plane, or from one lateral border to the other in the sagittal plane. During these scans, the peripheral zone should be carefully examined for focal areas of hypoechogenicity. All hypoechoic lesions (Figure 48.1) should be included in the biopsy specimen. Biopsy positive hypoechoic lesions visible on gray-scale ultrasonography have been shown to have a higher Gleason grade[24] and are less likely to be organ confined[25] than isoechoic tumors.

Unfortunately, only 60% to 70% of prostate tumors are identifiable as hypoechoic lesions on conventional gray-scale TRUS.[26] Prostate tumors have been recently shown to over-express the proangiogenic growth factors vascular endothelial growth factor (VEGF), epidermal growth factor (EGF), and basic fibroblast growth factor (bFGF),[27] all of which have been implicated in the process of malignant angioneogenesis.[28–30] The angioneogenic capabilities of prostate cancer have been confirmed by pathologic examinations of radical prostatectomy specimens, which demonstrate increased microvessel density within prostate tumors compared with surrounding benign tissue.[31]

Imaging of the blood flow within these aberrant tumor vessels on color and power Doppler imaging provides additional sonographic modalities for identifying prostate cancer. Halpern and Strup demonstrated that 17% (35 of 211) of prostate tumors could be prospectively identified as malignancies on Doppler imaging.[32] Ismail et al found that tumors with increased color Doppler signals at the time of TRUS biopsy were more likely to have a higher Gleason score, seminal vesical (SV) invasion, and extracapsular disease in the radical prostatectomy specimen than those

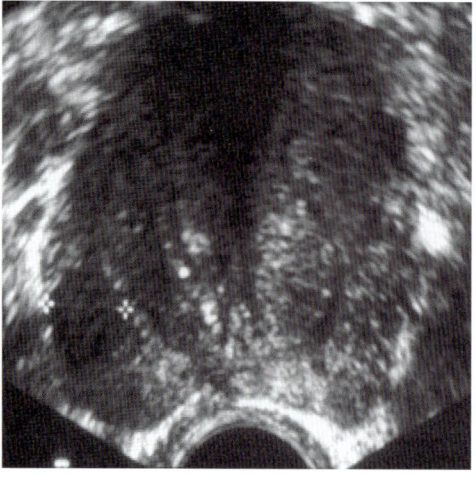

Fig. 48.1
Hypoechoic nodule visualized in the right base. Final pathology identified Gleason 3 + 4 adenocarcinoma of the prostate at this site.

tumors without noticeable Doppler flow.[33] More recent studies using color and power Doppler to target suspicious regions for biopsy have shown improved positive core rates versus sextant biopsy but have not succeeded in eliminating false negative results.[34–40] While considerable investigation remains to be conducted in this area, the neovascularity associated with prostate cancer appears to be a promising target for both its diagnosis and treatment.

ULTRASOUND-GUIDED BIOPSY TECHNIQUES

PREPARING THE PATIENT

As with any invasive procedure all anticoagulants (aspirin, nonsteroidal anti-inflammatory drugs [NSAIDs], herbal supplements) should be ceased 1 week prior to undergoing prostate biopsy. For patients on coumadin, do not perform biopsy until the INR is less than 1.5. The authors prefer to have patients self-administer a cleansing enema prior to presenting for biopsy. This decreases the amount of feces in the rectal vault, thereby producing a superior acoustic window for imaging the prostate; this, however, is not universally practiced. All patients receive antibiotic prophylaxis as this has been shown to decrease the risk of subsequent infection.[41] Typically an oral fluoroquinolone is given 30 to 60 minutes prior to the procedure and continued for 2 to 3 days post-biopsy. In patients at risk for endocarditis, intravenous antibiotics should be given preoperatively. Transrectal biopsies under gray-scale imaging may be performed with the patient in either dorsal lithotomy or lateral decubitus position.

ANALGESIA

Topical lidocaine jelly has been used with some success but may not provide optimal pain relief.[42] A local prostate

block is easily performed by injecting 5 mL of 2% lidocaine through a spinal needle (such as 7 inch 22 gauge) under ultrasound guidance using the needle biopsy guide. The anesthetic may be infiltrated along the entire length of the prostate. Our practice is to inject only at the level of the seminal vesicles near the bladder base. Local anesthesia for transperineal biopsies should include lidocaine infiltration of the skin and subcutaneous tissues of the perineum. Deeper tissues may be anesthetized under ultrasound-guided injection of local anesthetic along the anticipated biopsy needle tracts.

RANDOM SYSTEMATIC PROSTATE BIOPSY

Following the administration of local anesthesia and complete sonographic examination of the prostate, systematic biopsies of the peripheral zone may be taken, ensuring that any region of sonographic abnormality is included in the biopsy specimens. A spring loaded biopsy needle (typically 18 gauge) helps insure an adequate core sample has been taken with minimal discomfort. Fine needle aspiration is no longer commonly used in the diagnosis of prostate cancer. Since the introduction of the sextant biopsy protocol in 1989, several modifications and alternative strategies have been developed. Levine et al found that taking six additional biopsy cores improved cancer detection by 30%.[43] Additional studies have published improved cancer detection rates taking anywhere from 8 to 13 cores.[44–49] In a prospective study involving 483 consecutive patients, Presti et al addressed both increasing the biopsy number and altering its location. In this study, the technique involved lateral biopsies of the peripheral zone at the base and mid gland in addition to routine sextant biopsy regimen, for a total of 10 systematic cores. Patients with prostate volumes greater than 50 mL also underwent systematic sextant biopsies in the transition zone. Traditional sextant biopsy scheme missed about 20% of the cancers. The 10-core biopsy scheme detected 96% of the cancers by Presti et al and is shown in Figure 48.2 compared with other commonly used schemes.[46]

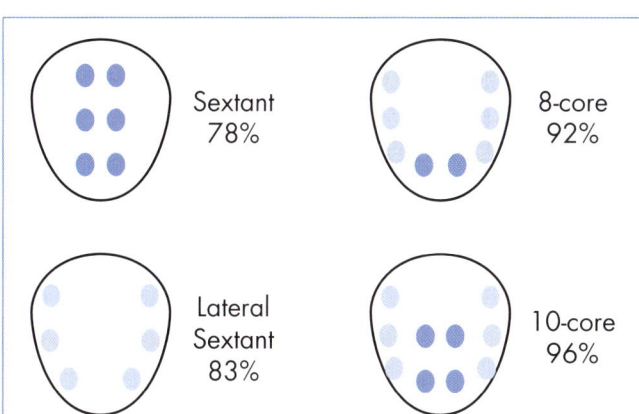

Fig. 48.2
Transrectal biopsy schemes compared relative to prostate cancer yield. Contemporary practice suggests at a minimum 8–10 cores should be performed with emphasis on the laterally directed cores. (After Presti et al references 44 and 46).

While the optimal number of cores to take from the peripheral zone remains an area of active investigation, it is generally agreed that biopsy from the transition zone and seminal vesicles is not routinely necessary as cores from these regions have been repeatedly shown to have low yields.[50,51] In patients with persistently elevated PSA levels and negative systematic biopsies, more extensive, "saturation" techniques have shown significantly improved cancer detection rates[52–54] compared with the declining returns seen with repetitive sextant biopsies.[55] These saturation biopsies often number greater than 20 to 30 samples and often require more extensive anesthesia (Figure 48.3). TUR biopsy is not longer commonly used on patients with repeat biopsy, but remains an option.

Transperineal biopsy must be performed with the patient in the dorsal lithotomy position. Once positioned, the perineum is shaved and prepared with a topical antiseptic solution and the biopsy is subsequently performed under sterile technique. This approach is generally reserved for patients that lack a rectum, as visualization of the prostate from the transrectal approach is markedly better than from the perineum. Using an end-fire ultrasound transducer, the prostate should be imaged in both the coronal and sagittal planes to calculate the gland volume.

From the transperineal vantage point, focal peripheral zone hypoechoic lesions are difficult to identify, as are the seminal vesicles. The urethra will appear as a hypoechoic midline structure and may be readily identified by following the corpus spongiosum proximally. Once the boundaries of the gland have been clearly identified in the coronal plane, six cores should be taken, three from either side of midline.

In a study by Vis et al, the diagnostic yield of TRUS was compared to that of the transperineal approach. In a simulation experiment (radical prostatectomy specimens with TRUS-detected prostate cancer), the transperineal (longitudinal) approach detected 82.5% of the cancers compared with 72.5% detected by the transrectal (transverse) approach. These investigators postulated that the transperineal procedure, in which the biopsy needle enters the prostate at the apex in the longitudinal direction, may more efficiently sample the peripheral zone. However, since this was an ex-vivo study design, caution should be observed in extrapolating the results to patient settings.

COMPLICATIONS

Using appropriate patient screening and techniques, the complication rates of contemporary TRUS-guided prostate biopsy are acceptable and usually minor. Major complications are rare, with complications from a large contemporary series summarized in Box 48.2.[57]

FUTURE DIRECTIONS FOR PROSTATE CANCER IMAGING

Given that patients with positive Doppler flow at the time of TRUS biopsy appear to be at a 10-fold increased risk of PSA recurrence following radical prostatectomy,[40] improved detection of flow within tumors may allow more accurate assessment of a given tumor's malignant potential. The microvessels associated with prostate tumors range in diameter from 10 to 50 μm; this is below the resolution limits of conventional color Doppler imaging. Contrast-enhanced (CE) TRUS utilizes microbubble contrast agents to amplify Doppler

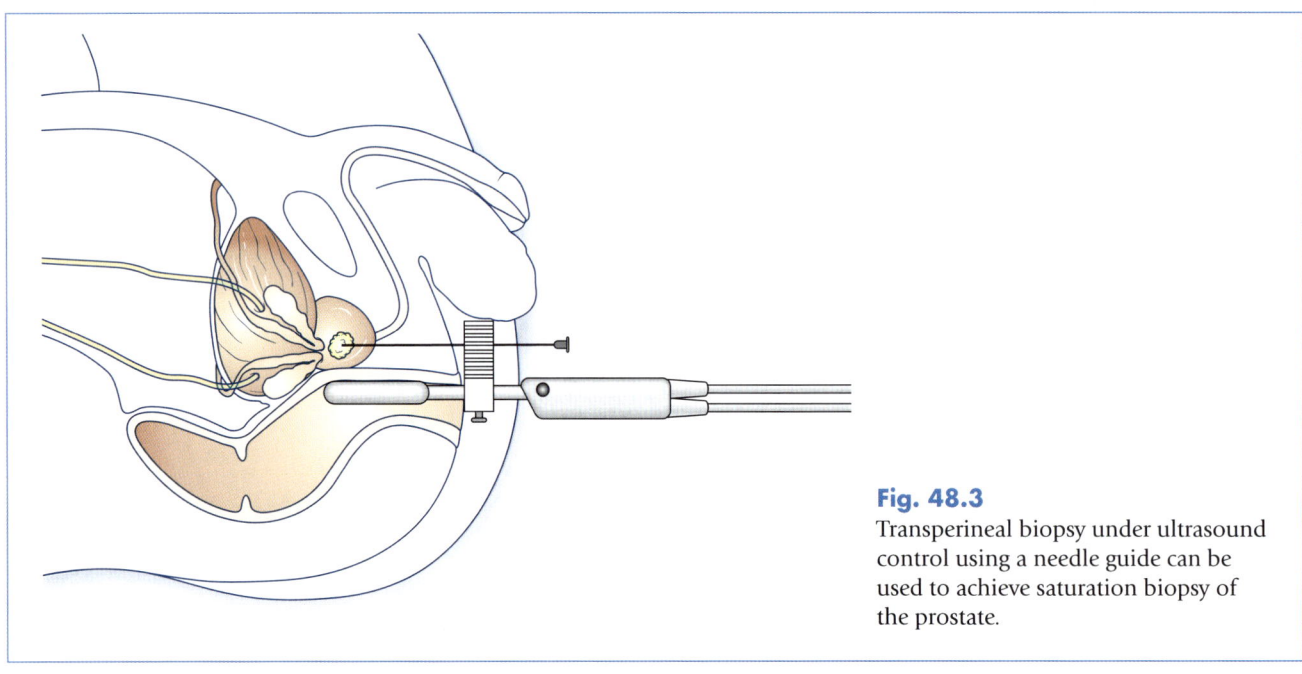

Fig. 48.3
Transperineal biopsy under ultrasound control using a needle guide can be used to achieve saturation biopsy of the prostate.

signals within these microvascular beds to selectively image prostate tumors. Using CE-TRUS, Frauscher et al were able to show an increase in the sensitivity of color and power Doppler imaging from 37% to 53% without significantly altering specificity.[58] Subsequent studies by our group and others have found significantly improved positive core rates using CE-TRUS to target biopsies.[59–62] Thus, CE-TRUS and other functional imaging studies may offer not only improved cancer detection rates but also aid in determining the appropriate treatment for individual patients. Prostate biopsies directed by MRI remain an investigational tool as well.

REFERENCES

1. Wantanabe H, Kato H, Kato T, et al. Diagnostic application of the ultrasonotomography for the prostate. Jpn J Urol 1968;59:273–279.
2. Terris MK. Ultrasonography and biopsy of the prostate. In Walsh PC, Retik AB, Vaughan ED, Wein AJ (eds): Campbell's Urology, 8th ed. Philadelphia: Saunders, 2002, pp 3038–3054.
3. Hodge KK, McNeal JE, Terris MK, et al. Random systematic versus directed ultrasound guided transrectal core biopsies of the prostate. J Urol 1989;142:71–75.
4. Jemal A, Tiwari RC, Murray T, et al. Cancer statistics, 2004. CA Cancer J Clin 2004;54:8–29.
5. Catalona WJ, Smith DS, Ratliff TL, et al. Detection of organ-confined prostate cancer is increased through prostate specific antigen-based screening. JAMA 1993;270:948–954.
6. Brawer MK, Chetner MP, Beatie J, et al. Screening for prostatic carcinoma with prostate specific antigen. J Urol 1992;147:841–841.
7. Bretton PR, Prostate-specific antigen and digital rectal examination in screening for prostate cancer: a community-based study. South Med J 1994;87:720–723.
8. Catalona WJ, Richie JP, Ahmann FR, et al. Comparison of digital rectal examination and serum prostate specific antigen in the early detection of prostate cancer: results of a multicenter clinical trial of 6630 men. J Urol 1994;151:1283-1290.
9. Coley CM, Barry MJ, Fleming C, et al. Early detection of prostate cancer. Ann Intern Med 1997;126:394–406.
10. Thompson IM, Pauler DK, Goodman PJ, et al. Prevalence of prostate cancer among men with a prostate-specific antigen level < 4.0 ng per milliliter. N Engl J Med 2004;350:2239–2246.
11. Krumholtz JS, Carvalhal GF, Ramos CG, et al. Prostate-specific antigen cutoff of 2.6 ng/mL for prostate cancer screening is associated with favorable pathologic tumor features. Urology 2002;60:469–473; discussion 473–474.
12. American Urological Association: Prostate-specific antigen (PSA) best practice policy. Oncology 2000;14:267.
13. Derweesh IH, Rabets JC, Patel A, Jones JS, Zippe C. Prostate biopsy: evolving indications and techniques. Contemp Urol 2004;16:28–44.
14. Leinonen J, Lovgren T, Vornanen T, et al. Double-label time-resolved imunofluorometric assay of prostate-specific antigen and of its complex with alpha-1-antichymotrypsin. Clin Chem 1993;39:2098–2103.
15. Lilja H. Significance of different molecular forms of serum PSA; the free, non-complexed form of PSA versus that complexed to alpha-1-antichymotrypsin. Urol Clin North Am 1993;681–686.
16. Stenman UH, Hakama M, Knekt P, et al. Serum concentrations of prostate specific antigen and its complex with alpha-1-antichymotrypsin before diagnosis of prostate cancer. Lancet 1994;344:1594–1598.
17. Catalona WJ, Partin AW, Slawin KM, et al. Use of the percentage of free prostate-specific antigen to enhance differentiation of prostate cancer from benign prostatic disease: a prospective multicenter clinical trial. JAMA 1998;279:1542–1547.
18. Davidson D, Bostwick D, Qian J, et al. Prostatic intraepithelial neoplasia is a risk factor for adenocarcinoma: predictive accuracy in needle biopsies. J Urol 1995;154:1295–1299.
19. O'Dowd GJ, Miller MC, Orozco R, et al. Repeat biopsy cancer incidence rates following a negative, high grade prostatic intraepithelial neoplasia, or suspicious diagnosis. J Urol 1999;161:73.
20. Kronz JD, Allan CH, Shaikh AA, et al. Predicting cancer following a diagnosis of high grade prostatic intraepithelial neoplasia on needle biopsy: data on men with more than one follow-up biopsy. Am J Surg Pathol 2001;25:1079–1085.
21. Iczkowski KA, Bassler TJ, Schwob VS, et al. Diagnosis of "suspicious for malignancy" in prostate biopsies: predictive value for cancer. Urology 1998;51:749–757.
22. Ouyang RC, Kenwright DN, Nacey JN, et al B. The presence of atypical small acinar proliferation in prostate needle biopsy is predictive of carcinoma on subsequent biopsy. BJU Int 2001;87:70–74.
23. Halpern EJ, Gray-scale evaluation of prostate cancer. In Halpern EJ, Cochlin DL, Goldberg BB (eds): Imaging of the Prostate. London: Martin Dunitz, 2002. pp 27–38.
24. Cornud F, Hamida K, Flam T, et al. Endorectal color Doppler sonography and endorectal MR imaging features of nonpalpable prostate cancer: correlation with radical prostatectomy findings. AJR Am J Roentgenol 2000;175:1161–1168.
25. Ohori M, Wheeler TM, Scardino PT. The New American Joint Committee on Cancer and International Union Against Cancer TNM classification of prostate cancer. Clinicopathologic correlations. Cancer 1994;74:104–114.
26. Purohit RS, Shinohara K, Meng MV, et al. Imaging clinically localized prostate cancer. Urol Clin North Am 2003;30:279–293.
27. Trojan L, Thomas D, Knoll T, et al. Expression of pro-angiogenic growth factors VEGF, EGF, and bFGF and their topographical relation to neovascularization in prostate cancer. Urol Res 2004;32:97–103.
28. Chodak GW, Haudenschild C, Gittes RF, et al. Angiogenic activity as a marker of neoplastic and preneoplastic lesions of the human bladder. Ann Surg 1980;192:762–771.
29. Sillman F, Boyce J, Fruchter R. The significance of atypical vessels and neovascularization in cervical neoplasia. Am J Obstet Gynecol 1981;139:154–159.
30. Wiedner N, Carroll PR, Flax J, et al. Tumor angiogenesis correlates with metastasis in invasive prostate carcinoma. Am J Pathol 1993;142:401–409.
31. Bigler SA, Deering RE, Brawer MK. Comparison of microscopic vascularity in benign and malignant prostate tissue. Hum Pathol 1993;24:220–226.
32. Halpern EJ, Strup SE. Using gray-scale and color and power Doppler sonography to detect prostatic cancer. AJR Am J Roentgenol 2000;174:623–627.
33. Kelly IMG, Lees WR, Rickards D. Prostate cancer and the role of color Doppler US. Radiology 1993;189:153–156.

34. Okihara K, Kojuma M, Nakanouchi T, et al. Transrectal power Doppler imaging in the detection of prostate cancer. BJU Int 2000;85:1053–1057.

35. Newman JS, Bree RL, Rubin JM. Prostate cancer: diagnosis with color Doppler sonography with histologic correlation of each biopsy site. Radiology 1995;195:86–90.

36. Rifkin MD, Sudakoff GS, Alexander AA. Prostate: techniques, results, and potential applications of color Doppler US scanning. Radiology 1993;186:509–513.

37. Shigeno K, Igawa H, Shiina H, et al. The role of colour Doppler ultrasonography in detecting prostate cancer. BJU Int 2000;86:229–233.

38. Sakarya ME, Arslan H, Unal O, et al. The role of power Doppler ultrasonography in the diagnosis of prostate cancer: a preliminary study. Br J Urol 1998;82:386–388.

39. Halpern EJ, Frauscher F, Strup SE, et al. Prostate: high-frequency Doppler US imaging for cancer detection. Radiology 2002;225:71–77.

40. Ismail M, Petersen RO, Alexander AA, et al. Color Doppler imaging in predicting the biologic behavior of prostate cancer: correlation with disease-free survival. Urology 1997;50:906–912.

41. Aron M, Rajeev TP, Gupta NP. Antibiotic prophylaxis for transrectal needle biopsy of the prostate: a randomized controlled study. BJU Int 2000;85:682–685.

42. Obek C, Ozkan B, Tunc B, et al. Comparison of 3 different methods of anesthesia before transrectal prostate biopsy: a prospective randomized trial. J Urol 2004;172:502–505.

43. Levine MA, Ittman M, Melamed J, et al. Two consecutive sets of transrectal ultrasound guided sextant biopsies of the prostate for the detection of prostate cancer. J Urol 1998;159:471–476.

44. Presti JC, Chang JJ, Bhargava V, et al. The optimal systematic prostate biopsy scheme should include 8 rather than 6 biopsies: results of a prospective clinical trial, J Urol 2000;163:163–167.

45. Fink KG, Hutarew G, Pytel A, et al. One 10-core biopsy is superior to two sets of sextant prostate biopsies. BJU Int 2003;92:385–388.

46. Presti JC Jr, O'Dowd GJ, Miller MC, et al. Extended peripheral zone biopsy schemes increase cancer detection rates and minimize variance in prostate specific antigen and age related cancer rates: results of a community multi-practice study. J Urol 2003;169:125–129.

47. Brossner C, Bayer G, Madersbacher S, et al. Twelve prostate biopsies detect significant cancer volumes (>0.5 mL). BJU Int 2000;85:705–707.

48. Durkan GC, Sheikh N, Johnson P, et al. Improving prostate cancer detection with an extended-core transrectal ultrasonography-guided prostate biopsy protocol. BJU Int 2002;89:33–39.

49. Eskew LA, Bare RL, McCullough DL. Systematic 5 region prostate biopsy is superior to sextant method for diagnosing carcinoma of the prostate J Urol;157:199–203.

50. Lui PD, Terris MK, McNeal JE, et al. Indications for ultrasound guided transition zone biopsies in the detection of prostate cancer. J Urol 1995;153:1000–1003.

51. Terris MK, Pham TQ, Issa MM, et al. Routine transition zone and seminal vesicle biopsies in all patients undergoing transrectal ultrasound guided prostate biopsies are not indicated. J Urol 1997;157:204–206.

52. Stewart CS, Leibovich BC, Weaver AL, et al. Prostate cancer diagnosis using a saturation needle biopsy technique after previous negative sextant biopsies. J Urol 2001;166:86–92.

53. Fleshner N, Klotz L. Role of "saturation biopsy" in the detection of prostate cancer among difficult diagnostic cases. Urology 2002;60:93–97.

54. Borboroglu PG, Comer SW, Riffenburgh RH, et al. Extensive repeat transrectal ultrasound guided prostate biopsy in patients with previous benign sextant biopsies. J Urol 2000;163:158–162.

55. Keetch DW, Catalona WJ, Smith DS. Serial prostatic biopsies in men with persistently elevated serum prostate specific antigen values. J Urol 1994;151:1571–1574.

56. Vis AN, Boerma MO, Ciatto S, et al. Detection of prostate cancer: a comparative study of the diagnostic efficacy of sextant transrectal versus sextant transperineal biopsy. Urology 2000;56:617–621.

57. Djavan B, Waldert M, Zlotta A, et al. Safety and morbidity of first and repeat transrectal ultrasound guided prostate needle biopsies: results of a prospective European prostate cancer detection study. J Urol 2001;166:856–860.

58. Frauscher F, Klauser A, Halpern EJ, et al. Detection of prostate cancer with a microbubble ultrasound contrast agent. Lancet 2001;357:1849–1850.

59. Halpern EJ, Rosenberg M, Gomella LG. Prostate cancer: contrast-enhanced US for detection. Radiology 2001;219:219–225.

60. Halpern EJ, Frauscher F, Rosenberg M, et al. Directed biopsy during contrast-enhanced sonography of the prostate. AJR Am J Roentgenol 2002;178:915–919.

61. Roy C, Buy X, Lang H, et al. Contrast enhanced color Doppler endorectal sonography of the prostate: efficiency for detecting peripheral zone tumors and role for biopsy procedure. J Urol 2003;170:69–72.

Multivariate models for decreasing unnecessary biopsies for prostate cancer

49

Carsten Stephan, Henning Cammann, Klaus Jung, Stefan A Loening

INTRODUCTION

This review gives an overview of the use of prostate-specific antigen (PSA) and percent free PSA (%fPSA)-based artificial neural networks (ANNs) and logistic regression (LR) models to eliminate unnecessary prostate biopsies.

All available studies and ongoing studies have been included to summarize the recent scientific knowledge regarding the use of ANNs and LR models. Additionally, the questions of whether different total PSA (tPSA) and fPSA assays may influence the outcome of ANNs as well as new serum markers within ANNs have been analyzed using receiver operating characteristic (ROC) analysis and cutoff calculations at 95% specificity or sensitivity.

There is a clear advantage of including clinically available data like age, digital rectal examination (DRE) and transrectal ultrasonography (TRUS) variables like prostate volume, PSA density, or prostate transition zone volume as additional factors to tPSA and %fPSA within ANNs and LR models. There is also an impact of the tPSA and fPSA assay on the outcome of ANNs but only parallel measurement with different PSA assays may finally solve the question of whether a general ANN can be established for use with any PSA assay combination. New markers show additional value within ANNs but, to prove their clinical usefulness, further testing is necessary.

PROSTATE-SPECIFIC ANTIGEN: MOLECULAR FORMS AND INFLUENCING FACTORS

Prostate cancer (PCa) is the most common malignancy in the western world, and its detection is considerably enhanced by measurement of PSA.[1] Since PSA is mostly organ-specific but not cancer-specific, elevated PSA concentrations are also observed in benign prostate hyperplasia (BPH), prostatic intraepithelial neoplasia (PIN), acute or chronic prostatitis, and other nonmalignant prostatic diseases.[2] This leads to a high number of false-positive findings in up to 65% of prostate biopsies, thus demonstrating the inability of PSA alone to discriminate between PCa and benign diseases. Various methods like PSA density, PSA transition zone density, PSA velocity, and age- or race-specific reference ranges have been developed to reduce the false-negative and false-positive rates but could not always come up to the expectations.[1,3–5]

Especially in the 4 to 10 ng/mL PSA "gray zone," PSA alone cannot distinguish between PCa and BPH, because only approximately 25% to 30% of men with these PSA concentrations undergoing a biopsy do have cancer.[6] In addition, PSA values less than 4 ng/mL do not indicate the absence of PCa, because 20% to 30% of patients with PCa show PSA concentrations in this low range.[7] A large screening study with a final number of 2950 biopsied men, after 7 years follow-up with PSA concentrations below 4 ng/mL, had an increasing incidence of PCa with increasing PSA: 0 to 0.5, 0.6 to 1, 1.1 to 2, 2.1 to 3, and 3.1 to 4 ng/mL ranges with rates of 6.6%, 10.1%, 17%, 23.9%, 26.9%, respectively. Therefore, the PSA range 2 to 4 ng/mL is comparable to the 4 to 10 ng/mL range regarding PCa detection rates.

Measurements of the molecular forms of PSA have been shown to improve specificity over tPSA alone.[8,9] Using the ratio of fPSA to tPSA (×100, %fPSA) in the tPSA range of 4 to 10 ng/mL, approximately 20% to 25% of unnecessary biopsies can be avoided.[10–12] For tPSA values less than 4 ng/mL the use of %fPSA has also been reported to increase specificity.[13–15] Others described a limited use of %fPSA at this low tPSA concentrations, but a better PCa risk assessment[16] or increased prediction of tumor aggressiveness.[17]

Although prostate biopsy is required for the diagnosis of PCa, this invasive and expensive procedure should be avoided in men with a low probability of harboring PCa. The %fPSA has been proposed as a primary decision tool for first time biopsy in men with unsuspicious DRE within the tPSA range 4 to 10 ng/mL, as well as for lower tPSA values.[18,19] It is known that %fPSA and tPSA are also influenced by prostate volume[10,12,20–22] and age.[12,21,23]

Using the knowledge about these above-mentioned relationships between tPSA, %fPSA, age, and prostate volume, different multivariate LR models[24,25] and ANNs[26–30] including these or similar parameters have been introduced to improve cancer detection specificity.

This review gives an overview of the Medline-available studies using ANN or LR models for diagnosis of PCa. Other studies for staging or prognosis of PCa have been reviewed recently.[31]

Another way of using an ANN to avoid unnecessary biopsies is an analysis of TRUS images in an attempt to obtain existing subvisual information, other than the gray scale, from conventional TRUS to enhance the ability to diagnose prostate cancer.[32] The authors significantly reduced the number of false-positive results in the 381 benign cases to about 1%. In the 119 PCa patients the rate of false-negative was 21%.[32] However, the authors stated that prospective real-time studies are needed to validate this TRUS-ANN model, which have not been published so far.[32] Also biopsy technique was not addressed in this review since a minimum of sextant biopsy was performed in all studies and different settings (8- to 12-fold) may have more impact on the achieved detection rate than other factors.

ARTIFICIAL NEURAL NETWORKS AND LOGISTIC REGRESSION MODELS

In general, ANNs are able to model complex biologic systems by revealing relationships among the input data that cannot always be recognized by conventional analyses.[33] The basic principles of ANNs, the description of the multilayer perceptron (MLP) as one of the most common ANN models and the "back-propagation learning algorithm" are already described elsewhere.[31,34] In 1994, Snow et al[35] described a tPSA-based ANN for PCa diagnosis and prognosis with an accuracy of 87% and 90%, respectively. A tPSA-based ANN called "ProstAsureIndex" used tPSA, prostatic acid phosphatase, and creatine kinase to assess the risk of PCa and was used in the mid-1990s.[34]

After %fPSA became clinically available, Carlson et al[24] developed an LR model using patient age, tPSA, and %fPSA to assign a probability of prostate cancer. Data analysis on 3773 urologically referred patients, including 1234 PCa and 2539 histologically proven BPH patients with serum PSA values between 4 and 20 ng/mL yielded an 11% increase in specificity from 23% for %fPSA alone compared with 34% (LR) at 95% sensitivity (Table 49.1).[24] The authors concluded that PCa probability based on age, tPSA, and %fPSA is more effective than %fPSA alone in differentiating benign prostate disease from PCa.[24] Results from the DRE (suspect or not suspect) from 1746 patients (46%) revealed DRE as significant variable for the LR model, but combining DRE with others decreased the discriminatory power of the LR model.[24]

Virtanen et al[25] compared LR with MLP in 212 men (53 PCa and 159 non-PCa) with tPSA from 3 to 10 ng/mL taken from a screening population of 974 men using the input variables tPSA, fPSA, %fPSA, DRE, age, family history, and findings (suspicious or not) on TRUS. Logistic regression models performed better than MLP and %fPSA; DRE status and heredity were found to be independent predictors of PCa, whereas tPSA, fPSA, age, and findings on TRUS were not.[25] By using receiver operation characteristic (ROC) analysis the LR with the input parameters tPSA, %fPSA, and DRE status reached an area under the curve (AUC) of 0.81 for all patients (n = 241) with a tPSA greater than or equal to 3 ng/mL.[25] The authors argued the slightly better performance of LR compared with the ANN in a relatively small number of patients.

COMPARISON OF ARTIFICIAL NEURAL NETWORKS

In 2000, Finne et al[28] compared MLP and LR models using tPSA, %fPSA, DRE, and prostate volume in 656 men taken from the randomized prostate cancer screening study in Finland aged 55 to 67 years within the tPSA range of 4 to 10 ng/mL. The MLP and LR models were validated using the "leave-one-out" method. At the 95% sensitivity level, specificity levels for %fPSA, LR, and MLP were 19%, 24% and 33% (P < 0.001). Additionally, the accuracy of the MLP and LR models was significantly higher than that of %fPSA. This study shows that MLP and LR models based on tPSA, %fPSA, DRE, and prostate volume could reduce the number of unnecessary biopsies significantly better than %fPSA alone at tPSA levels from 4 to 10 ng/mL.[28] Age, within this relatively narrow range, and heredity were not useful diagnostic variables within the MLP. The most powerful predictors of the MLP were %fPSA followed by prostate volume, whereas DRE and tPSA had a lower impact on prediction of PCa.[28] This is only partially in concordance with the data obtained by Virtanen et al,[25] who found heredity and DRE to be independent predictors of PCa while age did not contribute much in both studies.[28]

Table 49.1 Comparison of artificial neural network (ANN) and logistic regression (LR) studies for diagnosis of prostate cancer

Author	Year	Screening	Model (ranking)	PSA assays (company)	tPSA range (ng/mL)	Contributing factors (if numbered, then by value)	AUC	Specificity at 95% sensitivity
Carlson	1998	no	LR	Tosoh (Dianon)	4–20	1. %fPSA; 2. age; 3. tPSA	n.a.	34 (LR) 23 (%fPSA)
Virtanen	1999	yes	1.LR 2. ANN (MLP)	ProStatus (Wallac)	3–10 (3–45)	1. %fPSA; 2. DRE; 3. heredity	0.81 (LR for tPSA 3–45) %fPSA n.a.	n.a.
Finne	2000	yes	1.MLP (LOO) 2.LR	ProStatus (Wallac)	4–10	1. %fPSA 2. volume; 3. DRE; 4. tPSA	n.a.	33 (MLP) 24 (LR) 19 (%fPSA)
Babaian	2000	yes	ANN	Tandem R (Beckman Coulter)	2.5–4	%fPSA, tPSA, age, PAP, CK	0.74 ANN (0.64 %fPSA)	51 (ANN) 39 (PSAD) 10 (%fPSA)
Horninger	2001	yes	ANN LR	Abbot IMX (Abbott)	n.a. PSA>4 or DRE+	age, tPSA, %fPSA, DRE, volume, PSAD, PSAD-TZ, TZ-volume	n.a.	~27 (ANN) ~13 (%fPSA) ~13 (tPSA)
Stephan	2002	no	ANN LR	IMMULITE (DPC)	2–20	1. DRE; 2. %fPSA; 3. volume; 4. tPSA; 5. age	0.86 (ANN) 0.75 (%fPSA)	43 (ANN) 26 (%fPSA)
Djavan	2002	no	1.ANN (MLP) 2.LR	AxSYM (Abbott)	2.5-4 4–10	1. PSAD-TZ; 2. %fPSA; 3. PSAD 4. volume (2.5–4) 1. %fPSA; 2. PSAD-TZ; 3. PSAV; 4. tPSA; 5. TZ-volume; 6. tPSA; 7. PSAD	0.876 (ANN) 0.75 (%fPSA) 0.913 (ANN) 0.81 (%fPSA)	59 (ANN)* 33 (%fPSA)* 67 (ANN) 40 (%fPSA)
Kalra	2003	yes	1.ANN 2.LR	Immuno 1 (Bayer)	n.a. PSA>4 or DRE+	age, ethnicity, heredity, IPSS, DRE, tPSA, cPSA	0.825 (ANN) 0.678 (tPSA) 0.697 (cPSA)	n.a.
Remzi	2003	no	ANN, LR	AxSYM (Abbott)	4–10	tPSA, %fPSA, volume, PSAD, PSAD-TZ, TZ-volume	0.83 (ANN) 0.79 (LR) 0.745 (%fPSA)	68 (ANN) 54 (LR) 33.5 (%fPSA)
Finne	2004	yes	1.LR 2.ANN (MLP)	ProStatus (Wallac)	4–10	1. DRE; 2. %fPSA; 3. volume; 4. tPSA	0.764 (LR) 0.760 (MLP) 0.718 (%fPSA)	22 (LR) 19 (MLP) 17 (%fPSA)
Garzotto	2004	no	LR	AxSYM (Abbott)	<10	PSAD, DRE, age, TRUS findings	0.73 (LR) 0.62 (tPSA)	n.a.

ANN, artificial neural network; AUC, area under receiver operating characteristic curve; DRE, digital rectal examination; fPSA, free PSA; LR, logistic regression; PSA; prostate-specific antigen; MLP, multilayer perceptron; PSAD, PSA density; %fPSA, percent free PSA; tPSA, total PSA; TRUS, transrectal ultrasound; TZ, transition zone; n.a. not available.

*Sensitivity at 95% specificity.

Babaian et al[26] developed a neural network algorithm named prostate cancer detection index (PCD-I) with tPSA, %fPSA, creatine kinase, prostatic acid phosphatase, and age as input variables and compared this with PSA density (ratio of PSA to prostate volume, PSAD), transition zone density (PSAD-TZ), and %fPSA. They tested this neural network combination of three different ANNs (impact of the respective parameters on final ANN result is not given) on 37 PCa and 114 non-PCa patients with a tPSA between 2.5 and 4 ng/mL. The AUC comparison did not show significant differences between the PCD-I (0.74), PSAD (0.74), PSAD-TZ (0.75) or %fPSA (0.64). However, at 95% sensitivity the PCD-I reached a specificity of 51% whereas PSA density and %fPSA had only specificities of 39% and 10%, respectively. Thus, the advantage of PCD-I compared with %fPSA was at high sensitivities between 95% and 90%, more than 40% increase in specificity. The authors stated, that despite the insignificant differences regarding the AUCs, the benefit of PCD-I is clinically significant.

To develop risk profiles, in 2001 Horninger et al[36] used multivariate LR analysis in 2054 men and an ANN in 3474 men who were part of the Tyrol PSA Screening Project and who had undergone prostate biopsy. At sensitivity levels of 90% to 95%, the ANN was 150% to 200% more specific than the standard cutoff points. For screened volunteers with tPSA levels below 4 ng/mL, ANN showed a lower cancer predictive ability than for volunteers with total PSA levels above 4 ng/mL.[36] As in all other studies at high sensitivity levels, ANN increased the specificity for prostate carcinoma detection in a PSA-based screened population.[36] Unfortunately, the impact of each of the eight input factors as well as the AUCs were not given.

In 2002, Djavan et al[27] published data on 272 (24% of them with PCa) and 974 (35% PCa) referred patients within the tPSA ranges 2.5 to 4 and 4 to 10 ng/mL. The authors developed two ANNs for these tPSA ranges with the input data tPSA, fPSA, %fPSA, PSA velocity (PSAV, which is PSA change within time, three measurements were performed within 12 months), age, DRE, and the 4 TRUS variables PSAD, PSAD-TZ, TZ-volume, and prostate volume. For the low tPSA range (2.5–4 ng/mL) the contributing variables for the ANN were, in order of importance, PSAD-TZ, %fPSA, PSAD, and prostate volume, whereas tPSA, age, DRE, PSAV, and TZ-volume did not contribute and were excluded from the final ANN.[27] For these low tPSA concentrations the authors had chosen a high specificity to avoid as many unnecessary biopsies as possible. Thus, at 95% specificity the sensitivity increased from 33% (%fPSA and LR) to 59% (ANN). The AUCs for the ANN (0.876) and LR (0.85) were comparable and both were significantly larger than the AUC for %fPSA (0.75).[27] The most contributing variables for the ANN model at tPSA 4 to 10 ng/mL were %fPSA, PSAD-TZ, PSAV, fPSA,

TZ-volume, tPSA, and PSAD, whereas age, DRE, and prostate volume were excluded.[27] At 95% sensitivity the specificity increased from 40% for %fPSA to 60% for LR and 67% for the ANN model and the AUCs increased from 0.81 for %fPSA to 0.90 and 0.913 for LR and ANN, respectively.[27]

Also in 2002, Stephan et al[30] published data on 859 urologically referred patients (65% with PCa) with tPSA concentrations from 2 to 20 ng/mL with available data for tPSA, fPSA, age, prostate volume, and DRE. The authors compared different ANN models with LR, %fPSA, and PSA and developed an easily accessible ANN program named "ProstataClass" which is downloadable or online usable at *www.charite.de/ch/uro* (Figure 49.1). Within the low tPSA range of 2 to 4 ng/mL, the authors also wanted to have a high specificity to avoid general biopsies in most presumably healthy men and at 90% specificity the sensitivity increased from 0% for tPSA to 7.5% for %fPSA, and to 28.3% for the ANN.[30] A significant increase was also achieved for the AUCs with values of 0.55, 0.70, and 0.84 for tPSA, %fPSA, and ANN, respectively.[30] The same behavior was seen for the tPSA ranges 4 to 10 and 10 to 20 ng/mL, where the AUCs as well as the specificities at 90% sensitivity significantly increased from tPSA to %fPSA and the ANN. There was no statistical difference in the outcome of both statistical approaches, both LR and ANN identifying approximately 80% of all patients correctly. This is in concordance with a comprehensive comparison between ANN and LR, where in the eight largest studies (out of 26) ANN and LR performed equal in seven cases.[37] The most contributing variables for the ANN models were DRE, followed by %fPSA and prostate volume, whereas tPSA and age had only small influence on the

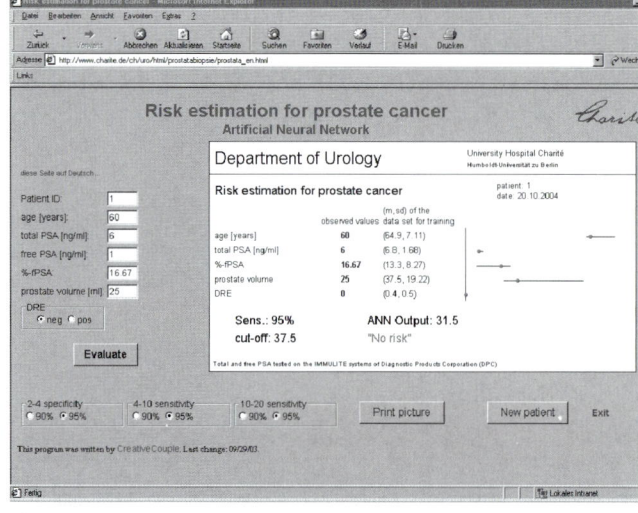

Fig. 49.1
Program "ProstataClass" window. Examples of the artificial neural network output indicating "no risk" at the 95% sensitivity level.

performance of the ANN.[30] This is in contrast to the study by Djavan et al[27] where DRE was excluded from both ANN models for tPSA 2.5 to 4 and 4 to 10 ng/mL and prostate volume was excluded in the 4 to 10 ng/mL tPSA range ANN model since these parameters did not contribute to the outcome of the ANN.

Stephan et al[38] initiated the first ANN multicenter study with six participating centers from three different countries on the basis of the above mentioned study.[30] All 1188 patients of this study were histologically confirmed, had a tPSA and fPSA measurement with the same assay (IMMULITE) and complete data for prostate volume, age, and DRE available. The authors confirmed their results with a significant improvement of %fPSA by using the ANN regarding AUC and at the cutoffs at 95% sensitivity (tPSA 4–10 and 10–20 ng/mL) and 95% specificity for the tPSA range 2 to 4 ng/mL (see Table 49.1). They recommended a first time biopsy within the tPSA range 2 to 4 ng/mL at a specificity of 95%, where the ANN increases sensitivity from 10% (%fPSA) to 65% (ANN).[38] For the tPSA range 4 to 10 ng/mL, a first time biopsy should be performed on the basis of a 95% sensitivity where specificity increases from 21% (%fPSA) to 41% by using the ANN.[38] At the tPSA range 10 to 20 ng/mL, the authors recommend using the ANN to indicate repeat biopsies on the basis of a 95% sensitivity.[38]

Remzi et al[39] focused in a study in 820 men taken from the Vienna-based multicenter European referral database for early PCa detection with a tPSA of 4 to 10 ng/mL on the prediction of the outcome of repeat prostate biopsies by using an advanced multilayer perceptron ANN. The input variables were, as in the study by Djavan et al,[27] age, tPSA, %fPSA, DRE status, PSA velocity, and the four TRUS variables prostate volume, PSAD, TZ-volume, and PSAD-TZ. The repeat biopsy PCa detection rate was 10% (n = 83). At 95% sensitivity, the specificity for the ANN was 68% compared with 54%, 33.5%, 21.4%, 14.7%, and 8.3% for LR, %fPSA, PSAD-TZ, PSAD, and tPSA, respectively. The AUC was 83% for the ANN versus 79%, 74.5%, 69.1%, 61.8%, and 60.5% for LR, %fPSA, PSAD-TZ, PSAD, and tPSA, respectively. Combining the individual clinical and biochemical markers into the ANN allows fore more accurate and individual counseling of patients with a negative initial biopsy.[39]

Also in 2003, Kalra et al[29] published data on 348 patients (unknown tPSA range and unknown amount of PCa detected) with prostate biopsy due to abnormal DRE or tPSA greater than 4 ng/mL. By using the input factors tPSA, complexed PSA (Immuno 1, Bayer) age, DRE, ethnicity, family history, and the International Prostate Symptom Score (IPSS), but not %fPSA, they achieved an AUC of 0.825 for their ANN model named "neUROn."[29] This was significantly larger than for complexed PSA (AUC: 0.697) and tPSA (0.678). All seven input factors of which at least six were always available, contributed significantly to the ANN model

(no ranking given).[29] However, this is in contrast to most of the other cited studies, since age and also tPSA usually had a lower impact on the ANN outcome.

Garzotto et al[40] performed a LR analysis in 1237 referred men with tPSA levels less than 10 ng/mL and a prostate biopsy. Variables analyzed were age, race, family history, referral indication(s), prior vasectomy, DRE, tPSA, PSAD, and TRUS findings, but not %fPSA.[40] Independent predictors of a positive biopsy result included elevated PSAD, abnormal DRE, hypoechoic TRUS finding, and age 75 years or older.[40] The AUC for the LR model was 0.73, which was significantly higher than the prediction based on tPSA alone (0.62). The application of this model to the biopsy decision could result in a 24% reduction in unnecessary biopsy procedures.[40] Stephan et al[41] recommended to the authors to include also %fPSA to further improve the outcome of the LR model. However, Garzotto et al[41] replied that PSAD as the strongest PCa predictor in their model has been shown in other studies to perform equal to %fPSA.

In 2004, Finne et al[42] investigated in a total of 1775 consecutive men aged 55 to 67 years taken from the European Randomized Study of Screening for Prostate Cancer (ERSCP) with a serum tPSA of 4 to 10 ng/mL whether multivariate algorithms like LR or a MLP neural network with Bayesian regularization (BR-MLP) can outperform %fPSA at 95% sensitivity. With the input variables tPSA, %fPSA, age, DRE, and prostate volume, the authors simulated a prospective setting by dividing the data set into one set for training and validation (67%, n = 1183) and one test set (33%, n = 592). At a fixed sensitivity of 95% in the test set, the LR model eliminated significantly more false-positive PSA results (22%) than %fPSA alone (17%), whereas the BR-MLP model did not (19%) (P = 0.178). The AUC was larger for the LR model (0.764, P = 0.030) and the BR-MLP model (0.760, P = 0.049) than for the %fPSA (0.718). The authors concluded that multivariate algorithms should be used in screening populations to reduce unnecessary prostate biopsies more effectively than with %fPSA alone.[42] A practical program can be used at *www.finne.info* (Figure 49.2) to estimate the risk of PCa and to decide on the necessity of a prostate biopsy. Different from the data of the Finnish arm of the ERSCP obtained also by Finne et al,[28] where %fPSA and prostate volume were the most powerful predictors of PCa, this study demonstrated DRE and %fPSA to be the strongest predictors of PCa.[42]

EFFECT OF DIFFERENT COMMERCIAL ASSAYS ON ARTIFICIAL NEURAL NETWORK MODELS

Practical experience within the last 8 to 10 years confirmed that the results from different commercial tPSA and fPSA

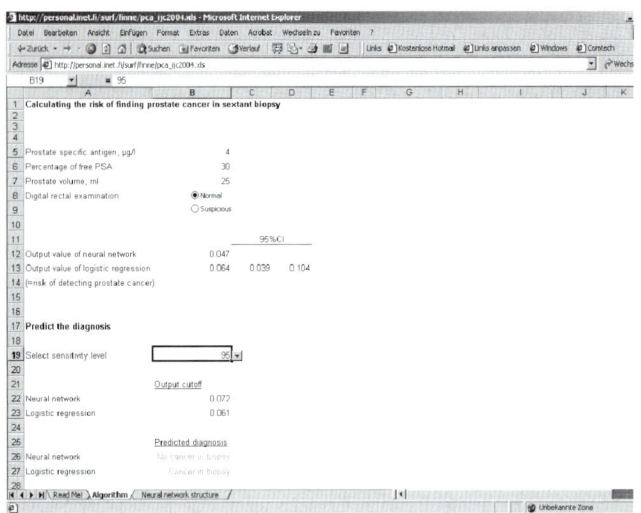

Fig. 49.2

The program at www.finne.info to estimate the risk of prostate cancer based on artificial neural network and logistic regression model at the 95% sensitivity level.

tests can vary widely.[43,44] It has been published that the use of different tPSA and fPSA assays does have an impact on the number of recommended prostate biopsies and consequently detected PCa.[45] Another recent study in 2304 screened men who underwent tPSA and fPSA measurement with two or three (when PSA was >2.5 ng/mL) different assays (Bayer, Beckman, DPC) confirmed that if assays with consistently lower tPSA values (Bayer and DPC) were used about 19% of all patients with tPSA concentrations greater than 2.5 ng/mL and a nonsuspicious DRE would not meet the criteria for a biopsy, whereas the tPSA by using the Beckman assay was greater than 4 ng/mL, indicating a biopsy.[46]

These data and the fact that the ANN studies by the different working groups used five different tPSA and fPSA assays (see Table 49.1) raise the question of whether different assays influence the outcome of the ANN models. So far, only Stephan et al[47] has addressed this topic. For 4480 patients from five different centers (two provided screening data) with five different tPSA and fPSA assays and available data on age, prostate volume, and DRE of all patients, the outcome of an IMMULITE tPSA and fPSA-based ANN (iANN) was compared with newly tPSA adapted neural networks (nANNs). Within the three different tPSA ranges 2 to 4, 4 to 10, and 2 to 10 ng/mL, the iANN reached significance compared with %fPSA in 11 of 15 comparisons of the AUC and in 6 of 15 comparisons of specificities at 95% sensitivity. This demonstrated, with some limitations, a general advantage of the externally tested iANN compared with %fPSA, regardless of the assay used. However, the new ANN models, which were internally trained and validated with the data of the respective patient cohort, showed a further advantage in all 15 AUC comparisons and in 12 of 15 comparisons at 95% sensitivity compared with %fPSA. Furthermore, the

comparison of both ANNs revealed a significant advantage in 12 of 15 and in 14 of 15 comparisons regarding the AUC and at 95% sensitivity for the respective tPSA specific nANNs compared with iANN. It seems to be necessary to separately create ANNs for each population and each different tPSA and fPSA assay. However, to exclude the factor of different populations, only parallel measurements of different tPSA and fPSA assays in one large study group and the subsequent comparison of nANNs to the iANN can solve the problem, whether different tPSA assay adapted ANNs or one (some) general ANN(s) are necessary. This conclusion is even more important, since tPSA alone will obviously not be used as clinical decision point in the future[48] and the single use of %fPSA for biopsy decision also gives contrary results regarding a specificity improvement compared with tPSA especially at lower tPSA concentration (<4 ng/mL).

NEW SERUM MARKERS WITHIN ARTIFICIAL NEURAL NETWORKS

Human glandular kallikrein 2 (hK2), another member of the human kallikrein family with the highest homology to PSA with about 80% identity at the amino acid and DNA level, has been reported to have additional value, especially for early detection of PCa. This has been reviewed recently.[49] It has been shown that the ratio of hK2 to free PSA as well as the combination of %fPSA and hK2/fPSA within the PSA ranges 2 to 4 and 4 to 10 ng/mL enhances the discrimination between PCa and BPH patients.[50] Other studies have confirmed the advantage of using hK2 and its ratios in addition to fPSA and %fPSA, especially at low PSA concentrations, for detection of prostate cancer.[51-53] To the authors' knowledge, no study has been published to date about the use of hK2 within an ANN. Own data by Stephan et al[54] on 475 patients with tPSA concentrations of 1 to 20 ng/mL show that the ANN performance was better than %fPSA except in the 4 to 10 ng/mL tPSA range. However, hK2 to %fPSA ratio almost always achieved equal results to the hk2 and %fPSA-based ANN regarding AUC comparisons and at 90% or 95% sensitivity. Despite some advantages for the ANN models in the lower tPSA ranges (<4 ng/mL) compared with %fPSA, the advantage of the hK2 and %fPSA-based ANN was only marginal compared with the hK2 to %fPSA ratio.[54]

In another recent study, the outcome of three promising serum markers for PCa was evaluated within an %fPSA-based ANN on 371 patients (135 PCa, 236 BPH) within the PSA range 0.5 to 20 ng/mL.[58] Promising data for improved PCa detection have been recently described by using the newly developed serum assays for human kallikrein 11 (hK11),[55] macrophage inhibitor cytokine 1 (MIC1),[56] and migration inhibitor factor (MIF).[57] Despite the significant lower concentrations for hK11 and MIC1 but not MIF (P = 0.065) in PCa patients compared with BPH patients, the AUCs for the three new serum markers when tPSA is in the range 2 to 10 ng/mL were smaller (0.56 to 0.61) than those for tPSA (0.66) and %fPSA (0.79).[58] However, an ANN and LR (AUC: each 0.83) with inclusion of all these new markers gave a significant improvement compared with %fPSA (P = 0.004) but %fPSA, ANN, and LR were equal at 90% and 95% sensitivity.[58] Additional inclusion of prostate volume resulted in a much better performance of the ANN model regarding AUC and cutoff comparison compared with %fPSA.[58]

Other newly described molecular forms—especially of fPSA-like intact fPSA, BPH PSA (BPSA) or the different forms of proenzyme PSA (proPSA)—show an interesting improvement for differentiation of PCa from BPH or a better detection of aggressive cancer.[31,59–62] If these new serum markers should become commercially available, an inclusion into multivariate ANN or LR models may further improve the PCa detection rate.

CONCLUSIONS

The use of PSA-based and %fPSA-based artificial neural networks (ANNs) and logistic regression (LR) models with clinically available data like age, DRE, and TRUS variables like prostate volume, PSA density, or TZ volume could clearly demonstrate an advantage to eliminate unnecessary prostate biopsies. At high sensitivity levels, improvement of specificity by 11% to 49% support these findings beside the significant larger AUCs for most multivariate models compared with %fPSA. The impact of the source of the tPSA and fPSA assays on the outcome of ANNs was demonstrated but only parallel measurement with different PSA assays may finally solve the problem, if a general ANN can be established for use with any PSA assay combination. New markers have additional value within ANNs but, so far, are not useful as single tests.

ACKNOWLEDGMENTS

This work was partly supported by the Mildred-Scheel-Foundation (Grant 70-3295-ST1 to C.S.), the Berliner Sparkassenstiftung (to C.S., H.C. and S.A.L.) and by the SONNENFELD-Stiftung (to S.A.L.).

REFERENCES

1. Polascik TJ, Oesterling JE, Partin AW. Prostate specific antigen: a decade of discovery—what we have learned and where we are going. J Urol 1999;162:293–306.
2. Bunting PS. A guide to the interpretation of serum prostate specific antigen levels. Clin Biochem 1995;28:221–41.
3. Brawer MK. Prostate-specific antigen. Semin Surg Oncol 2000;18:3–9.
4. Nixon RG, Brawer MK. Enhancing the specificity of prostate-specific antigen (PSA): an overview of PSA density, velocity and age-specific reference ranges. Br J Urol 1997;79:61–67.
5. Ukimura O, Durrani O, Babaian RJ. Role of PSA and its indices in determining the need for repeat prostate biopsies. Urology 1997;50:66–72.
6. Catalona WJ, Richie JP, Ahmann FR, et al. Comparison of digital rectal examination and serum prostate specific antigen in the early detection of prostate cancer: results of a multicenter clinical trial of 6,630 men. J Urol 1994;151:1283–1290.
7. Catalona WJ, Smith DS, Ratliff TL, et al. Measurement of prostate-specific antigen in serum as a screening test for prostate cancer. N Engl J Med 1991;324:1156–1161.
8. Lilja H, Christensson A, Dahlen U, et al. Prostate-specific antigen in serum occurs predominantly in complex with alpha 1-antichymotrypsin. Clin Chem 1991;37:1618–1625.
9. Stenman UH, Leinonen J, Alfthan H, et al. A complex between prostate-specific antigen and alpha 1-antichymotrypsin is the major form of prostate-specific antigen in serum of patients with prostate cancer: assay of the complex improves clinical sensitivity for cancer. Cancer Res 1991;51:222–226.
10. Catalona WJ, Smith DS, Wolfert RL, et al. Evaluation of percentage of free serum prostate-specific antigen to improve specificity of prostate cancer screening. JAMA 1995;274:1214–1220.
11. Catalona WJ, Partin AW, Slawin KM, et al. Use of the percentage of free prostate-specific antigen to enhance differentiation of prostate cancer from benign prostatic disease: a prospective multicenter clinical trial. JAMA 1998;279:1542–1547.
12. Partin AW, Catalona WJ, Southwick PC, et al. Analysis of percent free prostate-specific antigen (PSA) for prostate cancer detection: influence of total PSA, prostate volume, and age. Urology 1996;48:55–61.
13. Catalona WJ, Partin AW, Finlay JA, et al. Use of percentage of free prostate-specific antigen to identify men at high risk of prostate cancer when PSA levels are 2.51 to 4 ng/mL and digital rectal examination is not suspicious for prostate cancer: an alternative model. Urology 1999;54:220–224.
14. Djavan B, Zlotta A, Kratzik C, et al. PSA, PSA density, PSA density of transition zone, free/total PSA ratio, and PSA velocity for early detection of prostate cancer in men with serum PSA 2.5 to 4.0 ng/mL. Urology 1999;54:517–522.
15. Jung K, Stephan C, Elgeti U, et al. Molecular forms of prostate-specific antigen in serum with concentrations of total prostate-specific antigen <4 μg/l – are they useful tools for early detection and screening of prostate cancer? Int J Cancer 2001;93:759–765.
16. Roehl KA, Antenor JA, Catalona WJ. Robustness of free prostate specific antigen measurements to reduce unnecessary biopsies in the 2.6 to 4.0 ng/ml range. J Urol 2002;168:922–925.
17. Raaijmakers R, Blijenberg BG, Finlay JA, et al. Prostate cancer detection in the prostate specific antigen range of 2.0 to 3.9 ng/ml: value of percent free prostate specific antigen on tumor detection and tumor aggressiveness. J Urol 2004;171:2245–2249.
18. Lee CT, Scardino PT. Percent free prostate-specific antigen for first-time prostate biopsy. Urology 2001;57:594–598.
19. Stephan C, Lein M, Jung K, et al. Can prostate specific antigen derivatives reduce the frequency of unnecessary prostate biopsies? [Letter]. J Urol 1997;157:1371.
20. Haese A, Graefen M, Noldus J, et al. Prostatic volume and ratio of free-to-total prostate specific antigen in patients with prostatic cancer or benign prostatic hyperplasia. J Urol 1997;158:2188–2192.
21. Mettlin C, Chesley AE, Murphy GP, et al. Association of free PSA percent, total PSA, age, and gland volume in the detection of prostate cancer. Prostate 1999;39:153–158.
22. Stephan C, Lein M, Jung K, et al. The influence of prostate volume on the ratio of free to total prostate specific antigen in serum of patients with prostate carcinoma and benign prostate hyperplasia. Cancer 1997;79:104–109.
23. Lein M, Koenig F, Jung K, et al. The percentage of free prostate specific antigen is an age-independent tumour marker for prostate cancer: establishment of reference ranges in a large population of healthy men. Br J Urol 1998;82:231–236.

24. Carlson GD, Calvanese CB, Partin AW. An algorithm combining age, total prostate-specific antigen (PSA), and percent free PSA to predict prostate cancer: results on 4298 cases. Urology 1998;52:455–461.

25. Virtanen A, Gomari M, Kranse R, et al. Estimation of prostate cancer probability by logistic regression: free and total prostate-specific antigen, digital rectal examination, and heredity are significant variables. Clin Chem 1999;45:987–994.

26. Babaian RJ, Fritsche H, Ayala A, et al. Performance of a neural network in detecting prostate cancer in the prostate-specific antigen reflex range of 2.5 to 4.0 ng/mL. Urology 2000;56:1000–1006.

27. Djavan B, Remzi M, Zlotta A, et al. Novel artificial neural network for early detection of prostate cancer. J Clin Oncol 2002;20:921–929.

28. Finne P, Finne R, Auvinen A, et al. Predicting the outcome of prostate biopsy in screen-positive men by a multilayer perceptron network. Urology 2000;56:418–422.

29. Kalra P, Togami J, Bansal BSG, et al. A neurocomputational model for prostate carcinoma detection. Cancer 2003;98:1849–1854.

30. Stephan C, Jung K, Cammann H, et al. An artificial neural network considerably improves the diagnostic power of percent free prostate-specific antigen in prostate cancer diagnosis: Results of a 5-year investigation. Int J Cancer 2002;99:466–473.

31. Anagnostou T, Remzi M, Lykourinas M, et al. Artificial neural networks for decision-making in urologic oncology. Eur Urol 2003;43:596–603.

32. Loch T, Leuschner I, Genberg C, et al. [Improvement of transrectal ultrasound. Artificial neural network analysis (ANNA) in detection and staging of prostatic carcinoma]. Urologe A 2000;39:341–347.

33. Partin AW, Murphy GP, Brawer MK. Report on prostate cancer tumor marker workshop 1999. Cancer 2000;88:955–963.

34. Wei JT, Zhang Z, Barnhill SD, et al. Understanding artificial neural networks and exploring their potential applications for the practicing urologist. Urology 1998;52:161–172.

35. Snow PB, Smith DS, Catalona WJ. Artificial neural networks in the diagnosis and prognosis of prostate cancer: a pilot study. J Urol 1994;152:1923–1926.

36. Horninger W, Bartsch G, Snow PB, et al. The problem of cutoff levels in a screened population. Cancer 2001;91:1667–1672.

37. Sargent DJ. Comparison of artificial neural networks with other statistical approaches. Cancer 2001;91:1636–1642.

38. Stephan C, Cammann H, Semjonow A, et al. Multicenter evaluation of an artificial neural network to increase prostate cancer detection rate and reduce unnecessary biopsies. Clin Chem 2002;48:1279–1287.

39. Remzi M, Anagnostou T, Ravery V, et al. An artificial neural network to predict the outcome of repeat prostate biopsies. Urology 2003;62:456–460.

40. Garzotto M, Hudson RG, Peters L, et al. Predictive modeling for the presence of prostate carcinoma using clinical, laboratory, and ultrasound parameters in patients with prostate specific antigen levels < or = 10 ng/mL. Cancer 2003;98:1417–1422.

41. Stephan C, Jung K, Cammann H. Re: Predictive modeling for the presence of prostate carcinoma using clinical, laboratory, and ultrasound parameters in patients with prostate-specific antigen levels < or = 10 ng/ml. Cancer 2004;100:1988–1990.

42. Finne P, Finne R, Bangma C, et al. Algorithms based on prostate-specific antigen (PSA), free PSA, digital rectal examination and prostate volume reduce false-positive PSA results in prostate cancer screening. Int J Cancer 2004;111:310–315.

43. Jung K, Stephan C, Lein M, et al. Analytical performance and clinical validity of two free prostate-specific antigen assays compared. Clin Chem 1996;42:1026–1033.

44. Semjonow A, Oberpenning F, Brandt B, et al. Impact of free prostate-specific antigen on discordant measurement results of assays for total prostate-specific antigen. Urology 1996;48 (Suppl):10–15.

45. Yurdakul G, Bangma C, Blijenberg B, et al. Different PSA assays lead to detection of prostate cancers with identical histological features. Eur Urol 2002;42:154.

46. Link RE, Shariat SF, Nguyen CV, et al. Variation in prostate specific antigen results from 2 different assay platforms: clinical impact on 2304 patients undergoing prostate cancer screening. J Urol 2004;171:2234–2238.

47. Stephan C, Xu C, Cammann H, et al. Assay-specific artificial neural networks for 5 different PSA assays and populations with PSA 2-10 ng/mL in 4480 men. Int J Cancer; submitted, November, 2005.

48. Stamey TA, Caldwell M, McNeal JE, et al. The prostate specific antigen era in the United States is over for prostate cancer: What happened in the last 20 years? J Urol 2004;172:1297–301.

49. Stephan C, Jung K, Sinha P. Tumor markers for prostatic cancer – which way in this millenium? Res Adv Cancer 2002;2:147–157.

50. Partin AW, Catalona WJ, Finlay JA, et al. Use of human glandular kallikrein 2 for the detection of prostate cancer: preliminary analysis. Urology 1999;54:839–845.

51. Becker C, Piironen T, Pettersson K, et al. Discrimination of men with prostate cancer from those with benign disease by measurements of human glandular kallikrein 2 (HK2) in serum. J Urol 2000;163:311–316.

52. Magklara A, Scorilas A, Catalona WJ, et al. The combination of human glandular kallikrein and free prostate-specific antigen (PSA) enhances discrimination between prostate cancer and benign prostatic hyperplasia in patients with moderately increased total PSA. Clin Chem 1999;45:1960–1966.

53. Nam RK, Diamandis EP, Toi A, et al. Serum human glandular kallikrein-2 protease levels predict the presence of prostate cancer among men with elevated prostate-specific antigen. J Clin Oncol 2000;18:1036–1042.

54. Stephan C, Jung K, Soosaipillai AR, et al. Clinical usefulness of human glandular kallikrein 2 (hK2) within a neural network for prostate cancer detection. BJU Int, 2005;96:521–527.

55. Nakamura T, Scorilas A, Stephan C, et al. The usefulness of serum human kallikrein II for discriminating between prostate cancer and benign prostatic hyperplasia. Cancer Res 2003;63:6543–6546.

56. Brown DA, Stephan C, Ward RL, et al. Serum macrophage inhibitory cytokine (MIC-1) levels for the diagnosis and tumor grading of prostate cancer. Clin Cancer ResOncol; submitted 2005.

57. Meyer-Siegler KL, Bellino MA, Tannenbaum M. Macrophage migration inhibitory factor evaluation compared with prostate specific antigen as a biomarker in patients with prostate carcinoma. Cancer 2002;94:1449–1456.

58. Stephan C, Xu C, Kishi T, et al. Artificial neural network based on PSA, percent free PSA, and three new prostate cancer biomarkers. Proc Am Assoc Cancer Res 2004;45:#4478.

59. Catalona WJ, Bartsch G, Rittenhouse HG, et al. Serum pro-prostate specific antigen preferentially detects aggressive prostate cancers in men with 2 to 4 ng/ml prostate specific antigen. J Urol 2004;171:2239–2244.

60. Mikolajczyk SD, Marks LS, Partin AW, Rittenhouse HG. Free prostate-specific antigen in serum is becoming more complex. Urology 2002;59:797–802.

61. Mikolajczyk SD, Catalona WJ, Evans CL, et al. Proenzyme forms of prostate-specific antigen in serum improve the detection of prostate cancer. Clin Chem 2004;50:1017–1025.

62. Steuber T, Nurmikko P, Haese A, et al. Discrimination of benign from malignant prostatic disease by selective measurements of single chain, intact free prostate specific antigen. J Urol 2002;168:1917–1922.

MR imaging (MRI) and MR spectroscopic imaging (MRSI) in the diagnosis and staging of prostate cancer

50

John F Donohue, Hedvig Hricak

INTRODUCTION

Optimal management of prostate cancer remains elusive. At every stage on the patient pathway from diagnosis, localization, staging, and treatment planning to follow-up, there is a need to maximize information. This would allow better decision-making for both clinician and patient as, given the heterogeneous nature of prostate cancer, radical treatment and its associated sequelae must be balanced against active surveillance. In this chapter, we will discuss how magnetic resonance imaging (MRI) and magnetic resonance spectroscopic imaging (MRSI) can help in this decision-making. At present, the American Urological Association recommends that MRI be performed when the prostate-specific antigen (PSA) is over 25 ng/mL.[1] We aim to show, however, that, with recent developments, magnetic imaging should be undertaken more often than currently recommended.

BASIC SCIENCE

The science behind MRI is complex and beyond the scope of this chapter. However, while physicians do not need to be acquainted with the details, a brief outline of the basis of MRI, to allow better understand advantages and limitations of the modality, is given.

MAGNETIC RESONANCE

The MR machine is composed of a magnet and a radiofrequency (RF) coil, which can transmit and receive pulses of energy. This coil can be built into the main frame, placed on the surface (e.g., pelvic phased array coil used for MR images) or inside the body as in the case of an endorectal coil. Current magnets in clinical use can generate a range of fields up to 4 tesla (T). To appreciate this scale, 1 T equals 10 kiloGauss (kG) and the earth's magnetic field is 0.6 Gauss, therefore, these systems can produce magnetic fields approximately 66,000 times stronger than that of the earth.

Within the body, all tissues contain large amounts of hydrogen. The nucleus of each hydrogen atom has an intrinsic spin. This spinning nucleus with its electrical charge generates a small magnetic field so each nucleus behaves like a small bar magnet. The alignment of these multiple small magnets is random. However, when these nuclei are exposed to a large external magnetic field, they lose their random orientation and align themselves parallel to the force of the applied magnetic field. Energy is added to the nuclei in the form of an RF pulse, and this raises the nuclei to a higher energy level. They remain in this state until the RF pulse is turned off, at which stage they return to their previous equilibrium within the magnetic field. While returning to this state, they give off energy, which can be recorded in a waveform and transcribed in a spatial localization to generate an image. This is the basis of MRI. T1 and T2 are parameters used to describe this return of the nuclei to the resting state. Tissues in the body have various proportions of hydrogen and, thus, different signals are recorded allowing for soft tissue contrast and subsequent images to be processed.

MAGNETIC RESONANCE SPECTROSCOPY

Magnetic resonance spectroscopy (MRS) allows for the non-invasive assessment of tissue metabolism. In MRS, the nuclei of particular nuclides such as ^{1}H, ^{13}C, ^{31}P, and ^{19}F are excited with an RF pulse in the presence of a magnetic field. Different nuclei have various resonance frequencies and, by tuning in, different concentrations can be measured. Although other nuclei have been studied, to date only the clinical use of hydrogen has been demonstrated. As described above, the waveform elicited from the hydrogen proton is utilized and the signal intensity is recorded. The signal intensities from various molecules containing hydrogen are sufficiently different to allow them to be distinguished from each other. This is known as chemical shift. This enables a spectrum of signal intensity versus frequency (concentration) to be produced in a spatial manner for the prostate. The MRI image of the prostate is divided into small volumes of interest called voxels in a grid pattern. This allows for assessment of different areas of the gland. The chemicals used with regard to the prostate are choline, creatine, and citrate.

IMAGING TECHNIQUES

PATIENT PREPARATION

Combined MRI and MRS requires approximately 1 hour to perform. The patient should be advised that the process may be noisy and claustrophobic. The use of an expandable endorectal coil is essential for MRS and it helps improve the accuracy of MRI interpretation.[2] Contraindications for the use of the endorectal coil include a recent history of rectal surgery, inflammatory bowel disease, radiation therapy to the pelvis within the last 6 weeks, and the use of anticoagulation drugs. T1-weighted axial images of the pelvic region are used for the detection of nodal disease, bone metastases, and post-biopsy hemorrhage. Thin-section T2-weighted images in the axial, sagittal, and coronal planes are used for tumor detection, localization, and staging. To avoid under- and overestimation of tumor location and extent, MRI should be delayed for at least 8 weeks after prostate biopsy.[3]

NORMAL ANATOMY

MRI

On T1-weighted images, the prostate demonstrates homogeneous intermediate-to-low signal intensity. As with computed tomography (CT), the soft tissue contrast resolution is not sufficient for the visualization of the intraprostatic anatomy or pathology. The zonal anatomy of the prostate gland is best depicted on T2-weighted images (Figure 50.1). These images demonstrate the normal peripheral zone with high signal intensity. A thin rim of low signal intensity, which

represents the anatomic or true capsule, surrounds the peripheral zone, which is often incomplete especially at the apex, reflecting what is found on pathologic specimens. The neurovascular bundles can be identified as low-signal-intensity foci posterolateral to the capsule. The central and transition zones have similar appearances and can be distinguished from the peripheral zone by their respective anatomical locations. The anterior fibromuscular stroma demonstrates low signal intensity. The proximal urethra is rarely identifiable, unless a Foley catheter is present or a transurethral resection has been performed. On T2-weighted images, the distal prostatic urethra below the verumontanum can be seen as a low-signal-intensity ring similar to a doughnut. The vas deferens and seminal vesicles, which have grape-like configurations, demonstrate high signal intensity on T2-weighted images and are readily identifiable (Figure 50.2).

SPECTROSCOPY

Normal prostate tissue contains high levels of citrate, which are higher in the peripheral zone than in the central and transition zones, and low levels of choline. Glandular hyperplastic nodules, however, can demonstrate citrate levels as high as those observed in the peripheral zone.

DETECTING PROSTATE CANCER

MRI

On T2-weighted images, prostate cancer most commonly demonstrates low signal intensity in contrast to the high signal intensity of the normal peripheral zone (Figure 50.3). However, care is required, as low signal intensity in the peripheral zone on T2-weighted images can also be seen in several benign conditions, such as post-biopsy hemorrhage, prostatitis, or hyperplastic nodules. A low-signal-intensity tumor extending into the vesicles from the base of the gland can identify seminal vesicle invasion.

SPECTROSCOPY

In the presence of prostate cancer, the citrate level is diminished, or not detectable, because of a conversion from citrate-producing to citrate-oxidizing metabolism. The choline is elevated due to a high phospholipid cell membrane turnover in the proliferating malignant tissue. Hence, this method of depicting tumors is based on an increased choline/citrate ratio. Because the creatine peak is next to the choline peak on the spectral trace, the two may be inseparable. Therefore, there are

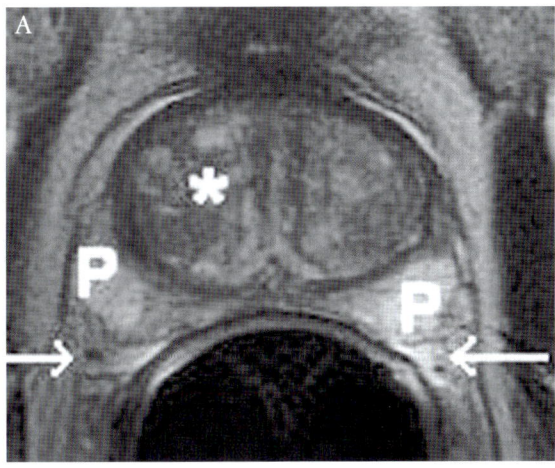
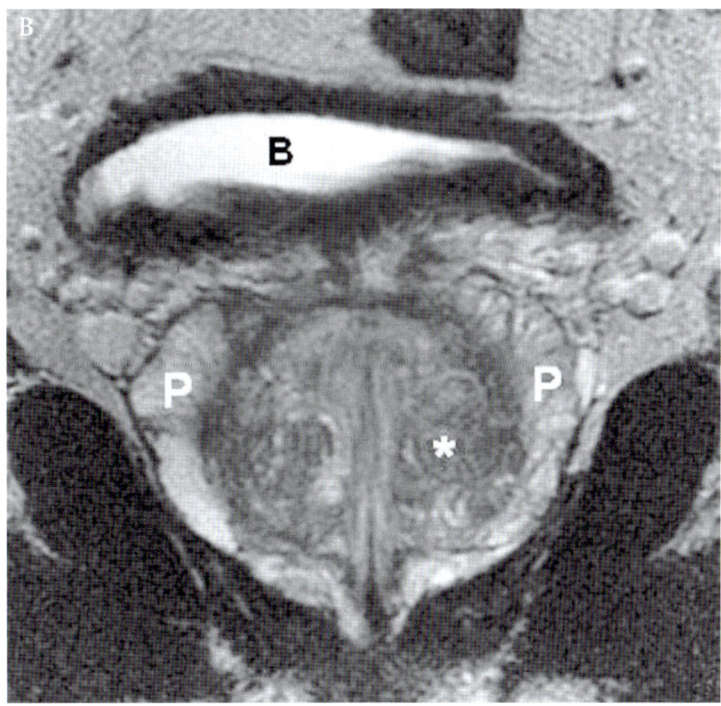

Fig. 50.1
Normal anatomy of prostate, T2-weighted image. *A,* Axial image showing the transition zone that demonstrates heterogeneous signal intensity due to benign prostatic hypertrophy *(*)* and can be distinguished from the homogenous high-signal-intensity peripheral zone (P). The neurovascular bundles *(arrows)* are seen posteriorly with the black area representing vessels. *B,* Coronal image showing the heterogeneous transition zone *(*)* surrounded by the higher-signal-intensity peripheral zone (P) with urinary bladder (B) above.

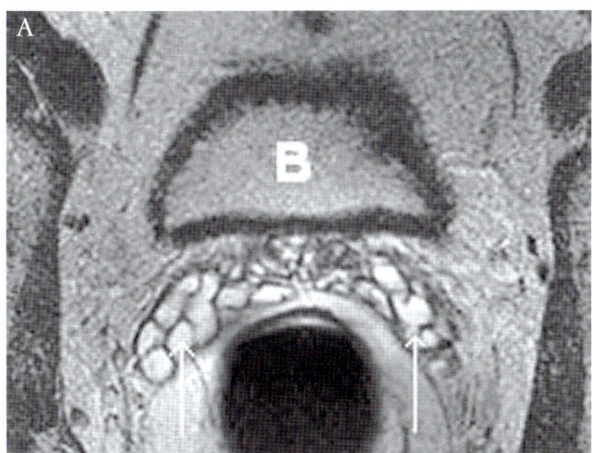
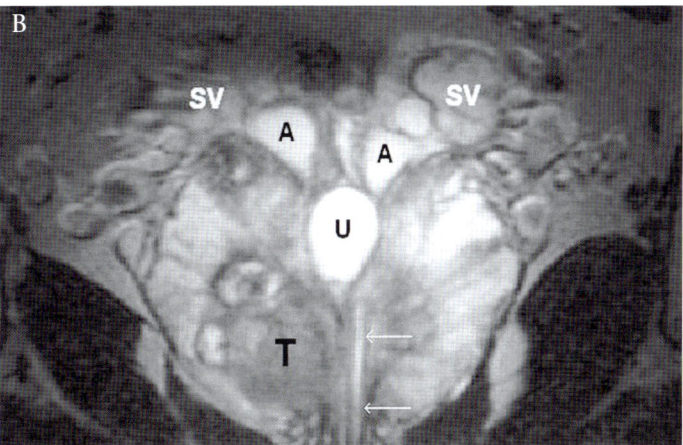

Fig. 50.2
Normal anatomy of seminal vesicles, T2-weighted images. *A,* Axial image showing the grape-like appearance of the seminal vesicles *(arrows)* lying posterior to the bladder (B). *B,* Coronal image of the ampulla (A) and seminal vesicle (SV) in a patient with a right-sided tumor (T) abutting into the urethra *(arrows)*. The prostatic utricle (U) is also noted.

no units to express the absolute metabolite measurement and the individual ratio of choline and creatine to citrate is used for spectral analysis in the clinical setting[4] (Figure 50.4).

The exciting aspect of this technique is that the preliminary results obtained show that the ratio of choline and creatine to citrate relates to the Gleason score and tumor aggressiveness.[5] At present, the relative size of the voxels is large in proportion to the prostate so that radiological virtual biopsies for diagnosis are not appropriate. Thus, MRSI detection of prostate cancer is based on the alteration of the choline to citrate ratio with an increase in the choline peak and a reduction in the citrate peak. It should be noted, however, that, while the citrate level falls in prostate cancer, it is also reduced by prostatitis and post-biopsy haemorrhage.[6]

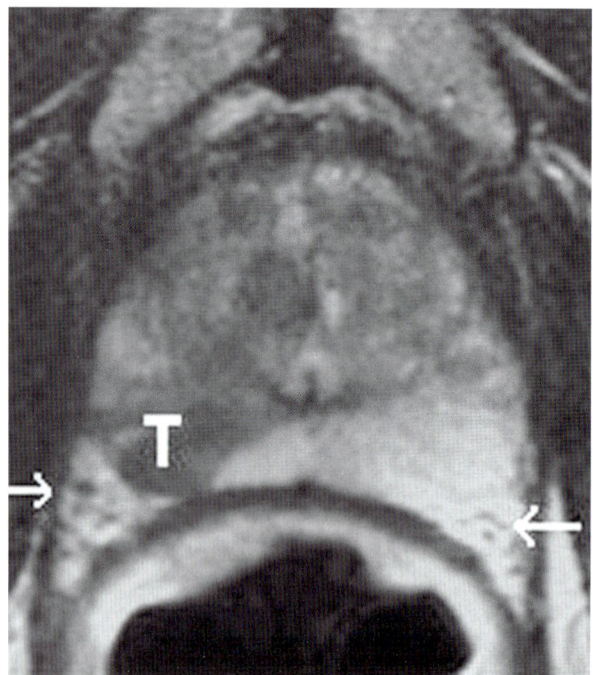

Fig. 50.3
Organ-confined tumor, T2-weighted images. Axial image demonstrating tumor (T) in the right peripheral zone. The neurovascular bundles *(arrows)*, containing multiple vessels seen as black areas, can clearly be distinguished from the tumor.

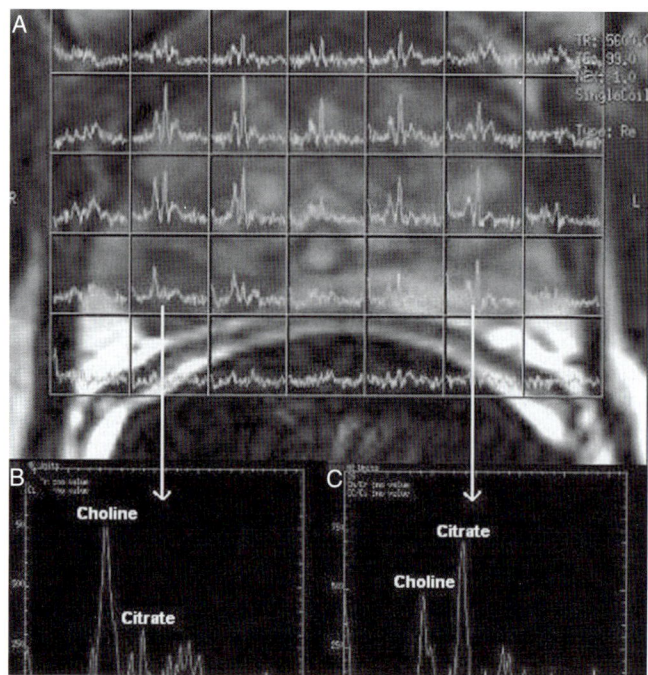

Fig. 50.4
Magnetic resonance spectroscopic imaging. This image shows an axial T2-weighted MR image of a right-sided tumor with the spectroscopic voxels overlaid *(A)*. The corresponding enlarged voxels below show an elevated choline peak with no accompanying citrate peak *(B)*. Compare that with a normal voxel from the left side with a normal choline–citrate relationship *(C)*.

THE ROLE OF MRI AND MRSI IN PROSTATE CANCER

Prostate cancer is not homogenous and tumor characteristics vary greatly amongst patients. Thus, every opportunity should be taken to obtain the maximum information regarding the tumor. The various roles of MRI and spectroscopy are outlined below.

DIAGNOSIS

The diagnosis of prostate cancer is usually obtained histologically following biopsy or transurethral resection of the prostate (TURP). MRI is reserved only for those patients in whom there is a clinical suspicion of cancer, often in the situation of an elevated PSA with one or more negative biopsies.

The utility of using MRI to give additional information so as to aid biopsy targeting or quantify the need for further biopsies was demonstrated in a study that showed a sensitivity of 83% for MRI diagnosed lesions in patients undergoing repeat transrectal ultrasonography (TRUS)-guided biopsy following previous negative biopsies.[7] Perrotti et al used MRI to stratify patients as being at low, intermediate, or high risk of having prostate cancer on repeat biopsy, and demonstrated a sensitivity of 70% in the high-risk

group.[8] In a pilot study by Yeun et al, 24 patients, with at least one prior negative biopsy, underwent combined MRI and MRSI before repeat biopsy. Prostate cancer was diagnosed in 7 of the 24 patients giving a sensitivity of 100% and specificity of 71%. Two cases were found as a result of additional targeted biopsy suggested by the imaging.[9] However, in this study, equivocal readings were regarded as test negative.

The routine use of MRI in the diagnosis of prostate cancer is certainly not appropriate, but in certain cases, as outlined above, there is a role for it, and the use of MRSI to more accurately grade tumors is an exciting development.

LOCALIZATION

Information regarding the location of a tumor can be gained from digital rectal examination (DRE), TRUS images, and the biopsy results depending on whether the biopsies were separately labeled. However, there are limitations to this approach.[10, 11]

Recently, this has been shown in a retrospective study comparing the ability of these modalities and MRI to locate a tumor within the prostate gland. In 106 consecutive patients who underwent radical prostatectomy, step section pathology was compared against MRI, DRE, and TRUS-guided biopsy. A single reader ranked the likelihood of tumor on a 5-point scale in each of 14 locations within the gland. They found that MRI was superior to DRE for localization of tumor in all regions of the prostate. There was no difference between MRI and TRUS with regard to detecting apical tumors, but MRI was better in all other areas of the prostate.[12]

The additional benefit of spectroscopy added to MRI information was evaluated by Scheidler et al, when they reported on the efficacy of two radiologists using MRI alone and in combination with MRSI to localize prostate cancer in 53 patients who were imaged prior to radical prostatectomy.[13] Using the histologic specimens as reference, they showed that while the sensitivity decreased slightly from 77% and 81% to 68% and 73% for the two readers, respectively, there was a marked improvement in the specificity from 46% and 61% to 70% and 80%, respectively. Radiological requests should always be accompanied with pertinent clinical information. However, Dhingsa et al showed that, while the radiologist's knowledge of sextant biopsy results, DRE findings, and PSA level increased the sensitivity, there was no overall improvement in accuracy, since there was an accompanied increase in the number of false-positive readings.[14]

While the majority of tumors arise in the peripheral zone, up to 30% can originate in the transition zone or central zone.[15] Radiological evaluation of the transition zone is difficult because of the heterogeneous appearance of BPH.[16,17] Unfortunately, at present, the metabolite spectrum from MRSI for transition zone cancer cannot be confidently differentiated from that for benign tissue.[18]

In the assessment of a newly diagnosed patient with prostate cancer, imaging can be hindered by post-biopsy hemorrhage or if the patient has already been commenced on neoadjuvant hormones. All metabolites detected by MRSI will decrease in a time-dependent manner, but citrate levels will fall faster than choline and creatine,[19] thus allowing the detection of tumor if MRSI is performed within 4 months after the initiation of hormone therapy.[20] Post-biopsy hemorrhagic areas have the same T2-weighted low signal intensity as cancer; however, Kaji et al showed that the addition of spectroscopy to MRI increased the sensitivity from 52% to 75% and the specificity from 26% to 66% in differentiating cancer from haemorrhage.[6]

TUMOUR AGGRESSIVENESS

The degree of differentiation of a tumor, as given by the Gleason score, is a strong predictor of outcome and has been incorporated into nomograms to give a prediction of final pathology and recurrence risk.[21,22]

However, there is often a disparity between the biopsy and final pathologic Gleason scores, and upgrading has been reported in as many as 54% of cases.[23] The choline

to citrate ratio increases with the Gleason score,[5] and this property of spectroscopy was used to correlate the preoperative MRSI against the final pathologic whole mount specimens of 123 patients who had a radical prostatectomy. Overall, MRSI sensitivity was 56% for tumor detection, increasing from 44% in Gleason pattern 3 + 3 to 89% in lesions with Gleason pattern of 4 + 4 lesions. This study confirmed the significant correlation between the choline to citrate ratio and the Gleason pattern.[24]

It is expected that 230,000 men will be diagnosed with prostate cancer in the United States in 2004.[25] However, some of these cancers will prove to be so small, low grade and non-invasive as not to pose any risk.[26] This has led to an interest in trying to identify these so called "indolent" tumors, and Kattan et al have developed nomograms to attempt to achieve this.[27] Their pathologic definition of an indolent tumor was an organ-confined cancer with volume less than 0.5 mL and no elements of Gleason grade 4 or 5. The nomogram variables include PSA, clinical stage, Gleason grade, proportion of cancer in a biopsy, and prostate volume on ultrasound. While the sensitivity of MRI to detect tumor volumes less than 0.5 mL is poor[28,29] and the choline to citrate ratio measured spectroscopically is proportional to the Gleason grade, the addition of MRI and spectroscopy to the nomogram significantly increased its discrimination (area under the receiver operating characteristic [ROC] curve) to 0.86 from 0.79.[30] While this information on its own is not sufficient to place a patient into a surveillance program, it will assist with patient counseling and decision making. Indeed, it could be more useful in ruling out indolent tumors and identifying aggressive tumors.

STAGING

The ability to accurately stage prostate cancer preoperatively with MRI and MRSI is the focus of much ongoing research. The ability to determine the presence or absence of extracapsular extension (ECE), seminal vesicle involvement, or lymph node or bone metastases is needed in the pretreatment setting to allow for more accurate prognostic and pathologic estimations and thus more confident patient counseling and "evidence based" treatment decisions.

Extra-capsular extension

A meta-analysis by Engelbrecht examining the performance of MRI in staging prostate cancer from 1984 to 2000 revealed an accuracy variance from 50% to 92%.[31] A retrospective review of preoperative MR images, by Yu et al in 77 patients who had pathologic T2 or T3 disease, found, on multivariate analysis, that obliteration of the rectoprostatic angle and asymmetry of the neurovascular bundles where the MRI features most indicative of ECE.[32] They did note that the

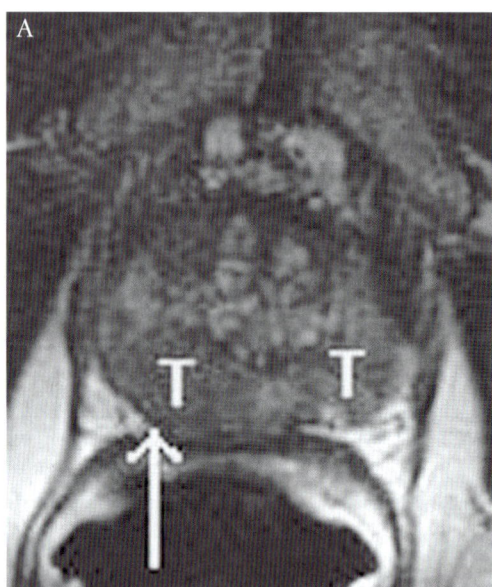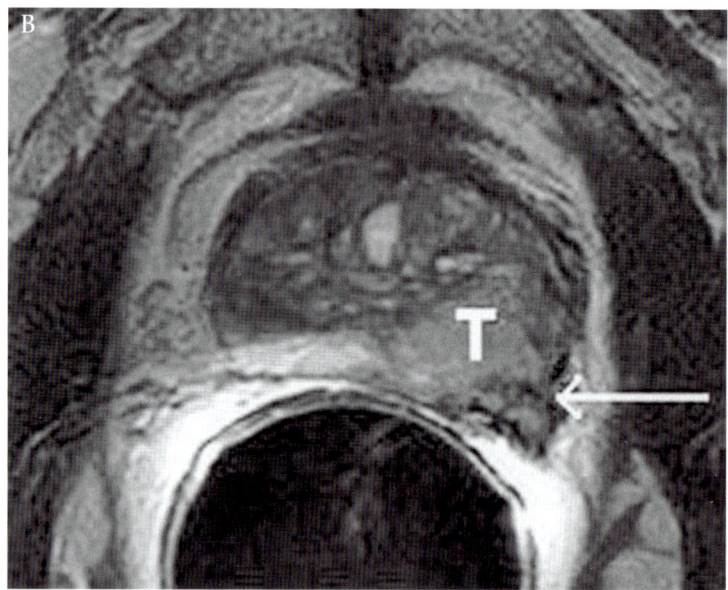

Fig. 50.5

Extracapsular extension in two different patients, T2-weighted images. *A*, Axial image showing bilateral tumors (T) with extracapsular extension on the right, shown by a focal bulge and obliteration of the rectoprostatic angle *(arrow)*. *B*, Axial image showing a left-sided tumor (T) with direct extension into the left neurovascular bundle *(arrow)*.

experience of the reader played an important role in the ability to interpret MRI and contributed to interobserver variability (Figure 50.5). The importance of interobserver variability has always been a factor and was noted in 1994 with the introduction of the endorectal coil, where initial results were poorer than with the conventional body coil.[33]

A recent study by Mullerad et al has shown the importance of using dedicated radiologists to analyze prostate images. The study demonstrated that genitourinary MR radiologists were significantly better at predicting ECE on MRI than general body MR specialists.[34] The addition of MRSI assists the reader, significantly improving the accuracy of the less experienced reader and reducing interobserver variability.[35] Wang et al compared the preoperative MRI report with the pathologic specimen in 344 consecutive patients who underwent a radical prostatectomy, of whom 216 also had MRSI.[36] The overall sensitivity, specificity, and positive and negative predictive values of MRI for ECE were 42%, 95%, 75%, and 84% respectively. There was a further, but not statistically significant, improvement with the addition of spectroscopy. Multivariate analysis of MRI and other preoperative variables (PSA, clinical stage, Gleason score, % cancer in biopsy cores, perineural invasion) showed that the addition of MRI findings significantly increased the area under the ROC curve from 0.77 to 0.84 in the prediction of ECE (p=0.022).

Seminal vesicle invasion

Since seminal vesicle invasion (SVI) and lymph node metastases are strong predictors of progression,[37] preoperative identification of these conditions is desirable (Figure 50.6). Bernstein et al reviewed 124 patients with T1c disease who were imaged by MRI prior to surgery.[38] While at multivariate analysis they didn't find any benefit from MRI in diagnosing ECE, they found that MRI and preoperative PSA levels were predictors of SVI. A recent study of 411 consecutive patients undergoing radical prostatectomy with preoperative MRI compared with the pathologic specimen reported positive and negative predictive value for detecting seminal vesicle invasion of 78% and 94% respectively.[39]

Lymph node invasion

The conventional imaging criterion for metastatic lymph node detection is 7 mm (Figure 50.7). However, given the shortcomings of present imaging modalities, MR lymphography to image lymph nodes is an exciting prospect. Nanoparticles containing iron oxide are injected intravenously 24 hours before MRI. These nanoparticles are slowly extravasated into the interstitial space and are transported to lymph nodes via the lymphatics, where they are internalized by macrophages. These iron-containing particles cause magnetic changes detectable by MRI, and disturbances in lymph node architecture caused by metastasis can be distinguished from normal lymph nodes. Initial work reported a sensitivity of 100% and specificity of 80%.[40] Harisinghani et al investigated 80 patients with prostate cancer (clinical stage T1–T3) who underwent lymph node resection or biopsy after MR lymphography.[41] There were 334 lymph nodes histologically assessed, of which 63 (19%) nodes from 33 (41%) patients had metastatic deposits. The sensitivity of this technique was 91% compared with 35% for conventional MRI. The main advantage of MR

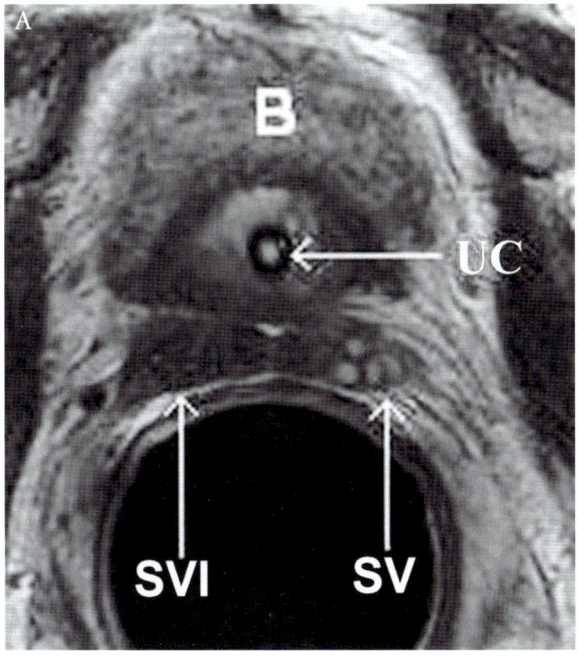

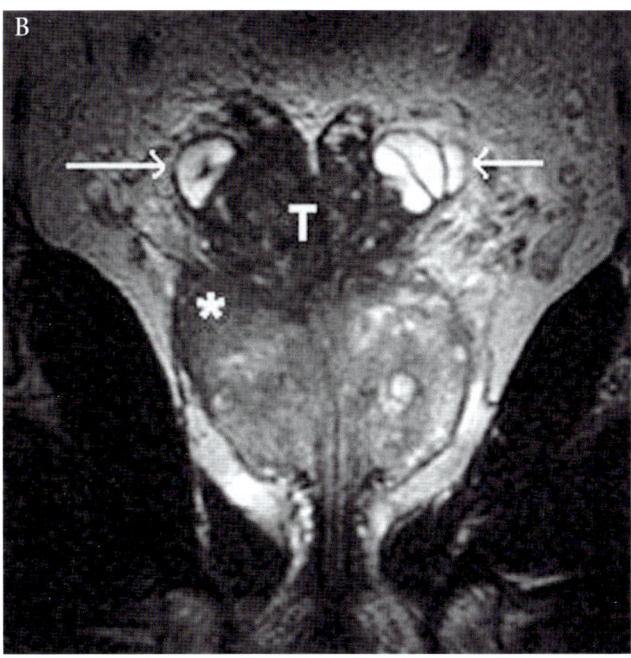

Fig. 50.6
Seminal vesicle invasion in two different patients, T2-weighted images. *A*, Axial image showing gross right-sided seminal vesicle invasion (SVI) and partial involvement on the left. The tip of the seminal vesicle on the left is normal (SV). Note the urethral catheter (UC) within the intravesicular portion of the prostate (median lobe) as it pushes into the bladder (B). *B*, Coronal image of a right-sided tumor (*) with extracapsular extension showing bilateral invasion of the seminal vesicles (T). Note that the tips are not involved *(arrows)*.

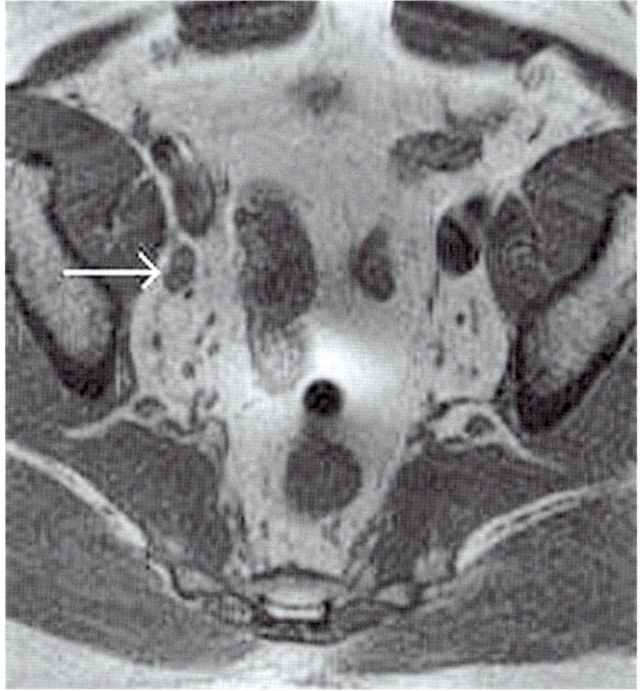

Fig. 50.7
Lymph node metastasis, T1-weighted image. Axial image showing a metastatic lymph node *(arrow)* lying below the external iliac vessels on the right side.

lymphography is its ability to detect metastatic deposits in normal size nodes, which is significant given that 75% of all the positive nodes were small enough (less than 8–10 mm) so as not to meet usual MRI radiological criteria. The approach of using this method in intermediate to high-risk patients has been shown to have net cost savings.[42]

Bone metastases

The confident prediction of bone metastasis is often difficult, with abnormalities on bone scintigraphy from noncancerous sources causing uncertainty. There is no doubt that MRI is superior to bone scan in detecting bone metastasis in the spine,[43] and is, therefore, often useful for resolving equivocal bone scans in this region.[44] Yet MRI may fail to detect peripheral bone lesions. Traill et al explored using MRI imaging of the axial skeleton as the initial investigation in place of bone scintigraphy.[45] In 200 patients with histologically proven prostate or breast cancer, only 4 patients (2%) had peripheral bone metastases, which would have been missed by MRI. However, 3 of these were painful and so would have prompted plain radiographs, so these would likely, given the clinical setting and a high index of suspicion, have been diagnosed anyway.

While at present bone scintigraphy remains the mainstay for the detection of bone metastases, rapid development of MR techniques and MR bone marrow survey may change this in the future.

TREATMENT PLANNING

Accurate staging of any cancer is essential, especially when therapeutic interventions are considered. It is even more important, given that many of these treatments have considerable morbidity, to have as much information as possible so as to maximize the benefit. The routine use of MRI and MRSI in staging, according to risk groups, needs to be clarified. However, there is evidence that magnetic resonance also has a role in treatment planning.

The neurovascular bundles (NVBs) are found posterolaterally to the prostate, which is often the site of ECE.[46–48] Therefore, to avoid positive surgical margins, it is often necessary to resect the NVBs.[49,50] A recent paper investigated whether MRI could influence a surgeon's decision with regard to the NVBs.[51] A decision on whether to preserve or resect the NVBs was made by a surgeon before and after reviewing the MRI with a radiologist. Histologic examination revealed that NVB resection was warranted in 44 of 270 NVBs (16%). Surgical planning changed in 39% of cases as a result of MRI findings and, when the pathologic specimens were examined, it was found that more aggressive or conservative surgery were the correct options in 67% and 90% of cases respectively. For patients considered at high risk of ECE, surgical management of the NVBs was changed as a result of MRI in 78% of cases, which was appropriate for 93% (Figure 50.8).

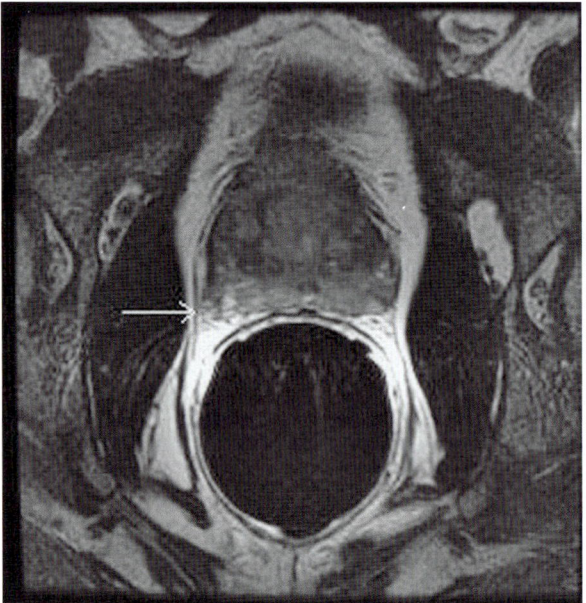

Fig. 50.8
Surgical planning for extracapsular extension, T2-weighted image. Axial image showing right-sided extracapsular extension *(arrow)*. Note the interruption in the capsule compared with the left side where the neurovascular bundle can be clearly visualized. This would suggest that a nerve-sparing procedure could be performed on the left with a wider margin taken on the right.

Other studies have shown that the length of the membranous urethra measured by MRI is predictive of return to continence,[52] and the prominence of the periprostatic veins on MRI is associated with greater intraoperative blood loss during radical prostatectomy.[53]

Imaging is essential when planning radiation treatment. It has been shown that CT overestimates the prostate volume by 32% to 34% compared with MRI,[54,55] which suggests that the use of MRI would result in the reduction of the radiation field to surrounding structures. In patients receiving brachytherapy, studies have shown the utility of giving higher radiation doses to areas of the prostate considered suspicious of containing tumor on MRSI.[56] Clarke et al reported on 390 patients who underwent brachytherapy, of whom 327 were staged by MRI.[57] Seed distribution was modified in 56% of cases as a result of more extensive disease on MRI and 18% had their treatment plan altered, with most receiving additional external beam radiotherapy. A Cox regression analysis was performed on known variables, including whether a patient had a pretreatment MRI to predict post-treatment biochemical failure. The Cox analysis showed that only failure to have an MRI and the percentage of positive cores were statistically significant.

FOLLOW-UP

A common problem for clinicians, in the presence of a rising PSA after curative treatment, is attempting to diagnose local or distant recurrence. Present diagnostic modalities, excluding MRI, have been disappointing.[58] Sella et al evaluated the role of MRI to diagnose local recurrence in patients following radical prostatectomy.[59] In 48 patients with a postoperative rising PSA, 41 were considered to have local recurrence based on the absence of bone metastases, regression of the PSA following pelvic radiotherapy, positive biopsy, or increasing size of tumor volume on serial MRIs. The sensitivity and specificity of MRI to diagnose local recurrence was 95% and 100% respectively. All tumors were hyperintense in relation to surrounding pelvic muscles on T2-weighted images (Figure 50.9). A similar study by Silverman et al found 100% sensitivity and specificity.[60]

In patients with biochemical failure after external beam radiotherapy, Coakley et al showed that MRSI gave sensitivity and specificity of 87% and 72% respectively.[61] There was a 100% negative predictive value for the exclusion of local recurrent tumor if there was no metabolic activity on spectroscopy. In patients who have had cryotherapy, MRSI has been shown to be superior to MRI or TRUS in determining local recurrence.[62,63]

SHORTCOMINGS AND CHALLENGES

The use of MRI and MRSI is not the panacea that it appears. The majority of literature comes from major

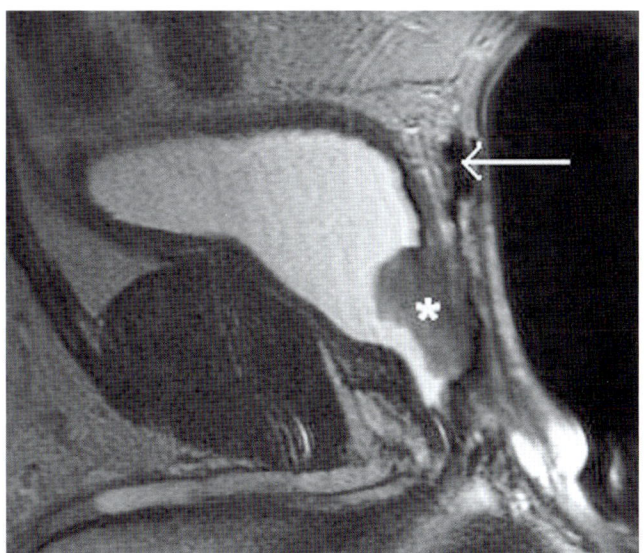

Fig. 50.9
Tumor recurrence, T2-weighted image. Sagittal image of a recurrence following radical prostatectomy lying behind and involving the bladder (*). Surgical clips are identified by the black areas *(arrow)* used during dissection of the seminal vesicles.

institutions with a great depth of experience in these modalities and a large patient profile. The ongoing challenge is to disseminate knowledge and standardize practice.

The technical aspect of performing and interpreting the radiological information becomes more difficult with further advances. While the introduction of the endorectal coil improved the imaging quality, it increased the complexity of data acquisition and initially reader accuracy dropped.[33] There is no doubt that there is a steep learning curve involved and that dedicated uroradiologists perform better.

Spectroscopy, while an exciting addition to the radiological armamentarium, still requires further research. Presently, it cannot be used to assess the seminal vesicles, since they do not contain citrate. Moreover, the whole prostate gland is problematic to assess, since the base, anterior portion, and apex are not covered. The changes in signal intensity occurring in the prostate as a result of phytotherapeutics have not yet been assessed.

CONCLUSION

We believe that MRI and MRSI are road maps allowing for more accurate assessment of tumor location and extent, which potentially leads to better, more patient-specific therapy. Magnetic resonance has been shown to be beneficial not just in staging but in other situations where precise knowledge of a tumor's anatomic and spectral properties are helpful. At present, most of the published work has come from major institutions with

expertise. However, considering the patient benefits that have already been shown, the skills required should be translated into routine use. Further research is required to define which clinical scenarios will benefit maximally given the fiscal costs involved.

REFERENCES

1. Prostate-specific antigen (PSA) best practice policy. American Urological Association (AUA). Oncology (Hunting) 2000;14:267–272, 277–278, 280 passim.
2. Hricak H, White S, Vigneron D, et al. Carcinoma of the prostate gland: MR imaging with pelvic phased-array coils versus integrated endorectal–pelvic phased-array coils. Radiology 1994;193:703–709.
3. Qayyum A, Coakley FV, Lu Y, et al. Organ-confined prostate cancer: effect of prior transrectal biopsy on endorectal MRI and MR spectroscopic imaging. AJR Am J Roentgenol 2004;183:1079–1083.
4. Kurhanewicz J, Vigneron DB, Hricak H, et al. Three-dimensional H-1 MR spectroscopic imaging of the in situ human prostate with high (0.24–0.7-cm³) spatial resolution. Radiology 1996;198:795–805.
5. Kurhanewicz J, Vigneron DB, Nelson SJ. Three-dimensional magnetic resonance spectroscopic imaging of brain and prostate cancer. Neoplasia 2000;2:166–189.
6. Kaji Y, Kurhanewicz J, Hricak H, et al. Localizing prostate cancer in the presence of postbiopsy changes on MR images: role of proton MR spectroscopic imaging. Radiology 1998;206:785–790.
7. Beyersdorff D, Taupitz M, Winkelmann B, et al. Patients with a history of elevated prostate-specific antigen levels and negative transrectal US-guided quadrant or sextant biopsy results: value of MR imaging. Radiology 2002;224:701–706.
8. Perrotti M, Han KR, Epstein RE, et al. Prospective evaluation of endorectal magnetic resonance imaging to detect tumor foci in men with prior negative prostatic biopsy: a pilot study. J Urol 1999;162:1314–1317.
9. Yuen JS, Thng CH, Tan PH, et al. Endorectal magnetic resonance imaging and spectroscopy for the detection of tumor foci in men with prior negative transrectal ultrasound prostate biopsy. J Urol 2004;171:1482–1486.
10. Obek C, Louis P, Civantos F, et al. Comparison of digital rectal examination and biopsy results with the radical prostatectomy specimen. J Urol 1999;161:494–498.
11. Salomon L, Colombel M, Patard JJ, et al. Value of ultrasound-guided systematic sextant biopsies in prostate tumor mapping. Eur Urol 1999;35:289–293.
12. Mullerad M, Hricak H, Kuroiwa K, et al. Comparison on endorectal magnetic resonance imaging, guided prostate biopsy and digital rectal examination in the pre-operative anatomical localization of prostate cancer. J. Urol (in press).
13. Scheidler J, Hricak H, Vigneron DB, et al. Prostate cancer: localization with three-dimensional proton MR spectroscopic imaging— clinicopathologic study. Radiology 1999;213:473–480.
14. Dhingsa R, Qayyum A, Coakley FV, et al. Prostate cancer localization with endorectal MR imaging and MR spectroscopic imaging: effect of clinical data on reader accuracy. Radiology 2004;230:215–220.
15. McNeal JE, Redwine EA, Freiha FS, et al. Zonal distribution of prostatic adenocarcinoma. Correlation with histologic pattern and direction of spread. Am J Surg Pathol 1988;12:897–906.
16. Ikonen S, Kivisaari L, Tervahartiala P, et al. Prostatic MR imaging. Accuracy in differentiating cancer from other prostatic disorders [see comment]. Acta Radiologica 2001;42:348–354.
17. Noguchi M, Stamey TA, Neal JE, et al. An analysis of 148 consecutive transition zone cancers: clinical and histological characteristics. J Urol 2000;163:1751–1755.
18. Zakian KL, Eberhardt S, Hricak H, et al. Transition zone prostate cancer: metabolic characteristics at 1H MR spectroscopic imaging— initial results. Radiology 2003;229:241–247.
19. Mueller-Lisse UG, Swanson MG, Vigneron DB, et al. Time-dependent effects of hormone-deprivation therapy on prostate metabolism as detected by combined magnetic resonance imaging and 3D magnetic resonance spectroscopic imaging. Magn Reson Med 2001;46:49–57.

20. Mueller-Lisse UG, Vigneron DB, Hricak H, et al. Localized prostate cancer: effect of hormone deprivation therapy measured by using combined three-dimensional 1H MR spectroscopy and MR imaging: clinicopathologic case-controlled study. Radiology 2001;221:380–390.

21. Kattan MW, Eastham JA, Stapleton AM, et al. A preoperative nomogram for disease recurrence following radical prostatectomy for prostate cancer. J Natl Cancer Inst 1998;90:766–771.

22. Partin AW, Kattan MW, Subong EN, et al. Combination of prostate-specific antigen, clinical stage, and Gleason score to predict pathological stage of localized prostate cancer. A multi-institutional update. JAMA 1997;278:1445–1451.

23. Cookson MS, Fleshner NE, Soloway SM, et al. Correlation between Gleason score of needle biopsy and radical prostatectomy specimen: accuracy and clinical implications. J Urol 1997;157:559–562.

24. Zakian KL, Sircar K, Hricak H, et al. Correlation of proton MR spectroscopic imaging with Gleason score based on step section pathology after radical prostatectomy. Radiology, 2005;234:804–814.

25. Jemal A, Tiwari RC, Murray T, et al. Cancer statistics, 2004. CA Cancer J Clin 2004;54:8–29.

26. Ohori M, Wheeler TM, Dunn JK, et al. The pathological features and prognosis of prostate cancer detectable with current diagnostic tests. J Urol 1994;152:1714–1720.

27. Kattan MW, Eastham JA, Wheeler TM, et al. Counseling men with prostate cancer: a nomogram for predicting the presence of small, moderately differentiated, confined tumors. J Urol 2003;170:1792–1797.

28. Coakley FV, Kurhanewicz J, Lu Y, et al. Prostate cancer tumor volume: measurement with endorectal MR and MR spectroscopic imaging. Radiology 2002;223:91–97.

29. Ikonen S, Karkkainen P, Kivisaari L, et al. Magnetic resonance imaging of clinically localized prostatic cancer. J Urol 1998;159:915–919.

30. Shulka-Dave A, Hricak H, Pucar D, et al. Indolent prostate cancer – predication by magnetic resonance imaging and spectroscopy, thirteeth annual meeting of international society of magnetic resonance in medicine (Proc. Intl. Soc. Magn. Reson. Med.) 262, May 2005, Florida. [Abstract]

31. Engelbrecht MR, Jager GJ, Laheij RJ, et al. Local staging of prostate cancer using magnetic resonance imaging: a meta-analysis. Eur Radiol 2002;12:2294–2302.

32. Yu KK, Hricak H, Alagappan R, et al. Detection of extracapsular extension of prostate carcinoma with endorectal and phased-array coil MR imaging: multivariate feature analysis. Radiology 1997;202:697–702.

33. Tempany CM, Zhou X, Zerhouni EA, et al. Staging of prostate cancer: results of Radiology Diagnostic Oncology Group project comparison of three MR imaging techniques. Radiology 1994;192:47–54.

34. Mullerad M, Hricak H, Wang L, et al. Prostate cancer: detection of extracapsular extension by genitourinary and general body radiologists at MR imaging. Radiology 2004;232:140–146.

35. Yu KK, Scheidler J, Hricak H, et al. Prostate cancer: prediction of extracapsular extension with endorectal MR imaging and three-dimensional proton MR spectroscopic imaging. Radiology 1999;213:481–488.

36. Wang L, Mullerad M, Chen HN, et al. Prostate cancer: incremental value of endorectal MR imaging findings for prediction of extracapsular extension. Radiology 2004;232:133–139.

37. Hull GW, Rabbani F, Abbas F, et al. Cancer control with radical prostatectomy alone in 1,000 consecutive patients. J Urol 2002;167:528–534.

38. Bernstein MR, Cangiano T, D'Amico A, et al. Endorectal coil magnetic resonance imaging and clinicopathologic findings in T1c adenocarcinoma of the prostate. Urol Oncol 2000;5:104–107.

39. Wang L, Hricak H, Eberhardt S, et al. Prostate cancer – value of 3D endorectal MR imaging in the evaluation of seminal vesicle invasion in patients treated by radical prostatectomy. AJR Am J Roentgenol (Suppl);182:67.

40. Bellin MF, Roy C, Kinkel K, et al. Lymph node metastases: safety and effectiveness of MR imaging with ultrasmall superparamagnetic iron oxide particles—initial clinical experience. Radiology 1998;207:799–808.

41. Harisinghani MG, Barentsz J, Hahn PF, et al. Noninvasive detection of clinically occult lymph-node metastases in prostate cancer. N Engl J Med 2003;348:2491–2499.

42. Hovels AM, Heesakkers RA, Adang EM, et al. Cost-analysis of staging methods for lymph nodes in patients with prostate cancer: MRI with a lymph node-specific contrast agent compared to pelvic lymph node dissection or CT. Eur Radiol 2004;14:1707–1712.

43. Algra PR, Bloem JL, Tissing H, et al. Detection of vertebral metastases: comparison between MR imaging and bone scintigraphy. Radiographics 1991;11:219–232.

44. Turner JW, Hawes DR, Williams RD. Magnetic resonance imaging for detection of prostate cancer metastatic to bone. J Urol 1993;149:1482–1484.

45. Traill ZC, Talbot D, Golding S, et al. Magnetic resonance imaging versus radionuclide scintigraphy in screening for bone metastases. Clin Radiol 1999;54:448–451.

46. McNeal JE. Cancer volume and site of origin of adenocarcinoma in the prostate: relationship to local and distant spread. Hum Pathol 1992;23:258–266.

47. Eastham JA, Scardino PT. Early diagnosis and treatment of prostate cancer. Dis Mon 2001;47:421–459.

48. Rosen MA, Goldstone L, Lapin S, et al. Frequency and location of extracapsular extension and positive surgical margins in radical prostatectomy specimens. J Urol 1992;148:331–337.

49. Kim ED, Nath R, Slawin KM, et al. Bilateral nerve grafting during radical retropubic prostatectomy: extended follow-up. Urology 2001;58:983–987.

50. Sofer M, Hamilton-Nelson KL, Schlesselman JJ, et al. Risk of positive margins and biochemical recurrence in relation to nerve-sparing radical prostatectomy. J Clin Oncol 1853;20:1853–1858.

51. Hricak H, Wang L, Wei DC, et al. The role of preoperative endorectal magnetic resonance imaging in the decision regarding whether to preserve or resect neurovascular bundles during radical retropubic prostatectomy. Cancer 2004;100:2655–2663.

52. Coakley FV, Eberhardt S, Kattan MW, et al. Urinary continence after radical retropubic prostatectomy: relationship with membranous urethral length on preoperative endorectal magnetic resonance imaging. J Urol 2002;168:1032–1035.

53. Coakley FV, Eberhardt S, Wei DC, et al. Blood loss during radical retropubic prostatectomy: relationship to morphologic features on preoperative endorectal magnetic resonance imaging. Urology 2002;59:884–888.

54. Sannazzari GL, Ragona R, Ruo Redda MG, et al. CT-MRI image fusion for delineation of volumes in three-dimensional conformal radiation therapy in the treatment of localized prostate cancer. British Journal of Radiology 2002;75:603–607.

55. Roach M, 3rd, Faillace-Akazawa P, Malfatti C, et al. Prostate volumes defined by magnetic resonance imaging and computerized tomographic scans for three-dimensional conformal radiotherapy. Int J Radiat Oncol Biol Phys 1996;35:1011–1018.

56. DiBiase SJ, Hosseinzadeh K, Gullapalli RP, et al. Magnetic resonance spectroscopic imaging-guided brachytherapy for localized prostate cancer. Int J Radiat Oncol Biol Phys 2002;52:429–438.

57. Clarke DH, Banks SJ, Wiederhorn AR, et al. The role of endorectal coil MRI in patient selection and treatment planning for prostate seed implants. Int J Radiat Oncol Biol Phys 2002;52:903–910.

58. Jhaveri FM, Klein EA. How to explore the patient with a rising PSA after radical prostatectomy: defining local versus systemic failure. Semin Urol Oncol 1999;17:130–134.

59. Sella T, Schwartz LH, Swindle PW, et al. Suspected local recurrence after radical prostatectomy: endorectal coil MR imaging. Radiology 2004;231:379–385.

60. Silverman JM, Krebs TL. MR imaging evaluation with a transrectal surface coil of local recurrence of prostatic cancer in men who have undergone radical prostatectomy. AJR Am J Roentgenol 1997;168:379–385.

61. Coakley FV, Teh HS, Qayyum A, et al. Endorectal MR imaging and MR spectroscopic imaging for locally recurrent prostate cancer after external beam radiation therapy: preliminary experience. Radiology 2004;233:441–448.

62. Kurhanewicz J, Vigneron DB, Hricak H, et al. Prostate cancer: metabolic response to cryosurgery as detected with 3D H-1 MR spectroscopic imaging. Radiology 1996;200:489–496.

63. Parivar F, Hricak H, Shinohara K, et al. Detection of locally recurrent prostate cancer after cryosurgery: evaluation by transrectal ultrasound, magnetic resonance imaging, and three-dimensional proton magnetic resonance spectroscopy. Urology 1996;48:594–599.

Radioimmunoscintigraphy for imaging prostate cancer 51

*D Bruce Sodee, A Dennis Nelson, Peter F Faulhaber,
Gregory T MacLennan, Martin I Resnick, George Bakale*

SCOPE

The intent of this review is to describe the current state of radioimmunoscintigraphy (RIS) as applied to imaging prostate cancer in order to enable urologists and oncologists to identify cases where it can be used to facilitate staging of their patients' disease. The focus of study is fusion of functional images of prostate cancer and metastases on anatomically detailed images obtained from computed tomography (CT) or magnetic resonance imaging (MRI) in order to facilitate optimally delineating the extent of disease. The functional modalities discussed are positron emission tomography (PET) and single photon emission computed tomography (SPECT). In its most widely used oncologic application, PET is based on identifying the enhanced metabolic activity that generally accompanies carcinogenesis by using 2-[F-18]fluoro-2-deoxy-D-glucose (FDG) as the marker of metabolic activity. In contrast, SPECT imaging of prostate cancer is based on localizing the uptake of the monoclonal antibody (MAB) capromab pendetide, which targets prostate-specific membrane antigen (PSMA), an antigen that is strongly associated with prostate cancer. Functional images of FDG or capromab pendetide uptake superimposed on CT or MRI images provide a map of prostate cancer localization both within and external to the prostate. This map greatly facilitates staging the cancer, and thereby permits optimum treatment of the disease. The same map can also be used to guide radiation therapy, lymphadenectomy, or biopsy. The key to the success of this fused imaging technology is optimizing each step of the imaging process from patient preparation to image acquisition, processing, fusing, and interpretation. A range of illustrative case reports are presented to demonstrate various aspects of applying RIS to characterize prostate cancer and sites of its metastasis.

BACKGROUND: IMAGING CHALLENGES PRESENTED BY THE PROSTATE-SPECIFIC ANTIGEN ERA

The number of new cases of prostate cancer that were projected in the United States in 2004 is 230,110 and the number of deaths is estimated to be 29,900.[1] Although these projections indicate the gravity of the problem, the silver lining is the more than seven-fold difference between incidence and mortality, which indicates that prostate cancer is a treatable disease. This conclusion, combined with the variety of treatment options that are available, underscores the importance of selecting the most judicious treatment; and the fact that each treatment modality has therapeutic and morbidity characteristics associated with it that significantly influence the patient's subsequent quality of life further highlights the need to make every effort to identify and accurately stage prostate cancer.

Paradoxically, staging prostate cancer was made more difficult with the dawning of the prostate-specific antigen (PSA) era, which brought an increased awareness of prostate cancer that encouraged men to seek digital rectal examination (DRE) and PSA testing at earlier ages and with increasing frequency. This resulted in earlier discovery of prostate cancer, which had distinctive costs and benefits with the latter being diagnosis at an earlier stage at the cost of an increased number of negative biopsies. A far more important cost, however, is the understaging that occurred in a significant fraction of the cases for whom disease was assumed to be, but was not, confined to the prostate. In our multicenter study of ProstaScint imaging of 487 pretherapy patients with biopsy-proven prostate cancer, 26.5% were found to have pelvic node involvement.[2] Burkhard et al similarly reported that 109 of 463 (24%) of prostate cancer patients who underwent a lymphadenectomy had lymph node metastasis.[3] This problem of understaging prostate cancer has long been recognized[4] as having the morbidity and quality of life issues associated with the different treatment regimens of prostate cancer.[5] Thus, the need to establish if cancer is confined to the prostate or has metastasized to the pelvic nodes or beyond cannot be overstated and should be a high priority in managing limited healthcare resources. This is especially true in view of baby-boomer males now reaching the age where prostate cancer incidence increases.[6]

Finding prostate cancer at an earlier stage has exacerbated the difficulty of applying conventional anatomy-based imaging modalities such as CT or MRI to identify prostate cancer and its metastasis; consequently, the cost/benefit ratio of applying these modalities to detect prostate cancer has increased to an unacceptable level. This is reflected in the review by Albertsen et al in their analysis of 5667 men with newly diagnosed prostate cancer in the Surveillance, Epidemiology, and End Results Program.[7] In that study, men with PSA values ranging from 4 to 20 ng/mL were found to have positive bone scans and CT scans in less than 5% and 12% of the cases, respectively. Carroll et al also recently recommended in Part II of their "PSA Best Practice Policy" that bone scans, CT, and MRI should not be routinely recommended for staging asymptomatic men with clinically localized prostate cancer and a PSA level less than 20 ng/mL.[8] Similarly, Flanigan et al concluded. "we could not find any justification for routine preoperative CT scanning in patients with a PSA of less than 25 ng/mL" and they, therefore, recommended "abandoning the practice of routine CT scanning for lymph node metastasis in all patients with newly diagnosed prostate cancer."[9]

If CT and MRI cannot provide the information needed to stage newly diagnosed prostate cancer, what imaging modalities are available to do so? In contrast to the anatomic imaging modalities, functional imaging provides information pertinent to identifying various diseases provided that a characteristic marker is available that targets the disease and can be labeled with a radioactive isotope. An example of a functional modality is PET, which in its most widely used oncologic application is based on identifying the enhanced metabolic activity that generally occurs concomitantly with carcinogenesis. The marker of metabolic activity most commonly used is FDG, a

derivative of glucose labeled with positron-emitting fluorine-18 which accumulates at the site of metabolism upon phosphorylation. Although PET-FDG imaging can be used to image prostate cancer and its metastasis, doing so requires stringent cleansing of the patient's bladder to preclude occlusion of cancer by adventitious urine.[10,11] If rigorous bladder-cleansing precautions are not done, inconsistent results are obtained,[12,13] which we have described elsewhere.[14] Recognition of the shortcomings of PET-FDG to the routine imaging of prostate cancer in the clinical setting[15] has prompted the search for targeting agents that are more sensitive and/or specific than FDG; and several candidate agents have emerged, such as choline labeled with carbon-11[16] or fluorine-18[17] as well as [C-11]-acetate[18,19] and 16β-[F-18]-fluoro-5-dihydrotestosterone.[20] Two rapidly growing applications of PET imaging are PET/CT and molecular imaging, with the latter providing a means to translate key information at the molecular level to unlock the multifaceted intricacies of various cancers including prostate cancer,[21] whereas PET/CT illustrates the clinical value that the fusion of functional and anatomical imaging offers diagnostic medicine.[22]

The clinical success of PET-FDG/CT introduces RIS and the focus of this work, viz. fused SPECT-capromab pendetide/CT imaging, and, just as CT facilitates reading PET-FDG images,[14] fusing capromab pendetide images obtained with SPECT onto corresponding CT images analogously facilitates identifying abnormal uptake of capromab pendetide. This analogy, however, does not extend to the targeting agent of the two functional modalities. Whereas FDG targets the ubiquitous process of glucose metabolism, capromab pendetide specifically targets PSMA, which is strongly associated with prostate cancer (*vide infra*). Generally, labeled disease-specific MABs constitute the basis of RIS, and among the myriad of MABs that are used in RIS, capromab pendetide is the one that has been most intensively studied to image prostate cancer. Capromab pendetide is commercially available in the USA as ProstaScint® (Cytogen Corp., Princeton, NJ), which is labeled with gamma-emitting [111]indium. ProstaScint is the only MAB that has been approved by the US Food and Drug Administration (FDA) for two indications: 1) detection of metastatic disease in high-risk pretreatment patients with biopsy-confirmed prostate cancer; and 2) detection of prostate cancer recurrence and/or metastasis in post-treatment patients with a rising PSA.[23] As noted by Rosenthal et al in their review of capromab pendetide imaging, the clinical trials on which FDA approval was based were conducted using suboptimal technology and methodology, relative to today's standards.[24] Thus, technologic and methodologic advances since the 1996 FDA approval should have significantly enhanced the accuracy of capromab pendetide imaging. The fused SPECT-capromab pendetide/CT imaging that we have strongly advocated for several years[25] represents another quantum advance toward optimized imaging of prostate cancer. Before presenting details on the fusion technique that we endorse, attention is focused on the correlation between PSMA uptake and prostate cancer, which is the basis of capromab pendetide or ProstaScint imaging.

PROSTATE-SPECIFIC MEMBRANE ANTIGEN: KEY TO CAPROMAB PENDETIDE IMAGING OF PROSTATE CANCER

The target of capromab pendetide is PSMA which is a type II transmembrane glycoprotein (~100 kDa) that numerous studies have shown to be associated with prostate cancer and its metastasis.[23,26–32] The MAB used initially in these studies to identify PSMA was 7E11-C5.3, which was derived from the human prostate cancer cell line LNCaP. As the name implies, PSMA was assumed to be anchored to the cellular membrane and, therefore, was also assumed to be a stationary imaging target. This markedly contrasts with PSA, which is distributed in the circulatory system from secretory vesicles of normal and malignant prostate tissue as well as from benign prostatic hyperplasia (BPH).[31] Subsequent studies of PSMA in which more sensitive PSMA-detecting techniques such as Western blot analysis, flow cytometry and reverse-transcription polymerase chain reaction (RT-PCR) were used found that PSMA is also in the blood and serum of prostate cancer patients[33–40] as well as in other subjects including healthy young men and women.[37,39] Reports of this nature raise questions that are analogous to questions that have been raised regarding the clinical significance of micrometastases of other cancers,[41,42] and in both cases caution should be exercised in view of the exquisite sensitivity of these techniques that are reported to detect as few as two molecules of PSMA/mL blood.[40] Analytical techniques with sensitivities in this range are prone to false-positive results unless extreme precautions are taken.[42] In addition to these studies demonstrating that PSMA is not a stationary target as had been generally assumed, other studies have shown that PSMA is also produced in tumor-associated neovasculature of nonprostatic cancers[43] and, therefore, is a less specific indicator of prostate cancer than had been initially assumed. This association of PSMA with neovasculature suggests that capromab pendetide could be exploited to identify various types of cancers, which has been discussed by others.[43–48]

Another question regarding the association between PSMA and prostate cancer concerns the location of the epitope of PSMA that capromab pendetide targets—i.e., is the target extra- or intracellular?[49,50] If the latter, the implication is that PSMA is accessible to capromab pendetide only if prostate cancer cells have undergone necrosis or apoptosis. Contradictory results regarding the location of the epitope of PSMA that capromab pendetide targets were reported by Barren et al, who used fluorescein isothiocyanate labeling of capromab pendetide to show that the LNCaP cell membrane is permeable to 7E11-C5.3 and thus binding of capromab pendetide to viable prostatic cancer cells does occur.[51] This issue has been discussed in numerous reviews,[44–48,52–60] which combined with the plethora of clinical reports in which capromab pendetide was used to image prostate cancer[2,23–26,61–85] strongly implies that capromab pendetide indeed targets PSMA in vivo. In our studies of correlating capromab pendetide imaging of prostate cancer with the histopathology of the tissues imaged, negligible evidence of necrosis or apoptosis was observed in more than 15 cases studied (GT MacLennan, private communication), which indirectly indicates that capromab pendetide targets PSMA in viable prostate cancer cells in humans. This result and the clinical studies cited imply that the 4-day time of interaction between capromab pendetide and target PSMA that occurs in imaging prostate cancer in the clinical setting is not accurately simulated in some in vitro studies.

STAGING PROSTATE CANCER WITH CT/SPECT

Fusion of capromab pendetide uptake with anatomically detailed CT or MR images provides information on risk factors that strongly influence the prognosis and staging of prostate cancer, which includes factors both within and beyond the prostate. Among the former are mapping the location of prostate cancer and distinguishing between peripheral and transitional zone cancer, the implications of which have been discussed by Augustin et al.[86] Similarly, capromab pendetide uptake can be used to identify whether extracapsular extension (ECE) and perineural invasion[87] or involvement of the seminal vesicles[88,89] has occurred. Risk factors beyond the prostate include the FDA-approved application of identifying lymphatic metastases. In addition, two of the case reports that follow demonstrate that capromab pendetide uptake also identifies skeletal metastasis, which is one of the most prevalent sites of prostate cancer metastasis.[90] Examples of applying fused capromab pendetide imaging to identifying the aforementioned risk factors are illustrated in the five case reports that follow.

CASE REPORTS

The following five case reports show several salient points that vividly illustrate the value of fused capromab pendetide/CT imaging to localize and stage prostate cancer and its metastasis. These cases were chosen to illustrate specific points on the value of capromab pendetide/CT imaging from more than 600 cases that we have done using fused SPECT/CT. The cases described represent a broad spectrum of pre- and post-therapy prostate cancer patients with involvement ranging from prostate-confined prostate cancer to cases involving pelvic and abdominal nodes as well as bone metastasis.

CASE I

Case I is a 73-year old pretherapy patient with PSA of 10 ng/mL and Gleason score of 7. The three images illustrated in Figure 51.1 are axial views of the CT image, the SPECT image of capromab pendetide uptake at the same slice, and the SPECT image fused or coeregistered on the CT image. Comparison of Figures 51.1B and 51.1C vividly illustrate the advantages of fusing the SPECT image of capromab pendetide uptake on CT to facilitate identifying landmarks such as the femurs that the anatomic detail of CT provides. Figure 51.1C clearly shows ECE into the neurovascular bundle that is not evident in the SPECT-only image. Additional views of the same case but at the high-mid level are shown in Figure 51.2 in which ECE is shown. The dominant activity seen in Figure 51.2C is in the rectum *(green arrow)*, which could be misinterpreted as a false-positive without anatomic correlation. The uptake observed at this level is peripherally localized and extends into the low-mid quadrant, shown in Figure 51.3B *(white arrow)* while Figure 51.3A is an additional axial view of the base that shows ECE into the transition zone *(blue arrow)* and neurovascular bundle *(white arrow)*. No abnormal uptake was seen in the seminal vesicles nor in the pelvic or abdominal nodes. The preceding information is summarized and illustrated schematically in the sketch in Figure 51.4. A sketch of this type in which abnormal capromab pendetide is mapped at the four major quadrants of the prostate and in the pelvic and abdominal nodes is prepared for every case to facilitate comprehension of the imaging results by the patient and referring physician.

CASE II

Case II was 66-years-old at time of imaging and had a radical prostatectomy (RP) 9 years prior to imaging with a Gleason score of 3 + 3 and PSA of 10.3 ng/mL. Seminal vesicle involvement and ECE but no positive nodes were found at RP, and these adverse risk factors appear to have presaged the recurrence 9 years later. Post-RP, the nadir PSA was 0.1 ng/mL which had increased to 50 ng/mL at the time of imaging. Surgical clips from the RP are seen in Figure 51.5A, and fused SPECT/CT capromab pendetide imaging showed abnormal uptake in the left prostate bed (Figure 51.5B). Capromab pendetide

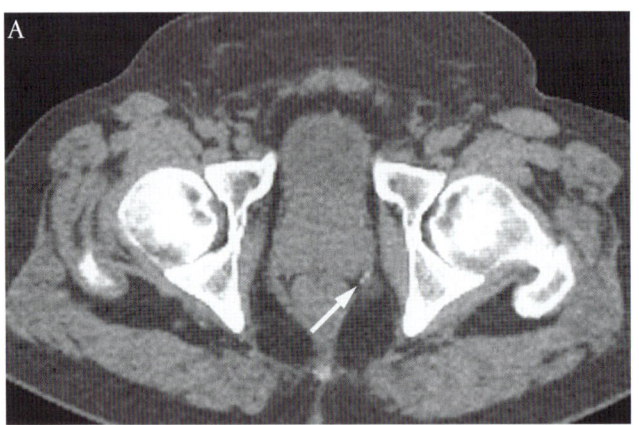

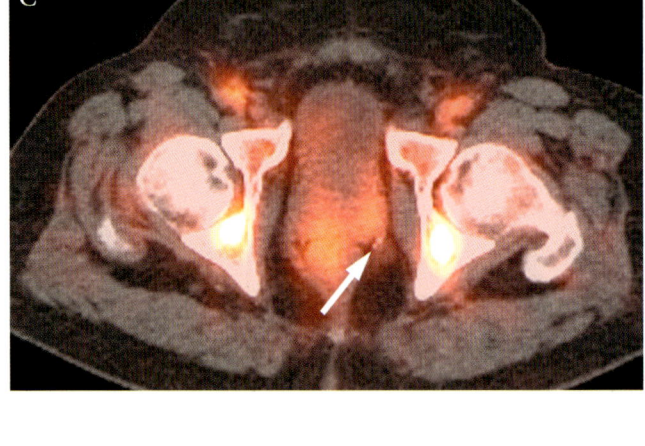

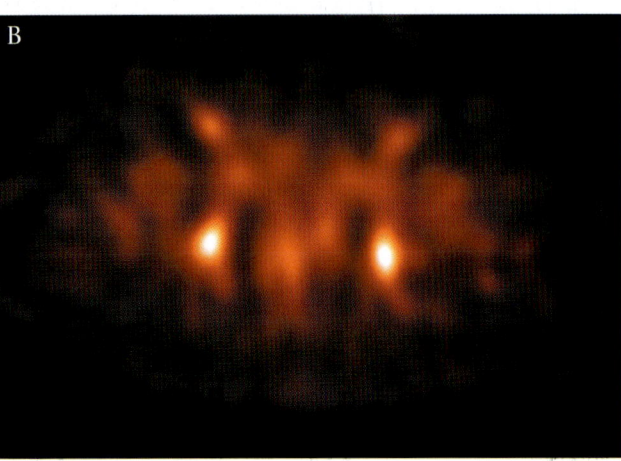

Fig. 51.1
Axial views of mid prostate of Case I imaged with *A*, CT, *B*, SPECT showing capromab pendetide uptake, and *C*, the same SPECT image fused on CT. *Arrow* indicates extension into neurovascular bundle.

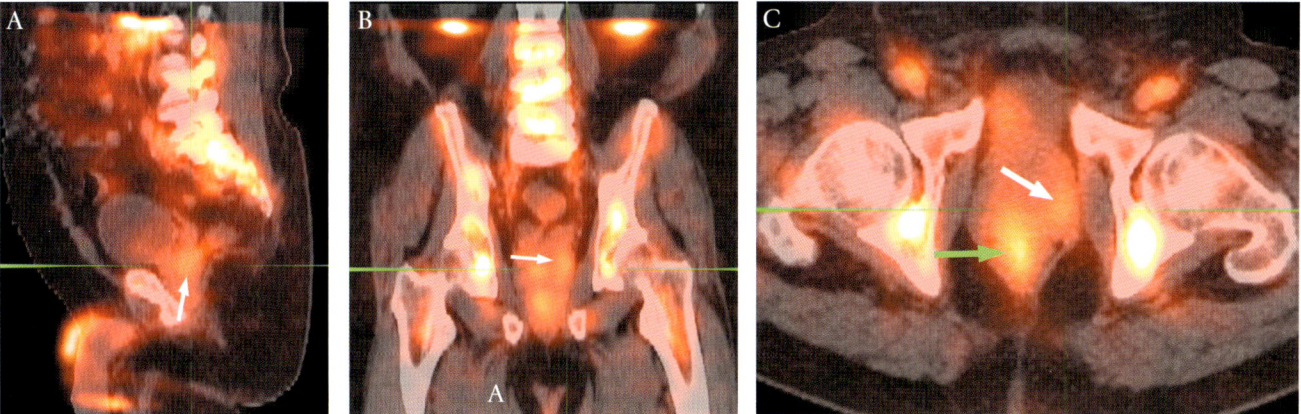

Fig. 51.2
A, Sagittal, B, coronal and C, axial views of mid-peripheral prostate of Case I with *white arrows* indicating extension into the neurovascular bundle. *Green arrow* in C indicates rectum.

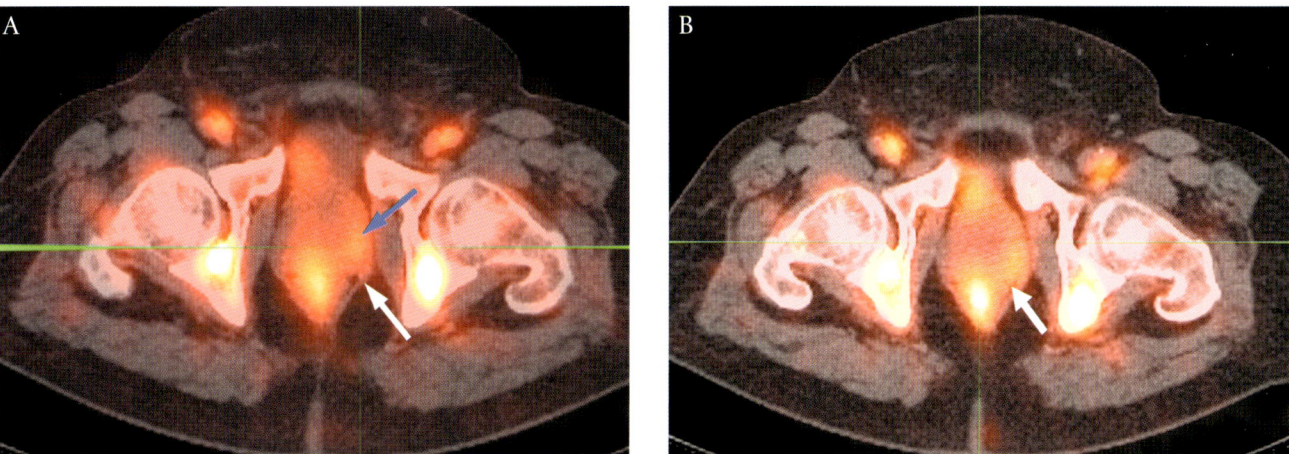

Fig. 51.3
Capromab pendetide uptake observed for Case I at: A, the base where extension into neurovascular bundle *(white arrow)* and transitional zone *(blue arrow)* are illustrated; and B, peripheral uptake in low-mid quadrant *(white arrow)*.

planar images showed no abnormal uptake in the prostate bed nor in regional or distal nodes.

CASE III

Case III is a 49-year-old patient with PSA of 5 ng/mL and Gleason score of 9 who had hormone therapy (Lupron®) initiated 4 months prior to imaging, during which time the PSA decreased to 0.2 ng/mL. Two bone scans were done prior to capromab pendetide imaging and were negative. Capromab pendetide planar images showed uptake in area of the prostate fossa and the left femoral lymph nodes. SPECT/CT capromab pendetide imaging showed abnormal accumulation in the right internal iliac lymph node measuring approximately 1 cm (Figure 51.6). Abnormal uptake was also observed in the left internal iliac node and in two left femoral lymph nodes measuring approximately 5.4 mm and 5 mm. Abnormal capromab pendetide uptake was also seen in the prostate from the base to the high-mid prostate.

CASE IV

Case IV is a 55-year-old with an unknown Gleason score and a PSA value of 6 ng/mL at time of imaging which was 4 years post-radiation therapy. A bone scan done immediately prior to the injection of capromab pendetide showed abnormal uptake in the left femoral neck and the right frontal sinus. Planar capromab pendetide images were negative, but fused SPECT/CT imaging showed abnormal capromab pendetide uptake in the left femoral neck and the prostate bed, which extends into the left external obturator muscle and the left seminal vesicle (Figure 51.7).

CASE V

Case V is a 51-year-old patient with PSA of 9.3 ng/mL and Gleason score of 9 (4 + 5) who had transurethral resection of the prostate (TURP) 2 months prior to imaging, and hormonal therapy (Casodex/Zolodex®), which decreased

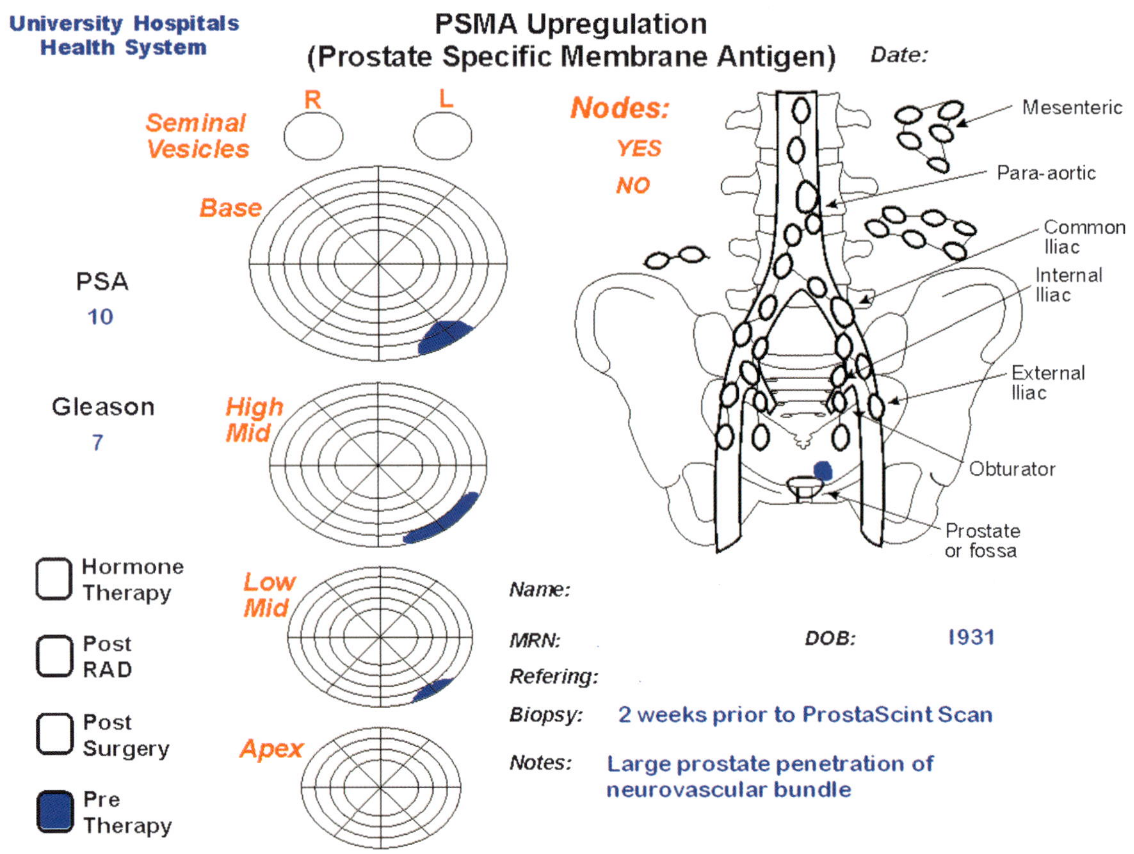

University Hospitals Health System

PSMA Upregulation (Prostate Specific Membrane Antigen)   *Date:*

Seminal Vesicles   R   L

Base

PSA 10

Gleason 7

High Mid

Low Mid

Apex

Hormone Therapy

Post RAD

Post Surgery

Pre Therapy

Nodes:
YES
NO

Mesenteric
Para-aortic
Common Iliac
Internal Iliac
External Iliac
Obturator
Prostate or fossa

Name:
MRN: *DOB:*   1931
Refering:
Biopsy: 2 weeks prior to ProstaScint Scan
Notes: Large prostate penetration of neurovascular bundle

Fig. 51.4
Schematic illustration of capromab pendetide uptake in four major quadrants of prostate and nodal chain for Case I. The only uptake observed beyond the prostate was penetration into neurovascular bundle.

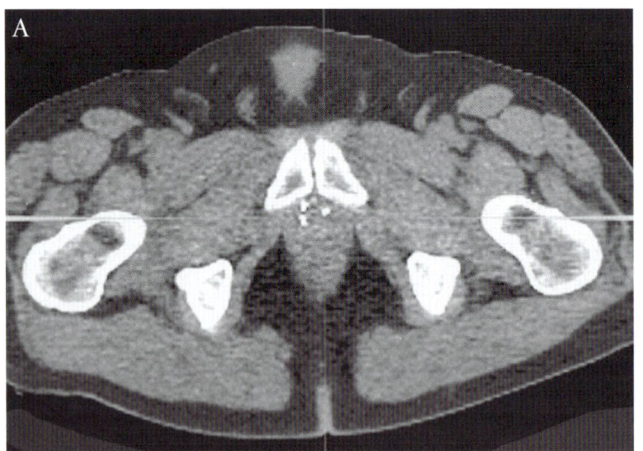
A

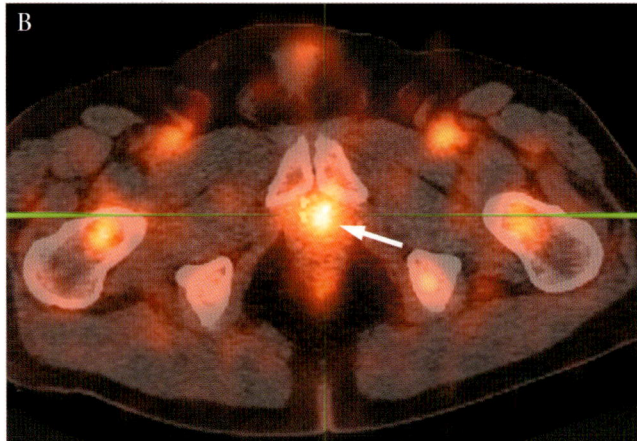
B

Fig. 51.5
Axial views of Case II. *A*, CT and *B*, SPECT fused on same CT showing extensive capromab pendetide uptake in left prostate bed as indicated by *arrow*.

PSA to 2.4 ng/mL at the time of imaging. Magnetic resonance imaging 1 month post-TURP showed abnormal intensity in the right acetabulum, bilateral ischium, and distal aspect of sacrum. A bone scan done immediately prior to the injection of capromab pendetide showed abnormal uptake in the sacrum. Abnormal capromab pendetide was also seen in the sacrum and right acetabulum with uptake ratios of target/background in these two regions being 9.6 and 6.4, respectively. Abnormal capromab pendetide was also seen in the prostate from apex to base at the right peripheral zone, and in the transition and central zones, as well as in the right seminal vesicle. The capromab pendetide uptake in the right acetabulum, right and left illum, and the. mid-sacrum are shown in Figure 51.8.

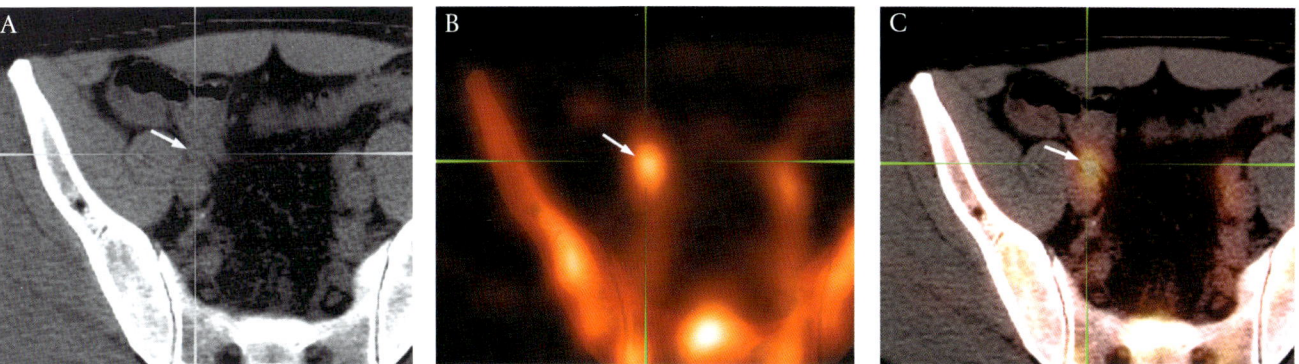

Fig. 51.6
A, CT, *B*, SPECT/capromab pendetide and *C*, the same image of *B* fused on *A* showing abnormal uptake in right internal iliac node of Case III.

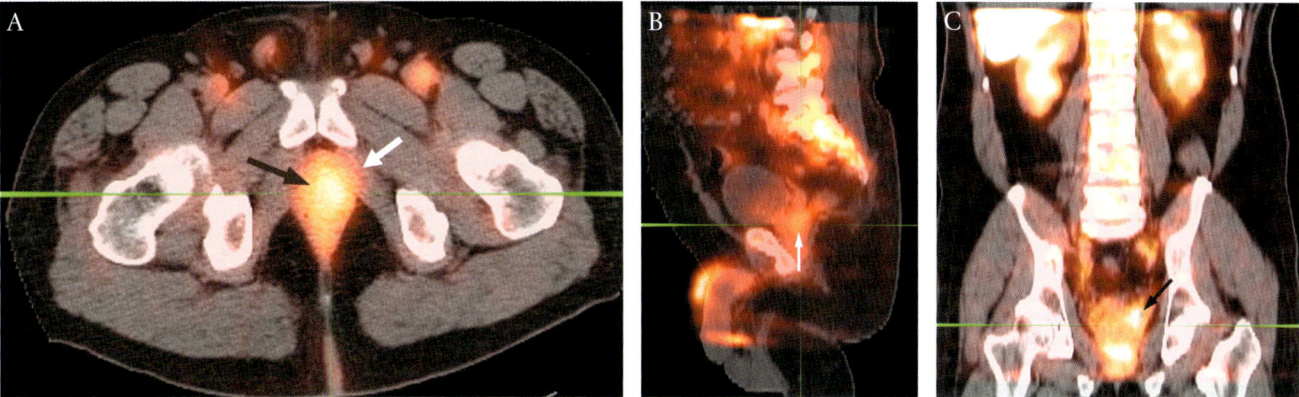

Fig. 51.7
Capromab pendetide uptake observed in *A*, axial, *B*, sagittal, and *C*, coronal fused SPECT/CT images of Case IV illustrating abnormal uptake in prostate in *A* and *C* by black arrow and left external obturator muscle by *white arrow* in A and B. Area of uptake inferior to prostate is rectum.

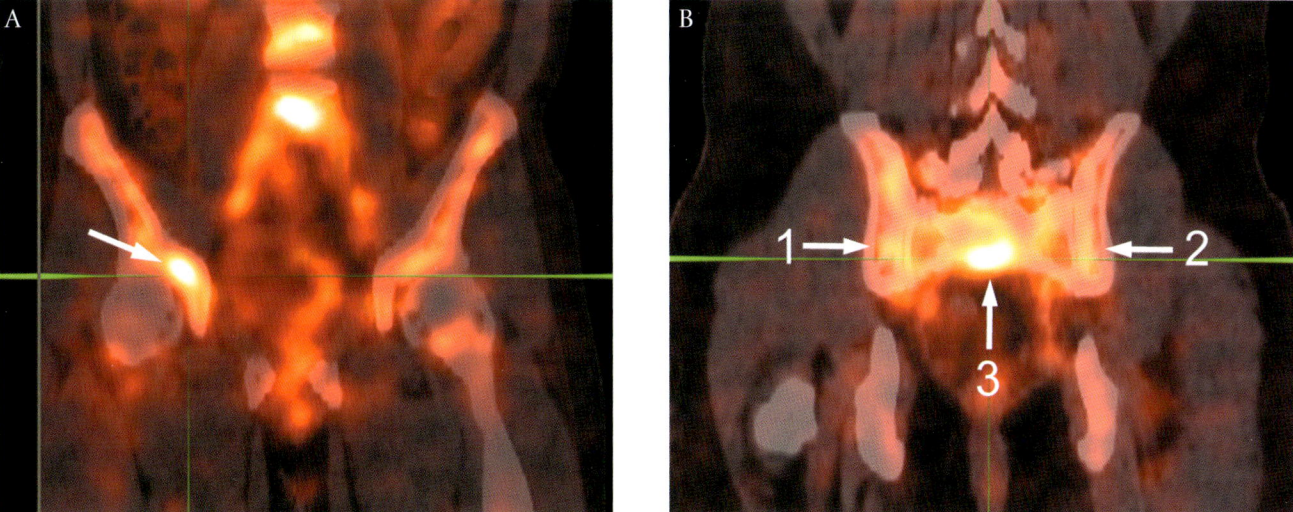

Fig. 51.8
Coronal views of Case V illustrating capromab pendetide uptake in *A*, acetabulum *(arrow)* and *B*, 1 and 2 denote right and left ileum, respectively, and 3 mid-sacrum.

DISCUSSION

The preceding case reports illustrate several points that vividly demonstrate the value of fused capromab pendetide/CT imaging to localize and stage prostate cancer and its metastasis. We have strongly advocated this fused multimodality imaging technique for several years,[2,25,77,91–94] and the value of this imaging methodology is being applied by others to noninvasively improve staging[95] and to guide the treatment of prostate cancer by radiation therapy (RT).[83,84,96–99] One of these capromab pendetide-guided RT studies, that of Shettino et al, dramatically illustrates the value of fused imaging in that 25 of 58 patients who were assumed to have regional or distal metastasis based on capromab pendetide imaging were found to have only local recurrence after fused capromab pendetide/CT imaging was done.[95] This change illustrates the value of fused imaging in decreasing the number of false-positive results, which has been one of the prevalent criticisms of capromab pendetide imaging.

Utilizing fused capromab pendetide/CT imaging to map prostate-confined prostate cancer is well illustrated by Case I for whom the images in Figures 51.1 to 51.3 could be used to optimize radiation therapy if that were chosen as the mode of treatment. As noted above, our fused capromab pendetide/CT imaging has been used in collaborations with radiation oncologists to guide RT which has been described by Ellis et al.[96–98] Case I also illustrates that fused capromab pendetide/CT imaging provides information on the risk factors of zonal location and ECE into the neurovascular bundle, which have been discussed by Augustin et al[86] and Beard et al,[87] respectively. Other significant staging information that capromab pendetide/CT imaging provides in Case I is the absence of metastasis to the lymph nodes. A final note on Case I is the sketch of capromab pendetide uptake depicted qualitatively in Figure 51.4. Sketches of this type are prepared from numerous fused images of each patient to provide the referring urologist or oncologist with an easily understood overview of the extent of prostate cancer to facilitate staging and formulating prognosis. The same sketch is also valuable in conveying the location and extent of disease to the patient.

Case II illustrates recurrence in a patient 9 years post-RP for whom planar images showed no abnormal uptake in the prostate bed or nodes, but fused SPECT/CT capromab pendetide imaging showed uptake in the left prostate bed. The recurrence is consistent with the seminal vesicle involvement and ECE found at RP. As noted earlier, involvement of the seminal vesicles is a well-established adverse prognostic factor,[87] which some view as tantamount to indicating that metastasis has occurred.[89]

Case III is of special interest in illustrating that capromab pendetide uptake was seen although the patient's PSA value was 0.2 ng/mL at the time of imaging. Referring urologists and oncologists frequently ask if capromab pendetide imaging is sufficiently sensitive to detect uptake when hormone or other therapy has depressed the PSA to less than 0.5 ng/mL, and Case III indicates an affirmative answer. Of the 620 patients whom we have imaged with fused capromab pendetide/CT, 22 had a PSA value of 0.1 ng/mL or less, and of these 15 had positive imaging results. For this case, abnormal capromab pendetide planar was seen in the prostate bed from the base to the high mid-prostate, the right and left internal iliac lymph nodes and two left femoral lymph nodes which suggests that the extent of disease is not reflected by the low value of PSA. Abnormal uptake in the right internal iliac node is also seen.

Case IV illustrates the general complementary value between bone scans and capromab pendetide imaging. Whereas a bone scan showed abnormal uptake in the left femoral neck and right frontal sinus, the planar capromab pendetide images were negative. Fused SPECT/CT imaging, however, showed capromab pendetide uptake in the prostate bed extending into the left external obturator muscle and seminal vesicle (see Figure 51.7) which, of course, was not seen on the bone scan.

The Gleason score of 9 for Case V combined with a pretherapy PSA value of 9.3 ng/mL suggest a poor prognosis prior to imaging which was borne out by both a bone scan and capromab pendetide imaging. The former showed abnormal uptake in the sacrum that was also seen with capromab pendetide imaging which also showed abnormal uptake in the right acetabulum, which illustrates that capromab pendetide imaging sometimes identifies bone metastasis that is not seen with bone scans. More significantly, abnormal capromab pendetide was also seen in the entire prostate and the right seminal vesicle which further diminishes the options available to the oncologist or therapist who is selecting treatment.

CONCLUSION

The preceding five cases demonstrate the clinical value of fused capromab pendetide/CT imaging in localizing and staging prostate cancer and its metastasis. The new generation of PSMA derivatives that are designed to target the extracellular domain of PSMA, which are actively being developed by several groups,[43–48] may offer increased sensitivity and specificity relative to capromab pendetide. When these newly developed MABs become available for clinical use, the fused imaging procedures described herein can be readily applied to these new targeting agents.

REFERENCES

1. Jemal A, Tiwari RC, Murray T, et al. Cancer Statistics, 2004. CA Cancer J Clin 2004;54:8–29.
2. Sodee DB, Malguria N, Faulhaber PF, et al. Multi-center ProstaScint imaging results in 2154 prostate cancer patients. Urol 2000;56:988–993.

3. Burkhard FC, Bader P, Schneider E, et al. Reliability of preoperative values to determine the need for lymphadenectomy in patients with prostate cancer and meticulous lymph node dissection. Eur Urol 2002;42:84–90.

4. Catalona WJ, Stein AJ. Staging errors in clinically localized prostatic cancer. J Urol 1982;127:452–456.

5. Bacon CG, Giovannucci, E, Testa M, et al. The association of treatment-related symptoms with quality-of-life outcomes for localized prostate carcinoma patients. Cancer 2002;94:862–871.

6. Metlin C. The American Cancer Society National Prostate Cancer Detection Project and national patterns of prostate cancer detection and treatment. Cancer J Clin 1997;47:265–272.

7. Albertsen PC, Hanley JA, Harlan LC, et al. The positive yield of imaging studies in the evaluation of men with newly diagnosed prostate cancer: A population based analysis. J Urol 2000;163:1138–1143.

8. Carroll P, Coley C, McLeod D, et al. Prostate-specific antigen best practice policy — part II: prostate cancer staging and post-treatment follow-up. Urol 2001;57:225–229.

9. Flanigan RC, McKay TC, Olson M, et al. Limited efficacy of preoperative computed tomographic scanning for the evaluation of lymph node metastasis in patients before radical prostatectomy. Urol 1996;48:428–432.

10. Leisure GP, Vesselle HJ, Faulhaber PF, et al. Technical improvements in fluorine-18-FDG PET imaging of the abdomen and pelvis. J Nucl Med Technol 1997;25:115–119.

11. Oyama N, Akino H, Suzuki Y, et al. Prognostic value of 2-deoxy-2-[F-18]fluoro-D-glucose positron emission tomography imaging for patients with prostate cancer. Mol Imag Biol 2002;4:99–104.

12. Hofer C, Laubenbacher C, Block T, et al. Fluorine-18-fluorodeoxyglucose positron emission tomography is useless for the detection of local recurrence after radical prostatectomy. Eur Urol 1999;36:31–35.

13. Sung J, Espiritu JI, Segall GM, et al. Fluorodeoxyglucose positron emission tomography studies in the diagnosis and staging of clinically advanced prostate cancer. BJU Int 2003;92:24–27.

14. Faulhaber PF, Mehta L, Echt EA, et al. Perfecting the practice of FDG-PET: Pitfalls and artifacts. In LM Freeman (ed): Nuclear Medicine Annual 2002, New York: Lippincott, Williams & Wilkins, 2002 pp 109–138.

15. Kotzerke J, Gschwend JE, Neumaier B. PET for prostate cancer imaging: Still a quandary or the ultimate solution? J Nucl Med 2002;43:200–202.

16. de Jong IJ, Pruim J, Elsinga PH et al. Visualization of prostate cancer with ^{11}C-choline positron emission tomography. Eur Urol 2002;42:18–23.

17. DeGrado TR, Coleman RE, Wang SY. Synthesis and evaluation of F-18-labeled choline as an oncologic tracer for positron emission tomography: Initial findings in prostate cancer. Cancer Res 2001;61:110–117.

18. Kotzerke J, Volkmer BG, Neumaier B. et al. Carbon-11 acetate positron emission tomography can detect local recurrence of prostate cancer. Eur J Nucl Med 2002;29:1380–1384.

19. Oyama N, Miller TR, Dehdashti F, et al. ^{11}C-Acetate PET imaging of prostate cancer: Detection of recurrent disease at PSA relapse. J Nucl Med 2003;44:549–555.

20. Larson SM, Morris M, Gunther I, et al. Tumor localization of 16β-^{18}F-fluoro-5-dihydrotestosterone versus ^{18}F-FDG in patients with progressive, metastatic prostate cancer. J Nucl Med 2004;45:366–373.

21. Czernin J, Weber W. Translational molecular imaging. Mol Imaging Biol 2004;6:181–182.

22. Townsend DW, Cherry SR. Combining anatomy and function: The path to true image fusion. Eur Radiol 2001;11:1968–1974.

23. Troyer JK, Beckett ML, Wright GL. Detection and characterization of the prostate-specific membrane antigen (PSMA) in tissue extracts and body fluids. Int J Cancer 1995;62:552–558.

24. Rosenthal SA, Haseman MK, Polascik TJ. Utility of capromab pendetide (ProstaScint) imaging in the management of prostate cancer. Tech Urol 2001;7:27–37.

25. Sodee DB, Faulhaber PF, Nelson AD, et al. Optimizing prostate cancer imaging: A new nuclear medicine technique improves prostate cancer diagnosis, staging, and therapy. Medscape/Radiology 2001;2: http://www.medscape.com/viewarticle/408705

26. Horoszewicz JS, Kawinski E, Murphy GP. Monoclonal-antibodies to a new antigenic marker in epithelial prostatic cells and serum of prostatic-cancer patients. Anticancer Res 1987;7:927–936.

27. Israeli RS, Powell CT, Fair WR, et al. Molecular cloning of a complementary DNA encoding a prostate-specific membrane antigen. Cancer Res 1993;53:227–230.

28. Wright GE Jr, Haley C, Beckett ML, et al. Expression of prostate-specific membrane antigen in normal, benign and malignant prostate tissues. Urol Oncol 1995;1:18–28.

29. Fair WR, Israeli RS, Heston WD. Prostate-specific membrane antigen. Prostate 1997;32:140–148.

30. Silver DA, Pellicer I, Fair WR, et al. Prostate-specific membrane antigen expression in normal and malignant human prostate tissues. Clin Cancer Res 1997;3:81–85.

31. Murphy GP, Elgamal AA, Su SL, et al. Current evaluation of the tissue localization and diagnostic utility of prostate specific membrane antigen. Cancer 1998;83:2259–2269.

32. Sweat SD, Pacelli A, Murphy GP, et al. Prostate-specific membrane antigen expression is greatest in prostate adenocarcinoma and lymph node metastases. Urol 1998;52:637–640.

33. Rochon YP, Horoszewicz JS, Boynton AL, et al. Western-blot assay for prostate specific membrane antigen in serum of prostate cancer patients. Prostate 1994;25:219–223.

34. Loric S, Dumas F, Eschwege P, et al. Enhanced detection of hematogenous circulating prostatic cells in patients with prostate adenocarcinoma by using nested reverse transcription polymerase chain reaction assay based on prostate-specific membrane antigen. Clin Chem 1995;41:1698–1704.

35. Lucotte G, Mercier G, Burckel A. The use of nested RT-PCR of prostate-specific membrane antigen in blood cells: Implications for the detection of haematogenous neoplastic cells in patients with prostate adenocarcinoma. Mol Cell Probes 1998;12:421–425.

36. Barren RJ, Holmes EH, Boynton AL, et al. Method for identifying prostate cells in semen using flow cytometry. Prostate 1998;36:181–188.

37. Beckett ML, Cazares LH, Vlahou A, et al. Prostate-specific membrane antigen levels in sera from healthy men and patients with benign prostate hyperplasia or prostate cancer. Clin Cancer Res 1999;5:4034–4040.

38. Su SL, Boynton AL, Holmes EH, et al. Detection of extraprostatic prostate cells utilizing reverse transcription-polymerase chain reaction. Semin Surg Oncol 2000;18:17–28.

39. Thomas J, Gupta M, Grasso Y, et al. Preoperative combined nested reverse transcriptase polymerase chain reaction for prostate-specific antigen and prostate-specific membrane antigen does not correlate with pathologic stage or biochemical failure in patients with localized prostate cancer undergoing radical prostatectomy. J Clin Oncol 2002;20:3213–3218.

40. Schmidt B, Anastasiadis AG, Seifert HH, et al. Detection of circulating prostate cells during radical prostatectomy by standardized PSMA RT-PCR: Association with positive lymph nodes and high malignant grade. Anticancer Res 2003;23:3991–3999.

41. Hosch SB, Braun S, Pantel K. Characterization of disseminated tumor cells. Semin Surg Oncol 2001;20:265–271.

42. Ghossein RA, Bhattacharya S. Molecular detection and characterization of circulating tumor cells and micrometastases in prostatic, urothelial, and renal cell carcinomas. Semin Surg Oncol 2001;20:304–311.

43. Chang SS, O'Keefe DS, Bacich DJ, et al. Prostate-specific membrane antigen is produced in tumor-associated neovasculature. Clin Cancer Res 1999;5:2674–2681.

44. Gong MC, Chang SS, Sadelain M, et al. Prostate-specific membrane antigen (PSMA)-specific monoclonal antibodies in the treatment of prostate and other cancers. Cancer Metastasis Rev 1999;18:483–490.

45. Chang SS, Gaudin PB, Reuter VE, et al. Prostate-specific membrane antigen: Much more than a prostate cancer marker. Mol Urol 1999;3:313–320.

46. Elgamal AA, Holmes EH, Su S, et al. Prostate-specific membrane antigen (PSMA): Current benefits and future value. Semin Surg Oncol 2000;18:10–16.

47. Chang SS, Bander NH, Heston DW. Monoclonal antibodies: Will they become an integral part of the evaluation and treatment of prostate

cancer—focus on prostate-specific membrane antigen. Curr Opin Urol 1999;9:391–395.

48. Chang SS, Heston WD. The clinical role of prostate-specific membrane antigen (PSMA). Urol Oncol 2002;7:7–12.

49. Troyer JK, Feng Q, Beckett ML, et al. Biochemical characterization and mapping of the 7E11-C5.3 epitope of the prostate-specific membrane antigen. Urol Oncol 1995;1:29–37.

50. Troyer JK, Beckett ML, Wright GL Jr. Location of prostate-specific membrane antigen in the LNCaP prostate carcinoma cell line. Prostate 1997;30:232–242.

51. Barren RJ, Holmes EH, Boynton AL, et al. Monoclonal antibody 7E11.C5 staining of viable LNCaP cells. Prostate 1997;30:65–68.

52. Maraj BH, Whelan P, Markham AF. Prostate-specific membrane antigen. Br J Urol 1998;81:521–528.

53. Lamb HM, Faulds D. Capromab pendetide — A review of its use as an imaging agent in prostate cancer. Drugs Aging 1998;12:293–304.

54. Haseman MK, Rosenthal SA, Polascik TJ. Capromab pendetide imaging of prostate cancer. Cancer Biother Radiopharm 2000;15:131–140.

55. Holmes EH. PSMA specific antibodies and their diagnostic and therapeutic use. Expert Opin Investig Drugs 2001;10:511–519.

56. Han M, Partin AW. Current clinical applications of the ¹¹¹In-capromab pendetide scan (ProstaScint Scan, Cyt-356). Reviews in Urology 2001;3:165–171.

57. Britton KE, Feneley MR, Jan H, et al. Prostate cancer: The contribution of nuclear medicine. BJU Int 2000;86:135–142.

58. Yao D, Trabulsi EJ, Kostakoglu L, et al. The utility of monoclonal antibodies in the imaging of prostate cancer. Semin Urol Oncol 2002;20:211–218.

59. Freeman LM, Krynyckyi BR, Li Y, et al. The role of ¹¹¹In capromab pendetide (Prosta-Scint®) immunoscintigraphy in the management of prostate cancer. Q J Nucl Med 2002;46:131–137.

60. Chang SS, Bander NH, Heston DW. Biology of PSMA as a diagnostic and therapeutic target. In Klein EA (ed): Current Clinical Urology: Management of Prostate Cancer, 2nd ed. Totowa, NJ: Humana Press, 2004, pp 609–630.

61. Abdel-Nabi H, Wright GL, Gulfo JV, et al. Monoclonal antibodies and radioimmuno-conjugates in the diagnosis and treatment of prostate cancer. Semin Urol 1992;10:45–54.

62. Babaian RJ, Sayer J, Podoloff DA, et al. Radioimmunoscintigraphy of pelvic lymph nodes with ¹¹¹Indium-labeled monoclonal antibody CYT-356. J Urol 1994;152:1952–1955.

63. Kahn D, Williams RD, Seklin DW, et al. Radioimmunoscintigraphy with ¹¹¹Indium labeled CYT-356 for the detection of occult prostate cancer recurrence. J Urol 1994;152:1490–1495.

64. Sanford E, Grzonka R, Heal A, et al. Prostate cancer imaging with a new monoclonal antibody: A preliminary report. Ann Surg Oncol 1994;1:400–404.

65. Haseman MK, Reed NL, Rosenthal SA. Monoclonal antibody imaging of occult prostate cancer in patients with elevated prostate-specific antigen positron emission tomography and biopsy correlation. Clin Nucl Med 1996;21:704–713.

66. Murphy GP, Maguire RT, Rogers B, et al. Comparison of serum PSMA, PSA levels with results of Cytogen-356 ProstaScint scanning in prostate cancer patients. Prostate 1997;33:281–285.

67. Hinkle GH, Burgers JK, Neal CE, et al. Multicenter radioimmunoscintigraphic evaluation of patients with prostate carcinoma using Indium-111 capromab pendetide. Cancer 1998;83:739–747.

68. Texter JH Jr, Neal CE. The role of monoclonal antibody in the management of prostate adenocarcinoma. J Urol 1998;160:2393–2395

69. Kahn D, Williams RD, Manyak MJ, et al. ProstaScint Study Group: ¹¹¹Indium-capromab pendetide in the evaluation of patients with residual or recurrent prostate cancer after radical prostatectomy. J Urol 1998;159:2041–2047.

70. Elgamal AA, Troychak MJ, Murphy GP. ProstaScint scan may enhance identification of prostate cancer recurrences after prostatectomy, radiation or hormone therapy: Analysis of 136 scans of 100 patients. Prostate 1998;37:261–269.

71. Kahn D, Williams RD, Hasemann MK, et al. Radioimmunoscintigraphy with In-111-labeled capromab pendetide predicts prostate cancer response to salvage radiotherapy after failed radical prostatectomy. J Clin Oncol 1998;16:284–289.

72. Levesque PE, Nieh PT, Zinman LN, et al. Radiolabeled monoclonal antibody indium 111-labeled CYT-356 localizes extraprostatic recurrent carcinoma after prostatectomy. Urol 1998;51:978–984.

73. Polascik TJ, Manyak MJ, Haseman MK, et al. Comparison of clinical staging algorithms and ¹¹¹indium-capromab pendetide immunoscintigraphy in the prediction of lymph node involvement in high risk prostate carcinoma patients. Cancer 1999;85:1586–1592.

74. Moul JW. Indium-111 capromab pendetide (ProstaScint) for the evaluation of prostate-specific antigen-only progression of prostate cancer. New Developments in Prostate Cancer Treatment 1999;4:42–45.

75. Murphy GP, Elgamal AA, Troychak MJ, et al. Follow-up ProstScint scans verify detection of occult soft-tissue recurrence after failure of primary prostate cancer therapy. Prostate 2000;42:315–317.

76. Fenely MR, Jan H, Granowska M, et al. Imaging with prostate-specific membrane antigen (PSMA) in prostate cancer. Prostate Cancer Prostatic Dis 2000;3:47–52.

77. Blend MJ, Sodee DB, ProstaScint: An update. In LM Freeman (ed): Nuclear Medicine Annual 2001. New York: Lippincott, Williams, & Wilkins, 2001, pp 109–138.

78. Sartor O, McLeod D. Indium-111 capromab pendetide scans: An important test relevant to clinical decision making. Urology 2001;57:399–401.

79. Moul JW, Kane CJ, Malkowicz SB. The role of imaging studies and molecular markers for selecting candidates for radical prostatectomy. Urol Clin North Am 2001;28:459–472.

80. Raj GV, Partin AW, Polascik TJ. Clinical utility of Indium-111-capromab pendetide immunoscintigraphy in the detection of early recurrent prostate carcinoma after radical prostatectomy. Cancer 2002;94:987–996.

81. Benaron DA. The future of cancer imaging. Cancer Metastasis Rev 2002;21:45–78.

82. Ross JS, Sheehan CE, Fisher HA, et al. Correlation of primary tumor prostate-specific membrane antigen expression with disease recurrence in prostate cancer. Clin Cancer Res 2003;9:6357–6362.

83. Jani AB, Blend MJ, Hamilton R, et al. Influence of radioimmunoscintigraphy on post-prostatectomy radiotherapy treatment decision-making. J Nucl Med 2004;45:571–578.

84. Jani AB, Spelbring D, Hamilton R. et al. Impact of radioimmunoscintigraphy on definition of clinical target volume for radiotherapy after prostatectomy. J Nucl Med 2004;45:238–246.

85. Wilkinson S, Chodak G. The role of ¹¹¹indium-capromab pendetide imaging for assessing biochemical failure after radical prostatectomy. J Urol 2004;172:133–136.

86. Augustin H, Hammerer PG, Blonski J, et al. Zonal location of prostate cancer: Significance for disease-free survival after radical prostatectomy. Urology 2003;62:79–85.

87. Beard CJ, Chen MH, Cote K, et al. Perineural invasion is associated with increased relapse after external beam radiotherapy for men with low-risk prostate cancer and may be a marker for occult, high-grade cancer. Int J Radiat Oncol Biol Phys 2004;58:19–24.

88. Ahlering TE, Skarecky DW, McLaren CE, et al. Seminal vesicle involvement in patients with D1 disease predicts early prostate specific antigen recurrence and metastasis after radical prostatectomy and early androgen ablation. Cancer 2002;94:1648–1653.

89. Johnson CW, McKiernan JM, Anastasiadis AG, et al. Prognostic indicators for long term outcome following radical retropubic prostatectomy for prostate cancer involving the seminal vesicles. Urol Oncol 2004;22:107–111.

90. Keller ET, Zhang J, Cooper CR, et al. Prostate carcinoma skeletal metastases: Cross-talk between tumor and bone. Cancer Metastasis Rev 2001;20:333–349.

91. Sodee DB, Malguria, N, Nelson AD, et al. Optimization of ProstaScint sensitivity in the diagnosis and staging of prostate cancer. J Nucl Med 2000;41:116P.

92. Sodee DB. Prostate cancer imaging 2002: Correlation with prostate cancer histology, In Pienta KJ, Getzenberg RH, Coffey (eds): Proceedings of AACR Conference: New Discoveries in Prostate Cancer Biology and Treatment. Naples, FL: 2001.

93. Sodee DB, Faulhaber PF, Nelson AD, et al. Multimodality imaging of prostate cancer. Mol Imaging Biol 2002;4:S50 [abstract].

94. Sodee DB, Bone, PET and ProstaScint scans. In Crawford ED (ed): Proceedings of the 13th Annual Prostate Cancer Update. Vail, CO: International Center for Postgraduate Education, 2003.

95. Schettino CJ, Kramer EL, Noz ME, et al. Impact of fusion of Indium-111 capromab pendetide volume data sets with those from MRI or CT in patients with recurrent prostate cancer. AJR Am J Roentgenol 2004;183:519–524.

96. Ellis RJ, Sodee DB, Spirnak JP, et al. Feasibility and acute toxicities of radioimmuno-guided prostate brachytherapy. Int J Radiat Oncol Biol Phys 2000;48:683–687.

97. Ellis RJ, Kim EY, Conant R, et al. Radioimmunoguided imaging of prostate cancer foci with histopathological correlation. Int J Radiat Oncol Biol Phys 2001;49:1281–1286.

98. Ellis RJ, Vertocnik A, Sodee B, et al. Combination conformal radiotherapy and radioimmunoguided transperineal 103Pd implantation for patients with intermediate and unfavorable risk prostate adenocarcinoma. Brachytherapy 2003;2:215–222.

99. DeWyngaert JK, Noz ME, Ellerin B et al. Procedure for unmasking localization information from ProstaScint scans for prostate radiation therapy treatment planning. Int J Radiat Oncol Biol Phys 2004;60:654–662.

Clinical applications of immunoscintigraphy for prostate cancer

Badrinath R Konety, Daniel Kahn, Richard D Williams

INTRODUCTION

Assessment of the stage of prostate cancer is critical in determining optimal therapy for the disease. Accurate staging is more important in patients with a high likelihood of extraprostatic spread, such as those with a prostate-specific antigen (PSA) greater than 10 ng/mL, Gleason 8 to 10 tumors, or with clinical stage T3 disease. Nuclear scintigraphy (bone scan) has been routinely utilized to assess bone involvement, while computed tomography (CT) scans and, more recently, endorectal magnetic resonance imaging (MRI), has been used to assess lymph node and soft tissue involvement as well as periprostatic extension. Traditional imaging methods such as CT and MRI utilize size criteria (>1 cm) to designate a lymph node as clinically significant and substantively underestimate stage, which may lead to false-negative scans in many individuals with small volume nodal metastases. Hence, currently, there are few options available to confirm metastatic sites even in patients who have a high likelihood of extraprostatic disease as predicted by commonly used preoperative predictive algorithms.[1] Identification of residual or recurrent disease following primary therapy such as radical prostatectomy or radiation therapy is also problematic. It is estimated that long-term biochemical failure after primary therapy can occur in as many as 40% of patients.[2] Determination of the extent of disease (local versus nodal versus extrapelvic) is critical in this situation as it will direct further therapy and impact prognosis. Traditional staging using CT, MRI, or bone scan have not always been very accurate in this setting, particularly in patients with small volume recurrence or metastases. These shortcomings of traditional radiologic techniques have prompted the search for better methods to image extraprostatic disease, both before primary therapy has been applied and to assess recurrent disease.

Monoclonal antibody-based imaging is one option that is conceptually attractive and has the potential to be highly sensitive and specific, allowing for the detection of even small volume disease. This approach has been investigated as a possible alternative to traditional imaging techniques for more precise staging evaluation of prostate cancer. Radiolabeled monoclonal antibodies to PSA and to prostatic acid phosphatase (PAP) have been used with limited success to image prostate cancer with metastases.[3,4] More recently, radiolabeled monoclonal antibody to the prostate specific membrane antigen (PSMA) has been widely investigated as this antigen is more ubiquitously expressed and retained in prostate cancer cells.

RADIOIMMUNOCONJUGATES

Radioimmunoscintigraphy (RIS) is based on employing antibodies directed against a tumor-associated antigen to facilitate detection of tumor deposits. To be used in RIS, the antibody must first be radiolabeled. Most whole anticancer antibodies used for RIS (including those used in patients with prostate cancer) are labeled with either [131]I (half-life, 8 days) or [111]In (half-life, 2.8 days). The isotope [99m]Tc (half-life, 6 hours) can be used with whole antibodies, but poses special problems in terms of the chemical labeling procedure and, due to the isotope's relatively short half-life, is not optimal for imaging whole antibodies. Protein labeling with ^{131}I is relatively simple using techniques such as the cholamine-T or

Iodogen methods. The principal disadvantages of RIS with ^{131}I-labeled antibodies are the dehalogenation that occurs and the lower dose of ^{131}I that must be used for safety concerns (both of which degrade image quality). Compared with iodinated antibodies, ^{111}In-labeled immunoconjugates offer the advantage of quality images (single photon emission computed tomography [SPECT]) when about 5 mCi is administered, substantially more stable binding of the radioatom to the protein, and a physical half-life that is approximately equal to the biologic serum half-life of many murine whole monoclonal antibodies. The main drawbacks of ^{111}In are that considerably more complex chemistry procedures are required for antibody labeling, and, unlike radio-iodinated antibodies, a significantly higher fraction of the injected dose normally accumulates in the liver, bone marrow, and other normal organs. This accumulation of activity degrades the lesion-to-background ratio such that tumor metastases in the bone and liver are often not detectable.

IMAGING TECHNIQUE

Following intravenous injection, most [131]I- or ^{111}In-radiolabeled whole antibodies have blood clearance half-times in excess of 24 hours; imaging, therefore, is typically delayed for at least 48 hours following injection. Imaging in patients receiving ^{99m}Tc-labeled proteins or peptides is often started by 4 to 6 hours and completed by 18 to 24 hours. In either case, the principal reason for the delay between the time of injection and scanning is to permit the activity in the blood (and, therefore, in normal body tissues) to decline so that antibody that is preferentially attached to the target site (e.g., tumor) can be detected.

Imaging has routinely been carried out using conventional nuclear medicine gamma cameras. Typically a planar, whole-body set of images is obtained so as to evaluate the entire body for sites of disease (Figure 52.1). The patient will have multiplanar tomography performed of the region(s) of the body which is (are) most likely to have disease present. Single photon emission computed tomography is more accurate than planar imaging when studying patients with cancer, and must be performed in all cases. The principal advantage of SPECT is attributable to the gain in lesion contrast. Consequently, smaller lesions that are otherwise obscured by radioactivity in adjacent sites are detected using this tomographic technique. Current gamma-camera technology has advanced to the point that larger field-of-view cameras are required, which are multi-headed and can have the camera head's orbit programmed to match a particular patient's body habitus. The newest generation of gamma cameras has a fully integrated CT unit. A CT/SPECT unit provides two data sets that are accurately registered to each other.

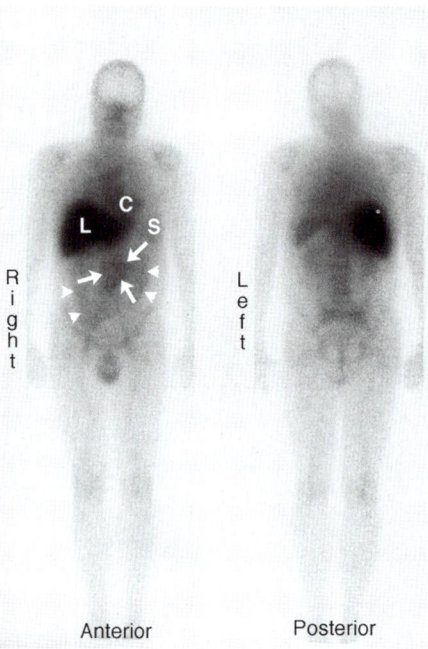

Fig. 52.1
Patient is status post-radical prostatectomy and has increasing serum prostate-specific antigen (PSA). Whole-body planar anterior and posterior images obtained 5 days after the injection of 5 mCi of ^{111}In-capromab pendetide. L and S represent normal activity in liver and spleen, respectively, and C is cardiac blood pool activity. Normal activity is also seen in colon *(arrowheads)*, bone marrow, kidney, large vessels and scrotum. Abnormal activity in the mid- and upper abdomen *(arrows)* is metastatic prostate cancer.

Fusion of the anatomic data (CT) with the functional specificity data of the antibody scan (SPECT) is routinely and easily obtained. The combined data set will permit interpreters of the studies to co-localize scan abnormalities with much greater confidence (Figure 52.2).

IMAGING ANTI-PROSTATE CANCER RADIOIMMUNOCONJUGATES IN HUMANS

In 1975, Kohler and Milstein first reported producing a monoclonal antibody through the use of their hybridoma system.[5] Until their method of producing "pure" murine antibodies became available, polyclonal antibodies had been used in clinical practice since about 1948, when Pressman and Keighley reported on their investigations of the murine kidney in vivo.[6] In the years that followed this work, a number of studies were performed using radio-iodinated polyclonal antibodies directed against a variety of tissues, including the pioneering work in tumors by Goldenberg et al[7] and Mach et al[8] in the late 1970s. The first report of RIS in patients with prostate cancer was published in 1983 by

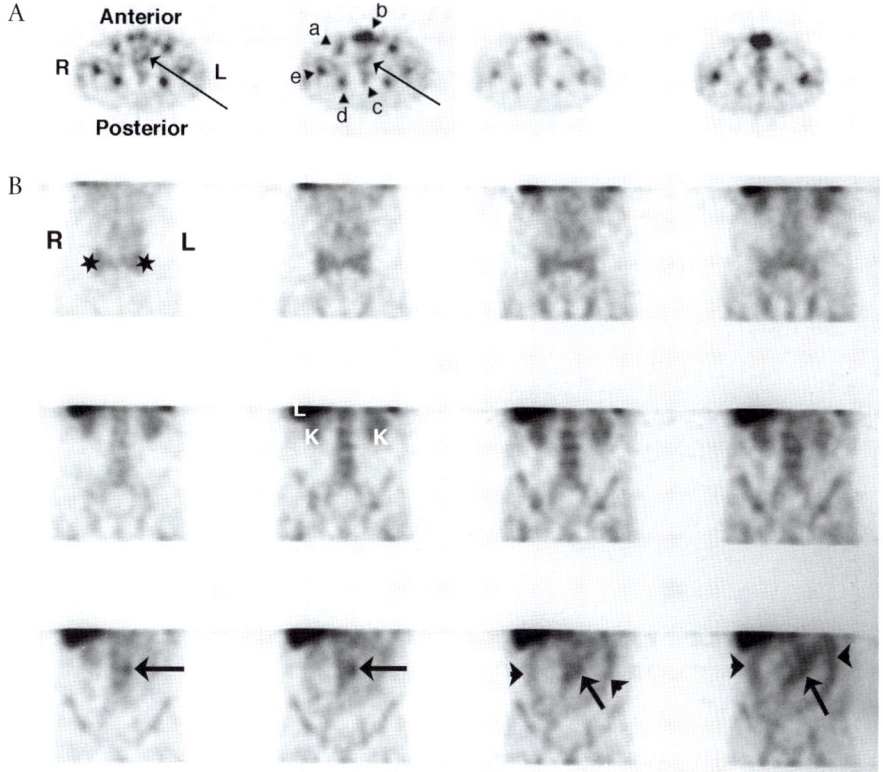

Fig. 52.2

A, Transaxial single photon emission computed tomography (SPECT) images from the patient in Figure 52.1. For reference, normal activity is seen in the following landmarks: external iliac (a) vessel, blood pool in base of penis (b), rectum (c), bone marrow in ischium and proximal femur (d and e, respectively). Abnormal focal activity *(arrows)* seen in prostate fossa region indicative of tumor. *B,* Coronal SPECT images from same patient. Slices move from posterior (top left) to anterior (bottom right). Normal activity seen in SI joints (*), kidneys (K), liver (L), colon *(arrowheads)* and in bone marrow. Abnormal activity, indicating tumor metastases, is seen in periaortic node region (bottom left two images, *arrows*) extending into mesenteric region (bottom right two images, *arrow*). (L, left; R, right.)

Goldenberg and DeLand[3] who later expanded their work in a larger group of patients with prostate cancer using the same polyclonal anti-PAP antibodies[9] (see Table 52.1). Prostate cancer soft tissue lesions were successfully imaged with these radioimmunoconjugates, and the authors concluded that RIS with this agent was safe and reasonably effective. Notably, bone lesions were not detected with this radioimmunoconjugate.

MONOCLONAL RADIOIMMUNOCONJUGATES

ANTI-PSA AND ANTI-PAP ANTIBODIES (Table 52.1)

Vihko and coworkers employed [111]In- or ^{99m}Tc-labeled monoclonal antibodies of murine origin or fragments against PAP.[10] They injected varying doses of protein and radionuclide in to four patients with prostate cancer. All sites of tumor, including the prostate gland, were seen with these immunoconjugates. They also reported five patients who, prior to scheduled prostatectomy and lymphadenectomy, had 1 mg of ^{99m}Tc-labeled F(ab)$_2$′ directed against PAP injected percutaneously into the

periprostatic space.[11] In one patient, abnormal activity was detected in multiple lymph nodes, including periaortic nodes. Histopathologic examination of multiple nodes in the obturator, iliac, and periaortic regions confirmed the scan findings in the single scan-positive patient, and confirmed the negative scan in the other four patients. The authors concluded from their preliminary data that lymphoscintigraphy may accurately determine the extent of regional spread of prostate cancer before prostatectomy.

Dillman et al studied nine patients, four with an anti-PSA monoclonal antibody (^{111}In-labeled PSA-399) and five with an anti-PAP antibody (^{111}In-labeled PAY-276).[4] With all doses administered, the fraction of tumor sites detected was 55% and 16% for the ^{111}In-labeled PSA-399 and the ^{111}In-labeled PAY-276, respectively. The results of this limited trial led the authors to conclude that antibodies directed against PSA were more promising than those directed against PAP. This same group confirmed their experience with anti-PAP radio-immunoscintigraphy in 10 patients following ^{111}In-labeled PAY-276 infusion.[12]

Babaian et al, using the same anti-PAP monoclonal antibody (^{111}In-labeled PAY-276), studied a larger series

Table 52.1 Monoclonal antibody-based imaging for prostate cancer

Authors	No. of patients	Antigen	Antibody	Results
Goldenberg et al[3]	2	PAP	Polyclonal	Bone lesions not seen; primary tumor imaged
Vihko et al[10]	4	PAP	Monoclonal	Primary tumor and extraprostatic sites imaged
	5	PAP	Monoclonal	Periprostatic injection; one patient with positive lymph node imaged 4/4 true negatives
Dillman et al[4]	4	PSA	PSA-399 (monoclonal)	55% of tumor sites imaged
	5	PAP	PAY-276 (monoclonal)	16% of tumor sites imaged
Halpern et al[12]	10	PAP	PAY-276	15% of tumor metastases imaged with high dose
Babaian et al[13]	25	PAP	PAY-276	Bone sensitivity with high dose 75%; lymph node metastases not detected

Modified from Kahn D, Williams RD.[13]

PAP, prostatic acid phosphatase; PSA, prostate-specific antigen

of patients (n = 25) with escalating doses of unlabeled antibody and 1 mg of the radioimmunoconjugate.[14] All patients had metastatic disease. The authors reported a high incidence of human anti-mouse-antibody (HAMA) formation in 8 of 16 tested, but no other adverse reactions. The sensitivity of the scan in detecting individual bone lesions (lesion sensitivity) as well as the presence or absence of bony metastases in any given patient (patient sensitivity) improved markedly in those cases receiving higher doses of unlabeled antibody (20–80 mg). Patient sensitivity increased from 40% to 100% while lesion sensitivity increased from 23% to 75%. The enhanced lesion sensitivity in this report, compared with series reported by Halpern et al,[12] is possibly explained by the dose of unlabeled antibody. In many of the patients in the series reported by Babaian et al, the dose was considerably higher than the dose used by Halpern et al. Notably however, lymph node metastases were not detected with this agent.

7E11-C5.3

The murine monoclonal antibody 7E11-C5.3 is an IgG1 protein. It is produced from a hybridoma using the human prostate cancer cell line LNCaP originally described by Horoszewicz et al in 1987.[15] This antibody recognizes a transmembrane prostate-specific glycoprotein (PSMA) that is only expressed by prostatic epithelial cells (benign and malignant) and whose DNA coding sequence has significant homology to that of the human transferrin receptor.[16] The monoclonal antibody 7E11-C5.3 underwent site-specific conjugation with the linker-chelator glycyl-tyrosyl-(N, e-diethylenetriaminepentaacetic acid)-lysine (GYK-DTPA) using the procedure developed by Rodwell et al.[17] The resulting immunoconjugate, 7E11-C5.3-GYK-DTPA labeled with [111]In (^{111}In-CYT-356/^{111}In-capromab pendetide

[ProstaScint®, Cytogen, Princeton, New Jersey, USA]) has been investigated in prostate cancer patients prior to or following radical prostatectomy. The 7E11-C5.3 antibody specifically recognizes an intracytoplasmic epitope of PSMA. This epitope is usually masked and can only be detected once exposed as in degenerated or lysed cells. Hence areas of necrotic prostate cancer are most likely to be detected by ^{111}In capromab pendetide.[18] It is a murine monoclonal antibody and hence prone to the generation of human anti-mouse antibodies (HAMA) when injected into humans. More recently, monoclonal antibodies to the extracellular epitope of PSMA have been developed in the mouse and have been humanized by replacing large portions of the mouse amino acid sequences with homologous, non-immunogenic, human amino acid sequences, while leaving the key antigen binding sequences undisturbed. This can be expected to decrease the likelihood of a HAMA response.

RESULTS OF ^{111}In-CAPROMAB PENDETIDE IMAGING

IN PREOPERATIVE PATIENTS

Several studies have examined the ability of ^{111}In-capromab pendetide imaging to identify biopsy confirmed primary tumor in the prostate. It has been noted that processing can image normal prostate tissue bearing the PSMA antigen as well. Hinkle et al identified uptake in the prostate in 47 of 51 patients before primary therapy for a sensitivity of 92% and positive predictive value of 100%.[19] Others have demonstrated a lower sensitivity: 88%[20] and 79%.[21]

A phase I/II trial using ^{111}In-capromab pendetide in patients with prostate cancer was reported by Abdel-Nabi et al.[22] Two types of patients were scanned: a group of men with no detectable metastatic disease prior to staging pelvic lymphadenectomy (n = 28) and a group of patients with known metastatic prostate cancer (n = 40). There were no significant adverse effects. Results of RIS demonstrated that 2 of 4 surgically-proven pelvic lymph node metastases were detected with the scan. The scan was correctly negative in 25 of 27 histologically confirmed negative lymph nodes. Sixteen of the 27 prostate glands (with confirmed cancer) were detected with the scan. In those patients with metastatic disease, 38 of 40 had bony lesions, which had been documented using conventional radiographic modalities. The antibody scan detected some lesions in 55% of these patients, but in only a minority of the patients were all bony lesions detected. Biopsy confirmation of bone lesions, particularly those that were discordant with the scan, were not obtained. In 4 of 6 patients with extraprostatic soft tissue lesions the scan was also positive. Overall, ^{111}In-capromab pendetide appeared to be safe, able to detect soft tissue lesions, but had only modest sensitivity for bone lesions.

Babaian et al assessed the diagnostic accuracy of ^{111}In-capromab pendetide for the detection of prostate cancer in the pelvic lymph nodes prior to bilateral pelvic lymph node dissection.[23] Whole-body scanning and SPECT were performed in 19 men two times, between 48 and 120 hours after ^{111}In-capromab pendetide administration. Titers of HAMA were not detected in any of the men

during follow-up. Results of the scan were compared with the histopathologic findings and the conventional radiographic appearance of the pelvic lymph nodes. Eight of the 19 patients had pathologic evidence of metastatic disease to the pelvic lymph nodes, with the scan detecting four of these cases. Abnormalities were detected in only 1 of the 8 patients using CT and MR imaging. The scan was normal in 9 of 11 patients who did not have metastatic cancer to the pelvic nodes.

Results on the largest group of preoperative patients who later underwent lymphadenectomy were reported by Maguire et al.[24] In 217 patients, a sensitivity of 60% was achieved for detecting lymph node metastases and the primary tumor was also identified on scan in 90% of cases. Results of other preoperative studies are shown in Table 52.2. Reported sensitivity and specificity range from 17% to 91% and 72% to 92%, respectively. Figure 52.3 demonstrates an algorithm that incorporates pre-treatment capromab pendetide scanning in the work-up of patients newly diagnosed with prostate cancer that we routinely follow.

IN PATIENTS WITH SUSPECTED RECURRENT PROSTATE CANCER

As part of the multicenter phase II and phase III trials, we and many other authors have studied patients following bilateral pelvic lymph node dissections and radical

Table 52.2 Results of CYT 356 capromab pendetide (ProstaScint®) imaging in patients with untreated prostate cancer

Authors	No. of patients	Sensitivity (%)	Specificity (%)	Positive predictive value (%)	Negative predictive value (%)	Pathologic confirmation	Comments
Babaian et al[22]	19	44	86	50	83	Yes	Each side of the pelvic lymphadenectomy assessed separately. Nine sets of nodes in 8 patients were histologically positive for cancer
Maguire RT[23] (abstract, J Nuc Med)	217	60	80	72	76	Yes	Primary tumor localized in 90%. 51/85 with pathologically confirmed metastases had positive scan
Sodee et al (1998)[56]	23	91	92	82	96	Yes	Study correlated scan results with sites of tumor on prostate biopsy
Hinkle et al (1998)[19]	48	75	86	79	83	Yes	Results are for prediction of extraprostatic disease
Polascik et al[43] (Cancer, 1999)	198	62	80	67	76	Yes	
Manyak et al[19] (Urology)	152	62	72	62	72	Yes	This pool of patients is included in the larger series by Polascik et al.
Ponsky et al[72] (Prostate Cancer Prost Dis)	22	17	90	11	94	Yes	Extended lymphadenectomy performed in all
Haseman et al*[35]	14	86	43	60	75	Yes	Assumed all negative biopsies were true negatives

*None of these patients received adjuvant hormonal therapy.

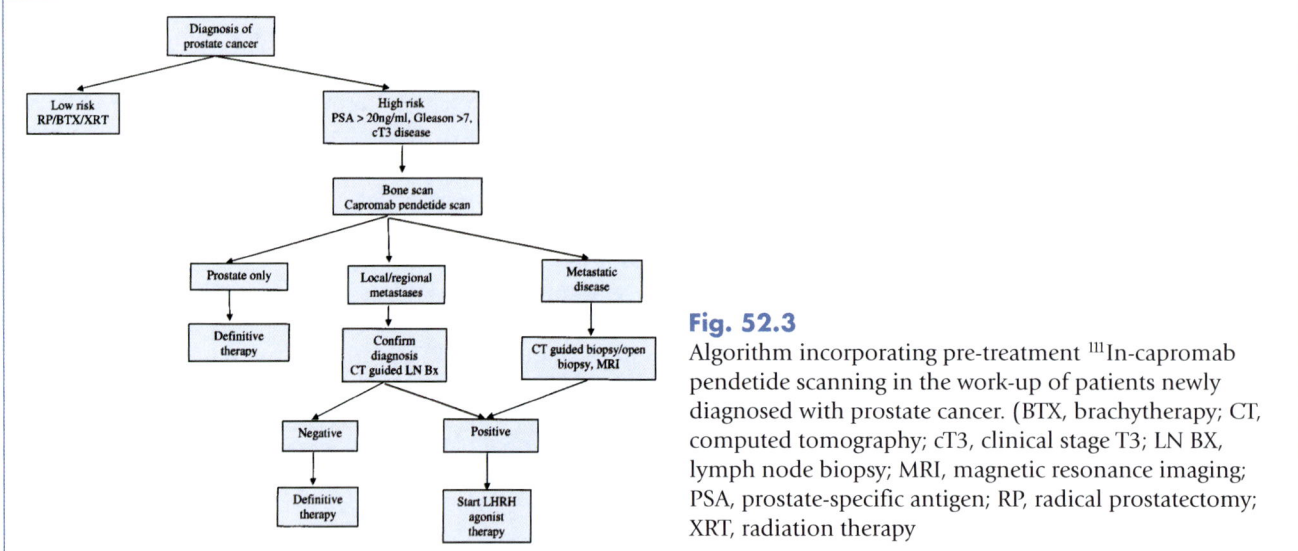

Fig. 52.3

Algorithm incorporating pre-treatment ^{111}In-capromab pendetide scanning in the work-up of patients newly diagnosed with prostate cancer. (BTX, brachytherapy; CT, computed tomography; cT3, clinical stage T3; LN BX, lymph node biopsy; MRI, magnetic resonance imaging; PSA, prostate-specific antigen; RP, radical prostatectomy; XRT, radiation therapy

prostatectomy with curative intent (see Table 52.2). All of the patients had evidence of residual or recurrent cancer as evidenced by abnormally elevated PSA (defined as "occult prostate cancer recurrence"). The patient's physical examination and all other tests, such as bone scans, CT, MRI, or transrectal ultrasound (TRUS) were negative for evidence of recurrent prostate cancer. We reported data from our institution and the Lahey Clinic Medical Center (Burlington, MA) obtained during the phase II trial of the first 27 subjects with occult prostate cancer recurrence.[25] In this series, we studied 27 men with 5 mCi of ^{111}In-capromab pendetide from 9 to 141 months (range) following radical prostatectomy. We did not detect a significant correlation between the serum PSA and the likelihood of detecting scan abnormalities. However, the initial pathologic grade of the tumor was related to the probability of an abnormal scan: those with disease confined to the prostate gland were statistically less likely to have disease seen on scan compared with those with unconfined disease (64% versus 94%). Based on scan findings from the initial infusion data, 22 of the 27 subjects had abnormalities seen in the prostatic fossa and/or extra-fossa sites. In 11 of 22 patients, some of the abnormalities were confirmed by CT or MRI or by fossa biopsy. Included in this group are subjects with abnormalities seen in the prostate fossa (biopsy confirmed, n = 8), mediastinum (radiographically confirmed, n = 2), abdominal lymph nodes (unconfirmed, n = 5), and lumbar spine (radiographically confirmed, n = 1). None of the subjects developed detectable HAMA titers during at least 8 weeks of follow-up. This preliminary data, like the data from the phase I/II trials described above, suggested that ^{111}In-capromab pendetide imaging was able to detect prostatic fossa cancer recurrence and that extra-fossa sites of soft tissue disease was also being seen.

In a subsequent multicenter phase III trial, 0.5 mg of ^{111}In-capromab pendetide was administered to patients with occult prostate cancer recurrence as defined

above.[26] This trial had the same entry criteria as did the phase II trial described above, except that all men had a TRUS-guided needle biopsy of the prostatic fossa within 8 weeks after the scan. Of 183 men, 181 had interpretable scans, of which 158 (87%) underwent a prostatic fossa biopsy. Scan abnormalities were seen in 108 of 181 (60%), and 18%, 17%, and 25% were seen, respectively, in the fossa only, the fossa plus extraprostatic fossa sites and extraprostatic sites only. Using the fossa biopsy as the standard, the sensitivity of ^{111}In-capromab pendetide (with 95% confidence intervals) was 49% (41–57%) and the specificity was 71% (63–78%). Examinations by CT or MRI were performed in 48 of the 76 (63%) men with scan evidence of extra-fossa abnormalities. In only 7 men were these scan abnormalities confirmed. We concluded that the relatively low accuracy of the scan was at least in part due to the diagnostic inaccuracy of a single fossa biopsy.[27–29] Abnormalities seen outside the prostatic fossa region, as in the phase II trial reported above, remain largely unconfirmed. While proof of accuracy is lacking, from our data it appears that, in patients who were treated with radical prostatectomy with curative intent, ^{111}In-capromab pendetide is able to detect prostate fossa recurrences with reasonable accuracy. The scan was certainly superior to reports of conventional techniques such as CT scanning, which has been shown to be relatively inaccurate.[30] More recently, pooled data from multiple institutions of 255 men with isolated biochemical recurrence following radical prostatectomy supported earlier findings that ^{111}In-capromab pendetide may localize sites of early recurrence.[31] When examining a subset of 95 of these patients who had known sites of disease recurrence, they found the sensitivity, specificity and positive predictive value of ^{111}In-capromab pendetide scan results to be 73%, 53%, and 89%, respectively, for site of disease. Values for regional disease (n = 60) determination were 76% sensitivity, 54% specificity, and 90% positive predictive value

(PPV). Corresponding values for distant disease identification (n = 46) were 69% sensitivity, 58% specificity, and 90% PPV. The comparable values for a positive CT scan or bone scan (n = 20) were 21% sensitivity, 63% specificity, and 65% PPV. Bone scan and CT scan results were not available in all patients. Importantly, the PSA value did not correlate with the likelihood of a scan abnormality, with no minimum abnormal PSA value necessary for a positive scan. As results from multiple studies indicate, the sensitivity of ^{111}In-capromab pendetide imaging ranges from 49% to 94% (Table 52.3). These results are based on studies in which biopsies were performed of the prostatic fossa or of the sites positive on the ^{111}In-capromab pendetide scan. It assumes that such biopsies detect all cancer present at that location, which may not necessarily be accurate, especially in the case of prostatic fossa biopsies. It is hard to interpret data from several other studies which report findings of ^{111}In-capromab pendetide scanning without any histologic correlation.[32,33] Figure 52.4 illustrates an algorithm we typically follow to decide when to obtain a capromab pendetide scan in a patient with rising PSA after primary therapy such as radical prostatectomy.

Jani et al analyzed the impact of ^{111}In-capromab pendetide imaging findings on clinical decision making and found that scan results altered clinical decisions in 18.5% of 54 post-radical prostatectomy patients referred for salvage radiotherapy.[34] In 11.1% of patients the radiation field was altered and in 7.4% of patients hormonal therapy was chosen instead of radiation, as the disease was suspected to be outside the pelvis based on scan results.

SIDE EFFECTS

The CYT 356 (7E11-C5.3) monoclonal antibody was developed in mice. Hence, one of the major concerns with the use of this antibody has been the development of HAMA, which in theory could elicit a strong hypersensitivity reaction on re-exposure. Most trials that measured serum levels of HAMA during the study report a rise in titers in 3% to 6% of patients,[20,26] which

Table 52.3 Results of CYT 356 capromab pendetide (ProstaScint®) imaging in patients with suspected recurrent prostate cancer

Authors	No. of patients	Sensitivity (%)	Specificity (%)	Positive predictive value (%)	Negative predictive value (%)	Pathologic confirmation	Comments
Kahn et al*[25]	181	49	71	50	70	Yes	Prostatic fossa biopsy assumed to detect all disease
Bermejo et al*[65]	31	94	42	53	92	Yes	Results are for 43 sites in 31 patients
Elgamal et al[34]	100	89	67	89	N/A	Yes	Only 33 patients underwent biopsy of suspicious lesions

*None of these patients received adjuvant hormonal therapy.

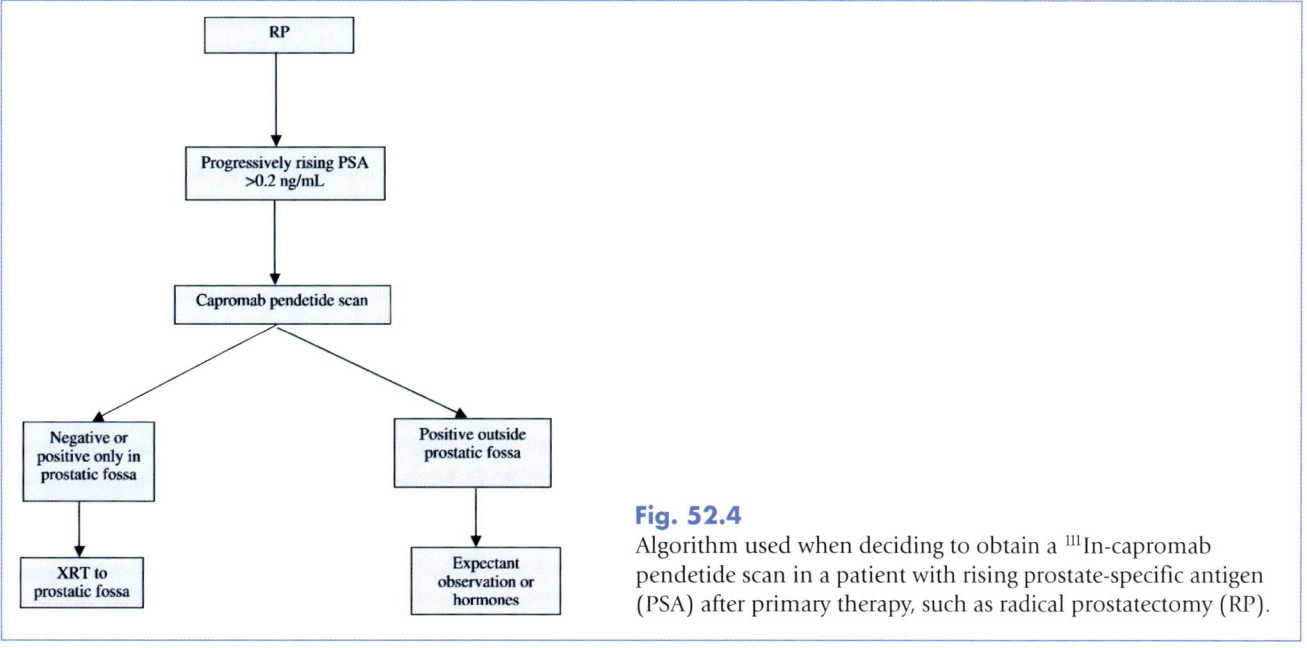

Fig. 52.4
Algorithm used when deciding to obtain a ^{111}In-capromab pendetide scan in a patient with rising prostate-specific antigen (PSA) after primary therapy, such as radical prostatectomy (RP).

typically revert back to baseline levels about 6 weeks to 6 months later. ^{111}In-capromab pendetide is generally well tolerated, with other side effects rarely being observed (hypertension, headache, reversible hyperbilirubinemia, rash, myalgia, eosinophilia, and paresthesias). It is reassuring to note that the threat of HAMA is not substantial as patients can undergo as many as four repeat scans without any reactions.[35]

COMPARISON OF ^{111}In-CAPROMAB PENDETIDE WITH OTHER IMAGING MODALITIES

Studies comparing the sensitivity and specificity of ^{111}In-capromab pendetide imaging to traditional methods to staging such as CT, MRI, and positron emission tomography (PET) scanning have yielded conflicting results. In a direct comparison between ^{111}In-capromab pendetide and 2-[F-18]fluoro-2-deoxy-D-glucose (FDG) PET imaging in 10 of 14 patients with recurrent prostate cancer, Haseman et al found that the sensitivity of ^{111}In-capromab pendetide was better than that of PET scanning (86% versus 17%).[36] Specificity was slightly higher with PET scanning than ^{111}In-capromab pendetide (50% versus 43%). All patients in this study underwent biopsy of the prostate bed within 8 weeks of ^{111}In-capromab pendetide scanning. In a similar study, Seltzer et al compared CT scanning, PET scanning, and ^{111}In-capromab pendetide scanning in 21 of 45 patients who had developed PSA recurrence following primary surgery, radiation or cryotherapy.[37] Only those lymph nodes considered abnormal on CT scan (>1 cm) were biopsied as long as they were accessible. Results of the three modalities were concordantly negative in 10 of 21 patients (48%). In the remaining 11 patients, 3 had a positive ^{111}In-capromab pendetide scan, 6 had a positive PET scan, and 10 had a positive CT scan. Upon biopsy of 6 of 10 patients with a positive CT scan, the authors found that CT scanning was more useful in identifying patients with lymph node metastases. However, there was obvious inherent bias in this study towards CT scanning since none of the patients with only positive PET or ^{111}In-capromab pendetide findings underwent a biopsy. Hinkle et al compared the combined sensitivities of traditional imaging modalities such as CT scan, MRI, or ultrasound to ^{111}In-capromab pendetide imaging in 51 patients scheduled to undergo pelvic lymphadenectomy.[19] They discovered that the sensitivity of ^{111}In-capromab pendetide for detecting biopsy-proven cancer in the prostate was better than that of the other imaging modalities (92% versus 51%). For detection of extraprostatic disease in the lymph nodes, sensitivity of ^{111}In-capromab pendetide imaging was higher than traditional imaging methods (75% versus 20%) while also yielding higher specificity (86% versus 68%). They also point out that in two of their patients, skip

metastases at the level of the aortic bifurcation with negative pelvic nodes were detected on ^{111}In-capromab pendetide imaging and confirmed histologically. While most studies report similar results of the improved sensitivity of ^{111}In-capromab pendetide imaging for detecting extraprostatic disease, traditional imaging modalities such as CT scan and MRI may be more specific.[20]

[111]In-capromab pendetide imaging appears to correlate poorly with other imaging results, with only 11.5% and 16.3% of patients having results on bone scan or CT scan, respectively, that matched with results on ^{111}In-capromab pendetide imaging.[31] Positive CT scan results are more likely to match with ^{111}In-capromab pendetide results than positive results on bone scan. Not unexpectedly, given the poor lesion-to-background contrast in bone, ^{111}In-capromab pendetide imaging was only able to identify 57% of the abnormalities on bone scan in one study.[35] Other studies indicate that ^{111}In-capromab pendetide imaging identifies metastatic lesions visible on bone scan in 13% and 55% of cases.[38,39] Even in cases with multiple lesions visible on bone scan, ^{111}In-capromab pendetide imaging was only able to identify one of these lesions in most patients.[38] Based on an artificial neural network algorithm that examined the accuracy of various serum parameters in predicting bone scan results in men with advanced prostate cancer, ^{111}In-capromab pendetide scan results were more predictive of bone scan results than serum PSA, free PSA, or PSMA.[40]

CORRELATION OF ^{111}In-CAPROMAB PENDETIDE AND LEVELS OF SERUM MARKERS

[111]In-capromab pendetide results do tend to correlate with tissue level expression of PSMA based on histochemical staining studies.[19] Foci of tumor as small as 4 to 7 mm can be detected on imaging that have later been confirmed histologically.[41] They do not however, appear to correlate well with serum levels of PSMA. This is not surprising given that the antibody is directed against the intracellular epitope of PSMA and the antigen is not secreted by the cancer cells. Murphy et al examined correlations between ^{111}In-capromab pendetide findings and serum PSA levels (Hybritech® Tandem-R assay, Beckman Coulter, Inc., Fullerton, California, USA) and serum PSMA levels determined by western blot densitometry.[42] Levels of PSMA were expressed as relative intensity levels and ranged from 0.1384 to 0.2198 in normal healthy volunteers 35 to 55 years of age. In preoperative patients with intact prostates, serum PSA correlated weakly with ^{111}In-capromab pendetide results, while serum PSMA levels only correlated with primary stage but not scan results. In this study, positive results in the prostate bed were

deemed negative in patients with intact prostates, which may confound the results. In patients who were post-prostatectomy but had not yet received secondary treatment, serum PSMA levels demonstrated a weak correlation with ^{111}In-capromab pendetide results. These findings were confirmed in a study of 100 patients and, again, it was discovered that correlation between serum PSMA and ^{111}In-capromab pendetide results were strongest in post-radical prostatectomy patients who had not yet received hormonal therapy.[35] These authors do acknowledge that the western blot assay for PSMA is not strictly comparable to a sandwich enzyme-linked immunosorbent assay (ELISA) assay used for PSA determination. The availability of an ELISA assay for PSMA may allow serum PSMA levels to be used as a guide to obtain ^{111}In-capromab pendetide imaging. Patients with elevated levels of serum PSMA may be better candidates for scanning than those with low PSMA levels. This group has also used ^{111}In-capromab pendetide scanning to assess response to immunotherapy in patients with recurrent prostate cancer and found disappearance or regression of scan detected lesions along with a decline in serum PSA levels in some patients.[43]

Many of the original studies that examined the value of ^{111}In-capromab pendetide imaging as a staging tool prior to primary curative therapy enrolled patients at high risk for extraprostatic disease.[19,20,44] Though many of these studies demonstrated that ^{111}In-capromab pendetide imaging had higher sensitivity than traditional staging methods for detecting extraprostatic disease, particularly in the lymph nodes, there is some concern if similar results could be obtained in patients who are at low to intermediate risk with lower volume of metastases. Many published algorithms[44–48] can predict the likelihood of pelvic lymph node involvement based on clinical variables such as serum PSA, clinical stage, and biopsy Gleason score with reasonably high sensitivity. In a direct comparison study conducted by Polascik et al, ^{111}In-capromab pendetide had a sensitivity of 61% compared with those of four clinical algorithms, which ranged from 87% to 98%, but the specificity of ^{111}In-capromab pendetide (80%) was far superior to that of the clinical algorithms, which ranged from 6% to 35%.[43] These authors also concluded that the inclusion of ^{111}In-capromab pendetide in the algorithms enhanced their predictive ability. There is no minimum level of serum PSA necessary to yield positive results on ^{111}In-capromab pendetide imaging, with levels less than 0.5 ng/mL yielding positive scan results in 68% of patients in one study.[29] ^{111}In-capromab pendetide imaging results are also consistent and repeat scanning in the same patient yielded similar results in 79% of cases and biochemical progression correlated with progression on ^{111}In-capromab pendetide in 24 of 34 (71%) patients.[40] Results of repeat ^{111}In-capromab pendetide scanning appear to correlate with clinical response to local radiation with disappearance of prior scan findings in the prostate fossa being reported following biochemical response to radiation.[49]

^{111}In-CAPROMAB PENDETIDE IMAGING AND RESULTS OF RADIATION THERAPY

Some of the strongest evidence to support the utility of ^{111}In-capromab pendetide imaging is derived from studies describing the outcome from local radiation for post-radical prostatectomy patients with biochemical failure based on positive scan results. Kahn et al retrospectively evaluated 32 post-radical prostatectomy patients with elevated serum PSA (1.1–2.4 ng/mL) who had positive results on ^{111}In-capromab pendetide imaging.[50] All of these men underwent salvage radiotherapy to the prostatic fossa and pelvis (a treatment decision made independently of the scan results) with curative intent. Prostatic fossa biopsies were positive in 62% of men with positive scans in the prostate bed. These men had PSA follow-up for a median of 13 months. In 16 of 23 (70%) patients with a negative scan, the PSA declined to less than or equal to 0.3 ng/mL and remained at or below this level for at least 6 months and at last follow-up (defined as a durable complete response). However, in men with scan evidence of disease outside the region of the prostatic fossa, only 2 of 9 (22%) had a durable complete response (difference significant, $P = 0.0225$). No other clinical variables were found to be predictive of a durable complete response. These results were updated with a follow-up evaluation at 55 months, at which time information was available on 29 of the original 32 patients. Sixty percent of men with a completely negative baseline scan and 44% with a scan positive in the prostatic fossa only continued to have undetectable serum PSA levels (<0.3 ng/mL) at 55 months following radiation therapy to the prostatic bed. There was essentially no change in the number of men who originally demonstrated positive results outside the prostatic fossa and remained PSA recurrence free after the longer duration of follow-up (22% versus 25%).[51] These findings indicate that scan results can predict the success or failure of salvage pelvic radiotherapy using PSA criteria. In a study by Levesque et al, response to salvage radiation was assessed in 13 of 48 post-radical prostatectomy patients with biochemical failure.[52] A favorable PSA response (<0.2 ng/mL) was achieved in 5 of 7 men (71%) who had positive scans confined to the radiation field, while 4 of 6 patients (67%) who had scans positive outside the radiation field experienced PSA failure in spite of radiation therapy to the prostate bed or pelvis. Wilkinson and Chodak retrospectively reviewed their experience in 42 patients believed to have recurrent prostate cancer after primary therapy.[53]

Fifteen patients received local salvage radiation after being found to have a positive ^{111}In-capromab pendetide scan isolated to the prostatic fossa. Ten of these patients (66.7%) experienced a PSA response to radiation therapy and in seven (46.7%) this response persisted at an average follow-up of 20.4 months.

At least one more recent study appears to contradict these earlier positive findings. Thomas et al retrospectively analyzed the results of salvage radiotherapy in 30 men who experienced biochemical failure post-radical prostatectomy.[54] They did not find any correlation between scan results and response to local radiotherapy with a median follow-up of 34.5 months. Only 1 of 4 of these patients had a prostatic fossa biopsy based on an abnormal digital rectal examination that revealed poorly differentiated prostate cancer. These authors also utilized the ASTRO criteria for judging post radiotherapy response. Alternative analysis using various PSA cutoffs of 0.2, 0.3, or 0.4 ng/mL did not alter the results of the study. Some potential proposed explanations for the difference in findings between studies pertain to the difference in imaging technique and lack of co-registration using CT scanning to better localize uptake to anatomic structures. As is evident from the conflicting results, further studies with tissue confirmation and long follow-up are required to better ascertain the value of ^{111}In-capromab pendetide imaging in identifying patients who would respond to local salvage radiation.

[111]In-capromab pendetide imaging has also been utilized to tailor transperineal brachytherapy. Areas of increased uptake on scan are targeted with higher dose (up to 150% of prescription dose). Using this approach, Ellis et al obtained a 4-year biochemical disease-free survival rate of 100% in 60 patients with low risk disease, which they argue is better than that reported by most other studies.[55] However, their follow-up was shorter than that of most other comparable brachytherapy series and they did not discuss their complications. Combination units that can obtain SPECT/CT images along with ^{111}In capromab-pendetide can be used in this setting with favorable results. In their series, 16% of patients also received either neoadjuvant or concomitant androgen ablation therapy and this could have also potentially influenced their results.

POTENTIAL CONFOUNDERS OF SCAN RESULTS AND STRATEGIES TO IMPROVE RESULTS

Potential reasons for false positive results could be vascular pooling particularly in the pelvis. Use of 3D imaging as well as dual isotope imaging with ^{99m}Tc-labeled red blood cells (RBC) to allow subtraction of vascular images may help obviate this problem.[56] Use of

a laxative or enema prior to obtaining the images will also avoid interference from tracer retained in the distal large bowel. Another approach to increase the specificity of ^{111}In-capromab pendetide imaging is to determine concentration of agent in the prostate relative to background of pelvic musculature. Sodee et al determined that a prostate to muscle ratio (P/M) of greater than 3.0 enhanced the predictive accuracy of the scan (see Table 52.2).[57] Most clinical studies of ^{111}In-capromab pendetide rely on the assumed accuracy of biopsies to verify the results of the ^{111}In-capromab pendetide scans. However, deposits of tumor that are not identified on initial biopsy but found on ^{111}In-capromab pendetide imaging may yet be detected by repeat biopsies of the same area and this may occur in as many as 20% to 40% of patients.[58]

Feneley et al investigated the ^{99m}Tc-labeled form of 7E.11-C5.3 (^{99m}Tc-CYT-351) in 22 patients prior to and after prostatectomy.[59] Their patients included a mixture of those with incidental carcinoma following prostatectomy for apparently benign disease through patients with metastatic cancer. Based on results from small subgroups of these patients, the authors conclude that this agent is able to detect cancer in the prostate fossa and in lymph node regions. However, only 1 of the 5 men with bone metastases documented by bone scan showed abnormal accumulation of this agent. While the data using ^{99m}Tc-CYT-351 is sparse, the ^{99m}Tc-labeled antibody offers potential advantages over the ^{111}In-labeled form, including study completion time (1 day versus 3–5 days for ^{111}In-capromab pendetide) and possible improved image quality. Further investigations with this agent seem warranted.

More recently, monoclonal antibodies have been developed to the extracellular epitope of PSMA.[60,61] Four of these IgG antibodies (J591, J415, J533, and E99) can recognize at least two distinct extracellular epitopes of PSMA. One of these antibodies (J591) has been humanized—by removing the mouse immunogenic amino acid sequences and replacing them with human amino acid sequences—and bound to ^{111}In-DOTA or ^{177}Lu-DOTA and used in two phase I trials for the treatment of metastatic prostate cancer.[62,63] Comparison of identification of metastatic deposits by J591 in these studies suggests that this antibody can identify up to 94% of all bony metastatic deposits identifiable on standard bone scans. This is a much higher percentage than identifiable by ^{111}In-capromab pendetide imaging where, at best, only about 57% are identifiable.[35] Identification of soft tissue lesions is slightly lower with 72% of patients demonstrating extrahepatic soft tissue metastases on CT scans being identified by J591 imaging.[62] In the preliminary analysis by Bander et al it does appear that targeting with the ^{177}Lu-J591 or ^{111}In-DOTA antibody demonstrated better correlation with standard imaging modalities (CT scan, bone scan) than with the ^{111}In-J591 antibody. The J591 antibody has been conjugated with Yttrium-90 for targeted radiotherapy of metastatic prostate cancer in a phase I study.[63] Prostate-specific antigen responses were observed in 2 of 21 patients treated and no human-anti-human antibody (HAHA) responses were observed, eliminating one of the concerns attendant upon using the murine antibody in CYT-356 for repeat therapies. Further studies both for imaging and targeted radiotherapy are underway with the J591 antibody, which will better define its utility in diagnosing and treating prostate cancer.

Other tumors, such as renal cell carcinoma,[64] adrenal myelolipoma,[65] meningioma,[66] non-Hodgkin lymphoma,[67] and neurofibroma[68] can also be inadvertently identified by ^{111}In-capromab pendetide scans. Presence of a pelvic kidney can confuse the results, particularly in the presence of a primary prostate tumor, as the kidney can appear as a site with significant uptake of antibody.[69] However, ^{111}In-capromab pendetide imaging may help identify uncommon sites of prostate cancer metastases such as the brain[70] or supraclavicular nodes,[71] which may help avoid needless exploration.

REFERENCES

1. Partin AW, Subong ENP, Walsh PC, et al. Combination of prostate-specific antigen, clinical stage and Gleason score to predict pathological stage of localized prostate cancer: a multi-institutional update. JAMA 1997;277:1445–1451.

2. Han M, Partin AW, Zahurak M, et al. Biochemical (prostate specific antigen) recurrence probability following radical prostatectomy for clinically localized prostate cancer. J Urol 2003;169:517–523.

3. Goldenberg DM, DeLand F, Kim E, et al. Use of radiolabeled antibodies to carcinoembryonic antigen for the detection and localization of diverse cancers by external photoscanning. N Engl J Med 1978;298:1384–1386.

4. Dillman RO, Beauregard J, Ryan KP, et al. Radioimmunodetection of cancer with the use of indium-[111]labeled monoclonal antibodies. NCI Monogr 1987;3:33–36.

5. Kohler G, Milstein C. Continuous cultures of fused cells secreting antibody of predefined specificity. Nature 1975;256:495–497.

6. Pressman D, Keighley G. The zone of activity of antibodies as determined by the use of radioactive tracers: the zone of activity of nephrotoxic antikidney serum. J Immunol 1948;59:141–146.

7. Goldenberg DM, DeLand FH, Bennett SJ, et al. Radioimmunodetection of prostate cancer. In vivo use of radioactive antibodies against prostatic acid phosphatase for diagnosis and detection of prostatic cancer by nuclear imaging. JAMA 1983;250:630–635.

8. Mach JP, Carrel S, Forni M, et al. Tumor localization of radiolabeled antibodies against carcinoembryonic antigen in patients with carcinoma. N Engl J Med 1980;305:5–10.

9. Goldenberg DM, DeLand FH. Clinical studies of prostatic cancer imaging with radiolabeled antibodies against prostatic acid phosphatase. Urol Clin North Am 1984;11:277–281.

10. Vihko P, Kontturi M, Lukkarinem O, et al. Radioimaging of prostate and metastases of prostate carcinoma with Tc 99m-labeled prostatic acid phosphatase-specific antibodies and their Fab fragments. Am Clin Res 1984;16:51–52.

11. Vihko P, Kontturi M, Lukkarinen O, et al. Immunoscintigraphic evaluation of lymph node involvement in prostate carcinoma. Prostate 1987;11:51–57.

12. Halpern SE, Haindl W, Beauregard J, et al. Scintigraphy with indium-labeled monoclonal antibodies: kinetics, biodistribution, and tumor detection. Radiology 1988;168:529–536.

13. Kahn D, Williams RD. Radioimmunoscintigraphy and Radioimmunotherapy in Cancer of the Prostate. In Petrovich Z, Baert

L, Brady LW (eds): Carcinoma of the Prostate: Diagnositc Imaging. Berlin: Springer-Verlag, pp 55–64, 1996.

14. Babaian RJ, Murray JL, Lamki LM, et al. Radioimmunological imaging of metastatic prostatic cancer with [111]Indium-labeled monoclonal antibody PAY-276. J Urol 1987;137:439–443.

15. Horoszewicz JS, Kawinski E, Murphy GP. Monoclonal antibodies to a new antigenic marker in epithelial prostatic cells and serum of prostatic cancer patients. Anticancer Res 1987;7:927–936.

16. Israeli RS, Powel CT, Fair WR, et al. Molecular cloning of a complementary DNA encoding a prostate-specific membrane antigen. Cancer Res 1993;53:227–230.

17. Rodwell JD, Alvarez VL, Lee C, et al. Site-specific covalent modification of monoclonal antibodies: in vitro and in vivo evaluations. Proc Natl Acad Sci USA 1986;83:2632–2636.

18. Smith-Jones PM, Vallabhajosula S, Navaro V, Bastidas D, Goldsmith SJ, Bander NH. Radiolabeled monoclonal antibodies specific to the extracellular domain of prostate specific membrane antigen: preclinical studies in nude mice bearing LnCaP human prostate tumor. J Nucl Med 2003;44:610.

19. Hinkle GH, Burgers JK, Neal CE, et al. Multicenter radioimmunoscintigraphic evaluation of patients with prostate carcinoma using indium-111 capromab pendetide. Cancer 1998;83:739–747.

20. Manyak MJ, Hinkle GH, Olsen JO, et al, For the ProstaScint Study Group. Immunoscintigraphy with indium-[111]capromab pendetide: evaluation before definitive therapy in patients with prostate cancer. Urology 1999;54:1058–1063.

21. Ellis RJ, Kim EY, Conant R, et al. Radioimmunoguided imaging of prostate cancer foci with histopathological correlation. Int J Radiat Oncol Biol Phys 2001;49:1281–1286.

22. Abdel-Nabi H, Wright GL, Gulfo JV, et al. Monoclonal antibodies and radioimmunoconjugates in the diagnosis and treatment of prostate cancer. Sem Urol 1992;10:45–54.

23. Babaian RJ, Sayer J, Podoloff DA, et al. Radioimmunoscintigraphy of pelvic lymph nodes with In-111-labeled monoclonal antibody CYT-356. J Urol 1994;152:1952–1955.

24. Maguire RT and the Capromab Pendetide Study Group. In-111 Capromab Pendetide (111In-capromab pendetide) for presurgical staging of patients with prostate cancer. J Nuc Med Proceedings of the 42nd Annual Meeting. 1995;10P (#29).

25. Kahn D, Williams RD, Seldin DW, et al. Radioimmunoscintigraphy with [111]Indium labeled CTY-356 for the detection of occult prostate cancer recurrence. J Urol 1994;152:1490–1495.

26. Kahn D, Williams RD, Manyak MJ, et al. In-111 capromab pendetide in the evaluation of patients with residual or recurrent prostate after radical prostatectomy. J Urol 1998;159:2041–2047.

27. Abi-Aad AS, MacFarlane MT, Stein A, et al. Detection of local recurrence after radical prostatectomy by prostate specific antigen and transrectal ultrasound. J Urol 1992;147:952.

28. Lightner DJ, Lange PH, Reddy PK, et al. Prostate specific antigen and local recurrence after radical prostatectomy. J Urol 1990;144:921–926.

29. Foster LS, Jajodia P, Fournier G, et al. The value of prostate specific antigen and transrectal ultrasound guided biopsy in detecting prostatic fossa recurrences following radical prostatectomy. J Urol 1993;149:1024–1028.

30. Platt JF, Bree RL, Schwab RE. The accuracy of CT in the staging of carcinoma of the prostate. AJR 1987;149:315–318.

31. Raj GV, Partin AW, Polsascik TJ. Clinical utility of indium-111-capromab pendetide immunoscintigraphy in the detection of early, recurrent prostate carcinoma after radical prostatectomy. Cancer 2002;94:987–996.

32. Sodee DB, Malguria N, Faulhaber P, et al. and the ProstaScint Imaging Centers. Multicenter ProstaScint imaging findings in 2154 patients with prostate cancer. Urology 2000;56:988–993.

33. Feneley MR, Jan H, Granowska M, et al. Imaging with prostate-specific membrane antigen (PSMA) in prostate cancer. Prost Cancer Prost Dis 2000;3:47–52.

34. Jani AB, Blend MJ, Hamilton R, et al. Influence of radioimmunoscintigraphy on postprostatectomy radiotherapy treatment decision making. J Nuc Med 2004;45:571–578.

35. Elgamal AA, Troychak MJ, Murphy GP. ProstaScint® scan may enhance identification of prostate cancer recurrences after prostatectomy, radiation or hormone therapy: analysis of 136 scans of 100 patients. Prostate 1998;37:261–269.

36. Haseman MK, Reed NL, Rosenthal SA. Monoclonal antibody imaging of occult prostate cancer in patients with elevated prostate-specific antigen positron emission tomography and biopsy correlation. Clin Nuc Med 1996;21:704–713.

37. Seltzer MA, Barbaric Z, Belldegrun A, et al. Comparison of helical computerized tomography, positron emission tomography and monoclonal antibody scans for evaluation of lymph node metastases in patients with prostate specific antigen relapse after treatment for localized prostate cancer. J Urol 1999;162:1322–1328.

38. Wynant GE, Murphy GP, Horoszewicz JS, et al. Immunoscintigraphy of prostatic cancer: preliminary results with ^{111}In-labeled monoclonal antibody 7E11-C5.3 (CYT-356). Prostate 1991;18:229–241.

39. Deb N, Goris M, Trisler K, et al. Treatment of hormone-refractory prostate cancer with 90Y-CYT-356 monoclonal antibody. Clin Cancer Res 1996;2:1289–1297.

40. Murphy GP, Snow PB, Elgamal AA, et al. Evaluation of prostate cancer patients receiving multiple staging tests, including ProstaScint scans. Prostate 2000;42:145–149.

41. Lau HY, Kindrachuk G, Carter M, et al. Surgical confirmation of ProstaScint® abnormalities in two patients with high risk prostate cancer. Can J Urol 2001;8:1199–1202.

42. Murphy GP, Maguire RT, Rogers B, et al. Comparison of serum PSMA, PSA levels with results of Cytogen-356 ProstaScint® scanning in prostatic cancer patients. Prostate 1997;33:281–285.

43. Murphy GP, Elgamal AA, Troychak MJ, et al. Follow-up ProstaScint scans verify detection of occult soft-tissue recurrence after failure of primary prostate cancer therapy. Prostate 2000;42:315–317.

44. Polascik TJ, Manyak MJ, Haseman MK, et al. Comparison of clinical staging algorithms and [111]indium-capromab pendetide immunoscintigraphy in the prediction of lymph node involvement in high risk prostate carcinoma patients. Cancer 1999;85:1586–1592.

45. Partin AW, Subong ENP, Walsh PC, et al. Combination of prostate-specific antigen, clinical stage, and Gleason score to predict pathological stage of localized prostate cancer: a multi-institutional update. JAMA 1997;277:1445–1451.

46. Bluestein DL, Bostwick DG, Bergsrath EJ, et al. Eliminating the need for bilateral pelvic lymphadenectomy in select patients with prostate cancer. J Urol 1994;151:1315–1320.

47. Roach M III, Marquez C, Hae-Sook Y, et al. Predicting the risk of lymph node involvement using pre-treatment prostate-specific antigen and Gleason score in men with clinically localized prostate cancer. Int J Radiat Oncol Biol Phys 1994;28:33–37.

48. Sands ME, Zagars GK, Pollack A, et al. Serum prostate-specific antigen, clinical stage, pathologic grade, and the incidence of nodal metastases in prostate cancer. Urology 1994;44:215–220.

49. Welsh JS, Yanez MH, Chin BB, et al. Indium-111 Capromab Pendetide (ProstaScint) Images Before and After Salvage Radiation Therapy. Clin Nuc Med 1999;12:983.

50. Kahn D, Williams RD, Haseman MK, et al. Radioimmunoscintigraphy with ^{111}In-capromab pendetide predicts prostate cancer response to salvage after failed radical prostatectomy. J Clin Onc 1998;16:284–289.

51. Hodroff M, Austin JC, Haseman M, et al. [111]In Capromab Pendetide MAB scan to predict radiotherapy response of tumor recurrence following radical prostatectomy: long-term follow-up. J Urol 2001;165:232 [Abstract #958].

52. Levesque PE, Nieh PT, Zinman LN, et al. Radiolabeled monoclonal antibody indium 111-labeled CYT-356 localizes extraprostatic recurrent carcinoma after prostatectomy. Urology 1998;51:978–984.

53. Wilkinson S, Chodak G. The role of [111]indium-capromab pendetide imaging for assessing biochemical failure after radical prostatectomy. J Urol 2004;172:133–136.

54. Thomas CT, Bradshaw PT, Pollock BH, et al. Indium-111-capromab pendetide radioimmunoscintigraphy and prognosis for durable biochemical response to salvage radiation therapy in men after failed prostatectomy. J Clin Oncol 2003;21:1715–1721.

55. Ellis RJ, Vertocnik A, Kin E, et al. Four-year biochemical outcome after radioimmunoguided transperineal brachytherapy for patients with prostate adenocarcinoma. Int J Radiat Oncol Biol Phys 2003;57:362–370.

56. Quintana JC, Blend MJ. The dual-isotope prostascint imaging procedure. Clin Nuc Med 2000;25:33–40.

57. Sodee DB, Ellis RJ, Samuels MA, et al. prostate cancer and prostate bed SPECT imaging with ProstaScint®: semi-quantitative correlation with prostatic biopsy results. Prostate 1998;37:140–148.

58. Fang DX, Stock RG, Stone NN, et al. Use of radioimmunoscintigraphy with indium-111-labeled CYT-356 (ProstaScint) scan for evaluation of patients for salvage brachytherapy. Techniques Urol 2000;6:146–150.

59. Feneley MR, Chengazi VU, Kirby RS, et al. Prostatic radioimmunoscintigraphy: preliminary results using technetium-labeled monoclonal antibody, CYT-351. Br J Urol 1996;77:373–381.

60. Liu H, Moy P, Kim S, et al. Monoclonal antibodies to the extracellular domain of prostate specific membrane antigen also react with tumor vascular endothelium. Cancer Res 1997; 3629–3634.

61. Liu H, Rajasekaran AK, Moy P, et al. Constitutive and antibody induced internalization of prostate specific membrane antigen. Cancer Res. 1998;58:4055–4060.

62. Bander NH, Trabulsi EJ, Kostakoglu L, et al. Targeting metastatic prostate cancer with radiolabeled monoclonal antibody J591 to the extracellular domain of prostate specific membrane antigen. J Urol 2003;170:1717–1721.

63. Milowsky MI, Nanus DM, Kostakoglu L, et al. Phase I trial of Yttrium-90 labeled anti-prostate-specific membrane antigen monoclonal antibody J591 for androgen independent prostate cancer. J Clin Oncol 2004;22:2522–2531.

64. Michaels EK, Blend M, Quintana JC. [111]Indium-capromab pendetide unexpectedly localizes to renal cell carcinoma. J Urol 1999;161:597–598.

65. Scott DL, Halkar RH, Fischer A, et al. False positive [111]indium capromab pendetide scan due to benign myelolipoma. J Urol 2001;165:901–911.

66. Bermejo CE, Coursey J, Basler J, et al. Histologic Confirmation of lesions identified by ProstaScint® scan following definitive treatment. Urol Oncol 2003;21:349–353.

67. Zanzi I, Stark R. Detection of a non-Hodgkin's lymphoma by capromab pendetide scintigraphy (ProstaScint) in a patient with prostate carcinoma. Urology 2002;60:514.

68. Khan K, Caride V. Indium-111 capromab pendetide (ProstaScint) uptake in neurofibromatosis. Urology 2000;56:154xxii–154xxiv.

69. Valliappan S, Joyce JM, Myers DT. Possible false-positive metastatic prostate cancer on an In-111 capromab pendetide scan as a result of a pelvic kidney. Clin Nuc Med 1999;24:984–985.

70. Garcia-Morales F, Chengazi VU, O'Mara RE. Detection of brain metastasis with indium-111-capromab pendetide (ProstaScint) due to prostatic carcinoma. Urology 2000;55:286xiii–286xv.

71. Anderson RS, Eifert B, Tartt S, et al. Radioimmunoguided surgery using indium-111 capromab pendetide (ProstaScint) to diagnose supraclavicular metastasis from prostate cancer. Urology 2000;56:669xii–669xiv.

72. Ponsky LE, Cherullo EE, Starkey R, et al. Evaluation of pre-operative ProstaScint scans in the prediction of nodal disease. Prostate Cancer Prostatic Dis 2002;5:132–135.

Future directions in imaging prostate cancer 53

Michael J Manyak, John H Makari

INTRODUCTION

Determination of disease extent is one of the most crucial issues for both the patient and the physician in the selection of appropriate therapy for prostate cancer. Neither digital rectal exam (DRE) nor transrectal ultrasound (TRUS), alone or in combination, are reliable for either initial disease diagnosis or for detection of recurrence.[1,2] Combining information about histopathologic tumor characteristics and tumor markers such as prostate-specific antigen (PSA), especially in their extremes, allows some prediction of disease stage. In cases where recurrent disease is suspected, it is quite clear that PSA elevation precedes radiographic or physical detection of recurrence by at least several months, but PSA does not distinguish between local recurrence and more widespread disease.

Noninvasive imaging has been utilized to evaluate patients with prostate cancer, but the clinical utility of current imaging studies is limited because a relatively large volume of disease is required for detection. Consequently, conventional cross-sectional radiographic imaging has substantial limitations for identification of local disease extent or regional and distant metastatic involvement. Refinements in magnetic resonance imaging (MRI), selective use of monoclonal antibody-derived radioimmunoscintigraphy, and introduction of novel imaging agents for existing cross-sectional and sonographic technology may improve diagnostic capabilities.[3–5] However, the lack of reliable, cost effective imaging has led to an increased reliance on clinical and serologic parameters to guide treatment decisions.

The convergence of technology in the fields of material science, the defense and communications industries, and biology has led to widely diverse technical approaches for evaluation of tissue and biologic processes (Box 53.1).[6] In addition, the complex cascade of molecular events in the evolution from normal to neoplastic tissue and then metastasis has provided biomolecular targets for evaluation at every stage of prostate cancer. Technologic improvements in image resolution for existing modalities continue to refine our capability to discern abnormal from normal growth. Furthermore, the use of highly sophisticated signal processing provided by advances in computational technology, such as the quantum computer, will allow real time evaluation of large amounts of data, making it possible to fuse information that collectively may yield much more information about tumor biology and prognosis.

All of these advances suggest that rapid coregistration of images from a variety of sources will be possible to compile a very detailed composite about an individual tumor biology. Coregistration superimposes radiographic images to further define specific anatomic areas of interest. As currently used in treatment planning and dosimetric assessment for radiotherapy, coregistration of computed tomography (CT) and MRI has shown superiority over use of pelvic bony reference marks.[7] The addition of functional imaging to anatomic information from CT and ultrasound is now being utilized for intraprostatic dose escalation strategies and for confirmation of 3D energy delivery.[8] This combination of functional and anatomic imaging with MRI and MR spectroscopic imaging (MRSI) to provide high-resolution spatiovascular information in prostate cancer is also under review.[9,10] Furthermore, coregistration of radiolabeled monoclonal antibody scans with both CT and MRI have improved specificity for both newly-diagnosed prostate cancer and recurrent disease.[11,12]

Box 53.1 Technical approaches for evaluation of tissue and biologic processes

Molecular-based imaging
- Radioimmunoscintigraphy
- X-ray diffraction
- Electron microscopy
- Autoradiography
- Magnetic resonance imaging (MRI)
- Electron paramagnetic resonance (EPR)
- Positron emission tomography (PET)

Diagnostic light technologies
- Fluorescent detection
- Hyperspectral spectroscopy
- Photon migration
- Laser Doppler
- Diffuse reflectance spectroscopy
- Optical coherence tomography (OCT)

ADVANCES IN EXISTING TECHNOLOGIES

ULTRASOUND

Established clinical applications of gray-scale TRUS in prostate cancer include biopsy guidance, placement of radioactive seeds, and assessment of response to therapy. Despite the advantages of a relatively inexpensive, fast, and minimally invasive imaging technology, TRUS has shown very limited benefit for detection and staging of prostate cancer and is not recommended for screening. It has a relatively low sensitivity and specificity because most hypoechoic peripheral zone lesions are not malignant, and up to 56% of carcinomas are isoechoic.[13] Likewise, TRUS is not very sensitive for detection of seminal vesicle invasion and is more suited as a guide for biopsy in those cases suspected of seminal vesicle involvement.[14]

Recent advances in ultrasound technology have attempted to address the limitations of TRUS in prostate cancer detection and staging. The two-fold increase of microvessel density in prostate cancer compared with benign prostatic hyperplasia suggests that Color Doppler ultrasonography (CDUS) may be useful for diagnosis.[15] However, the false-positive rate (and corresponding unnecessary biopsies) remain high.[16] Power Doppler (PD) ultrasound, with its 3D images and where blood flow direction is independent of ultrasound transmission, may have more potential to demonstrate tumor hypervascularity, though dynamic contrast-enhanced MRI may be superior to either.[17] Another report in 282 men with elevated PSA has

similar sensitivities for TRUS and PD (87.9% and 92.4%, respectively) but a significantly higher negative predictive value for PD (80.6%).[18] Compared with TRUS, flow sonography increased detection rates from 61% to 86% in 70 whole-mount radical prostatectomy specimens.[19] A fluorocarbon microbubble contrast agent has been used with CDUS to enhance sensitivity (CE-CD). The contrast-enhanced CD-guided biopsies provided a 2.6 times greater chance of detecting cancer in the 230 patients tested.[20]

Specificity for malignancy, however, has been less encouraging in many of these studies, with PD specificity ranging from 61% to 77%.[17,18] Another study compared detection rates by DRE, serum markers, TRUS, CDUS, and CE-CD in 34 patients scheduled for transperineal extended biopsy. All three sonographic modalities had equally low specificities (TRUS, 56.2%; CDUS, 56.2%; CE-CD, 54%) and were all less specific than DRE (72%) and free PSA ratio (88.8%).[21] The use of these enhanced ultrasound modalities for staging remains inconclusive.

CROSS-SECTIONAL IMAGING

The limitations of both CT and MRI to detect prostate cancer and lymph node metastasis are recognized. Although CT resolution has improved with technologic advances, the threshold for CT detection of lymph node involvement is between 1.0 cm and 1.5 cm.[22] Computed tomography may fail to detect lymphadenopathy because the nodes are beneath the size threshold for detection, may contain microscopic tumor foci without enlargement, or because of technical performance of the scan and interobserver variability in interpretation.[23] When adenopathy is detected, CT does not distinguish between inflammatory and neoplastic involvement, and CT sensitivity has ranged from 2.5% to 75%.[24] In one of the few studies with tissue confirmation of radiographic findings, CT had a sensitivity of 4% in a cohort of intermediate-to-high-risk patients.[4] Therefore CT is best reserved for patients with clinical stage T3 or T4 disease and for radiotherapy pretreatment planning.[3] It also remains useful as a conformal study for image coregistration.

Magnetic resonance imaging has been used as an imaging modality in prostate cancer for local evaluation with a widely variable accuracy ranging from 54% to 90%.[25] The accuracy varies with the type of coil used, the type of spin sequence used, the site of extraprostatic extension (extracapsular versus seminal vesicle), and the degree of radiologist subspecialization.[26–28] However, MRI has not proven to be significantly better than CT for evaluation of nodal involvement, with pooled data from four series with more than 50 patients demonstrating an overall sensitivity of 42% and specificity of 98%.[29] The only useful criterion so far has been size, which obviously results in the failure to detect microscopic disease. This criterion may vary with the anatomic location of lymph node structures, however, because the 95th percentile value for normal lymph node size has been suggested to be 7 mm for internal iliac, 8 mm for obturator, 9 mm for common iliac, and 10 mm for external iliac lymph nodes.[22]

The utility of MRI may be significantly enhanced by the use of ultrasmall superparamagnetic iron oxide particles, first reported in a murine model in 1990.[30] The 20 nm hexagonal iron oxide cores coated with dextran are injected intravenously and filtered through the lymphatic system. High-intensity signal is noted in all lymph nodes, but macrophage phagocytosis in normal lymph nodes eliminates signal on repeat MRI 24 hours later. Lymph nodes with metastatic disease demonstrate continued high-intensity signal in areas of tumor. In the recently published study on incidence of lymph node involvement with prostate cancer, performance characteristics of the MRI with lymphotrophic particles compared with MRI alone were (sensitivity, 96% versus 29%; specificity, 99% versus 87%; positive predictive value, 96% versus 29%; negative predictive value, 99% versus 87%) in lymph nodes between 5 mm and 1 cm, while in lymph nodes less than 5 mm, sensitivity and positive predictive value were 41% and 78%, respectively versus 0% for MRI alone.[5] Furthermore, several noncontiguous positive lymph nodes were detected, corroborating previous work that reported up to 17% of patients with a solitary iliac metastasis and 7% to 14% of patients with a solitary presacral or presciatic metastasis outside of the conventional area for lymph node dissection.[31,32] The tissue-confirmed results of this study are striking and strongly suggest that this modality will be highly useful to determine treatment regimens. This changes the paradigm for evaluation of lymph nodes from one of size alone to one of signal-intensity characteristics denoting functional activity regardless of size.

POSITRON EMISSION TOMOGRAPHY

Positron emission tomography (PET) measures metabolism of a radiolabeled analog in tissue with the higher metabolic rate of neoplasia registering an increased scintigraphic signal, especially noted in rapidly progressive tumors. Although the most commonly used radiotracer for PET is ^{18}F-fluoro-2-deoxyglucose (FDG), this analog is not particularly useful in evaluation of prostate cancer.[33] In addition to not being able to differentiate between tumor and hyperplasia, PET is also not as good as bone scintigraphy for detection of osseous metastases.[33] Variable results have been shown for lymph node assessment with FDG-PET, and its use may be hampered because of relatively low glycolytic rate in prostate cancer and its metastases.[34]

The recently developed analogs ^{11}C-choline and ^{11}C-acetate do show greater promise for use in prostate cancer metastatic lymph node detection. Positron emission tomography with ^{11}C-choline yielded a sensitivity of 80%, specificity of 96%, and accuracy of 93% in one study of 67 patients.[35] In another report using ^{11}C-acetate, this analog significantly outperformed both FDG-PET and CT.[36] While these studies are encouraging, perhaps the next major leap for use of PET imaging will occur with the introduction of small high-resolution PET scanners for the prostate (Figure 53.1), which have achieved a three-fold increase in resolution over conventional PET scanners (Weinberg IN, Naviscan PET Systems, Rockville, MD, personal communication). This prototype scanner has two heads, similar to standard PET scanners, but one of the gamma camera heads is highly miniaturized so that it is handheld and can be inserted into the rectum. This unit employs specialized proprietary Monte Carlo-based computer algorithms that incorporate position-sensing technology needed to obtain images from the handheld PET geometry.

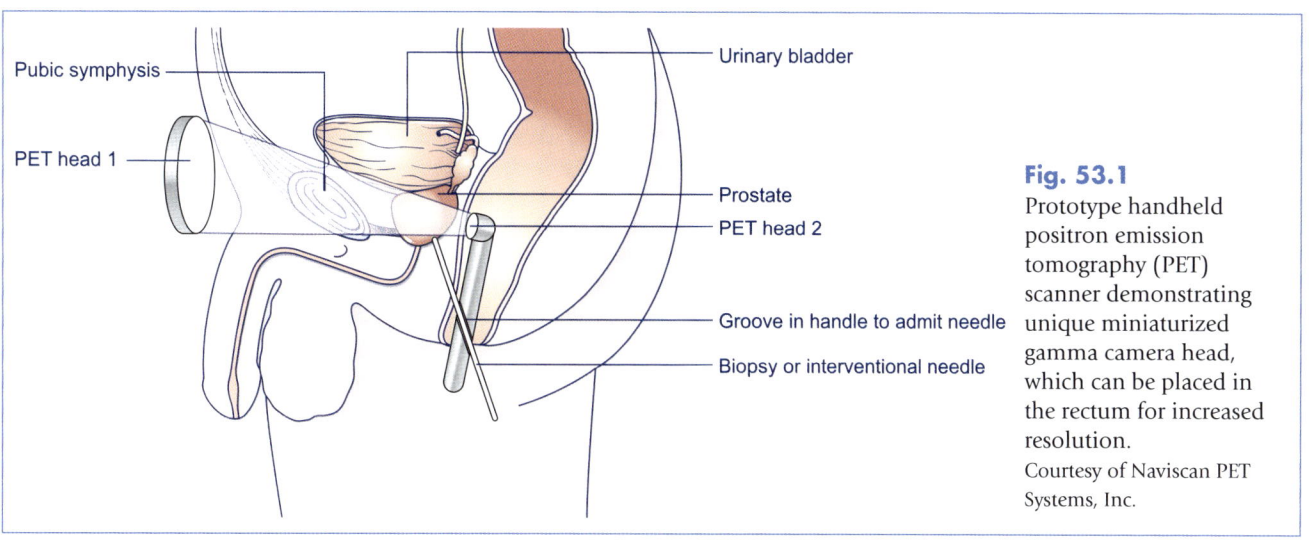

Pubic symphysis

PET head 1

Urinary bladder

Prostate

PET head 2

Groove in handle to admit needle

Biopsy or interventional needle

Fig. 53.1
Prototype handheld positron emission tomography (PET) scanner demonstrating unique miniaturized gamma camera head, which can be placed in the rectum for increased resolution.
Courtesy of Naviscan PET Systems, Inc.

TECHNOLOGIES ON THE HORIZON

ELECTRON PARAMAGNETIC RESONANCE

Another very interesting functional imaging modality that is promising for prostate cancer evaluation utilizes electron paramagnetic resonance (EPR) to determine tumor hypoxia. It has been reported that localized prostate cancer is characterized by marked hypoxia and significant heterogeneity in oxygenation.[37-39] Overhauser-enhanced MRImaging (OMRI) combines two spectroscopic techniques, nuclear magnetic resonance (NMR) and EPR to provide high-resolution MR images at low magnetic fields ($\sim$10 mT). While NMR detects species with magnetic nuclei such as water protons, EPR detects species with unpaired electrons such as paramagnetic molecules. Infusion with the paramagnetic agent before scanning with both the EPR frequency and the NMR frequency yields MR images with high spatial resolution.[38] Image resolution is poor without the contrast agent, consistent with the low magnetic fields employed, but significantly enhanced resolution is evident after infusion with the paramagnetic agent (Figure 53.2). Very small probes are used that require about 650-fold less energy than standard MRI. In-vivo studies demonstrate that tumor accumulates significant amounts of the contrast agent yet large areas of the tumor are severely hypoxic. This unique, small, portable OMRI technique is capable of providing anatomically coregistered images of oxygen distribution.

DIAGNOSTIC LIGHT TECHNOLOGY

Light is increasingly being used in various forms to gather information about biologic systems with implications for

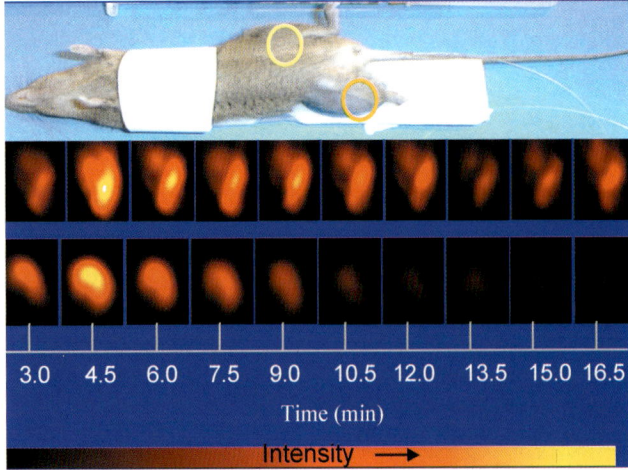

Fig. 53.2
Electron paramagnetic resonance (EPR) of normal and tumor-bearing areas with contrast agent demonstrating severe intra-tumor hypoxia. Electron paramagnetic resonance requires 650 times less energy than standard magnetic resonance imaging.

use in prostate cancer. Diagnosis using light varies in one fundamental respect from therapeutic applications of light sources, such as lasers. Therapeutic uses of light are determined by the *effect of light* on tissue while diagnostic uses generally detect changes which result from the *effect of tissue* on light.[40] The rapid, noninvasive determination of tissue characteristics, such as scattering and absorption, is essential to process information received from the light interaction in tissue during a diagnostic procedure. These are the fundamental principles governing diagnostic light use in tissue for the emerging modalities such as optical coherence tomography and hyperspectral imaging (see Box 53.1).

OPTICAL COHERENCE TOMOGRAPHY

Optical coherence tomography (OCT) is an intriguing application of diffuse reflectance spectroscopy, the same principle used in pulse oximetry, and was originally used to image human tissue in 1991. It employs continuous wave light (instead of sound waves) to obtain images in a manner analogous to B-mode ultrasonography. Reflected light, generated in the near infrared spectrum by a superluminescent diode, is measured by interferometry to produce two-dimensional images. Optical coherence tomography images tissue in situ and in real time, providing resolution on the order of 5 to 20 μm, which is comparable to traditional microscopic analysis. Cellular features detected by OCT include mitotic activity, nuclear-to-cytoplasmic ratios and cellular migration.[41] Optical coherence tomography does not require a conducting medium and can, therefore, image through air or water with far greater resolution than ultrasound.[42] In addition, OCT is relatively inexpensive, portable, and can be used with existing endoscopic instrumentation.[43]

Initially, OCT technology was used to image the transparent ocular structures in vitro. Expansion of this technique included imaging of the retina and macula in vivo, with resolution of 10 μm.[44,45] After initial studies demonstrated the ability to image the nearly transparent ocular structures with OCT, efforts focused on imaging solid tissue.[46] In-vivo imaging of dermatologic structures was performed successfully, followed by endoluminal imaging of vascular tissue components.[47] Compared with high-frequency intravascular ultrasound, OCT produced resolution over six times greater than the highest frequency imaging modality available.[48] Improvements in the ability to obtain OCT images strongly suggest that greater depth of tissue penetration will be possible with greater implications for solid tissue evaluation.

Endoscopic application of OCT also has been demonstrated in the human gastrointestinal tract. Compared with histologic specimens, OCT has demonstrated promise in discriminating inflammatory, neoplastic, metaplastic and cancerous processes of the esophagus, colon, and endometrium.[49,50]

Optical coherence tomography imaging of human genitourinary tissue was first demonstrated in 1997. In-vitro OCT images from biopsies of prostate, bladder, and ureter were obtained and compared with standard preparations with hematoxylin and eosin staining. The OCT images demonstrated differentiation between the prostatic urethra and prostate, visualization of the neurovascular bundle and the prostate-adipose border, visualization of the prostatic capsule, and differentiation of the anatomic layers in the bladder and ureter with axial resolution of 16 μm.[51] A recent report has demonstrated the feasibility and high sensitivity for determination of early bladder tumor invasion (Figure 53.3).[52] Currently, OCT is being used to evaluate effects on prostate tissue from ionizing radiation and to locate neurovascular tissue during radical prostatectomy.

HYPERSPECTRAL IMAGING

Diffuse reflectance spectroscopy from different wavelengths of light can be used to gather a composite image of tissue and identify abnormalities. This type of diagnostic light technology is referred to as hyperspectral imaging (Figure 53.4) and has been used for evaluation of diverse problems ranging from oxygen saturation and

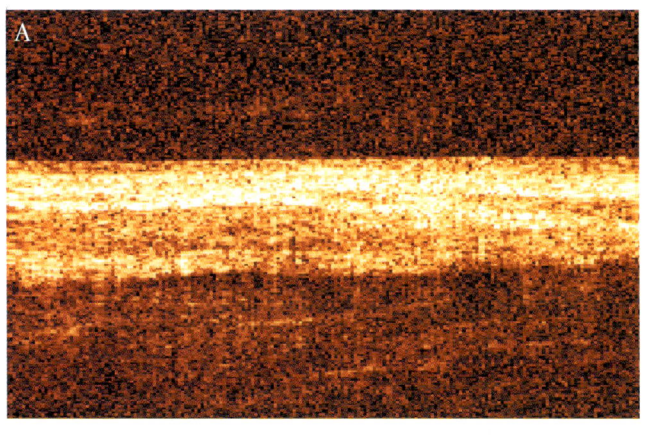

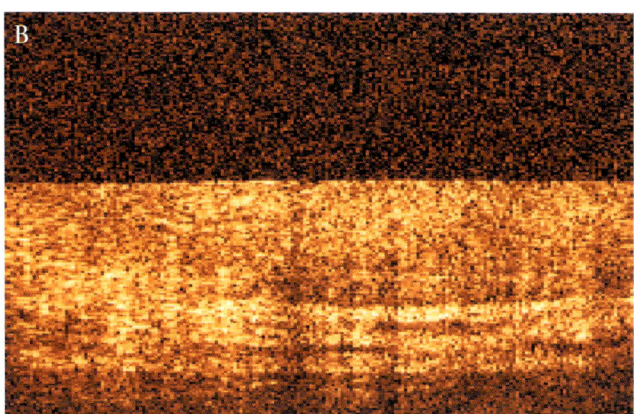

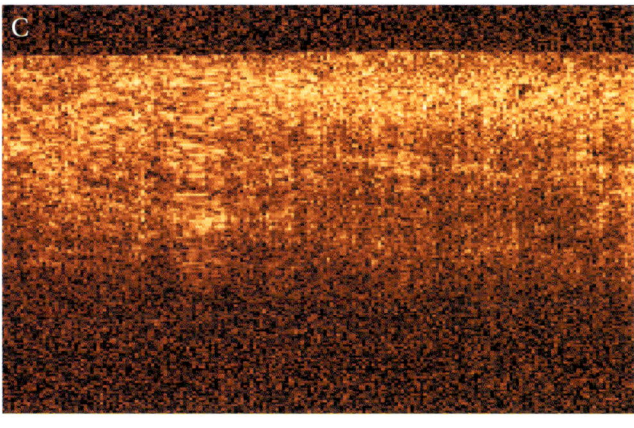

Fig. 53.3
Optical coherence tomography (OCT) of *A*, normal bladder epithelium, *B*, carcinoma in situ, and *C*, invasive transitional cell carcinoma. Optical coherence tomography is under evaluation for radiation damage and identification of neurovascular periprostatic tissue.

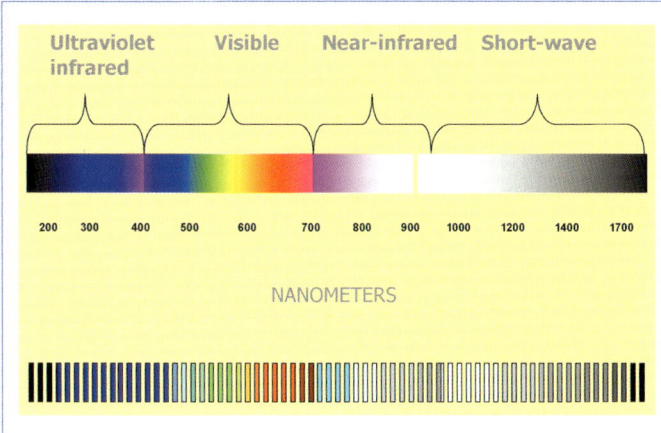

Fig. 53.4
Electromagnetic spectrum demonstrating wavelengths used for hyperspectral image analysis. Multiple wavelengths provide different signal by diffuse reflectance spectroscopy.
Courtesy of Institute for Technology Development, Stennis Space Center, MS.

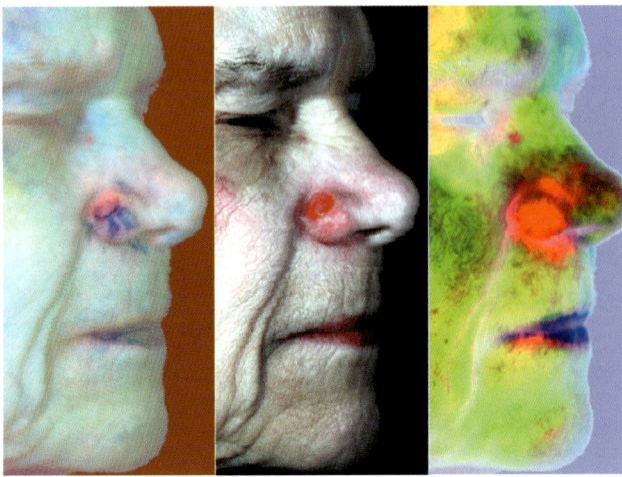

Fig. 53.5
Hyperspectral analysis of epidermal carcinoma demonstrating distinct spectral signature highly consistent with pathologic findings.
Courtesy of Institute for Technology Development, Stennis Space Center, MS.

tissue perfusion to wound extent and neoplasia.[53-56] In cases of cutaneous lesions (Figure 53.5), analysis of full-thickness dermal specimens yielded distinct spectral signatures for regions of interest including the epidermis, normal dermis, and abnormal dermal areas. The scanning of the regional surface area using these hyperspectral signatures revealed an exclusionary, pseudo-color pattern, which consistently defined a central abnormal area with a unique spectral signature. An algorithm compared abnormal hyperspectral areas with histopathologic findings, which showed no significant variation from standard bright-field microscopy. These data indicate that hyperspectral analysis may provide a high-throughput alternative for tissue evaluation that approximates standard bright-field image analysis. While use for this technology for prostate cancer has not yet been attempted, the ability to perturb tissue with a variety of wavelengths delivered by an optical fiber holds promise for solid tissue evaluation, especially in combination with other minimally invasive diagnostic imaging technologies. It is the combination of these types of diagnostic techniques with other imaging information that is the wave of the future.

REFERENCES

1. Schroder FH, van der Maas P, Beemsterboer P, et al. Evaluation of the digital rectal examination as a screening test for prostate cancer. Rotterdam section of the European Randomized Study of Screening for Prostate Cancer. J Natl Cancer Inst 1998;90:1817–1823.

2. Gustafsson O, Carlsson P, Norming U, et al. Cost-effectiveness analysis in early detection of prostate cancer: an evaluation of six screening strategies in a randomly selected population of 2,400 men. Prostate 1995;26:299–309.

3. Purohit RS, Shinhara K, Meng MV, et al. Imaging clinically localized prostate cancer. Urol Clin North Am 2003;30:279–293.

4. Manyak MJ, Hinkle GH, Chiacchierini RP, et al. Immunoscintigraphy with ^{111}In-capromab pendetide: evaluation before definitive therapy in patients with prostate cancer. Urology 1999;54:1058–1063.

5. Harisinghani MG, Barentsz J, Hahn PF, et al. Noninvasive detection of clinically occult lymph-node metastases in prostate cancer. N Engl J Med 2003;348:2491–2499.

6. Manyak MJ. The light at the end of the tunnel: one view of laparoscopic future. Sem Urol 1992;10:205–212.

7. Servois V, Chauveinc L, El Khoury C, et al. CT and MR image fusion using two different methods after prostate brachytherapy: impact on post-implant dosimetric assessment. Cancer Radiother 2003;7:9–16.

8. Mizowaki T, Cohen GN, Fung AY, et al. Towards integrating functional imaging in the treatment of prostate cancer with radiation: the registration of the MR spectroscopy imaging to ultrasound/CT images and its implementation in treatment planning. Int J Radiat Oncol Biol Phys 2002;54:1558–1564.

9. van Dorsten FA, van der Graaf M, Engelbrecht MR, et al Combined quantitative dynamic contrast-enhanced MR imaging and MR spectroscopic imaging of human prostate cancer. J Magn Reson Imaging 2004;20:279–87.

10. Claus FG, Hricak H, Hattery RR. Pretreatment evaluation of prostate cancer: role of MR imaging and 1H MR spectroscopy. Radiographics 2004;24:S167–180.

11. Haseman MK, Rosenthal SA, Polascik TJ. Capromab pendetide imaging of prostate cancer. Cancer Biother Radiopharm 2000;15:131–140.

12. Schettino CJ, Kramer EL, Noz ME, et al. Impact of fusion of indium-111 capromab pendetide volume data sets with those from MRI or CT in patients with recurrent prostate cancer. AJR Am J Roentgenol 2004;183:519–524.

13. Sanders LM: Ultrasound of the Prostate. In: Lang EK (ed): Medical Radiology: Diagnostic Imaging and Radiation Oncology. New York: Springer-Verlag, 1994, pp 185–194.

14. Wymenga LF, Duisterwinkel FJ, Groenier K, Mensink HJ. Ultrasound-guided seminal vesicle biopsies in prostate cancer. Prostate Cancer Prostatic Dis 2000;3:100–106.

15. Sedelaar JP, van Leenders GJ, Hulsbergen-van de Kaa CA, et al. Microvessel density: correlation between contrast ultrasonography and histology of prostate cancer. Eur Urol 2001;40:285–293.

16. Okihara K, Miki T, Babaian RJ. Clinical efficacy of prostate cancer detection using power doppler imaging in American and Japanese men. J Clin Ultrasound 2002;30:213–221.

17. Ito H, Kamoi K, Yokoyama K, et al. Visualization of prostate cancer using dynamic contrast-enhanced MRI: comparison with transrectal power Doppler ultrasound. Br J Radiol 2003;76:617–624.

18. Sauvain JL, Palascak P, Bourscheid D, et al. Value of power Doppler and 3D vascular sonography as a method for diagnosis and staging of prostate cancer. Eur Urol 2003;44:21–30.

19. Sedelaar JP, van Leenders GJ, Goossen TE, et al. Value of contrast ultrasonography in the detection of significant prostate cancer: correlation with radical prostatectomy specimens. Prostate 2002;53:246–253.

20. Frauscher F, Klauser A, Volgger H, et al. Comparison of contrast enhanced color Doppler targeted biopsy with conventional systematic biopsy: impact on prostate cancer detection. J Urol 2002;167:1648–1652.

21. Pepe P, Patane D, Panella P, et al. Does ecographic contrast medium Levovist improve the detection rate of prostate cancer? Prost CA and Prost Dis 2003;6:159–162.

22. Manyak MJ, Javitt MC. The role of computerized tomography, magnetic resonance imaging, bone scan, and monoclonal antibody nuclear scan for prognosis prediction in prostate cancer. Sem Urol Oncol 1998;16:145–152.

23. Ferguson JK, Oesterling JE. Patient evaluation if prostate-specific antigen becomes elevated following radical prostatectomy or radiation therapy. Urol Clin North Am 1994;21:677–685.

24. Platt JF, Bree RL, Schwab RE. The accuracy of CT in the staging of cancer of the prostate. Am J Radiol 1987;149:315–320.

25. Swanson MG, Vigneron DB, Tran TK, et al. Magnetic resonance imaging and spectroscopic imaging of prostate cancer. Cancer Invest 2001;19:510–23.

26. Nakashima J, Tanimoto A, Imai Y, et al. Endorectal MRI for prediction of tumor site, tumor size, and local extension of prostate cancer. Urology 2004;64:101–105.

27. Cornud F, Belin X, Flam T, et al. Local staging of prostate cancer by endorectal MRI using fast spin-echo sequences: prospective correlation with pathological findings after radical prostatectomy. Br J Urol 1996;77:843–850.

28. Bates TS, Gillatt DA, Cavanagh PM, et al. A comparison of endorectal magnetic resonance imaging and transrectal ultrasonography in the local staging of prostate cancer with histopathological correlation. Br J Urol 1997;79:927–932.

29. David V. MR imaging of the prostate and seminal vesicles. MRI Clin North Am 1996;4:497–518.

30. Weissleder R, Elizondo G, Wittenberg J, et al. Ultrasmall superparamagnetic iron oxide: an intravenous contrast agent for assessing lymph nodes with MR imaging. Radiolog 1990;175:494–498.

31. McLaughlin AP, Saltzstein SL, McCullough DL, et al. Prostatic carcinoma: incidence and location of unsuspected lymphatic metastases. J Urol 1976;115:89–94.

32. Golimbu M, Morales P, Al-Askari S, et al. Extended pelvic lymphadenectomy for prostate cancer. J Urol 1979;121:617–620.

33. Hain SF, Maisey MN. Positron emission tomography for urological tumours. BJU Int 2003;92:159–164.

34. Shvarts O, Han KR, Seltzer M, et al. Positron emission tomography in urologic oncology. Cancer Control 2002;9:335–342.

35. de Jong IJ, Pruim J, Elsinga PH, et al. Preoperative staging of pelvic lymph nodes in prostate cancer by 11C-choline PET. J Nucl Med 2003;44:331–335.

36. Oyama N, Miller TR, Dehdashti F, et al. 11C-acetate PET imaging of prostate cancer: detection of recurrent disease at PSA relapse. J Nucl Med 2003;44:549–555.

37. Parker C, Milosevic M, Toi A, et al. Polarographic electrode study of tumor oxygenation in clinically localized prostate cancer. Int J Radiat Oncol Biol Phys 2004;58: 750–757.

38. Krishna MC, English S, Yamada K, et al. Overhauser enhanced magnetic resonance imaging for tumor oximetry: coregistration of tumor anatomy and tissue oxygen concentration. Proc Natl Acad Sci USA 2002;99:2216–2221.

39. Zhao D, Ran S, Constantinescu A, et al. Tumor oxygen dynamics: correlation of in vivo MRI with histological findings. Neoplasia 2003;5:308–318.

40. Parrish JA, Wilson BC. Current and future trends in laser medicine. Photochem Photobiol 1991;53:731–738.

41. Boppart SA, Bouma BE, Pitris C, Southern JF, Brezinski ME, Fujimoto JG. In vivo cellular optical coherence tomography imaging. Nat Med 1998;4:861–865.

42. Feldchtein FI, Gelikonov GV, Gelikonov VM, et al. Endoscopic applications of optical coherence tomography. Optics Express 1998;3:257–260.

43. Manyak MJ, Warner JW. An update on laser use in urology. Contemp Urol 2003;15:13–28.

44. Hee MR, Izatt JA, Swanson EA, et al. Optical coherence tomography of the human retina. Arch Ophthalmol 1995;113:325–332.

45. Puliafito CA, Hee MR, Lin CP, et al. Imaging of macular diseases with optical coherence tomography. Ophthalmology 1995;102:217–229.

46. Schmitt JM, Knüttel A, Yadlowsky M, et al. Optical-coherence tomography of a dense tissue: statistics of attenuation and backscattering. Phys Med Biol 1994;39:1705–1720.

47. Brezinski ME, Tearney GJ, Bouma BE, et al. Optical coherence tomography for optical biopsy. Properties and demonstration of vascular pathology. Circulation 1996;93:1206–1213.

48. Brezinski ME, Tearney GJ, Weissman NJ, et al. Assessing atherosclerotic plaque morphology: comparison of optical coherence tomography and high frequency intravascular ultrasound. Heart 1997;77:397–403.

49. Jackle S, Gladkova N, Feldchtein F, et al. In vivo endoscopic optical coherence tomography of the human gastrointestinal tract—toward optical biopsy. Endoscopy 2000;32:743–749.

50. Pitris C, Goodman A, Boppart SA, et al. High-resolution imaging of gynecologic neoplasms using optical coherence tomography. Obstet Gynecol 1999;93:135–139.

51. Tearney GJ, Brezinski ME, Southern JF, et al. Optical biopsy in human urologic tissue using optical coherence tomography. J Urol 1997;157:1915–1919.

52. Manyak MJ, Gladkova ND, Makari JH, et al. Evaluation of superficial bladder transitional cell carcinoma by optical coherence tomography. J Endourol 2005;19:570–574.

53. Khoobehi B, Beach JM, Kawano H. Hyperspectral imaging for measurement of oxygen saturation in the optic nerve head. Invest Ophthalmol Vis Sci 2004;45:1464–1472.

54. Zuzak KJ, Gladwin MT, Cannon RO 3rd, et al. Imaging hemoglobin oxygen saturation in sickle cell disease patients using noninvasive visible reflectance hyperspectral techniques: effects of nitric oxide. Am J Physiol Heart Circ Physiol 2003;285: H1183–1189.

55. Shah SA, Bachrach N, Spear SJ, et al. Cutaneous wound analysis using hyperspectral imaging. Biotechniques 2003;34:408–413.

56. Zuzak KJ, Schaeberle MD, Lewis EN, et al. Visible reflectance hyperspectral imaging: characterization of a noninvasive, in vivo system for determining tissue perfusion. Anal Chem 2002;74:2021–2028.

Local therapy for prostate-specific antigen recurrence after definitive treatment

54

Maxwell V Meng, Peter R Carroll

INTRODUCTION

The use of prostate-specific antigen (PSA) screening in conjunction with digital rectal examination (DRE) and transrectal ultrasound (TRUS) has resulted in earlier cancer diagnosis and increased opportunities for cure. Nevertheless, disease recurrence after local therapy for prostate cancer is increasingly common. In part this is due to clinical understaging of the cancer, which occurs in up to 50% of patients undergoing radical prostatectomy, although the contemporary incidence is likely closer to 20%.[1,2] An analysis of patients enrolled in a disease registry of prostate cancer patients demonstrated that 22% of patients who received initial treatment with radical prostatectomy, radiation therapy, or cryotherapy required a second form of prostate cancer treatment within 3 years of initial therapy.[3] Most of these treatments were administered in a nonadjuvant (therapeutic) fashion for apparent evidence of disease recurrence. Patients managed with radical prostatectomy had the lowest rate of second cancer treatment. Similar results have been reported by others, with at least 16% to 35% of radical prostatectomy patients and 24% of radiotherapy patients receiving second cancer treatments within 5 years of primary treatment.[4–6] Currently, failure of therapy is most often manifest solely by a rising PSA level. Moul estimated that up to 50,000 men per year may have PSA-only recurrence after definitive treatment.[7] However, there are no adequate studies comparing outcomes of these secondary treatments, and the specific indications and optimal timing for additional therapy are equally undefined. Herein, we discuss the various treatment options with definitive, curative intent in patients whose cancers recur locally after radical prostatectomy, radiation therapy, or cryotherapy.

RISK FACTORS FOR RECURRENCE

Multiple studies have examined predictors of recurrence after definitive treatment for prostate cancer. Most of this data is derived from analysis of outcomes of patients treated by radical prostatectomy (Box 54.1). Pretreatment clinical features that correlate with prognosis include T stage, biopsy Gleason score, and serum PSA level.[23] As one would expect, higher stage, the presence of Gleason pattern 4 or greater or a Gleason sum greater than 7, and PSA levels exceeding 10 ng/mL are associated with an increased risk of progression after surgery. These elements have been combined in order to more accurately predict tumor extent, or pathologic stage, and, therefore, prognosis; such probability tables and multivariate models have been based on a larger number of men who have undergone radical

---

Box 54.1 Risk factors for recurrence after radical prostatectomy

Pretreatment features
- Higher stage[8–14]
- Biopsy Gleason grade (any pattern 4, sum >7)[8–14]
- Preoperative PSA (>10 ng/mL)[8–14]
- Greater number of positive biopsies[15]

Pathologic features
- Higher stage (seminal vesicle, lymph node involvement)[8,11,13,16,17]
- Higher tumor Gleason grade[8,9,16,18]
- Positive surgical margin[8,16,19,20]
- DNA ploidy[21]
- Vascular invasion[22]

prostatectomy.[24–26] Pathologic criteria that are independent factors include tumor grade, surgical margin status, and the presence of extracapsular disease, seminal vesicle invasion, or involvement of pelvic lymph nodes (i.e., pathologic stage greater than T2N0M0).[27] A recent analysis of clinicopathologic factors confirmed that pathologic category, based on tumor extent and margin status, was the variable most strongly associated with biochemical failure.[22] Interestingly, vascular invasion was the only other variable significantly associated with failure after radical prostatectomy. Similarly, in patients receiving radiation therapy and cryotherapy, risks of recurrence are associated with pretreatment serum PSA, tumor grade, and clinical stage. In addition, PSA nadir following treatment predicts risk for treatment failure.[28] Thus, multiple predictors are available to help identify patients receiving definitive therapy for localized prostate cancer who are at increased risk for disease recurrence.

IDENTIFYING RECURRENCE AND ITS SITE

PROSTATE-SPECIFIC ANTIGEN

Prostate-specific antigen is a powerful tool in the monitoring of patients after definitive treatment of clinically localized prostate cancer. Typically, biochemical failure precedes clinical disease recurrence by 6 to 48 months.[29] Pound et al characterized disease progression after PSA elevation in patients undergoing radical prostatectomy.[30] Actuarial time to metastases was 8 years from the time of PSA failure and was predicted by time from surgery to biochemical failure, Gleason score, and PSA doubling time. The serum PSA of patients after radical prostatectomy should fall to undetectable levels and initial testing should begin at 2 to 3 months. Serial PSA measurements provide the most reliable method in detecting recurrence, as tumor progression rarely occurs in the absence of PSA elevation. Currently, the precise threshold defining "PSA failure" remains unclear. Lange et al suggested a cut-off of 0.4 ng/mL, with clinical recurrence evident in all men with PSA greater than this level.[29] Amling et al also concluded that biochemical recurrence be defined as PSA greater than or equal to 0.4 ng/mL.[31] This was based on the fact that PSA progression at 3 years was observed in 72% of the cohort, compared with lower rates of progression with lower thresholds (62% for 0.3 ng/mL and 49% for 0.2 ng/mL). However, contemporary clinical practice typically defines biochemical relapse when postoperative PSA reaches 0.2 ng/mL on at least two successive evaluations. Freedland et al reported that

all patients (95% confidence interval [CI], 87–100%) demonstrated PSA progression at 3 years if the PSA was greater than 0.2 ng/mL.[32] The role and impact of ultrasensitive PSA assays, with the ability to detect levels of 0.001 ng/mL, remain to be determined.

Likewise, PSA is used as an endpoint in monitoring outcomes after radiotherapy. In these cases, however, PSA declines to low but often detectable levels and the PSA response to treatment is unpredictable.[33] As a result, definitions of treatment success and failure are variable, and no consensus exists. Recent recommendations from the American Society of Therapeutic Radiology and Oncology (ASTRO) define recurrence after radiotherapy as three consecutive rises in serum PSA independent of PSA nadir.[34] Only a single study has validated this definition by correlation with clinical outcomes.[35] Critz et al propose a PSA nadir of 0.5 ng/mL or more to define brachytherapy treatment failure, demonstrating a significant likelihood of disease-free survival at 5 and 10 years in those with nadir PSA values less than 0.5 ng/mL.[36,37] However, the prognostic value of this nadir depends on most men achieving a nadir of 0.2 ng/mL or less.[38,39] Time to reach PSA nadir varies with treatment modality. A PSA nadir is typically achieved within 6 weeks after radical prostatectomy. Following radiation therapy, time to PSA nadir ranges from 8 to 18 months and even longer with brachytherapy. Ragde et al reported an average of 42 months to PSA nadir in a series of 152 patients receiving brachytherapy.[40] In a cohort of 539 men achieving a PSA nadir of 0.2 ng/mL or less, Critz reported a 27 month median time to nadir, with 99% reaching this level by 60 months.[41] Patterns of PSA failure, such as time to failure, nadir PSA reached, time to nadir PSA level, and PSA velocity, are current methods to further evaluate for treatment failure.[36,37,42,43] Another confounding factor in patients treated with radiation therapy is the concomitant use of androgen deprivation. No standard regimens or recommendations exist to address the optimal timing and duration of neoadjuvant or adjuvant hormonal therapy, resulting in difficulty assessing treatment success, degree of recurrence, and efficacy (i.e., disease-specific survival) of initial or salvage therapy. Thus, despite the widespread use of PSA to monitor disease activity after radiotherapy, controversy exists regarding exact definitions of treatment failure. In addition, it is important to keep in mind that most studies use PSA failure as a surrogate endpoint for cancer-specific survival. While PSA may be a sensitive indicator of recurrent or residual disease, it may not accurately reflect the more relevant outcome of survival.[44] The development of alternative intermediate endpoint biomarkers is needed. Recent studies demonstrate serum acid phosphatase and quantitative nuclear grade as independent predictors of post-prostatectomy biochemical progression and suggest potential use as novel biomarkers of treatment outcome.[45,46]

Distinguishing between local recurrence and distant failure is important in making subsequent treatment decisions (Figure 54.1). Physical examination of the prostate or surgical bed by DRE is neither sensitive nor specific in detection or localization of low-volume disease recurrence because of irradiated and post-surgical changes in the prostatic fossa.[47,48] One study of 1916 men after prostatectomy demonstrated that all recurrences, both local and distant, were associated with elevated PSA levels; thus, DRE was unnecessary in those with undetectable PSA. Changes in serial examinations over time, however, may help to detect local disease.[49] More recently, the need for anastomotic biopsy has been questioned. Data from our patients receiving radiotherapy after prostatectomy show no differences in outcomes between those treated for biochemical failure alone and those treated for biopsy proven recurrence, suggesting that biopsy may not be necessary to define patients most appropriate for salvage local therapy.[50]

In conjunction with pathologic stage and Gleason grade, PSA kinetics may provide the best means of identifying the location of tumor failure. Patients with low-grade disease generally have local recurrence, while those with seminal vesicle invasion or positive lymph nodes are more likely to fail distantly. A PSA velocity of less than 0.75 ng/mL/year was observed in 94% of patients with local recurrence.[51] Conversely, over 50% of men with metastatic disease had a PSA velocity greater than 0.75 ng/mL/year. In the same study, earlier postoperative elevations in PSA, within 2 years, were associated with distant disease. Clearly, a PSA doubling time of less than 6 months suggests distant disease. Trapasso et al described a median PSA doubling time of 4.3 months in patients ultimately progressing with distant failure, while those patients with clinically detected local failure or biochemical failure only had a PSA doubling time of 11.7 months.[52] Shorter PSA doubling times also predict increased risk for and shorter time to the appearance of clinical disease.[53,54]

IMAGING

Imaging studies complement clinical and pathologic information in localizing primary treatment failure. These modalities include TRUS, bone scan, pelvic computed tomography (CT) and magnetic resonance imaging (MRI), positron emission tomography (PET), and single-photon-emission computerized tomography (SPECT; i.e. ProstaScint).

The probability of a positive anastomotic biopsy performed for an elevated PSA is between 40% and 50% and is *not* dependent on rectal examination findings.[55–57] Transrectal ultrasound alone does not increase detection of local recurrence but guides needle placement to the vesicourethral anastomosis (Figure 54.2). Pelvic anatomy after radical prostatectomy is well described.[57–59] Bladder neck tissue can be seen as a homogeneous, hyperechoic ring at the level of the anastomosis. Recurrent disease is typically seen as a hypoechoic mass posterior or posterolateral to the anastomosis; recurrences elsewhere are less common.[57] Nonmalignant postoperative tissue may also appear hypoechoic, decreasing the sensitivity and specificity for identifying local recurrence. In addition, up to a third of recurrences may have an isoechoic appearance. A recent study addressed some of these issues.[60] Of 99 patients with PSA failure after prostatectomy, 41 cases of local recurrence were detected using TRUS-guided biopsies. Most were at the anastomosis and bladder neck (82%), although lesions noted in the retrovesical space were likely to represent recurrent disease. Overall sensitivity of TRUS was 76% with a specificity of 67% (Table 54.1).

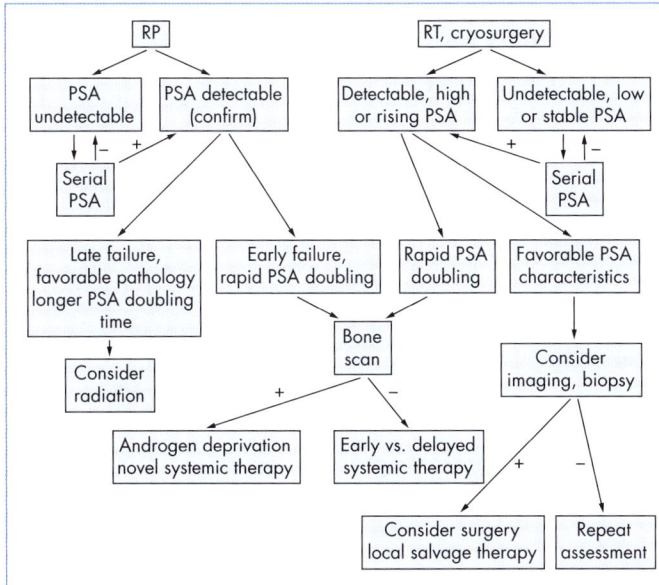

Fig. 54.1

Algorithm for evaluation, diagnosis, and treatment of recurrent prostate cancer. (PSA, prostate specific antigen; RP, radical prostatectomy; RT, radiotherapy.)

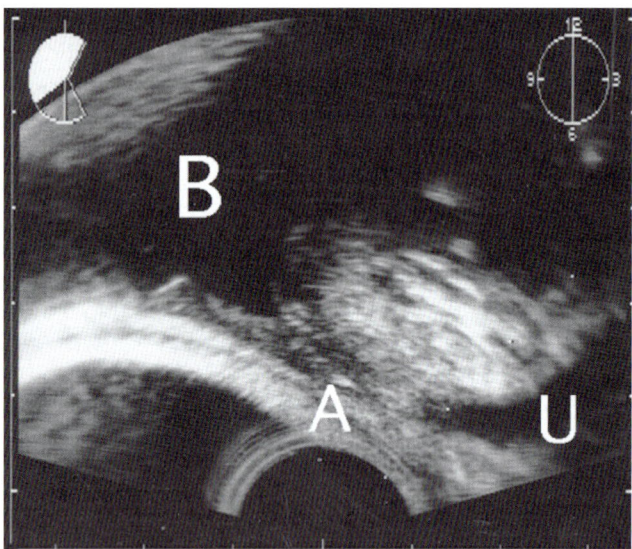

Fig. 54.2
Transrectal ultrasound after radical prostatectomy in the mid-sagittal plane demonstrating normal anatomy. A, urethrovesical anastomosis; B, bladder; U, bulbar urethra.

Table 54.1 Studies of transrectal ultrasound-guided biopsy after prostatectomy

Study	Number of patients	Ultrasound finding (%)	% Positive biopsy	Mean PSA (ng/mL)*
Saleem[61]	91	Positive (49)	52	7.8
		Negative (51)	25	
Shekarriz[62]	45	Positive (76)	65	5.2
		Negative (24)	18	
Leventis[60]	99	Positive (51)	62	2.4
		Negative (49)	20	
Scattoni[63]	119	Positive (54)	67	1.6
		Negative (46)	34	

*In those with positive biopsy

PSA, prostate-specific antigen.

Post-treatment changes of the in-situ organ after radiation or cryotherapy make the use of TRUS even more difficult in the detection of local recurrence. Radiation creates a small, hyperechoic gland with distortion of normal tissue planes; after cryotherapy, the prostate appears "fuzzy."[55] Nevertheless, local recurrences can be visualized as peripheral hypoechoic lesions. As mentioned earlier, TRUS-guided biopsies may not be necessary after radical prostatectomy to confirm local recurrence. In a cohort of 67 patients receiving radiation therapy after radical prostatectomy, outcomes were equivalent in those undergoing treatment for PSA-only recurrence and those with biopsy-proven disease.[50] Indications for TRUS guided biopsy after radiation and cryotherapy are also not clear. Most would agree that biopsies should be considered in

patients who show serial elevations in serum PSA after reaching a PSA nadir. Nadir levels of PSA are usually reached within 8 to 18 months after radiation and within 3 months after cryotherapy.

Most patients with evidence of disease recurrence undergo both bone scan and CT; however, the utility of these tests is unclear in patients with PSA-only progression. Oesterling suggested that radionucleotide bone scintigraphy is not cost effective in those with minimal PSA elevation after prostatectomy.[64] Cher et al reported that bone scans are rarely positive (5%) until PSA reaches 30 to 40 ng/mL; most patients who fail are detected at significantly lower PSA levels.[65] Bone scans are most useful in patients with rapidly rising PSA (5 ng/mL/month) or new skeletal symptoms. Likewise, cross-sectional imaging to detect local recurrence or lymphadenopathy is fairly insensitive (60% and 30–80%, respectively) and plays a greater role in men with higher PSA elevations and shorter PSA doubling time.[66,67] Endorectal MRI increases resolution to 3 mm, appreciably greater than TRUS.[68,69] Most recurrences after surgery appear on T1-weighted images as isointense lesions relative to the surrounding levator ani muscles, and as areas of reduced signal intensity on T2-weighted images in the normally high signal intensity peripheral zone (Figure 54.3). After radiotherapy, tumor recurrences have similar characteristics—hyperintense on T2-weighted images when compared to the levator ani muscles but hypointense relative to the peripheral zone (Figure 54.4). As technology in high-resolution CT and MRI spectroscopy evolves, so too will their roles in visualizing local and distant recurrence.

Positron emission tomography is not well-characterized in prostate cancer. Imaging takes advantage of differential cellular uptake and metabolism of a radiolabeled compound, such as the glucose analog ^{18}F-fluoro-2-deoxyglucose (FDG).[70] Theoretically the increased positron emission by tumor cells is detected and allows localization. Early studies report sensitivity and specificity of 75% and 67%, respectively, in detecting lymph node metastases, although the utility of PET in recurrent prostate cancer especially after radiotherapy and cryotherapy is unclear.[71]

The ProstaScint scan is based on a murine monoclonal antibody, recognizing prostate-specific membrane antigen (PSMA), conjugated to a linker-chelator and the radioisotope ^{111}Indium.[72] The test has been approved by the FDA for use in men with PSA-only recurrence after radical prostatectomy. Early data do not indicate a clear role for the capromab penditide immunoscintigraphy, but it appears to detect prostatic fossa recurrence with reasonable accuracy.[73] Kahn et al reported on SPECT findings and ability to predict response to salvage radiotherapy in 32 patients.[74] Seventy percent of those patients with a normal scan or evidence of only local disease had a durable, complete response to radiotherapy while only 22% with

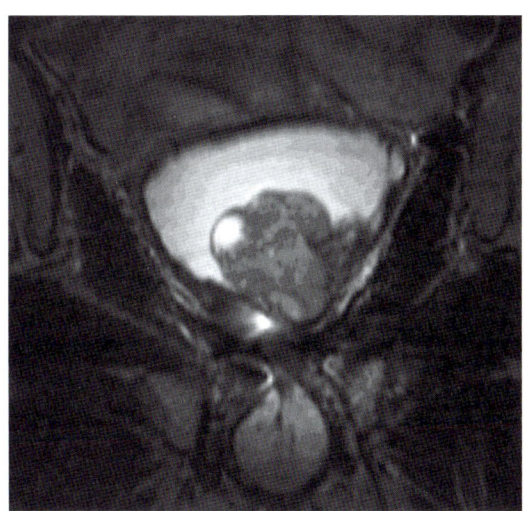

Fig. 54.3
Coronal T2-weighted MRI demonstrating recurrent prostate cancer after radical prostatectomy, extending into the bladder.

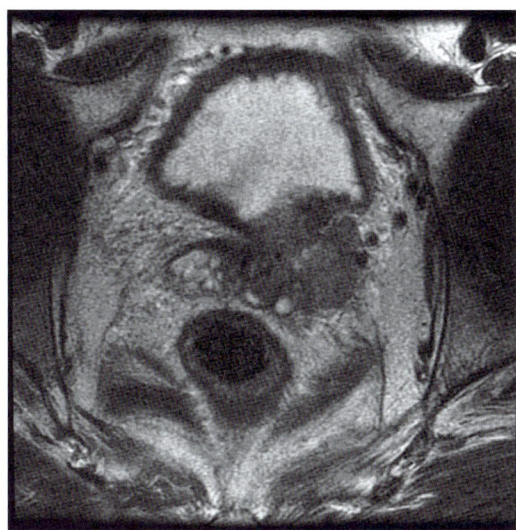

Fig. 54.4
Axial T2-weighted MRI showing recurrent tumor after radiation therapy involving the seminal vesicle, bladder base, extending into the adjacent fat.

capromab pendetide findings outside the prostatic fossa responded. Others have reported conflicting data, with ProstaScint findings not predictive to outcomes after salvage radiation therapy.[75] Thomas et al studied 30 men after with PSA recurrence after surgery undergoing ProstaScint scanning and radiotherapy.[76] At median follow-up of 35 months, biochemical control at 2 years was comparable in those with negative (31%) and positive (38%) scan. However, in men with evidence of disease in the prostatic bed only, response was poor (13%), whereas men with a positive scan elsewhere exhibited a better (60%) response. Novel techniques may improve the ability to assess recurrent prostate cancer. Schettino et al reported promising results of fusing data obtained from cross-sectional imaging (CT or MRI) and ProstaScint in men with evidence of bio-

chemical failure.[77] A 46% reduction in false-positive findings was noted due to the identification of physiologic uptake by normal structures, such as the bowel and vessels. In men thought to harbor non-localized disease, the combined scans suggested local recurrence in 43%. Of this group, 71% had decreasing PSA levels after local radiotherapy with the implication of improved negative predictive value of the fused images.

RECURRENCE AFTER RADICAL PROSTATECTOMY

Despite earlier diagnosis, improved patient selection, and evolution in surgical technique, as many as 35% to 50% of patients undergoing radical prostatectomy develop biochemical recurrence after treatment. Up to half of these men have local recurrence, with the remainder having distant disease alone or combined local and distant failure.[78] Therefore, it is important to define the role of regional therapy in patients after radical prostatectomy who may potentially benefit from further treatment.

Treatment of biochemical disease recurrence with radiation can often result in an undetectable PSA. In general, freedom from biochemical recurrence has been reported in 30% to 65% of men following therapeutic, or salvage, radiotherapy (Table 54.2).[79–88] Schild et al reported an overall 50% disease-free survival at 3 years; however, 78% of those patients with a pre-radiation PSA less than 1.0 ng/mL were disease-free while only 18% of men with PSA greater than 1.0 ng/mL remained disease-free.[79] Forman et al also reported improved disease-free survival in patients with lower pre-radiation PSA (<2.0 ng/mL).[84] More recently, in a cohort of 166 patients treated with radiotherapy after prostatectomy, 46% were free of biochemical relapse at 5 years of follow-up.[85] Multivariate analysis identified pathologic stage, tumor grade, and pre-radiation PSA as independent factors associated with PSA relapse. Leventis et al studied response to salvage radiation in a group of 49 men with biopsy-proven recurrence after prostatectomy.[89] Pre-radiation PSA and post-recurrence PSA doubling time before radiation were the only predictors of response to secondary therapy. In our series of 34 men with biopsy-proven recurrence after radical prostatectomy, 47% achieved favorable PSA response (<0.1 ng/mL or stable PSA <0.5 ng/mL) at a mean of 38.3 months after salvage external beam radiotherapy.[90] Predictors of secondary treatment success included prostatectomy Gleason sum less than 7 and pre-radiation PSA less than or equal to 4.0 ng/mL. Other investigators have reported no differences between adjuvant and therapeutic radiotherapy in patients with initially undetectable PSA after surgery.[91] Similarly, Coetzee et al noted a more durable response to radiation in men who failed after an

Table 54.2 Results of therapeutic radiotherapy after prostatectomy

Study	Number of patients	Percent with undetectable PSA	Length of follow-up
Hudson[80]	21	29	12.6 months
Schild[79]	46	50	5 years
Wu[83]	53	23	2 years
McCarthy[86]	37	54	27.5–36 months
Morris[87]	48	47	3 years
Forman[84]	47	73	36 months
Cadeddu[94]	30	37	at least 2 years
vander Kooy[81]	30	56	8 years
Coetzee[82]	45	51	33 months
Nudell[92]	47	41	3 years
Pisansky[85]	166	46	5 years
Stephenson[93]	501	45	4 years

PSA, prostate-specific antigen.

initial undetectable PSA when compared to men with a persistently detectable PSA (66% at 40 months versus 20% at 12 months, respectively).[82] We recently evaluated our experience with radiation following radical prostatectomy in 105 patients at the University of California San Francisco.[92] The overall 5-year disease-free survival rate was 43%, with failure after radiation defined as PSA greater than 0.2 ng/mL. Outcomes were equivalent in those men receiving adjuvant and salvage radiotherapy when therapeutic radiation was initiated with a low serum PSA (<1.0 ng/mL) (Figure 54.5). There were no differences between the adjuvant and salvage radiotherapy groups with respect to pre-prostatectomy PSA, tumor grade, or pathologic stage. In univariate analyses, low stage prior to prostatectomy and low Gleason sum predicted a response to radiotherapy in multivariate analysis pre-prostatectomy PSA under 20 ng/mL predicted radiotherapy success. Our data, as well

as those from Vicini et al, also demonstrate that the indication for radiotherapy (adjuvant versus therapeutic) was an independent prognostic factor associated with biochemical control.[88] However, no other clinical, pathologic, or treatment-related factors were associated with 5-year outcome in their patients. Stephenson et al reported the outcomes of salvage radiotherapy for recurrent prostate cancer after radical prostatectomy in 501 patients from five tertiary centers.[93] The 4-year progression-free survival was 45% (95% CI, 40–50%), with 10% developing distant metastases. Predictors of progression after radiotherapy included Gleason score of 8 to 10 (hazard ratio [HR], 2.6; 95% CI, 1.7–4.1), negative surgical margins (HR, 1.9; 95% CI, 1.4–2.5), seminal vesicle invasion (HR, 1.4; 95% CI, 1.1–1.9), PSA greater than 2.0 ng/mL at the time of radiation therapy (HR, 2.3; 95% CI, 1.7–3.2), and PSA doubling time of 10 months (HR, 1.7; 95% CI, 1.2–2.2). Nevertheless, some men with these adverse features could achieve a durable response to salvage therapy. Patients with higher Gleason sum and positive surgical margin receiving early radiotherapy (PSA ≤ 2.0 ng/mL) had 4-year progression-free probability of 81% when the PSA doubling time was more than 10 months, but only 37% when doubling time was 10 months. Cadeddu et al present more pessimistic data.[94] Only 21% of men had an undetectable PSA for over 2 years after therapeutic radiation following prostatectomy. No patients with Gleason score 9 or greater, positive seminal vesicles, or positive lymph nodes had undetectable PSA levels greater than 2 years. Finally, early treatment at lower PSA or isolated PSA elevation without documented local recurrence did not predict a favorable response to therapy. Thus, while it appears that adjuvant radiotherapy is a viable option in patients at higher risk for local recurrence, radiation may be utilized with efficacy in a therapeutic fashion when tumor volume, as reflected by serum PSA, is low. Patients most likely to benefit from salvage radiation after prostatectomy include those with low-to-moderate grade tumors with an undetectable postoperative PSA that rises more than 1

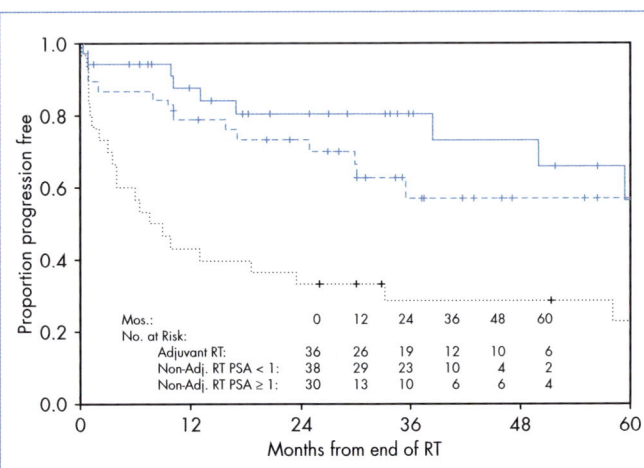

Fig. 54.5
Prostate-specific antigen (PSA) progression-free survival by pre-radiotherapy PSA. Comparison of the interval to biochemical disease recurrence in patients after radical prostatectomy treated with adjuvant radiotherapy (RT), therapeutic RT with pre-RT PSA less than 1.0 ng/mL, and therapeutic RT with pre-RT PSA greater than or equal to 1.0 ng/mL. The number of patients at risk according to the indication for RT is given below the curves.
From Nudell DM, Grossfeld GD, Weinberg VK, et al. Radiotherapy after radical prostatectomy: treatment outcomes and failure patterns. Urology 1999;54:1049–1057.

year after surgery. The exact timing of radiation has yet to be determined, although a PSA cut-point of 2.0 ng/mL currently appears reasonable. The recent ASTRO consensus panel recommendations regarding salvage radiotherapy include a dose of at least 6400 cGy given, with 1.8 or 2 Gy per fraction, when PSA is less than 1.5 ng/mL.[95] Interestingly, the ASTRO recommendations state that use of androgen deprivation is not standard in patients receiving secondary radiation therapy.

Other forms of treatment for locally recurrent disease after radical prostatectomy have been reported but are not well characterized. These include brachytherapy and cryosurgical ablation. Kotrouvelis et al treated five patients with salvage brachytherapy after prostatectomy with acceptable morbidity and results.[96] At UCSF, we have treated three cases of local recurrence after prostatectomy with cryoablation; one patient has had an undetectable PSA for 3 years. Another patient had salvage brachytherapy after prostatectomy, and 18 months after the procedure his PSA is 0.03 ng/mL. However, further studies are required before their routine use after radical prostatectomy can be recommended.

A caveat has been raised regarding residual benign prostate glands as a potential source for post-prostatectomy elevations in PSA. Djavan et al found benign prostatic glands in the surgical margins of 95 of 351 prostatectomy specimens (27%).[97] These were found most commonly in the posterior and lateral areas. A large fraction (79%) of patients with pT2 disease and benign glands at the surgical margin had detectable postoperative PSA, ranging from 0.6 to 2.0 ng/mL. They concluded that remaining benign prostate glands may be a cause of apparent biochemical failure after surgery. More recently, Shah et al reported a significantly lower incidence of benign prostatic glands at the surgical margins.[98] A prospective analysis of 119 consecutive prostatectomy specimens was performed with whole-mount sectioning at 3 mm intervals. Only 13 cases (11%) demonstrated benign glands, with most focally involving the apex. Higher Gleason score and larger prostate gland volume were significantly associated with the finding of benign glands on the surgical margins. No patients with benign glands on the inked margins had PSA recurrences; however, follow-up was relatively short with a median of 2 months. Thus, one may consider benign prostate glands as a source for detectable PSA after surgery but recurrent or persistent cancer must be sought and presumed to be present in those with high-risk disease characteristics or progressive rise in PSA.

RECURRENCE AFTER RADIATION THERAPY

Radiation therapy, both external beam and brachytherapy, is increasingly used for patients with organ-confined cancers.[99] A certain percentage of patients receiving radiation will fail locally due to either inadequate localization of the target, inadequate dose, or radiation resistance. Therefore, issues of detection and localization of recurrence after radiation and subsequent treatment options are important to elucidate.

As discussed, various definitions of PSA failure after radiation have been used. Nevertheless, any rising PSA level after radiation therapy may signal active, residual disease. An exception may be those who have been treated with neoadjuvant hormonal therapy, where androgen levels and PSA may rise after ceasing androgen deprivation. In addition, an interesting phenomenon has been noted in about one third of patients who receive brachytherapy, but not other forms of radiation. A self-limited, temporary rise in serum PSA often occurs 12 to 18 months after the procedure ("PSA bounce"); this benign PSA flare is unrelated to tumor progression.[40] In a report of 591 men treated with brachytherapy, a significant fraction exhibited a temporary increase in post-treatment PSA (between 0.3 and 3.4 ng/mL) at a mean of 24.8 months after implant.[100] Importantly, this spiking of PSA was not associated with a higher risk of subsequent clinical failure nor risk factors for recurrent disease.

As many as one third of patients may demonstrate rising PSA at 3 years, and as many as half may fail clinically within 5 to 7 years after radiotherapy.[101–103] Recurrence rates may have decreased with the use of techniques that target the prostate better and allow for delivery of higher doses. In those patients with recurrent or persistent localized disease, the curative options traditionally included salvage prostatectomy or cryoablation. Most commonly, however, androgen ablation is instituted with post-irradiation recurrence. We found that androgen deprivation is the most common form (88%) of secondary treatment after radiotherapy, suggesting limited curative options for those patients currently failing initial radiation.[3]

Salvage prostatectomy after radiotherapy has been approached with caution in the past. It is often technically difficult but has been demonstrated to be feasible with acceptable morbidity and cure rates. Overall, cancer-specific survival and disease-free rates have ranged from 70% to 90% and 30% to 50% at 8 to 10 years, respectively.[104–106] Pathologically, organ-confined disease is found in 20% to 50% of cases and is an important prognostic factor. Tefilli et al reported that all patients with organ-confined disease were disease free at 34 months.[107] Amling et al reported a 10-year disease free survival of 43% in 108 patients, similar to results from Rogers et al and Moul et al.[106,108,109] Both DNA ploidy and preoperative serum PSA were significant predictors of outcome following surgery. Another study also reported radical prostatectomy Gleason score as an independent predictor of cancer-specific survival.[110] Other factors influencing outcomes of salvage prostatectomy include pre-radiation clinical stage and preoperative PSA.[111] Data suggest that PSA levels less than 10 ng/mL prior to surgery may predict pathologically localized disease and reduced recurrence. In general, salvage prostatectomy after radiation should be reserved for men with few co-morbidities and a 10-year life expectancy in whom recurrence is not locally advanced. Parameters guiding the decision include Gleason sum less than 7, PSA less than 10 ng/mL, and clinical stage T2 or less at the time of both radiation and surgery. However, accurate presurgical staging is often difficult after radiation and may make appropriate patient selection difficult.

Interest in both primary and salvage cryosurgical ablation of the prostate has reemerged with technical innovations and the desire for minimally-invasive procedures. High-resolution TRUS allows precise placement of the probes and real-time visualization of the freezing process. In addition, freezing may cause greater tumor destruction of a heterogeneous, radioresistant cell population, even outside the prostate in adjacent tissue, when compared with other modalities. Reported results of salvage cryotherapy have been modest with the largest series of patients treated at M.D. Anderson Cancer Center.[112] Seventy seven percent of patients had negative sextant biopsies 6 months after cryoablation, but only 45 of 150 patients (31%) had persistently undetectable PSA with a mean follow-up for 13.5 months. A double freeze-thaw cycle appeared more effective than a single cycle in reducing both positive post-treatment biopsy and biochemical failure rates. In multivariate analyses, the number of probes and post-cryotherapy PSA nadir predicted positive post-cryotherapy biosies.[113] Bales et al noted only a 9% disease-free rate after salvage cryotherapy.[114] The recent report from Columbia University on salvage cryotherapy found a 66% PSA-free survival in 43 patients at 12 months; PSA nadir (>0.1 ng/mL) was the only independent predictor of biochemical recurrence.[115] A second large cohort has been reported by Chin et al.[116] The study analyzed 118 patients receiving cryoablation for proven local recurrence after full dose radiotherapy. Although few patients had positive post-cryotherapy biopsies, actuarial freedom from biochemical failure was 68%, 55%, and 34% at PSA thresholds of 4, 2, and 0.5 ng/mL, respectively. Predictors of adverse PSA outcomes included pre-cryotherapy PSA greater than 10 ng/mL, pre-cryotherapy stage T3/T4, and initial Gleason score greater than 7. Prostate -specific antigen characteristics in monitoring outcome following cryotherapy, either primary or salvage, are not well defined. Early evidence suggests that PSA nadir (>0.5 ng/mL) is currently the best prognostic indicator of biochemical and biopsy proved failure. Furthermore, it was noted that even small fluctuations in PSA may signify subsequent biochemical failure.[117] Other variables, such as initial clinical stage,

number of probes, and operator experience, may play a role in salvage outcomes.

Salvage brachytherapy after primary radiotherapy has been proposed as a promising treatment modality.[118] In the past, concerns centered on the risk of injury to the urethra, bladder, and rectum with additional radiation as well as the questionable biologic response in a tumor with possible radioresistant elements, given failure of standard external beam radiotherapy. Further investigation is warranted given improvements in treatment planning and delivery methods, as well as the documented morbidity of alternatives (i.e., prostatectomy and cryoablation). Grado et al followed 49 patients treated with brachytherapy after biopsy-proven, primary radiotherapy failure.[118] Actuarial biochemical-free survival was 34% at 5 years and was associated with a post-salvage PSA nadir below 0.5 ng/mL. Local disease control was 98%. These results are encouraging, especially given the treatment population. The median age was 73.3 years and 71% had locally advanced disease at initial presentation; 90% of the cancers were moderately to poorly differentiated on pre-brachytherapy biopsies. Complications were similar to those of patients undergoing primary brachytherapy and much lower than for salvage prostatectomy and cryotherapy. Beyer reported a comparable 5-year actuarial freedom from relapse rate (53%) for salvage brachytherapy. PSA-free survival was associated with tumor grade and pre-brachytherapy PSA, but neither factor reached statistical significance due to the small number of patients.[119]

Innovative forms of therapy are being developed that may play a role in salvage therapy. Both high intensity focused ultrasound (HIFU) and radiofrequency interstitial ablation are being studied and appear to have promise in local control of prostate cancer.[120–122] In preliminary studies, primary HIFU achieved local control in 60% to 80% of patients.[123] Radiofrequency ablation was able to produce predictable lesions in prostates in vivo prior to radical prostatectomy.

We have preliminary data on the use of a novel palladium–cobalt alloy to treat local recurrence using thermal ablation.[124] These ThermoRods™ are permanent, biocompatible rods designed to produce precise and specific local tissue temperatures when placed in a magnetic field. In 10 patients with biopsy proved recurrence after external beam radiation therapy, ThermaRods™ were placed throughout the prostate under TRUS guidance and subsequently induced for 1 hour. Eight patients achieved post-thermotherapy PSA less than 0.1 ng/mL at a mean follow-up of 7 months. Measurement of temperatures demonstrated average prostate temperatures above, but urethral and rectal temperatures below, the cytotoxic 46°C threshold. Urethral sloughing and urinary tract infections were the most common complications, occurring in 40% of patients. Further investigation is needed to reduce treatment morbidity and confirm duration of the PSA response.

RECURRENCE AFTER CRYOTHERAPY

Cryosurgical ablation of the prostate has evolved over the past 30 years. Early experience revealed limited local and overall control with significant treatment morbidity. More contemporary data provide a better understanding of the technique. We have performed cryoablation in 176 patients over a 5-year period with a mean follow-up of 31 months.[125] Nadir PSA was undetectable in almost half of the patients, but biopsies were positive in 38%. Treatment success, defined as PSA nadir less than 0.5 ng/mL that did not rise by more than 0.2 ng/mL on two consecutive measurements, was seen in 43% of men. Pre-treatment PSA less than 10 ng/mL and undetectable PSA nadir after cryotherapy predicted for biochemical recurrence-free survival. Similar results have been reported by Long et al[126] Although it appears that a substantial number of patients fail cryotherapy, the majority were at high risk for disease recurrence based on pre-treatment stage, serum PSA, and Gleason grade. Results of cryotherapy may be more comparable to other forms of primary therapy when accounting for the unfavorable patient population.

For those patients whose cancers recur after cryotherapy, the choice of secondary treatment is not well defined. Repeat freezing has been reported, as well as salvage prostatectomy. In the subset of patients at UCSF who underwent multiple cryotherapy procedures, 67% had no cancer on subsequent biopsies, but only 33% achieved long-term, favorable PSA values.[125] Grampas et al successfully performed radical perineal prostatectomy in six patients after initial cryotherapy.[127] Pisters et al used cryotherapy in a neoadjuvant fashion in conjunction with radical prostatectomy in patients with locally advanced cancer.[128] Of seven patients treated, only one failed by PSA criteria, one had positive surgical margins, and four had stage pT0. Burton et al report the only experience with salvage radiotherapy after initial cryosurgical prostate ablation.[129] The overall biochemical control rate (PSA nadir < 1.0 ng/mL) was 61% at a mean follow-up of 32 months. Those with PSA less than 2.5 ng/mL prior to salvage radiation and a dose greater than 64 Gy had improved biochemical response. Thus, post-cryotherapy radiation appears feasible but further investigation is warranted to assess cancer outcomes and morbidity.

MORBIDITY FROM SECONDARY TREATMENT

In evaluating additional treatments for prostate cancer recurrence, both local and distant, factors other than PSA-free or overall survival must be considered. All modalities, including salvage surgery, radiation, cryotherapy, and traditional hormonal therapy, have significant side effects and morbidity. Nevertheless, few studies carefully address these points. Tefilli et al examined quality of life in 68 men undergoing salvage procedures.[130] They reported significantly worse outcomes in urinary continence and physical well-being after salvage prostatectomy; however, similar satisfaction with respect to overall quality of life and potency was found after salvage prostatectomy and salvage radiotherapy.

Morbidity of therapeutic external beam radiation after radical prostatectomy has not been carefully reported. Typically 45 to 65 Gy is delivered to the prostatic bed and is generally well tolerated. Short-term complications, including bowel and bladder irritability, are seen in approximately 10% of patients, whereas long-term and significant complications are less well defined but approach 20% of the population.[131,132] A retrospective study of 294 men analyzed the effects of adjuvant external beam radiation on urinary continence and potency after nerve-sparing prostatectomy.[133] With a median follow-up of 2.6 years, no significant impact of postoperative radiation was seen on urinary continence or erectile dysfunction. However, a more recent study suggests that primary external beam radiation therapy may lead to hypogonadism, with lower testosterone, free testosterone, and dihydrotestosterone levels as well as increase leuteinizing and follicle-stimulating hormone levels.[134] Although lower doses of radiation may be administered as secondary therapy, this report suggests that salvage radiotherapy may potentially cause testicular damage and resultant hypogonadism.

Complications of salvage prostatectomy are more common when compared with primary prostatectomy. Urinary incontinence is seen in 20% to 60% of patients, bladder neck contracture in approximately 20%, and impotence is virtually universal. Rectal injury may occur in fewer than 10% of patients but rarely necessitates fecal diversion.[104,106,135,136] Contemporary series report better outcomes owing to improved patient selection, earlier identification of failure, and improved surgical techniques. Vaidya and Soloway performed salvage prostatectomy in six patients with isolated local recurrence after radiotherapy.[137] Although all were rendered impotent, five were continent and operative morbidity was excellent, with mean operative time of 195 minutes, blood loss of 680 mL, and hospitalization of 3.2 days. Nevertheless, patients must be informed of all potential outcomes, including cystoprostatectomy and urinary diversion, temporary diverting colostomy, and inoperability due to pelvic desmoplasia. Some have proposed planned cystoprostatectomy with urinary diversion at the time of salvage surgery to maximize subsequent lower urinary tract function.[138-140] Careful preoperative evaluation is necessary to identify manifestations of radiation injury, such as intractable hematuria, low-volume bladder, and irritative lower urinary tract symptoms, which may alter treatment decisions.

A study of salvage cryotherapy has recently been published.[141] The data support the importance of urethral warming with respect to several aspects of quality of life and the authors conclude that salvage cryotherapy is not superior to salvage prostatectomy when considering morbidity. Patients should be made aware of these issues and the decision-making process should weigh these factors against potential benefits in prognosis. Moreover, additional studies are necessary to clarify questions of morbidity and quality of life in secondary treatments for recurrent prostate cancer.

NATURAL HISTORY OF RECURRENCE

Currently, evidence of biochemical recurrence after definitive therapy is utilized as an end point for defining outcome after treatment. Although PSA is accepted as a surrogate marker of disease status and elevations lead to subsequent evaluation and intervention, the true clinical significance of biochemical "failure" remains uncertain. As mentioned previously, the time from PSA progression to the development of metastasis is lengthy, with reports of a median of 7.5 years.[142] It remains to be determined whether the early institution of therapy, either local or systemic (i.e., androgen deprivation), improves cancer-related mortality. Similarly, a study of 1132 men after radical prostatectomy at the Cleveland Clinic suggested that biochemical failure did not predict survival.[44] The 10-year survival in those with and without PSA failure (defined as ≥ 0.2 ng/mL) was 88% and 93%, respectively ($P = 0.94$). In men receiving secondary treatment, the 10-year overall survival was 86%.

Rogers et al recently examined the outcome in 160 men who failed to reach an undetectable PSA (<0.1 ng/mL) after radical prostatectomy but did not receive adjuvant therapy.[143] Distant metastasis-free survival was 68%, 49%, and 22% at 3, 5, and 10 years, respectively. Forty seven percent of men ultimately developed distant metastases at a median time of 5 years (range 0.5–13 years). Predictors of outcome included Gleason score in the prostatectomy specimen and pathologic stage (i.e. pT3 and N+), as well as PSA velocity during the year following surgery (≥ 0.05 ng/mL). Thus, a significant number of men remain without metastatic disease after radical prostatectomy, for an extended period, despite a persistently detectable PSA level.

Further indirect evidence is present from the study of D'Amico et al, where a cohort of 8669 patients were treated with either surgery or external beam radiation therapy.[144] Of the 611 men with biochemical failure after surgery, only 36 (6%) deaths were observed during a 7 year median follow-up; of these, 73% were prostate cancer-related. Of the 840 men with biochemical failure after radiotherapy, there were 188 deaths (14%) of which 84 (71%) were from prostate cancer. The authors also found that PSA doubling time was a surrogate for prostate cancer-specific mortality after both prostatectomy and radiation. A post-treatment PSA doubling time less than 3 months was a direct correlate to death from prostate cancer, and once this endpoint was reached, death was independent of other interventions.

CONCLUSIONS

Recurrence after definitive treatment for prostate cancer is a significant problem. Few studies exist examining the optimal diagnostic and therapeutic strategies following either radical prostatectomy or radiation therapy where there is evidence of local disease. Limited curative options are available in many situations. We await the development of more efficacious and less morbid treatment options.

Promising areas of research include molecular characterization and earlier detection of prostate cancer relapse. Pathologic and immunohistochemical markers may add information to determine prognosis. It remains to be determined if genetic markers can predict disease recurrence or metastatic potential. If found, this information could direct the type and timing of additional treatments. Moreover, it may be recognized that not all patients who fail initial therapy as evidenced by biochemical relapse will suffer disease-specific morbidity or mortality. Identification of such patients would spare them the inconvenience, cost, and morbidity of complex testing and/or treatment. Earlier determination of PSA failure and prompt institution of salvage therapy may be possible with the ultrasensitive PSA assay. The lead-time may increase the efficacy of second treatments, such as radiotherapy after prostatectomy, by minimizing tumor burden. Finally, patients may fail both primary and salvage therapy because of undetected metastatic, or micrometastatic, disease. Development of better diagnostic techniques and systemic treatments may address this issue by affecting both local and distant prostate cancer cells. New approaches currently undergoing evaluation, such as antiangiogenesis agents or gene therapy, may revolutionize therapy of prostate cancer.

REFERENCES

1. Johansson JE, Holmberg L, Johansson S, et al. Fifteen-year survival in prostate cancer. A prospective, population-based study in Sweden. JAMA 1997;277:467–471.

2. Grossfeld GD, Chang JJ, Broering JM, et al. Under staging and under grading in a contemporary series of patients undergoing radical prostatectomy: results from the Cancer of the Prostate Strategic Urologic Research Endeavor database. J Urol 2001;165:851–856.

3. Grossfeld GD, Stier DM, Flanders SC, et al. Use of second treatment following definitive local therapy for prostate cancer: data from the CaPSURE database. J Urol 1998;160:1398–1404.

4. Lu-Yao GL, Potosky AL, Albertsen PC, et al. Follow-up prostate cancer treatments after radical prostatectomy: a population-based study. J Natl Cancer Inst 1996;88:166–173.

5. Fowler FL Jr, Barry MJ, Lu-Yao G, et al. Patient-reported complications and follow-up treatment after radical prostatectomy. The National Medicare Experience: 1988–1990 (updated June 1993). Urology 1993;42:622–629.

6. Fowler FJ Jr, Barry MJ, Lu-Yao G, et al. Outcomes of external-beam radiation therapy for prostate cancer: a study of Medicare beneficiaries in three surveillance, epidemiology, and end results areas. J Clin Oncol 1996;14:2258–2265.

7. Moul JW. Prostate specific antigen only progression of prostate cancer. J Urol 2000;163:1632–1642.

8. Eastham JA and Scardino PT. Radical prostatectomy. In Walsh PC, Retik AB, Vaughan ED, Jr, Wein AJ (eds): Campbell's Urology, 7th ed. Philadelphia: WB Saunders, 1998, pp 2547–2564.

9. Partin AW, Pound CR, Clemens JQ, et al. Prostate-specific antigen after anatomic radical prostatectomy: The Johns Hopkins experience after ten years. Urol Clin North Am 1993;20:713–725.

10. Zincke H, Oesterling JE, Blute ML, et al. Long-term (15 years) results after radical prostatectomy for clinically localized (stage T2c or lower) prostate cancer. J Urol 1994;152:1850–1857.

11. D'Amico AV, Whittington R, Malkowicz SB, et al. A multivariate analysis of clinical and pathological factors that predict for prostate specific antigen failure after radical prostatectomy. J Urol 1995;154:131–138.

12. Zietman AL, Edelstein RA, Coen JJ, et al. Radical prostatectomy for adenocarcinoma of the prostate: The influence of preoperative and pathologic findings on biochemical disease-free outcome. Urology 1994;43:828–833.

13. Catalona WJ and Smith DJ. Five-year tumor recurrence rates after anatomic radical retropubic prostatectomy for prostate cancer. J Urol 1994;152:1837–1842.

14. Ohori M, Goad JR, Wheeler TM, et al. Can radical prostatectomy alter the progression of poorly differentiated prostate cancer? J Urol 1994;152:1843–1849.

15. Presti JC Jr, Shinohara K, Bacchetti P, et al. Positive fraction of systematic biopsies predicts risk of relapse after radical prostatectomy. Urology 1998;52:1079–1084.

16. Epstein JI, Pizov G, Walsh PC. Correlation of pathologic findings with progression after radical retropubic prostatectomy. Cancer 1993; 71:3582–3543.

17. Epstein JI, Partin AW, Sauvageot J, et al. Prediction of progression following radical prostatectomy: A multivariate analysis of 721 men with long-term follow-up. Am J Surg Pathol 1996;20:286–292.

18. Epstein JI, CarMichael MJ, Pizov G, et al. Influence of capsular penetration on progression following radical prostatectomy: A study of 196 cases with long-term follow-up. J Urol 1993;150:135–141.

19. Ohori M, Wheeler TM, Kattan MW, et al. Prognostic significance of positive surgical margins in radical prostatectomy specimens. J Urol 1995;154:1818–1824.

20. Montie JE. Significance and treatment of positive margins or seminal vesicle invasion after radical prostatectomy. Urol Clin North Am 1990;17:803–812.

21. CarMichael MJ, Veltri RW, Partin AW, et al. Deoxyribonucleic acid ploidy analysis as a predictor of recurrence following radical prostatectomy for stage T2 disease. J Urol 1995;153:1015–1019.

22. Babaian RJ, Troncoso P, Bhadkamkar VA, et al. Analysis of clinicopathologic factors predicting outcome after radical prostatectomy. Cancer 2001;91:1414–1422.

23. Nasseri KK and Austenfeld MS. PSA recurrence after definitive treatment of clinically localized prostate cancer. AUA Update Series 1997;16:82–87.

24. Partin AW, Subong ENP, Walsh PC, et al. Combination of prostate-specific antigen, clinical stage, and Gleason score to predict pathological stage of localized prostate cancer: a multi-institutional update. JAMA 1997;277:1445–1451.

25. Kattan MW, Wheeler TM, Scardino PT. Postoperative nomogram for disease recurrence after radical prostatectomy for prostate cancer. J Clin Oncol 1999;17:1499–1507.

26. D'Amico AV, Chang H, Holoupka E. Calculated prostate cancer volume: the optimal predictor of the actual prostate cancer volume. Urology 1997;49:385–391.

27. Epstein JI. Pathology of adenocarcinoma of the prostate. In Walsh PC, Retik AB, Vaughan ED Jr, Wein AJ (eds): Campbell's Urology, 7th ed. Philadelphia: WB Saunders, 1998, pp 2497–2505.

28. Goad JR, Chang SJ, Ohori M, et al. PSA after definitive radiotherapy for clinically localized prostate cancer. Urol Clin North Am 1993;20:727–736.

29. Lange PH, Ercole CJ, Lightner DJ, et al. The value of serum prostate specific antigen determinations before and after radical prostatectomy. J Urol 1989;141:873–879.

30. Pound CR, Partin AW, Eisenberger MA, et al. Natural history of progression after PSA elevation following radical prostatectomy. JAMA 1999;281:1591–1597.

31. Amling CL, Bergstralh EJ, Blute ML, et al. Defining prostate specific antigen progression after radical prostatectomy: what is the most appropriate cut point? J Urol 2001;165:1146–1451.

32. Freedland SJ, Sutter ME, Dorey F, et al. Defining the ideal cutpoint for determining PSA recurrence after radical prostatectomy. Prostate-specific antigen. Urology 2003;61:365–369.

33. Polascik TJ, Oesterling JE, Partin AW. Prostate-specific antigen 1998: What we have learned and where we are going. Part II: Detection, staging, and monitoring of prostate cancer. AUA Update Series 1998;17:218–223.

34. American Society for Therapeutic Radiology and Oncology Consensus Panel. Consensus statement: Guidelines for PSA following radiation therapy. Int J Radiat Oncol Biol Phys 1997;37:1035–1041.

35. Horwitz EM, Vicini FA, Ziaja EL, et al. The correlation between the ASTRO consensus panel definition of biochemical failure and clinical outcome for patients with prostate cancer treated with external beam irradiation. American Society of Therapeutic Radiology and Oncology. Int J Radiat Oncol Biol Phys 1998;41:267–272.

36. Critz FA, Levinson AK, Holladay D, et al. Prostate-specific antigen nadir of 0.5 ng/mL or less defines disease freedom for surgically staged men irradiated for prostate cancer. Urology 1997;49:668–672.

37. Critz FA, Levinson AK, Williams WH, et al. The PSA nadir that indicates potential cure after radiotherapy for prostate cancer. Urology 1997;49:322–326.

38. Critz FA, Levinson AK, Williams WH, et al. Prostate specific antigen nadir achieved by men apparently cured of prostate cancer by radiotherapy. J Urol 1999;161:1199–1203.

39. Critz FA, Williams WH, Holladay CT, et al. Post-treatment PSA < or = 0.2 ng/mL defines disease freedom after radiotherapy for prostate cancer using modern techniques. Urology 1999;54:968–971.

40. Ragde H, Elgamal AA, Snow PB, et al. Ten-year free survival after transperineal sonography-guided iodine-125 brachytherapy with or without 45-gray external beam irradiation in the treatment of patients with clinically localized, low to high Gleason grade prostate carcinoma. Cancer 1998;83:989–1001.

41. Critz FA. Time to achieve a prostate specific antigen nadir of 0.2 ng/ml after simultaneous irradiation for prostate cancer. J Urol 2002;168:2434–2438.

42. Zagars GK. Serum PSA as a tumor marker for patients undergoing definitive radiation therapy. Urol Clin North Am 1993;20:737–747.

43. Goad JR, Chang S, Ohori M, et al. PSA after definitive radiotherapy for clinically localized prostate cancer. Urol Clin North Am 1993;20:727–736.

44. Jhaveri FM, Zippe CD, Klein EA, et al. Biochemical failure does not predict overall survival after radical prostatectomy for localized prostate cancer: 10-year results. Urology 1999;54:884–890.

45. Han M, Piantadosi S, Zahurak ML, et al. Serum acid phosphatase level and biochemical recurrence following radical prostatectomy for men with clinically localized prostate cancer. Urology 2001;57:707–711.

46. Veltri RW, Miller MC, An G. Standardization, analytical validation, and quality control of intermediate endpoint biomarkers. Urology 2001;57:164–170.

47. Pound CR, Christens-Barry OW, Gurganus RT, et al. Digital rectal examination and imaging studies are unnecessary in men with undetectable prostate specific antigen following radical prostatectomy. J Urol 1999;162:1337–1340.

48. Johnstone PA, McFarland JT, Riffenburgh RH, et al. Efficacy of digital rectal examination after radiotherapy for prostate cancer. J Urol 2001;166:1684–1687.

49. Schellhammer PF, Kuban DA, el-Mahdi AM. Local failure after definitive radiation or surgical therapy for carcinoma of the prostate and options for prevention and therapy. Urol Clin North Am 1991;18:485–499.

50. Koppie TM, Grossfeld GD, Nudell DM, et al. Is anastomotic biopsy necessary before radiotherapy after radical prostatectomy? J Urol 2001;166:111–115.

51. Partin AW, Pearson JD, Landis PK, et al. Evaluation of serum prostate-specific antigen velocity after radical prostatectomy to distinguish local recurrence from distant metastases. Urology1994; 43:649–659.

52. Trapasso JG, deKernion JB, Smith RB, et al. The incidence and significance of detectable levels of serum prostate serum antigen after radical prostatectomy. J Urol 1994;152:1821–1825.

53. Patel A, Dorey F, Franklin J, et al. Recurrence patterns after radical retropubic prostatectomy: clinical usefulness of prostate specific antigen doubling times and log slope prostate specific antigen. J Urol 1997;158:1441–1445.

54. Roberts SG, Blute ML, Bergstralh EJ, et al. PSA doubling time as a predictor of clinical progression after biochemical failure following radical prostatectomy for prostate cancer. Mayo Clin Proc 2001;76:576–581.

55. Lightner DJ, Lange PH, Reddy PK, et al. Prostate specific antigen and local recurrence after radical prostatectomy. J Urol 1990;144:921–926.

56. Foster LS, Jajodia P, Fournier G, et al. The value of prostate specific antigen and transrectal ultrasound guided biopsy in detecting prostatic fossa recurrence following radical prostatectomy. J Urol 1993;149:1024–1028.

57. Connolly JA, Shinohara K, Presti JC Jr, et al. Local recurrence after radical prostatectomy: characteristics in size, location, and relationship to prostate-specific antigen and surgical margins. Urology 1996;47:225–231.

58. Goldenberg SL, Carter M, Dashefsky S, et al. Sonographic characteristics of the urethrovesical anastomosis in the early post-radical prostatectomy patient. J Urol 1992;147:1307–1309.

59. Parra RO, Wolf RM, Huben RP. The use of transrectal ultrasound in the detection and evaluation of local pelvic recurrences after a radical urological pelvic operation. J Urol 1990;144:707–709.

60. Leventis AK, Shariat SF, Slawin KM. Local recurrence after radical prostatectomy: correlation of US features with prostatic fossa biopsy findings. Radiology 2001;219:432–439.

61. Saleem MD, Sanders H, Abu El Naser M, et al. Factors predicting cancer detection in biopsy of the prostatic fossa after radical prostatectomy. Urology 1998;51:283–286.

62. Shekarriz B, Upadhyay J, Wood DP Jr, et al. Vesicourethral anastomosis biopsy after radical prostatectomy: predictive value of prostate-specific antigen and pathologic stage. Urology 1999;54:1044–1048.

63. Scattoni V, Roscigno M, Raber M, et al. Multiple vesico-urethral biopsies following radical prostatectomy: the predictive roles of TRUS, DRE, PSA and the pathological stage. Eur Urol 2003;44:407–414.

64. Oesterling JE. Using PSA to eliminate the staging radionuclide bone scan. Significant economic implications. Urol Clin North Am 1993;20:705–711.

65. Cher ML, Bianco FJ Jr, Lam JS, et al. Limited role of radionuclide bone scintigraphy in patients with prostate specific antigen elevations after radical prostatectomy. J Urol 1998;160:1387–1391.

66. Oyen RH, Van Poppel HP, Ameye FE, et al. Lymph node staging of localized prostatic carcinoma with CT and CT-guided fine-needle aspiration biopsy: prospective study of 285 patients. Radiology 1994;190:315–322.

67. Kramer S, Gorich J, Gottfried HW, et al. Sensitivity of computed tomography in detecting local recurrence of prostatic carcinoma following radical prostatectomy. Br J Radiol 1997;70:995–999.

68. Huch Boni RA, Meyenberger C, Lundquist JP, et al. Value of endorectal coil versus body coil MRI for diagnosis of recurrent pelvic malignancies. Abdom Imaging 1996;21:345–352.

69. Silverman JM and Krebs TL. MR imaging evaluation with transrectal surface coil of local recurrence of prostatic cancer in men who have undergone radical prostatectomy. Am J Radiol 1997;168:379–385.

70. Hoh CK, Seltzer MR, Franklin J, et al. Positron emission tomography in urological oncology. J Urol 1998;159:347–356.

71. Selzer MA, Cangiano T, Rosen P, et al. Comparison of computed tomography, positron emission tomography, and monoclonal antibody scan for evaluation of lymph node metastases in patients with PSA relapse after treatment for localized prostate cancer. J Urol 1999;162:1322–1328.

72. Texter JH, Jr and Neal CE. The role of monoclonal antibody in the management of prostate adenocarcinoma. J Urol 1998;160:2393–2395.

73. Elgamal AA, Troychak MJ, Murphy GP. ProstaScint scan may enhance identification of prostate cancer recurrences after prostatectomy, radiation, or hormone therapy: analysis of 136 scans of 100 patients. Prostate 1998;37:261–269.

74. Kahn D, Williams RD, Haseman MK, et al. Radioimmunoscintigraphy with In-111-labeled capromab pendetide predicts prostate cancer response to salvage radiotherapy after failed radical prostatectomy. J Clin Oncol 1998;16:284–289.

75. Mohideen N, Flanigan RJ, Dillehay G, et al. Role of prostascint scan in the assessment of patients who undergo radiotherapy for biochemical failure after radical prostatectomy for prostate cancer. J Urol 2002;167S:174.

76. Thomas CT, Bradshaw PT, Pollock BH, et al. Indium-111-Caprom pendetide radioimmunoscintigraphy and prognosis for durable biochemical response to salvage radiation therapy in men after failed prostatectomy. J Clin Oncol 2003;21:1715–1721.

77. Schettino CJ, Kramer EL, Noz ME, et al. Impact of fusion of indium-111 capromab pendetide volume data sets with those from MRI or CT in patients with recurrent prostate cancer. AJR Am J Roentgenol 2004;183:519–524.

78. Partin AW, Oesterling JE. The clinical usefulness of prostate specific antigen: update 1994. J Urol 1994;152:1358–1368.

79. Schild SE, Buskirk SJ, Won WW, et al. The use of radiotherapy for patients with isolated elevation of serum prostate specific antigen following radical prostatectomy. J Urol 1996;156:1725–1729.

80. Hudson MA and Catalona WJ. Effect of adjuvant radiation therapy on prostate specific antigen following radical prostatectomy. J Urol 1990;143:1174–1177.

81. vander Kooy MJ, Pisanski TM, Cha SS, Blute ML. Irradiation for locally recurrent carcinoma of the prostate following radical prostatectomy. Urology 1997;49:65–70.

82. Coetzee LJ, Hars V, Paulson DF. Postoperative prostate-specific antigen as a prognostic indication in patients with margin-positive prostate cancer, undergoing adjuvant radiotherapy after radical prostatectomy. Urology 1996;47:232–235.

83. Wu JJ, King SC, Montana GS, et al. The efficacy of postprostatectomy radiotherapy in patients with an isolated elevation of serum prostate-specific antigen. Int J Radiat Oncol Biol Phys 1995;32:317–323.

84. Forman JD, Wharam MD, Lee DJ, et al. Definitive radiotherapy following prostatectomy: results and complications. Int J Radiat Oncol Biol Phys 1986;12:185–189.

85. Pisansky TM, Kozelsky TF, Myers RP, et al. Radiotherapy for isolated serum prostate specific antigen elevation after prostatectomy for prostate cancer. J Urol 2000;163:845–850.

86. McCarthy JF, Catalona WJ, Hudson MA. Effect of radiation therapy on detectable serum prostate specific antigen levels following radical prostatectomy: early versus delayed treatment. J Urol 1994;151:1575–1578.

87. Morris MM, Dallow KC, Zietman AL, et al. Adjuvant and salvage irradiation following radical prostatectomy for prostate cancer. Int J Radiat Oncol Biol Phys 1997;38:731–736.

88. Vicini FA, Ziaja EL, Kestin LL, et al. Treatment outcome with adjuvant and salvage irradiation after radical prostatectomy for prostate cancer. Urology 1999;54:111–117.

89. Leventis AK, Shariat SF, Kattan MW, et al. Prediction of response to salvage radiation therapy in patients with prostate cancer recurrence after radical prostatectomy. J Clin Oncol 2001;19:1030–1039.

90. Rogers R, Grossfeld GD, Roach M 3rd, et al. Radiation therapy for the management of biopsy proved local recurrence after radical prostatectomy. J Urol 1998;160:1748–1753.

91. Forman JD and Velasco J. Therapeutic radiation in patients with a rising post-prostatectomy PSA level. Oncology 1998;12:33–39.

92. Nudell DM, Grossfeld GD, Weinberg VK, et al. Radiotherapy after radical prostatectomy: treatment outcomes and failure patterns. Urology 1999;54:1049–1057.

93. Stephenson AJ, Shariat SF, Zelefsky MJ, et al. Salvage radiotherapy for recurrent prostate cancer after radical prostatectomy. JAMA 2004;291:1325–1332.

94. Cadeddu JA, Partin AW, DeWeese TL, et al. Long-term results of radiation therapy for prostate cancer recurrence following radical prostatectomy. J Urol 1998;159:173–177.

95. Cox JD, Gallagher MJ, Hammond EH, et al. Consensus statements on radiation therapy of prostate cancer: guidelines for prostate re-biopsy after radiation and for radiation therapy with rising prostate-specific antigen levels after radical prostatectomy. American Society for Therapeutic Radiology and Oncology Consensus Panel. J Clin Oncol 1999;17:1155–1163.

96. Kotrouvelis PG, Katz SE, Lailas N, et al. Salvage CT guided brachytherapy for recurrent prostate cancer. J Urol 1999;161:297A.

97. Djavan B, Sesterhann I, Hruby S, et al. Benign prostatic glands in the surgical margin of radical retropubic prostatectomies: redefining PSA nadir. J Urol 2000;163:142A.

98. Shah R, Bassily N, Wei J, et al. Benign prostatic glands at surgical margins of radical prostatectomy specimens: frequency and associated risk factors. Urology 2000;56:721–725.

99. Mettlin C. The American Cancer Society National Prostate Cancer Detection Project and national patterns of prostate cancer detection and treatment. CA Cancer J Clin 1997;47:265–272.

100. Cavanagh W, Blasko JC, Grimm PD, et al. Transient elevation of serum prostate-specific antigen following (125)I/(103)Pd brachytherapy for localized prostate cancer. Semin Urol Oncol 2000;18:160–165.

101. Lee WR, Hanlon AL, Hanks GE. Prostate specific antigen nadir following external beam radiation therapy for clinically localized prostate cancer: the relationship between nadir level and disease free survival. J Urol 1996;156:450–453.

102. Stamey TA, Ferrari MK, Schmid HP. The value of serial prostate specific antigen determinations 5 years after radiotherapy: steeply increasing values characterize 80 percent of patients. J Urol 1993;150:1856–1859.

103. Zietman AL, Coen JJ, Dallow KC, et al. The treatment of prostate cancer by conventional radiation therapy: an analysis of long-term outcome. Int J Radiat Oncol Biol Phys 1995;32:287–292.

104. Lerner SE, Blute ML, Zincke H. Critical evaluation of salvage surgery for radiorecurrent/resistant prostate cancer. J Urol 1995;154:1103–1109.

105. Pontes JE. Role of surgery in managing local recurrence following external-beam radiation therapy. Urol Clin North Am 1994;21:701–706.

106. Rogers E, Ohori M, Kassabian VS, et al. Salvage radical prostatectomy: outcome measure by serum prostate specific antigen levels. J Urol 1995;153:104–110.

107. Tefilli MV, Gheiler EL, Tiguert R, et al. Salvage surgery or salvage radiotherapy for locally recurrent prostate cancer. Urology 1998;52:224–229.

108. Moul JW, Paulson DF. The role of radical surgery in the management of radiation recurrent and large volume prostate cancer. Cancer 1991;68:1265–1271.

109. Amling CL, Lerner SE, Martin SK, et al. Deoxyribonucleic acid ploidy and serum prostate specific antigen predict outcome following salvage prostatectomy for radiation refractory prostate cancer. J Urol 1999;161:857–862.

110. Cheng L, Sebo TJ, Slezak J, et al. Predictors of survival for prostate carcinoma patients treated with salvage radical prostatectomy after radiation therapy. Cancer 1998;83:2164–2171.

111. Gheiler EL, Tefilli MV, Tiguert R, et al. Predictors for maximal outcome in patients undergoing salvage surgery for radio-recurrent prostate cancer. Urology 1998 51:789–795.

112. Pister LL, Von Eschenbach AC, Scott SM, et al. The efficacy and complications of salvage cryotherapy of the prostate. J Urol 1997;157:921–925.

113. Izawa JI, Perrotte P, Greene GF, et al. Local tumor control with salvage cryotherapy for locally recurrent prostate cancer after external beam radiotherapy. J Urol 2001;165:867–870.

114. Bales GT, Williams MJ, Sinner M, et al. Short-term outcomes after cryosurgical ablation of the prostate in men with recurrent prostate carcinoma following radiation therapy. Urology 1995;46:676–680.

115. de la Taille A, Hayek O, Benson MC, et al. Salvage cryotherapy for recurrent prostate cancer after radiation therapy: The Columbia experience. Urology 2000;55:79–84.

116. Chin JL, Pautler SE, Mouraviev V, et al. Results of salvage cryoablation of the prostate after radiation: identifying predictors of treatment failure and complications. J Urol 2001;165:1937–1941.

117. Greene GF, Pisters LL, Scott SM, et al. Predictive value of prostate specific antigen nadir after salvage cryotherapy. J Urol 1998;160:86–90.

118. Grado GL, Collins JM, Kriegshauser JS, et al. Salvage brachytherapy for localized prostate cancer after radiotherapy failure. Urology 1999;53:2–10.

119. Beyer DC. Permanent brachytherapy as salvage treatment for recurrent prostate cancer. Urology 1999;54:880–883.

120. Madersbacher S, Pedevilla M, Vingers L, et al. Effect of high-intensity focused ultrasound on human prostate cancer in vivo. Cancer Res 1995;55:3346–3351.

121. Beerlage HP, van Leenders GJ, Oosterhof GO, et al. High-intensity focused ultrasound (HIFU) followed after one to two weeks by radical retropubic prostatectomy: results of a prospective study. Prostate 1999;39:41–46.

122. Zlotta AR, Djavan B, Matos C, et al. Percutaneous transperineal radiofrequency ablation of prostate tumour: safety, feasibility and pathological effects of human prostate cancer. Br J Urol 1998;81:265–275.

123. Gelet A, Chapelon JY, Bouvier R, et al. Local control of prostate cancer by transrectal high intensity focused ultrasound therapy: preliminary results. J Urol 1999;161:156–161.

124. Master VA, Shinohara K, Carroll PR. Ferromagnetic thermal ablation of locally recurrent prostate cancer: prostate specific antigen results and immediate/intermediate morbidities. J Urol 2004;172:2197–202.

125. Koppie TM, Shinohara K, Grossfeld GD, et al. The efficacy of cryosurgical ablation of prostate cancer: the University of California, San Francisco experience. J Urol 1999;162:427–432.

126. Long JP, Fallick ML, LaRock DR, Rand W. Preliminary outcomes following cryosurgical ablation of the prostate in patients with clinically localized prostate carcinoma. J Urol 1998;159:477–484.

127. Grampsas SA, Miller GJ, Crawford ED. Salvage radical prostatectomy after failed transperineal cryotherapy: histologic findings from prostate whole-mount specimens correlated with intraoperative transrectal ultrasound images. Urology 1995;45:936–941.

128. Pisters LL, Dinney CP, Pettaway CA, et al. A feasibility study of cryotherapy followed by radical prostatectomy for locally advanced prostate cancer. J Urol 1999;161:509–514.

129. Burton S, Brown DM, Colonias A. Salvage radiotherapy for prostate cancer recurrence after cryosurgical ablation. Urology 2000;56:833–838.

130. Tefilli MV, Gheiler EL, Tiguert R, et al. Quality of life in patients undergoing salvage procedures for locally recurrent prostate cancer. J Surg Oncol 1998;69:156–161.

131. Ornstein DK, Oh J, Herschman JD, Andriole GL. Evaluation and management of the man who has failed primary curative therapy for prostate cancer. Urol Clin North Am 1998;25:591–601.

132. Grossfeld GD, Tigrani VS, Nudell D, et al. Management of a positive surgical margin after radical prostatectomy: decision analysis. J Urol 2000;164:93–99.

133. Formenti SC, Lieskovsky G, Simoneau AR, et al. Impact of moderate dose of postoperative radiation on urinary continence and potency in patients with prostate cancer treated with nerve sparing prostatectomy. J Urol 1996;155:616–619.

134. Daniell HW, Clark JC. Pereira SE, Hypogonadism following prostate-bed radiation therapy for prostate carcinoma. Cancer 2001;91:1889–1895.

135. Pontes JE, Montie J, Klein E, Huben R. Salvage surgery for radiation failure in prostate cancer. Cancer 1993;71:976–980.

136. Zincke H. Radical prostatectomy and exenterative procedures for local failure after radiotherapy with curative intent: comparison of outcomes. J Urol 1992;147:894–899.

137. Vaidya A and Soloway MS. Salvage radical prostatectomy for radiorecurrent prostate cancer: morbidity revisited. J Urol 2000;164:1998–2001.

138. Bochner BH, Figueroa AJ, Skinner EC, et al. Salvage radical cystoprostatectomy and orthotopic urinary diversion following radiation failure. J Urol 1998;160:29–33.

139. Gheiler EL, Wood DP, Jr., Montie JE, et al. Orthotopic urinary diversion is a viable option in patient undergoing salvage cystoprostatectomy for recurrent prostate cancer after definitive radiation therapy. Urology 1997;50:580–584.

140. Pisters LL, English SF, Dinney CPN, et al. Salvage prostatectomy with continent catheterizable urinary reconstruction: a novel approach to recurrent prostate cancer following radiation therapy. J Urol 1999;161:335A.

141. Perrotte P, Litwin MS, McGuire EJ, et al. Quality of life after salvage cryotherapy: the impact of treatment parameters. J Urol 1999;162:398–402.

142. Eisenberger MA, Partin AW, Pound C, Van Roostelaar C, et al. Natural history of patients with biochemical (PSA) relapse following radical prostatectomy: update. Proc Am Soc Clin Oncol 2003;22:380.

143. Rogers CG, Khan MA, Craig Miller M, et al. Natural history of disease progression in patients who fail to achieve an undetectable prostate-specific antigen level after undergoing radical prostatectomy. Cancer 2004;101:2549–2556.

144. D'Amico AV, Moul JW, Carroll PR, Sun L, et al. Surrogate end point for prostate cancer-specific mortality after radical prostatectomy or radiation therapy. J Natl Cancer Inst 2003;95:1376–1383.

Multivariate models for predicting pathologic stage

55

Misop Han, Alan W Partin

INTRODUCTION

When newly diagnosed with prostate cancer, a patient has to decide whether to be treated and which treatment modality to undergo. These decisions depend on many factors including the patient's clinical tumor stage, tumor grade from a biopsy specimen, serum prostate-specific antigen (PSA) level, overall health status, life expectancy, and the potential outcomes of treatment modality.

Pathologic stage of prostate cancer is a crucial piece of information that a patient and a physician can incorporate into the treatment decision-making process. In men with locally advanced or metastatic prostate cancer, local therapy alone may not be an ideal treatment choice. On the other hand, in men with organ-confined prostate cancer, local therapy, such as surgery or radiation therapy, will likely achieve a cure. However, true pathologic staging information is only available after the pathologic examination of a surgical specimen.

Although many individual preoperative parameters are shown to be associated with pathologic stage, a physician usually incorporates those parameters together to predict the likely outcome of pathologic stage. A physician can make a treatment recommendation based on a heuristic learning process with clinical experience and acumen. However, a physician's personal biases will invariably play an important role in the decision-making. Multivariate prediction models for pathologic stage were developed to accurately predict the pathologic outcome without human bias, prior to a definitive therapy for clinically localized prostate cancer.

Ideally, the prediction model should be accurate and easy to use. If a physician can reliably and correctly predict the pathologic stage of tumor, he or she can recommend more rational treatment modality. Numerous prediction models have been developed based on large surgical series.[1] In this chapter, we review several multivariate prediction models that predict comprehensive or specific pathologic stage of clinically localized prostate cancer. Then, we discuss potential problems associated with multivariate prediction models on pathologic stage.

MODELS PREDICTING COMPREHENSIVE PATHOLOGIC STAGE

In 1987, Oesterling et al reported that a multivariate logistic regression model using a combination of clinical stage, serum prostatic acid phosphatase level, and biopsy Gleason grade performed better than individual variables in predicting final pathologic stage in 275 men with prostate cancer.[2] Subsequently, Narayan et al used preoperative serum PSA level, biopsy Gleason score, and transrectal ultrasound-guided biopsy-based staging information in their prediction models.[3] They generated probability graphs to predict pathologic stage.[3] However, neither prediction model was subsequently validated.

In 1993, as the serum PSA test became widely available and used in screening men for prostate cancer, Partin et al developed nomograms based on PSA, clinical stage, and biopsy Gleason score to predict the likelihood of various final pathologic stages.[4] These nomograms, also known as the "Partin nomograms," provided the probabilities of organ-confined disease, extraprostatic extension, seminal vesicle and lymph node involvement status based on a cohort of 703 men from a single institution.[4] Subsequently, these nomograms were validated using an external cohort.[5] In 1997, those nomograms were updated and internally validated by incorporating cohorts from three academic institutions.[6] Since the nomograms only required three readily available parameters at the time of diagnosis to predict pathologic stage probability, they became widely used in urology. They have been extensively validated using the US and European patient cohorts.[7-10] Most recently, these nomograms were updated and validated to reflect the stage migration in men presenting with prostate cancer in the modern era.[10,11]

MODELS PREDICTING ORGAN CONFINEMENT/EXTRAPROSTATIC EXTENSION STATUS

Organ confinement and extraprostatic extension status are important pathologic information in prostate cancer management. Badalament et al developed a probability formula for organ confinement status based on biopsy Gleason score, nuclear grade, PSA, and total percent tumor involvement.[12] Extraprostatic extension status prediction models were developed using biopsy Gleason score, PSA, percent tumor involvement, and patient age.[13,14] Because these models required specific parameters, such as nuclear grade or percent tumor involvement, they never became widely used.

MODELS PREDICTING SEMINAL VESICLE/ LYMPH NODE INVOLVEMENT STATUS

Advanced pathologic features such as seminal vesicle or lymph node involvement are associated with a poor prognosis.[15] In men with cancerous involvement of seminal vesicle or lymph node, a local monotherapy with surgery or radiation therapy will not likely achieve a cure. Therefore, when there is a high likelihood of seminal vesicle or lymph node involvement, adjuvant therapy can be considered as a part of the treatment strategy. There are several predictive models estimating the probabilities of advanced prostate cancer with seminal vesicle invasion[13,16] or lymph node involvement.[17-19] However, the role of these prediction models for advanced prostate cancer may diminish as more men present with earlier stage and grade disease in the modern era.[20,21]

MODELS PREDICTING SURGICAL MARGIN STATUS

Surgical margin status is an important predictor of recurrence following radical prostatectomy.[22,23] Theoretically, the information can be used in identifying men at increased risk for positive surgical margins, then technical modifications can be considered to avoid possible surgical margins. However, the surgical margin status depends on the pathologic stage of the cancer as well as the surgical technique. With more men diagnosed with organ-confined disease, the positive surgical margin rate should continue to decrease. In addition, no predictive model for surgical margin status has been validated.[19,24]

POTENTIAL PROBLEMS OF MULTIVARIATE PREDICTION MODELS

There are several potential problems to be considered while using currently available multivariate prediction models. First, multivariate models predicting pathologic stage are generated from a retrospective review of large radical prostatectomy series. Therefore, the models may not be as applicable in men considering nonsurgical treatment as in men undergoing radical prostatectomy. Second, many prediction models, with the exception of the "Partin nomograms," have not been validated. In addition, only a few studies have compared prediction models with each other or with a physician's heuristic decision making.[10,25] For example, Ross et al compared the performances between human and nomograms on prostate cancer outcomes, although they included clinicians with different levels of experience. They concluded that nomograms do not seem to diminish the predictive accuracy of a physician, and they may be of significant benefit in certain clinical decision making settings.[25] Third, these models provide the probability of pathologic stage, which is an intermediate outcome in prostate cancer patients. More important outcome measures include recurrence-free or cancer-specific survival probability and comorbidity outcomes following treatment.[22,26,27] Finally, as new and improved predictors of pathologic stage are discovered, the predictive models will have to be continually updated or revised to include those predictors.

CONCLUSIONS

Several prediction models exist that estimate the likelihood of the pathologic stages based on pretreatment parameters. Because of their ease of use and multiple validation studies, the "Partin nomograms" have been used most widely to predict the pathologic stage of prostate cancer. Until a radiographic study becomes available that can delineate the accurate pathologic stage, multivariate prediction models will continue to be used to assist clinical decision making process in men with clinically localized prostate cancer.

REFERENCES

1. Ross PL, Scardino PT, Kattan MW. A catalog of prostate cancer nomograms. J Urol 2001;165:1562–1568.
2. Oesterling JE, Brendler CB, Epstein JI, et al. Correlation of clinical stage, serum prostatic acid phosphatase and preoperative Gleason grade with final pathological stage in 275 patients with clinically localized adenocarcinoma of the prostate. J Urol 1987;138:92–98.
3. Narayan P, Gajendran V, Taylor SP, et al. The role of transrectal ultrasound-guided biopsy-based staging, preoperative serum prostate-specific antigen, and biopsy Gleason score in prediction of final pathologic diagnosis in prostate cancer. Urology 1995;46:205–212.
4. Partin AW, Yoo J, Carter HB, et al. The use of prostate specific antigen, clinical stage and Gleason score to predict pathological stage in men with localized prostate cancer. J Urol 1993;150:110–114.
5. Kattan MW, Stapleton AM, Wheeler TM, et al. Evaluation of a nomogram used to predict the pathologic stage of clinically localized prostate carcinoma. Cancer 1997;79:528–537.
6. Partin AW, Kattan MW, Subong EN, et al. Combination of prostate-specific antigen, clinical stage, and Gleason score to predict pathological stage of localized prostate cancer. A multi-institutional update [see comments] [published erratum appears in JAMA 1997;278:118]. JAMA 1997;277:1445–1451.
7. Blute ML, Bergstralh EJ, Partin AW, et al. Validation of Partin tables for predicting pathological stage of clinically localized prostate cancer. J Urol 2000;164:1591–1595.
8. Graefen M, Augustin H, Karakiewicz PI, et al. Can predictive models for prostate cancer patients derived in the United States of America be utilized in European patients? A validation study of the Partin tables. Eur Urol 2003;43:6–10; discussion 11.
9. Penson DF, Grossfeld GD, Li YP, Henning JM, et al. How well does the Partin nomogram predict pathological stage after radical prostatectomy in a community based population? Results of the cancer of the prostate strategic urological research endeavor. J Urol 2002;167:1653–1657; discussion 1657–1658.
10. Augustin H, Eggert T, Wenske S, et al. Comparison of accuracy between the Partin tables of 1997 and 2001 to predict final pathological stage in clinically localized prostate cancer. J Urol 2004;171:177–181.
11. Partin AW, Mangold LA, Lamm DM, Walsh PC, et al. Contemporary update of prostate cancer staging nomograms (Partin Tables) for the new millennium. Urology 2001;58:843–848.
12. Badalament RA, Miller MC, Peller PA, et al. An algorithm for predicting nonorgan confined prostate cancer using the results obtained from sextant core biopsies with prostate specific antigen level. J Urol 1996;156:1375–1380.
13. Bostwick DG, Qian J, Bergstralh E, et al. Prediction of capsular perforation and seminal vesicle invasion in prostate cancer. J Urol 1996;155:1361–1367.
14. Gilliland FD, Hoffman RM, Hamilton A, et al. Predicting extracapsular extension of prostate cancer in men treated with radical prostatectomy: results from the population based prostate cancer outcomes study [see comments] [published erratum appears in J Urol 2000 May;163:1526]. J Urol 1999;162:1341–1345.
15. Han M, Partin AW, Pound CR, Epstein JI, Walsh PC. Long-term biochemical disease-free and cancer-specific survival following anatomic radical retropubic prostatectomy. The 15-year Johns Hopkins experience. Urol Clin North Am 2001;28:555–565.
16. Pisansky TM, Blute ML, Suman VJ, et al. Correlation of pretherapy prostate cancer characteristics with seminal vesicle invasion in radical prostatectomy specimens. Int J Radiat Oncol Biol Phys 1996;36:585–591.
17. Bluestein DL, Bostwick DG, Bergstralh EJ, et al. Eliminating the need for bilateral pelvic lymphadenectomy in select patients with prostate cancer. J Urol 1994;151:1315–1320.
18. Roach M, 3rd, Marquez C, Yuo HS, et al. Predicting the risk of lymph node involvement using the pre-treatment prostate specific antigen and Gleason score in men with clinically localized prostate cancer. Int J Radiat Oncol Biol Phys 1994;28:33–37.
19. Ackerman DA, Barry JM, Wicklund RA, et al. Analysis of risk factors associated with prostate cancer extension to the surgical margin and pelvic node metastasis at radical prostatectomy. J Urol 1993;150:1845–1850.
20. Han M, Partin AW, Piantadosi S, et al. Era specific biochemical recurrence-free survival following radical prostatectomy for clinically localized prostate cancer. J Urol 2001;166:416–419.
21. Petros JA, Catalona WJ. Lower incidence of unsuspected lymph node metastases in 521 consecutive patients with clinically localized prostate cancer. J Urol 1992;147:1574–1575.
22. Kattan MW, Wheeler TM, Scardino PT. Postoperative nomogram for disease recurrence after radical prostatectomy for prostate cancer. J Clin Oncol 1999;17:1499–1507.
23. Khan MA, Partin AW, Mangold LA, Epstein JI, Walsh PC. Probability of biochemical recurrence by analysis of pathologic stage, Gleason score, and margin status for localized prostate cancer. Urology 2003;62:866–871.
24. Rabbani F, Bastar A, Fair WR. Site specific predictors of positive margins at radical prostatectomy: an argument for risk based modification of technique. J Urol 1998;160:1727–1733.
25. Ross PL, Gerigk C, Gonen M, et al. Comparisons of nomograms and urologists' predictions in prostate cancer. Semin Urol Oncol 2002;20:82–88.
26. Kattan MW, Eastham JA, Stapleton AM, et al. A preoperative nomogram for disease recurrence following radical prostatectomy for prostate cancer. J Natl Cancer Inst 1998;90:766–771.
27. Han M, Partin AW, Zahurak M, et al. Biochemical (prostate specific antigen) recurrence probability following radical prostatectomy for clinically localized prostate cancer. J Urol 2003;169:517–523.

Multivariate models for predicting biochemical recurrence after definitive local therapy

56

Kozhaya N Mallah, Michael W Kattan

INTRODUCTION

With the use of transrectal ultrasound (TRUS) and prostate-specific antigen (PSA) testing, an increasingly large number of nonpalpable tumors are being discovered in the prostate.[1] Some of these tumors are indolent but many are clinically significant, and deciding the most appropriate treatment strategy has been a challenge for both physicians and patients. Whatever the treatment option, whether watchful waiting, radical prostatectomy, brachytherapy, or external-beam radiation therapy (EBRT), the patient needs to be able to make an informed decision based on his predicted probability of survival, as well as his perception of his future quality of life. Prostate cancer is a classic example of a disease in which quality of life is as important as survival time, if not more so.[2] A tool that aids in the decision-making process is of great value for the patient who must weigh various treatment strategies against their possible complications and comorbidities.[3] Several instruments do exist,[4,5] the most common of which are risk-grouping tables and specialized prediction models called nomograms. Risk-grouping tables place patients into categories based on the overall prognosis of the group. Nomograms, on the other hand, focus on the risk for the individual patient, and thus maximize predictive accuracy. Although risk-grouping tables are usually more paper-friendly, their construction is often flawed, resulting in loss of homogeneity in the group.[6,7] In this chapter, we will outline the models available for predicting biochemical recurrence after local definitive therapy with radical prostatectomy, brachytherapy, and EBRT. Because many of the models that we will discuss in detail are nomograms, we will provide a description of the construction of nomograms, as well as their uses and limitations.

NOMOGRAMS

Good patient counseling requires the ability to predict probabilities of future outcomes (Figure 56.1). Because the human mind is poor at probability computations, nomograms have outperformed clinicians even after the latter were informed of the nomograms' predictions.[8] Nomograms are also better than risk-group tables in conserving the homogeneity of strata of patients.[7] Although most patients in traditional high-risk groups have increased probability of failure, a few patients in those groups might not have.[9] To avoid their being miscategorized and subsequently unable to make well-informed decisions regarding treatment, all patients

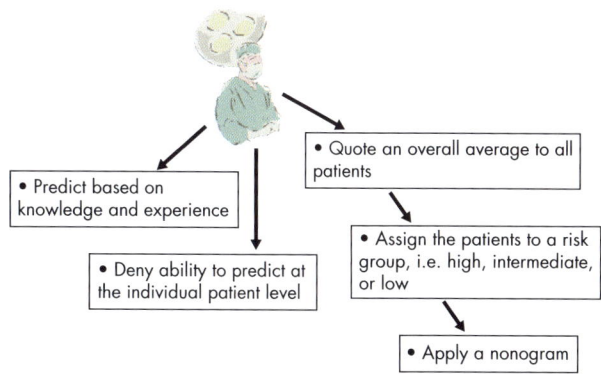

Fig. 56.1
When the patient wants a prediction, what options does the clinician have?

should have predicted probabilities tailored to their individual parameters, and not to those of a group. Figure 56.2 is an illustration of a real data set subjected to the predictions of a risk-grouping table and a nomogram.

NOMOGRAM DEFINITION

Nomograms are specialized prediction models that use algorithms incorporating many variables to calculate the predicted probability that a patient will reach a particular endpoint.[10] A nomogram is composed of a series of axes that vary according to purpose and a set of non-variable axes: the Points Axis, the Total Points Axis, and the Predicted Probability Axis. Each variable axis is a scale on which a value corresponds to a particular number on the Points Axis. Next, all the corresponding calculated numbers on the Points Axis are added and the result is plotted on the Total Points Axis. Finally, a line is drawn from the plotted point on the Total Points Axis to the Predicted Probability Axis, and the intersection shows the probability that a patient will reach a particular endpoint.

NOMOGRAM APPLICATION

The key importance of nomograms lies in patient counseling.[6,10] For a patient diagnosed with clinically localized prostate cancer, nomograms help the physician explain the risks and benefits of different treatment options.[9,11,12] As mentioned above, both the quantity and quality of life should be considered when comparing treatments.[3] An inappropriately aggressive treatment might prolong survival but decrease the quality of life. By using a patient's clinical and pathologic features after definitive therapy, nomograms

assist physicians and patients in the decision regarding adjuvant therapy.[13] Moreover, nomograms can guide treatment strategies for patients who have biochemical recurrence after local definitive therapy.[14,15] However, one should keep in mind that nomograms are to be used to provide input into the decision-making process, not as a substitute.[16]

Another valuable use of nomograms is in clinical trials.[4,6,17] By providing a standard variable to compare patients—the predicted probability—nomograms ensure a homogenous stratification of patients by risk, and promote balance between the two arms of a study. This helps to avoid an erroneously successful phase II trial.[18] Nomograms can accurately predict patients who are at high risk of failure to justify their involvement in potentially harmful phase III trials. In addition, nomograms can maximize the number of events and increase the statistical power of the study.[18] Nomograms can also be used to appropriately schedule follow-ups tailored to likelihood of recurrence.[19] Finally, an important measure of outcome in prostate cancer treatment is informed consent.[17,20] If informed of his treatment efficacy based on his individual parameters, the patient is less likely to regret his choice of treatment.

NOMOGRAM LIMITATIONS

Nomograms do not directly make treatment recommendations.[17] Because current clinical endpoints do not incorporate survival adjusted for quality-of-life variables, and because progression can have a different meaning across different clinical settings, the patient and physician cannot simply pick the treatment whose nomogram calculates the highest prediction score.

Nomograms are often designed based on a majority of white patients treated at academic centers.[9,11–13,21,22] Nonetheless, many have been shown to be accurate

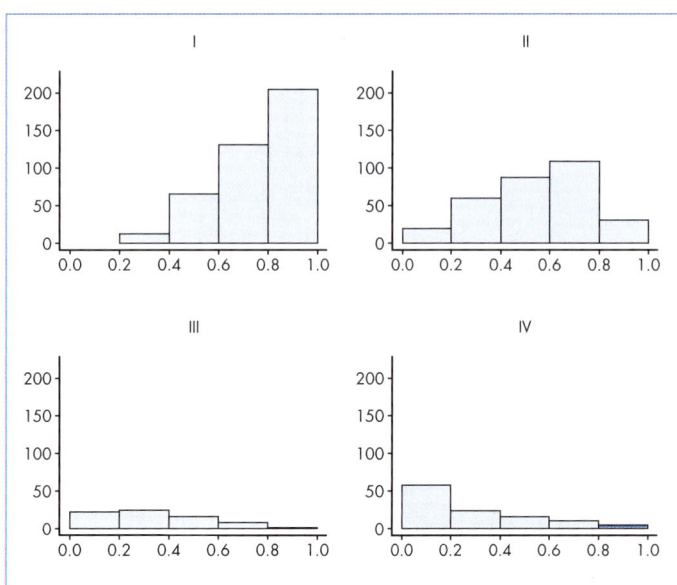

Fig. 56.2
Nomogram predictions within each level of risk stratification, I (most favorable) through IV (least favorable).[15] Within each risk-group quadrant is a histogram of the nomogram-predicted probabilities (x-axis) of freedom from recurrence.
Adapted from Kattan MW, Zelefsky MJ, Kupelian PA, Scardino PT, Fuks Z, Leibel SA. Pretreatment nomogram for predicting the outcome of three-dimensional conformal radiotherapy in prostate cancer. J Clin Oncol 2000;18:3352–3359.

when applied in community settings,[23] as well as in the black patient population.[24]

Current nomograms use correlate measures of treatment failure (e.g., PSA rise) rather than disease-specific survival.[17] Although most patients develop PSA recurrence before eventually developing metastasis and/or dying,[25] it might take years before a patient with biochemical recurrence develops metastasis or dies from prostate cancer.

A RECOMMENDED APPROACH TO NOMOGRAM DEVELOPMENT

Many nomograms are based on Cox proportional hazards regression analysis incorporating restricted cubic splines. Restricted cubic splines avoid forcing linear effects onto the continuous variables and limiting the flexibility of the nomogram and its predictive accuracy.[4,6] Nomogram validation usually requires two measures: accuracy (internal validity) and generalizability (external validity).

Accuracy refers to the degree to which predicted outcomes match observed outcomes.[26] It is divided into discrimination and calibration.

Discrimination is the ability to correctly identify which patients will and will not achieve a particular endpoint. A common approach is to measure the concordance index—the probability that, in a randomly chosen pair of cases, the case that recurs first has the higher predicted probability of failure. The concordance index is calculated by first forming all possible pairs of patients, and removing those pairs in which the patient with shorter follow-up time is censored; then, of the remaining pairs, the concordance index is the percentage of pairs in which the prediction method predicted lower survival for the case that failed first.[5] The concordance index ranges from 0.5 (chance) to 1.0 (perfect discrimination). Additionally, subjecting the nomogram to bootstrapping by resampling many times reduces bias.[27] Of note, the concordance index is the same concept as the area under the receiver operating curve but it is more appropriate for time-to-event cases.

For a comparison of the nomogram's predicted probability of recurrence to the actual recurrence, calibration is commonly performed by dividing the sample into subcohorts based on the predicted risk of the nomogram. Furthermore, the predicted risk in each subcohort is compared with the actual fraction of patients free of disease progression at the desired time interval.[9,11–13]

Nomogram validation also requires generalizability. This is the ability of the nomogram to provide accurate predictions in a new sample of patients. It is divided into reproducibility and transportability.

Whereas reproducibility refers to the nomogram's accuracy when applied to a sample of patients not included in the original model used in developing the nomogram, but from an identical population,[9,11–13] transportability refers to the accuracy of the nomogram when applied to a different population.[23,24,28–30]

MODELS FOR PREDICTING BIOCHEMICAL RECURRENCE AFTER DEFINITIVE THERAPY

Only the models that have been validated at outside institutions or have been based on multi-institution datasets will be discussed in detail.

PRETREATMENT PREDICTION MODELS: RADICAL PROSTATECTOMY

KATTAN NOMOGRAM

A Kattan nomogram that predicts 5-year PSA recurrence was developed in 1998. This nomogram (Figure 56.3) was based on 983 patients treated at the Baylor College of Medicine (BCM) between 1983 and 1996 by a single surgeon.[11] Kattan et al used three widely available prognostic variables (clinical stage, pretreatment PSA, biopsy Gleason sum) in the Cox regression analysis described earlier to predict treatment failure. The clinical stage was assigned based on the 1992 TNM (tumor-node-metastasis) classification system, and ranged from T1ab to T3a NxM0. Biopsy Gleason scores were combined into 6 groups ($\leq 2 + \leq 2$; $\leq 2 + 3$, $3 + \leq 2$; $3 + 3$; $\leq 3 + \geq 4$; and $\geq 4 + \geq 3$) and treated as a categorical variable. The pretreatment PSA was modeled as a restricted cubic spline of its natural logarithm for reasons mentioned above.[4] Treatment failure was defined as the *first* occurrence of one of the following: biochemical recurrence (BCR), treatment with secondary therapy in the form of radiation or hormonal agents, or clinical evidence of cancer recurrence without a PSA rise. Biochemical recurrence was defined as a serum PSA level of 0.4 ng/mL or more followed by a rise. Patients for whom radical prostatectomy was aborted because of cancer invasion of the lymph nodes were considered immediate failures. This nomogram discriminated well; the concordance indices without and with bootstrapping were 0.76 and 0.74 respectively. Calibration of this nomogram with bootstrap analysis showed that it performed within 10% of actual outcome. This nomogram was validated (at BCM) on a separate sample of 168 patients and the concordance index measured 0.79. External validation of this nomogram was performed across three continents and the concordance index ranged from 0.70 to 0.77 with good calibration.[29] On further studies, this nomogram

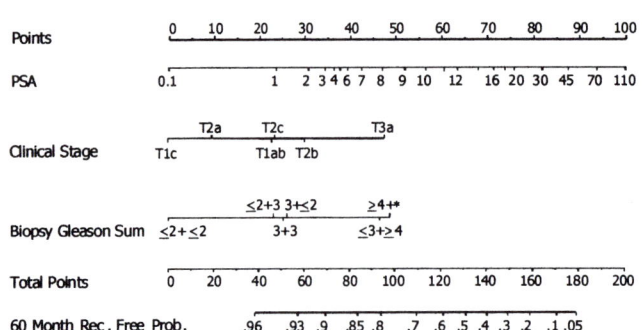

Fig. 56.3

Preoperative nomogram for prostate cancer recurrence.

Instructions for physician: Locate the patient's prostate-specific antigen (PSA, ng/mL) on the **PSA Axis**. Draw a line straight upwards to the **Points Axis** to determine how many points towards recurrence the patient receives for his PSA. Repeat this process for the other axes, each time drawing straight upward to the **Points Axis**. Add the points achieved for each predictor and locate this sum on the **Total Points Axis**. Draw a line straight down to find the patient's probability of remaining recurrence free for 60 months, assuming he does not die of another cause first. Note: This nomogram is not applicable to a man who is not otherwise a candidate for radical prostatectomy. You can use this only on a man who has already selected radical prostatectomy as treatment for his prostate cancer.

Instruction to patient: "Mr. X, if we had 100 men exactly like you, we would expect between [predicted percentage from nomogram –10%] and [predicted percentage + 10%] to remain free of their disease at 5 years following radical prostatectomy, and recurrence after 5 years is very rare."

©1997 Michael W. Kattan and Peter T. Scardino, Scott Department of Urology. Adapted from Kattan MW, Eastham JA, Stapleton AM, Wheeler TM, Scardino PT. A preoperative nomogram for disease recurrence following radical prostatectomy for prostate cancer. J Natl Cancer Inst 1998;90:766–771. By permission of Oxford University Press.

was validated in a cohort of black men; the concordance index measured 0.74 and calibration was excellent.[24] Recently, this nomogram was validated in a community-based setting, where the concordance index measured 0.68. It tended to overestimate survival in patients in the low-risk category, but the nomogram is still appropriate for use in community hospitals.[23] The addition of interleukin 6 soluble receptor (IL6SR) and transforming growth factor-β1 (TGFβ1), even though these are not routinely measured, to the other clinical variables increased the concordance index from 0.75 to 0.83 in a newer nomogram by Kattan et al.[22]

D'AMICO PREDICTION TABLES

D'Amico prediction tables predict 2-year PSA recurrence. The developers of these tables (Table 56.1) used a sample of 892 patients treated at the Hospital of the University of Pennsylvania between 1989 and 1997 with radical retropubic prostatectomy and bilateral lymph node sampling.[31] As in the Kattan nomograms, preoperative variables incorporated in the model included clinical stage (AJCC 1992 staging system), PSA, and biopsy Gleason score. Similarly, a Cox regression analysis was performed. Clinical stage was treated as a categorical variable and included T1c, T2a, T2b, and T2c. The biopsy Gleason score was ordered into 4 rankings (2–4, 5–6, 7, 8–10). Pretreatment PSA was treated as a continuous variable, and PSA failure was defined as three consecutive increasing PSA values after an undetectable value. Patients whose PSA level never became undetectable, as

well as those whose lymph nodes were positive on pathology, were considered immediate failures. This definition limited these prediction tables, as approximately 20% of patients with positive lymph nodes on radical prostatectomy pathology remain free from biochemical progression after 5 years.[32] The probabilities of 2-year recurrence were calculated from the coefficients of the Cox model.[31] These tables have been validated externally and the area under the receiver operating curve (AUC) was 0.80.[30] A direct comparison with the Kattan nomogram was done on a sample of 932 patients who fit the criteria for both models; the Kattan nomogram was statistically superior (AUC, 0.81; p = 0.027),[30] taking into consideration the predicted time of failure (2 years, D' Amico; 5 years, Kattan).

HAN ET AL PREDICTION TABLES

Han et al prediction tables[33] have not been validated in outside institutions.

PRETREATMENT PREDICTION MODELS: EXTERNAL-BEAM RADIATION THERAPY

KATTAN NOMOGRAM

A Kattan nomogram that predicts 5-year PSA recurrence was developed in 2000. This nomogram (Figure 56.4) was based on 1042 patients treated with three-dimensional conformal radiotherapy[34] (3D-CRT) at

Table 56.1 Preoperative and pre-radiation treatment tables—percent prostate-specific antigen (PSA) failure at 2 years (and 95% confidence intervals [CI]), stratified by pretreatment PSA, AJCC clinical stage, and biopsy Gleason score

Pretreatment PSA, ng/mL	Biopsy Gleason score	Clinical stage			
		T1c, % (CI)	T2a, % (CI)	T2b, % (CI)	T2c, % (CI)
Surgically managed patients at Hospital of the University of Pennsylvania, n = 892					
0–4.0	2–4	4 (2–7)	5 (3–7)	8 (4–13)	10 (6–17)
	5	8 (5–11)	9 (6–11)	15 (8–21)	18 (12–25)
	6	10 (6–15)	11 (8–14)	19 (11–27)	24 (17–31)
	7	14 (8–20)	15 (11–19)	25 (15–35)	31 (22–40)
	8–10	24 (13–37)	26 (16–36)	42 (24–59)	50 (34–65)
4.1–10.0	2–4	5 (3–8)	6 (4–9)	10 (5–16)	13 (8–20)
	5	10 (6–14)	11 (8–13)	18 (11–25)	22 (16–30)
	6	13 (8–18)	14 (11–17)	24 (15–32)	29 (22–37)
	7	17 (11–24)	19 (14–23)	31 (20–42)	37 (28–46)
	8–10	29 (17–44)	32 (20–44)	50 (31–67)	58 (43–72)
10.1–20.0	2–4	7 (4–12)	8 (5–13)	15 (8–23)	18 (11–29)
	5	14 (9–20)	15 (11–19)	25 (17–34)	31 (23–40)
	6	18 (11–26)	20 (15–25)	33 (22–43)	39 (31–48)
	7	24 (15–34)	26 (20–33)	42 (29–54)	49 (40–59)
	8–10	39 (24–58)	43 (29–58)	63 (44–80)	72 (56–84)
20.1–50.0	2–4	18 (10–34)	20 (12–36)	33 (19–54)	40 (25–64)
	5	31 (18–52)	34 (23–53)	52 (36–73)	61 (46–81)
	6	40 (24–63)	43 (30–63)	63 (47–83)	72 (60–88)
	7	50 (32–74)	53 (39–75)	75 (58–91)	82 (71–95)
	8–10	72 (48–94)	76 (57–94)	92 (77–99)	96 (88–100)
Radiation-managed patients at Joint Center for Radiation Therapy, n = 762					
0–4.0	2–4	3 (1–5)	4 (2–7)	5 (3–9)	6 (3–9)
	5	7 (4–10)	8 (5–12)	11 (7–16)	12 (7–17)
	6	10 (6–14)	12 (8–17)	16 (10–23)	17 (11–24)
	7	14 (9–20)	18 (11–25)	23 (15–34)	25 (17–35)
	8–10	29 (17–46)	36 (21–55)	45 (27–68)	48 (29–69)
4.1–10.0	2–4	4 (2–6)	5 (2–8)	6 (3–10)	7 (3–11)
	5	8 (5–11)	10 (6–14)	13 (8–18)	14 (9–20)
	6	11 (7–15)	14 (9–19)	18 (12–26)	20 (13–27)
	7	16 (11–23)	20 (13–28)	26 (17–37)	28 (19–39)
	8–10	33 (20–50)	40 (24–59)	50 (31–72)	52 (33–74)
10.1–20.0	2–4	4 (2–8)	5 (3–10)	7 (4–13)	8 (4–14)
	5	9 (6–14)	12 (7–17)	16 (10–22)	17 (11–24)
	6	14 (9–19)	17 (11–24)	22 (15–31)	24 (17–33)
	7	20 (13–27)	25 (16–34)	32 (22–44)	34 (24–46)
	8–10	39 (25–57)	47 (30–67)	58 (38–79)	61 (40–81)
20.1–50.0	2–4	7 (3–14)	9 (4–18)	12 (6–23)	13 (7–24)
	5	16 (10–24)	20 (13–30)	26 (16–37)	27 (17–39)
	6	23 (15–32)	28 (20–39)	36 (25–49)	38 (27–51)
	7	32 (23–42)	39 (28–51)	49 (36–64)	51 (38–66)
	8–10	58 (41–76)	67 (49–85)	78 (58–93)	80 (62–94)

Adapted from D'Amico et al.[31]

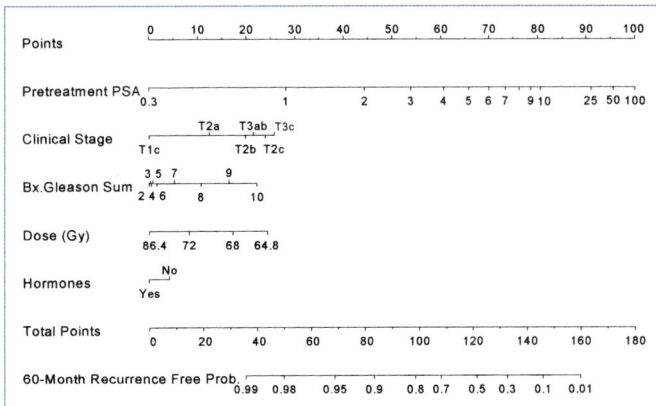

Fig. 56.4

Three-dimensional conformal radiation therapy nomogram for prostate-specific antigen (PSA) recurrence, based on 1042 patients treated at Memorial Sloan-Kettering Cancer Center.

Instructions for physician and instruction to patient: see legend for Figure 56.3.

Adapted from Kattan MW, Zelefsky MJ, Kupelian PA, Scardino PT, Fuks Z, Leibel SA. Pretreatment nomogram for predicting the outcome of three-dimensional conformal radiotherapy in prostate cancer. J Clin Oncol 2000;18:3352–3359. Reprinted with permission from the American Society of Clinical Oncology.

Memorial Sloan-Kettering Cancer Center between 1988 and 1998. Kattan et al[19] used five widely available prognostic variables (clinical stage, pretreatment PSA, biopsy Gleason sum, treatment with neoadjuvant hormones, and the required radiation dose) in the Cox regression analysis described earlier to predict treatment failure. The clinical stage was assigned by three different radiation oncologists based on the 1992 TNM classification system and ranged from T1c to T3c NxM0. Biopsy Gleason score was simply the sum of the primary and secondary Gleason grades. The pretreatment PSA was modeled as a restricted cubic spline of its natural logarithm.[4] Treatment failure was defined according to the methods of Shipley et al,[35] a modification of the American Society of Therapeutic Radiation Oncology (ASTRO) definition[36] (see next section). This nomogram discriminated well; the bootstrapped concordance index measured 0.73. Calibration of this nomogram with bootstrap analysis showed that it performed within 10% of actual outcome. This nomogram was externally validated on a separate sample of 912 patients treated with EBRT (n = 529) or 3D-CRT (n = 383) at the Cleveland Clinic and the concordance index was 0.76.

SHIPLEY ET AL PREDICTION TABLE

Shipley et al prediction table predicts 5-year PSA recurrence. Developed in 1999, this model was based on 1607 patients treated with EBRT alone (no androgen-deprivation treatment) between 1988 and 1995 at five different institutions; 51% of patients were treated with 3D-CRT.[35] Shipley et al included three common prognostic variables (clinical stage, pretreatment PSA, and biopsy Gleason sum) in the Cox regression analysis to predict treatment failure, a modified version[35] of the ASTRO consensus.[36] Essentially, three consecutive rises in PSA or any rise great enough to prompt adjuvant hormonal therapy with backdating (i.e., time of failure considered to be the midpoint between last non-rising and first rising value). They further used recursive partitioning to determine the optimal cut-points between the Kaplan–Meier curves in identifying their subgroups.

OTHER MODELS

Other models that predict PSA recurrence after radiotherapy have been created but remain to be validated in outside institutions[31,37] (see Table 56.1).

PRE-TREATMENT PREDICTION MODEL: BRACHYTHERAPY

KATTAN NOMOGRAM

A Kattan nomogram that predicts 5-year PSA recurrence was developed in 2001. This nomogram (Figure 56.5) was based on 920 patients treated with permanent prostate brachytherapy at Memorial Sloan-Kettering Cancer Center between 1992 and 2000.[12] Kattan et al used four prognostic variables (clinical stage, pretreatment PSA, biopsy Gleason sum, and treatment with EBRT) in the Cox regression analysis to predict treatment failure. The clinical stage was assigned based on the 1997 TNM classification system[38] and ranged from T1c to T2 N0M0. The pretreatment PSA was modeled as a restricted cubic spline of its natural logarithm.[4] Treatment failure was defined according to the ASTRO definition,[36] with two conservative modifications.[39] This nomogram discriminated significantly better than chance (p < 0.0001) and was externally validated at the Seattle Prostate Institute (c-index, 0.61) and Arizona Oncology Services (c-index, 0.64). Upon calibration at these two institutions, the Kattan nomogram predictions were within 5% worse and 30% better than the actual outcome. Although the predictive accuracy of this nomogram is imperfect, it might be the best that prediction models can offer to patients selecting brachytherapy as their treatment of choice.

POST-TREATMENT PREDICTION MODELS: EXIST ONLY FOR RADICAL PROSTATECTOMY

KATTAN NOMOGRAM

A Kattan nomogram that predicts 7-year PSA recurrence was developed in 1999. This nomogram (Figure 56.6)

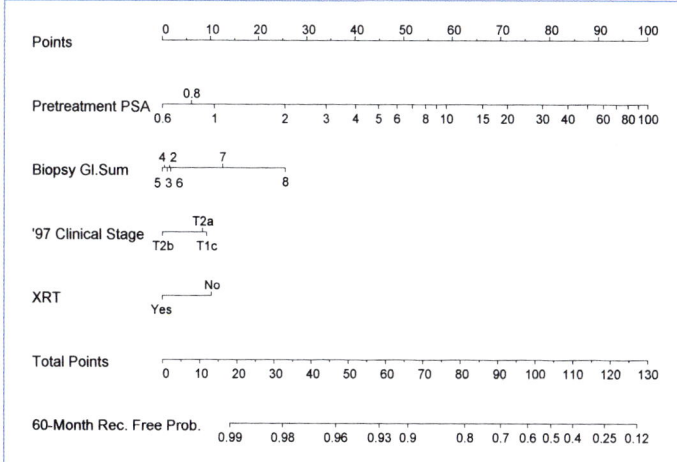

Fig. 56.5

Nomogram for predicting 5-year freedom from prostate-specific antigen (PSA) recurrence after permanent prostate brachytherapy without neoadjuvant androgen ablative therapy.

Instructions for physician and instruction to patient: see legend for Figure 56.3.

Reprinted from Urology, 58, Kattan MW, Potters L, Blasko JC, et al. Pretreatment nomogram for predicting freedom from recurrence after permanent prostate brachytherapy in prostate cancer, 393–399, copyright 2001, with permission from Elsevier.

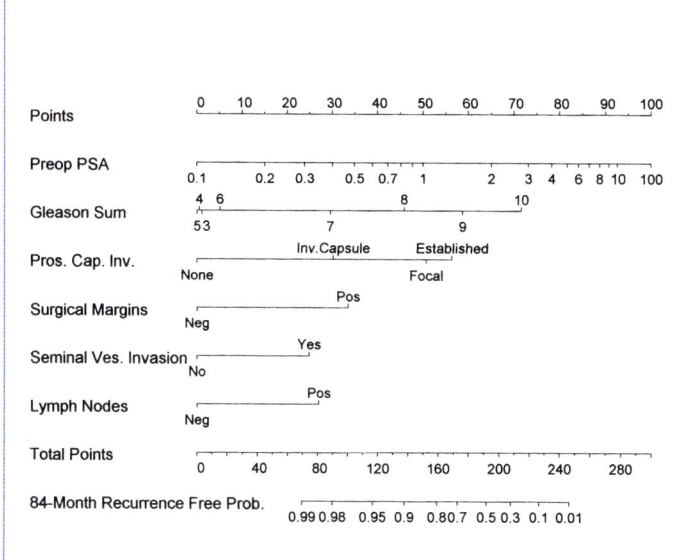

Fig. 56.6

Postoperative nomogram for prostate cancer recurrence.

Instructions for physician: Locate the patient's PSA on the **PSA Axis**. Draw a line straight upwards to the **Points Axis** to determine how many points towards recurrence the patient receives for his PSA. Repeat this process for the other axes, each time drawing straight upward to the **Points Axis**. Sum the points achieved for each predictor and locate this sum on the **Total Points Axis**. Draw a line straight down to find the patient's probability of remaining recurrence free for 84 months, assuming he does not die of another cause first.

Instruction to patient: "Mr. X, if we had 100 men exactly like you, we would expect between [predicted percentage from nomogram –10%] and [predicted percentage + 10%] to remain free of their disease at 7 years following radical prostatectomy, and recurrence after 7 years is very rare."

© 1998 Michael W. Kattan and Peter T. Scardino, MSKCC Division of Urology. Adapted from Kattan MW, Wheeler TM, Scardino PT. Postoperative nomogram for disease recurrence after radical prostatectomy for prostate cancer. J Clin Oncol 1999;17:1499–1507. Reprinted with permission from the American Society of Clinical Oncology.

was based on 996 patients treated with radical prostatectomy at BCM between 1983 and 1997 by a single surgeon.[13] Kattan et al used six widely available clinicopathologic variables (pretreatment PSA, pathology Gleason sum, capsular invasion of the prostate, surgical margin status, seminal vesicle invasion, and lymph node involvement) in the Cox regression analysis described earlier to predict treatment failure. They analyzed pretreatment PSA as its natural logarithm. Pathology Gleason score was simply the sum of the primary and secondary Gleason grades in the surgical specimen. Because they suspected nonlinear effects, Kattan et al modeled both PSA and Gleason sum with restricted cubic splines.[4] They grouped prostate capsular invasion into four categories: no invasion, capsular invasion, focal, and established extracapsular extension. Cancer within the muscular coat of the seminal vesicle and not in the surrounding fat was considered invasion.[40] Treatment failure was defined as the *first* occurrence of one of the following: BCR,

treatment with secondary therapy in the form of radiation or hormonal agents, death from prostate cancer, or clinical evidence of cancer recurrence without a PSA rise. Biochemical recurrence was defined as a serum PSA level of 0.4 ng/mL or more followed by a rise. Patients for whom radical prostatectomy was aborted because of cancer invasion of the lymph nodes were excluded from the study. This nomogram discriminated very well; the concordance index both without and with bootstrapping, was 0.88. Calibration of this nomogram with bootstrap analysis showed that it performed within 10% of actual outcome. This nomogram's predictions were calculated in a separate sample of 322 patients and the concordance index measured 0.89. External validation of this nomogram was performed across three continents and the concordance index ranged from 0.77 to 0.82 with good calibration.[28] On further studies, this nomogram was validated in a cohort of black men: the concordance index measured 0.83. Although it overestimated freedom from recurrence during calibration, the Kattan postoperative nomogram is still appropriate for use with black men.[24]

MOUL ET AL PREDICTION TABLE

The Moul et al prediction table that predicts 3-, 5-, and 7-year PSA recurrence[41] was developed in 2001. This model is a modification of the earlier version designed by Bauer et al.[42] It was based on 1515 patients either treated at the Walter Reed Army Medical Center (n = 503) or part of the Cancer of the Prostate Strategic Urologic Research Endeavor (CaPSURE; n = 1012), a large multicenter community-based prostate cancer database. The developers used four clinicopathologic variables which included postoperative Gleason sum (G), pretreatment PSA (PSA), race (R), and pathologic stage (S) in the Cox regression analysis to predict the relative risk (RR) of disease recurrence defined as two successive PSA measurements greater than 0.2 ng/mL.

$$RR = \text{exponent (exp)}[0.54R + 0.05PSA_{ST} + 0.23G + 0.69S]$$

Where PSA_{ST} represents the sigmoidal transformation of PSA calculated as:

$$PSA_{ST} = 10/(1+e^{6.8704 - 0.9815 \times PSA})$$

Race was 0 for whites and 1 for blacks. G represents the sum of the primary and secondary Gleason grades in the prostatectomy specimen. S was 0 if prostate cancer was organ confined and 1 if it penetrated the capsule.

Based on the RR value, the patients were partitioned into eight risk groups that were later combined to form four summary risk groups based on the Kaplan–Meier survival curves predicted probabilities. These risk groups included very low, low, high, and very high.

PARTIN ET AL PREDICTION TABLE

The Partin et al prediction table predicts 5-year PSA recurrence. Developed in 1995, this model[43] represents the foundation for those subsequently built by Bauer et al[42] and Moul et al.[41] The developers of these tables used a cohort of 216 patients with clinical stages T2b and T2c treated at the Johns Hopkins University School of Medicine between 1984 and 1991 with radical retropubic prostatectomy. The developers included three clinicopathologic variables (pretreatment PSA [PSA], prostatectomy Gleason sum [G], and pathologic stage [S]) in the proportional hazards regression analysis to predict the risk of disease recurrence defined as a sustained PSA of more than 0.2 ng/mL. The patients were grouped into three categories (low, intermediate, and high risk) based on the values of the logarithm of the relative risk (Rw), where $Rw = 0.06PSA_{ST} + 0.54G + 1.87S$. The variables G, S, and PSA_{ST} were defined as previously stated in Moul et al. A validation of this model in a cohort of 214 men treated at two different

institutions showed it to be accurate only for the high-risk subset.

OTHER POSTOPERATIVE MODELS

Other postoperative models include Han et al,[33] Bauer et al,[42] Blute et al,[44] and D'Amico et al.[45]

CONCLUSION

Prediction models are valuable tools that aid physicians in making more accurate prognostic assessments. Of many existing models, nomograms have outperformed traditional risk groups. Although a few prediction models have been validated in outside institutions, most still lack generalizability, which makes clinicians hesitant to use them. Furthermore, better predictor variables are needed to improve predictive accuracy, and there is a need for development of additional models representing different outcomes, such as cancer-specific survival and survival adjusted for quality of life.

REFERENCES

1. Ohori M, Wheeler TM, Dunn JK, et al. The pathological features and prognosis of prostate cancer detectable with current diagnostic tests. J Urol 1994;152:1714–1720.

2. Cowen ME, Miles BJ, Cahill DF, et al. The danger of applying group-level utilities in decision analyses of the treatment of localized prostate cancer in individual patients. Med Decis Making 1998;18:376–380.

3. Kattan MW. Comparing treatment outcomes using utility assessment for health-related quality of life. Oncology (Huntingt) 2003;17:1687–1693; discussion 1693–1694, 1697, 1701.

4. Harrell FE Jr, Lee KL, Mark DB. Multivariable prognostic models: issues in developing models, evaluating assumptions and adequacy, and measuring and reducing errors. Stat Med 1996;15:361–387.

5. Kattan MW. Comparison of Cox regression with other methods for determining prediction models and nomograms. J Urol 2003;170:S6–9; discussion S10.

6. Kattan MW, Scardino PT. Prediction of progression: nomograms of clinical utility. Clin Prostate Cancer 2002;1:90–96.

7. Kattan MW. Nomograms are superior to staging and risk grouping systems for identifying high-risk patients: preoperative application in prostate cancer. Curr Opin Urol 2003;13:111–116.

8. Ross PL, Gerigk C, Gonen M, et al. Comparisons of nomograms and urologists' predictions in prostate cancer. Semin Urol Oncol 2002;20:82–88.

9. Kattan MW, Zelefsky MJ, Kupelian PA, et al. Pretreatment nomogram for predicting the outcome of three-dimensional conformal radiotherapy in prostate cancer. J Clin Oncol 2000;18:3352–3359.

10. Diblasio CJ, Kattan MW. Use of nomograms to predict the risk of disease recurrence after definitive local therapy for prostate cancer. Urology 2003;62 (Suppl 1):9–18.

11. Kattan MW, Eastham JA, Stapleton AM, et al. A preoperative nomogram for disease recurrence following radical prostatectomy for prostate cancer. J Natl Cancer Inst 1998;90:766–771.

12. Kattan MW, Potters L, Blasko JC, et al. Pretreatment nomogram for predicting freedom from recurrence after permanent prostate brachytherapy in prostate cancer. Urology 2001;58:393–399.

13. Kattan MW, Wheeler TM, Scardino PT. Postoperative nomogram for disease recurrence after radical prostatectomy for prostate cancer. J Clin Oncol 1999;17:1499–1507.

14. Halabi S, Small EJ, Kantoff PW, et al. Prognostic model for predicting survival in men with hormone-refractory metastatic prostate cancer. J Clin Oncol 2003;21:1232–1237.

15. Smaletz O, Scher HI, Small EJ, et al. Nomogram for overall survival of patients with progressive metastatic prostate cancer after castration. J Clin Oncol 2002;20:3972–3982.

16. Hull GW, Rabbani F, Abbas F, et al. Cancer control with radical prostatectomy alone in 1,000 consecutive patients. J Urol 2002;167:528–534.

17. Kattan MW, Eastham J. Algorithms for prostate-specific antigen recurrence after treatment of localized prostate cancer. Clin Prostate Cancer 2003;1:221–226.

18. Kattan MW, Vickers AJ. Incorporating predictions of individual patient risk in clinical trials. Urol Oncol 2004;22:348–351.

19. Ross PL, Scardino PT, Kattan MW. A catalog of prostate cancer nomograms. J Urol 2001;165:1562–1568.

20. Miles BJ, Giesler B, Kattan MW. Recall and attitudes in patients with prostate cancer. Urology 1999;53:169–174.

21. Kattan MW, Zelefsky MJ, Kupelian PA, et al. Pretreatment nomogram that predicts 5-year probability of metastasis following three-dimensional conformal radiation therapy for localized prostate cancer. J Clin Oncol 2003;21:4568–4571.

22. Kattan MW, Eastham J. Algorithms for prostate-specific antigen recurrence after treatment of localized prostate cancer. Clin Prostate Cancer 2003;1:221–226.

23. Greene KL, Meng MV, Elkin EP, et al. Validation of the Kattan Preoperative Nomogram for Prostate Cancer Recurrence Using a Community Based Cohort: Results from Cancer of the Prostate Strategic Urological Research Endeavor (Capsure). J Urol 2004;171:2255–2259.

24. Bianco FJ, Jr., Kattan MW, Scardino PT, et al. Radical prostatectomy nomograms in black American men: accuracy and applicability. J Urol 2003;170:73–76;discussion 76–77.

25. D'Amico AV, Cote K, Loffredo M, et al. Pretreatment predictors of time to cancer specific death after prostate specific antigen failure. J Urol 2003;169:1320–1324.

26. Justice AC, Covinsky KE, Berlin JA. Assessing the generalizability of prognostic information. Ann Intern Med 1999;130:515–524.

27. Efron B, Tibshirani R. An introduction to the bootstrap. New York: Chapman & Hall, 1993:xvi, p. 436.

28. Graefen M, Karakiewicz PI, Cagiannos I, et al. Validation study of the accuracy of a postoperative nomogram for recurrence after radical prostatectomy for localized prostate cancer. J Clin Oncol 2002;20:951–956.

29. Graefen M, Karakiewicz PI, Cagiannos I, et al. International validation of a preoperative nomogram for prostate cancer recurrence after radical prostatectomy. J Clin Oncol 2002;20:3206–3212.

30. Graefen M, Karakiewicz PI, Cagiannos I, et al. A validation of two preoperative nomograms predicting recurrence following radical prostatectomy in a cohort of European men. Urol Oncol 2002;7:141–146.

31. D'Amico AV, Whittington R, Malkowicz SB, et al. Pretreatment nomogram for prostate-specific antigen recurrence after radical prostatectomy or external-beam radiation therapy for clinically localized prostate cancer. J Clin Oncol 1999;17:168–172.

32. Hull GW, Rabbani F, Abbas F, et al. Cancer control with radical prostatectomy alone in 1,000 consecutive patients. J Urol 2002;167:528–534.

33. Han M, Partin AW, Zahurak M, et al. Biochemical (prostate specific antigen) recurrence probability following radical prostatectomy for clinically localized prostate cancer. J Urol 2003;169:517–523.

34. Leibel SA, Zelefsky MJ, Kutcher GJ, et al. The biological basis and clinical application of three-dimensional conformal external beam radiation therapy in carcinoma of the prostate. Semin Oncol 1994;21:580–597.

35. Shipley WU, Thames HD, Sandler HM, et al. Radiation therapy for clinically localized prostate cancer: a multi-institutional pooled analysis. JAMA 1999;281:1598–1604.

36. Consensus statement: guidelines for PSA following radiation therapy. American Society for Therapeutic Radiology and Oncology Consensus Panel. Int J Radiat Oncol Biol Phys 1997;37:1035–1041.

37. Roach M, Lu J, Pilepich MV, et al. Four prognostic groups predict long-term survival from prostate cancer following radiotherapy alone on Radiation Therapy Oncology Group clinical trials. Int J Radiat Oncol Biol Phys 2000;47:609–615.

38. Fleming ID, American Joint Committee on Cancer, National Cancer Institute (U.S.), et al. AJCC cancer staging manual. Philadelphia: Lippincott-Raven, 1997:xv, p. 294.

39. Kattan MW, Fearn PA, Leibel S, et al. The definition of biochemical failure in patients treated with definitive radiotherapy. Int J Radiat Oncol Biol Phys 2000;48:1469–1474.

40. Ohori M, Scardino PT, Lapin SL, et al. The mechanisms and prognostic significance of seminal vesicle involvement by prostate cancer. Am J Surg Pathol 1993;17:1252–1261.

41. Moul JW, Connelly RR, Lubeck DP, et al. Predicting risk of prostate specific antigen recurrence after radical prostatectomy with the Center for Prostate Disease Research and Cancer of the Prostate Strategic Urologic Research Endeavor databases. J Urol 2001;166:1322–1327.

42. Bauer JJ, Connelly RR, Seterhenn IA, et al. Biostatistical modeling using traditional preoperative and pathological prognostic variables in the selection of men at high risk for disease recurrence after radical prostatectomy for prostate cancer. J Urol 1998;159:929–933.

43. Partin AW, Piantadosi S, Sanda MG, et al. Selection of men at high risk for disease recurrence for experimental adjuvant therapy following radical prostatectomy. Urology 1995;45:831–838.

44. Blute ML, Bergstralh EJ, Iocca A, et al. Use of Gleason score, prostate specific antigen, seminal vesicle and margin status to predict biochemical failure after radical prostatectomy. J Urol 2001;165:119–125.

45. D'Amico AV, Whittington R, Malkowicz SB, et al. The combination of preoperative prostate specific antigen and postoperative pathological findings to predict prostate specific antigen outcome in clinically localized prostate cancer. J Urol 1998;160:2096–2101.

Clinical interpretation of prostate biopsy reports

57

J Kellogg Parsons, Alan W Partin

INTRODUCTION

The prostate needle biopsy is the gold standard for the tissue diagnosis of prostate cancer and provides data vital to clinical decision-making. Now that the majority of prostate cancers are detected with serum prostate-specific antigen (PSA) screening and transrectal ultrasound-guided biopsy, accurate interpretation of needle biopsy reports is particularly important for informed care guidance in asymptomatic men with localized disease. In this chapter, we outline the information contained in needle biopsy reports and explain how to apply this information to clinical practice. We do not discuss the indications for and techniques of prostate needle biopsy, as these are topics featured in other chapters.

Our discussion is in three parts: 1) interpretation and management of nonmalignant lesions; 2) interpretation of immunohistochemical markers for distinguishing between nonmalignant and malignant glands; and 3) interpretation of adenocarcinoma.

CLINICAL INTERPRETATION AND MANAGEMENT OF SELECT NONMALIGNANT LESIONS ON NEEDLE BIOPSY

There are three nonmalignant lesions on needle biopsy associated with prostate cancer with which the clinician should be familiar.

FOCAL ATROPHY

Focal atrophy is a term for benign regions of prostate glandular and stromal volume reduction. There are several morphologic patterns of focal prostate atrophy, including simple atrophy, post-atrophic hyperplasia, and partial atrophy. Since most focal atrophy lesions are actively proliferating and are associated with inflammation, De Marzo et al prefer the term proliferative inflammatory atrophy (PIA).[1]

There is emerging evidence that focal atrophy lesions in the prostate may potentially be associated with prostate carcinogenesis.[1,2] However, there are currently no clinical data to suggest that an isolated finding of focal atrophy on prostate biopsy is associated with an increased incidence of adenocarcinoma on subsequent biopsies. Indeed, since some forms of focal atrophy are so common on needle biopsy, many pathologists will not consistently report on either its presence or absence. In the future, ongoing studies should provide information as to clinical significance of these lesions.

Currently, rebiopsy for isolated atrophy is not indicated. For a finding of isolated atrophy on needle biopsy, the clinician should determine the appropriate next step in management based upon consideration of other clinical parameters: race, age, family history, digital rectal examination (DRE), total and free prostate-specific antige (PSA) values, and PSA kinetics (velocity and/or doubling time).

ATYPIA

Atypia is a nonspecific term for small, proliferative acini or foci that are suspicious for, but not diagnostic of, adenocarcinoma. Phrases used to describe these lesions include "atypical glands suspicious for carcinoma,"[3] "suspicious, atypical focus," and, most commonly, "atypical small acinar proliferation (ASAP)."[4]

An atypical focus is not a distinct premalignant lesion but rather a suspicious finding that represents one of two possibilities: 1) an adenocarcinoma that lacks the architectural and/or cytologic criteria needed to definitively diagnose malignancy; or 2) a nonmalignant glandular focus that appears abnormal in the biopsy specimen.[3] The frequency of atypia in published case series ranges from 1.5% to 23.4%, with a median frequency of 4.5%.[3-5]

An isolated finding of atypia is associated with a diagnosis of adenocarcinoma on subsequent biopsy in approximately 50% of cases.[3,4,6] Therefore, repeat biopsy for atypia should be performed within three months of the initial biopsy[6-8] and include increased sampling of the atypical site and adjacent areas.[3,6,8] The probability of cancer detection in subsequent biopsies after a diagnosis of atypia is not associated with DRE results or serum PSA concentration.[3,5]

If no cancer is found on rebiopsy, consideration should be given to close follow-up with digital rectal exam, serum PSA, and periodic extended-pattern biopsy.[8] Data from sextant biopsy series suggest that 2 additional biopsies following an initial atypical biopsy are sufficient for detecting the majority of lesions.[4] The applicability of these data to the current practice of extended-pattern biopsy, however, is unclear.

PROSTATIC INTRAEPITHELIAL NEOPLASIA

Prostatic intraepithelial neoplasia (PIN) is a lesion characterized by structurally benign glands and ducts lined by atypical cells. There is much evidence to support the concept that PIN is a precursor to prostate cancer. As a diagnosis, PIN represents a spectrum of neoplastic changes and was originally conceived as two different lesions: low and high grade. However, current opinion is that low-grade PIN should not be documented as a separate diagnosis, since it lacks reproducibility among different pathologists and is associated with a risk of cancer in subsequent biopsies comparable to benign tissue.[5]

The frequency of high-grade PIN on needle biopsy ranges from 1.5% to 24%, with a median frequency of 5% to 6%.[5] In early series of sextant biopsies, an isolated finding of high-grade PIN was associated with a diagnosis of adenocarcinoma on subsequent biopsy in approximately 30% of cases.[5] However, recent data from extended-pattern biopsy series suggest that this risk is much lower.[10,11] Therefore, if high-grade PIN was detected on an initial sextant biopsy, immediate rebiopsy using an extended-pattern technique is indicated. If high-grade PIN was detected on an initial extended-pattern biopsy, then close follow-up with DRE and serum PSA is indicated.[8]

CLINICAL INTERPRETATION OF IMMUNOHISTOCHEMISTRY ON NEEDLE BIOPSY

Pathologists frequently utilize immunohistochemistry as an adjunct to standard diagnosis with hematoxylin and eosin (H&E) stain in order to help establish whether an indeterminate or suspicious epithelial lesion is malignant. There are at least four common immunohistochemical markers currently used in needle biopsies to distinguish between nonmalignant and malignant prostate glands with which the clinician should be familiar (Table 57,1). Issues regarding sensitivity, specificity, and predictive values of these markers are not discussed, as they relate specifically to pathologic diagnosis rather than clinical practice.[2]

ANTI-CYTOKERATINS

Cytokeratins 5 and 14 are structural proteins selectively and constitutively expressed in the basal cells of prostate epithelium and are frequently identified using the monoclonal antibody 34βE12, which is also known as keratin 903. Since basal cells are absent in prostate cancer, the majority of cancers do not express cytokeratins 5 and 14. A positive stain for these cytokeratins, therefore, supports the *absence* of malignancy.[12-14]

ANTI-P63

The p63 protein is a homolog of the tumor suppressor p53 that is selectively and constitutively expressed in the basal cells of normal epithelium, benign prostatic hyperplasia (BPH), atrophy, and high-grade PIN. Although its exact function remains to be elucidated, it

Table 57.1 Immunohistochemical markers for prostate cancer on needle biopsy

Protein	Expression	Interpretation
Cytokeratin 5 Cytokeratin 14 Cytokeratin 903 (34βE12)	↓ in cancer[12-14]	+ stain suggests *no* malignancy
p63	↓ in cancer[15,16]	+ stain suggests *no* malignancy
AMACR	↑ in cancer[17,18]	+ stain suggests malignancy

AMACR, alpha-methylacyl-CoA racemase.

is believed to be a stem cell marker and transcription factor that is required for prostate development.[15] Signoretti et al first reported the absence of p63 protein in prostate cancer[15] and Parsons et al first demonstrated the clinical usefulness of p63 immunostaining for aiding in the diagnosis of prostate cancer in needle biopsies.[16] Unlike benign and premalignant prostate tissue, at least 90% of prostate adenocarcinomas do not express p63.[16] Therefore, a positive stain for p63 supports the *absence* of malignancy.

ANTI-ALPHA-METHYLACYL-COA RACEMASE

Alpha-methylacyl-CoA racemase (AMACR) is an enzyme that plays an integral role in the metabolism of dietary branched-chain fatty acids and bile acid intermediates.[17] Compared with its levels in benign tissue, BPH, atrophy, and high-grade PIN, AMACR is overexpressed in the majority of prostate cancer cells.[17-20] Therefore, a positive stain for AMACR supports the *presence* of malignancy.

ANTI-P63/ALPHA-METHYLACYL-COA RACEMASE COCKTAIL

De Marzo et al first described using antibodies for p63 and AMACR in combination in needle biopsies to facilitate the diagnosis of cancer.[17] When used together, the two different antibodies produce the same immunostaining reactions that each produces separately (i.e., overexpression of AMACR and lack of expression of p63). The patterns are complementary and provide a more vivid staining pattern for facilitating detection of prostate cancer cells.[17,21] A simultaneous positive stain for AMACR and negative stain for p63 supports the *presence* of malignancy.

CLINICAL INTERPRETATION OF ADENOCARCINOMA ON NEEDLE BIOPSY

GLEASON SCORE

The Gleason grading system is the predominant system for grading prostate adenocarcinoma. The system assigns a score from 1 to 5 for each area of cancer based upon the histopathologic pattern of the tumor: 1 for a well-differentiated and 5 for a poorly differentiated pattern. The Gleason score, also called the Gleason sum, is the predominant method of reporting Gleason patterns in pathology reports. It represents the sum of two numbers: 1) the most prevalent Gleason pattern;

and 2) the second most prevalent pattern. Thus, if a biopsy contains a large tumor area of pattern 4 and a smaller area of pattern 3, the Gleason score is 4 + 3 = 7. If the tumor in the specimen contains only one type of pattern, the pattern number is doubled. Thus, the Gleason score of a tumor containing only a Gleason 4 pattern is 4 + 4 = 8.

Gleason scores of 2 to 4 are classified as "well differentiated," 5 to 6 as "moderately differentiated," 7 as "moderately-to-poorly differentiated," and 8 to 10 as "poorly differentiated".[5] Recent opinion is that Gleason scores of 2 to 4, which are primarily observed in transurethral resection specimens, should not be documented on needle biopsy, since the majority of them are reclassified as 5 to 6 on review by a genitourinary pathologist and may inappropriately lead to under treatment.[5,22,23]

Gleason score is associated with cancer aggressiveness and remains a fundamental component of every major predictive instrument used for clinical prognostication from needle biopsies (i.e., the Partin tables and Kattan nomograms). These predictive instruments generate probabilities for final pathologic stage and biochemical recurrence and disease progression after definitive local therapy with surgery or radiation. They are an important component of patient counseling following needle biopsy.

Although the statistical contribution of the Gleason score to disease risk assessment varies depending upon the predictive model, the clinician may assume a few general principles about the association between biopsy Gleason score and the aggressiveness of the tumor. A Gleason score of less than 7 generally indicates less aggressive disease and is one of the pathologic criteria for considering a patient with a nonpalpable tumor for expectant management.[24,25] A Gleason score of 7 or more indicates more aggressive disease. Men with localized prostate cancer and biopsy scores 7 to 10 have a high probability of dying from prostate cancer, even at older ages.[26]

A frequently raised issue in the interpretation of needle biopsy Gleason score, associated primarily with sampling error, is lack of correlation with final pathologic score. Lack of correlation may potentially result in under grading: in general, while a high Gleason score in the needle biopsy reliably predicts a high Gleason score in the prostatectomy specimen, a low Gleason score in the biopsy does not reliably predict a low score in the final specimen.[22] In radical prostatectomy series, 30% to 50% of biopsy Gleason scores less than 7 had a final pathologic Gleason score greater than or equal to 7.[27-30] In contrast, in one large series, 87.5% of patients with Gleason score of 7 or more had the same score on final pathology.[27]

Because of the potential for under grading, we recommend that clinicians recognize the prognostic limitations of the needle Gleason score and consider additional clinical parameters when counseling patients by using validated, appropriate predictive instruments. Biopsy Gleason score is but one variable in these instruments, which also incorporate PSA, clinical stage, and quantification of cancer.[31]

CANCER QUANTIFICATION

There are at least five methods for quantifying the amount of cancer detected on needle biopsy: 1) the total number of cores containing cancer; 2) the percentage of each individual core that involves cancer; 3) the largest percentage of cancer in any one core; 4) the total percentage of cancer in all cores combined; and 5) the total length in millimeters of cancer in all cores combined.

Although no one method has proven superior, two of the most common methods used are the number of positive cores and the percentage of each positive core that involves cancer.[22] Epstein et al advocate the use of a reporting system that combines the number of positive cores with a quantitative assessment of the amount of cancer present in each positive core.[5] Differences in quantification methods not withstanding, numerous studies of prostatectomy series have demonstrated that the amount of cancer present in the biopsy specimen is positively associated with extraprostatic extension,[32–38] seminal vesicle invasion,[34,38,39] and positive surgical margins.[37,40,41] However, the clinical significance of biopsy tumor volume in predicting disease outcomes independent of other clinical parameters is unclear. Therefore, we recommend that, as with Gleason score, clinicians consider the biopsy tumor volume in association with other clinical parameters when counseling patients.

CANCER LOCATION

There has been debate as to whether location of the cancer in the needle biopsy specimen will predict pathologic stage[32,42] or the probability of extraprostatic extension on the ipsilateral side.[43,44] Proof of the latter would favor using this information to identify patients who would potentially benefit from ipsilateral excision of the neurovascular bundle at surgery. At this time, however, there is no definitive evidence that tumor location in the biopsy specimen provides useful information for guiding treatment decisions.

There has also been debate as to whether each biopsy core should be individually labeled by sextant site (base, mid, apex) and side or, since it is more cost-effective, only by side.[22,44] Since additional sampling of areas around atypia and high-grade PIN maximizes the potential for detecting occult cancer in repeat biopsies, we recommend precise labeling of all cores at an initial

biopsy in order to direct the performance of repeat biopsies.[5]

PERINEURAL INVASION

Perineural invasion (PNI) refers to the tracking of prostate cancer cells along or around a nerve, and is a major mechanism by which prostate cancer cells spread from the prostate into periprostatic soft tissue.[5] This feature has prompted study as to the prognostic significance of PNI identified in pathologic specimens. Although PNI in a radical prostatectomy specimen is not significant,[5] PNI in a needle biopsy is associated with extraprostatic extension[35,45–47] and biochemical recurrence after radical prostatectomy.[48] But definitive evidence is lacking that PNI independently predicts extraprostatic extension or biochemical recurrence—or adds anything to prognostication and patient management—when PSA, clinical stage, and needle biopsy Gleason score are also included in the analysis.[22,45,46,49]

There are also data to suggest that, when PNI is present on biopsy, excision of one or both neurovascular bundles during radical prostatectomy may result in decreased incidence and extent of positive surgical margins: an observation prompting the recommendation that selected men with PNI should be considered for neurovascular bundle excision.[50] It should be noted, however, that these are single institution data that have not been independently confirmed.

Although there is no formal consensus regarding the prognostic value of PNI on needle biopsy, the results of a recent survey of members of the Society of Urologic Oncology provide an indication of current practice patterns among a select group of academic urologic oncologists. The majority of respondents (57%) to this survey did not believe the presence of PNI was important for planning treatment.[51]

NEEDLE BIOPSY CRITERIA FOR DEFINING CLINICALLY INSIGNIFICANT STAGE T1C CANCER

One additional component of the information obtained from prostate biopsy reports merits discussion. In 1994, Epstein et al proposed criteria, based on needle biopsy and PSA density, for identifying patients with nonpalpable tumors (clinical stage T1c) who have small volume, clinically insignificant disease: 1) Gleason score less than 7; 2) cancer involving less than three cores; 3) cancer involving less than 50% of any single core; and 4) PSA density (PSA divided by transrectal ultrasound determined prostate volume) less than 0.15 ng/mL/cm^3.[25] Carter et al later confirmed the predictive value of these criteria[52] and have applied them, with favorable results, in the identification of appropriate candidates for expectant management with intent to cure. Patients over 65 years of age who meet these criteria are reasonable candidates for expectant management.[24,53]

SUMMARY

Focal atrophy, atypia, and high-grade PIN are three non-malignant diagnoses detected on needle biopsy. For atypia, rebiopsy within three months of the initial biopsy— including increased sampling of the atypical site and adjacent areas—is indicated. If no cancer is found on rebiopsy, consideration should be given to close follow-up with digital rectal exam, serum PSA, and periodic extended-pattern biopsy. For high-grade PIN, immediate rebiopsy using an extended-pattern technique is recommended only if a sextant pattern was used initially. If an extended-pattern was used initially, then close follow-up with DRE and serum PSA is recommended.

Immunohistochemistry in needle biopsies may help detect prostate cancer cells and determine if a suspicious gland is malignant. Positive stains for cytokeratins and p63 suggest the absence of malignancy. A positive stain for AMACR suggests the presence of malignancy. Antibodies to p63 and AMACR may be combined into a single assay.

Gleason score, cancer quantification, cancer location, and PNI are all features used to characterize adenocarcinoma detected on needle biopsy. Gleason score is associated with cancer aggressiveness and provides vital information for guiding treatment. The prognostic value of cancer quantification is unproven, but may be considered with other clinical parameters. The prognostic value of cancer location is unproven; however, we recommend precise labeling of all cores at an initial biopsy in case repeat biopsy is later indicated for atypia or high-grade PIN. The prognostic value of reporting PNI in needle biopsy is unproven. A majority of academic urologic oncologists responding to a recent survey indicated that PNI is not important for planning treatment.

Patients over 65 years of age with nonpalpable tumors, needle biopsy Gleason score less than 7, cancer involving less than three biopsy cores, cancer involving less than 50% of any single biopsy core, and PSA density less than 0.15 ng/mL/cm^3 are reasonable candidates for expectant management with intent to cure.

REFERENCES

1. De Marzo AM, Marchi VL, Epstein JI, et al. Proliferative inflammatory atrophy of the prostate: implications for prostatic carcinogenesis. Am J Pathol. 1999;155:1985–1992.

2. DeMarzo AM, Nelson WG, Isaacs WB, et al. Pathological and molecular aspects of prostate cancer. Lancet. 2003;361:955–964.

3. Chan TY and Epstein JI. Follow-up of atypical prostate needle biopsies suspicious for cancer. Urology. 1999;53:351–355.

4. Iczkowski KA, Bassler TJ, Schwob VS, et al. Diagnosis of "suspicious for malignancy" in prostate biopsies: predictive value for cancer. Urology. 1998;51:749–757 discussion 757–8, 1998.

5. Epstein JI and Potter SR. The pathological interpretation and significance of prostate needle biopsy findings: implications and current controversies. J Urol. 2001;166:402–410.

6. Park S, Shinohara K, Grossfeld GD, et al. Prostate cancer detection in men with prior high grade prostatic intraepithelial neoplasia or atypical prostate biopsy. J Urol. 2001;165:1409–1414.

7. Borboroglu PG, Sur RL, Roberts JL, et al. Repeat biopsy strategy in patients with atypical small acinar proliferation or high grade prostatic intraepithelial neoplasia on initial prostate needle biopsy. J Urol. 2001;166:866–870.

8. Network NCC. Practice Guidelines in Oncology--v.2.2005: Clinical Practice Guidelines in Oncology, 2005.

9. Allen EA, Kahane H, Epstein JI. Repeat biopsy strategies for men with atypical diagnoses on initial prostate needle biopsy. Urology. 1998;52:803–807.

10. Lefkowitz GK, Sidhu GS, Torre P, et al. Is repeat prostate biopsy for high-grade prostatic intraepithelial neoplasia necessary after routine 12-core sampling? Urology. 2001;58:999–1003.

11. O'Dowd G J, Miller MC, Orozco R, et al. Analysis of repeated biopsy results within 1 year after a noncancer diagnosis. Urology. 2000;55:553–539.

12. Gown AM and Vogel AM. Monoclonal antibodies to intermediate filament proteins of human cells: unique and cross-reacting antibodies. J Cell Biol. 1982;95:414–424.

13. Yang Y, Hao J, Liu X, et al. Differential expression of cytokeratin mRNA and protein in normal prostate, prostatic intraepithelial neoplasia, and invasive carcinoma. Am J Pathol. 1997;150:693–704.

14. Nagle RB, Ahmann FR, McDaniel KM, et al. Cytokeratin characterization of human prostatic carcinoma and its derived cell lines. Cancer Res. 1987;47:281–286.

15. Signoretti S, Waltregny D, Dilks J,et al. p63 is a prostate basal cell marker and is required for prostate development. Am J Pathol. 2000;157:1769–1775.

16. Parsons JK, Gage WR, Nelson WG, et al. p63 protein expression is rare in prostate adenocarcinoma: implications for cancer diagnosis and carcinogenesis. Urology. 2001;58:619–624.

17. Luo J, Zha S, Gage WR,et al. Alpha-methylacyl-CoA racemase: a new molecular marker for prostate cancer. Cancer Res. 2002;62:2220–2226.

18. Rubin MA, Zhou M, Dhanasekaran SM, et al. alpha-Methylacyl coenzyme A racemase as a tissue biomarker for prostate cancer. Jama. 2002;287:1662–1670.

19. Xu J, Stolk JA, Zhang X, et al. Identification of differentially expressed genes in human prostate cancer using subtraction and microarray. Cancer Res. 2000;60:1677–1682.

20. Jiang Z, Woda BA, Rock KL, et al. P504S: a new molecular marker for the detection of prostate carcinoma. Am J Surg Pathol. 2001;25:1397–1404.

21. Sanderson SO, Sebo TJ, Murphy LM, et al. An analysis of the p63/alpha-methylacyl coenzyme A racemase immunohistochemical cocktail stain in prostate needle biopsy specimens and tissue microarrays. Am J Clin Pathol. 2004;121:220–225.

22. Zhou M and Epstein JI. The reporting of prostate cancer on needle biopsy: prognostic and therapeutic implications and the utility of diagnostic markers. Pathology. 2003;35:472–479.

23. Epstein JI. Gleason score 2-4 adenocarcinoma of the prostate on needle biopsy: a diagnosis that should not be made. Am J Surg Pathol. 2000;24:477–478.

24. Carter HB, Walsh PC, Landis P, et al. Expectant management of nonpalpable prostate cancer with curative intent: preliminary results. J Urol. 2002;167:1231–1234.

25. Epstein JI, Walsh PC, Carmichael M, et al. Pathologic and clinical findings to predict tumor extent of nonpalpable (stage T1c) prostate cancer. Jama. 1994;271:368–374.

26. Albertsen PC, Hanley JA, Gleason DF, et al. Competing risk analysis of men aged 55 to 74 years at diagnosis managed conservatively for clinically localized prostate cancer. Jama. 1998;280:975–980.

27. Steinberg DM, Sauvageot J, Piantadosi S, et al. Correlation of prostate needle biopsy and radical prostatectomy Gleason grade in academic and community settings. Am J Surg Pathol. 1997;21:566–576.

28. Spires SE, Cibull ML, Wood DP, et al. Gleason histologic grading in prostatic carcinoma. Correlation of 18-gauge core biopsy with prostatectomy. Arch Pathol Lab Med. 1994;118:705–708.

29. Grossfeld GD, Chang JJ, Broering JM, et al. Under staging and under grading in a contemporary series of patients undergoing radical prostatectomy: results from the Cancer of the Prostate Strategic Urologic Research Endeavor database. J Urol. 2001;165:851–856.

30. Sved PD, Gomez P, Manoharan M, et al. Limitations of biopsy Gleason grade: implications for counseling patients with biopsy Gleason score 6 prostate cancer. J Urol. 2004;172:98–102.

31. D'Amico AV, Whittington R, Malkowicz SB, et al. Clinical utility of the percentage of positive prostate biopsies in defining biochemical outcome after radical prostatectomy for patients with clinically localized prostate cancer. J Clin Oncol. 2000 ;18:1164–1172.

32. Badalament RA, Miller MC, Peller PA,et al. An algorithm for predicting nonorgan confined prostate cancer using the results obtained from sextant core biopsies with prostate specific antigen level. J Urol. 1996 ;156:1375–1380.

33. Wills ML, Sauvageot J, Partin AW,et al. Ability of sextant biopsies to predict radical prostatectomy stage. Urology. 1998;51:759–764.

34. Bostwick DG, Qian J, Bergstralh E,et al. Prediction of capsular perforation and seminal vesicle invasion in prostate cancer. J Urol. 1996;155:1361–1367.

35. Ukimura O, Troncoso P, Ramirez EI, et al. Prostate cancer staging: correlation between ultrasound determined tumor contact length and pathologically confirmed extraprostatic extension. J Urol. 1998;159:1251–1259.

36. Ravery V, Schmid HP, Toublanc M, et al. Is the percentage of cancer in biopsy cores predictive of extracapsular disease in T1-T2 prostate carcinoma? Cancer. 1996;78:1079–1084.

37. Terris MK, Haney DJ, Johnstone IM, et al. Prediction of prostate cancer volume using prostate-specific antigen levels, transrectal ultrasound, and systematic sextant biopsies. Urology. 1995;45:75–80.

38. Freedland SJ, Aronson WJ, Csathy GS, et al. Comparison of percentage of total prostate needle biopsy tissue with cancer to percentage of cores with cancer for predicting PSA recurrence after radical prostatectomy: results from the SEARCH database. Urology. 2003;61:742–747.

39. Peller PA, Young DC, Marmaduke DP, et al. Sextant prostate biopsies. A histopathologic correlation with radical prostatectomy specimens. Cancer. 1995;75:530–538.

40. Bismar TA, Lewis JS, Jr., Vollmer RT, et al. Multiple measures of carcinoma extent versus perineural invasion in prostate needle biopsy tissue in prediction of pathologic stage in a screening population. Am J Surg Pathol. 2003;27:432–440.

41. Tigrani VS, Bhargava V, Shinohara K, et al. Number of positive systematic sextant biopsies predicts surgical margin status at radical prostatectomy. Urology. 1999;54:689–693.

42. Rogatsch H, Horninger W, Volgger H, et al. Radical prostatectomy: the value of preoperative, individually labeled apical biopsies. J Urol. 2000;164:754-7; discussion 757–758.

43. Taneja SS, Penson DF, Epelbaum A, et al. Does site specific labeling of sextant biopsy cores predict the site of extracapsular extension in radical prostatectomy surgical specimen. J Urol. 1999;162:1352-7; discussion 1357–1378.

44. Elliott SP, Shinohara K, Logan SL, et al. Sextant prostate biopsies predict side and sextant site of extracapsular extension of prostate cancer. J Urol. 2002;168:105–109.

45. Vargas SO, Jiroutek M, Welch WR, et al. Perineural invasion in prostate needle biopsy specimens. Correlation with extraprostatic extension at resection. Am J Clin Pathol. 1999;111:223–228.

46. Egan AJ and Bostwick DG. Prediction of extraprostatic extension of prostate cancer based on needle biopsy findings: perineural invasion lacks significance on multivariate analysis. Am J Surg Pathol. 1997;21:1496–1500.

47. de la Taille A, Katz A, Bagiella E, et al. Perineural invasion on prostate needle biopsy: an independent predictor of final pathologic stage. Urology. 1999;54:1039–1043.

48. de la Taille A, Rubin MA, Bagiella E, et al. Can perineural invasion on prostate needle biopsy predict prostate specific antigen recurrence after radical prostatectomy? J Urol. 1999;162:103–106.

49. Epstein JI. The role of perineural invasion and other biopsy characteristics as prognostic markers for localized prostate cancer. Sem Urol Oncol. 1998;16:124.

50. Holmes GF, Walsh PC, Pound CR, et al. Excision of the neurovascular bundle at radical prostatectomy in cases with perineural invasion on needle biopsy. Urology. 1999;53:752–756.

51. Rubin MA, Bismar TA, Curtis S, et al. Prostate needle biopsy reporting: how are the surgical members of the Society of Urologic Oncology using pathology reports to guide treatment of prostate cancer patients? Am J Surg Pathol. 2004;28:946–952.

52. Carter HB, Sauvageot J, Walsh PC, et al. Prospective evaluation of men with stage T1C adenocarcinoma of the prostate. J Urol. 1997;157:2206–2209.

53. Khan MA, Carter HB, Epstein JI, et al. Can prostate specific antigen derivatives and pathological parameters predict significant change in expectant management criteria for prostate cancer? J Urol. 2003;170:2274–2278.

Urine-based diagnostic tests for prostate cancer

58

Yves Fradet

INTRODUCTION

Serum prostate-specific antigen (PSA) testing and digital rectal examination (DRE) of the prostate have been accepted as effective methods for early detection of prostate cancer since the beginning of the 1990s. However, as late as 2002, the US Preventive Services Task Force did not recommend routine screening, in good part because of the potential harm resulting from the lack of specificity of PSA screening methods.[1] The true sensitivity of PSA testing has also been more recently challenged by studies showing a very high incidence of prostate cancer in men with PSA in the normal range.[2] Of even more concern are the findings that high-grade cancers are more prevalent in the latter group of patients, thus challenging the rationale of current detection strategies. Therefore, there is clearly an urgent need for new detection methods that would be both sensitive and specific for the biologically significant prostate cancer. The detection of prostate cancer cells or nucleic acid fragments using highly sensitive nucleic acid amplification techniques offers great promises for noninvasive detection of prostate cancer. We review herein the recently published results of tests based on the analysis of nucleic acid-based prostate cancer markers in the urine after DRE of the prostate showing significant improvement in accuracy over that of serum PSA levels and its various forms.

CURRENT CLINICAL DILEMMAS OF PROSTATE CANCER DETECTION

Screening for prostate cancer using serum total PSA level has evolved significantly over the last decade. One of the most important advances in increasing the specificity of this approach was the use of a more aggressive biopsy policy raising the number of biopsies from 6 to between 10 and 12 cores using transrectal ultrasound (TRUS) guided biopsies of the prostate. Even with this approach, two out of three men with a serum PSA level of 4 ng/mL or greater will have negative biopsies and as many as 15% to 20% of those men will have cancer detected on subsequent biopsies. These findings highlight one of the main limitations of serum PSA screening for prostate cancer: the lack of specificity and the high number of unnecessary biopsies required along with the anxiety generated by such practice. Nevertheless, the approach has been widely accepted in USA and, to a lesser extent, in Canada and Europe, leading to a marked increase in the incidence of prostate cancer diagnosis. As a consequence the proportion of men likely to die of the disease over those diagnosed has significantly been reduced. Identifying those cancers that are more likely to progress and kill the host has become a primary challenge for the oncology community. To date, in the absence of molecular fingerprints of such biologic behavior, the Gleason grade of the tumor is the most accurate predictor of the risk of death by cancer in patients undergoing a watchful waiting policy.[3]

In most recent years, studies performed in men with PSA level of 2.5 to 4 ng/mL and undergoing systematic prostate biopsies have shown a cancer incidence ranging from 20% to 23%.[4,5] Preliminary results of the European screening studies have estimated that approximately half of the tumors missed in men with PSA level from 0 to 4 ng/mL had aggressive characteristics (high Gleason grade) and were organ-confined.[6] By contrast, similar high-grade cancers found in men with PSA above 4 ng/mL were most frequently extracapsular and, therefore, had a lower chance of being cured by surgery or other modalities. While approximately 7% of men over the age of 50 years have a serum PSA level of 4 ng/mL and above, up to 16% of men in the same age group have a PSA level between 2.5 and 4 ng/mL. Lowering the threshold for biopsy to 2.5 ng/mL would almost triple the number of men at risk of biopsy and would significantly raise the number of negative or unnecessary biopsies.[7]

A devastating finding was recently published by Thompson et al resulting from their analysis of biopsy results from 2950 men in the placebo arm of the Prostate Cancer Prevention Trial (PCPT).[2] These men had an average of 7.9 serum PSA measurements over a 7-year period and remained within the normal range of PSA level (<4 ng/mL). All accepted to undergo sextant prostate biopsies and 15.2% of those men were found to have cancer. While high-grade cancer is found in approximately 19% of men with serum PSA of 4 ng/mL or above, up to 15% of men with PSA of less than 4 ng/mL had high-grade cancer. Based on these results and as shown in Table 58.1, screening 10,000 men for prostate cancer with a PSA cut-off of 4 ng/mL would detect 36 high-grade cancers, while up to 208 high-grade cancers are found in men with PSA of less than 4 ng/mL. If our goal is to detect high-grade cancers while they are highly curable, new strategies must be designed to detect more selectively these cancers without picking up lesions of lower malignant potential that may remain clinically insignificant for the life of the patients.

To date, only modest improvements in specificity have been observed using tests to measure the various forms of free and complexed PSA or proPSA.[8–10] A promising novel approach is the molecular detection of prostate cancer cells in urine obtained after prostatic massage: an equivalent to a molecular cytology sampling of the prostate. The concept is based on the detection of prostate cancer-specific nucleic acid markers using highly sensitive amplification technologies that are widely used for the detection of human immunodeficiency virus (HIV) and hepatitis B and C RNA viruses in the blood, or other infectious agents in the urine.

Table 58.1 Estimated proportion of cancer in a population of 10,000 men over 50 years old*

Serum PSA (ng/mL)	Total number (%)	Number with positive biopsy (%)	Number with high-grade cancer (%)
≥4	760 (7.6)	190 (25)	**36** (19)
<4	9241 (92.4)	1386 (25)	**208** (15)

*Adapted from Thompson IM, Pauler DK, Goodman PJ, Tangen CM, Lucia MS, Parnes HL, et al. Prevalence of prostate cancer among men with a prostate-specific antigen level ≤4.0 ng per milliliter. N Engl J Med 2004;350:2239–2246.

DETECTION OF TELOMERASE ACTIVITY OR TELOMERASE RNA IN URINE

The cytologic examination of ejaculates and voided urine after prostatic massage had shown that cancer cells could be present, although in low concentration, thus yielding a low sensitivity for cancer detection.[11] The ability to detect these cells with highly sensitive methods using rare event detection of targets overexpressed in prostate cancer cells appears to be a logical concept. Several specific alterations have been identified in prostate cancer cells that could be used as targets for the detection of neoplastic cells in clinical samples.

Telomerase is a ribonucleoprotein that sensitizes and repairs telomeres, which protect the ends of chromosomes from degradation and fusion with other chromosomes. Telomerase activity is required to prevent cells from senescence and has been found to be repressed in normal human somatic tissues but reactivated in the majority of cancers. A sensitive polymerase chain reaction (PCR) based method was developed to detect telomerase activity by the amplification of telomeric repeats. Studies have shown that at least 90% of prostate cancers express telomerase activity. Meid et al reported on experiments measuring telomerase activity by PCR in voided urine obtained after prostatic massage from patients undergoing prostate biopsies for suspicion of cancer. Their assay used gel-based detection of PCR products according to the TRAP (telomerase repeat amplification protocol) method assessed visually.[12] They showed that telomerase activity was detected in 14/24 patients with known prostate cancer (sensitivity 58%) and was not found in 12 cases without histologic evidence of carcinoma (specificity 100%). Telomerase activity uses an internal RNA to template the synthesis of telomeric DNA by reverse transcription. This human telomerase RNA (hTERT) is an essential requirement for telomerase activity and several studies have shown that hTERT mRNA expression levels correlate well with the incidence of invasive tumors in multiple cancers including prostate cancer. Crocitto et al recently published results of a study of hTERT expression by reverse transcriptase PCR performed on 49 samples of expressed prostatic secretions from men being evaluated for prostate cancer.[13] Expressed prostatic secretions could be obtained from 86% of subjects tested and, of those, 90% of the samples yielded sufficient RNA for measurements. In 49 samples, hTERT expression provided a 36% sensitivity and 66% specificity for the presence of prostate cancer on the subsequent biopsy. Table 58.2 summarizes the clinical performances of molecular prostate cancer urine tests based on different targets.

Table 58.2 Summary of clinical performances of molecular prostate cancer urine tests based on different targets

Molecular target	Study	Patient number	Adequacy (%)	Sensitivity (%)	Specificity (%)
Telomerase	Meid et al[12]	36	—	58	100
	Crocitto et al[13]	49	80	36	66
Hypermethylation of GSTP1	Goessl et al[15]	11	—	40	—
	Cairns et al[16]	22	—	27	—
	Gonzalgo et al[17]	45	80	58	67
	Crocitto et al[13]	58	—	46	56
	Goessl et al[18]	45	100	75	98
PCA3[DD3]/uPM3 test	Hessels et al[27]	108	—	67	83
	Fradet et al[28]	517	86	66	89
	Tinzl et al[29]	201	79	82	76

GSTP1, glutathione S-transferase P1; PCA3[DD3]/uPM3, prostate cancer-specific gene of unknown function.

DETECTION OF HYPERMETHYLATION OF GLUTATHIONE S-TRANSFERASE P1 GENE PROMOTER IN URINE

Hypermethylation of the normally unmethylated CpG highlands in the promoter regions of tumor suppressor genes correlates with loss of gene expression in human tumors. Glutathione S-transferase P1 (GSTP1) is part of the GST superfamily of enzymes responsible for detoxification of a wide range of xenobiotics. Hypermethylation of the promoter of the GSTP1 gene locus is found in over 90% of primary prostate carcinoma but not in normal prostatic tissues or other normal tissues.[14] Initial studies of *GSTP1* methylation status in prostate cancer were performed using the standard Southern blot analysis that requires significant amount of nucleic acid. This epigenetic DNA alteration can be reliably detected by methylation-specific PCR, a method capable of identifying hypermethylated alleles from tumor DNA within 10^4 to 10^5-fold excess amounts of unmethylated alleles from normal DNA. This new method uses a DNA modification step before PCR amplification to determine the presence or absence of methylation of a gene locus, it is more sensitive and requires less DNA and, thus, could be applied to voided urine collected from patients with prostate cancer.

Goessl et al were first to report results using fluorescent methylation-specific PCR reaction for DNA-based detection of prostate cancer in bodily fluids.[15] While their test was negative in tissues and bodily fluid from patients with benign prostate hypertrophy, they found 16/17 (94%) tumor tissues positive and 4/8 (50%) ejaculate and 4/11 (36%) urine samples from patients with prostate cancer positive with their assay. Cairns et al reported the detection of *GSTP1* methylation in urine-sediment DNA in 6/22 (26%) prostate cancer cases where *GSTP1* methylation was

found on the biopsy.[16] Gonzalgo et al used a similar assay in urine obtained after prostate biopsy from 45 patients and the test was informative in 36 (80%).[17] *GSTP1* methylation was detected in 7/18 (39%) patients with adenocarcinoma of the prostate but 58% of those informative cases. The test was also positive in 7/21 (33%) patients without cancer on biopsy and 4/6 (67%) with atypia or high-grade prostatic intraepithelial neoplasia (HGPIN). Crocitto et al analyzed *GSTP1* methylation in 58 samples of expressed prostate secretions and showed a 46% sensitivity and 56% specificity for the detection of prostate cancer.[13] These studies on a limited number of cases using nonquantitative research laboratory methods have showed the feasibility of detecting prostate cancer cells using nucleic amplification methodologies.

More recently, Goessl et al reported results of another study in 45 patients using an improved method for RNA and DNA isolation from urine samples.[18] The sensitivity of their assay was improved to 73% compared with 36% in their first study. Moreover, they showed a detection rate of 68% for early-stage prostate cancer using a method similar to that of Cairns et al,[16] who reported only 27% detection in urine obtained without prior prostate massage. These results highlight the potential of technical improvements in the design of a more sensitive assays while retaining the specificity provided by the cancer-specific target gene. They also emphasize the potential benefit provided by prostate massage that increases the shedding of cells and the sampling of the gland for the presence of prostate cancer cells. Although the quality of the prostate massage could influence the accuracy of the test, most of our diagnostic methods, including prostate TRUS-guided biopsy, are to a certain extent operator dependent.

A better understanding of the molecular mechanisms of prostate cancer oncogenesis combined with improved analytic techniques have identified a number of other genes specifically expressed in prostate cancer. Elevated expression of the prostate-specific membrane antigen (PSMA) has long been correlated with poor prognosis particularly in metastatic disease.[19] Other overexpressed targets include NKX3.1,[20] an androgen-regulated homeobox gene, prostate stem cell antigen (PSCA),[21] prostate tumor inducing gene 1 (PTI),[22] α-methylacyl coenzyme A racemase (AMACR)[23] and prostate cancer gene 1 (PCGEM1).[24] So far, no diagnosis based on the expression of these prostate-specific genes has been described but they represent so many more potential targets for the future.

PCA3[DD3] RNA DETECTION IN URINE

PCA3[DD3] is the most prostate cancer specific gene described so far. This gene was initially identified by differential display hence its first name *DD3*, which was changed to *PCA3* in the official database.[25] This gene located on chromosome 9q21-22 was found to be 10- to 100-fold overexpressed in 53 of 56 human prostate cancer tissues using Northern blot analysis, whereas it was not expressed by the same technique in adjacent nonmalignant prostate tissues. Using the more sensitive reverse transcription polymerase chain reaction (RT-PCR), no PCA3 transcript was demonstrated in a wide range of normal tissues and other human malignant tumors but the gene was detectable in normal prostate at low level. The current understanding is that the PCA3 gene expresses a noncoding RNA that may have functions other than synthesizing a protein.

de Kok et al analyzed the expression of PCA3 and hTERT gene (telomerase) expression in prostate cancers and nonmalignant adjacent tissues using RT-PCR.[26] While the median hTERT expression level was 1.7 in normal tissues and 10.1 in tumor tissues, PCA3 median normalized expression was 174 in nonmalignant tissues and 5849 in malignant prostate tissues. Thus the median upregulation of PCA3 from normal to tumor tissues was 34-fold compared with 6-fold for hTERT. These results suggested that diagnostic tests based on the detection of PCA3 molecular target may be more sensitive than other gene-based assays.

Using the same quantitative time-resolved fluorescence-based RT-PCR assay, Hessels et al tested tissues from prostatectomy specimen to determine relative levels of PCA3 expression.[27] As shown in Figure 58.1, the median upregulation of PCA3 was 11-fold in 13 prostate tissue samples containing less than 10% tumor cells compared with normal prostate tissue, while it was 66-fold in 26 tumor samples containing more than 10% prostate cancer tissue. They also tested for PCA3 level in urinary sediments obtained after prostate massage in patients undergoing biopsy. Quantitative RT-PCR testing for PSA transcripts was used as a reflection of the number of prostate cells (benign or malignant) present in the urinary sediment. The PCA3:PSA ratio was then used as the diagnostic tool in a cohort of 108 consecutive patients undergoing prostate biopsies based on serum-PSA levels of more than 3 ng/mL. The receiver operating characteristic (ROC) curve developed had an area under the curve of 0.72. Based on the ROC curve, the cut-off for positivity gave a sensitivity for the assay of 67% and a specificity was 83%. The negative predictive value (NPV) based on their cohort of patients was 90%.

The uPM3 assay was developed to detect PCA3 and PSA RNA simultaneously with a real-time resolved fluorescence detection. In this assay, PCA3 and PSA RNA are amplified in the same tube using the nucleic acid sequence-based amplification (NASBA) technology. This technique is designed to amplify directly RNA using a set of three enzymes and is performed at a constant temperature of 41°C instead of the cycling reaction required for PCR. Several studies have shown this technique to be equivalent in sensitivity to the RT-PCR methodology for the detection of RNA viruses in the blood. The amplification of the target is detected by specific Beacon probes to PSA and PCA3 products. The

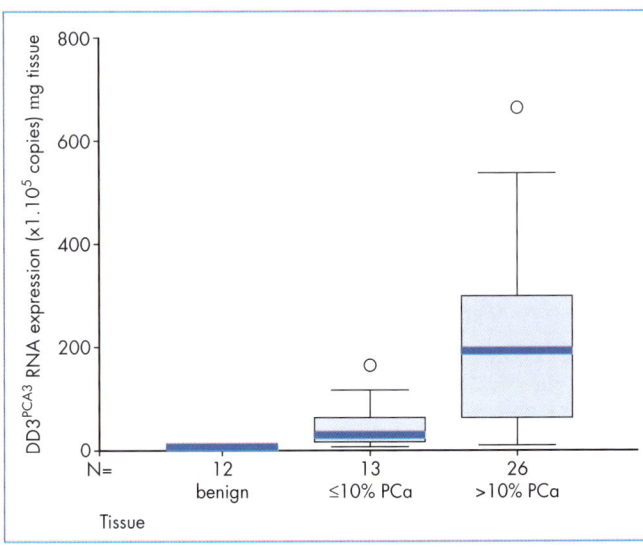

Fig. 58.1

Expression (in copies/μg of tissue) of PCA3[DD3] RNA in benign prostate tissue, prostate tissue containing 10% or less cancer and prostate tissue containing more than 10% cancer. The median expression is shown by the thick black horizontal line.
Reprinted from Eur Urol, 44, Hessels D, Klein Gunnewick JM, van Oort I, Karthaus HFM, van Leenders GJL, van Balken B, et al. DD2(PCA3)–based molecular urine auaylsis for the diagnoses of prostate cancer, 8–16, 2003, with permission from the European Association of Urology.

reaction is read kinetically during a 2 hour period in a thermostated spectrofluorometer detecting green fluorescence for PCA3 marker and red fluorescence for PSA. The curves were analyzed using logistic curve fitting. ROC curves of sensitivity and specificity were determined and provided an area under the curve of 0.86 (Figure 58.2). Depending on the cut-off used for positivity, sensitivity could go up from 43% to 94% and specificity go down from 95% to 43%.

This assay was then tested in a multicenter study to evaluate the clinical performance of the uPM3 test in 517 men undergoing TRUS-guided prostate biopsies at five medical centers of the Province of Quebec.[28] The first voided urine sample was obtained after an attentive DRE performed by one of nine different physicians with instruction of doing a thorough prostate palpation for 15 to 30 seconds. Urines were collected and mixed with an equal volume of phosphate buffer (pH 7) and stored and shipped at 2° to 8°C. The assay was performed within 3 days of collection.

Of the 517 subjects recruited, 443 (86%) provided samples with sufficient PSA RNA signal for analysis of PCA3 RNA. Table 58.3 summarizes the results obtained according to the different groups of patients based on total serum PSA value. The overall sensitivity was 66% with a specificity of 89% in the 443 patients. Interestingly, in the 94 patients with PSA less than 4 ng/mL, sensitivity was 74% and specificity was 91%. This resulted in an overall NPV of 84% and a positive predictive value (PPV) of 75%.[67–82] The overall accuracy of the assay was 81%[77–84] compared with 43%[39–48] for serum PSA greater than 2.5 ng/mL and 47%[42–52] for PSA greater than or equal to 4 ng/mL. Within this group of 443 patients with evaluable clinical samples, 91 were undergoing a subsequent biopsy after one or more previous negative biopsies. In these patients, the uPM3 test had 74% sensitivity and 87% specificity corresponding to a NPV of 87% and PPV of 74%. These results suggest that such an assay could be of particular benefit in helping patients and physicians to decide on the need for subsequent biopsies. This multicenter study provided the first evidence of the feasibility of such type of nucleic-acid based test in routine clinical practice.

Using the same UPM3 assay to detect PCA3 RNA in urine, Tinzl et al reported similar results on a study performed in 201 patients undergoing TRUS-guided biopsies[29] (see Tables 58.2 and 58.3). In this study, samples were collected in Vienna, snap-frozen, stored and shipped on ice to Canada for performing the testing. Despite these difficult conditions, 79% of the samples were adequate for analysis. Cancer was found in 62 (39%) of the evaluable patients. The overall sensitivity of the assay in their cohort of patients using a similar cut-off point was 82% with a specificity of 76% while the specificity of total serum PSA at a cut-off of 2.5 ng/mL was 5% only and 16% for PSA at cut-off of 4 ng/mL. Of their 158 evaluable patients, 24 had a PSA of less than 4 ng/mL of which 11/24 had a positive biopsy. The uPM3 assay showed a sensitivity of 73% and a specificity of 61% in this subgroup of patients.

Results of these two studies suggest that assays can be developed for routine clinical testing based on nucleic acid amplification of molecular targets highly overex-

Table 58.3 Sensitivity and specificity of the uPM3 test by serum total prostate-specific antigen (tPSA) range

tPSA range (ng/mL)	Number	Sensitivity (%)	Specificity (%)
Fradet et al[28]			
<4	94	74	91
4–10	243	58	91
>10	106	79	80
Tinzl et al[29]			
<4	24	73	61
4–10	98	84	80
>10	36	84	70

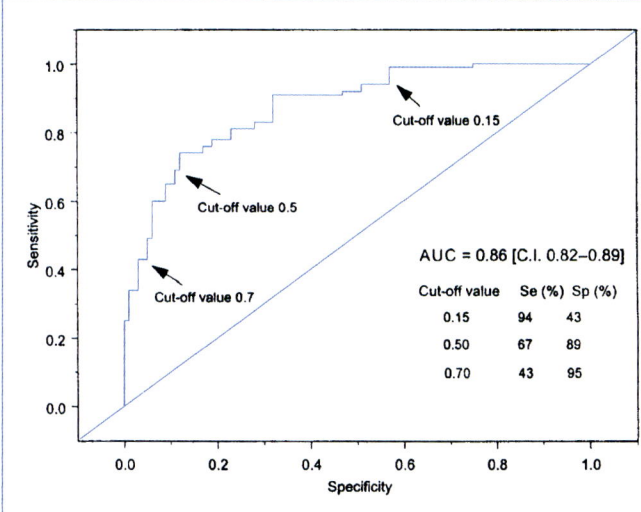

AUC = 0.86 [C.I. 0.82–0.89]

Cut-off value	Se (%)	Sp (%)
0.15	94	43
0.50	67	89
0.70	43	95

Fig. 58.2
Receiver operator characteristic (ROC) curve of sensitivity and specificity of prediction probability of cancer obtained by the analysis of amplification curves compared with biopsy results.
Reprinted from Urology, 64, Fradet Y, Saad F, Aprikian A, Dessureault J, Elhilali M, Trudel C, et al. uPM3, a new molecular urine test for the detection of prostate cancer, 64, 2004, with permission from Elsevier.

pressed in prostate cancer cells compared to normal prostate cells. One limitation of all the studies described using this approach is the proportion of samples where the test cannot be evaluable due to insufficient material. With the uPM3 assay, this was approximately 86% adequacy. The adequacy problem can be related to the quality of the DRE. However, although the extent of the prostate massage varied among investigators of the three PCA3 studies, the adequacy was relatively constant between all three studies. It is also possible that the technical improvement in the assay may increase its sensitivity in the future. A urine test based on the PCA3:PSA RNA ratio is currently being developed by Gen Probe of San Diego. In their assay, the RNA is extracted and stabilized within the collecting tubes. Moreover, although their TMA nucleic acid amplification technique used in their product is similar to the NASBA concept, they also use a specific capture probe to enrich the target to be amplified as well as chemoluminescence detection of the amplification product. These technologic improvements have shown a 100% adequacy of all samples tested in a development phase and are, therefore, very promising for the future use of this test. An important and unresolved issue is whether such tests would be able to detect more selectively the higher grade cancers. Preliminary information from the group of Nijmegen University suggest that most of the cancers missed by a PCA3 urine test are Gleason 6 and lower, while all higher grade cancers seem to be detected (J Schalken, personal communication).

FUTURE PERSPECTIVES

A salient feature of post-DRE urine tests based on the molecular detection of rare cancer cells is their higher specificity as demonstrated in most studies performed to date. Given the high proportion of negative biopsies required to detect cancers in men with PSA in the normal range, a urine test with performances comparable to those observed in the two uPM3 studies in a limited number of these men would be a most logical first step in this population. Moreover, it is tempting to speculate that the average smaller prostate found in men with normal PSA would potentially yield cancer cells more easily than larger prostate with a benign prostatic hyperplasia (BPH) component that might compress the ducts and thus decrease prostate cancer yield in the urine. These hypotheses will obviously need to be tested in a large-scale study once fully developed assays become commercially available. Similarly it is likely that, with the number of genes selectively overexpressed in prostate cancer, a phenotype more specific to the high-risk cancers will be identified in the future.

The progress made in the management of prostate cancer patients during the last 20 years was mostly due to the introduction of a simple blood test (PSA), which in the end appears to be more related to the size of the prostate gland than to the presence of cancer for diagnostic purposes. The concurrent availability of TRUS and of the biopsy gun allowing for easy multiple samplings of the prostate gland in a tolerable way has been a major advance in our understanding of the true incidence of prostate cancer. The initial fears that prostate cancer screening would detect small tumors found at autopsy in men dying of other causes seems to become a reality as prostate biopsies are performed more aggressively in men with lower PSA. The biggest challenge ahead is now to develop screening assays that would selectively detect high-risk cancers at a time where they are highly curable, that is in men with serum PSA in the normal range. Based on the results obtained to date with post-DRE urine nucleic acid tests, this approach likely represents one of the main hopes for the near future.

REFERENCES

1. Harris R, Lohr KN. Screening for prostate cancer: an update of the evidence for the U.S. Preventive Services Task Force. Ann Intern Med 2002;137:917–929.
2. Thompson IM, Pauler DK, Goodman PJ, et al. Prevalence of prostate cancer among men with a prostate-specific antigen level < or = 4.0 ng per milliliter. N Engl J Med 2004;350:2239–2246.
3. Albertsen PC, Hanley JA, Gleason DF, et al. Competing risk analysis of men aged 55 to 74 years at diagnosis managed conservatively for clinically localized prostate cancer. JAMA 1998;280:975–980.
4. Babaian RJ, Johnston DA, Naccarato W, et al. The incidence of prostate cancer in a screening population with a serum prostate specific antigen between 2.5 and 4.0 ng/ml: relation to biopsy strategy. J Urol 2001;165:757–760.
5. Catalona WJ, Smith DS, Ornstein DK. Prostate cancer detection in men with serum PSA concentrations of 2.6 to 4.0 ng/mL and benign prostate examination: enhancement of specificity with free PSA measurements. JAMA 1997;277:1452–1455.
6. Schroder FH, van der Cruijsen-Koeter I, de Koning HJ, et al. Prostate cancer detection at low prostate specific antigen. J Urol 2000;63:806–812.
7. De Koning HJ, Auvinen A, Berenguer Sanchez A, et al. Large-scale randomized prostate cancer screening trials: program performances in the European Randomized Screening for Prostate Cancer Trial and the prostate, lung, colorectal and ovary cancer trial. Int J Cancer 2002;97:237–244.
8. Mikolajczyk SD, Marks LS, Partin AW, et al. Free prostate-specific antigen in serum is becoming more complex. Urology 2002;59:797–802.
9. Sokoll LJ, Chan DW, Mikolajczyk SD, et al. Proenzyme PSA for the early detection of prostate cancer in the 2.5-4.0 ng/ml total PSA range: preliminary analysis. Urology 2003;61:274–276.
10. Roehl KA, Antenor JAV, Catalona WJ. Robustness of free prostate specific antigen measurements to reduce unnecessary biopsies in the 2.6 to 4.0 ng/ml range. J Urol 2002;168:922–925.
11. Garrett M, Jassie M. Cytologic examination of post prostatic massage specimens as an aid in diagnosis of carcinoma of the prostate. Acta Cytol 1976;20:126.
12. Meid FH, Gygi CM, Leisinger HJ, et al. The use of telomerase activity for the detection of prostatic cancer cells after prostatic massage. J Urol 2001;165:1802–1805.
13. Crocitto LE, Korns D, Kretzner L, et al. Prostate cancer molecular markers GSTP1 and hTERT in expressed prostatic secretions as predictors of biopsy results. Urology 2004;64:821–825.
14. Brooks JD, Weinstein M, Lin X, et al. CG island methylation changes near the GSTP1 gene in prostatic intraepithelial neoplasia. Cancer Epidemiol Biomark Prev 1998;7:531–536.

15. Goessl C, Krause H, Müller M, et al. Fluorescent methylation-specific polymerase chain reaction for DNA-based detection of prostate cancer in bodily fluids. Cancer Res. 2000;60:5941–5945.

16. Cairns P, Esteller M, Herman JG, et al. Molecular detection of prostate cancer in urine by GSTP1 hypermethylation. Clin Cancer Res 2001;7:2727–2730.

17. Gonzalgo ML, Pavlovich CP, Lee SM, et al. Prostate cancer detection by GSTP1 methylation analysis of postbiopsy urine specimens. Clin Cancer Res 2003;9:2673–2677.

18. Goessl C, Müller M, Heicappell R, et al. DANN-based detection of prostate cancer in urine after prostatic massage. Urology 2001;58:335–338.

19. Murphy GP, Barren RJ, Erickson SJ, et al. Evaluation and comparison of two new prostate carcinoma markers. Free-prostate specific antigen and prostate specific membrane antigen. Cancer 1996;78:809–818.

20. Xu LL, Srikantan V, Sesterhenn IA, et al. Expression profile of an androgen regulated prostate specific homeobox gene NKX3.1 in primary prostate cancer. J Urol 2000;163:972–979.

21. Gu Z, Thomas G, Yamashiro J, et al. Prostate stem cell antigen (PSCA) expression increases with high Gleason score, advanced stage and bone metastasis in prostate cancer. Oncogene 2000;19:1288–1296.

22. Sun Y, Lin J, Katz AE, et al. Human prostatic carcinoma oncogene PTI-1 is expressed in human tumor cell lines and prostate carcinoma patient blood samples. Cancer Res 1997;57:18–23.

23. Luo J, Zha S, Gage WR, et al. Alpha-methylacyl-CoA racemase:a new molecular marker for prostate cancer. Cancer Res 2002;62:2220–2226.

24. Srikantan V, Zou Z, Petrovics G, et al. PCGEM1, a prostate-specific gene, is overexpressed in prostate cancer. Proc Natl Acad Sci USA 2000;97:12216–12221.

25. Bussemakers MJG, van Bokhoven A, Verhaegh GW, et al. DD3: a new prostate-specific gene highly overexpressed in prostate cancer. Cancer Res 1999;59:5975–5979.

26. de Kok JB, Verhaegh GW, Roelofs RW, et al. DD3(PCA3), a very sensitive and specific marker to detect prostate tumors. Cancer Res 2002;62:2695–2698.

27. Hessels D, Klein Gunnewiek JMT, van Oort I, et al. DD2(PCA3)-based molecular urine analysis for the diagnosis of prostate cancer. Eur Urol 2003;44:8–16.

28. Fradet Y, Saad F, Aprikian A, et al. uPM3, a new molecular urine test for the detection of prostate cancer. Urology 2004;64:311–314.

29. Tinzl M, Marberger M, Horvath S, et al. DDA(PCA3) RNA analysis in urine—a new perspective for detecting prostate cancer. Eur Urol 2004;46:182–187.

Diagnostic tests for prostate cancer: future directions

59

Alexandre R Zlotta, Brian J Duggan

INTRODUCTION

Since the mid-1980's, urologists have been very lucky to rely on one of the best serum markers available in medicine, prostate-specific antigen (PSA), for the diagnosis of the most common solid cancer in men, prostate cancer. There is, however, a critical need to improve the specificity of serum PSA in order to decrease the number of unnecessary prostate biopsies. Indeed, currently most men with serum PSA levels between 2.5 and 10 ng/mL, depending on their age and percent free PSA are recommended for a biopsy, even though 65% to 75% of them do not have prostate cancer.[1]

The unparalleled success of the human genome project has resulted in an array of new approaches to the diagnosis and treatment of human disease. These approaches can be roughly divided into two categories: those that are *DNA-based (functional genomics)* and those that are *protein-based (proteomics)*.[2] The most well-known example of functional genomics is the use of microarrays or DNA chips that simultaneously monitor the expression levels of thousands of genes in cells or tissues. This technology has been successfully employed to obtain genetic expression profiles, or signatures, that are useful in distinguishing normal from diseased samples, and to characterize diseases in terms of clinical classification, prognosis, or response to therapy. Additionally, gene profiling can be used to identify specific genes or sets of genes that may serve as useful diagnostic markers or potential therapeutic targets.

Although gene profiling represents a major benefit of the human genome project, it is becoming increasingly clear that such information, in spite of its complexity, does not adequately reflect human physiology or pathology. This is due to three major factors:

1. Relatively small changes in gene expression that are not defined as significant in gene profiling experiments may have important physiological consequences.[2]
2. Concordance between changes in gene expression (i.e., mRNA levels assessed by arrays, chips, or more standard techniques) and changes in the levels of the gene product is, in fact, rather poor.
3. The capacity of many genes to encode a range of gene products via alternative splicing and post-translational modifications such as phosphorylation, acetylation, proteolysis, etc. Thus, the human genome that comprises approximately *50,000 genes* may have the capacity to generate *more than 1,000,000 distinct gene products*. These 50,000 genes are far fewer than had been predicted. Cancer largely involves protein abnormalities, including abnormal structure, location in the cell, synthesis, turnover, interactions with other proteins and molecules, and modifications such as the addition of phosphate groups (phosphorylation) or sugar residues (glycosylation).

Having successfully deciphered the human genome, researchers are now shifting focus to solve the riddle of human proteome—that is proteins—the ultimate product of gene expression.

We have, therefore, witnessed a transition from genome-based to proteome-based discovery research. The proteome is the complete set of proteins encoded by the genome, and proteomics aims to identify, characterize, and quantify protein dynamics in healthy tissues and pathologic conditions such as cancer. The profiling of differentially expressed proteins in healthy and diseased conditions thus represents proteomics.

Proteomics identifies small amounts of proteins, peptides, and other small molecules in a patient's blood serum using mass spectrometry. Recent evidence indicates that patterns of these molecules are specific and sensitive for a variety of cancers, including prostate, ovarian, and many others. The idea is to detect patterns of proteins rather than individual biomarkers for cancer.

The particular techniques used range from profiling approaches such as two-dimensional gel electrophoresis and surface-enhanced laser desorption-ionization time-of-flight analysis (SELDI-TOF) to identification and microsequencing on matrix-assisted laser desorption-ionization (MALDI)-TOF and tandem mass spectrometric platforms. As with functional genomics, the goal of proteomics is the definition of disease-specific protein profiles and the identification of specific proteins as diagnostic markers and/or therapeutic targets. This, in turn, is aiding the discovery of protein-based biomarkers that are expected to play a major role in drug discovery, molecular diagnostics, and personalized medicine.

The investigation of single molecular targets has yielded important information, but this remains limited in its extension to clinical practice.[3,4] Single gene analysis has usually not given clinicians conclusive data regarding diagnosis or prognosis. The relationship between a gene mutation and the expression level of that gene or its protein and disease etiology or extent of disease is often complex. This is not surprising considering that a single gene can encode many proteins through differential splicing. Furthermore, the functionality of the protein will depend on post-translational modifications. It is, therefore, not that surprising that a laborious, single gene-by-gene analysis or single protein-by-protein analysis yields limited information. This problem is now being addressed by using novel molecular and biochemical techniques together with bioinformatics and data analysis systems that facilitate multiparameter analysis.

Comprehensive global analysis of both mRNA and proteins can be achieved using microarrays and proteomics.[5–7] It might be possible to identify genes and biochemical pathways that are deregulated in tumors, and prostate cancer is a good example of how this process may be used for diagnostic purposes as well.[8] Using molecular profiling (MP) and proteomics, it will be possible to generate a global view of DNA alterations, mRNA and proteins in single small samples of tissue.[8]

MOLECULAR PROFILING TECHNOLOGIES: MRNA ANALYSIS, AND MICROARRAYS

The aim of microarrays is to highlight biologically relevant and differentially expressed markers not only for

diagnosis but also for predicting recurrence, progression, and drug resistance by assessing tumor cell mRNA.[2,8] The sequence complementarity of the DNA duplex has been used in successive ways since Ed Southern used labeled nucleic acids to interrogate nucleic acids on a solid support. Southern and Northern blots that examine DNA and RNA fragments, respectively, and other methods, including in-situ hybridization, have allowed one gene sequence at a time to be examined. Although since the mid-1980s vast amounts of data in terms of sequencing, which has increased understanding of biologic function of many genes, their use was limited for the clinician. Since the mid-1990s the latest extension of exploitation of the chemical complementarity of bases to look at the expression of multiple genes at once has been developed via arrays of immobilized nucleic acids.

A microarray is the reverse of the Southern blot. Known nucleic acid sequences are fixed to a support at defined positions. These are interrogated with cDNA probes synthesized from the mRNA extracted from the sample population of interest.[8] Extraction of a sufficient quantity of good quality RNA is imperative to the rest of the procedure. A variety of standard methods are currently used in laboratories, and there are also many kits available commercially, with Affimatrix being one of the first. The RNA is treated with an enzyme DNase to remove contaminating DNA. Purity of RNA can be verified most simply on an agarose gel. A reaction facilitated by reverse transcriptase is carried out, during which a marker (either radioactive or fluorescent) is incorporated to form a cDNA probe. In a hybridization chamber, the probe, which has been synthesized from the RNA of interest, is mixed with the target nucleic acids, which are present on the array. Hybridization will occur if there is a complementary sequence between the analyzed labeled sample and the target nucleic acid, which in turn, allows generation of a detectable signal. The differential expression can then be analyzed in paired samples—for example, normal and tumor; treated and untreated; and responsive and nonresponsive. Microarrays are broadly either cDNA microchips or oligonucleotide chips. The latter include short (<25 bases) oligonucleotides that can be used for both RNA expression studies and sequence analysis. Using light directed chemistry methods, synthesis of these is fabricated in situ to produce high-density arrays (Figure 59.1). In-situ synthesis allows consistent high yields over the surface. Thousands of nucleic acid sequences may be immobilized for analysis. These require high-resolution detection, and so fluorochromes are the preferred detection system (see Figure 59.1). A major development is the use of a nonporous support glass, which allows use of fluorescent markers. This minimizes background and gives a high resolution facilitating miniaturization.

Complementary DNA (cDNA) arrays use a larger size of nucleic acids (>100) and are used in RNA expression

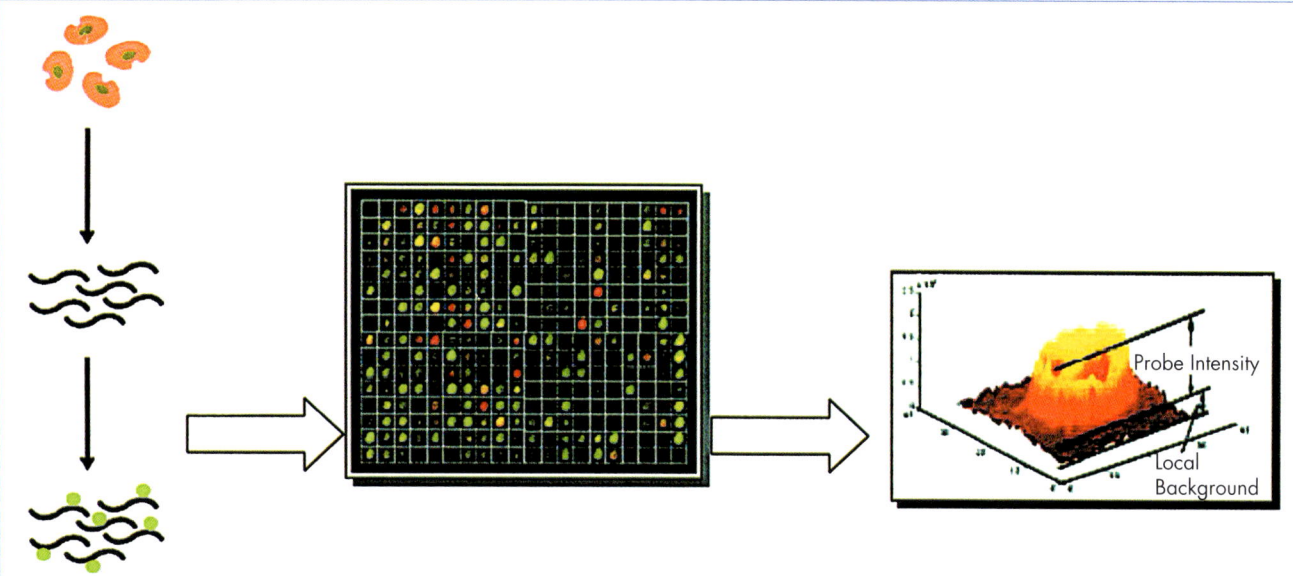

Fig. 59.1

Microarray chips have a range of cDNA sequences arranged so that complementary binding to the specific target site takes place if the gene is present in the test sample. The level of hybridization is then assayed on the microarray plate by assessing the intensity of fluorescence. Higher fluorescence detected for a well of the plate reflects increased mRNA expression for that specific gene in the tumor sample. Reprinted from Clin Cancer Res, 9, Duggan et al, The need to embrace molecular profiling of tumor cells in prostate and bladder cancer, 1240–1247, 2003, with permission.

studies. In this instance, the targets are labeled radioactively with ^{32}P or ^{33}P that is incorporated during first strand synthesis of the reverse transcriptase reaction. The microarrays are usually nylon membranes containing robotically spotted cDNAs or polymerase chain reaction (PCR) products.

Single nucleotide polymorphisms are variations that occur when a single nucleotide is altered in the genome sequence. Tumor DNA can be derived from urine, serum, or plasma in patients with urologic malignancies and this affords minimally invasive access to material for microarrays.[9] In urologic malignancies, different polymorphisms have been investigated, for example, the polymorphisms at the androgen receptor and PSA genes have been examined to assess their association with PSA levels.[10] Investigation by array methods are gradually replacing current laborious methods to detect allelic imbalances in individual diseases.[10]

However, genes are large, and mutations may be small and scattered, and are thus difficult to find and characterize even with microarrays, the principle of which relies on gain or loss of hybridization signals.

Differential gene expression in disease compared with normal states, tumor versus histologically normal tissue, and early versus late carcinogenesis can be determined. In cancers, this data may generate signatures for diagnostic purposes and is likely to reveal new insights into tumorigenesis. Most array methods have been validated by Northern blots of the sample. As an internal control, arrays incorporate housekeeping genes and mismatch control probes that are often a perfect match minus 1 base.

LASER CAPTURE MICROSCOPY

Laser capture microscopy isolates histologically defined cells of interest from stained clinical tissue samples using an infrared laser.[12] Laser capture microdissection has helped in sampling specific cell populations directly from tissue sections without causing any mechanical disruption while maintaining cell viability. The procedure involves the use of a thermosensitive polymer film layered over the targeted cells. The film is then melted by an infrared laser, forming a solid composite with the target, and lifted from the rest of the tissue without disruption to the cellular dynamics or tissue morphology. Laser capture microdissection enriches cell populations at speed, and this is beneficial because RNA degrades rapidly and also some proteins are labile. Microdissected cells from a tissue section are captured on membranes and analyzed. If at least 50,000 cells are microdissected, direct cDNA probe synthesis may be carried out. Unfortunately, often only a small number of cells are available.

PROTEIN ANALYSIS: PROTEOMICS

Proteomics complements genomic-based approaches in the study of cancer. Proteins are the functional output of a cell and form an intrinsic part of its dynamic network. Their expression, activities, and location can be changed any time through post-translation modifications.

The proteome is the complete set of proteins encoded by the genome, and proteomics aims to identify, characterize, and quantify protein dynamics in healthy tissues and during their response to stress and pathologic conditions. Since 1975, two-dimensional gel electrophoresis (2DE) has been the workhorse in quantitative proteomics.[13] Typically, protein samples are denatured and separated on the basis of their charge through isoelectric focusing. Immobilized pH gradients have greatly enhanced reproducibility in resolving almost the complete spectrum of basic to acidic proteins and have allowed both analytical and preparative amounts of proteins to be resolved. Narrow-range pH gradients are helping increase protein detection.[14] A range of 1 pH unit was demonstrated to resolve 1000 protein spots. The proteins are further separated by migration in a polyacrylamide gel on the basis of their molecular weights. By use of silver staining techniques, 3000 proteins can be visualized on a single gel. Fluorescent dyes are being developed to overcome some of the drawbacks of silver staining in making the protein samples more amenable to mass spectrometry. Stained gels can then be scanned at different resolutions with laser densitometers, and data can be analyzed with software systems for spot detection and quantification.[14] A process of subtraction of gels aided by software allows comparison between two samples. Labeling peptides with isotope-coded affinity tags allows accurate quantitation of levels of differences in expression of proteins. Ratio analysis is used to detect quantitative changes in proteins between two samples. Mass spectrometry (MS) has provided a powerful means for obtaining peptide mass fingerprints for proteins resolved in 2DE gels. Protein databases and reference maps have been built to catalog proteins resolved by 2DE from various cell types both in healthy and diseased states. Specialized software then allows an investigator to compare 2D gel patterns with one another and with reference maps on the internet, allowing both quantitative and qualitative differences in protein profiles to be detected for biomarker identification.

Affinity-based MS techniques present a novel proteomic approach for the identification and measurement of cancer-associated biomarkers. Surface-enhanced laser desorption/ionization-TOF/MS is a novel combination of chromatography and MS in which small amounts of complex protein mixtures are enriched and can then be identified in a very short time.[15] Cell lysates or body fluids are directly applied onto bait spots. Each spot contains either a chemically or biochemically treated surface. Surfaces treated chemically react with whole classes of proteins, whereas biochemically treated surfaces react with affinity reagents such as antibodies, receptors, or enzymes. After enrichment, peptides are ionized and brought into a gaseous phase for analysis of their mass-to charge ratios using MS. Ionized proteins and peptides travel down the vacuum tube in times that vary according to their size. Smaller molecules will have a shorter TOF (Figure 59.2). Ciphergen Biosystems, Inc. has developed the SELDI ProteinChip® MS technology platform.

Using cell lysates, SELDI has been used to separate benign prostatic hyperplasia (BPH) from prostatic intraepithelial neoplasia (PIN) and prostate cancer[16] (Figures 59.3 and 59.4); it has also been used to quantify prostate-specific membrane antigen (PSMA) from serum for differential diagnosis of prostate cancer.[17] Using samples from a serum bank and utilizing SELDI as an immunoassay platform, Wright's group demonstrated that PSMA in combination with PSA could discriminate between BPH patients and prostate cancer patients.

Protein array technology allows high-throughput screening for gene expression and molecular interactions. Protein arrays appear as new tools in functional genomics, enabling the translation of gene expression patterns of normal and diseased tissues into a protein

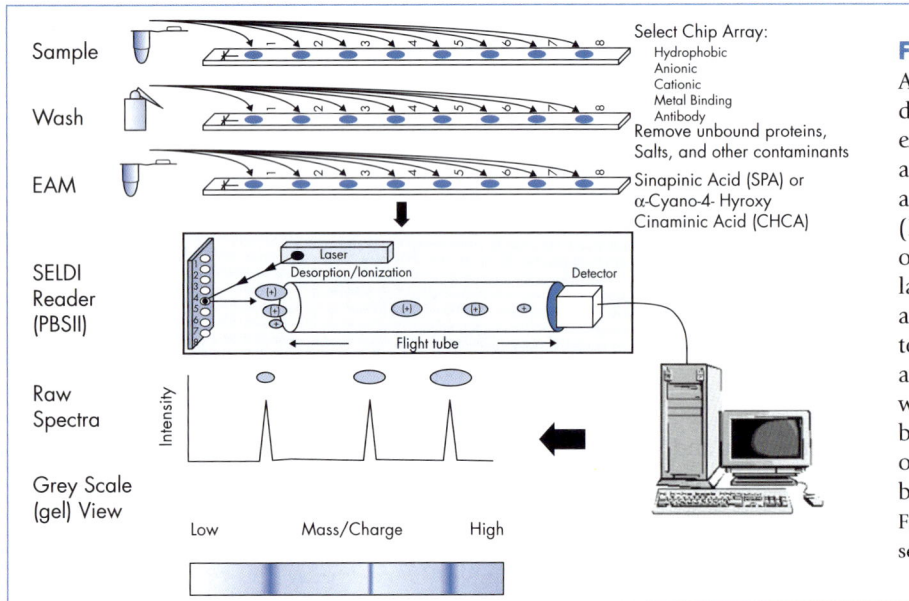

Fig. 59.2

A typical surface-enhanced laser desorption and ionization (SELDI) experiment. Chip processing—i.e., adding the protein sample, washing, adding the energy adsorbing molecule (EAM)—can either be done manually or by using a robotic workstation. The latter becomes essential when analyzing a large number of samples to maximize reproducibility. The chips are then processed in the mass reader where the bound proteins are liberated by ionization, and fly through a "time-of-flight" tube where they separate based on mass and charge.

From http://www.evms.edu/vpc/seldi/seldiprocess/fig2.jpg.

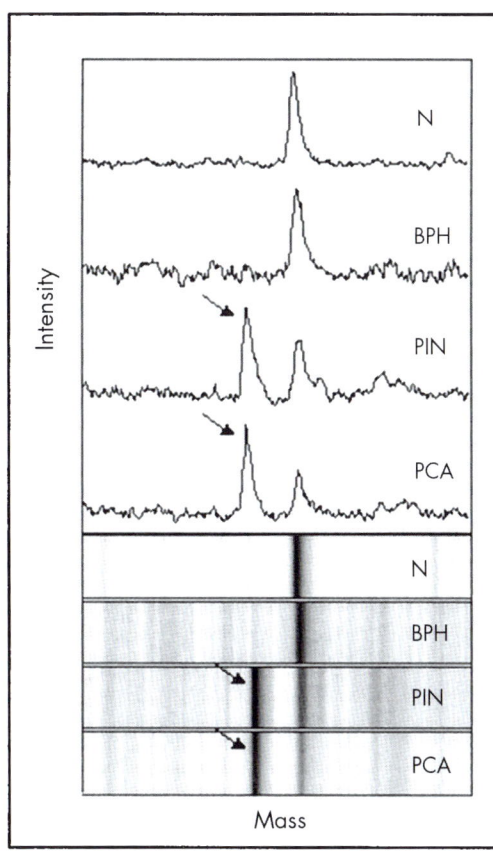

Fig. 59.3
Surface-enhanced laser desorption-ionization (SELDI) analysis of cell lysates prepared from pure cell populations obtained by laser capture microdissection. Mass spectra of nondiseased (N) epithelial cells, benign prostatic hyperplasia (BPH), prostate intraepithelial neoplasia (PIN), and prostate cancer (PCA) obtained from a single surgical tissue specimen. The top four panels are the raw spectra and the bottom four are the gray scale or gel views. The arrows identify a protein that is overexpressed in both PIN and PCA. Taken from Srinivas PR et al, with permission.[16]

product catalog. Protein function, such as enzyme activity, antibody specificity, and other ligand-receptor interactions and binding of nucleic acids or small molecules can be analyzed on a whole-genome level.

As the array technology develops, an ever-increasing variety of formats become available (e.g., nanoplates, patterned arrays, three-dimensional pads, flat-surface spot arrays, microfluidic chips), and proteins can be arrayed onto different surfaces (e.g., membrane filters, polystyrene film, glass, silane, gold). Various techniques are being developed for producing arrays, and robot-controlled, pin-based, or ink-jet printing heads are the preferred tools for manufacturing protein arrays. CCD cameras or laser scanners are used for signal detection; atomic force microscopy and mass spectrometry are upcoming options. The emerging future array systems will be used for high-throughput functional annotation of gene products. Of all the applications for protein microarrays, molecular diagnostics is most clinically relevant. Different proteins such as antibodies, antigens, and enzymes can be immobilized within protein microchips. Miniaturized and highly parallel immunoassays will greatly improve efficiency by increasing the amount of information acquired with single examination and will reduce cost by decreasing reagent consumption.

At present, these technologies are still research tools that are used to investigate potential biomarkers, for example, identifying protein fingerprints that could be used to distinguish clinically significant and insignificant carcinomas of the prostate.[18,19] In the not too distant future, it is conceivable cancer patients will be fingerprinted from their sera or cells, their profiles will be interpreted using bioinformatic software and the management of their disease will be individualized.

DATA ANALYSIS: BIOINFORMATICS

Molecular profiling is aimed at generating a large amount of data from a given sample of tissue. This potentially represents an enormous multidimensional dataset that needs to be explored to remove redundant features and uncover useful biomarkers of clinical outcome. Having identified useful and robust biomarkers (there may be many), one then needs to combine these in such a way as to obtain a reliable tumor signature that can be used in clinical management of patients.

Handling and making sense of these enormous and complex datasets requires a range of multivariate statistical and mathematical techniques, and sufficient computing resources are needed to store the data and run the analyses. This field, which combines the use of computing, mathematics, and biology, is termed *bioinformatics*. It encompasses the development of database software to manage molecular data; the design and use of database search engines to identify annotated sequences such as contigs, promoter sites, and open reading frames; the use of three-dimensional modeling of molecules and its impact on functional genomics; the use of statistical methods, such as cluster analysis, to identify related features and reduce dimensionality of the data; and the development of artificial intelligence techniques such as neural networks and decision support systems for classification of molecular profiles.[20,21]

PROTEOMICS AND MOLECULAR PROFILING IN PROSTATE CANCER

CLINICAL APPLICATION: NEAR-FUTURE OPPORTUNITIES

Initial results are emerging for the diagnosis of prostate cancer using the proteomics technology. The major

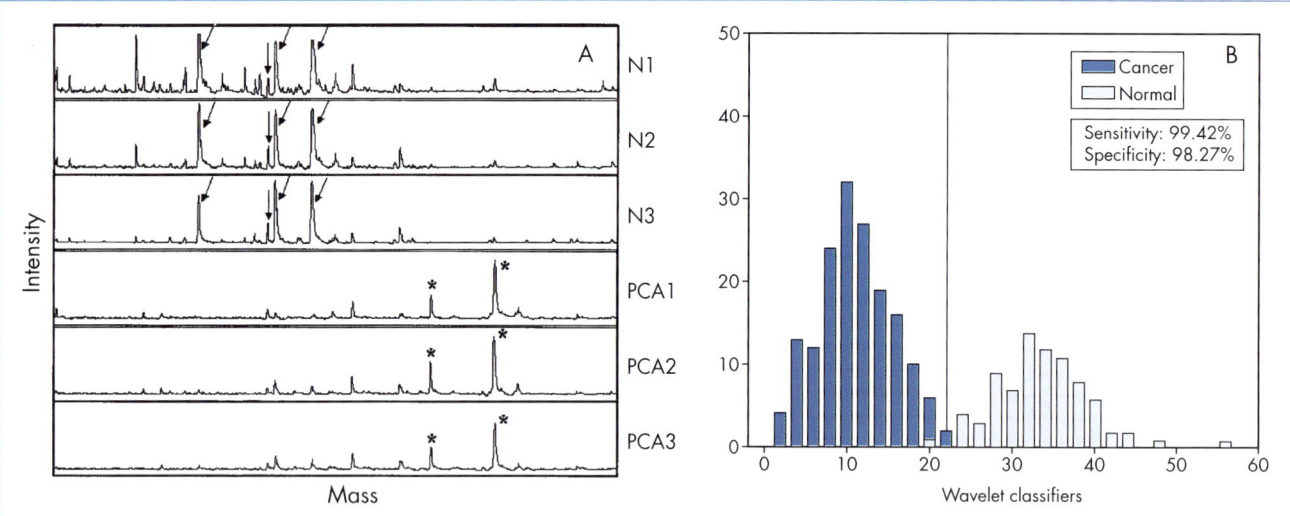

Fig. 59.4

Surface-enhanced laser desorption-ionization (SELDI) protein profiling of serum from nondiseased, age-matched men (N1, N2, N3) and patients with prostate cancer (PCA1, PCA2, PCA3). *A*, Representative example of the raw spectra. The arrows identify proteins that are underexpressed in the three prostate cancer samples, and the asterisks identify proteins overexpressed in the cancer patient sera. *B*, Example of the output from the Wavelet transform learning algorithm. The vertical line is the cutoff point of 22.23. The distributions of the classifier scores for prostate cancer are clearly different from those for the nondiseased population. Taken from Srinivas PR et al, with permission.[16]

problem of these studies is that they have to be supported by data from other centers and duplicated by the authors themselves. There are also obviously still some problems in the reliability of the proteomics technology. However, this field is certainly an exciting one.

Serum proteomic mass spectra was used with a bioinformatics tool to reveal the most fit pattern that discriminated the training set of sera of men with a histopathologic diagnosis of prostate cancer (PSA ≥4 ng/mL) from those men without prostate cancer (serum PSA level <1 ng/mL). Mass spectra of blinded sera (N = 266) from a test set derived from men with prostate cancer or men without prostate cancer were matched against the discriminating pattern revealed by the training set. The proteomic pattern correctly predicted 36 of 38 patients with prostate cancer, while 177 of 228 patients were correctly classified as having benign conditions.[22]

A series of 345 men (a cancer group of 246 men who underwent radical prostatectomy and a noncancer group including 99 men with no histologic evidence of prostate cancer on biopsy) who had an archival serum sample available were included in a proteomics study at Johns Hopkins Hospital.[23] Serum proteomics mass spectra of these patients were generated using ProteinChip arrays and a ProteinChip Biomarker System II SELDI-TOF mass spectrometer (Ciphergen Biosystems, Inc., Fremont, California). The cases and controls were randomly split into training and testing groups by a stratified sampling procedure. A combination of bioinformatics tools was used to reveal

the optimal panel of biomarkers for maximum separation of the prostate cancer and the benign prostate disease cohorts. A panel of three proteins (PC-1, PC-2 and PC-3) was selected using the training data. The area under the curve for PSA, PC-1, PC-2, PC-3 and PC-com3 (all three proteins) was 0.542, 0.585, 0.600, 0.636 and 0.643, respectively. The benefit brought by the use of proteomics was relatively modest compared with PSA alone, but worth further investigations.

Adam et al described the use of proteomics on serum samples whereby they distinguished prostate cancer patients from healthy controls. They reported that the sensitivity and specificity of the proteomics test was 83% and 97%, respectively, and stated that they obtained a positive predictive value of 96% for the study population.[18]

In a letter, Stattin and Hakama downplayed somehow the exciting results of the use of proteomics in the diagnosis of prostate cancer.[24] These authors noted that the predictive value depends not only on the sensitivity and specificity (validity) but also on the prevalence of disease in the study population. The case-control ratio of the above-mentioned study was roughly one control per case (i.e., a prevalence of 50%), a ratio that is not attained even in high-risk populations. Had the authors chosen to have 10 controls per case, the positive predictive value would have decreased from 96% to 75%, although the validity of the test would have remained the same.

Assuming a prevalence of 2%, the application of proteomics test with the cited validity would result in a positive predictive value of 36%. In comparison, the corresponding value for PSA testing has been 30% when applied to a population with the same prevalence.

In a recent study, artificial intelligence based pattern recognition has been developed to analyze complex serum proteomic data streams generated by SELDI-TOF mass spectroscopy. Ornstein et al collected serum samples from 154 men with serum PSA of 2.5 to 15.0 ng/mL and/or abnormal DRE prior to transrectal ultrasound (TRUS) biopsies.[25] Serum samples were applied to WCX2 (a weak cation exchange protein chip) protein arrays by a robotic liquid handler. Low-molecular-weight proteomic patterns were generated with the API QSTAR Pulsar i LC/MS/MS system. High-resolution mass spectra were analyzed with a pattern recognition bioinformatics tool in order to identify key discriminating ion signatures. Serum samples from 63 men were used to train the diagnostic algorithm, the remaining 91 samples being analyzed in a blinded fashion. Testing those 91 men, the model used yielded a 100% sensitivity for a 67% specificity. Therefore 67% negative biopsies would have been avoided while no cancers would have been missed.

As the authors pointed out themselves, there are several limitations to this study. The best models were selected, and so the ability of these models to discriminate men with prostate cancer in a general population remains to be tested. On top of that, the models used were generated with only 30 cancer and 33 benign samples, which is extremely reduced. Larger samples and additional data should confirm these preliminary results.

CURRENT DEVELOPMENTS

The National Cancer Institute (NCI) has taken a lead role in this regard by creating the Early Detection Research Network. This network brings together national and international experts from academia and industry to promote biomarker discovery and validation and help translation into clinical practice. The Cancer Genome Anatomy Project, a large multi-institutional effort, was initiated by the NCI in the United States to identify all abnormal genes in prostate cancer. Prostate cancer cells from radical prostatectomy specimens are processed through a number of steps to identify and sequence the genes expressed.

Aldehyde-based fixatives (e.g., formalin) damage mRNA and other biomolecules. Conversely, frozen tissue specimens permit the study of mRNA from dissected cell populations. Frozen sections are technically difficult, and it requires skill to avoid destruction of the histology. In addition, the frozen sample contains only a limited portion of the tumor. The goal is to develop a universal protocol that is robust but protective of DNA, RNA, and protein while maintaining histological detail. The NCI Prostate Group has developed a three-dimensional

prostate model prototype for this purpose. Prostatectomy specimens are processed with a nonaldehyde fixative and a low temperature embedding compound that preserves histologic detail and protects mRNA. Whole mount cross-sections of the entire prostate gland are present in the x- and y-dimensions for viewing and microdissection. Several hundred adjacent serial recut slides are prepared from the tissue blocks at a thickness of 8 μm, and all of the normal histology and pathology in the z-dimension are recreated into a three-dimensional view of the prostate. Thus, it is possible to determine the exact physical relationship of the normal ducts, premalignant lesions, and tumor(s) and overlay this with the gene expression data.

The NCI have several other initiatives as well, including research on the abnormal proteins expressed in prostate cancer (Proteomics Project) and karyotypic abnormalities in prostate cancer (Cancer Chromosome Abnormality Project).

The European Bioinformatics Institute (EMBL.EBI), the Swiss Institute of Bioinformatics (SIB) and Georgetown University Medical Center's Protein Information Resource (PIR) have launched UniProt, a protein resource that is a comprehensive catalog of information on proteins.[26] Protein sequence databases have become a crucial resource for molecular biologists, allowing them to analyze the proteomes of newly sequenced organisms, to make intelligent predictions about the functions of newly identified proteins, and to move towards understanding how proteins interact to create pathways, networks, and entire systems. To do this efficiently, they need access to a defined set of features describing all the proteins that are known to exist or have been predicted to exist by extrapolation from their gene sequences.

Other complementary databases exist such as Swiss-Prot, the TrEMBL (a large database in which information on protein function is derived computationally by comparison with other proteins), and the PIR International Protein Sequence Database (PIR-PSD), the world's first database of classified and functionally annotated proteins. These databases hold different, but overlapping, subsets of proteins. This unification was made possible by funding from the US National Institutes of Health. The National Human Genome Research Institute (NHGRI) is the primary funding institute. RESID Database of Protein Modifications is a comprehensive collection of annotations and structures for protein modifications and cross-links including pre-, co-, and post-translational modifications

Underpinning the entire project is the UniProt archive, an accessible non-redundant protein sequence database available. Protein sequences are loaded daily from the public databases, including not only Swiss-Prot, TrEMBL, and PIR-PSD, but also the EMBL.Bank/DDBJ/GenBank nucleotide sequence databases, the Ensembl database of animal genomes, the International Protein Index (IPI), the Protein Data Bank (PDB), the NCBI's Reference Sequence Collection (RefSeq), model organism databases such as FlyBase and WormBase, and protein sequences from the European, American, and Japanese Patent Offices. Researchers will also be able to submit protein sequences directly to the Knowledgebase of UniProt using a new web-based submission tool.

Table 59.1 summarizes some applications in proteomics diagnostics, such as protein biochips for high-throughput applications for instance. Many others are on launch or already started.

ADVANTAGES AND LIMITATIONS OF MOLECULAR PROFILING AND PROTEOMICS

Techniques to enable efficient and highly parallel identification, measurement, and analysis of proteins remain a bottleneck. A platform technology that makes collection and analysis of proteomic data as accessible as genomic data has unfortunately yet to be developed. Sensitive and highly parallel technologies analogous to the nucleic acid biochip, for example, do not exist for protein analysis. Given the promise of proteomic technologies, there are also limitations that need to be overcome to increase the sensitivity and enhance information capture. The identification of low-abundance proteins may often be hindered by the highly abundant ones, which mask them. Important biomarker information could thus be lost because there is no PCR equivalent available to amplify proteins. Furthermore, given the complex nature of carcinogenesis and the heterogeneous nature of cellular interaction within the microenvironment of a tumor, analysis of appropriate cell population is necessary to obtain meaningful proteomic output and screen out background noise. This can be achieved by obtaining protein profiles from specific cell populations to avoid potential contamination from sources not related to the onset or progression of the cancer.

Stability and reproducibility also remain a major issue, as for instance the stability of the SELDI procedure over multiple experiments.[27] Baggerly et al compared SELDI proteomic spectra from serum from three experiments by the same group on separating ovarian cancer from normal tissue. These spectra are available on the web at http://clinicalproteomics.stem.com. In

Table 59.1 Example of potential applications of molecular profiling and proteomics		
Company/institute	**Method**	**Applications**
Aclara (Mountain View, CA)	eTag reporter detection by microfluidic capillary electrophoresis	Protein expression profiling
Adaptive Screening (Cambridge, UK)	Surrogate proteome on a chip measures the complex binding relationships of compounds or proteins	Prediction of adverse drug reactions
Biacore (Uppsala, Sweden)	Biomolecular interaction analysis (BIA) and surface plasmon resonance (SPR). BIA-mass spectrometry (BIA-MS)	Immunodiagnostics, biomedical research and drug discovery
Biosite Diagnostics (San Diego, CA)	Microfluidics protein biochip with antibody arrays	Diagnostic proteomics
BioTraces Inc. (Herndon, VA)	Multiphoton detection permits quantitation of sub-zeptomole amounts of proteins	Diagnostic proteomics
Caliper/Agilent Technologies (Palo Alto, CA)	LabChip Lab-on-a-chip: a miniaturized and integrated liquid handling and biochemical processing device for computer-aided analytical laboratory procedures that can be performed automatically in seconds	DNA amplification, automated nucleic acid analysis, genome sequencing, proteomics.
Ciphergen (San Diego, CA)	ProteinChip for monitoring of differential protein expression. Rapid and sensitive analysis of proteins directly from crude biological samples	Discovery and characterization of disease marker proteins and drug target proteins
Intrinsic Bioprobes (Tempe, AZ)	Biosensor chip mass spectrometry	Diagnostic proteomics
Phylos Inc. (Lexington, MA)	Trinectin Proteome chip: based on automated protein selection platform (PROfusion) for production of high-affinity capture proteins	A protein biochip for high-throughput applications
Quantum Dot Corp. (Hayward, CA)	QBEAD system, using microspheres that are bar coded with different colors of quantum dots	Proteomics and gene expression.
SurroMed (Mountain View, CA).	Detection of proteins captured on nanoparticles	To improve 2D microarrays for protein profiling
Zyomyx Inc. (Hayward, CA)	High-density protein microarrays for quantification of proteins. Immobilization of exactly defined quantities of proteins on each spot while retaining the full activity of the protein	Multiplexed immunoassay to analyze expression levels of multiple serum proteins in complex mixtures

general, the results were not reproducible across experiments! Baseline correction prevented reproduction of the results for two of the experiments. In one experiment, there was evidence of a major shift in protocol mid-experiment, which could bias the results. In another, structure in the noise regions of the spectra allowed us to distinguish normal from cancer, suggesting that the normals and cancers were processed differently. Sets of features found to discriminate well in one experiment did not generalize to other experiments. Taken together, these and other concerns suggested that part of the structure uncovered in these experiments could be due to artifacts of sample processing, not to the underlying biology of cancer.

Serious questions about SELDI-TOF technology for protein profiling thus remain unanswered. It is possible that the data obtained using this technology are biased by artifacts of sample collection, storage and processing patients selection and analytical methods.[28]

There has been great progress in the proteomic analysis of multiprotein complexes and subcellular organelles. However, routine, in-depth proteome analyses of whole-cell lysates, tissue samples, and plasma still elude the dynamic-range capabilities and sensitivity of the instruments that are available at present.

CONCLUSION AND PERSPECTIVES

The application of proteomics in prostate cancer diagnosis is novel and promising, and it may improve early prostate cancer detection. However numerous refinements have to be brought to bring this exciting technology into daily clinical practice. At this stage, it is still investigational. If the cited validity of proteomics could be preserved when applied to serum samples from men selected for intermediately elevated levels of PSA (e.g., range, 3–10 ng/mL, a range in which one of four men has cancer on subsequent prostate biopsies), this could translate into a large reduction in the number of negative prostatic biopsies without decreasing sensitivity for prostate cancer detection.

Exciting information is expected to emerge from several collaborative efforts that can ultimately be applied to population screening for the early detection and diagnosis of cancer.

REFERENCES

1. Djavan B, Remzi M, Zlotta A, et al. Novel artificial neural network for early detection of prostate cancer. J Clin Oncol 2002;20:921–929.

2. Duggan BJ, McKnight JJ, Williamson KE, et al. The need to embrace molecular profiling of tumor cells in prostate and bladder cancer. Clin Cancer Res 2003;9:1240–1247.

3. Zlotta AR, Schulman CC. Biological markers in superficial bladder tumors and their prognostic significance. Urol Clin N Am 2000;27:179–189.

4. Duggan BJ, Kelly JD, Keane PF, et al. Belfast Uro-oncology Research Group. Molecular targets for the therapeutic manipulation of apoptosis in bladder cancer. J Urol 2001;165:946–954.

5. Emmert-Buck MR, Strausberg RL, Krizman DB, et al. Molecular profiling of clinical tissue specimens: feasibility and applications. Am J Pathol 2000;156:1109–1115.

6. Steen H, Mann M. The ABC's (and XYZ's) of peptide sequencing. Nat Rev Mol Cell Biol 2004;5:699–711.

7. Diehn M, Alizadeh AA, Brown PO. Examining the living genome in health and disease with DNA microarrays. JAMA 2000;283:2298–2299.

8. Dhanasekaran SM, Barrette TR, Ghosh D, et al. Delineation of prognostic biomarkers in prostate cancer. Nature 2001;412:822–826.

9. Goessl C, Muller M, Straub B, et al. DNA alterations in body fluids as molecular tumor markers for urological malignancies. Eur Urol 2002;41:668–676.

10. Xu J, Meyers DA, Sterling DA, et al. Association studies of serum prostate-specific antigen levels and the genetic polymorphisms at the androgen receptor and prostate-specific antigen genes. Cancer Epidemiol Biomark Prev 2002;11:664–669.

11. Primdahl H, Wikman FP, von der Maase H, et al. Allelic imbalances in human bladder cancer: genome-wide detection with high-density single-nucleotide polymorphism arrays. J Natl Cancer Inst 2002;94:216–223.

12. Paweletz CP, Liotta LA, Petricoin EF. New technologies for biomarker analysis of prostate cancer progression: laser capture microdissection and tissue proteomics. Urology 2001;57:160–161.

13. O'Farrell PH. High resolution two-dimensional electrophoresis of proteins. J Biol Chem, 1975;250:4007–4021.

14. Srinivas PR, Verma M, Zhao Y, Srivastava S. Proteomics for cancer biomarker discovery. Clin Chem 2002;48:1160–1169.

15. Issaq HJ, Veenstra TD, Conrads TP, et al. The SELDI-TOF MS approach to proteomics: protein profiling and biomarker identification. Biochem Biophys Res Commun 2002;292:587–592.

16. Srinivas PR, Srivastava S, Hanash S, Wright GL Jr. Proteomics in early detection of cancer. Clin Chem 2001;47:1901–1911.

17. Xiao Z, Adam BL, Cazares LH, et al. Quantitation of serum prostate-specific membrane antigen by a novel protein biochip immunoassay discriminates benign from malignant prostate disease. Cancer Res 2001;61:6029–6033.

18. Cazares LH, Adam BL, Ward MD, et al. Normal, benign, preneoplastic, and malignant prostate cells have distinct protein expression profiles resolved by surface enhanced laser desorption/ionization mass spectrometry. Clin Cancer Res 2002;8:2541–2552.

19. Adam BL, Qu Y, Davis JW, et al. Serum protein fingerprinting coupled with a pattern-matching algorithm distinguishes prostate cancer from benign prostate hyperplasia and healthy men. Cancer Res 2002;62:3609–3614.

20. Khan J, Wei JS, Ringner M, et al. Classification and diagnostic prediction of cancers using gene expression profiling and artificial neural networks. Nat Med 2001;7:673–679.

21. Cole KA, Krizman DB, Emmert-Buck MR. The genetics of cancer: a 3D model. Nat Genet 1999;21:38–41.

22. Petricoin EF 3rd, Ornstein DK, Paweletz CP, et al. Serum proteomic patterns for detection of prostate cancer. J Natl Cancer Inst 2002;94:1576–1578.

23. Li J, White N, Zhang Z, et al. Detection of prostate cancer using serum proteomics pattern in a histologically confirmed population. J Urol 2004;171:1782–1787.

24. Stattin P, Hakama M. Correspondence re: B-L. Adam et al., Serum protein fingerprinting coupled with a pattern-matching algorithm distinguishes prostate cancer from benign prostate hyperplasia and healthy men. Cancer Res 62: 3609–3614, 2002. Cancer Res 2003;63:2701; author reply 2701–2702.

25. Ornstein DK, Rayford W, Fusaro VA, et al. Serum proteomic profiling can discriminate prostate cancer from benign prostates in men with total prostate specific antigen levels between 2.5 and 15.0 ng/ml. J Urol 2004;172:1302–1305.

26. Garavelli JS. The RESID Database of Protein Modifications as a resource and annotation tool. Proteomics 2004;4:1527–1533.

27. Baggerly KA, Morris JS, Coombes KR. Reproducibility of SELDI-TOF protein patterns in serum: comparing datasets from different experiments. Bioinformatics 2004;20:777–785.

28. Diamandis EP. Commentary – Analysis off serum proteomic patterns for early cancer diagnosis: Drawing attention to potential problems. J Nal Cancer Inst 2004;96:5353–5356.

Treatment of early stage prostate cancer

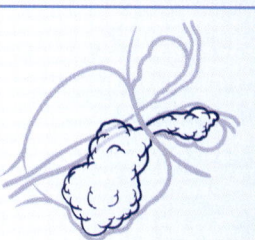

Coping with a diagnosis of prostate cancer: the patient and family perspective

60

Brian Wells

INTRODUCTION

Prostate cancer kills men from all socioeconomic groups, races, and cultures. Some are retired, others are at the peak of their careers, usually with wives/partners and often with (sometimes young) children.

The prostate remains something of a mystery to the public, although general awareness is being raised by organized campaigns, celebrity cases reported by the media, and the enhanced profile of "men's wellness" generally, although it still falls a long way behind that of women.

A diagnosis of prostate cancer, no matter how it is revealed and presented, is likely to have a profound emotional effect on the patient and his family, as well as others in close contact, such as work colleagues. This should be remembered and treated in an appropriate context, which will vary according to the age, nationality, culture, and resources of the patient, as well as the healthcare systems available. Few of these systems are well equipped to deal comprehensively, rapidly, and effectively with the myriad of potential problems that may arise. There is much ignorance and confusion about prostate cancer, and the overall experience can be traumatic or relatively trouble free.

Relevant factors include:

- Prostate cancer is only found in men ("manhood" issues, responsibilities, etc).
- TNM stage of the disease.
- Lifestyle of the family (this can be complicated).
- Philosophical, spiritual/religious, and other values involved.
- Family system and dynamics (there may be 20 years of "baggage" between husband and wife, or the

relationship may be "healthy" and highly supportive).
- "What goes on" at home and at work (this is often difficult for clinicians to appreciate when patients are seen in hospitals and clinics).
- Previous family experience of illness, doctors, and treatments.

EXAMPLE CASES

CASE 1

Patient X is a 57-year-old managing director of a company that employs 70 staff in northern England. He has been married for 30 years and has three mature children who have left home. A routine annual visit to his family doctor reveals an asymptomatic prostate-specific antigen (PSA) of 6 ng/ml with an unremarkable digital rectal examination (DRE). He is referred to a local urologist who organizes a transrectal ultrasonography (TRUS) biopsy, which he finds uncomfortable and "messy" to say the least. He waits for the results, is told that he has a Gleason score of 7, adenocarcinoma of the prostate, and is referred for an MRI and bone scan. At this point he tells his wife and children. Again, they wait for results and are told that "the tumor seems to be localized" and that if he has appropriate treatment, there is a "good chance of complete cure."

His wife (an intelligent former nurse) has talked to friends, explored the Internet, and begun to reach a stage of "information overload." She worries about her anxious husband, treatment options, side effects, and what the future holds, but both are relieved that he is unlikely to die of prostate cancer.

Neither feels inspired by the urologist who has an abrupt manner and seems too busy. Despite assurances that a radical prostatectomy is likely to lead to cure, the couple remains concerned about possible complications.

Their 25-year-old son phones a friend whose father is a cardiologist in Los Angeles. The friend reports back that, compared to radical prostatectomy, brachytherapy is "far more popular on the west coast," has a similar success rate, is less invasive, and is unlikely to cause incontinence or erectile dysfunction. However, should the disease recur (15–20% chance), further radiotherapy will not be an option, and surgery will be virtually excluded due to tissue damage caused by the radioactive seeds. Various transatlantic phone calls take place; patient X and his supportive wife visit a total of five "experts" (they have a health insurance scheme that allows for some flexibility) and talk to former patients who share their experiences.

Eight weeks after the diagnosis has been presented, they opt for a radical prostatectomy in London, under the care of a surgical team that has been recommended as "the best," and in which they have confidence. Another 8 weeks postop, patient X returns to work, but feels tired, irritable, and bored with the problems presented to him, and over the ensuing 6 months arranges to take early retirement.

Two years later (having required a dilatation 3 months postop), his PSA is unreadable. He and his wife have developed an intimacy that is deeper than previously (including adequate erectile function with the aid of PD5 inhibitors). They travel, enjoy mutual interests, exercise together, and the family, which now includes two grandchildren, look back on the entire process as having been traumatic but subsequently life-enhancing. Patient X is determined to "give something back." He makes regular donations to prostate-related charities and declares himself available to share his experiences with other patients, either by telephone or in a group setting.

CASE 2

Patient Y is a 47-year-old Islamic international businessman from the Lebanon. He has three wives, is deeply religious, and wishes to have more children. His active sexual life is of great importance and he is distraught at having been diagnosed with prostate cancer at so young an age. After consulting a multitude of professionals in various countries, he eventually decides to visit a sperm bank and opts for brachytherapy. He keeps his diagnosis a secret from everyone (including his wives who are baffled by the sudden use of condoms) because he is concerned that the stigma of "cancer" will be used to his disadvantage by business competitors.

Four months post-treatment he begins to experience erectile dysfunction and becomes depressed. This leads to a short admission at a psychiatric facility where he improves, following culturally sensitive counseling and antidepressant pharmacotherapy. He remains under the care of an Arabic-speaking psychiatrist, and 1-year post-brachytherapy is considering in vitro fertilization (IVF) with one of his wives.

CASE 3

Patient Z is a 64-year-old alcoholic divorcee, living alone in Ohio, having previously served in Vietnam. His three adult children all live in different cities and the family tries to get together, complete with grandchildren, at Thanksgiving and Christmas. Over a 3-year period, he becomes aware of worsening symptoms. His local Veterans Administration hospital finds a PSA in excess of 300 ng/ml with secondary tumors in the lower spine. Hormone therapy is commenced and after 3 months a concomitant 8-week course of external beam radiotherapy is undertaken. Subsequently, when family members call on the phone, he is usually drunk, sometimes aggressively minimizing his loneliness and the extent of his bone pain. The family is by now used to "Dad's alcoholism" and unpredictable nature. All members have been affected by his drinking over the previous 30 years. Feelings are mixed, and support is offered in a variable and sometimes ambivalent manner by family members who have problems of their own; one being divorced, another following a "recovery" program resulting from his own addiction to drugs and alcohol, consequences of which included an 18-month jail sentence.

THE PATIENT AND FAMILY JOURNEY

These three examples serve to illustrate a tip of the emotional icebergs that can accompany prostate cancer. "Emotional language" is often difficult to articulate, as emotions are experiential, and sometimes difficult to describe. Some patients and family members are "psychologically sophisticated" and can express feelings more comprehensively than others. Cultures vary in the manner that emotions are expressed and just as some patients have higher and lower thresholds to physical pain, the same is true for emotional pain.

Many adverse life events (deaths, robberies, accidents, etc.) lead to a *grief reaction*. It can be helpful for the patient and his family to be aware of the psychological components of this often subconscious series of defences. Not only is it healthy to progress through these phases, it is important in order to survive traumatic experiences. The phases are not necessarily in strict order, or of the same intensity, but are likely to be experienced by the patient and his significant others at various stages of "the journey":[1]

- Denial.
- Anger (often displaced).
- Bargaining (if only the doctors knew more).
- Depression (rarely requires psychiatric treatment in this context).
- Acceptance.

Prostate cancer, if diagnosed early, is highly treatable with a good prognosis. The patient journey, however, will vary according to:

- Patient and family confidence in their healthcare professionals (families are often more distressed than the index patient).
- "Mid-life" issues (awareness of mortality, financial stability, activities, and interests other than work, etc.).
- Appointment schedules (sometimes complicated), poor communication, sitting in waiting rooms, delayed results, attitudes and personalities of staff (including secretaries).
- Sensitivity of staff to potentially traumatic procedures such as TRUS biopsies (which can produce negative results despite a rising PSA).
- Postoperative care in the short-, medium-, and long-term.
- Feelings of "violation" (manhood having been affected, etc.).

- Competent advice regarding catheters, bladder control, future erectile dysfunction, etc.

Conflicting advice, "anti-doctor" attitudes found on websites and "chat rooms," as well as a need for greater research clarity, can make decision-making difficult (See Chapter 61). "Fuzzy indicators," such as PSA results, can confuse. Professional competition, financial incentives, and an overall absence of culturally-sensitive understanding and support from within the profession, can lead patients and families to feel isolated. Some institutions offer emotional help by making use of volunteers and "survivors of cancer" (support groups, etc). However, professional supervision and guidance in this area is generally lacking. While relatively few patients and families require the services of a psychiatrist, basic counseling skills do involve an element of training.

As technology advances, research results appear, and professionals become increasingly skilled with new equipment, there are good reasons for future optimism.

At the time of writing, it is interesting for a psychiatrist to witness the professional and political conflicts that currently surround the diagnosis and management of prostate cancer. Controversy over routine PSA testing, watchful waiting (active surveillance) versus curative treatments, and passionate debate on future quality of life issues, make prostate cancer a rich source of technical, scientific, and emotional material.

REFERENCES

1. Kubler Ross E. On Death and Dying 1970 Collier Paperbacks.

Decision-making for men with prostate cancer 61

Mark R Feneley, Leslie Moffat, Charlotte Rees

INTRODUCTION

Decision-making is complex and involves processes comprising highly variable components; often these are unique to the individuals involved. It would be fair to say that the scientific analysis of decision-making by patients is in its infancy. Traditional expectations would pre-suppose that all patients receive the same factual information, that clinicians explaining treatment options would have only disinterested perceptions of best treatment, and that patients would have equivalent interests and expectations. Even in such rational and unbiased circumstances, decisions may be expected to differ. Outcomes, though notoriously variable for men with prostate cancer, are to some extent related to decisions and the factors that influence them. This chapter will consider factors that may influence decisions concerning prostate cancer management from medical, educational, and economic perspectives, as well as how "best" decisions may be facilitated.

PATIENT DECISION-MAKING

Men with prostate cancer are faced with growing choices and increased involvement in decision-making for their disease management. There is a growing awareness that the "best choice" perceived by increasingly empowered patients may not necessarily be their physician's recommendation. Decisions regarding prostate cancer management should be reached by taking into consideration the best available evidence, but they are also influenced by other factors, such as the type of doctor–patient relationship, availability and use of

information, individual circumstances, and personal values.

An expanding body of evidence, addressed in this chapter, indicates the importance of patient involvement in the medical decision-making process. Important (but often forgotten) issues that arise from facilitating such involvement relate to the ability of patients to make particular decisions, the extent of their willingness to engage in decisions, and the consequences arising when a patient's decisions differ from the recommendations of healthcare professionals. These considerations may influence substantially the presentation, content, and use of educational material required by patients.

PATIENT ENGAGEMENT IN HEALTHCARE

For the patient with prostate cancer who is faced with therapeutic alternatives, involvement in decision-making is often not his first opportunity for choice in matters of prostate health, particularly when the disease was diagnosed through involvement in a healthcare program such as screening. Ethical consideration demands that prior to participation in a program of screening or early diagnosis, an individual should be reliably informed of the implications of test results.

Information and views acquired through the screening process may influence a patient's subsequent presentation to specialists after a diagnosis of prostate cancer. Hanna et al[1] observed that the specialty of the physician to whom patients were initially referred reflected subsequent treatment. Fowler et al[2] showed that individual oncologists and surgeons tend to favor the treatment they themselves deliver. These studies suggest potentially significant decisional bias. From the first healthcare contact, a patient's involvement in decision-making may be influenced significantly by the patient–doctor relationship.

DOCTOR–PATIENT RELATIONSHIPS

The importance of the doctor–patient relationship in decision-making is continually emphasized. Morgan[3] outlined four types of relationship—paternalism, mutuality, consumerism, and default—and describes them as follows. A *paternalistic* relationship involves high physician control over decision-making but low patient control. Here, the doctor acts as a trusted parent and makes decisions for the good of his/her patient. This relationship is vital in contexts such as emergency medicine where patients may be incapable of participating in decision-making processes. The *consumerist* relationship reverses this power association, and involves high patient control over decision-making but low physician control. This relationship is seen most keenly in settings such as private healthcare. A *mutual* relationship is characterized by a partnership between the patient and doctor, with the patient and doctor having active involvement in decisions. In this situation, the doctor and patient bring different expertise to the consultation. The patient comes as an expert on his experiences, beliefs, feelings, and expectations and the doctor brings his/her clinical experience to the consultation. The final type of doctor–patient relationship, *default*, occurs when doctors reduce their control within the consultation but patients continue to adopt a passive role in decision-making.

SHARED DECISION-MAKING

Shared decision-making is a widely used descriptive term, but the concept is often applied without precise definition. General definitions refer to increasing patient involvement in medical decisions,[4] and more specific definitions include the notion that professionals and patients contribute equally to decisions about treatment.[5] In shared decision-making, control is not vested entirely in the patient as in an informed choice model.[5]

Patients of course differ in their preferences for involvement in decision-making.[6] In a decision analysis study based in general practice, physical problems, older age, and lower social class were shown to be positively correlated with patients preferring a more directed approach over a shared approach.[7] However, other assumed factors, such as gender and perceived chronic health, were not found to predict preferences for a directed approach.[7] In addition, other studies emphasize a correlation between a preference for shared decision-making and a higher level of education. The value of the shared decision-making model and its various components requires further exploration and research, and the term should therefore be understood in the context of its given definition.

INFORMATION CONTENT

Patients' effective participation in decision-making requires that they are offered the most relevant information, and this is presented optimally for their understanding. Obligatory information must include the future impact of their disease, its likely response to treatment, and the potential side effects of treatment.[8] Details, however, may be perceived subjectively in relation to decision-making, and treatment outcomes cannot be predicted with absolute accuracy. There is large variation in the information required by individuals with early prostate cancer for decision-making, and this needs to be accommodated in the process of informing patients.[9]

The content utilized by individuals may vary according to the type of doctor–patient relationship, with more detailed information on treatments and impact on quality of life required in collaborative decision-making than if the patient takes an active or a passive role.[10] The conditions for balanced decisions will always be difficult to standardize. Also, the distinction between a patient's desire for information and his wish to assume responsibility for decision-making is important.[11] A patient's desire to participate actively in decision-making should therefore not be assumed on the basis of his need for information.

Information is frequently sought by patients following diagnosis and used in anticipation of specialist consultation. Davison et al[12] have shown that a computerized prostate cancer information program can provide men newly diagnosed with prostate cancer and their partners with individualized information that supports subsequent decision-making while also reducing psychological distress. This and other studies have shown that information provided at this early stage may empower the patient and facilitate his preferred more active or collaborative decision-making style within the consultation, as well as improving his subsequent recall of the consultation.[13–15]

The need for content and quality of standardized information resources to add benefit in terms of patient preferences and satisfaction has been pointed out by Rimer et al.[16] Importantly, but frequently assumed, the possible negative consequences of using standardized information should also be avoided.[16] As yet, the provision of information has not been linked to decisional regret following treatment, but this has not been evaluated sufficiently and further longitudinal study is required.[17,18] Appropriate tools for studying decisional regret need to be developed and validated,[19] particularly for long-term follow-up of prostate cancer decisions.

Patients now have access to vast amounts of information, selected and viewed from a wide variety of resources. The process tends to be nonsystematic and biased by individual interests. Content and quality may be inadequate, even in material prepared and provided by healthcare professionals.[20,21] Content generally considered imperative for men with prostate cancer includes prostate biology, anatomy, physiology, prostate specific antigen (PSA) testing, tumor biology, including grading and staging, description of standard management options, and outcomes. This medical information must be presented in a style appropriate to the patient in terms of educational level and literacy. Additional content helping the patient and his family to understand and live with the disease, cope with its potential impact on personal relationships, family, employment, and social life, as well as provide resources for support is essential, and must not be undervalued. The distinction between the need for information and the desire to participate in decision-making has been emphasized above,[11] and is important in the selection of content and its evaluation.

The particular sources and content of information that ultimately influence individual treatment decisions vary considerably. Healthcare professionals need to ensure that patients are appropriately informed of their choices and have a balanced understanding prior to decision-making. The patient's own views may nevertheless differ from a professional's assessment. This potential conflict emphasizes the need for a balance between a patient's quality of life, dignity, and autonomy on one side, and medical evidence and compassion on the other.

Educational material provided prior to consultation may be more effective when combined with additional individualized interventions. For instance, Davison and Degner[22] showed that an empowerment intervention supplementing the provision of brochures on prostate cancer resulted in patients taking a more active role during the consultation. This additional individualized and patient-orientated intervention included a review of a list of questions for discussion, an option to record on audiotape the subsequent consultation, and encouragement to bring significant others to accompany the patient.

TREATMENT DECISIONS FOR MEN WITH PROSTATE CANCER

All patients do not perform equally in making choices, regardless of the value or a right or wrong attribute of an individual decision. Patients also vary in their desire to

make choices and have different perceptions of what might constitute their best treatment choice. Patients differ in their self-interest and may be influenced by others, including the experiences of friends, relatives, significant others, and professionals.

Self-interested behavior has been described by Sen[23] to be characterised by three features:

- Self-centred welfare: a person's welfare depends only on his/her own consumption.
- Self-welfare goals: a person's goal is to maximize his/her own welfare and—given uncertainty—the probability-weighted expected value of that welfare.
- Self-goal choice: each act of choice of a person is guided immediately by the pursuit of his/her own goal.

Differences in self-interest may influence how individuals differently perceive risk versus benefit, and incorporate assessment of such trade-offs in deciding between available choices.

For men first diagnosed with early prostate cancer, immediate treatment choices include radical prostatectomy, various forms of radiation therapy, or active monitoring (with no immediate treatment). Alternatively, interventions employing developing technologies (i.e. those without long-term outcome data) may be considered. How the "best" medical decision is to be made will vary between patients. Its complexity is increased by the lack of any contemporary randomized trials demonstrating overall statistically significant survival differences between the three principal management choices (or the alternatives). Various trials of treatment are in progress, including the ProtecT (prostate testing for cancer and treatment) study in the UK, which importantly includes active monitoring in its randomization.[24]

Decisions may be strongly influenced, therefore, by the relative value placed on the impact of the disease versus the durability of treatment response, its side effects and impact on quality of life. Value assessments may reflect an individual's personality and experiences, and this may contribute to absolute differences in decision outcomes between patients and between patients and their healthcare advisors. For instance, the impact of incontinence may be over- or under-played by patient and doctor alike, depending on its impact, acceptability, and individual factors. Where none of the prospective options can be shown to be of comparative benefit by robust evidence, the predominating values of individuals and the nature of doctor–patient relationships will ultimately drive medical decisions.

An ethical view has arisen concerning the status of no immediate treatment (i.e. active monitoring) as an equivalent choice.[25-27] Views on equivalence may be influenced by information provided by healthcare professionals,[28] but there may be other considerations. Receiving no immediate treatment is not always considered objectively to be equivalent to effective treatment, either by the patient or by healthcare professionals. Furthermore, significant practical difficulties can face patients for whom watchful waiting may be a reasonable option.[29,30] The lack of perceived decisional equivalence may prevail in spite of the risk and implications of over-treatment (i.e. treatment of disease that would not impact the patient's future health). It seems likely that future studies will define increasing numbers of patients with early stage low-risk prostate cancer for whom active treatment may be appropriately deferred.

Wider ethical issues concern choices to which patients do not have equal opportunity, reflecting both individual entitlement and distribution of healthcare. Furthermore, given the finite budget of any healthcare system, there will be trade-offs between equity and efficiency endangering what could loosely be termed "fairness." Equity can be defined as equality of access for equal needs, whereas efficiency is the efficient allocation of resource where such resource is forced to be limited. The concept of efficiency is borrowed from the private sector.[31] If social and economic inequalities are to be arranged for an overall advantage to everyone, as suggested by the philosopher John Rawls, then ethical concerns will arise in healthcare.[32]

DECISION TOOLS

Decision tools may facilitate the complex process of decision-making. They must, however, be applied and integrated carefully within healthcare systems, and subjected to rigorous evaluation. Tools have been developed in a variety of settings for patients with prostate cancer, other malignancies, nonmalignant conditions, and prostate cancer screening.[33,34] Mostly, they have been evaluated for their impact on decision-making itself, and few studies have examined their effect on subsequent outcomes.

The various components and processes in decision-making, and extrinsic factors that may influence decisions indirectly, give rise to a wide range in the utility of decision tools and other materials. Some tools are designed to facilitate the task of decision-making by reducing decisional conflict, mostly in an interactive setting.[35] These tools need to be distinguished from educational materials or programs that facilitate treatment decisions by other means. Any or all of these approaches need to be validated, and applied according to their specific design and purpose.

Educational material can be provided for patients with a variety of purposes, including as a decision-aid.[36] A wide range of information-containing media for use as decision aids has been described in relation to prostate cancer, but with limited evaluation of their utility. Indeed, much of the available patient educational material fails to address adequately components of decision-making other than disease, and therefore may perform poorly as decision aids.[20] Examples of the range of media include paper-based pamphlets, video tools,[13,37] CD-ROMs,[38] websites on the Internet,[39–41] and hypermedia programs.[42] Such products are widely distributed and supported by charities, government agencies, professional organizations, and other bodies.[43–45] Web-based programs can be accessed widely and updated appropriately. The information tends to be standardized rather than individualized.[12] Media that specifically allow patient interaction offer the means for individualized information requirements to be met, and they may be supported by print. Further research is required to assure the effectiveness and value of different approaches.

The facilitation of understanding via particular media varies between individuals, owing to differences in need, perception, and application (use) of the information offered. For example, patients differ significantly in their predisposition to monitoring (wanting voluminous information) or blunting (avoiding information) to facilitate coping processes.[46] Also, the degree of empowerment provided and its impact on the balance of the doctor–patient relationship may be highly variable.[47] The impact on decisions (and ultimately outcomes) of the availability of large volumes of information and various media is, however, poorly understood.[48]

Perceptions of prostate cancer diagnosis and involvement in treatment decisions may differ significantly between patients and their partners.[49] For example, Davison et al[50] found differences in the need for content-related information and preferences for decision-making, with patients preferring active roles and partners preferring collaborative roles. Appropriate information may also alter involvement of both patient and partner in decision-making.[12] These observations serve to illustrate the influence of relatives in decision-making and, therefore, their vital role.[51,52] This was exemplified in a Dutch study of shared decision-making in patients with prostate cancer.[53] Most patients (76%) were found to have had some influence in decision-making, and those who did not were more likely to be older and not to have a partner.[53]

Rees et al[44] examined the quality of 31 patient information leaflets widely available in the UK and which discuss treatment options. The leaflets were assessed for quality, readability, and suitability using the DISCERN instrument, Flesch formula, and Suitability Assessment of Materials (SAM) instrument. Despite scores on all measures varying between leaflets, it was possible to identity the best five leaflets across the conditions, including those produced for Cancer BACUP, the Prostate Cancer Charity, and the Covent

Garden Cancer Research Trust. The study also examined their acceptability to patients, but not their effectiveness in aiding treatment decision-making.

Feldman-Stewart et al[54] reported on the use of a question-and-answer booklet aimed at addressing the distinct requirements of patients and their families wanting to understand early-stage prostate cancer. They showed that information is used differently by patients and family. Patients were more inclined to want help for decision-making and planning, while family tended to seek help for providing support. Due to the design of the study, however, it is impossible to say whether this booklet was effective in helping to make treatment decisions. Feldman-Stewart and Brundage[33] subsequently explored the challenges for designing and implementing decision aids with three illustrative examples. One of these was their decision aid to help patients with treatment decisions for early-stage prostate cancer. They observed that the design and implementation of such aids require critical assessment in definition of content, presentation of information, and application into decision-making, and may challenge preconceived assumptions.

Some educational programs aim to reduce anxiety associated with newly diagnosed cancer, particularly where ongoing distress may impair understanding and coping as well as decision-making itself.[55] Anxiety may also be influenced by personal relationships, educational background, and cultural differences.[56-59] Perceptions of "best" choice may also be significantly influenced by peer experience and opinion.[60] Conflict may also arise where decisions do not relate to the wider objectives of healthcare systems.

As mentioned above, important distinctions should be made between a patient's desire for information and his desire or ability to participate in decision-making. Understanding is essential for decision-making and this may be difficult to achieve when highly complex information is presented. Individual decision-making incorporates the utility of alternatives with characteristics of self-interested behavior. Patients' and doctors' judgements may also be biased, particularly by selective processing of information, and patients tend not to use available material either comprehensively or systematically.[61]

All these factors may have an unpredictable impact on patient-centered decision-making. For instance, in a study showing that paper-based decision aids increased men's knowledge of the advantages and disadvantages of screening, this benefit could not be related to men's decision to undergo screening.[34] This illustrates the importance of taking into consideration the many factors other than information that influence decision-making and outcomes, and the need to incorporate these in the critical evaluation of decision tools.

Evaluating an early prostate cancer treatment decision tool against disease-specific and quality-of-life outcomes is currently fraught with difficulties associated with lack of prospective data, changing clinical practice, and unavoidable bias in the observation of clinical outcomes. Decision tools to predict clinically useful endpoints have, however, been used for conditions other than prostate cancer. Dowding et al[62] reported on the development and preliminary evaluation of computerized decision aids for two nonmalignant conditions, including benign prostatic hyperplasia. This program is based on decision analysis using decision trees as a means to provide users with information about the probability of various outcomes and guidance on what might be the "best" option for the individual.[62]

Decision tools are likely to be developed and used by patients with prostate cancer at various stages of disease and may challenge medical recommendations and concepts in healthcare. Research and well-designed prospective longitudinal studies are required to exclude long-term negative impact from decisional regret, interpersonal conflict or discordance with professionals, as well as demonstrate reproducible advantages and benefits from the use of appropriately designed tools.

CONCLUSION

Educational material may be sought by patients, or provided by healthcare professionals, to give information necessary for patients to understand their condition and participate in medical decision-making. The balance between understanding and participation may vary considerably according to ability and desire, as well as personal values and relationships. Choices that face patients may not be equal, particularly in relation to inequalities in distribution and the therapeutic efficiency of alternative interventions, and thereby are subject to sociopolitical and ethical considerations.

Decision tools can facilitate specific aspects of medical decision-making and reduce anxiety or distress arising following diagnosis. The role and behavior of the patient and healthcare professional in specific decision-making may be altered with wider and longer-term potential benefits, such as concordance, and improved physical and psychological outcomes. Further research is needed to develop and validate programs to improve therapeutic decision-making and demonstrate advantage in long-term medical, physical, psychological, and social outcomes.

REFERENCES

1. Hanna CL, Mason MD, Donovan JL, et al. Clinical oncologists favour radical radiotherapy for localized prostate cancer: a questionnaire survey. BJU Int 2002;90:558–560.
2. Fowler FJ Jr, McNaughton Collins M, et al. Comparison of recommendations by urologists and radiation oncologists for treatment of clinically localized prostate cancer. JAMA 2000;283:3217–3222.

3. Morgan M. The doctor–patient relationship. In Scambler G (ed): Sociology as Applied to Medicine, 4th ed. Edinburgh: WB Saunders, 1997, pp 47–62.

4. Malis R, Makoul G. Definitions of "shared decision making" evident in the medical literature. Paper presented at the International Conference on Communication in Healthcare, Sept 14–17, 2004, Bruges, Belgium.

5. Edwards A, Elwyn G. The potential benefits of decision aids in clinical medicine. JAMA 1999;282:779–780.

6. Degner LF, Kristjanson LJ, Bowman D, et al. Information needs and decisional preferences in women with breast cancer. JAMA 1997;277:1485–1492.

7. McKinstry B. Do patients wish to be involved in decision making in the consultation? A cross sectional survey with video vignettes. BMJ 2000;321:867–871.

8. Davison BJ, Keyes M, Elliott S, et al. Preferences for sexual information resources in patients treated for early-stage prostate cancer with either radical prostatectomy or brachytherapy. BJU Int 2004;93:965–969.

9. Feldman-Stewart D, Brundage MD, et al. The information required by patients with early-stage prostate cancer in choosing their treatment. BJU Int 2001;87:218–223.

10. Davison BJ, Parker PA, Goldenberg SL. Patients' preferences for communicating a prostate cancer diagnosis and participating in medical decision-making. BJU Int 2004;93:47–51.

11. Fallowfield L. Participation of patients in decisions about treatment for cancer. BMJ 2001;323:1144.

12. Davison BJ, Goldenberg SL, Gleave ME, et al. Provision of individualized information to men and their partners to facilitate treatment decision making in prostate cancer. Oncol Nurs Forum 2003;30:107–114.

13. McGregor S. Information on video format can help patients with localised prostate cancer to be partners in decision making. Patient Educ Couns 2003;49:279–283.

14. Schapira MM, Meade C, Nattinger AB. Enhanced decision-making: the use of a videotape decision-aid for patients with prostate cancer. Patient Educ Couns 1997;30:119–127.

15. Auvinen A, Hakama M, Ala-Opas M, et al. A randomized trial of choice of treatment in prostate cancer: the effect of intervention on the treatment chosen. BJU Int 2004;93:52–56.

16. Rimer BK, Briss PA, Zeller PK, et al. Informed decision making: what is its role in cancer screening? Cancer 2004;101(5 Suppl):1214–1228.

17. Davison BJ, Goldenberg SL. Decisional regret and quality of life after participating in medical decision-making for early-stage prostate cancer. BJU Int 2003;91:14–17.

18. Diefenbach MA, Dorsey J, Uzzo RG, et al. Decision-making strategies for patients with localized prostate cancer. Semin Urol Oncol 2002;20:55–62.

19. Brehaut JC, O'Connor AM, Wood TJ, et al. Validation of a decision regret scale. Med Decis Making 2003;23:281–292.

20. Fagerlin A, Rovner D, Stableford S, et al. Patient education materials about the treatment of early-stage prostate cancer: a critical review. Ann Intern Med 2004;140:721–728.

21. Walling AM, Maliski S, Bogorad A, et al. Assessment of content completeness and accuracy of prostate cancer patient education materials. Patient Educ Couns 2004;54:337–343.

22. Davison BJ, Degner LF. Empowerment of men newly diagnosed with prostate cancer. Cancer Nurs 1997;20:187–196.

23. Sen AK. On Ethics and Economics. Oxford: Blackwell, 1987.

24. Neal DE, Donovan JL. Prostate cancer: to screen or not to screen? Lancet Oncol 2000;1:17–24.

25. Lilford RJ. Ethics of clinical trials from a bayesian and decision analytic perspective: whose equipoise is it anyway? BMJ 2003;326:980–981.

26. Frankel S, Sterne J, Ebrahim S. Ethics of clinical trials from bayesian perspective: Medical decision making should use posteriors, not priors. BMJ 2003;326:1456.

27. Hamdy FC, Donovan JL, Lane JA, et al. Ethics of clinical trials from bayesian perspective: Randomisation to clinical trials may solve dilemma of treatment choice in prostate cancer. BMJ 2003;326:1456.

28. Donovan J, Mills N, Smith M, et al. Quality improvement report: Improving design and conduct of randomised trials by embedding them in qualitative research: ProtecT (prostate testing for cancer and treatment) study. Commentary: presenting unbiased information to patients can be difficult. BMJ 2002;325:766–770.

29. Chapple A, Ziebland S, Herxheimer A, et al. Is 'watchful waiting' a real choice for men with prostate cancer? A qualitative study. BJU Int 2002;90:257–264.

30. Holmboe ES, Concato J. Treatment decisions for localized prostate cancer: asking men what's important. J Gen Intern Med 2000;15:694–701.

31. Mooney G. Economics, Medicine and Health Care. London: Wheatsheaf, 1992.

32. Rawls J. A Theory of Justice. Oxford: Oxford University Press, 1999.

33. Feldman-Stewart D, Brundage MD. Challenges for designing and implementing decision aids. Patient Educ Couns 2004;54:265–273.

34. Sheridan SL, Felix K, Pignone MP, et al. Information needs of men regarding prostate cancer screening and the effect of a brief decision aid. Patient Educ Couns 2004;54:345–351.

35. Deyo RA. A key medical decision maker: the patient. BMJ 2001;323:466–467.

36. O'Connor AM, Stacey D, Entwistle V, et al. Decision aids for people facing health treatment or screening decisions. Cochrane Database Syst Rev 2003;(2):CD001431.

37. Gomella LG, Albertsen PC, Benson MC, et al. The use of video-based patient education for shared decision-making in the treatment of prostate cancer. Semin Urol Oncol 2000;18:182–187.

38. DePalma A. Prostate cancer shared decision: a CD-ROM educational and decision-assisting tool for men with prostate cancer. Semin Urol Oncol 2000;18:178–181.

39. Lipp ER. Web resources for patients with prostate cancer: a starting point. Semin Urol Oncol 2002;20:32–38.

40. Pautler SE, Tan JK, Dugas GR, et al. Use of the internet for self-education by patients with prostate cancer. Urology 2001;57:230–233.

41. Moul JW, Esther TA, Bauer JJ. Implementation of a web-based prostate cancer decision site. Semin Urol Oncol 2000;18:241–244.

42. Jenkinson J, Wilson-Pauwels L, Jewett MA, et al. Development of a hypermedia program designed to assist patients with localized prostate cancer in making treatment decisions. J Biocommun 1998;25:2–11.

43. Godolphin W, Towle A, McKendry R. Evaluation of the quality of patient information to support informed shared decision-making. Health Expect 2001;4:235–242.

44. Rees CE, Ford JE, Sheard CE. Patient information leaflets for prostate cancer: which leaflets should healthcare professionals recommend? Patient Educ Couns 2003;49:263–272.

45. Rees CE, Ford JE, Sheard CE. Evaluating the reliability of DISCERN: a tool for assessing the quality of written patient information on treatment choices. Patient Educ Couns 2002;47:273–275.

46. Miller SM. Monitoring versus blunting styles of coping with cancer influence the information patients want and need about their disease. Implications for cancer screening and management. Cancer 1995;76:167–177.

47. Wong F, Stewart DE, Dancey J, et al. Men with prostate cancer: influence of psychological factors on informational needs and decision making. J Psychosom Res 2000;49:13–19.

48. Patel HR, Mirsadraee S, Emberton M. The patient's dilemma: prostate cancer treatment choices. J Urol 2003;169:828–833.

49. Boehmer U, Clark JA. Married couples' perspectives on prostate cancer diagnosis and treatment decision-making. Psychooncology 2001;10:147–155.

50. Davison BJ, Gleave ME, Goldenberg SL, et al. Assessing information and decision preferences of men with prostate cancer and their partners. Cancer Nurs 2002;25:42–49.

51. Srirangam SJ, Pearson E, Grose C, et al. Partner's influence on patient preference for treatment in early prostate cancer. BJU Int 2003;92:365–369.

52. Carlson LE, Ottenbreit N, St Pierre M, et al. Partner understanding of the breast and prostate cancer experience. Cancer Nurs 2001;24:231–239.

53. Fischer MJ, Visser AP, Voerman B, et al. Who decides? Information and shared decision making in prostate cancer in the Netherlands. Paper presented at the International Conference on Communication in Healthcare, 14–17th Sept, 2004, Bruges, Belgium.

54. Feldman-Stewart D, Brundage MD, Van Manen L, et al. Evaluation of a question-and-answer booklet on early-stage prostate-cancer. Patient Educ Couns 2003;49:115–124.

55. Flynn D, Van Schaik P, Van Wersch A, et al. The utility of a multimedia education program for prostate cancer patients: a formative evaluation. Br J Cancer 2004;91:855–860.

56. Kim SP, Knight SJ, Tomori C, et al. Health literacy and shared decision making for prostate cancer patients with low socioeconomic status. Cancer Invest 2001;19:684–691.

57. Taylor KL, Turner RO, Davis JL, III, et al. Improving knowledge of the prostate cancer screening dilemma among African American men: an academic-community partnership in Washington, DC. Public Health Rep 2001;116:590–598.

58. Myers RE. African American men, prostate cancer early detection examination use, and informed decision-making. Semin Oncol 1999;26:375–381.

59. Guidry JJ, Aday LA, Zhang D, et al. Information sources and barriers to cancer treatment by racial/ethnic minority status of patients. J Cancer Educ 1998;13:43–48.

60. Berry DL, Ellis WJ, Woods NF, et al. Treatment decision-making by men with localized prostate cancer: the influence of personal factors. Urol Oncol 2003;21:93–100.

61. Steginga SK, Occhipinti S, Gardiner RA, et al. Making decisions about treatment for localized prostate cancer. BJU Int 2002;89:255–260.

62. Dowding D, Swanson V, Bland R, et al. The development and preliminary evaluation of a decision aid based on decision analysis for two treatment conditions: benign prostatic hyperplasia and hypertension. Patient Educ Couns 2004;52:209–215.

Reflections on prostate cancer: personal experiences of two urologic oncologists

62

Paul H Lange, Paul F Schellhammer

INTRODUCTION

This chapter aims to enhance urologists' understanding of certain subjective events surrounding radical prostatectomy. We both had radical prostatectomies several years ago and were emotionally, and in one case practically, involved in each other's surgical process (Paul H Lange (PHL) performed the radical prostatectomy on Paul F Schellhammer (PFS)). We are urologists whose practical and academic interests (and accomplishments) have principally centered on prostate cancer. Also, we have been close friends for many years and thus have had frequent occasions to reflect on and discuss many facets of prostate cancer in relation to our own experiences. We will individually describe the experiences surrounding our diagnoses, surgeries, and subsequent events, using them as discussion points for academic commentaries. Finally, we will present our mutual insights about these experiences. While this effort is highly personal, for a variety of reasons we have chosen to say very little about the sexual aspects of our experiences other than to state that the outcome has been satisfactory to both of us: PHL had a bilateral nerve-sparing prostatectomy and has no problem, and PFS had a unilateral nerve-sparing prostatectomy and uses some assistance. In the realm of sexual performance and urinary function, satisfactory post-treatment outcomes are very much predicated on pretreatment knowledge and expectations. In brief, we both were very much aware of what we were getting into and were very satisfied with the quality of life afterwards. The key word is "awareness." Unrealistic expectations that life will not be altered after treatment can lead to a dissatisfied patient.

REFLECTIONS OF PHL

Though we had known of each other early in our academic careers, the friendship between PFS and I deepened over events involving prostate cancer in my family. Briefly, my father-in-law, who lived in the Norfolk area, had a transurethral resection of the prostate (TURP) for benign disease carried out by PFS's partner, Charles Devine. When Charles retired, PFS took over my father-in-law's routine care, and we then began to communicate regularly about that care. Several years later I got a letter from PFS apologizing that my father-in-law, now 82 years old, had been given a PSA blood test by mistake. I was informed that his PSA level was 20 ng/ml, and, because I had by then started speaking and publishing on the use of PSA,[1] PFS asked for my advice. Of course, we did not then appreciate the importance of a PSA of 20 ng/ml and, while healthy, my father-in-law was 82! I do remember enquiring of some of my urologic oncology friends, and particularly remember one very famous one who looked at me as if I were crazy to even contemplate following up on the PSA. So I advised (and PFS agreed) that nothing be done or even followed, and I thwarted off the confusions of my wife and my extended family about why I was not concerned, if PSA was so important and prostate cancer so serious. PFS did confirm that my father-in-law's digital rectal examination (DGE) was unremarkable for a post-TURP patient.

Over the next 2 years my father-in-law watched his brother-in-law and two of his close golfing partners die from prostate cancer. During this time I tried to educate him about length and lead-time biases over diagnosis and so forth. He was very intelligent but had a business man "bottom line" personality at heart. He kept asking, given that prostate cancer was a possibility, didn't I want to diagnose and possibly treat it, especially since his mother was still alive at 102. Finally, PFS and I acquiesced, got a PSA, which now was 30 ng/ml, caved in to a biopsy in this benign feeling gland, and got a diagnosis of grade 4/3 prostate cancer. His staging studies were negative. My father-in-law had recently lost his wife, was uninterested in sexual activity, and was adamant about beginning therapy, which was hormone ablation. This therapy lasted for 13 years, his PSA remained undetectable, and he had no serious obvious complications from the therapy. He died recently of cardiac failure at 97 years. My wife's family (and my father-in-law when he was alive) were incredulous that anyone would say that this aggressive approach to diagnosis and therapy did not extend his life, and I must admit that I am hard pressed to deny their position.

During this time, PFS and I used this management dilemma and my yearly visits to the Norfolk area to visit family to deepen our relationship and conversations about prostate cancer in general. Little did we suspect that later in our acquaintance this subject would become more personally important.

PFS PERSPECTIVE

As the urologist to whom PHL's family looked for counseling and care, I shared the misgivings of "attacking" prostate cancer in an asymptomatic octogenarian. When treatment was begun and the PSA level plummeted to and remained undetectable, the patient's anxiety and apprehension vanished, and his energy seemed primed at each visit, which yielded a normal DRE and an undetectable PSA level. I was providing medicine that was certainly good for his soul and wellbeing, regardless of how operative it was in extending survival. I also achieved a somewhat heroic status as a healer and was so recognized at the large family reunions I was fortunate to attend. As physicians we are privileged to enjoy this respect but must be cautious not to become enamored and entitled by it.

RADICAL PROSTATECTOMY

I was involved in the early elucidation of the clinical value of serum PSA,[1] and I first measured my own PSA when I was in my early 40s in 1984 as part of these experimental efforts. The level was 0.7 ng/ml. I was reassured; that value was considered normal. Of course, today we have a different perspective. For example, in the Prostate Cancer Prevention Trial (PCPT), as many as 15% of men with a PSA level less than 4 ng/ml over a 7-year period were found to have prostate cancer, and 5% of these cancers were found when the PSA was less than 0.5 ng/ml. Also, some of these cancers in the PCPT controls were of intermediate or high grade.[2] It is now

known that the median PSA level for a 40-year old is less than 0.7 ng/ml.[3] Indeed, the draft of the new National Comprehensive Cancer Network (NCCN) clinical care pathway for prostate cancer diagnosis is hotly debated as it proposes to measure PSAs at age 40 in all men, and if this is greater than 0.6 ng/ml, for yearly PSAs and DREs to be performed, and for biopsies to be taken if the PSA or DRE becomes "suspicious."[4] Conversely, Stamey, who brought PSA to the attention of the general medical community over 20 years ago by correlating serum PSA levels with tumor volume,[5] now claims that levels between 2 and 10 ng/ml are attributed primarily to benign hyperplasia and are not related to cancer.[6]

Over the years I regularly determined my PSA value and noted that very gradually, and in a somewhat "saw tooth" fashion, the values rose. When it "hit" 3.0 ng/ml, I remember reassuring myself that the slope was less than 0.75 ng/ml, which according to Carter et al[7] was a good sign. Then, about 2 years later, it was 3.7 ng/ml— still a reassuring velocity. However, by then there was talk from my good friend Bill Catalona about lowering the normal cut-off to 2.5 ng/ml,[8] and because my prostate was small (I had yearly DREs that were normal), suggesting a worrisome PSA density, I somewhat whimsically decided to have a biopsy, confidently expecting it to be negative for the above reasons and because there was no prostate cancer in my very large family of primary relatives. The sextant biopsy was preformed by my colleague Bill Ellis somewhat secretly (only he, my nurse, and our main prostate pathologist Larry True knew). I also remember remarking that the biopsy was not as uncomfortable as a sigmoidoscopy but that local anesthesia (then not given or studied) might be very useful here (especially if more than six biopsies were taken). That prediction was based on my observations years before when we conducted our trial of TURPs under local anesthesia.[9] I was shocked when pathologic analysis revealed 1 mm of Gleason 5 (it would be the ubiquitous 6 now) on the left side in one of six cores.

What to do? I pondered, reread the literature, reflected especially on watch and wait, and flirted with denial. I even called my friend Martin Gleave who was leading the neoadjuvant androgen ablation trial in Canada,[10] obfuscating the problem by stating that "I had a patient who wanted to know about....," and asked what the pathologic no-tumor (P_0) rate was after 8 months of hormone therapy. When he told me it was less than 10%, I abandoned the escapist solution of going on hormone therapy for 8 months (keeping up a tan and a strict diet to avert suspicion) and then getting periodic PSAs and biopsies to delay or infinitely postpone aggressive treatment.

Finally, I decided to have a second biopsy and again 1 mm of Gleason 5 was found in about the same place. That was it! I wanted to be treated despite all my scholastic ruminations about watch and wait, length and lead-time biases, and the turtles and birds.[11] Deciding what treatment I should have was not a problem. However, contemplating my treatment choice did highlight my intellectual realization that despite my surgical orientation and practice, the relative value of surgery versus radiation therapy regarding quality of life and survival is unknown, and I remember feeling ashamed that it was not, and gaining more sympathy for the layman patient who has to decide amidst this intellectual and entrepreneurial confusion.

Surgery was my only option for several reasons. First, if I had had radiation therapy, the opprobrium from my colleagues would have been too much. However, John Blasko later commented that if I had gotten radiation therapy, I would have received many speaking invitations and honorariums for radiation oncology meetings. He also said that in similar circumstances he, for the same reasons of loyalty to his procedure and profession, could hardly have considered surgery and would have had the "seed" option. More seriously, with my experience I had little fear of the surgery, and with my personality I just wanted to know what was in there and to get the problem behind me if possible. This, I have come to realize, is the main legitimate reason for a surgical choice and is what I seek to hear from those of my patients who chose surgery.

I was surprised by the amount of trepidation I experienced. I thought that with all my experience I would embrace this necessity with aplomb. I was wrong. With my cancer parameters, I feared impotence and incontinence, not diminished survival. This was despite the realization that most of my patients did very well on those scores. "When it's you, it's different" now had a more poignant meaning.

Who was going to do my surgery was not a very difficult problem once analyzed. I realized that going somewhere else to "keep it quiet" would be impossible. Also, I knew that my associate Bill Ellis did the operation pretty much as I did (so it seemed almost like fulfilling a cocky surgeon's dream of using a mirror), and I trusted him. He agreed to do it and did a wonderful job under what must have been some significant pressure. I realized that the comfortable and very personal sense of trust and reassurance of "home ground," in addition to expertise, were more important elements than I had heretofore acknowledged.

While awaiting surgery, I was running an errand and passed an alternative medicine store which I had passed many times before. I must admit I had been very vocal in my criticism of alternative medicine approaches, believing that medicine needed to defend its hard-won evidence-based position. Yet, I entered the store and was enthralled with all the optimistic advertisements and comforting labels with pictures of fruit and such on the bottles of pills. Before I knew it, I walked out with two bottles (one was selenium and the other I forget). When I realized what I had done, I had a good laugh at myself,

and never used them. However, the weekend before my surgery I thought I was getting a cold. The prospect of having to reschedule was overwhelming. Thus, I literally snuck into a drug store and bought a bottle of Echinacea. I did not get a cold and I had my surgery. I began to wonder about Echinacea's validity and then had to laugh at myself once again when the randomized study on Echinacea's effectiveness for preventing colds was announced 6 months later and was negative.[12] However, I realized that empowering the patient to do something for himself, even if through the use of yet unproven remedies, has merit. Also, I realized that medicine must determine better ways to retain the placebo effect without lying to the patient, and to teach these to future practitioners in a more systematic way. Finally, it reinforced a lesson that I had gleaned years before from my association with Michael Milken; namely, waiting for 100% proof is not a good way to make business decisions and possibly not scientific ones when it comes to prostate cancer.[13]

The recovery was relatively easy: pain was manageable, the catheter was more bothersome than I had imagined, and the only real surprise was the degree of fatigue that I experienced over a 3- to 4-week period. This was not from blood loss (I lost very little), but something else hard to define. Yet I was playing tennis at 4 weeks, though with less effectiveness than usual. I look forward to a scientific analysis of laparoscopic radical prostatectomy in that regard; I suspect the fatigue factor will be much less.

My pathology was good (vida infra) and the catheter was removed at 2 weeks. Its discomfort has pushed me to try to shorten that period even further in most of my patients. For 3 weeks I was not continent and I was very unhappy. Like any good Northern European Lutheran, I feared the worst. I did learn that once accepted, pads, at least temporarily, are not that odious. Thereafter, I gained continence quickly. I am now firmly ensconced in the continent group by any definition. Yet I am not as continent as I was before surgery. Though I use no pads or such, there are times when I do leak a little though almost never to the point of social embarrassment; these times include such events as the need to pass flatus, an overly full bladder precipitated by coffee, sexual anticipation, more than my usual alcoholic intake, or when extremely fatigued. Yet leakage with these events is unpredictable and rare. I have now begun to question my heretofore continent patients in ways I never did before and found similar though never quite the same stories. Of course, when I queried them why they had not told me this before, it was because I never asked. I have come to believe that almost no post-radical prostatectomy patient is totally continent and that current quality-of-life questionnaires need further refinement. Furthermore, there are more physiologic factors related to continence in this context then we realize, and these factors have little to do with how the radical prostatectomy is performed and/or how the patient heals. For years now I have told my patients that they can generally expect social continence but I cannot promise that they will be "trampoline dry."

My PSA has remained undetectable for over 6 years now, emotionally I have dismissed prostate cancer as a worry, and I admit to neglecting getting my PSA in a timely fashion. Yet initially and even now, waiting for the PSAs to come back gives me some anxiety.

I am almost glad I had this experience with prostate cancer. In ways that are hard to articulate, I think it has made me a better urologist when it comes to dealing with patients with the disease. I listen more; I am more empathetic; I have better insight into the morbidities of the surgery and yet more confidence that surgery offers a very good therapeutic solution. As an academic surgeon scientist, I have a greater sense of purpose in conducting and administrating research on prostate cancer. I have often been asked "would I do it again; would I have surgery if I were not a urologist; would I have more seriously considered watch and wait with a Gleason 6, 1-mm cancer?" One academic urologist who has made many contributions to prostate cancer, even expounded that I should not have had a biopsy. Also, if I had been so unwise as to have a biopsy, he explained, I should not have had the surgery even if I had known what my surgical pathology revealed; namely, 1 cm^3 of low-grade cancer with negative margins. He furthered explained that: 1) theoretically by half life considerations, it would have taken almost 20 to 30 years to reach "lethal" volumes; and 2) I could have at least waited another 10 years. No way! Taking a chance on the surgery was infinitely less fearsome than taking a chance on cancer theory. Besides, I won: no real morbidities, I am probably cured, and it has made me a better servant in the fight against this disease.

REFLECTIONS OF PFS

When PHL was approached concerning this chapter, I could not resist. We have known each other for 30 years. As described above, the cementing of our friendship and prostate cancer relationship was originally based on the fact that PHL's father-in-law, who resided in my city, had prostate cancer, and was a patient. On his visits East, our mutual interest—prostate cancer—was often a subject of discussion and became even more so after PHL's diagnosis and surgery in 1999, and my diagnosis and surgery by him in 2000. We often concluded our discussions with the promise that we needed to write a book or at least a chapter on the subject. PHL, ever energetic, did write that book—Prostate Cancer for Dummies[14]—and when the opportunity for this chapter arose, he kindly asked me to participate.

In writing of my personal experience, I recognize two important principles. First, you cannot place yourself in another's shoes when walking a decision pathway since each individual processes and acts on information based on certain genetic predispositions and environmental conditioning. Even the closest of biologic and environmental human experiments, identical twins, will not process and react identically on each and every issue. I am married to an identical twin and can testify to this. Second, the ability of an individual to conclusively state his decisions relative to a hypothetical event, in this case the diagnosis and treatment of prostate cancer, might find that position quite altered when confronted with the reality of the diagnosis. To use a military analogy, there is a huge difference between boot camp and the battlefield, or a sporting analogy, between the practice and playing field.

I had started Proscar in 1998 due to urinary symptoms. A PSA in 2000 was 2.5 ng/ml (corrected to 5.0 ng/ml), which represented a significant rise from my prior levels. That I had prostate cancer was intuitively very clear to me. My annual PSA readings, beginning at age 50, had been very stable at 2.0 to 2.5 ng/ml between 1990 and 1998 (a cardiac event [see below] interfered with my 1999 annual draw). I was very content with these PSA levels, but they have since been shown to be associated with a five-fold increase in cancer risk.[15] Furthermore, at age 50 to 60, a PSA of greater than 0.7 ng/ml when compared to a PSA less than 0.7 ng/ml is associated with a 3.5-fold increase in risk for prostate cancer by age 70.[3] The PCPT has demonstrated a 23% incidence of prostate cancer at PSA levels between 2 and 3 ng/ml.[2] A PSA of 5.0 ng/ml was abnormal by any standard for a 60-year old.

Several strategies materialized in my mind. I decided I would have numerous biopsies (about 25) initially, not the then routine 6, to avoid repeat sessions to clarify the etiology of the PSA elevation. I did not want to come back to the biopsy scenario again and again. I presumed a Gleason 3 + 3 cancer since it was the grade most commonly found among patients with a diagnosis in this PSA range and which I diagnose on almost a daily basis.

RADICAL PROSTATECTOMY

What treatment approach? As a surgeon, I was viscerally inclined to surgery, although intellectually, I could not identify radiation by either interstitial implant of external beam as any less effective. I was also attracted to a definitive pathology report. I put erectile dysfunction and incontinence in perspective and had the advantage of first-hand knowledge of intervention that could soften their impact. Having been to France to observe a new laparoscopic approach and being adventurous in nature, I considered this option for the anticipated 3 + 3 low-risk cancer. The biopsy session was uneventful and I was correct in my first hunch—prostate cancer was found. Only 3 (all unilateral) of the 25 cores were positive, and I was certainly pleased that I had chosen the multiple biopsy approach. Fewer cores might have missed the cancer. However, my second hunch, that the cancer would be scored Gleason 3 + 3 was incorrect. All biopsies had predominant pattern 4. Bone and CT scan were normal. I put aside the adventure of a laparoscopic procedure for the tried and true open prostatectomy. Should I have the operation in my home hospital by my partner or take the "monkey off the locals back" and go elsewhere? I consulted with my good friend, PHL, who had had a prostatectomy, and we had operated together. He kindly agreed to do the surgery. I traveled to the University of Washington. The Gleason pattern influenced my attitude of weighing surgical side effects with benefits. My focus was on benefit (life centered) and the risk of urinary and sexual dysfunction became very secondary. This contrasts with PHL's primary concern about side effects when dealing with focal 3 + 3 cancer. I did not favor unilateral nerve-sparing on the biopsy-negative side, unless, at surgery, all circumstances (prostate size, adherence, consistency, ease of dissection) permitted it. A radical retropubic prostatectomy with pelvic node dissection was performed by PHL. The pathology report brought the good news of absence of lymph node involvement, a unilateral pT2 lesion with negative margins. The Gleason pattern 4 + 3 was confirmed but also with some Gleason 5 tertiary pattern. Gleason 4 + 3 + 5 has been plotted on the biochemical no evidence of disease (NED) curve and very much parallels the 4 + 4 curve.[16] A second pathologic opinion by an expert labeled the tumor as 4 + 5 with tertiary 3. Histopathology can be subjective! Also my 2-year course of Proscar may have caused a grading artifact. At least this is one of the explanations used to reconcile the PCPT results.[17]

We decided initially against adjuvant radiotherapy. However, a year after surgery, PSA "creep" began and the menu of uncertainty addressing salvage strategies was brought to my table. Anticipating a PSA failure, I had obtained frequent PSA assays and watched them rise through 0.1 and 0.2. When my PSA exceeded 0.2 ng/ml on two occasions (0.27 and 0.34) I chose to initiate external beam radiation therapy to the prostate bed with neoadjuvant and adjuvant androgen deprivation for 6 months. Androgen deprivation was a choice based on extrapolation of the studies aimed at primary therapy and the apparent synergistic or at least additive benefit of androgen deprivation when combined with radiation. It has been reported with salvage protocols as well.[18] While salvage radiation likely achieves better results with increasing time interval from surgery to PSA rise, and a lower Gleason sum cancer, the potential of a 5-year biochemical control, when initiated "early" (i.e. a PSA <1.0 ng/ml or even 0.6 ng/ml) is quite reasonable for a salvage therapy.[19] The opportunity for a "second chance," whether 10% or substantially more, was very attractive.

Now, two and a half years after restoration of my testosterone level, I anticipate each periodic PSA check with apprehension. I find myself scheduling the blood draw after important events like weddings, holidays, and family visits, so as not to risk blunting the joie de vie associated with these events. I am well, modifying the pace of life, and now appreciate more the interesting future that prostate cancer presents—a cancer that is chronic, that mimics life with its slow and steady attrition but, thankfully, permits rather extended life with good quality. However, the blessing and curse of PSA, especially the latter, can not be underestimated. Even in the elderly male, for whom life-expectancy is limited, the knowledge that a particular process is measurable and that increases, however small, indicate disease activity focuses attention almost exclusively on that disease to the extent that other more debilitating and life-threatening issues are relegated to secondary importance or ignored completely. The ticking clock, regardless of how slow the tick, still is an audible and repetitive reminder of the limitations of life. Yes, we all are subject to the ticking clock, but there is something quite powerful in seeing its face as cancer and envisioning a disabling terminus.

A brief comment regarding urinary function and bother is applicable here. The return of continence was prolonged in part due to a psoas abscess and the vesicle irritation that it produced. Briefly, I began experiencing some mild intermittent right leg pain and toe numbness about 12 days after surgery, which was not very bothersome until I experienced fever and chills 6 weeks after surgery. A CT diagnosed a psoas abscess, which was percutaneously drained and all problems quickly resolved.

I have achieved a very satisfactory continence status which requires one small pad (a liner) daily; I could indeed get by many days without protection but the uncertainty of leaking with a sudden cough, sneeze or positional change, especially at day's end, make protection insurance wise. I agree with PHL that return to the state described as "trampoline dry" is probably quite rare post-prostatectomy, and relying on a patient interview to assess and report perfect continence is a trap for the unwary urologist. When my surgeon asks me if I am continent, I respond with a strong "yes." Only if specifically asked and coached to a detailed description will I state the exact situation and do this to provide academic information and not to describe bother or displeasure. However, I am not perfectly continent and, if I had been promised so as a patient, I would feel disappointed.

PHL COMMENTS

I was of course flattered when PFS asked me to do his surgery. Being a professional, the surgery was not particularly stressful for me or my team and it went very well in all respects. I was very aggressive on the side of his cancer with the lymphadenectomy; no wider surgical margin was technically possible, and on the other side, I reflected on PFS's wishes but saved the nerves nonetheless. I was very happy with the procedure as we closed and while he recuperated at my house. I was pleased that the margins were negative and that there was no cancer on the unilateral nerve-sparing side.

However, after surgery I took every event in PFS's recovery and clinical course very personally. I have never had a patient with a psoas abscess postoperatively and cannot think of a surgical cause for this one. Yet this result and the rising PSA continue to elicit that irrational response: I could have done better. I would want it no other way; for him and in fact for all our patients.

FURTHER REFLECTIONS BY PFS

Approximately 2 years prior to the diagnosis of prostate cancer, I experienced an event which, like prostate cancer, only even more so, comprises the rite of passage for the aging male. Sudden crushing chest pain brought me to my knees. Fortunately, it occurred at home rather than in a hotel room, car, or airplane. A prompt angioplasty and stent corrected the obstruction of the left anterior descending coronary artery. There are several reasons for mentioning this event. Prior to transfer from the emergency room to the angio suite, the cardiologist outlined for me a four-arm clinical trial for which he advised my participation. The trial randomized to angioplasty ± stent with anticoagulation A or B. I am sure every individual addresses instant information and decisions differently. I am also certain that most individuals, myself included, would ask the consenting physician, in this circumstance, "do you think this is a good idea and should I participate?" In this urgent situation, an affirmative from the physician invariably results in consent to the proposed trial. And so I consented. I can only contrast this process with the laborious explanations, interactions, and reviews with patients and significant others that was required to inform and encourage patients to consider the SPIRIT trial. This trial was initiated by the American College of Surgeons Oncology Group in the US and Canada and was a randomized trial between brachytherapy and radical prostatectomy for low-risk disease. Both PHL and I spent many months in helping getting this trial started, but we were ultimately unsuccessful (see below). The deck is certainly stacked, at least in this situation, in favor of a cardiology intervention trial versus a prostate cancer intervention trial. This was so despite the fact that both arms of the prostate trial had a proven track record of success, whereas the cardiology trial was constructed to measure the unknown of adding a new stent procedure to angioplasty. The trial playing field is overwhelmingly tipped in favor of cardiology intervention based on urgency and ultimate "at the mercy of the MD and situation" status of a cardiac event.

Another reason for mentioning this cardiac event is to compare the visceral response and emotion associated with the diagnosis of cardiac disease and prostate cancer. After my coronary occlusion, during and after rehabilitation (parenthetically the rehabilitation experience in the company of fellow patients cemented the concept that group interaction is good for both body and soul, and supports participation in post-prostate cancer treatment support groups), my mindset was one of establishing a program of understanding of and cooperation with my heart. Through diet modifications, exercise, and other strategies, I committed to a partnership for mutual recovery. This was satisfying and comforting to implement. My reactions generated by a prostate cancer diagnosis were totally different. A sense of betrayal and hostility toward the betraying organ were overpowering and were followed by a committed investment to destroy it by whatever means.

The emerging field of psychoneuroimmunology or mind–body interaction lends support to a relationship between mental attitude and physical recovery. Prayer and meditation tend to relax the mind and body, offset stress, and exert many positive influences. They are receiving more attention and study.[20,21] As we learn more about these disciplines or approaches, it becomes evident that responses to therapy, in addition to the application of the traditional modalities of allopathic medicine, depend on the patient's state of mind. The astute diagnostician William Osler recognized this interaction when he stated that it was more important to know about the patient who had the disease than about the disease the patient had. I therefore concur with PHL's comments about exploiting the placebo effect.

FINAL REFLECTIONS AND CONCLUSION (PHL AND PFS)

Although much has already been written about personal reactions to the events surrounding radical prostatectomy, we hope our accounts have been interesting if not informative, perhaps because they were experienced by men who have had long careers treating prostate cancer. In reflecting on our individual and somewhat different situations and reactions, we find several common themes that deserve reemphasis.

FEAR

We were both surprised at the degree of fear we felt despite our familiarity with the disease and its management. The objects of this fear are of course survival, suffering, loss of control, and the morbidities of incontinence and impotence. We experienced them in different proportions, but we were both humbled by their disruptive power.

UNCERTAINTY

Of course, one cause of fear is the uncertainty surrounding the relative effectiveness of the various local treatments. We were both ashamed that our specialty had not worked harder to remedy this deficiency. In fact, we were heavily involved in launching the so-called SPIRIT Trial—a randomized comparison of brachytherapy versus radical prostatectomy for low-risk prostate cancer. We were sobered by the difficulties we had in randomizing these men but learned many things about how to do it, primarily from the Canadians who were actually quite successful. However, in the US we found meager support both among radiotherapists and surgeons for this effort. The trial was eventually dropped by the National Cancer Institute. There was of course great skepticism initially about its feasibility; PFS has already commented on why such trials are particularly difficult, but the greatest barrier was the lack of will and lack of culture in urology to do difficult randomized clinical trials. We believe this lack does not exist as much among practitioners of other cancers and in other diseases. In our opinion this must change if urology is to maintain its place as a leader in prostate cancer management.

QUALITY OF LIFE

Urinary, sexual, and bowel function can be impacted substantially by local therapies. Much has already been written about this subject. However, how an individual patient will react to this alteration will depend on two factors, namely the degree of alteration and the patient's attitude towards it. We believe that there is a general underestimation and reporting of the impact of side effects. The resilience of the human spirit generates an attitude to deal with dysfunction. In this setting physicians need to be wary that they do not become overconfident in their ability to return the patient to his preoperative state. There are some patients for whom this assurance can have a devastating effect postoperatively because of unrealistic expectations.

We have several particular observations about incontinence. First, wearing pads is not as bad as we anticipated once we got used to it. It could be that familiarizing men to wearing them before the surgery may have merit despite its negative connotations. Also, continence after radical prostatectomy is relative and rarely absolutely achieved. Thus, the current quality-of-life surveys may need modification, especially regarding mild incontinence. We believe the use of so-called safety pads, such as "panty liners," should be included in the assessments. This is because most pads can absorb as much as 60 ml with the wearer never really feeling wet, while liners can tolerate little more than a few drops. In our view acceptable continence after radical prostatectomy is no pads or just one liner a day, since the difference between these groups regarding continence is small (or even nonexistent) while "one pad" can cover many different degrees of incontinence, almost all of which are "limiting."

Also, it appears that the precipitating events surrounding what causes mild incontinent episodes vary greatly between men, and often it is not the usual events associated with stress incontinence such as lifting and straining. Some men leak upon wiping after defecation, others do not; some with significant alcohol intake, but not everyone; some with sexual foreplay or just mental anticipation; many but not all when passing flatus. We believe this suggests that men differ significantly in some neurologic aspects of continence, and we need to better understand these differences if we are to continue to strive to understand and improve continence after radical prostatectomy.

ALTERNATIVE/COMPLEMENTARY/INTEGRATIVE MEDICINE AND PATIENT CONTROL

We both learned the power of the complementary/integrative medicine movement. We must work harder to legitimately interface with that world and develop better ways to empower patients to participate substantially in their disease management. If nothing else, the placebo effect must not be labeled as a nefarious phenomenon, but exploited honestly to the patients benefit.

PSA ANXIETY

Of course, PSA anxiety varies among patients and with the severity of disease, but it exists in almost all. This burden is mostly unavoidable and an acceptable price for the value of PSA monitoring, but perhaps it can be lessened by giving the patient more control over when he has the test and more importantly how he gets the result. Waiting for a doctor or nurse to call or return a call produces stress. Perhaps some web-based system allowing more patient control could be developed. Undoubtedly, there are other methods in other areas besides PSA anxiety and alternative/complementary medicine whereby the patient can have more control over the experiences surrounding surgery.

PSA RECURRENCE

The options for treating PSA failure carry as much or even more uncertainty than those involved with the discussion of primary therapy. The patient recognizes that, with failure of primary therapy, there is diminishing likelihood of cure, and his apprehension is heightened. Practitioners should make every effort to couch their explanations and directions with a sense of assurance and hope. To do otherwise would risk the patient's emotional state and compound the negative impact of recurrent disease.

As previously implied, both of us are in retrospect thankful we had this experience because it has made us more empathetic in many ways, some of which are hard to convey. We are certainly more effective (and we think more even handed) at initial orientation. We are better listeners. Also, we both have developed more effective ways of relating to patients during their management. We appreciate more the need to provide hope, to develop trust, and to encourage a sense of control. Finally, we have become more passionate about facilitating progress in prostate cancer diagnosis and cure.

REFERENCES

1. Ercole CJ, Lange PH, Mathisen M, et al. Prostatic specific antigen and prostatic acid phosphatase in the monitoring and staging of patients with prostatic cancer. J Urol 1987;138:1181–1184.

2. Thompson IM, Goodman PJ, Tangen CM, et al. The influence of finasteride on the development of prostate cancer. N Engl J Med 2003;349:215–224.

3. Fang J, Metter EJ, Landis P, et al. Low level of prostate specific antigen predict long-term risk of prostate cancer: results from the Baltimore Longitudinal Study Aging. Urology 2001;58:411–426.

4. National Comprehensive Cancer Network (NCCN). Clinical Practice Guidelines in Oncology. Prostate Cancer Early Detection, vol 1, 2004. www.nccn.org

5. Stamey TA, Yang N, Hay AR, et al. Prostate-specific antigen as a serum marker for adenocarcinoma of the prostate. N Engl J Med 1987;317:909–916.

6. Stamey TA, Caldwell M, McNeal JE, et al. The prostate specific antigen era in the United States is over for prostate cancer: what happened in the last 20 years? J Urol 2004;172:1297–1301.

7. Carter HB, Pearson JD, Metter EJ, et al. Longitudinal evaluation of prostate-specific antigen levels in men with and without prostate disease. JAMA 1992;267:2215–2220.

8. Krumholtz JS, Carvalhal GF, Ramos CG, et al. Prostate-specific antigen cutoff of 2.6 ng/ml for prostate cancer screening is associated with favorable pathologic tumor features. Urology 2002;60:469–474.

9. Sinha B, Haikel G, Lange PH, et al. Transurethral resection of the prostate with local anesthesia in 100 patients. J Urol 1986;135:719–721.

10. Gleave ME, Goldenberg SL, Chin JL, et al. Randomized comparative study of 3 versus 8-month neoadjuvant hormonal therapy before radical prostatectomy: biochemical and pathological effects. J Urol 2001;166:500–506, discussion 506–597.

11. Lange PH. Future studies in localized prostate cancer. What should we think? What can we do? J Urol 1994;152:1932–1938.

12. Taylor JA, Weber W, Standish L, et al. Efficacy and safety of Echinacea in treating upper respiratory tract infections in children: a randomized controlled trial. JAMA 2003;290:2824–2830.

13. Daniels C. Beating cancer: the man who changed medicine. Fortune Mag 2004;150:90–112.

14. Lange PH, Adamec C. Prostate Cancer for Dummies. New York: Wiley Publishing, 2003.

15. Gann PH, Hennekens CH, Stampfer MJ. A prospective evaluation of plasma prostate-specific antigen for detection of prostatic cancer. JAMA 2004;172:1297–1301.

16. Pan CC, Potter S, Partin AW, et al. The prognostic significance of tertiary Gleason patterns of higher grade in radical prostatectomy specimens: a proposal to modify the Gleason grading system. Am J Surg Path 2000;24:563–569.

17. Thompson IM, Goodman PH, Tangen CM, et al. The influence of finateride on the development of prostate cancer. N Engl J Med 2003;349:215–224.

18. Jani AB, Sokoloff M, Shalhav A, et al. Androgen ablation adjuvant to postprostatectomy radiotherapy: complication-adjusted number needed to treat analysis. Urology 2004;64:976–981.

19. Stephenson AJ, Shariat SF, Zelefski MJ, et al. Salvage radiotherapy for recurrent prostate cancer after radical prostatectomy. JAMA 2004;291:1325–1332.

20. Holland JC, Lewis S. The Human Side of Cancer. New York: Harper Collins Publishers, 2000.

21. Dossey L. Healing Words: The Power of Prayer and the Practice of Medicine. New York: Harper Collins Publishers, 1993.

Role of the primary care professional in the care of the patient with prostate cancer: a UK perspective

63

Michael Kirby

There is growing recognition of the importance of the primary care physician in decision-making, diagnosis and management of patients with prostate cancer. This chapter describes the general practitioners' perspective within the UK in the context of international advances. With growing numbers of men diagnosed with this cancer and their increasing life expectancy, there is an increasing need for primary care health providers to be actively involved in shared care programs.

Prostate cancer is one of the most common forms of cancer among men in Western societies and, after lung cancer, is the second most common cause of death in men in the UK, accounting for 20,000 new cancer cases and about 10,000 deaths per year.[1] Prostate cancer is identified microscopically in 30% to 50% of men at postmortem,[2] so clearly some men are dying with, rather than as a result of, prostate cancer. Prostate cancer occurs rarely in men under 50 years of age, but the incidence increases rapidly in men between 60 and 80 years of age. More than 75% of cases are diagnosed in men over 65 years of age.[3]

Prostate cancer has a relatively high survival rate, approximately 50% at 5 years[4]; however, it still rates second in male cancer mortality in both Europe and the US.[5-7] A general practice in the UK with a list size of 7000 patients can expect at least two new diagnoses of prostate cancer each year.[8] Also, with the death rates for competitive mortalities falling and the incidence of clinical prostate cancer rising, the challenge in primary care is to identify and treat the life-threatening lesions in the most effective manner.

The causes of prostate cancer remain largely unknown and no single risk factor can explain the majority of cases. It is known that the tumor requires the presence of testosterone to grow, and the overall risk of developing the disease may be affected by hereditary, race, and environmental and dietary factors.[9]

Survival rates in patients with prostate cancer vary widely according to the stage and grade of disease at diagnosis. Favorable treatment outcomes, including cure or long-term disease-free survival, are more likely if the disease is detected and treated early. Unfortunately, men are notoriously reticent about seeking help for their health problems, especially any they consider embarrassing, and many men do not seek medical attention until the disease has spread beyond the prostate.

Increasing awareness of the symptoms of early prostate cancer, and the importance of seeking medical attention for these symptoms, is a major public health challenge, and those of us working in primary care have an important role to play in this. Men who are at risk of developing prostate cancer are likely to visit their primary healthcare practitioner (PHCP) for routine health checks or for the treatment of chronic conditions such as hypertension. PHCPs are likely to be the first point of contact in the event of any health concerns. They are, therefore, in an ideal situation to be proactive in providing advice about prostate cancer, its prevalence, symptoms, and treatment, as well as being in a prime position to detect the disease in its early stages.

PHCPs will refer patients with suspected prostate cancer to a urologist to confirm diagnosis. Tumor grade, established by biopsy, determines prognosis. If a patient is particularly frail, there are strong contraindications to transurethral biopsy, the prostate-specific antigen (PSA) is less than 10 ng/ml, there are no bothersome symptoms, and life expectancy is less than 10 years, nonreferral is an option. However, if a firm diagnosis would alter management, the patient should be referred.

DIAGNOSTIC DILEMMA

The diagnostic challenge for the PHCP is distinguishing prostate cancer from benign prostatic hyperplasia (BPH), because they commonly coexist. Both the PHCP and patient may initially consider prostate cancer as a cause of the lower urinary tract symptoms (LUTS) and many cancers of the prostate in the UK are diagnosed after presentation with LUTS. Studies have shown minimal association between BPH and cancer.[10-12] A man with obstructive urinary symptoms, such as frequency, hesitancy, and poor stream, is most likely to have BPH or detrusor instability.[13]

Because most men presenting to their PHCP with LUTS will have a rectal examination and their PSA tested, some cancers will be found, even though the tumors in these cases are often not responsible for the symptoms. Having BPH may be protective in that it increases the chances of discovering an incidental tumor.[14]

It is probable that T1 and T2 tumors may be symptomless and BPH is more likely to be the cause of LUTS. However, no urinary symptoms are sufficiently sensitive and specific to enable the PHCP to diagnose prostate cancer from these alone.[15]

It is not possible to distinguish precisely between the tumors that will progress to clinical disease and those that will remain latent for the patient's lifetime. Studies of carcinomas found by chance and diagnosed following transurethral resection of the prostate (TURP) indicate that the average time to progression for T1a tumors (well differentiated, low volume tumors) is 13.5 years, compared to 4.75 years for T1b tumors (moderately or poorly differentiated tumors of high volume). Therefore, a younger man with T1b disease is likely to benefit from more aggressive, potentially curative therapy, whereas an elderly man with T1a tumors may be best managed by watchful waiting alone.[16]

SCREENING

The introduction of screening programs to aid early detection, when the chances of survival are greatest, would have considerable resource and training implications for any healthcare service. To cope with this situation in the UK, the National Screening Committee has recognized that many men are now asking for a PSA test and that previous policies have not given clear guidance on how to respond. As a result health ministers made the decision that men who ask for a PSA test are now eligible to have it performed, together with any subsequent follow-up deemed necessary within the NHS. The National Screening Committee has recommended, therefore, that the first response to a request for a test should be to provide the patient with full information to ensure an informed choice. A website has been developed for those who wish to explore the subject in depth (www.nelh.nhs.uk/psatesting).

The value of screening asymptomatic men for prostate cancer is controversial because there is much discrepancy between the incidence of clinically significant disease and the presence of microscopic disease. In addition, the science for identifying patients in whom disease progression is probable is imprecise. The positive aspects of screening include the availability of simple tests (PSA and digital rectal examination [DRE]), detection of early lesions, reassurance of those screened as negative, and in theory, reduction in prostate cancer morbidity and mortality. The negative aspects of screening are that it may detect slow-growing tumors and some of the cancers detected may have never presented clinically. The efficacy of screening in reducing mortality is not proven, false-positive tests create stress and anxiety, it is expensive and time-consuming, and the transrectal ultrasound (TRUS)-guided biopsy carries a small risk of serious infection.

SCREENING RATE IN ENGLAND AND WALES

There are no routinely collected data in the UK with which to monitor or study the extent to which men are being tested for prostate cancer. An independent investigation of the rate of PSA measurement in primary care in England and Wales was funded by The Policy Research Programme of the Department of Health. The study was conducted by the Cancer Screening Evaluation Unit at The Institute of Cancer Research in association with 28 pathology laboratories and over 300 general practices.[17]

The aim of the study was to investigate the rate of PSA testing in asymptomatic men and to study factors associated with variation in the rate of testing within general practice. Taking part in the study were 443 practices (32% of which were potentially eligible). These practices had a total male population of 1,483,937. Retrospective data on PSA tests were collected from each laboratory's computerized database over a 2-year period, November 19, 1999 to November 18, 2001. Prospective data on PSA tests were collected from each laboratory and general practice from November 19, 2001 to May 31, 2002.

There were a total of 65,258 and 18,545 PSA records in the retrospective and prospective periods, respectively. The overall annual rate of testing in men with no prior diagnosis of prostate cancer was estimated to be 6.0 per 100 men, of which the annual rates of asymptomatic testing, symptomatic testing, and retesting were 2.0, 2.8, and 1.2 per 100 men, respectively, after adjusting for missing values. The rate decreased with increasing social deprivation and increasing proportions of black and Asian populations.

The overall rate of PSA testing increased significantly from 1999 to 2002. The number of PSA requests submitted to the researchers by laboratories (from general practices not participating in the study, but not the total number), rose from 35,695 (November 1999–May 2000) to 50,703 (December 2001–May 2002), a 42% rise.

If the NHS Prostate Cancer Risk Management Programme recommendations were applied, 14% of the asymptomatic tests and 23% of the symptomatic tests would be referred. Because the rate of PSA testing is rising and the benefits of screening are still unclear, monitoring of the workload and costs in primary care must be performed.

Clinical best practice guidelines have been issued to ensure there is a specific quality standard of PSA testing and a systematic and standardized pathway of follow-up available for those whose test result is above the threshold.

PROSTATE CANCER RISK MANAGEMENT PROGRAM (PCRMP)

As part of the NHS prostate cancer program, the prostate cancer risk management program (PCRMP) was officially launched on July 4, 2001 by Yvette Cooper, Health Minister. Because more and more men are requesting PSA tests from their PHCP, the program was initiated to ensure that all men considering a PSA test are given an informed choice and information on the benefits, risks, and limitations of the test. General practitioners, practice nurses, urologists, and pathologists received information packs containing evidence-based material to aid this.

The packs are a useful aid for general practitioners and practice nurses to use in counseling men who do not have symptoms but are worried about prostate cancer. The packs contain a tear-off pad which men can take home to read in their own time, allowing them to make an informed choice about whether or not to proceed with a PSA test. If they decide they would like a test, it is available free on the NHS.

PCRMP NURSE PROJECT

Practice nurses are often ideally placed to advise the often difficult-to-assess older male population through chronic disease clinics. Hence, the program encourages the use of PCRMP packs among practice nurses in primary care. It is hoped that practice nurses will enquire about LUTS, especially urine outflow obstruction, in men over 45 years, exclude urinary tract infection (UTI) (recheck after treatment if positive), and discuss the pros, cons, and limitations of the PSA test using the information pack. The program also includes nurses taking blood from those requesting a PSA test as part of an informed choice, and discussing with them the results of the test, arranging repeat tests if necessary, or a DRE or urgent urologic referral. Practice nurses will also be involved in informing, educating, and advising younger, asymptomatic men about prostate cancer.

DIAGNOSIS

SYMPTOMS

Because prostate tumors are relatively slow growing, men may live with the disease for many years without experiencing any symptoms. Symptoms may only occur once the disease has progressed beyond the periphery of the prostate gland, when the cancer has grown to compress the urethra or invade the sphincter or neurovascular bundle (Table 63.1).[18,19]

HISTORY

The first step in making a diagnosis is taking a good history. Because men may feel embarrassed to raise the issue, early symptoms of prostate disease may be revealed by asking the patient three questions as part of a well-man check:

● Are you bothered by any urinary symptoms?
● Have you noticed any deterioration in your urinary flow?
● Do you get up at night to pass urine?

African men appear to be at highest risk of prostate cancer, whereas Asian men have the lowest incidence. Family history is important as an affected first-degree relative raises the chance of clinical disease by two- to three-fold; if two first-degree relatives are affected, the risk is raised four-fold. Increasing age parallels an increased risk of prostate cancer. Men under 40 years of age have a 1 in 10,000 chance of invasive prostate cancer, whereas in men aged 60 to 79 years the risk rises to 1 in 8.[1]

For the man with LUTS, the initial enquiry may then lead on to a structured approach to investigation and treatment.[20]

INVESTIGATION

Diagnosis of prostate cancer requires a methodical and multitechnical approach. Although not perfect, modern techniques provide useful information that helps distinguish between benign conditions and those more likely to be malignant.

Table 63.1 Symptoms of prostate cancer

Localized or locally advanced	Advanced (additional symptoms)
Prostatism (obstructive or irritative)	Loin pain, anuria and/or uremia due to obstruction of the ureters by lymph nodes
Cystitis	Impotence (neurovascular bundle involvement)
Urinary retention	General malaise or nausea
Hematuria (seminal vesicle involvement)	Bone pain (metastases and/or pathologic fracture)
Painful ejaculation	Spinal cord compression
Reduced ejaculatory volume	Paraplegia secondary to spinal cord compression
Blood in semen	Hypercalcemia (constipation, dehydration, confusion, low mood)
Perineal and suprapubic pain	Thrombosis or phlebitis
	Lymph node enlargement
	Anorexia
	Weight loss
	Incontinence
	Renal failure
	Rectal symptoms, including tenesmus
	Lymphoedema, especially in lower limbs

A general physical examination, including blood pressure measurement, is important in patients with prostatic disease, as men beyond middle age often suffer from other co-morbidities, such as hypertension, diabetes, and chronic obstructive airways disease. The abdomen should be examined in all patients with suspected prostate cancer to detect a palpable bladder or kidneys. Other symptomatic areas should also be examined, such as vertebral tenderness, and a focused neurologic examination will identify most significant neurologic diseases, which may be causing lower urinary tract symptoms. A number of techniques are used to detect the presence of prostate cancer, with the four most common being DRE, PSA, TRUS, and prostate biopsy.

DIGITAL RECTAL EXAMINATION

The DRE is the cornerstone of the physical assessment for prostate disease. It is the most simple and cost-effective method of assessing prostate health and has almost no morbidity. Studies have shown high levels of interobserver agreement for DRE which increases its value in diagnosis.[21,22]

The normal prostate is roughly the size of a chestnut and has the same rubbery consistency as the tip of the nose. BPH results in symmetrical enlargement with little alteration in consistency and preservation of the midline sulcus. Prostate cancer, by contrast, results in stony induration of the prostate that often starts as a palpable nodule and progresses to asymmetry of one lobe of the gland, with eventual involvement and fixation of adjacent structures, especially the seminal vesicles which are normally impalpable (Table 63.2).

PROSTATE-SPECIFIC ANTIGEN TEST

PSA is not a definitive test for prostate cancer and elevated levels may also be found in men with prostatitis and BPH, hence the debate regarding the use of the test as a screening tool. The PSA test can often be justified by the fact that prostate cancer will be treated differently from BPH and in some cases it will lead to the accurate diagnosis and treatment of locally advanced cancers. However, one disadvantage is that, like screening, it may detect early, stage T1 cancers that would not have given rise to symptoms in the patient's lifetime.[24] The use of age-related PSA, free/total PSA, PSA velocity, and PSA density may provide more precise methods to aid diagnosis, but the relative merits of these measures are still debated. However, PSA measurements are useful for monitoring response to treatment and can act as an early warning of tumor recurrence. Patients should receive counseling with respect to the pros and cons of PSA testing, prior to requesting the investigation.

TRANSRECTAL ULTRASONOGRAPHY

This procedure serves several purposes:

- Imaging of the internal structure of the gland and periprostatic tissues and the seminal vesicles.
- Estimation of prostate volume.
- Facilitation and aiming of ultrasound-guided prostate biopsy.

TRUS sometimes allows estimation of the local stage of a prostate cancer because asymmetry and irregularity of the capsule are associated with extracapsular spread of adenocarcinoma,[25] and prostatic blood flow can be

Table 63.2 Clinical parameters that may be assessed by digital rectal examination[23]

Size	Transverse and longitudinal dimension estimated, as well as posterior protrusion. The normal gland is the size of a chestnut (20 g). In benign prostatic hyperplasia, the gland progressively enlarges to the size of a satsuma (>50 g)
Consistency	Slight pressure applied smoothly while gliding over the surface of the gland to detect whether: Smooth or elastic (normal) Hard or woody (may indicate cancer) Tender (suggests prostatitis)
Mobility	Attempts to move the prostate up and down or to the sides. A malignant gland may be fixed to adjacent tissue
Anatomic limits	Finger used to try and reach lateral and cranial borders; medial sulcus palpated carefully. The seminal vesicles should be impalpable; induration of these suggests malignancy

evaluated with color Doppler ultrasound imaging incorporated into TRUS technology. Following the administration of a covering dose of antibiotics, which should be continued for several days, TRUS-guided biopsy of the prostate may be done, usually under local anesthesia.

MANAGEMENT DECISIONS

Knowledge of the treatment options is essential when counseling the patient with prostate cancer, and discussion should include possible side effects and complications.

EARLY DISEASE

The management of early prostate cancer remains controversial and many patients will attend their general practitioner to discuss the therapeutic options. Patients with clinically localized prostate cancer, i.e. biopsy-proven disease with no evidence of extraprostatic extension, should be informed about the advantages and disadvantages of the following options.

WATCHFUL WAITING

Active surveillance is most appropriate for men with low volume, less aggressive disease and in those with a life expectancy of less than 10 years. Regular PSA checks are recommended and active treatment initiated if the disease progresses.

RADICAL PROSTATECTOMY

This is considered by many to be the gold standard of treatment. Radical prostatectomy involves the removal of the entire prostate gland. Provided that all cancer tissue is excised, and all surgical margins, seminal vesicles, and lymph nodes are clear, then life expectancy is equivalent to that of an age-matched individual who has never had cancer. Side effects include a low risk

(<2–3%) of stress incontinence and a higher risk (>50%) of erectile dysfunction. However, both these problems improve with time and can often be treated effectively. If the entire prostate and all cancer has been excised the postoperative PSA should fall to less than 0.1 ng/ml, which aids follow-up and early identification of tumor recurrence. More recently, laparoscopic radical prostatectomy has been developed which, in expert hands, results in less bleeding and shorter hospital stays.

EXTERNAL BEAM RADIOTHERAPY

External beam radiotherapy (EBRT) is an effective form of therapy in early disease. Neoadjuvant androgen ablation, usually with a luteinizing hormone-releasing hormone (LHRH) analog, enhances results. Side effects include proctitis and rectal bleeding due to the anterior rectal wall being included in the treatment field. However, side effects may be reduced by focusing more accurately on the prostate with the use of conformal technology.

BRACHYTHERAPY

This involves the transperineal implantation of radioactive seeds into the prostate under light anesthesia.[26] LUTS may worsen for some time following this procedure due to swelling of the gland, so it should be used with caution in patients with preexisting severe bladder outflow obstruction. Brachytherapy may be used in conjunction with EBRT in patients who are considered at high risk of disease recurrence. Men who have previously undergone TURP are generally not suitable for brachytherapy because the seeds are not satisfactorily retained in the prostate.

CRYOTHERAPY

Growing in popularity but still regarded as experimental, so-called third-generation cryotherapy involves the insertion of between 10 and 20 needles into the prostate and the creation of an ice ball within the gland.[27]

ADVANCED DISEASE

Patients are considered to have advanced disease if they have prostate cancer involving lymph nodes, other soft tissues or the skeleton. In these cases cure is not possible but androgen withdrawal will, in most cases, result in a remission that may be maintained for 24 to 36 months, depending on the extent of the metastatic burden at presentation.

A proportion of patients with prostate cancer present with extraprostatic extension, but no evidence of distant metastases. Radical surgery is inappropriate because of the high local and distant recurrence rates. Radiotherapy is usually the preferred treatment option.

TREATMENT OF METASTASES

The proportion of patients with localized disease at the time of diagnosis is now rising, probably as a result of PSA testing. Depriving the cancer cells of the androgens necessary for their growth can be accomplished by a variety of means, both medical and surgical.

Four antiandrogenic agents have been extensively evaluated clinically for the treatment of metastatic prostate cancer: cyproterone acetate, flutamide, nilutamide, and bicalutamide. The addition of such an agent to achieve maximal androgen blockade may possibly increase both the time to disease progression and provide a survival advantage in some patients with good performance status and less advanced metastatic disease, although this is still controversial. Some aspects of sexual function may be preserved with the use of antiandrogens such as bicalutamide. However, the Committee on Safety of Medicines recommends that bicalutamide is not used as a primary treatment of clinically organ confined in prostate cancer. This is because data has suggested a possible increased mortality rate in men with localized prostate cancer treated with bicalutamide alone compared to placebo (5-year mortality 25.5% vs 20.5% with placebo; hazard ratio 1.2; 95% CI 1.0–1,5).[28]

Androgen ablation can be achieved either by bilateral orchidectomy or the use of depot LHRH analog.

POTENTIAL SIDE EFFECTS

Potential side effects of prostate cancer treatments include:

- Complete or partial loss of sexual functioning.
- Erectile dysfunction.
- Bladder problems.
- Bowel problems.
- Reduction of bone mineral density.
- Change in body shape/weight gain.
- Breast enlargement/tenderness.
- Hot flushes.
- Lethargy.

PALLIATIVE CARE

Considerable distress is experienced by the majority of cancer patients and their carers before death.[29] This aspect is often unrecognized or overlooked by services focusing on the terminal phase of the illness and it is important to identify and alleviate this suffering as much as possible.

One important initiative is gaining momentum within primary care. The Gold Standards framework is a resource for organizing proactive palliative care in the community. It is supported by funding from the National Lottery, Cancer Services Collaborative, and Macmillan Cancer Relief.[30] The framework provides a detailed guide to providing patient-centered care and facilitates effective, holistic care in the community. Other recently initiated mechanisms for the improvement of primary palliative care include the training of general practitioners with a special interest in palliative care and the new end of life initiative in England to improve palliative care provision.[31]

Because primary care teams often know patients over long periods of time, they may be in a prime position, using chronic disease or cancer registers, to identify patients who would benefit from an early palliative care approach. PHCPs may be able to identify such patients by asking themselves one simple question, "Would I be surprised if this patient were to die in the next 12 months?"[32] This proactive approach in the early identification of such patients would facilitate active treatment and patient-centered support, through a team with which many patients and their carers establish a valued long-term relationship. For such an approach to be initiated, the goals of care need to be established and agreed, and management plans adjusted to suit the patent's specific situation. The effective control of symptoms and the maintenance of quality of life must be prioritized.

LOOKING TO THE FUTURE

The optimal management of prostate cancer now requires care to be shared between urologist and family practitioner. The initial treatment strategy should be devised by a specialist on the basis of tissue diagnosis and careful staging. Radiotherapy or prostatectomy are obviously the province of the hospital-based team but the initial diagnosis and follow-up may be the joint responsibility of the urologist and family practitioner. Metastatic disease is increasingly managed by monthly or 3-monthly depo injections of LHRH analogs, and there is now evidence to support the early introduction of endocrine therapy at the time of diagnosis rather than waiting for symptoms to develop.[33]

In future it may be possible to predict a subgroup of patients in whom total androgen blockade rather than antiandrogen therapy may offer a definite survival advantage. Newer and more effective first- and second-line curative pharmacotherapies also need to be developed. These challenges may be added to the many others that must be overcome to reduce the morbidity and mortality of this prevalent and insidious disease. Measures for the future might include:

- Early detection—using more accurate tumor markers to improve the ability of clinicians to distinguish early prostate cancer from BPH.
- Better staging—enhanced imaging and molecular staging.
- Prognostic indicators—molecular prognostic indicators, e.g. E-cadherin expression, are currently the subject of intense research.
- New therapies—laparoscopic radical prostatectomy, cryosurgery, high-intensity focused ultrasound, specific inhibitors of growth factors, and possibly gene therapy.

Antiprostate cancer vaccines are also now a not too distant prospect. Eventually, oncogenes could be neutralized or deleted or tumor suppressor genes reinserted by any of the several vector methods currently under development.

REFERENCES

1. Office for National Statistics. Registrations of cancer diagnosed in 1994–1997, England and Wales. Health Statistics Quarterly 2000;7:71–82.
2. Selby M. Prostate cancer. Urology Update 2004;24 Sept:110–117.
3. Reis LAG, Eisner MP, Kosary CL, et al (eds). Seer Cancer Statistics Review 1973–1998, Bethesda, MD: National Cancer Institute, 2001.
4. Quinn M, Babb P, Brock A, et al. Cancer trends in England and Wales 1950–1999. London: The Stationary Office, 2001. http://www.statistics.gov.uk/statbase.
5. Lu Yao GL, Greenberg ER. Changes in prostate cancer incidence and treatment in the USA. Lancet 1994;343:251–254.
6. Edwards B, Howe H, Reis L, et al. Annual report to the nation on the status of cancer, 1973–1999 featuring implications of age and aging on US cancer burden. Cancer 2002;94:2766–2792.
7. Chu K, Tarone RE, Freeman H. Trends in prostatic cancer mortality among black men and white men in the United States. Cancer 2003;97:1507–1516.
8. Gronberg H. Prostate cancer epidemiology. Lancet 2003;361:859–364.
9. Steinberg GD, Carter BS, Beaty TH, et al. Family history and the risk of prostate cancer. Prostate 1990;17:337–347.
10. Guess HA. Benign prostatic hyperplasia and prostate cancer. Epidemiol Rev 2001;23:152–158.
11. Coley CM, Barry MJ, Fleming C, et al. Early detection of prostate cancer. Part II: Estimating the risks, benefits and costs. American College of Physicians. Ann Intern Med 1997;126:468–479.
12. Greenwald P, Kirmss V, Polan AK, et al. Cancer of the prostate among men with benign prostatic hyperplasia. J Natl Cancer Inst 1974;53:335–340.
13. Verhamme K, Dieleman J, Bleumink G, et al. Incidence and prevalence of lower urinary tract symptoms suggestive of benign prostatic hyperplasia in primary care—The TRIUMPH Project. Eur Urol 2002;42:232–328.
14. Hamilton W, Sharp D. Symptomatic diagnosis of prostate cancer in primary care: a structured review. Br J Gen Pract 2004;54:617–621.
15. Department of Health. Referral Guidelines for Suspected Cancer. London: Department of Health, 2000. http://www.dh.gov.uk/assetRoot/04/01/44/21/04014421.pdf.
16. Kirby RS, Oesterling JE, Denis LJ. Prostate Cancer: Fast Facts. Oxford: Health Press, 1996.
17. Melia J, Moss S, John L, and contributors in the participating laboratories. Rates of prostate specific antigen testing in general practice in England and Wales in asymptomatic and symptomatic patients: A cross sectional study. BJU Int 2004;94:51–56.
18. Horwich A, Waxman J, Abel P, et al. Tumours of the prostate. In: Souhami R, Tannock I, Hohenberger P, Horiot JC (eds): The Oxford Textbook of Oncology, 2nd ed. Oxford. Oxford University Press, 2001, pp 1939–1971.
19. Guess HA. Benign prostatic hyperplasia and prostate cancer. Epidemiol Rev 2001;23:152–158.
20. Speakman M, Kirby R, Joyce S, et al. Guidelines for the primary care management of male lower urinary tract symptoms. BJU Int 2004;93:985–990.
21. Herranz Amo F, Verdu Tartajo F, Diez Cordero JM, et al. Variability of rectal examination of the prostate among various groups of observers. Actas Urol Esp 1996;20:873–876.
22. Roehrborn CG, Sech S, Montoya J, et al. Interexaminer reliability and validity of a three-dimensional model to assess prostate volume by digital rectal examination. Urology 2001;57:1087–1092.
23. Kirby R, Fitzpatrick J, Kirby M, et al. Shared Care for Prostatic Diseases, 2nd ed. ISIS Medical Media, Oxford, 2000.
24. Etzioni R, Cha R, Feuer EJ, et al. Asymptomatic incidence and duration of prostate cancer. Am J Epidemiol 1998;148:775–785.
25. Ohori M, Egawa S, Shinohara K, et al. Detection of microscopic extracapsular extension prior to radical prostatectomy for clinically localised prostate cancer. Br J Urol 1994;74:72–79.
26. Ragde H, Elgamal A, Snow PB, et al. Ten year disease free survival after transperineal sonography-guided iodine 125 brachytherapy with or without 45 Gray external beam irradiation in the treatment of patients with clinically localised, low to high Gleason grade prostate carcinoma. Cancer 1998;83:989–1001.
27. Donnelly BJ, Saliken JC, Ernst DS, et al. Prospective trial of cryosurgical ablation of the prostate: 5 year results. Urology 2002;60:645–649.
28. Committee on Safety of Medicines. Casodex 150 mg (bicalutamide): no longer indicated for treatment of localised prostate cancer. http://www.mca.gov.uk/ourwork/monitorsafequalmed/safetymessages/casodex.
29. Murray SA, Kendall M, Boyd K, et al. Exploring the spiritual needs of people dying of lung cancer or heart failure: a prospective qualitative interview study of patients and their carers. Palliat Med 2004;18:39–45.
30. Thomas K. Caring for the Dying at Home: Companions on a Journey. Oxford: Radcliffe Medical Press, 2003.
31. Murray SA, Boyd K, Sheikh A, et al. Developing primary palliative care. BMJ 2004;329:1056–1057.
32. Lynn J. Serving patients who may die soon and their families: the role of hospice and other services. JAMA 2001;285:925–932.
33. The Medical Research Council Prostate Cancer Working Party Investigators Group. Immediate versus deferred treatment for advanced prostate cancer. Initial results of the Medical Research Council Trial. Br J Urol 1997;79:235–246.

Natural history and expectant management of prostate cancer

64

Jonathan R Osborn, Gerald W Chodak

INTRODUCTION

Adenocarcinoma of the prostate is a growing health problem in the US, and is now the most common solid tumor in adult men. Unlike most malignancies, there is a wide disparity between the prevalence and mortality of this disease; prostate cancer is present in approximately 30% of 50-year-old men, and over 50% of 80-year-old men,[1] yet only a small percentage of men actually die from the disease.[2,3] Although one in every six men living in the US will be diagnosed with prostate cancer during his lifetime,[4] the risk of dying is only 3%.[2] In 2004, the number of prostate cancer-related deaths is predicted to be 30,000.[4]

The advent of the prostate-specific antigen (PSA) blood test, combined with the increased testing of asymptomatic men and the use of more core biopsies in each patient, has increased the chances of finding clinically insignificant cancers. Up to a third of men in PSA-screened populations, diagnosed with nonpalpable prostate cancer and undergoing radical prostatectomy, have small (<0.5 cm^3) low-grade (Gleason 6 or less) tumors.[5,6] Such tumors are associated with a long natural history and are unlikely to affect the lifespan of select older men.[7] The median time from diagnosis to death from prostate cancer for men diagnosed with nonpalpable disease in the pre-PSA era was approximately 17 years.[7] Since the US male life-expectancy at 65 years of age is estimated at 15 years, it is unlikely that aggressive treatment is going to add significantly to the average lifespan of most men.[8] Thus, PSA overdetects prostate cancer and may subject many patients to the morbidity of treatment with only a small, if any, measurable gain. The challenge is to identify those patients who harbor non-life-threatening tumors and those whose tumor is progressing rapidly.

Because of the unusual biology of prostate cancer, *watchful waiting* (also called active surveillance or expectant management) has received increased attention as an option for patients with early-stage disease. Traditionally, this strategy followed patients with small volume low-grade prostate cancer without immediate local treatment. If and when progression occurred, androgen ablation was administered. Clearly, watchful waiting was not a curative therapy; however, the risks from this therapy are more than offset by avoiding the complications that result from definitive therapies.

The advent of PSA, however, has led to a change in watchful waiting. Now patients are followed and monitored to identify those cases with early progression. When that occurs, watchful waiting is abandoned and local therapy often is instituted. Men with slowly progressive disease continue on watchful waiting. To understand why conservative therapy is appropriate for the management of some patients, the outcomes from this approach must be reviewed.

RESULTS OF CONSERVATIVE THERAPY

One of the earliest reports on conservative management was published in 1969 by Barnes.[9] He reviewed the outcomes of patients presenting to his institution between 1930 and 1958 and identified 86 patients who were treated conservatively and who were thought to have localized disease based on digital rectal examination (DRE). Only 50% of these patients survived 10 years and only 30% survived 15 years. Barnes noted that over two-thirds of these patients died from competing medical conditions rather than prostate cancer. He recognized that concurrent medical conditions were equally important as tumor stage and grade when selecting therapy and that prostate cancer often was a slowly progressive disease, which could recur more than 10 years after seemingly curative treatment. Barnes concluded that "conservative therapy" was indicated for patients with an expected survival of 10 years or less.

From 1970 to 1990, several cohort series were published on the outcome from watchful waiting. In 1994, Chodak et al[10] assembled a cohort of 828 patients from six of these reports that included patients from throughout Europe, North America, and Israel.[10] They showed that patients with poorly differentiated carcinomas have a 10-fold greater risk of death from prostate cancer compared to men with well-differentiated disease. Specifically, men with poorly differentiated prostate cancer had a 10-year cause-specific survival of only 34% compared to men with well- or moderately-differentiated disease, who have a cause-specific survival of 87%. These findings demonstrated that for the latter group of men, the outcomes from watchful waiting might not differ significantly from aggressive therapy. At the very least, watchful waiting should be offered to patients at the time a well- or moderately-differentiated prostate cancer is diagnosed.

In 1997, Lu-Yao and Yao[11] evaluated long-term overall survival and cause-specific survival for patients treated with surgery, radiation, and conservative management. Using the Surveillance Epidemiology and End Results database, the outcome of 59,876 patients diagnosed with prostate cancer over a 10-year period was reviewed retrospectively. Patients had been treated according to the preferences of the physicians and patients. The authors concluded that the overall survival for men with well- or moderately-differentiated cancers did not differ substantially from the survival observed for men treated by radiation therapy. Small differences were seen when watchful waiting was compared to radical prostatectomy; however, this could be explained by methodologic differences—the tumor grade for men treated by watchful waiting or radiation therapy was based on the initial biopsy, whereas the tumor grade for the surgery patients was based on the final pathology. Studies have clearly demonstrated that biopsy grade underestimates actual tumor grade. As a result, some men in the surgery group with a biopsy showing moderately-differentiated cancer would have been moved to the higher grade group, thus making the survival for those with moderately-differentiated cancers appear better.

To date, only one sizeable prospective study has compared the outcomes of patients managed aggressively to those managed by watchful waiting. Holmberg et al[12] performed a prospective randomized trial comparing watchful waiting (followed by palliative therapy) and radical prostatectomy. A total of 675 patients were enrolled in 14 Scandinavian hospitals between 1988 and 1998. Patients had T1B, T1C or T2 disease that was judged to be well- or moderately-differentiated at enrollment. All patients had a PSA less than 50 ng/ml and a negative baseline bone scan. Patients were randomized to radical prostatectomy or watchful waiting. Recommended treatment for local progression was transurethral resection of the prostate in the watchful waiting arm, and androgen ablation in the radical prostatectomy arm. The primary outcome measure was disease-specific mortality, with overall mortality, time to metastasis, and local progression being secondary endpoints. A blinded independent endpoint committee determined cause of death, with prostate cancer deaths being autopsy diagnosed or associated with evidence of progressive metastatic disease, with a mean duration of follow-up of 6.2 years. The authors reported a statistically significant decreased risk of death from prostate cancer in patients treated with radical prostatectomy versus those followed expectantly (4.6% vs 8.9% respectively, $P = 0.02$). Additionally, the risk of metastases was significantly increased in the watchful waiting group. The overall survival, however, was not statistically different between these two groups. A more recent follow-up shows a small but significant difference in overall survival at 10 years and a difference in cancer-specific survival holding at approximately 5%.

One potential problem with this study is the unequal distribution of higher grade tumors with 13 more men in the watchful waiting group having Gleason 7 disease. Given the worse natural history of these men compared with Gleason 5 or 6 cancers, the true difference in survival actually might be smaller. A second problem is that the average PSA at diagnosis was substantially higher than found for patients in the US, where the average PSA is less than 10 ng/ml at diagnosis. Had patients with PSA levels similar to those diagnosed in the US been enrolled, the difference also would have been smaller, at least for the same, relatively short follow-up. A third problem is that the primary endpoint is of some concern, as discussed by Alibhai and Klotz.[13] They argue that determination of cause of death is difficult, even by an independent, blinded committee, and that if the six excess noncancer deaths in the surgery arm are added to the 16 prostate cancer deaths, then the benefit from surgery is attenuated.

The advent of PSA testing appears to have advanced the date of diagnosis of prostate cancer (the "lead time") by 5 years or more, and the onset of secondary treatment by a similar amount.[14–16] Therefore, it is reasonable to suggest that our current knowledge base underestimates rather than overestimates a man's survival, if diagnosed with localized prostate cancer by PSA and managed by watchful waiting.

IMPACT OF COMPETING MEDICAL HAZARDS

Albertsen et al[17,18] have written extensively on the impact of concomitant medical conditions on survival. They showed that men with well-differentiated disease managed by watchful waiting experienced little if any loss of life compared to men with no evidence of prostate cancer. In contrast, men with moderately-differentiated prostate cancer lost an average of 4 to 5 years of life, while men with poorly-differentiated disease lost approximately 6 to 8 years of life, in comparison to age-matched controls. A multiple stepwise regression analysis in men treated conservatively demonstrated that the grade of tumor was the most powerful predictor of survival, followed by co-morbidities. Among all men diagnosed with clinically localized disease, 40% died of competing medical conditions rather than prostate cancer within 10 years of diagnosis.[17,18]

IDENTIFYING MEN FOR DELAYED LOCAL THERAPY

Given the variable natural history of prostate cancer, one of the most important questions to answer is, which tumors will progress slowly and which will progress rapidly? One approach is to use changes in PSA and the findings on prostate biopsy. In 1994 Epstein et al[6] retrospectively examined the use of PSA criteria and needle biopsy findings to predict small volume tumors in patients with clinical T1C prostate cancer. Using PSA density and identifying favorable (Gleason 6 or less, fewer than three cores containing cancer, ≤50% of any core involving cancer) and adverse needle biopsy findings (Gleason score 7 or higher, more than two cores containing cancer, >50% cancer involvement in any core), this study correlated the pathologic extent of disease to already existing pretreatment parameters. Seventy-nine percent of patients with a PSA density less than 0.15 ng/ml/cm^3 and favorable needle biopsy findings had a tumor of total volume 0.5 cm^3 or smaller, which was not of high grade and was organ confined. In contrast, 83% of men with a PSA density of 0.15 ng/ml/cm^3 or greater or adverse findings on needle biopsy had tumors of volume 0.5 cm^3, or which were high grade or nonorgan confined. A subsequent prospective study validated these parameters as accurate predictors of tumor volume.[19]

Choo et al[20] described PSA doubling time as a useful predictor of progression to guide treatment intervention for patients managed with watchful waiting. While PSA doubling time varies wildly between patients, a doubling time of less than 2 years shows a high risk of local progression, with a doubling time of 3 years being the suggested threshold for initiation of curative treatment. El-Geneidy et al[21] confirmed the predictive power of PSA doubling time, and also found that age and percentage positive biopsy cores were independent predictors of delayed therapy.

The dedifferentiation of prostate cancer grade with time in men undergoing watchful waiting has recently been studied.[22] Almost 13% showed a significant change in grade from Gleason 6 or less to Gleason 7 or more. It is interesting to note that in all but one of the upgraded cases the change occurred within 15 months of the initial biopsy, with no difference in initial PSA level, percent-free PSA or PSA density and velocity between the upgrading and grade-stable groups. Therefore, it is possible that these tumors did not progress, but that the area of higher grade was missed in the initial biopsy. One conclusion from these data is that men with a Gleason 6 cancer who are considering conservative therapy might undergo a repeat biopsy to rule out higher grade disease that might have been missed on the original biopsy.

Taking a delayed approach initially, Choo et al[23] reported that 23% of patients received delayed curative therapy after a median follow-up of 2.4 years. Other investigators reported somewhat lower incidences of such therapy in contemporary watchful-waiting patients,[24–26] although the follow-up was less than 2 years. Zeitman et al[27] reported 57% of such patients receiving curative therapy within 5 years and 74% within 7 years (median follow-up 3.4 years). They also commented that 81% of patients perceived the therapy was initiated by physicians, due to increasing PSA or the presence of a nodule, while physicians believed that they advocated treatment in only 24% of cases. This might be a function of anxiety regarding sequential PSA levels ("PSA-itis").[28] Each of these approaches has some merit, but the optimal approach for selecting men for delayed therapy has not yet been defined.

COUNSELING PATIENTS ABOUT WATCHFUL WAITING

After all the benefits and risks have been presented, a common question asked by patients is, "What would you do if you were in my position?" Not surprisingly urologists would mostly select prostatectomy, and radiation oncologists would select radiation therapy.[29] Both physicians and patients should be aware of this possible bias when they are being counseled about therapy. Ultimately, the patient should make decisions by prioritizing his goals, with help from the physician to ensure he is in possession of accurate information and has no misconceptions.

All patients should understand that watchful waiting is an option that has its own set of risks and benefits, which are different from those for radiation therapy or radical prostatectomy. Clearly, if a patient wishes to maximize his survival and minimize the chance that prostate cancer will cause him pain or suffering, then aggressive therapy should be selected. On the other hand, if the patient views the potential complication rates as too high, or the relative gains from treatment as too low to warrant the risk of the various complications, or if he wants to maximize his immediate quality of life even if it potentially means a shorter survival, then watchful waiting is the best choice.

The two most important factors for a patient to consider when making his decision are the grade of tumor and his anticipated lifespan. Watchful waiting poses the least risk to a man with a well- or moderately-differentiated palpable tumor and a life-expectancy of 10 years or less. For a man whose cancer was detected by PSA (stage T1C) and is nonpalpable, watchful waiting may be equally reasonable, even if his life-expectancy approaches 15 years due to the lead time (the time between screen detection and predicted clinical detection) of diagnosis associated with this test. Essentially, watchful waiting represents a throw of the dice with the degree of risk dependent on the growth rate of the tumor and the lifespan of the patient, neither of which can be reliably predicted for an individual. In the end, the decision for the patient is about balancing risk versus benefit.

THE FUTURE FOR WATCHFUL WAITING WITH DELAYED THERAPY

As the average age of the population gradually increases, it is likely that watchful waiting with delayed curative therapy will become an increasingly important option for patients. It is generally assumed that the rate of PSA increase remains stable over time in men with prostate cancer; however, it has been clearly documented that some patients have sudden and rapid increases in PSA after long periods of stability (PSA acceleration). It is unknown at which stage in the natural history of prostate cancer these accelerations occur. Perhaps acceleration is related either to a change in tumor grade or the growth of tumor beyond the prostate. Studying the long-term outcome of patients after delayed therapy and the value of periodic repeat biopsies will be important in furthering our understanding of prostate cancer.

CONCLUSION

With the recent dramatic increase in the detection of prostate cancer, there has been the enormous challenge to recommend the best treatment for patients with localized prostate cancer. This challenge has been difficult because of the absence of well-conducted comparative trials. Since the primary goal of the urologist is to "cure" prostate cancer and prolong life, the concept of watchful waiting seems somewhat inappropriate. However, few other diseases have treatments that can so negatively impact on a man's daily quality of life. In addition, the natural history of this cancer, in contrast to many others, does not invariably lead to metastasis or death during the normal lifespan of most patients. Therefore, many patients may wish to maximize their quality of life rather than their duration of survival. This choice depends on the probability of the good and bad outcomes that are possible with each treatment option. Watchful waiting is a reasonable option for many patients. The key is to determine when cancers are becoming life-threatening, and to intervene in these, while observing the remainder. Physicians would do well to be mindful of Hippocrates' maxim, *primum non nocere* (first, do no harm). Ultimately, it is the patient's choice to make, with help and unbiased guidance from his physician.

REFERENCES

1. Scardino PT. Early detection of prostate cancer. Urol Clin North Am 1989;16:635–655.
2. Sakr WA, Grignon DJ. Prostate cancer: indicators of aggressiveness. Eur Urol 1997;32(Suppl 3):15–23.
3. Franks LM. Proceedings: etiology, epidemiology, and pathology of prostatic cancer. Cancer 1973;32:1092–1095.
4. Jemal A, Murray T, Samuels A, et al. Cancer statistics, 2003. CA Cancer J Clin 2003;53:5–26.
5. Humphrey PA, Keetch DW, Smith DS, et al. Prospective characterization of pathological features of prostatic carcinomas detected via serum prostate specific antigen based screening. J Urol 1996;155:816–820.
6. Epstein JI, Walsh PC, Carmichael M, et al. Pathologic and clinical findings to predict tumor extent of nonpalpable (stage T1c) prostate cancer. JAMA 1994;271:368–374.
7. Horan AH, McGehee M. Mean time to cancer-specific death of apparently clinically localized prostate cancer: policy implications for threshold ages in prostate-specific antigen screening and ablative therapy. BJU Int 2000;85:1063–1066.
8. Minino AM, Arias E, Kochanek KD, et al. Deaths: final data for 2000. Natl Vital Stat Rep 2002;50:1–119.
9. Barnes RW. Survival with conservative therapy. JAMA 1969;210:331–332.
10. Chodak GW, Thisted RA, Gerber GS, et al. Results of conservative management of clinically localized prostate cancer. N Engl J Med 1994;330:242–248.
11. Lu-Yao GL, Yao SL. Population-based study of long-term survival in patients with clinically localised prostate cancer. Lancet 1997;349:906–910.
12. Holmberg L, Bill-Axelson A, Helgesen F, et al. A randomized trial comparing radical prostatectomy with watchful waiting in early prostate cancer. N Engl J Med 2002;347:781–789.
13. Alibhai SM, Klotz LH. A systematic review of randomized trials in localized prostate cancer. Can J Urol 2004;11:2110–2117.
14. Draisma G, Boer R, Otto SJ, et al. Lead times and overdetection due to prostate-specific antigen screening: estimates from the European Randomized Study of Screening for Prostate Cancer. J Natl Cancer Inst 2003;95:868–878.
15. Gann PH, Hennekens CH, Stampfer MJ. A prospective evaluation of plasma prostate-specific antigen for detection of prostatic cancer. JAMA 1995;273:289–294.

16. Tornblom M, Eriksson H, Franzen S, et al. Lead time associated with screening for prostate cancer. Int J Cancer 2004;108:122–129.

17. Albertsen PC, Fryback DG, Storer BE, et al. Long-term survival among men with conservatively treated localized prostate cancer. JAMA 1995;274:626–631.

18. Albertsen PC, Fryback DG, Storer BE, et al. The impact of co-morbidity on life expectancy among men with localized prostate cancer. J Urol 1996;156:127–132.

19. Carter HB, Sauvageot J, Walsh PC, et al. Prospective evaluation of men with stage T1C adenocarcinoma of the prostate. J Urol 1997;157:2206–2209.

20. Choo R, DeBoer G, Klotz L, et al. PSA doubling time of prostate carcinoma managed with watchful observation alone. Int J Radiat Oncol Biol Phys 2001;50:615–620.

21. El-Geneidy M, Garzotto M, Panagiotou I, et al. Delayed therapy with curative intent in a contemporary prostate cancer watchful-waiting cohort. BJU Int 2004;93:510–515.

22. Epstein JI, Walsh PC, Carter HB. Dedifferentiation of prostate cancer grade with time in men followed expectantly for stage T1c disease. J Urol 2001;166:1688–1691.

23. Choo R, Klotz L, Danjoux C, et al. Feasibility study: watchful waiting for localized low to intermediate grade prostate carcinoma with selective delayed intervention based on prostate specific antigen, histological and/or clinical progression. J Urol 2002;167:1664–1669.

24. Carter HB, Walsh PC, Landis P, et al. Expectant management of nonpalpable prostate cancer with curative intent: preliminary results. J Urol 2002;167:1231–1234.

25. Koppie TM, Grossfeld GD, Miller D, et al. Patterns of treatment of patients with prostate cancer initially managed with surveillance: results from The CaPSURE database. Cancer of the Prostate Strategic Urological Research Endeavor. J Urol 2000;164:81–88.

26. McLaren DB, McKenzie M, Duncan G, et al. Watchful waiting or watchful progression?: Prostate specific antigen doubling times and clinical behavior in patients with early untreated prostate carcinoma. Cancer 1998;82:342–348.

27. Zeitman AL, Thakral H, Wilson L, et al P. Conservative management of prostate cancer in the prostate specific antigen era: the incidence and time course of subsequent therapy. J Urol 2001;166:1702–1706.

28. Lofters A, Juffs HG, Pond GR, Tannock IF. "PSA-itis": knowledge of serum prostate specific antigen and other causes of anxiety in men with metastatic prostate cancer. J Urol 2002;168:2516–2520.

29. Moore MJ, O'Sullivan B, Tannock IF. How expert physicians would wish to be treated if they had genitourinary cancer. J Clin Oncol 1988;6:1736–1745.

Clinical trials comparing expectant management to definitive treatment of prostate cancer

65

Chris Parker

INTRODUCTION

For cancers of other primary sites, it would be unethical to even contemplate the idea of clinical trials comparing expectant management with definitive treatment. Expectant management of most cancers would lead to certain disease progression, disfigurement, and death. Prostate cancer is different. While prostate cancer *can* follow an aggressive and ultimately fatal course, similar to that of other cancers, a significant proportion of cases will behave in an indolent fashion, and have no effect either on health or longevity. For these patients, definitive treatment is both unnecessary and potentially harmful. Furthermore, there has been much uncertainty as to whether definitive treatment of the more aggressive, potentially lethal, prostate cancers does in fact prolong survival.

It is for these reasons that, in the case of prostate cancer, comparison between expectant management and definitive treatment is a vitally important issue. Given that it is so important, it is unfortunate that there is such a paucity of quality data comparing the outcome of expectant management with that of definitive treatment. Furthermore, almost all available data relate to cases typical of the pre-prostate-specific antigen (PSA) era, and such data may not be generalizable to contemporary, PSA screen-detected disease.

RETROSPECTIVE COMPARISONS OF EXPECTANT MANAGEMENT AND DEFINITIVE TREATMENT

Retrospective comparisons between expectant management and definitive treatment are of very limited value,

given the possibility (indeed the likelihood) of significant confounding variables. That said, two retrospective comparisons merit consideration, not least because they generate the hypothesis that the magnitude of any benefit for definitive treatment will vary with tumor grade.

The population-based study of outcome from the SEER database was based on data for 59,876 cancer-registry patients aged between 50 and 79 years who had clinically localized prostate cancer diagnosed between 1982 and 1992.[1] Overall and disease-specific survival were analyzed by grade and by type of treatment (Table 65.1). By the intention-to-treat approach, 10-year prostate cancer-specific survival for grade 1 cancer was 94% (95% CI, 91–95) after prostatectomy, 90% (87–92) after radiotherapy, and 93% (91–94) after conservative management. The corresponding survival figures for grade 2 cancers were 87% (85–89), 76% (72–79), and 77% (74–80); those for grade 3 cancer were 67% (62–71), 53% (47–58), and 45% (40–51).

It is no surprise that disease-specific mortality increases with tumor grade. Nor is it any surprise, given the likely differences in co-morbidities, quite apart from

Table 65.1 Actuarial 10-year disease-specific mortality (DSM) in men with localized prostate cancer by type of treatment according to the SEER population-based retrospective study.[1]

	Radical prostatectomy		Watchful waiting	
	n	10-year DSM (%)	n	10-year DSM (%)
Grade 1	3854	6 (5–9)	9804	7 (6–9)
Grade 2	14,287	13 (11–15)	6198	23 (20–26)
Grade 3	5133	33 (29–38)	2236	55 (49–60)

anything else, that survival following definitive treatment appears better than that for watchful waiting. It is, however, interesting to note that the apparent benefit of radical treatment varies markedly with tumor grade. The absolute difference in 10-year disease-specific survival between radical prostatectomy and watchful waiting was 1%, 10%, and 22% for grade 1, 2 and 3 disease, respectively. Although the watchful waiting patients no doubt differ markedly from the radical prostatectomy patients in terms of co-morbidity as well as in other important respects, it is at least arguable that such differences would be similar regardless of cancer grade. Thus, this study generates the hypothesis that the magnitude of any benefit for definitive treatment will vary with tumor grade.

This possibility is supported by another retrospective comparison of expectant management and definitive treatment. Albertsen et al[2] reported a watchful waiting series that has been held in high regard on account of its size, the maturity of the outcome data, and the use of centralized pathology review with the Gleason scoring system. The Albertsen series included men aged 55 to 74 years, diagnosed with prostate cancer between 1971 and 1984, who were identified from the Connecticut Tumor Registry. Cases were excluded if they were known to have metastatic disease at presentation, or if they had undergone radical treatment. Of 767 evaluable cases, 610 were known to have died at the time of analysis. Mean follow-up for the remaining 157 patients was 15 years. Outcome, expressed in terms of 15-year mortality from prostate cancer, was derived from a regression-based competing risks model. Subsequently, an analysis from the Mayo Clinic of long-term outcome following radical prostatectomy was designed to be as comparable as possible to the Albertsen data set.[3] This surgical series was based on 751 men with clinically localized disease, also aged between 55 and 74, who underwent radical prostatectomy during the same time period (1971–1984). The outcome in terms of 15-year mortality from prostate cancer was derived using the same competing risks methodology. Figure 65.1 shows the results of the two studies for men aged between 60 and 64 at diagnosis. It must be remembered that these are two different series, from two very different

healthcare settings, and that any comparison between them should be interpreted with great caution. With that strong proviso, it is interesting to note that the apparent benefit of radical treatment over watchful waiting is modest for Gleason scores less than or equal to 6, and becomes larger for the more poorly-differentiated cancers. Specifically, the absolute difference in 15-year disease-specific mortality between radical prostatectomy and watchful waiting was 0% for Gleason scores 2 to 4, –1% for Gleason score 5, 10% for Gleason score 6, 37% for Gleason score 7, and 49% for Gleason scores 8 to 10.

These retrospective comparisons suggest that subgroup analysis by tumor grade should be an important part of randomized trials which compare expectant management and definitive treatment.

RANDOMIZED COMPARISONS OF EXPECTANT MANAGEMENT AND DEFINITIVE TREATMENT

There are just two published randomized controlled trials comparing expectant management and definitive treatment of prostate cancer. Of these, one, which included just 142 patients, is too small for meaningful analysis.[4] The other, the Scandinavian Prostatic Cancer Group Study, randomized almost 700 men with localized disease between radical prostatectomy and watchful waiting, and the first results were published in 2002.[5] Interpretation of these results has varied widely. According to Patrick Walsh, "for the first time we have clear evidence that surgical treatment reduces the risk of death from prostate cancer."[6] In contrast, the British Medical Journal's account of the same data appeared under the heading, "Watchful waiting as good as surgery for prostate cancer." While interpretations may differ, there is wide agreement that this trial provides the best available data comparing expectant management and definitive treatment.

The Scandinavian trial was designed in 1988, with the main aim of comparing prostate cancer mortality following radical prostatectomy and watchful waiting.

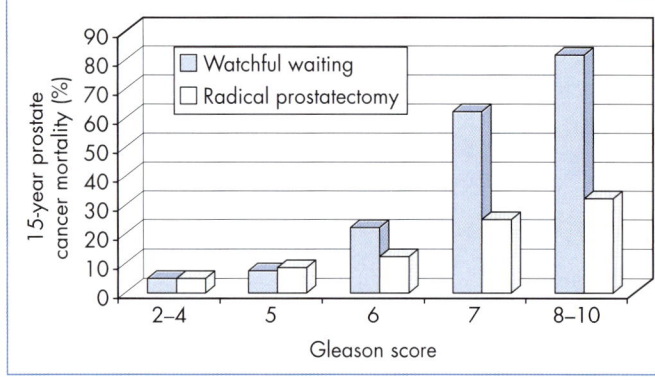

Fig. 65.1
Fifteen-year prostate cancer mortality for men aged 60–64 at diagnosis: comparison of Mayo Clinic radical prostatectomy series[3] with Albertsen et al watchful waiting data.[2]

Eligible patients were younger than 75 years, with newly diagnosed, clinically localized prostate cancer, with a negative bone scan, a PSA of less than 50 ng/ml, and a life-expectancy of at least 10 years. Cases were graded according to the World Health Organization (WHO) classification, and those with either well- or moderately (but not poorly)-differentiated tumors were included. Gleason scoring was also used, and eligibility was restricted to patients in whom less than 25% of the tumor tissue examined was Gleason grade 4 and less than 5% was Gleason grade 5. Patients were randomized between watchful waiting and radical prostatectomy. Following surgery, adjuvant treatment was not used. For patients on watchful waiting, transurethral resection was recommended for local progression. Patients were followed up with PSA levels and annual bone scans. The study accrued 695 patients from 14 centers between 1989 and 1999. Thirty of 348 patients (9%) randomized to watchful waiting received treatment with curative intent, and 25 of 347 patients (7%) randomized to surgery were in fact managed by watchful waiting (in addition to 23 patients who were found to be node positive at the time of surgery and did not proceed to radical prostatectomy). All analyses were performed according to intention to treat, rather than treatment received.

Results were obtained at a median follow-up of 6.2 years, and so must be regarded as preliminary, with just 115 (17%) of the 695 patients having died. Forty-seven (41%) of the deaths were attributed to prostate cancer, and 68 (59%) to other causes. Randomization to radical prostatectomy was associated with improved disease-specific mortality, with a hazard ratio of 0.50 (95% CI, 0.27–0.9; $P = 0.02$), which translated into an absolute benefit of 6.6% (95% CI, 2.1–11.1) at 8 years. While this is an important endpoint, it is not beyond criticism, because ascertainment of cause of death in patients with prostate cancer can be problematic. In terms of overall mortality, a statistically nonsignificant trend was seen in favor of radical prostatectomy with a hazard ratio of 0.83 (95% CI, 0.57–1.20). It seems likely that a significant overall survival advantage will emerge with longer follow-up, given that radical prostatectomy was associated with a reduction in the risk of metastatic disease (hazard ratio 0.63; 95% CI, 0.41–0.96). The main outcomes are shown in Figures 65.2 to 65.4.

Although the Scandinavian trial provides the best available data comparing expectant management and definitive treatment, there are obvious, major differences between Scandinavian practice during the early 1990s and contemporary, state-of-the-art clinical practice. First, the case-mix is certainly not representative of screen-detected prostate cancer—only 11% of patients in the trial had stage T1C disease, and the mean initial PSA level was as high as 13 ng/ml, with 18% of patients having a PSA greater than 20 ng/ml. Second, traditional watchful waiting as practiced in the trial, with palliative treatment for symptomatic progression, is very different from expectant management as it is now widely practiced, with radical treatment for those patients with biochemical or histologic progression. Third, radical prostatectomy in the trial was used as a sole modality of treatment, rather than with adjuvant or early salvage radiation and/or hormonal therapy.

The differences in outcome between the two arms of the trial are usually attributed to the effects of surgery. However, an alternative, and apparently plausible, explanation is that the benefits in the surgical arm were due, at least in part, to the earlier use of hormone therapy. Data on the timing of hormone therapy are not publicly available. However, it seems likely that the 23 patients (7%) randomized to radical prostatectomy but found to

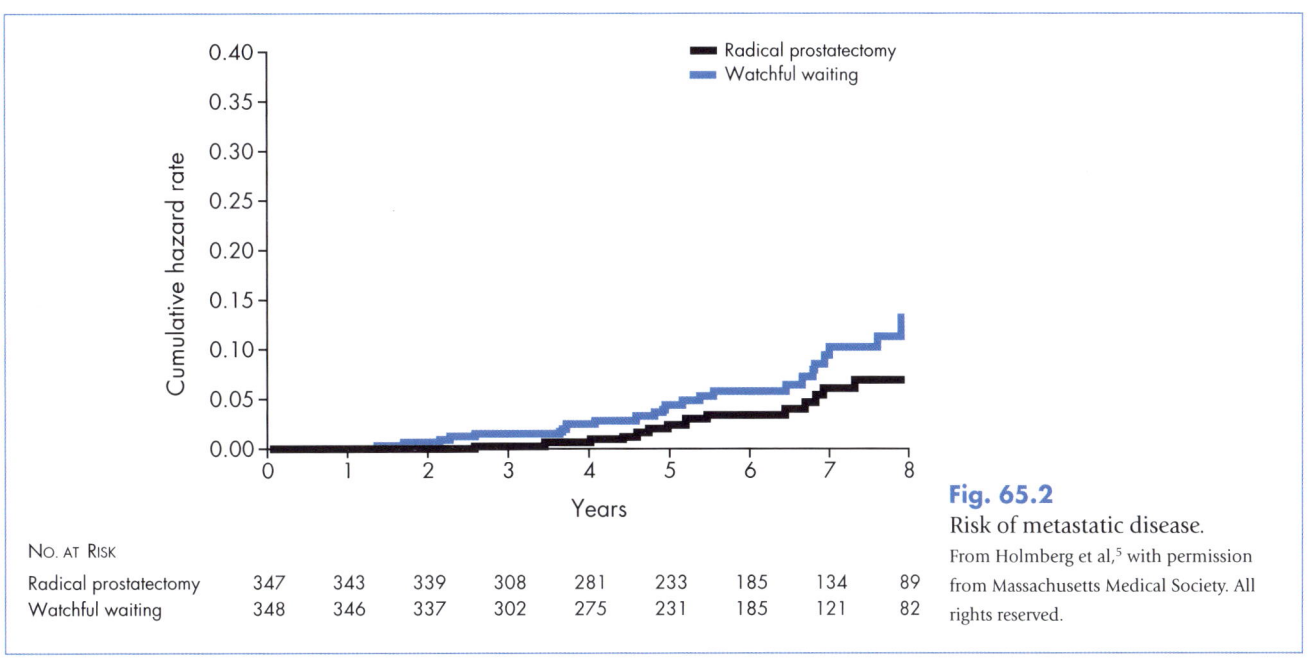

Fig. 65.2
Risk of metastatic disease.

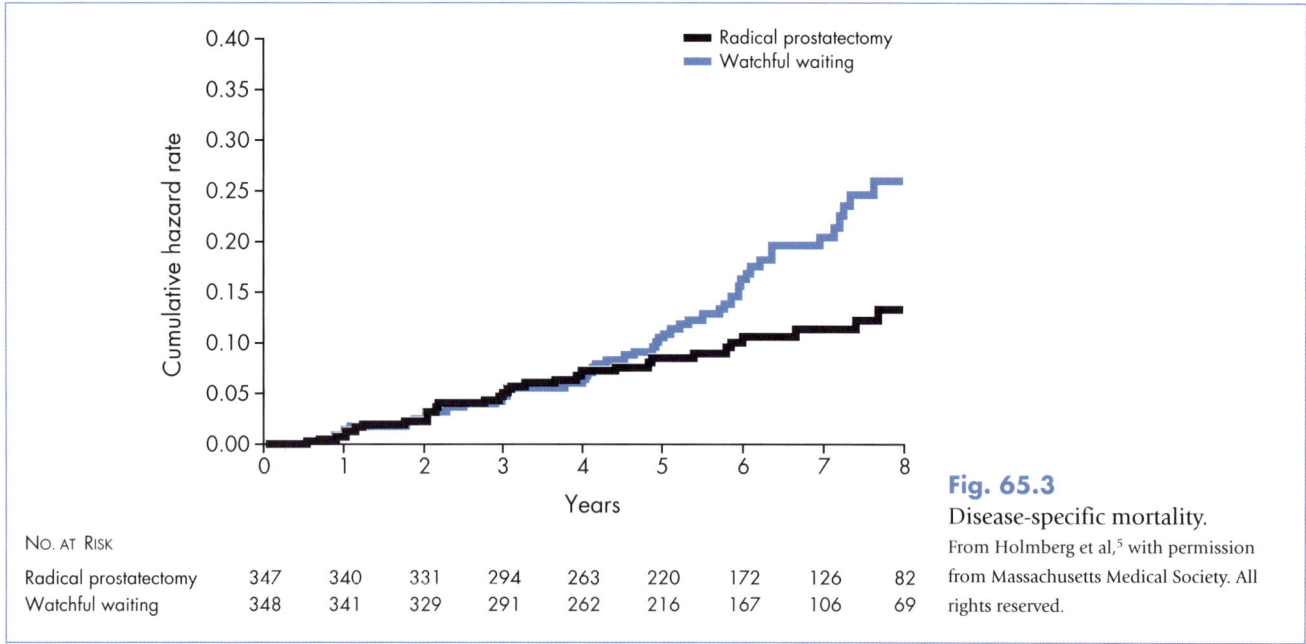

Fig. 65.3
Disease-specific mortality.

No. at Risk									
Radical prostatectomy	347	340	331	294	263	220	172	126	82
Watchful waiting	348	341	329	291	262	216	167	106	69

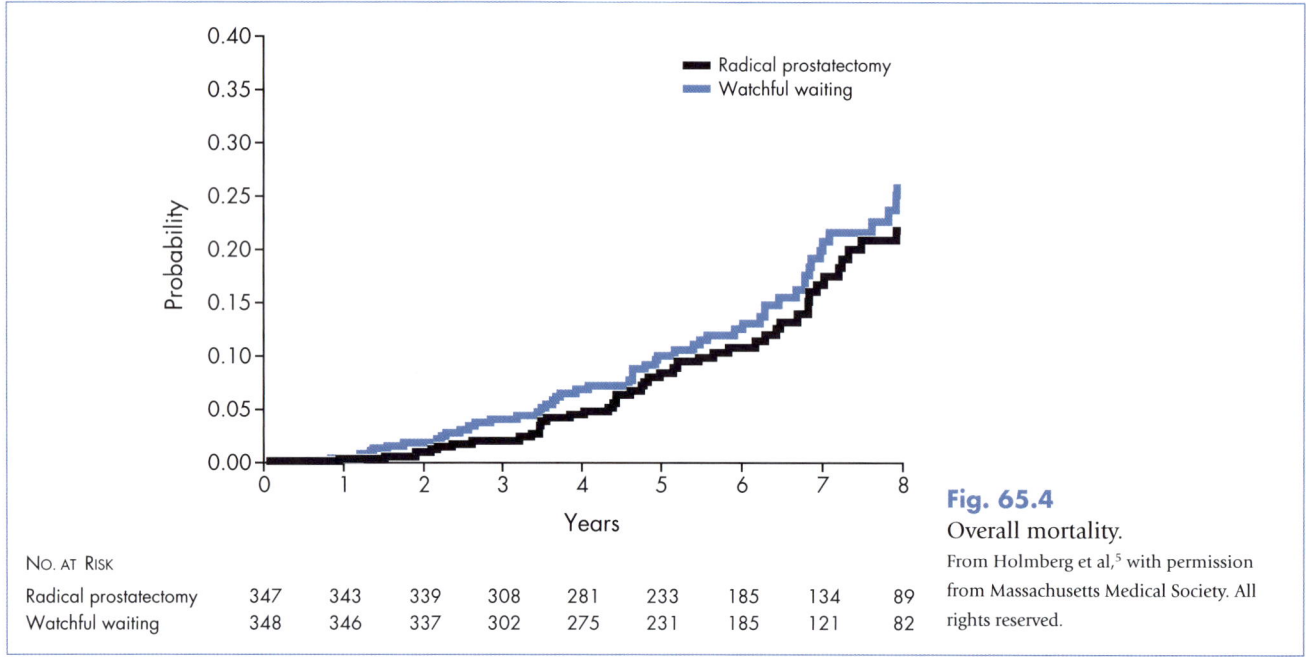

Fig. 65.4
Overall mortality.

No. at Risk									
Radical prostatectomy	347	343	339	308	281	233	185	134	89
Watchful waiting	348	346	337	302	275	231	185	121	82

be node positive at the time of surgery, commenced hormone therapy at that time. Furthermore, hormonal therapy was recommended for patients with local recurrence after radical prostatectomy, but not for patients with local progression on watchful waiting. It is conceivable that differences in the timing of hormone therapy between the two arms of the trial could have introduced a bias, delaying the development of metastatic disease in patients randomized to radical prostatectomy.

Notwithstanding these limitations, the Scandinavian trial remains a very important study. It is now known that treating localized prostate cancer is not always a waste of time and effort. It is now hard to argue that traditional watchful waiting is as effective as surgery for all patients with localized disease. The reduction in the

risk of metastatic prostate cancer, even in the absence of an overall survival benefit, is a clinically meaningful benefit of treatment. The challenge now is to identify *which* patients stand to benefit from curative treatment.

In addition to the efficacy data described above, the Scandinavian trial also provides the only randomized comparison of quality of life following expectant management and definitive intervention.[7] Of the 695 patients in the main trial, those who were recruited either in Finland or after February 1996, were excluded from the quality-of-life comparison, leaving 376 eligible patients. Self-reported data were obtained using a study-specific 77-item questionnaire that was mailed to patients following an introductory letter and telephone call. The response rate was impressive, with 87% of questionnaires returned, suggesting that the findings are likely to be representative of the entire cohort. It is important to note that, as in the main trial, a minority (6%) of the patients randomized to watchful waiting actually received radical prostatectomy, and 20% of patients randomized to surgery did not in fact undergo radical prostatectomy. The data reported were analysed by intention to treat.

Radical prostatectomy was associated with increased sexual dysfunction. For example, erectile function "seldom or never sufficient for intercourse" was reported by 80% in the surgical arm, versus 45% of those randomized to watchful waiting (relative risk 1.8; 95% CI, 1.5–2.2). Distress caused by decline in sexual function was also greater among patients randomized to radical prostatectomy (56% vs 40%). A contrasting pattern of urinary dysfunction was seen in the two groups, with bladder emptying problems more common in the watchful waiting group, and urinary leakage more common in the radical prostatectomy group. For example, bladder emptying difficulty, defined as an American Urological Association symptom index score of greater than 7, was reported by 35% in the radical prostatectomy group versus 49% in the watchful waiting group (relative risk 0.7; 95% CI, 0.5–0.9). Whereas moderate or severe urinary leakage was reported by 18% of patients assigned to radical prostatectomy and 2% of those assigned to watchful waiting (relative risk 9.3; 95% CI, 2.9–29.9). No significant differences were seen between the two groups in terms of either bowel function or psychological symptoms.

These are extremely important data since they are patient- rather than physician-reported, collected prospectively in the context of a randomized trial, and with an excellent compliance rate. The risks of impotence and incontinence associated with radical prostatectomy are much higher than those quoted in series from individual surgeons at academic institutions in the US.[8] It is not clear to what extent this difference reflects disparities in case selection and methods of data collection, and to what extent the morbidity of radical prostatectomy is operator-dependent. However, the data from the Scandinavian trial likely provide a better indication of surgical morbidity for most patients managed in routine clinical practice. That being the case, it is even more important to determine which patients stand to benefit from definitive treatment, and which patients can safely avoid the associated risks of impotence and incontinence.

ONGOING RANDOMIZED COMPARISONS OF EXPECTANT MANAGEMENT AND DEFINITIVE TREATMENT

There are two ongoing randomized trials which aim to compare definitive treatment with expectant management

in PSA screen-detected disease. The Prostate Cancer Intervention versus Observation Trial (PIVOT) compares radical prostatectomy versus watchful waiting, and has completed enrolment with 731 patients.[9] The Prostate testing for cancer and Treatment (ProtecT) study compares radical prostatectomy, external beam radiotherapy, and active monitoring, and aims to recruit over 2000 patients.[10] The results of these trials will be critically important in helping to determine the relative merits of definitive treatment and expectant management of early prostate cancer.

PIVOT opened to recruitment in 1994 under the auspices of the Department of Veterans Affairs and the National Cancer Institute. Eligible patients were younger than 75 years, with biopsy-proven localized prostate cancer of any grade, a serum PSA less than 50 ng/ml, and a life-expectancy of 10 years or more. Strengths of the trial design include the collection of baseline co-morbidity data and the use of a centralized pathology review. The trial compares two different general approaches to management, rather than two specific interventions. Patients randomized to radical prostatectomy were therefore able to receive adjuvant or salvage postoperative radiation and/or hormone therapy as clinically indicated. Patients randomized to expectant management were managed according to the general principle of using palliative therapies with low morbidity for symptomatic or metastatic progression. Radical prostatectomy, "definitive" radiation, early hormone therapy or treatment for an asymptomatic rising PSA were proscribed for patients in this arm of the trial. Interestingly, patients on expectant management and their physicians were blinded to PSA results in order to minimize intervention for asymptomatic biochemical progression. The main endpoint is overall mortality, and the initial accrual target was 2000 cases. Unfortunately, this target proved unattainable, and the trial closed to recruitment with 731 patients entered, with the plan to analyse the outcome data after 15 years of follow-up.

PIVOT is in many ways similar to the Scandinavian trial of radical prostatectomy versus watchful waiting, but involves a different patient population. On the one hand, PIVOT will likely include a greater proportion of men with PSA screen-detected cancers with a more favorable natural history and less potential to benefit from definitive treatment. On the other, patients with high grade disease for whom the opposite is true were eligible for PIVOT, but not for the Scandinavian trial. The results of exploratory subgroup analyses by tumor grade will be of interest, although the final accrual of just 731 patients will be a limiting factor in such analyses. One important limitation of PIVOT, which it shares with the Scandinavian trial, is that the approach to expectant management, with palliative treatment for symptomatic progression, is very different from expectant management as it is now widely practiced, with radical treatment for those patients with biochemical or histologic progression. If radical treatment for all patients turns out to improve survival compared with radical treatment for none, it will beg the question as to whether radical treatment for some, selected for example according to PSA kinetics, would have been as effective, but less morbid.

It is not surprising that PIVOT failed to reach its target accrual. It is recognized that patients and clinicians may find it difficult to accept the concept of randomization between two such different approaches to treatment. The ProtecT study opened in 1999, supported by the UK Department of Health, with an unusual recruitment methodology designed to address this problem. Individuals are invited, by letter from their general practitioner, to attend a prostate check clinic. Those who agree to attend the clinic are informed about the significance of prostate cancer, and about the randomized trial of treatment options. At this stage men who wish to participate are asked to give informed consent, and have a PSA test. Transrectal ultrasound biopsy is performed in those with a PSA level greater than 3 ng/ml, and those found to have clinically localized prostate cancer are potentially eligible for the treatment randomization, for which a separate informed consent is required. By informing the subjects about the uncertainties of prostate cancer management, and about the treatment trial before, rather than after, diagnosis, it is hoped that randomization between the different treatments will be easier. This approach has been successful in that approximately 70% of eligible patients have agreed to three-way randomization between active monitoring, radical prostatectomy, and radical radiotherapy.[11] However, just as in the Holmberg et al trial,[5] among those who have been randomized, not all patients accept their allocated treatment. One concern is that this approach to recruitment could lead to an increased rate of "crossover" from the allocated treatment, since this could significantly reduce the power of the trial to detect differences in outcome using an intention-to-treat analysis.

Patients randomized to active monitoring are being followed with PSA tests every 3 months in the first year and then at 3- to 6-monthly intervals. Repeat prostate biopsies are not routinely performed. PSA progression is suspected if there is a 50% increase in PSA level within any 12-month period. Suspected progression will prompt restaging investigations, and the decision whether to proceed to curative treatment will be "based on full participant information and joint decision-making." It will be interesting to see what proportion of patients in the active monitoring arm do proceed to curative treatment. A 50% increase in PSA within 12 months is the equivalent of a PSA doubling time of less than 20 months. Only a very small proportion of patients with localized prostate cancer will have such a rapid rate of rise of PSA level,[12] suggesting that this active monitoring policy may be similar in effect to traditional watchful waiting. While there is no evidence-based definition of the criteria that should be used to define disease progression requiring radical treatment, this approach differs from published series of active monitoring in which 25% to 33% of patients receive radical treatment.[13,14]

ProtecT is on course to recruit over 2000 patients by 2006, which will be an outstanding achievement. It promises to be the single most important trial comparing expectant management and definitive treatment of PSA screen-detected prostate cancer. In addition, since the participating general practices represent a random sample of practices within a defined area, and since background rates of PSA screening in nonparticipating general practices remains relatively low, this program will also provide data on the value of PSA screening. Put another way, ProtecT represents the intervention arm of a randomized trial of PSA screening, with those practices not invited to take part acting as the control arm.

The long-term mortality outcomes from PIVOT and the ProtecT trial will provide the best data comparing expectant management and definitive treatment, but will not be available for several years. In the meantime, it is tempting to speculate as to what those results will be. If it is assumed that the 15-year survival for early prostate cancer in the PSA era managed by watchful waiting is that predicted by Nicholson and Harland,[15] and that the improvement in prostate cancer mortality with radical treatment matches the improvement seen in the 8-year risk of metastasis observed in the Scandinavian Prostatic Cancer Group study (hazard ratio, 0.63; confidence interval, 0.41–0.96),[5] then the size of the survival benefit of radical treatment can be guesstimated (Table 65.2). These estimates of the potential survival benefit of radical treatment must be regarded with some caution. There is uncertainty with regard to both the predicted natural history of PSA-detected early prostate cancer, and the impact of radical treatment on prostate cancer mortality. However, based on the assumptions stated above, the potential 15-year survival benefit of radical treatment for PSA-detected early prostate cancer appears modest. For example, for men aged 70 at diagnosis, radical treatment is estimated to result in a 1.6% absolute benefit in 15-year survival (number needed to treat [NNT], 62.5), and for men aged 60, the estimated absolute benefit is 2.8% (NNT, 35.7). These results serve as a reminder that, in the absence of good data from randomized trials, the decision whether or not to have radical treatment is a value judgement, comparing the known morbidity of treatment with the unknown, but potential, survival benefit. Faced with a 50% risk of treatment-related impotence and a 2% potential survival benefit, a significant proportion of men will likely elect for expectant management in preference to definitive treatment.

Table 65.2 Estimated 15-year outcome for PSA screen-detected early prostate cancer managed by watchful waiting (WW) versus radical treatment (RRx).

Age at diagnosis	Alive		Dead from prostate cancer		Dead from other causes	
	WW (%)	RRx (%)	WW (%)	RRx (%)	WW (%)	RRx (%)
50	72.1	75.9 (72.5–78.2)	12.2	7.7 (5.0–11.7)	15.7	16.4 (15.8–16.8)
55	65.2	68.5 (65.6–70.5)	11.6	7.3 (4.8–11.1)	23.2	24.2 (23.3–24.8)
60	56.3	59.1 (56.6–60.7)	11.1	7.0 (4.6–10.7)	32.6	33.9 (32.7–34.7)
65	44.7	47.0 (44.9–48.4)	11.1	7.0 (4.6–10.7)	44.2	46.0 (44.4–47.1)
70	31.4	33.0 (31.5–34.0)	10.5	6.6 (4.3–10.1)	58.1	60.4 (58.3–61.7)
75	7.9	8.3 (7.9–8.6)	7.4	4.7 (3.0–7.1)	84.7	87.0 (85.0–88.4)
80	2.2	2.3 (2.2–2.3)	4.0	2.5 (1.6–3.8)	93.8	95.2 (94.0–96.0)

The estimate for outcome of watchful waiting is taken from Nicholson and Harland.[15] The ranges shown correspond to a range of hazard ratios for effect of RRx on prostate cancer mortality of 0.41–0.96.

THE FUTURE FOR TRIALS OF EXPECTANT MANAGEMENT VERSUS DEFINITIVE TREATMENT

This chapter has focused on trials of watchful waiting versus definitive treatment with either surgery or radiotherapy. Such trials will leave other important questions to be addressed. First, newer definitive treatments such as brachytherapy, cryotherapy, and high intensity focussed ultrasound (HIFU) offer the promise of less morbidity and greater convenience than either surgery or radiotherapy. Such modalities have the potential to shift the balance of risks and benefits further in favor of definitive treatment. After all, if definitive treatment were effective and had no morbidity, then there would be no case for expectant management.

Second, just as there are advances in definitive treatment techniques over time, so the approach to expectant management is also evolving. At present, there is no consensus on the optimum approach to expectant management. Uncertainties include the frequency of PSA testing, the need for repeat biopsies, the role of imaging investigations, and the criteria used to define disease progression requiring radical treatment. As the approach to active surveillance is optimized, so the ability to target treatment to those who stand to benefit should improve. In future, it can be envisaged that active surveillance could be combined with low-toxicity interventions designed, not to eradicate the disease, but to alter its natural history. This is an attractive possibility, not least because "incidental" prostate cancer is an extremely common postmortem finding even in countries with the lowest rates of clinically significant disease,[16] suggesting that environmental factors, such as diet, may influence prostate cancer progression, rather than initiation. Nutritional interventions require further study, but could become a middle way between definitive treatment and traditional approaches to expectant management.

The long-standing debate concerning the relative merits of expectant management and definitive intervention rests to a large extent on the extraordinary degree of interpatient variation in prostate cancer behavior, together with the inability to predict that behavior in individual cases. While it is known beyond reasonable doubt that half the men diagnosed with early prostate cancer do not need treatment, it is not known which these patients are. As understanding of the molecular pathology of prostate cancer advances, it is likely that new and better predictors of prostate cancer behavior will be identified. In the long-term, the use of such biologic predictors could revolutionize the ability to select patients for definitive treatment on the one hand, or expectant management on the other.

REFERENCES

1. Lu-Yao G, Yao S. Population-based study of long-term survival in patients with clinically localised prostate cancer. Lancet 1997;349:906–910.

2. Albertsen, P, Gleason D, Barry M. Competing risk analysis of men aged 55 to 74 years at diagnosis managed conservatively for clinically localized prostate cancer. JAMA 1998;280:975–980.

3. Sweat SD, Bergstralh EJ, Slezak J, et al. Competing risk analysis after radical prostatectomy for clinically nonmetastatic prostate

adenocarcinoma according to clinical Gleason score and patient age. J Urol 2002;168:525–529.

4. Iversen P, Madsen PO, Corle DK. Radical prostatectomy versus expectant treatment for early carcinoma of the prostate. Twenty-three year follow-up of a prospective randomized study. Scand J Urol Nephrol 1995;172(Suppl):65–72.

5. Holmberg L, Bill-Axelson A, Helgesen F, et al. A randomized trial comparing radical prostatectomy with watchful waiting in early prostate cancer. N Engl J Med 2002;347:781–789.

6. Walsh PC. A randomized trial comparing radical prostatectomy with watchful waiting in early prostate cancer. J Urol 2003;169:1588–1589.

7. Steineck G, Helgesen F, Adolfsson J, et al. Quality of life after radical prostatectomy or watchful waiting. N Engl J Med 2002;347:790–796.

8. Walsh P. Radical prostatectomy for localized prostate cancer provides durable cancer control with excellent quality of life: a structured debate. J Urol 2000;163:1802–1807.

9. Wilt TJ, Brawer MK. The Prostate Cancer Intervention Versus Observation Trial (PIVOT): A randomized trial comparing radical prostatectomy versus expectant management for the treatment of clinically localised prostate cancer. Cancer 1995;75(Suppl7):1963–1968.

10. Donovan J, Hamdy F, Neal D, et al. Prostate testing for cancer and treatment (ProtecT) feasibility study. Health Technol Assess 2003;7:1–88.

11. Donovan J, Mills M, Smith M, et al. Quality improvement report: Improving design and conduct of randomised trials by embedding them in qualitative research: ProtecT (prostate testing for cancer and treatment) study. Commentary: presenting unbiased information to patients can be difficult. BMJ 2002;325:766–770.

12. Choo R, DeBoer G, Klotz L, et al. PSA doubling time of prostate carcinoma managed with watchful observation alone. Int J Radiat Oncol Biol Phys 2001;50:615–620.

13. Choo R, Klotz L, Danjoux C, et al. Feasibility study: watchful waiting for localized low to intermediate grade prostate carcinoma with selective delayed intervention based on prostate specific antigen, histological and/or clinical progression. J Urol 2002;167:1664–1669.

14. Carter HB, Walsh PC, Landis P, et al. Expectant management of nonpalpable prostate cancer with curative intent: preliminary results. J Urol 2002;167:1231–1234.

15. Nicholson PW, Harland SJ. Survival prospects after screen-detection of prostate cancer. BJU Int 2002;90:686–693.

16. Yatani R, et al. Trends in frequency of latent prostate carcinoma in Japan from 1965–1979 to 1982–1986. J Natl Cancer Inst 1988;80:683–687.

Practical and realistic lifestyle changes and supplements for the man concerned about prostate cancer: What do I tell my patients?

66

Mark A Moyad

ABSTRACT

It is critical to remember that the primary cause of death in the United States and in most countries around the world is cardiovascular disease (CVD), and it is also the number 1 or 2 cause of death in prostate cancer prevention trials, and in untreated and treated prostate cancer patients. These findings serve to place the overall risk of death in men into its proper perspective, and it does not serve to belittle the seriousness of prostate cancer or another disease or condition. Generally speaking, what has been found to be heart healthy has been tantamount to prostate healthy, and there may even be a relationship between the two conditions. Therefore, clinicians need to provide a simplistic and realistic set of lifestyle changes to patients to not only attempt to reduce prostate cancer risk and mortality, but to attempt to impact all-cause mortality. A list of recommendations are provided in this chapter to assist the clinician and patient in their discussion of simple and practical changes that may not only be accomplished in a short period of time, but should provide at least some type of tangible overall benefit for the man concerned about prostate cancer.

INTRODUCTION

Some simplistic and practical observations need mentioning to place lifestyle recommendations in their proper perspective. Cardiovascular disease continues to be the number 1 cause of death in the United States and in other industrialized countries,[1] and it is now the primary cause of mortality worldwide. The World Health Organization (WHO) has documented that CVD is the number one cause of mortality in every region of the world with the exception of sub-Saharan Africa, and it is predicted that this disease will surpass the number 1 cause of death in that specific region, infectious disease, within the next decade.[2–5]

Recently the media was replete with reports indicating that cancer has now surpassed heart disease as the leading cause of death in Americans.[6] This was an interesting new finding, but it was not entirely correct. In 2002, the latest year for which mortality data are available, cancer was responsible for 478,082 deaths and heart disease was responsible for 446,727 deaths in individuals younger than the age of 85. Therefore, cancer was reported as the number 1 killer for Americans younger than 85 years of age. If this age consideration was not categorized in this manner then heart disease is still the number 1 killer of Americans—in 2002, 696,947 individuals in the US died of heart disease versus 557,271 deaths from cancer. Heart disease is the primary cause or mortality in those aged 85 and older. In fact, in this older age group, heart disease was responsible for three times more deaths (>250,000) compared with cancer (~80,000 deaths) in 2002. Additionally, if one actually compares CVD (heart disease and diseases of the blood vessels, including strokes) with cancer, an entirely different picture of the situation is revealed. Cardiovascular disease is responsible for 38% of all deaths and is responsible for more deaths than the next five leading causes of death combined. Death rates from all cancers combined have been slowly declining over the past decade (1.5% per year since 1993 for men and 0.8% per year for women since 1992). However, the death rate from heart disease has been falling for a greater period of time, since the mid-1970s. Therefore, even in 1999, cancer deaths outnumbered heart disease deaths in individuals younger than 85 years. Even in individuals over the age of 85 years, heart disease deaths have declined compared with cancer. The notable improvements in mortality rates for both prominent diseases apparently were partially due to a decrease in smoking rates in the US. For example, in women, lung cancer deaths have stabilized after increasing for several decades, and death rates from breast and colorectal cancer have decreased. In men, the death rate has also continued to fall for the three most prevalent cancers (colorectal, lung, and prostate).

Some of the largest US cancer prevention trials and cancer screening studies demonstrate the impact of the observations presented above. The recent results of the Prostate Cancer Prevention Trial (PCPT) seem to have generated a lot of interest and controversy regarding the use of daily finasteride to reduce the risk of prostate cancer.[7–9] Finasteride was responsible for an approximate and significant 25% reduction in the number of prostate cancer cases during 7 years of study, but an apparent higher risk of aggressive prostate cancer was also found in the finasteride arm of the trial. Interestingly, as the debate over the advantages and disadvantages of finasteride continue, several important observations from this trial have not received much attention in the medical literature. Over 18,000 men were included in this randomized trial, and 5 men died from prostate cancer in the finasteride arm and 5 men died of prostate cancer in the placebo arm, but over 1100 men died in this study. Thus, prostate cancer was responsible for less than 1% of the deaths in this trial, while the majority of the deaths were apparently due to CVD. Thus, the results of the first large-scale prostate cancer prevention trial ever conducted in medicine demonstrated that CVD is indeed the primary cause of death in men, but again this finding has received little attention until now. Does this finding reduce the seriousness or impact of prostate cancer prevention utilizing a prostate-specific chemoprevention agent? Obviously not; but again it places the overall risk of mortality in it's proper perspective. Men inquiring about the benefits and detriments of finasteride for prostate cancer prevention should be told first that the number 1 risk to them, in general, is CVD, and then the potential prostate cancer risk-specific consultation should take place after the first point is discussed and emphasized.

Observations taken from the well-known selenium supplementation randomized trial that noted a significant reduction in the number of prostate cancer cases with the use of 200 µg/day selenium versus placebo seems to have generated much interest in utilizing selenium supplements to reduce the risk of prostate cancer. However, despite men in this trial having a higher mean risk of cancer, the number 1 cause of death in this randomized trial was still CVD.[10]

Additionally, the past and recent observation that the primary or secondary cause of death in patients with prostate cancer seems to be CVD[12] continues to emphasize the past non-emphasized discussion that clinicians and patients need to give more attention to the impact of CVD on overall mortality. Also, a study of the macrophage scavenging receptor gene 1 (*MSR1*) revealed that a mutation in this gene not only increases the risk of atherosclerosis, but it also appears to increase the risk of prostate cancer.[13] Some of the potential mechanisms involved in increasing a man's risk for heart disease may also increase his risk for prostate cancer,[14,15] and other chronic disease risk may also be increased with an abnormal cardiovascular risk[16,17] or lipid mutation, for example.[18] If the clinician were to highlight lifestyle changes that may impact one or ideally both conditions (CVD and cancer) favorably this would seem like the wisest and most practical and realistic clinical approach for the patient both before being diagnosed with prostate cancer and after being diagnosed or treated for this disease.[19]

These observations and general findings are not mentioned to belittle or reduce the seriousness of prostate cancer, but they place the average risk of death for a man in its proper perspective. Dietary or lifestyle changes to reduce the risk of CVD just make realistic and practical sense when examining the larger overall mortality picture. In other words a so-called "forest over the tree" approach seems most appropriate when discussing options with patients. Clinicians should not solely emphasize a prostate cancer-specific diet or prostate-specific lifestyle change only because this would ignore the previous important but seemingly unstressed findings from the past studies of prostate cancer. Heart healthy seems to be prostate healthy, and this should be constantly and consistently reiterated and emphasized to the man concerned about prostate cancer. The simplistic lifestyle recommendations proffered in this chapter serve not only to impact prostate cancer, but CVD as well. Therefore, patients may now be offered lifestyle changes that can potentially impact all-cause mortality rather than the more myopic focus or attention on disease-specific mortality.

CARDIOVASCULAR RISKS AND ASSESSMENT MARKERS

Recommendation #1: Men should know their lipid profile, and other cardiovascular risks and assessment markers as well as they know their PSA values and the other results from their prostate exam.

In my experience, many patients seem to be well aware of their past prostate-specific antigen (PSA) values, but have either never had a cholesterol test, or are unaware of their latest values, or how to correctly construe these values. This observation seems initially frustrating, because again the number 1 or 2 cause of death in these patients is CVD.[1,7,10,11] This lack of comprehensive knowledge is not only prevalent in some prostate populations, but surveys of the general population indicate that a majority of individuals do not know their cholesterol values, or they have a lack of understanding of what they actually represent.[20] Clinicians need to emphasize the dual concern of CVD and cancer risk. In my experience, when this is emphasized, patients begin to become familiar with all of their clinical values or numbers. A simplistic clinical change and discussion or explanation seems to be very effective in these cases. Initially, it would seem appropriate to conduct a cholesterol/blood-pressure screening and prostate cancer screening on the same day at any institution. Second, patients should be educated regularly on the normal values of a cholesterol panel and blood pressure test, because these have recently been updated twice according to the expert panel from the National Cholesterol Education Program (NCEP).[21,22]

Ideally, for most men a total cholesterol (TC) level of less than 200 mg/dL and a low-density lipoprotein (LDL or "bad cholesterol") level of less than 100 mg/dL are optimal, but for some high-risk men (for example, those with documented CVD or a CVD past event), an LDL less than 70 mg/dL is optimal. A high-density lipoprotein (HDL or "good cholesterol") of 40 mg/dL or higher is good but 60 mg/dL or higher is optimal, and a triglyceride level of less than 150 mg/dL is optimal. It should also be kept in mind that a fasting (9–12 hours) cholesterol level is best, but in the case of prostate cancer screenings this is difficult, so a non-fasting test can be drawn and if certain levels of TC, HDL, or LDL are not ideal than a follow-up fasting test should be suggested.

Clinicians should also discuss other potential risks for CVD, which is also affected by lifestyle risk factors such as overweight and obesity, physical inactivity, and an atherogenic diet. Other emerging risk factors or risk markers should ideally be discussed because despite the cholesterol test being a good test for predicting future cardiovascular problems, it is not a perfect test. This should be similar to the clinician's approach to a PSA test—it is a good test for potential risk or recurrence following definitive therapy, but it is not a perfect test. Other newer cardiovascular markers, such as C-reactive protein (CRP),[21,23–26] homocysteine,[21,27] lipoprotein (a) or Lp(a),[21,28,29] impaired fasting glucose, or hemoglobin A1c,[21] and evidence of subclinical atherosclerotic disease[21] should also be discussed with the patient. A referral to a cardiologist may be appropriate in other cases because some of these markers may also be related to overall mortality as well as CVD risk. Several other advantages may occur for the patient and clinician that

continue to follow these overall cardiovascular markers. For example, cholesterol levels are an excellent indicator of how well a patient may be adopting lifestyle changes following a PSA test or after definitive therapy. If these numbers improve, it may be more likely that the patient is adhering to a prostate-healthy lifestyle program. The HDL level may be a good indicator of the overall amount of exercise a patient is getting following a PSA test. The HDL tends to rise, and at times substantially, with a greater amount of physical activity,[30] and a higher HDL may be correlated with a lower risk of abnormal prostate conditions.[31]

On the other hand, in a minority of patients that follow a healthy lifestyle, a less than optimal change in cholesterol may occur, but these patients can then be referred to a specialist for potential drug and more aggressive lifestyle therapy. Blood pressure values should also be emphasized as much as the cholesterol and PSA values. Recently, the Joint National Committee on Prevention, Detection, Evaluation, and Treatment of High Blood Pressure also altered the criteria for what constitutes a healthy blood pressure.[32] Men should be informed that normal blood pressure is less than 120/80 mmHg and individuals with a systolic blood pressure of 120 to 139 mmHg or diastolic blood pressure of 80 to 89 mmHg are actually considered to be "prehypertensive," and lifestyle changes should be advocated in these individuals. Blood pressure tends to decrease with a healthier lifestyle[33] and again is a good indicator of lifestyle compliance; and a healthy blood pressure may also lower the risk of abnormal prostate conditions.[31] A minority of patients may not reduce their blood pressure with lifestyle changes, but these men can be referred to a specialist. Men that adopt lifestyle changes that do not result in a PSA change should still be given encouragement to continue these changes because of the other potential profound impacts these behaviors may have on overall health. For example, my experience has demonstrated that a man who does not reduce his PSA after lifestyle change still seems very much encouraged to continue these behaviors after he is told, for example, that his blood pressure has been reduced along with cholesterol values. In other words, the glass is very much half-full for patients who adopt healthy lifestyle changes and follow cardiovascular risk markers in addition to the PSA test.

There is one other recent pertinent example that highlights the problem with isolated PSA screenings without offering comprehensive screening and education. We conducted two large PSA screenings of African-American men in 2004 in two large metropolitan areas.[34] In the past, these screenings only offered PSA testing. However, we also offered cholesterol and other types of screenings in these settings and we were surprised to find that although PSA abnormalities were observed in less than 10% of these men, the rate of dyslipidemia was over 50% at both sites! Again, this drives home the point that more comprehensive screening and education seems to be the best potential approach for men concerned about prostate disease.

BODY-FAT INDICATORS

Recommendation #2: The clinician needs to measure the patient's body mass index (BMI), and/or waist-to-hip ratio (WHR), or waist circumference (WC), and it should become a regular part of the clinical record.

The negative impact of being overweight or obese on overall health and mortality is well known. Less known is the impact of weight on prostate cancer risk, but it seems that its impact may be just as detrimental.[35] Body mass index is a fairly reliable and fast method to determine who may be overweight or obese.[36] It is defined as the weight in kilograms divided by the square of the height in meters (kg/m^2). Another method to calculate the BMI is to take weight in pounds and divide it by the height in inches squared and to multiply this number by 704 (pounds/inches^2 × 704). A BMI of less than 25 is considered normal by the World Health Organization (WHO), whereas 25 to 29 is overweight, 30 or more than is defined as obese, and 35 or more is considered morbidly obese. Several recent large randomized trials have demonstrated that most individuals in these studies are overweight,[37] and this includes dietary trials to prevent prostate cancer or reduce PSA.[38]

Waist-to-hip ratio may be another simple measurement to determine obesity.[36] Individuals must stand during the entire measurement of WHR. This more precisely measures abdominal adipose circumference or tissue and fat distribution. The waist is defined as the abdominal circumference midway between the costal margin and the iliac crest. The hip is defined as the largest circumference just below the iliac crest. For men, a WHR of more than 0.90 is a fairly accurate indicator of an increased risk for obesity-related conditions, independent of BMI.

Waist circumference is perhaps the simplest and fastest method to currently access obesity. WC is rapidly gaining acceptance as one of the best predictors of a future cardiovascular event, regardless of the ethnic group studied.[39] Recent evidence also suggests that it may be a better predictor of early mortality from prostate cancer than other methods of weight measurement.[40] Regardless, WC has been one of the criteria to access metabolic syndrome. A WC of 35 inches or greater has been suggested as "overweight" and 40 or more is considered obese. Interestingly, a WC of 40 or more is also one of the five specific criteria of metabolic syndrome.

Also noteworthy is that dual energy X-ray absorptiometry (DEXA) has become the gold standard of measuring bone mineral density and determining the future risk of fracture in women and men.[41] However, in 2005 to 2006, it may be one of the most accurate predictors of body fat. Clinicians should advise patients who will be receiving a DEXA scan in the future for osteoporosis risk to also inquire about an overall body fat measurement. Utilizing the proper software, the DEXA scan allows an accurate determination of overall fat-free mass, but the ability to specifically quantify belly fat is more controversial.

Investigations of weight and prostate cancer are preliminary and not conclusive,[42] but some of the largest studies to date suggest a potential serious negative impact, especially post-diagnosis and treatment. For example, a large cohort study by Andersson et al followed 135,000 Swedish construction workers.[43] It included one of the largest numbers of prostate cancer cases (2368), prostate cancer deaths (708), and one of the longest follow-up periods to date (18 years). All of the anthropometric measurements were correlated with the risk of prostate cancer, but there was a stronger relation to mortality than to incidence. The risk of mortality from prostate cancer demonstrated statistical significance in all of the BMI subsets above the reference. This investigation represented a young cohort, because more than 50% of these men were under 40 years of age at entry into this investigation.

The Netherlands Cohort Study was one of the largest prospective studies to evaluate diet and lifestyle and the risk of prostate cancer.[44] This study found no associations between larger intakes of overall dietary fat and prostate cancer incidence; however, these same researchers also recorded BMIs, and it seems that this part of the study did not receive as much publicity.[45] A total of 58,279 men aged 55 to 69 years were followed. A total of 681 cases new cases of prostate cancer were diagnosed during 6.3 years of follow-up. There was a moderate association observed for BMI and prostate cancer (relative risk [RR] = 1.33) if a man was obese at a younger age, which was stronger for localized cancers than for advanced cancer.

One of the few large-scale randomized trials to report on obesity and prostate cancer risk was from a study whose primary endpoint was lung cancer incidence after taking vitamin E, β-carotene, both, or neither.[46,47] Prostate cancer incidence and mortality was a secondary endpoint of the trial. This study was known as the "Alpha-Tocopherol Beta-Carotene" (ATBC) Trial, and it documented 579 cases of prostate cancer with an 11-year follow-up. No relation between prostate cancer risk and BMI was noted in the moderate-to-overweight BMI ranges.[46] Researchers discovered later that men in the highest weight and BMI category had a 40% increased risk of developing prostate cancer compared with men with a normal BMI.[47] This was an interesting later discovery of the trial, because it was this same study that found that men consuming 50 mg/day vitamin E as a supplement had a 32% reduction in prostate cancer risk.[46] The results with the vitamin E supplement seemed to garner the most publicity in most major media outlets. Yet, another way of perceiving the results of this study was that the potential negative impact of being obese was greater than the positive impact of taking a vitamin E supplement, though few if any media sources have publicized this finding from the trial. Men were not only obese but smoked a mean of 20 cigarettes per day over several decades. This negative synergism of being obese and having a chronic heavy smoking history, or having other significant unhealthy habits, may lead to a greater risk and progression of prostate cancer. It seems critical for the clinician to explain to the patient that two of the largest dietary and supplement studies to analyze the risk of prostate cancer essentially both arrived at the same conclusion—that obesity can negatively impact prostate cancer risk or progression. This seems to provide a convincing argument that men need to maintain a healthy weight before or after a prostate cancer diagnosis.

One of the largest prospective epidemiologic investigations to evaluate the impact of obesity on cancer mortality was also published.[48] More than 900,000 US adults (404,576 men) who did not have cancer at baseline in 1982 were included in this 16-year follow-up study. Higher cancer mortality was associated with increasing BMIs and this included prostate cancer mortality. A significant ($p < 0.001$) increased risk of prostate cancer mortality was associated with increasing BMI from 25 to 29.9 (RR = 1.08), 30 to 34.9 (RR = 1.20), and 35 to 39.9 (RR = 1.34) for the 4004 deaths from prostate carcinoma that were documented.

Post-diagnosis studies are also providing some concerns for the man being treated for prostate cancer. Two large retrospective pooled multi-institutional analyses arrived at somewhat similar conclusions after evaluating patients following radical prostatectomy.[49,50] The first study included 3162 patients and found that a higher BMI was a significant independent predictor of a higher Gleason score, and a higher BMI was significantly associated with a higher risk of biochemical recurrence.[49] African-American men had significantly higher BMIs than white men, and also had significantly higher prostate cancer recurrence rates, which could provide a partial explanation of racial differences sometimes observed with this disease. The second study compared 1106 men treated with radical prostatectomy from 1998 to 2002. A BMI of over 35 was associated with a significant risk of biochemical recurrence after treatment even when controlling for surgical margin status.[50] Interestingly, the percentage of obese men undergoing surgery in this data set doubled in the last decade, and obesity was associated with higher-grade prostate cancers, a trend toward an increased risk of positive surgical margins, and higher biochemical failure rates.

Another recent epidemiologic study (Health Professionals Follow-Up Study) that published incidence but not mortality data from prostate cancer found a significantly lower risk of prostate cancer in men with higher BMIs if they were younger (<60 years) or had a family history of prostate cancer.[51] However, men with more sporadic cancers seemed to have a higher risk of prostate cancer with an increasing BMI. This observation led researchers of this study to hypothesize that, since obesity is associated with lower testosterone levels or partial androgen suppression, this could have resulted in a lower risk of prostate cancer in the early-onset or hereditary prostate cancers in these men compared with the more sporadic cancers. Obese men could theoretically also harbor prostate tumors, but have lower PSA levels, which could lead to the clinician falsely considering these men to be cancer free, and this may explain why some have been identified to have more advanced disease at the time of diagnosis and treatment.[49,50]

The proper perspective to the patient should be constantly emphasized, even if these recent alternative findings are accurate. Prostate cancer recurrence and mortality, and especially early mortality in general have been highly correlated with an increasing BMI. Whether or not obesity impacts just the incidence of prostate cancer should not be the primary focus for any man, because this observation simply fails to see the forest over the single tree when discussing the overall effect of obesity on general health.[35] For example, two of the largest prospective epidemiologic studies examining the issue of BMI and overall mortality had similar findings.[52,53] Both studies utilized data from the American Cancer Society. The first investigation was the American Cancer Society's Cancer Prevention Study I.[52] Over 62,000 men were included, and these men had no smoking history, no history of heart disease, stroke, or cancer (other than skin carcinoma), and no history of recent involuntary weight loss at baseline. Overall mortality was measured over 12 years. The second study was the Cancer Prevention Study II.[53] This was a study of 457,000 men observed for 14 years. Both studies documented that men with a BMI of approximately 25 to 30 had an increased mortality of 10% to 25%.[52,53] Individuals with a BMI of 30 or more had a 50% to 100% increased mortality compared with those with a BMI less than 25. The second study not only included more men but also looked at general cancer mortality.[53] The men within the highest BMI category (>35) had a 40% to 80% increased risk of mortality from cancer, and no evidence of any increased risk was found among the leanest individuals (BMI <20). Past studies completed in the US indicate that only a minority of adults (less than 8%) have a BMI of less than 20, and more than 50% of men in the US have a BMI over 25.[54]

Numerous cancers seem to be at least somewhat associated with a higher BMI, but renal cell carcinoma has demonstrated perhaps the strongest correlation with BMI compared with all the cancers studied to date.[55] Also, recent research suggesting increased risks of erectile dysfunction[56,57] and kidney stones[58] with obesity should be discussed with patients. Healthcare professionals working in the field of urology should constantly emphasize the negative overall impact of obesity. Clinicians need to let their patients know that maintaining a healthy weight should be one of the primary goals. For example, placing a BMI chart in the clinic office and always making BMI or WHR or WC a part of the individual clinical record should be a goal for every patient, regardless of his or her concern of a specific disease risk, because early mortality from all-causes is associated with increasing BMI. Clinicians should also refer patients on a regular basis to nutritionists, therapists, and to a variety of professional weight-loss programs. Clinicians should be able to provide the name and number of these individuals and organizations to the patient at the time of the urologic appointment in order to improve compliance, convey enthusiasm, and the immediacy or importance of this lifestyle change.

FITNESS FIRST

Recommendation #3: Always encourage fitness and overall health first in patients by telling them to get approximately 30 minutes of physical activity a day or more depending on individual need, and to lift weights or perform resistance exercises several times/week. Aerobic and resistance exercise should be emphasized equally; one is not more vital than the other. Weight loss should not be the initial goal.

The impact of exercise or regular physical activity on prostate cancer is controversial, but, like most lifestyle changes, it will always be deemed so due to the lack of long-term randomized trials, which will probably not be performed any time soon. A large review of the epidemiologic evidence pointed toward a "probable" reduction in risk with regular physical activity,[59] but keep in mind that prostate cancer mortality and obesity are related. Recently, higher levels of physical activity were associated with a lower risk of being diagnosed with a more aggressive prostate cancer, and a potential for improved survival in the Health Professionals Follow-up Study.[60]

Physical activity reduces CVD and mortality, and the data is profound, and weight lifting also seems to provide benefits. Additional data from the Health Professionals' Follow-up Study prospectively followed over 44,000 men for 12 years.[61] Men who ran for 1 hour or more per week had a 42% reduction (RR = 0.58; p < 0.001 for trend) in the risk of coronary heart disease (CHD), and those who just walked for 30 minutes or

more per day or who were involved in other physical activities also had a risk reduction in CHD versus those who did not engage in these activities. Surprisingly, men who trained with weights for just 30 minutes or more per week experienced a 23% risk reduction (RR = 0.77; p = 0.03 for trend) in CHD. This was a unique observation because previous prospective studies have not addressed this issue. Weight training can increase fat-free mass, lean body weight, and resting metabolic rate, and potentially reduce the risk of abdominal fat deposition.[62] Weight training or resistance training also seems to improve glucose control or increase insulin sensitivity,[63] improve lipid levels,[64] and reduce hypertension.[65]

The first randomized study of resistance exercise for men receiving androgen deprivation therapy or luteinizing hormone-releasing hormone (LHRH) therapy for prostate cancer was completed several years ago.[66] The trial was only 12 weeks in duration (n = 155) and men either lifted weights 3 times per week, or were assigned to a non-lifting group. Body composition did not change during this short study, but the significant reduction in fatigue and improved quality of life with weight training should probably make this a standard lifestyle change for men receiving this type of treatment in the future, especially for those without bone metastasis. Men with bone metastasis should be told to check with several physicians in order to receive the approval of a resistance program due to the theoretical possibility of an increased risk for fracture with osteoblastic bone lesions.

Physical activity may reduce the risk of other urologic conditions, such as benign prostatic hyperplasia (BPH)[67] and erectile dysfunction (ED).[68] This unique and recent 2-year randomized trial of vigorous exercise to improve ED needs to garner more attention.[69] Approximately one third of the men reporting ED regained normal erectile function in this trial, but the majority of men experienced at least some tangible improvement in function and in reducing the risk of common CVD markers.[68] Also, the potential to impact the risk of several major cancers, such as colorectal carcinoma, should make exercise itself a lifelong priority for most men.[70]

Mental health benefits of physical activity seem to be just as acute preliminarily as the physical health benefits. A 6-month follow-up study of 156 adult volunteers with major depressive disorder (MDD) who were randomly assigned to a 4-month course of aerobic exercise (30 minutes 3 times/week), sertraline therapy, or a combination of exercise and sertraline was completed.[71,72] After 4 months, patients in all three groups demonstrated significant mental improvement. However, after 10 months, individuals in the exercise group had significantly lower recurrence rates than individuals in the medication arm of the study. Exercising during the follow-up period was associated with a 51% reduction in the risk of a diagnosis of depression at the end of the investigation. Men need to be instructed that regular physical activity and resistance training have such profound physical and mental health benefits that not performing these activities certainly limits the potential for improved overall health. I often tell patients that if the overall results from physical activity studies were viewed similar to a pharmacologic intervention then it would have already garnered a Nobel prize in medicine.

Again, the initial goal for men should be to achieve fitness or wellness before assessing success in terms of weight loss. In other words, many men considered overweight or obese may reduce the risk of overall early mortality by just performing regular physical activity and not losing any weight. Men who exercise should be told that weight loss is not initially needed in order to obtain clinically relevant benefits. These findings have already been well documented in large prospective studies of women who have not lost weight, but who exercise on a regular basis.[73]

LIFESTYLE CHANGES TAILORED TO EACH PERSON

Recommendation #4: Emphasize to patients that there is no single ideal weight loss diet or intervention. Help patients choose a diet or lifestyle change and interventions that are tailored to their own personality. Remember, the end result may actually justify the means, and most diets and interventions consist of several consistent and overall related healthy messages.

Low-fat diets, low-carbohydrate diets, drug therapy, surgery—the list of potential methods to reduce weight continues to abound, confuse, and at times frustrate many men.[36] The potential to lose sight of one of the primary goals is always a risk when dealing with a patient attempting to lose weight. A similar analogy exists for smoking cessation, whereby numerous potential credible interventions are now available rather than a single intervention.[74] Some dietary interventions involving men with prostate cancer, such as reducing overall dietary fat have been beneficial in terms of a PSA response,[75] while other longer randomized trials have not demonstrated such a benefit for men without prostate cancer.[38] Low-carbohydrate diets have provided some sustained weight loss in recent randomized trials, and it is a novel dietary method, but compliance rates in just 1 year approach 50% and PSA and prostate cancer risk data are needed.[76,77] Higher insulin or glucose levels from a variety of etiologies, such as diet and obesity, have been preliminarily associated with a higher prostate cancer risk, cancer-specific mortality, and overall mortality.[78–81]

A truly unique recently randomized published study comparing the effects of a variety of fad diets on weight loss and cardiovascular risk should provide the impetus for any clinician dealing with any patient attempting to lose weight with a more practical perspective on weight loss itself. A total of 160 overweight or obese men and women (mean BMI = 35) were randomized to one of the following diets for 1-year: low carbohydrate (Atkins®), low fat (Ornish®), low glycemic load (Zone®), or a calorie-restricted (Weight Watchers®) dietary program.[82] All of the diets were associated with weight loss and a reduced risk of coronary heart disease from Framingham risk scores in participants that were able to adhere to their respective allocated diets. However, drop-out rates within just 1 year of this study were notable. The drop out rates were 48% with the Atkins diet, 50% with the Ornish diet, 35% for the Zone diet, and 35% for Weight Watchers. Compliance is difficult, but for those who can adhere to these diets, the benefits may outweigh the negatives when considering the impact of obesity on all-cause mortality. All of these so-called "fad" diets carry consistent themes, such as reducing overall caloric intake and increasing physical activity levels. Most fad diets consist of a delicate balancing act between caloric control and additional exercise. The consistent simple mantra of caloric restriction should be emphasized. Food and beverage sizes have increased in recent years with obesity rates, and greater portion sizes and access to fast foods appear to at least encourage greater caloric intake.[83,84] Some studies have found an increased risk of prostate cancer in men with higher caloric intakes over time; regardless of whether these calories were mostly derived from fat, protein, or carbohydrate.[85] Simple caloric control may be one method of effective weight loss and disease prevention, and the research derived from the centenarians and schoolchildren on the island of Okinawa (Japan) have been a model for the benefits of caloric restriction and its potential impact on all-cause mortality.[86] Simply reducing total fat intake cannot be the only viable, realistic, or even practical solution, and the effectiveness over just caloric restriction has been questioned recently in meta-analysis,[87] especially since greater caloric concentrations can now be found in a variety of carbohydrate sources, for example.[88] Diet should indeed fit personality.

The most extensive animal studies to date examining the correlation between prostate cancer and fat and energy intakes may have revealed the most insight on energy restriction and cancer progression.[89] Researchers utilized androgen-sensitive prostate tumors from donor rats, transplanted them to other rats, and fed them either fat-restricted or carbohydrate-restricted diets. Severe combined immunodeficient mice (SCID) mice were injected with LNCaP human prostate cancer cells to generate tumors, and then ingested similar diets. Researchers restricted energy intake by reducing energy from fat or carbohydrate, or simply reducing total energy from all sources, while at all times keeping other nutrients constant. Cancer proliferation was observed to be independent of the percentage of fat in the diet, as long as the total energy was restricted. The reduction in cancer growth was even identical in all types of energy-restricted laboratory animals. The findings of this experiment suggest that a reduction in overall energy intake, and not just fat, reduced the risk or progression of prostate cancer.[89,90]

Again, another perspective on weight loss that can be proffered to patients is highlighted by the results of a unique recent prospective cohort. A total of 6391 overweight and obese individuals who were at least 35 years of age were followed for 9 years.[91] Compared with individuals not trying to lose weight and reporting no weight change, those individuals reporting intentional weight loss had a 24% reduced mortality rate. Mortality rates were reduced in individuals who reported attempting to lose weight compared with those not attempting to lose weight, independent of the actual weight change. Compared with individuals not attempting to lose weight and reporting no weight change, individuals attempting to lose weight had the following hazard rate ratios (HRR): no weight change (HRR = 0.80), lost weight (HRR = 0.76), and gained weight (HRR = 0.94). Attempted weight loss was associated with lower all-cause mortality; independent or regardless of the actual weight change. This study stresses an important overall issue; again weight loss is not necessarily the ultimate goal but at least attempting weight loss through whatever method seems to impact health. The current concern over which diet or exercise program has the most data, or which dietary method is best may not be the most effective realistic and practical approach. Men should be allowed to choose a fairly safe method of weight loss because the end may justify the means. A patient willing to simply attempt a weight loss program should provide encouragement to the clinician. In my practice, if a man is motivated to try a low-carbohydrate diet, low-fat, or another type of diet, drug therapy or even surgery; a proper review of the data is provided but ultimately whatever method the patient ultimately chooses, we will work with them to achieve the first goal of becoming more healthy or fit, and hopefully the second goal of losing weight. If the second goal is not immediately, or ever, achieved then we do not believe that this is tantamount to a lack of success, because other cardiovascular markers have demonstrated that the first of the two goals is by far the most important. Effort counts, and the result may not ideally match the effort, but generally, in some capacity, the results are affected at least minimally by the effort. The concept of being overweight or obese and simultaneously healthy is plausible. Other individuals make no attempt or a feeble attempt to reduce weight regardless of their current status. It seems appropriate to encourage and applaud the consistent weight loss effort,

and clinicians may play a primary role in monitoring and motivating patients, but only if regular contact between the patient and practitioner over a long duration is possible.[92] The clinician's role is to provide the range of possible of interventions, from least to most invasive, and the risks and benefits of each intervention. Ultimately the patient makes the choice and we monitor these patients and always encourage regular physical activity with the intervention to achieve the best potential result. I recommend certain dietary or lifestyle interventions more than others for most patients seeking advice, and they provide a foundation that other interventions can build upon and utilize to some degree. Some of these basic lifestyle interventions are listed in the rest of the following chapter.

SATURATED, TRANS-FATTY ACIDS AND CHOLESTEROL

Recommendation #5: Replace saturated, trans-fatty acids, and even cholesterol with more healthy types of monounsaturated or polyunsaturated fat. Total fat intake should not be the initial concern, but the specific types of dietary fat consumed. In addition, the utilization of commercial plant sterol/stanol products may also be heart and prostate healthy.

Saturated fat (SF) is also simply known as "hydrogenated fat," and it reduces LDL receptor expression and increases LDL serum levels[21]—LDL increases by 2% for every 1% increase in total calories from SF. The NCEP (Adult Treatment Panel III or ATP III) recommends that SF be reduced to less than 7% of total calories to reduce the risk of CVD. The average US adult intake of SF is 11% of total calories. Some non-lean meats, high-fat dairy products (whole milk, butter, cheese, ice cream, and cream), tropical oils (palm oil, coconut oil, and palm kernel oil), baked products, and mixed dishes with dairy fats and shortenings are some of the primary sources of SF. Many foods that contain high levels of SF also contain high levels of trans-fat ("partially hydrogenated fat").

Epidemiologic studies have found that the consumption of a high concentration of SF and cholesterol may significantly increase the risk for CHD.[93] A meta-analysis that included 6356 person-years of follow-up has documented that reducing serum cholesterol by reducing SF intake reduces the risk of CHD by 24%.[94,95] A 21% reduction in coronary mortality and a 6% reduction in total mortality were also observed. No increase in non-CVD mortality was observed.

Past lifestyle changes and prostate cancer risk studies revolve around primary prevention, but there have been several studies of men post-treatment, and these should also be discussed.[96] A Canadian prospective study of men with prostate cancer observed a total of 384 men for a median of 5.2 years.[97] Compared with the men consuming the lowest levels of SF, those consuming the highest amount had a significant increase in risk of mortality from prostate cancer (RR = 3.1). Total fat and other subtypes of fat (except saturated) did not show any correlation between prostate cancer and mortality. A collaborative analysis of five prospective studies compared death rates from diseases of vegetarians versus non-vegetarians with similar lifestyles.[98] Data on more than 76,000 men and women documented 8330 deaths with a mean of 10.6 years of follow-up. There were no significant differences in death between vegetarians and non-vegetarians from prostate cancer, breast cancer, colorectal cancer, lung cancer, stomach cancer, or all other causes combined. However, mortality from ischemic heart disease was significantly lowered by 24% in vegetarians. This lower mortality from ischemic heart disease was greater at younger ages and was limited to those who had followed this diet for a longer period of time (>5 years). Further subset analyses of vegetarian versus non-vegetarian diets found that ischemic heart disease was 20% lower in occasional meat eaters, 34% lower in those that ate fish but not meat, 34% lower in lactoovovegetarians, and 26% lower in vegans when compared with regular meat eaters. Reducing all saturated fat in an individual's diet is not necessarily a practical and healthy dietary lifestyle change. The current cardiovascular goal of obtaining less than 7% of calories from saturated fat seems almost ideal from past studies, because getting zero calories from saturated fat not only seems too excessive, but can actually decrease levels of HDL.[99] Therefore, the old adage "everything in moderation" applies to this lifestyle recommendation.

All three primary classes of fatty acids: saturated, monounsaturated, and polyunsaturated can increase HDL when they substitute for carbohydrates in the diet and this effect is slightly greater for saturated fat, and monounsaturated fat is slightly greater than polyunsaturated fat (saturated>monounsaturated>polyunsaturated).[100] Saturated fats increase LDL and monounsaturated and polyunsaturated fat slightly decrease LDL. Dietary fatty acids replaced by carbohydrates cause an increase in triglyceride levels. Replacing saturated fat with carbohydrates proportionally reduces both HDL and LDL, and has minimal impact on the LDL/HDL ratio and increases triglycerides. Thus, this type of dietary change would be expected to have a minimal impact on the risk of CHD. When mono- or polyunsaturated fats are utilized or replace saturated fat, LDL is reduced and HDL changes minimally. Additionally, utilizing polyunsaturated instead of saturated fat could have numerous health benefits, for example, increasing insulin sensitivity and decreasing the risk of type II diabetes.[101,102]

Trans-fatty acids are also known as "partially hydrogenated" fatty acids.[103,104] They are found in higher concentrations in a variety of foods such as doughnuts, cake mixes, fast foods, potato chips, and many other products. Many of these compounds were placed in the food supply over a decade ago to increase the shelf-life of numerous popular food items. Some trans-fats are also found naturally in other foods. However, recent cardiovascular investigations have demonstrated a general health concern with these types of fatty acids.[105-108] These compounds seem to demonstrate a unique and dual negative effect because not only do they raise levels of LDL, but they can also reduce levels of HDL. In fact, the increase in the ratio of total/HDL cholesterol for these fats are approximately double that found for saturated fat.[109] Some specific unhealthy changes associated with greater intakes of trans-fat are increases in lipoprotein a,[110,111] increases in triglycerides,[107] impaired vasodilation,[112] increases in sudden cardiac death,[105] increased insulin resistance[113] and type II diabetes,[112] and adverse effects on the metabolism of healthy polyunsaturated fats through the inhibition of delta-6 desaturase.[114,115]

The association of trans-fat with cancer is unknown because some past and recent epidemiologic studies have not found an association,[44,116] but interestingly some other recent studies have suggested that these fatty acids may encourage cancer growth[117-119] and increase the risk of prostate cancer, and so the simple rule of what is heart healthy/unhealthy is also prostate healthy/unhealthy may also be applicable to these specific types of fatty acids. The observation that trans-fat is heart unhealthy makes the recommendation to reduce the intake of these fatty acids a priority.

Some food manufacturers tend to include large concentrations of these trans-fats in their products and others tend to include small concentrations or none at all. Men should be generally encouraged to consume items low in trans- or saturated fat. The Danish government decided that oils and fat with more than 2% industrially produced trans-fatty acids would no longer be sold in Denmark after January 1, 2004,[120] and the United States Food and Drug Administration (FDA) will require that the actual amount of trans-fat be reported on all food labels by January 1, 2006.[121] The FDA predicts that by 3 years after that date, the labeling of trans-fat will have prevented from 600 to 1200 additional cases of CHD and approximately 250 to 500 deaths per year. When this occurs, patients should simply compare several similar food items and choose the one lower in trans-fat. Consumer and economic pressure should lead to a general reduction or elimination of these fatty acids in the diet.

It is a fairly simple method to just rapidly and simply compare food labels and choose a similar dietary item that has a reduced quantity of saturated fat. Patients should be instructed to compare several milks, meats, potato chips, and any other items and choose the one that is lower in saturated fat. For example, when comparing whole milk to 2% fat, 1% fat, and skim milk one will quickly learn that all of these milk types compared with skim milk contain many more grams of saturated fat, and a higher amount of overall calories.

Again, the simple past suggestion of just reducing overall dietary fat intake, instead of sub-types of fat has not been supported recently in the prostate cancer or CVD literature,[38,122,123] especially in regards to mortality data.[123] Clinicians need to emphasize that the types of fat ingested seem to influence disease risk overall more than just dietary fat intake. In the worst case scenario, this tends to decrease cholesterol and reduce the risk of CVD, which is why this recommendation makes the most practical sense to any man concerned about prostate cancer.

Dietary cholesterol increases serum cholesterol, but not as significantly as saturated fat. A total of 100 mg of dietary cholesterol increases serum cholesterol approximately 10 mg/dL per 1000 kcal.[21] Daily mean cholesterol intake is greater for men in the US (331 mg) than women (213 mg). Foods high in cholesterol include eggs, animal and dairy products, poultry, and shellfish. Sterols or the marine equivalent of cholesterol in shellfish and shrimp do not greatly impact human serum cholesterol unless cooked in butter, fried, or consumed in high quantities.[124,125] Dietary cholesterol ingestion should be encouraged to be less than 200 mg/day to impact or lower LDL cholesterol.[21] The impact of dietary cholesterol on prostate cancer is unknown, but it is known that prostate cancer cells tend to utilize large amounts of cholesterol in their cellular membranes,[126] and this is especially notable with a greater extent or progression (metastases) of the disease itself.[127] Reducing dietary cholesterol just makes practical sense from a cardiovascular risk standpoint.

Plant sterols/stanols or the plant equivalent of cholesterol is found in higher concentrations in vegetarian diets.[128,129] These compounds inhibit the intestinal absorption of dietary and biliary cholesterol and are most effective in individuals with high cholesterol absorption and low cholesterol synthesis. Patients with apolipoprotein (apo) E4 experience greater cholesterol absorption and may respond more favorably to these compounds.[130] A total of 2 to 3 g/day of plant-derived sterols/stanols decreases LDL cholesterol in most individuals by 6% to 15% without changing HDL or triglyceride levels.[21,131-137] These products are now available in grocery stores as regular and low-fat margarines (Benecol®, Take Charge®) and may soon be widely available in other products such as orange juice, yogurt, and some dietary supplements.[128,129] Clinicians can encourage patients with higher cholesterol levels to consume 2 to 3 g/day of these compounds, but the current high price of these products is an issue,[21] and their impact on prostate cancer is not known. Interestingly, one of the main sources of these compounds is actually soybean oil, so the utilization of this oil in cooking is theoretically another option.

FRUIT AND VEGETABLES

Recommendation #6: Encourage the regular consumption of a diversity of fruits and vegetables for CVD risk reduction, and not just tomato products and lycopene. Lycopene dietary supplements should not be recommended at this time for most patients.

Few topics in prostate cancer prevention have garnered as much attention as lycopene, tomato products, and their potential benefits. Numerous studies support the intake of tomatoes and tomato products, but numerous other investigations have not found a relationship. For example, a well-referenced analysis of over 80 epidemiologic studies was completed on tomatoes and cancer risk several years ago.[138] Half of the studies analyzed support the consumption of tomato products at least once a day to reduce the risk of a variety of cancers including prostate cancer, but a large number of studies in this same analysis failed to detect a correlation. Another important finding was that no investigations to date have indicated that a greater consumption of tomato products significantly increases the risk of cancer, but the overall recommendation of the author was to increase the consumption of fruits and vegetables and not just tomato products! The ongoing research of tomatoes and lycopene continues to moderately support the potential for these products to impact prostate cancer risk or progression.[139-141]

One of the largest animal studies utilized lycopene or tomato powder or a calorie-restricted diet and found some interesting results.[142] The consumption of tomato powder but not lycopene inhibited prostate carcinogenesis, which suggests that tomato products contain compounds in addition to lycopene that can potentially inhibit the growth of prostate tumors. Reducing overall caloric intake also reduced the risk of prostate cancer and increased survival in these male rats.

Tomatoes are not the only source of lycopene. A variety of other healthy foods contain this compound, including apricots, guava, pink grapefruit, and watermelon.[96] Indeed, a recent dietary case-control study from China that observed one of the largest reductions in prostate cancer risk in the literature (odds ratio = 0.18) found watermelon consumption may have been partially responsible, but the impact of pumpkin, spinach, tomatoes, and citrus intake was also notable even after adjusting for a variety of confounders such as fat and total caloric intake.[143]

The initial focus and ongoing interest in lycopene and its sources may actually stem from a potential reduced risk of CVD with a greater intake of this compound from dietary sources.[144-147] Again, heart health seems to potentially promote prostate health.

However, a variety of fruits and especially vegetables have been associated with a reduced risk of prostate cancer.[148] For example, members of the Brassica vegetable group such as: broccoli, Brussels sprouts, cabbage, cauliflower, kale, watercress, and many others may reduce the risk of prostate cancer.[149] The Allium vegetables have also been associated with a reduced risk of prostate cancer, and this group includes chives, garlic, leeks, onions, and scallions.[150] The interpretation of the sum of the data thus far is lucid—it advocates the increased consumption of fruits and vegetables to potentially impact prostate cancer, but the data currently supports the reduction in CVD risk and mortality. If a patient desires to focus only on the consumption of tomato products, it represents a myopic and not necessarily plausible choice in many cases because compliance can become a major issue after a period of time, and this behavior is not consistent with the overall research that supports that many fruits and vegetables have combined unique and shared anticancer and anti-heart disease compounds that contribute to improved overall health.[148]

It is disappointing and surprising to many currently that the largest prospective epidemiologic studies recently have not found a correlation for the increased consumption of fruits and vegetables and a reduced risk of most cancers or mortality from cancer,[151–155] and this includes prostate cancer. Clinicians need to be candid with patients and explain that, currently at least, a CVD risk reduction may occur, but the data is not as profound in cancer or survival from cancer.

Lycopene dietary supplements always seem to draw attention, but long-term data with these pills are lacking. In addition, a recent 1-year pilot trial of small to large intakes (15–120 mg/day) of lycopene pills for rising PSA following failed local therapy in 36 men also failed to demonstrate any initial PSA or clinical benefits.[156] Therefore, intake from dietary sources at this time continues to remain the wisest and cheapest choice.

DIETARY FIBER

Recommendation #7: Encourage the consumption of more total dietary fiber (25–30 g/day) from food and even supplements, especially viscous ("soluble") fiber, but insoluble fiber is also beneficial.

The diverse health benefits derived from consuming dietary fiber have been well referenced in the medical literature and include a decrease in CHD risk.[157–161] Most recent pooled analysis of past cohort studies of dietary fiber for the reduction of CHD included data from 10 studies from the US and Europe.[162] Over a period of 6 to 10 years of follow-up, a total of 5249 total coronary cases and 2011 coronary deaths were observed among over 91,000 men and 245,000 women. After researchers adjusted for demographics, BMI, and behavioral changes, each 10 g/day increase of calorie-adjusted total dietary fiber was correlated with a 14% reduction in the risk of total coronary events (RR = 0.86) and a 27% reduction in risk of coronary death (RR = 0.73). Cereal, fruit, and vegetable fiber consumption demonstrated a relative risk reduction of 0.90, 0.84, and 1.00 for total coronary events, and 0.75, 0.70, and 1.00 for coronary deaths with each 10 g/day increase of calorie-adjusted total dietary fiber from these sources. The findings were similar for both sexes. There was obviously minimal support for an inverse relationship between vegetable fiber consumption and risk of CHD, which was potentially explained by these researchers by the potential of some vegetables to lack many nutrients and/or that have the ability to dramatically increase glucose levels (potatoes), especially with the common starchy and highly processed vegetables (corn, peas, etc). Researchers from the pooled analysis also attempted to determine whether the decrease in risk of CHD was from soluble (viscous) and/or insoluble fiber. Past studies have not found a consistent benefit with one class of fiber over the other.[163–166] However, in this recent pooled analysis,[162] inverse associations occurred for both soluble and insoluble fiber, but the reductions in risk were greater for soluble fiber (RR = 0.46) and coronary death for each 10-g increment in intake. Soluble fiber has the ability to increase the concentration of intraluminal viscosity of the small intestine, and this can reduce nutrient absorption and encourage binding to bile acids.[167] This impact may reduce insulin production and improve glucose control,[168] reduce serum cholesterol,[169] and may even reduce blood pressure.[170] Viscous or "soluble" fiber from oats, barley, guar, pectin, beans, and psyllium (Metamucil®, etc) for example, has consistently demonstrated the ability to reduce LDL cholesterol levels compared with insoluble fiber.[21]

The addition of only 15 g of psyllium (soluble fiber) daily with a 10 mg statin (simvastatin) was demonstrated to be as effective as 20 mg of statin alone in lowering cholesterol in a recent small pilot placebo study of 68 patients over 12 weeks.[171]

Another recent meta-analysis of 24 randomized placebo-controlled trials of fiber supplementation found a consistent impact on blood pressure.[172] Supplementation with just small amounts of fiber (mean dose, 11.5 g/day) reduced systolic blood pressure by 1.13 mmHg and diastolic pressure by 1.26 mmHg. These reductions were greater in individuals over the age of 40 years and in hypertensive individuals compared with younger and normotensive subjects. It is of interest that the daily intake of fiber in the US and many other Western countries is only around 15 g/day, which is approximately only 50% of the amount consistently recommended by the American Heart Association (25 to 30 g/day).[173]

The data on fiber intake and cancer prevention are not consistent or without controversy, especially in the area of polyp formation and colorectal cancer risk.[161,174,175] In addition, the impact of dietary fiber on PSA levels has not been thoroughly evaluated. A recent randomized trial of a combination of a low-fat and high fiber diet over a 4-year period failed to find a reduction in PSA and prostate cancer risk in white and African-American men.[38,176] However, one of the largest case-control studies was published from Italy and found a moderate reduced risk of prostate cancer with increased consumption of dietary fiber, especially soluble fiber, cellulose, and vegetable fiber.[177] One of the only clinical studies of soluble versus insoluble fiber only for PSA reduction was published several years ago.[178] This small study (n = 14) of short duration (4 months) included men with hyperlipidemia and without cancer. Researchers found a small but statistically lower PSA in men consuming soluble fiber compared with insoluble fiber (25–30 g per 1000 kcal). Similar minimal clinical benefits in another short clinical controlled study of men with prostate cancer was noteworthy when utilizing only foods with higher fiber intakes such as rye-bran bread,[179] but whether the soluble fiber in these foods or the synergistic interaction of other nutrients with and without fiber were the reason for the benefit is not known. Again, soluble fiber can reduce cholesterol levels (LDL) compared with insoluble fiber. Thus, the increase of fiber and especially viscous fiber to 25 to 30 g/day makes sense in terms of potentially lowering LDL and the risk of CHD,[21] and this can be achieved with the combination of foods and supplements, or with food by itself.

In my experience, costly commercial products that contain modified citrus pectin (MCP) are popular with some patients with prostate cancer because some laboratory studies,[180,181] and one small (n = 13) clinical study of limited duration has suggested that this compound may inhibit the growth of a variety of cancers and may increase PSA doubling time after recurrent prostate cancer.[182] It is notable that the vast majority of the MCP is composed of soluble fiber. Recommending MCP or in my opinion just increasing amounts of soluble fiber from food or cheaper supplements, for example psyllium, seems to make more sense.

"PLANT ESTROGEN" PRODUCTS

Recommendation #8: Encourage the use of moderate amounts of traditional cheap dietary soy and other so-called "plant estrogen" products, such as flaxseed, because they also contain much more than just "plant estrogens."

Ischemic heart disease reductions have been correlated with a higher consumption of traditional soy products. International comparison studies have observed a reduced rate of this disease in Asian countries along with a higher consumption of soy products versus Western countries.[183] Although this correlation is most likely confounded by other dietary and lifestyle factors, such as a lower overall intake of saturated fat; laboratory and clinical studies have been fairly consistent in supporting the cardiovascular benefits of soy.[184–189] Soy protein may increase LDL uptake and removal, and increase the activity of hydroxymethylglutaryl-coenzyme A reductase and cholesterol 7α-hydroxylase, which further eliminates cholesterol in bile acids. Soy may contain additional benefits beyond its protein and phytoestrogen content, such as an adequate concentration of omega fatty acids, fiber, and vitamin E.[190] A past and more recent meta-analysis of clinical studies suggests that 2 to 3 servings per day of soy protein (approximately 25 g) or greater may be sufficient to significantly decrease cholesterol levels in men and women.[191,192] Although, the FDA has supported this finding, it is important to understand that this benefit is enhanced when soy protein consumption is increased and saturated fat consumption is decreased because otherwise the beneficial effects may not be as tangible. The FDA did not provide support for the plant estrogen content of soy and cardiovascular protection because the majority of the evidence demonstrated that the soy protein content has been more closely related to cholesterol reduction.

Biochanin A, a genistein precursor (from soy), and genistein itself have demonstrated the ability to inhibit the proliferation of both hormone-sensitive and hormone-insensitive cancer cell lines,[193,194] and both compounds have decreased PSA levels of LNCaP cells in vitro.[195] Genistein may inhibit the growth of prostate cancer through a variety of mechanisms, such as interfering with tyrosine kinase growth factor and other similar growth factors and receptors,[196–199] affecting topoisomerase II,[200] inhibiting angiogenesis,[201] and promoting apoptosis.[202] However, significant reductions in testosterone have not been observed in Japanese men consuming these products.[203] Perhaps partial suppression of a variety of hormones over several months, years or even decades may be sufficient to delay the onset of clinically significant prostate cancer or a recurrence.[204] Other potential benefits of genistein and other soy compounds may occur because of their estrogenic activity, the ability to inhibit 5α-reductase and/or the aromatase enzyme, and overall antioxidant free radical scavenger properties.[205] Clinical trials utilizing soy and its various isolated compounds, such as genistein, at a variety of dosages are required to determine if the in-vitro and epidemiologic data correlate to an actual clinical response. Clinical trials utilizing soy or soy products are currently being conducted at numerous institutions.[206,207] Early results from some small pilot trials have observed some benefits for genistein supplementation in men with prostate cancer undergoing watchful waiting, but not as an adjunct to or after conventional treatment.[208] Another smaller randomized trial did not find a significant impact with soy isoflavones on PSA, but increasing dosages of soy protein were not studied.[209]

Soy was a part of a randomized trial of men undergoing a combination lifestyle and supplement regimen after being diagnosed with prostate cancer, and after 1 year of study the results have been encouraging in men with lower Gleason scores (less than 7) or well-differentiated tumors.[75] Men without prostate cancer or those with minimal and less aggressive disease may potentially have the most to gain from including soy in their diet. Regardless, the cardiovascular benefits of soy seem adequate to recommend these products to most men. For example, the cholesterol lowering benefits of incorporating soy products in the diet seem reason enough to encourage their consumption.[210] Clinicians should recommend products that are high in soy protein or that have retained the characteristics of the traditional soy products such as soybeans, tofu, tempeh, soy protein powder, soy oil, soy nuts that are low in saturated fats, and in some cases, soy milk.[96,211] Soy protein bars are popular but, in our opinion, most contain too many calories; therefore, most of these products should be avoided. Soy pills are also a concern since they have not demonstrated a consistent ability to reduce hot flashes,[212] which may be an indicator of poor potency, and they do not contain the numerous other compounds available in the traditional dietary sources of soy.[96]

Clinical research and recommendations should not be limited to soy, because of the potential benefit of numerous other phytoestrogens in nature.

Flaxseed, also known as "linseed" has demonstrated a fairly consistent ability to lower cholesterol in normolipidemic and hyperlipidemic individuals.[213–217] Flaxseed contains an unusually high content of plant estrogen called "lignans," an omega-3 fatty acid (α-linolenic acid [ALA]), and soluble fiber; and it is low in cost.[96] Interestingly, crushed or grounded flaxseed has also demonstrated an ability to reduce menopausal symptoms as well as moderate doses of estrogen and progesterone in a cross-over 4-month total study trial of hypercholesterolemic menopausal women.[218] This same study demonstrated a minimal impact on cholesterol, but an ability to reduce glucose and insulin levels.

Again, ALA is an omega-3 fatty acid found in high concentrations in flaxseed and flaxseed oil, canola oil, and soybean oils, and this compound can be partially converted to eicosapentaenoic acid (EPA) and docosahexaenoic acid (DHA) in humans; interestingly, EPA and DHA are the primary omega-3 oils found in fish, which have demonstrated past significant cardiovascular benefits.[219] Randomized trials utilizing foods high in ALA have consistently reduced the risk of CHD and have favorably impacted all-cause mortality despite no significant changes in serum cholesterol.[220-222]

Lignans, another type of phytoestrogen found in high concentrations in flaxseed, and other components in flaxseed (ALA) have demonstrated potent anticancer properties in laboratory studies utilizing breast and prostate cancer cell lines.[223,224] The largest cohort study examining the correlation between fat intake and prostate cancer risk was the Netherlands Cohort Study.[225] Approximately 58,000 men were followed for more than 6 years, and 642 cases of prostate cancer were documented. An extensive 150-item food frequency questionnaire was utilized. No correlations were found between total fat and other subtypes of fat and prostate cancer risk. There was an association between a reduced risk of prostate cancer and an increased intake of ALA. This was a notable observation because several past prospective investigations observed the opposite trend with this fatty acid.[226,227] The first trial of flaxseed in men with prostate cancer was published several years ago. This pilot study of men consuming flaxseed and a low-fat diet 4 weeks before radical prostatectomy demonstrated that flaxseed (about 3 round tablespoons/day of ground seed) may have provided a clinical benefit via hormone suppression and via other mechanisms, such as reducing the proliferation index of cancer cells in the prostate and encouraging apoptosis, especially for men with lower Gleason scores (6 or less), before and after this conventional treatment versus historic controls.[228] Also, the mean reduction in total cholesterol over the 4-week study was an impressive 27 points. A similar and almost identical recent study was performed by some of the same researchers. Men at higher-risk for prostate cancer (negative biopsy patients) also observed an apparent risk reduction and decreased cholesterol with just a 6-month course of daily flaxseed powder and a low-fat diet.[229]

Clinicians need to remind patients that cheap ground flaxseed itself has received the most research, while straight flaxseed oil and pills have received little research in humans.[96] In addition, flaxseed should be ingested 2 to 3 hours before or after taking a prescription drug(s) or dietary supplement(s) because the high concentration of fiber could theoretically reduce the absorption of these agents, as is the potential case with any product or supplement high in fiber. Moderate intakes are also important (1–3 tablespoons/day) along with water consumption with flaxseed because of the potential for impaction and/or laxative effects. Again, the potential for CVD risk reduction should be emphasized because the prostate benefits are preliminary.

FISH

Recommendation #9: Encourage the consumption of moderate weekly intakes of canned, broiled, baked,

and raw fish (not fried), and other healthy sources of omega-3 fatty acids (for example, fish oil supplements, nuts, and cooking oils), dietary selenium, vitamin D, and vitamin E.

Soy and especially flaxseed are good sources of omega-3 fatty acids, but fish also contain high concentrations of omega-3 fatty acids (EPA and DHA) and in addition, vitamin D.[96] These compounds have demonstrated numerous benefits in terms of reducing the risk of a variety of prevalent chronic diseases,[230] especially CVD.[231,232] Some of the observed mechanisms of action for fish and fish oil include a reduction in triglycerides,[233] blood pressure,[234] platelet aggregation,[235] and arrhythmias.[236] However, the primary focus of their benefit has been their potential ability to reduce the risk of sudden cardiac death.[237–239]

Fish oils have also been shown to inhibit the growth of prostate tumors in the laboratory.[240] Several epidemiologic and pilot studies also support the consumption of fish or fish oils to reduce the incidence and progression of prostate cancer,[241,242] and the ability to reduce cyclooxygenase II (COX2) in patients may be one of the many apparent benefits.[242] Although an epidemiologic review of fish and marine fatty acids concluded that no consistent reduction in prostate cancer risk has been observed in past studies,[243] the results of a large recent prospective study published after this analysis may tip the balance in favor of prevention. The Health Professionals Follow-up Study included over 47,000 men with 12-years of follow-up.[244] During this study, a total of 2482 cases of prostate cancer were diagnosed, and 617 of these cases were diagnosed as advanced prostate cancer, including 278 metastatic prostate cancers. Researchers found that consuming fish more than 3 times per week compared with less than twice per month was associated with a reduced risk of prostate cancer, and the strongest relationship was for metastatic disease (44% reduction). Fish consumption in this study consisted of canned tuna, dark meat fish (mackerel, salmon, sardines, bluefish, and swordfish), and other unspecified fish dishes. The consumption of seafood such as shrimp, lobster, and scallops were not associated with prostate cancer risk.

Clinicians need to tell their patients that many fish contain high levels of omega-3 fatty acids and vitamin D—salmon, tuna, sardines, and a variety of other baked, broiled, raw, but not fried fish are potentially beneficial.[96] Variety should be encouraged to increase compliance. Overall, the beneficial effects of fish consumption on prostate cancer risk remain to be proven, but its role in reducing cardiovascular risk or all-cause mortality is extremely strong as mentioned before and as observed from clinical trials encouraging fish[245] or fish oil consumption[246,247] in patients with a history of CHD. A recent concern over mercury levels of fish has been expressed by the FDA and in the overall medical literature, but the preliminary data is controversial, and

it is not known at this time what kind of clinical impact these mercury levels may have on the individual.[248,249] Four types of large predatory fish (king mackerel, shark, swordfish, and tilefish) have caused most concern because these fish retain greater concentrations of methyl-mercury. Regardless, moderate consumption (2–3 times/week) of most fish should have little impact on overall human mercury serum levels, but more ongoing research in this area should soon provide better clarity of the clinical impact of this concern. Interestingly, a recent large investigation of moderate mercury serum levels in older individuals found little to no negative long-term impacts on neurobehavioral parameters.[250] In any event, the positive impact of consuming fish seems to outweigh the negative impact in the majority of individuals with the exception of women considering pregnancy or who are pregnant.

A variety of nuts share some similar clinical positive impacts to omega-3 oils found in fish. For example, a consistent reduction in the risk of CHD and/or sudden cardiac death has been associated with an increased consumption of nuts in prospective studies.[251–256] Nuts contain a variety of potential beneficial compounds, such as ALA, other polyunsaturated fats, mono-unsaturated fats, vitamin E, magnesium, potassium, flavonoids,[251] and potentially selenium, for example, from Brazil nuts.[96] Some of these and other compounds from a variety of foods, but not necessarily dietary supplement sources, have been associated with a lower risk of prostate cancer, for example, vitamin E,[257] ALA,[225] and selenium.[96] However, more research is needed in this area.

A variety of cooking oils such as soybean, canola, and olive oil also contain a high concentration of omega-3 fatty acids, monounsaturated fat, and numerous other vitamins and minerals including vitamin E.[96,219,258] Consumption of a variety of these nuts and oils could also be encouraged to the patient concerned about prostate cancer, but again most of the evidence surrounding their use is for cardiovascular protection. Patients need to keep in mind that most cooking oils contain 120 calories per tablespoon; therefore, moderation is again the foundation of good health.

Recent reviews of healthy omega-3 fatty acids can be found in the literature.[259,260] Reviews such as this one continue to emphasize the general health benefits of certain diets and supplements without just a focus on prostate cancer itself. These publications continue to suggest that heart healthy products have some of the best potential to produce a prostate healthy situation.

COMMON SENSE CHANGES

Recommendation #10: Always emphasize the obvious changes such as smoking cessation, moderate alcohol

consumption, daily multivitamin, reduced supplement intake, especially vitamin E, and appropriate heart healthy drug intervention when needed because of the potential impacts on prostate and general health.

Numerous other lifestyle modifications and supplements should be discussed by clinicians such as smoking cessation to reduce all-cause mortality including cancer,[261,262] and potentially to reduce the risk of prostate cancer,[263] or the risk of advanced or aggressive prostate cancer.[264,265] Alcohol consumption in moderation seems to reduce cardiovascular events,[266] and its impact at this level of consumption has not been positive or negative in regards to prostate cancer risk.[96]

Most men may derive a benefit from taking a cheap low-dose multivitamin daily to eliminate basic nutritional deficiencies and improve overall health, and a recent 7.5 year randomized trial confirmed the potential benefits of this simplistic recommendation.[267] In addition, patients that qualify for a low-dose aspirin,[268] statin,[269] or other heart protective medications for CVD reduction[270] may be surprised to learn that even these products have been associated with prostate health.[267–270] Along the same line of thinking, patients should currently stay away from individual vitamin E supplements (apart from the low-dose-50 IU or less in a multivitamin) due to recent concerning data observed in randomized cardiovascular,[271,272] and cancer trials.[273]

CONCLUSIONS

This chapter may provide a strong foundation for men with a desire to incorporate lifestyle changes to not only reduce the risk of prostate cancer, but, more importantly, to impact all-cause mortality. Minimal time is needed to suggest these changes in an office encounter. These recommendations may seem simplistic; nevertheless, past studies have clearly demonstrated that very few men (less than 5%) report adherence to numerous healthy behaviors at one time.[274] It seems to be more common in the past to follow one healthy change in excess, rather than multiple changes in moderation. This may be the result of past studies focusing on one lifestyle change to produce an overall impact on disease risk, poor compliance, lack of attention, time, or understanding, or a lack of motivation. Regardless of the multiple potential reasons for minimal adherence, investigations of combined moderate lifestyle changes continue to demonstrate that it is more the sum of what you do, rather than one or two specific behavioral changes, that can impact cardiovascular markers, cancer, and all-cause mortality.[275]

Recommending a pill is the simple answer, but few supplements for prostate cancer prevention or total mortality reduction can be recommended at this time.[96,276–278] Moreover, compliance is also an issue over a long period of time with any agent. Additionally, potential supplements that may increase the risk of prostate cancer or interfere with conventional treatment continues to be a concern,[273,279,280] and no dietary supplement has ever come close to matching the reduction in all-cause mortality observed in clinical trials of lifestyle changes.[96] The time seems more than ripe to redirect our attention toward lifestyle changes with regard to prostate cancer. Indeed, what is turning out to be heart healthy seems tantamount to prostate healthy, and this is the best potential practical and realistic recommendation that has worked in my consulting practice for over 10 years. It also seems that larger health organizations are beginning to apply this same concept,[281] and this is truly exciting, because "the forest has to take precedence over the tree" when it comes to this important subject.

REFERENCES

1. Bonow RO, Smaha LA, Smith SC, et al. The international burden of cardiovascular disease: responding to the emerging epidemic. Circulation 2002;106:1602–1605.

2. World Heart Federation web site. Available at: http://www.world-heart.org/introduction/call_to_action.html. Accessed August 20, 2002.

3. World Health Report. Mental Health: New Understanding, New Hope. Geneva, Switzerland: World Health Organization, 2001, pp 144–149.

4. Michaud CM, Murray CJL, Bloom BR. Burden of disease: implications for future research. JAMA 2001;285:535–539.

5. Murray CJL, Lopez AD. Mortality by cause for eight regions of the world: Global Burden of Disease Study. Lancet 1997;349:1269–1276.

6. Twombly, R. Cancer surpasses heart disease as leading cause of death for all but the very elderly. J Natl Cancer Inst 2005;97:330–331.

7. Thompson IM, Goodman PJ, Tangen CM, et al. The influence of finasteride on the development of prostate cancer. N Engl J Med 2003;349:215–224.

8. Scardino PT. The prevention of prostate cancer-The dilemma continues. N Engl J Med 2003;349:297–299.

9. Reynolds T. Prostate cancer prevention trial yields positive results, but with a few cautions. J Natl Cancer Inst 2003;95:1030–1031.

10. Clark LC, Combs GF Jr, Turnbull BW, et al. Effects of selenium supplementation for cancer prevention in patients with carcinoma of the skin. A randomized controlled trial. Nutritional Prevention of Cancer Study Group. JAMA 1996; 276:1957–1963.

11. Newschaffer CJ, Otani K, McDonald MK, et al. Causes of death in elderly prostate cancer patients and in a comparison nonprostate cancer cohort. J Natl Cancer Inst 2000;92:613–621.

12. Groome PA, Rohland SL, Brundage MD, et al. The relative risk of early death from comorbid illnesses among prostate cancer patients receiving curative treatment. J Urol 2005;173 (Suppl.):53 [abstract 193].

13. Senior K. Atherosclerosis gene increases susceptibility to prostate cancer. Lancet 2002;360:928.

14. Neugut AI, Rosenberg DJ, Ahsan H, et al. Association between coronary heart disease and cancers of the breast, prostate, and colon. Cancer Epidemiol Biomarkers Prev 1998;7:869–873.

15. Peterson HI. Tumor angiogenesis inhibition by prostaglandin synthetase inhibitors. Anticancer Res 1986;6:251.

16. Sandfeldt L, Hahn RG. Cardiovascular risk factors correlate with prostate size in men with bladder outlet obstruction. BJU Intl 2003;92:64–68.

17. Solomon H, Man JW, Wierzbicki AS, et al. Relation of erectile dysfunction to angiographic coronary artery disease. Am J Cardiol 2003;91:230–231.

18. Clark CM, Karlawish JHT. Alzheimer disease: Current concepts and emerging diagnostic and therapeutic strategies. Ann Intern Med 2003;138:400–410.

19. Moyad MA. Emphasizing and promoting overall health and nontraditional treatments after a prostate cancer diagnosis. Semin Urol Oncol 1999;17:119–124.

20. Nash IS, Mosca L, Blumenthal RS, et al. Contemporary awareness and understanding of cholesterol as a risk factor: Results of an American Heart Association National Survey. Arch Intern Med 2003;163:1597–1600.

21. The Expert Panel. Executive summary of the Third Report of the National Cholesterol Education Program (NCEP). Expert Panel on Detection, Evaluation, and Treatment of High Blood Cholesterol in Adults (Adult Treatment Panel III). JAMA 2001;285:2486–2498.

22. Grundy SM, Cleeman JI, Marz NB, et al. Implications of recent clinical trials for the National Cholesterol Education Program Adult Treatment Panel III Guidelines. Circulation 2004;110:227–239.

23. Mosca L. C-reactive protein-to screen or not screen? N Engl J Med 2002;347:1615–1616.

24. Ridker PM. Clinical application of C-reactive protein for cardiovascular disease detection and prevention. Circulation 2003;107:363–369.

25. Nissen SE, Tuzcu EM, Schoenhagen P, et al. for the Reversal of Atherosclerosis with Aggressive Lipid Lowering (REVERSAL) Investigators. Statin therapy, LDL cholesterol, C-reactive protein, and coronary heart disease. N Engl J Med 2005;352:29–38.

26. Ridker PM, Cannon CP, Morrow D, et al. C-reactive protein levels and outcomes after statin therapy. N Engl J Med 2005;352:20–28.

27. The Homocysteine Studies Collaboration. Homocysteine and risk of ischemic heart disease and stroke. A meta-analysis. JAMA 2002; 288:2015–2022.

28. Kostner KM, Kostner GM. Lipoprotein(a): still an enigma? Curr Opin Lipidol 2002;13:391–396.

29. Ariyo AA, Thach C, Tracy R, for the Cardiovascular Health Study Investigators. Lp(a) lipoprotein, vascular disease, and mortality in the elderly. N Engl J Med 2003;349:2108–2115.

30. Kraus WE, Houmard JA, Duscha BD, et al. Effects of the amount and intensity of exercise on plasma lipoproteins. N Engl J Med 2002;347:1483–1492.

31. Hammarsten J, Hogstedt B. Hyperinsulinaemia as a risk factor for developing benign prostatic hyperplasia. Eur Urol 2001;39:151–158.

32. Chobanian AV, Bakris GL, Black HR, et al. for the Joint National Committee on Prevention, Detection, Evaluation, and Treatment of High Blood Pressure. National Heart, Lung, and Blood Institute; National High Blood Pressure Education Program Coordinating Committee. Hypertension 2003;42:1206–1252.

33. Whelton SP, Chin A, Xin X, et al. Effect of aerobic exercise on blood pressure: a meta-analysis of randomized, controlled trials. Ann Intern Med 2002; 136:493–503.

34. Moyad MA, Giacherio D, National Prostate Cancer Coalition (NPCC), Montie J. African-American men, high cholesterol & hs-CRP & alternative medicine use documented at a prostate cancer screening: A unique opportunity for a complete men's health intervention. Proceedings of the American Society of Clinical Oncology (ASCO) 2005;23(16S, part I of II):408s [abstract 4623].

35. Moyad MA. Is obesity a risk factor for prostate cancer, and does it even matter? A hypothesis and different perspective. Urology 2002; 59 (Suppl 4A):41–50.

36. Moyad MA. Current methods used for defining, measuring, and treating obesity. Semin Urol Oncol 2001;19:247–256.

37. Writing Group for the Women's Health Initiative Investigators. Risks and benefits of estrogen plus progestin in healthy postmenopausal women: principal results from the Women's Health Initiative randomized controlled trial. JAMA 2002;288:321–333.

38. Shike M, Latkany L, Riedel E, et al. Lack of effect of a low-fat, high-fruit, -vegetable, and -fiber diet on serum prostate-specific antigen of men without prostate cancer: results from a randomized trial. J Clin Oncol 2002;20:3592–3598.

39. Zhu S, Heymsfield SB, Toyoshima H, et al. Race-ethnicity-specific waist circumference cutoffs for identifying cardiovascular disease risk factors. Am J Clin Nutr 2005;81:409–415.

40. Marcella S, Rhoads GG. Waist size and mortality from prostate cancer. Proceedings of the American Society of Clinical Oncology (ASCO) 2005;23:409 [abstract 4626].

41. Moyad MA. Osteoporosis: a rapid review of risk factors and screening methods. Urol Oncol: Seminars and Original Investigations 2003;21:375–379.

42. Freedland SJ, Aronson WJ. Obesity and prostate cancer. Urology 2005;65:433–439.

43. Andersson SO, Wolk A, Bergstrom R, et al. Body size and prostate cancer: a 20-year follow-up study among 135,006 Swedish construction workers. J Natl Cancer Inst 1997;89:385–389.

44. Schuurman AG, van den Brandt PA, Dorant E, et al. Association of energy and fat intake with prostate carcinoma risk: results from the Netherlands Cohort Study. Cancer 1999;86:1019–1027.

45. Schuurman AG, Goldbohm RA, Dorant E, et al. Anthropometry in relation to prostate cancer risk in the Netherlands Cohort Study. Am J Epidemiol 2000;151:541–549.

46. Heinonen OP, Albanes D, Virtamo J, et al. Prostate cancer and supplementation with alpha-tocopherol and beta-carotene: incidence and mortality in a controlled trial. J Natl Cancer Inst 1998;90:440–446.

47. Aziz NM, Hartman T, Barrett M, et al. Weight and prostate cancer in the Alpha-Tocopherol Beta-Carotene Cancer Prevention (ATBC) Trial. ASCO 2000;19:647a.

48. Calle EE, Rodriguez C, Walker-Thurmond K, et al. Overweight, obesity, and mortality from cancer in a prospectively studied cohort of U.S. adults. N Engl J Med 2003;348:1625–1638.

49. Amling CL, Riffenburgh RH, Sun L, et al. Pathologic variables and recurrence rates as related to obesity and race in men with prostate cancer undergoing radical prostatectomy. J Clin Oncol 2004;22:439–445.

50. Freedland SJ, Aronson WJ, Kane CJ, et al. Impact of obesity on biochemical control after radical prostatectomy for clinically localized prostate cancer: A report by the Shared Equal Access Regional Cancer Hospital Database Study Group. J Clin Oncol 2004;22:446–453.

51. Giovannucci E, Rimm EB, Liu Y, et al. Body mass index and risk of prostate cancer in U.S. health professionals. J Natl Cancer Inst 2003;95:1240–1244.

52. Stevens J, Cai J, Pamuk ER, et al. The effect of age on the association between body-mass index and mortality. N Engl J Med 1998;338:1–7.

53. Calle EE, Thun MJ, Petrelli JM, et al. Body-mass index and mortality in a prospective cohort of US adults. N Engl J Med 1997;341:1097–1105.

54. Kuczmarski RJ, Carroll MD, Flegal KM, et al. Varying body mass index cutoff points to describe overweight prevalence among US adults: NHANES III (1988 to 1994). Obes Res 1997;5:542–548.

55. Moyad MA. Obesity, interrelated mechanisms, and exposures and kidney cancer. Semin Urol Oncol 2001;19:270–279.

56. Bacon CG, Mittleman MA, Kawachi I, et al. Sexual function in men older than 50 years of age: results from the Health Professionals Follow-up Study. Ann Intern Med 2003;139:161–168.

57. Walczak MK, Lokhandwala N, Hodge MB, et al. Prevalence of cardiovascular risk factors in erectile dysfunction. J Gend Specif Med 2002;5:19–24.

58. Taylor EN, Stampfer MJ, Curhan GC. Obesity, weight gain, and the risk of kidney stones. JAMA 2005;293:455–462.

59. Friedenreich CM. Physical activity and cancer prevention: from observational to intervention research. Cancer Epidemiol Biomark Prev 2001;10:287–301.

60. Giovannucci EL, Liu Y, Leitzmann MF, et al. A prospective study of physical activity and incident and fatal prostate cancer. Arch Intern Med 2005;165:1005–1010.

61. Tanasescu M, Leitzmann MF, Rimm EB, et al. Exercise type and intensity in relation to coronary heart disease in men. JAMA 2002; 288:1994–2000.

62. Poehlman ET, Melby C. Resistance training and energy balance. Int J Sport Nutr 1998;8:143–159.

63. Poehlman ET, Dvorak RV, DeNino WF, et al. Effects of resistance training and endurance training on insulin sensitivity in nonobese, young women. J Clin Endocrinol Metab 2000;85:2463–2468.

64. Prabhakaran B, Dowling EA, Branch JD, et al. Effect of 14 weeks of resistance training on lipid profile and body fat percentage in premenopausal women. Br J Sports Med 1999;33:190–195.

65. Hurley BF, Roth SM. Strength training in the elderly. Sports Med 2000;30:249–268.

66. Segal RJ, Reid RD, Courneya KS, et al. Resistance training in men receiving androgen deprivation therapy for prostate cancer. J Clin Oncol 2003;21:1653–1659.

67. Platz EA, Kawachi I, Rimm EB, et al. Physical activity and benign prostatic hyperplasia. Arch Intern Med 1998;158:2349–2356.

68. Esposito K, Giugliano F, Di Palo C, et al. Effect of lifestyle changes on erectile dysfunction in obese men: a randomized controlled trial. JAMA 2004;291:2978–2984.

69. Saigal CS. Obesity and erectile dysfunction: common problems, common solution? JAMA 2004,291.3011–3012.

70. Slattery ML, Edwards S, Curtin K, et al. Physical activity and colorectal cancer. Am J Epidemiol 2003;158:214–224.

71. Blumenthal JA, Babyak MA, Moore KA, et al. Effects of exercise training on older patients with major depression. Arch Intern Med 1999;159:2349–2356.

72. Babyak M, Blumenthal JA, Herman S, et al. Exercise treatment for major depression: maintenance of therapeutic benefit at 10 months. Psychosom Med 2000;62:633–638.

73. Hu FB, Willett WC, Li T, et al. Adiposity as compared with physical activity in predicting mortality among women. N Engl J Med 2004;351:2694–2703.

74. Grable JC, Ternullo S. Smoking cessation from office to bedside. An evidence-based, practical approach. Postgrad Med 2003;114:45–48,51–54.

75. Ornish D, Fair W, Pettengill E, et al. Can lifestyle changes reverse prostate cancer? J Urol 2003;169:74 [abstract 286].

76. Samaha FF, Iqbal N, Seshadri P, et al. A low-carbohydrate as compared with a low-fat diet in severe obesity. N Engl J Med 2003;348:2074–2081.

77. Foster GD, Wyatt HR, Hill JO, et al. A randomized trial of a low-carbohydrate diet for obesity. N Engl J Med 2003;348:2082–2090.

78. Hsing AW, Chua S Jr, Gao YT, et al. Prostate cancer risk and serum levels of insulin and leptin: a population-based study. J Natl Cancer Inst 2001;93:783–789.

79. Augustin LS, Franceschi S, Jenkins DJA, et al. Glycemic index in chronic disease: a review. Eur J Clin Nutr 2002;56:1049–1071.

80. Hsing AW, Gao Y-T, Chua S Jr, et al. Insulin resistance and prostate cancer risk. J Natl Cancer Inst 2003;95:67–71.

81. Jee SH, Ohrr H, Sull JW, et al. Fasting serum glucose level and cancer risk in Korean men and women. JAMA 2005;293:194–202.

82. Dansinger ML, Gleason JA, Griffith JL, et al. Comparison of the Atkins, Ornish, Weight Watchers, and Zone Diets for weight loss and heart disease risk reduction: a randomized trial. JAMA 2005;293:43–53.

83. Rolls BJ, Morris EL, Roe LS. Portion size of food affects energy intake in normal-weight and overweight men and women. Am J Clin Nutr 2002;76:1207–1213.

84. Pereira MA, Kartashov AI, Ebbeling CB, et al. Fast-food habits, weight gain, and insulin resistance (the CARDIA study): 15-year prospective analysis. Lancet 2005;365:36–42.

85. Hsieh LJ, Carter B, Landis PK, et al. Association of energy intake with prostate cancer in a long-term aging study: Baltimore Longitudinal Study of Aging (United States). Urology 2003;61:297–301.

86. Heilbronn LK, Ravussin E. Calorie restriction and aging: review of the literature and implications for studies in humans. Am J Clin Nutr 2003;78:361–369.

87. Pirozzo S, Summerbell C, Cameron C, et al. Advice on low-fat diets for obesity. Cochrane Database Syst Rev 2002;2:CD003640.

88. Hill JO, Peters JC. Environmental contributions to the obesity epidemic. Science 1998;280:1371–1374.

89. Mukherjee P, Sotnikov AV, Mangian HJ, et al. Energy intake and prostate tumor growth, angiogenesis, and vascular endothelial growth factor expression. J Natl Cancer Inst 1999;91:512–523.

90. Bosland MC, Oakley-Girvan I, Whittemore AS. Dietary fat, calories, and prostate cancer risk. J Natl Cancer Inst 1999;91:489–491.

91. Gregg EW, Gerzoff RB, Thompson TJ, et al. Intentional weight loss and death in overweight and obese U.S. adults 35 years of age and older. Ann Intern Med 2003;138:383–389.

92. Clinical guidelines on the identification, evaluation, and treatment of overweight and obesity in adults. www.nhlbi.nih.gov/guidelines/obesity/ob_home.htm. Accessed September 2002.

93. Keys A, Menotti A, Karvonen MJ, et al. The diet and 15-year death rate in the Seven Countries Study. Am J Epidemiol 1986;124:903–915.

94. Gordon DJ. Cholesterol and mortality: what can meta-analysis tell us? In: Gallo LL (ed.): Cardiovascular disease 2: cellular and molecular mechanisms, prevention, and treatment. New York: Plenum Press, 1995, pp 333–340.

95. Gordon DJ. Cholesterol lowering and total mortality. In: Rifkind BM (ed.): Lowering cholesterol in high-risk individuals and populations. New York: Marcel Dekker, 1995, pp 333–348.

96. Moyad MA. The ABCs of nutrition and supplements for prostate cancer. Ann Arbor, MI: JW Edwards Publishing, 2000.

97. Meyer F, Bairati I, Shadmani R, et al. Dietary fat and prostate cancer survival. Cancer Causes Control 1999;10:245–251.

98. Key TJ, Fraser GE, Thorogood M, et al. Mortality in vegetarians and non-vegetarians: detailed findings from a collaborative analysis of 5 prospective studies. Am J Clin Nutr 1999;70 (suppl):516S-524S.

99. Yu JN, Cunningham JA, Rosenberg Thouin S, et al. Hyperlipidemia. Primary Care 2000;27:541–587.

100. Mensink RP, Katan MB. Effect of dietary fatty acids on serum lipids and lipoproteins: a meta-analysis of 27 trials. Arterioscler Thromb 1992;12:911–919.

101. Hu FB, van Dam RM, Liu S. Diet and risk of type II diabetes: the role of types of fat and carbohydrate. Diabetologia 2001;44:805–817.

102. Salmeron J, Hu FB, Manson JE, et al. Dietary fat intake and risk of type 2 diabetes in women. Am J Clin Nutr 2001;73:1019–1026.

103. Innis SM, Green TJ, Halsey TK. Variability in the trans fatty acid content of foods within a food category: implications for estimation of dietary trans fatty acid intakes. J Am Coll Nutr 1999;18:255–260.

104. Clandinin MT, Wilke MS. Do trans fatty acids increase the incidence of type 2 diabetes? Am J Clin Nutr 2001;73:1001–1002.

105. Lemaitre RN, King IB, Raghunathan TE, et al. Cell membrane trans-fatty acids and the risk of primary cardiac arrest. Circulation 2002;105:697–701.

106. Nelson GJ. Dietary fat, trans fatty acids, and risk of coronary heart disease. Nutr Rev 1998;56:250–252.

107. Katan MB. Trans fatty acids and plasma lipoproteins. Nutr Rev 2000;58:188–191.

108. Mensink RP, Katan MB. Effect of dietary trans fatty acids on high-density and low-density lipoprotein cholesterol levels in healthy subjects. N Engl J Med 1990;323:439–445.

109. Ascherio A, Katan MB, Zock PL, et al. Trans fatty acids and coronary heart disease. N Engl J Med 1999;340:1994–1998.

110. Nestel P, Noakes M, Belling BE. Plasma lipoprotein and Lp(a) changes with substitution of elaidic acid for oleic acid in the diet. J Lipid Res 1992;33:1029–1036.

111. Sundram K, Ismail A, Hays KC, et al. Trans (elaidic) fatty acids adversely affect the lipoprotein profile relative to specific saturated fatty acids in humans. J Nutr 1997;127:514S–520S.

112. de Roos NM, Bots ML, Siebelink E, Schouten E, Katan MB. Flow-mediated vasodilation is not impaired when HDL-cholesterol is lowered by substituting carbohydrates for monounsaturated fat. Br J Nutr 2001;86:181–188.

113. Lovejoy JC. Dietary fatty acids and insulin resistance. Curr Atheroscler Rep 1999;1:215–220.

114. Kinsella JE, Bruckner G, Mai J, et al. Metabolism of trans fatty acids with emphasis on the effects of trans, trans-octadecadienoate on lipid composition, essential fatty acid, and prostaglandins: an overview. Am J Clin Nutr 1981;34:2307–2318.

115. Hill EG, Johnson SB, Lawson LD, et al. Perturbation of the metabolism of essential fatty acids by dietary hydrogenated vegetable oil. Proc Natl Acad Sci USA 1982;79:953–957.

116. Byrne C, Rockett H, Holmes MD. Dietary fat, fat subtypes, and breast cancer risk: lack of an association among postmenopausal women with no history of benign breast disease. Cancer Epidemiol Biomarkers Prev 2002;11:261–265.

117. Slattery ML, Benson J, Ma KN, et al. Trans-fatty acids and colon cancer. Nutr Cancer 2001; 39:170–175.

118. Voorrips LE, Brants HA, Kardinaal AF, et al. Intake of conjugated linoleic acid, fat, and other fatty acids in relation to postmenopausal breast cancer: the Netherlands Cohort Study on Diet and Cancer. Am J Clin Nutr 2002; 76:873–882.

119. King IB, Kristal AR, Schaffer S, et al. Serum trans-fatty acids are associated with risk of prostate cancer in beta-carotene and retinol efficacy trial. Cancer Epidemiol Biomarkers Prev 2005;14:988–992.

120. Stender S, Dyerberg J. Influence of trans fatty acids on health. Ann Nutr Metab 2004;48:61–66.

121. United States Food and Drug Administration web site. Available at: http://www.fda.gov/oc/initiatives/transfat. Accessed February 15, 2004.

122. Moyad MA. Dietary fat reduction to reduce prostate cancer risk: controlled enthusiasm, learning a lesson from breast or other cancers, and the big picture. Urology 2002;59 (Suppl 4A):51–62.

123. Laaksonen DE, Nyyssonen K, Niskanen L, et al. Prediction of cardiovascular mortality in middle-aged men by dietary and serum linoleic and polyunsaturated fatty acids. Arch Intern Med 2005;165:193–199.

124. Connor WE, Lin DS. The effect of shellfish in the diet upon the plasma lipid levels in humans. Metabolism 1982;31:1046–1051.

125. Childs MT, Dorsett CS, Failor A, et al. Effect of shellfish consumption on cholesterol absorption in normolipidemic men. Metabolism 1987;36:31–35.

126. Zhuang L, Kim J, Adam RM, et al. Cholesterol targeting alters lipid raft composition and cell survival in prostate cancer cells and xenografts. J Clin Invest 2005;115:959–968.

127. Henriksson P, Eriksson M, Ericsson S, et al. Hypocholesterolaemia and increased elimination of low-density lipoproteins in metastatic cancer of the prostate. Lancet 1989;2:1178–1180.

128. Wong NCW. The beneficial effects of plant sterols on serum cholesterol. Can J Cardiol 2001;17:715–721.

129. Katan MB, Grundy SM, Jones P, et al. For the Stresa Workshop Participants. Efficacy and safety of plant stanols and sterols in the management of blood cholesterol levels. Mayo Clin Proc 2003;78:965–978.

130. Schaefer EJ. Lipoproteins, nutrition, and heart disease. Am J Clin Nutr 2002;75:191–212.

131. Vuorio AF, Gylling H, Turtola H, et al. Stanol ester margarine alone and with simvastatin lowers serum cholesterol in families with familial hypercholesterolemia caused by the FH-North Karelia mutation. Arterio Thromb Vasc Biol 2000;20:500–506.

132. Gylling H, Miettinen TA. Cholesterol reduction by different plant stanol mixtures and with variable fat intake. Metabolism 1999;48:575–580.

133. Hallikainen MA, Uusitupa MI. Effects of 2 low-fat stanol ester-containing margarines on serum cholesterol concentrations as part of a low-fat diet in hypercholesterolemic subjects. Am J Clin Nutr 1999;69:403–410.

134. Hendriks HFJ, Weststrate JA, van Vliet T, et al. Spreads enriched with three different levels of vegetable oil sterols and the degree of cholesterol lowering in normocholesterolaemic and mildly hypercholesterolaemic subjects. Eur J Clin Nutr 1999;53:319–327.

135. Gylling H, Radhakrishnan R, Miettinen TA. Reduction of serum cholesterol in postmenopausal women with previous myocardial infarction and cholesterol malabsorption induced by dietary sitostanol ester margarine: women and dietary sitostanol. Circulation 1997;96:4226–4231.

136. Miettinen TA, Puska P, Gylling H, et al. Reduction of serum cholesterol with sitostanol-ester margarine in a mildly hypercholesterolemic population. N Engl J Med 1995;333:1308–1312.

137. Vanhanen HT, Blomqvist S, Ehnholm C, et al. Serum cholesterol, cholesterol precursors, and plant sterols in hypercholesterolemic subjects with different apoE phenotypes during dietary sitostanol ester treatment. J Lipid Res 1993;34:1535–1544.

138. Giovannucci E. Tomatoes, tomato-based products, lycopene, and cancer: review of the epidemiologic literature. J Natl Cancer Inst 1999;91:317–331.

139. Mucci LA, Tamimi R, Lagiou P, et al. Are dietary influences on the risk of prostate cancer mediated through the insulin-like growth factor system? Brit J Urol Intl 2001;87:814–820.

140. Chen L, Stacewicz-Sapuntzakis M, Duncan C, et al. Oxidative DNA damage in prostate cancer patients consuming tomato sauce-based entrees as a whole-food intervention. J Natl Cancer Inst 2001;93:1872–1879.

141. Etminan M, Takkouche B, Caamano-Isorna F. The role of tomato products and lycopene in the prevention of prostate cancer: a meta-analysis of observational studies. Cancer Epidemiol Biomarkers Prev 2004;13:340–345.

142. Boileau TWM, Liao Z, Kim S, et al. Prostate carcinogenesis in N-methyl-N-nitrosurea (NMU)-testosterone-treated rats fed tomato powder, lycopene, or energy-restricted diets. J Natl Cancer Inst 2003;95:1578–1586.

143. Jian L, Du CJ, Lee AH, et al. Do dietary lycopene and other carotenoids protect against prostate cancer? Int J Cancer 2005;113:1010–1014.

144. Street DA, Comstock GW, Salkeld RM, et al. Serum antioxidants and myocardial infarction. Are low levels of carotenoids and alpha-tocopherol risk factors for myocardial infarction? Circulation 1994;90:1154–1161.

145. Arab L, Steck S. Lycopene and cardiovascular disease. Am J Clin Nutr 2000;71(suppl):1691S–1695S.

146. Rissanen TH, Voutilainen S, Nyyssonen K, et al. Serum lycopene concentrations and carotid atherosclerosis: the Kuopio Ischaemic Heart Disease Risk Factor Study. Am J Clin Nutr 2003;77:133–138.

147. Sesso HD, Buring JE, Norkus EP, et al. Plasma lycopene, other carotenoids, and retinol and the risk of cardiovascular disease in women. Am J Clin Nutr 2004;79:47–53.

148. Cohen JH, Kristal AR, Stanford JL. Fruit and vegetable intakes and prostate cancer risk. J Natl Cancer Inst 2000;92:61–68.

149. Kristal AR, Lampe JW. Brassica vegetables and prostate cancer risk: a review of the epidemiological evidence. Nutr Cancer 2002;42:1–9.

150. Hsing AW, Chokkalingam AP, Gao Y-T, et al. Allium vegetables and risk of prostate cancer: a population-based study. J Natl Cancer Inst 2002;94:1648–1651.

151. van Gils CH, Peeters PHM, Bueno-de-Mesquita HB, et al. Consumption of vegetables and fruits and risk of breast cancer. JAMA 2005;293:183–193.

152. Hung H-C, Joshipura KJ, Jiang R, et al. Fruit and vegetable intake and risk of major chronic disease. J Natl Cancer Inst 2004;96:1577–1584.

153. Sesso HD, Buring JE, Zhang SM, et al. Dietary and plasma lycopene and the risk of breast cancer. Cancer Epidemiol Biomarkers Prev 2005;14:1074–1081.

154. Vastag B. Recent studies show limited association of fruit and vegetable consumption and cancer risk. J Natl Cancer Inst 2005;97:474–475.

155. Michaud DS, Skinner HG, Wu K, et al. Dietary patterns and pancreatic cancer risk in men and women. J Natl Cancer Inst 2005;97:518–524.

156. Borden LS Jr., Clark PE, Miller A, et al. Prospective dose-escalation trial of lycopene in men with recurrent prostate cancer following definitive local therapy. Proceedings of the American Urologic Association Annual Meeting 2005;173:275 [abstract 1014].

157. Van Horn L. Fiber, lipids, and coronary heart disease. Nutrition Committee Advisory. Circulation 1997;95:2701–2704.

158. U.S. Department of Health and Human Services. Food and Drug Administration. Food labeling: health claims; soluble fiber from certain foods and coronary heart disease: final rule. Federal Register 1998;63:8103–8121.

159. U.S. Department of Health and Human Services. Food and Drug Administration. Food labeling: health claims; soluble fiber from certain foods and coronary heart disease: proposed rule. Federal Register 1997;62:28234–28245.

160. Brown L, Rosner B, Willett WW, et al. Cholesterol-lowering effects of dietary fiber: a meta-analysis. Am J Clin Nutr 1999;69:30–42.

161. Lieberman DA, Prindiville S, Weiss DG, et al. Risk factors for advanced colonic neoplasia and hyperplastic polyps in asymptomatic individuals. JAMA 2003;290:2959–2967.

162. Pereira MA, O'Reilly E, Augustsson K, et al. Dietary fiber and risk of coronary heart disease: a pooled analysis of cohort studies. Arch Intern Med 2004;164:370–376.

163. Liu S, Buring J, Sesso H, et al. A prospective study of dietary fiber intake and risk of cardiovascular disease among women. J Am Coll Cardiol 2002;39:49–56.

164. Wolk A, Manson ME, Stampfer MJ, et al. Long-term intake of dietary fiber and decreased risk of coronary heart disease among women. JAMA 1999;281:1998–2002.

165. Pietinen P, Rimm EB, Korhonen P, et al. Intake of dietary fiber and risk of coronary heart disease in a cohort of Finnish men: the Alpha-Tocopherol, Beta-Carotene Cancer Prevention Study. Circulation 1996;94:2720–2727.

166. Rimm EB, Ascherio A, Giovannucci E, et al. Vegetable, fruit, and cereal fiber intake and risk of coronary heart disease among men. JAMA 1996;275:447–451.

167. Marlett JA, Hosig KB, Vollendorf NW, et al. Mechanism of serum cholesterol reduction by oat bran. Hepatology 1994;20:1450–1457.

168. Chandalia M, Garg A, Lutjohann D, et al. Beneficial effects of high dietary fiber intake in patients with type 2 diabetes mellitus. N Engl J Med 2000;342:1392–1398.

169. Leinonen KS, Poutanen KS, Mykkanen HM. Rye bread decreases serum total and LDL cholesterol in men with moderately elevated serum cholesterol. J Nutr 2000;130:164–170

170. Keenan JM, Pins JJ, Frazel C, et al. Oat ingestion reduces systolic and diastolic blood pressure among moderate hypertensives: a pilot trial. J Fam Pract 2002;51:369.

171. Moreyra AE, Wilson AC, Koraym A. Effect of combining psyllium fiber with simvastatin in lowering cholesterol. Arch Intern Med 2005;165:1161–1166.

172. Streppel MT, Arends LR, van't Veer P, Grobbee DE, Geleijnse JM. Dietary fiber and blood pressure: a meta-analysis of randomized placebo-controlled trials. Arch Intern Med 2005;165:150–156.

173. Marlett JA, McBurney MI, Slavin JL, for the American Dietetic Association. Position of the American Dietetic Association: health implications of dietary fiber. J Am Diet Assoc 2002;102:993–1000.

174. Schatzkin A, Lanza E, Corle D, et al, and the Polyp Prevention Trial Study Group. Lack of effect of a low-fat, high-fiber diet on the recurrence of colorectal adenomas. N Engl J Med 2000;342:1149–1155.

175. Alberts DS, Martinez ME, Roe DJ, et al. Lack of effect of high-fiber cereal supplement on the recurrence of colorectal adenomas. N Engl J Med 2000;342:1156–1162.

176. Eastham JA, Riedel E, Latkany L, et al. for the Polyp Prevention Trial Study Group. Dietary manipulation, ethnicity, and serum PSA levels. Urology 2003;62:677–682.

177. Pelucchi C, Talamini R, Galeone C, et al. Fibre intake and prostate cancer risk. Int J Cancer 2004;109:278–280.

178. Tariq N, Jenkins DJ, Vidgen E, et al. Effect of soluble and insoluble fiber diets on serum prostate specific antigen in men. J Urol 2000;163:114–118.

179. Bylund A, Lundin E, Zhang JX, et al. Randomised controlled short-term intervention pilot study on rye bran bread in prostate cancer. Eur J Cancer Prev 2003;12:407–415.

180. Pienta KJ, Naik H, Akhtar A, et al. Inhibition of spontaneous metastasis in a rat prostate cancer model by oral administration of modified citrus pectin. J Natl Cancer Inst 1995;87:348–353.

181. Hayashi A, Gillen AC, Lott JR. Effects of daily oral administration of quercetin chalcone and modified citrus pectin on implanted colon-25 tumor growth in Balb-c mice. Altern Med Rev 2000;5:546–552.

182. Guess BW, Scholz MC, Strum SB, et al. Modified citrus pectin (MCP) increases the prostate-specific antigen doubling time in men with prostate cancer: a phase II pilot study. Prostate Cancer Prostatic Dis 2003;6:301–304.

183. Moyad MA, Sakr WA, Hirano D, et al. Complementary medicine for prostate cancer: effects of soy and fat consumption. Reviews in Urology 2001;3 (Suppl 2):S20–S30.

184. Sirtori CR, Galli G, Lovati MR, et al. Effects of dietary proteins on the regulation of liver lipoprotein receptors in rats. J Nutr 1984;114:1493–1500.

185. Khosla P, Sammam S, Carrol KK. Decreased receptor-mediated LDL catabolism in casein-fed rabbits precedes the increase in plasma cholesterol levels. J Nutr Biochem 1991;2:203–209.

186. Potter SM. Soy protein and serum lipids. Curr Opin Lipidol 1996;7:260–264.

187. Potter SM. Overview of possible mechanisms for the hypocholesterolemic effect of soy protein. J Nutr 1995;125:606S–611S.

188. U.S. Department of Health and Human Services. Food and Drug Administration. Food labeling: health claims; soy protein and coronary heart disease: proposed rule. Federal Register 1998;63:62977–63015.

189. U.S Department of Health and Human Services. Food and Drug Administration. Food labeling: health claims; soy protein and coronary heart disease: final rule. Federal Register 1999;64:57699–57733.

190. Potter SM. Soy protein and cardiovascular disease: the impact of bioactive components in soy. Nutr Rev 1998;56:231–235.

191. Anderson JW, Johnstone BM, Cook-Newell ME. Meta-analysis of the effects of soy protein intake on serum lipids. N Engl J Med 1995;333:276–282.

192. Zhan S, Ho SC. Meta-analysis of the effects of soy protein containing isoflavones on the lipid profile. Am J Clin Nutr 2005;81:397–408.

193. Peterson G, Barnes S. Genistein and biochanin-A inhibit the growth of human prostate cancer cells but not epidermal growth factor receptor tyrosine autophosphorylation. Prostate 1993;22:335–345.

194. Rokhlin OW, Cohen MB. Differential sensitivity of human prostatic cancer cell lines to the effects of protein kinase and phosphatase inhibitors. Cancer Lett 1995;98:103–110.

195. Adlercreutz H, Makela S, Pylkkanen L, et al. Dietary phytoestrogens and prostate cancer. Proc Am Assoc Cancer Res 1995;36:687 [abstract 41].

196. Akiyama T, Ishida J, Nakagawa S, et al. Genistein, a specific inhibitor of tyrosine-specific protein kinases. J Biol Chem 1987;262:5592–5595.

197. Linnassier C, Pierre M, Le Pecq JB, et al. Mechanisms of action in NIH-3T3 cells of genistein, an inhibitor of EGF receptor kinase activity. Biochem Pharmacol 1990;39:187–193.

198. Nishimura J, Huang JS, Deuel TF. Platelet-derived growth factor stimulates tyrosine-specific protein kinase activity in Swiss mouse 3T3 cell membranes. Proc Natl Acad Sci USA 1982;79:4303–4307.

199. Rubin JB, Shia MA, Pilch PF. Stimulation of tyrosine-specific phosphorylation in vitro by insulin-like growth factor I. Nature 1983;305:438–440.

200. Okura A, Arakawa H, Oka H, et al. Effect of genistein on topoisomerase activity and on the growth of (VAL 12)Ha-ras-transformed NIH 3T3 cells. Biochem Biophys Res Commun 1988;157:183–189.

201. Fotsis T, Pepper M, Adlercreutz H, et al. Genistein, a dietary ingested isoflavonoid, inhibits cell proliferation and in vitro angiogenesis. J Nutr 1995;125:S790–S797.

202. Kyle E, Neckers L, Takimoto C, et al. Genistein-induced apoptosis of prostate cancer cells is preceded by a specific decrease in focal adhesion kinase activity. Mol Pharmacol 1997;51:193–200.

203. Nagata C, Inaba S, Kawakami N, et al. Inverse association of soy product intake with serum androgen and estrogen concentrations in Japanese men. Nutr Cancer 2000;36:14–18.

204. Moyad MA. Lifestyle/dietary supplement partial androgen suppression and/or estrogen manipulation: A novel PSA reducer and preventive/treatment option for prostate cancer? Urol Clin N Amer 2002;29:115–124.

205. Morton MS, Turkes A, Denis L, et al. Can dietary factors influence prostatic disease? BJU International 1999;84:549–554.

206. Ornish DM, Lee KL, Fair WR, et al. Dietary trial in prostate cancer: early experience and implications for clinical trial design. Urology 2001;57 (Suppl 4A):200–201.

207. Bosland MC, Kato I, Melamed J, et al. Chemoprevention trials in men with prostate-specific antigen failure or at high risk for recurrence after radical prostatectomy: application to efficacy assessment of soy protein. Urology 2001;57 (Suppl 4A):202–204.

208. DeVere White RW, Hackman RM, Soares SE, et al. Effects of a genistein-rich extract on PSA levels in men with a history of prostate cancer. Urology 2004;63:259–263.

209. Adams KF, Chen Chu, Newton KM, et al. Soy isoflavones do not modulate prostate-specific antigen concentrations in older men in a

randomized controlled trial. Cancer Epidemiol Biomarkers Prev 2004;13:644–648.

210. Lichtenstein AH, Ausman LM, Jalbert SM, et al. Effects of different forms of dietary hydrogenated fats on serum lipoprotein cholesterol levels. N Engl J Med 1999;340:1933–1940.

211. Tham DM, Gardner CD, Haskell WL. Potential health benefits of dietary phytoestrogens: a review of the clinical, epidemiological, and mechanistic evidence. J Clin Endocrinol Metab 1998;83:2223–2235.

212. Kronenberg F, Fugh-Berman A. Complementary and alternative medicine for menopausal symptoms: a review of randomized, controlled trials. Ann Intern Med 2002;137:805–813.

213. Cunnane SC, Ganguli S, Menard C, et al. High alpha-linolenic acid flaxseed (Linum usitatissimum): Some nutritional properties in humans. Br J Nutr 1993;69:443–453.

214. Bierenbaum ML, Reichstein R, Watkins TR. Reducing atherogenic risk in hyperlipemic humans with flax seed supplementation: A preliminary report. J Am Coll Nutr 1993;12:501–504.

215. Arjmandi BH, Khan DA, Juma S, et al. Whole flaxseed consumption lowers serum LDL-cholesterol and lipoprotein(a) concentrations in postmenopausal women. Nutr Res 1998;18:1203–1214.

216. Jenkins DJ, Kendall CW, Vidgen E, et al. Health aspects of partially defatted flaxseed, including effects on serum lipids, oxidative measures, and ex vivo androgen and progestin activity: A controlled crossover trial. Am J Clin Nutr 1999;69:395–402.

217. Bloedon LT, Szapary PO. Flaxseed and cardiovascular risk. Nut Rev 2004;62:18–27.

218. Lemay A, Dodin S, Kadri N, et al. Flaxseed dietary supplement versus hormone replacement therapy in hypercholesterolemic menopausal women. Obstet Gynecol 2002;100:495–504.

219. Hu FB, Willett WC. Optimal diets for prevention of coronary heart disease. JAMA 2002;288:2569–2578.

220. Singh RB, Niaz MA, Sharma JP, et al. Randomized, double-blind, placebo-controlled trial of fish oil and mustard oil in patients with suspected acute myocardial infarction: the Indian Experiment of Infarct Survival 4. Cardiovasc Drugs Ther 1997;11:485–491.

221. de Lorgeril M, Renaud S, Mamelle N, et al. Mediterranean alpha-linolenic acid-rich diet in secondary prevention of coronary heart disease. Lancet 1994;343:1454–1459.

222. de Lorgeril M, Salen P, Martin JL, et al. Mediterranean diet, traditional risk factors, and the rate of cardiovascular complications after myocardial infarction: final report of the Lyon Diet Heart Study. Circulation 1999;99:779–785.

223. Dabrosin C, Chen J, Wang L, et al. Flaxseed inhibits metastasis and decreases extracellular vascular endothelial growth factor in human breast cancer xenografts. Cancer Lett 2002;185:31–37.

224. Lin X, Gingrich JR, Bao W, et al. Effect of flaxseed supplementation on prostatic carcinoma in transgenic mice. Urology 2002;60:919–924.

225. Schuurman AG, van den Brandt PA, Dorant E, et al. Association of energy and fat intake with prostate carcinoma risk: results from the Netherlands Cohort Study. Cancer 1999;86:1019–1027.

226. Giovannucci E, Rimm EB, Colditz GA, et al. A prospective study of dietary fat and risk of prostate cancer. J Natl Cancer Inst 1993;85:1571–1579.

227. Gann PH, Hennekens CH, Sacks FM, et al. Prospective study of plasma fatty acids and risk of prostate cancer. J Natl Cancer Inst 1994;86:281–286.

228. Demark-Wahnefried W, Price DT, Polascik TJ, et al. Pilot study of dietary fat restriction and flaxseed supplementation in men with prostate cancer before surgery: exploring the effects on hormonal levels, prostate-specific antigen, and histopathologic features. Urology 2001;58:47–52.

229. Demark-Wahnefried W, Robertson CN, Walther PJ, et al. Pilot study to explore effects of low-fat, flaxseed-supplemented diet on proliferation of benign prostatic epithelium and prostate-specific antigen. Urology 2004;63:900–904.

230. Morris MC, Evans DA, Bienias JL, et al. Consumption of fish and n-3 fatty acids and risk of incident Alzheimer disease. Arch Neurol 2003;940–946.

231. Bucher HC, Hengstler P, Schindler C, et al. N-3 polyunsaturated fatty acids in coronary heart disease: a meta-analysis of randomized controlled trials. Am J Med 2002;112:298–304.

232. Kris-Etherton PM, Harris WS, Appel LJ, for the Nutrition Committee. Fish consumption, fish oil, omega-3 fatty acids, and cardiovascular disease. Circulation 2002;106:2747–2757.

233. Harris WS. N-3 fatty acids and serum lipoproteins: human studies. Am J Clin Nutr 1997;65(5 Suppl):1645S–1654S.

234. Morris MC, Sacks F, Rosner B. Does fish oil lower blood pressure? A meta-analysis of controlled trials. Circulation 1993;88:523–533.

235. Mori TA, Beilin LJ, Burke V, et al. Interactions between dietary fat, fish, and fish oils and their effects on platelet function in men at risk of cardiovascular disease. Arterioscler Thromb Vasc Biol 1997;17:279–286.

236. Christensen JH, Korup E, Aaroe J, et al. Fish consumption, n-3 fatty acids in cell membranes, and heart rate variability in survivors of myocardial infarction with left ventricular dysfunction. Am J Cardiol 1997;79:1670–1673.

237. Leaf A, Kang JX, Xiao Y-F, et al. Clinical prevention of sudden cardiac death by n-3 polyunsaturated fatty acids and mechanism of prevention of arrhythmias by n-3 fish oils. Circulation 2003;107:2646–2652.

238. Albert CM, Campos H, Stampfer MJ, et al. Blood levels of long-chain n-3 fatty acids and the risk of sudden death. N Engl J Med 2002;346:1113–1118.

239. Kromhout D. Fish consumption and sudden cardiac death. JAMA 1998;279:65–66.

240. Chung BH, Mitchell SH, Zhang SS, et al. Effects of docosahexaenoic acid and eicosapentaenoic acid on androgen-mediated cell growth and gene expression in LNCaP prostate cancer cells. Carcinogenesis 2001;22:1201–1206.

241. Terry P, Lichtenstein P, Feychting M, et al. Fatty fish consumption and risk of prostate cancer. Lancet 2001;357:1764–1766.

242. Aronson WJ, Glapsy JA, Reddy ST, et al. Modulation of omega-3/omega-6 polyunsaturated ratios with dietary fish oils in men with prostate cancer. Urology 2001;58:283–288.

243. Terry PD, Rohan TE, Wolk A. Intakes of fish and marine fatty acids and the risks of cancers of the breast and prostate and of other hormone-related cancers: a review of the epidemiologic evidence. Am J Clin Nutr 2003;77:532–543.

244. Augustsson K, Michaud DS, Rimm EB, et al. A prospective study of intake of fish and marine fatty acids and prostate cancer. Cancer Epidemiol Biomark Prev 2003;12:64–67.

245. Burr ML, Fehily AM, Gilbert JF, et al. Effects of changes in fat, fish, and fibre intakes on death and myocardial reinfarction: Diet and Reinfarction Trial (DART). Lancet 1989;2:757–761.

246. GISSI-Prevenzione Investigators. Dietary supplementation with n-3 polyunsaturated fatty acids and vitamin E after myocardial infarction: results from the GISSI-Prevenzione trial. Lancet 1999;354:447–455.

247. Marchioli R, Barzi F, Bomba E, et al. Early protection against sudden cardiac death by n-3 polyunsaturated fatty acids after myocardial infarction: time-course analysis of the results of the Gruppo Italiano per lo Studio della Sopravvivenza nell'Infarto Miocardico (GISSI)-Prevenzione. Circulation 2002;105:1897–1903.

248. Guallar E, Sanz-Gallardo MI, van't Veer P, et al. Mercury, fish oils, and the risk of myocardial infarction. N Engl J Med 2002;347:1747–1754.

249. Yoshizawa K, Rimm EB, Morris JJ, et al. Mercury and the risk of coronary heart disease in men. N Engl J Med 2002;347:1755–1760.

250. Weil M, Bressler J, Parsons P, et al. Blood mercury levels and neurobehavioral function. JAMA 2005;293:1875–1882.

251. Albert CM, Gaziano JM, Willett WC, et al. Nut consumption and decreased risk of sudden cardiac death in the physicians' health study. Arch Intern Med 2002;162:1382–1387.

252. Ellsworth JL, Kushi LH, Folsom AR. Frequent nut intake and risk of death from coronary heart disease and all causes in postmenopausal women: the Iowa Women's Health Study. Nutr Metab Cardiovasc Dis 2001;11:372–377.

253. Brown L, Sacks F, Rosner B, et al. Nut consumption and risk of coronary heart disease in patients with myocardial infarction. FASEB J 1999;13:A4332 [abstract].

254. Hu FB, Stampfer MJ, Manson JE, et al. Frequent nut consumption and risk of coronary heart disease: prospective cohort study. BMJ 1998;317:1341–1345.

255. Fraser GE, Shavlik DJ. Risk factors for all-cause and coronary heart disease mortality in the oldest-old: the Adventist Health Study. Arch Intern Med 1997;157:2249–2258.

256. Fraser GE, Sabate J, Beeson WL, et al. A possible protective effect of nut consumption on risk of coronary heart disease: the Adventist Health Study. Arch Intern Med 1992;152:1416–1424.

257. Helzlsouer KJ, Huang H-Y, Alberg AJ, et al. Association between alpha-tocopherol, gamma-tocopherol, selenium, and subsequent prostate cancer. J Natl Cancer Inst 2000;92:2018–2023.

258. Hu FB, Manson JE, Willett WC. Types of dietary fat and risk of coronary heart disease: A critical review. J Am Coll Nutr 2001;20:5–19.

259. Moyad MA. An introduction to dietary/supplemental omega-3 fatty acids for general health and prevention: Part I. Urol Oncol 2005;23:28–35.

260. Moyad MA. An introduction to dietary/supplemental omega-3 fatty acids for general health and prevention: Part II. Urol Oncol 2005;23:36–48.

261. Critchley JA, Capewell S. Mortality risk reduction associated with smoking cessation in patients with coronary heart disease: a systematic review. JAMA 2003;290:86–97.

262. Yu GP, Ostroff JS, Zhang ZF, et al. Smoking history and cancer patient survival: a hospital cancer registry study. Cancer Detect Prev 1997;21:497–509.

263. Plaskon LA, Penson DF, Vaughan TL, et al. Cigarette smoking and risk of prostate cancer in middle-aged men. Cancer Epidemiol Biomarkers Prev 2003;12:604–609.

264. Roberts WW, Platz EA, Walsh PC. Association of cigarette smoking with extraprostatic prostate cancer in young men. J Urol 2003;169:512–516.

265. Rodriguez C, Tatham LM, Thun MJ, et al. Smoking and fatal prostate cancer in a large cohort of adult men. Am J Epidemiol 1997;145:466–475.

266. Mukamal KJ, Conigrave KM, Mittleman MA, et al. Roles of drinking pattern and type of alcohol consumed in coronary heart disease in men. N Engl J Med 2003;348:109–118.

267. Hercberg S, Galan P, Preziosi P, et al. The SU.VI.MAX Study: a randomized, placebo-controlled trial of the health effects of antioxidant vitamins and minerals. Arch Intern Med 2004;164:2335–2342.

268. Basler JW, Piazza GA. Nonsteroidal anti-inflammatory drugs and cyclooxygenase-2 selective inhibitors for prostate cancer chemoprevention. J Urol 2004;171:S59–S63.

269. Moyad MA, Merrick GS. Statins and cholesterol lowering after a cancer diagnosis: Why not? Urol Oncol 2005;23:49–55.

270. Debes JD, Roberts RO, Jacobson DJ, et al. Inverse association between prostate cancer and the use of calcium channel blockers. Cancer Epidemiol Biomarkers Prev 2004;13:255–259.

271. The Hope and Hope-Too Trial Investigators. Effects of long-term vitamin E supplementation on cardiovascular events and cancer. JAMA 2005;293:1338–1347.

272. Miller ER III, Pastor-Barriuso R, Dalal D, et al. Meta-analysis: High-dosage vitamin E supplementation may increase all-cause mortality. Ann Intern Med 2005;142:37–46.

273. Bairati I, Meyer F, Gelinas M, et al. A randomized trial of antioxidant vitamins to prevent second primary cancers in head and neck cancer patients. J Natl Cancer Inst 2005;97:481–488.

274. Platz EA, Willet WC, Colditz GA, et al. Proportion of colon cancer risk that might be preventable in a cohort of middle-aged US men. Cancer Causes Control 2000;11:579–588.

275. Trichopoulou A, Costacou T, Bamia C, et al. Adherence to a Mediterranean diet and survival in a Greek population. N Engl J Med 2003;348:2599–2608.

276. Morris CD, Carson S. Routine vitamin supplementation to prevent cardiovascular disease: a summary of the evidence for the U.S. Preventive Services Task Force. Ann Intern Med 2003;139:56–70.

277. U.S. Preventive Services Task Force. Routine vitamin supplementation to prevent cancer and cardiovascular disease: Recommendations and rationale. Ann Intern Med 2003;139:51–55.

278. Leitzmann MF, Stampfer MJ, Wu K, et al. Zinc supplement use and risk of prostate cancer. J Natl Cancer Inst 2003;95:1004–1007.

279. Markowitz JS, Donovan JL, DeVane CL, et al. Effect of St John's wort on drug metabolism by induction of cytochrome P450 3A4 enzyme. JAMA 2003;290:1500–1504.

280. Ang-Lee MK, Moss J, Yuan C-S. Herbal medicines and perioperative care. JAMA 2001;286:208–216.

281. Eyre H, Kahn R, Robertson RM, et al. for the ACS/ADA/AHA Collaborative Writing Committee Members. Preventing cancer, cardiovascular disease, and diabetes: A common agenda for the American Cancer Society, the American Diabetes Association, and the American Heart Association. Circulation 2004;109:3244–3255.

Mortality trends in prostate cancer 67

Peter C Albertsen

With the exception of skin cancers, prostate cancer is the most commonly diagnosed cancer among men and the second leading cause of cancer death in many industrialized nations. In 2004, the American Cancer Society estimates that 29,900 American men will die from prostate cancer and 230,110 will be diagnosed with this disease.[1] Until the late 1980s the incidence and mortality of prostate cancer was rising in most western countries. During the past decade, death rates have declined in some parts of the world while rising in others (Table 67.1). Epidemiologists have closely followed these trends with great interest because they provide insight into the efficacy of screening for prostate cancer using prostate-specific antigen (PSA).

Whether the decline in prostate cancer mortality can be attributed to early diagnosis and treatment is the subject of much controversy and debate. This chapter will examine recent trends in prostate cancer mortality and explore potential explanations for these changes.

DATA COLLECTION, ANALYSIS, AND PRESENTATION

Information regarding prostate cancer incidence and mortality often comes from different sources. Accurate incident rates require an organized tumor registry system in which all new diagnoses of cancers are recorded. In the US, information concerning newly diagnosed cancers is collected by the National Cancer Institute's Surveillance, Epidemiology, and End Results (SEER) program.[2] The SEER program was created following passage of the National Cancer Act in 1971 and is mandated to collect, analyze, and disseminate information that is useful in preventing, diagnosing, and treating cancer. The geographic area comprising the SEER program's database includes approximately 15% of the US population and consists of 11 population-based tumor registries located throughout the country. Similar tumor registries exist in other western countries. Some countries record 100% of cancer diagnoses, while others use an organized system to sample a representative portion of the population. A few tumor registries were organized before World War II; most have been organized more recently.

Information regarding prostate cancer deaths is obtained from death certificates. Several decades ago the

Table 67.1 Contemporary trends in age-standardized prostate cancer mortality rates (age 50–79 years)

Increasing	Decreasing	Unchanged
Australia	Austria	Belgium
Bulgaria	Canada	Finland
Greece	France	Hungary
Ireland	Germany	Norway
Israel	Italy	
Japan	UK	
Netherlands	US	
New Zealand		
Poland		
Portugal		
Romania		
Spain		
Sweden		

World Health Organization (WHO) developed a standardized death certificate that is utilized by most industrialized countries (Figure 67.1). In the US, death certificates are collected and filed by state health departments and vital statistics offices. Each state subsequently forwards the information recorded on the certificate to the National Center for Health Statistics. The underlying cause of death is selected for tabulation following procedures specified by the WHO in the relevant Manual of the International Classification of Diseases, Injuries, and Causes of Death.[3] Similar reporting mechanisms have been developed by most industrialized nations. The information compiled by each country is subsequently reported to the WHO for analysis.

Cancer incidence and mortality rates are often reported either as actual counts at a given point in time or are expressed as age-adjusted rates. Reporting the raw number of new cases annually provides some information concerning the magnitude of disease incidence and mortality within a country, but it does not take into account the demographic profile of the country. Since countries or regions within the US differ in the number of older men that reside within the geographic boundary of the tumor registry, absolute counts need to be divided by the number of men residing in a region who are at risk of developing prostate cancer. Western countries generally have a greater number of elderly men compared to most developing nations. As men live longer, their risk of developing prostate cancer increases. As a consequence, the absolute number of new cancer cases may increase, but the relative incidence or mortality rate may increase, decrease or remain the same.

To identify trends in cancer incidence and mortality, epidemiologists adjust rates by the age of the men at risk. This facilitates comparisons across differing geographic regions or time periods. In the US, the Bureau of Vital Statistics adjusts incidence and mortality rates to fit the US population age distribution present during a census year. Rates are usually reported as an age-adjusted rate per 100,000 men.

Although the systems for collecting and recording information vary throughout the world, the results can be viewed with a reasonable degree of confidence. In the US data collection takes approximately 3 to 4 years. The widely quoted projections reported annually by the American Cancer Society are derived from data available from the US Census Bureau and the cancer incidence rates collected by the SEER program. Estimates of new cancer cases are calculated using a three-step procedure. First, the annual age-specific cancer incidence rates for a 15-year period are multiplied by the age-appropriate US Census Bureau population projections for the same years to estimate the number of cancer cases diagnosed annually for a 15-year period. These annual cancer case estimates are then fitted to an autoregressive quadratic model. This method is used to predict the following year's rates, and the rates are subsequently extrapolated 3 to 4 years into the future.

Trends in prostate cancer mortality rates are frequently calculated using join-point regression techniques.[4,5] This is a form of regression analysis in which trend data can be described by a number of contiguous linear segments and "join points," a point at which trends change. Usually the statistics derived from these models are the annual percent change (APC) in rates associated with each line segment. Regression models are usually estimated using weighted least squares. A full description of the use of join point regression in the analysis of trends in cancer rates, with special reference to prostate cancer, is given by Kim et al.[5]

INTERNATIONAL TRENDS IN PROSTATE CANCER MORTALITY RATES

Oliver et al have published age-standardized prostate cancer mortality rates for each of 24 countries (Figure 67.2).[6] The figures are derived from data compiled by the WHO between 1979 and 1997. There is a greater than five-fold difference between rates in Japan

PART 1. DEATH WAS CAUSED BY (ENTER ONLY ONE CAUSE PER LINE FOR (a), (b) AND (c))		APPROXIMATE INTERVAL BETWEEN ONSET AND DEATH
30	IMMEDIATE CAUSE	
CONDITIONS, IF ANY WHICH GAVE RISE TO IMMEDIATE CAUSE (a) STATING THE UNDERLYING CAUSE LAST.	(a)	
	DUE TO, OR AS A CONSEQUENCE OF:	
	(b)	
	DUE TO, OR AS A CONSEQUENCE OF:	
	(c)	
PART II. OTHER SIGNIFICANT CONDITIONS: CONDITIONS CONTRIBUTING TO DEATH BUT NOT RELATED TO CAUSE	AUTOPSY ☐ Y ☐ N	IF YES, Were findings considered in determining cause of death
31	32	33
NURSE PRONOUNCEMENT TYPE OR PRINT NAME	DEGREE	SIGNATURE	DATE AND TIME PRONOUNCED MONTH	DAY	YEAR	TIME ☐ A.M. ☐ P.M.

Fig. 67.1
Death certificate.

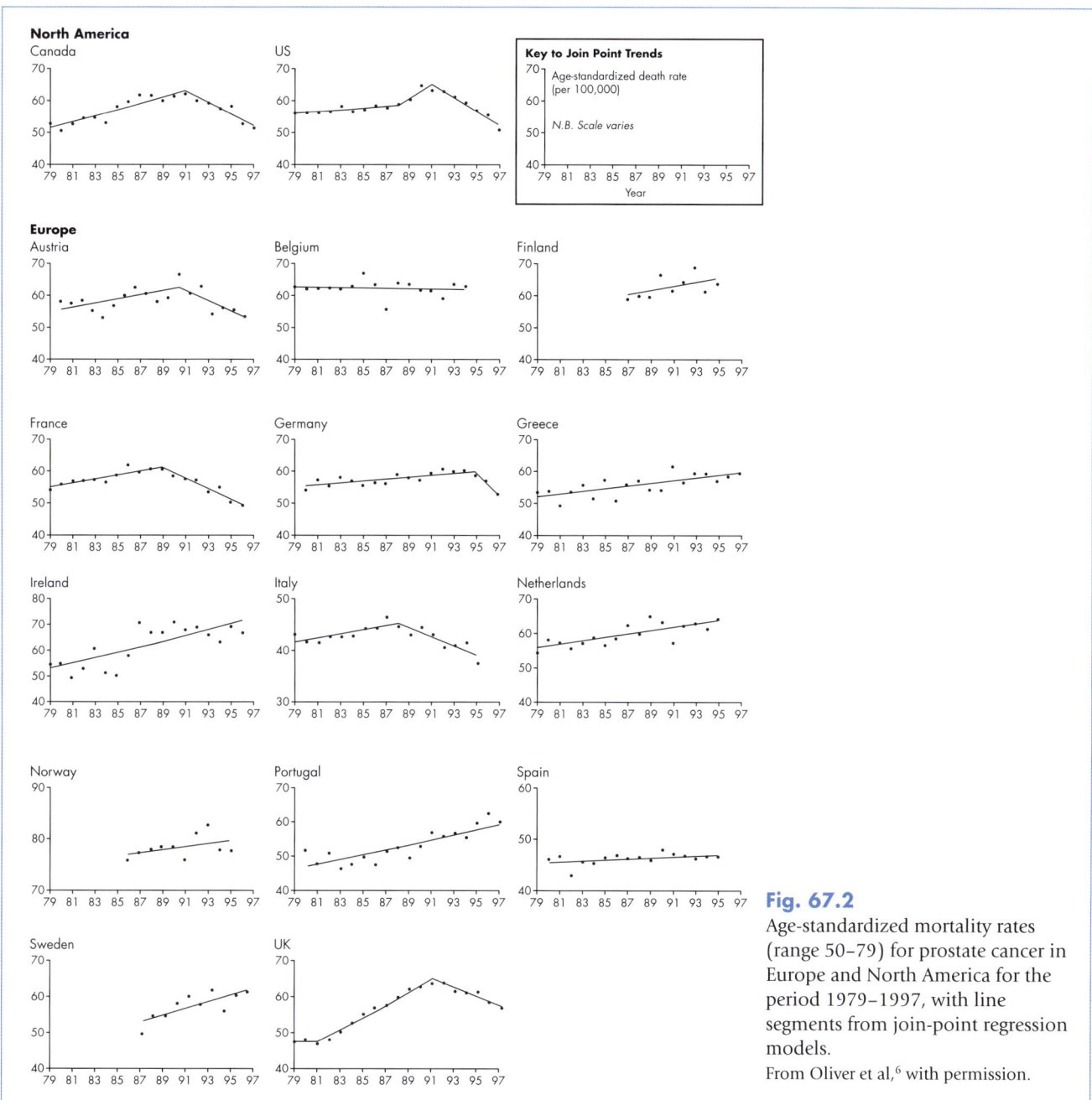

Fig. 67.2
Age-standardized mortality rates (range 50–79) for prostate cancer in Europe and North America for the period 1979–1997, with line segments from join-point regression models.
From Oliver et al,[6] with permission.

(15 prostate cancer deaths/100,000) and Sweden (82/100,000). The highest death rates are in Scandinavia and the lowest in Japan and southern Europe. There has been a constant increase in prostate cancer mortality during most of the period studied. Prostate cancer mortality rates have increased an average of 1% to 2% annually. Although, Japan has one of the lowest prostate cancer mortality rates, it has had one of the highest rates of increase. Downward trends in prostate cancer have been seen in Canada, the US, Austria, France, Germany, Italy, and the UK. Rates in Belgium and Hungary have remained static. Most of these downward trends became established around 1988 to 1991 and have generally decreased annually by 2.1% to 6.0%. Downward trends have been seen in all age groups in those countries

experiencing a decrease in prostate cancer mortality with the exception of Germany and Austria, where decreases have been concentrated primarily in the age group 74 to 79 years (Figure 67.3).

EFFECT OF PSA SCREENING AND RESULTING AGGRESSIVE TREATMENT

Researchers have advanced several theories to explain the observed changes in prostate cancer mortality during the past two decades. Proponents of PSA screening frequently cite the recent declines in prostate cancer mortality rates as proof that PSA testing and subsequent treatment is efficacious.[7–13] Unfortunately, some of the

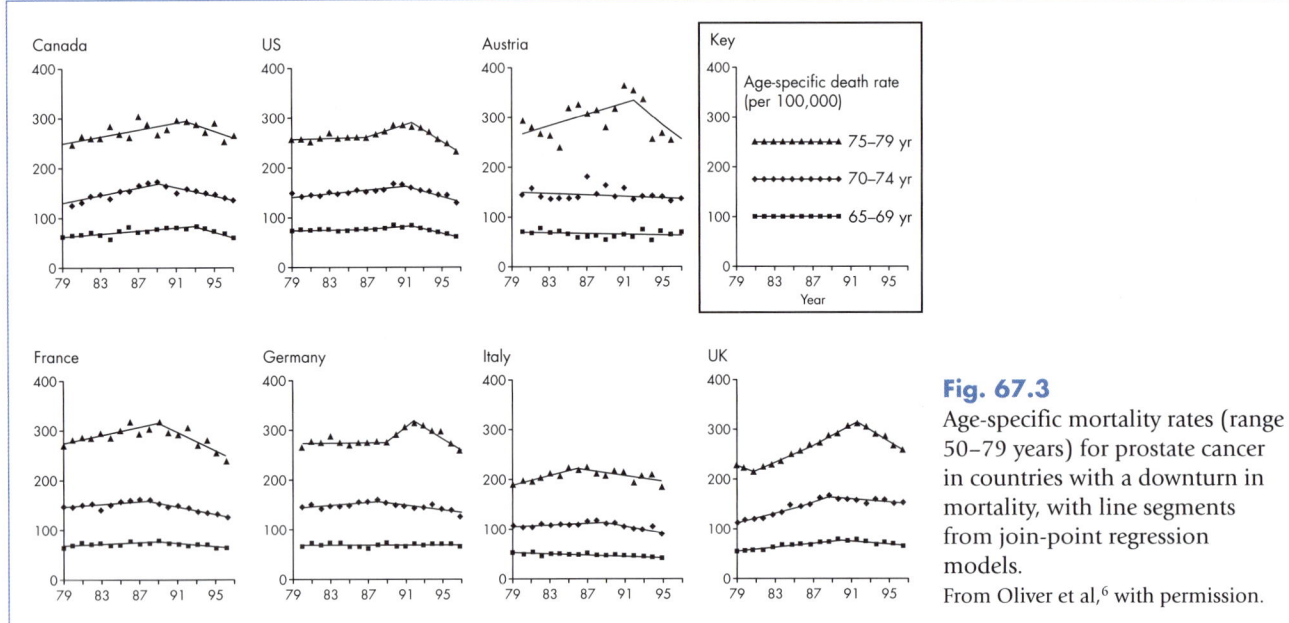

Fig. 67.3

Age-specific mortality rates (range 50–79 years) for prostate cancer in countries with a downturn in mortality, with line segments from join-point regression models.

From Oliver et al,[6] with permission.

conclusions result from several biases and flawed analyses.[13] Others hypothesize a cause-and-effect relationship that is too short considering the natural history of localized prostate cancer.[7] Even in the US it is difficult to attribute major population effects to treatment without making implausibly optimistic assumptions.[14]

The explanation that falling mortality rates are the result of PSA testing and aggressive treatment of localized disease does not account for the fact that prostate cancer mortality rates are falling both in regions where there is a high prevalence of screening and treatment and in regions were aggressive PSA testing is not practiced. The UK, for example, has recently witnessed declines in prostate cancer mortality during a period of time when there has been no widespread PSA testing.[15] We recently conducted a comparison of prostate cancer mortality rates in two SEER regions, Connecticut and Seattle.[16] We documented that the physicians in the greater Seattle/King County region were much more aggressive in adopting PSA testing in the late 1980s compared with their Connecticut colleagues. Despite much higher rates of screening, biopsy, and treatment with radical prostatectomy and radiation therapy in Seattle, no differences were noted in the prostate cancer mortality rates in the two regions during 10 years of follow-up. Interestingly, both regions showed similar declines in prostate cancer mortality beginning around 1991.

EFFECT OF ATTRIBUTION BIAS

Feuer et al[17] explored the possibility that incorrect attribution of cause of death may have contributed to the recent trends in prostate cancer mortality. The large

pool of undiagnosed prostate disease identified through autopsy studies makes the reported incidence of prostate cancer particularly susceptible to changes in the use of medical interventions such as PSA testing. The increased number of prostate cancer cases detected as a result of screening efforts drives up the observed pool of prevalent cases and yields a large population of men whose death may potentially be attributed to prostate cancer. Because prostate cancers are often slow growing and men with this disease commonly die of other causes, there is likely to be a certain number of men who die of causes other than prostate cancer but who mistakenly have had their underlying cause of death attributed to prostate cancer merely because they were labeled as having the disease as a result of screening.

To test this hypothesis Feuer et al[17] analyzed incidence-based mortality rates beginning before 1987, when PSA testing began in the US, and for several years afterwards. They noted that after 1987 incidence-based prostate cancer mortality rates rose above the baseline level, but returned to this level by 1994. They concluded that the rise and fall in prostate cancer mortality observed since the introduction of testing in the general population was consistent with the hypothesis that a fixed percent of the rising and falling pool of recently diagnosed patients who died of other causes were mislabeled as dying of prostate cancer.

In two separate studies, we explored the possibility of misattribution bias as a possible confounding effect when interpreting prostate cancer mortality rates. The first explored cause of death determination in Connecticut in two time periods, 1985 and 1995, dates that overlapped the introduction of PSA testing.[18] We found a high level of agreement concerning the underlying cause of death after a review of the information in hospital medical records and on death certificates for men who had previously been diagnosed with prostate cancer. The International Classification of Diseases-9 coding rules concerning cause of death attribution favored over- rather than under-reporting of prostate cancer deaths, but the effect was very modest. More importantly, the cause of death determination did not appear to have changed after the introduction of PSA testing.

A second study involving a review of clinical information and death certificates in King County, Washington confirmed these findings.[19] There was excellent agreement between the underlying cause of death from death certificates and medical records in prostate cancer patients. Prostate cancer patients with concurrent cardiovascular disease were less likely to be coded as having died of prostate cancer than if they had other co-morbidities. Patients with other cancers, such as colon or lung cancer, were also subject to misclassification, but there did not appear to be any systematic bias in either over- or under-diagnosing prostate cancer.

EFFECT OF ANTIANDROGEN THERAPY

Another plausible explanation for the recent decline in prostate cancer mortality rates is the early use of antiandrogen therapy in the treatment of this disease. PSA has been used not only to screen for prostate cancer, but also to monitor disease recurrence following definitive surgery or radiation. Prior to the advent of PSA testing, urologists usually waited for symptomatic metastases before initiating antiandrogen therapy. Rising PSA values have alerted urologists to the presence of residual disease and have led many to initiate antiandrogen therapy before metastases can be identified. The report by Crawford et al in 1989[20] concerning the use of leuprolide and flutamide among men with very early metastatic disease, spurred an enormous increase in the use of antiandrogen therapy that has persisted throughout the past decade.[21]

The strongest evidence supporting the hypothesis that early antiandrogen therapy can increase survival, and thereby lower prostate cancer mortality rates, comes from the phase III EORTC randomized trial comparing external radiation alone with external radiation combined with antiandrogen therapy in men with advanced localized disease. After a median follow-up of 66 months this trial has demonstrated a significant cancer-specific and all-cause survival advantage for men receiving 3 years of antiandrogen therapy.[22] Other evidence comes from the prospective trial conducted by the Eastern Cooperative Oncology Group that randomized 100 men with node-positive disease at the time of radical prostatectomy to receive either immediate or delayed antiandrogen therapy.[23] After a median follow-up of 7.1 years, men who received immediate antiandrogen therapy had a significant cause-specific and all-cause survival advantage.

The declines in prostate cancer mortality rates documented in several countries also support this hypothesis. Although screening for prostate cancer is not widely supported in the UK, the early use of antiandrogen therapy for men with evidence of systemic disease has paralleled practices in North America. Both geographic regions first witnessed a decline in prostate cancer mortality rates in 1991, shortly after the practice of maximum androgen blockade became widespread. The decline in prostate cancer mortality noted in Quebec is also difficult to ascribe to PSA screening when trends within birth cohorts are analyzed, but the results could be explained by the widespread early use of antiandrogen therapy.[24] Despite significantly different practice patterns in regard to PSA screening, we noted similar declines in prostate cancer mortality rates in Connecticut and Seattle, beginning in 1991.[16] Both regions adopted the practice of maximum androgen blockade around 1990. The evidence of declining prostate cancer mortality rates in Austria also support this hypothesis.[7] The time from the initiation of widespread PSA testing to the subsequent decline in prostate cancer mortality rates is too short to be explained by surgical intervention. The widespread use of early antiandrogen therapy, however, may have had an impact on mortality rates in a much shorter timeframe.

SUMMARY

Before the 1980s prostate cancer mortality was increasing in most industrialized countries.[25] Between 1988 and 1991 rates began to turn downward in a number of different regions. Several hypotheses have been advanced to explain these findings.[26] Some believe that the downturn in prostate cancer mortality rates is a direct response to aggressive PSA screening and treatment with surgery or radiation. Arguing against this explanation is the observation that mortality rates have declined both in regions where screening is aggressively practiced, such as the US and Canada, *and* in regions were screening with PSA is not practiced, such as the UK. Furthermore, some regions with aggressive PSA screening programs, such as Australia, have not seen a subsequent decline in prostate cancer mortality rates. Even within the US, a region with very aggressive screening and treatment practices, Seattle, saw declines in prostate cancer mortality similar to a region, Connecticut, where PSA testing was not adopted as rapidly.

Another explanation for these findings is a possible systematic misattribution of prostate cancer to many men dying *with* this disease rather than *of* this disease. We have examined this problem and found that death certificates appear to be a reasonably accurate tool for identifying patients who die from prostate cancer. Problems arise in approximately 10% of cases and usually occur when men have other malignancies, such as lung or colon cancer, or suffer from significant co-morbidities, especially cardiac disease. Furthermore, we found no change in cause-of-death attribution when records from before and after the introduction of PSA testing were compared.

One potential explanation for the observed decline in prostate cancer mortality is the widespread use of early antiandrogen therapy. Two randomized trials have documented a survival benefit for those patients placed on antiandrogen therapy very early in the course of their disease. By prolonging life in an older male population many potential prostate cancer deaths may have been converted to deaths from other causes.

Unfortunately observational data are only capable of generating hypotheses. Linking declines in prostate cancer mortality with a specific cause requires a randomized trial. For this reason, clinical trials to determine whether PSA screening can reduce prostate cancer mortality continue in Europe and the US, and are expected to yield results by 2009. Should these trials prove negative, the efficacy of early antiandrogen therapy to lower prostate cancer mortality should be reinvestigated.

REFERENCES

1. Jemal A, Tiwari RC, Murray T, et al. Cancer statistics, 2004. CA Cancer J Clin 2004;54:8–29.

2. Ries LAG, Kosary CL, Hankey BF, et al (eds). SEER Cancer Statistics Review, 1973–1995 (NIH Publication No. 98–2789). Bethesda, MD: National Cancer Institute, 1998.

3. World Health Organization. World Health Statistics Annual 1996. Geneva: World Health Organization, 1998.

4. Hinkley DV. Inference in two–phase regression. J Am Stat Assoc 1971;66:736–743.

5. Kim HJ, Fay MP, Feuer EJ, et al. Permutation tests for joinpoint regression with applications to cancer rates. Stat Med 2000;19:335–351.

6. Oliver SE, May MT, Gunnell D. International trends in prostate cancer mortality in the "PSA era". Int J Cancer 2001;92:893–898.

7. Bartsch G, Horninger W, Klocker H, et al. Prostate cancer mortality after introduction of prostate-specific antigen mass screening in the federal state of Tyrol, Austria. Urology 2001;58:417–424.

8. Hankey BF, Feuer EJ, Clegg LX, et al. Cancer surveillance series: Interpreting trends in prostate cancer – Part I: Evidence of the effects of screening in recent prostate cancer incidence, mortality and survival rates. J Natl Cancer Inst 1999;91:1017–1024.

9. Farkas A, Schneider D, Perrotti M, et al. National trends in the epidemiology of prostate cancer, to 1994: evidence for the effectiveness of PSA screening. Urology 1995;52:444–448.

10. Littrup PJ. Future benefits and cost-effectiveness of prostate carcinoma screening. Cancer 1997;80:1864–1870.

11. Hoeksema MJ, Law C. Cancer mortality rates fall: a turning point for the nation. J Natl Cancer Inst 1996;88:1706–1707.

12. Horninger W, Reissigl A, Rogatsch H, et al. Prostate cancer screening in the Tyrol, Austria: experience and results. Eur J Cancer 2000;36:1322–1335.

13. Labrie F, Candas B, Dupont A, et al. Screening decreases prostate cancer death. First analysis of the 1988 Quebec prospective randomized controlled trial. Prostate 1999;38:83–91.

14. Etzioni R, Legler JM, Feuer EJ, et al. Cancer surveillance series: Interpreting trends in prostate cancer – Part III: Quantifying the link between population prostate-specific antigen testing and recent declines in prostate cancer mortality. J Natl Cancer Inst 1999;91:1033–1039.

15. Oliver SE, Gunnell D, Donovan JL. Comparison of trends in prostate cancer mortality in England and Wales and the USA. Lancet 2000;355:1788–1789.

16. Lu-Yao G, Albertsen PC, Stanford JL, et al. Natural experiment examining the impact of aggressive screening and treatment on prostate cancer mortality in two fixed cohorts from Seattle area and Connecticut. BMJ 2002;325:740.

17. Feuer EJ, Merrill RM, Hankey BF. Cancer surveillance series: Interpreting trends in prostate cancer. Part II. Cause of death misclassification and the recent rise and fall in prostate cancer mortality. J Natl Cancer Inst 1999;91:1025–1032.

18. Albertsen PC, Walters S, Hanley JA. A comparison of cause of death determination in men previously diagnosed with prostate cancer who died in 1985 or 1995. J Urol 2000;163:519–523.

19. Penson DF, Albertsen PC, Nelson PS, et al. Determining cause of death in prostate cancer: are death certificates valid? J Natl Cancer Inst 2001;93:1822–1823.

20. Crawford ED, Eisenberger MA, McLeod DG, et al. A controlled trial of leuprolide with and without flutamide in prostatic cancer. N Engl J Med 1989;321:419–424.

21. Cooperberg MR, Grossfeld GD, Lubeck DP, et al. National practice patterns and time trends in androgen ablation for localized prostate cancer. J Natl Cancer Inst 2003;95:981–989.

22. Bolla M, Collette L, Blank L, et al. Long-term results with immediate androgen suppression and external radiation in patients with locally advanced prostate cancer (an EORTC study): a phase III randomized trial. Lancet 2002;360:103–108.

23. Messing EM, Manola J, Sarosdy M, et al. Immediate hormonal therapy compared with observation after radical prostatectomy and pelvic lymphadenectomy in men with node-positive prostate cancer. N Engl J Med 1999;341:1781–1788.

24. Perron L, Moore L, Bairati I, et al. PSA screening and prostate cancer mortality. Can Med Assoc J 2002;166:586–591.

25. Hsing A, Tsao L, Devesa SS. International trends and patterns of prostate cancer incidence and mortality. Int J Cancer 2000;85:60–67.

26. Frankel S, Smith GD, Donovan J, et al. Screening for prostate cancer. Lancet 2003;361:1122–1128.

Preservation of sexual function after treatment for prostate cancer 68

James A Eastham

INTRODUCTION

Patients diagnosed with a clinically localized prostate cancer face a daunting variety of management choices, including deferred treatment with observation, brachytherapy and/or external beam irradiation therapy with or without neoadjuvant hormonal therapy, cryotherapy, and radical prostatectomy. Physicians have long sought to guide patients through these choices based on their best judgment about the threat posed by the cancer, the effectiveness of treatment, the life-expectancy of the patient, as well as the potential for complications. Because screening programs have resulted in the identification of cancers much earlier in their natural history, the expection is that an individual patient will have a prolonged life-expectancy. In weighing treatment options, the patient and physician must consider the ability of the treatment to provide a durable cure while minimizing any negative impact on quality of life.

The most favorable outcome that can be achieved after local therapy for prostate cancer is complete eradication of the cancer with full recovery of urinary, bowel, and sexual function. These goals are inextricably linked and at times may appear to conflict with one another in that achieving one goal may occur at the expense of the others. The technical challenge of local treatment for prostate cancer is to treat sufficient periprostatic tissue to achieve cure, while at the same time preserving the cavernosal nerves required for erectile function, and the neuromusculature required for normal urinary and bowel function. This chapter will review the preservation of sexual function following local treatment for prostate cancer.

RADICAL PROSTATECTOMY

Potency is defined as the ability to obtain an erection that is sufficient for vaginal penetration and sexual intercourse. Before the 1980s, most patients permanently lost erectile function after radical prostatectomy. Then, Walsh et al[1,2] developed a technique for radical retropubic prostatectomy based on identification of the anatomic structures surrounding the prostate, including the autonomic nerves that control blood flow to the penis. Current surgical techniques are based on a more precise understanding of the autonomic innervation of the corpora cavernosa, allowing preservation of sexual function in the majority of men undergoing radical prostatectomy. Quinlan et al[3] demonstrated that recovery of potency is quantitatively related to the preservation of nerves. They identified three factors associated with recovery of potency after radical prostatectomy: age, clinical and pathologic stage, and preservation of the neurovascular bundles. In their series, approximately 90% of men younger than 50 were potent if either one or both neurovascular bundles were preserved. For men older than 50, return of potency was more likely if both neurovascular bundles were preserved rather than only one. Catalona et al[4] reported potency in 68% of patients when both nerves were preserved and 47% when just one nerve was spared. They also demonstrated a strong correlation between preservation of potency and age.

Rabbani et al[5] have developed a nomogram to predict the return of potency based on a series of 314 previously potent patients treated since 1993 with radical prostatectomy for T1C to T3A prostate cancer (Table 68.1). Factors significantly associated with recovery of

Table 68.1 Probability of recovery of potency by 24 and 36 months based on a combination of pre- and post-operative parameters.[5]

Preoperative potency	Probability (%) of recovery of potency by 24 months (36 months)		
	Age ≤60	Age 60.1–65	Age >65
Bilateral nerve sparing			
Full erection	70 (76)	49 (55)	43 (49)
Full erection, recently diminished	53 (59)	34 (39)	30 (35)
Partial erection	43 (49)	27 (31)	23 (27)
Unilateral or bilateral neurovascular bundle damage			
Full erection	60 (67)	40 (46)	35 (41)
Full erection, recently diminished	44 (50)	28 (32)	24 (28)
Partial erection	35 (40)	21 (25)	18 (21)
Unilateral neurovascular bundle resection			
Full erection	26 (30)	15 (18)	13 (15)
Full erection, recently diminished	17 (20)	10 (12)	8.5 (10)
Partial erection	13 (15)	7.5 (8.8)	6.3 (7.5)

spontaneous erections satisfactory for intercourse included age of the patient, quality of erections before the operation, and degree of preservation of the neurovascular bundles. Time after surgery is also an important factor in the recovery of potency. The median time to recovery of an international index of erectile function (IIEF) score greater than or equal to 17 was 24 months, while 42 months was required to reach an IIEF of greater than or equal to 26 (Figure 68.1).

In addition to preservation of the autonomic innervation to the corpora cavernosa (i.e. the neurovascular bundles), preservation of the vascular branches to the corpora cavernosa has been reported to affect the recovery of erectile function after radical prostatectomy.[6–8] Accessory arterial branches that supply the corpora have been described.[7,8] When these branches are preserved, a normal arterial inflow to the penis will be maintained after surgery. Adequate arterial inflow may enable a patient to remain potent or, for a patient who is impotent, it will ensure an adequate response to medical treatment.

PRESERVATION OF THE NEUROVASCULAR BUNDLES

Radical prostatectomy is among the most complex operations performed by urologists, and challenges surgeons because outcomes are highly sensitive to fine details in surgical technique. Modern outcomes research has repeatedly documented that the results and complications of this operation vary markedly, not only with surgeons' experience, but even more so among experienced surgeons. The elusive goals of modern radical prostatectomy are to remove the cancer completely with negative surgical margins, minimal blood loss, no serious perioperative complications, and complete recovery of continence and potency. No surgeon achieves such results uniformly. This section provides surgeons with details about one approach to this operation, which has been modified frequently in a continual effort to improve results. The technique described here is not the only successful approach; various other techniques work as well. The hope is that the reader will discern the important anatomic and surgical principles that will allow him/her to improve his/her own technique and patient outcomes.

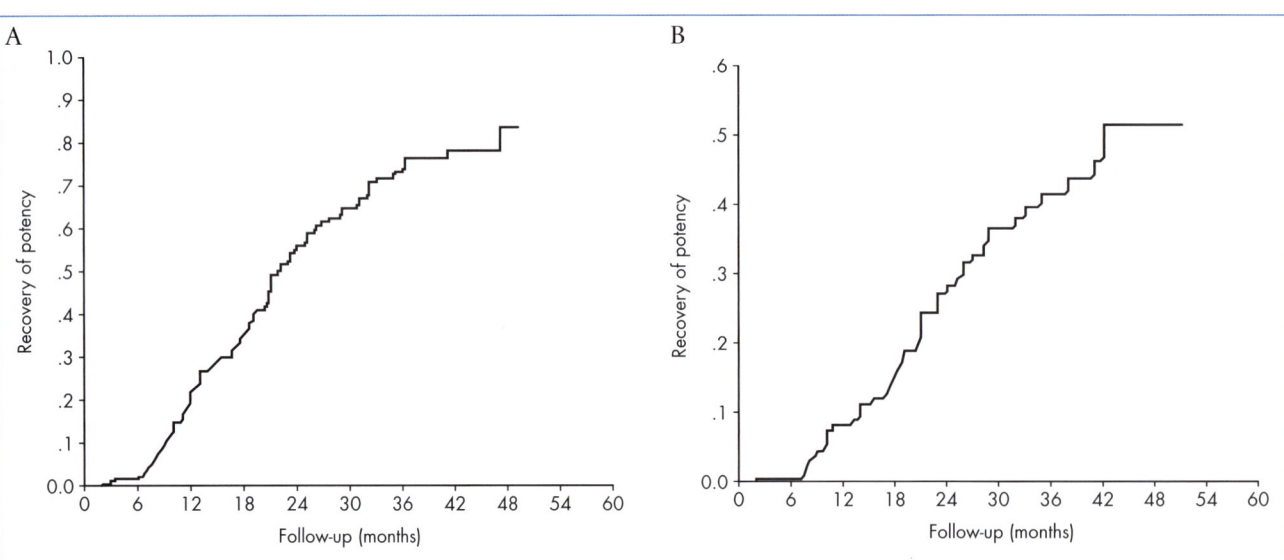

Fig. 68.1
Probability of recovery of potency over time after bilateral nerve-sparing radical prostatectomy. *A*, International index of erectile function (IIEF) ≥17, and *B*, IIEF ≥26.

A lateral approach to the neurovascular bundles (Fig. 68.2) allows wide exposure of the apex so that the apical tissue can be completely resected. The lateral pelvic fascia over the neurovascular bundle can be incised more medially or laterally to the nerve, depending on the extent or location of the tumor and whether the nerves are to be preserved (see Figure 68.2A, B). A "peanut," or Kitner, dissector is used to gently sweep the nerves laterally away from the prostate. Denonvilliers' fascia must be deliberately incised, releasing the neurovascular bundle laterally and allowing a deep plane of dissection along the fat of the anterior rectal wall (see Figure 68.2C–E). The risk of a positive surgical margin will be greatly reduced if this layer of fascia is included in the excised specimen. This apical dissection is performed without a catheter in the prostate to give the prostate

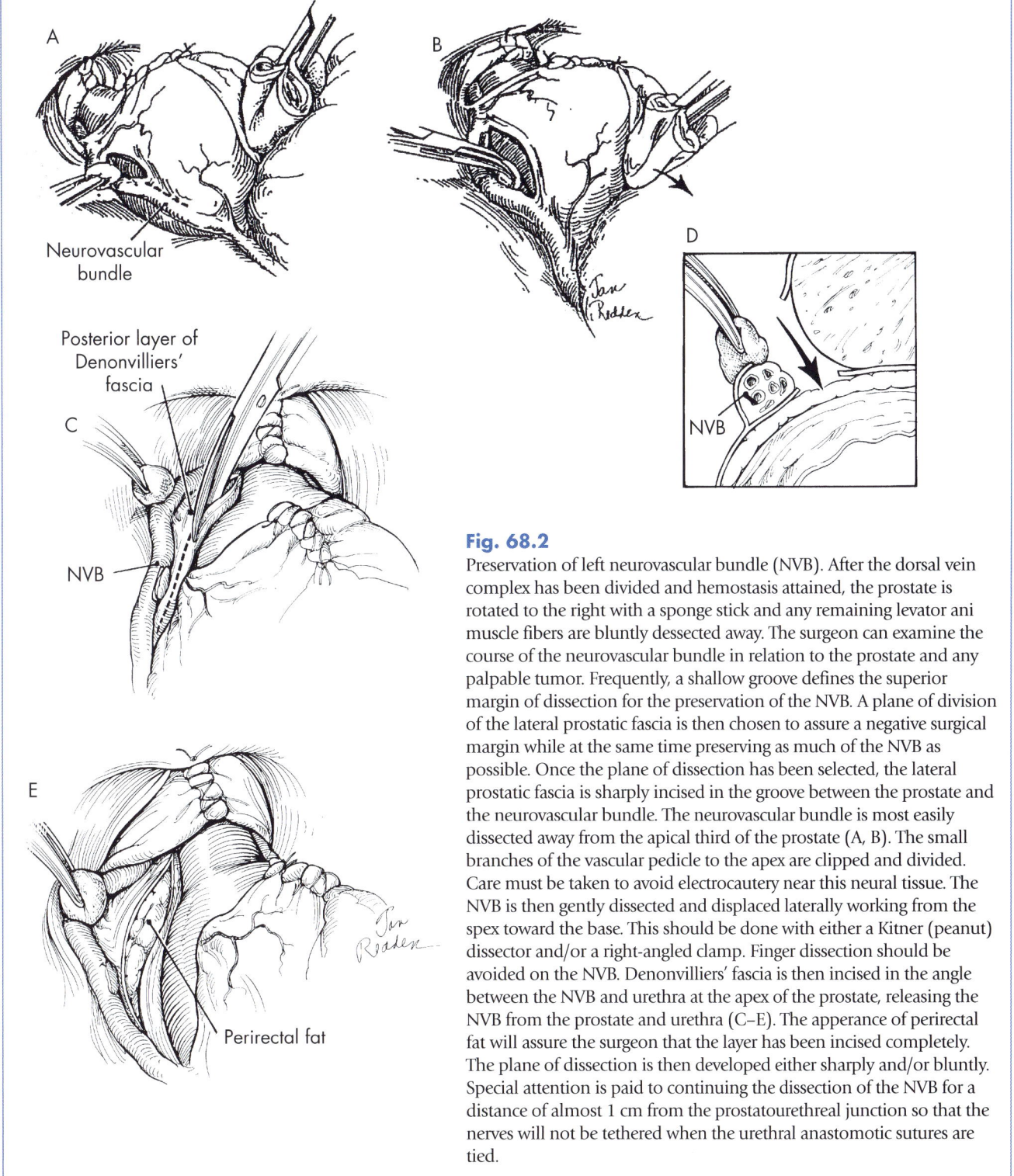

Fig. 68.2

Preservation of left neurovascular bundle (NVB). After the dorsal vein complex has been divided and hemostasis attained, the prostate is rotated to the right with a sponge stick and any remaining levator ani muscle fibers are bluntly dessected away. The surgeon can examine the course of the neurovascular bundle in relation to the prostate and any palpable tumor. Frequently, a shallow groove defines the superior margin of dissection for the preservation of the NVB. A plane of division of the lateral prostatic fascia is then chosen to assure a negative surgical margin while at the same time preserving as much of the NVB as possible. Once the plane of dissection has been selected, the lateral prostatic fascia is sharply incised in the groove between the prostate and the neurovascular bundle. The neurovascular bundle is most easily dissected away from the apical third of the prostate (A, B). The small branches of the vascular pedicle to the apex are clipped and divided. Care must be taken to avoid electrocautery near this neural tissue. The NVB is then gently dissected and displaced laterally working from the spex toward the base. This should be done with either a Kitner (peanut) dissector and/or a right-angled clamp. Finger dissection should be avoided on the NVB. Denonvilliers' fascia is then incised in the angle between the NVB and urethra at the apex of the prostate, releasing the NVB from the prostate and urethra (C–E). The apperance of perirectal fat will assure the surgeon that the layer has been incised completely. The plane of dissection is then developed either sharply and/or bluntly. Special attention is paid to continuing the dissection of the NVB for a distance of almost 1 cm from the prostatourethreal junction so that the nerves will not be tethered when the urethral anastomotic sutures are tied.

more mobility. Small clips placed parallel to the neurovascular bundle are used to control the small vascular bands that are usually present, particularly near the apex of the prostate. Once the neurovascular bundles have been mobilized off the prostate at the apex and mid gland, the urethra can be safely divided and the anastomotic sutures placed. The initial incisions in Denonvilliers' fascia are connected across the midline beneath the apex of the prostate.

Once the apex is completely mobilized, a catheter is placed through the urethra to facilitate dissection. Traction on this catheter allows the remaining neurovascular bundles to be dissected away bluntly as the prostate is dissected off the rectum, beneath Denonvilliers' fascia.

The nerves lie close to the prostate near the base. Dissection too close to the prostate will result in a positive margin in this area, shown to be associated with an increased risk of recurrence. We have been successful in preserving most or all of both neurovascular bundles in the majority of patients using this lateral approach, while still allowing a wider dissection around the apex of the prostate, especially posteriorly.

When resection of one or both neurovascular bundles is necessary, we use a technique for placing interposition grafts from the sural or genitofemoral nerve to one or both neurovascular bundles (Figure 68.3).[9,10] Surgeons have performed nerve grafts successfully for decades to replace damaged or transected peripheral sensorimotor nerves. The basis for nerve regeneration, and consequently for nerve grafting, is the ability of axons to produce axon sprouts. After nerve transection, axon sprouts will invariably grow, forming a neuroma if they do not come into contact with an environment that channels their growth. The cut end of a nerve sprouts minifascicles

that contain axon sprouts, fibroblasts, Schwann cells, and capillaries. The minifascicles grow haphazardly for a limited distance and then form a neuroma. However, if the axons encounter an empty nerve sheath, growth becomes organized and directed, resulting in a new nerve. A nerve graft functions to provide a conduit through which regenerating nerve fibers are directed to meet with the distal end of the transected nerve. These concepts support the hypothesis that cavernous nerve grafts may restore penile autonomic innervation and the ability to achieve spontaneous erections after deliberate neurovascular bundle resection during radical prostatectomy. With bilateral nerve grafts, one-third of patients with bilateral nerve resection have had spontaneous, medically unassisted erections sufficient for sexual intercourse. The greatest return of function is observed 14 to 18 months after surgery. In our experience, nerve grafts provide one solution to a common surgical dilemma: in a patient with a large, high grade cancer located adjacent to the posterolateral capsule, should the surgeon dissect close to the prostate to preserve the nerve or dissect close to the nerve, risking recovery of potency? Over the past 3 years, we have performed nerve grafts in about 15% of all previously untreated patients. The risks were very low: there was only one graft-related complication (cellulitis), and the overall operative time, blood loss, and hospital stays were identical in grafted and nongrafted patients. Final proof of the efficacy of nerve grafts must await completion of a prospective randomized trial comparing nerve grafts to no grafts after unilateral neurovascular bundle resection. Until then, surgeons must use sound judgment and informed consent to decide, along with their patients, whether a nerve graft is indicated when a neurovascular bundle is damaged or resected during radical prostatectomy.

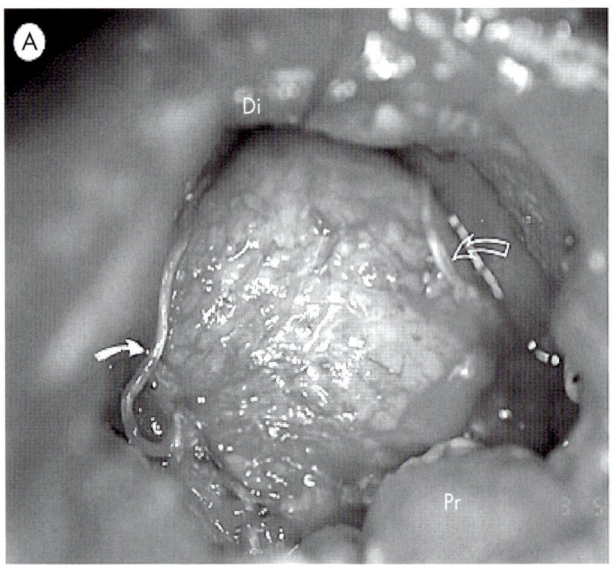
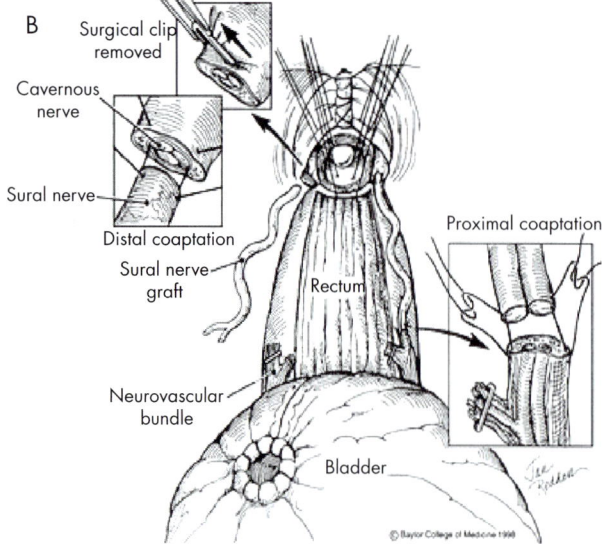

Fig. 68.3
Sural nerve graft interposed between severed ends of each cavernosal nerve.

STRATEGIES TO IMPROVE SEXUAL FUNCTION AFTER RADICAL PROSTATECTOMY

EARLY USE OF INTRACAVERNOSAL AGENTS

Montorsi et al[11] prospectively assessed the effect of postoperative intracavernous injections of alprostadil on the recovery of spontaneous erectile function after nerve-sparing radical prostatectomy. Thirty preoperatively potent patients underwent bilateral nerve-sparing radical prostatectomy and were subsequently randomized to alprostadil injections three times per week for 12 weeks or observation without any treatment. Eight of 15 (53%) patients receiving alprostadil injections compared to 3 of 15 (20%) untreated men reported recovery of spontaneous erections at 6 months sufficient for satisfactory sexual intercourse. The investigators hypothesized that alprostadil injections improve cavernosal oxygenation, thereby limiting hypoxia-induced tissue damage.

EARLY USE OF PHOSPHODIESTERASE-5 INHIBITORS

Levine et al[12] examined 54 men with normal preoperative erectile function who underwent bilateral nerve-sparing radical prostatectomy. Patients were randomized to either sildenafil citrate (50 mg, n = 17; 100 mg, n = 18) or placebo (n = 19) 4 weeks post surgery and entered a 36-week, double-blind treatment period with nightly drug administration. Assessment 48 weeks after surgery demonstrated that 10 of 35 (29%) men given sildenafil citrate but only 5% of the control group had spontaneous erectile function as determined by nocturnal penile tumescence and rigidity testing. The investigators concluded that early postoperative treatment with a phosphodiesterase-5 inhibitor improves long-term recovery of erectile function and supports the concept of early rehabilitation of erectile function.

PERIOPERATIVE IMMUNOPHILIN LIGAND THERAPY

Immunophilin ligands have shown neuroprotective activity in several animal models of nerve injury, including damage to sciatic, facial, and optic nerves assayed by nerve regeneration and/or functional recovery.[13,14] Histopathologically, axonal cross-sectional areas in animals with crushed nerves were significantly greater in those treated with immunophilin ligands compared to placebo. In addition, animals receiving placebo after nerve-crush injury had a greater than 90% decrease in myelination levels, while treated animals regained 30% to 40% of their original myelination levels.

Recently, the immunophilin ligand FK506 and its nonimmunosuppressive derivative GPI1046 have been investigated in a model of cavernous nerve injury.[15] In treated animals, the recovery of erections was significantly greater than in animals receiving placebo. Immunohistochemical studies demonstrated that the immunophilin ligand-treated animals had preserved cavernosal tissue histology. The authors suggested that the neurotrophic effects of these agents may decrease the extent of cavernosal nerve degeneration and improve the recovery of erectile function after radical prostatectomy. These agents are being evaluated in clinical trials to determine their potential role as neuroprotective agents following radical prostatectomy.

CRYOSURGERY

Technologic advances in cryosurgery as primary treatment for localized prostate cancer, including transrectal ultrasound guidance, urethral warmers, and argon-based cryomachines, have substantially reduced morbidity and improved quality-of-life outcomes after this procedure. Several years ago, erectile dysfunction was a universally expected outcome after cryosurgery, but current technology and treatment delivery permit a minority of men to regain potency after treatment. Ellis[16] reported results from his series of 75 patients with newly diagnosed, clinically localized prostate cancer treated between 2000 and 2001 by a double freeze–thaw cycle. Of the 34 patients who were potent preoperatively, 6 (18%) regained potency after surgery. Robinson et al[17] reported 3-year quality-of-life outcomes using patient-reported questionnaires after cryosurgery. At 36 months, 5 of 38 (13%) preoperatively potent patients had recovered erectile function. Bahn et al[18] reported their 7-year efficacy and safety results with targeted cryotherapy in 590 consecutive patients with newly diagnosed prostate cancer. Of the 373 men who were potent before the procedure, 95% were impotent after surgery. The average recovery time was 16.4 months. Clearly, the majority of men treated with cryosurgery will be impotent after the procedure, and potent men with clinically localized prostate cancer considering this option must be appropriately counseled.

RADIATION THERAPY

The mechanism of erectile dysfunction after radiation therapy is not well defined. Radiation damage to the nerve bundles and vascular structures has been proposed as the cause.[19] However, the ability to decrease dose to these structures is limited by the proximity of the neurovascular bundles to the peripheral zone of the prostate, an area where cancer commonly is located and which thus requires the full prescription dose. In addition, total radiation dose, the use of concurrent/adjuvant hormonal therapy, and time since treatment may influence post-radiation potency. To date, there has been little study of neuroprotective agents or the early use of either intracavernosal injection therapy or phosphodiesterase type-5 inhibitors during and after radiation therapy, but these may improve outcomes in the future.

PROSTATE BRACHYTHERAPY

Prostate brachytherapy is an increasingly common treatment for early-stage prostate cancer; its biochemical outcomes for low-risk patients are similar to those of external beam radiation therapy and radical prostatectomy at 5 and 10 years after treatment. As seen in radical prostatectomy, there is emerging evidence that erectile dysfunction induced by prostate brachytherapy is technique related and may be minimized by careful attention to source placement. Merrick and Butler[19] recently reviewed published reports to identify factors associated with post-brachytherapy erectile dysfunction. They found no data that either the radiation dose to the neurovascular bundle or choice of isotope was associated with brachytherapy-induced erectile dysfunction, while conflicting data have been reported regarding radiation dose to the prostate and the use of supplemental external beam radiation therapy. They concluded that the available data support the proximal penis as an important site-specific structure, and that refinements in implant technique will result in lower doses to this area with potential improvement in potency preservation.

In an attempt to improve preimplantation planning, Wright et al[20] examined factors associated with brachytherapy-induced erectile dysfunction. They concluded that increasing the dose to the penile bulb may increase the risk of erectile dysfunction, but increasing the dose to the neurovascular bundle did not appear to. Similarly, Merrick et al[21] studied 46 potent men with clinically localized prostate cancer, 23 of whom developed post-brachytherapy erectile dysfunction. The mean volume of the penile bulb was greater in the potent men than in the impotent patients. Impotent men had received approximately twice the radiation dose of the potent men in each area of the bulb that was examined. While the penile bulb is not believed to play a role in the development of an erection,[22] it is easily recognized on prostate imaging and may serve as a surrogate for another structure involved in erectile function.

Reported rates of potency following prostate brachytherapy are summarized in Table 68.2.[23-25] Stock et al[23] treated 313 potent men with prostate brachytherapy alone between 1990 and 1998. The

actuarial preservation of potency was 79% and 59% at 3 and 6 years, respectively. In this series, potency was assessed by physician interview and excluded the use of oral medications. Merrick et al[24] examined outcomes for 209 potent men following prostate brachytherapy. At 6-year follow-up, 39% maintained potency; including men using sildenafil citrate, this increased to 54%. Factors associated with postimplant erectile dysfunction were preimplant potency score, use of supplemental external beam radiation therapy, and diabetes. Potters et al[25] evaluated 482 men treated with prostate brachytherapy, including combination treatment with external beam radiation therapy and/or neoadjuvant hormonal therapy. Potency was preserved in 311 of the 482 patients, with a 5-year actuarial potency rate of 52.7%. The potency rate was better for those receiving monotherapy (76%) than those receiving combination therapy (see Table 68.2). Of 84 patients treated with sildenafil citrate, 52 had a successful result (62%), although the response to sildenafil citrate was significantly better in those patients not treated with neoadjuvant hormonal therapy. Taken together, these studies suggest that potency can be preserved in the majority of patients treated with prostate brachytherapy. Most patients with erectile dysfunction respond to oral medications such as sildenafil citrate. Potency outcomes appear to be worse when brachytherapy is combined with external beam radiation therapy and/or hormonal therapy. Lastly, time appears to be a critical factor as well, with potency rates decreasing over time.

EXTERNAL BEAM RADIATION THERAPY

As with prostate brachytherapy, both experimental and clinical evidence suggest that the radiation dose to the bulb of the penis is critical to the maintenance of

Table 68.2 Potency rates following radiation therapy

Series	Type of radiation	Time after treatment	Potency (%)
Stock et al[23]	PPB	36 months	79
Stock et al[23]	PPB	72 months	59
Merrick et al[24]	PPB	6 year actuarial	54
Potters et al[25]	PPB	5 year actuarial	76
Potters et al[25]	PPB + EBT	5 year actuarial	56
Potters et al[25]	PPB + NAAD	5 year actuarial	52
Potters et al[25]	PPB + EBT + NAAD	5 year actuarial	29
Wilder et al[29]	EBT	3 year actuarial	63
Mantz et al[30]	EBT	5 year actuarial	53
Chen et al[31]	EBT	12 months	58

EBT, external beam radiation; NAAD, neoadjuvant androgen deprivation; PPB, permanent prostate brachytherapy.

potency after external beam radiation therapy.[26-28] This again suggests that the technique used to deliver treatment, be it radical prostatectomy, prostate brachytherapy or external beam radiation therapy, significantly impacts recovery of erectile function after treatment. Careful pretreatment planning and treatment delivery will improve outcomes following any treatment for clinically localized prostate cancer.

Potency after external beam radiation therapy is shown in Table 68.2.[29-31] Wilder et al[29] reported potency preservation after three-dimensional conformal radiation therapy in 35 potent men with prostate cancer. Total dose to the prostate ranged from 66 to 79.2 Gy. Kaplan-Meier estimates of the potency preservation rates at 1, 2, and 3 years after treatment were 100%, 83%, and 63%, respectively. Mantz et al[30] performed a retrospective review of 287 men with clinically localized prostate cancer treated with conformal techniques to 62 to 73.8 Gy.[30] Actuarial potency rates at 40 and 60 months were 59% and 53%, respectively. Factors identified as significant predictors of erectile dysfunction after external beam radiation therapy included pretreatment potency status, diabetes, coronary artery disease, and antiandrogen usage. To further examine the potential effects of concomitant hormonal therapy and external beam radiation therapy, Chen et al[31] evaluated sexual function using self-administered patient questionnaires in 144 men (55 of whom also received hormonal therapy) before and after three-dimensional conformal radiation therapy for clinically localized prostate cancer. Before radiation therapy, 87 (60%) of the patients were potent compared to 47% at 12 months after treatment. Of 60 men who were completely potent before treatment and were followed for at least 1 year, 58% retained their baseline function. Patients who had radiation alone were more likely to be potent at 1 year than those receiving radiation and hormonal therapy (56% vs 31%, respectively).

Several studies have demonstrated that many men with erectile dysfunction after radiation therapy (brachytherapy or external beam) will respond to sildenafil citrate.[32-34] Incrocci et al[34] performed a randomized, double-blind, placebo-controlled cross-over study to determine the efficacy of sildenafil citrate in treating erectile dysfunction in men treated with three-dimensional conformal radiation therapy. The study included 60 patients who had completed radiation therapy at least 6 months earlier. They received 2 weeks' treatment with 50 mg of sildenafil citrate or placebo; at week 2 the dose was increased to 100 mg if there was an unsatisfactory response. At week 6, patients crossed over to the alternative treatment. Data were collected using the IIEF questionnaire. Successful intercourse was reported in 55% of patients after sildenafil citrate versus 18% after placebo. Most patients (90%) required an increase in the dose of sildenafil citrate to 100 mg. Whether or not earlier use of sildenafil citrate would improve these outcomes is unknown.

CONCLUSION

A better understanding of periprostatic anatomy and the factors associated with the development of post-treatment erectile dysfunction should result in a continued improvement in functional outcomes after radical prostatectomy, cryotherapy, prostate brachytherapy, and external beam radiation therapy for clinically localized prostate cancer. Each of these treatment options appears to be sensitive to the fine details of delivery of the therapy. While the technical aspects of neurovascular bundle preservation and the role of the surgeon in preserving potency at the time of radical prostatectomy have received considerable attention, outcomes after radiation therapy also appear to be sensitive to how treatment is delivered. In particular, the dose of radiation delivered to the bulb of the penis appears to be intimately associated with the preservation of erectile function after both prostate brachytherapy and external beam radiation therapy. While the role of neoadjuvant and/or adjuvant phosphodiesterase-5 inhibitors or immunophilin ligands in preserving potency certainly needs further study, careful attention to the fine details of delivery of any of the treatment options should improve outcomes in the short term.

REFERENCES

1. Walsh PC. Anatomic radical prostatectomy: evolution of the surgical technique. J Urol 1998;160:2418–2424.

2. Walsh PC, Donker PJ. Impotence following radical prostatectomy: insight into etiology and prevention. J Urol 1982;128:492–497.

3. Quinlan DM, Epstein JI, Carter BS, et al. Sexual function following radical prostatectomy: influence of preservation of neurovascular bundles. J Urol 1991;145:998–1003.

4. Catalona WJ, Carvalhal GF, Mager DE, et al. Potency, continence and complication rates in 1,870 consecutive radical retropubic prostatectomies. J Urol 1999;162:433–438.

5. Rabbani F, Stapleton AM, Kattan MW, et al. Factors predicting recovery of erections after radical prostatectomy. J Urol 2000;164:1929–1934.

6. Rogers CG, Trock BP, Walsh PC. Preservation of accessory pudendal arteries during radical retropubic prostatectomy: surgical technique and results. Urology 2004;64:148–151.

7. Bahnson RR, Catalona WJ. Papaverine testing of impotent patients following nerve sparing radical prostatectomy. J Urol 1988;139:773–774.

8. Breza J, Aboseif SR, Orvis BR, et al. Detailed anatomy of penile neurovascular structures: surgical significance. J Urol 1989;141:437–443.

9. Kim ED, Scardino PT, Hampel O, et al. Interposition of sural nerve restores function of cavernous nerves resected during radical prostatectomy. J Urol 1999;161:188–192.

10. Kim ED, Nath R, Slawin KM, et al. Bilateral nerve grafting during radical retropubic prostatectomy: extended follow-up. Urology 2001;8:983–987.

11. Montorsi F, Guazzoni G, Strambi LF, et al. Recovery of spontaneous erectile function after nerve-sparing radical retropubic prostatectomy with and without early intracavernous injections of alprostadil: results of a prospective, randomized trial. J Urol 1997;158:1408–1410.

12. Levine LA, McCullough AR, Padma-Nathan H. Longitudinal randomized placebo-controlled study of the return of nocturnal erections after nerve-sparing radical prostatectomy in men treated with nightly sildenafil citrate. J Urol 2004;171:231–232 (abstract).

13. Gold BG, Katoh K, Storm-Dickerson T. The immunosuppressant FK506 increases the rate of axonal regeneration in rat sciatic nerve. J Neurosci 1995;15:7509–7516.

14. Freeman EE, Grosskreutz CL. The effects of FK506 on retinal ganglion cells after optic nerve crush. Invest Ophthalmol Vis Sci 2000; 41:1111–1115.

15. Burnett AL, Becker RE. Immunophilin ligands promote penile neurogenesis and erection recovery after cavernous nerve injury. J Urol 2004;171:495–500.

16. Ellis DS. Cryosurgery as primary treatment for localized prostate cancer: a community hospital experience. Urology 2002;60:34–39.

17. Robinson JW, Donnelly BJ, Saliken JC, et al. Quality of life and sexuality of men with prostate cancer 3 years after cryosurgery. Urology 2002;60(2 Suppl 1):12–18.

18. Bahn DK, Lee F, Badalament R, et al. Targeted cryoablation of the prostate: 7-year outcomes in the primary treatment of prostate cancer. Urology 2002;60(2 Suppl 1):3–11.

19. Merrick GS, Butler WM. The dosimetry of brachytherapy-induced erectile dysfunction. Med Dosim 2003;28:271–274.

20. Wright JL, Newhouse JH, Laguna JL, et al. Localization of neurovascular bundles on pelvic CT and evaluation of radiation dose to structures putatively involved in erectile dysfunction after prostate brachytherapy. Int J Radiat Oncol Biol Phys 2004;59:426–435.

21. Merrick GS, Butler WM, Wallner KE, et al. The importance of radiation doses to the penile bulb vs. crura in the development of postbrachytherapy erectile dysfunction. Int J Radiat Oncol Biol Phys 2002;54:1055–1062.

22. Mulhall JP, Yanover PM, Correlation of radiation dose and impotence risk after three-dimensional conformal radiotherapy for prostate cancer. Urology 2001;58:828.

23. Stock RG, Kao J, Stone NN. Penile erectile function after permanent radioactive seed implantation for treatment of prostate cancer. J Urol 2001;165:436–439.

24. Merrick GS, Butler WM, Galbreath RW, et al. Erectile function after permanent prostate brachytherapy. Int J Radiat Oncol Biol Phys 2002;52:893–902.

25. Potters L, Torre T, Fearn PA, et al. Potency after permanent prostate brachytherapy for localized prostate cancer. Int J Radiat Oncol Biol Phys 2001;50:1235–1242.

26. Carrier S, Hricak H, Lee SS, et al. Radiation-induced decrease in nitric oxide synthase-containing nerves in the rat penis. Radiology 1995;195:95–99.

27. Fisch BM, Pickett B, Weinberg V, et al. Dose of radiation received by the bulb of the penis correlates with risk of impotence after three-dimensional conformal radiotherapy for prostate cancer. Urology 2001;57:955–999.

28. Merrick GS, Wallner K, Butler WM, et al. A comparison of radiation dose to the bulb of the penis in men with and without prostate brachytherapy-induced erectile dysfunction. Int J Radiat Oncol Biol Phys 2001;50:597–604.

29. Wilder RB, Chou RH, Ryu JK, et al. Potency preservation after three-dimensional conformal radiotherapy for prostate cancer: preliminary results. Am J Clin Oncol 2000;23:330–333.

30. Mantz CA, Nautiyal J, Awan A, et al. Potency preservation following conformal radiotherapy for localized prostate cancer: impact of neoadjuvant androgen blockade, treatment technique, and patient-related factors. Cancer J Sci Am 1999;5:230–236.

31. Chen CT, Valicenti RK, Lu J, et al. Does hormonal therapy influence sexual function in men receiving 3D conformal radiation therapy for prostate cancer? Int J Radiat Oncol Biol Phys 2001;50:591–595.

32. Zelefsky MJ, McKee AB, Lee H, et al. Efficacy of oral sildenafil in patients with erectile dysfunction after radiotherapy for carcinoma of the prostate. Urology 1999;53:775–778.

33. Weber DC, Bieri S, Kurtz JM, et al. Prospective pilot study of sildenafil for treatment of postradiotherapy erectile dysfunction in patients with prostate cancer. J Clin Oncol 1999;17:3444–3449.

34. Incrocci L, Koper PC, Hop WC, et al. Sildenafil citrate (Viagra) and erectile dysfunction following external beam radiotherapy for prostate cancer: a randomized, double-blind, placebo-controlled, cross-over study. Int J Radiat Oncol Biol Phys 2001;51:1190–1195.

Quality-of-life instruments for prostate cancer

69

Marcus L Quek, David F Penson

INTRODUCTION

Quality of life has become an increasingly important concern in clinical decision-making for patients with prostate cancer. With the advent of screening programs utilizing serum prostate-specific antigen (PSA) testing, prostate cancer appears to be diagnosed at an earlier stage than in the pre-PSA era. Whether early treatment has translated into improved survival rates or has increased the burden of treatment of clinically-insignificant cancers is debatable. What is certain, however, is that due to this stage migration, more patients are treated for prostate cancer and are thus living longer with their disease.[1]

Whereas traditional outcome measures of overall and recurrence-free survival rates have been used to directly compare various therapeutic modalities, focus on "non-traditional" quality-of-life outcomes may further allow patients to make truly informed decisions regarding their treatment. This is especially true for localized prostate cancer in which none of the standard therapies—radical prostatectomy, radiotherapy—has been shown to date to have a clear survival difference in observational studies,[2] and in which novel therapeutic modalities continue to emerge touting less impact on a patients' quality of life. In fact, the American Urological Association's practice guidelines committee has stressed the importance of measuring quality of life as an outcome in the management of this condition.[3]

For many patients, quality of life is the primary outcome of interest when selecting among the available options. Helgason et al asked 299 prostate cancer patients if they would undergo a treatment that could possibly lengthen life expectancy at the expense of complete loss of sexual function. Forty-seven percent were either unwilling to accept treatment regardless of the survival benefit or would only accept the treatment if it provided a greater than 10 year improvement in life expectancy over no treatment.[4] Obviously quality of life is an important factor that clinicians must recognize when discussing therapeutic options with their patients. In advanced disease, where hormone ablation remains the mainstay of therapy, quality of life issues are particularly salient, since hormone therapy does not offer cure and may significantly impact daily functioning and sense of well-being.

Health-related quality of life (HRQOL) is a novel variable from the field of public health research that encompasses a wide range of human experience, including necessities of daily living, intrapersonal and interpersonal responses to illness, and activities associated with professional fulfillment and personal happiness. Perhaps more importantly, HRQOL involves the patient's own perceptions of personal health, the ability to function in life, and the overall sense of satisfaction with life's experiences.[5] The degree of bother or distress associated with the functional limitations or symptoms resulting either from the disease itself or its treatment are also important considerations in this concept of quality of life. Health-related quality of life is a patient-centered outcome that should not be estimated from a physician's report. The impact of quality of life on therapeutic decision-making is now considered so important that some suggest that clinical cancer trial design should routinely include an assessment of HRQOL as a measure of outcome.[6]

The goal of this chapter is to review the basic tenets of HRQOL assessment and introduce several established instruments currently in practice.

MEASURING HEALTH-RELATED QUALITY OF LIFE IN MEN WITH PROSTATE CANCER

Utilizing principles of psychometric test theory, standardized questionnaires (also known as "instruments" or "tools") are administered directly to patients (or a neutral third party interviewer) in order to objectively quantify HRQOL. These instruments typically contain questions, or items, that are organized into scales. Each scale measures a different aspect, or domain of HRQOL, which may be generic or disease-specific. Generic HRQOL domains address general aspects relevant to all persons regardless of their disease, and typically include overall sense of well-being and self-perceptions, and functionality in physical, emotional, and social arenas. Disease-specific HRQOL domains focus on the symptoms and/or concerns directly relevant to a particular condition or its treatment, such as anxiety about cancer recurrence, hot flashes, bladder irritability, bowel dysfunction, sexual dysfunction, and urinary incontinence.

Both generic and disease-specific domains need to be addressed in order to obtain the most complete "portrait" of the patient's experience. A recent study of men treated for early-stage prostate cancer noted that those who demonstrated dysfunction in the disease-specific domains also experienced small but significant changes in the generic domains, when compared with patients with no or minimal disease-specific dysfunction.[7] Hence, it is necessary to employ a multidimensional approach when assessing quality-of-life outcomes following prostate cancer treatment.

As HRQOL is a patient-centered outcome, it is critical that this outcome be measured directly from the patient, using either a self-administered survey or a third-party objective interviewer, as opposed to an invested healthcare provider. Many clinicians mistakenly underestimate the degree of symptoms and their impairment on HRQOL, introducing significant measurement error. In a large study of 2252 men, patients' self-assessment of HRQOL was compared with urologists' views, which significantly differed in all disease-specific domains, including urinary, sexual and bowel function, fatigue, and bone pain.[8] Other studies[9,10] have shown similar differences in assessment of HRQOL between patients and clinicians.

All HRQOL instruments must undergo arduous pilot testing and statistical analyses to ensure the psychometric properties of validity and reliability.[11] Reliability refers to the scale's reproducibility. In other words, what proportion of a patient's test score is true and what proportion is due to individual variation. There are different forms of reliability, which are routinely assessed during instrument development. Test-retest reliability is a measure of response stability over time. It is assessed by administering scales to patients at two separate time points, typically 1 month apart. The correlation coefficients between the two scores reflect the stability of responses. Internal consistency reliability is a measure of the similarity of an individual's responses across several items, indicating the homogeneity of a scale.[11]

Validity refers to how well the scale or instrument measures the attribute it is intended to measure. Validity provides evidence to support drawing inferences about HRQOL from the scale scores. Like reliability, there are different forms of validity, which are assessed during instrument development. Content validity involves a non-quantitative assessment of the scope and completeness of a proposed scale. Criterion validity is a more quantitative approach to assessing the performance of scales and instruments. It requires the correlation of scales scores with other measurable health outcomes (predictive validity) and with results from other established tests (concurrent validity). For example, the predictive validity of a new HRQOL scale for urinary incontinence might be correlated with the number of pads used per day. Alternatively, the concurrent validity of a new erectile dysfunction instrument might be correlated with an existing validated instrument, such as the International Index of Erectile Function.[12] Generally accepted standards dictate that validity statistics should exceed 0.70. Construct validity is a measure of how meaningful the scale or survey instrument is when in practical use. Often, it is not calculated as a quantifiable statistic. Rather, it is frequently seen as a gestalt of how well a survey instrument performs in a multitude of settings and populations over a number of years.

Given the fact the instrument development is quite an onerous task and that there are an increasing number of studies on HRQOL in urologic cancers, it is always preferable to use existing validated instruments that are established in the literature when assessing HRQOL in prostate cancer. In doing so, one can compare HRQOL from the current study cohort to prior reports and draw more meaningful conclusions that may ultimately assist patients when choosing therapy for this disease.

HEALTH-RELATED QUALITY-OF-LIFE INSTRUMENTS IN PROSTATE CANCER

Several HRQOL instruments have been developed for patients with prostate cancer (Table 69.1), including the University of California Los Angeles Prostate Cancer Index (UCLA PCI), the Expanded Prostate Cancer Index Composite (EPIC), the European Organization for Research and Treatment of Cancer Core Quality of Life Questionnaire (EORTC QLQ-C30) with its 25-item prostate cancer specific module (QLQ-PR25), the

Table 69.1 Comparison of commonly utilized instruments to assess health-related quality of life in patients with prostate cancer

Instrument	Reference	Number of items	Mode of administration	Time recall	Est. completion time	Score report	Score direction	Bother assessed	Target population
UCLA-PCI (+ SF-36)	Litwin et al[12]	20 (+ 36)	Self	Past 4 wks	15–20 min	Individual domains	Higher = Better	Yes	Localized
EORTC QLQ-PR25 (+ EORTC QLQ-C30)	Borghede et al[19]	25 (+ 30)	Self	Past 1 wk	Not reported	Global summary	Lower = Better	No	Localized; metastatic
FACT-P (+ FACT-G)	Esper et al[23]	12 (+ 34)	Self	Past 1 wk	8–10 min	Global summary	Higher = Better	No	Metastatic
EPIC	Wei et al[16]	50	Self	Past 1 wk	15 min	Individual domains	Higher = Better	Yes	Localized; metastatic
PROSQOLI	Stockler et al[25]	10	Self	Past 24 hrs	Not reported	Global summary	Higher = Better	No	Hormone refractory

Functional Assessment of Cancer Therapy-Prostate Instrument (FACT-P), and the Prostate Cancer Specific Quality of Life Instrument (PROSQOLI). All of these validated instruments provide an objective assessment of both generic and disease-specific domains. While this is not a complete list of the available validated HRQOL instruments for prostate cancer, it represents the most commonly used instruments and provides the reader with a reasonable overview of the available tools.

UCLA PROSTATE CANCER INDEX

The UCLA PCI was the first validated instrument designed specifically to measure HRQOL in patients with localized prostate cancer.[13,14] General HRQOL domains are addressed in the first 36 questions, which are taken from the Medical Outcomes Study Short Form (SF-36), considered by many to be the "gold standard" questionnaire for general HRQOL.[15] The following 20 questions address six prostate-specific domains— urinary function and bother, sexual function and bother, and bowel function and bother. It has been applied to men with localized and metastatic disease and has been validated in other languages.[16] As the level of dysfunction does not necessarily correlate with the degree of bother experienced by the patient, the UCLA PCI attempts to distinguish between these two aspects of disease-specific quality of life.

EXPANDED PROSTATE CANCER INDEX COMPOSITE

Wei et al modified the UCLA-PCI to create the EPIC instrument which includes 12 generic HRQOL items as well as items that address the impact of hormone therapy and irritative voiding symptoms.[17] Whereas the UCLA-PCI urinary domain focuses primarily on incontinence, the EPIC also captures irritative voiding complaints, thereby expanding EPIC's utility in evaluating the impact of interstitial brachytherapy and external bean radiotherapy. Questions related to hot flashes and fatigue, commonly associated with hormone ablative therapy, are also included in the EPIC.

EORTC CORE QUALITY OF LIFE QUESTIONNAIRE

The QLQ-C30 is a 30-item quality-of-life survey developed to assess domains significant to cancer patients, regardless of the site of the malignancy.[18] It incorporates five general function scales (physical, role, emotional, cognitive, and social), a global health scale, three symptom scales (fatigue, nausea/vomiting, and pain), and six items dealing with dyspnea, insomnia, appetite loss, constipation, diarrhea, and financial difficulties associated with the disease. In response to the lack of prostate-specific domains, the EORTC QLQ-PR25, an additional 25-item prostate cancer module was developed to include scales for bowel, urinary, and sexual symptoms.[19] The validity and reliability of this instrument has been tested in men with both localized and metastatic prostate cancer.[20–22] Although the EORTC QLQ-C30 and QLQ-PR25 do not distinguish between function and bother as in the UCLA PCI and the EPIC, the QLQ-C30 may be a better measure of HRQOL in patients with advanced disease given its unique symptom scales.

FUNCTIONAL ASSESSMENT OF CANCER THERAPY—PROSTATE

The generic portion of this instrument (FACT-G) contains 28 items covering four domains—physical, social/family, emotional, and functional well-being.[23] Like the EORTC QLQ-C30, the FACT-G also was developed to specifically assess HRQOL in cancer patients. The accompanying prostate-specific module (FACT-P) consists of a 12-item scale pertaining to appetite, weight loss, urinary difficulties, and erectile dysfunction.[24,25] A single summary score is generated, which unlike the UCLA PCI or EPIC does not capture symptom bother nor individual scores for specific areas, such as the urinary or sexual domain.

PROSTATE CANCER SPECIFIC QUALITY-OF-LIFE INSTRUMENT

This instrument utilizes linear analog self-assessment scales to measure pain, fatigue, appetite, constipation, physical activity, mood, family/marital relationships, urinary difficulty, and overall well-being. Designed specifically for use with advanced hormone-refractory prostate cancer, the PROSQOLI is relatively easy to administer and may be most suitable if the focus is on simple physical symptoms and function, rather than more complex psychosocial issues.[26]

CONCLUSION

Several validated and reliable disease-specific HRQOL instruments are now available for use in patients with all stages of prostate cancer. These instruments provide a means to quantify the effects of prostate cancer and its treatment on physical, emotional, and social functioning. As all current and emerging therapies have an effect on patients' quality of life, it is important that clinicians and researchers alike use these tools to assess outcomes in their patient with prostate cancer. By using these instruments and being aware of the literature on HRQOL outcomes in prostate cancer, clinicians will be better equipped to counsel their patients to make more informed treatment decisions.

REFERENCES

1. Stephenson RF. Population-based prostate cancer trends in the PSA era: data from the SEER program. Monographs in Urology, vol. 91. 1998, pp 1.

2. Klein EA. Radiation therapy versus radical prostatectomy in the PSA era: a urologist's view. Semin Radiat Oncol 1998;8:87.

3. Schellhammer P, Cockett A, Boccon-Gibod L, et al. Assessment of endpoints for clinical trials for localized prostate cancer. Urology 1997;49(4A Suppl):27.

4. Helgason AR, Adolfsson J, Dickman P, et al. Waning sexual function—the most important disease-specific distress for patients with prostate cancer. Br J Cancer 1996;73:1417.

5. Patrick DL, Erickson P. Assessing health-related quality of life for clinical decision-making. In: Quality of Life Assessment: Key Issues in the 1990's. Walker SR, RM Rosser (eds): Boston: Kluwer Academic Publishers, 1993, pp 11.

6. Altwein J, Ekman P, Barry M, et al. How is quality of life in prostate cancer patients influenced by modern treatment? The Wallenberg Symposium. Urology 1997;49(4A Suppl):66.

7. Clark JA, Rieker P, Propert KJ, et al. Changes in quality of life following treatment for early prostate cancer. Urology 1999;53:161.

8. Litwin MS, Lubeck DP, Henning JM, et al. Differences in urologist and patient assessments of health related quality of life in men with prostate cancer: results from the Capsure database. J Urol 1998;159:1988.

9. Bennett CL, Chapman G, Elstein AS, et al. A comparison of perspectives on prostate cancer: analysis of utility assessments of patients and physicians. Eur Urol 1997;32 (Suppl 3):86.

10. Crawford ED, Bennett CL, Stone NN, et al. Comparison of perspectives on prostate cancer analyses of survey data. Urology 1997;50:366.

11. Tulsky DS. An introduction to test theory. Oncology 1990;4:43.

12. Rosen RC, Riley A, Wagner G, et al. The International Index of Erectile Function(IIEF): A Multidimensional Scale for Assessment of Erectile Dysfunction. Urology 1997;49:822.

13. Litwin MS, Hays RD, Fink A, et al. The UCLA Prostate Cancer Index: development, reliability, and validity of a health-related quality of life measure. Med Care 1998;36:1002.

14. Litwin MS, Hays RD, Fink A, et al. Quality-of-life outcomes in men treated for localized prostate cancer. JAMA 1995;273:129.

15. Ware JE. SF-36 Health Survey: Manual and Interpretation Guide, 2nd ed. Boston: The Health Institute, 1977.

16. Krongrad A, Perczek RE, Burke MA, et al. Reliability of Spanish translations of select urological quality of life instruments. J Urol 158: 493, 1997.

17. Wei JT, Dunn RL, Litwin MS, et al. Development and validation of the expanded prostate cancer index composite (EPIC) for comprehensive assessment of health-related quality of life in men with prostate cancer. Urology 2000;56:899.

18. Aaronson NK, Ahmedzai S, Bergman B, et al. The European Organization for Research and Treatment of Cancer QLQ-C30: a quality of life instrument for use in international clinical trials in oncology. J Natl Cancer Inst 1993;85:365.

19. Aaronson NK, van Andel G. EORTC Protocol 15011-30011: an international field study of the reliability and validity of the EORTC QLQ-C30 version 3 and a disease-specific questionnaire module (QLQ-PR25) for assessing the quality of life of patients with prostate cancer. Brussels: EORTC Data Center, 2001.

20. Borghede G, Sullivan M. Measurement of quality of life in localized prostatic cancer patients treated with radiotherapy. Development of a prostate cancer-specific module supplementing the EORTC QLQ-C30. Qual Life Res 1996;5:212.

21. Borghede G, Karlsson J, Sullivan M. Quality of life in patients with prostatic cancer: results from a Swedish population study. J Urol 1997;158:1477.

22. Albertsen PC, Aaronson NK, Muller MJ, et al. Health-related quality of life among patients with metastatic prostate cancer. Urology 1997;49:207.

23. Cella DF, Tulsky DS, Gray G, et al. The Functional Assessment of Cancer Therapy scale: development and validation of the general measure. J Clin Oncol 1993;11:570.

24. Esper P, Mo F, Chodak G, et al. Measuring quality of life in men with prostate cancer using the functional assessment of cancer therapy-prostate instrument. Urology 1997;50:920.

25. Esper P, Hampton JN, Smith DC, et al. Quality-of-life evaluation in patients receiving treatment for advanced prostate cancer. Oncol Nurs Forum 1999;26:107.

26. Stockler MR, Osoba D, Goodwin P, et al. Responsiveness to change in health-related quality of life in a randomized clinical trial: a comparison of the Prostate Cancer Specific Quality of Life Instrument (PROSQOLI) with analogous scales from the EORTC QLQ-C30 and a trial specific module. European Organization for Research and Treatment of Cancer. J Clin Epidemiol 1998;51:137.

Comparison of treatment modalities for localized prostate cancer using quality-of-life measures

70

David Miller, John T Wei

The physician's primary responsibility in caring for a patient with prostate cancer is to address the patient's concerns regarding treatment and prognosis. Currently, the most common therapeutic options for localized prostate cancer are radical prostatectomy, external radiation, and interstitial brachytherapy. Each of these interventions has undergone significant refinement in the past 10 years and can independently achieve higher than 95% cancer-specific survival at 5 years following primary treatment.[1-6] Therefore, the vast majority of patients with prostate cancer can anticipate post-therapy survival that is measured in years or even decades and, in many cases, prostate cancer can reasonably be characterized as a "chronic" disease of aging.[7] As with most chronic diseases, health-related quality of life (HRQOL) is often a primary concern for the patient and, as a result, there is now an increased emphasis on the importance of HRQOL outcomes after prostate cancer therapy. Indeed, the use of HRQOL endpoints is now commonplace in prostate cancer trials and research, and clinicians often identify HRQOL outcomes as a means for distinguishing between treatment options that are generally equivalent with regard to cancer control.[8-13] To date, studies of prostate cancer HRQOL have focused on two distinct, but complementary, priorities: 1) developing and utilizing validated instruments to more precisely and reliably characterize the prevalence and severity of adverse urinary, sexual, and bowel HRQOL effects after prostate cancer treatment; and 2) establishing patient-, rather than physician-, report data as the standard methodology for characterizing the HRQOL effects of prostate cancer and its treatment.[10,14-16]

Available instruments for measuring HRQOL among prostate cancer survivors, as well as their relative merits and pitfalls, are described in Chapter 69. The aim of this chapter is to review several "state of the art" concepts underlying the assessment of HRQOL and to summarize the contemporary literature that examines and compares patient-report HRQOL changes and outcomes following contemporary therapies for localized prostate cancer (e.g. radical prostatectomy, external beam radiation therapy, and brachytherapy), with emphasis on knowledge gained from studies that employ one or more validated HRQOL instruments.

HEALTH-RELATED QUALITY OF LIFE

The utilization of rigorous HRQOL methods to evaluate prostate cancer outcomes is a relatively recent development.[12,15,17,18] The term "quality of life" in the urologic literature has been used as a "catch phrase" to include studies of urinary symptoms and health function; however, more appropriately, HRQOL should represent the functional effects and impairment that an illness or its therapies have on a patient as perceived by that patient. This definition is particularly appropriate given that it is usually the therapies for prostate cancer that negatively impact patient quality of life, rather than the manifestations of the disease. Increasingly, HRQOL endpoints are being included in clinical trials and studies. In many cases, funding agencies for large prostate cancer clinical research efforts require assessment of HRQOL, and a growing number of measures have been developed and validated to meet these demands.[18-24] Research over the past decade has laid the foundation for HRQOL assessments in prostate cancer, and the HRQOL literature on prostate cancer has grown exponentially. Consequently, clinicians and scientists alike must become familiar with this discipline.

The common goal of HRQOL assessment is to measure changes or differences in physical, functional, psychological, and social health. A frequent application of HRQOL assessments is the evaluation of new programs or interventions.[25] While the measurement of HRQOL is relevant to most clinical research, findings should be considered in the context of a broader research paradigm that includes clinical outcomes, such as biologic and physiologic measures.[26] As described by Wilson and Cleary,[26] health assessments should be considered on a continuum of biologic and physiologic factors that arise from the diagnosis and treatment of prostate cancer. Specifically, symptoms resulting from prostate cancer, or associated treatment, may affect physiologic functions (e.g. urinary or sexual function) that then lead to impairment of normal activities. In turn, these individual and collective processes will impact a patient's overall HRQOL. Hence, simultaneous assessment of symptoms, functions, and impairment will enhance the validity of HRQOL evaluations. Furthermore, various personal, motivational, and psychosocial factors may affect elements of this continuum. For example, post-prostatectomy urinary incontinence is quite distressing to most men; however, the use of adaptive behaviors such as a small continence pad may decrease the level of impairment associated with this symptom. As the goal of healthcare in general is to improve patient outcomes, the design of clinical research studies should attempt to identify the causal links within this continuum. As such, reliable assessments of HRQOL are necessary to complement traditional clinical endpoints, such as cancer control and survival.

HRQOL AND PROSTATE CANCER

Measurement and interpretation of HRQOL among men with prostate cancer is complex and should not be undertaken lightly. One factor that must be considered when interpreting HRQOL outcomes among prostate cancer survivors is the timing of the assessment along the prostate cancer treatment continuum. Whereas prostate cancer typically has a slowly progressive natural history, most therapies will acutely alter HRQOL and health status. As a result, some effects are short-lived,[27] while others persist even among long-term survivors. In a longitudinal cohort study, Litwin et al[28] evaluated the rate of HRQOL recovery in men following RP. Using the University of California, Los Angeles prostate cancer index (UCLA PCI), they found that bowel function was the first symptom to return to baseline level (mean, 4.8 months); sexual function was the last (mean, 11.3 months); and urinary function was intermediate (mean,

7.7 months). Therefore, survey time point(s) should be based on the specific question being asked (e.g. early vs long-term recovery of function after RP).[29] As a corollary, the investigator should statistically adjust for the duration of follow-up after therapy if data are collected over a range of follow-up time points, to account for potential confounding effects.

Socioeconomic factors (e.g. patient age, race, education, income, insurance status, and marital status) must also be assessed concomitant with HRQOL. In addition to disease factors, various indicators of socioeconomic status have been found to be associated with HRQOL outcomes. Lubeck et al[30] have examined the question of racial disparity in prostate cancer HRQOL using the Cancer of the Prostate Strategic Urologic Research Endeavor (CaPSURE) dataset. They observed that black men generally had lower pretreatment HRQOL scores as measured by the SF-36 instrument and the UCLA PCI. Moreover, post-treatment recovery in a number of health domains was prolonged for black patients compared to white patients. Other social factors, including lower income and health insurance status, have also been associated with less favorable post-treatment HRQOL.[31] Eton et al[32] also explored the role of psychosocial factors on HRQOL among men who have recently completed therapy for prostate cancer. They observed that a higher level of spousal support was associated with better urinary and mental functioning in patients. In the same study, researchers evaluated demographic factors and found that African American men were more likely to report poorer urinary and sexual function following therapy, even after adjustment for age. In general, nonuniform distributions of these socioeconomic factors are likely to have an important impact on HRQOL, and adjustment for these potentially confounding factors must be undertaken in the analysis and interpretation of all HRQOL findings.

Finally, assessment of HRQOL among men with prostate cancer should be based on validated measures of generic HRQOL, cancer-specific aspects of quality of life, and prostate-specific quality of life.[33] The most common approach taken by researchers is to administer validated survey instruments (questionnaires or tools) that contain items (individual questions) that have been formulated to capture one or more of these aspects of a patient's quality of life (see Chapter 69). Whenever possible, HRQOL instruments should have demonstrable validity and reliability to ensure meaningful interpretation of the findings.[34] In survey work, *reliability* is an estimate of the consistency in the measurements. In other words, reliability is a measure of the likelihood an instrument will yield the same result on repeated trials without any significant changes in the clinical condition. *Validity* is the concept that an instrument will measure the attributes that it was designed to measure. The validity of a measure is more difficult to assess than reliability, particularly in the absence of an external criterion or "gold standard." There are several forms of validity (face validity, content validity, convergent validity, criterion validity, concurrent validity, and construct validity) and reliability (test–retest reliability, internal consistency, interobserver reliability, and intraobserver reliability). In the ideal sense, all survey instruments will have demonstrated all aspects of validity and reliability; however, this is seldom accomplished without years of instrument application and continued research. Practically speaking, a "valid" instrument is one that has demonstrated robust properties in several forms of validity and reliability, but not necessarily all.[34] Those reading the literature must be cognizant of the many HRQOL studies that are based on homegrown questionnaires that lack reliability and validity.[35] The practice of applying a subset of items from a previously validated instrument is fundamentally flawed, as the validity of the instrument will be necessarily reduced and the individual items may not perform reliably when taken out of context. Currently, all properly designed clinical protocols should strive to utilize only validated instruments and it is the results of such studies that will be emphasized in this chapter.

HRQOL IN LOCALIZED PROSTATE CANCER

IMPACT OF RADICAL PROSTATECTOMY

Data from the National Cancer Institute's Surveillance, Epidemiology and End Results (SEER) database, as well as from the American College of Surgeons National Cancer Database, consistently report surgery as the most commonly employed therapy for localized prostate cancer.[36–38] The composite results of existing studies have consistently shown that declines in both urinary incontinence and sexual HRQOL are common in the first 2 years after radical prostatectomy.[8,9,12,39] In contrast, radical prostatectomy has limited, if any, impact on urinary irritative and bowel HRQOL.[8,9]

In a cross-sectional study from our institution, the Expanded Prostate Cancer Index Composite (EPIC) instrument was employed to examine postsurgical HRQOL among 672 men treated with radical prostatectomy; outcomes for surgical patients were compared with concurrent HRQOL among an age-matched control group.[9] Based on the SF-36 instrument, general HRQOL scores did not differ between surgical patients and controls; however, EPIC urinary incontinence and sexual domain summary scores were significantly lower (poorer health state) for the radical prostatectomy group.[9]

In a longitudinal study of radical prostatectomy outcomes that employed the UCLA PCI, Litwin et al[28] prospectively observed that recovery of baseline urinary function occurred in only 56% of patients at 12 months postoperatively, with little additional recovery beyond 18 months. Sexual function had returned to baseline in only one-third of patients by 12 months post-radical prostatectomy; however, ongoing improvements in sexual HRQOL were noted beyond 24 months of follow-up as well.

In a population-based sample from the Prostate Cancer Outcomes Study (PCOS), Stanford et al[39] noted frequent leakage or no urinary control in 8.4% of men treated surgically; moreover, more than 20% of patients reported wearing one or more pads per day even up to 24 months after surgery. In this sample, post-radical prostatectomy sexual dysfunction was even more prevalent with nearly 60% of patients reporting the absence of erections adequate for intercourse at 24 months postoperatively. Based on the PCOS instrument, mean urinary incontinence and sexual function summary scores were significantly lower at 24 months post-radical prostatectomy compared with baseline levels of function.

More recently, Hu et al[40] prospectively studied 372 men from the CaPSURE database and reported that, 1 year after radical prostatectomy, only 63% and 20% of patients had returned to baseline continence and potency, respectively, based on the UCLA PCI urinary and sexual function domain summary scores. During this same interval, more than 80% of patients had returned to baseline physical and mental health. Notably, younger patient age was the most robust predictor of return to baseline urinary and sexual function.

Finally, in a recent randomized, controlled trial from Sweden, self-reported symptoms were compared among men treated with radical prostatectomy versus those managed expectantly.[41] The investigators demonstrated a significantly higher prevalence of distressful erectile dysfunction and urinary leakage among surgical patients versus those assigned to watchful waiting. However, measures of general HRQOL, including physical and psychological well-being and subjective quality of life were similar between the two groups.

Taken together, these data support the assertion that adverse sexual and urinary HRQOL outcomes are frequently observed following radical prostatectomy for localized prostate cancer.

In this context, nerve-sparing surgery has become a common practice among urologists in the hope of improving functional outcomes after prostatectomy (see Chapter 68).[42] This approach has been shown to decrease the time to recovery for both erectile function and urinary continence after RP.[39,42–44] Indeed, in the population-based PCOS sample, Stanford et al[39] reported that potency preservation was significantly more common among men receiving a bilateral nerve-sparing procedure versus a non-nerve sparing approach. The purported benefits of nerve-sparing techniques are further supported by a prospective observational study that examined the impact of nerve sparing on sexual function.[45] In this study, potency was defined as erection sufficient for intercourse, and a significant benefit was noted for the bilateral nerve-sparing technique (21% vs 0%). An effect of unilateral nerve sparing was not found at 12 months following surgery; however, the study was severely underpowered with an evaluable cohort size of only 49 subjects. In cases where nerve sparing cannot be performed for fear of compromising cancer control, sural nerve grafting has the theoretical ability to permit regeneration of the peripheral nerves necessary for erectile function.[46–48] In a study of 28 men who had undergone bilateral neurovascular bundle resection, 26% of patients had spontaneous return of erections sufficient for sexual intercourse at nearly 2 years of follow-up. Another 26% reported partial erections using a visual analog scale. Although this technique may have promise, further investigation using validated HRQOL instruments will be necessary before its widespread application.[46–48]

Recently, laparoscopic and robotic surgical techniques have emerged, with the purported potential for improving postoperative functional outcomes.[49–54] To date, implementation and utilization of these techniques has been driven by a combination of patient demand and individual surgeon interest. Notably, there remains a paucity of validated HRQOL data that demonstrate superior outcomes compared with conventional open radical prostatectomy. A preliminary study reported spontaneous erections in 45% of men who had preoperative erections, but a validated instrument was not used in this study.[55] Another group of investigators examined urinary continence at 1, 3, 6, and 12 months following laparoscopic prostatectomy.[56] As expected, urinary control improved over the course of the first year and daytime control, defined as needing no pads and reporting no leakage at all, was observed in 56.8% of patients at 12 months follow-up. These data suggest that recovery of urinary and sexual function is feasible with contemporary laparoscopic approaches; however, comparative HRQOL studies between laparoscopic and standard open radical prostatectomy techniques using validated instruments will be necessary to justify the increased expense that accompanies the use of this new technology. By and large, these data are immature and further experience with longer follow-up will be necessary for both sural nerve grafting and laparoscopic techniques in order to adequately determine the marginal benefit of these techniques over standard nerve-sparing techniques.

IMPACT OF EXTERNAL BEAM RADIATION THERAPY

External beam radiation therapy (EBRT) is the second most commonly employed modality for the treatment of localized prostate cancer. Over the years, treatment techniques for EBRT have continued to evolve towards higher therapeutic doses, while minimizing concurrent toxicity to adjacent normal tissues.[57,58] A randomized trial comparing conformal to conventional EBRT demonstrated a lower incidence of proctitis and rectal bleeding in the conformal group at 2 years of follow-up.[59] Persistence of bladder and bowel symptoms was also evident with longer follow-up in one cross-sectional study of conformal EBRT.[60] Additional radiation to the entire pelvis was also found to decrease HRQOL in this study. Moreover, the manifestation of toxicities for EBRT patients may occur in a delayed fashion, and use of neoadjuvant and adjuvant androgen deprivation therapies are common.[61] Hence, there is a need to be mindful of the treatment technique and duration of follow-up in HRQOL studies of patients undergoing EBRT.

In a randomized trial of 108 men with localized-stage prostate cancer, EBRT was found to have significantly poorer outcomes for generic HRQOL (social functioning and limitations in daily activities) compared to expectant management as measured by the QLQ-C30 and QUFW94 instruments.[62,63] The median dose received in this study was only 64.8 Gy, and subjects received either conventional or conformal techniques. With a median follow-up of more than 30 months, urinary incontinence, hematuria, stool frequency, stool soilage, and other bowel symptoms were also found to be significantly higher in men receiving EBRT compared to expectant management. More immediate effects of EBRT on urinary, sexual, and bowel function, and cancer-specific HRQOL have been well documented.[63–66] Caffo et al[67] described the primary side effects of radiation therapy to be urinary and sexual impairment. More globally, physical and psychological functions were found to remain relatively high.

In a comprehensive evaluation based on the PCOS sample and HRQOL instrument, Hamilton et al[66] reported significant declines in disease-specific domains among 497 men with clinically localized disease treated with external beam radiation monotherapy. At 24 months of follow-up, 7.4% of men reported having frequent bowel movements on a daily basis, 14% reported pain on at least some days, and 8.9% described bowel function as being a moderate to severe problem. Urinary function was affected to a much lesser degree with severe urinary incontinence being an uncommon occurrence. Significant declines in sexual function are an additional important concern following EBRT, as the neurovascular bundles are immediately adjacent to the posterolateral limits of the prostate gland. To completely treat the peripheral zone where the prostate cancer is likely to be, EBRT must, by definition, also include the neurovascular bundles in the radiated field. The potential for collateral injury to the neurovascular bundle(s) is supported by HRQOL findings of decreased frequency of sexual activity, decreased penile rigidity, and decreased ability to maintain an erection following EBRT.[66] Moreover, 40% of men complained of a moderate to severe problem with sexual function at 24 months compared to 26% at baseline. An age effect of EBRT on post-treatment sexual HRQOL was also observed, with older men reporting significantly worse function in multiple sexual health domains. This finding may have particular clinical relevance, as the average age of men undergoing EBRT tends to be significantly older than for other active therapies. Overall, significant advances in EBRT techniques have improved HRQOL outcomes. Nonetheless, significant effects on disease-specific HRQOL remain apparent after EBRT.

IMPACT OF BRACHYTHERAPY

Brachytherapy, which is often presented as a less invasive alternative to radical prostatectomy and EBRT, is now recognized as a standard treatment option for men with low-risk prostate cancer.[68,69] Recently, HRQOL studies following contemporary brachytherapy techniques have identified urinary, bowel, and sexual HRQOL concerns among men treated with interstitial seed implantation.[9,70–73] With regard to post-brachytherapy urinary HRQOL, it is now increasingly recognized that urinary irritative and/or obstructive symptoms (e.g. pain/burning on urination, urinary frequency, hematuria, incomplete bladder emptying) are an important HRQOL concern following interstitial brachytherapy.[8,9,74,75] In general, this constellation of lower urinary tract symptoms, as measured by the American Urological Association symptom index (AUASI) or international prostate symptom score (IPSS), is most pronounced in the early postimplant period and tends to improve toward baseline with longer follow-up. Indeed, several prospective studies, using the AUASI/IPSS, have suggested that most brachytherapy patients experience new-onset or progressive urinary irritative and/or obstructive symptomatology, but that improvement in this domain may be anticipated within 1–2 years from the time of implantation.[75–77] Moreover, recent data from our institution suggest that significant and bothersome declines in urinary irritative/obstructive HRQOL (as measured by the EPIC instrument) may be primarily limited to the first 2 years after brachytherapy. With time, these post-brachytherapy urinary irritative and obstructive concerns diminish and, in fact, may continue to improve for up to 8 years following treatment.[9,78]

In addition to irritative/obstructive concerns, brachytherapy may also adversely affect urinary incontinence HRQOL. In a cross-sectional study with long-term (median, 5.2 years) follow-up, Talcott et al[70] observed that 40% of brachytherapy patients reported some degree of urinary leakage when queried regarding their urinary control during the prior week. However, this study has been criticized for its liberal definition of incontinence and, in contrast, Merrick et al[72] reported no differences in long-term (median follow-up, 64 months) urinary control, based on EPIC urinary incontinence domain summary scores, when brachytherapy survivors were compared with a group of newly diagnosed (but untreated) patients with prostate cancer. Ultimately, reconciliation of these disparate outcomes will require multi-institutional, prospective studies of post-brachytherapy urinary HRQOL that not only measure baseline urinary control, but also consider the potential impact of various technical factors, including treatment planning and urethral dosimetry.[72]

Deterioration in sexual and bowel HRQOL has also been reported following interstitial brachytherapy for adenocarcinoma of the prostate. Using an adaptation of a validated patient-report survey instrument, Talcott et al[70] observed that 73% of long-term brachytherapy survivors reported erections that were not firm enough for penetration without manual assistance. In a more recent study that utilized questions from the validated international index of erectile function (IIEF), Merrick et al[79] noted that only 40% of patients treated with brachytherapy monotherapy reported satisfactory erectile function (IIEF score ≥ 11) at more than 5 years from the time of therapy. Similar findings have been noted at our institution, where men treated with brachytherapy (median follow-up, 5.4 years) reported significantly lower EPIC sexual domain summary scores compared with a sample of age-matched, prostate cancer-free controls.[78] Several studies have now demonstrated that bowel dysfunction, including diarrhea, painful bowel movements, and rectal bleeding, may also manifest as an important short-term HRQOL concern following seed implantation.[8,9] In general, however, post-brachytherapy rectal morbidity subsides with time and the long-term effects on bowel HRQOL may be less pronounced.[71]

An important caveat to the interpretation of studies evaluating post-brachytherapy HRQOL is the clinical reality that many patients classified as receiving brachytherapy may have actually been treated with a combination of brachytherapy and EBRT. This practice pattern is particularly common for patients considered "high risk" based on various pretreatment parameters, including clinical stage, prostate-specific antigen level, and biopsy Gleason sum. Among patients receiving such combination therapy, the administration of an EBRT "boost" may result in adverse HRQOL outcomes that cannot be uniquely attributed to seed implantation. Indeed, several investigators have identified supplemental EBRT as an important determinant of unfavorable HRQOL outcomes following brachytherapy.[70,71,80] In their cross-sectional study of long-term BT survivors, Talcott et al[70] observed that bowel dysfunction was both more prevalent and more severe among men treated with combination therapy (brachytherapy plus EBRT). Using the validated rectal function assessment score, Merrick et al[71] also noted an inverse association between post-brachytherapy rectal HRQOL and the use of supplemental EBRT. The use of supplemental EBRT has also been associated with increased urinary morbidity and sexual dysfunction following brachytherapy.[80] As a result, it is important to keep in mind that the validity and precision of post-brachytherapy HRQOL assessments will depend on the application of one or more methodologic techniques that adjust for the effect of concurrent EBRT.

COMPARISONS OF TREATMENT-SPECIFIC HRQOLS

As mentioned above, patients with localized prostate cancer are faced with several treatment options and frequently ask their physician to discuss the side effect profiles of radical prostatectomy, EBRT, and brachytherapy. A number of recent studies have compared HRQOL outcomes following contemporary therapy for localized prostate cancer and may serve as a useful guide for addressing such concerns (Table 70.1). It is worth noting that, in many of these observational studies, men who receive EBRT are older and have less favorable cancers (e.g. slightly higher stage and grade of disease). As a result, it is important to be mindful of these differences (and the analyses should attempt to adjust for them) when comparing EBRT to other therapies. Brachytherapy patients, in contrast, generally have a demographic and disease profile similar to radical prostatectomy patients.

Many of the initial comparisons of treatment-specific HRQOL were based on cross-sectional studies from single institutions. In the first study to employ the UCLA PCI, Litwin et al[10] evaluated HRQOL outcomes among 214 patients with localized prostate cancer, as well as among 273 age-matched control patients. In this pioneering study, patients treated with radiation therapy or observation reported significantly better urinary function when compared to men treated with radical prostatectomy. This difference was explained primarily by treatment-specific variations in the frequency and severity of urinary incontinence; notably, patients undergoing radiation therapy were equally bothered by their current urinary function. In contrast to urinary function, Litwin et al[10] observed that radical prostatectomy patients were less likely to have bowel dysfunction when compared with men receiving EBRT. More recently, Davis et al[81] also utilized the UCLA PCI and SF-36 instruments to carry out a single-institution, cross-sectional comparison of HRQOL among men treated with surgery, EBRT, and brachytherapy. This study compared 269 brachytherapy patients with a

mean follow-up of 22 months, to 222 men treated with EBRT and 142 men treated with RP. Even after adjustment for patient age, follow-up time, and co-morbidity, EBRT patients tended to have poorer general health function as measured by the SF-36. In terms of disease-specific outcomes, the investigators observed more favorable sexual and urinary HRQOL among brachytherapy and EBRT patients, relative to men treated surgically. In contrast, radical prostatectomy was associated with more favorable bowel function. Using the EPIC instrument, a similar study of men undergoing radical prostatectomy, EBRT, and brachytherapy was conducted at our institution during the same period of time.[9] Relative to radical prostatectomy and EBRT, we observed less favorable urinary HRQOL among brachytherapy patients, primarily due to a greater prevalence of bothersome irritative and obstructive symptomatology. Similarly, bowel HRQOL was lowest among the brachytherapy group. Although these findings may be attributable to differences in patient selection or implantation technique, it seems likely that the observed declines in HRQOL for brachytherapy patients simply reflect the greater sensitivity of the EPIC instrument to irritative urinary and bowel symptoms.[9]

Although critical for hypothesis generation, cross-sectional studies are subject to a number of limitations including a lack of baseline HRQOL data. As a result, investigators are generally unable to control for unmeasured differences in baseline function that may explain the observed variations in HRQOL among the distinct therapy groups. Recognizing this limitation, a number of longitudinal prostate cancer HRQOL studies have been completed or are in progress, and provide valuable insight regarding the differential HRQOL impact of contemporary therapies. In a study with short-term follow-up, Lee et al[82] administered the FACT-P and the AUASI to a cohort of men treated with brachytherapy, EBRT or radical prostatectomy. In this analysis, in which HRQOL data were collected pretreatment and again at 1, 3, and 12 months post-therapy, clinically and statistically significant decreases in HRQOL were observed for all three treatment cohorts. The changes were greatest following prostate brachytherapy and radical prostatectomy, but the observed differences disappeared by 12 months. They also noted that moderate to severe urinary complaints persisted for at least 3 months following brachytherapy. Although the mean score for the AUASI was not statistically different from baseline, it is noteworthy that significantly lower (better) scores were evident for the radical prostatectomy and EBRT groups.

In a separate study based on prospectively collected data from the Health Professionals Follow-up Study, Bacon et al[83] examined the impact of cancer therapy on HRQOL in a sample of 1201 men with localized prostate cancer. General health function as measured by the SF-36 was highest for the surgery group and lowest

Table 70.1 Studies demonstrating differences in HRQOL across therapies.*

Author/reference	Study design	n	HRQOL instrument	Follow-up	Mean HRQOL scores by therapy			Statistically significant
					RP	EBRT	BT	
Lee et al[82]	Longitudinal	90	FACT P	1 month	117.7	129.5	120.5	Yes (RP vs EBRT and BT vs EBRT)
			AUASI		17.2	13.8	20.8	NR
Davis et al[81]	Cross-sectional	528	SF-36 domains:	5 years				
			Physical function		83.3	74.3	80.8	Yes (BT vs EBRT)
			Role limitation		74.6	58.6	69.1	Yes (RP vs EBRT)
			Bodily pain		82.9	78.0	78.8	NS
			General health		70.9	63.9	66.3	NS
			Vitality		67.8	65.5	62.5	Yes (RP vs EBRT)
			PCI domains:					
			Bowel function		85.5	76.8	82.5	Yes (RP vs EBRT and BT vs EBRT)
			Bowel bother		83.0	71.8	79.3	Yes (RP vs EBRT)
			Sexual function		17.9	26.0	32.2	Yes (RP vs EBRT and RP vs BT)
			Sexual bother		25.2	40.0	40.4	Yes (RP vs EBRT and RP vs BT)
			Urinary function		68.4	86.4	86.8	Yes (RP vs EBRT and RP vs BT)
			Urinary bother		73.9	82.6	76.8	Yes (RP vs EBRT)
Bacon et al[83]	Cross-sectional	842	SF-36 domains:	5 years				
			Physical function		90	83	90	NR
			Role limitation		86	72	79	NR
			Bodily pain		85	79	81	NR
			General health		80	74	78	NR
			Vitality		71	64	66	NR
			Social function		92	87	92	NR
			Emotional function		90	82	86	NR
			Mental health		84	81	84	NR
			Physical component		52	49	51	NR
			Mental component		55	53	54	NR
		752	CARES domains:					
			Physical		0.20	0.33	0.26	NR
			Psychosocial		0.36	0.43	0.37	NR
			Medical interaction		0.17	0.22	0.22	NR
			Sexual problems		1.04	1.09	0.93	NR

Table 70.1 *continued*

Author/reference	Study design	n	HRQOL instrument	Follow-up	RP	EBRT	BT	Statistically significant
		752	Marital interaction		0.41	0.43	0.45	NR
			Cancer rehabilitation		0.26	0.31	0.27	NR
			PCI domains:					
			Bowel function		86	81	80	NR
			Bowel bother		86	78	72	NR
			Sexual function		26	34	36	NR
			Sexual bother		43	51	54	NR
			Urinary function		76	89	87	NR
			Urinary bother		82	83	75	NR
Wei et al[9]	Cross-sectional	1014	EPIC summary measures:	4 years				
			Urinary irritative		89.6	84.2	71.5	Yes (all pairwise comparisons)
			Urinary incontinence		77.5	92.8	82.1	Yes (RP vs EBRT)
			Bowel		93.2	85.2	76.0	Yes (all pairwise comparisons)
			Sexual		33.9	38.8	26.9	Yes (EBRT vs BT)
			Hormonal		90.9	87.2	83.7	No
			FACT P		36.9	36.4	32.4	Yes (RP vs BT and BT vs EBRT)
Madalinska et al[84]	Prospective		PCI domains:	1 year				
			Bowel function		92	80	–	Yes
			Bowel bother		94	78	–	Yes
			Sexual function		NR	NR	–	–
			Sexual bother		NR	NR	–	–
			Urinary function		70	79	–	Yes
			Urinary bother		81	88	–	Yes
Talcott et al[8]	Prospective	391	Validated, study-specific instrument:	2 years				
			Urinary irritative		18.8	12.1	11.1	NR
			Urinary incontinence		23.9	15.7	15.1	NR
			Bowel		4.8	8.9	7.2	NR
			Sexual		68.5	69.2	45.0	NR
Downs et al[88]	Prospective (CaPSURE)		PCI domains:	2 years				
			Bowel function		88.3	–	89.5	NR
			Bowel bother		90.6	–	87.1	NR
			Sexual function		28.0	–	33.8	NR

Table 70.1 continued

Author/reference	Study design	n	HRQOL instrument	Follow-up	Mean HRQOL scores by therapy			Statistically significant
					RP	EBRT	BT	
			PCI domains:					
		752	Sexual bother		38.8	–	44.5	NR
			Urinary function		75.5	–	88.1	NR
			Urinary bother		83.6	–	85.6	NR
Litwin et al[89]	Prospective (CaPSURE)	452	SF-36 domains:	2 years				
			Mental health		85	75	–	Yes
			Role limitation		94	81	–	Yes
			Vitality		73	61	–	Yes
			Social function		100	86	–	Yes
Potosky et al[12]	Prospective	1591	PCOS domains:#	2 years				
			Incontinence bother		11.2%	2.3%	–	Yes
			Bowel bother		3.3%	8.4%	–	No
			Sexual bother, ages 55–59		59.4%	25.3%	–	Yes
			Sexual bother, ages 60–74		53.2%	46.1%	–	No

*Higher scores on the PCI, EPIC, SF-36 and FACT P represent better HRQOL, whereas lower scores on the CARES, AUASI, and instrument used by Talcott et al[8] represent better HRQOL.

#Percent of patients reporting being bothered for each domain.

BT, brachytherapy; EBRT, external beam radiation therapy; NR, not reported; RP, radical prostatectomy.

among EBRT patients, even after adjusting for differences in demographic features. However, surgical patients tended to report worse sexual bother and urinary function, as measured by the UCLA PCI. In contrast, EBRT patients experienced greater decrements in bowel HRQOL compared to the radical prostatectomy group. Although the brachytherapy group was small, these men did report general health function that was equivalent to surgical patients, but the disease-specific outcomes were more variable. Specifically, brachytherapy patients had less favorable bowel function and greater bowel bother than men treated surgically; moreover, urinary bother was more pronounced among brachytherapy patients than among the radical prostatectomy cohort.

In a more recent report, Talcott et al[8] prospectively assessed short-term, disease-specific HRQOL outcomes among a contemporary cohort of men receiving initial primary therapy with radical prostatectomy (n = 129), EBRT (n = 182) or brachytherapy (n = 80). After adjustment for baseline differences in socio-demographics, cancer severity, and disease-specific HRQOL, greater decrements were observed in urinary incontinence HRQOL in the first 12 months after radical prostatectomy relative to EBRT and brachytherapy. In contrast, brachytherapy and EBRT patients reported less favorable urinary irritative and bowel HRQOL in the first year after therapy. Sexual HRQOL declined substantially for all three treatment groups, although the magnitude was greatest for surgery patients. Moreover, minimal benefit was noted from nerve-sparing techniques with regard to preservation of postsurgical sexual HRQOL.

Another prospective cohort study worth noting is the Rotterdam Trial of the European Randomized Study of Screening for Prostate Cancer (ERSPC). In the framework of the ERSPC, Madalinska et al[84] prospectively compared HRQOL (UCLA PCI) at baseline, as well as at 6 and 12 months post-radical prostatectomy or EBRT among a large cohort of men with either screen-detected or clinically-diagnosed prostate cancers. Treatment-specific variations in HRQOL impairment were noted, with radical prostatectomy patients reporting significantly larger declines in sexual and urinary function versus men treated with EBRT. At the same time, the incidence of post-therapy bowel dysfunction was greater among the EBRT cohort.

To date, most prospective HRQOL studies using validated instruments have evaluated patients with relatively short-term (e.g. 2 years or less) follow-up and there has been limited data that examine patient-report HRQOL changes during the later survivorship phase (4–8 years) after radical prostatectomy, EBRT, and brachytherapy. To address this, we recently prospectively reassessed a large cohort (n=1008) of patients from our institution, at a time when the survivors of prostate

cancer treatment were a median of 6.2 years after primary treatment with radical prostatectomy, EBRT or brachytherapy.[78] During the interval between 2.6 and 6.2 years of median follow-up, no significant change in general HRQOL (measured with the SF-12 instrument) was observed for any treatment group. In contrast, treatment-specific changes in disease-specific HRQOL (as measured by the EPIC instrument) were evident during this extended follow-up period. Specifically, as patients transition from early to later stages of survivorship, significant improvement was observed for the urinary irritative–obstructive domain among brachytherapy patients, whereas urinary incontinence HRQOL actually worsened among both brachytherapy and three-dimensional EBRT patients. With longer follow-up, overall sexual HRQOL deteriorated for the EBRT patients. In contrast, bowel HRQOL improved among brachytherapy patients. Among radical prostatectomy patients, urinary, bowel, and sexual HRQOL were similar at long-term (median, 6.2 years) and earlier (median, 2.6 years) follow-up. Taken together, these data suggest that, whereas post-prostatectomy HRQOL remains relatively stable beyond 2 years after treatment, disease-specific HRQOL continues to evolve among men treated with brachytherapy and three-dimensional CRT, with improvements in some domains and deterioration in others.

Although the above prospective studies have furthered understanding of treatment-specific HRQOL outcomes, they often draw subjects exclusively from tertiary care centers and, therefore, may have limited generalizability to the entire population of men treated for localized prostate cancer. Therefore, it is particularly informative to consider HRQOL data gleaned from more population-based samples.

CaPSURE is a nationwide observational cohort comprising more than 10,000 patients with prostate cancer accrued at 31 primarily community-based sites across the US.[85] As part of the CaPSURE protocol, patient-report HRQOL is collected on multiple occasions, including pretreatment or baseline assessments, using the SF-36 and UCLA PCI instruments. Thus, data from CaPSURE have played an important role in advancing understanding, on a national level, of the HRQOL impact of various localized prostate cancer therapies.

In an early study from CaPSURE, Lubeck et al[86] prospectively compared changes in general and disease-specific HRQOL in the first 2 years following radical prostatectomy (n = 351) and EBRT (n = 75). Although immediate post-therapy outcomes were less favorable among surgical patients, men treated with radical prostatectomy generally reported significant improvements in urinary, sexual, and bowel HRQOL during the first year post-treatment. Sexual health recovery continued during the second postoperative year, while slight declines in urinary and bowel HRQOL were concurrently noted. Comparatively, short-term HRQOL changes were less pronounced following EBRT, although sexual function did decline over time. In subsequent studies, Litwin et al[11,87] again compared urinary and sexual HRQOL during the first 2 years after radical prostatectomy (nerve sparing and non-nerve sparing) and EBRT.[11,87] Once again, while short-term declines in sexual and urinary HRQOL were more prominent among surgical patients, subsequent improvements in disease-specific HRQOL among radical prostatectomy patients, combined with deteriorating and/or stable sexual and urinary function following EBRT, resulted in largely convergent HRQOL outcomes by 2 years after treatment.

In a more recent publication from the CaPSURE database, Downs et al[88] prospectively compared general and disease-specific HRQOL changes during the first 24 months following brachytherapy monotherapy and radical prostatectomy. No significant changes (from baseline) were detected in general HRQOL among patients more than 12 to 18 months after radical prostatectomy or brachytherapy. In contrast, using the PCI instrument, treatment-specific changes in disease-specific HRQOL were observed during this interval. Urinary function declined significantly for both treatment cohorts, although brachytherapy patients reported less substantial declines for this domain during the first 2 years post-therapy. Notably, and perhaps reflecting the limited sensitivity of the PCI for irritative and obstructive urinary concerns, post-therapy changes in urinary bother did not differ between treatment groups. In contrast to the stable outcomes for surgical patients, brachytherapy patients also experienced concurrent declines in bowel function during the first 12 months following implantation; by 2 years, however, bowel HRQOL had essentially returned to baseline for both therapy groups. Consistent with prior studies, Downs et al[88] also observed significant (and relatively large magnitude) declines in sexual HRQOL during the follow-up interval. While sexual HRQOL did not return to baseline for either cohort, it is worth noting that the magnitude of the observed declines in sexual function and bother were generally greater for men treated with radical prostatectomy.

In addition to this variation in disease-specific outcomes, the CaPSURE investigators have also observed significant differences in post-therapy mental health among 452 men treated with radical prostatectomy, EBRT, and watchful waiting.[89] Based on the mental health domains of the SF-36 instrument, Litwin et al[89] observed that mental health outcomes varied by therapy group, with surgical patients reporting more favorable mental health, vitality, and social function at 24 months post-therapy.

Like CaPSURE, the PCOS is a rich source of data regarding the HRQOL effects of localized prostate cancer therapy, and is both unique and exemplary in that a population-based sample was used, thereby greatly enhancing the generalizability of the analyses.[12,90] One limitation of the PCOS study design, which should be kept in mind when considering the findings from this study, is that baseline HRQOL was assessed via post-treatment patient recall rather than prospective, pretherapy assessment, and is therefore subject to potential recall bias.

In an early PCOS report, Potosky et al[12] compared the effects of radical prostatectomy and conventional EBRT on urinary, sexual, and bowel function among a population of patients treated in multiple and diverse healthcare settings. With an average of 2 years of follow-up, the PCOS investigators observed that both severe urinary incontinence (9.6% vs 3.5%) and impotence (79.6% vs 61.5%) were more common among radical prostatectomy patients compared to EBRT patients. In contrast, bowel dysfunction, including pain with bowel movements and rectal urgency, was more common for EBRT patients. In a subsequent report, Penson et al[91] examined general HRQOL outcomes (SF-36 instrument) following radical prostatectomy and EBRT and noted that type of therapy (e.g. radical prostatectomy vs EBRT) was not independently associated with general quality of life at 2 years after treatment. However, regardless of treatment, men with greater sexual and urinary dysfunction were noted to have less favorable general HRQOL, suggesting an indirect effect of treatment on long-term physical and emotional function. In future, the PCOS dataset will undoubtedly provide additional insight regarding the long-term HRQOL effects of radical prostatectomy and conventional EBRT.

SUMMARY

The composite results of existing studies suggest that general health-related quality of life is favorable following treatment for localized prostate cancer and does not differ substantially by therapy choice. In contrast, sexual, urinary, and bowel dysfunction are both prevalent and bothersome among men treated with radical prostatectomy, EBRT, and brachytherapy. A number of studies suggest that declines in urinary incontinence and sexual HRQOL are more pronounced in the first 2 years after radical prostatectomy compared with radiotherapeutic techniques, although this finding is not universal and differences in function do not always correlate with levels of bother. In contrast, urinary irritative concerns and lower gastrointestinal dysfunction compromise postradiation HRQOL to a greater extent than those reported by surgical patients. Although limited long-term data are available, there is some evidence that, while post-radical prostatectomy HRQOL remains stable beyond 2 years, post-radiation (brachytherapy and EBRT) HRQOL may continue to evolve and change.

Currently, there is insufficient evidence to support one treatment as superior with regard to preservation of urinary, sexual, and bowel HRQOL. Instead, patients should be counseled about the potential HRQOL effects of each treatment option and encouraged to choose a therapeutic option based on their own preferences and utilities. In future, urologists and radiation oncologists will undoubtedly continue to refine these therapeutic techniques such that cancer control is preserved, while the degree of collateral damage to surrounding tissues is diminished. In this context, progressive improvements in HRQOL can be anticipated for patients with prostate cancer patients, regardless of choice of therapy.

CONCLUSION

HRQOL assessment for prostate cancer is a rapidly evolving field. Choice of therapy has been shown to have a significant and measurable effect on a patient's HRQOL after treatment for localized prostate cancer. In spite of recent progress in the evaluation of prostate cancer-related HRQOL, more research is still necessary. Several prospective studies that seek to compare HRQOL between therapies are underway, including a multicenter observational study (PROST-QA) that will provide a detailed examination of HRQOL and satisfaction with cancer care in men who self-selected treatment with radical prostatecomy, EBRT or brachytherapy.

In considering HRQOL as an endpoint, it is important to be cognizant of other factors that affect HRQOL, including disease and sociodemographic factors, as well as technical aspects of the treatment provided (e.g. nerve-sparing radical prostatectomy and urethral-sparing brachytherapy). Such confounding factors may have measurable effects on HRQOL and must be controlled for in the analyses of future comparative studies. Moreover, investigators should select HRQOL tools that are reliable, valid, and meet the needs of their study objectives. In some studies, generic HRQOL would suffice, whereas cancer-specific and prostate cancer-specific HRQOL assessments may be desirable in others. With the proliferation of HRQOL tools, it must be kept in mind that these tools generally only provide summary scores and do not in and of themselves quantify urinary incontinence and sexual impotence. Results from such evaluations must be considered together with the clinical condition of the patient. Assessments of HRQOL are an established component of prostate cancer clinical research and are poised to become a valuable addition to the clinical care of patients with prostate cancer.

REFERENCES

1. Roehl KA, Han M, Ramos CG, et al. Cancer progression and survival rates following anatomical radical retropubic prostatectomy in 3,478 consecutive patients: long-term results. J Urol 2004;172:910–914.

2. Blasko JC, Mate T, Sylvester JE, et al. Brachytherapy for carcinoma of the prostate: techniques, patient selection, and clinical outcomes. Semin Radiat Oncol 2002;12:81–94.

3. Blasko JC, Wallner K, Grimm PD, et al. Prostate specific antigen based disease control following ultrasound guided ^{125}iodine implantation for stage T1/T2 prostatic carcinoma. J Urol 1995;154:1096–1099.

4. Gerber GS, Thisted RA, Scardino PT, et al. Results of radical prostatectomy in men with clinically localized prostate cancer. JAMA 1996;276:615–619.

5. Pound CR, Partin AW, Eisenberger MA, et al. Natural history of progression after PSA elevation following radical prostatectomy. JAMA 1999;281:1591–1597.

6. Blasko JC, Ragde H, Luse RW, et al. Should brachytherapy be considered a therapeutic option in localized prostate cancer? Urol Clin N Am 1996;23:633–650.

7. Albertsen PC, Hanley JA, Gleason DF, et al. Competing risk analysis of men aged 55 to 74 years at diagnosis managed conservatively for clinically localized prostate cancer. JAMA 1998;280:975–980.

8. Talcott JA, Manola J, Clark JA, et al. Time course and predictors of symptoms after primary prostate cancer therapy. J Clin Oncol 2003;21:3979–3986.

9. Wei JT, Dunn RL, Sandler HM, et al. Comprehensive comparison of health-related quality of life after contemporary therapies for localized prostate cancer. J Clin Oncol 2002;20:557–566.

10. Litwin MS, Hays RD, Fink A, et al. Quality-of-life outcomes in men treated for localized prostate cancer. JAMA 1995;273:129–135.

11. Litwin MS, Pasta DJ, Yu J, et al. Urinary function and bother after radical prostatectomy or radiation for prostate cancer: a longitudinal, multivariate quality of life analysis from the Cancer of the Prostate Strategic Urologic Research Endeavor. J Urol 2000;164:1973–1977.

12. Potosky AL, Legler J, Albertsen PC, et al. Health outcomes after prostatectomy or radiotherapy for prostate cancer: results from the Prostate Cancer Outcomes Study. J Natl Cancer Inst 2000;92:1582–1592.

13. Schapira MM, Lawrence WF, Katz DA, et al. Effect of treatment on quality of life among men with clinically localized prostate cancer. Med Care 2001;39:243–253.

14. Wei JT, Dunn RL, Litwin MS, et al. Development and validation of the expanded prostate cancer index composite (EPIC) for comprehensive assessment of health-related quality of life in men with prostate cancer. Urology 2000;6:899–905.

15. Penson DF, Litwin MS, Aaronson NK. Health related quality of life in men with prostate cancer. J Urol 2003;169:1653–1661.

16. Krupski TL, Saigal CS, Litwin MS. Variation in continence and potency by definition. J Urol 2003;170: 1291–1294.

17. Ware JE Jr, Brook RH, Davies AR, et al. Choosing measures of health status for individuals in general populations. Am J Public Health 1981;71:620–625.

18. Barry MJ. Quality of life and prostate cancer treatment. J Urol 1999;162:407.

19. Moinpour CM, Lovato LC. Ensuring the quality of quality of life data: the Southwest Oncology Group experience. Stat Med 1998;17:641–651.

20. Moinpour CM, Lovato LC, Thompson IM Jr, et al. Profile of men randomized to the prostate cancer prevention trial: baseline health-related quality of life, urinary and sexual functioning, and health behaviors. J Clin Oncol 2000;18:1942–1953.

21. Ganz PA, Moinpour CM, Cella DF, et al. Quality-of-life assessment in cancer clinical trials: a status report. J Natl Cancer Inst 1992;84:994–995.

22. Sloan JA, Varricchio C. Quality of life endpoints in prostate chemoprevention trials. Urology 2001;57(4 Suppl 1):235–240.

23. Sloan JA, Loprinzi CL, Kuross SA, et al. Randomized comparison of four tools measuring overall quality of life in patients with advanced cancer. J Clin Oncol 1998;16:3662–3673.

24. Moinpour CM, Hayden KA, Thompson IM, et al. Quality of life assessment in Southwest Oncology Group trials. Oncology 1990;4:79–84, 89, discussion 104.

25. Testa MA, Simonson DC. Assessment of quality-of-life outcomes. N Engl J Med 1996;334:835–840.

26. Wilson IB, Cleary PD. Linking clinical variables with health-related quality of life. A conceptual model of patient outcomes. JAMA 1995;273:59–65.

27. Kielb S, Dunn RL, Rashid MG, et al. Assessment of early continence recovery after radical prostatectomy: patient reported symptoms and impairment. J Urol 2001;166:958–961.

28. Litwin MS, Melmed GY, Nakazon T. Life after radical prostatectomy: a longitudinal study. J Urol 2001;166:587–592.

29. Melmed GY, Kwan L, Reid K, et al. Quality of life at the end of life: trends in patients with metastatic prostate cancer. Urology 2002;59:103–109.

30. Lubeck DP, Kim H, Grossfeld G, et al. Health related quality of life differences between black and white men with prostate cancer: data from the cancer of the prostate strategic urologic research endeavor. J Urol 2001;166:2281–2285.

31. Penson DF, Stoddard ML, Pasta DJ, et al. The association between socioeconomic status, health insurance coverage, and quality of life in men with prostate cancer. J Clin Epidemiol 2001;54:350–358.

32. Eton DT, Lepore SJ, Helgeson VS. Early quality of life in patients with localized prostate carcinoma: an examination of treatment-related, demographic, and psychosocial factors. Cancer 2001;92:1451–1459.

33. Macdonagh R. Quality of life and its assessment in urology. Br J Urol 1996;78:485–496.

34. Streiner DL, Norman J. Health Measurement Scales. New York: Oxford University Press, 1995.

35. Yarbro CH, Ferrans CE. Quality of life of patients with prostate cancer treated with surgery or radiation therapy. Oncol Nurs Forum 1998;25:685–693.

36. Ellison LM, Heaney JA, Birkmeyer JD. Trends in the use of radical prostatectomy for treatment of prostate cancer. Effective Clin Practice 1999;2:228–233.

37. Mettlin CJ, Murphy GP, Cunningham MP, et al. The National Cancer Data Base report on race, age, and region variations in prostate cancer treatment. Cancer 1997;80:1261–1266.

38. Mettlin C. Changes in patterns of prostate cancer care in the United States: results of American College of Surgeons Commission on Cancer studies, 1974–1993. Prostate 1997;32:221–226.

39. Stanford JL, Feng Z, Hamilton AS, et al. Urinary and sexual function after radical prostatectomy for clinically localized prostate cancer: the Prostate Cancer Outcomes Study. JAMA 2000;283:354–360.

40. Hu JC, Elkin EP, Pasta DJ, et al. Predicting quality of life after radical prostatectomy: results from CaPSURE. J Urol 2004;171:703–707, discussion 707–708.

41. Steineck G, Helgesen F, Adolfsson J, et al. Quality of life after radical prostatectomy or watchful waiting. N Engl J Med 2002;347:790–796.

42. Steiner MS, Morton RA, Walsh PC. Impact of anatomical radical prostatectomy on urinary continence. J Urol 1991;145:512–514.

43. Wei JT, Dunn RL, Marcovich R, et al. Prospective assessment of patient reported urinary continence after radical prostatectomy. J Urol 2000;164:744–748.

44. Eastham JA, Kattan MW, Rogers E, et al. Risk factors for urinary incontinence after radical prostatectomy. J Urol 1996;156:1707–1713.

45. Talcott JA, Rieker P, Propert KJ, et al. Patient-reported impotence and incontinence after nerve-sparing radical prostatectomy. J Natl Cancer Inst 1997;89:1117–1123.

46. Kim ED, Nath R, Slawin KM, et al. Bilateral nerve grafting during radical retropubic prostatectomy: extended follow-up. Urology 2001;58:983–987.

47. Kim ED, Scardino PT, Kadmon D, et al. Interposition sural nerve grafting during radical retropubic prostatectomy. Urology 2001;57:211–216.

48. Scardino PT, Kim ED. Rationale for and results of nerve grafting during radical prostatectomy. Urology 2001;57:1016–1019.

49. Guillonneau B, Cathelineau X, Doublet JD, et al. Laparoscopic radical prostatectomy: assessment after 550 procedures. Crit Rev Oncol Hematol 2002;43:123–133.

50. Guillonneau B, el Fettouh H, Baumert H, et al. Laparoscopic radical prostatectomy: oncological evaluation after 1,000 cases a Montsouris Institute. J Urol 2003;169:1261–1266.

51. Tewari A, Peabody JO, Fischer M, et al. An operative and anatomic study to help in nerve sparing during laparoscopic and robotic radical prostatectomy. Eur Urol 2003;43:444–454.

52. Tewari A, Gamito EJ, Crawford ED, et al. Biochemical recurrence and survival prediction models for the management of clinically localized prostate cancer. Clin Prostate Cancer 2004;2:220–227.

53. Menon M, Shrivastava A, Sarle R, et al. Vattikuti Institute Prostatectomy: a single-team experience of 100 cases. J Endourol 2003;17:785–790.

54. Guillonneau B, Vallancien G. Laparoscopic radical prostatectomy: the Montsouris technique. J Urol 2000;163:1643–1649.

55. Guillonneau B, Vallancien G. Laparoscopic radical prostatectomy: the Montsouris technique. J Urol 2000;163:1643–1649.

56. Olsson LE, Salomon L, Nadu A, et al. Prospective patient-reported continence after laparoscopic radical prostatectomy. Urology 2001;58:570–572.

57. Michalski JM, Winter K, Purdy JA, et al. Trade-off to low-grade toxicity with conformal radiation therapy for prostate cancer on Radiation Therapy Oncology Group 9406. Semin Radiat Oncol 2002;12(Suppl):75–80.

58. Sandler HM, Dunn RL, McLaughlin PW, et al. Overall survival after prostate-specific-antigen-detected recurrence following conformal radiation therapy. Int J Radiat Oncol Biol Phys 2000;48:629–633.

59. Dearnaley DP, Khoo VS, Norman AR, et al. Comparison of radiation side-effects of conformal and conventional radiotherapy in prostate cancer: a randomised trial. Lancet 1999;353:267–72.

60. Hanlon AL, Watkins Bruner D, Peter R, et al. Quality of life study in prostate cancer patients treated with three-dimensional conformal radiation therapy: comparing late bowel and bladder quality of life symptoms to that of the normal population. Int J Radiat Oncol Biol Phys 2001;49:51–59.

61. Nguyen LN, Pollack A, Zagars GK. Late effects after radiotherapy for prostate cancer in a randomized dose-response study: results of a self-assessment questionnaire. Urology 1988;51:991–997.

62. Fransson P, Damber JE, Tomic R, et al. Quality of life and symptoms in a randomized trial of radiotherapy versus deferred treatment of localized prostate carcinoma. Cancer 2001;92:3111–3119.

63. Widmark A, Fransson P, Tavelin B. Self-assessment questionnaire for evaluating urinary and intestinal late side effects after pelvic radiotherapy in patients with prostate cancer compared with an age-matched control population. Cancer 1994;74:2520–2532.

64. Janda M, Gerstner N, Obermair A, et al. Quality of life changes during conformal radiation therapy for prostate carcinoma. Cancer 2000;89:1322–1328.

65. Michalski JM, Purdy JA, Winter K, et al. Preliminary report of toxicity following 3D radiation therapy for prostate cancer on 3DOG/RTOG 9406. Int J Radiat Oncol Biol Phys 2000;46:391–402.

66. Hamilton AS, Stanford JL, Gilliland FD, et al. Health outcomes after external-beam radiation therapy for clinically localized prostate cancer: results from the Prostate Cancer Outcomes Study. J Clin Oncol 2001;19:2517–2526.

67. Caffo O, Fellin G, Graffer U, et al. Assessment of quality of life after radical radiotherapy for prostate cancer. Br J Urol 1996;78:557–563.

68. Mettlin CJ, Murphy GP, McDonald CJ, et al. The National Cancer Database Report on increased use of brachytherapy for the treatment of patients with prostate carcinoma in the U.S. Cancer 1999;86:1877–1882.

69. D'Amico AV, Vogelzang NJ. Prostate brachytherapy: increasing demand for the procedure despite the lack of standardized quality assurance and long term outcome data. Cancer 1999;86:1632–1634.

70. Talcott JA, Clark JA, Stark PC, et al. Long-term treatment related complications of brachytherapy for early prostate cancer: a survey of patients previously treated. J Urol 2001;166:494–499.

71. Merrick GS, Butler WM, Wallner KE, et al. Late rectal function after prostate brachytherapy. Int J Radiat Oncol Biol Phys 2003;57:42–48.

72. Merrick GS, Butler WM, Wallner KE, et al. Long-term urinary quality of life after permanent prostate brachytherapy. Int J Radiat Oncol Biol Phys 2003;56:454–461.

73. Merrick GS, Wallner KE, Butler WM. Management of sexual dysfunction after prostate brachytherapy. Oncology (Huntington) 2003;17:52–62; discussion 62, 67–70, 73.

74. Merrick, GS, Butler, WM, Wallner KE, et al. Dysuria after permanent prostate brachytherapy. Int J Radiat Oncol Biol Phys 2003;55:979–985.

75. Lee WR, McQuellon RP, Harris-Henderson K, et al. A preliminary analysis of health-related quality of life in the first year after permanent source interstitial brachytherapy (PIB) for clinically localized prostate cancer. Int J Radiat Oncol Biol Phys 2000;46:77–81.

76. Al Booz H, Ash D, Bottomley DM, et al. Short-term morbidity and acceptability of 125iodine implantation for localized carcinoma of the prostate. BJU Int 1999;83:53–56.

77. Henderson A, Cahill D, Laing RW, et al. (125)Iodine prostate brachytherapy: outcome from the first 100 consecutive patients and selection strategies incorporating urodynamics. BJU Int 2002;90:567–572.

78. Miller DC, Sanda MG, Dunn RL, et al. Long-term outcomes among localized prostate cancer survivors: health-related quality-of-life changes 4 to 8 years following brachytherapy, external radiation and radical prostatectomy. J Clin Oncol 2005;23:2772–2780.

79. Merrick GS, Butler WM, Galbreath RW, et al. Erectile function after permanent prostate brachytherapy. Int J Radiat Oncol Biol Phys 2002;52:893–902.

80. Merrick GS, Wallner KE, Butler WM. Minimizing prostate brachytherapy-related morbidity. Urology 2003;62:786–792.

81. Davis JW, Kuban DA, Lynch DF, et al. Quality of life after treatment for localized prostate cancer: differences based on treatment modality. J Urol 200;166:947–952.

82. Lee WR, Hall MC, McQuellon RP, et al. A prospective quality-of-life study in men with clinically localized prostate carcinoma treated with radical prostatectomy, external beam radiotherapy, or interstitial brachytherapy. Int J Radiat Oncol Biol Phys 2001;51:614–623.

83. Bacon CG, Giovannucci E, Testa M, et al. The impact of cancer treatment on quality of life outcomes for patients with localized prostate cancer. J Urol 2001;166:1804–1810.

84. Madalinska JB, Essink-Bot ML, de Koning HJ, et al. Health-related quality-of-life effects of radical prostatectomy and primary radiotherapy for screen-detected or clinically diagnosed localized prostate cancer. J Clin Oncol 2001;19:1619–1628.

85. Cooperberg MR, Broering JM, Litwin MS, et al. The contemporary management of prostate cancer in the United States: lessons from the cancer of the prostate strategic urologic research endeavor (CaPSURE), a national disease registry. J Urol 2004;171:1393–1401.

86. Lubeck DP, Litwin MS, Henning JM, et al. Changes in health-related quality of life in the first year after treatment for prostate cancer: results from CaPSURE. Urology 1999;53:180–186.

87. Litwin MS, Flanders SC, Pasta DJ, et al. Sexual function and bother after radical prostatectomy or radiation for prostate cancer: multivariate quality-of-life analysis from CaPSURE. Cancer of the Prostate Strategic Urologic Research Endeavor. Urology 1999;54:503–508.

88. Downs TM, Sadetsky N, Pasta DJ, et al. Health related quality of life patterns in patients treated with interstitial prostate brachytherapy for localized prostate cancer—data from CaPSURE. J Urol 2003;170:1822–1827.

89. Litwin MS, Lubeck DP, Spitalny GM, et al. Mental health in men treated for early stage prostate carcinoma: a posttreatment, longitudinal quality of life analysis from the Cancer of the Prostate Strategic Urologic Research Endeavor. Cancer 2002;95:54–60.

90. Potosky AL, Harlan LC, Stanford JL, et al. Prostate cancer practice patterns and quality of life: the Prostate Cancer Outcomes Study. J Natl Cancer Inst 1999;91:1719–1724.

91. Penson DF, Feng Z, Kuniyuki A, et al. General quality of life 2 years following treatment for prostate cancer: what influences outcomes? Results from the prostate cancer outcomes study. J Clin Oncol 2003;21:1147–1154.

Anatomic considerations in radical prostatectomy

71

Robert P Myers, Arnauld Villers

This chapter covers what we believe to be the most important anatomic points for successful radical prostatectomy by whatever method, retropubic or perineal. Illustrations have been fastidiously created by using of specimens from fresh autopsy material, magnetic resonance images of pelvic floor anatomy before radical prostatectomy, and intraoperative photography. On the basis of anatomy, practical observations related to the conduct of surgery are also described.

PELVIC FASCIA, PARIETAL AND VISCERAL, AND ITS SURGICAL IMPORTANCE

Radical prostatectomy must be performed with a clear understanding of the fascia that helps to identify the correct planes of surgical dissection. The pelvic fascia is either *parietal* or *visceral* (fascia pelvis parietalis, fascia pelvis visceralis, TA*).[1] The parietal component (also commonly called endopelvic fascia) covers the levator ani laterally, and the visceral component covers the bladder, prostate, seminal vesicles, rectum, and pudendal vasculature, the latter coursing anteriorly and superiorly from the dorsal vascular (veins and arteries) complex of the penis. The surgical removal of prostate cancer and the adjacent fasciae in an en-bloc package lessens the risk of local recurrence due to residual tumor.

When the abdominal wall entry is made en route to the prostate in the retropubic approach, the first layer of fascia encountered is the transversalis fascia, extending distally from the posterior rectus abdominis sheath as a prominent thin sheet, which must be incised or penetrated bluntly. Once this is accomplished, there is then an amorphous fascia of loose connective tissue encountered in developing the retropubic and paravesical spaces, the latter space for pelvic lymphadenectomy. This amorphous tissue has no more substance than thin cotton candy.

For a full view of the pelvic fascia, all the retropubic adipose tissue must be teased away. The parietal and visceral components of the pelvic fascia meet in a thickened, curvilinear white line, the fascial tendinous arch of the pelvis (arcus tendineus fasciae pelvis, TA), which stretches from the pubovesical (puboprostatic) ligaments to the ischial spine. The whiteness is due to the thickened nature of the fascia along this line. When the levator ani (parietal or endopelvic) fascia is incised just lateral to the fascial tendinous arch of the pelvis, the bare levator ani muscle that overlies the obturator internus above and the ischioanal fossa below appears laterally.

As the levator muscle is displaced laterally to expose the lateral surfaces of the prostate, its fascia remains abandoned and adherent to the outer lateral surfaces of the prostate. This remnant levator fascia overlying the outer surface of the prostate (Walsh's lateral pelvic fascia)[2] extends in a posterior direction continuously over the neurovascular bundle (NVB) and the rectum, and distally over the prostatourethral junction and its surrounding vessels. In the retropubic operation, this remnant levator fascia, which is transferred to a visceral location on the lateral surface of the prostate at this point, must be incised anterior and parallel to the NVB in order to preserve it. For wide resection to include the NVBs and the prostatoseminal vesicular (Denonvilliers') fascia (see below) together with the specimen, this fascia

---

* TA = Terminologia Anatomica, New York: Thieme Stuttgart, 1998.

must be incised posterior and parallel to the nerve bundle.

Underneath the remnant levator fascia on the lateral surfaces of the prostate, the prostate visceral fascia, where multilayered, contains fat, smooth muscle, and collagen fibers. It is easier to identify grossly when nerves and vessels run among its layers. It consists of three subdivisions (according to its location): 1) anterior prostate visceral fascia, associated with the isthmus or anterior commissure of the prostate; 2) lateral prostate visceral fascia, which covers the lateral glandular prostate; and 3) posterior prostate visceral fascia, known eponymically as Denonvilliers' fascia (septum rectovesicale, *TA*).

The current terminology used above does not capture the continuous sweep of the fascia from the posterior surface of the prostate superiorly over the posterior surfaces of the seminal vesicles. In keeping with the policy of most medical schools currently not to teach eponyms, we propose herein "*prostatoseminal vesicular fascia*" (PSVF) to describe anatomically this posterior fascia, which is neither rectal nor a septum. The PSVF is separated from the rectal fascia propria by a prerectal cleavage plane, which trails distally from the variable distal endpoint of the peritoneal cul-de-sac (rectovesical pouch) (Figure 71.1). This cleavage plane is a remnant of the two peritoneal layers that fused and disappeared before birth. On the posterior surface of the prostate, the PSVF has no macroscopically discernible layers.[3,4] Distally, the PSVF thickens and is demonstrably multilayered just distal to the prostatourethral junction. The PSVF extends posterior to the prostate apex and sphincteric (membranous) urethra and, as a terminal plate,[5] has direct continuity with the midline raphe ending in the perineal body or central tendon of the perineum.

In contrast to the posterior surface of the prostate, the PSVF is frequently multilayered over the seminal vesicles (predominance of smooth muscle fibers), but is, with only very rare exception, a single layer of fascia over the immediate posterior surface of the prostate.[3,6–8] It has been suggested to distinguish a fascial leaf anterior to the seminal vesicles and a fascial leaf posterior to the seminal vesicles and prostate.[9]

Posterolaterally, the NVB is bounded by PSVF, which splits to pass above and below the bundle, and the levator fascia, which passes lateral to the bundle (Figure 71.1B). Thus, in axial or transverse histologic section, the NVB is bounded by a triangle of fascia.[10]

On the basis of these observations, we propose, from an anatomic standpoint with respect to surgical dissection of the prostate, that an *extrafascial plane of dissection* would define the prostate removed with all layers of visceral fascia present on the specimen (wide resection).

Furthermore, an *intrafascial plane of dissection* would define some portion of the visceral fascia being absent from the specimen with prostate capsular and glandular tissue at the margin. In this type of dissection, as the prostate is excised, a triangular layer of PSVF will remain on the posterior surface of the prostate, but the posterolateral surfaces of the prostate where the NVBs resided will be bare of PSVF. Because the PSVF abuts the NVBs laterally and cavernous nerves run in the lateral PSVF, NVB-preserving surgery may injure the nerves associated with the PSVF. Fascia then will be left covering the medial aspect of the NVB as the NVB is dissected away from the posterolateral prostate (Figure 71.1B, inset).

Finally, an *interfascial plane of dissection* would define PSVF covering the entire posterior prostate but not the medial aspect of the NVB (Figure 71.1B). In this case, a safety zone of complete visceral fascial covering will be present on the specimen, thereby reducing the risk of positive posterolateral surgical margins. This is important because perineural tumor extension has been shown to involve microscopic posterolateral nerves to the prostate in the area of the NVB; this is the main mechanism of extraprostatic extension and an important factor for positive margins.[5,8,11]

DORSAL VASCULAR COMPLEX (DORSAL VEIN COMPLEX, SANTORINI'S PLEXUS, PUDENDAL PLEXUS)

The corpus spongiosum and flanking corpora cavernosa of the penis (corpora) have a rich blood supply that, in part, intimately invests the prostate. Prostate removal cannot be accomplished without some disruption of this blood supply, which is less with the properly performed perineal operation and more with the open retropubic operation. More than veins are involved; the pudendal arteries are multiple and of variable caliber and approach the corpora from below or above the pelvic diaphragm. In some cases, the main arterial supply is found exclusively above the pelvic diaphragm with main, large (e.g. 4 mm in diameter), aberrant pudendal arteries coursing along the pelvic sidewall and diving, immediately posterior to the symphysis pubis, into tissue that sits anterior to the prostatourethral junction. In a cadaveric preparation, Benoit et al[12] illustrated the corpora being subserved by a single, large, aberrant pudendal artery with division into two branches just anterior to the prostatourethral junction. Sacrifice of some arterial blood supply during dorsal vascular complex (DVC) control could contribute directly to postoperative erectile dysfunction.

The pudendal veins course from the DVC in three ways: 1) anterior to the prostate in a hyperbolic path along the lateral edges of the detrusor apron (see below) to enter the vascular pedicle at the junction of

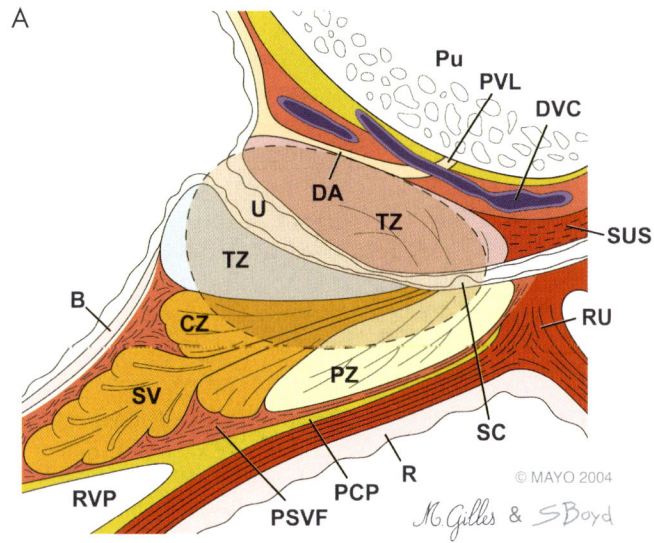

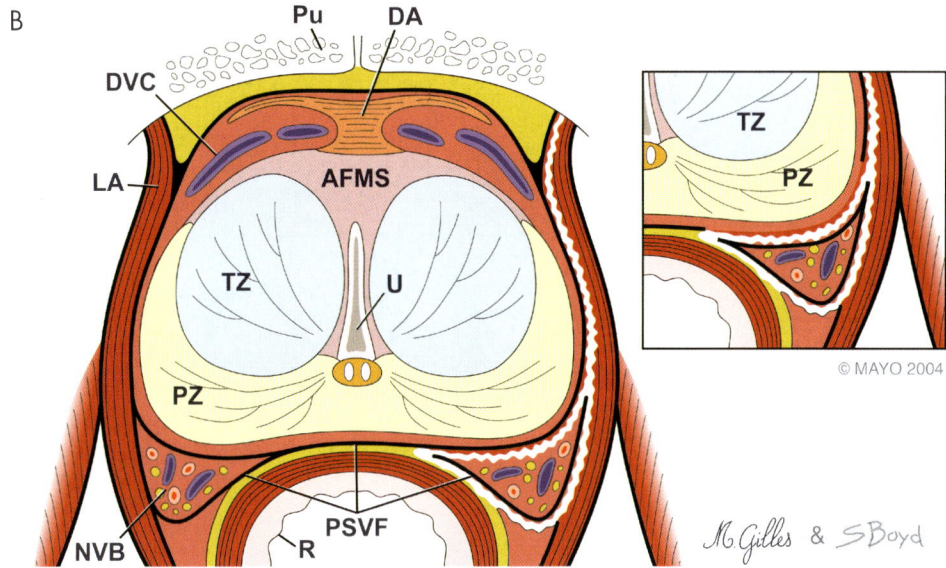

Fig. 71.1

Fascial anatomy. *A*, Sagittal and *B*, transverse section of interfascial dissection of neurovascular bundle (NVB). Extrafascial dissection (not shown) would encompass all layers of the periprostatic fascia. AFMS, anterior fibromuscular stroma of McNeal; B, urinary bladder; CZ, central zone; DA, detrusor apron; DVC, dorsal vascular complex; LA, levator ani; PCP, prerectal cleavage plane; PSVF, prostatoseminal vesicular (Denonvilliers') fascia; Pu, pubis; PVL, pubovesical (puboprostatic) ligament; PZ, peripheral zone; R, rectum; RU, rectourethralis; RVP, rectovesical pouch; SC, seminal colliculus; SUS, striated urethral sphincter; SV, seminal vesicle; TZ, transition zone benign prostatic hyperplasia; U, urethra. Courtesy of Mayo Foundation for Medical Education and Research.

the bladder and prostate laterally; 2) posterolateral to the prostate in conjunction with the NVBs; and 3) below the pelvic diaphragm, as the pudendal vein runoff within each ischioanal fossa. Anastomosis between these three main groups is common and variable with respect to quantity, size, and distribution. The unpredictable nature in individual cases can make surgical control of the DVC in the retropubic operation a formidable challenge because failure to understand the nature of the DVC in any one patient and to control bleeding could be rapidly life-threatening. In the perineal operation, the prostate, with care, is shelled away from the overlying DVC when the plane of dissection from the prostatourethral junction to the bladder neck is taken posterior to the visceral preprostatic fascia and the detrusor apron (see below). Serious bleeding in the perineal operation should be very rare if the DVC is not violated.

RELATION OF THE URINARY BLADDER TO THE PROSTATE

DETRUSOR APRON

From the bladder neck to approximately the mid-anterior commissure of the prostate, the anterior surface of the prostate is covered by outer longitudinal smooth muscle of the bladder in a layer, the detrusor apron, that extends distally to end as two pubovesical (officially "puboprostatic") ligaments on either side of the pubic symphysis (Figure 71.2).[13] Because the core of each ligament contains smooth muscle from the detrusor apron, the ligaments are essentially pubovesical in men, just as they are in women. However, because the smooth muscle stroma of the prostate merges imperceptibly with the inferior surface of the detrusor apron at the vesicoprostatic junction, the ligaments also have a puboprostatic basis. The detrusor apron is just one component of McNeal's anterior fibromuscular stroma.[14,15] In radical prostatectomy, it is useful anatomically to separate the detrusor apron component from McNeal's anterior fibromuscular stroma, as originally illustrated,[14] because it is so intimately involved in control of the DVC. Pubourethral association of the ligaments (pubourethral ligaments) is recognized;[16] this concept has much to do with the continuity of these ligaments and the periurethral levator fascia.

The detrusor apron can serve as a buttress to compress and tamponade with clamp or suture the large flanking, often multiple, anterolateral pudendal veins that emanate from the DVC (Figures 71.1B and 71.2).[17]

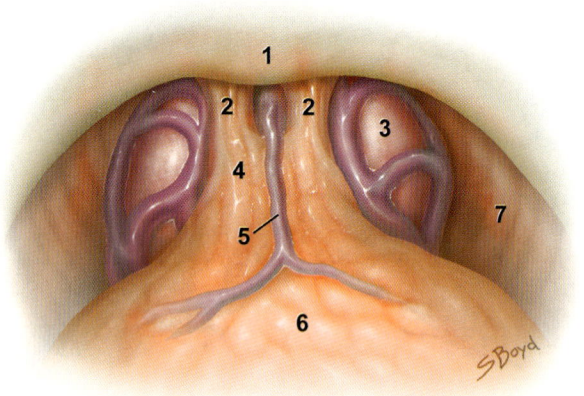

© MAYO 2004

Fig. 71.2
Retropubic view after endopelvic fascia is incised and levator fascia (lateral pelvic fascia of Walsh) is removed from lateral surfaces of prostate to allow bulging of pudendal veins emanating from dorsal vascular complex. 1, pubis; 2, pubovesical (puboprostatic) ligaments; 3, prostate; 4, detrusor apron; 5, superficial vein; 6, urinary bladder; 7, levator ani.
Courtesy of Mayo Foundation for Medical Education and Research.

These veins, bulging and situated in loose connective tissue (fascia), are decompressed when bunched together. This bunching maneuver over the anterior commissure of the prostate allows hemostasis of the anterolateral pudendal plexus and significantly increases visibility of the adjacent anterolateral surfaces of the prostate for the purpose of subsequent NVB preservation. Furthermore, the bunching facilitates control of any anastomotic veins (and there is pronounced variability) traversing the lateral surface of the prostate from NVBs to the anterolateral plexus.

BUNDLE OF HEISS

Relatively thick bundles of the outer longitudinal smooth muscle sweep distally from the lateral surfaces of the bladder and then pass anterolaterally in a loop across the vesicoprostatic junction. This loop was described by Heiss in 1916,[18] illustrated by Wesson in 1920,[19] and emphasized by Woodburne in 1968.[20] It is separate and posterior in relation to the anterior longitudinal muscle that courses off the anterior surface of the bladder to form the detrusor apron. The wall of the bladder is typically much thinner superior to the bundle of Heiss. Anatomically, the bundle of Heiss adheres closely to the prostate and is easily sacrificed in radical prostatectomy when the bladder is entered anteriorly in the process of resecting the prostate. If the bundle of Heiss is preserved, it then can be incorporated in racquet plication and, because of its relative thickness, some passive continence often may be observed if the caliber of the reconstructed bladder neck is no larger than 24 to 26 Charrière and the bladder mucosa is everted (personal observation, RPM).

PROXIMAL BLADDER NECK SPHINCTER AT THE INTERNAL URETHRAL MEATUS

The inner circular smooth muscle of the bladder neck forms a sphincteric ring of smooth muscle that may extend distally to the veru as the preprostatic sphincter in the absence of benign prostatic hyperplasia (BPH). When nodules of BPH begin within the wall of the preprostatic sphincter distal to the bladder neck as well as outside the preprostatic sphincter, the sphincteric function from the bladder neck to the veru progressively disappears. Whether there are one or two sphincters at the bladder neck has been a matter of controversy. Grossly, during radical prostatectomy, it is our observation that there is only one sphincter at the bladder neck and its function must be very much dependent on circular smooth muscle integrity. Loss of anatomic integrity and compromised neural innervation must then contribute to the observation that the bladder neck never regains normal sphincteric function postoperatively. After healing takes place, the bladder neck is always fixed and open.

PROSTATE SHAPE

Variation in prostate appearance includes 1) size; 2) presence or absence of BPH; 3) degree of prostate urethral angulation at the veru (verumontanum, seminal colliculus); 4) size of the anterior commissure (isthmus); and 5) apical configuration. We ascribe McNeal's prostate components as peripheral zone, central zone, transition zone, and anterior fibromuscular stroma.[21] We include also the anterior commissure or isthmus and the detrusor apron.

SIZE

Radical prostatectomy specimens may vary in weight from as little as 10 g to as much as 200 g (personal experience, RPM). The primary contributor to this considerable range is BPH, but there is variation in size and configuration without BPH, and a phenotypic difference can be appreciated in teenagers.[22]

PROSTATE URETHRAL ANGULATION

McNeal[23] emphasized a 35° bend at the verumontanum (veru, seminal colliculus) in the prostatic urethra. Rarely, it is 0°, and on occasion it may subtend at a 90° angle even in young men.[24] It is in the latter case that "rigid cystoscopy" is difficult, and the introduction of "flexible cystoscopy" has brought peace and comfort to awake patients.

VARIABLE ANTERIOR COMMISSURE

The anterior commissure (isthmus) is the bridge of prostate tissue anterior to the urethra that connects the left and right sides of the prostate. It varies from narrow to broad, which means the distance from the bladder to the prostatourethral junction may be very short or relatively long, especially in the presence of BPH. *The practical application of this concept is that the sphincter and neurovascular tissue may be damaged if the technique to secure the DVC is the use of a large right-angle forceps in the presence of a narrow anterior commissure.* The narrow anterior commissure is most often associated with small prostates.

APICAL CONFIGURATION

Variations in apical configuration of the prostate affect the exit of the sphincteric (membranous) urethra from the prostate. Many variations manifest (Figure 71.3). Variations in apical configuration will be completely overlooked by surgeons who blindly transect the urethra at the apex without allowing for the phenomenon of overlap of the sphincter by prostate at the prostatourethral junction. Overlap was emphasized by Turner Warwick[25] and has been confirmed in coronal section in phosphotungstic acid-hematoxylin stain.[26] Overlap varies from 1) circumferential; 2) symmetrically bilateral; 3) asymmetrically unilateral; 4) anterior only; 5) posterior only in the not uncommon posterior lip configuration;[27] and 6) absent. Whatever the apical configuration, the net result of urethral transection should be the delivery of a cylindrical urethral stump that protrudes proximally from the surrounding NVBs (Figure 71.3). If overlap is present but not appreciated and not dealt with properly, urethral transection may leave the patient with a urethral stump far too short for urinary control. In the perineal operation, in order to obtain a more proximal point for urethral transection, Hudson[28] used a scalpel handle to retract proximally the posterior apex. In the retropubic operation, a vein retractor can be used effectively to hold the parenchyma slightly cephalad and thereby to expose precisely the point where the striated sphincter ends and the smooth muscle of the urethral wall begins at the apex.[27] After transection of the anterior half of the urethra, the veru can be appreciated in relation to the point of transection. Also, if the urethra is transected just distal to the veru, the same boundary will be respected as in transurethral resection of the prostate, wherein resection distal to the veru often results in urinary incontinence. *This principle is no different in radical prostatectomy.*

Although the urethra can be separated from the adjacent prostate apex, it must be emphasized that the prostate apex is the most treacherous and common site for the occurrence of positive resection margins. Ukimura et al[29] recently recommended the use of realtime ultrasonography during laparoscopic radical prostatectomy to assess apical configuration, including the important posterior lip variant mentioned above.

URETHRAL STUMP (SPHINCTERIC URETHRA, MEMBRANOUS URETHRA) PRESERVATION

URETHRAL SUPPORT

As a column of tissue, the membranous urethra with its striated sphincter is supported by its attachment to the prostate proximally and corpus spongiosum of the penis distally. Anteriorly and distally, the transverse ligament of the perineum fixes the base of the striated sphincter. Laterally, thickened fascial band components of the

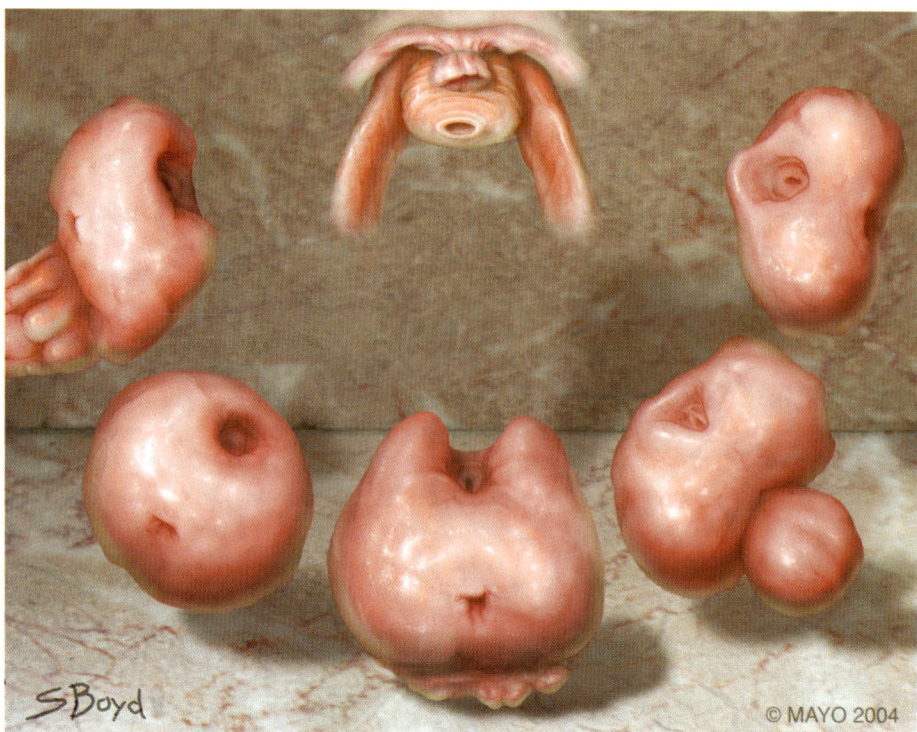

Fig. 71.3
Diversity of prostate shape, including apices. Regardless of shape, the prostate has to be removed so that the intact cylindrical urethral stump protrudes proximally with intact flanking neurovascular bundles (NVB) (*center top*) in the NVB-preserving operation.
Courtesy of Mayo Foundation for Medical Education and Research.

DVC (Walsh's pillars,[30] Müller's ischioprostatic ligaments[31]) provide insertion for the anterior layer of the striated sphincter (Figure 71.4). Posteriorly, there is a variably thick fibrous tissue raphe into which is inserted the circular component fibers of the striated sphincter (Figure 71.5). The degree of circumferentiality of the striated sphincter is variable depending on the thickness of the raphe. Even when the sphincter appears to be circumferential grossly during transection, a raphe will be identifiable histologically in axial section, should one be obtained. This then gives rise to the concept that the striated sphincter is essentially horseshoe-shaped in axial section.[27,32] However, the actual transverse or axial shape is difficult to describe because the striated sphincter changes configuration in serial axial section from the apex of the prostate to the bulb of the penis. *The lateral bands and posterior raphe, however, are constant anatomic features that contribute to support of the residual urethral stump in the male adult age group that undergoes radical prostatectomy.*

UROGENITAL HIATUS VERSUS UROGENITAL DIAPHRAGM

In coronal sections of the pelvis, the sphincteric (membranous) urethra is flanked by the anterior levator

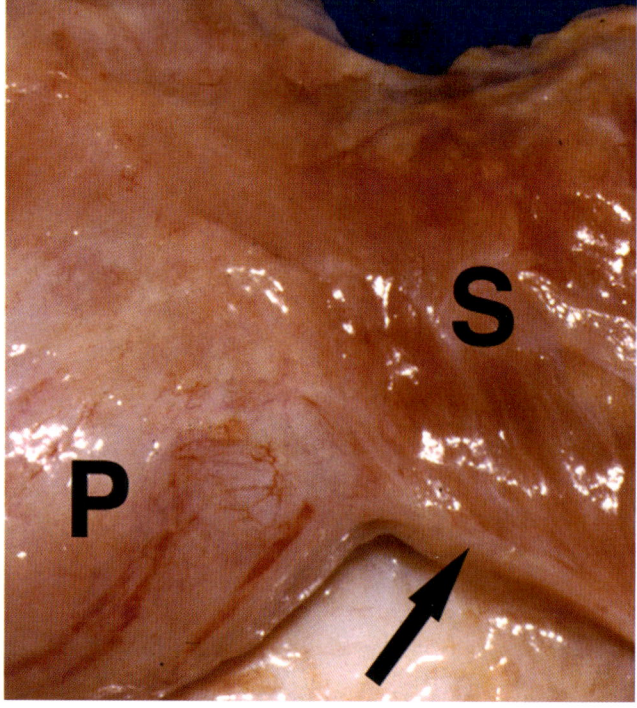

Fig. 71.4
Prostatosphincteric urethral junction (gross cadaveric dissection). P, prostate; S, striated urethral sphincter with its superficial layer inserting into lateral fascial band (Walsh's pillar, Müller's ischioprostatic ligament) (*arrow*).

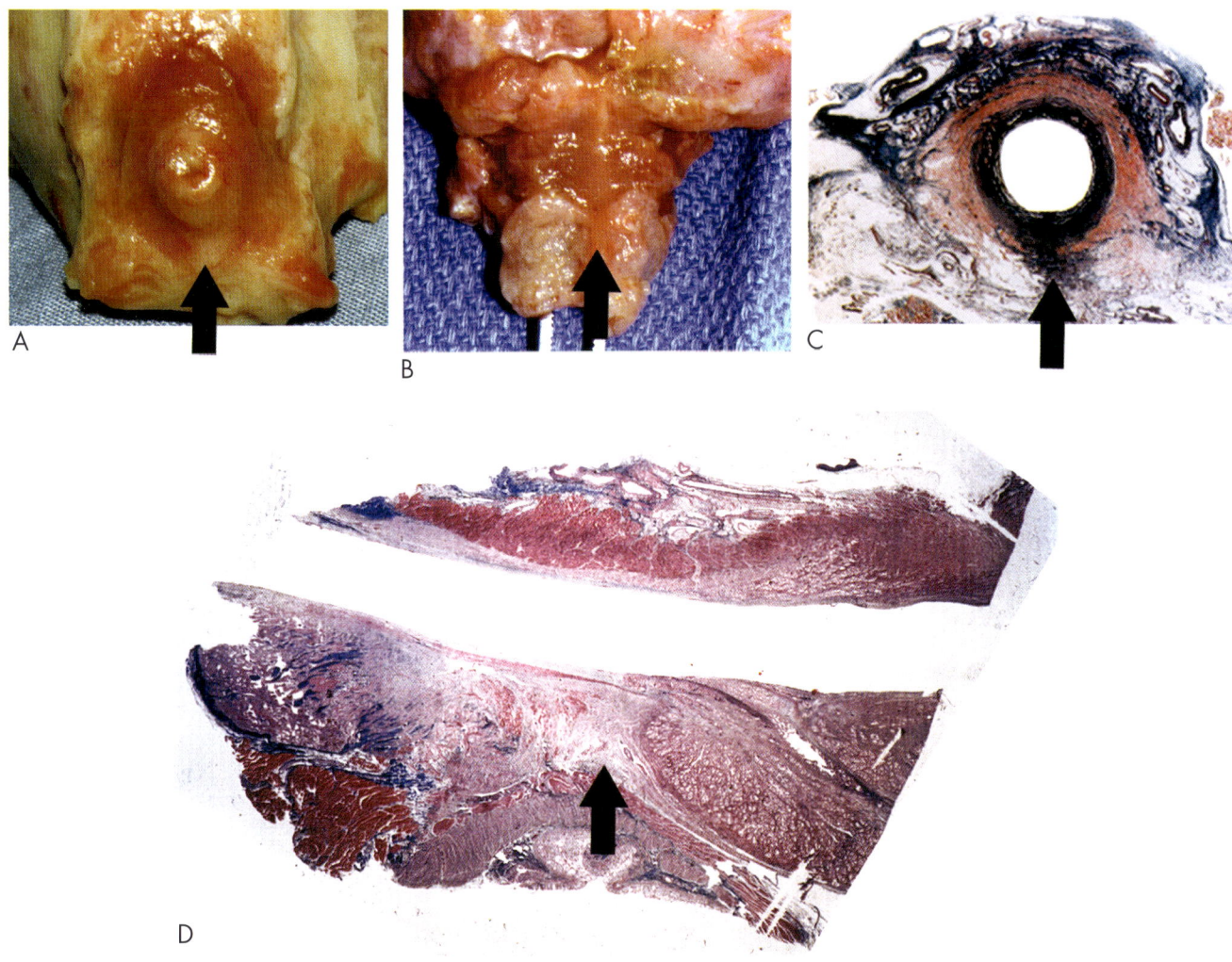

Fig. 71.5
Posterior urethral raphe (*arrows*) to confirm horseshoe configuration of striated urethral sphincter. *A*, Cadaveric specimen, gross axial section through mid-membranous urethra. *B*, Cadaveric specimen, posterior view of raphe from apex of prostate above to paired bulbourethral glands below. *C*, Histologic section through mid-membranous urethra. (Masson-trichrome.) *D*, Histologic sagittal section from penile bulb on left to prostate on right to anorectal junction at bottom (Masson-trichrome).

(urogenital) hiatus proximally (Figure 71.6). Between the levator hiatus and the corpus spongiosum, the urethra is flanked by the fibrofatty and vascular recesses of the ischioanal fossae. By magnetic resonance imaging (MRI) in coronal section, it is the combination of the perineal membrane and penile corporal body complex bridging the ischiopubic rami that forms an irregular, thick urogenital diaphragm. Importantly, the urethral stump after urethral transection will not be part of a urogenital diaphragm, as illustrated by Netter.[33] Netter illustrated, at the apex of the prostate, a mythical plate of muscle spanning the ischiopubic rami, containing the striated sphincter. He sandwiched his muscle plate between a superior and inferior fascia (of a urogenital diaphragm) from which he suspended the corpora cavernosa and corpus spongiosum. There is no evidence from gross dissection, histologic section, or MRI to support Netter's illustrated urogenital diaphragm.

URETHRAL STUMP FUNCTION FROM AN ANATOMIC STANDPOINT

When the prostate is removed, only the sphincter of the urethral stump functions to provide urinary control. As described above, the proximal or bladder neck smooth muscle urethral sphincter at the internal meatus is destroyed. As readily confirmed endoscopically in the postoperative period and reiterated here, the bladder neck always becomes fixed and open regardless of what is done to preserve, plicate, or intussuscept it.[34]

Turner Warwick[25] used "distal sphincter mechanism" to describe the functional system of the residual urethra and periurethral tissue. In this "mechanism," urinary continence depends on six anatomic elements. From urethral stump lumen outward, these six elements

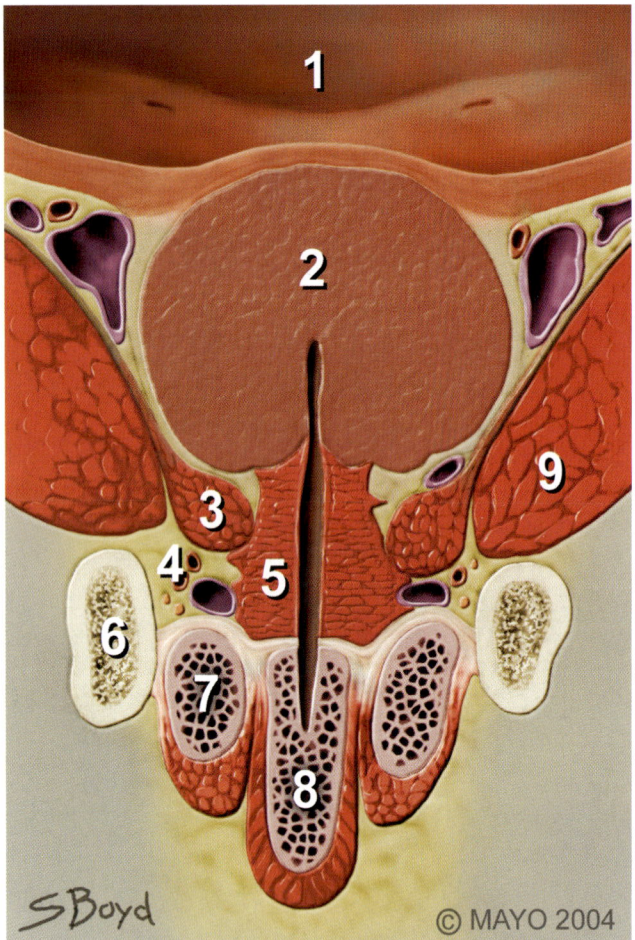

Fig. 71.6
Anatomy of radical prostatectomy, coronal section through midprostate (2) and striated urethral sphincter (5), adapted from magnetic resonance image of a 52-year-old man. 1, urinary bladder; 3, levator ani; 4, anterior recess of ischioanal fossa; 6, ischiopubic ramus; 7, corpus cavernosum; 8, corpus spongiosum; 9, obturator internus.
Courtesy of Mayo Foundation for Medical Education and Research.

consist of 1) the mucosal seal; 2) urethral wall smooth muscle and elastic tissue; 3) striated urethral sphincter; 4) puboperineal portion of the levator ani; 5) associated autonomic and somatic nerves, and 6) blood vessels.

MUCOSAL SEAL

A delicate mucosa with numerous luminal invaginations is apparent in cross-sections of the membranous urethra. The mucosa is thus subject to injury from prolonged flattening from an indwelling Foley catheter and disruption from rotations of a grooved sound. To protect the mucosal seal, surgeons should use only a small-caliber smooth sound for anastomotic suture placement and the smallest diameter catheter that can function properly.

URETHRAL WALL SMOOTH MUSCLE AND ELASTIC TISSUE (LISSOSPHINCTER, INTRINSIC SPHINCTER)

This element is the single most important component of the distal sphincter mechanism. If this element is not intact, the patient will be rendered incontinent. It extends the entire length of the urethral stump and from the verumontanum (veru, seminal colliculus) to the penile bulb or corpus spongiosum when the prostate is intact. Injury occurs if its full functioning length is shortened by surgical transection that sacrifices the length necessary for urinary control. How much residual urethral length is necessary? The normal membranous urethra is of variable length and, in one MRI study, was measured in a range of 1.5 to 2.4 cm, with 2 cm on average.[35] Study by endorectal coil MRI before surgery has shown that the longer the membranous portion of the urethra before surgery, the more rapid the return of urinary continence.[36] Although not fully established, patients probably need at least 1 cm of functioning residual membranous urethral length to be continent. Thus, a patient with a 1.5-cm membranous urethra before transection cannot tolerate sacrifice of as much length as a patient with a 2.4-cm membranous urethra. Because the prostate gland may overlap the membranous urethra up to approximately 1 cm, urethral transection made without knowledge of the placement of the veru may result in serious risk of subsequent urinary leakage.

Another variable factor is the placement of the veru with respect to the posterior apical extent of the prostate. The veru may sit exactly at the posterior apex or as much as 1 cm proximal to the apex with prostate posterior to the membranous urethra. If the veru is situated right at the apex, it will have no urethral crest distal to it. In this case, transection of the posterior apex will not sacrifice the membranous urethral stump length. If the veru is proximal to the posterior apex margin and urethral transection is made at the apex, variable urethral stump length will be lost. Technique to optimize residual urethral stump length then might involve preoperative retrograde urethrography to measure the distance from veru to corpus spongiosum to determine whether it is unduly short. Additionally, midline sagittal T_2-weighted MRI can be used to assess urethral stump length and the presence or absence of posterior lip of prostate beneath the membranous urethra. Such studies allow preoperative assessment of prostate apical and urethral stump variability and potentially can help in planning the operation. If patients have positive results of apical biopsy, this assessment could prove to be particularly worthwhile and preoperatively allow the patient to be informed of a pending challenging dissection.

STRIATED URETHRAL SPHINCTER (RHABDOSPHINCTER, SPHINCTER URETHRAE, TA)

Composed of unique striated fibers (smaller with primarily slow-twitch capacity), the striated urethral sphincter most probably functions to assist passive continence during bladder filling or in the absence of micturition. The striated urethral sphincter covers the critical smooth muscle urethral wall and functions in the male from the apex of the prostate to the bulb. In Caine and Edwards' classic study,[37] when the pelvic floor musculature was paralyzed, subjects maintained urinary continence. Krahn and Morales[38] found the same phenomenon after transurethral resection of the prostate when proximal bladder neck sphincter function had been destroyed.

The striated urethral sphincter is much bulkier in young men undergoing the retropubic operation; older patients often have visible age-related sphincter atrophy. Older patients often also have BPH with detrusor hypertrophy, as evidenced by trabeculation, cellule, and diverticula formation, and this produces detrusor instability. If the prostate is removed, the combination of sphincter atrophy plus detrusor instability makes the older patient more vulnerable to pad usage despite meticulous preservation of all the continence components of the urethral stump. Preoperative older patients should be counseled accordingly.

PUBOPERINEAL PORTION OF THE LEVATOR ANI (PUBOURETHRALIS, LEVATOR URETHRAE, "QUICK STOP MUSCLE" OF GOSLING)

As mentioned above, the striated sphincter is flanked by the thickened anteromedial edges of the anterior levator ani, or what Oelrich called the urogenital hiatus (Figure 71.6).[39] This anterior levator hiatus begins posterior to the urethra at the level of and anteriorly adjacent to the anorectal junction and perineal body. As the puboperineal portion of the levatores ani,[40] the medial fibers of the puborectalis sling do not follow its outer fibers around the anorectal junction; they descend diagonally downward on either side of the sphincteric (membranous) urethra to insert in the midline perineal body anterior to the anorectal junction. Thus, they form an incomplete sling behind the urethra. On contraction, they forcefully propel the prostate, prostatourethral junction, and striated sphincter upward and forward toward the posterior pubis. Santorini[41] called these thickenings "projectors," and their action has been confirmed in dynamic MRI.[42] This action then allows the quick stop of urination.[43] The upward, forward

movement is countered by the horseshoe-shaped striated sphincter, which contracts downward and backward toward the perineal body. This counter-contraction of the striated sphincter has been corroborated by transluminal urethral ultrasonography during pelvic floor contraction.[44] Thus, there is an opposing active loop system: outer levator ani loop upward and forward, and striated sphincter loop backward and downward. The bladder neck is thought to function similarly, but the opposing loops, outer longitudinal detrusor (bundle of Heiss) and inner circular detrusor, are both smooth muscle loops, whereas the distal sphincter mechanism is essentially opposing striated muscle loops.

INTACT BLOOD VESSELS AND NERVES

Urethral length and integrity of the urinary continence tissue components of mucosa, urethral wall, smooth muscle, elastic tissue, and striated sphincter are moot if the blood vessels and nerves are significantly injured during dissection. How can this occur? Somatic branches of the pudendal nerve innervate the levator ani muscle superiorly and inferiorly. Practically speaking, this means that there are significant branches on the inner surface of the levator ani during lateral mobilization of the levator ani in the retropubic operation and on the undersurface of the levator ani in the perineal operation. Branches from above and below the pelvic diaphragm also supply the striated sphincter. Autonomic innervation is also thought to be dual. Whether above or below the pelvic diaphragm, somatic and autonomic fibers predominate at the 5- and 7-o'clock positions in relationship to the striated sphincter. Some fibers travel in the NVBs. Not all autonomic fibers are destined for the cavernous bodies of the penis. In 1982, Walsh and Donker[45] elucidated the nature of the cavernous nerve supply to the penis with respect to the prostate and clarified why men subject to radical prostatectomy were virtually always rendered impotent. Walsh et al[2] then showed how the cavernous nerves in the NVB could be saved and the patient rendered potent on a consistent basis. Walsh's monumental work paved the way for significant evolution in surgical technique. Of interest, in 1975, Finkle et al[46] reported potency preservation in four of five patients undergoing the perineal operation, but did not explain why. Cavernous nerves are multiple in each bundle and originally were characterized as major and minor.[31] In a study of one NVB, the nerves varied in diameter from approximately 0.04 to 0.37 mm, averaging 0.12 mm.[47]

Takenaka et al[48] recently performed cadaveric dissections and showed the "spray-like" entry of pelvic splanchnic nerve components as they join hypogastric nerve components to the nerve bundle distal to the vesicoprostatic junction. Their findings may be of significance with respect to sural nerve graft interposition in replacing a resected NVB.

In radical prostatectomy, it is possible to find a plane between the NVB and periprostatic "visceral" fascia overlying the capsule (interfascial dissection). Of anatomic importance, the nerves may travel very close to the medial surface of the NVB; when they also travel in close proximity to small arteries and veins that bleed, hemostasis by metal clip or suture may damage these tiny nerve fibers. The nerve bundles in cross-section subtend a crescentic shape as they hug the posterolateral aspect of the prostate. Autonomic nerves, some of which are destined for the cavernous bodies, are distributed throughout the NVB, and those situated at the tips of the crescent are particularly vulnerable to injury. The anterior tip of the crescent often contains veins and associated small arteries, as mentioned above, and the posterior tip of the crescent runs along the lateral aspect of the line of division of the PSVF. More recent studies[10,49] corroborate significant numbers of autonomic nerves in the lateral aspects of the PSVF. These PSVF-associated nerve fibers then are vulnerable to injury and sacrifice as a result of freeing the NVB from the adjacent prostate.

The NVB is delicate and tolerates little shear without breaking. It is tethered along the posterolateral prostate by fine capsular vessels that may angulate the NVB at the prostatourethral junction.[50] From an anatomic and surgical standpoint, release of these vessels from the adjacent prostate fascia then allows release of the NVB. The result of release at the apex of the prostate is the creation of an anatomic triangle formed by the NVB laterally and the prostate and urethra medially as the two additional legs of the triangle immediately adjacent to the prostatourethral junction. This relationship does not become apparent until the fibrous bands (ischioprostatic ligaments, Walsh's pillar tissue) are severed at their prostate junction, as mentioned above.

In the region of the vascular pedicle to the prostate at the vesicoprostatic junction laterally, the NVB is relatively thick.[50] The reason for this is that the pedicle contains, in addition to the inferior vessels to the bladder, numerous ganglia and branch points for autonomic nerves supplying the seminal vesicles, vasa deferentia, and bladder.[31,48,49,51] From the pedicle running distally toward the apex of the prostate, there is notable narrowing of the bundle.

LEVATORES ANI AND ANAL SPHINCTERS

Radical prostatectomy by any route is impossible without mobilization of the levator ani, whose muscle fibers embrace the lateral surfaces of the prostate,

urethra, and anorectal junction. Fecal soiling after radical prostatectomy is a serious health-related quality-of-life issue. Determination of its frequency requires a validated prospective questionnaire like the UCLA prostate cancer index, which measures both bowel function (dysfunction) and bother (distress).[52] If a surgeon denies that it happens in his practice, he simply may not have asked his patients about an embarrassing subject. Reduced anal manometry pressures and fecal soiling have been reported after both perineal and retropubic operations.[53] The cause is very likely damage to the levator ani and its nerve supply.

RETROPUBIC OPERATION

The levatores ani, which form a conical pelvic diaphragm,[54] are first encountered after the endopelvic fascia is incised 3 to 5 mm lateral to the fascial tendinous arch (arcus tendineus fasciae pelvis, TA). This muscle bulges medially on each side because it overlies the inner convex surface of the underlying obturator internus superiorly and adipose tissue to the underlying ischioanal fossae inferiorly (Figure 71.6). (The obturator internus is covered and usually not seen in this maneuver unless there is the rare convergence of the fascial and muscular tendinous arches of the pelvis.[55]) Fibers of the levator ani that comprise its puborectalis (puboanalis) portion pass posteriorly toward the anorectal junction where the anal canal, situated below the pelvic diaphragm, meets the rectum above the pelvic diaphragm (Figure 71.7).

During dissection of the prostate, the first fibers of the levator ani laterally to be disturbed are those of the pubococcygeus, which tightly embrace the lateral surface of the prostate in a very thin sheet. In the retropubic operation, these fibers are displaced laterally with an instrument or index finger in order to see the lateral surfaces of the prostate; it is this maneuver that may disrupt muscle fiber integrity as well as pelvic nerve innervation along the superior surface of the pelvic diaphragm.[56]

As the prostatourethral junction is exposed, the thickened anteromedial edges of the anterior levator hiatus are evident immediately adjacent to the insertion of the pubovesical (puboprostatic) ligaments. The pubic insertion points of the levator ani are tiny but serve as the take-off for the sling (puborectalis, puboanalis[35]) around the anorectal junction that is so important to fecal control. The deep external anal sphincter fuses to the puborectalis posteriorly, and together they are primarily responsible for fecal continence (Figure 71.7). The tiny tendinous insertion points of the puborectalis sling are situated only 1.3 cm lateral to the midline.[57] *Because these points of insertion are immediately adjacent to the insertion points of the pubovesical (puboprostatic) ligaments, they are subject to inadvertent transection if the*

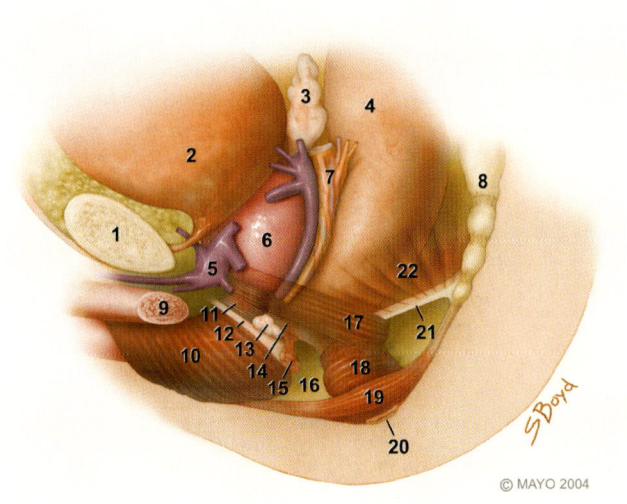

Fig. 71.7

Anatomy of radical prostatectomy, three-dimensional side view of male pelvis, developed from sagittal magnetic resonance image. 1, pubis; 2, urinary bladder with pubovesical (puboprostatic) ligament; 3, seminal vesicle; 4, rectum; 5, dorsal vein complex with venous sinus; 6, prostate; 7, neurovascular bundle; 8, coccyx; 9, corpus cavernosum; 10, bulbospongiosus; 11, striated urethral sphincter; 12, perineal membrane; 13, bulbourethral gland; 14, "rectourethralis;" 15, transverse superficial perinei; 16, retrobulbar "space;" 17, puboanalis (puborectalis); 18, deep external anal sphincter; 19, superficial external anal sphincter; 20, anus; 21, anococcygeal ligament; 22, pubococcygeus, iliococcygeus, and coccygeus components of pelvic diaphragm (from anterior to posterior).
Courtesy of Mayo Foundation for Medical Education and Research.

pubovesical ligaments are transected at their pubic attachment. If this happens, the patient might experience compromised fecal control.

PERINEAL OPERATION

Once the perineal skin incision is made, the first sphincter to be encountered is the superficial external anal sphincter (superficial sphincter). It has prominent bow-shaped extensions (bows) on either side of the anus. Anteriorly, the bows converge in the midline tendinous insertion into the midline raphe of the bulb along its inferior surface. *The insertion point of this muscle is not into the perineal body, as commonly illustrated.* It is the anterior insertion point into the bottom of the bulb of the penis that allows the creation of a retrobulbar space with an index finger (Figure 71.8). With the finger so placed, the sphincter can be taken down at its bulbar insertion point, or divided transversely anterior to the anus in what is known as the Young technique of dividing the "central tendon."[58] It is not commonly appreciated that the anterior bowlike extensions of the superficial sphincter may be transected along with the

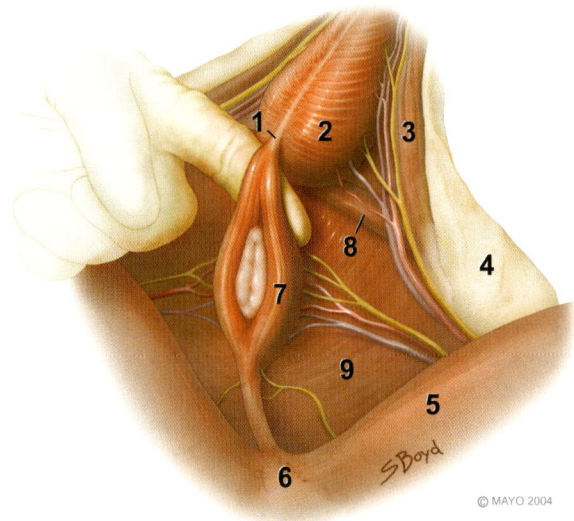

Fig. 71.8

Anatomy of radical perineal prostatectomy, initial index finger development of retrobulbar space beneath anterior extension of the superficial external anal sphincter (7). 1, central tendon; 2, bulbospongiosus; 3, ischiocavernosus; 4, ischial tuberosity; 5, gluteus maximus; 6, coccyx; 8, superficial transverse perinei; 9, levator ani.
Courtesy of Mayo Foundation for Medical Education and Research.

midline fibrous tissue. Alternatively, the superficial sphincter is so situated that entry into the retrobulbar space can be achieved by retraction of the bows anterolaterally in what is known as the Belt technique.[59] The superficial sphincter has perianal subcutaneous attachment as the bows pass the anus, and this is sometimes illustrated as a separate cutaneous sphincter. However, in gross dissection, the cutaneous fibers are not separate but an integral part of the superficial sphincter. Posteriorly, the bows converge into tendinous attachment to the tip of the coccyx. Importantly, the superficial sphincter is not essential to anal continence. Some of its anterior fibers have been diagrammed converging with the bulbospongiosus and the superficial transverse perinei muscles.[60]

Just superior to the superficial sphincter is the deep external anal sphincter (Figure 71.7), which is closely bound to the anterior wall of the anal canal. In the perineal operation, it should be passed over without disturbance in progressing from the retrobulbar space to the rectourethralis attachment at the anorectal junction. As noted above, the deep sphincter fuses posteriorly with the puborectalis and is absolutely essential for anal continence. In the perineal operation, the recto-urethralis attachment to the perineal body, which centers on the midline posterior aspect of the perineal membrane at the superior backside of the bulb, is transected. Transecting the rectourethralis allows the anorectal junction to lose its sharp anterior angulation and to drop away posteriorly. The anal canal (3–4-cm long in the adult male) has a thick wall due to the presence of the smooth muscle internal anal sphincter. The wall of the rectum superior to the rectourethralis is much thinner. It is at this junction of thick anal canal wall to thin rectal wall that provides the opportunity for inadvertent rectotomy.

After takedown of the rectourethralis, the posterior prostatourethral junction is first exposed. The levator ani muscle that must be retracted laterally to expose the prostate is first the puborectalis sling and more deeply the pubococcygeus. The puborectalis is a misnomer in the sense that its sling passes behind the anococcygeal ligament; it is literally more puboanalis than puborectalis. Some of its inferior fibers insert directly into the wall of the anal canal intercalating with fibers of the smooth muscle internal sphincter, the conjoined longitudinal fibers.[61]

RECTOURETHRALIS

The rectourethralis is a fibromuscular complex that produces anterior angulation of the anorectal junction, as noted above. It consists primarily of a dominant (more substantial) midline component of smooth muscle from the anterior wall of the anal canal coming from below (anoperinealis, *TA*) and a less dominant midline component of smooth muscle from the anterior wall of the rectum coming from above (rectoperinealis, *TA*). These two components then converge from below and above, respectively, and insert into the perineal body (central tendon of the perineum). There is no direct urethral attachment. Importantly, the attachment anteriorly is distal to the posterior apex of the prostate, and therefore *the rectourethralis is not part of the retropubic operation as it is in the perineal operation*. Descriptions of the retropubic operation often mistakenly describe transection of the rectourethralis after urethral transection, when what is being described is actually transection of the termination of the PSVF as it joins the midline fibrous tissue raphe of the perineal body. The rectourethralis attachment varies considerably in bulk from thick to thin.

REFERENCES

1. Federative Committee on Anatomical Terminology. Terminologia Anatomica: International Anatomical Terminology/FCAT. Stuttgart: Thieme, 1998.
2. Walsh PC, Lepor H, Eggleston JC. Radical prostatectomy with preservation of sexual function: anatomical and pathological considerations. Prostate 1983;4:473–485.
3. Silver PH. The role of the peritoneum in the formation of the septum recto-vesicale. J Anat 1956;90:538–546.
4. Lindsey I, Guy RJ, Warren BF, et al. Anatomy of Denonvilliers' fascia and pelvic nerves, impotence, and implications for the colorectal surgeon. Br J Surg 2000;87:1288–1299.
5. Villers A, Stamey TA, Yemoto C, et al. Modified extrafascial radical retropubic prostatectomy technique decreases frequency of positive surgical margins in T2 cancers <2 cm³. Eur Urol 2000;38:64–73.
6. Benoit G, Delmas V, Quillard J, et al. Surgical significance of Denonvilliers' aponeurosis [French]. Ann Urol (Paris) 1984;18:284–287.
7. van Ophoven A, Roth S. The anatomy and embryological origins of the fascia of Denonvilliers: a medico-historical debate. J Urol 1997;157:3–9.
8. Villers A, McNeal JE, Freiha FS, et al. Invasion of Denonvilliers' fascia in radical prostatectomy specimens. J Urol 1993;149:793–798.
9. Vordos D, Delmas V, Hermieu JF, et al. Can a precise vesiculectomy be performed during radical prostatectomy? [French]. Prog Urol 2001;11:1259–1263.
10. Kourambas J, Angus DG, Hosking P, et al. A histological study of Denonvilliers' fascia and its relationship to the neurovascular bundle. Br J Urol 1998;82:408–410.
11. Stamey TA, Villers AA, McNeal JE, et al. Positive surgical margins at radical prostatectomy: importance of the apical dissection. J Urol 1990;143:1166–1172.
12. Benoit G, Droupy S, Quillard J, et al. Supra and infralevator neurovascular pathways to the penile corpora cavernosa. J Anat 1999;195:605–615.
13. Myers RP. Detrusor apron, associated vascular plexus, and avascular plane: relevance to radical retropubic prostatectomy: anatomic and surgical commentary. Urology 2002;59:472–479.
14. McNeal JE. The prostate and prostatic urethra: a morphologic synthesis. J Urol 1972;107:1008–1016.
15. McNeal JE. New morphologic findings relevant to the origin and evolution of carcinoma of the prostate and BPH. UICC Technical Rep Series 1979;48:24–37.
16. Steiner MS. The puboprostatic ligament and the male urethral suspensory mechanism: an anatomic study. Urology 1994;44:530–534.
17. Myers RP. The surgical management of prostate cancer: radical retropubic and radical perineal prostatectomy. In Lepor H (ed): Prostatic Diseases. Philadelphia: WB Saunders, 2000, pp 410–443.
18. Heiss R. Über den Sphincter vesicae internus. Archiv Anat Physiol 1916;24:367–384.
19. Wesson MB. Anatomical, embryological and physiological studies of the trigone and neck of the bladder. J Urol 1920;4:279–315.
20. Woodburne RT. Anatomy of the bladder and bladder outlet. J Urol 1968;100:474–487.
21. McNeal JE. Normal histology of the prostate. Am J Surg Pathol 1988;12:619–633.
22. Myers RP. An anatomic approach to the pelvis in the male. In Crawford ED, Das S (eds): Current Genitourinary Cancer Surgery, 2nd ed. Baltimore: Williams & Wilkins, 1997, pp 155–169.
23. McNeal JE. The zonal anatomy of the prostate. Prostate 1981;2:35–49.
24. Glenister TW. The development of the utricle and of the so-called 'middle' or 'median' lobe of the human prostate. J Anat 1962;96:443–455.
25. Turner Warwick R. The sphincter mechanisms: their relation to prostatic enlargement and its treatment. In Hinman F Jr (ed): Benign Prostatic Hypertrophy. New York: Springer-Verlag, 1983, pp 809–828.
26. Blacklock NJ. Surgical anatomy of the prostate. In Williams DI, Chisholm GD (eds): Scientific Foundations of Urology, vol 2. London: William Heinemann Medical Books, 1976, pp 113–125.
27. Myers RP. Male urethral sphincteric anatomy and radical prostatectomy. Urol Clin North Am 1991;18:211–227.
28. Hudson PB. Perineal prostatectomy. In Campbell MF, Harrison JH (eds): Urology, vol 3, 3rd edn. Philadelphia: WB Saunders, 1970, p 2436.
29. Ukimura O, Gill IS, Desai MM, et al. Real-time transrectal ultrasonography during laparoscopic radical prostatectomy. J Urol 2004;172:112–118.
30. Walsh PC. Radical prostatectomy, preservation of sexual function, cancer control: the controversy. Urol Clin North Am 1987;14:663–673.
31. Müller J. Ueber die organischen Nerven der erektilen männlichen Geschlechtsorgane des Menschen und der Säugethiere. Berlin: F Dümmler, 1836.

32. Yucel S, Baskin LS. An anatomical description of the male and female urethral sphincter complex. J Urol 2004;171:1890–1897.

33. Netter FH. Atlas of Human Anatomy, Pelvis and Perineum. Summit, NJ: Ciba-Geigy, 1989, Plate 361.

34. Walsh PC, Marschke PL. Intussusception of the reconstructed bladder neck leads to earlier continence after radical prostatectomy. Urology 2002;59:934–938.

35. Myers RP, Cahill DR, Devine RM, et al. Anatomy of radical prostatectomy as defined by magnetic resonance imaging, J Urol 1998;159:2148–2158.

36. Coakley FV, Eberhardt S, Kattan MW, et al. Urinary continence after radical retropubic prostatectomy: relationship with membranous urethral length on preoperative endorectal magnetic resonance imaging. J Urol 2002;168:1032–1035.

37. Caine M, Edwards D. The peripheral control of micturition: a cine-radiographic study. Br J Urol 1958;30:34–42.

38. Krahn MD, Mahoney JE, Eckman MH, et al. Screening for prostate cancer: a decision analytic view. JAMA 1994;272:773–780.

39. Oelrich TM. The urethral sphincter muscle in the male. Am J Anat 1980;158:229–246.

40. Myers RP, Cahill DR, Kay PA, et al. Puboperineales: muscular boundaries of the male urogenital hiatus in 3D from magnetic resonance imaging. J Urol 2000;164:1412–1415.

41. Santorini GD. Observationes Anatomicae. Venetiis: JB Recurti, 1724, pp173–205.

42. Mikuma N, Tamagawa M, Morita K, et al. Magnetic resonance imaging of the male pelvic floor: the anatomical configuration and dynamic movement in healthy men. Neurourol Urodyn 1998;17:591–597.

43. Gosling JA, Dixon JS, Critchley HO, et al. A comparative study of the human external sphincter and periurethral levator ani muscles. Br J Urol 1981;53:35–41.

44. Strasser H, Poisel S, Stenzl A, et al. Anatomy and innervation of the male urethra, the rhabdosphincter, and the corpora cavernosa (Lesson 16). AUA Update Series 2001;20:122–127.

45. Walsh PC, Donker PJ. Impotence following radical prostatectomy: insight into etiology and prevention. J Urol 1982;128:492–497.

46. Finkle JE, Finkle PS, Finkle AL. Encouraging preservation of sexual function postprostatectomy. Urology 1975;6:697–702.

47. Myers RP. Gross and applied anatomy of the prostate. In Kantoff PW, Carroll PR, D'Amico AV (eds): Prostate Cancer: Principles and Practice. Philadelphia: Lippincott Williams & Wilkins, 2002, pp 3–15.

48. Takenaka A, Murakami G, Soga H, et al. Anatomical analysis of the neurovascular bundle supplying penile cavernous tissue to ensure a reliable nerve graft after radical prostatectomy. J Urol 2004;172:1032–1035.

49. Costello A, Brooks M, Cole OJ. Anatomical studies of the neurovascular bundle and cavernous nerves. BJU Int 2004;94:1071–1076.

50. Walsh PC. Anatomic radical retropubic prostatectomy. In Walsh PC, Retik AB, Vaughan ED Jr, Wein AJ (eds): Campbell's Urology, 8th edn. Philadelphia: WB Saunders, 2002, pp 3107–3129.

51. Lepor H, Gregerman M, Crosby R, et al. Precise localization of the autonomic nerves from the pelvic plexus to the corpora cavernosa: a detailed anatomical study of the adult male pelvis. J Urol 1985;133:207–212.

52. Litwin MS, Sadetsky N, Pasta DJ, et al. Bowel function and bother after treatment for early stage prostate cancer: a longitudinal quality of life analysis from CaPSURE. J Urol 2004;172:515–519.

53. Bishoff JT, Motley G, Optenberg SA, et al. Incidence of fecal and urinary incontinence following radical perineal and retropubic prostatectomy in a national population. J Urol 1998;160:454–458.

54. Brooks JD, Chao WM, Kerr J. Male pelvic anatomy reconstructed from the visible human data set. J Urol 1998;159:868–872.

55. Thompson P. On the arrangement of the fasciae of the pelvis and their relationship to the levator ani. J Anat Physiol 1901;35:127–141.

56. Hollabaugh RS Jr, Dmochowski RR, Steiner MS. Neuroanatomy of the male rhabdosphincter. Urology 1997;49:426–434.

57. Uhlenhuth ECA. Problems in the Anatomy of the Pelvis. Philadelphia: Lippincott, 1953.

58. Young HH, Davis DM. Young's Practice of Urology: Based on a Study of 12,500 Cases, vol 2. Philadelphia: WB Saunders, 1926, pp 414–512.

59. Belt E, Ebert CE, Surber AC Jr. New anatomic approach in perineal prostatectomy. J Urol 1939;41:482–497.

60. Roux C. Beiträge zur Kenntniss der Aftermuskulatur des Menschen [German]. Archiv Mikr Anat 1880–1881;19:721–733.

61. Lawson JO. Pelvic anatomy: I: pelvic floor muscles. Ann R Coll Surg Engl 1974;54:244–252.

Anatomic radical retropubic prostatectomy

72

J Kellogg Parsons, Alan W Partin, Patrick C Walsh

INTRODUCTION

Since its initial description by Walsh, anatomic radical retropubic prostatectomy (RRP) has become the gold standard to which all other therapies for localized prostate cancer are compared. The first surgical procedure to provide definitive therapy with acceptably low rates of morbidity, RRP has transformed prostate cancer treatment paradigms and galvanized basic science research by making available for study previously unprecedented amounts of prostate tissue. In this chapter, the evolution, preoperative evaluation, surgical technique, and postoperative management of RRP for treatment of clinically localized prostate cancer are discussed.

EVOLUTION OF RADICAL RETROPUBIC PROSTATECTOMY

The modern RRP developed from two distinct but complementary insights: first, that prostate removal is technically feasible; second, that prostate removal may potentially benefit patients with prostate cancer. Kuchler[1] reported the earliest documented prostatectomy in 1858 via a perineal approach. Forty years later, Young[2] both refined the technical performance of the radical perineal prostatectomy and conceived of its application to prostate cancer. In 1947, Millin[3] first described the retropubic approach for radical prostatectomy and the removal of benign adenomas. Over the next decade, a number of investigators modified Millin's technique.[4–8] The radical

retropubic approach, however, failed to gain widespread acceptance due to its associations with severe intraoperative hemorrhage and inappropriately high rates of postoperative urinary incontinence and impotence.

During the late 1970s and early 1980s, a series of seminal observations provided three key insights into periprostatic anatomy that vastly improved the surgeon's ability to radically excise the prostate with substantially reduced morbidity. First, detailed anatomic characterization of the dorsal vein improved intraoperative hemostasis and permitted more precise dissection in a relatively bloodless field,[9,10] which in turn resulted in fewer transfusions, shorter hospital stays, substantially improved postoperative urinary continence,[11–13] and superior cancer control. Second, elucidation of the anatomy of the pelvic nerve plexus and its structural relationship to sexual function led to precise modifications in surgical technique that, for the first time, made it possible to systematically preserve this plexus and thereby maintain potency in appropriately selected men.[10] Third, Oelrich's descriptions[14] of striated urethral sphincter structure allowed for greater preservation of urinary continence. Thereafter, RRP was widely adopted as a primary therapy for localized prostate cancer.

PREOPERATIVE EVALUATION

Preoperative evaluation should include clinical staging when indicated (see Chapter 43) and discussion of the risks, complications, and expected benefits of the procedure. Surgery should be deferred for a minimum of

4 to 6 weeks following prostate biopsy or transurethral resection of the prostate. This delay, which will not compromise long-term cancer control,[15] allows for resolution of inflammatory adhesions or hematomas that may obscure visualization of the anatomic relationships between the prostate and adjacent structures.

During the preoperative period, patients may elect to donate 2 or 3 units of blood to decrease the risk of receiving a perioperative homologous transfusion. The relative costs and benefits of preoperative autologous transfusion, however, remain a focus of debate. Although some investigators have observed significantly lower rates of homologous transfusion among preoperative autologous blood donors,[16,17] others have not,[18] while still others have noted that a majority of autologous units are either discarded[19] or inappropriately given to patients with low cardiac risk.[20] In counseling these patients, therefore, the surgeon may wish to consider two pieces of information. First, the probability of receiving a perioperative homologous blood transfusion among those who do not donate blood appears to be low: 2.4% to 3.8% at three high-volume university hospitals.[18,21,22] Second, the following variables have been associated with increased risk of homologous transfusion: a low-volume surgeon (defined as <15 RRPs performed annually) (OR, 8.63; 95% CI, 3.95–18.86), neoadjuvant hormonal therapy (OR, 3.35; 95% CI, 1.51–7.44), general anesthesia (OR, 2.22; 95% CI, 1.12–4.41), and prostate volume greater than 50 g (OR, 1.74; 95% CI, 1.33–2.29).[22]

Another potential option to lower the risk of homologous transfusion is preoperative administration of erythropoietin (Epoetin alfa). Lepor et al[23–25] have observed that preoperative erythropoietin increases serum hemoglobin concentration and is associated with rates of perioperative homologous transfusion comparable to patients who donate autologous blood. However, it is unclear if preoperative erythropoietin decreases the risk of homologous transfusion among men who do not donate autologous blood.

Regardless of preoperative transfusion status, patients should be counseled to avoid medications with potential antiplatelet effects—including vitamin E greater than 400 IU/day, aspirin, clopidogrel (Plavix®), and nonaspirin nonsteroidal anti-inflammatory drugs—for at least 1 week prior to donating blood or having surgery.

We recommend restriction to a clear liquid diet on the day before surgery, oral ingestion of magnesium citrate 250 ml the evening before surgery, and administration of a Fleets® enema early in the morning on the day of surgery. We also recommend administration of standard preoperative antibiotic prophylaxis and application of thromboembolic deterrent stockings and sequential compression devices to the lower extremities prior to beginning the procedure.

SURGICAL TECHNIQUE

INSTRUMENTS AND POSITIONING

RRP requires few special instruments. We recommend use of a fiberoptic headlight, which facilitates illumination of the retropubic space; a Balfour retractor with narrow and standard wide malleable blades for retraction of the peritoneum; coagulating forceps; and 2.5 to 4.5 power loupes to enhance visualization of the neurovascular bundles (NVBs).

Preexisting medical conditions and anesthesiologist and patient preferences should dictate choice of anesthesia. General, spinal or epidural anesthetics are all acceptable alternatives. Data suggest that regional (spinal or epidural) anesthesia may be associated with less operative blood loss,[17,22,26,27] but not with decreased postoperative morbidity.[28]

The patient is placed supine and flat on the operative table. After skin preparation and sterile draping, a 16-Fr Foley catheter is passed into the bladder, the balloon inflated with 20 ml of saline, and the catheter connected to sterile, closed, continuous drainage.

INCISION AND PELVIC LYMPH NODE DISSECTION

A midline, infraumbilical incision is extended from the pubis to the umbilicus. The rectus muscles are separated along the midline and the transversalis fascia is opened sharply without violation of the peritoneal cavity. The anterior fascia is incised inferiorly to the pubis, while the posterior fascia is left intact. The space of Retzius is developed manually, and the peritoneum is mobilized off the external iliac vessels—with care taken not to disturb the tissue overlying the external iliac artery—just caudal to the vas deferens to allow for placement of the narrow retractor blade. We do not recommend isolation and/or division of the vasa, nor development of the retroperitoneal space, as these maneuvers do not facilitate subsequent performance of the operation.

Next, after the Balfour retractor is placed, a narrow malleable blade is used to expose the iliac vessels and provide visualization of the lateral pelvis for staging pelvic lymph node dissection. If necessary, a deep Deaver retractor may provide additional medial retraction of the bladder. Lymph node dissection is initiated on the side of the dominant tumor. Careful division of the adventitia over the external iliac vein with Metzenbaum scissors facilitates access to the obturator fossa and allows for development of the space immediately posterior to the external iliac vein (Figure 72.1). A Gil-Vernet or similar retractor is placed under the external iliac vein to provide gentle anterior

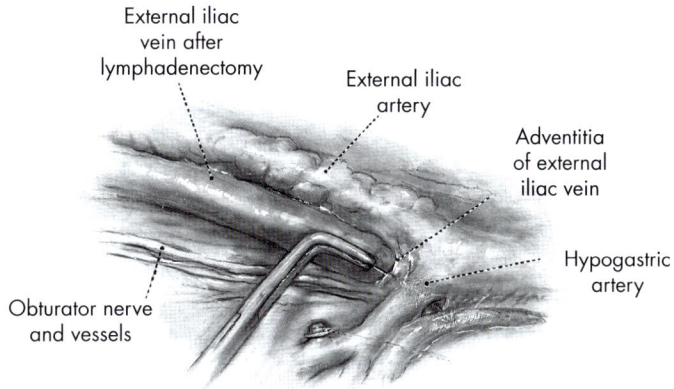

Fig. 72.1
View of the right pelvis after completion of the staging lymph node dissection. Note that the fibroadipose tissue around the obturator nerve and vessels—but not that overlying the external iliac artery—has been removed.
Courtesy of the Brady Urological Institute.

retraction. The dissection then moves inferiorly toward the femoral canal, with the surgeon bluntly sweeping the nodal package away from the pelvic sidewall while simultaneously identifying the obturator nerve. The nodal tissue should be ligated distal to Cloquet's node, with care taken not to injure the obturator nerve.

The dissection then proceeds superiorly along the pelvic side wall to the bifurcation of the common iliac artery, where the lymph nodes lying in the angle between the external iliac and hypogastric arteries are removed. Posteriorly, the dissection is carried down to the hypogastric veins.[29] The adventitia overlying the external iliac artery should be preserved to maintain lymphatic drainage from the lower extremities. Next, the obturator lymph nodes are removed with care taken to avoid injury to the obturator nerve, artery, and vein. The narrow retractor blade is then removed and the dissection is repeated on the contralateral side. We do not routinely perform frozen-section analyses unless there are palpable nodal abnormalities.

INCISION OF THE ENDOPELVIC FASCIA

Once the nodal dissection is completed, we recommend that the surgeon utilizes 2.5 to 4.5 power loupes for the remainder of the operation. To expose the anterior surface of the prostate, the peritoneum is gently retracted superiorly with the wide malleable Balfour blade.

The fibroadipose tissue covering the anterior and anterolateral surfaces of the prostate is cleared with forceps to expose the pelvic fascia, puboprostatic ligaments, and superficial branches of the dorsal vein. The superficial branch of the dorsal vein complex medial to the puboprostatic ligaments is coagulated and divided. The endopelvic fascia is entered sharply with Metzenbaum scissors at its reflection over the pelvic sidewall, well away from the attachments to the bladder

and prostate (Figure 72.2). Here, the endopelvic fascia fibers are translucent and should allow for visualization of the underlying levator ani musculature. After entering the endopelvic fascia, care should be taken not to injure the lateral aspect of the venous plexus of Santorini, which may be appreciated medially. The incision in the endopelvic fascia is extended anteromedially toward the puboprostatic ligaments. During this step, small arterial and venous branches of the pudendal vessels may be encountered as they emerge from the pelvic musculature to supply the prostate. To avoid coagulation injury to the pudendal artery and nerve, located just deep to the muscle along the pubic ramus, these vessels should be ligated with clips.

After division of the endopelvic fascia bilaterally, a sponge stick is used to displace the prostate posteriorly, and the puboprostatic ligaments are sharply divided bilaterally with Metzenbaum scissors (Figure 72.3A). We suggest only dividing the ligaments enough to expose the apical surface of the prostate. The pubourethral

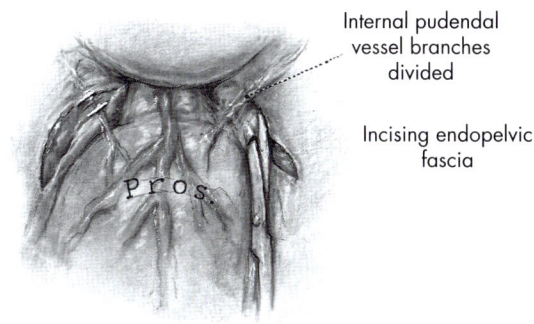

Fig. 72.2
Incision in the endopelvic fascia is made at the junction with the pelvic sidewall, well away from the bladder and prostate. Small anterior branches from the internal pudendal vessels are often encountered, and should be clipped and divided. Pros, prostate.
Courtesy of the Brady Urological Institute.

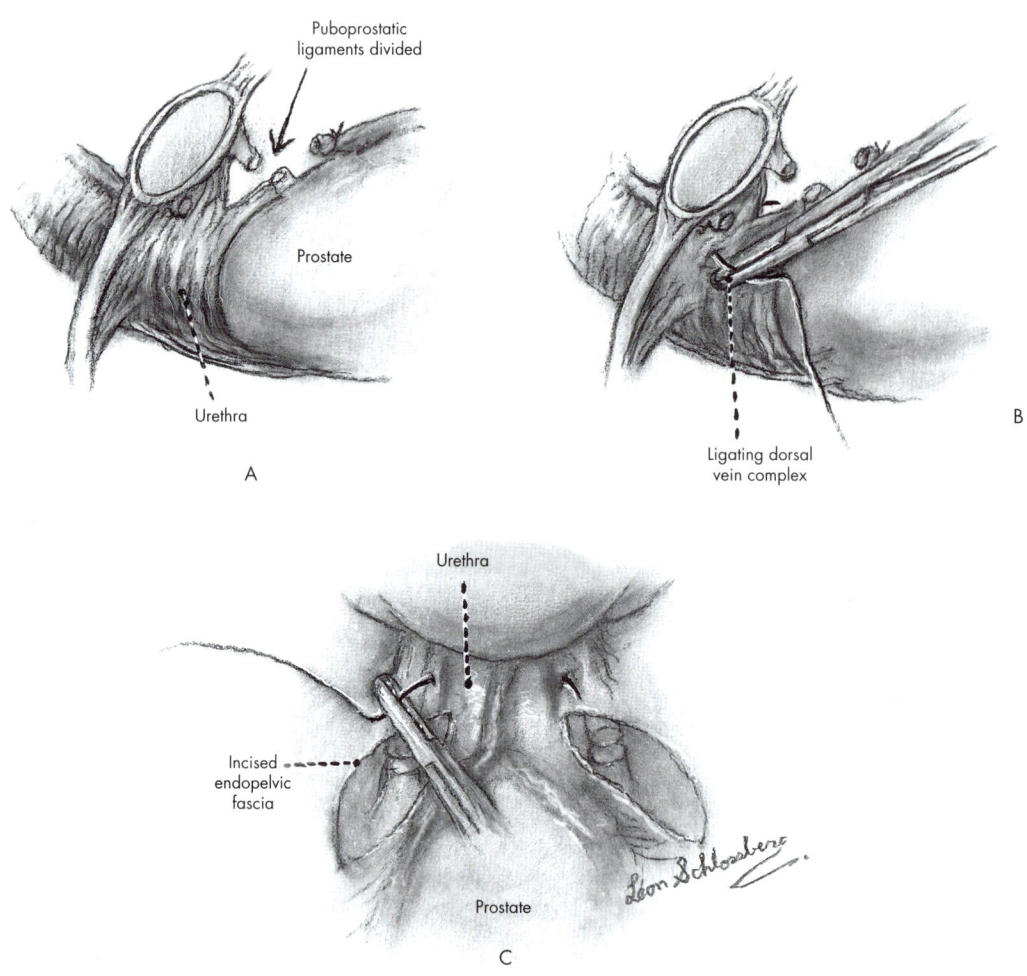

Puboprostatic
ligaments divided

Prostate

Urethra

A

Ligating dorsal
vein complex

B

Urethra

Incised
endopelvic
fascia

Prostate

C

Fig. 72.3
Steps in division of the dorsal vein complex. A, Superficial puboprostatic ligaments are sharply divided, exposing the junction between the apex of the prostate and the anterior surface of the dorsal vein complex. The pubourethral component of the complex should remain intact. B and C, 3-0 Monofilament suture is passed superficially through the dorsal vein complex just distal to the apex of the prostate. D and E, Needle is then reversed, and the same suture is placed through the perichondrium of the pubic symphysis. F, This horizontal suture is tied. G, Striated sphincter dorsal vein complex is then divided using Metzenbaum sutures.
Courtesy of the Brady Urological Institute.

component of the complex should remain intact to preserve the anterior fixation of the striated urethral sphincter to the pubis.[30]

DIVISION OF THE DORSAL COMPLEX AND URETHRA

While displacing the prostate posteriorly with a sponge stick, a 3-0 monofilament suture on a 5/8 circle needle is passed anterior to the urethra through the dorsal vein complex just distal to the apex of the prostate (Figure 72.3B and C). Next, the needle is reversed in the needle driver and placed through the perichondrium of the pubic symphysis. This maneuver is repeated as a figure-of-eight suture and tied (Figure 72.3D and E), which

accomplishes two objectives: first, because it elevates the distal complex, it enables the surgeon to visualize the plane on the anterior apex of the prostate during division of the dorsal vein complex; and second, it provides superior hemostasis (Figure 72.3F).

While again displacing the prostate posteriorly with a sponge stick, Metzenbaum scissors or a No 15 blade on a long handle are used to completely divide the dorsal vein complex (Figure 72.3G). Absolute hemostatic control of the complex is mandatory to provide a bloodless field for the remainder of the procedure. To achieve hemostasis, the same 3-0 monofilament suture placed through the pubic perichondrium during the previous step is used to oversew the superficial edges of the complex (Figure 72.4). In addition, clips may be used to control bleeding from circumflex veins often

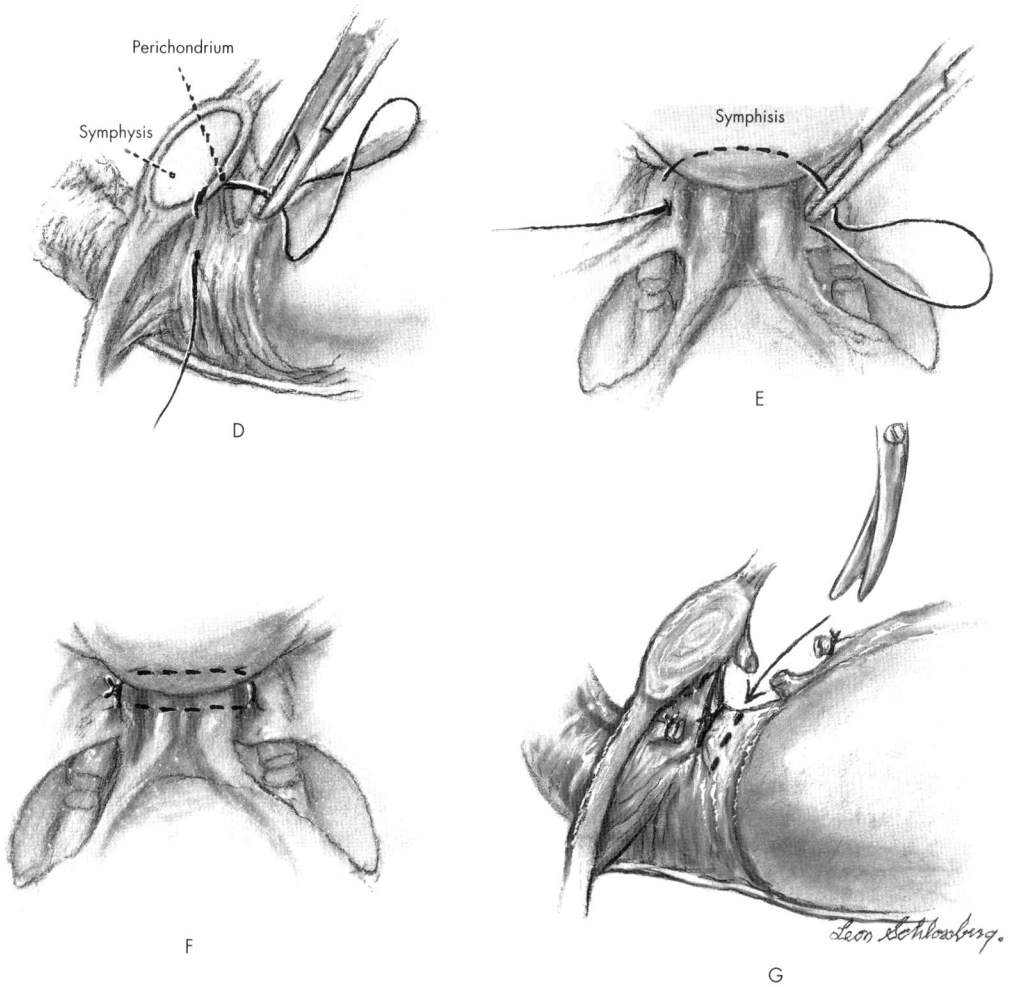

present at the posterior edges of the complex at 5 and 7 o'clock. The proximal dorsal vein on the anterior surface of the prostate is oversewn with a 2-0 absorbable suture (Figure 72.4).

Once the vein is oversewn, attention is turned toward urethral division. Gentle posterior displacement of the prostate with a sponge stick should provide excellent visualization of the prostatourethral junction. A right-angle clamp should be passed immediately posterior to the urethral smooth muscle near the apex of the prostate to ensure that the urethra is transected as close to the apex as possible. The anterior urethra is then sharply divided with care taken to avoid entering the Foley catheter (Figure 72.4C). This should provide excellent exposure for urethral suture placement. If additional exposure is necessary, however, the anterior surface of the lateral bands of the striated urethral sphincter may be divided at their midpoint beyond the apex of the prostate.

Five 3-0 monofilament sutures on 5/8 circle tapered needles are then placed, from outside to inside, through the urethra at the following positions: 12, 2, 5, 7, and 10 o'clock. Each suture should incorporate the urethral mucosa and submucosa but exclude the smooth muscle

of the sphincter (Figure 72.5). The 2 o'clock suture should be placed first, as it will elevate the urethral mucosa and submucosa, and thus facilitate placement of the remaining sutures. After placement, the sutures are tagged and covered with towels to avoid inadvertent traction or displacement. The Foley catheter is removed. A single suture is then placed through the urethra at the 6 o'clock position in the same manner as the previous five (Figure 72.6A), and the posterior wall of the urethra sharply divided (Figure 72.6B).

To divide the posterior portion of the sphincter complex and develop the plane between the prostate and rectum, the right-angle clamp is placed immediately posterior to the left edge of the complex at a point midway between the prostatic apex and the distal urethra (Figure 72.7). At this midway point, the NVBs are relatively posterior and thus should lie deep to the clamp.[31] Placement of the clamp too close to the prostatic apex may result in NVB damage.

The left border of the complex exposed by the clamp is sharply divided. Next, the right-angle clamp is placed immediately posterior to the right edge of the complex at the midway point (Figure 72.8, top) and the remaining complex is sharply divided (Figure 72.8,

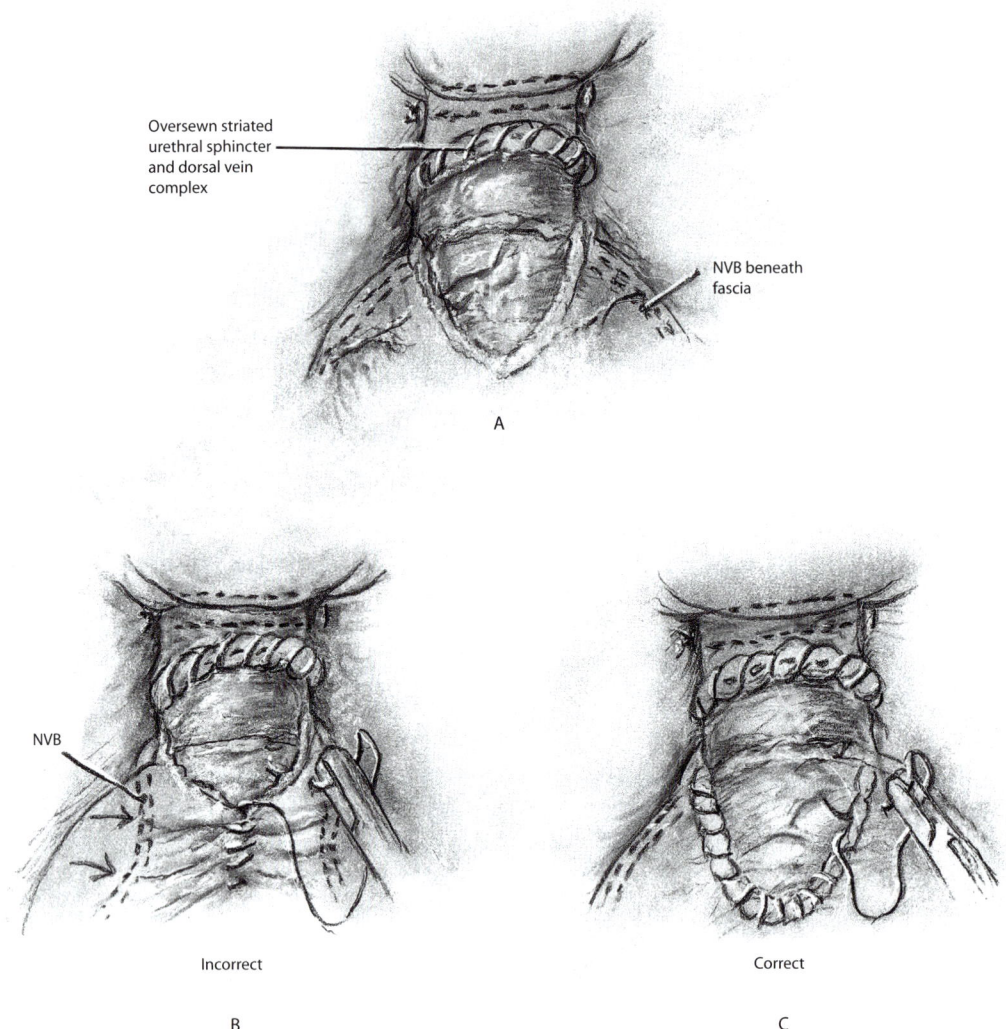

Oversewn striated
urethral sphincter
and dorsal vein
complex

NVB beneath
fascia

A

NVB

Incorrect

Correct

B

C

Fig. 72.4

Ligation of the dorsal vein complex. *A*, Superficial edges of the distal striated urethral sphincter–dorsal vein complex have been oversewn utilizing the same 3-0 monofilament suture illustrated in Fig. 72.3B and C. The edges of the proximal dorsal vein over the prostate are oversewn. If they are pulled together in the midline (*B*), the neurovascular bundles (NVBs) may be advanced too far anteriorly on the prostate, and thus may be in harm's way. Instead, the edges are oversewn in the shape of a "V" using a running 2-0 absorbable suture (*C*).

Courtesy of the Brady Urological Institute.

bottom). Division of the complex in this manner—lateral to medial on each side—minimizes the potential for inadvertent injury to the NVBs or rectum.

INCISION OF THE SUPERFICIAL LATERAL PELVIC FASCIA AND APICAL DISSECTION OF THE NEUROVASCULAR BUNDLE

During initial dissection of the NVBs, there should be no upward traction placed on the prostate; exposure should instead be accomplished by rolling the prostate from side to side with the sponge stick. The superficial layers of the lateral pelvic fascia are first released with

the right-angle clamp at the bladder neck where the fibers coalesce into a thick band (Figure 72.9). Division of this band should immediately increase prostate mobility. The remainder of the superficial lateral pelvic fascia is then divided from the bladder neck to the apex (Figure 72.10). This maneuver, performed on each side, releases the NVBs laterally, which in turn facilitates performance of the next step—posterior release of the NVBs at the apex.

Division of the superficial lateral pelvic fascia should reveal the subtle groove on the posterolateral edge of the prostate that marks the location of the NVB. Beginning at the apex, each bundle is released by gently rolling the prostate to the contralateral side and spreading with the right angle (Figure 72.11). Initial release of the bundles

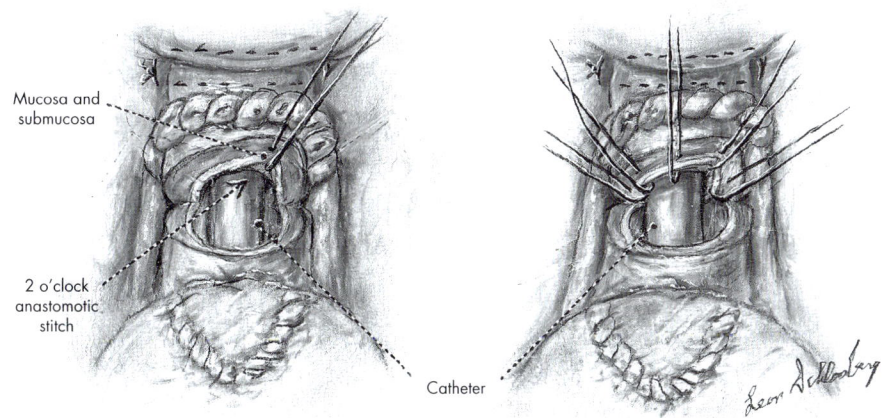

Fig. 72.5
Placement of urethral anastomotic sutures and division of the posterior urethra. 3-0 Monofilament sutures on 5/8 circle tapered needles are placed in the distal urethral segment, from outside to inside, at 12, 2, 5, 7, and 10 o'clock. The suture should incorporate only the mucosa and submucosa of the urethra. Placement of the 2 o'clock suture first facilitates placement of the other four.
Courtesy of the Brady Urological Institute.

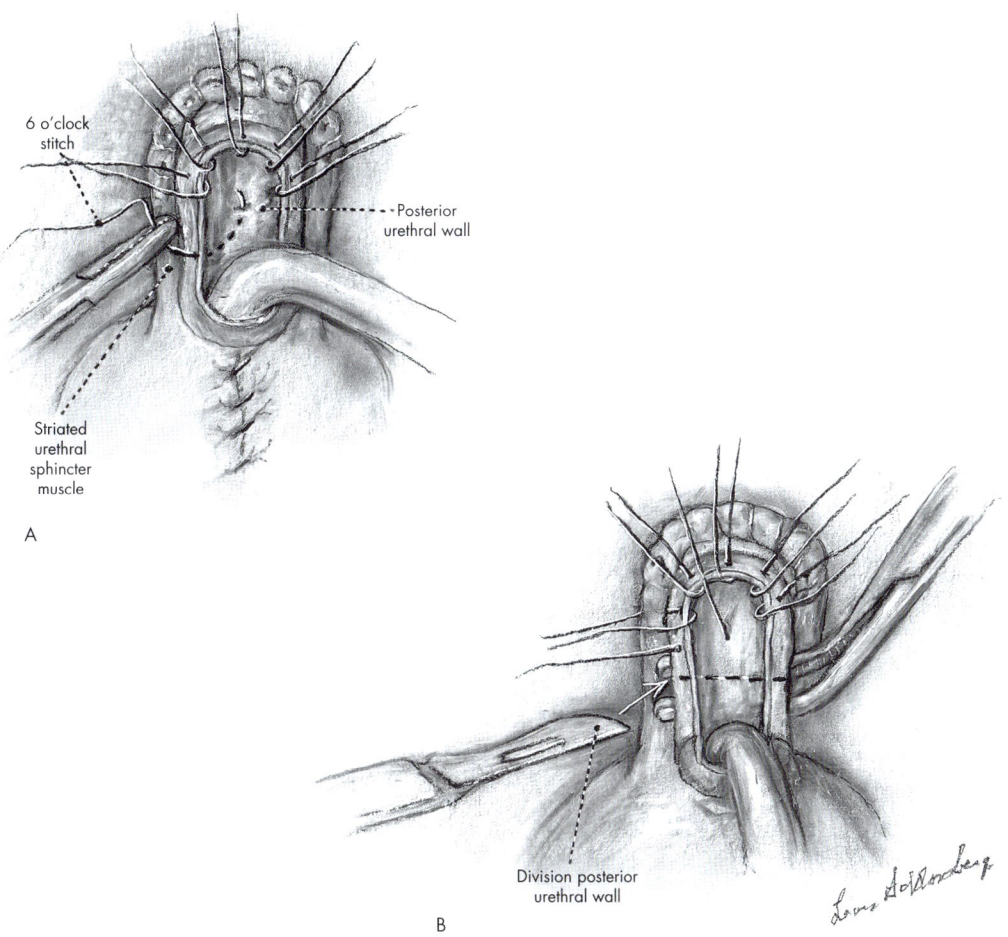

Fig. 72.6
A, After Foley catheter removal, a single 3-0 monofilament suture on a 5/8 circle tapered needle is placed at 6 o'clock in the same manner as the previous five. B, Posterior wall of the urethra is divided.
Courtesy of the Brady Urological Institute.

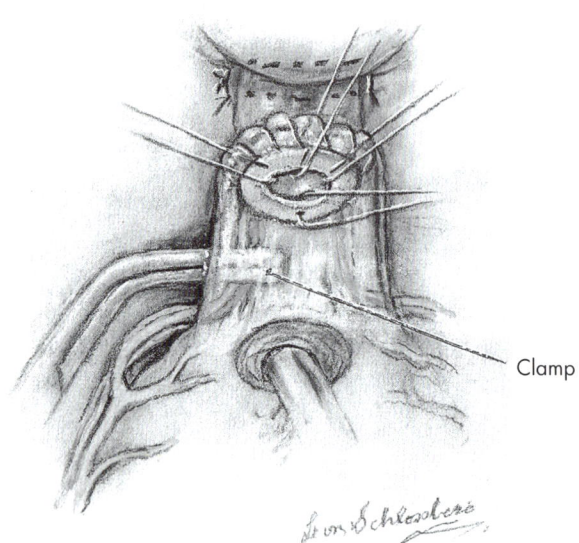

Clamp

Lon Schlossberg

Fig. 72.7
Right-angle clamp is passed immediately posterior to the left edge of the striated urethral sphincter complex, anterior to the neurovascular bundle (NVB), midway between the prostatic apex and the distal urethra.
Courtesy of the Brady Urological Institute.

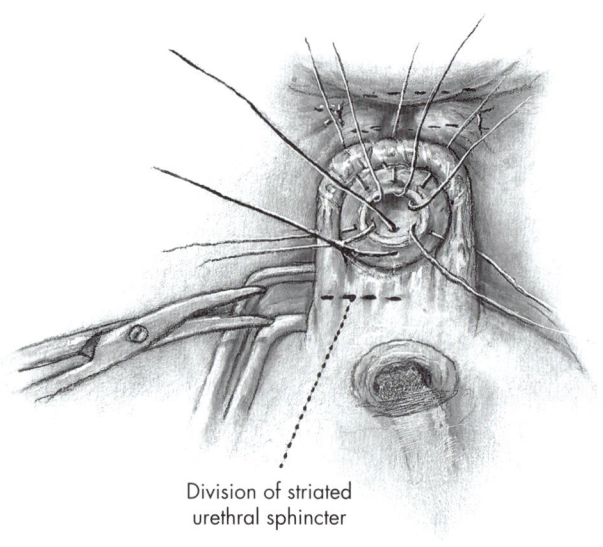

Division of striated
urethral sphincter

Fig. 72.8
Division of the remaining striated urethral sphincter complex. A right-angle clamp is passed posterior to the right edge of the striated urethral sphincter complex midway between the prostatic apex and the distal urethra, and the complex is sharply divided.
Courtesy of the Brady Urological Institute.

at the apex mitigates two potential difficulties that may be encountered. First, in patients in whom the bundle lies more anterior, apical release reduces the likelihood of confusing the groove with the potential space lying between the prostate and rectum. Second, in most patients, it facilitates identification and management of veins on the lateral surface of the prostate that run between Santorini's plexus anteriorly and the NVBs posteriorly. The dissection should proceed toward the base along the plane that leaves Denonvilliers' fascia and the prostatic fascia intact on the prostate but releases the residual fragments of the levator fascia laterally. If the NVBs do not fall easily from the prostate, there may be small apical vessels tethering it in place (Figures 72.12 and 72.13). These are best controlled with small clips placed parallel to the bundle followed by sharp division with fine scissors. Due to the potential for nerve injury, electrocoagulation should never be used on the bundle or its branches.[32] If fixation of a bundle to the prostate cannot be explained by vascular tethering, then tumor-induced desmoplasia should be suspected and the bundle excised.

EXCISION OF THE LATERAL PELVIC FASCIA AND THE NEUROVASCULAR BUNDLE

Excision of the lateral pelvic fascia and NVBs on one or both sides may be necessary. The decision to excise should be based on preoperative evaluation and intraoperative findings. It is important to note that the

bundle should not always be excised on the side of the positive biopsy or palpable lesion.[33,34]

Preoperative evaluation should include assessment of sexual function, lesion location (apex versus base), Partin Table probability of capsular extension, and presence of perineural invasion. These criteria should not be used as absolute indications. For example, when considering NVB excision in impotent men, it should be remembered that innervation from the NVBs to the smooth musculature of the urethra may play a role in the recovery of urinary control.[11,35]

There are three intraoperative findings which favor wide excision of the NVB: induration in the lateral pelvic fascia, adherence of the NVB to the prostate during release, and inadequate tissue covering the posterolateral surface of the prostate after prostate removal. This last point is important—the decision to excise or preserve the NVB may be made after prostate removal, and if there is insufficient soft tissue covering the prostate, secondary wide excision of the NVB may be performed.

It is almost never necessary to excise both NVBs.[34,36] Before performing unilateral NVB excision, the contralateral NVB should be freed from the prostate starting at the apex to avoid traction injury. The NVB to be excised is identified at the apex and isolated with a right-angle clamp, which is passed from medial to lateral immediately on the anterior surface of the rectum (Figure 72.14). To maximize the amount of soft tissue excised, the bundle is divided without ligation; if necessary, the distal end may be clipped later for hemostasis.

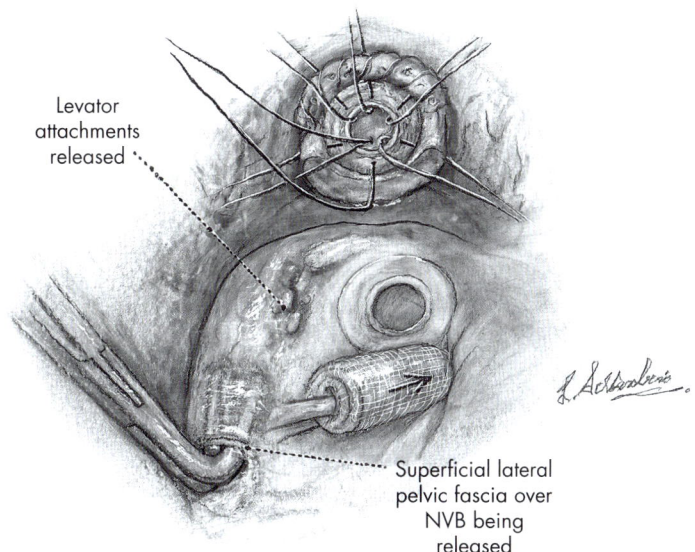

Levator
attachments
released

Superficial lateral
pelvic fascia over
NVB being
released

Fig. 72.9
Incision of the superficial lateral pelvic fascia and exposure of the neurovascular bundle (NVB) grooves. The superficial layers of
the lateral pelvic fascia are released with a right-angle clamp where the fibers coalesce into a thick broad surface.
Courtesy of the Brady Urological Institute.

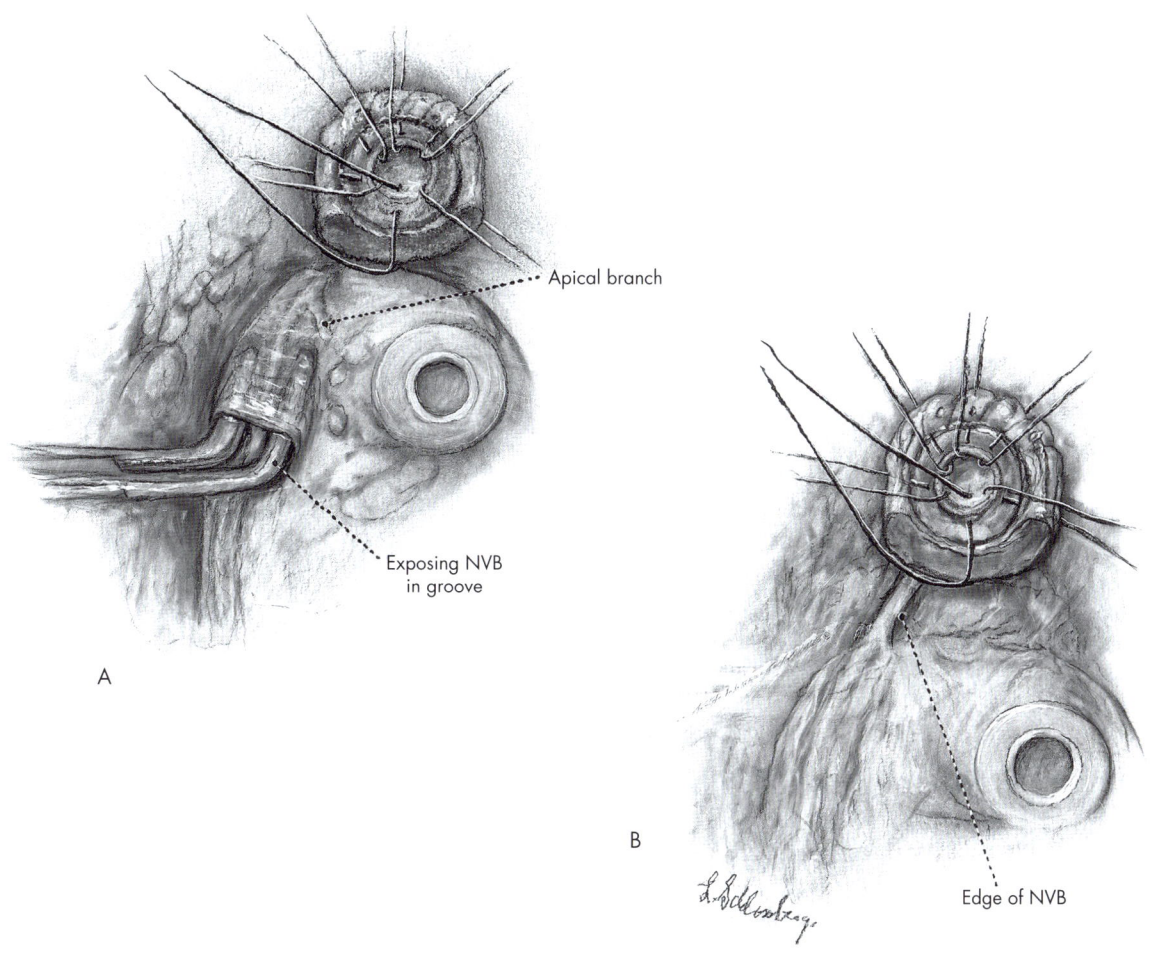

Apical branch

Exposing NVB
in groove

A

B

Edge of NVB

Fig. 72.10
A and *B*, Remainder of the superficial lateral pelvic fascia is divided from the bladder neck to the apex. NVB, neurovascular bundle.
Courtesy of the Brady Urological Institute.

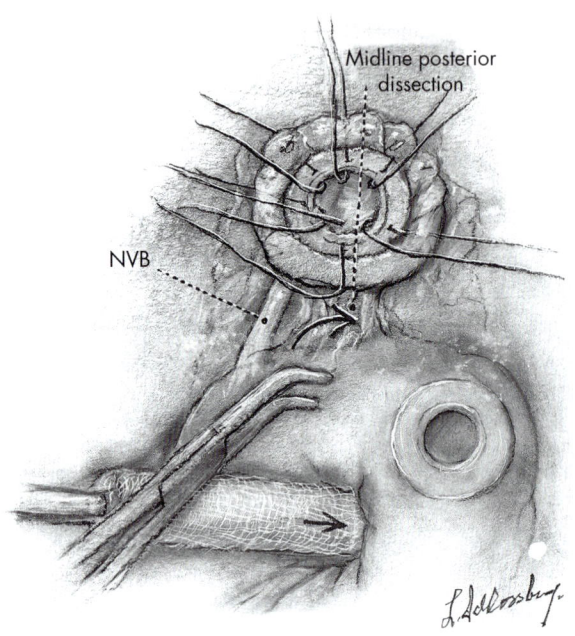

Fig. 72.11
Apical dissection of the neurovascular bundle (NVB). Each
bundle is released by gently rolling the prostate to the
contralateral side and spreading with the right angle.
Courtesy of the Brady Urological Institute.

The dissection is then continued by dividing the
fascia on the lateral surface of the rectum from the
apex to the base; this allows for the NVB and
abundant fascial tissue to be included in the
specimen. This procedure is performed under direct
vision, with the dissection terminating at the tip of the
seminal vesicle, where the NVB is ligated and divided
(Figure 72.15)

POSTERIOR DISSECTION AND DIVISION OF THE LATERAL PEDICLES

Once the NVBs have been released from the apex to the
midpoint of the prostate or widely excised, the catheter
is replaced. Because the NVBs have been released from
the caudal aspect of the prostate, cephalad-directed
traction may now be applied to the catheter to maximize
exposure of the prostatic base and seminal vesicles.
While holding cephalad-directed traction on the
catheter, the attachment of Denonvilliers' fascia to the
rectum is sharply divided in the midline posteriorly.
Denonvilliers' fascia overlying the seminal vesicles
should be left intact (Figure 72.16A). Next, a prominent
arterial branch arising from the NVB and running over
the seminal vesicles to supply the base of the prostate
should be identified. This vessel should be ligated on
each side and divided (Figure 72.16B). Division should
cause each bundle to fall away posteriorly from the
prostate and thus allow for safe division of the lateral

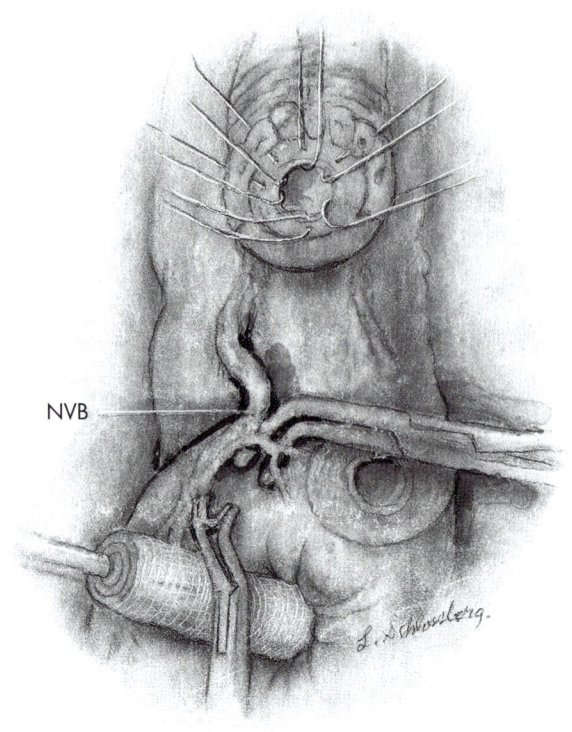

Fig. 72.12
Using the plane that was established posteriorly, the vessels
should be released beginning at the apex. There is often an
apical vessel near the midline that tethers the neurovascular
bundle (NVB), causing it to kink as the prostate is pushed on
its side. Once these apical vessels are released, the bundle
straightens out, and the plane along the posterolateral surface
of the prostate becomes clearer.
Courtesy of the Brady Urological Institute.

pedicle on the lateral surface of the seminal vesicles
without bundle injury (Figure 72.17).

The plane between the lateral edge of the seminal
vesicles and the overlying lateral pelvic fascia is
developed, and then each of the lateral pedicles is
divided without ligation: superficial layers first,
followed by the deeper layers. Arterial bleeders are
controlled with clips. In this manner, the dissection
proceeds superiorly onto the anterolateral surface at the
junction between the bladder and prostate.
Denonvilliers' fascia is then divided over the tips of the
seminal vesicles. If preferred, division of the vasa
deferentia and mobilization of the seminal vesicles may
be performed at this point.

DIVISION OF THE BLADDER NECK AND EXCISION OF THE SEMINAL VESICLES

Now that the prostate is nearly completely mobilized,
the bladder neck is incised along the anterior
prostatovesicular junction (Figure 72.18). The incision
is carried through the mucosa. The Foley balloon is

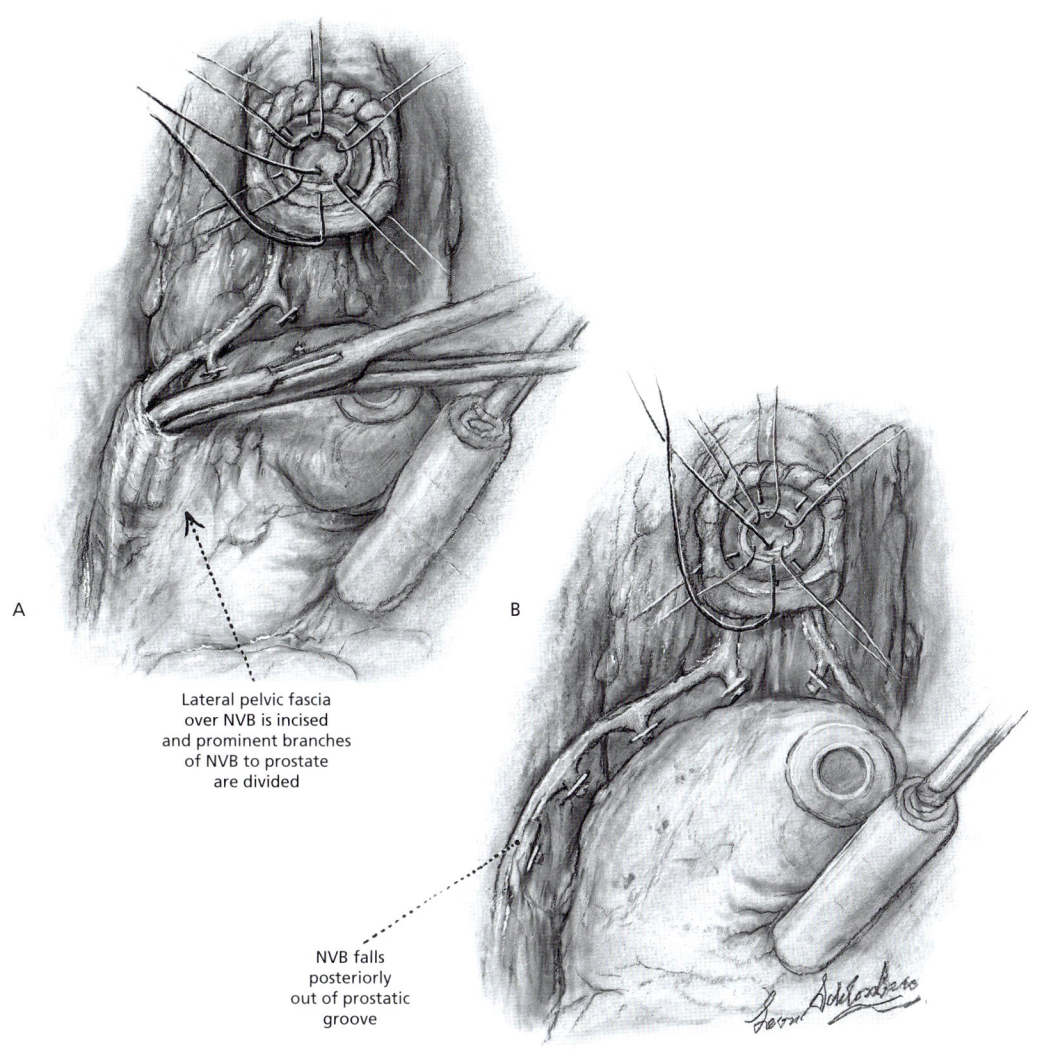

A

Lateral pelvic fascia
over NVB is incised
and prominent branches
of NVB to prostate
are divided

B

NVB falls
posteriorly
out of prostatic
groove

Fig. 72.13
A, Small arterial and venous branches at the apex are divided using clips. *B*, Once the bundle has been identified and released at
the apex, it should be released up to the mid-portion of the prostate.
Courtesy of the Brady Urological Institute.

deflated, and the two ends of the catheter are clamped together to provide traction. As the incision in the bladder neck is widened, vessels running from the inferior vesical pedicle to the prostate will be encountered at 5 and 7 o'clock (Figure 72.19). Division of these vessels should reveal the plane lying between the anterior surface of the seminal vesicles and the posterior wall of the bladder. The posterior bladder neck is safely divided by using scissor dissection that hugs the anterior surface of the seminal vesicles, with attention paid to the location of the ureteral orifices (Figure 72.20).

After dividing the posterior bladder wall, the bladder neck is retracted with an Allis clamp. If not performed prior to division of the bladder neck, the vasa deferentia are now ligated with clips and divided, and the seminal vesicles are dissected free from surrounding structures

(Figure 72.21). Since the pelvic plexus is located on the lateral surface of the seminal vesicles, as the tips of the seminal vesicles are freed, small arterial branches should be identified, ligated, and divided with care to avoid pelvic plexus injury. Any residual attachments of Denonvilliers' fascia are then divided, and the specimen is removed. The specimen is inspected carefully to identify any areas where the margin of resection is uncertain. If there is any concern about either of the margins on the posterolateral surfaces of the prostate, the NVB on that side should be excised.

The operative site is inspected carefully for bleeding. Small bleeding vessels near the NVB should be clipped—not cauterized—in order to avoid nerve injury.[32] Hemostatic control of these vessels is important for preventing hematoma development between the bladder and rectum.

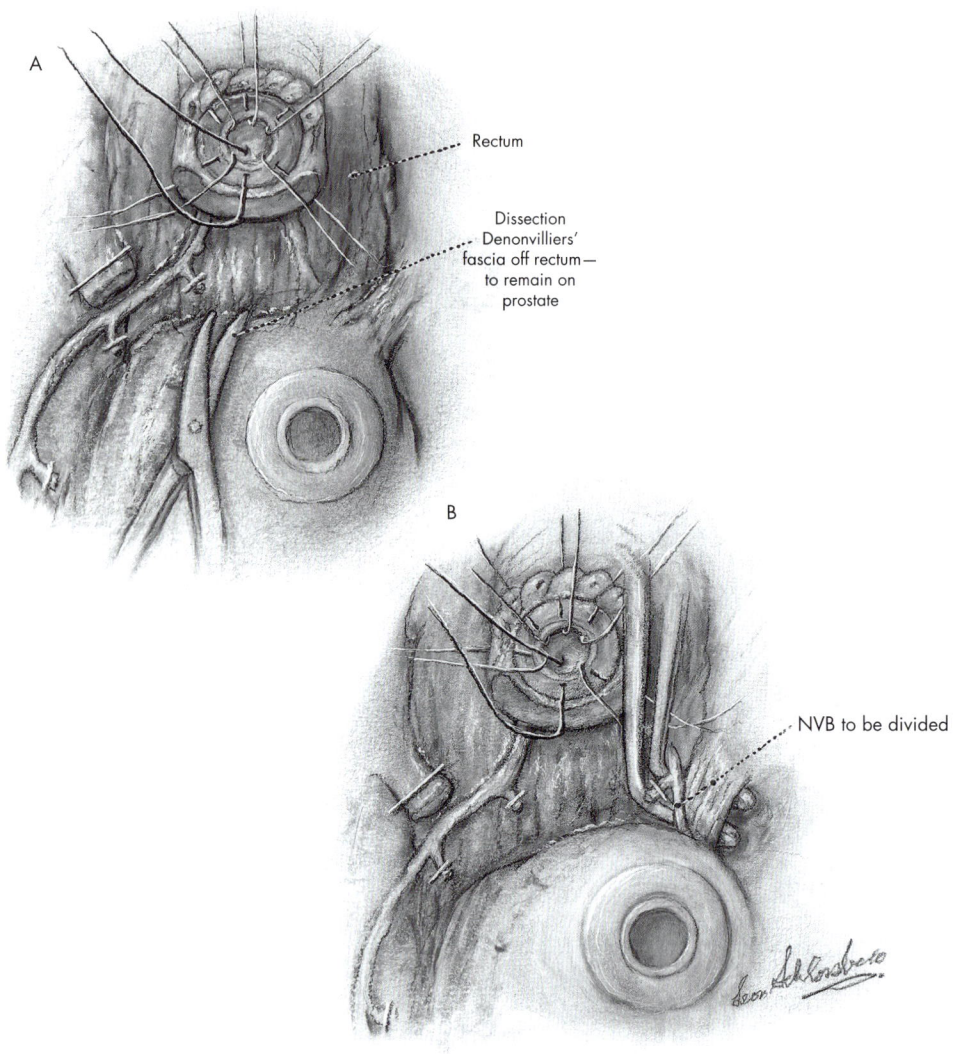

Fig. 72.14
A, Residual attachments of the apex of the prostate in the midline are sharply released in preparation for wide excision of the right neurovascular bundle (NVB). *B*, Right-angle clamp is passed directly on the anterior surface of the rectum from medial to lateral, which minimizes the potential for rectal injury.
Courtesy of the Brady Urological Institute.

BLADDER NECK CLOSURE AND URETHRAL ANASTOMOSIS

The bladder neck is reconstructed using a running suture or interrupted sutures of 3-0 monofilament incorporating full-thickness muscularis and mucosa. A tennis-racket configuration is formed by initiating the closure in the posterior midline and proceeding anterior until the bladder neck is narrowed to the approximate the diameter of the urethra. To facilitate construction of a mucosa-to-mucosa urethrovesical anastomosis, three interrupted 4-0 monofilament sutures should be used to advance the mucosa over the raw musculature of the bladder neck (Figure 72.22). One of these sutures should be placed at the 6 o'clock position and left long to facilitate later placement of the urethral sutures.

To hasten the recovery of urinary control, Walsh has suggested the use of two additional buttressing sutures that intussuscept the bladder neck and prevent it from pulling open as the bladder fills.[37] These sutures are placed in three steps (Figure 72.23). First, a 2-0 monofilamanet suture is placed through the edges of the posterior bladder wall, approximately 2 cm posterior to the reconstructed bladder neck, where the bladder was previously attached to the prostate. This suture is tied in the midline. Second, tension on the anterior bladder wall is released by loosening the malleable blade. This maneuver helps identify the loose perivesical tissue that should be incorporated in the next stitch. Third, another 2-0 monofilament suture is placed as a figure-of-eight approximately 2 cm lateral to the bladder neck on each side and tied loosely. The bladder neck should now lie beneath the

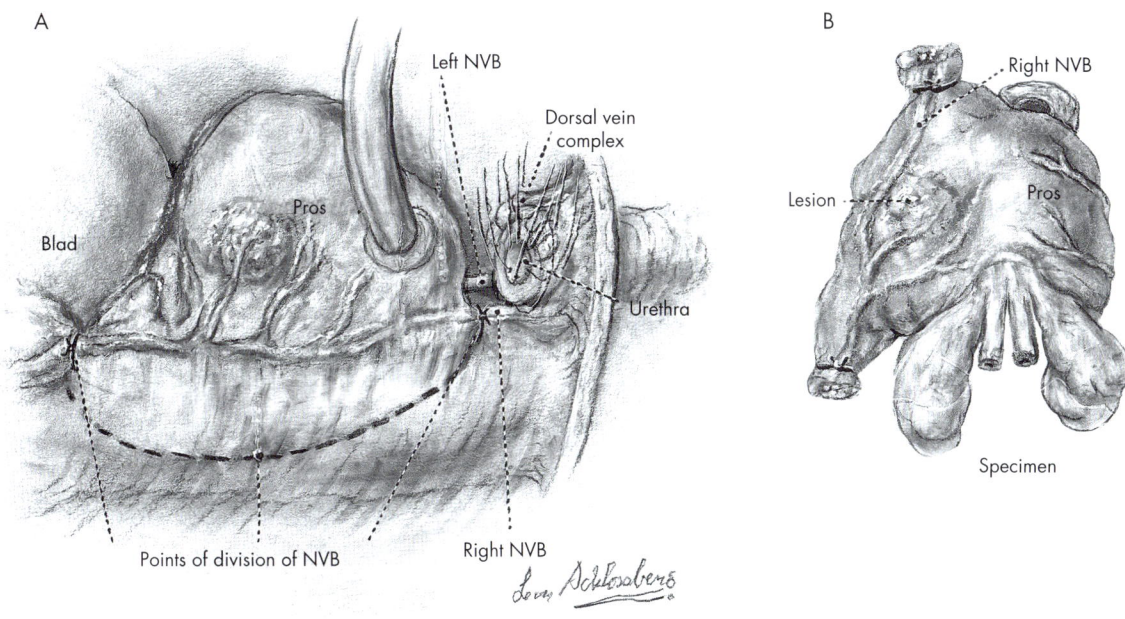

Fig. 72.15

A, Lateral extent of neurovascular bundle (NVB) excision from the apex to the tip of the seminal vesicle, where the neurovascular bundle is ligated. *B,* Neurovascular bundle excision provides extensive soft tissue covering the primary lesion.

Courtesy of the Brady Urological Institute.

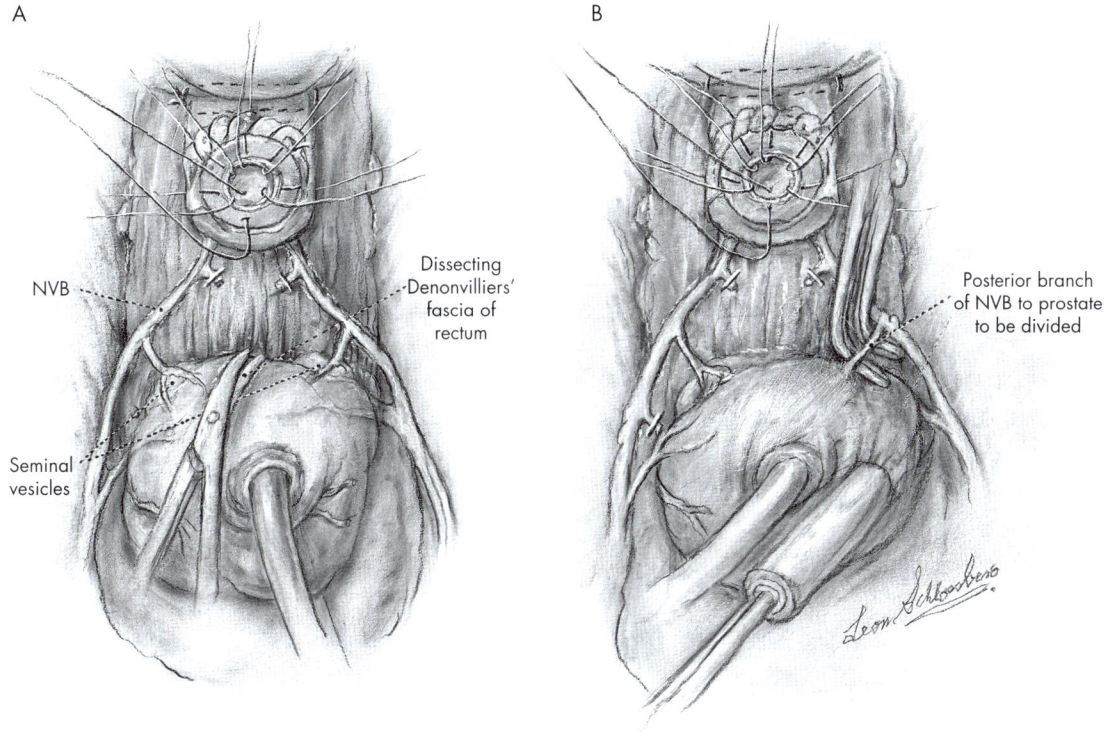

Fig. 72.16

Posterior dissection. *A,* Attachment of Denonvilliers' fascia to the rectum is released. Denonvilliers' fascia overlying the posterior surface of the seminal vesicles should be left intact. *B,* Arterial branch arising from the neurovascular bundle and running over the seminal vesicles to supply the base of the prostate is identified, ligated, and divided.

Courtesy of the Brady Urological Institute.

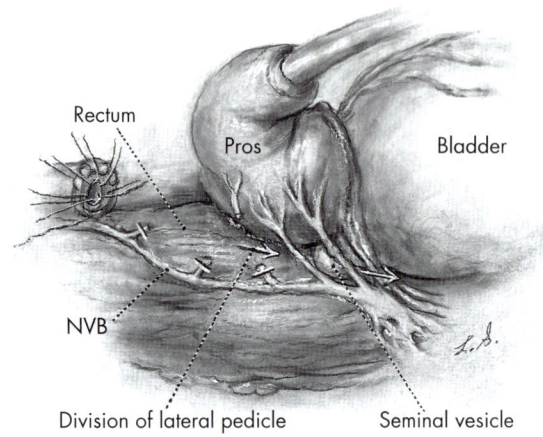

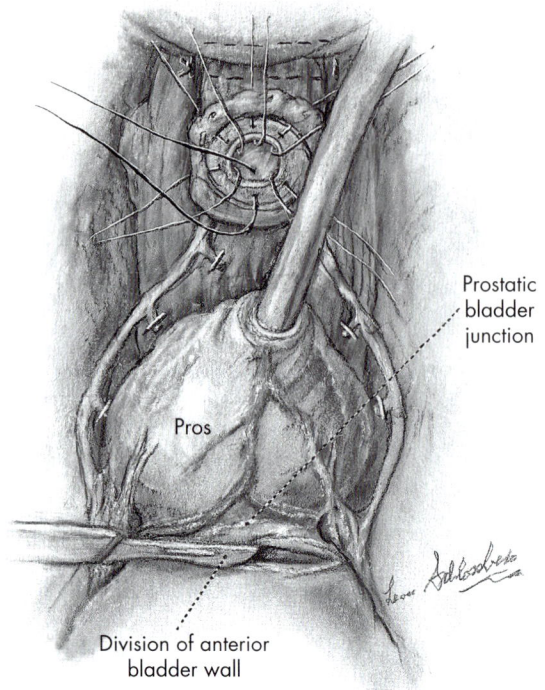

Fig. 72.17

Lateral view demonstrating location of the neurovascular bundle (NVB) following ligation of the posterior branch to the prostate. Division of this posterior branch should free the NVB and allow it to fall away. Pros, prostate.

Courtesy of the Brady Urological Institute.

Fig. 72.18

Anterior bladder neck is incised along the anterior prostatovesicular junction.

Courtesy of the Brady Urological Institute.

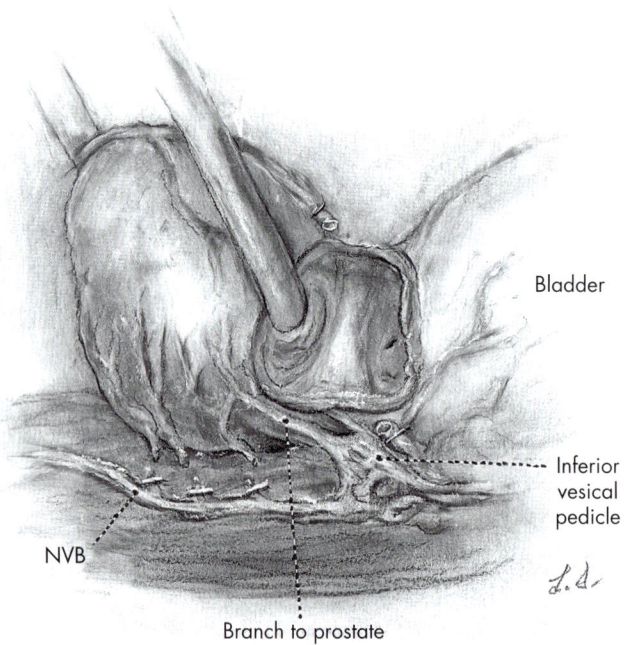

Fig. 72.19

As the incision in the anterior bladder neck is extended, vessels running from the inferior vesical pedicle to the prostate will be encountered at 5 and 7 o'clock. Division of these vessels should reveal the plane lying between the anterior surface of the seminal vesicles and the posterior wall of the bladder.

Courtesy of the Brady Urological Institute.

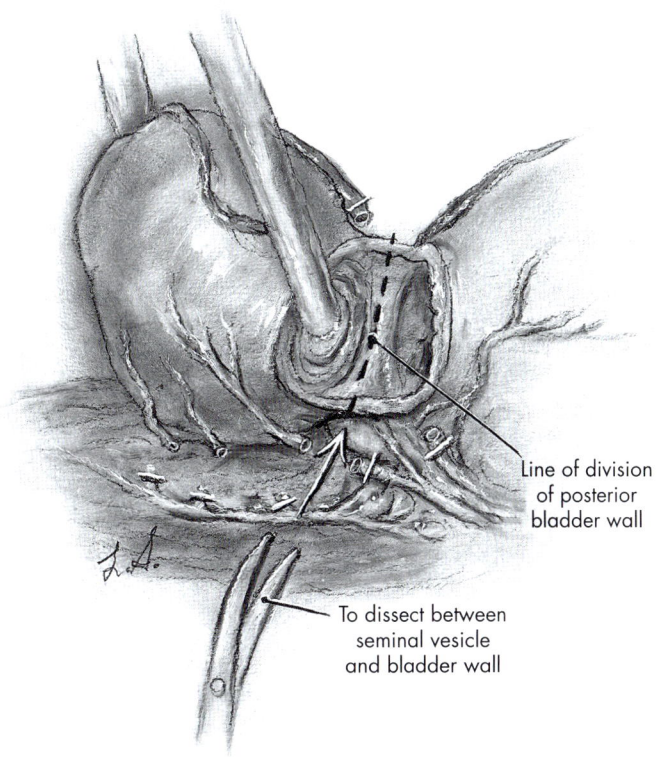

Fig. 72.20
Posterior bladder neck is divided with careful scissor dissection.
Courtesy of the Brady Urological Institute.

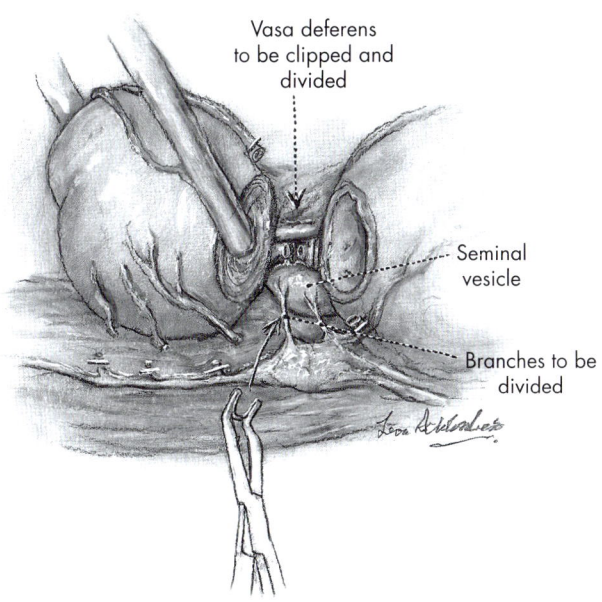

Fig. 72.21
Vasa deferentia are ligated and divided, and the seminal vesicles dissected free from the pelvic plexus with direct visualization and ligation of the small arterial branches.
Courtesy of the Brady Urological Institute.

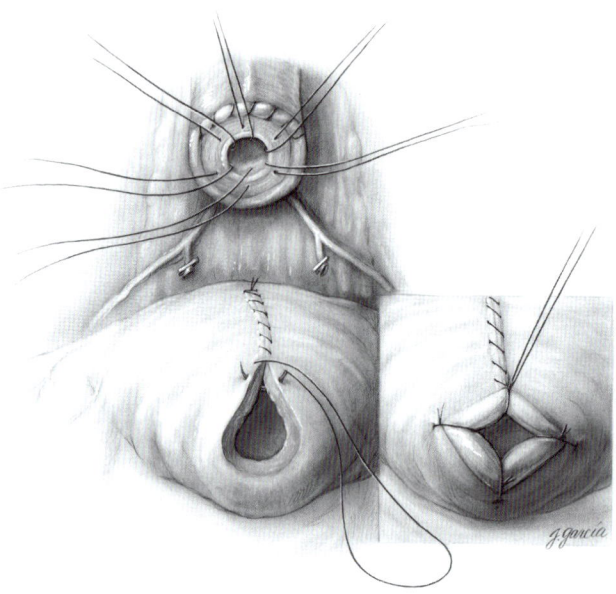

Fig. 72.22
Tennis-racket closure of bladder neck using running 2-0 monofilament suture incorporating all layers of the bladder wall. The suture is tied and left long. *Inset*, Three interrupted 4-0 monofilament sutures are used to advance the mucosa over the raw musculature of the bladder neck.
Courtesy of the Brady Urological Institute.

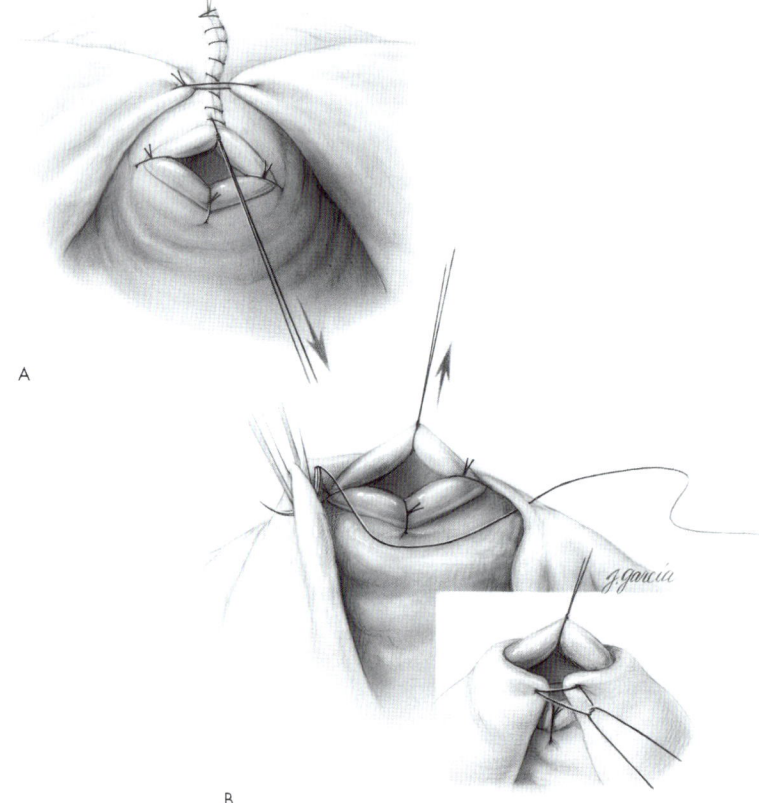

A

B

Fig. 72.23
Intussusception of the bladder neck. *A*, 2-0 Chromic catgut suture is placed in the edges of the posterior bladder wall, about 2 cm from the reconstructed bladder neck, and is tied loosely in the midline. *B*, A second 2-0 monofilament suture is placed as a figure-of-eight approximately 2 cm lateral to the bladder neck on each side and is tied (*inset*).
Courtesy of the Brady Urological Institute.

anterior hood of tissue created by the anterior stitch, resembling a turtle that has pulled its head inside its shell.

The operative site is inspected carefully for bleeding. A new silicone Foley catheter (16-Fr, 5-ml balloon) is placed through the urethra and into the pelvis. Traction on the long ends of the mucosal advancement suture at the 6 o'clock position may now be used to expose the bladder neck. The six 3-0 monofilament sutures that were previously placed in the distal urethra are now placed in their corresponding positions through the bladder neck, from inside to outside and incorporating only the mucosa and submucosa (Figure 72.24). The catheter is irrigated free of clots, the balloon is tested, and the catheter is placed through the bladder neck and inflated with 15 ml of saline.

To ensure that the bladder neck remains in close approximation to the urethra during tying of the sutures, the bladder should be pushed down to the urethra with a Babcock positioned on its anterior surface and held there while the sutures are tied. The anterior suture is initially tied without tension. If tension is present, the bladder should be released from the peritoneum prior to tying the remaining sutures. The sutures are then tied in the following sequence: 2, 5, 10, 7, and 6 o'clock. To ensure that no sutures have entrapped the catheter, the catheter should be rotated through 360° after tying each suture.

The catheter is then irrigated with saline to eliminate clots. A small suction drain is placed through the anterior rectus sheath on one side of the midline. The drain should run between (not through) the rectus muscles with the tip sited in the operative bed in the midline. The incision is closed with a running number 2 nylon suture and skin clips. The catheter is carefully fixed to the thigh with tape or a catheter strap.

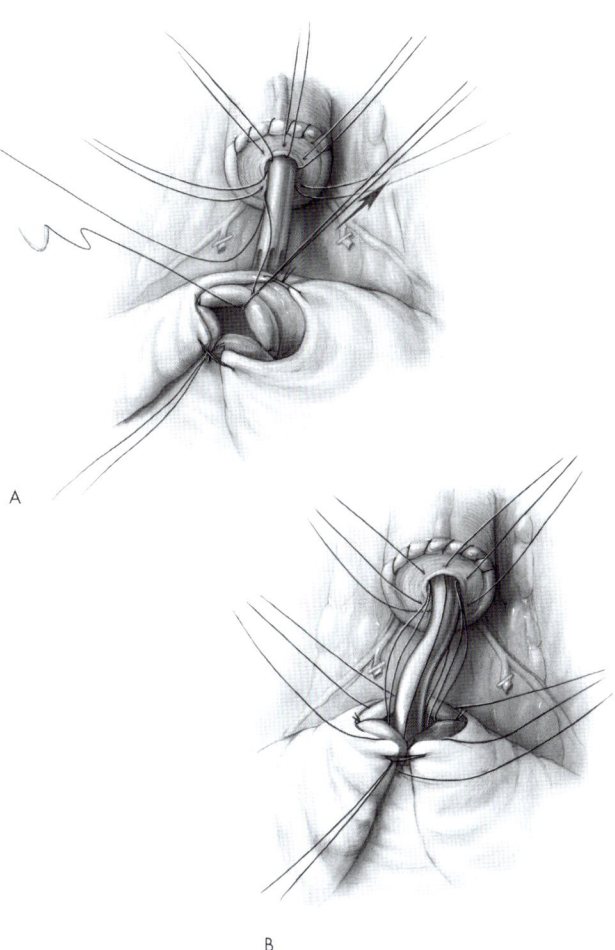

Fig. 72.24
A and *B*, Final anastomosis is performed by placing the six 3-0 monofilament sutures previously placed in the distal urethra through their corresponding positions in the bladder neck, from inside to outside and incorporating only the mucosa and submucosa. The anterior sutures are tied first.
Courtesy of the Brady Urological Institute.

POSTOPERATIVE MANAGEMENT

The postoperative recovery of men who undergo radical retropubic prostatectomy is usually uneventful. Patients should ambulate the morning after the procedure. For the first 12 h, pain control is achieved with intravenous patient-controlled narcotic analgesia. Thereafter, nonaspirin nonsteroidal anti-inflammatory drugs—intravenous ketorolac or oral agents—may reduce narcotic analgesic requirements, postoperative nausea, and ileus. Patients are fed a regular diet on the evening of the first postoperative day. Closed-suction drains are left in place until output is minimal. Patients are discharged from hospital on the second postoperative day with a Foley catheter in place and return 10 to 14 days after surgery for catheter removal. Management of postoperative complications is discussed in detail in Chapter 80.

SUMMARY

The development and dissemination of anatomic RRP has had a major impact on the treatment of localized prostate cancer. Its operative principles have proven durable: novel, minimally invasive techniques for radical prostatectomy utilizing laparoscopy and robot-assistance are firmly grounded in the same fundamental anatomic and surgical techniques. More than that, though, RRP remains an ideal form of treatment for younger men with localized disease, offering a standard of durable cancer-free survival with acceptably low morbidity to which other primary treatments for prostate cancer—both surgical and nonsurgical—are compared. It will likely continue as such for some time.

REFERENCES

1. Kuchler H. Uber prostatavergrosserungh. Deutsch Klin 1866;18:458.

2. Young HH. The early diagnosis and radical cure of carcinoma of the prostate: a study of 40 cases and presentation of a radical operation which was carried out in four cases. Johns Hopkins Hosp Bull 1905;16:315–321.

3. Millin T. Retropubic Urinary Surgery. Baltimore: Williams and Wilkins, 1947.

4. Ansell JS. Radical transvesical prostatectomy: preliminary report on an approach to surgical excision of localized prostate malignancy. J Urol 1959;82:373–374.

5. Campbell EW. Total prostatectomy with preliminary ligation of the vascular pedicle. J Urol 1959;81:464–467.

6. Chute R. Radical retropubic prostatectomy for cancer. J Urol 1954;71:347–372.

7. Lich R, Grant O, Maurer JE. Extravesical prostatectomy: a comparison of retropubic and perineal prostatectomy. J Urol 1949;61:930.

8. Memmelaar J. Total prostatovesiculectomy: retropubic approach. J Urol 1949;62:349.

9. Reiner WG, Walsh PC. An anatomical approach to the surgical management of the dorsal vein and Santorini's plexus during radical retropubic surgery. J Urol 1979;121:198–200.

10. Walsh PC. Anatomic radical prostatectomy: evolution of the surgical technique. J Urol 1998;160:2418–2424.

11. Steiner MS, Morton RA, Walsh PC. Impact of anatomical radical prostatectomy on urinary continence. J Urol 1991;145:512–514; discussion 514–515.

12. Walsh PC, Quinlan DM, Morton RA, et al. Radical retropubic prostatectomy. Improved anastomosis and urinary continence. Urol Clin North Am 1990;17:679–684.

13. Walsh PC, Marschke P, Ricker D, et al. Patient-reported urinary continence and sexual function after anatomic radical prostatectomy. Urology 2000;55:58–61.

14. Oelrich TM. The urethral sphincter muscle in the male. Am J Anat 1980;158:229–246.

15. Khan MA, Mangold LA, Epstein JI, et al. Impact of surgical delay on long-term cancer control for clinically localized prostate cancer. J Urol 2004;172:1835–1839.

16. Nash PA, Schrepferman CG, Rowland RG, et al. The impact of pre-donated autologous blood and intra-operative isovolaemic haemodilution on the outcome of transfusion in patients undergoing radical retropubic prostatectomy. Br J Urol 1996;77:856–860.

17. Peters CA, Walsh PC. Blood transfusion and anesthetic practices in radical retropubic prostatectomy. J Urol 1985;134:81–83.

18. Goldschlag B, Afzal N, Carter HB, et al. Is preoperative donation of autologous blood rational for radical retropubic prostatectomy? J Urol 2000;164:1968–1972.

19. Goh M, Kleer CG, Kielczewski P, et al. Autologous blood donation prior to anatomical radical retropubic prostatectomy: is it necessary? Urology 1997;49:569–573, discussion 574.

20. O'Hara JF Jr, Sprung J, Klein EA, et al. Use of preoperative autologous blood donation in patients undergoing radical retropubic prostatectomy. Urology 1999;54:130–134.

21. Koch MO, Smith JA Jr. Blood loss during radical retropubic prostatectomy: is preoperative autologous blood donation indicated? J Urol 1996;156:1077–1079; discussion 1079–1080.

22. Dash A, Dunn RL, Resh J, et al. Patient, surgeon, and treatment characteristics associated with homologous blood transfusion requirement during radical retropubic prostatectomy: multivariate nomogram to assist patient counseling. Urology 2004;64:117–122.

23. Chun TY, Martin S, Lepor H. Preoperative recombinant human erythropoietin injection versus preoperative autologous blood donation in patients undergoing radical retropubic prostatectomy. Urology 1997;50:727–732.

24. Nieder AM, Rosenblum N, et al. Comparison of two different doses of preoperative recombinant erythropoietin in men undergoing radical retropubic prostatectomy. Urology 2001;57:737–741.

25. Rosenblum N, Levine MA, Handler T, et al. The role of preoperative epoetin alfa in men undergoing radical retropubic prostatectomy. J Urol 2000;163:829–833.

26. Salonia A, Crescenti A, Suardi N, et al. General versus spinal anesthesia in patients undergoing radical retropubic prostatectomy: results of a prospective, randomized study. Urology 2004;64:95–100.

27. Shir Y, Raja SN, Frank SM, et al. Intraoperative blood loss during radical retropubic prostatectomy: epidural versus general anesthesia. Urology 1995;45:993–999.

28. Shir Y, Frank SM, Brendler CB, et al. Postoperative morbidity is similar in patients anesthetized with epidural and general anesthesia for radical prostatectomy. Urology 1994;44:232–236.

29. Allaf ME, Palapattu GS, Trock BJ, et al. Anatomical extent of lymph node dissection: impact on men with clinically localized prostate cancer. J Urol 2004;172:1840–1844.

30. Burnett AL, Mostwin JL. In situ anatomical study of the male urethral sphincteric complex: relevance to continence preservation following major pelvic surgery. J Urol 1998;160:1301–1306.

31. Walsh PC, Marschke P, Ricker D, et al. Use of intraoperative video documentation to improve sexual function after radical retropubic prostatectomy. Urology 2000;55:62–67.

32. Ong AM, Su LM, Varkarakis I, et al. Nerve sparing radical prostatectomy: effects of hemostatic energy sources on the recovery of cavernous nerve function in a canine model. J Urol 2004;172:1318–1322.

33. Rogatsch H, Horninger W, Volgger H, et al. Radical prostatectomy: the value of preoperative, individually labeled apical biopsies. J Urol 2000;164:754–757; discussion 757–758.

34. Walsh PC. Re: Radical prostatectomy: the value of preoperative, individually labeled apical biopsies. J Urol 2001;165:915.

35. Wei JT, Dunn RL, Marcovich R, et al. Prospective assessment of patient reported urinary continence after radical prostatectomy. J Urol 2000;164:744–748.

36. Walsh PC. Nerve grafts are rarely necessary and are unlikely to improve sexual function in men undergoing anatomic radical prostatectomy. Urology 2001;57:1020–1024.

37. Walsh PC, Marschke PL. Intussusception of the reconstructed bladder neck leads to earlier continence after radical prostatectomy. Urology 2002;59:934–938.

Radical retropubic prostatectomy: contemporary modifications

73

Murugesan Manoharan, Mark Soloway

INTRODUCTION

Retropubic radical prostatectomy (RRP) was first described by Millin in 1947,[1] but never gained popularity because of significant morbidity and mortality. This trend changed following the description of the anatomic retropubic prostatectomy by Walsh.[2] In the past two decades, it has become one of the most common oncologic procedures performed in the US.[3] Better understanding of the structural and functional anatomy of the pelvic floor, including the cavernosal nerves, dorsal venous complex, sphincter muscles, and puboprostatic ligaments has led to several modifications which result in better oncologic and functional outcome with a dramatic reduction in perioperative morbidity. This chapter summarizes various contemporary modifications to RRP.

MODIFIED PFANNENSTEIL APPROACH

RRP is traditionally performed using a vertical midline incision. However, a transverse Pfannensteil incision[4] is commonly used by gynecologists for a variety of pelvic procedures. We have modified this incision,[5] and over the past 2 years have performed every RRPs using a modified Pfannensteil approach that provides excellent exposure and better cosmetic results than a vertical incision.

SURGICAL TECHNIQUE

The patient is placed in a supine position with the antero-superior iliac spine at the level of the kidney bridge. The bridge is raised and the operating table flexed to provide better access to the pelvis. A transverse curvilinear incision, approximately 8- to 10-cm long, is made along the pubic hairline centered over the pubic symphysis (Fig. 73.1A). The superficial and deep fasciae are divided along the line of the skin incision to the level of the rectus sheath.

A V-shaped incision is initially made in the rectus sheath, with the midpoint of the V situated 2 cm above the symphysis pubis (Fig. 73.1B). The limbs of the V are directed superiorly and laterally at a 30° angle to the skin incision. This avoids entering the inguinal canal inadvertently. The rectus sheath is opened on either side up to the lateral border of the rectus muscle.

The superior leaflet of the rectus sheath is reflected off the rectus muscle for a distance of 3 to 4 cm. To achieve

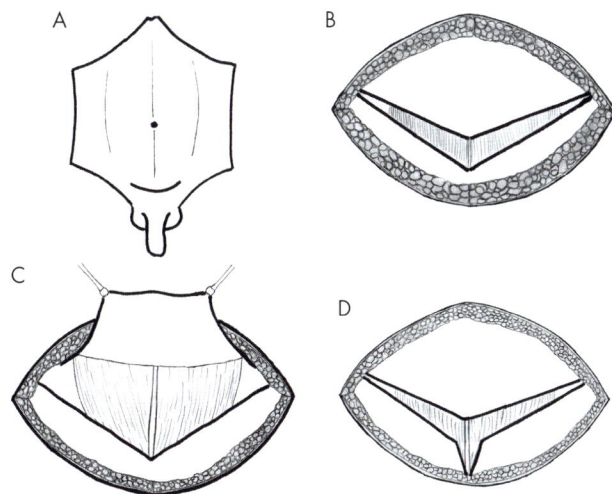

Fig. 73.1
A, Skin incision. *B*, V-shaped incision of rectus sheath.
C, Reflection of superior leaflet of rectus sheath. *D*, V to Y conversion of rectus sheath incision.

this, two Allis clamps are applied to the superior leaflet of the rectus sheath on either side of the midline, and gentle traction is exerted. The rectus sheath is connected to the rectus muscle only by loose areolar tissue laterally and fibrous tissue along the midline. This is separated easily by a combination of blunt dissection and electrocautery (Fig. 73.1C). A few small branches of the inferior epigastric artery pierce the rectus muscle and supply the rectus sheath. These should be identified and cauterized, because they may be avulsed easily and retract into the rectus muscle, possibly leading to a rectus hematoma.

The V incision is converted to a Y incision by making a vertical incision on the inferior leaflet of the rectus sheath along the midline up to the pubic symphysis (Fig. 73.1D). It is not necessary to reflect the inferior leaflet of the rectus sheath off the rectus muscle.

The rectus and pyramidalis muscles are then exposed and are separated in the midline. The transversalis fascia is incised close to the pubis, and the retropubic space of Retzius is entered. By gentle blunt dissection, the peritoneum is mobilized superiorly from the pelvis. A Buckwalter self-retaining retractor is used to expose the wound. Two lateral blades are applied over the rectus muscle to retract the wound laterally. A small Richardson retractor is placed inferiorly to retract the skin and fatty tissue. A 16-F Foley catheter is inserted into the bladder, and the balloon inflated with 30 ml of water. The grooved Holtgrewe-Yu retractor is applied over the balloon, and the bladder neck is retracted superiorly (Fig. 73.2A). This provides excellent exposure of the prostate. A standard RRP is performed. The transverse incision provides excellent exposure for a pelvic lymph node dissection. A malleable retractor is fitted to the Buckwalter frame to retract the bladder and facilitate exposure of the external iliac vessels and pelvic lymph nodes.

After completion of the RRP, the rectus muscle is approximated with absorbable suture. The rectus sheath is closed with a 0 Vicryl suture. The subcutaneous layers are closed with 3-0 chromic catgut. The skin is closed with a 4-0 Monocryl subcuticular technique (Fig. 73.2B).

This incision is well accepted by patients because of the better cosmetic results and wound healing. We have performed more than 200 consecutive RRPs using this approach. The exposure is not dependent on the patient's body habitus. This incision provides excellent access to the inguinal canal. Five to 10% of patients with clinically localized prostate cancer have a detectable inguinal hernia. The modified Pfannensteil approach allows for concurrent mesh repair of the inguinal hernia without the need for a separate incision.[6]

ANESTHESIA AND ANALGESICS

The administration of analgesia prior to a painful stimulus reduces short- and long-term analgesic requirements and permits earlier resumption of normal

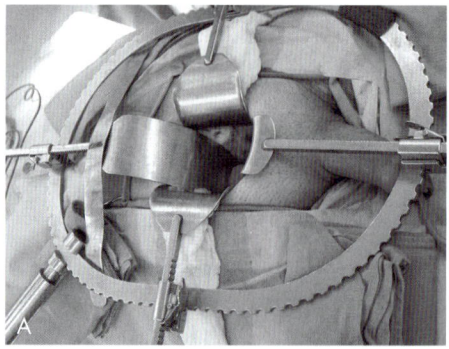
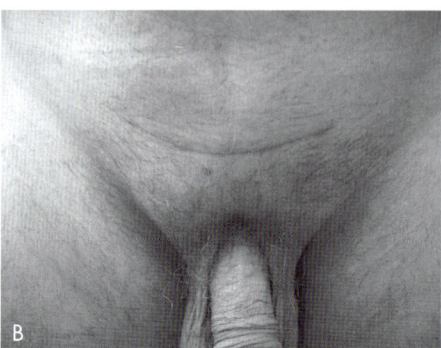

Fig. 73.2
A, Wound exposure with self-retaining Buckwalter retractor. *B*, Healed incision.

activities.[7] Such "preemptive" analgesia may act via a reduction in central nervous system sensitization before the nociceptive input.

In a prospective randomized trial, Gottschalk et al[8] showed that preoperative epidural analgesia significantly decreased postoperative pain during hospitalization and long after discharge in patients undergoing radical prostatectomy. RRP has been successfully performed under epidural anesthesia in many centers. However, intrathecal administration of the anesthetic has some advantages over epidural anesthesia.[7,9] It allows faster onset of action and is technically easier than epidural anesthesia.[9] Failure rates of 2% to 5% have been reported for epidural administration of analgesia due to misplacement of the epidural catheter. In addition, intrathecal administration of opioids is less expensive than epidural analgesia when drug costs, delivery tubing, and administration trays are considered.[7,10]

In a retrospective analysis of factors affecting length of stay after radical prostatectomy, Gardner et al[11] showed that patients receiving epidural analgesia combined with general anesthesia had longer hospital stays compared to those not receiving epidural analgesia. This was believed to be the result of delayed ambulation and prolonged administration of epidural analgesia. Such factors are eliminated with a single preoperative dose of intrathecal opioid.

The safety of intrathecal opioids has been confirmed by Gwirtz et al,[10] who reported a series of approximately 6000 patients who received intrathecal morphine immediately following a variety of operative procedures. The efficacy of preoperative intrathecal morphine for reducing pain after radical prostatectomy has been evaluated by Eandi et al.[7] In a retrospective study of 62 patients who received a single dose of intrathecal morphine sulfate prior to RRP, 45% did not require postoperative narcotics and 95% were satisfied with their postoperative pain control. Mean hospital stay was 2.3 ± 0.3 days and patients resumed normal activities by a mean of 5.3 weeks after surgery.

In a prospective study involving 103 patients, Sved et al[12] demonstrated that RRP can be performed safely with spinal anesthesia and a single dose of intrathecal long-acting morphine. In their series, the mean times to tolerate oral fluids and unassisted ambulation were 11 and 20 h, respectively. Forty-three percent of patients were discharged on the first postoperative day and mean length of stay was 37.5 ± 11.8 h. The average narcotic requirements were 7.4 morphine equivalents (ME) prior to discharge and 28.1 ME in the first week after discharge. Mean visual analog pain score was 4.47 at the time of discharge and fell significantly to 1.6 by the time of catheter removal on postoperative day 7 to 8.

It is recommended that, whenever feasible, the RRP be performed under spinal anesthesia and intrathecal opioids. This provides better pain control and early ambulation of the patient.

SURGICAL TECHNIQUES FOR IMPROVED CONTINENCE

Continence rates following RRP range from 85% to 100% depending on subtle differences in surgical technique.[13–16] In 1982, Walsh and Donker[17] described the anatomic or nerve-sparing RRP with early control of the dorsal vein complex, careful apical dissection, precise urethral–vesical anastomosis, and preservation of the neurovascular bundles. Since then, many modifications have been described to improve post-prostatectomy continence further, including bladder neck preservation, meticulous dissection of the rhabdosphincter, puboprostatic ligament preservation, and maximal urethral preservation with dissection within the prostate to maintain the integrity of the proximal continence mechanism (posterior urethral segment sparing technique).

The puboprostatic "complex" consists of three components. The *pyramidal portion* (also called the puboprostatic ligament) lies between the base of the prostate and the pubic symphysis, and extends laterally into the endopelvic fascia that covers the lateral pelvic muscles (levator ani, internal obturator) constituting the dense medial part of the endopelvic fascia. The *dorsal vein complex* (Santorini plexus) lies below the first portion and behind the pubic symphysis in the retropubic fat, and is separated from the prostate by

fibromuscular and soft connective tissue. The *fibromuscular and soft connective tissue* attach the prostate to the pubic arch in the median plane, forming the intermediate pubourethral ligament that inserts at the anterior commissure of the prostate, the isthmus prostate. The anterior urethral ligament and the urethra lie at the distal margin of this third portion.

Preservation of the distal striated sphincter is the most critical aspect for maintaining urinary continence following RRP.[18,19] In addition, supporting structures of the external striated urethral sphincter, such as the puboprostatic ligaments, may play a role in normal continence by maintaining the normal position of the urethra in the pelvic floor.[15,20] This is the anatomic principle underlying the placement of the suture that ligates the dorsal vein to the symphysis pubis[21] or the preservation of the supporting puboprostatic ligaments.[15]

Complete cancer removal remains the goal of RRP and modifications in the surgical technique should not compromise the pathologic outcome. It is conceivable that by preserving the bladder neck, cancer at the base of the prostate may be left behind with increased incidence of positive margin rates. On a similar note, puboprostatic ligament sparing not only makes the ligation of the Santorini venous plexus difficult, but might also leave the apical prostatic tissue behind with a high incidence of positive apical surgical margin rate. Myers et al[19] demonstrated that the posterior lip of the prostate extends more caudally and an inappropriate urethral dissection might result in dissection through the posterior prostatic tissue at the level of the prostatic apex. In addition, the risk of positive margins exists anteriorly during the dissection between the dorsal vein complex and the prostate.[14]

Maintenance of the integrity of the external striated muscle urethral sphincter and its attachments is of paramount importance for continence. Presti et al[22] demonstrated that continence rates correlate with the mean functional urethral length and maximal urethral closure pressure following RRP. Sphincteric integrity of the pelvic floor has been found to be more important for continence than retubularization of the bladder neck.[19] It is, therefore, very important to preserve, as far as possible, the integrity of the periurethral tissues that form the posterior urethral plate.

BLADDER NECK PRESERVATION

The so-called "bladder neck preservation" technique involves careful sharp and blunt dissection between the circular fibers of the bladder neck and base of the prostate.[13,23] Deliveliotis et al,[18] Braslis et al,[24] Lowe,[25] Gaker et al,[26] and Klein[27] reported improved early (3–6 months) continence rates following bladder neck preservation, and suggested that the early return of continence is the result of the added passive outlet resistance from the unaltered bladder neck. The reported continence rates are variable and may be due to the differing definitions of continence.[4,13] Following the initial period, the external sphincter becomes stronger and recovers from the surgery, playing a more important role in continence and, therefore, masking the effect of the bladder neck preservation. At 9 and 12 months most patients have similar excellent continence rates whether the bladder neck has been preserved or not.

Deliveliotis et al[18] reported similar cancer control rates in terms of positive margins following bladder neck preservation (21%), puboprostatic ligament sparing (18%), and both (22%) in patients with a final Gleason score of greater than 7, similar to the rates reported by Braslis et al[24] in patients with a prostate-specific antigen (PSA) level of less than 10 ng/ml. Bladder neck dissection could have avoided positive margins in 5 of 149 (3%) patients. In contrast, Srougi et al[16] demonstrated in a randomized, prospective study that, although the positive margin rates were similar following bladder neck preservation or wide bladder neck resection, margins were positive only at the bladder neck in 10% of the preservation group, whereas no patients in the bladder neck resection group had a positive bladder neck margin.

Bladder neck preservation avoids the need for bladder neck reconstruction and mucosal eversion, and in our experience reduces the incidence of vesicourethral anastomotic strictures.[13] However, care should be exercised in using this modification in patients with high volume, high-grade cancers at the base of the prostate. Bianco et al[28] found positive margins at the apex and bladder neck in 104 (19%) and 13 (2%) patients, respectively, of 555 patients. Of those with a positive bladder neck margin, eight had a Gleason score of 7 or greater, three had seminal vesicle invasion, and two had nodal disease. Only two patients had a positive bladder neck margin as the sole adverse pathologic feature. Significant independent predictors of survival in their study included Gleason score, PSA, pathologic stage, and presence of positive margins in more than one location. Marcovich et al[29] reported that bladder neck preservation can be associated with an increased rate of positive surgical margins in a pT3A cancer subset with focal penetration through the prostatic capsule, with an associated trend toward decreased PSA-free survival.

PUBOPROSTATIC LIGAMENT PRESERVATION

Puboprostatic ligament (PL) preservation during RRP entails division of the ligaments adjacent to the prostate rather than the pubis, and is believed to preserve the tissues that provide support to the proximal urethra and striated sphincter complex.[14,15]

Poore et al[14] reported earlier return of continence following PL-sparing prostatectomy. However, final outcome was similar to non–PL-sparing techniques. Deliveliotis et al[18] did not find any advantage with the PL-sparing prostatectomy, and the discrepancies can be attributed to the definition of continence (no need for pads[14] vs use of one pad daily[17]). Noh et al[3] demonstrated that mean time to recovery of continence was similar for bladder reconstruction (2.3 months) and bladder neck preservation (2.9 months) but was significantly longer (P = <0.05) for bladder neck and PL preservation (4.3 months). None of their patients had "bladder neck-only positive margins," although 9% had positive margins.

It remains unclear whether PL preservation improves the continence both in the short- and long-term.

POSTERIOR URETRHAL SPARING TECHNIQUE

Urethral length at the time of anastomosis has been shown to correlate with continence rates.[30,31] The modified technique of RRP with urethral preservation entails preservation of 1 to 1.5 cm of the posterior urethra, which should be circumferentially intact. Proximal urethral dissection is performed at the time of bladder neck preservation. The tissue plane between the bladder base and prostate is identified, and the proximal urethra is carefully separated from the prostate by blunt dissection. Exposure to the area of dissection is the primary challenge, as the surrounding prostate limits visualization. The preserved urethra includes mucosa and immediate periurethral tissue for 1 to 1.5 cm distal to the bladder neck. Splitting of the anterior fibromuscular septum of the prostate allows direct visualization of the prostatic urethra with an improved angle of dissection. Using this technique, Tongco et al[32] demonstrated positive margins in 5 of 12 (41.66%) patients with a PSA greater than 10 ng/ml and/or a Gleason score of greater than 7. They found residual prostate adenoma on the dissected urethral specimens. Gaker et al[26] performed true urethra-urethrostomy in 24 patients, sparing the distal urethra to the level of the verumontanum by blunt dissection of the apical urethra from the surrounding prostatic tissue. Proximal urethral dissection was performed to the proximal verumontanum (average length, 2.0 cm), sparing the prostatic and periurethral musculature. Two of the 24 patients had positive margins, but none of the urethral biopsies had benign or malignant prostatic tissue. Eighty-three percent of patients were continent by 7 weeks following prostatectomy. There were no anastomotic complications.

There is no unequivocal evidence that this technique improves continence rates significantly. There are no large series to confirm the long-term benefits and oncologic safety of this technique and hence this technique is not recommended at present.

In conclusion, 1-year continence rates after bladder neck preservation and/or PL sparing do not differ. Using strict continence definition criteria, bladder neck preservation achieves earlier return to continence. PL preservation has been found to be associated with slower recovery of continence and does not alter the long-term continence rates. Bladder neck sparing can safely be performed to obtain earlier return to continence without compromising cancer control. Bladder neck preservation further improves morbidity with fewer incidences of anastomotic strictures.

OTHER MODIFICATIONS

ROLE OF PELVIC DRAIN

Though it is a common practice to drain the pelvis following a RRP, Savoie et al[33] reported that routine drainage of the pelvis is not required in all cases. In their series, after the RRP was performed and the anastomotic sutures were tied, the bladder was filled with saline through the urethral catheter. If there was no significant leakage, a drain was not placed (73% of 116 consecutive patients who underwent RRP). None had clinical evidence of lymphocele, hematoma or infection. One patient developed an urinoma that required percutaneous drainage without any sequelae. We have performed 397 consecutive radical prostatectomies in the past 3 years and have not placed a drain in 76% of these, with excellent outcome.

If the bladder neck is preserved or meticulously reconstructed, there may be little or no extravasation and, thus, routine drainage may be unnecessary. Moreover, studies from other specialties have demonstrated several disadvantages associated with wound drains, including drain site pain, retained drains, infection, and cost.[34] In properly selected cases, morbidity is not increased by omitting a drain from the pelvic cavity after RRP.

BLOOD TRANSFUSION AND CELL SAVER

Transfusion rates during RRP have decreased steadily over the past several years as increasing surgeon skill and familiarity with the operation have reduced estimated blood loss (EBL). An analysis of the Department of Defense Center for Prostate Disease Research Multicenter National Research Database of 2918 patients undergoing radical prostatectomy showed statistically significant decreases in the median EBL (from 1800 to 800 ml), rates of preoperative blood donation (from 81.7% to 10.9%), and transfusion rates (from 93.2% to 13.7%) from 1985 to 2000.[35] Other recent studies have reported homologous blood transfusion rates of 4.6%, 7.1%, and 9.7%.[36-38] Thus, although the likelihood of a patient receiving blood is relatively low, the risk is still present.

Different means of managing blood loss include preoperative donation of autologous blood, preoperative recombinant erythropoeitin injection, intraoperative hemodilution, allogenic blood transfusion, and intraoperative cell salvage (IOCS). IOCS, commonly referred to as "cell saver," is an attractive blood management strategy since it is relatively inexpensive, obviates a trip to the blood bank, and prevents the risks associated with allogeneic blood transfusion, such as viral infection.

Many oncologic surgeons have been reluctant to utilize IOCS because of the theoretical risk of tumor dissemination. Davis et al[39] published our institutional experience with IOCS between 1992 and 1998 and reported no short-term increased risk of biochemical recurrence among 408 patients. We further evaluated 1038 patients from our database and there was no significant difference in the biochemical recurrence rate between those who did and those who did not receive cell salvaged blood. Further stratification of our patients according to low, intermediate, and high risk did not demonstrate any significant differences in the biochemical recurrence rate between the cohorts.[40]

The use of IOCS is a safe and valuable technique of blood management for patients undergoing RRP and decreases the need for allogenic transfusion.

INSTRUMENTATION

Various advances in the field of medical instrumentation have facilitated the ease of performing RRP and improved outcome. Several surgeons routinely use magnifying optical loupes and headlight to improve the visualization and dissection of the apex of the prostate and neurovascular bundle.[41] We use 2.5X loupes but do not routinely use headlights.

Devices such as Ligasure and vascular staplers have been reported to facilitate the dorsal venous complex control.[42] These devices, however, have not gained widespread acceptance as most surgeons are comfortable with suture ligation of the dorsal venous complex. The harmonic scalpel is another useful device that can be used to secure the vascular pedicles of the prostate. We routinely use this device and find it reliable.

CONCLUSION

With the perceived benefits of reduced postoperative morbidity, earlier return to normal activity, and improved cosmesis, minimally invasive surgical options for localized prostate cancer, such as laparoscopic radical prostatectomy (LRP) and robot-assisted prostatectomy (RAP) have gained popularity in recent years. However, these procedures are expensive and technically difficult, with a steep learning curve. The total operating time is usually longer than with a standard RRP. Moreover, these technologies are not available universally and many centers cannot afford them.

On the other hand, simple modifications to the standard RRP (Table 73.1) have resulted in dramatic improvement in patient outcome without any significant increase in cost. These modifications can be easily adapted by urologists, both in the community and in referral centers.

The contemporary RRP offers a viable alternative treatment option to the expensive and technically challenging minimally invasive procedures.

Table 73.1 "University of Miami approach" to retropubic radical prostatectomy.

- Spinal anesthesia and intrathecal long-acting morphine ± laryngeal mask

- Intermittent compression device prior to induction, no routine use of heparin or heparinoid prophylaxis

- Intraoperative cell salvage (IOCS) system and salvaged red cells transfused as required

- Supine position, bridge elevated at the level of the anterior superior iliac spine and the table is flexed to provide better exposure to the pelvis

- Modified Pfannensteil incision, Buckwalter retractor to expose the wound

- Bilateral pelvic lymph node dissection performed routinely, but not obligatory

- Standard retropubic prostatectomy, preservation of neurovascular bundles, bladder neck preservation, no routine mucosal eversion

- Pelvic drain not routinely used

- Early mobilization and routine discharge from the hospital within 36–48 h

- Foley catheter for 7 days, no routine cystogram prior to removal of the catheter

---

REFERENCES

1. Millin T. Retropubic Urinary Surgery. London: Livingstone, 1947.

2. Walsh PC. Radical prostatectomy for the treatment of localized prostatic carcinoma. Urol Clin North Am 1980;3:583–591.

3. Noh C, Kshirsagar A, Mohler JL. Outcome after radical retropubic prostatectomy. Urology 2003;61:412–416.

4. Griffiths DA. A reappraisal of the Pfannensteil incision. BJU Int 1976; 48: 469–474.

5. Manoharan M, Gomez P, Sved P, Soloway MS. Modified Pfannensteil approach for radical retropubic prostatectomy. Urology 2004;64:369–371.

6. Manoharan M, Gomez P, Soloway MS. Concurrent radical retropubic prostatectomy and inguinal hernia repair through a modified Pfannensteil incision. BJU Int 2004;93:1203–1206.

7. Eandi JA, de Vere White RW, Tunuguntla HS, et al. Can single dose preoperative intrathecal morphine sulfate provide cost-effective postoperative analgesia and patient satisfaction during radical prostatectomy in the current era of cost containment. Pros Can Pros Dis 2002;5:226–230.

8. Gottschalk A, Smith DS, Jobes DR, et al. Preemptive epidural analgesia and recovery from radical prostatectomy. JAMA 1998;279:1076–1082.

9. Stoelting RK. Intrathecal morphine: an understood combination for postoperative pain management. Anesth Analg 1989;68:707–709.

10. Gwirtz KH, Young JV, Byers RS, et al. The safety and efficacy of intrathecal opioid analgesia for acute postoperative pain: Seven years' experience with 5969 surgical patients at Indiana University Hospital. Anesth Analg 1999;88:599–604.

11. Gardner TA, Bissonette EA, Petroni GR, et al. Surgical and postoperative factors affecting length of stay after radical prostatectomy. Cancer 2000;89:424–430.

12. Sved PD, Nieder AM, Manoharan M, et al. Evaluation of analgesic requirements and postoperative recovery after radical retropubic prostatectomy using long-acting spinal anesthesia. Uroloy 2005;65:509–512.

13. Shelfo SW, Obek C, Soloway M. Update on bladder neck preservation during radical retropubic prostatectomy: impact on pathologic outcome, anastomotic strictures, and continence. Urology 1998;51:73–78.

14. Poore RE, McCullough DL, Jarow JP. Puboprostatic ligament sparing improves urinary continence after radical retropubic prostatectomy. Urology 1998;51:67–72.

15. Jarow JP. Puboprostatic ligament sparing radical retropubic prostatectomy. Semin Urol Oncol 2000;18:28–32.

16. Srougi M, Nesrallah LJ, Kauffmann JR, et al. Urinary continence and pathological outcome after bladder neck preservation during radical retropubic prostatectomy: a randomized prospective trial. J Urol 2001;165:815–818.

17. Walsh PC, Donker PJ. Impotence following radical prostatectomy: insight into etiology and prevention. J Urol 1982;128:492–497.

18. Deliveliotis C, Protogerou V, Alargof E, Varkarakis J. Radical prostatectomy: bladder neck preservation and puboprostatic ligament sparing-effects on continence and positive margins. Urology 2002;60:855–858.

19. Myers RP. Male urethral sphincgteric anatomy and radical prostatectomy. Urol Clin North Am 1991;18:211–227.

20. Steiner MS. Anatomic basis for the continence-preserving radical retropubic prostatectomy. Semin Urol Oncol 2000;18:9–18.

21. Eastham JA, Kattan MW, Rogers E, et al. Risk factors for urinary incontinence after radical prostatectomy. J Urol 1996;156:1707–1713.

22. Presti JC Jr, Schmidt RA, Narayan PA, et al. Pathophysiology of urinary incontinence after radical prostatectomy. J Urol 1990;143:975–978.

23. Soloway MS, Neulander E. Bladder-neck preservation during radical retropubic prostatectomy. Semin Urol Oncol 2000;18:51–56.

24. Braslis KG, Petsch M, Lim A, et al. Bladder neck preservation following radical prostatectomy: continence and margins. Eur Urol 1995;28:202–208.

25. Lowe BA. Comparison of bladder neck preservation to bladder neck resection in maintaining postprostatectomy urinary incontinence. Urology 1996;48:889–893.

26. Gaker DL, Gaker LB, Stewart JF, et al. Radical prostatectomy with preservation of urinary continence. J Urol 1996;156:445–449.

27. Klein EA. Early continence after radical prostatectomy. J Urol 1992;148:92–95.

28. Bianco FJ Jr, Grignon DJ, Sakr WA, et al. Radical prostatectomy with bladder neck preservation: impact on positive margins. Eur Urol 2003;43:461–466.

29. Marcovich R, Wojno KJ, Wei JT, Rubin MA, Montie JE, Sanda MG. Bladder neck-sparing modification of radical prostatectomy adversely affects surgical margins in pathologic T3a prostate cancer. Urology 2000;55:904–908.

30. Levy JB, Seay TM, Wein AJ. Postprostatectomy incontinence. In Ball TP (ed): AUA Update Series, vol XV, Lesson 8. Houston: American Urologic Association, 1996.

31. McGuire EJ. Urethral sphincter mechanisms. Urol Clin North Am 1979;6:39–49.

32. Tongco WP, Wehner MS, Basler JW. Does urethral-sparing prostatectomy risk residual prostate cancer? Urology 2001;57:495–498.

33. Savoie M, Soloway MS, Kim SS, Monoharan M. A pelvic drain may be avoided after radical retropubic prostatectomy. J Urol 2003;170:112–114.

34. Scott H, Brown AC. Is routine drainage of pelvic anastomosis necessary? Am Surg 1996;62:452–457.

35. Moul JW, Sun L, Wu H, et al. Factors associated with blood loss during radical prostatectomy for localized prostate cancer in the prostate-specific antigen (PSA)-era: an overview of the Department of Defence (DOD) Center for Prostate Disease Research (CPDR) national database. Urol Oncol 2003;21:447–455.

36. Lepor H, Kaci L. Contemporary evaluation of operative parameters and complications related to open radical retropubic prostatectomy. Urology 2003;62:702–706.

37. Nuttall GA, Cragum MD, Hill DL, et al. Radical retropubic prostatectomy and blood transfusion. Mayo Clin Proc 2002;77:1301–1305.

38. Lepor H, Nieder AM, Ferrandino MN. Intraoperative and postoperative complications of radical retropubic prostatectomy in a conservative series of 1,000 cases. J Urol 2001;166:1729–1733.

39. Davis M, Sofer M, Gomez-Marin O, Bruck D, Soloway MS. The use of cell salvage during radical retropubic prostatectomy: does it influence cancer recurrence? BJU Int 2003;91:474–476.

40. Nieder AM, Manoharan M, Soloway MS, et al. Intraoperative cell salvage during radical prostatectomy is not associated with greater biochemical recurrence. Urology 2005;65:730–734.

41. Altwein JE. Enhancing the efficacy of radical prostatectomy in locally advanced prostate cancer. Urol Int 1998;60(Suppl):2–10.

42. Daskalopoulos G, Karyotis I, Heretis I, Delakas D. Electrothermal bipolar coagulation for radical prostatectomies and cystectomies: a preliminary case-controlled study. Int Urol Nephrol 2004;36:181-185.

Role of lymphadenectomy in prostate cancer 74

Fiona C Burkhard, Martin Schumacher, Natalie Tschan, Urs E Studer

INTRODUCTION

When and to what extent lymphadenectomy should be performed in patients undergoing radical prostatectomy remains a matter of intense debate. Lymphadenectomy provides important information for prognosis (number of nodes involved, tumor volume, capsular perforation) that is not matched by any other procedures. Whether, in addition, a potential therapeutic effect of extended lymph node dissection with removal of all diseased nodes can be expected has still not been fully documented, due to the relatively benign course of this disease. In contrast, in other malignancies such as gastric, breast, colorectal, and cervical cancer, and in recent years also bladder cancer, it has become apparent that survival and accuracy of staging improve with the number of nodes removed and therefore the extent of lymph node dissection.[1–6]

PELVIC LYMPHADENECTOMY AS A STAGING PROCEDURE

Precise tumor staging is the basis for optimal therapeutic management. In prostate cancer the availability of biochemical markers and preoperative biopsies allows a differentiated staging. Based on these, nomograms have been developed to help decide which patients will benefit from pelvic lymphadenectomy and in which it can be avoided.[7] To date all nomograms are based on standard lymph node dissection and with the increasing awareness of possible lymph node metastasis outside the region of standard dissection, these nomograms may prove increasingly inadequate.

Classic imaging modalities, such as computerized tomography (CT) and magnetic resonance imaging (MRI), are relatively insensitive for the detection of lymph node metastasis in the pelvis and are of no value in deciding therapeutic strategies.[8–10] Newer developments such as sentinel node lymphoscintigraphy with gamma probe detection and high-resolution MRI with magnetic nanoparticles are emerging. If these are only a slight improvement over available methods or are truly of advantage with high sensitivity and specificity remains to be determined. For the time being, a meticulous pelvic lymph node dissection remains the most accurate and cost-efficient solution, requiring only minor additional surgical time.

Lymphatic drainage from the prostate shows large variability, with sentinel nodes found mainly along the external iliac vein, in the obturator fossa, or along the internal iliac vessels.[11] Single sentinel nodes have not been identified. For this reason, dissection should include all primary drainage areas from the diseased organ (Figs 74.1 and 74.2). Accordingly, the boundaries for extended lymphadenectomy are: laterally, the upper limit of the external iliac vein (leaving the periarteric tissue untouched); distally, the femoral canal; proximally, the bifurcation of the common iliac artery; medially, the side wall of the bladder; and inferiorly, the floor of the obturator fossa and the internal iliac (hypogastric) vessels. Tissue medial to the internal iliac artery should be included, which some may describe as the presacral/pararectal area.

With these templates in our series at the University of Bern a median of 21 (range 6–50) nodes were removed in 365 patients with prostate cancer.[12] The number of removed nodes corresponds well with the

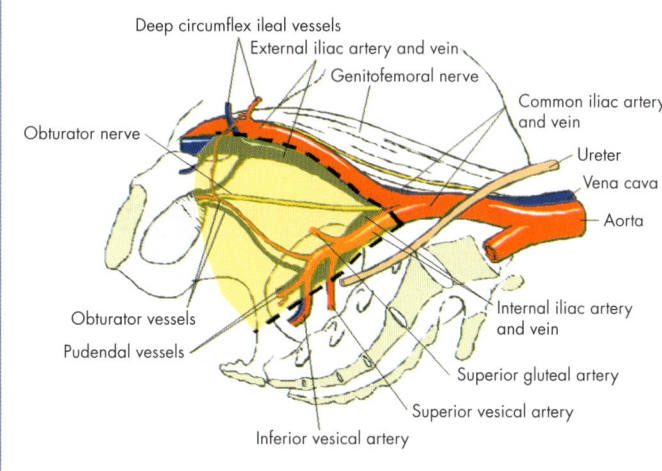

Fig. 74.1

Boundaries of extended lymph node dissection and subdivision into three different locations, including the external iliac vein, obturator fossa, and internal iliac artery. Note that tissue medial to the internal iliac artery is also removed.

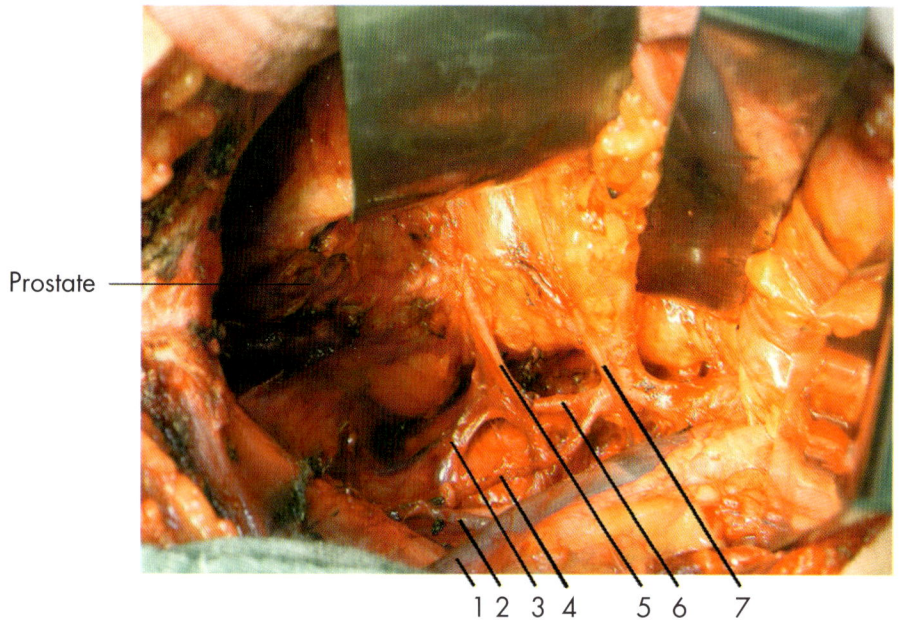

1. External iliac vein
2. Obturator vein
3. Pudendal vessels
4. Obturator artery
5. Inferior vesical artery
6. Internal iliac artery
7. Superior vesical artery

Fig. 74.2

Intraoperative photograph after extended lymph node dissection. The pubis is on the left and the bladder on the right. All tissue has been removed from the external iliac vein, the obturator fossa, and along the internal iliac artery.

results of an anatomic study by Weingaertner et al,[13] who determined that approximately 20 removed lymph nodes can be considered a representative pelvic lymphadenectomy. Stone et al[14] compared 150 patients with modified and 39 with extended laparoscopic lymph node dissection; not only did they find, as to be expected, a significant difference in the number of nodes removed (9.3 vs 17.8 [P = <0.05]), but also three times as many patients with lymph node metastasis (7.3% versus 23.1% [P = 0.02]). This was confirmed by Heidenreich et al[15] in a study comparing a historical control group with standard lymph node dissection (external iliac vein and obturator fossa) and a contemporary group with extended lymph node dissection (external iliac vein, obturator fossa, internal iliac artery, common iliac vessels, and presacral). A median of 11 (6–19) and 28 (21–46) nodes were removed for standard and extended lymph node dissection, respectively. At the same time, the number of patients with diseased nodes increased from 12 of 100 to 27 of 103. The authors concluded that as only three of all the positive nodes were found along the common iliac vessels and in the presacral area, removing lymphatic tissue from these regions could be neglected. In our prospective study of 365 patients undergoing extended lymph node dissection, we detected positive nodes in 24%.[12]

These percentages are significantly higher than the 5% to 10% positive nodes described in other, albeit not necessarily comparable, series without extended lymph node dissection.[16–18] One explanation for the noticeably higher percentage of positive nodes in our series may be that a significant number of nodes were found outside the standard area of dissection and the importance of removing nodes along the internal iliac vessels is becoming increasingly clear. Indeed, when performing extended lymphadenectomy, almost two-thirds of all patients with lymph node metastasis have positive nodes along the internal iliac vessels and approximately one-fifth of these patients have them solely at this location.[12,19] The proportion of patients with positive nodes either exclusively in this area or in combination with another location was 59% in our series and 67% in a series by Tenaglia and Ianucci.[20] Not only would a significant number of patients be understaged if the internal iliac nodes were not removed, but many would also be left with diseased nodes. Considering the fact that many urologists do not remove nodes in this region, this may seem quite astonishing. Despite support from evolving highly sensitive detection techniques for the existence of lymph node metastasis outside the standard area of dissection, controversy still persists concerning the extent of dissection.

A study by Clark et al[21] appears to support those who consider standard dissection to be adequate. They performed a randomized prospective evaluation of extended versus limited lymph node dissection in 100 patients with clinically localized prostate cancer and found no difference between these two groups concerning metastatic disease. However, they did describe a significantly higher rate of complications after extended versus lymph node dissection in 123. This study, although addressing an important subject, does have some limitations, which may explain why the findings are in contrast to most other studies. The number of patients is too small to test for equivalence. In the low-risk patient groups, the majority would not have required lymph node dissection, which further limits the power of the trial. In addition, the researchers randomly assigned patients to extended lymph-adenectomy on one side only, independent of tumor localization, thus introducing a large risk of lymph node dissection on the non–tumor-bearing side. They also did not define the pathologic work-up or the number of nodes removed.

COMPLICATIONS OF LYMPH NODE DISSECTION

The typical complications associated with lymph node dissection are lymphoceles, lymphedema, venous thrombosis, and pulmonary embolism. Reported complication rates for patients with prostate cancer range from 4% to 50%.[22] Clark et al[21] described a total complication rate of 13 of 123 (10.5%) patients, with

75% of complications occurring on the side of extended pelvic lymphadenectomy. Heidenreich et al,[19] however, found no statistical difference concerning intraoperative complications, postoperative complications, blood loss, and lymphocele formation. In our series of 463 patients, the incidence of prolonged hospitalization or rehospitalization attributable to extended lymph node dissection was as low as 2% and only one patient developed persisting lymphedema. We ascribe this low rate of complications to a meticulous surgical technique: 1) ligation, instead of clipping, of all the lymphatics from the lower extremities—hemoclips have a tendency to be torn away during subsequent surgery; 2) placement of two drains instead of one, with one on each side of the pelvis where lymphadenectomy was performed—these are not removed until the total amount drained is less than 50 ml/24 h; and 3) injection of low molecular heparin into the upper arm instead of the thigh.

INDICATION FOR EXTENDED LYMPHADENECTOMY

Is extended lymph node dissection necessary in all patients? In general, we feel that all patients requiring lymph node dissection need extended dissection, including nodes along the internal iliac artery. Many urologists now consider patients with a clinically localized tumor, a prostate-specific antigen (PSA) level of less than 10 ng/ml to be at low risk for metastatic disease. In our series, we found positive nodes in 11% of patients in this low-risk group. Only patients with a PSA of less then 10 ng/ml and a Gleason score less than 6 have a minimal chance of node metastasis.[23] However, as approximately 30% of preoperative biopsies are understaged, it is difficult to recognize this low-risk group with certainty preoperatively. Therefore, we feel that extended lymphadenectomy should be performed in all patients.

POSSIBLE ADVANTAGE OF EXTENDED LYMPHADENECTOMY IN PROSTATE CANCER

Prostate cancer generally has quite a benign course. In contemporary series, the 10-year cancer-specific survival rates are approximately 85% for watchful waiting and 90% to 94% for radical retropubic prostatectomy in patients with clinically localized prostate cancer (Table 74.1). A high rate of biochemical failure has been reported after radical prostatectomy, but the interpretation of biochemical failure remains controversial and may not have an impact on survival in the majority of patients.[24]

Lymph node metastasis, however, does have a negative impact on prognosis. This is not as obvious after 5 years (Table 74.1 vs Table 74.2) as after 10 years, when recurrence/metastasis-free rates (without immediate hormonal therapy) range from 10% to 68%,[25–29] and cancer-specific survival rates from 56% to 62% (Table 74.2).[26,28,30–32] For this reason it is often stated that once patients have node-positive disease, this should be considered systemic and treated accordingly, and that removal of further nodes shows no benefit for the patient. However, there are findings suggesting that in certain patients treatment can be curative even in lymph node-positive prostate cancer. In Catalona et al's[33] relatively small series of 12 patients with minimal lymph node involvement (micrometastasis and only one positive node) and no adjuvant therapy, no tumor was detectable at 5 and 10 years in 75% and 58% of patients, respectively. In Pound et al's[34] in patients with lymph node metastasis found in a 10-year metastasis-free survival rate of 68%,

again without adjuvant therapy. After a 60- and 80-month follow-up, 83% and 68% of patients were free of detectable tumor in Steinberg et al's[28] series of 64 patients. Golimbu et al[35] reported on 42 patients with lymph node metastasis with a mean follow-up of 5 years. Their patients with microscopic metastatic disease or fewer than one positive node had an 85% 5-year and a 50% 10-year survival free of disease. In a more recent series by Bader et al,[26] 74% of patients with only one positive node remained free of tumor progression and only 14% have died to date. Daneshmand et al[37] observed a clinical recurrence-free survival rate of 70% and 73% in patients with one or two positive nodes versus 49% in those with more than five positive nodes. In Steinberg et al's[30] study, the number of positive nodes did not have a significant prognostic value. However, in Frazier et al's[30] series patients with two or fewer positive nodes showed improved cancer-specific survival compared to patients with more than two positive nodes. In our series of 92 patients with lymph node metastasis, time to progression was significantly correlated with the number of positive

Table 74.1 Survival rates following radical retropubic prostatectomy (RRP) for prostate cancer, including patients with positive nodes.

	Number of patients	Median follow-up (years)	Treatment	Projected metastasis-free survival (%)		Projected cancer-specific survival (%)	
				5 years	10 years	5 years	10 years
Jhaveri et al[24]	1132	2.8	RRP	–	–	–	90†
Pound et al[34]	1997	5.3	RRP	–	87	99	94
Han et al[25]	2404	6.3	RRP	84‡	74‡	–	–

*8-year follow-up.

†Overall survival.

‡Recurrence free

Table 74.2 Survival rates in node-positive patients without immediate hormonal therapy

	Number of patients	Median follow-up (years)	Treatment	Metastasis-free survival (%)		Cancer-specific survival (%)	
				5 years	10 years	5 years	10 years
Han et al[25]	135	6.3	RRP	26‡	10‡	–	–
Bader et al[26]	92	3.75	RRP	~50	~25	74	~ 62
Catalona et al[35]	12	≥7	RRP	75	58§	–	–
Steinberg et al[28]	64	3.75	RRP	83	68	97	62
Caddedu et al[33]	19*	5.5	RRP	–	–	93	56
Messing et al[34]	51	10	RRP	–	–	–	57

‡Recurrence free.

§7-year follow-up.

*33% with hormonal therapy, 3% with radiation therapy

nodes.[26] Allaf et al[38] reported a survival difference in men with less than 15% of positive nodes, the 5-year PSA-free survival rate was 43% versus 10% for extended versus limited lymph node dissection, respectively.

In contrast, Dimarco et al[39] detected no survival advantage after extended lymphadenectomy for prostate cancer. In their study, the median number of nodes removed decreased from 14 between 1987 and 1989 to 5 between 1999 and 2000. Interestingly, removing more nodes in the earlier period led to similar results for disease progression and survival as removing fewer nodes in the later period. As T-stage migration is an accepted phenomenon these results may imply that, thanks to the more extended lymphadenectomy, patients with a higher T-stage had comparable survival chances to the more recent population with earlier stage disease.

The need for extended lymphadenectomy is further supported by Di Blasio et al's[40] analysis showing that the number of nodes removed is associated with progression. Removal of 13 nodes had the lowest risk of disease progression, regardless of nodal disease status. Bader et al[38] reported similar findings, with 16%, 12%, 8%, and 8% of patients showing disease progression after removing 0 to 4, 5 to 9, 10 to 14 and more than 14 nodes for pT1/pT2N0 prostate cancer, respectively.

There are few reports concerning the percentage of positive nodes in prostate cancer. In a univariate and multivariate analysis, Steinberg et al[28] found the percentage of positive nodes to have a significant prognostic value. In a series from the John Hopkins Universtiy, 52% of patients with less then 15% positive nodes, Gleason score less than 7, and negative seminal vesicle invasion remained free of progression at 5 years.[38,41] In agreement with this, Daneshmand et al[37] reported that patients with a lymph node density (number of positive nodes removed/total number of removed nodes) of 20% or greater were at higher risk for progression than those with a density of less than 20%.

Overall, there does seem to be a subset of patients with a good chance of asymptomatic long-term survival in the presence of minimal lymph node metastasis (two or fewer positive nodes, low metastatic volume), most likely as a consequence of having the diseased nodes removed.

CONCLUSION

Lymph node dissection remains the only reliable method for exact staging. Extended lymphadenectomy, including tissue along the external iliac vein, obturator fossa, and internal iliac vessels, should be performed in all patients undergoing radical prostatectomy. There is an increasing amount of data suggesting that removal of all diseased nodes that contain minimal metastatic disease may have a positive impact on disease-free and,

perhaps, overall survival. Due to the relatively benign course of prostate cancer, longer follow-up is still necessary before a definitive statement can be made.

REFERENCES

1. Mathiesen O, Carl J, Bonderup O, et al. Axillary sampling and the risk of erroneous staging of breast cancer. An analysis of 960 consecutive patients. Acta Oncol 1990;29:721–725.

2. Siewert JR, Böttcher K, Stein HJ, et al. Relevant prognostic factors in gastric cancer. Ann Surg 1998;228:449–461.

3. Friedberg V. Results of 108 exenteration operations in advanced gynecologic cancers [German]. Geburtshilfe Frauenheilkd 1989;49:423–427.

4. Caplin S, Cerottini JP, Bosman FT, et al. For patients with Duke's B (TNM Stage II) colorectal carcinoma, examination of six or fewer lymph nodes is related to poor prognosis. Cancer 1998;83:666–672.

5. Mills RD, Turner WH, Fleischmann A, et al. Pelvic lymph node metastases from bladder cancer: outcome in 83 patients after radical cystectomy and pelvic lymphadenectomy. J Urol 2001;166:19–23.

6. Leissner J, Hohenfellner R, Thüroff JW, et al. Lymphadenectomy in patients with transitional cell carcinoma of the urinary bladder; significance for staging and prognosis. Br J Urol 2000;85:817–823.

7. Partin AW, Mangold LA, Lamm DM, et al. Contemporary update of prostate cancer staging nomograms (Partin Tables) for the new millennium. Urology 2001;58:843–848.

8. Wolf JS Jr, Cher M, Dall'era M, et al. The use and accuracy of cross-sectional imaging and fine needle aspiration cytology for detection of pelvic lymph node metastases before radical prostatectomy. J Urol 1995;153:993–999.

9. Paik ML, Scolieri MJ, Brown SL, et al. Limitations of computerized tomography in staging invasive bladder cancer before radical cystectomy. J Urol 2000;163:1693–1696.

10. Tempany CM, McNeil BJ. Advances in biomedical imaging. JAMA 2001;285:562–567.

11. Wawroschek F, Vogt H, Wengenmair H, et al. Prostate lymphoscintigraphy and radio-guided surgery for sentinel lymph node identification in prostate cancer. Technique and results of the first 350 cases. Urol Int 2003;70:303–310.

12. Bader P, Burkhard FC, Markwalder R, et al. Is a limited lymph node dissection an adequate staging procedure for prostate cancer? J Urol 2002;168:514–518, discussion 518.

13. Weingaertner K, Ramaswamy A, Bittinger A, et al. Anatomical basis for pelvic lymphadenectomy in prostate cancer: results of an autopsy study and implications for the clinic. J Urol 1996;156:1969–1971.

14. Stone NN, Stock RG, Unger P. Laparoscopic pelvic lymph nodes dissection for prostate cancer: comparison of the extended and modified techniques. J Urol 1997;158:1891–1894.

15. Heidenreich A, Varga Z, Von Knobloch R. Extended pelvic lymphadenectomy in patients undergoing radical prostatectomy: high incidence of lymph node metastasis. J Urol 2002;167:1681–1686.

16. Bluestein DL, Bostwick DG, Bergstralh EJ, et al. Eliminating the need for bilateral pelvic lymphadenectomy in select patients with prostate cancer. J Urol 1994;151:1315–1320.

17. Petros JA, Catalona WJ. Lower incidence of unsuspected lymph node metastases in 521 consecutive patients with clinically localized prostate cancer. J Urol 1992;147:1574–1575.

18. Bishoff JT, Reyes A, Thompson IM, et al. Pelvic lymphadenectomy can be omitted in selected patients with carcinoma of the prostate: development of a system of patient selection. Urology 1995;45:270–274.

19. Heidenreich A, Von Knobloch R, Varga Z, et al. Extended pelvic lymphadenectomy in men undergoing radical retropubic prostatectomy (RRP) — an update on >300 cases. J Urol 2004;171:312 (A1183).

20. Tenaglia JL, Iannucci M. Extended pelvic lymphadenectomy for the treatment of localized prostate carcinoma. Eur Urol Today 2004;15.

21. Clark T, Parekh DJ, Cookson MS, et al. Randomized prospective evaluation of extended versus limited lymph node dissection in

patients with clinically localized prostate cancer. J Urol 2003;169:145–147, discussion 147–148.

22. Link RE, Morton RA: Indications for pelvic lymphadenectomy in prostate cancer. Urol Clin North Am 2001;28:491–498.

23. Burkhard FC, Schumacher M, Thalmann GN, et al. Is pelvic lymphadenectomy really necessary in patients with a serum prostate-specific antigen level of <10 ng/ml undergoing radical prostatectomy for prostate cancer? BJU Int 2005;95:275–278.

24. Jhaveri FM, Zippe CD, Klein EA, et al. Biochemical failure does not predict overall survival after radical prostatectomy for localized prostate cancer: 10-year results. Urology 1999;54:884–890.

25. Han M, Partin AW, Pound CR, et al. Long-term biochemical disease-free and cancer-specific survival following anatomic radical retropubic prostatectomy. The 15-year Johns Hopkins experience. Urol Clin North Am 2001;28:555–565.

26. Bader P, Burkhard FC, Markwalder R, et al. Disease progression and survival of patients with positive lymph nodes after radical prostatectomy. Is there a chance of cure? J Urol 2003;169:849–854.

27. Roehl KA, Han M, Ramos CG, et al. Cancer progression and survival rates following anatomical radical retropubic prostatectomy in 3,478 consecutive patients: long-term results. J Urol 2004;172:910–914.

28. Steinberg GD, Epstein JI, Piantadosi S, et al. Management of stage D1 adenocarcinoma of the prostate: the Johns Hopkins experience 1974 to 1987. J Urol 1990;144:1425–1432.

29. Zwergel U, Lehmann J, Wullich B, et al. Lymph node positive prostate cancer: long-term survival data after radical prostatectomy. J Urol 2004;171:1128–1131.

30. Frazier HA, 2nd, Robertson JE, Paulson DF. Does radical prostatectomy in the presence of positive pelvic lymph nodes enhance survival? World J Urol 1994;12:308–312.

31. Cadeddu JA, Partin AW, Epstein JI, et al: Stage D1 (T1–3, N1–3, M0) prostate cancer: a case-controlled comparison of conservative treatment versus radical prostatectomy. Urology 1997;50:251–255.

32. Messing E, Manola J, Sarosdy M, et al. Immediate hormonal therapy compared with observation after radical prostatectomy and pelvic lymphadenectomy in men with node positive prostate cancer; Results at 10 years of EST 3886. J Urol 2003;169:396.

33. Catalona WJ, Miller DR, Kavoussi LR. Intermediate-term survival results in clinically understaged prostate cancer patients following radical prostatectomy. J Urol 1988;140:540–543.

34. Pound CR, Partin AW, Eisenberger MA, et al. Natural history of progression after PSA elevation following radical prostatectomy. JAMA 1999;281:1591–1597.

35. Golimbu M, Provet J, Al-Askari S. Radical prostatectomy for stage D1 prostate cancer. Urology 1987;30:427–435.

36. Bader P, Spahn M, Huber R, et al. Limited lymph node dissection in prostate cancer may miss lymph node metastasis and determines outcome of apparently pN0 prostate cancer. Eur Urol 2004;3:16 (A55).

37. Daneshmand S, Quek ML, Stein JP, et al. Prognosis of patients with lymph node positive prostate cancer following radical prostatectomy: long-term results. J Urol 2004;172:2252–2255.

38. Allaf ME, Palapattu GS, Trock BJ, et al. Anatomical extent of lymph node dissection: impact on men with clinically localized prostate cancer. J Urol 2004;172:1840–1844.

39. Dimarco DS, Zincke H, Slezak JM, et al. Does the extent of lymphadenectomy impact disease free survival in prostate cancer? J Urol 2003;169:295 (A1145).

40. Di Blasio CJ, Fearn P, Seo HS, et al. Association between number of lymph nodes removed and freedom from disease progression in patients receiving pelvic lymph node dissection during radical prostatectomy. J Urol 2003;169:456 (A1708).

41. Palapattu GS, Allaf ME, Trock BJ, et al. Prostate specific antigen progression in men with lymph node metastases following radical prostatectomy: results of long-term followup. J Urol 2004;172:1860–1864.

Clinical management of rising prostate-specific antigen after radical retropubic prostatectomy

75

J Kellogg Parsons, Alan W Partin

INTRODUCTION

Approximately 40% of men diagnosed with prostate cancer will undergo radical prostatectomy.[1] Of these, 15% to 46% will manifest an isolated, asymptomatic rise in postoperative PSA within 15 years. This phenomenon is referred to as biochemical recurrence. Since an estimated 75,000 radical prostatectomies are performed annually in the US, biochemical recurrence after prostatectomy represents a healthcare issue of considerable magnitude, affecting several thousand men each year.[2]

This chapter reviews the definition, natural history, diagnosis, and treatment of biochemical recurrence after radical prostatectomy, emphasizing practical considerations in the management of these patients.

DEFINITION OF BIOCHEMICAL RECURRENCE

APPROPRIATE PROSTATE-SPECIFIC ANTIGEN ASSAYS

The gold standard for detecting biochemical recurrence after surgery is measurement of total prostate-specific antigen (PSA). Subsequent statements regarding PSA in this chapter are in reference only to total PSA.

Ultrasensitive assays for total PSA, capable of detection thresholds of 0.001 to 0.01 ng/ml, are not recommended for routine surveillance since they are of unproven clinical value,[3] may detect minute amounts of PSA originating from nonmalignant extraprostatic sources,[4] and may generate problems with false-positive results.[5]

TIMING OF POSTOPERATIVE PROSTATE-SPECIFIC ANTIGEN SURVEILLANCE

The oncologic goal of radical prostatectomy is removal of all prostatic tissue. Since the half-life of PSA is 3.15 days,[6] serum PSA should fall to undetectable levels within 21 to 30 days after successful surgery.[7]

There are no uniform standards for the timing of postoperative PSA surveillance. Practice patterns vary considerably. Typically, PSA is drawn every 3 months during the first year, every 6 months during the second through fifth years, and every 12 months thereafter, unless there is clinical or laboratory evidence of recurrent disease.[8]

There are also no uniform standards for the required duration of follow-up for patients with a persistently undetectable PSA. Although some investigators have observed that biochemical recurrence after 7 years is rare,[9] other data suggest that it may occur in a substantial number of patients up to10 years after surgery.[10,11]

DEFINITION OF RECURRENCE: PROSTATE-SPECIFIC ANTIGEN LEVEL

There has been considerable debate as to what level of PSA constitutes true biochemical failure. Recommendations for cut-off values range from 0.2 to 0.5 ng/ml.[3,9–16] If postoperative PSA never falls below 0.2 to 0.4 ng/ml, the presence of systemic disease should be strongly considered. If postoperative PSA is initially undetectable but then rises above 0.2 to 0.4 ng/ml, the presence of local recurrence and/or systemic disease should be strongly considered. In 2004, the Group on Clinical Trials in the State of a Rising PSA defined a cut-off of 0.4 ng/ml for eligibility for enrollment in clinical trials.[17]

Rarely, PSA will fail to reach undetectable levels after surgery but remains stable at levels less than 0.4 ng/ml.[16] Should this occur, it is reasonable to consider retained benign tissue as a potential etiology,[15] and expectant management with serial PSAs is an acceptable treatment option. If a persistently detectable PSA rises above 0.4 ng/ml within 3 years of surgery, the presence of recurrent local or systemic disease should be considered.[16]

NATURAL HISTORY OF BIOCHEMICAL RECURRENCE

INCIDENCE

Among patients who undergo radical retropubic prostatectomy (RRP), biochemical failure will eventually occur in about one-third, with 15-year PSA-free actuarial survival ranging from 54% to 85%.[5,9,10,13,18–20] PSA-free survival varies depending upon pathologic stage of tumor, grade, margin status, and institutional series.

Data on the incidence of biochemical failure after perineal prostatectomy are considerably less extensive but appear to be similar when compared by equivalent stage, grade, and margin status.[21,22] Data from laparoscopic radical prostatectomy are not yet mature, but at least one institution has observed 3-year recurrence rates comparable to some retropubic series.[23]

PREDICTION OF BIOCHEMICAL RECURRENCE

A number of equations, graphs, and tables have been developed to predict which patients are most likely to develop biochemical recurrence.[24] The clinical goal of these prediction instruments is to improve the delivery of care by providing clinicians and patients with additional information on which to base treatment decisions.

In the case of biochemical recurrence, stratifying patients by risk identifies those who would potentially benefit from adjuvant treatment *before* biochemical recurrence occurs. The rationale is to delay or prevent biochemical recurrence in those patients most likely to develop it.

There are at least 16 models for predicting the likelihood of biochemical recurrence after radical prostatectomy (Table 75.1). Consistently, the most important variables in these models are preoperative PSA, Gleason score, specimen confinement status, and

seminal vesicle or lymph node involvement.[15] Although a number of other variables independently predict biochemical recurrence,[25,26] it is not yet clear whether these individual markers add anything to existing predictive models.[27]

There is no consensus as to how these nomograms should be applied to clinical practice, nor any data to support the hypothesis that adjuvant treatment of patients likely to experience biochemical recurrence improves cancer-specific survival. Nevertheless, our institution and others[9,15] recommend the use of validated nomograms to direct at-risk patients into appropriate clinical trials or more rigorous surveillance programs.

PREDICTION OF TIME TO METASTASES AND DEATH

The natural history of progression to frank metastases and death after biochemical recurrence is variable but is generally prolonged.[10,28,29] Among 304 patients with biochemical recurrence followed for up to 15 years, 34% progressed to metastases over a median period of 8 years. Of those who progressed, median time to cancer-specific death after documented metastases was 5 years.[10]

The challenge in clinical practice has been to identify the minority of men who will progress rapidly after the onset of biochemical recurrence. PSA kinetics, the study of changes in PSA over time, has been useful in this regard. Three measures are associated with rapid clinical progression after biochemical recurrence: time to biochemical recurrence (time between surgery and onset of biochemical recurrence), PSA velocity (PSAV; change in PSA/unit time), and PSA doubling time (PSADT; time it takes for serum PSA levels to double).

Shorter time to recurrence is associated with faster progression. Men who recur within 1 to 3 years of surgery will progress more quickly to metastases and death.[10,16,30,31] Larger PSAV is associated with faster progression. A PSAV greater than or equal to 0.75 ng/ml/year at 1 year after surgery is associated with an increased likelihood of early metastatic disease.[6]

PSADT is calculated by: 1) log-transforming longitudinal PSA levels to create a linear relationship between serum PSA level and time; 2) determining the slope of this log-transformed curve; and 3) multiplying the slope of the log-transformed curve by the inverse of the natural log of 2.[32] Shorter PSADT is associated with decreased time to metastases[10,31–33] and increased prostate cancer-specific mortality.[28,34] The advantage of PSADT over time to recurrence or PSAV at 1 year is that it predicts metastatic progression independently of the number of years since surgery.[11,32] PSADT cut-off values for stratifying patients into low- and high-risk groups for metastatic progression and death range from 3[28] to 6[32,33] to 12 months.[34]

Table 75.1 Models for prediction of biochemical recurrence after radical retropubic prostatectomy

Reference	Year	Number of patients	Prediction instrument	Prediction variables	Validated?
Partin et al[66]	1995	216	Equation categorizing men into low-, intermediate-, and high-risk groups	PSA, specimen Gleason score, specimen confinement status	Yes
Bauer et al[67]	1997	132	Equation categorizing men into low-, intermediate-, and high-risk groups	*BCL2* status, p53 status, PSA, race, specimen confinement status	No
Bauer et al[68]	1998	378	Equation categorizing men into low-, intermediate-, and high-risk groups	PSA, race, specimen confinement status, specimen Gleason score	Yes
D'Amico et al[69]	1998	862	Probability graph	Pathologic stage, PSA specimen Gleason score, surgical margin status	No
Kattan et al[70]	1998	983	Probability nomogram	Biopsy Gleason score, clinical stage, PSA	Yes
D'Amico et al[71]	1999	892	Probability nomogram	Biopsy Gleason score clinical stage, PSA	Yes
Graefen et al[72]	1999	318	Quantitative analysis of high-grade cancer categorizing men into low- and high- risk groups	Biopsy Gleason score, number of positive biopsy cores, pathologic stage, PSA, specimen Gleason score	No
Kattan et al[9]	1999	996	Probability nomogram	Lymph node invasion, PSA, seminal vesicle invasion, specimen confinement status, specimen Gleason score	Yes
Potter et al[73]	1999	214	Neural network	DNA ploidy, patient age, quantified nuclear grade, specimen confinement status, specimen Gleason score	Yes
D'Amico et al[74]	2000	823	Percent of positive biopsy cores categorizing men into risk groups	Biopsy Gleason grade, Clinical stage, Percentage of positive biopsy cores, PSA	Yes
Stamey et al[75]	2000	326	Equation for probability of biochemical failure	Gleason score, lymph node invasion, percent of intraductal cancer, prostate weight, PSA, tumor volume, vascular invasion	Yes
Blute et al[76]	2001	2518	Equation categorizing men into low- and high-risk groups	Adjuvant therapy, Gleason score, PSA, seminal vesicle invasion, surgical margin status	Yes
Moul et al[25]	2001	1012	Equation categorizing men into four different risk groups	PSA, race, specimen confinement status, specimen Gleason score	Yes
Roberts et al[77]	2001	904	Equation categorizing men into low- and high-risk groups	Gleason score, lymph node invasion, seminal vesicle invasion, surgical margin status	Yes
Khan et al[78]	2003	1955	Probability nomogram	Gleason score, pathologic stage, surgical margin status	No
Freedland et al[79]	2004	459	Model categorizing men into low-, intermediate-, high-, and very high-risk groups	Gleason score, percent of positive biopsy cores, PSA	No

DIAGNOSIS OF BIOCHEMICAL RECURRENCE: LOCAL VERSUS SYSTEMIC DISEASE

One of the most problematic aspects of evaluating patients with biochemical recurrence is determining whether the source of the PSA is localized or metastatic disease. Ideally, identifying isolated localized disease allows for therapy to be directed towards the prostatic fossa. Estimates for the incidence of isolated local recurrence vary from 4% to 53%, reflecting the difficulty in establishing this diagnosis.[5,35–38]

Current diagnostic modalities for distinguishing between local and systemic disease remain limited. Available options (Tables 75.2 and 75.3) are described below.

Table 75.2 Prostate-specific antigen (PSA) and pathologic variables for distinguishing between local and systemic disease in patients with biochemical recurrence after radical prostatectomy

Variable	Local recurrence	Systemic recurrence
Gleason score[30]	≤7	>7
Lymph node invasion[30]	No	Yes
PSA doubling time (PSADT)[10,28,32–34]	≥3–12 months	<3–12 months
PSA velocity at 1 year[6,30]	<0.75 ng/ml/year	≥0.75 ng/ml/year
Seminal vesicle invasion[30]	No	Yes
Time to PSA recurrence[6,31,32,39]	>1–2 years	<1–2 years

Table 75.3 Diagnostic modalities for distinguishing between local and systemic disease in patients with biochemical recurrence after radical prostatectomy

Diagnostic modality	Clinical usefulness
Digital rectal examination	None
Ultrasound-guided biopsy	None
Computed tomography	Marginal. May consider if PSA >10 ng/ml or PSA doubling time (PSADT) <6 months
Magnetic resonance imaging	Under investigation
Bone scan	Marginal. May consider if PSA >10–50 ng/ml or PSADT <6 months
Radiolabeled antibody to PSMA	Potentially useful. Further trials needed in setting of biochemical recurrence
Positron emission tomography	Under investigation

PSMA, prostate-specific membrane antigen.

PROSTATE-SPECIFIC ANTIGEN KINETICS AND TUMOR PATHOLOGY

PSA kinetics and tumor pathology are the most useful parameters for estimating the likelihood that systemic disease is present.[3] With respect to the three PSA kinetic measurements mentioned above, the following criteria suggest the presence of systemic disease: 1) time to biochemical recurrence of less than 1 to 2 years,[6,31,32,39] 2) a PSAV at 1 year greater than or equal to 0.75 ng/ml/year,[6] and 3) a PSADT less than 3 to 12 months.[10,28,32–34]

Higher tumor grade and advanced stage also suggest the presence of systemic disease.[30] Table 75.3 summarizes the PSA and pathologic criteria associated with an increased likelihood of distant disease. Table 75.4 presents data for predicting the probability of metastasis-free survival at 3, 5, and 7 years with Gleason score, time to biochemical recurrence, and PSADT.[5,10]

DIGITAL RECTAL EXAMINATION

Digital rectal examination should be performed with the recognition that its diagnostic utility is limited. The postoperative contour of the prostatic fossa is highly variable and is not consistently associated with the presence of local recurrence.[36,40–42] Management decisions, therefore, should not be based on examination findings alone.

ULTRASOUND-GUIDED BIOPSY

We do not recommend routine biopsy of the prostatic fossa or vesicourethral anastomosis. Despite some favorable initial reports,[36] there are at least four substantial problems with biopsy as a diagnostic tool for guiding therapy in this setting. First, the true sensitivity of ultrasound in detecting local recurrence is not known. Second, since the true false-negative rate is not known,[2,3] negative biopsy does not preclude the presence of local disease. Third, distant disease may exist concomitantly with local disease.[3,39] Fourth, post-biopsy salvage radiation therapy to the prostatic bed has produced similar results regardless of whether the biopsy was positive or negative.[43,44]

COMPUTED TOMOGRAPHY

Computed tomography (CT) of the abdomen and pelvis has poor yield for identifying either local or metastatic disease after prostatectomy.[45–49] Its clinical usefulness is particularly limited in asymptomatic patients with a PSA of less than 10 ng/ml. It may hold limited value in patients with a PSADT of less than 6 months.[49]

MAGNETIC RESONANCE IMAGING

The primary role for endorectal magnetic resonance imaging (MRI) is to rule out osseous metastases after an equivocal bone scan.[3] The efficacy of MRI in identifying soft-tissue and nodal disease is unclear and is under study.[50]

BONE SCAN

Bone scan also possesses limited clinical usefulness in asymptomatic men with biochemical recurrence and low PSA.[3,15,49,51] For asymptomatic patients, most investigators recommend bone scan only for select patients with a serum PSA of greater than 10 to 50 ng/ml and/or a PSADT of less than 6 months.[3,15,49,51]

Table 75.4 Estimation of metastasis-free survival following biochemical recurrence after radical prostatectomy

| | | | Percent with metastasis-free survival (95% CI) | | |
			3 years	5 years	7 years
All patients			78 (73–84)	63 (56–70)	52 (44–60)
Gleason score 5–7	Recurrence >2 years	PSADT >10 months	95 (83–96)	86 (74–92)	82 (69–90)
		PSADT ≤10 years	82 (54–94)	69 (40–86)	60 (32–80)
	Recurrence ≤2 years	PSADT >10 months	79 (65–88)	76 (61–86)	59 (40–73)
		PSADT ≤10 years	81 (57–93)	35 (16–56)	15 (4–33)
Gleason score 8–10	Recurrence >2 years		77 (55–89)	60 (33–79)	47 (17–72)
	Recurrence ≤2 years		53 (39–66)	31 (17–45)	21 (9–35)

Data adapted from Pound et al[5] and Laufer et al.[10]

PSADT, PSA doubling time.

RADIOLABELED ANTIBODY TO PROSTATE-SPECIFIC ANTIGEN (PROSTASCINT)

Prostate-specific membrane antigen (PSMA) is a prostate-restricted cell-surface antigen expressed by all prostate cancers. Expression tends to be increased in poorly differentiated, metastatic, and hormone refractory tumors. Capromab pendetide (ProstaScint, Cytogen Corporation, Princeton, NJ) is a monoclonal, radiolabeled anti-PSMA antibody that is FDA-approved for imaging of soft-tissue metastases. Sensitivities for capromab pendetide for the detection of metastatic prostate cancer range from 62% to 75%.[52,53] Although it may potentially distinguish local from systemic disease in patients with a PSA as low as 0.5 ng/ml,[54] more prospective trials are needed to evaluate its usefulness in post-prostatectomy patients.

POSITRON EMISSION TOMOGRAPHY

Positron emission tomography (PET) scanning, which utilizes a radiolabeled glucose analog to identify areas of increased tumor activity, has only a limited role in the evaluation of biochemical recurrence.[55,56] Studies of newer radiotracers are ongoing.[57]

TREATMENT OF BIOCHEMICAL RECURRENCE

Discussion of the management of biochemical recurrence after prostatectomy merits contemplation of one important caveat: currently, there are no prospective data as to whether treatment of biochemical recurrence, at any time point or with any modality, improves cancer specific survival. While many current treatment modalities are effective at returning serum PSA to undetectable levels, it is unclear as to whether or not this alters the natural history of the disease.

EXPECTANT MANAGEMENT

Since there is no definitive evidence that treatment of biochemical recurrence will improve cancer-specific mortality, and since the median time for the onset of metastases in untreated patients after an initial rise in PSA is 8 years,[10] expectant management may be an appropriate treatment option in older patients with significant co-morbidity and/or a lower probability of disease progression. These patients may be followed closely, with treatment reserved for those with a PSADT of less than 3 to 12 months or clinical symptoms.

SALVAGE RADIOTHERAPY

Salvage radiotherapy is radiotherapy applied to the prostatic bed with curative intent for postoperative biochemical recurrence.[58] It should be considered if PSA kinetics, pathologic variables, and/or radiologic imaging suggest an isolated local recurrence.

The efficacy of salvage radiotherapy at improving cancer-specific survival remains unproven. In most studies, the primary outcome is a PSA response to treatment. Although 60% to 90% of patients may initially achieve an undetectable PSA after radiation, only 10% to 45% remain free of PSA recurrence 5 years later.[58–60]

The single most important prognostic factor in predicting objective PSA response to salvage radiotherapy is pretreatment PSA. A lower PSA is associated with increased likelihood of response.[60–63] Accordingly, in 1999 the American Society for Therapeutic Radiology and Oncology (ASTRO) consensus panel recommended that treatment be initiated at a PSA of less than 1.5 ng/ml with a minimum dose of 64 to 65 Gy.[58]

The benefit of adjuvant hormonal therapy with salvage radiotherapy is also unproven. Although retrospective data suggest that hormonal therapy may improve PSA response,[64] there are no prospective data. The Radiation Therapy Oncology Group is conducting a study (RTOG 96-01) randomizing patients with biochemical recurrence after radical prostatectomy to radiotherapy alone versus radiotherapy plus bicalutamide 150 mg/day.[60]

In summary, salvage radiotherapy is effective at lowering PSA. It should be considered in patients in whom isolated local recurrence is suspected. Treatment when PSA is less than 1.5 ng/ml maximizes the potential response. Studies are ongoing as to whether adjuvant hormonal therapy will improve response.

HORMONAL THERAPY

The rationale for treating biochemical recurrence with androgen ablation is that, in the absence of isolated local recurrence, biochemical recurrence represents systemic disease. The appropriate timing of androgen ablation in the treatment of advanced prostate cancer—early versus late—is disputed. In the post-prostatectomy patient, androgen ablation for asymptomatic biochemical recurrence represents early therapy, while ablation for symptomatic metastases represents late therapy.

Regardless of timing, androgen ablation will reduce serum PSA levels in men with biochemical recurrence after radical prostatectomy.[65] Retrospective data suggest that select men with aggressive disease who receive early hormonal therapy for biochemical recurrence have improved PSA progression-free survival and increased time to the onset of metastases.[65] However, there is no evidence that either early or late androgen ablation improves cancer-specific survival.

Other means by which the androgen axis may be manipulated include maximum androgen blockade, oral androgen antagonists, and 5-alpha reductase inhibitors. There are no conclusive data on the benefits of any of these modalities for the treatment of biochemical recurrence.

SUMMARY

The most appropriate assay for diagnosing biochemical recurrence is serum total PSA, which should be checked every 3 months for the first year after surgery and at least every 12 months thereafter for a minimum of 10 years. Definitions for the diagnosis of biochemical recurrence after radical prostatectomy range from 0.2 to 0.4 ng/ml. A multidisciplinary group has recommended a cut-off of

0.4 ng/ml as a criterion for inclusion in clinical trials. Persistent, stable levels below 0.4 ng/ml for up to 3 years following surgery may be followed expectantly.

Fifteen-year PSA-free actuarial survival rates vary from 54% to 85%. Several validated prediction models exist for predicting biochemical recurrence. Disease progression following biochemical recurrence is generally indolent. Time to recurrence, PSAV, PSADT, and tumor pathology are all associated with the risk of progression to metastases and death.

In distinguishing between patients with local and systemic recurrence, PSA kinetics and tumor features remain the most valuable clinical parameters. Digital rectal examination should be performed, but its usefulness at planning therapy is limited. Ultrasound-guided biopsy of the prostatic fossa is not recommended. CT and bone scan have marginal clinical utility. MRI, ProstaScint, and PET scanning are investigational modalities at this time.

Expectant management should be considered in patients with an onset of recurrence more than 2 years after surgery, a PSADT of greater than 3 to 12 months, and no evidence of clinical disease. Salvage radiotherapy is efficacious at lowering serum PSA in men suspected of having isolated local recurrence, particularly with a PSA of less than 1.5 ng/ml. However, it is unclear whether it improves survival. Early hormonal therapy will lower PSA and, in men with aggressive disease, potentially increase time to metastases. However, there is no evidence that either early or delayed hormonal therapy will improve cancer-specific survival.

REFERENCES

1. Burkhardt JH, Litwin MS, Rose CM, et al. Comparing the costs of radiation therapy and radical prostatectomy for the initial treatment of early-stage prostate cancer. J Clin Oncol 2002;20:2869–2875.

2. Moul JW. Prostate specific antigen only progression of prostate cancer. J Urol 2000;163:1632–1642.

3. Swindle PW, Kattan MW, Scardino PT. Markers and meaning of primary treatment failure. Urol Clin North Am 2003;30:377–401.

4. Diamandis EP, Yu H. Nonprostatic sources of prostate-specific antigen. Urol Clin North Am 1997;24:275–282.

5. Laufer M, Pound CR, Carducci MA, et al. Management of patients with rising prostate-specific antigen after radical prostatectomy. Urology 2000;55:309–315.

6. Partin AW, Oesterling JE. The clinical usefulness of prostate specific antigen: update 1994. J Urol 1994;152:1358–1368.

7. Oesterling JE, Chan DW, Epstein JI, et al. Prostate specific antigen in the preoperative and postoperative evaluation of localized prostatic cancer treated with radical prostatectomy. J Urol 1988;139:766–772.

8. Oh J, Colberg JW, Ornstein DK, et al. Current followup strategies after radical prostatectomy: a survey of American Urological Association urologists. J Urol 1999;161:520–523.

9. Kattan MW, Wheeler TM, Scardino PT. Postoperative nomogram for disease recurrence after radical prostatectomy for prostate cancer. J Clin Oncol 1999;17:1499–1507.

10. Pound CR, Partin AW, Eisenberger MA, et al. Natural history of progression after PSA elevation following radical prostatectomy. JAMA 1999;281:1591–1597.

11. Ward JF, Blute ML, Slezak J, et al. The long-term clinical impact of biochemical recurrence of prostate cancer 5 or more years after radical prostatectomy. J Urol 2003;170:1872–1876.

12. Moul JW, Douglas TH, McCarthy WF, et al. Black race is an adverse prognostic factor for prostate cancer recurrence following radical prostatectomy in an equal access health care setting. J Urol 1996;155:1667–1673.

13. Zincke H, Oesterling JE, Blute ML, et al. Long-term (15 years) results after radical prostatectomy for clinically localized (stage T2c or lower) prostate cancer. J Urol 1994;152:1850–1857.

14. Freedland SJ, Sutter ME, Dorey F, et al. Defining the ideal cutpoint for determining PSA recurrence after radical prostatectomy. Prostate-specific antigen. Urology 2003;61:365–369.

15. Moul JW. Variables in predicting survival based on treating "PSA-only" relapse. Urol Oncol 2003;21:292–304.

16. Amling CL, Bergstralh EJ, Blute ML, et al. Defining prostate specific antigen progression after radical prostatectomy: what is the most appropriate cut point? J Urol 2001;165:1146–1151.

17. Scher HI, Eisenberger M, D'Amico AV, et al. Eligibility and outcomes reporting guidelines for clinical trials for patients in the state of a rising prostate-specific antigen: recommendations from the Prostate-Specific Antigen Working Group. J Clin Oncol 2004;22:537–556.

18. Catalona WJ, Smith DS. 5-year tumor recurrence rates after anatomical radical retropubic prostatectomy for prostate cancer. J Urol 1994;152:1837–1842.

19. Khan MA, Han M, Partin AW, et al. Long-term cancer control of radical prostatectomy in men younger than 50 years of age: update 2003. Urology 2003;62:86–91, discussion 91–92.

20. Trapasso JG, deKernion JB, Smith RB, et al. The incidence and significance of detectable levels of serum prostate specific antigen after radical prostatectomy. J Urol 1994;152:1821–1825.

21. Iselin CE, Robertson JE, Paulson DF. Radical perineal prostatectomy: oncological outcome during a 20-year period. J Urol 1999;161:163–168.

22. Harris MJ. Radical perineal prostatectomy: cost efficient, outcome effective, minimally invasive prostate cancer management. Eur Urol 2003;44:303–308, discussion 308.

23. Guillonneau B, el-Fettouh H, Baumert H, et al. Laparoscopic radical prostatectomy: oncological evaluation after 1,000 cases a Montsouris Institute. J Urol 2003;169:1261–1266.

24. Ross PL, Scardino PT, Kattan MW. A catalog of prostate cancer nomograms. J Urol 2001;165:1562–1568.

25. Moul JW, Connelly RR, Lubeck DP, et al. Predicting risk of prostate specific antigen recurrence after radical prostatectomy with the Center for Prostate Disease Research and Cancer of the Prostate Strategic Urologic Research Endeavor databases. J Urol 2001;166:1322–1327.

26. Rhodes DR, Sanda MG, Otte AP, et al. Multiplex biomarker approach for determining risk of prostate-specific antigen-defined recurrence of prostate cancer. J Natl Cancer Inst 2003;95:661–668.

27. Kattan MW. Judging new markers by their ability to improve predictive accuracy. J Natl Cancer Inst 2003;95:634–635.

28. D'Amico AV, Moul JW, Carroll PR, et al. Surrogate end point for prostate cancer-specific mortality after radical prostatectomy or radiation therapy. J Natl Cancer Inst 2003;95:1376–1383.

29. Jhaveri FM, Zippe CD, Klein EA, Kupelian PA. Biochemical failure does not predict overall survival after radical prostatectomy for localized prostate cancer: 10-year results. Urology 1999;54:884–890.

30. Partin AW, Pearson JD, Landis PK, et al. Evaluation of serum prostate-specific antigen velocity after radical prostatectomy to distinguish local recurrence from distant metastases. Urology 1994;43:649–659.

31. Amling CL, Blute ML, Bergstralh EJ, et al. TM, Slezak J, Zincke H. Long-term hazard of progression after radical prostatectomy for clinically localized prostate cancer: continued risk of biochemical failure after 5 years. J Urol 2000;164:101–105.

32. Patel A, Dorey F, Franklin J, et al. Recurrence patterns after radical retropubic prostatectomy: clinical usefulness of prostate specific antigen doubling times and log slope prostate specific antigen. J Urol 1997;158:1441–1445.

33. Roberts SG, Blute ML, Bergstralh EJ, et al. PSA doubling time as a predictor of clinical progression after biochemical failure following radical prostatectomy for prostate cancer. Mayo Clin Proc 2001;76:576–581.

34. Albertsen PC, Hanley JA, Penson DF, et al. Validation of increasing prostate specific antigen as a predictor of prostate cancer death after treatment of localized prostate cancer with surgery or radiation. J Urol 2004;171:2221–2225.

35. Han M, Partin AW, Pound CR, et al. Long-term biochemical disease-free and cancer-specific survival following anatomic radical retropubic prostatectomy. The 15-year Johns Hopkins experience. Urol Clin North Am 2001;28:555–565.

36. Foster LS, Jajodia P, Fournier G Jr, et al. The value of prostate specific antigen and transrectal ultrasound guided biopsy in detecting prostatic fossa recurrences following radical prostatectomy. J Urol 1993;149:1024–1028.

37. Connolly JA, Shinohara K, Presti JC Jr, et al. Local recurrence after radical prostatectomy: characteristics in size, location, and relationship to prostate-specific antigen and surgical margins. Urology 1996;47:225–231.

38. Zietman AL, Shipley WU, Willett CG. Residual disease after radical surgery or radiation therapy for prostate cancer. Clinical significance and therapeutic implications. Cancer 1993;71(3 Suppl):959–969.

39. Pound CR, Partin AW, Epstein JI, et al. Prostate-specific antigen after anatomic radical retropubic prostatectomy. Patterns of recurrence and cancer control. Urol Clin North Am 1997;24:395–406.

40. Saleem MD, Sanders H, Abu El Naser M, et al. Factors predicting cancer detection in biopsy of the prostatic fossa after radical prostatectomy. Urology 1998;51:283–286.

41. Fowler JE, Jr., Brooks J, Pandey P, et al. Variable histology of anastomotic biopsies with detectable prostate specific antigen after radical prostatectomy. J Urol 1995;153:1011–1014.

42. Lightner DJ, Lange PH, Reddy PK, et al. Prostate specific antigen and local recurrence after radical prostatectomy. J Urol 1990;144:921–926.

43. Cadeddu JA, Partin AW, DeWeese TL, et al. Long-term results of radiation therapy for prostate cancer recurrence following radical prostatectomy. J Urol 1998;159:173–177, discussion 177–178.

44. Koppie TM, Grossfeld GD, Nudell DM, et al. Is anastomotic biopsy necessary before radiotherapy after radical prostatectomy? J Urol 2001;166:111–115.

45. Seltzer MA, Barbaric Z, Belldegrun A, et al. Comparison of helical computerized tomography, positron emission tomography and monoclonal antibody scans for evaluation of lymph node metastases in patients with prostate specific antigen relapse after treatment for localized prostate cancer. J Urol 1999;162:1322–1328.

46. Kramer S, Gorich J, Gottfried HW, et al. Sensitivity of computed tomography in detecting local recurrence of prostatic carcinoma following radical prostatectomy. Br J Radiol 1997;70:995–999.

47. Johnson PAS. Yield of imaging and scintigraphy assessing bNED failure in prostate cancer patients. Urol Oncol 1997;70:995.

48. Kane CJ, Amling CL, Johnstone PA, et al. Limited value of bone scintigraphy and computed tomography in assessing biochemical failure after radical prostatectomy. Urology 2003;61:607–611.

49. Okotie OT, Aronson WJ, Wieder JA, et al. Predictors of metastatic disease in men with biochemical failure following radical prostatectomy. J Urol 2004;171:2260–2264.

50. Harisinghani MG, Barentsz J, Hahn PF, et al. Noninvasive detection of clinically occult lymph–node metastases in prostate cancer. N Engl J Med 2003;348:2491–2499.

51. Cher ML, Bianco FJ Jr, Lam JS, et al. Limited role of radionuclide bone scintigraphy in patients with prostate specific antigen elevations after radical prostatectomy. J Urol 1998;160:1387–1391.

52. Quintana JC, Blend MJ. The dual-isotope ProstaScint imaging procedure: clinical experience and staging results in 145 patients. Clin Nucl Med 2000;25:33–40.

53. Hinkle GH, Burgers JK, Neal CE, et al. Multicenter radioimmunoscintigraphic evaluation of patients with prostate carcinoma using indium-111 capromab pendetide. Cancer 1998;83:739–747.

54. Raj GV, Partin AW, Polascik TJ. Clinical utility of indium 111-capromab pendetide immunoscintigraphy in the detection of early, recurrent prostate carcinoma after radical prostatectomy. Cancer 2002;94:987–996.

55. Hofer C, Laubenbacher C, Block T, et al. Fluorine-18-fluorodeoxyglucose positron emission tomography is useless for the detection of local recurrence after radical prostatectomy. Eur Urol 1999;36:31–35.

56. Effert PJ, Bares R, Handt S, et al. Metabolic imaging of untreated prostate cancer by positron emission tomography with 18fluorine-labeled deoxyglucose. J Urol 1996;155:994–998.

57. Hricak H, Schoder H, Pucar D, et al. Advances in imaging in the postoperative patient with a rising prostate-specific antigen level. Semin Oncol 2003;30:616–634.

58. Cox JD, Gallagher MJ, Hammond EH, et al. Consensus statements on radiation therapy of prostate cancer: guidelines for prostate re-biopsy after radiation and for radiation therapy with rising prostate-specific antigen levels after radical prostatectomy. American Society for Therapeutic Radiology and Oncology Consensus Panel. J Clin Oncol 1999;17:1155.

59. Forman JD, Velasco J. Therapeutic radiation in patients with a rising post-prostatectomy PSA level. Oncology (Huntingt) 1998;12:33–39, discussion 39, 43–44, 47.

60. Macdonald OK, Schild SE, Vora SA, et al. Radiotherapy for men with isolated increase in serum prostate specific antigen after radical prostatectomy. J Urol 2003;170:1833–1837.

61. Anscher MS, Clough R, Dodge R. Radiotherapy for a rising prostate-specific antigen after radical prostatectomy: the first 10 years. Int J Radiat Oncol Biol Phys 2000;48:369–375.

62. Song DY, Thompson TL, Ramakrishnan V, et al. Salvage radiotherapy for rising or persistent PSA after radical prostatectomy. Urology 2002;60:281–287.

63. Liauw SL, Webster WS, Pistenmaa DA, et al. Salvage radiotherapy for biochemical failure of radical prostatectomy: a single-institution experience. Urology 2003;61:1204–1210.

64. Eulau SM, Tate DJ, Stamey TA, et al. Effect of combined transient androgen deprivation and irradiation following radical prostatectomy for prostatic cancer. Int J Radiat Oncol Biol Phys 1998;41:735–740.

65. Moul JW, Wu H, Sun L, et al. Early versus delayed hormonal therapy for prostate specific antigen only recurrence of prostate cancer after radical prostatectomy. J Urol 2004;171:1141–1147.

66. Partin AW, Piantadosi S, Sanda MG, et al. Selection of men at high risk for disease recurrence for experimental adjuvant therapy following radical prostatectomy. Urology 1995;45:831–838.

67. Bauer JJ, Connelly RR, Sesterhenn IA, et al. Biostatistical modeling using traditional variables and genetic biomarkers for predicting the risk of prostate carcinoma recurrence after radical prostatectomy. Cancer 1997;79:952–962.

68. Bauer JJ, Connelly RR, Seterhenn IA, et al. Biostatistical modeling using traditional preoperative and pathological prognostic variables in the selection of men at high risk for disease recurrence after radical prostatectomy for prostate cancer. J Urol 1998;159:929–933.

69. D'Amico AV, Whittington R, Malkowicz SB, et al. The combination of preoperative prostate specific antigen and postoperative pathological findings to predict prostate specific antigen outcome in clinically localized prostate cancer. J Urol 1998;160:2096–2101.

70. Kattan MW, Eastham JA, Stapleton AM, et al. A preoperative nomogram for disease recurrence following radical prostatectomy for prostate cancer. J Natl Cancer Inst 1998;90:766–771.

71. D'Amico AV, Whittington R, Malkowicz SB, et al. Pretreatment nomogram for prostate-specific antigen recurrence after radical prostatectomy or external-beam radiation therapy for clinically localized prostate cancer. J Clin Oncol 1999;17:168–172.

72. Graefen M, Noldus J, Pichlmeier U, et al. Early prostate-specific antigen relapse after radical retropubic prostatectomy: prediction on the basis of preoperative and postoperative tumor characteristics. Eur Urol 1999;36:21–30.

73. Potter SR, Miller MC, Mangold LA, et al. Genetically engineered neural networks for predicting prostate cancer progression after radical prostatectomy. Urology 1999;54:791–795.

74. D'Amico AV, Whittington R, Malkowicz SB, et al. Clinical utility of the percentage of positive prostate biopsies in defining biochemical outcome after radical prostatectomy for patients with clinically localized prostate cancer. J Clin Oncol 2000;18:1164–1172.

75. Stamey TA, Yemoto CM, McNeal JE, et al. Prostate cancer is highly predictable: a prognostic equation based on all morphological variables in radical prostatectomy specimens. J Urol 2000;163:1155–1160.

76. Blute ML, Bergstralh EJ, Iocca A, et al. Use of Gleason score, prostate specific antigen, seminal vesicle and margin status to predict biochemical failure after radical prostatectomy. J Urol 2001;165:119–125.

77. Roberts WW, Bergstralh EJ, Blute ML, et al. Contemporary identification of patients at high risk of early prostate cancer recurrence after radical retropubic prostatectomy. Urology 2001;57:1033–1037.

78. Khan MA, Partin AW, Mangold LA, et al. Probability of biochemical recurrence by analysis of pathologic stage, Gleason score, and margin status for localized prostate cancer. Urology 2003;62:866–871.

79. Freedland SJ, Terris MK, Csathy GS, et al. Preoperative model for predicting prostate specific antigen recurrence after radical prostatectomy using percent of biopsy tissue with cancer, biopsy Gleason grade and serum prostate specific antigen. J Urol 2004;171:2215–2220.

Radical perineal prostatectomy 76

David M Hartke, Martin I Resnick

INTRODUCTION

Prostate cancer is the most frequently diagnosed noncutaneous cancer in American men and the second leading cause of cancer death. Fortunately, we are in an era of early detection and men are diagnosed with and present for treatment of adenocarcinoma of the prostate at earlier stages. Though various methods of therapy are available, over the last century, surgical cure has been a mainstay of prostate cancer therapy. Hugh Hampton Young, the first Chairman of Urology at Johns Hopkins School of Medicine, is credited with performing the first radical perineal prostatectomy for treatment of cancer.[1] In 1939, Belt modified the procedure by introducing a subsphincteric dissection as a means of improving exposure of the prostate.[2] For years, many surgeons adopted this approach, which was the principle method for treating those patients with localized prostate malignancies. In 1945, the retropubic prostatectomy was first introduced by Dr Terrence Millin, however, due to the large intra-operative blood loss and high morbidity, the perineal approach remained the accepted method of treatment.[3] In the late 1970s, the importance of pelvic lymphadenectomy for accurate disease staging was understood and the retropubic approach and concomitant pelvic lymph node dissection through the same incision replaced the perineal prostatectomy as the more popular approach. Furthermore, the works of Dr Patrick Walsh improved upon Millin's technique, demonstrating functional anatomic relationships that reduced the intraoperative blood loss and improved outcomes of impotence and urinary incontinence.[4,5,6] Thus, the radical retropubic prostatectomy has been the most common surgical approach over the last two decades.

Recently, there has been a resurgence of interest in the radical perineal prostatectomy. The reason for increased popularity is multifactorial. First, the work of Partin et al. has allowed for a relatively accurate prediction of disease stage and pelvic lymph node involvement through analysis of PSA level, clinical stage, and Gleason pathologic score.[7] This work has allowed for a more selective use of staging lymphadenectomy.[8] Moreover, the advancement of laparoscopy has allowed for a combined laparoscopic pelvic lymphadenectomy and standard radical perineal prostatectomy in those patients who require staging lymph node analysis.[8,9,10] Thus, with the need for an abdominal incision obviated, and due to advancements in technique,[11] the perineal prostatectomy offers patients a cost-effective operation, with shorter hospital stays, shorter time to reconvalescence, low morbidity, and cancer control as effective as with the retropubic approach. Moreover, the perineal prostatectomy may have an easier learning curve than the retropubic approach.[12]

PATIENT SELECTION

Radical curative surgery is offered to those patients with an expected non-cancer survival of greater than 15 years who demonstrate a high likelihood of organ-confined disease. Those with a biopsy Gleason score of 8 or less, a PSA level below 20 ng/ml and are without palpable bilateral disease are eligible candidates; patients with higher values tend to have more advanced disease and are not eligible for the procedure. Laparoscopic pelvic lymphadenectomy is deemed unnecessary because of the low likelihood of nodal disease if the biopsy Gleason score is less than 7 in the presence of unilateral disease and the serum PSA level is less than 10 ng/ml. When required, the laparoscopic lymphadenectomy is usually carried out immediately prior to prostatectomy.[10] While the lymph nodes specimens are processed as frozen sections, the patient is repositioned. RPP is aborted if the lymph nodes are positive for metastatic disease.

In patients with localized prostate cancer, there are few contraindications to this procedure. Patients with severe ankylosis of the hips or spine and those with unstable artificial hip replacements may not tolerate the exaggerated lithotomy position. However, common degenerative disc disease is not a contra-indication to positioning. Furthermore, patients with extreme obesity may not be eligible secondary to the restrictive force upon ventilation generated by excessive weight on the diaphragm. These extremely obese patients are poor candidates for the retropubic approach as well and are often offered non-surgical treatment. Some patients, such as those having a renal transplant or those with severe inflammation secondary to placement of synthetic mesh for repair of a hernia may not be amenable to a retropubic approach but typically can have the prostate removed perineally without incident.

PREOPERATIVE CARE

A full bowel preparation is administered the day prior to surgery. Although the patient may consume a regular diet, he is instructed to consume 4 L of polyethylene glycol in the afternoon prior to the surgery. Also, 1.0 g of neomycin is administered orally at 12:00, 2:00, 4:00, 6:00, 8:00 and 10:00 pm. This bowel prep allows for primary closure of any inadvertent rectal injury at the time of surgery.

A blood type and antibody screen is obtained from all patients in the days or hours prior to surgery. Because blood loss is minimal and transfusions rarely required, a cross-match is unnecessary.

In the preoperative holding area, knee-high antithromboembolic surgical stockings are placed without the need for sequential compression devices. The patient is given 1.0 g of intravenous cefazolin in the operating room. Patients with cephalosporin allergy are administered intravenous gentamicin at a dose of 2 to 5 mg/kg body weight.

ANESTHESIA

Anesthetic options are discussed with the patient pre-operatively. Although regional anesthetics such as spinal or epidural anesthesia are possible, they are somewhat limited by the exaggerated lithotomy positioning of the patient. Thus, most patients elect to receive a general anesthetic.

POSITION

After the induction of anesthesia, the patient is positioned supine so that when the leg portion of the operating table is lowered, the buttocks are extended beyond the table edge. Allen® stirrups are stationed 2 inches cranially on the rail so that there is ample room for the attachment of the self-retaining retractor. The patient's feet are placed in the Allen® stirrups with the stirrups at the level of his legs. The stirrups are then simultaneously elevated into a modified exaggerated dorsal lithotomy position such that the upper thigh is at a 75° angle with the spine. The perineum is at a right angle to the floor (Figure 76.1). The perineum, anus, and scrotum are shaved and the anterior abdomen inferior to the umbilicus, penis, scrotum, perineum, anus, and both thighs are painted with povidone-iodine in the standard sterile fashion. After gowning, a sterile towel is sewn from the 9 o'clock to the 3 o'clock position around the anus at the mucocutaneous pigmentation line with silk suture. Leg and perineal drapes are placed. The upright of the self-retaining retractor is secured to the table rail on the patient's left while maintaining the sterility of the upright. A headlight is adorned to supplement the overhead lighting.

EXPOSURE OF THE PROSTATE

A curved Lowsley tractor is placed transurethrally into the bladder and its wings are opened. A curvilinear incision is made from a position just medial to the right ischial tuberosity to a position just medial to the left ischial tuberosity. The incision should not extend posteriorly beyond the 3 and 9 o'clock positions relative to the anus (Figure 76.2). Subcutaneous tissues and Colle's fascia are then sharply incised along the same direction as the incision. Electrocautery and blunt dissection are employed to open and develop each ischiorectal fossa lateral to the central tendon. The central tendon is then divided using electrocautery. The fibers of the superficial external anal sphincter are dissected and retracted anteriorly using an appendiceal retractor (Belt modification).[2] The longitudinal muscle fibers of the rectum are identified and gentle traction is placed dorsally on the rectum using a dampened sponge. The plane is developed leading to the rectourethralis muscle, which is formed by fascicles of the rectal muscle, connecting the rectum to the perineal body. It appears as a strap of muscle tenting the rectum ventrally (Figure 76.3). For the next step, traction should not be placed on the Lowsley tractor to avoid rectal injury. The rectourethralis muscle is divided close to the apex of the prostate using vertically oriented scissors or electrocautery, allowing the rectum to fall dorsally;

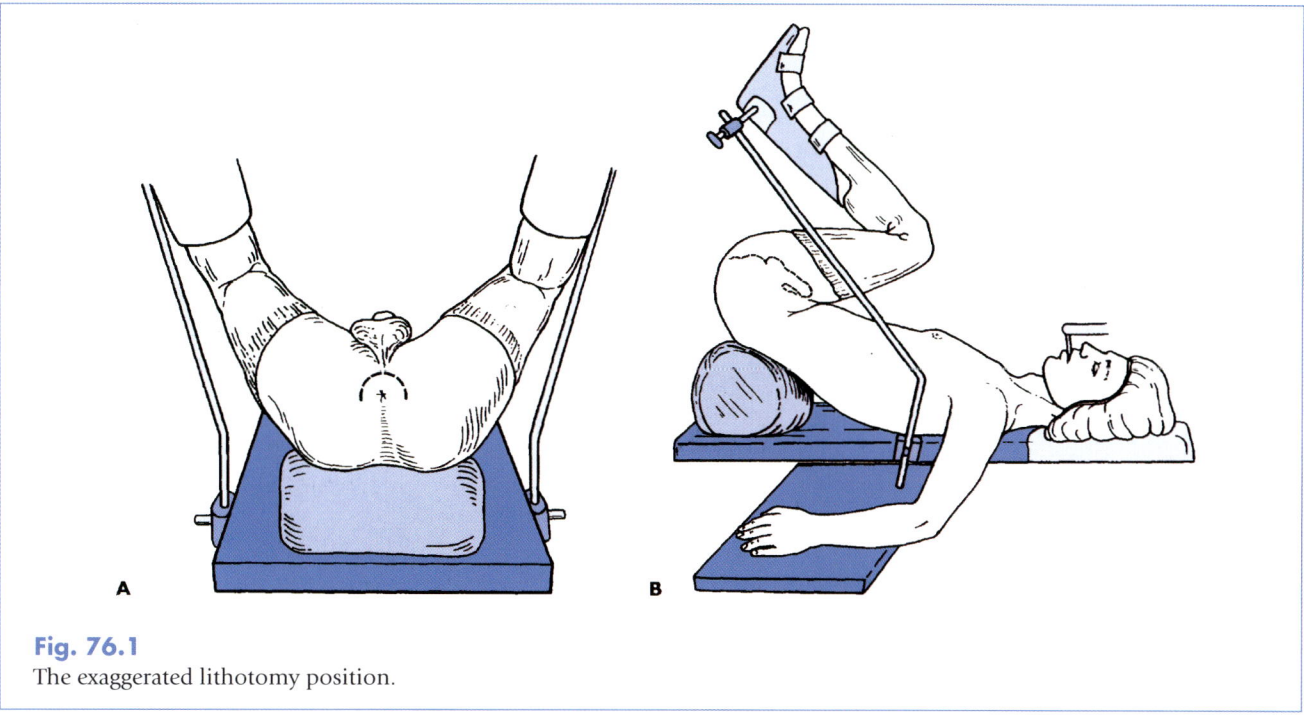

Fig. 76.1
The exaggerated lithotomy position.

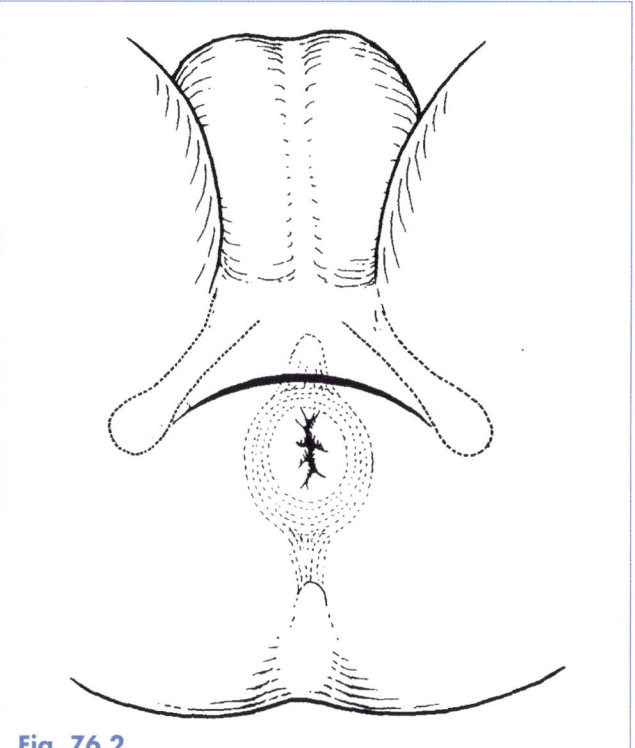

Fig. 76.2
The curvilinear skin incision is made approximately 1 to 2 cm above anal verge.[35]

caution must be exercised to prevent rectal injury at this point of the procedure. Gentle pressure is applied on the Lowsley tractor toward the anterior abdominal wall. This maneuver delivers the prostate well into the field of view and allows the blunt, digital dissection of the prostate from the rectum in a cephalad direction until the base of the prostate is identified at the vesicoprostatic junction. The proper plane is between the anterior and posterior leafs of Denonvillier's fascia.[35]

NERVE-SPARING DISSECTON

Resumed traction on the Lowsley tractor toward the anterior abdominal wall again brings the prostate into the incision. If preservation of the neurovascular bundles is intended, the exposed anterior layer of Denonvillier's fascia is incised vertically in the midline from the vesicoprostatic junction to the apex of the prostate using a number 15-blade scalpel. Careful lateral dissection with gentle lateral traction preserves the neurovascular bundles as they course between the leaves of Denonvillier's fascia at the posterolateral edge of the prostate. The fascia and enclosed nerves must be mobilized sufficiently to allow for eventual extraction of the prostate without stretching or damaging the bundles.

Attention is then directed toward the prostatic apex and urethra. The Lowsley tractor can be palpated within the urethra and a right-angle clamp is placed with the open points facing cephalad on either side of the urethra to dissect the neurovascular bundles off of the urethra as they course distally. The number 15 blade scalpel is again used to incise the posterior aspect of the urethra over the Lowsley tractor. The curved Lowsley tractor is then replaced by a straight Lowsley tractor and the wings opened. With moderate traction on the Lowsley tractor, and the right-angle clamp beneath the remaining intact urethra, the anterior aspect of the membranous urethra is transected from the prostatic apex using scissors.

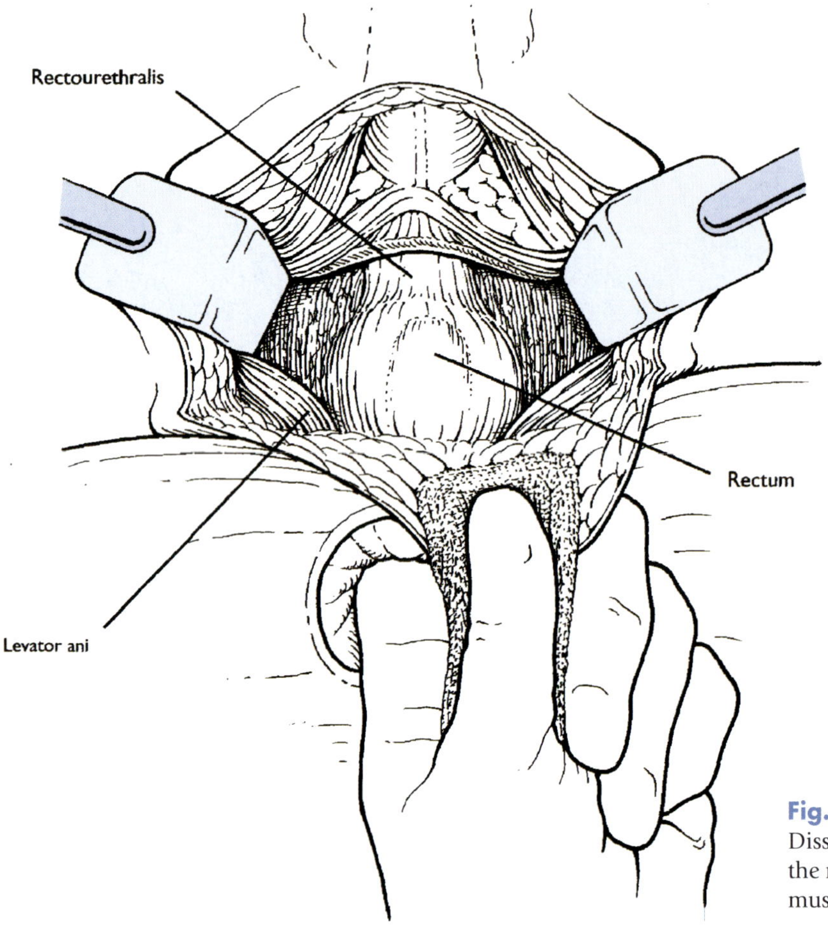

Rectourethralis

Rectum

Levator ani

Fig. 76.3
Dissection along the longitudinal fibers of the rectal wall exposes the rectourethralis muscle.[35]

The self-retaining retractor is attached to the previously placed upright and blades are placed in the 6, 9, 12, and 3 o'clock positions. Dissection is then directed over the anterior prostate from the apex toward the bladder neck. Traction on the Lowsley tractor aids in this portion by bringing the prostate into the incision. The surgeon must be mindful not to dissect too far ventrally and come upon the dorsal venous complex. The puboprostatic ligaments are encountered during this dissection and are divided with scissors, not avulsed.

The junction of the bladder neck and prostate base is then identified by palpating the wings of the Lowsley tractor. This junction is then further developed with blunt and sharp dissections, preserving the bladder neck. This dissection is continued and the bladder entered anteriorly using a scalpel (Figure 76.4). The Lowsley tractor is removed from the urethra and a long right-angle clamp is passed retrograde through the prostatic urethra and bladder neck. A 14-French red rubber catheter is then fed into the open right angle clamp and pulled through the prostatic urethra; the ends are clamped together with a Kelly clamp. Traction on the catheter further delivers the prostate into the incision and dissection of the anterior bladder neck is continued circumferentially around the prostate base.

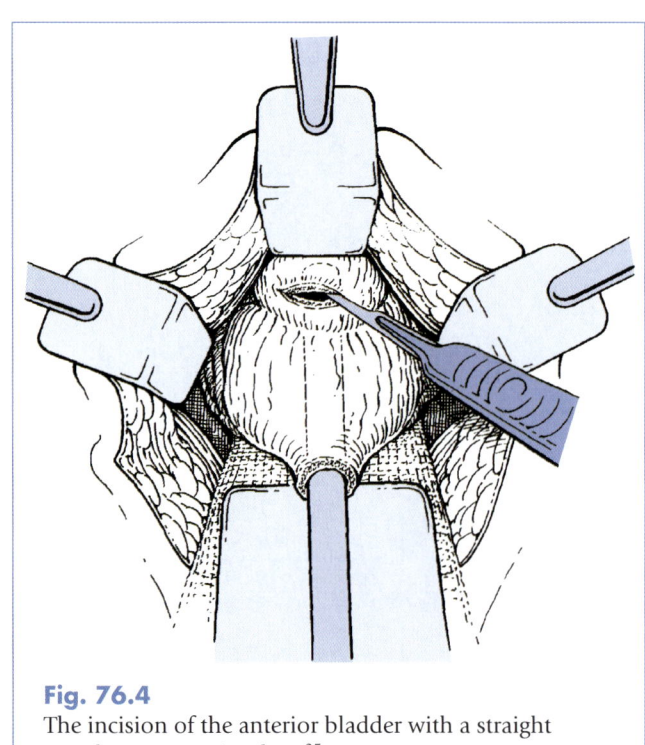

Fig. 76.4
The incision of the anterior bladder with a straight Lowsley retractor in place.[35]

Identification of the ureteral orifices is generally unnecessary unless the dissection inadvertently involves the trigone posteriorly. The lateral attachments and vascular pedicles are found coursing toward the base of the prostate and are dissected, sharply divided between right-angle clamps, and secured using 3-0 absorbable ties. To preserve the neurovascular bundles, the lateral pedicles should be divided close to the prostate, taking care not to compromise the surgical margin. Electrocautery is avoided during this phase.

The dissection is continued posteriorly at the bladder neck to separate it completely from the prostate. The red-rubber catheter is then removed and a right-angle clamp is passed along the midline posterior surface of the prostate with tips directed toward the base. The 14-French red-rubber is passed through the open tips of the right-angle clamp, pulled through, and ends secured together with a Kelly clamp. Traction can then be applied around the entirety of the prostate toward the incision, exposing the vasa deferentia and seminal vesicles (Figure 76.5). Each vas deferens is grasped with a right-angle clamp, bluntly dissected, and divided with electrocautery. Each seminal vesicle is similarly grasped with a right-angle clamp, bluntly dissected and divided, ligating the seminal vesicle artery with 3-0 absorbable ties. The complete surgical specimen is removed and passed-off for pathologic examination.

VESICOURETHRAL ANASTOMOSIS

Occasionally, it may be necessary to reconstruct the bladder neck using simple interrupted absorbable suture placed posteriorly in a tennis racquet fashion. The ureteral orifices should be identified and care should be taken to prevent harm.

The retractor placed at the 12 o'clock position is removed and a 12-French red-rubber catheter is placed retrograde through the penile urethra and grasped at the glans with a Kelly clamp. This catheter aids in the ability to identify the membranous urethra and prevents risk of damage to a catheter balloon. A 3-0 polyglycolic acid suture is placed from outside the anterior bladder neck at the 12 o'clock position and from inside to outside the membranous urethra at the same position and tied. While the assistant places traction on the red-rubber catheter toward the contralateral side, the surgeon places sutures at the 2 and 10 o'clock positions. The red-rubber catheter is removed and a 22-French silastic Foley catheter is carefully passed retrograde from the penile urethra and into the bladder. The 5-ml balloon is inflated with 15-mL of sterile water. Sutures are then placed at the 4, 6, and 8 o'clock positions and tied, completing the anastomosis.

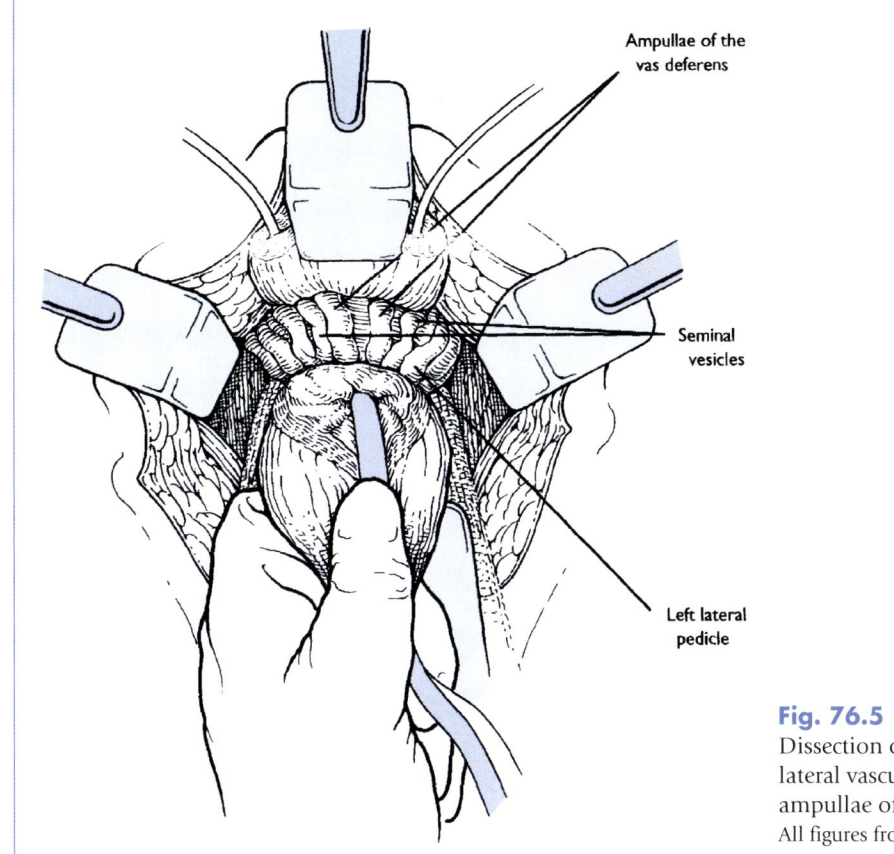

Fig. 76.5
Dissection of the posterolateral prostate reveals the lateral vascular pedicles, seminal vesicles, and ampullae of the vas deferens.
All figures from Haas and Resnick[35]

CLOSURE

The field is inspected for hemostasis and again for rectal injury. A penrose drain is positioned near the vesicourethral anastomosis and brought through the incision. The levator ani are reapproximated using 2-0 absorbable sutures, avoiding damage to the neurovascular bundles and penrose drain. The central tendon and Colles' fascia is reapproximated respectively with 2-0 absorbable sutures. The skin is closed with 4-0 caprosyn suture interrupted in a vertical mattress fashion. The penrose drain is sutured to the skin with a simple stitch. The wound is dressed with a fluffed gauze dressing.

POSTOPERATIVE CARE

Regardless of whether the patient underwent a laparoscopic lymph node dissection at the time of prostatectomy, the postoperative care remains the same. Patients are started on a clear liquid diet on the day of surgery and are advanced to a regular diet by the first postoperative day. Patients are encouraged to ambulate routinely beginning the evening of surgery and at least 4 times per day thereafter. Lower-extremity sequential compression devices are used while in bed. Likewise, incentive spirometry is encouraged every hour while in bed to prevent atelectasis. Rectal stimulation, instrumentation, and medication insertion is prohibited. Furthermore, gentle irrigation of the catheter is performed only when absolutely necessary and only by a physician. The patients are provided oral narcotic analgesia; intravenous narcotics are given only for breakthrough pain. Docusate is prescribed until the patient no longer requires the oral narcotic. All patients are maintained on a prophylactic oral antibiotic until the catheter is removed. The Penrose drain is typically removed on postoperative day 1 and the urethral catheter is removed in the office 2 to 3 weeks after the day of surgery. The majority of patients are discharged on post-operative day number 2; however, nearly one-third are discharged on the first postoperative day.

PERIOPERATIVE MORBIDITY

Without the need for an abdominal incision and as a result of relatively short operative times,[13] perioperative morbidity is low. Weldon and colleagues reported that 18% of their perineal prostatectomies experienced adverse events. However, most events were not serious and no deaths were reported.[14] Patients are typically administered general anesthetic and may have comorbidities such as hypertension, atherosclerosis, and diabetes; they are at risk of perioperative myocardial

infarction, stroke, and death. Given a relatively low operative blood loss and short operative time, these serious risks are small.[10,14,15] Anastomotic strictures which can usually be managed with urethral dilatations under local anesthetic or direct vision urethrotomy occur from 1% to 8% and often occur within the first 4 months of surgery.[10,14,16,17] The incidence of transient lower extremity neurapraxia increases with increased operative time in the extended lithotomy position as reported by Price, noting a 21% incidence with a mean operative time of 188 min.[18] Keller reported a 0% incidence of neurapraxia in 284 prostatectomies with a mean operative time of 99 minutes.[13] Other series note a neurapraxia incidence rate of less than 2%.[14,15,16] Keller postulates that operative times with a patient in the exaggerated lithotomy position of less than 180 minutes is paramount to prevention of neurapraxia.[13]

BLOOD LOSS

Blood loss incurred during a radical perineal prostatectomy is less than that during a radical retropubic prostatectomy.[17,19] This is attributed to the fact the dorsal venous complex is merely reflected from the specimen during the perineal approach whereas it is transected during a retropubic prostatectomy. A review of the literature supports an average blood loss from perineal prostatectomy between 400 and 800 ml and the need for red blood cell transfusions is found to vary from 1–11%.[10,14–17,19–21] Ruiz-Deya et al. report that, over time, their transfusion rates improved from 11% to 5%.[15]

RECTAL INJURY

Rectal injuries have been reported to occur during 0.6–11% of perineal prostatectomies.[10,14,16,19,22,23] When recognized at the time of surgery and repaired primarily with a two layer closure, clinical sequelae are typically avoided. If unrecognized, or when occurring in concert with postoperative urinary extravasation, a rectocutaneous or rectourethral fistula may develop. These fistulas can usually be managed conservatively with a short period of bowel rest followed by a low-residue diet. If spontaneous closure does not occur, the fistula must be explored and excised. In rare cases, a temporary diverting colostomy is required.

FECAL INCONTINENCE

As with rectal injury, fecal incontinence occurs at a higher rate following a radical perineal prostatectomy than retropubic prostatectomy. Bishoff et al. surveyed 227 patients 12 months following radical prostatectomy and report 18% of perineal patients had new onset of fecal incontinence compared with only 5% in the retropubic group.[24] In a prospective longitudinal assessment by Dahm and colleagues, rectal urgency was the most common complaint and symptoms resolved over time; only 2.9% of patients reported involuntary stool leakage by 12 months after radical perineal prostatectomy.[25] Of note, less than 50% of incontinent patients in the Bishoff study had mentioned this problem to their surgeon.[24] Thus, surgeons may be underestimating this problem in their practices.

OUTCOMES

URINARY CONTINENCE

Postoperative urinary continence is an outcome that has garnered much attention due to its impact on quality of life. As a result of the excellent exposure of the bladder neck and prostatic apex enjoyed through the perineal approach, it is generally believed to offer a higher percentage of urinary continence to patients. In a survey by Bishoff, a higher rate of urinary continence and a faster time to continence postoperatively were supported.[24] Unfortunately, controlled studies are lacking. Furthermore, the different definitions of incontinence employed among the various studies make comparisons difficult. It is of the authors' opinion that the 2 procedures are comparable in this regard and that has been shown in several studies.[19,26]

Based on a number of series, the rate of incontinence following radical perineal prostatectomy is reported to range from 4 to 8%.[14,17,20] In Weldon's experience of 220 consecutive perineal cases where incontinence was described as the use of daily pads, continence returned in 23% of patients by 1 month, in 56% by 3 months, in 90% by 6 months and in 95% by 10 months. The only variable significantly related to continence status was age greater than 69; all men in the incontinent group after 10 months were older than 69 years of age.[14] Thus, patients are counseled that final continence status may not be achieved until 1 year after surgery and evaluation for treatment is limited only to those patients who remain incontinent at that time.

POTENCY

In 1988, Weldon applied the nerve-sparing technique previously unique to the retropubic approach to the radical perineal prostatectomy.[11] In the time since, it has been established that potency is preserved at rates similar to those achieved using a retropubic approach. Patients are instructed that potency may be regained up to 24 months after nerve-sparing surgery and that,

although they may have an erection sufficient for vaginal penetration, the overall quality is likely to be diminished. Potent men following radical retropubic prostatectomy were reported by Walsh and colleagues to have erection quality at 60% to 95% of their preoperative state.[27] Moreover, patients who were impotent prior to surgery will remain so post-operatively and those with decreased sexual function preoperatively are at a higher risk for impotence. Investigations are currently under way to assess the benefit of early, regimented use of phosphodiesterase inhibitors in the post-prostatectomy patients. It has been shown that regimented use of sildenafil may help to preserve and increase intrcorporeal smooth muscle content, maintaining the pro-erectile ultrastructure of post-prostatectomy patients.[28] Improved nocturnal erections were demonstrated in post-prostatectomy patients who were administered nightly sildenafil compared to those given placebo.[29] As our understanding of pharmacotherapy improves, so may potency outcomes.

In the series by Weldon and colleagues, post-operative potency was reported in 70% of the 50 patients who met preoperative criteria for nerve-sparing dissection (preoperative potency, unlikely compromise of posterolateral margins) and had follow-up for a minimum of 18 months.[14] 50% of Weldon's patients achieved potency at 1 year and 70% at 2 years. Preservation of only a unilateral neurovascular bundle did not produce significantly different results from a bilateral nerve-sparing operation (68% versus 73%).[14] These results are similar to the 68% potency rates following radical retropubic prostatectomy reported by Walsh et al.[27] However, it is reported that, with older patients, bilateral nerve preservation may afford improved potency compared to only unilateral nerve-sparing operation.[30]

CANCER CONTROL

Although outcomes of potency and urinary continence are exceedingly important for patient satisfaction, radical perineal prostatectomy is foremost an operation to treat cancer. Lance et al. reviewed 1382 men treated by radical retropubic prostatectomy and 316 by radical perineal prostatectomy.[19] To eliminate the selection bias of men with higher preoperative PSA and Gleason score in the retropubic group, patients were matched by race, preoperative PSA level, and Gleason sum. Results did not show any differences among the numbers of organ confined, specimen confined and margin positive disease. As expected by the different exposures afforded, there were higher instances of posterior margin-positive disease in the radical retropubic group, while the perineal group revealed a higher incidence of positive margins at the bladder neck and anterior surface.[19] In

Weldon's series of patients with T1 and T2 disease, the rate of positive margins was 44%.[31] The rate of positive margins was 7%, 16%, and 25% for the apex, posterolateral, and anterior prostate respectively. Korman and colleagues reviewed the pathology specimens from 60 radical retropubic and 40 perineal prostatectomies and did not find a statistically significant difference in the 2 groups: positive margins were apparent in 16% of the retropubic patients and 22% of the perineal patients (p = 0.53) and the capsular incision rate was 4% in each group.[32] Likewise, Frazier and co-workers did not find a difference in the positive margins between retropubic and perineal approaches.[17] In the experience of 508 consecutive radical perineal prostatectomies in the PSA-era, Harris reported 36% of patients had extracapsular disease, but only 18% of cases had margin-positive disease.[33] Clearly, the literature supports radical perineal prostatectomy as an excellent operation for cancer control.

In general, cancer outcomes following surgery are favorable. In the 20-year experience of Paulson whereby radical perineal prostatectomy was performed on 1,242 men with clinically confined andenocarcinoma of the prostate the median time to non-cancer death was 19.3 years.[34] Median cancer-associated death was not reached for patients with organ and specimen confined disease, but it was 12.7% in those with positive margins at time of excision. After 5 years, PSA failure (defined by PSA > 0.5 ng/ml) occurred in 8%, 35%, and 65% of men with organ confined, specimen confined, and margin positive disease respectively. In patients with positive margins, the median time to PSA failure was 2.4 years. Approximately 20% of patients with positive margins did not have biochemical failure. Cancer-associated death occurred approximately 10 years following the time of PSA failure.[34]

SUMMARY

The resurgence of the radical perineal prostatectomy for the treatment of localized prostate cancer has been facilitated by the current emphasis on reducing medical costs, the identification of prostate cancer at earlier stages, and the selected use of laparoscopic lymph node sampling. This technique offers cancer control for localized prostate cancer as efficacious as the radical retropubic prostatectomy in a manner that is cost-effective, and with low morbidity.

REFERENCES

1. Young HH. The early diagnosis and radical cure of carcinoma of the prostate: being a study of 40 cases and presentation of a radical operation which was carried out in 4 cases. Bull Johns Hopkins 1905;16:315.

2. Belt E, Ebert CE, Surber AC. A new anatomic approach in perineal prostatectomy. J Urol 1939;41:482.

3. Millen T. Retropubic Prostatectomy. A new extravesical technique: report of 20 cases. Lancet 1945;2:693–6.

4. Reiner WJ, Walsh PC. An anatomic approach to the surgical management of the dorsal vein and Santorini's plexus during radical retropubic surgery. J Urol 1979;147:1574.

5. Walsh PC, Donker PJ. Impotence following radical prostatectomy: insight into etiology and prevention. J Urol 1982;128:492–494.

6. Walsh PC, Lepor H, Eggleston JC. Radical prostatectomy with preservation of sexual function: anatomical and pathological considerations. Prostate 1983;4:473.

7. Partin AW, Kattan MW, Subong EN, et al. Combination of prostate-specific antigen, clinical stage, and Gleason score to predict pathological stage of localized prostate cancer. J Am Med Assoc 1997;277:1445–1451.

8. Parra RO, Isorna S, Perez MG, et al. Radical perineal prostatectomy without pelvic lymphadenectomy: selection criteria and early results. J Urol 1996;155:612–615.

9. Lerner SE, Fleischmann J, Taub HC, et al. Combined laparoscopic lymph node dissection and modified Belt radical perineal prostatectomy for localized prostate adenocarcinoma. Urology 1994;43:493–498.

10. Levy DA, Resnick MI. Laparoscopic Pelvic Lymphadenectomy and radical perineal prostatectomy: a viable alternative to radical retropubic prostatectomy. J Urol 1994;151:905–908.

11. Weldon VE, Tavel FR. Potency-sparing radical perineal prostatectomy: anatomy, surgical technique, and initial results. J Urol 1988;140:559–562.

12. Mokulis J, Thompson I. Radical prostatectomy: is the perineal approach more difficult to learn? J Urol 1997;157:230–232.

13. Keller H. Comment: Re: Transient lower extremity neurapraxia associated with radical perineal prostatectomy. A complication of exaggerated lithotomy position. J Urol 1999;162:171.

14. Weldon VE, Tavel FR, Neuwirth H. Continence, potency and morbidity after radical perineal prostatectomy. J Urol 1997;158:1470–1475.

15. Ruiz-Deya G, Davis R, Srivastav SK, et al. Outpatient radical prostatectomy: impact of standard perineal approach on patient outcome. J Urol 2001;166:581–586.

16. Gillitzer R, Thuroff JW. Relative advantages and disadvantages of radical perineal prostatectomy versus radical retropubic prostatectomy. Crit Rev Oncol Hematol 2002;43:167–190.

17. Frazier HA, Robertson JE, Paulson DF. Radical prostatectomy: the pros and cons of the perineal versus retropubic approach. J Urol 1992;147:888–890.

18. Price DT, Vieweg J, Roland F, et al. Transient lower extremity neurapraxia associated with perineal prostatectomy. A complication of the exaggerated lithotomy position. J Urol 1998;160:1376–1378.

19. Lance RS, Freidrichs PA, Kane C, et al. A comparison of radical retropubic with perineal prostatectomy for localized prostate cancer within the Uniformed Services Urology Research Group. BJU 2001;87:61–65.

20. Boczko J, Melman A. Radical perineal prostatectomy in obese patients. Urology 2003;62:467–469.

21. Parra RO, Boullier JA, Rauscher JA, et al. The value of laparoscopic lymphadenectomy in conjunction with radical perineal or retropubic prostatectomy. J Urol 1994;151:1599–1602.

22. Lassen PM, Kearse WS. Rectal injuries during radical perineal prostatectomy. Urology 1995;45:266–269.

23. Zincke H, Oesterling JE, Blute ML, et al. Long-term (15 years) results after radical prostatectomy for clinically localized (stage T2c or lower) prostate cancer. J Urol 1994;152:1850–1857.

24. Bishoff JT, Motley G, Optenberg SA, et al. Incidence of fecal and urinary incontinence following radical perineal and retropubic prostatectomy in a national population. J Urol 1998;160:454–458.

25. Dahm P, Silverstein AD, Weizer AZ, et al. A longitudinal assessment of bowel related symptoms and fecal incontinence following radical perineal prostatectomy. J Urol 203;169:2220–2224.

26. Gray M, Petroni GR, Theodorescu D. Urinary function after radical prostatectomy: a comparison of the retropubic and perineal approaches. Urology 1999;53:881–891.

27. Walsh PC, Partin AW, Epstein JI. Cancer control and quality of life following anatomical radical retropubic prostatectomy: results at 10 years. J Urol 1994;152:1831–1836.

28. Schwartz EJ, Wong P, Graydon RJ. Sildenafil preserves intracorporeal smooth muscle after radical retropubic prostatectomy. J Urol 2004;171:771–774.

29. Levine LA, McCullough AR, Padma-Nathan H. Longitudinal randomized placebo-controlled study of the return of nocturnal erections after nerve-sparing radical prostatectomy in men treated with nightly sildenafil citrate. J Urol Abstracts 2004;171:231 (Abstract)

30. Quinlan DM, Epstein JI, Carter BS, et al. Sexual function following radical prostatectomy: influence of preservation of neurovascular bundles. J Urol 1991;145:998–1002.

31. Weldon VE, Travel FR, Neuwirth H, et al. Patterns of positive specimen margins and detectable prostate-specific antigen after radical perineal prostatectomy. J Urol 1995;153:1565–1569.

32. Korman HJ, Leu PB, Huang RR, et al. A centralized comparison of radical perineal and retropubic prostatectomy specimens: Is there a difference according to the surgical approach? J Urol 2002;168:991–994.

33. Harris MJ. Radical perineal prostatectomy: cost efficient, outcome effective, minimally invasive prostate cancer management. European Urology 2003;44:303–308.

34. Iselin CE, Robertson JE, Paulson DF. Radical perineal prostatectomy: oncological outcome during a 20-year period. J Urol 1999;161:163–168.

35. Haas CA, Resnick MI. Radical perineal prostatectomy: late division of seminal vesicles. In: Resnick MI, Thompson IM, Eds. Surgery of the Prostate. New York: Churchill Livingstone, 1998:131–148. Figures reprinted with permission from Elsevier.

Laparoscopic and robotic radical prostatectomy 77

Xavier Cathelineau, Carlos Arroyo, Marc Galiano,
Francois Rozet, Eric Barret, Guy Vallancien

INTRODUCTION

Laparoscopic surgery dates back to 1901 when Kelling performed a "celioscopic procedure" by inserting a cystoscope into an air insufflated abdomen of a dog to inspect the abdominal viscera. However, it was not until the 1940s, that laparoscopic surgery was actually developed in the field of gynecology, and afterwards in gastrointestinal surgery from 1986 onwards. There was a significant delay in its use in urologic procedures if we consider that it was not until 1990 that the first laparoscopic nephrectomy was performed by Ralph Clayman, and 2 years later Schuessler et al reported the first attempt to perform a laparoscopic prostatectomy; then, in 1997, they published 9 cases of laparoscopic radical prostatectomy finding it a difficult procedure with no advantages over open surgery.[1] During that same year, Raboy published a case of an extraperitoneal radical prostatectomy.[2] By December that same year, Richard Gaston (Bordeaux, France), in a personal communication, indicated that he had performed a transperitoneal radical prostatectomy in less than 6 hours. Six weeks later, Bertrand Guillonneau and Guy Vallancien started to perform their first radical prostatectomies;[3,4] followed 5 months later by Claude Abbou.[5] Nowadays, virtually all of the urologic oncologic surgeries can be performed by a laparoscopic approach.[6]

Current progress in robotic manipulators is encouraging for laparoscopic surgery because it could make the procedures easier. The first group includes robots that assist the surgeon by actively positioning the laparoscope, such as the robotic arm AESOP™ that uses speech recognition to maneuver the endoscope to place the camera where it is required. The second group involves what we consider robotic-assisted surgery—this involves a computer-enhanced master–slave telemanipulator, which allows a remote manipulation of the instruments in the operative field; however, they are not really robots.

In the last few years, laparoscopic radical prostatectomy has gained popularity, with a significant increase in the number of procedures performed worldwide.[7] Part of this increase can be explained because minimally invasive surgery is appealing to patients[8] and surgeons, because by maintaining the oncologic results of open surgery it offers the benefit of a minimally invasive technique that should reduce the postoperative pain, shorten the convalescence time, and improve the quality of the procedure by perfecting the urethrovesical anastomosis and preservation of neurovascular bundles.

Currently our experience in the Institut Montsouris adds up to over 2000 laparoscopic radical prostatectomies, performed from 1998 to 2004, distributed as follows: 1400 transperitoneal and 600 extraperitoneal, including over 120 have been robot assisted (70 transperitoneal and 50 extraperitoneal). In this chapter we will discuss the indications, techniques, complications, and results of laparoscopic and robotic radical prostatectomy.

INDICATIONS AND CONTRAINDICATIONS

Concerning the indications of laparoscopic or robotic radical prostatectomy, there is no debate because they are exactly the same as in open radical prostatectomy. However, as in open surgery, the adequate selection of the patients who are candidates for a surgical treatment will impact on the results obtained with either approach. The best indication for a radical prostatectomy would be a young patient, without any serious co-morbidity, a PSA lower than 15 ng/mL, clinical stage T1, with less than 50% of biopsies positive and a Gleason score of less than 8.

However, just as in open surgery, laparoscopic radical prostatectomy can be performed in selected T3N0M0 stages, without neurovascular bundle preservation, but always cautioning the patient of the risk of residual disease that may require complementary treatment. Also, salvage laparoscopic radical prostatectomy after radiotherapy or brachytherapy can be done; however, it is important to keep in mind that this surgery involves a high risk of damage to the rectum whether it is performed by open surgery or a laparoscopic approach.

There are some absolute anesthetic contraindications that are shared with any laparoscopic approach, involving high intracranial pressure of whatever etiology. Abdominal laparoscopic surgery, especially in an extraperitoneal approach, causes an increased partial pressure of carbon dioxide (P_{CO_2}), that requires an increased minute ventilation, in order to maintain a P_{CO_2} between 30 and 35 mmHg (data to be published). This explains additional relative anesthetic contraindications that include, severe emphysema, cardiac insufficiency, atrioventricular defects, chronic respiratory disease, and severe glaucoma.

As in open radical prostatectomy, there are no anatomic contraindications for laparoscopic approach. However, there are some cases considered as potentially challenging, especially those circumstances in which tissues around the prostate are more difficult to dissect. These include a large volume prostate (over 100 g), neoadjuvant hormonotherapy, previous prostatic surgery (transurethral resection of the prostate [TURP] or adenomectomy), history of prostatitis, radiotherapy, brachytherapy, thermal ablation of the prostate (Ablatherm™) or previous major abdominopelvic surgery because of the formation of adhesions.[9–11] Finally, for an extraperitoneal approach the history of previous bilateral mesh hernia repair can make this approach difficult because of the formation of adhesions that can make the Retzius space dissection difficult..[12]

An important consideration for surgeons at the beginning of their learning curve is to carefully select their cases, because it has been shown that the surgeon's experience is inversely related to in-hospital complications and length of stay for open radical prostatectomy.[13] Importantly, always keep in mind that in laparoscopic surgery, conversion to open surgery is not a shame but a sign of wisdom.

PREOPERATIVE PREPARATION

The patient is admitted to the hospital the night before the surgery to start prophylactic anticoagulation with an injection of low-molecular-weight heparin, which is continued for at least 7 days postoperatively. Another measure to prevent thromboembolic complications is the systematic use of varicose vein stockings. We do not do any gastrointestinal or skin preparation (shaving), nor do we prescribe any antibiotic prophylaxis.

PATIENT INSTALLATION AND TROCAR PLACEMENT

PATIENT INSTALLATION

Laparoscopic radical prostatectomies by the transperitoneal or extraperitoneal approach are performed under general anesthesia, with the patient placed in a dorsal supine position. During the transperitoneal technique an exaggerated Trendelenburg position is preferred compared with a moderate position in the extraperitoneal approach. The lower limbs are in abduction for intraoperative access to the rectum. The upper limbs are positioned alongside the body to avoid the risk of stretch injuries to the brachial plexus. Two security belts are placed across the thorax in an "X" pattern, to ensure that there is no patient movement during surgery, and yet ensuring there is no risk of pressure injury in using shoulder rests.

The surgeon stands on the left side of the patient with the operating room nurse and instrument table, and the assistant stands on the right side of the operating table. The video column with the insufflator and light source are placed between the legs of the patient and the electrocautery and aspirator behind the assistant.

In the case of a robot-assisted technique, before the entry of the patient in the operative room the "robot" is set up. The system is started and performs a self-testing procedure, during which it recognizes its own spatial position and various components. The cameras are black and white, balanced, and calibrated. The patient positioning is the same except for a slight flexion of the lower limbs to allow the robot to approach as close as possible to the surgical table. The surgeon remains in the console for the entire procedure, and a scrub nurse and assistant remain on the left side of the patient.

TROCAR PLACEMENT

In case of laparoscopic radical prostatectomy, we routinely use five trocars, and they are the same with either approach, except for a slight displacement in the extraperitoneal approach, in which the trocars tend to be slightly lower than for the transperitoneal approach. They depend on the surgeons preferences and include:

The linear distribution, in which a 10 mm trocar is introduced in the umbilicus for the camera, the surgeon will work with two 5 mm trocars that are introduced— one above and medial to the iliac spine and another one lower and lateral to the umbilical port. The assistant will work with a 5 mm trocar that is placed above and medial to the right iliac spine, and a second 10 mm trocar between the umbilical and lateral ports on the right (Figure 77.1).

The triangular trocar variation involves placement of the surgeon's ports on the left side between the umbilical port and the left iliac spine and the other one two thirds of the distance between the umbilical port and the suprapubic rim along the midline (Figure 77.2).

In the case of a robot-assisted procedure, no matter if it is extra- or transperitoneal, the trocar distribution is as follows: a 12 mm trocar is introduced in the umbilicus for the camera, and two 8 mm trocars for the robot arms are placed on both sides five fingerbreadths lateral to the optic and slightly lower. Finally, for the assistant, a 5 mm trocar is introduced above and medial to the left iliac spine and a 10 mm trocar for the suture introduction is placed slightly higher between the optic and right robot trocar (Figure 77.3).

TECHNIQUES

TRANSPERITONEAL APPROACH

This approach was the first one to be described for laparoscopic radical prostatectomy,[14,15] and it has been divided into the following six critical steps:

1. Incision of the posterior vesical peritoneum with dissection of the vasa deferens and seminal vesicles. Denonvilliers' fascia is also incised.
2. Dissection of the Retzius space. The intrapelvic fascia is incised with selective suture ligation of the Santorini's plexus.
3. Bladder neck is identified and dissected, with the seminal vesicles delivered.
4. The lateral surfaces of the prostate are dissected in the intrafascial plane in order to preserve the neurovascular bundles (when indicated).
5. Selective dissection of the urethra with the aid of a metal Béniqué dilator.
6. A urethrovesical anastomosis is performed with interupted or running vicryl sutures. Finally, the prostate is extracted using a laparoscopic bag.

There have been some variations described in the literature concerning the technique, such as the one

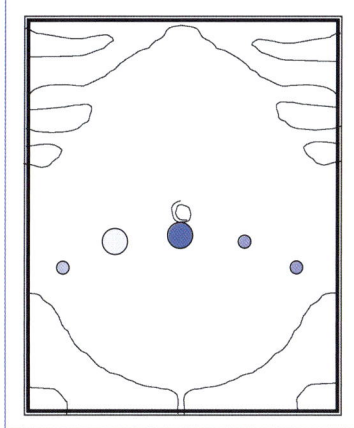

Optic 10 mm port
Assistant 10 mm port / surgeon during sutures
Assistant 5 mm port
Surgeon 5 mm ports

Fig. 77.1
The first trocar position variation involves placement of all the ports as high as possible with respect to the umbilicus; the left side ports are used by the surgeon and the right side for the assistant.

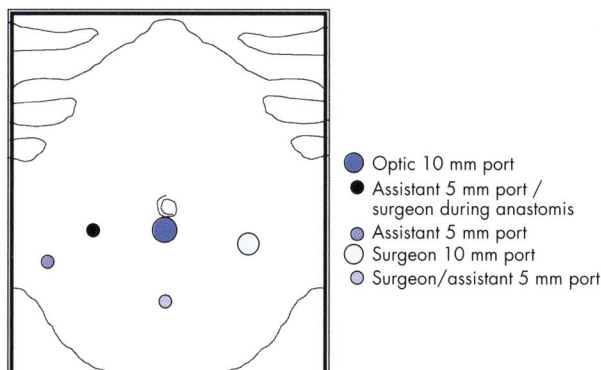

Optic 10 mm port
Assistant 5 mm port / surgeon during anastomis
Assistant 5 mm port
Surgeon 10 mm port
Surgeon/assistant 5 mm port

Fig. 77.2
The triangular trocar variation involves placement of the surgeon ports on the left side between the umbilical port and the left iliac spine and the other two thirds of the distance between the umbilical port and the suprapubic rim along the midline.

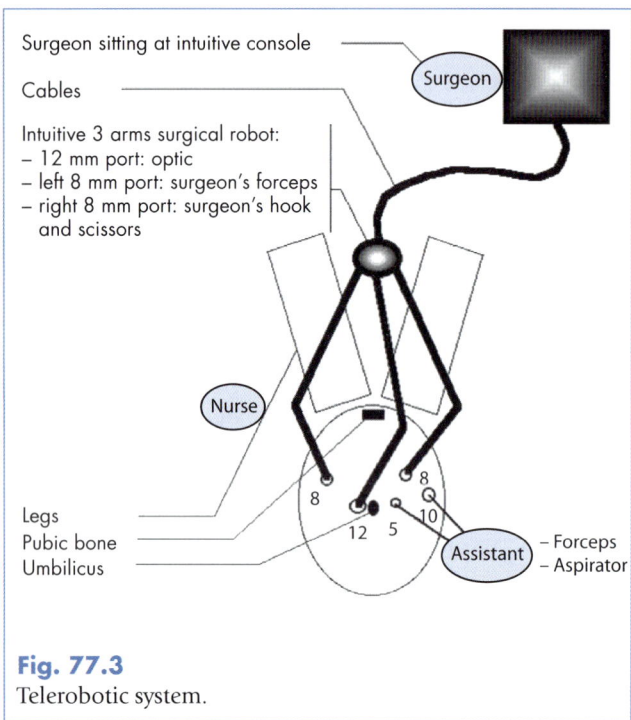

Surgeon sitting at intuitive console

Cables

Intuitive 3 arms surgical robot:
– 12 mm port: optic
– left 8 mm port: surgeon's forceps
– right 8 mm port: surgeon's hook and scissors

Surgeon

Nurse

Legs
Pubic bone
Umbilicus

8
8
12 5 10

Assistant
– Forceps
– Aspirator

Fig. 77.3
Telerobotic system.

proposed by Abbou et al,[16,17] in which he prefers to divide the Santorini's plexus after having opened the bladder neck, which is identified by palpation with scissors to distinguish a mobile bladder wall from solid prostatic substance. Another difference is that the urethrovesical anastomosis is performed with two hemicircumferential running sutures.

Rassweiler et al have also proposed the Heilbronn technique in which he places five trocars in a W-shaped distribution and starts the surgery by immediate access to the Retzius space. They recommend a 6th port for an optimal exposure and describe an ascending part as the incision of the endopelvic fascia and trans-section of the puboprostatic ligaments, and the dorsal vein complex with a previously placed suture, in order to gain access to the urethra at the level of the apex. The descending part of the surgery implies the traction of the prostate ventrally for the dissection of the bladder neck to gain access to the seminal vesicle by a retrovesical approach.[18]

These and other modifications only prove that the steps in the laparoscopic radical prostatectomy can be performed according to the surgeon's preferences, but always with the idea of making the technique more effective and to improve the functional results.

EXTRAPERITONEAL APPROACH

This approach has been previously described in the literature[19–21] and can be divided into steps similarly:

1. The dissection of the Retzius space is done by blunt dissection with the laparoscope or by the use of a balloon.

2. Opening of the intrapelvic fascia floor with the suture ligature of Santorini's plexus.
3. Bladder neck dissection, which reveals the initial plane of dissection of the seminal vesicles and the Denonvilliers' fascia.
4. The lateral surfaces of the prostate are dissected in the intrafascial plane in order to preserve the neurovascular bundles (when indicated).
5. The prostatic apex is dissected and mobilized for a selective section of the urethra.
6. A urethrovesical anastomosis is performed with interrupted or running vicryl sutures with extraction of the prostate with a laparoscopic bag.

This retropubic approach, described after the experience gained with the transperitoneal prostatectomy, has gained a lot of interest because it is argued that the anatomy is more comparable to the open technique,[22] with the added benefit that by avoiding the peritoneum, the danger of gastrointestinal damage is decreased.[23,24] What has been learned from experience is that it also allows a better identification of the hypogastric vessels, which is very helpful during the placement of the lateral ports. Also, if there is an anastomotic urinary leak, it can be managed better because there is no contact with the peritoneal organs.

TELEROBOTIC SURGICAL SYSTEM

The surgical technique varies only in the placement of the trocars and the equipment. The position of the patient is basically the same as in any laparoscopic radical prostatectomy; however, the umbilical port is a 12 mm trocar for the use of the 3D-endocamera that is attached to the medial arm of the robot. Both 8 mm lateral ports are for the introduction of the specially designed instruments for the robot, that feature the Endo-Wrist™ articulations and include the cautery hook, a short-tip grasper, a bipolar hemostatic grasper, and needle holders.[25] The fourth 10 mm port is for the introduction of the needles and instruments by the assistant, and, finally, the fifth 5 mm port will also be used by the assistant for conventional laparoscopic instruments (clip appliers, large grasper, and suction device).

Once all of the attachments and instruments are placed, the surgery is basically done following the steps mentioned in the transperitoneal or extraperitoneal approach. The da Vinci system™ is a master–slave type of surgical robot, that consists of a slave or work unit and a master or control unit, which are connected by a computer-based system. The master unit is located in the remote console and transmits the movements that the surgeons is performing to the slave unit, which will move the camera and two instruments. The role of the assistant is limited to exposing the operative field, assisting in hemostasis by suction and irrigation, and the application of clips.[26]

All of the above require a complete knowledge of the performance capabilities and steps in the attachment of the instruments by the assistant and the operating room nurse, in order to facilitate the introduction of the instruments and assist the surgeon to make it efficient.

The role of robotic technology in laparoscopic urologic surgery is becoming more widely accepted because of the advantages provided by this technology, which include: the improved visualization by the InSitte Vision System that provides a 3D-vision and 10-fold magnification; the handling of the laparoscopic tools that is facilitated by the Endo-Wrist instrument technology, which allows the surgeon to use instruments as in open surgery; and finally, the procedure can be undertaken in a relaxed working position at the console.[27]

The above has allowed not only the performance of radical prostatectomy, but other techniques associated with it, such as sural nerve grafting during the same procedure[28] or more complex procedures, including nerve-sparing radical cystoprostatectomy and urinary diversion.[29]

POSTOPERATIVE MANAGEMENT

The bladder catheter is left for 3 to 7 days depending on the quality of the suture evaluated by the surgeon. Postoperative cystogram is not routinely performed. Our analgesia scheme is limited to i.v. paracetamol during the first 24 hours, followed on day 1, by oral paracetamol/dextropropoxyphene if necessary. Major analgesics are administered if necessary. The intravenous perfusion is stopped on day 1, and oral fluids are started on the next morning after the surgery, and a normal diet can generally be resumed on day 2.

RESULTS

Since 1998 we have been performing laparoscopic radical prostatectomy, and our current experience adds up to over 2000 cases, which include: 1400 transperitoneal cases and 600 extraperitoneal cases. Among them we have performed 120 robot assisted laparoscopic radical prostatectomies, 70 transperitoneal and 50 by the extraperitoneal approach.

The patient characteristics are summarized in Table 77.1.

MORBIDITY

INTRAOPERATIVE COMPLICATIONS

The median blood loss during laparoscopic radical prostatectomy in our experience was 350 mL with a transfusion rate of 3%. Concerning retropubic radical prostatectomy, Catalona et al,[30] using the technique of hemodilution, reported that most of the patients received autologous transfusion during or after surgery; 9% also needed heterologous postoperative transfusion.

Gastrointestinal injuries are rare and directly related to the operator's experience and to the patient's history (especially previous radiotherapy). The rate of rectal injuries is similar regardless of the technique (retropubic or laparoscopic), ranging from 0.5% to 2%.[30]

EARLY POSTOPERATIVE COMPLICATIONS

Thromboembolic complications constitute the main cause of postoperative mortality in open procedures. Catalona et al[30] reported 2% of thromboembolic accidents, while Rassweiler[18] as in our experience[31] reported a thromboembolic accident rate of less than 0.5%. Prophylactic anticoagulation and early mobilization (especially after laparoscopic procedure) decrease the frequency of these complications.

Anastomotic leaks are often missed when minimal and correctly drained, and their incidence is, therefore, often underestimated.

Our complications are summarized in Table 77.2. To date, we have had neither deaths nor any cardiac complications.

FUNCTIONAL RESULTS

CONTINENCE

The quality of continence after radical prostatectomy is difficult to assess, as reflected by the marked variability of incontinence rates reported in the literature. This variability is related to three main factors: definition of incontinence, modalities of evaluation, and follow-up.

Table 77.1 Preoperative characteristics for 2000 patients who underwent laparoscopic radical prostatectomy

Median age	61 years
Median PSA	9.2 ng/mL
Gleason score	6.5
Number of positive biopsies	2.2

Table 77.2 Intraoperative and early postoperative complications in patients who underwent laparoscopic radical prostatectomy

Complication	Occurrence (%)
Transfusion rate	3.5
Prolonged urinary leakage	1.8
Rectal injury	0.8
Bowel injury	0.2
Lymphocele	0.2
Hematoma	0.2

In our department, the patient is sent a self questionnaire by regular mail. The median follow-up is at 12 months, and reports the continence rates—if they do not use any protection pads, if they are continent but prefer to use a precaution pad; and, finally, if they use one pad on a daily basis because of small urine leaks. Our results are encouraging with a continence rate higher than 84% with either approach (the patients report not using any pad) and only 8% to 14% use 1 pad daily for occasional urine leaks.

POTENCY

As for continence, objective evaluation of sexual potency encounters a number of difficulties: absence of a consensual definition of sexual potency, various methods of evaluation, and variable follow-up.

Currently, for two years, we have evaluated the erectile function with a self applied questionnaire that is mailed to our patients postoperatively. With a median follow-up of 6 months, in the preoperatively potent patients (IIEF5 >20), the erectile function was recovered for 64% with the bilateral nerve-sparing technique, and 43% with unilateral nerve preserving surgery. Longer follow-up is obviously needed.

ONCOLOGIC RESULTS

For patients with organ-confined disease treated with the open approach, at 3 years, Catalona et al[30] had a recurrence-free survival of 93%. Similar results are observed by the Johns Hopkins group, where their 5-years recurrence-free rate was 97% for organ-confined cancer. Concerning the positive margins in series using retropubic approach, the rate ranges between 10% and 40% depending on the experience of the team, the pathologic stage, and the preservation or not of the neurovascular bundles.

In our experience of laparoscopy and robotic radical prostatectomy, 92% of the patients with organ-confined disease had a PSA of less than 0.1 ng/mL at 5 years. The overall rate of positive margin was 14%. Up to now, no port seeding has been observed.[31,32]

DISCUSSION

Some of the benefits obtained with laparoscopic over open radical prostatectomy are the result of the excellent view and magnification provided by the laparoscope, which enables a more precise dissection, especially for the neurovascular bundles, and a more detailed suturing during the urethrovesical anastomosis.[33] Another advantage during laparoscopy is lower hemorrhage rate compared with open surgery. This is the result of the careful and inherent selective coagulation that is essential in this technique. Moreover, less postoperative pain induces quicker recovery, and the preliminary functional results are really encouraging.

In relation to the controversy between the transperitoneal and extraperitoneal laparoscopic approach, our experience, which includes over 1400 transperitoneal and 600 extraperitoneal radical prostatectomies, has shown both approaches to be equivalent in terms of operative, postoperative, and pathologic data. This is why we consider that there is no gold standard in terms of a technique or approach, but rather the outcome depends on the surgeon's experience.[33,34]

Finally, the most relevant difficulty in laparoscopic urologic surgery is the steep learning curve that has been described to be of a minimum of 50 surgeries, as well as the frequency issue, because it has to be done in a rather short period of time. However, this issue is still in debate, but it is clear that laparoscopic surgery does require a long and intensive training period in order to obtain the most out of this technique.

Concerning robot-assisted laparoscopic surgery, the robotically assisted prostatectomy has proven to be a feasible technique that is safe, associated with less blood-loss, and could shorten the hospital stay and catheterization time with the same oncologic and functional results as open surgery.[35] These results are in accordance with the over 120 prostatectomies (70 transperitoneal and 50 extraperitoneal) performed in our institute with the assistance of the da Vinci robot,[36] and they could be attributed to a better visualization, anatomical dissection, reduced blood loss, and improved ability to reconstruct the anatomy.[35,37]

Disadvantages of the robotic interface include the extremely high cost of the equipment, the limitations in the surgical instruments that are available, and the time involved with the positioning of the robot. However, we have also seen that if the same surgical team is routinely involved with the placement of the robot then the time for the complete preparation for the surgery can be decreased significantly (it currently takes between 20 and 25 minutes to start the surgery with the different ports in place).

Overall, the robotic assistance is a safe and effective procedure, which could be the result of the increased range of movements at the instrument tip and the 3D visualization that make a more precise anatomical dissection possible,[38] making this a promising technique.

However, today, for a surgeon experienced in laparoscopy, there are no real advantages for the patient in having a radical prostatectomy carried out by robot-assisted surgery compared with the "classical" laparoscopic approach. This technique is still under development, and improvement of the instrumentation and long-term studies are necessary, but it is already showing promise regarding ease of instrument handling, and we think that it is a matter of time for the full benefits to come to light.

CONCLUSIONS

The development of laparoscopy in surgery is a natural evolution toward a minimally invasive approach with better quality of surgery. The laparoscopic option, through still in evolution, provides a viable alternative with a steep learning curve. The laparoscopic radical prostatectomy remains one of the most technically demanding laparoscopic procedures in view of the difficulty of surgical access and the need for precise intracorporeal suturing. Today, computer-assisted surgery does not currently provide any significant benefit for the patient compared with laparoscopy, but developments are expected. The surgical and oncologic standards of open surgery are maintained by the minimally invasive techniques. Finally, the benefit of an excellent vision, and potential benefits for the patient provided by a laparoscopic approach, requires the surgeon to keep an open attitude for further improvement of the technique.

REFERENCES

1. Schuessler WW, Schulam PG, Clayman RV, et al. Laparoscopic radical prostatectomy: initial short-term experience. Urology 1997;50:854–857.

2. Raboy A, Ferzli G, Albert P. Initial experience with extraperitoneal endoscopic radical retropubic prostatectomy. Urology 1997;50:849–853.

3. Guillonneau B, Cathelineau X, Barret E, et al. Prostatectomie radical coelioscopique. Premier evaluation apres 28 interventions. Pess Med 1998;27:1570–1574.

4. Guillonneau B, Cathelineau X, Barret E, et al. Laparoscopic radical prostatectomy: Technical and early oncological assessment of 40 operations. Eur Urol 1999;36:14–20.

5. Abbou CC, Salomon L, Hoznek A, et al. Laparoscopic radical prostatectomy: preliminary results. Urology 2000;55:630–634.

6. Gomella LG. Editorial: Laparoscopy and urologic oncology – I now pronounce you man and wife. J Urol 2003;169:2057–2058.

7. Lu-Yao GL, McLerran D, Wasson J, et al. An assessment of radical prostatectomy: time trends, geographic variation and outcomes. JAMA 1993;269:2633–2636.

8. Hara I, Kawabata G, Miyake H, et al. Comparison of quality of life following laparoscopic and open prostatectomy for prostate cancer. J Urol 2003;169:2045–2048.

9. Seifman BD, Dunn RL, Wolf JS. Transperitoneal laparoscopy into the previously operated abdomen: effect on operative time, length of stay and complications. J Urol 2003;169:36–40.

10. Weibel MA, Majno G. Peritoneal adhesions and their relation to abdominal surgery. A postmortem study. Am J Surg 1973;126:345.

11. Parsons JK, Jarrett TJ, Chow GK, et al. The effect of previous abdominal surgery on urological laparoscopy. J Urol 2002;168:2387–2390.

12. Katz EE, Patel RV, Sokoloff MH, et al. Bilateral laparoscopic inguinal hernia repair can complicate subsequent radical retropubic prostatectomy. J Urol 2002;167:637–638.

13. Hu JC, Gold KF, Pashos CL, et al. Role of surgeon volume in radical prostatectomy outcomes. J Clin Oncol 2003;21:401–405.

14. Guillonneau B, Cathelineau X, Barret E, et al. Prostatectomie radical coelioscopique. Premier evaluation apres 28 interventions. Pess Med 1998;27:1570–1574.

15. Guillonneau B, Vallancien G. Laparoscopic radical prostatectomy: The Montsouris technique. J Urol 2000;163:1643–1649.

16. Hoznek A, Solomon L, Rabii R, et al. Vesicourethral anastomosis during laparoscopic radical prostatectomy: the running suture method. J Endourol 2001;14:749–753.

17. Hoznek A, Salomon L, Olsson LE, et al. Laparoscopic radical prostatectomy. The Creteil experience. Eur Urol 2001;40:38–45.

18. Rassweiler J, Sentker L, Seemann O, et al. Laparoscopic radical prostatectomy with the Heilbronn technique: an analysis of the first 180 cases. J Urol 2001;166:2101–2108.

19. Bollens R, Vanden Bossche M, Roumeguere T, et al. Extraperitoneal laparoscopic radical prostatectomy. Results after 20 cases. Eur Urol 2001;40:65–69.

20. Dubernard P, Enchetrit S, Hamza T, et al. Prostatectomie extra-peritoneale retrograde laparoscopique (P.E.R.L.) avec dissection premiere des bandelettes vasculo-nerveuses erectiles – technique simplifiee – a propos de 100 cas. Prog Urol 2003;13;163.

21. Vallancien G, Guillonneau B, Fournier G, et al. Laparoscopic Radical Prostatectomy, Technical Manual, 21st ed. In Vallancien G, Khoury S (eds): European School of Surgery Collection, 2002.

22. Bollens R, Bossche MV, Roumeguere T, et al. Extraperitoneal laparoscopic radical prostatectomy. Eur Urol 2001;40:65–69.

23. Bollens R, Roumeguere T, Vanden Bossche M, et al. Comparison of laparoscopic radical prostatectomy technique. Curr Urol Rep 2002;3:148–151.

24. Abreu SC, Gill IS, Kaouk JH, et al. Laparoscopic radical prostatectomy: comparison of transperitoneal laparoscopic radical prostatectomy. Urology 2003;61:617.

25. Guillonneau B, Cappele O, Martinez JB, et al. Robotic assisted laparoscopic pelvic lymph node dissection in humans. J Urol 2001;165:1078–1081.

26. Abbou CC, Hoznek A, Salomon L, et al. Laparoscopic radical prostatectomy with a remote controlled robot. J Urol 2001;165:1964–1966.

27. Binder J, Kramer W. Robotically-assisted laparoscopic radical prostatectomy. Br J Urol Int 2001;87:408–410.

28. Kaouk JH, Sesai MH, Abreu SC, et al. Robotic assisted laparoscopic sural nerve grafting during radical prostatectomy: initial experience. J Urol 2003;170:909–912.

29. Menon M, Hemal AK, Tewari A, et al. Nerve-sparing robot-assisted radical cystoprostatectomy and urinary diversion. Br J Urol Int 2003;92:232–236.

30. Catalona WJ, Carvalhal GF, Mager DE, et al. Potency, continence and complication rates in 1,870 consecutive radical retropubic prostatectomies. J Urol 1999;162:433–438.

31. Guillonneau B, Rozet F, Cathelineau X, et al. Perioperative complications of laparoscopic radical prostatectomy: the Montsouris 3 year experience. J Urol 2002;167:51–56.

32. Vallancien G, Cathelineau X, Baumert H, et al. Complications of transperitoneal laparoscopic surgery in urology: review of 1,311 procedures at a single center. J Urol 2002;168:23–26.

33. Cathelineau X, Arroyo C, Rozet F, et al. Laparoscopic radical prostatectomy: the new gold standard? Curr Urol Report 2004;5:108–114.

34. Cathelineau X, Cahill D, Widmer H, et al. Transperitoneal or extraperitoneal approach for laparoscopic radical prostatectomy: a false debate for a real challenge. J Urol 2004;171:714–716.

35. Tewari A, Srivasatava A, Menon M. A prospective comparison of radical retropubic and robot-assisted prostatectomy: experience in one institution. Br J Urol Int 2003;92:205–210.

36. Cathelineau X, Widmer H, Rozet F, et al. Telerobotic assisted prostatectomy. In Ballantyne GH, Marescaux J, Giulianotti PC (eds): Primer of Robotic and Telerobotic Surgery. Lippincott Williams Wilkins, 2004.

37. Ahlering TE, Skarecky D, Lee D, et al. Successful transfer of open surgical skills to a laparoscopic environment using a robotic interface: initial experience with laparoscopic radical prostatectomy. J Urol 2003;170:1738–1741.

38. Rassweiler J, Frede T. Robotics, telesurgery and telementoring: their position in modern laparoscopy. Arch Esp Urol 2002;55:610–628.

Vattikuti Institute prostatectomy: A robotic technique for the management of localized prostate cancer

78

James A Brown, Ashok K Hemal, Mani Menon

INTRODUCTION

In November 2000, the development of robotic radical prostatectomy using the da Vinci surgical system (Intuitive Surgical, Mountain View, CA) began at Henry Ford Hospital. The da Vinci™ combination of three-dimensional magnified vision and wristed instrumentation provided the rationale for incorporating this technology into radical prostatectomy surgery. A structured program was developed to accomplish this goal.[1] The first step was to gain experience with the laparoscopic radical prostatectomy techniques developed by Guillonneau and Vallencien.[2] Two surgeons from Henry Ford spent a month at L'Institut Mutualiste Montsouris learning laparoscopic skills from a trainer in the animal laboratory and observing 50 laparoscopic radical prostatectomy (LRP) cases performed without robotic assistance. The French surgeons then trained the Henry Ford team in Detroit for 50 additional LRP cases. Our initial robotic prostatectomy procedures closely mimicked the Montsouris laparoscopic procedure. We have, however, made several modifications to our technique over the past 4 years, the most significant being the abandonment of the initial dissection of the seminal vesicles, technique of apical dissection, neurovascular bundle dissection, and vesicourethral anastomosis.[3-5] To date, we have performed about 1200 robotic surgeries at our medical center, of which over 1000 have been Vattikuti Institute prostatectomy (VIP). We describe our current technique and provide insight into the lessons we have learned developing robotic radical prostatectomy.

ROBOTIC TECHNOLOGY

The da Vinci robotic system uses a sophisticated master–slave system. It provides three-dimensional stereoscopic vision, movement scaling, and wristed instrumentation with 7° of movement. A mobile control console houses two-finger controlled handles (masters) to control the robotic arms and foot pedals to control camera movement and electrocautery. The bedside tower has three (and an optional fourth) multijoint robotic arms. The first controls the binocular endoscope and the others the articulated instruments.[6] Instrument movement can be scaled from 1:1 to 1:3 and 1:5. The former setting allows exact finger-movement transmission to the instrument tip, while the latter two settings scale down the surgeon's movements; all with tremor filtration.

PATIENT SELECTION

Any patient meeting the requirements for open or laparoscopic radical prostatectomy is a candidate for robotic radical prostatectomy (VIP). The same factors that exclude a patient from open or laparoscopic surgery apply to robotic prostatectomy patient selection; namely, bleeding diatheses or inability to tolerate general anesthesia. In addition, the patient must be able to tolerate the dorsal lithotomy position placed in steep Trendelenburg. Therefore, patients with lower extremity contractures, severe pulmonary conditions (e.g. chronic obstructive pulmonary disease) or a history of cerebrovascular accident, indwelling ventriculoperitoneal shunt or cerebral aneurysm should be carefully evaluated or avoided. Previous abdominal surgery, including mesh inguinal herniorrhapy, and obesity up to a body mass index of 40 are not contraindications. However, patients who have had previous pelvic surgery should be evaluated prior to embarking on a robotic prostatectomy, given alternative therapeutic options (perineal prostatectomy and radiation therapy). Large prostate size is not a contraindication, as the wristed instruments and scope mobility of the da Vinci robot make this procedure an ideal surgical treatment option for these patients.

PREOPERATIVE MANAGEMENT

Anticoagulants, including aspirin, are discontinued 5 to 7 days prior to surgery. Patients with mandatory indications for coumadin are hospitalized for intravenous heparin conversion prior to surgery. Antibiotic prophylaxis, typically with a first-generation cephalosporin, and 5000 IU subcutaneous heparin are provided on call to the operating room. Lower extremity sequential compression devices are placed just prior to induction of general anesthesia and intravenous fluids are restricted at surgery to less than 800 ml, beginning the morning of surgery until the anastomosis is complete during the operation.

ROBOTIC PROSTATECTOMY TECHNIQUE

The steps and equipment needed in performing a robot-assisted radical prostatectomy are listed in Table 78.1. Table 78.2 gives tips and solutions to problems that may be encountered during the procedure.

POSITIONING

The patient is placed in the dorsal lithotomy position on a gel pad operative table, with the arms tucked along the sides. Cotton pads are used to protect the axilla and other pressure points. The elbows and hands are protected with egg crate foam padding. The shoulders and chest are also padded with egg crate foam and 3-inch tape and straps are criss-crossed across the chest to secure the patient to the table prior to placing him in the steep Trendelenburg position with the table fully lowered. The lower extremities are secured in Allen-type stirrups and the thighs abducted 45° and placed in line with the torso (Figure 78.1). The abdomen is prepped from the costal margin to the groin, and an 18-Fr Foley catheter is placed.

PORT PLACEMENT

A 20 mmHg pneumoperitoneum is established through a left lateral umbilical incision using a Veress needle

Table 78.1 Surgical steps in performing Vattikuti Institute prostatectomy				
Step	**Procedure**	**Lens**	**Right instrument**	**Left instrument**	**Equipment**
1	Extraperitoneal space development	30° up	Endowrist® permanent cautery hook	Endowrist® long tip forceps	Monopolar cautery setting 80–120
2	Apical exposure	0°	Endowrist® permanent cautery hook	Endowrist® long tip forceps	Monopolar cautery setting 80–120
3	Dorsal vein complex ligation	0°	Endowrist® needle driver	Endowrist® needle driver	0-Vicryl on CT-1 needle (6–7 inches)
4	Bladder neck transection	30° down	Endowrist® permanent cautery hook	Endowrist® long tip forceps	Monopolar cautery setting 80–120
5	Seminal vesical and initial posterior prostate dissection	30° down	Endowrist® permanent cautery hook (or Endowrist® round tip scissors)	Endowrist® long tip forceps (or Endowrist® precise bipolar)	Monopolar cautery setting 80–120 (or bipolar setting 25)
6	Posterior prostate, pedicle and neurovascular bundle dissection	30° down	Endowrist® round tip scissors	Endowrist® precise bipolar	Bipolar cautery setting 25
7	Apical dissection and urethral transaction	0°	Endowrist® round tip scissors	Endowrist® precise bipolar	Bipolar cautery setting 25
8	Pelvic lymphadenectomy	0°	Endowrist® round tip scissors	Endowrist® precise bipolar	Bipolar cautery setting 25
9	Urethrovesical anastomosis	0°	Endowrist® needle driver	Endowrist® needle driver (± Endowrist® long tip forceps for initial suture placement)	3-0 Monocryl on RB-1 needle (two dyed and undyed 7–8 inch tied together)

Table 78.2 Technical tips and troubleshooting caveats

Problem	Solution
Port placement for tall/short patients	Camera port placed infra- or supra-umbilical if much taller/shorter than 5 foot 10 inches
Port placement for narrow pelvis	Move ports medial to keep robotic port medial to anterior superior iliac spine
Bowel adhesions	Alter order of port placement to allow lysis of adhesions
Localizing bladder neck transection	Pull Foley balloon into and out of bladder neck to define, elevate prostate and keep tension on bladder in midline, angle dissection slightly inferiorly
Large intravesical median lobe	Elevate through bladder neck and incise mucosa at margin approximately 1 cm distal to ureteral orifices, dissect bladder neck of adenoma
Capacious bladder neck opening bleeding along neurovascular bundles or prostatic fossa	Narrow using figure-of-eight 2-0 vicryl on SH needle at inferolateral corners, use 8-inch 3-0 monocryl running suture, consider "tennis-racket" reconstruction of bladder neck
Inability to move robotic arm caudally/inferiorly in pelvis	Place "cottonoid" Codman surgical strip (Codman & Shurtleff Inc), consider FloSeal (FloSeal matrix hemostatic sealant, Baxter Inc)
Inability to move robotic arm laterally in pelvis	"Lengthen" robotic arm by clutching and further introducing robotic port 1–2 cm
Inability to rotate robotic arm further in a given direction	"Medialize" robotic arm by clutching and rotating arm in medial direction
Dorsal vein complex bleeding after division	Release handle and untwist arm 360°, then grasp master
Anastomotic extravasation	Cauterize with bipolar if ineffective monopolar current or relegate with 2-0 vicryl on RB-1 needle, place interrupted or figure-of-eight 2-0 vicryl sutures, consider redoing anastomosis or tacking bladder or peritoneum to sidewall to "reperitonealize" and take pressure of anastomosis
Postoperative ileus or abdominal pain	Abdominal CT scan to rule out urinary ascites, pelvic hematoma, hernia or ileus

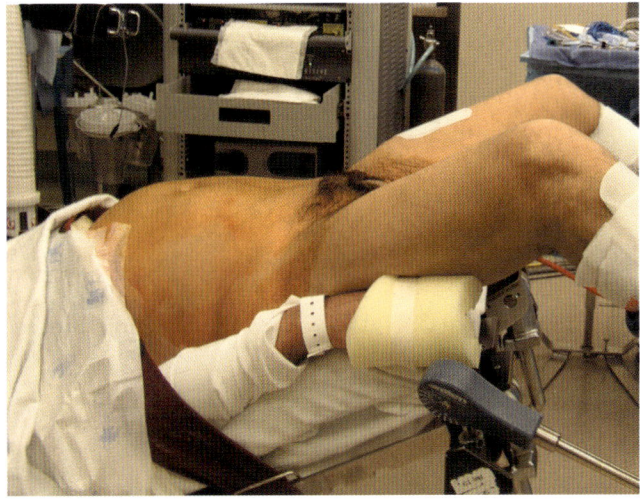

Fig. 78.1
Patient positioned in steep Trendelenburg, dorsal lithotomy position.

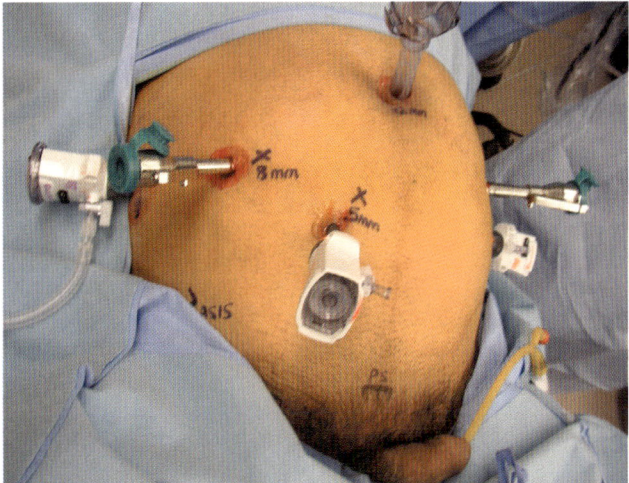

Fig. 78.2
Abdominal port locations.

(Ethicon Endo-Surgery, Albuquerque, NM). The pressure is reset to 14 mmHg after initial port placement. Six ports are then placed as configured in Figure 78.2. The periumbilical incision is typically made along the superior left lateral aspect of the umbilicus for a man 70 inches tall. For shorter men it is moved cephalad and for taller men caudad, approximately 1 to 2 cm. A 12-mm port is placed and the 30° upward lens is introduced. The peritoneum is inspected for injury, abnormalities or bowel adhesions. The right-sided 8-mm robotic port is introduced approximately 3 cm below the level of the umbilicus, 10 to 12 cm off the midline, 2 cm medial to

and three finger breadths superomedial to the anterior superior iliac spine. Two right-sided assistant ports are placed for suture introduction/extraction, suction, and tissue grasping. The first is a 12-mm radial dilating port placed two to three finger breadths above the iliac crest as far lateral along the abdominal wall as possible, entering just anterior to the ascending colon. The second is a 5-mm port placed midway between the camera port and the 8-mm right robotic port. It is placed approximately 2 to 3 cm inferior to the robotic port to allow instruments to reach the pelvis. The left-sided ports are then placed; an 8-mm robotic port in the mirror image location of the right and a 5-mm assistant port in a symmetrical position to the 12-mm right lateral assistant port. The robotic tower is then wheeled between the legs and carefully docked into position, with the right- and left-sided bedside assistant surgeons ensuring proper alignment and avoidance of leg, hand or abdominal skin contact or injury. It typically takes 15 min from Veress needle insufflation to completion of robot docking.

DEVELOPMENT OF EXTRAPERITONEAL SPACE

We have performed several completely extraperitoneal robotic prostatectomies after initially dilating the extraperitoneal space of Retzius with a balloon (Auto Suture, OMS-PDBS2), but we have found port placement to be more challenging than with the transperitoneal approach. Fewer than 50 cases have been done by extraperitoneal VIP technique. The 30° up endoscope is used with the Endowrist® permanent cautery hook (hook cautery) on the right and Endowrist® long tip forceps (long tip forceps) on the left. The cautery (Valley Lab Force FX, Medical Solutions Inc, Minneapolis, MN) power is set as follows: bipolar 25 (standard, medium), cut 50 (pure), and coagulation 80–120 (desiccate, low). Atraumatic graspers (Medtronic Xomed France, LePavillon, France) and the suction/irrigator are used by the assistants. The parietal peritoneum is incised just lateral to the medial umbilical ligament and just medial to the internal inguinal ring over the vas deferens. The latter is grasped and divided, cauterizing the deferential vessel. The dissection is carried anteriorly, 1 cm lateral to the medial umbilical ligament to above the bladder dome (Figure 78.3). The avascular plane of dissection is developed and carried inferiorly through predominantly aereolar

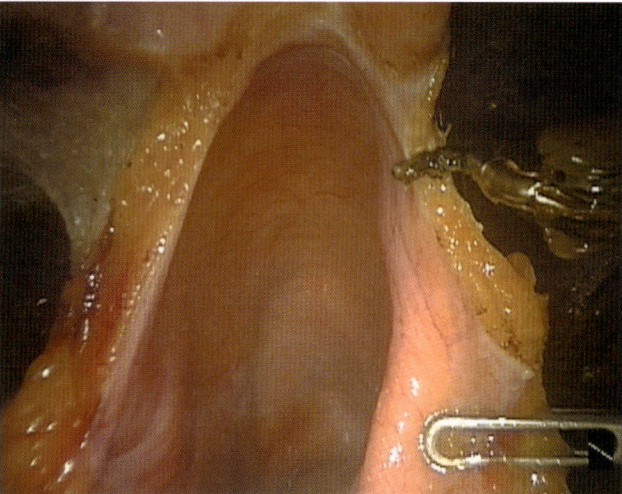

Fig. 78.3
Incisions lateral to the medial umbilical ligaments on either side, during development of the extravesical space.

tissue until the pubic arch is identified. Care is taken to identify and avoid injuring the iliac vessels just lateral to the plane of dissection. This procedure is repeated on the contralateral side. Subsequently, the medial umbilical ligaments are divided above the bladder, with the assistants providing posterior traction on the ligaments with graspers and anterior traction with suction. The dissection is carried medially, dividing the urachus and then reflecting the bladder posteriorly. Fat is dissected off the pubic arch and endopelvic fascia. The superficial dorsal vein is cauterized and divided and the anterior prostate cleaned of adherent fat.

PROSTATIC APICAL DISSECTION AND CONTROL OF DORSAL VENOUS COMPLEX

The 0° endoscope is introduced, and the endopelvic fascia is scored with a hook just lateral to the prostate. Blunt dissection allows exposure of the lateral surface of the prostate as the levator ani muscle fibers are bluntly dissected laterally. Care is taken to minimize use of cautery and avoid inadvertent neurovascular bundle injury. Dissection is carried distally until the urethra with its surrounding puboperinealis muscle is exposed.[7] The wristed action of the instruments allows for precise cephalad retraction of the prostate apex and caudad reflection of adjacent periprostatic levator ani muscle fibers and fascial attachments—a difficult dissection to perform with standard laparoscopic instruments. The puboprostatic ligaments are left intact. The dissection is carried superiorly until a tongue of retroperitoneal fat is identified at the prostatovesical junction. The robotic instruments are exchanged for Endowrist® needle drivers bilaterally and a vertical mattress 7-inch suture of zero polyglactin (0-vicryl) on a CT-1 taper needle is used to secure the dorsal vein complex. We prefer to place the suture without scaling and pass the suture behind the puboprostatic ligaments. The remainder of the suture is used to place a traction suture midway between the prostate apex and base.

BLADDER NECK TRANSECTION

The endoscope is changed to 30° down and the hook cautery is replaced on the right and the long tip forceps on the left. We have used Endowrist® round tip scissors (scissors) on the right and Endowrist® precise bipolar (bipolar) on the left, but have found this to be more time consuming and less hemostatic. The assistants sequentially lift the prostate anteriorly with the traction suture, while the surgeon identifies the prostatovesical junction as a shallow groove just cephalad to the prostate, and incises it lateral to the midline approximately 1 cm cephalad to the prostate. The previously identified tongue of retroperitoneal fat is a constant guide to the prostatovesical junction. Laterally, about 2 cm of fatty tissue separates the detrusor muscle from the prostate, and it is quite safe to incise at this location. If fat is not identified when the incision is made, it is likely that the surgeon is too close to the prostate. The transection follows the contour of the prostatovesical junction distally in the midline, where the bladder is entered anteriorly just cephalad to the prostate. The catheter balloon is deflated, grasped by the second assistant and used to provide anterior traction to expose the posterior bladder neck. The latter is incised and the plane between the prostate and bladder is developed inferiorly and laterally. If a prostatic median lobe is present, it is grasped and elevated out of the bladder, and its cephalad margin is incised 1 to 2 cm distal to the visualized ureteral orifices.

VAS DEFERENS, SEMINAL VESICLE AND POSTERIOR PROSTATIC DISSECTION

The posterior lip of the bladder neck is elevated and dissected off the prostate. The anterior layer of Denonvilliers' fascia is identified and incised, exposing the ampullas of the vas deferens and seminal vesicles. Often the vasa are easily visualized in the midline but may be widely separated with significant prostatic enlargement. Variations in seminal vesicle and vasal anatomy can be recognized more easily if the incision is made wide, before making it deep. Upward traction of the posterior prostate base by the left assistant is applied and the left vas is grasped, cleaned, and divided. The distal and proximal ends are grasped and retracted by the left and right assistants, respectively. The ipsilateral seminal vesicle tip is identified by mobilizing the proximal vas. The seminal vesicle is then skeletonized and freed, avoiding damage to the neurovascular bundle laterally. Subsequently both the left vas and seminal vesicle are grasped by the left assistant, and an identical procedure is performed on the right. The second assistant then grasps and elevates both seminal vesicles and the transected vasa, and the second layer of Denonvilliers' fascia is grasped approximately 1 cm from the prostate and retracted posteriorly. It is divided in the midline and careful blunt dissection allows visualization of the anterior perirectal fat. The plane of dissection between the prostate and rectum is continued with blunt and sharp dissection to the prostatic apex distally and laterally to the medial aspect of the prostatic pedicles. We have recently begun to dissect out the seminal vesicles in select patients using scissors and bipolar cautery in an effort to minimize neurovascular bundle electocautery damage. In addition, we preserve the seminal vesicles (with frozen-section control) in low-risk patients (Gleason score ≤6, clinical T1C, low volume, prostate-specific antigen [PSA] <10 ng/ml) to determine if this modification might improve potency preservation.

PROSTATIC PEDICLE CONTROL AND NEUROVASCULAR BUNDLE PRESERVATION

The scissors are placed on the right and the bipolar instrument on the left (coagulation setting 25). The prostatic pedicles, when discrete and thick, may be controlled with Hem-o-lock MLK clips (Weck Closure Systems, Research Triangle Park, NC) or may be divided sharply with bipolar cauterization of discreet bleeding vessels. The neurovascular bundles run along the posterolateral aspect of the prostate encircled by the inner (prostatic) and outer (levator) layers of periprostatic fascia and anterior layer of Denonvilliers' fascia posteriorly. After dividing the prostatic pedicle, the plane between the prostatic capsule and inner prostatic fascial layer covering the neurovascular bundle is developed at its cranial extent. With the assistants providing superomedial retraction on the prostate and lateral retraction of the neurovascular bundle, careful sharp and blunt dissection of the neurovascular bundle off the prostate is performed until the bundle is mobilized lateral to the prostatic apex. Bipolar cautery is used to coagulate vascular branches or micropedicles that enter the prostate. The wristed instrumentation facilitates this dissection, especially near the prostate apex.

"VEIL OF APHRODITE" LATERAL PERIPROSTATIC FASCIA DISSECTION

We hypothesize that preservation of the lateral periprostatic fascia along with the posterolateral neurovascular bundle might preserve additional accessory nerves and better preserve the vascular supply to the nerves. We, therefore, in February 2003 initiated preservation of the lateral periprostatic fascia ("veil of Aphrodite") in continuity with the posterolateral "neurovascular bundle" in selected sexually potent patients with low-risk disease (serum PSA <10 ng/ml, clinical T1C, Gleason score ≤6, and low-volume tumor) in an effort to determine if this surgical modification would improve erectile potency preservation. The neurovascular bundle is dissected free as described above but, in addition, all periprostatic fascia along the lateral aspect of the prostate up to and including the ipsilateral puboprostatic ligament is preserved in continuity. When performed properly, intact veils of periprostatic tissue, coined "veil of Aphrodite", hang from the puboprostatic ligament(s).

APICAL DISSECTION AND URETHRAL TRANSECTION

The 0° endoscope is used for this and the remainder of the operation. Any residual periapical rectal attachments are taken down and the neurovascular bundles are confirmed free. The Foley catheter is inserted and the dorsal vein complex is divided sharply with scissors, with bipolar used to cauterize any bleeders. The periurethral tissues are divided and the prostatic apex and apical notch identified. The anterior and subsequently lateral and posterior urethra is divided sharply, and the rectourethralis and any remaining prostatic attachments are divided (Figure 78.4). Urethral and apical biopsies are typically obtained and sent for frozen-section analysis, and selected biopsies along the neurovascular bundles and rectum are obtained if indicated.[4] The prostate is then entrapped in an EndoCatch (Auto Suture, Norwalk, CT) bag for later retrieval.

PELVIC LYMPHADENECTOMY

The stereoscopic vision and wristed instrumentation of the da Vinci robot make pelvic lymphadenectomy a much easier operation than its standard laparoscopic counterpart. The endoscopic scissors and bipolar are used to carefully tease the node packet away from the external iliac vein and any accessory vessels. The node packet is cauterized and divided just distal to the node of Cloquet. The obturator nerve is identified and additional distal attachments divided. The packet is mobilized off the obturator nerve and vein and divided proximally. For patients with higher risk disease (Gleason score ≥7, clinical stage T2, PSA ≥10 ng/ml), we perform an extended node dissection to include all fatty and lymphatic tissues posterior and medial to the obturator nerve up to the bifurcation of the iliac vein.

URETHROVESICAL ANASTOMOSIS

We initially performed an interrupted anastomosis but converted to a running anastomosis based on the principles described by Van Velthoven et al[8] for laparoscopic radical prostatectomy. The suture (the MVAC [Menon, Van Velthoven, Ahlering, Clayman] suture) is made by tying a 6 to 8 inch dyed to a similar undyed 3-0 monocryl suture on an RB-1 tapered needle. A needle driver is used on the right and long tip forceps on the left to start the anastomosis. The dyed suture is initially placed out-to-in at the 4 o'clock position of the bladder neck just lateral to the right ureteral orifice. It is run clockwise across the posterior urethra with two to three passes until the suture is just medial to the left ureteral orifice. The suture is cinched down with gentle caudad traction on the bladder (Figure 78.5). The needle driver is placed on the left and the anastomosis continued for two to three passes. It may be intermittently locked or tension may be maintained by the surgeon or assistant. At the 9 o'clock position, the suture is reversed and an additional two passes are performed out-to-in on the urethral and in-to-out on the bladder neck until approximately the 10 o'clock position is reached, where the left assistant holds the suture under tension. The undyed suture is then started by passing it out-to-in at the 4 o'clock position of the urethra and continuing in a counter-clockwise fashion until the anastomosis is complete. If the bladder neck is capacious, it may be closed in a tennis-racket fashion, with the anterior cystotomy closed after completing the anastomosis. A 20-Fr silicone-coated Foley catheter is positioned in the bladder with 20 ml placed in a 5 ml balloon. The bladder is filled to 120 ml to confirm the anastomosis is water-tight.

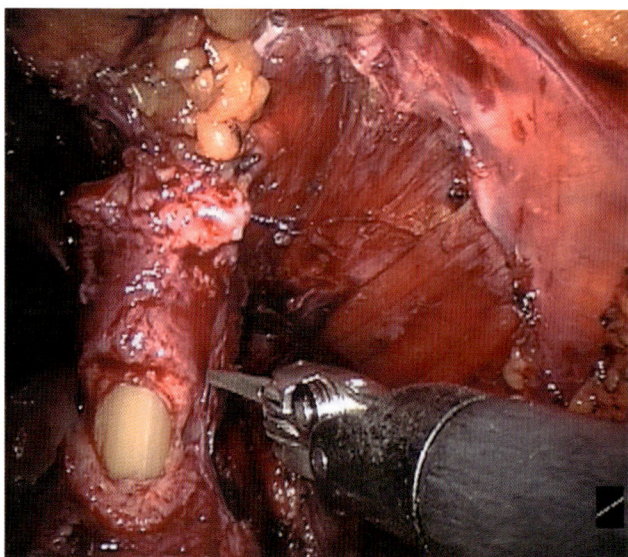

Fig. 78.4
Transection of the urethra.

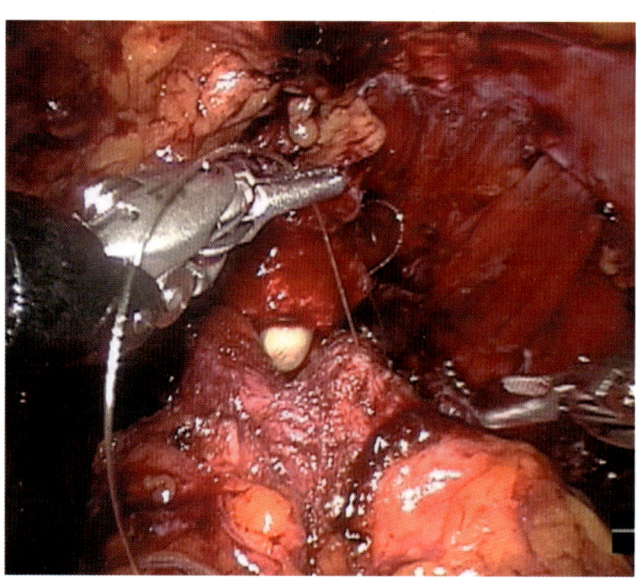

Fig. 78.5
Urethrovesical anastomosis.

SPECIMEN RETRIEVAL AND COMPLETION OF SURGERY

A 15-Fr Jackson-Pratt drain is placed through the left lateral 5-mm port and positioned in the pelvis. The robot is then dedocked and the specimen bag removed through the umbilical port site, enlarging it as necessary. The umbilical port is closed in layers, with 1-0 ethibond on a CTX needle for the fascia. The skin of all port sites is reapproximated with 4-0 vicryl subcuticular sutures and steristrips. Band-Aids or gauze covered with Tegaderm are applied. The drain and Foley catheter are secured, and the patient is transferred to the recovery room.

POSTOPERATIVE CARE

The patient is admitted for overnight observation, allowed to ambulate, and given clear liquids the evening of surgery. Pain management is provided with ketorolac and acetaminophen with codeine. He is discharged on postoperative day 1, typically after removal of the drain. A gravity cystogram is obtained on postoperative day 4 to 6, and the Foley catheter is removed if no anastomotic extravasation is noted. The patient resumes full activity 1 to 2 weeks postoperatively.

RESULTS

TECHNIQUE EVOLUTION

Our initial surgical technique included initial posterior dissection of the seminal vesicles,[2] division of the puboprostatic ligaments, use of a urethral sound, and performance of an interrupted anastomosis.[3] We subsequently abandoned initial posterior seminal vesicle dissection, puboprostatic ligament division, and use of a urethral sound, and incorporated use of a running anastomosis into our technique.[9] We have recently initiated preservation of the lateral prostatic fascia ("veil of Aphrodite") and selective preservation of the seminal vesicles in an effort to improve sexual potency preservation. We have completed our first 1000 VIPs and are now compiling and evaluating our results. We have reported results from our initial 100 patients[10] and subsequently our first 200 VIP patients.[11]

INITIAL EXPERIENCE

We have published the results of our first 100 cases performed between August 2001 and May 2002.[10] Mean patient age was 60 years, and mean body mass index was 27.5. Mean preoperative PSA level was 7.2 ng/ml and follow-up was 5.5 months. Thirty-eight patients had pelvic lymphadenectomy. Mean operative time was 195 ± 5.0 min. Mean blood loss was 149 ml and no patient required transfusion. Twenty-one, 64, 5, 9, and 1 tumors were pathologic stage pT2a, pT2b, pT3a, pT3b, and pT3BN1, respectively. Positive surgical margin rate was 15%. At 1, 3, and 6 months, the continence rates were 37%, 72%, and 92%, respectively, and the potency rates were 11%, 32%, and 59%. A significant improvement was noted between our initial 40 and subsequent 60 cases. Mean operative time decreased from 274 to 195 min, estimated blood loss (EBL) from 256 to 149 ml, and positive margin rate from 17.5% to 12%.

INTERIM EXPERIENCE: COMPARISON OF VIP AND RADICAL RETROPUBIC PROSTATECTOMY

We subsequently compared the results of our first 200 VIPs to a contemporary series of 100 radical retropubic prostatectomies (RRPs) performed at our institution.[11] No statistically significant difference in patient age, preoperative serum PSA level, body mass index, abdominal or pelvic surgery history, Charlson score or clinical grade or stage was noted. A significant difference favoring VIP was observed in terms of mean EBL (153 vs 910 ml), intraoperative blood transfusion (0% vs 67%), postoperative pain score (3 vs 7), discharge hemoglobin (130 vs 101 g/L), hospital stay (1.2 vs 3.5 days), catheterization time (7 vs 15.8 days), total positive margins (9% vs 23%) and extensive (>1 mm) positive margins (1% vs 15%) in pT2A to pT3A tumors. Analysis of functional outcomes demonstrated faster recovery of continence and potency for the VIP cohort.

ASSESSMENT OF RUNNING URETHROVESICAL ANASTOMOSIS

We evaluated the results of our first 120 running anastomoses performed by a single surgeon.[4] Mean time was 13 min. Ninety-six (80%) patients had their catheter removed 4 days after surgery after negative cystogram. The remainder had their Foley catheter removed at 7 days. Two patients developed urinary retention requiring recatheterization. Ninety-six percent of patients were continent (no pads) at 3 months follow-up. No patient developed a bladder neck contraction.

ASSESSMENT AND MODIFICATION OF NEUROVASCULAR BUNDLE PRESERVATION

In an effort to better understand the neurovascular anatomy, we performed a critical analysis of the neurovascular bundles using cadaver dissection.[5] More recently, we have developed the hypothesis that preservation of the lateral periprostatic fascia along with the posterolateral neurovascular bundle might preserve additional accessory nerves and better preserve the vascular supply to the nerves. As described above, we have initiated preservation of the lateral periprostatic fascia ("veil of Aphrodite") in continuity with the posterolateral "neurovascular bundle" in selected patients with low-risk disease in an effort to determine if these surgical modifications would improve erectile potency preservation. A follow-up (conducted by an independent third party) of 33 patients 1 year after surgery with a preoperative sexual function (SHIM) score of 20 or higher was performed. Twenty-two patients had undergone standard nerve preservation and 11 had preservation of the lateral periprostatic fascia ("veil of Aphrodite"). Seven (32%) patients who underwent standard bilateral nerve sparing and 9 (82%) who underwent the "veil of Aphrodite" reported 1-year SHIM scores of 20 or greater (P = <0.05). While the sample size is extremely small, we are encouraged that the return of potency and the quality of erections were superior in the cohort of patients undergoing the "veil of Aphrodite" modification of the VIP.

Our initial postoperative potency preservation results were not improved for patients in whom we spared the tips of the seminal vesicles. We have, therefore, also initiated sparing the entire seminal vesicle in "low-risk" patients. We look forward to analyzing these patients' results to determine if these surgical technique modifications result in improved postoperative outcomes.

SUMMARY

The development of the da Vinci robot has ushered in a new era of surgery.[12] We now have technology that allows us to combine the magnified view and minimally-invasive benefits of laparoscopy with the three-dimensional vision and wristed movements of open surgery. The surgeon is able to operate from a comfortable seated position and provide the patient with outcomes equivalent to or surpassing the best results of open and laparoscopic radical prostatectomy. One can only dream what the future holds for robotic surgery.

REFERENCES

1. Menon M, Shrivastava A, Tewari A, et al. Laparoscopic and robotic assisted radical prostatectomy: establishment of a structured program and preliminary analysis of outcomes. J Urol 2002;168:945–949.

2. Guillonneau B, Vallancien G. Laparoscopic radical prostatectomy: the Montsouris technique. J Urol 2000;163:1643–2649.

3. Tewari A, Peabody J, Sarle R, et al. Technique of da Vinci robot-assisted anatomic radical prostatectomy. Urology 2002;60:569–572.

4. Menon M, Hemal AK, Tewari A, et al. The technique of apical dissection of the prostate and urethrovesical anastomosis in robotic radical prostatectomy. BJU Int 2004;93:715–719.

5. Tewari A, Peabody JO, Fischer M, et al. An operative and anatomic study to help in nerve sparing during laparoscopic and robotic radical prostatectomy. Eur Urol 2003;43:444–454.

6. Menon M, Hemal AK . Laparoscopic surgery: Where is it going? Prous Science: Timely Topics in Medicine, Oct 10, 2003, ttmed.com (epub), www.prous.com.

7. Myers RP. Detrusor apron, associated vascular plexus, and avascular plane: relevance to radical retropubic prostatectomy—anatomic and surgical commentary. Urology 2002;59:472–9.

8. Van Velthoven RF, Ahlering TE, Peltier A, et al. Technique for laparoscopic running of urethrovesical anastomosis: the single knot method. Urology 2003;61:699–702.

9. Menon M, Tewari A, Peabody J. Vattikuti Institute Prostatectomy: Technique. J Urol 2003;169:2289–2292.

10. Menon M, Shrivastava A, Sarle R, et al. Vattikuti Institute prostatectomy: A single-team experience with 100 cases. J Endourology 2003;17:785–790.

11. Tewari A, Shrivastava A, Menon M. A prospective comparison of radical retropubic and robot-assisted prostatectomy: experience in one institution. BJU Int 2003;92:205–210.

12. Hemal AK, Menon M. Robotics in urology. Curr Opin Urol 2004;14:89–94.

Role of surgery in the management of high-risk localized prostate cancer

79

Laurence Klotz, Alessandro Volpe

INTRODUCTION

Prostate cancer is a heterogeneous disease with very different phenotypes. Defining the subgroup of patients who are at high risk for developing recurrence after local treatment is a priority.

Historically, initial risk assessment was based on clinical staging and anatomic extent of the disease, assessed by digital rectal examination (DRE) and imaging. However, a large proportion of patients with clinically organ-confined disease are subsequently found to have extracapsular disease at the time of surgery. Such patients are at high risk of recurrence. Partin et al[1] developed a nomogram which improves the ability to clinically predict pathologic stage, taking into account biopsy Gleason grade and prostate-specific antigen (PSA) level along with clinical stage.

Many studies reveal a significant association between an increased biopsy Gleason score and decreased disease-free survival after radical prostatectomy or radiation therapy.[2–4] Superior outcomes occur with a Gleason score of 6 or less, intermediate outcomes with a Gleason score of 7, and poorer outcomes with a Gleason score of 8 or more.[2,4–6] Pretreatment PSA is also a significant predictor of outcome either after surgery[2,3,7] or radiation therapy.[8,9]

Given the independent prognostic significance of pretreatment PSA, Gleason score, and clinical stage, various algorithms have been produced to establish the risk of PSA failure after local therapy of localized prostate cancer. Kattan et al[10] developed a nomogram to predict 5-year prognosis after radical prostatectomy. Similar nomograms have been developed for external beam radiation therapy[11] and brachytherapy.[12] These are widely used in clinical practice.

D'Amico et al[13,14] proposed stratifying patients with localized prostate cancer into categories with low (<25%), moderate (25–50%), and high risk (>50%) of PSA failure at 5 years from definitive local treatment. According to this classification, patients with AJCC clinical stage T2C, a PSA level of more than 20 ng/ml, or a biopsy Gleason score of 8 or more are considered at high risk of recurrence (Table 79.1).

In a recent paper, the same investigators[15] observed that patients presenting with all the characteristics used to define intermediate-risk cancers (Table 79.1) had a time to PSA failure and a prostate cancer-specific mortality after radical prostatectomy significantly shorter than patients whose definition was based on just one or two factors. This observation may support the shift of this group of intermediate-risk patients into the high-risk category.

Blute et al[7] developed a different scoring system called GSPM (Gleason score, Seminal vesicle, PSA, and Margin status) to predict the risk of biochemical failure after radical prostatectomy (Table 79.2). In their series, 5-year progression-free survival was 94% for a score lower than 5, 60% for a score of 10, and 32% for a score greater than 12.

Several studies have shown that the addition of information about the percentage of prostate biopsy

Table 79.1 Classification of localized prostate cancer in risk groups based on preoperative prognostic factors.[13,14]

	Low risk	Intermediate risk	High risk
AJCC clinical stage	T1 – T2a	T2b	T2c
Biopsy Gleason score	≤6	7	≥8
PSA level (ng/ml)	<10	10–20	> 20

Table 79.2 Mayo Clinic GSPM score system.[7]

Clinical feature	Score
Gleason score	Gleason score value
PSA 4–10 ng/ml	+1
PSA 10–20 ng/ml	+2
PSA >20 ng/ml	+3
Positive seminal vesicles	+2
Positive surgical margins	+2

High scores are associated with increased risk of biochemical recurrence.

cores involved by cancer can further stratify patients with respect to the probability of PSA failure.[16–20]

Some authors have used results from high-density tissue microarrays to define combinations of biomarkers associated with prostate cancer progression after radical prostatectomy.[21] Neural networks have also been utilized to predict the risk of biochemical failure after surgical treatment.[22]

ROLE OF RADICAL PROSTATECTOMY IN THE MANAGEMENT OF HIGH-RISK LOCALIZED DISEASE

The first goal in the management of patients diagnosed with localized prostate cancer is the selection of a treatment that can provide the best chance of cure with the least morbidity. Appropriately, high-risk patients who are aware of the life-threatening nature of their disease are more accepting of treatment morbidity. However, the side effects of radical prostatectomy are not increased in patients with high-risk disease.[23–25]

In a randomized trial comparing radical prostatectomy with watchful waiting in clinically localized prostate cancer, Bill-Axelson et al[26] observed a lower cancer-specific mortality in the surgical group at 5 to 10 years from diagnosis (Figure 79.1). According to Pound et al,[27] the median time to death from prostate cancer

in men who have had a radical prostatectomy is 16 years.[27] Thus, deaths from prostate cancer at 5 to 10 years from diagnosis reflect high-risk, aggressive disease. This suggests that the survival benefit in the Bill-Axelson et al study is a function of a survival benefit of radical prostatectomy in high-risk patients.

Other than the unique Holmberg et al trial,[26] determining the rational, evidence-based choice of treatment of localized prostate cancer has been hampered by the scarcity of unbiased data on outcome from randomized clinical trials. Few studies have been carried out outside specialized academic centers. However, a population-based approach has provided some convincing evidence for the role of surgery. In 1997, Lu-Yao and Yao[28] analyzed the data for 59,876 patients included in the Surveillance, Epidemiology and End Results (SEER) program database to establish overall and disease-specific survival in patients treated by surgery, radiotherapy or conservative management for clinically localized prostate cancer in diverse clinical settings. They observed that cancer grade significantly affects overall survival for all treatments, confirming its role as the most important predictor of survival. In each grade group, radical prostatectomy provided higher 10-year cancer-specific survival rates compared to radiation therapy or watchful waiting (Table 79.3). The benefit of surgery when compared to other treatments was greatest in patients with high-grade disease and therefore high risk of mortality; this benefit was apparent within 5 years of diagnosis. Though Lu-Yao and Yao's study[28] was not randomized, these findings support the view that surgical treatment can significantly improve long-term survival in patients with high-risk localized prostate cancer.

Menon et al[29] retrospectively evaluated long-term survival in 3159 men with clinically localized prostate cancer managed conservatively or treated definitively with either radiation therapy or radical prostatectomy. The overall adjusted survival rate was significantly increased in patients with high-grade cancers who underwent surgery when compared to patients treated with radiation therapy ($P = 0.009$), which was superior

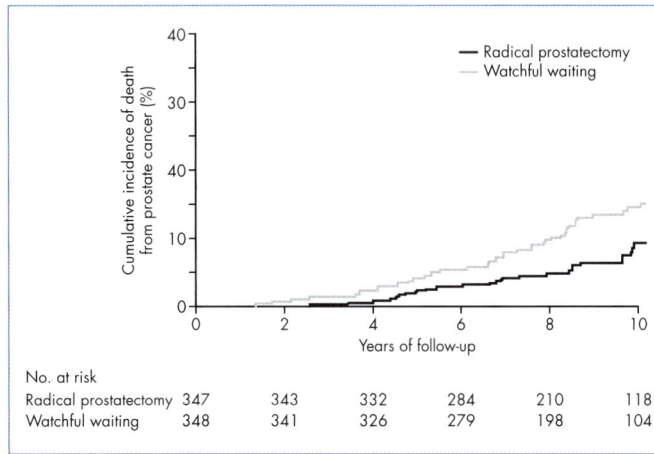

No. at risk
Radical prostatectomy	347	343	332	284	210	118
Watchful waiting	348	341	326	279	198	104

Fig. 79.1
Disease-specific cumulative incidence of death for patients with newly diagnosed, clinically localized prostate cancer who were randomly assigned to watchful waiting or radical prostatectomy.
From Bill-Axelson et al,[26] with permission

Table 79.3 Ten-year disease-specific survival in patients with clinically localized prostate cancer according to treatment received.[28]

Treatment	Gleason 2–4		Gleason 5–7		Gleason 8–10	
	n	% Survival (95% CI)	n	% Survival (95% CI)	n	% Survival (95% CI)
Radical prostatectomy	3402	**98** (97–99)	12,922	**91** (89–93)	4154	**76** (71–80)
Radiation therapy	4188	**89** (87–92)	8456	**74** (71–77)	2977	**52** (46–57)
Watchful waiting	10,133	**92** (90–93)	7046	**76** (73–78)	2834	**43** (38–48)

to conservative treatment (*P* = 0.023). The increase in the duration of survival was 4.6 years with radiation therapy and over 8.6 years with radical prostatectomy.[29]

In another retrospective study, D'Amico et al[13] used a multivariable time-to-PSA-failure analysis to compare PSA outcome after radical prostatectomy, external beam radiation therapy, and interstitial radiation therapy with or without neoadjuvant androgen deprivation for patients stratified by pretreatment risk group of recurrence. The group of patients at low risk for post-therapy PSA failure was estimated to derive equal benefit from the different treatments, while patients at high risk treated with radical prostatectomy had a significantly better 5-year PSA outcome compared to patients treated with seeds implant, and a higher 5-year PSA outcome compared to those treated with external beam radiation therapy, even though this difference was not statistically significant.

The impact on outcome of the improved surgical technique acquired in the PSA era has been reported in more recent series.[2,30,31] Eastham et al[32] identified the surgeon as the single most important independent variable predicting cancer recurrence after radical prostatectomy.

The 10-year postsurgical prostate cancer-specific mortality for high-risk patients in recent studies[2,30,31] is considerably lower than the mortality observed in high-grade cancer after treatment with external beam radiation therapy in the population-based study of Lu-Yao et al,[28] or the mortality observed after radiation therapy in the high-risk patients in the Boston radiotherapy cohort (Table 79.4).[33]

Clearly, current techniques of conformal radiation therapy may also provide better long-term cancer control rates than the radiation therapy modalities used 10 years ago. Other pitfalls exist in comparing the results of surgery to radiation, including different definitions of PSA failure.

MULTIMODALITY TREATMENT

Several studies have evaluated whether better outcomes can be achieved in high-risk patients with a multimodality treatment approach. Excellent survival rates with low treatment-related morbidity have been achieved at the Mayo Clinic by performing primary radical prostatectomy with different protocols of adjuvant therapy in a large series of patients with clinical stage T3 prostate cancer. Ten-year crude and cancer-specific survival rates were 70% and 80%, respectively.[24]

NEOADJUVANT THERAPY

Neoadjuvant therapy can provide cytoreduction for locally advanced disease and (in theory) early treatment for micrometastases. Several trials have randomized patients to 3 months of androgen blockade before radical prostatectomy versus surgery alone. A significant decrease in positive surgical margins was observed, but no study was able to show a benefit in term of PSA progression-free survival at 3 to 6 years of follow-up.[34–39] Importantly, none of these studies was enriched for high-risk patients, and none was powered to show a PSA progression difference. The only study to report follow up longer than 5 years found a PSA progression benefit in the patients with a PSA level greater than 20 ng/ml.[39]

Other recent studies suggest that a longer period of androgen deprivation (6–8 months) may be needed to obtain improved pathologic and clinical outcomes.[40,41] Gleave et al[40] randomized 547 patients with clinically localized prostate cancer to 3 versus 8 months of androgen deprivation before radical prostatectomy.

Table 79. 4 Ten-year prostate cancer-specific mortality with different treatment modalities.

	Low grade (%)	Intermediate grade (%)	High grade (%)
Population study[28]			
Radical prostectomy	2	9	**21**
Radiation therapy	11	26	**48**
Watchful waiting	8	24	57
Baylor College radical prostatectomy cohort[30]			
Radical prostatectomy	2	1	**18**
Boston radiotherapy cohort[33]			
Radiation therapy	0	6	**45**

They observed ongoing biochemical and pathologic regression of the tumors between 3 and 8 months of neoadjuvant hormonal therapy. These findings suggest that longer androgen blockade in high-risk patients may result in a benefit. A long-term neoadjuvant study in high-risk patients is required to test this hypothesis.

Several groups are studying the role of neoadjuvant chemotherapy in high-risk localized prostate cancer. Most available data come from small phase II trials.[42–45] A randomized phase III study of radical prostatectomy alone versus estramustin and docetaxel before radical prostatectomy has been initiated by the Cancer and Leukemia Group B (CALGB 90203) and will enrol approximately 700 men who will be observed for a follow-up of at least 7 years.[46] The use of more targeted and therefore less toxic drugs (growth factor inhibitors, angiogenesis inhibitors, antioxidants, and inducers of apoptosis) may also have a role in the neoadjuvant setting and have been studied in preliminary trials.[47,48]

ADJUVANT RADIATION THERAPY

For patients with residual disease after radical prostatectomy, therapy should be more effective shortly after removal of the primary tumor, when the number of malignant cells is low. An advantage of adjuvant therapy is that it does not delay definitive local treatment.

Adjuvant radiation therapy has been widely studied in patients with high risk of recurrence after radical prostatectomy. Retrospective series reported that the 5-year biochemical recurrence rate may be decreased with this approach in patients with positive margins or extracapsular extension,[7,49–54] but the effect on overall and cause-specific mortality is still unclear. Reports of 10-year survival rates range from 52% to 80% in patients without adjuvant radiation, to 60% to 76% in patients receiving adjuvant radiation.[55–58] A survival advantage related to better local control has been often suggested, but has not been confirmed by randomized trials. The Southwest Oncology Group (SWOG) and the European Organization for Research and Treatment of Cancer (EORTC) have completed accrual to two randomized adjuvant radiation studies (SWOG 8794 and EORTC 22911) that will help to clarify this issue. Until these results become available, adjuvant radiation therapy alone should be reserved for patients with positive surgical margins and without Gleason 8 to 10 disease or other poor prognostic features such as seminal vesicles invasion. These latter patients are at high risk for occult distant metastases and are less likely to benefit from further local therapy.

ADJUVANT HORMONAL THERAPY

Data regarding the use of adjuvant hormonal therapy after radical prostatectomy for high-risk localized disease are limited. Most published studies have enrolled patients with locally advanced or metastatic disease.[59–63] A recent large study by See et al[64] revealed a significant reduction in the risk of PSA progression after radical prostatectomy (hazard ratio, 0.49) with the administration of bicalutamide 150 mg/day in a large cohort of men with early prostate cancer. An obvious concern with this endpoint is that the patients progressing in the bicalutamide arm are not completely hormonally naïve; those in the placebo arm are. The progressing bicalutamide patients may have an increased component of hormone refractory disease. Thus, an improved time to progression may not translate into a disease-specific survival benefit.

Based on a review of their experience, Kupelian et al[65] suggested that patients with localized high-grade disease (Gleason score of 8 or above) but an initial PSA level less than or equal to 10 ng/ml might benefit from only 6 months of adjuvant androgen deprivation following local therapy. A two-fold reduction in mortality with the addition of 6 months of androgen suppression therapy to three-dimensional conformal radiation therapy for high-risk clinically localized prostate cancer has been recently observed by D'Amico et al[66] in a randomized controlled trial. This benefit is comparable to that reported by Bolla et al[67] with 3 years of androgen blockade after radiation therapy for locally advanced disease, and suggests that the benefit of adjuvant hormonal therapy may be achieved with a shorter duration of treatment.

ADJUVANT CHEMOTHERAPY

The identification of chemotherapeutic agents with promising activity in prostate cancer has led to some enthusiasm for the development of adjuvant chemotherapy trials in patients with high-risk disease. Data are still very limited.[68]

ADJUVANT RADIATION AND HORMONAL THERAPY

The use of hormonal ablation combined with adjuvant radiation therapy soon after surgical treatment has been studied in small cohorts of high-risk patients.

Akakura et al[69] reported a prospective randomized trial comparing the results of radical prostatectomy versus external beam radiation therapy (60–70 Gy) with the combination of endocrine therapy in both modalities in a total of 95 patients with stage B2 and C prostate cancer. The two groups were well balanced in terms of risk factors. The endocrine therapy, consisting in most patients of the daily administration of diethylstilbestrol diphosphate, was initiated approximately 8 weeks before surgery or radiation and continued indefinitely thereafter. The surgery group was associated with a significantly higher 5-year progression-free and cause-specific survival compared to the radiation group (Table 79.5; Figure 79.2). This study demonstrated that radical prostatectomy plus endocrine therapy may contribute to a survival benefit for patients with high-risk clinically localized and locally advanced prostate cancer. This approach is being evaluated in patients with clinically organ-confined prostate cancer in a randomized prospective trial by the Radiation Therapy Oncology Group (RTOG P-0011).

SALVAGE RADIATION AND HORMONAL THERAPY

Another approach is delayed salvage therapy with hormonal and/or radiation treatment at the time of biochemical failure. Androgen deprivation is often recommended in these cases because it is clinically challenging to identify the subgroup of patients who have disease confined to the prostate bed and might therefore receive radiation therapy alone.

Stephenson et al[70] reviewed a multicenter cohort of 501 patients who received radiation therapy for biochemical failure after radical prostatectomy. They observed that patients with a Gleason score of less than 8, positive surgical margins, preradiotherapy PSA level of less than 2 ng/ml, PSA doubling time of greater than 10 months, and absence of seminal vesicle invasion are more likely to have durable response with radiation therapy alone. Radiation therapy may prevent metastatic disease progression in patients at high risk if it is delivered early in the course of recurrent disease.

The survival benefit of combined salvage hormonal and radiation therapy is not yet well defined. The RTOG is conducting a phase III trial (RTOG 96-01) that will help to clarify this issue. Meanwhile, the results of several small series provide evidence of durable biochemical control in a significant percentage of patients.

Table 79.5 Five-year survival in patients with stage B2-C prostate cancer treated with radical prostatectomy or radiation therapy plus adjuvant hormonal treatment.[69]

	Progression-free survival (%)	Cause-specific survival (%)	Overall survival (%)
Radical prostatectomy	90.5	96.6	85.6
Radiation therapy	81.2	84.6	75.9
Significance	0.044	0.024	NS

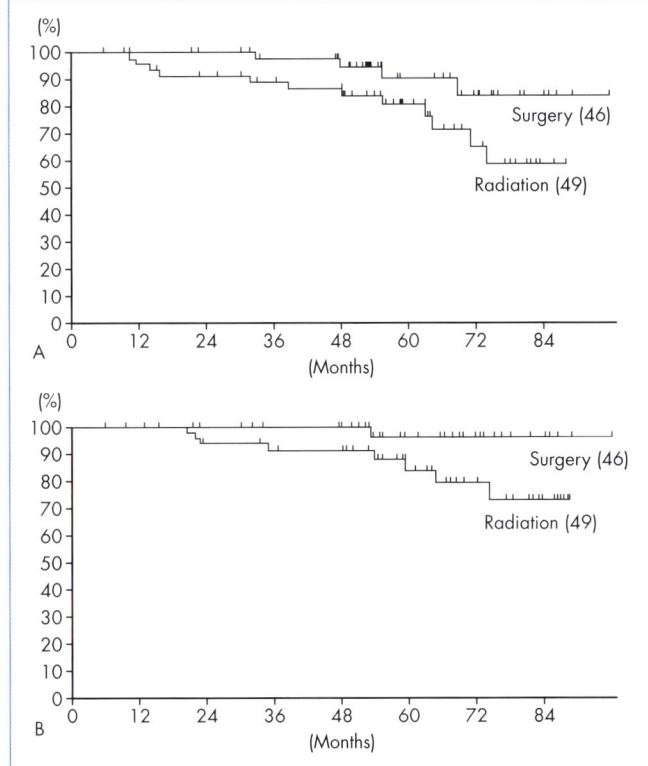

Fig. 79.2

A, Progression-free and B, cause-specific survival curves by treatment group for patients with clinical stage B2 and C prostate cancer who were randomly treated with radical prostatectomy or external beam radiation therapy with a common endocrine therapy in both modalities.
From Akakura et al,[69] with permission

Tiguert et al[71] retrospectively evaluated the benefit of androgen deprivation (3 months of injection of a LH–RH analog) administered before salvage external beam radiation therapy (median, 60 Gy) in 81 patients with biochemical failure following radical prostatectomy. The actuarial biochemical failure-free rate was 50% at 5 years.

Similar results are reported by Katz et al[72] who followed 115 patients treated with salvage three-dimensional conformal radiation therapy with or without neoadjuvant androgen deprivation. The 4-year PSA relapse-free survival rate was 39% for the 70 patients treated with radiation alone and 59% for the 45 patients who also received hormonal therapy. Androgen deprivation significantly improved PSA-free survival in patients with either negative surgical margins, absence of extracapsular extension, or presence of seminal vesicles invasion.

Finally, Eulau et al[73] reviewed the results of 105 consecutive patients treated with pelvic irradiation after radical prostatectomy for locally advanced disease, persistent or rising postoperative PSA or local recurrence. In their experience biochemical relapse-free survival and clinical relapse-free survival were significantly higher in patients who also received 6 months of androgen blockade before and during radiation therapy (56% vs 27% and 100% vs 70% at 5 years, respectively). The short-term use of androgen deprivation was the only significant predictor of biochemical failure at the multivariate analysis.

CONCLUSION

Randomized studies have shown that radical prostatectomy reduces cancer-specific mortality by 44% compared to watchful waiting.[26] This survival advantage is likely due to benefit in high-risk patients. The use of adjuvant treatments after surgery for high-risk disease can contribute to further decreases in the rate of local and distant failure. In high-risk patients, this likely translates into a survival benefit.

Radical prostatectomy in conjunction with adjuvant radiation and/or androgen deprivation should be considered in the management of young patients who are diagnosed with high-risk localized prostate cancer.

REFERENCES

1. Partin AW, Kattan MW, Subong EN, et al. Combination of prostate-specific antigen, clinical stage, and Gleason score to predict pathological stage of localized prostate cancer. A multi-institutional update. JAMA 1997;277:1445–1451.

2. Han M, Partin AW, Pound CR, et al. Long-term biochemical disease-free and cancer-specific survival following anatomic radical retropubic prostatectomy. The 15-year Johns Hopkins experience. Urol Clin North Am 2001;28:555–565.

3. Feneley MR, Partin AW. Indicators of pathologic stage of prostate cancer and their use in clinical practice. Urol Clin North Am 2001;28:443–458.

4. Roach M 3rd, Lu J, Pilepich MV, et al. Long-term survival after radiotherapy alone: radiation therapy oncology group prostate cancer trials. J Urol 1999;161:864–868.

5. Roach M, Lu J, Pilepich MV, et al. Four prognostic groups predict long-term survival from prostate cancer following radiotherapy alone on Radiation Therapy Oncology Group clinical trials. Int J Radiat Oncol Biol Phys 2000;47:609–615.

6. Epstein JI, Partin AW, Sauvageot J, et al. Prediction of progression following radical prostatectomy. A multivariate analysis of 721 men with long-term follow-up. Am J Surg Pathol 1996;20:286–292.

7. Blute ML, Bergstralh EJ, Iocca A, et al. Use of Gleason score, prostate specific antigen, seminal vesicle and margin status to predict biochemical failure after radical prostatectomy. J Urol 2001;165:119–125.

8. Shipley WU, Thames HD, Sandler HM, et al. Radiation therapy for clinically localized prostate cancer: a multi-institutional pooled analysis. JAMA 1999;281:1598–1604.

9. Zietman AL, Coen JJ, Shipley WU, et al. Radical radiation therapy in the management of prostatic adenocarcinoma: the initial prostate specific antigen value as a predictor of treatment outcome. J Urol 1994;151:640–645.

10. Kattan MW, Eastham JA, Stapleton AM, et al. A preoperative nomogram for disease recurrence following radical prostatectomy for prostate cancer. J Natl Cancer Inst 1998;90:766–771.

11. Kattan MW, Zelefsky MJ, Kupelian PA, et al. Pretreatment nomogram for predicting the outcome of three-dimensional conformal radiotherapy in prostate cancer. J Clin Oncol 2000;18:3352–3359.

12. Kattan MW, Potters L, Blasko JC, et al. Pretreatment nomogram for predicting freedom from recurrence after permanent prostate brachytherapy in prostate cancer. Urology 2001;58:393–399.

13. D'Amico AV, Whittington R, Malkowicz SB, et al. Biochemical outcome after radical prostatectomy, external beam radiation therapy, or interstitial radiation therapy for clinically localized prostate cancer. JAMA 1998;280:969–974.

14. D'Amico AV, Whittington R, Malkowicz SB, et al. Pretreatment nomogram for prostate-specific antigen recurrence after radical prostatectomy or external-beam radiation therapy for clinically localized prostate cancer. J Clin Oncol 1999;17:168–172.

15. D'Amico AV, Moul J, Carroll PR, et al. Cancer-specific mortality after surgery or radiation for patients with clinically localized prostate cancer managed during the prostate-specific antigen era. J Clin Oncol 2003;21:2163–2172.

16. Freedland SJ, Terris MK, Csathy GS, et al. Preoperative model for predicting prostate specific antigen recurrence after radical prostatectomy using percent of biopsy tissue with cancer, biopsy Gleason grade and serum prostate specific antigen. J Urol 2004;171:2215–2220.

17. D'Amico AV, Whittington R, Malkowicz SB, et al. Clinical utility of the percentage of positive prostate biopsies in defining biochemical outcome after radical prostatectomy for patients with clinically localized prostate cancer. J Clin Oncol 2000;18:1164–1172.

18. Grossfeld GD, Latini DM, Lubeck DP, et al. Predicting disease recurrence in intermediate and high-risk patients undergoing radical prostatectomy using percent positive biopsies: results from CaPSURE. Urology 2002;59:560–565.

19. D'Amico AV, Schultz D, Silver B, et al. The clinical utility of the percent of positive prostate biopsies in predicting biochemical outcome following external-beam radiation therapy for patients with clinically localized prostate cancer. Int J Radiat Oncol Biol Phys 2001;49:679–684.

20. Nelson CP, Dunn RL, Wei JT, et al. Contemporary preoperative parameters predict cancer-free survival after radical prostatectomy: a tool to facilitate treatment decisions. Urol Oncol 2003;21:213–218.

21. Rhodes DR, Sanda MG, Otte AP, et al. Multiplex biomarker approach for determining risk of prostate-specific antigen-defined recurrence of prostate cancer. J Natl Cancer Inst 2003;95:661–668.

22. Ziada AM, Lisle TC, Snow PB, et al. Impact of different variables on the outcome of patients with clinically confined prostate carcinoma: prediction of pathologic stage and biochemical failure using an artificial neural network. Cancer 2001;91(8 Suppl):1653–1660.

23. Fradet Y. Role of radical prostatectomy in high-risk prostate cancer. Can J Urol 2002;9(Suppl 1):8–13.

24. Lerner SE, Blute ML, Zincke H. Extended experience with radical prostatectomy for clinical stage T3 prostate cancer: outcome and contemporary morbidity. J Urol 1995;154:1447–1452.

25. van den Ouden D, Hop WC, Schroder FH. Progression in and survival of patients with locally advanced prostate cancer (T3) treated with radical prostatectomy as monotherapy. J Urol 1998;160:1392–1397.

26. Bill-Axelson A, Holmberg L, Ruutu M et al. Radical prostatectomy versus watchful waiting in early prostate cancer. N Engl J Med 2005 352:1977–1984.

27. Pound CR, Partin AW, Eisenberger MA, et al. Natural history of progression after PSA elevation following radical prostatectomy. JAMA 1999;281:1591–1597.

28. Lu-Yao GL, Yao SL. Population-based study of long-term survival in patients with clinically localised prostate cancer. Lancet 1997;349:906–910.

29. Menon M, Tewari A, Divine G, et al. Comparison of long-term survival in men with clinically localized prostate cancer managed conservatively, with definitive radiation or radical prostatectomy. J Urol 2001;165 (5 suppl):151–152 (abstract 621).

30. Hull GW, Rabbani F, Abbas F, et al. Cancer control with radical prostatectomy alone in 1,000 consecutive patients. J Urol 2002;167:528–534.

31. Roehl KA, Han M, Ramos CG, et al. Cancer progression and survival rates following anatomical radical retropubic prostatectomy in 3,478 consecutive patients: long-term results. J Urol 2004;172:910–914.

32. Eastham JA, Kattan MW, Riedel E, et al. Variations among individual surgeons in the rate of positive surgical margins in radical prostatectomy specimens. J Urol 2003;170:2292–2295.

33. D'Amico AV, Cote K, Loffredo M, et al. Determinants of prostate cancer-specific survival after radiation therapy for patients with clinically localized prostate cancer. J Clin Oncol 2002;20:4567–4573.

34. Soloway MS, Pareek K, Sharifi R, et al. Neoadjuvant androgen ablation before radical prostatectomy in cT2bNxMo prostate cancer: 5-year results. J Urol 2002;167:112–116.

35. Aus G, Abrahamsson PA, Ahlgren G, et al. Three-month neoadjuvant hormonal therapy before radical prostatectomy: a 7-year follow-up of a randomized controlled trial. BJU Int 2002;90:561–566.

36. Witjes WP, Schulman CC, Debruyne FM. Preliminary results of a prospective randomized study comparing radical prostatectomy versus radical prostatectomy associated with neoadjuvant hormonal combination therapy in T2–3 N0 M0 prostatic carcinoma. The European Study Group on Neoadjuvant Treatment of Prostate Cancer. Urology 1997;49(3A Suppl):65–69.

37. Schulman CC, Debruyne FM, Forster G, et al. 4-Year follow-up results of a European prospective randomized study on neoadjuvant hormonal therapy prior to radical prostatectomy in T2–3N0M0 prostate cancer. European Study Group on Neoadjuvant Treatment of Prostate Cancer. Eur Urol 2000;38:706–713.

38. Van Poppel H, De Ridder D, Elgamal AA, et al. Neoadjuvant hormonal therapy before radical prostatectomy decreases the number of positive surgical margins in stage T2 prostate cancer: interim results of a prospective randomized trial. The Belgian Uro-Oncological Study Group. J Urol 1995;154:429–434.

39. Klotz LH, Goldenberg SL, Jewett MA, et al. Long-term followup of a randomized trial of 0 versus 3 months of neoadjuvant androgen ablation before radical prostatectomy. J Urol 2003;170:791–794.

40. Gleave ME, Goldenberg SL, Chin JL, et al. Randomized comparative study of 3 versus 8-month neoadjuvant hormonal therapy before radical prostatectomy: biochemical and pathological effects. J Urol 2001;166:500–506; discussion 506–507.

41. Selli C, Montironi R, Bono A, et al. Effects of complete androgen blockade for 12 and 24 weeks on the pathological stage and resection margin status of prostate cancer. J Clin Pathol 2002;55:508–513.

42. Clark PE, Peereboom DM, Dreicer R, et al. Phase II trial of neoadjuvant estramustine and etoposide plus radical prostatectomy for locally advanced prostate cancer. Urology 2001;57:281–285.

43. Hussain M, Smith DC, El-Rayes BF, et al. Neoadjuvant docetaxel and estramustine chemotherapy in high-risk/locally advanced prostate cancer. Urology 2003;61:774–780.

44. Oh WK, George DJ, Kaufman DS, et al. Neoadjuvant docetaxel followed by radical prostatectomy in patients with high-risk localized prostate cancer: a preliminary report. Semin Oncol 2001;28(4 Suppl 15):40–44.

45. Konety BR, Eastham JA, Reuter VE, et al. Feasibility of radical prostatectomy after neoadjuvant chemohormonal therapy for patients with high risk or locally advanced prostate cancer: results of a phase I/II study. J Urol 2004;171:709–713.

46. Eastham JA, Kelly WK, Grossfeld GD, et al. Cancer and Leukemia Group B (CALGB) 90203: a randomized phase 3 study of radical prostatectomy alone versus estramustine and docetaxel before radical prostatectomy for patients with high-risk localized disease. Urology 2003;62(Suppl 1):55–62.

47. Kucuk O, Sarkar FH, Sakr W, et al. Phase II randomized clinical trial of lycopene supplementation before radical prostatectomy. Cancer Epidemiol Biomarkers Prev 2001;10:861–868.

48. Howe LR, Dannenberg AJ. A role for cyclooxygenase-2 inhibitors in the prevention and treatment of cancer. Semin Oncol 2002;29(3 Suppl 11):111–119.

49. Davis BJ, Pisansky TM, Leibovich BC. Adjuvant external radiation therapy following radical prostatectomy for node-negative prostate cancer. Curr Opin Urol 2003;13:117–122.

50. Leibovich BC, Engen DE, Patterson DE, et al. Benefit of adjuvant radiation therapy for localized prostate cancer with a positive surgical margin. J Urol 2000;163:1178–1182.

51. Do LV, Do TM, Smith R, et al. Postoperative radiotherapy for carcinoma of the prostate: impact on both local control and distant disease-free survival. Am J Clin Oncol 2002;25:1–8.

52. Valicenti RK, Gomella LG, Ismail M, et al. The efficacy of early adjuvant radiation therapy for pT3N0 prostate cancer: a matched-pair analysis. Int J Radiat Oncol Biol Phys 1999;45:53–58.

53. Petrovich Z, Lieskovsky G, Langholz B, et al. Postoperative radiotherapy in 423 patients with pT3N0 prostate cancer. Int J Radiat Oncol Biol Phys 2002;53:600–609.

54. Mayer R, Pummer K, Quehenberger F, et al. Postprostatectomy radiotherapy for high-risk prostate cancer. Urology 2002;59:732–739.

55. Paulson DF, Moul JW, Walther PJ. Radical prostatectomy for clinical stage T1–2N0M0 prostatic adenocarcinoma: long-term results. J Urol 1990;144:1180–1184.

56. Shevlin BE, Mittal BB, Brand WN, et al. The role of adjuvant irradiation following primary prostatectomy, based on histopathologic extent of tumor. Int J Radiat Oncol Biol Phys 1989;16:1425–1430.

57. Thompson IM, Paradelo JC, Crawford ED, et al. An opportunity to determine optimal treatment of pT3 prostate cancer: the window may be closing. Urology 1994;44:804–811.

58. Petrovich Z, Lieskovsky G, Stein JP, et al. Comparison of surgery alone with surgery and adjuvant radiotherapy for pT3N0 prostate cancer. BJU Int 2002;89:604–611.

59. Messing EM, Manola J, Sarosdy M, et al. Immediate hormonal therapy compared with observation after radical prostatectomy and pelvic lymphadenectomy in men with node-positive prostate cancer. N Engl J Med 1999;341:1781–1788.

60. Prayer-Galetti T, Zattoni F, Capizzi A, et al. Disease-free survival in patients with pathological C stage prostate cancer at radical prostatectomy submitted to adjuvant hormonal treatment. Eur Urol 2000;38:48 (abstract).

61. Ghavamian R, Bergstralh EJ, Blute ML, et al. Radical retropubic prostatectomy plus orchiectomy versus orchiectomy alone for pTxN+ prostate cancer: a matched comparison. J Urol 1999;161:1223–1227; discussion 1227–1228.

62. Myers RP, Larson-Keller JJ, Bergstralh EJ, et al. Hormonal treatment at time of radical retropubic prostatectomy for stage D1 prostate cancer: results of long-term followup. J Urol 1992;147:910–915.

63. Schmeller N, Lubos W. Early endocrine therapy versus radical prostatectomy combined with early endocrine therapy for stage D1 prostate cancer. Br J Urol 1997;79:226–234.

64. See W, Iversen P, Wirth M, et al. Immediate treatment with bicalutamide 150 mg as adjuvant therapy significantly reduces the risk of PSA progression in early prostate cancer. Eur Urol 2003;44:512–517; discussion 517–518.

65. Kupelian PA, Buchsbaum JC, Elshaikh M, et al. Factors affecting recurrence rates after prostatectomy or radiotherapy in localized prostate carcinoma patients with biopsy Gleason score 8 or above. Cancer 2002;95:2302–2307.

66. D'Amico AV, Manola J, Loffredo M, et al. 6-month androgen suppression plus radiation therapy vs radiation therapy alone for patients with clinically localized prostate cancer: a randomized controlled trial. JAMA 2004;292:821–827.

67. Bolla M, Gonzalez D, Warde P, et al. Improved survival in patients with locally advanced prostate cancer treated with radiotherapy and goserelin. N Engl J Med 1997;337:295–300.

68. Wang J, Halford S, Rigg A, et al. Adjuvant mitozantrone chemotherapy in advanced prostate cancer. BJU Int 2000;86:675–680.

69. Akakura K, Isaka S, Akimoto S, et al. Long-term results of a randomized trial for the treatment of Stages B2 and C prostate cancer: radical prostatectomy versus external beam radiation therapy with a common endocrine therapy in both modalities. Urology 1999;54:313–318.

70. Stephenson AJ, Shariat SF, Zelefsky MJ, et al. Salvage radiotherapy for recurrent prostate cancer after radical prostatectomy. JAMA 2004;291:1325–1332.

71. Tiguert R, Rigaud J, Lacombe L, et al. Neoadjuvant hormone therapy before salvage radiotherapy for an increasing post-radical prostatectomy serum prostate specific antigen level. Role of radical prostatectomy in high-risk prostate cancer. J Urol 2003;170:447–450.

72. Katz MS, Zelefsky MJ, Venkatraman ES, et al. Predictors of biochemical outcome with salvage conformal radiotherapy after radical prostatectomy for prostate cancer. J Clin Oncol 2003;21:483–489.

73. Eulau SM, Tate DJ, Stamey TA, et al. Effect of combined transient androgen deprivation and irradiation following radical prostatectomy for prostatic cancer. Int J Radiat Oncol Biol Phys 1998;41:735–740.

Prevention and management of complications associated with open radical retropubic prostatectomy

80

Herbert Lepor

INTRODUCTION

An anatomic approach to radical perineal prostatectomy was described by Young in 1905.[1] Forty years later, Millin described the retropubic approach for radical prostatectomy.[2] The primary advantage of the perineal approach was avoidance of the dorsal venous complex, resulting in less bleeding and a quicker recovery. Nevertheless, the radical retropubic prostatectomy (RRP) was preferred by most urologists since they were generally more familiar with retropubic anatomy and this approach provided the opportunity to perform a simultaneous staging pelvic lymphadenectomy through the single lower midline incision.[3]

Historically, radical perineal and radical retropubic prostatectomies were associated with significant morbidity and mortality.[4] In the modern era, radical prostatectomy performed by expert surgeons is associated with exceedingly rare mortality and minimal morbidity.[5] The dramatically lower complication rates in contemporary series can be attributed to greater experience of individual surgeons, improved surgical technique, younger surgical candidates with fewer co-morbidities, better anesthetic agents, and more sophisticated intraoperative monitoring.

Between 1986 and 2004, the author has performed over 2500 RRPs. Two thousand of these were performed between 1994 and 2004 at New York University (NYU) Medical Center. We have reported both a large retrospective and prospective outcomes assessment of 1000[6] and 500[7] cases, respectively. In both of these personal series, complication rates were exceedingly low. The low complication rates may be attributed to high surgical volume, thoughtful patient selection, rigorous preoperative assessment, meticulous surgical technique,

and compulsive postoperative management. This chapter focuses on the prevention and management of complications associated with open RRP, and draws on the personal experiences of the author.

CARDIOVASCULAR COMPLICATIONS

Cardiovascular complications associated with radical prostatectomy include myocardial infarction, cerebral vascular accidents, cardiac arrhythmias, pulmonary embolus, and deep venous thrombosis (DVT). These complications may occur intra- and post-operatively. In the modern era, these cardiovascular events are the primary cause of rare intra- and post-operative mortalities. For example, our only intra- or post-operative mortality occurred in an individual who experienced a myocardial infarction during his hospitalization and died at home within 30 days of surgery. The rates of DVT (0.2–2.7%), pulmonary embolus (0.3–2.0%), and other cardiovascular complications (myocardial infarction and arrhythmias) (0.1–0.7%) reported by experienced surgeons is exceedingly low (Table 80.1).[6–11]

A detailed preoperative review of systems, social history, and family history should focus on identifying significant cardiovascular disease or associated risk factors. Risk factors include hyperlipidemia, hypertension, diabetes, smoking, and a family history of atherosclerotic vascular disease. The presence of erectile dysfunction may represent an early indicator of occult systemic vascular disease. Men with known cardiovascular disease or high-risk factors should undergo a thorough preoperative cardiovascular evaluation, including auscultation for carotid bruits, an echocardiogram to

Table 80.1 Intraoperative technical complications during radical retropubic prostatectomy

Surgeon/ institution	Year	Number of patients	Rectal injury (%)	Ureteral injury (%)
Saint-Jean Cerou, Languedoc[11]	1992	620	0.5	0
Mayo Clinic[8]	1995	1000	0.6	0
Catalona[9]	1999	1870	0.05	0.05
Lepor[6]	2001	1000	0.5	0.10
Lepor[7]	2003	500	0	0.20

assess ejection fraction and cardiac wall motion, and an exercise stress test to identify cardiac ischemia.

Men with significant functional cardiac compromise or coronary artery disease generally should not be offered radical prostatectomy since their limited life-expectancy and increased surgical risks do not justify surgical attempts to cure the disease. Men with evidence of coronary artery disease who are deemed appropriate candidate for radical prostatectomy should be carefully monitored intraoperatively to avoid sustained hypotension. A lower threshold should be established for transfusing blood products if bleeding occurs in order to decrease myocardial ischemia. All men with preexisting coronary artery disease should undergo serial EKGs and cardiac enzyme monitoring immediately postoperatively, independent of their postoperative course. Identifying a myocardial infarction early in its course allows for immediate thrombolytic intervention, which may diminish mortality and damage to the myocardium associated with the event.

Any changes in mental status or extremity weakness should prompt immediate computerized tomography (CT) of the head with contrast in order to identify a cerebrovascular accident. A thromboembolic event arising from a plaque in the carotid or basilar arteries or an intimal dissection of these vessels may represent the etiology for an intra- or post-operative cerebrovascular accident. A thrombus arising from the left atrium in association with atrial fibrillation is another relatively common cause of postoperative cerebrovascular accident. A hypertensive crisis or a right-sided embolus passing to the left side of the heart via a septal defect is a rare etiology for a cerebrovascular accident. An echocardiogram should always be obtained to exclude the heart as the source of the thrombus. In some cases, prompt initiation of anticoagulation may decrease the extent of the final neurologic deficit.

Pulmonary embolus represents the most common life-threatening thromboembolic event associated with radical prostatectomy. The role of prophylaxis for preventing pulmonary embolus and deep venous thrombosis is highly controversial.[12] We do not recommend any routine pharmacologic or mechanical prophylaxis for deep venous thrombosis or pulmonary embolus with the exception of compression stockings. A personal or family history of DVT should trigger a hematology consultation and a more aggressive preventative strategy, including mechanical compression boots and administration of low molecular weight heparin immediately after surgery if there is no evidence of postoperative bleeding. In our recent series of 500 consecutive cases of RRP,[7] only 0.2% of men experienced a DVT and none a pulmonary embolus within 30 days of the surgical procedure. We attribute the extraordinarily low rates of DVT and pulmonary embolus to avoidance of staging a pelvic lymph node dissection in almost 70% of men with a Gleason score of 6 or less, a quick surgical procedure, early ambulation, short hospital stay, and encouragement for early return to activities.

INTRAOPERATIVE TECHNICAL COMPLICATIONS

RECTAL INJURY

The rate of rectal injury during radical prostatectomy in the modern era ranges between 0.5% and 3% (Table 80.2).[5] Rectal injury, if unrecognized, represents a very serious complication which may lead to sepsis and fistula formation.[13] In the setting where the rectal fistula is identified postoperatively and is associated with an abscess, a diverting colostomy is mandatory with incision and drainage of the associated abscess. The fistula, if persistent, can be closed at a later time and the colostomy taken down. Some smaller fistulas will close spontaneously.[14]

Historically, the standard of practice for all rectal injuries recognized intraoperatively was to primarily close the rectal injury and perform a diverting colostomy. Borland and Walsh[15] reported excellent outcomes with primary closure of the rectal injury and

Table 80.2 Postoperative complications following radical retropubic prostatectomy

Surgeon/ institution	Percent		
	Deep venous thrombosis	Pulmonary embolism	Cardiovascular (myocardial infarction and arrhythmia)
Saint-Jean Cerou Languedoc[11]	2.3	0.8	0.2
Mayo Clinic[8]	1.3	0.7	0.7
Catalona[9]	–	2.0	0.1
Lepor[6]	0.1	0.1	0.7
Lepor[7]	0.4	0	0.4

interposition of omentum between the rectal closure and the vesicourethral anastomosis. Excellent outcomes were achieved in men whose mechanical bowel preparation consisted only of Fleets enemas. It is often advisable to perform a colostomy if the rectal injury occurs in a previously radiated field.

In the recent personal series of 500 RRPs, only one intraoperative rectal injury was identified, which was small and closed primarily in two layers without interposition of omentum. An attempt was made to imbricate the adjacent perirectal soft tissue over the suture line. The wound was copiously irrigated and intravenous ampicillin and gentamicin were administered for 48 h. The anal sphincter was manually dilated and the patient's diet was limited to clear liquids for 48 h. A meticulous effort was made to achieve a water-tight vesicourethral anastomosis. Pelvic drains were removed per routine.

Rectal injury usually occurs while dissecting the apex of the prostate posteriorly. The injury is most likely to occur in men with small prostates since the apex may not be easily discernible. Prior radiation therapy, underlying bowel disease such as ulcerative colitis or diverticulitis, and multiple sets of transrectal biopsies are risk factors for rectal injury. In those cases with risk factors for rectal injury, the dissection of the apex should be initiated laterally rather than in the midline.

OBTURATOR NERVE INJURY

The obturator nerve is most vulnerable during the pelvic lymphadenectomy. Injury to it is associated with the inability to adduct the thigh. Injury can be avoided if the nerve is always identified prior to ligating the nodal package inferiorly. The obturator nerve must be identified early in the course of the lymphadenectomy. The first step in the lymphadenectomy should be to bluntly sweep the lymph node package off the pelvic sidewall and immediately identify the obturator nerve.

The author has no personal experience of injury to the obturator nerve. If identified intraoperatively, the nerve can be reapproximated using nonabsorbable sutures. Obturator nerve injuries are often recognized postoperatively when the patient complains of the inability to adduct the lower extremity. In these cases, the injury often spontaneously resolves with limited functional deficit. Physical therapy may facilitate the return of lower extremity function.

URETERAL INJURY

Ureteral injury is a rare complication occurring in between 0.05% and 1.6% of cases (Table 80.2).[5] Injury to the ureter may occur during an extended staging pelvic lymphadenectomy, during mobilization of the seminal vesicles, while dividing the prostatovesical junction, while obtaining hemostasis for brisk pelvic bleeding, or when performing the bladder neck reconstruction. Failure to observe a blue efflux from both ureteral orifices following administration of methylene blue or indigo carmine during the surgical procedure provides the opportunity to identify most ureteral injuries intraoperatively. If a blue efflux is not observed bilaterally, it is mandatory to pass a 5-Fr feeding tube in order to confirm that the ureter is intact and not ligated. Depending on the site and degree of injury, ureteroneocystotomy or ureterourererotomy should be performed. At times, deligation may be adequate. A ureteral ligation or transaction not detected intraoperatively typically present with flank pain, a slight and transient increase in the serum creatinine, or persistent urinary drainage from the pelvic drains. Any one of these events should trigger a renal ultrasound in order to identify hydronephrosis and/or a contrast imaging study to identify urinary extravasation. A very slight rise in creatinine may be attributed to a ureteral ligation whereas a marked rise suggests a ureteral transection with intraperitoneal extravasation owing to an associated peritonotomy.

The author has personally encountered three ureteral injuries. One injury was identified intraoperatively and occurred while mobilizing the seminal vesicle. An ureteroneocystotomy with a psoas hitch reimplantation was performed without sequelae. The second injury occurred in an individual from Kenya who failed to divulge a history of schistosomiasis. The prostate and bladder were encased in extensive fibrosis and the ureter was ligated just outside the bladder. This individual postoperatively experienced flank pain and a slight elevation of the serum creatinine. A renal ultrasound revealed hydronephrosis. A ureteroneocystotomy was also performed without sequelae. A third patient presented 3 years following an uncomplicated radical prostatectomy. An abdominal CT scan was performed following a motor vehicle accident which revealed an atrophic kidney. Subsequent imaging studies demonstrated the site of ureteral obstruction to be just outside the bladder wall. The patient never experienced flank pain postoperatively despite what appears to have been a complete ligation of the ureter. Since the hydronephrotic kidney was atrophic and asymptomatic, no treatment was recommended.

VASCULAR INJURY

Injury to the external iliac vesicles rarely occurs during radical prostatectomy. In cases where there is a laceration, the vessels should be repaired with appropriate vascular sutures. In rare cases when the external iliac artery or vein is inadvertently ligated, these structures must be repaired immediately to avoid ischemia to the lower extremity.

HEMORRHAGE

Historically, radical prostatectomy was associated with significant bleeding. The description of the dorsal venous complex by Reiner and Walsh and a technique for its early control has greatly diminished the likelihood of encountering life-threatening intraoperative bleeding.[16] Significant intraoperative bleeding is most likely to occur in men with very large prostates,[17] excessive perivesical and periprostatic venous tributaries, or an unrecognized coagulopathy.

If the prostate exceeds 100 g, a row of hemostatic prostatic capsular sutures are placed on the anterior surface of the prostate in order to reduce back-bleeding prior to ligating the dorsal venous complex distally. In some cases, the prostate is so large it is not feasible to suture/ligate the dorsal venous complex prior to dividing this structure. In these cases, the dorsal venous complex is sharply divided and hemostasis is secondarily achieved. The urethra is then divided without preplacement of the anastomotic sutures, and the apex is mobilized with care not to inadvertently enter the plane between the capsule and adenoma. The prostate is quickly mobilized off the rectum. With the Foley catheter retracted in a cephalad direction, the dorsal venous complex is controlled.

In cases where there are massive venous tributaries enveloping the bladder and prostate, attempts at achieving hemostasis with suture ligation may promote bleeding. Efforts to achieve hemostasis may become futile and the surgeon must proceed expeditiously to complete the prostatectomy. Packing of the pelvis with lap pads during the prostatectomy will significantly reduce blood loss.

In rare cases, the surgeon may encounter diffuse small vessel bleeding that is refractory to attempts at hemostasis. If the bleeding cannot be controlled with suture ligatures, empiric transfusion of platelets and clotting factors should be considered. The author recently experienced this scenario. An intraoperative coagulation profile was sent before the administration of platelets and clotting factors which revealed disseminated intravascular coagulopathy.

POSTOPERATIVE COMPLICATIONS

HEMORRHAGE

Significant and potentially life-threatening hemorrhage may occur during the immediate postoperative period. In many of these cases, the patient left the operating room after achieving meticulous hemostasis. The signs of life-threatening postoperative hemorrhage include hypotension, tachycardia, and low urine output. In the majority of cases, these signs of life-threatening postoperative bleeding occur in the first 2 to 4 h while the patient is in the recovery room. Central venous and arterial lines should be placed in order to facilitate monitoring of blood pressure and provide access for rapid volume replacement. If the hypotension, tachycardia, and low urine output do not respond rapidly to boluses of intravenous fluids, the surgeon should begin to make plans to return the patient to the operating room even if multiple units of blood products have not yet been transfused. If there is a transient response to fluid expansion, the patient must remain in a monitored setting. Serial hematocrits should be obtained. In cases of significant bleeding, the response to intravascular fluid replacement is often transient. The volume of pelvic drainage is a very unreliable indicator of significant bleeding. As the bleeding progresses, the abdomen becomes distended. The expanding hematoma exerts tension and may disrupt the anastomosis, which leads to greater abdominal distention as both urine and blood fill the pelvis. If the decision is made not to return the patient immediately to the operating room, the patient should remain or be transferred to a monitored setting with repeat hematocrits obtained until stabilization is demonstrated and hypotension resolves. In our experience, only six (0.2%) men have returned to the operating room for control of life-threatening bleeding. This is similar to Walsh et al's reported reoperation rate of 1% for the control of bleeding.[18] In our experience, the decision to return the patient to the operating room was always made within the first 8 postoperative hours. While it is difficult to provide absolute criteria for reoperation, this decision should be made before the patient has received extensive transfusions. As the amount of transfused blood products increases, the patient's clotting capacity further deteriorates. While significant bleeding may eventually subside, the pelvic hematoma will likely cause a protracted clinical course due to anastomotic disruption, ileus, infection, and clot retention. Re-exploration with evacuation of the hematoma and repair of the anastomosis often expedites recovery.

Prior to re-exploration, large-bore intravenous access must be obtained with restoration of intravascular volume. It is also prudent to place an arterial line for blood pressure monitoring. Depending on the volume of blood transfused, fresh frozen plasma, platelets, and calcium should be administered. In several cases requiring reoperation, we have identified an unrecognized coagulopathy such as factor II deficiency and von Willebrand disease. In these cases, no active bleeding site was identified in the operative field. Replacement of clotting factors was the primary requirement for achieving hemostasis.

The incision is reopened and blood clots evacuated. In many cases, the anastomosis is already disrupted due to the expanding hematoma. It is not possible to adequately explore the pelvis for bleeding with the anastomosis intact. Therefore, it is always taken down and meticulous hemostasis secured. In the rare case where bleeding is persistent and a specific site is not identified, the pelvis should be tightly packed and the incision closed with retention sutures. The author has resorted to this measure on only one occasion. The packing may be removed 24 h later when the patient is hemodynamically stabilized. In our cases where the decision to re-explore was made relatively early, patients were discharged within 48 h after the reoperation; and the catheter removed on the seventh postoperative day.

ANASTOMOTIC LEAKAGE

In the majority of cases, pelvic drains are removed by the second postoperative day.[6] Persistent drainage from the pelvic drains may be attributed to a lymphatic or urine leak. If drainage is excessive and not decreasing after 48 h, the drainage fluid should be tested for creatinine and glucose in order to differentiate between urine and serum (lymph).

If the fluid creatinine and glucose content is consistent with urine, an intravenous contrast imaging study should be performed to identify a ureteral injury. A cystogram should also be performed to exclude a bladder injury and to demonstrate that the catheter is indwelling within the bladder. The anastomotic leak may be attributed to a technically poor anastomosis, disruption of the bladder neck repair or a pelvic hematoma. The overwhelming majority of urine leaks due to partial disruption of the anastomosis will heal spontaneously with prolonged catheter drainage. If the catheter is not in the bladder, attempts should be made to reposition it endoscopically. If these endoscopic efforts are not successful, the patient should be brought to the operating theater for an open cystotomy.

A significant disruption of the anastomosis may exist despite no evidence of urinary extravasation from the pelvic drain sites. This phenomenon has been recognized more commonly since the routine use of cystograms to facilitate early removal of the catheter. In our experience, moderate or massive urinary extravasation was seen in only 10% of cases, 3 or 4 days after radical prostatectomy.[19] These men often have gross hematuria and blood emanating around the catheter while straining to have a bowel movement. The longest time to demonstrate a dry anastomosis in our experience is 6 weeks postoperatively. Men who develop significant postoperative bleeding not necessitating re-exploration are at greater risk for developing partial disruption of the anastomosis requiring prolonged catheter drainage. The catheter should not be removed in this setting until healing of the anastomosis is confirmed.

In the setting of persistent lymphatic drainage, the pelvic drain should be left indwelling until the drainage is less than 50 ml/day. It is advisable to release the suction on the closed drainage system. Premature removal of the pelvic drains may result in a lymphocele which will require percutaneous or open drainage.

A lymphocele may develop if a lymph leak is not recognized. This occurs following a staging pelvic lymphadenectomy. A lymphocele may present with lower extremity edema, flank pain due to hydronephrosis or scrotal edema. Percutaneous drainage with or without instillation of a sclerosing agent often is the initial management of a symptomatic lymphocele.[20,21] Historically, a recurrent or untreated lymphocele required open exploration with unroofing and drainage into the peritoneal cavity. In the modern era, a recurrent lymphocele is best managed laparoscopically.[21]

LONG-TERM COMPLICATIONS

BLADDER NECK CONTRACTURE

Bladder neck contracture is a relatively common complication following radical prostatectomy (Figure 80.1). The incidence has been reported to be as high as 27%.[22] The incidence of postoperative bladder neck contracture depends on surgical technique, the definition of a bladder neck contracture, and how aggressively the diagnosis is pursued. Lower rates exist among those experts who do not consider bladder outlet obstruction responding to a single dilation as a bladder neck contracture.

Bladder neck contractures almost always present within the first 3 months following radical prostatectomy.[23] A diminished urinary stream is the most common symptom of a bladder neck contracture. Deterioration of urinary continence also suggests a bladder neck contracture.

The etiology of a bladder neck contracture is likely multifactorial. Undoubtedly, technical issues must influence its development. Many experts recommend everting the bladder neck to facilitate a mucosa-to-mucosa apposition in order to decrease the incidence of a bladder neck contracture.[24] Catalona et al[9] reported that bladder neck contractures occurred more commonly when the bladder neck is reconstructed too tightly, which is consistent with the author's personal observations. We have reported that men who form keloids of the abdominal incision also have a greater risk of developing a bladder neck contracture, suggesting that in some cases the etiology is not technical but rather a generalized hypertrophic healing response.[23]

Some experts have speculated that the development of a bladder neck contracture is dependent on achieving a water-tight anastomosis.[25] Since February 2000, it has

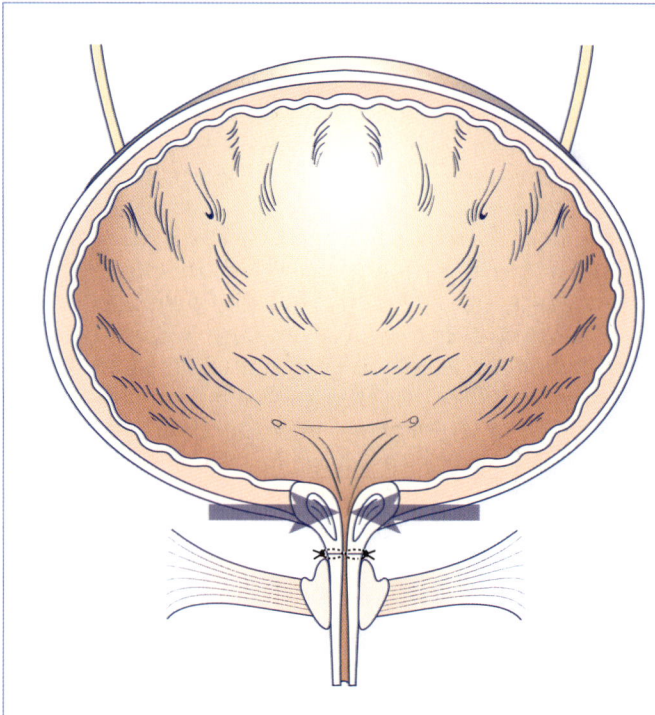

Fig. 80.1
Bladder neck contractures may develop after radical prostatectomy. The point of narrowing is usually just above the anastomosis and usually responds well to treatment.

been our practice to perform cystograms between 3 to 8 days postoperatively in order to facilitate early removal of the urinary catheter. In one series, 77%, 17%, 7%, and 3% of men were noted to have none, slight, moderate or severe extravasation on a cystogram performed 7 days following radical prostatectomy, respectively.[26] In men with moderate-to-severe extravasation, the urinary catheters were left indwelling until a follow-up cystogram showed complete resolution of the extravasation. In our experience, the incidence of bladder neck contracture is independent of the degree of extravasation on the initial cystogram. These observations suggest that urinary extravasation may have an impact on stricture formation only if the catheter is removed prematurely. Performing a cystogram between 3 and 8 days postoperatively not only provides the opportunity to remove the catheter early, but identifies the small cohort of men who likely benefit from prolonged catheter drainage.

Our bladder neck contracture rate in the year 2001 was 16.6%. To decrease this rate, we reconstructed the bladder neck to a caliber of 30 Fr instead of 20 Fr, and removed the catheter only in the absence of extravasation. We consider these measures lowered the bladder neck contracture rate in 2003 to 7.7%.

A bladder neck contracture is suspected when the patient complains of a poor urinary flow rate. It is important to determine whether the perceived decreased flow rate is due simply to small voided volumes or bladder outlet obstruction. Uroflowmetry, in cases of bladder neck contracture, will demonstrate a prolonged urinary flow pattern and a decreased flow rate. The bladder neck contracture is confirmed with flexible cystoscopy. The overwhelming majority of bladder neck

contractures will resolve following a simple dilation.[23] Under direct vision, a flexible guidewire is passed through the constricted urethral lumen and advanced into the bladder. The bladder neck contracture is dilated to an 18 Fr, using Nottingham dilating catheters. The anastomosis and bladder is inspected to ensure that a calculi has not formed on a retained anastomotic suture. The patient is instructed to self-catheterize using an 18-Fr red-rubber catheter once a day for a month, every other day the following month, and once a week for the next month. Refractory strictures will typically recur within 3 months of the initial dilation. In these cases, a second dilation is performed. Bladder neck contractures refractory to two dilations are treated with endoscopic incision or resection.

INCONTINENCE

Between 2.5% and 87% of men fail to regain continence following radical prostatectomy.[27] The broad range of continence rates may be attributed to varying expertise of surgeons, different definitions of continence, different methodologies for assessing continence, and the timing of reporting continence outcomes. Lepor et al,[28] utilizing a validated self-administered questionnaire, reported that 96% of men achieved urinary continence two years following radical prostatectomy.

Incontinence following radical prostatectomy is almost always stress induced and is caused by damage to the rhabdosphincter.[29] Therefore, every effort should be made to maximally preserve the rhabdosphincter while dividing the prostatourethral junction. In an effort to maximize urethral length and its surrounding periurethral smooth and skeletal muscle, the prostatourethral junction should be divided as close to the prostate as possible. A frozen section is sent from the urethral (apical) soft-tissue margin in order to minimize the likelihood that the cancer is not completely removed.[30]

We have shown that men who develop bladder neck contractures are more prone to develop incontinence.[23] Therefore, every effort should be made to prevent bladder neck contractures.

All men are encouraged to perform pelvic floor (Kegel) exercises immediately after the urinary catheter is removed. The NYU Continence Index is a useful instrument for predicting the time interval to regain continence and final continence status.[31] If the continence score is less than 14, we recommend initiating a formal biofeedback program immediately following catheter removal. By 3 months postoperatively, 80% of men will have regained their urinary continence.[28] For those men who fail to do so, uroflowmetry and a urine culture should be obtained to rule out bladder neck contracture and urinary tract infection (UTI), respectively. If uroflowmetry is normal and there is no UTI, a formal biofeedback program is initiated.

Continence may continue to improve over a 2-year interval.[28] Men with moderate-to-severe incontinence (more than two pads/day, moderate-to-severe bother, frequent or total incontinence) 1 year following radical prostatectomy, are encouraged to undergo a male sling (generally recommended for men with moderate incontinence) or placement of an artificial urinary sphincter (men with severe incontinence).

ERECTILE DYSFUNCTION

Erectile dysfunction is the most common complication confronting men following radical prostatectomy. The likelihood of preserving sexual function following radical prostatectomy is dependent on age, baseline sexual function, number of neurovascular bundles preserved (Figure 80.2), expertise of the surgeon, and baseline sexual activity. Overall preservation of erection following radical prostatectomy ranges between 20% and 65%.[32] The potency rates presented in the literature are highly variable and dependent on the skill and experience of the surgeon, methodology utilized for ascertaining potency, patient selection, definition of potency, number of neurovascular bundles preserved, and use of oral and intracavernous agents. Post-prostatectomy potency rates in the modern era have improved, presumably due to the development of the nerve-sparing technique,[24] and the availability of phosphodiesterase (PDE) inhibitors.[32] Several experts have reported and illustrated their techniques for performing nerve-sparing prostatectomy.[24,34]

Walsh et al[18] have provided compelling evidence that excision of a single neurovascular bundle significantly

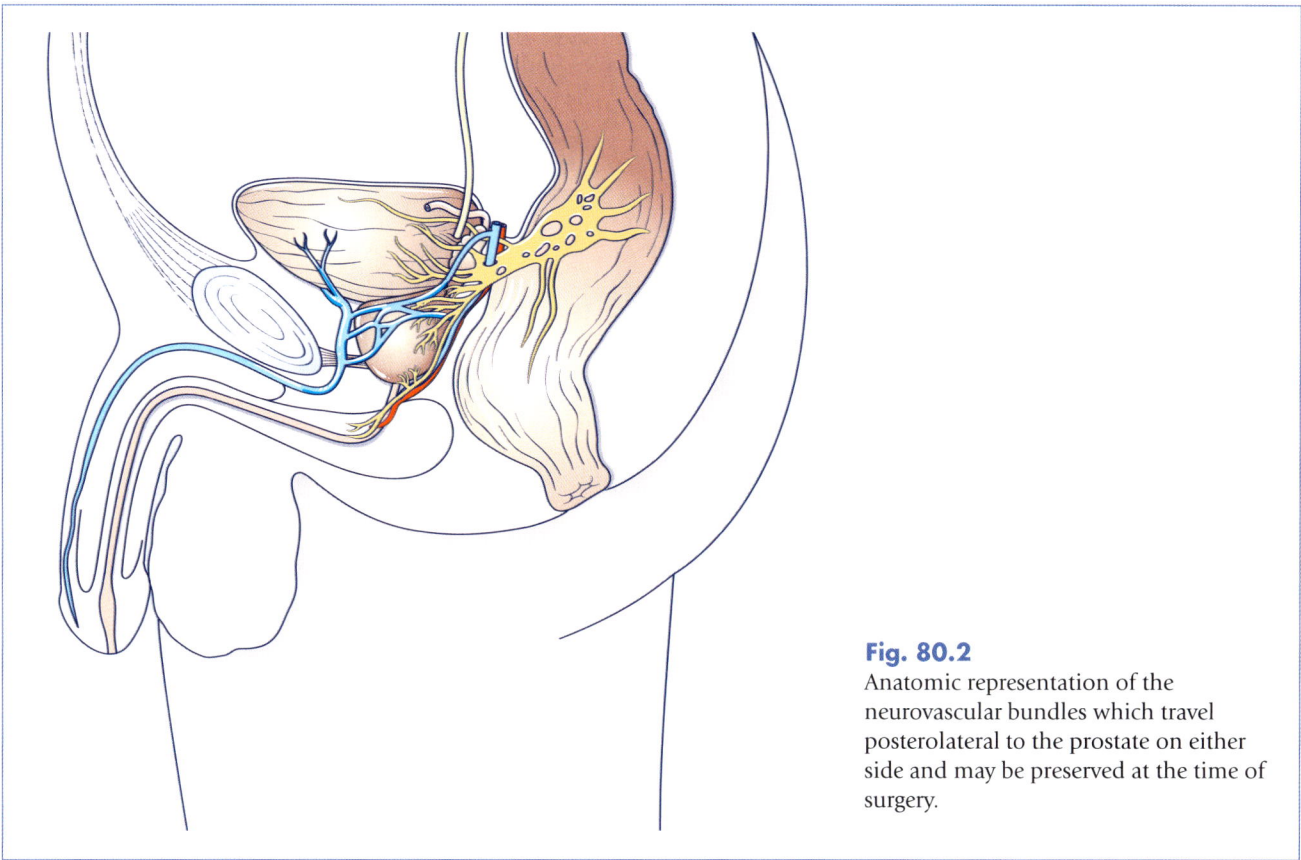

Fig. 80.2
Anatomic representation of the neurovascular bundles which travel posterolateral to the prostate on either side and may be preserved at the time of surgery.

lowers potency rates. Obviously, the surgeon must balance preserving potency against curing the cancer. A significant proportion of men with extracapsular extension do not develop progressive disease, especially when a negative margin is achieved.[35] Lepor et al[36] have proposed an algorithm for guiding decisions regarding preservation or excision of the neurovascular bundle based on preoperative Gleason score, presence of perineural invasion, and tumor volume.

There is reason to believe that administration of PDE inhibitors immediately after RRP may increase potency rates. Padma-Nathan et al[37] reported the results of a randomized placebo controlled trial comparing return of sexual function in men randomized to receive 50 mg/day of oral sildenafil versus placebo for 9 months following radical prostatectomy. Those men randomized to sildenafil achieved better sexual function off all treatment 1 year following radical prostatectomy. The rationale for daily sildenafil is to prevent cavernosal muscle soft-tissue atrophy by stimulating penile smooth muscle activity during nocturnal erections. Based on this study, we offer an oral PDE inhibitor immediately after catheter removal.

Men must be counseled that the return of erections may take up to 2 years. If substantial erectile function has returned 3 months following radical prostatectomy, men are not encouraged to pursue intracavernosal therapy since the ability to obtain erections adequate for intercourse will likely return imminently. If erectile function is minimal at 3 months, men interested in resuming sexual activity are encouraged to pursue a penile injection program. There is evidence that penile injection therapy not only restores erectile function but also increases the likelihood erections will return.[38]

The most significant way to impact potency rates following radical prostatectomy is to optimally perform the nerve-sparing technique. This mandates a bloodless surgical field. Care must be taken while dividing the prostatourethral junction not to injure the neurovascular bundle which is attenuated and in close proximity to the prostatourethral junction. In most cases, the author incises the visceral layer of the pelvic fascia beginning at the apex of the prostate and extending the incision toward the bladder neck. The incision in the visceral pelvic fascia is extended along the anterior surface of the prostate in cases with low volume disease in order to maximally preserve the autonomic innervation to the penis. In cases with significant fibrosis at the apex, the incision in the visceral pelvic fascia is started at the bladder neck and extended to the apex. The neurovascular bundle is sharply and/or bluntly mobilized off the prostate to the level of the vascular pedicle and only significant bleeders are controlled with surgical clips. The advantage of open versus laparoscopic radical prostatectomy is the ability to rely on palpation to ensure the prostate is not inadvertently incised. The Denonvilliers' fascia is then incised, exposing the vas

deferens and seminal vesicles. The medial margin of the vascular pedicle to the prostate is identified immediately lateral to the prostate. The lateral pedicle is then divided as close to the prostate as possible without entering the gland.

Several surgeons have advocated nerve grafting in order to improve potency rates following uni- or bilateral excision of the neurovascular bundles.[39,40] Unfortunately, these studies have serious methodologic design flaws and, therefore, the benefit of nerve grafting remains unanswered.

REFERENCES

1. Young HH. The early diagnosis and radical cure of carcinoma of the prostate: Being a study of 40 cases and presentation of a radical operation which was carried out in four cases. Bull Johns Hopkins Hosp 1905;16:315.
2. Millin T. Retropubic Urinary Surgery. London: Livingstone, 1947.
3. Walsh PC, Lepor H. The role of radical prostatectomy in the management of prostatic carcinoma. Cancer 1987;60(Suppl):526–537.
4. Catalona WJ, Scott WW. Carcinoma of the prostate. In Walsh PC, Gittes RF, Perlmutter AD, Stamey TA (eds): Campbell's Urology, vol 5. Philadelphia: WB Saunders, 1986, pp 1463–1534.
5. Shekarriz B, Upadhyay J, Wood PP. Intraoperative, perioperative and long-term complications of radical prostatectomy. Urol Clin North Am 2001;28:639–653.
6. Lepor H, Nieder AM, Ferrandino MN. The intraoperative and postoperative complications following radical retropubic prostatectomy in a consecutive series of 1,000 cases. J Urol 2001;166:1729–1733.
7. Lepor H, Kaci L. Contemporary evaluation of operative parameters and complications related to open radical retropubic prostatectomy. Urology 2003;62:702–706.
8. Lerner SE, Blute ML, Lieber MM, et al. Morbidity of contemporary radical retropubic prostatectomy for localized prostate cancer. Oncology (Williston Park) 1995;9:379–382, discussion 382, 385–386, 389.
9. Catalona WJ, Carvalhal GF, Mager DE, et al. Potency, continence and complication rates in 1870 consecutive radical retropubic prostatectomies. J Urol 1999;162:433–438.
10. Gheiler EL, Lovisolo JA, Tiguert R, et al. Results of a clinical care pathway for radical prostatectomy patients in an open hospital-multiphysician system. Eur Urol 1999;35:210–216.
11. Leandri P, Rossignol G, Gautier JR, et al. Radical retropubic prostatectomy: Morbidity and quality of life. Experience with 620 consecutive cases. J Urol 1992;147:883–887.
12. Hull RD, Pineo GF. Prophylaxis of deep venous thrombosis and pulmonary embolism. Med Clin North Am 1998;82:477–493.
13. Harpster LE, Rommel FM, Sieber PR, et al. The incidence and management of rectal injury associated with radical prostatectomy in a community based urology practice. J Urol 1995;154:1435–1438.
14. McLaren RH, Barrett DM, Zincke H. Rectal injury occurring at radical retropubic prostatectomy for prostate cancer: Etiology and treatment. Urology 1993;42:401–405.
15. Borland RN, Walsh PC. The management of rectal injury during radical retropubic prostatectomy. J Urol 1992;147:905–907.
16. Reiner WG, Walsh PC. An anatomical approach to the surgical management of the dorsal vein and Santorini's plexus during radical retropubic surgery. J Urol 1979;121:198–200.
17. Hsu EI, Hong EK, Lepor H. The influence of body weight and prostate volume on intraoperative, perioperative, and postoperative outcomes following radical retropubic prostatectomy. Urology 2003;61:601–606.
18. Walsh PC, Partin AW, Epstein JI. Cancer control and quality of life following anatomical radical retropubic prostatectomy: Results at 10 years. J Urol 1994;152:1831–1836.

19. Patel R, Lepor H. Removal of the urinary catheter on postoperative days 3 or 4 following radical retropubic prostatectomy. Urology 2003;61:156–160.

20. Gilliland JD, Spies JB, Brown SB, et al: Lymphoceles: Percutaneous treatment with povidone-iodine sclerosis. Radiology 1989;171:227–229.

21. Waples MJ, Wegenke JD, Vega RJ. Laparoscopic management of lymphocele after pelvic lymphadenectomy and radical retropubic prostatectomy. Urology 1992;39:82–84.

22. Surya BV, Provet J, Johanson KE, et al. Anastomotic strictures following radical prostatectomy: Risk factors and management. J Urol 1990;143:755–758.

23. Park R, Martin S, Lepor H. Anastomotic strictures following radical prostatectomy: Insights into incidence, effectiveness of intervention, impact on continence and factors predisposing to occurrence. Urology 2001;57:742–746.

24. Walsh PC. Anatomic radical retropubic prostatectomy. In Walsh PC, Retik AB, Vaughan ED, et al (eds): Campbell's Urology, ed 7. Philadelphia: WB Saunders, 1998, p 2565.

25. Novicki DE, Larson TR, Andrews PE, et al. Comparison of the modified vest and the direct anastomosis for radical retropubic prostatectomy. Urology 1997;49:732–736.

26. Lepor H, Nieder AM, Fraiman MC. Early removal of urinary catheter after radical retropubic prostatectomy is both feasible and desirable. Urology 2001;58:425–429.

27. Foote J, Yun S, Leach GE. Post prostatectomy incontinence. Pathology, evaluation and management. Urol Clin North Am 1991;18:229–241.

28. Lepor H, Kaci L. The impact of open radical retropubic prostatectomy on continence and lower urinary tract symptoms (LUTS): A prospective assessment using validated self-administered outcome instruments. J Urol 2004;171:1216–1219.

29. Ficazzola MA, Nitti VW. The etiology of post-radical prostatectomy incontinence and correlation of symptoms with urodynamic findings. J Urol 1998;160:1317–1320.

30. Lepor H, Kaci L. The role of intraoperative biopsies during radical retropubic prostatectomy. Urology 2004;63:499–502.

31. Twiss C, Martin S, Shore R, et al. A continence index predicts the early return of urinary continence following radical retropubic prostatectomy. J Urol 2000;164:1241–1247.

32. McCullough AR. Prevention and management of erectile dysfunction following radical prostatectomy. Urol Clin North Am 2001;28:613–627.

33. Marks LS, Duda C, Dorey FJ, et al. Treatment of erectile dysfunction with Sildenafil. Urology 1999;53:19–24.

34. Lepor H. Radical retropubic prostatectomy. Urol Clin North Am 2001;28:509–520.

35. Han, M, Partin AW, Pound CR, et al. Long-term biochemical disease-free and cancer-specific survival following anatomic radical retropubic prostatectomy. The 15-year Johns Hopkins Experience. Urol Clin North Am 2001;28:555–565.

36. Shah O, Robbins DA, Mani N, et al. The NYU nerve sparing algorithm decreases the rate of positive surgical margins following radical retropubic prostatectomy. J Urol 2003;169:2147–2159.

37. Padma-Nathan H, McCullough AR, Giuliano F, et al. Postoperative nightly administration of Sildenafil citrate significantly improves the return of normal spontaneous erectile function after bilateral nerve-sparing radical prostatectomy. J Urol 2003;169(Suppl):375–376.

38. Montorsi F, Guazzoni G, Strambi L, et al. Recovery of spontaneous erectile function after nerve-sparing radical retropubic prostatectomy with and without early intracavernous injections of alprostadil. J Urol 1997;158:1408–1410.

39. Kim ED, Scardino PT, Hampel O, et al. Interposition of sural nerves restores function of cavernous nerves resected during radical prostatectomy. J Urol 1999;161:188–192.

40. Sawin KM, Canto EI, Shariat SF, et al. Sural nerve interposition grafting during radical prostatectomy. Rev Urol 2002;4:12–23.

External beam radiotherapy for the treatment of prostate cancer

81

Vincent S Khoo, David P Dearnaley

INTRODUCTION

External beam radiotherapy is a commonly used modality in the radical treatment of both early and locally advanced prostate cancer. It also has a role in men with biochemical prostate-specific antigen (PSA) relapse following radical prostatectomy and in metastatic disease (see Chapters 73 and 101, respectively). This chapter will discuss the rationale, treatments, and outcomes for both early and locally advanced prostate cancer, briefly chronicle the technical developments in external beam irradiation, outline the methods underpinning modern radiotherapy, and address the treatment issues pertinent to external beam radiotherapy. New and future developments will be described including hypo-fractionation, image-guided radiotherapy, and treatment individualization.

TREATMENT SELECTION FOR PROSTATE CANCER

Careful clinical assessment and staging is essential to select the appropriate treatment for men presenting with prostate cancer. Patients with localized disease and no clinical evidence of metastatic disease are suitable for radical radiotherapy. Many factors need to be considered in the selection of treatment for the individual patient, including:

- Patient factors such as age, clinical symptoms, sexual function, co-morbid conditions such as inflammatory bowel disease, potential life-expectancy and individual preference

- Tumor factors such as tumor grade (Gleason scoring), tumor stage, and initial PSA value at presentation
- Treatment factors such as method of treatment, probability of local control, and morbidity profile of the therapy.

Currently, the optimal management in men with localized prostate cancer remains uncertain. This is because there is substantial biologic heterogeneity within each prostate cancer subgroup dictating local behavior and metastatic potential. This is reflected by the widely variable treatment outcomes for each individual disease stage. However, there is reasonable evidence to recommend rational guidelines for radiotherapy treatment. For men anticipated to have a life-expectancy of 10 or more years, it would be appropriate to offer curative treatment. This judgment is based on the balance of probability that the cancer is likely to progress during this timespan in these individuals. It is also reasonable to consider curative treatment for men with shorter life-expectancy (≥5 years) if they have poorly differentiated cancer,[1] as data from Chodak et al[2] suggest their disease is more likely to progress during this period.

CLINICAL PARAMETERS

The clinicopathologic factors used to estimate clinical outcomes, such as tumor grade (Gleason score), tumor stage, and initial PSA values at presentation, are discussed in earlier chapters. Using these factors, a variety of clinical algorithms or nomograms have been formulated to predict the extent of disease and clinical outcomes (see Chapters 55 and 56). Based on large surgical series, Partin's tables is one example of a nomogram that correlates clinical T stage, biopsy Gleason score, and presenting PSA for the prediction of final pathologic stage.[3] Nomograms are also available for men with clinically localized prostate cancer to classify patients into early and locally advanced disease groups, depending on the likelihood of pelvic lymph node involvement.[4] Nomograms are also available to predict PSA-based outcomes following external beam radiotherapy.[5,6] These algorithms can be used to tailor radiotherapy regimens to each clinical prognostic subgroup.

COMPARISON OF RADIOTHERAPY VERSUS SURGERY

The relative merits of radical external beam radiotherapy or surgery for the individual will depend on the factors mentioned above. There are no adequate large randomized trials comparing radical radiotherapy with radical prostatectomy. The only randomized trial comparing radiotherapy and radical prostatectomy showed superior results for radical prostatectomy in "time to first evidence of treatment failure."[7] However, this trial has been criticized for violations in randomization, inadequate staging and follow-up, and possible selection bias,[8] and was disregarded in the National Institutes of Health consensus recommendations.[9] This issue has fueled nonrandomized comparisons of men with early localized prostate cancer treated by radical radiotherapy techniques and radical surgery. However, issues that can hamper interpretation of retrospective and nonrandomized comparisons include case selection, lack of central pathologic review, uncertain quality assurance of treatment methods with variable lengths of follow-up and definitions of biochemical failure.

Recent comparisons have not shown any consistent differences between radical radiotherapy and prostatectomy approaches.[10–12] The largest comparison collated pooled data from six large US centers of 6877 men treated over a 10-year period between 1989 and 1998.[12] Although there was variation in outcomes within individual institutions using the same treatment, the overall 5-year PSA results were similar for patients within the same prognostic risk group regardless of the form of therapy. These data suggest that there is little difference between radical radiotherapy and radical prostatectomy for early-stage localized disease. In general, nomogram predictions give very similar outcomes for surgery and radiotherapy.

The situation is different for men with locally advanced prostate cancer (clinical stage T3/4). The results of radical prostatectomy alone are unsatisfactory.

Two large surgical series report pathologic evidence of extracapsular extension or seminal vesicle disease in 36% to 41% of cases, positive nodal involvement in 42%, and only 9% to 22% had pathologic T2 stage.[13,14] The high probability of positive resection margins and/or residual disease means that radical prostatectomy alone is inadequate to control disease in these patients. A multicenter analysis of 345 men with clinical T3 disease treated with radical prostatectomy alone reported actuarial 10-year metastatic-free survival rates of only 32%.[15] The results for clinical T3 patients treated with radiotherapy appear to be better than those for surgery. Zagars et al[16] treated 551 men with clinical stage T3 disease using external beam radiotherapy alone and reported 10-year actuarial disease-free survival and local control rates of 46% and 81%, respectively. It is important to note that a proportion of clinical T3 patients will not be cured by prostate radiotherapy even if pelvic volumes are treated because clinical outcome will be influenced by the presence of subclinical metastatic disease at the outset.

RESULTS OF EXTERNAL BEAM RADIOTHERAPY

The long-term survival of patients with T1 to T3 prostate cancer treated with external beam radiotherapy in the USA Patterns of Care (POC) study group, Radiation Therapy Oncology Group (RTOG) randomized studies, and other large single institute series are shown in Table 81.1. The POC and RTOG study group results represent national outcome averages for the US and provide reasonable estimation of treatment outcomes following conventional and more modern external beam radiotherapy techniques, respectively. It is also important to note that these results span a long period of time, during which both prescribed radiation dose and radiotherapy techniques have evolved considerably, and relate principally to clinically detected cancers in the pre-PSA era.

Local tumor control is related to clinical stage and is best for T1 disease and decreases with higher T stage (see Table 81.1). At 10 years, local control is reported at 92% to 96% for T1, 71% to 83% for T2, and 69% to 81% for T3 disease. Local control at 15 years is in the region of 83% for T1, decreasing to 65% to 68% for T2 and 44% to 75% for T3 disease. Tumor size can also influence local control rates. Analysis of the earlier RTOG studies revealed that tumors smaller than 25 cm³ have local control rates of up to 75% compared to tumors greater than 25 cm³ with local control rates of less than 50%.[17] Tumor sizes greater than 25 cm³ are also more likely to be advanced T stage disease.

PSA testing has revolutionized and standardized reporting of treatment outcome. Serum PSA estimations at disease presentation have been shown to be a useful

Table 81.1 External beam radiotherapy in prostate cancer: Long-term results from Patterns of Care studies, RTOG studies and large single institute series.[16,17,113,114]

	Number	Local recurrence (%)			Disease-free survival (%)			Overall survival (%)		
		5 year	10 year	15 year	5 year	10 year	15 year	5 year	10 year	15 year
T1Nx	583	3–6	4–8	17	84–85	52–68	39	83–95	52–76	41–46
T2Nx	1117	12–14	17–29	32–35	66–90	27–85	15–42	74–78	43–70	22–36
T3NX	2292	12–26	19–31	25–56	32–60	14–46	17–40	56–72	32–42	23–27

prognosticator, and PSA levels following radical radiotherapy can also be a sensitive indicator of disease recurrence. In a study of 120 patients treated with radical radiotherapy and mean follow-up of 12.6 years, Hanks et al[18] reported biochemical PSA control of up to 72% in T1 disease, 54% in T2A disease, and 28% in T3 disease. Additionally, low Gleason scores were associated with a 75% rate of PSA control compared to 18% for Gleason summed score of 7 and 0% in those cases with Gleason summed scores of 8 or 9. In a multi-institutional series of 1765 men with T1 and T2 cancers treated to a median dose of 69.4 Gy between 1988 and 1995, 5-year PSA control rates were 81%, 68%, 51%, and 31% for men with initial presenting PSA levels of less than 10 ng/ml, 10 to less than 20 ng/ml, 20 to less than 30 ng/ml, and 30 ng/ml or more, respectively. For the group with T1C cancers, PSA control rates were 87% and 47% for presenting PSA levels of less than 20 ng/ml and 20 ng/ml or more, respectively.[19]

There is emerging evidence that biochemical or clinical failures are less likely after 5 years if PSA levels remain controlled at this time point,[19–21] and that PSA control is a surrogate for clinically defined disease progression.[21]

RADIATION-RELATED COMPLICATIONS

The likelihood of radiation-related complications is dependent on the dose delivered, irradiation technique used, volume of normal tissues or organs-at-risk irradiated, and tolerance/radiosensitivity of the respective normal tissues. Radiotherapy-related complications can be divided into acute side effects (i.e. those occurring during and/or within 3 months of radiotherapy) and late side effects (i.e. those occurring >3 months following radiotherapy but usually developing months to years post-irradiation).

The RTOG and European Organization Research and Treatment of Cancer (EORTC) have collaborated to update toxicity grading criteria in order to provide a suitable framework for consistent reporting and thorough evaluation of late radiation complications—the late effects normal tissues (LENT) scoring system.[22] The RTOG grading scales for the assessment of acute and late radiation-related toxicity are shown in Tables 81.2 and 81.3, respectively.

Acute side-effects resulting from pelvic or prostate radiotherapy can include abdominal discomfort, rectal symptoms such as proctitis, diarrhea, bleeding, bladder symptoms such as urinary frequency, nocturia, dysuria, bleeding, and rarely skin reactions. The reported incidence of acute side effects range from 70% to 90% for mild symptoms, 20% to 45% for moderate, and 1% to 4% for severe or prolonged reactions.[23–25] The majority of acute complications resolve completely within 2 to 6 weeks following completion of external beam radiotherapy.

For external beam radiotherapy in prostate cancer, late rectal side effects are the major dose-limiting complications and include persistent rectal discharge,

Table 81.2 RTOG/EORTC grading criteria for acute effects.[22]

Grade	Gastrointestinal symptoms	Genitourinary symptoms
0	No change	No change
1	Increased frequency or change in quality of bowel habits not requiring medication, rectal discomfort not requiring analgesics	Frequency of urination or nocturia twice the pretreatment habit, dysuria, urgency not requiring medication
2	Diarrhea requiring antidiarrheal medication, mucus discharge not requiring pads, rectal or abdominal pain requiring analgesics	Frequency of urination or nocturia less frequent than every hour, dysuria, urgency, bladder spasm requiring local anesthetic
3	Diarrhea requiring parenteral support, mucus or blood discharge necessitating pads, abdominal distention	Frequency with urgency and nocturia hourly or more frequently, dysuria, pelvic plain or bladder spasm requiring regular narcotics, gross hematuria with or without clot passage
4	Acute or subacute obstruction, fistula or perforation, gastro-intestinal bleeding requiring transfusion, abdominal pain or tenesmus requiring tube decompression or bowel diversion	Hematuria requiring transfusion, acute bladder obstruction not secondary to clot passage, ulceration or necrosis

Table 81.3 RTOG/EORTC grading criteria for late effects.[22]

Grade	Gastrointestinal symptoms	Genitourinary symptoms
0	No change	No change
1	Mild diarrhea, mild cramping, bowel movements 5 times daily, slight rectal discharge or bleeding	Slight epithelial atrophy, minor telangiectasia, microscopic hematuria
2	Moderate diarrhea and colic, bowel movements >5 times daily, excessive mucus discharge or intermittent bleeding	Moderate frequency, generalized telangiectasia, intermittent microscopic hematuria
3	Obstruction or bleeding requiring surgery	Severe frequency and dysuria, severe telangiectasia (often with petechiae), frequent hematuria, reduction in bladder capacity (<150 ml)
4	Necrosis, perforation, fistula	Necrosis, contracted bladder (<100 ml), severe hemorrhagic cystitis

tenesmus and rectal urgency, and rectal bleeding, ulcer or stricture. Important late genitourinary complications include chronic cystitis, urinary incontinence, bladder ulceration, hematuria, urethral stricture, and impotence.

Late complications from conventional external beam radiotherapy have been reported by the POC study group. The overall incidence of major late complications, defined as those requiring hospital admission for investigation or management, was 4.5% (1.8% urologic and 2.8% gastrointestinal). These complications resulted from substandard radiotherapy techniques that are no longer used, such as very large fields or anteroposterior fields treating only one field each day.[26] The 10-year update from the POC study group reported actuarial 5- and 10-year major complication-free rates of 93% and 86%, respectively.[27]

The predominant type of late gastrointestinal complication is proctitis with grade 2 side effects occurring in 3% to 15% of cases.[28,29] Less than 1% of late rectal complications require colostomy.[28,30] The most common late urinary side effect is cystitis in 2% to 11% of cases, followed by urethral stricture in 2% to 10%, while urinary incontinence occurs in less than 1% to 2%.[28–31] The main predisposing factor for the development of urinary strictures and urinary incontinence is previous transurethral resections.[28–31]

An important prostate radiotherapy side effects is erectile dysfunction. Etiology of this complication is multifactorial and is influenced by factors such as pretreatment function, age, small vessel disease, and previous urologic surgery. Its incidence is estimated as between 30% and 40% of treated men.[32] Recent studies may be more reliable because of routine pre- and post-therapy evaluations of sexual function. Using quality-of-life questionnaires, up to 62% of men reported return of sexual function following conformal radiotherapy.[33] Similarly, a RTOG study revealed that 76% of sexually potent men reported return of function following radiotherapy.[34] However, the impact on different patient age groups can vary substantially, with 75% of men between 55 and 59 years and 53% between 60 and 74 years being bothered by sexual dysfunction following surgery compared to 40% and 47%, respectively, after radiotherapy.[35]

FACTORS INFLUENCING TREATMENT OUTCOME WITH RADIOTHERAPY

An important determinant of radiotherapy treatment outcome is local control. Lack of local control has been associated with higher biochemical PSA failure and metastatic rates.[36] At the Royal Marsden Hospital, London, analysis of radically irradiated patients with clinically locally controlled disease at 5 years revealed a 57% metastatic-free survival rate compared to 26% in patients who have developed local failure (P = <0.01). Multivariate analysis of metastatic-free and overall survival in this cohort of patients revealed that local control remains a highly significant parameter when included as a time-dependent variable (P = <0.01). This finding is consistent with reports from other series,[37,38] and is applicable to patients who present with bulky disease or higher stage (T3/4), higher initial PSA levels, and poorly differentiated grades.

Strategies to improve local control include an increase in the prescribed dose or the use of neoadjuvant and/or adjuvant androgen deprivation. The use of hormonal therapy is covered in Chapters 90 to 93 and will not be discussed further here. A dose–response relationship has been demonstrated for local control. Retrospective studies have reported lower local control rates of 62% to 63% when prescribed doses were less than 60 Gy, increasing to 74% to 80% for doses between 60 and 70 Gy, and 81% to 88% when doses were greater than 70 Gy.[39,40] There is potential for an increase in radiation-related complication rates when dose is increased. Using conventional external beam radiation techniques, the overall incidence of side-effects increased from 6% to 11% when patients received more than 65 Gy.[41] However, other investigators have not noted such a substantial increase in rectal complications with doses up to 70 Gy.[16,31] Studies suggest that the threshold for dose-limiting rectal complications is higher. The RTOG studies report a significant increase in late morbidity with doses greater than 70 Gy,[30] while other investigators note that when dose to the anterior rectal wall exceeds 75 Gy, the incidence of grade 2 or greater proctitis/bleeding rises from less than 20% to around 60%.[42] However, newer radiotherapy techniques (described below) may permit acceptable escalation of dose without an increase in late complications.

DEVELOPMENTS IN EXTERNAL BEAM RADIOTHERAPY

A major advance in pelvic external beam irradiation was the introduction of higher energy x-rays in the 1960s, which superseded the use of orthovoltage or deep x-ray beams of 200 kV to 300 kV. This heralded the modern era of prostate radiotherapy. Subsequently, megavoltage beams of greater 4 MeV (usually 10–18 MeV), produced by linear accelerators, delivered enhanced clinical depth–dose beam profiles that enable skin sparing and improved dose coverage of the prostate gland and seminal vesicles within the pelvis. Optimal visualization of the tumor volume and its surrounding anatomic structures is necessary for any cancer treatment delivered in a localized manner, such as radiotherapy. The use of computed tomography (CT) scanning has allowed clinicians to more accurately define treatment volumes. Initial studies assessing the value of CT scanning when it was first introduced recorded that geographic miss of the gross tumor can be avoided in up to 40% of cases.[43]

RADIOTHERAPY PLANNING NOMENCLATURE

Modern radiotherapy planning techniques, such as conformal radiotherapy (CFRT) and intensity-modulated

radiotherapy (IMRT), require definition of treatment volumes distinct from the simple visualization of gross tumor. The International Commission for Radiation Units (ICRU) Report 50 and 62 provides a series of definitions that incorporates parameters such as the extent of disease and its variation, organ motion due to physiologic activity, and uncertainties in patient and treatment set-up.[44,45] This nomenclature (Table 81.4; Figure 81.1) permits unambiguous specification of treatment volumes, uniformity in planning and treatment delivery, and consistency in reporting and comparison of results between different radiotherapy centers.

CROSS-SECTIONAL IMAGING AND CONFORMAL RADIOTHERAPY

Cross-sectional anatomic information has permitted the development of advanced radiotherapy techniques and is the basis of CFRT. CFRT uses CT to create three-dimensional (3D) models of the prostate gland and seminal vesicles in relation to their surrounding normal tissues or pelvic organs. This allows each radiotherapy beam to be shaped to the projected profile of the target within the axis of the beam (beams-eye-view, BEV) (Figure 81.2). By using multiple beams with each beam shaped in the BEV, the high dose region is made to conform to the shape of the planning target volume in 3D. This method can reduce unnecessary irradiation of the adjacent normal structures. Until recently, CT has been the main method of imaging for radiotherapy planning. Although CT provides geometrically stable images and electron density information needed for planning dose calculations, it is limited in defining soft tissues/organs in anatomic sites where there are many tissues/organs of similar electron densities, such as within the pelvis. As a result of the uncertainty in

Table 81.4 ICRU-50 and -62 treatment planning volumes.

Nomenclature	Definition
Gross target volume (GTV)	Radiologically visible or clinically palpable extent of tumor
Clinical target volume (CTV)	GTV with a margin that includes the presumed microscopic extent of disease or subclinical nodal involvement
Planning target volume (PTV)	CTV with a margin added to account for patient movement, internal organ and target motion, uncertainties in patient set-up, and treatment beam penumbra. This can be subdivided into the following: • Internal margin (IM) is that which is added for variations in position and/or shape and size of the CTV • Set-up margin (SM) is that which is added to account for all the variations and uncertainties in patient-beam positioning. Therefore CTV + IM + SM define the PTV.
Treated volume (TV)	Volume of tissue actually treated to the prescribed dose as specified by the clinician (e.g. 95% isodose volume)
Irradiated volume (IV)	Volume of tissue irradiated to a clinically significant dose in relation to normal tissue tolerance (e.g. 50% isodose volume)
Planning organ-at-risk volume (PRV)	Margin added to the organ-at-risk (OAR) to account for the positional/shape variation and uncertainties of the location of the OAR

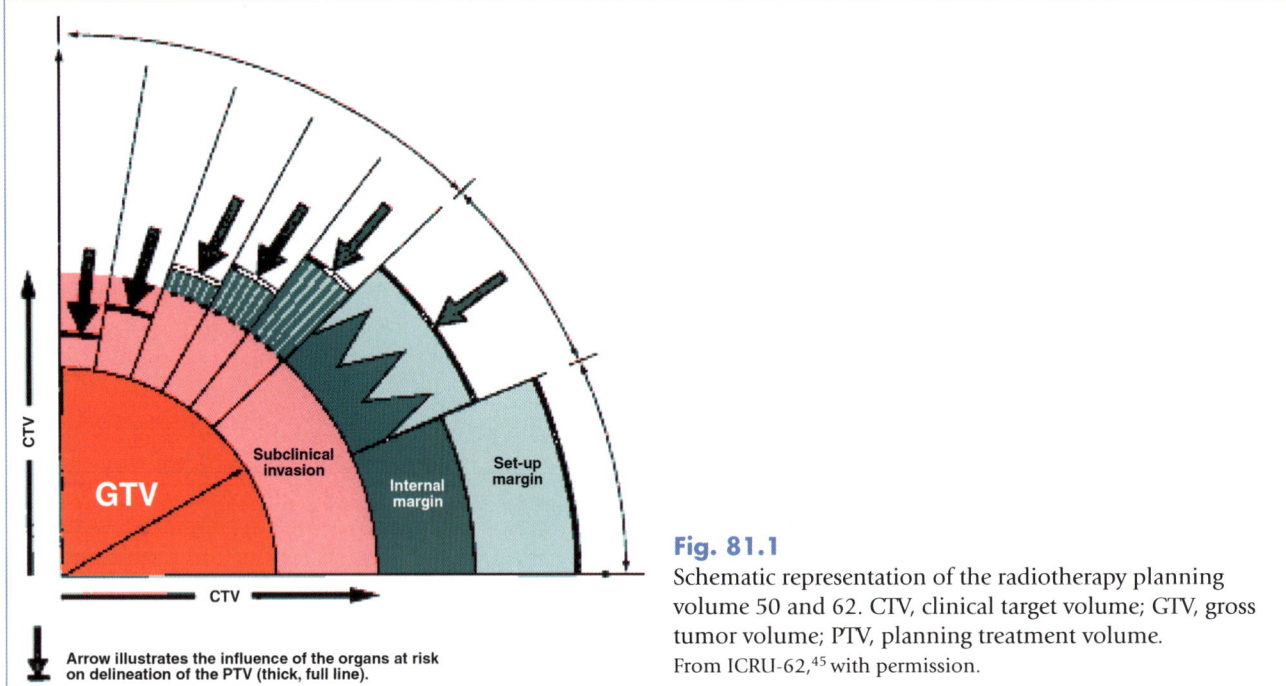

Fig. 81.1

Schematic representation of the radiotherapy planning volume 50 and 62. CTV, clinical target volume; GTV, gross tumor volume; PTV, planning treatment volume.

From ICRU-62,[45] with permission.

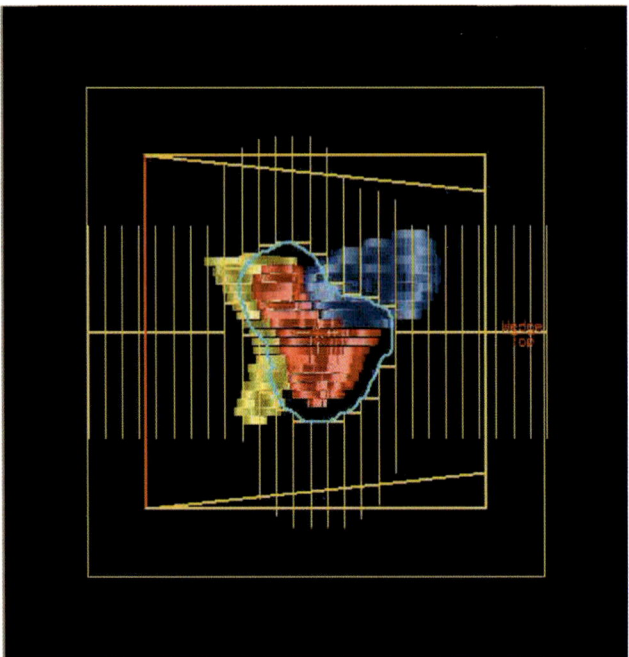

Fig. 81.2

Beams-eye-view (BEV) for a lateral prostate radiotherapy field. Prostate (red), rectum (yellow), bladder (blue).

accurately determining organ boundaries, clinicians often provide larger treatment volumes to compensate for this uncertainty.

The use of magnetic resonance imaging (MRI) can overcome some of the limitation of CT scanning and improve the definition of prostate treatment volumes. Its applications in radiotherapy have been reviewed.[46] The major advantage of MRI is its superior ability to distinguish between soft-tissue structures of similar tissue electron densities. This is particularly useful when

imaging structures such as the prostate gland, rectum, and bladder in the pelvis. Comparative MRI versus CT planning studies using MRI-defined prostate volumes as the gold standard have reported that CT-defined prostate volumes tend to overestimate the planning volume by as much as 40%.[47] Thus, the use of MR-based prostate planning volumes can result in smaller treatment volumes, leading to more appropriate shaping of the treatment fields and thereby reducing the risk of treatment-related complications. Although there are potential problems of image distortion with MRI, these technical issues can be effectively and reliably corrected or minimized.[46] The value of MR spectroscopy in defining tumor volumes within the prostate gland for radiotherapy is being investigated.[48,49] This procedure offers the opportunity to selectively boost identified clonagenic tumor regions for potentially better local control and subsequently improved survival. Other imaging methods under investigation are discussed in Chapters 50 to 53.

PLANNING FOR PROSTATE RADIOTHERAPY

CFRT is the minimum planning standard for prostate radiotherapy, providing reduced treatment-related toxicity compared to nonconformal techniques.[50] The radiotherapy treatment planning procedure involves a series of steps that start with obtaining 3D anatomic information of the patient in the treatment position, defining the target volumes, determining the optimal treatment plan, and implementing appropriate quality assurance, which includes treatment verification and monitoring of the patient during and following radiotherapy.

PATIENT POSITIONING AND IMMOBILIZATION

Patient positioning and immobilization are important to ensure that the patient can lie on the treatment table quietly and comfortably in a reliably immobile and reproducible manner for each treatment fraction. Usually, the patient lies supine and is supported with a foam head pad, and knee and ankle stocks help to maintain his position. Different treatment centers may use prone compared to supine positions, but a recent randomized trial demonstrated significantly less prostate motion and normal tissue irradiation with the supine position.[51]

Many immobilization devices are available to aid stabilization of the patient treatment position from body casts or cradles to ankle stocks. Although some investigators have shown that treatment set-up can be improved by immobilization of both the pelvis and legs,[52,53] a recent randomized trial revealed that the combination of knee supports and ankle stocks provided a high degree of accuracy, making pelvic immobilization unnecessary.[54]

PLANNING CT SCANNING

A CT scan in the treatment position is used to plan radiotherapy. Small skin tattoos are used to mark points on the patient's surface anteriorly and laterally. These skin points are used to align treatment room lasers for more reproducible patient set-up. The planning CT scan usually uses a slice interval of between 1 and 5 mm from below the ischial tuberosities to above the top of the bladder dome, or for the whole pelvis if pelvic treatment is intended.

The patient is usually instructed to keep his bladder comfortably "full" for the CT scan to reduce the proportion of the bladder and bowel within the planning target volume (PTV). At the Royal Marsden Hospital, patients are asked to empty their bladder 1 h prior to the start of the planning scan or treatment, and are asked to drink 300 to 400 ml of water during the waiting period. The bladder is thus partially filled but remains comfortable throughout scanning or treatment.

Rectal filling and emptying can influence prostate position during radiotherapy.[55] Strategies to achieve a more reliable rectal "state" include the use of daily laxatives or enemas prior to each radiotherapy fraction, endorectal balloons[56,57] or tensioned radioopaque marked urethral catheters.[58] These approaches have not been evaluated in controlled settings and some techniques may have issues with patient acceptability.

The position of the prostate may also be indirectly visualized using implanted intraprostatic markers. These radioopaque markers allow daily verification of the prostate location using electronic portal imaging devices, which can quantify the degree of positioning errors and permit online correction of these set-up errors.

Once the CT information has been obtained, these data are transferred to a radiotherapy planning workstation. It is important to ensure that all the relevant pelvic organs of interest for radiotherapy are adequately imaged so that they can be outlined for treatment planning and evaluation using dose–volume histograms. This is particularly crucial for IMRT to ensure that any organs to be treated or avoided can be optimized.

DEFINITION OF TARGET VOLUMES: PROSTATE, SEMINAL VESICLES, AND PELVIS

Treatment planning nomenclature based on ICRU-62 recommendations[45] is not always relevant for prostate radiotherapy. For example, the gross target volume (GTV) cannot be defined either by clinical examination or standard prostate imaging used for treatment planning. By definition it is not defined in T1 tumors. The clinical target volume (CTV) should include the whole prostate gland with all or part of the seminal vesicles, depending on clinical risk and an appropriate margin to account for subclinical disease spread. Multimodality imaging, particularly using MRI, may be used to improve definition of the target volumes.[46,59]

There is considerable controversy as to what forms appropriate coverage of the seminal vesicles, from some clinicians not including them in the treatment volume to complete coverage of the whole extent of the seminal vesicles. One pathologic series suggested seminal vesicle involvement was sequential in 96% of cases with direct extension through the prostatic capsule or spread along the ejaculatory ducts.[60] This sequential pattern of spread was also advocated by others who suggested that seminal vesicle coverage can be limited to the proximal 20 to 25 mm because in 90% of cases pathologic involvement was limited to the proximal 20 mm.[61] Our local institution policy is to include the proximal 20 mm of the seminal vesicles if they are to be treated. Table 81.5 lists the planning protocols in recent and ongoing major clinical trials for treatment margins and inclusion of the seminal vesicles.

When coverage of the pelvic lymph nodes is intended, the internal and external iliac nodal groups, including the presciatic, presacral, and obturator groups, are usually included in the treatment volume. These nodal groups are selected based on their likely microscopic involvement from surgical series.[62,63] Some clinicians may also include part of the common iliac lymph nodes.

DEFINITION OF TREATMENT MARGINS

PTV margins depend on local institution policy and relate to local experience as well as known thresholds for systematic and random errors that may manifest during treatment planning and delivery. All treatment margins need to be added in 3D to ensure adequate coverage, particularly where there is considerable variation in the size of the outline between consecutive CT slices.[64] PTV margins may be nonuniform, varying from 7 to 10 mm isotropically, with tighter posterior margins (0–5 mm) to limit dose to the anterior wall of the rectum depending on the prescribed dose. Treatment margins usually change for different phases of the treatment, particularly if different treatment volumes and dose escalation is used (see Table 81.5).

TREATMENT PLANNING

The use of Hounsfield units from the CT data allows for the assessment of tissue inhomogeneities and dose calculation. The number of treatment beams and their beam orientation largely depends on local facility expertise, experience, and protocols. Frequently three to four fields are used in Europe, while more than four fields are usually used in North America. The number of fields and their orientation may also change for different phases of the treatment. A recent comprehensive review for CFRT concluded that a three-field technique (an anterior and two wedged opposed lateral fields) gave equivalent or improved dose distributions.[65] For cases where there is asymmetry in the posterior extent of the

PTV, individual optimization of the beam orientations, such as substituting a posterior oblique field for one lateral field, may provide better coverage and this may be automated using optimization algorithms.[66] The use of non-coplanar CFRT plans may not provide substantial additional dosimetric gains compared to coplanar CFRT plans to warrant the increased efforts required for non-coplanar planning.[67]

Comparative studies of CFRT versus IMRT reveal that IMRT techniques can permit better dose distributions for irregularly shaped or concave target volumes, such as those found in seminal vesicles wrapping around the rectum, and improved avoidance or sparing of adjacent dose-limiting normal structures, such as the rectum.[68–70] When treating pelvic lymph nodes, IMRT techniques have been shown to permit better avoidance of bowel compared to CFRT, and allow escalation of dose to nodal regions while respecting bowel tolerances.[71] The tolerance of such a strategy is being assessed in a trial setting at the Royal Marsden Hospital. If an IMRT technique is used to treat the prostate and/or pelvis, five equally spaced coplanar fields can provide equivalent plans as more complex field arrangements.[71]

In the prostate treatment planning process, particularly with IMRT techniques, it is necessary to define minimum dose coverage of the target and/or limitations of dose to susceptible organs at risk (OARs),

Table 81.5 Contemporary prostate cancer radiotherapy trials showing details of radiotherapy technique.

Trial	Risk of SV involvement* (%)	Target + margin (mm)† Phase I	Phase II	Phase III	Dose‡ (Gy) Phase I	Phase II	Phase III	Total
Dutch	Low (<10)	P + 10	P + 5/0	–	68	0, 10	–	68, 78
	Mod (10–25)	P + SV + 10	P + 10	P + 5/0	50	18	0, 10	68, 78
	High (>25)	P + SV + 10	P + 5/0	–	68	0, 10	–	68, 78
	Involved	P + SV + 10	P + SV+ 5/0	–	68	0, 10	–	68, 78
PROTECT, UK	Low (<15)	P + bSV + 10/5	P + 0	–	56	18	–	74
	High (≥15)	P + SV	P + 0	–	56	18	–	74
RT-01, UK	Low (<15)	P + bSV + 10	P + 0	–	64	0, 10	–	64, 74
	High (≥15)	P + SV	P + 0	–	64	0, 10	–	64, 74
EORTC 22991	All	P + SV + 10 ± nodes	P + bSV + 10	P + 5/0	46	24	0, 4, 8	70, 74, 78 (not randomized)
RTOG P-0126	All	P + SV + 10/5	P + 10/5	–	58	15, 24	–	73, 82
RTOG 9406	Low (<15)	P + 5–10	P + 5–10	–	68	0, 6, 11	–	68, 74, 79
	High (≥15)	P + SV + 5–10	P + 5–10	–	56	12, 8, 23	–	68, 74, 79
	Involved	P + SV + 5–10	–	–	68, 74, 79	–	–	68, 74, 79
MSKCC	All	P + SV + 10/6	P + SV + 10/6 Rectal block	–	65, 70, 76, 76	0, 0, 0, 5	–	65, 70, 76, 81
CHHIP, UK (high-dose arm)	Low (<15)	P + bSV + 10	P + 10/5	P + 5/0	56	16	4	74
	High (≥15)	P + SV + 10	P + 10/5	P + 5/0	56	16	4	74

bSV, base of seminal vesicle; P, prostate; SV, seminal vesicle.

*Risk of SV based on Roach formula and Partin tables.

†"/" Indicates margin: all around prostate/prostate–rectum interface.

‡Multiple figures in each risk group indicate different dose arms of trials.

such as the rectum, bladder, bowel or femoral heads. These clinical planning dose thresholds may also be used to determine the "goodness" of the treatment plan. In evaluating the acceptability of any plan, treatment parameters, such as dose statistics (mean, minimum or maximum doses), dose–volume histograms, and visual inspection of the dose distribution on each transaxial slice of the treatment volume, are used to ensure appropriate coverage of the target and maximal avoidance of the OARs. Reported dose thresholds for both acute and late toxicity are available for a variety of OARs, such as rectum,[72–80] bladder,[81] bowel,[75,82] and femoral heads.[83] We have collated a set of suitable planning dose thresholds that guide our current assessment of plans for either prostate and/or pelvic radiotherapy at the Royal Marsden Hospital (Table 81.6). Future reporting of dose-related toxicity from randomized trials of dose escalation is likely to refine these dose thresholds.

VERIFICATION

Accurate and reliable delivery of radiation to the target is paramount for prostate radiotherapy. Treatment verification is needed to identify systematic and random errors in the treatment planning process in order to allow its correction. During treatment delivery, film-based portal x-rays or electronic portal images are used to compare patient positioning with reference simulator films or digitally reconstructed radiographs. Gross inaccuracies may be corrected by repositioning the patient in realtime.[84] However, these verification methods only permit identification of field boundaries

relative to bony landmarks and not the spatial location of the prostate or other internal organs. The use of radioopaque markers implanted in the prostate will allow daily quantification of the prostate position. More recent methods for visualizing the spatial location of targets and OARs during radiotherapy and image-guided treatment strategies will be discussed later.

RESULTS FROM CONFORMAL RADIOTHERAPY

The impact and value of CFRT was assessed in a randomized prostate radiotherapy trial at the Royal Marsden Hospital. This trial compared the use of conformal shaped fields versus conventional or unshaped rectangular fields at a dose of 64 Gy.[85] In men treated with CFRT, the incidence of clinically relevant late radiation sequelae, such as rectal proctitis requiring treatment (RTOG grade ≥ 2), was significantly reduced compared to conventional techniques (5% vs 15% respectively). More importantly, the close shaping of the conformal fields did not lead to any reduction in PSA-based local control between the randomized arms at a median follow-up of 3.6 years. These data set CFRT as the standard for prostate external beam irradiation. The use of CFRT to reduce the rate of treatment-related complications provides the potential for safe dose escalation. It has been postulated that if radiation dose can be safely escalated by 20%, this may result in demonstrable improvements in local tumor control rates by up to 10%.[86,87] This may subsequently increase the probability of cancer-specific survival for some cancer types such as prostate cancer.

The dose–response hypothesis fueled by data from the pre-PSA Patterns of Care analysis from the US suggested that higher doses provided improved disease-free intervals, especially for locally advanced disease.[26,88] However, depending on the level of dose escalation, radiotherapy using conventional techniques has been associated with an unreasonable and substantial increase in rectal bleeding, from 6% to 12% around 60 Gy to 11% to 20% with doses above 64 to 65 Gy.[26,31,41]

The result of dose escalation with CFRT was reviewed in a retrospective study from three USA institutions.[89] This study of 180 men reported a dose effect for men with high-grade T1/T2 disease with improved 5-year biochemical PSA control rates using doses of 70 Gy or greater. In a larger CFRT study of 743 patients with localized prostate cancer treated with escalating doses, PSA relapse-free survival rates in patients with intermediate or unfavorable prognosis (characterized by ≥ 1 or ≥ 2 higher prognostic indicators, respectively, i.e. $\geq$T3, PSA level >10 ng/ml, Gleason score >6) was significantly improved with doses of 75.6 Gy or greater ($P = <0.05$).[90]

Translation of improved local control into survival was reported for the first time by the RTOG.[91] The

Table 81.6 Suggested dose/volume thresholds for organs at risk used at the Royal Marsden Hospital

Dose (Gy) at 2 Gy/ fraction to 100%	Maximum volume (%)
Rectum*	
50	60
60	50
65	30
70	15
74	3
Bladder†	
50	50
60	25
74	5
Femoral heads‡	
50	50

*Rectum including outer wall and contents from rectosigmoid junction to ischial tuberosities.

†Defined as whole bladder including outer wall.

‡Defined as the round part of the femoral head.

outcomes from four randomized RTOG trials comprising 1465 men treated between 1975 and 1992 with a median follow-up of 8 years showed an improvement in 10-year disease-specific survival and overall survival rates for high-grade prostate cancers treated to doses of 66 Gy or greater. This was associated with a 29% lower relative risk of death from prostate cancer and 27% reduced mortality rate (P = <0.05). No neoadjuvant or adjuvant androgen deprivation therapy was used. These data suggest that increases in radiation dose alone can confer a survival benefit in men with localized prostate cancer but this may be limited to those with higher grade disease.

However, improvements in outcome during the PSA era may in part be due to a shift in presentation to low-risk disease and earlier detection of high-grade disease.[92] Caution is needed in the interpretation of results from sequentially treated cohorts of patient, such as those reported from phase I/II studies of dose-escalated prostate radiotherapy. Phase III randomized controlled trials are needed to properly define the use of higher dose radiotherapy, clinical prognostic parameters, reporting PSA control rates, and clinically important endpoints, including toxicity and quality-of-life data.

Two randomized controlled trials have reported results of dose escalation in prostate radiotherapy and the results of others are maturing. The first of these to report was from the MD Anderson Cancer Center; this randomized 305 men with T1 to T3 localized prostate cancer between 1993 and 1998 to either 70 or 78 Gy.[80] With a median follow-up of 60 months, the 6-year freedom-from-failure rates, including biochemical PSA failure rates, were 64% for 70 Gy and 70% for 78 Gy (P = 0.03). Subgroup multivariate analysis revealed that those patients with presenting a PSA level of greater than 10 ng/ml benefited from dose escalation with a freedom-from-failure rate of 62% compared to 43% in the 70-Gy arm (P = 0.01). However, late rectal side effects were also significantly increased in the 78-Gy arm with an actuarial risk of RTOG grade 2 or greater toxicity at 6 years of 26% compared to 12% in the 70-Gy arm (P = 0.001). This late complication was highly correlated to the volume of rectum treated beyond 70 Gy with a threshold at 25% of the irradiated rectal volume. This may be avoided by more stringent attention to limiting dose to the rectum by better radiation techniques.

The second trial to report results was from the Institute of Cancer Research/Royal Marsden Hospital, which in a randomized pilot study (which led into the UK Medical Research Council [MRC] RT-01 trial) included 125 men with T1 to T3 cancers treated for 3 to 6 months with neoadjuvant androgen suppression and then randomized to either 64 or 74 Gy.[93] This patient group had less favorable prognostic features than those patients included in the MD Anderson Cancer Center trial (e.g. initial presenting PSA level of 14 versus 8 ng/ml). After a median follow-up of 74 months, the 5-year PSA control rate was higher in the 74-Gy (71%) than in

the 64-Gy (59%) group (hazard ratio, 0.64; P = 0.10). Bowel and bladder side effects were also increased in the higher dose group, particularly in the subgroup of patients who in a second randomization had the phase I radiotherapy volume treated with a 15-mm rather than a 10-mm margin.[93] The PSA control rates were very similar for these groups and as the 15-mm margin increased toxicity without any apparent clinical benefit, a 10-mm margin was used in the subsequent MRC RT-01 trial.

The MRC RT-01 trial has now completed recruitment of over 850 men with localized prostate cancer in 2003.[94,95] The Netherlands CKVO 96-10 trial completed recruitment of approximately 670 men in 2003 and randomized patients to either 68 or 78 Gy, also using CFRT methods.[96] The use of neoadjuvant androgen deprivation therapy was allowed in this trial. The French Collaborative trial recruited 306 patients with localized prostate cancer to a randomized trial of 70 versus 80 Gy. No androgen deprivation therapy was used in this trial.[97] Outcomes for biochemical PSA control rates and incidence of late complications from these trials are awaited with much interest and will provide further clarification for optimization of patient management.

INTENSITY-MODULATED RADIOTHERAPY

Whether dose escalation is being considered or not, it is crucial to ensure that any potential treatment-related complications are minimized. Advances in technology have enabled the development of more sophisticated radiotherapy treatment methods. Such technical developments include multileaf collimators (MLC) that allow automatic shaping of the radiotherapy field and routine use of electronic portal imaging devices (EPID) that permit daily online verification of the treatment fields. These devices together with modern computational power for sophisticated 3D radiotherapy dose-cube calculations and "inverse" planning algorithms have enabled the refinement of conformal techniques into a new treatment paradigm, IMRT.

IMRT expands the concept of CFRT by enabling the high-dose regions to be shaped around "concave" targets and not just to the profile of the target in the BEV. IMRT can produce deliberate inhomogeneous dose distributions, such as to tumor regions as defined by MR spectroscopy, for boosting or to conformally avoid important OARs, such as the rectum in prostate radiotherapy. Compared to CFRT where the beam fluence is constant across each treatment field, in the IMRT technique, the intensity of the beam fluence is varied across each treatment field. The effect of IMRT is to produce a series of many smaller beamlets for each treatment field, each of which can be controlled individually to provide different dose fluences; these beamlets are then combined to generate the overall desired dose distribution. The conceptual difference in

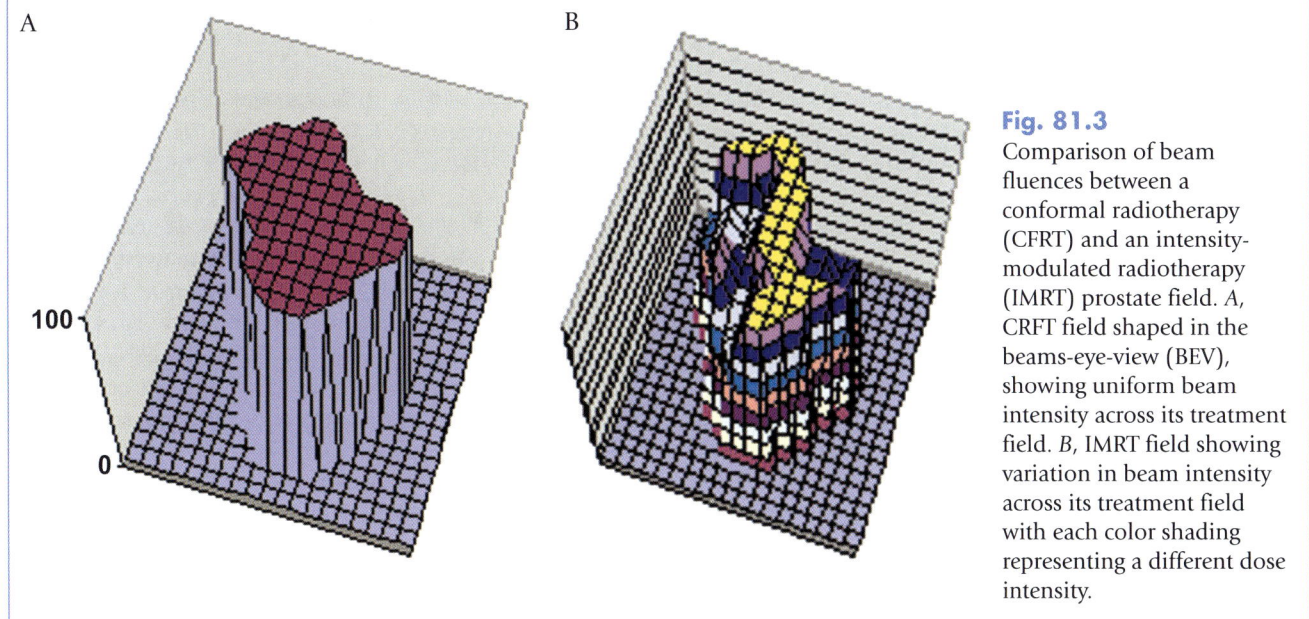

A   B

Fig. 81.3
Comparison of beam fluences between a conformal radiotherapy (CFRT) and an intensity-modulated radiotherapy (IMRT) prostate field. *A*, CRFT field shaped in the beams-eye-view (BEV), showing uniform beam intensity across its treatment field. *B*, IMRT field showing variation in beam intensity across its treatment field with each color shading representing a different dose intensity.

beam fluences between conformal and intensity-modulated fields is schematically shown in Figure 81.3A and B, respectively. Inverse planning algorithms are needed to create and optimize the IMRT plan. These algorithms avoid previous manual trial-and-error methods of producing appropriate prostate radiotherapy plans by using an iterative computational process based on cost functions and/or physical dose parameters to obtain the optimum plan from the desired projected dose distribution for the ideal prostate with or without seminal vesicles radiotherapy plan.

RESULTS

The delivery of appropriately designed nonuniform dose intensities with IMRT can produce better sculpturing of the high-dose region to complex irregular shapes, particularly concave-shaped target volumes such as the coverage of seminal vesicles or pelvic nodal volumes. One clinical example where IMRT is being used to cover a "U"-shaped target volume (Figure 81.4) to a relatively high dose (55–60 Gy) within the pelvis while dramatically sparing bowel dosage is our phase I/II trial of pelvic nodal irradiation in high-risk prostate cancer patients. Preliminary results from this study report acceptable early toxicity.[98]

IMRT plans can provide a very steep high-to-low-dose gradient at the edge of the target volume for improved avoidance of important adjacent normal structures in prostate radiotherapy, such as the rectum, bowel, and bladder. In this manner, external beam radiotherapy-related complications may be further reduced and higher dose escalation may be safely achieved compared to CFRT. Using this refined technique with appropriate and judicious shielding of the rectum, clinicians at the Memorial Sloan-Kettering Cancer Center treated 772 men to doses 81 Gy or greater and reported a relatively

low incidence of late rectal complications.[99] With a median follow-up of 24 months, the 3-year actuarial likelihood of greater than late grade 2 rectal toxicity was 4%.

NEW STRATEGIES FOR EXTERNAL BEAM RADIOTHERAPY

DEVELOPMENTS IN RADIOTHERAPY FRACTIONATION

External beam prostate radiotherapy is usually given by conventional fractionation (i.e. 1.8–2.0 Gy/fraction) in

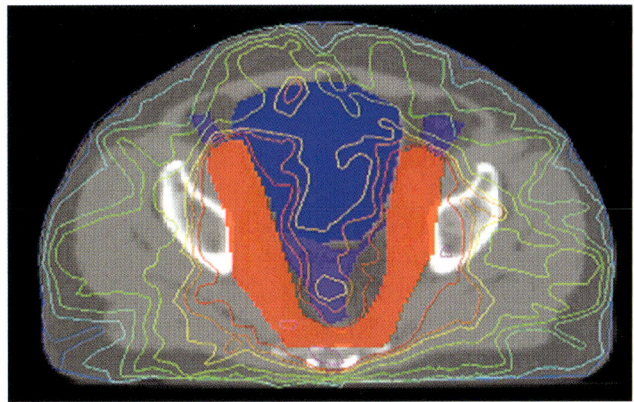

Fig. 81.4
Example of an intensity-modulated radiotherapy (IMRT) plan used to treat pelvic lymph nodes at the Royal Marsden Hospital. In the transaxial plane, the 90% isodose (red line) is shaped around the planning target volume (solid red) and spares doses to the organs at risk (OARs) located adjacent and centrally (solid purple and blue, respectively).

many parts of the world. The dogma of conventional fractionation for prostate cancer has been challenged recently by several investigators.[100,101] In radiobiology, the components of lethal radiation damage to the cell are expressed by the interrelationship of two measures, α and β, which can be modeled. The most commonly used radiobiologic model utilizing α and β values is the linear-quadratic formula and this can be used to guide the rationale for different fractionation schemes. It has been suggested that the α:β ratio for prostate cancer is much lower than previously thought, being around 1.2 to 1.5 Gy. This is lower than for other tumor types where the α:β ratio can range from 4 to 30 Gy; an "average" α:β ratio value of 10 Gy is generically assumed for most tumors. This lower predicted α:β ratio is consistent with the slower growth rates or low labeling indices of around 1% noted in prostate cancer compared to other tumor types that have labeling indices of around 3% to 5%.[102,103]

The low α:β ratio of prostate cancer implies that these cancers possess higher fractionation sensitivity similar to that for late-responding normal tissues. This means that the use of hypofractionation (i.e. larger dose/fraction and fewer fractions) in prostate external beam radiotherapy may provide an improved therapeutic ratio by reducing the probability of late radiation morbidity for the same level of local control. Early indications for this are provided by a recent Australian trial that reported on a randomized comparison of 64 Gy in 32 fractions (2 Gy/fraction) with 55 Gy in 20 fractions (2.75 Gy/fraction) in men with early stage (T1–2N0M0) prostate cancer.[104] The interim analysis of the first 120 patients with a median follow-up of 43.5 months revealed similar PSA relapse-free survival rates and toxicities between the two radiation schedules. The follow-up is still too short to determine long-term control but is reasonable for defining the potential safety or toxicity of the program. A larger study from the National Cancer Institute of Canada PR-5 trial randomized 936 patients with T1/T2 prostate cancer to either 66 Gy in 33 fractions or 52.5 Gy in 20 fractions between 1994 and 1998.[105] With a median follow-up of 59 months, preliminary results in abstracted form showed comparable late toxicity between the arms (hypofractionated 2.6% vs conventional 3.6%), but the 5-year failure probability was higher in the hypofractionated arm than in the conventional fractionation arm (55.6% vs 48.6%, respectively; hazards ratio, 1.20). One potential explanation may be that the arms were not biologically equivalent in dose. This result is compatible with a α:β ratio of 1.5 assuming a γ 50 value of approximately 2.0.[106]

Local control rates will vary when different prognostic groups are considered, particularly with locally advanced cases. The hypofractionated schedule can also be dose escalated to improve the likelihood of local control, while maintaining the same level of radiation morbidity expected from the use of higher dose prescriptions (>74–78 Gy) using conventional fractionation schemes.

A large UK series has recently reported on 703 patients from 1995 to 1998 with clinical staged T1–4N0M0 prostate cancer treated to 50 Gy in 16 daily fractions (3.13 Gy/fraction) without hormonal manipulation.[107] Using this hypofractionated scheme to a relatively low total dose, the reported overall 5-year PSA relapse-free survival and radiation morbidity rates are similar to those obtained with 65 to 70 Gy delivered using 1.8- to 2-Gy fractions. This study grouped the patients into three prognostic subsets based on PSA at presentation, clinical T stage, and Gleason score. The "good" group was defined as stage T1/2, PSA level of 10 ng/ml or less, and Gleason score less than 7; the "intermediate" group had one raised value; and the "poor" group had two or more raised values. With a median follow-up of 48 months, the 5-year PSA relapse-free survival rates were 82%, 56%, and 39% for the good, intermediate, and poor groups, respectively, with RTOG grade 2 or greater for bowel and bladder toxicity in 5% and 9%, respectively. These data on late complications confirms acceptable toxicity at this hypofractionated dose level and suggests that this is an acceptable regimen for good prognosis patients but may be less adequate for the other prognostic groups. The lower PSA relapse-free survival rates experienced by the intermediate and poor risk groups may be improved by dose escalation.

Several reservations have been directed towards the recent estimation for a much lower α:β ratio in prostate cancer:[108] the use of biochemical PSA-dependent results at 5 years which may not reflect long-term outcomes; data obtained at different centers and over time periods; estimations of the radiation damage repair half life and its effectiveness; as well as assumptions about the biologic and physical dose heterogeneity of the different patient groups. Nevertheless, the hypothesis is an attractive one not only for the potential improved therapeutic ratio but also for logistic and workflow issues. The advantages of hypofractionation are a shortened overall treatment time with reduced patient visits and departmental resources. This has prompted several groups around the world to reinvestigate the use of hypofractionation and dose escalation.

A variety of phase I/II studies are being undertaken to evaluate the use of hypofractionation regimens. One US collaborative study has reported on the use of 2.5 Gy/fraction prescribed to 70 Gy in 100 men with T1 to T3 prostate cancer.[109] With a median follow-up of 43 months, the overall biochemical PSA relapse-free survival at 4 years was reported to be 88%, with a 4-year actuarial late rectal RTOG grade 2 or 3 complication rate of 6%. Only 1 of the 100 patients suffered a grade 3 complication. The outcome from this study group demonstrated a favorable survival and toxicity profile.

At the Christie Hospital in Manchester, UK, Princess Margaret Hospital in Toronto and Notre-Dame Hospital in Montreal, Canada, 3 Gy/fraction to escalated doses of 60 to 66 Gy are being studied for different prognostic groups. A randomized phase III study comparing 74 Gy in 2 Gy/fraction with 57 Gy and 60 Gy using 3 Gy/fraction has begun at the Institute of Cancer Research/Royal Marsden Hospital, London, and with Department of Health support will aim to increase recruitment to a larger cohort of 450 men in a multicenter study. These centers have reported acceptable rates of toxicity in abstracted form and mature outcome for local control and late complication are awaited with much interest.

VERIFYING RADIOTHERAPY AND FOUR-DIMENSIONAL TREATMENT STRATEGIES

Currently, the technology for shaping treatment beam and radiation dose distributions far exceeds the ability to localize tumor extent and variability in internal target position using conventional means. Furthermore, there are inaccuracies in treatment and patient set-up during a fractionated course of radiotherapy that need to be addressed. Laser guidance systems and patient immobilization devices are often used to aid reproducibility of the treatment position. New approaches to these issues involve the development of systems that use patient surface or multiregion sensing with automated linkage to predefined topologic maps or treatment portals, and delivery simultaneously correlated to automated indexed treatment couches based on the realtime information gleaned from the patient on the therapy bed.

Traditional methods to verify static prostate radiation fields involved exposing radiographic film to a small test dose for each delivered field portal. Recently, this same task has been replaced by electronic portal imaging devices (EPIDs). This method conveniently avoids the need for film and provides digital advantages in terms of image processing, transfer, and storage. However, the disadvantage of these systems is that only the prostate radiation field shapes are verified. It is well known that the anatomic position of the prostate/seminal vesicles within the pelvis can vary from day to day and is influenced by the physiologic activity of the surrounding pelvic organs.[55] There is little information available from EPIDs to determine if the internal organs, such as the prostate and/or seminal vesicles, are within the treatment portal unless a radioopaque marker is implanted to provide a surrogate measure.

A variety of methods have been investigated to address the issue of prostate organ motion, each with their peculiar advantages and disadvantages. Some investigators have used rectal obturators or balloons,[57] while others have utilized special transurethral catheters with radioopaque markers[110] to help reproduce the treatment position. One disadvantage of these methods is the need for daily instrumentation, which may not be well tolerated by patients. Daily localization of the prostate gland can be performed using a portable ultrasound machine (BAT or B-mode acquisition targeting ultrasound system, Nomos Corporation), which provides spatial localization of the prostate correlated to the position of the patient on the therapy couch. This method relies heavily on operator expertise for reliability.

Another method is to use implanted markers within the prostate. The position of the radioopaque markers in relation to bony pelvic landmarks imaged using EPIDs can then be used to correct for errors in field placement. More recent approaches to this consider a four-dimensional (4D) strategy (with time as the fourth dimension) or the realtime element of the prostate position during radiation delivery. Again, implanted radioopaque markers in the prostate or body/pelvic surface contours with deformable organ modeling act as surrogates for prostate gland position to permit tracking and/or gating of radiation treatment in realtime. This approach is the subject of a research project, called ON-TARGET (ONline Tracking And Realtime Gated External beam Therapy), in several clinical subsites, including the prostate, at our institution. This ON-TARGET project uses the Elekta Synergy (Elekta Oncology Systems) in which an x-ray volumetric imager device capable of kilovoltage (kV) cone beam imaging forms part of the linear accelerator (LINAC). This digital kV flat panel device provides the opportunity for 3D cross-sectional and fluoroscopic imaging of the patient on a linear accelerator (Figure 81.5A). This system can also provide 3D information for treatment verification. Similar systems for 3D and kV imaging on the LINAC have been developed by Varian Oncology Systems with their On-Board Imager (Figure 81.5B) and by Siemens Artiste (Figure 81.5C). The latter system differs from both the Varian and Elekta systems by having its kV imager along the same axis as the gantry head instead of perpendicular to the irradiation axis. Another novel system that is in current usage incorporates a CT scanner within the LINAC, delivering treatment in a helical tomotherapy method (TomoTherapy Inc, Wisconsin).

Other available systems that can track the prostate include the system sponsored by Mitsubishi Electronics at the Hokkaido University School of Medicine and the CyberKnife (Accuray Inc, Sunnyvale, CA). The Hokkaido University system uses a linear accelerator synchronized with a fluoroscopic realtime tumor tracking system which has four sets of diagnostic x-ray television systems, each adjusted such that the central axis of the individual systems would cross at the isocenter of the linear accelerator (Figure 81.6). Together with a moving object recognition software system, this system has been reported to have an accuracy of ±1 mm in determining

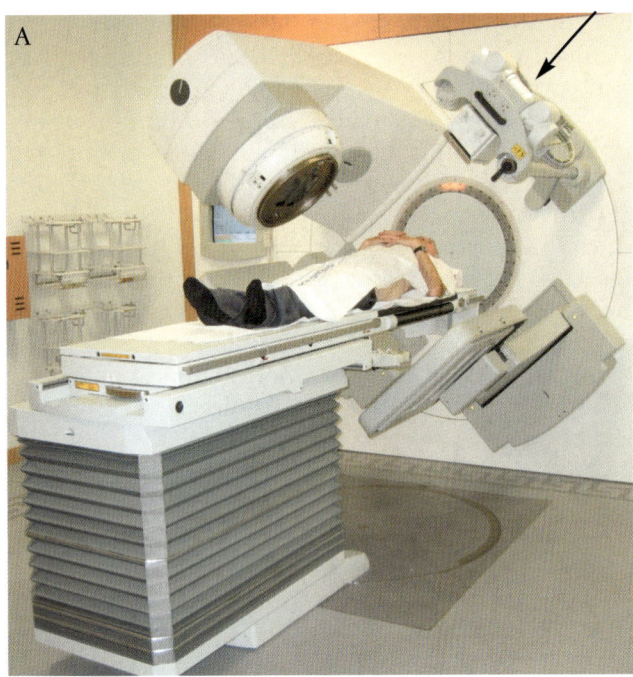

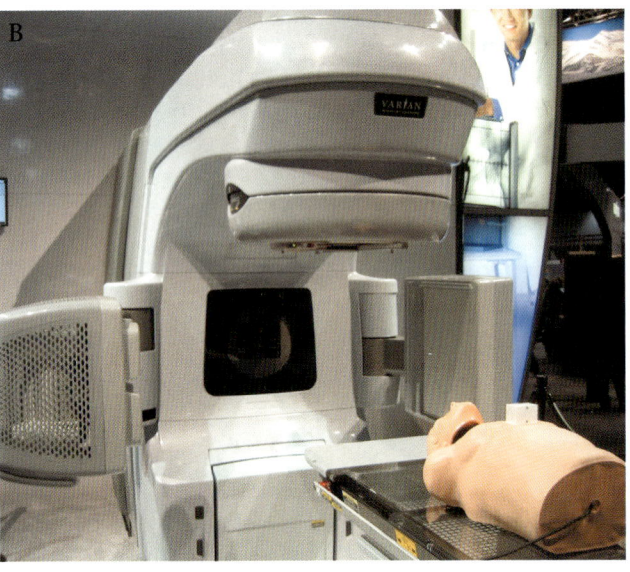

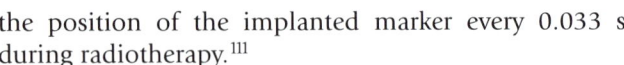

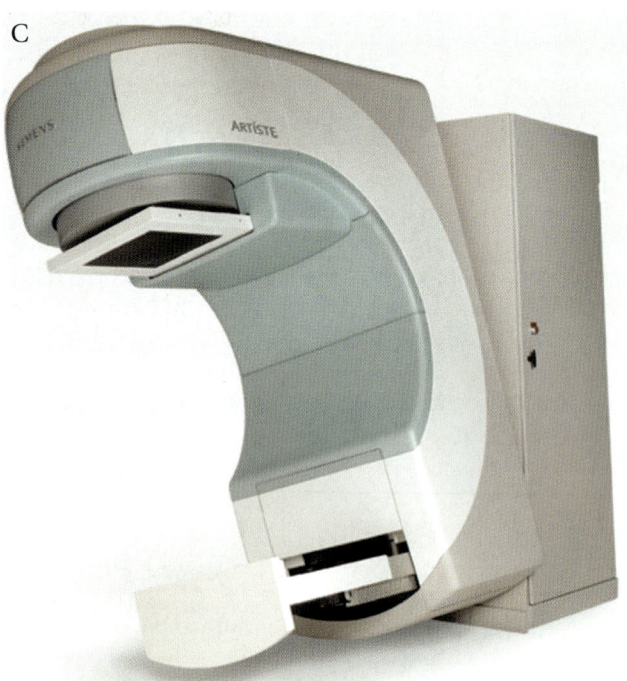

Fig. 81.5
A kilovoltage x-ray imager (arrow) capable of obtaining cross-sectional volumetric and fluoroscopic images is mounted perpendicular to the gantry head of a linear accelerator. Examples are shown of A, Elekta Synergy XVI system; B, Varian On-Board Imager system; and C, Siemens Artiste system.
Courtesy of Elekta Oncology Systems (A), Varian Medical Systems (B), and Siemens Medical Solutions (C).

the position of the implanted marker every 0.033 s during radiotherapy.[111]

The CyberKnife is a 6-MV linear accelerator mounted on a computer-controlled robotic arm and is equipped with an orthogonal pair of diagnostic quality digital x-ray imaging devices that monitor the position of implanted markers (Figure 81.7). It has been reported that the CyberKnife allows delivery with a precision of less than 0.5 mm and a tracking error of less than 1 mm to the position of the radioopaque markers.[112]

The guiding principle of all these systems is that by accurate localization to the actual position of the target at the time of delivery, either gated or not, geographic miss and set-up errors will be avoided, treatment margins can be reduced, and dose escalation can be safely delivered. However, regardless of the system used and its possible complexity, it is imperative that protocols and adequate quality assurance are present to ensure safety of the system for patient use.

SUMMARY

External beam irradiation is a well established curative treatment modality for men with nonmetastatic prostate cancer and additionally has a role in palliation of patients with metastatic disease. Recent technologic developments have changed prostate radiotherapy practice. The widespread availability of cross-sectional CT imaging with the development of software to reconstruct anatomy and manipulate 3D images, together with hardware such as MLC, has enabled the routine use of conformal radiotherapy. The addition of multimodality morphologic imaging, such as pelvic MRI, has enhanced volume definition for treatment planning in prostate cancer.

Sophisticated computing has allowed the development of IMRT. These developments and techniques have permitted the safe escalation of radiation dose in prostate cancer. The published data suggest a dose–response relationship for different

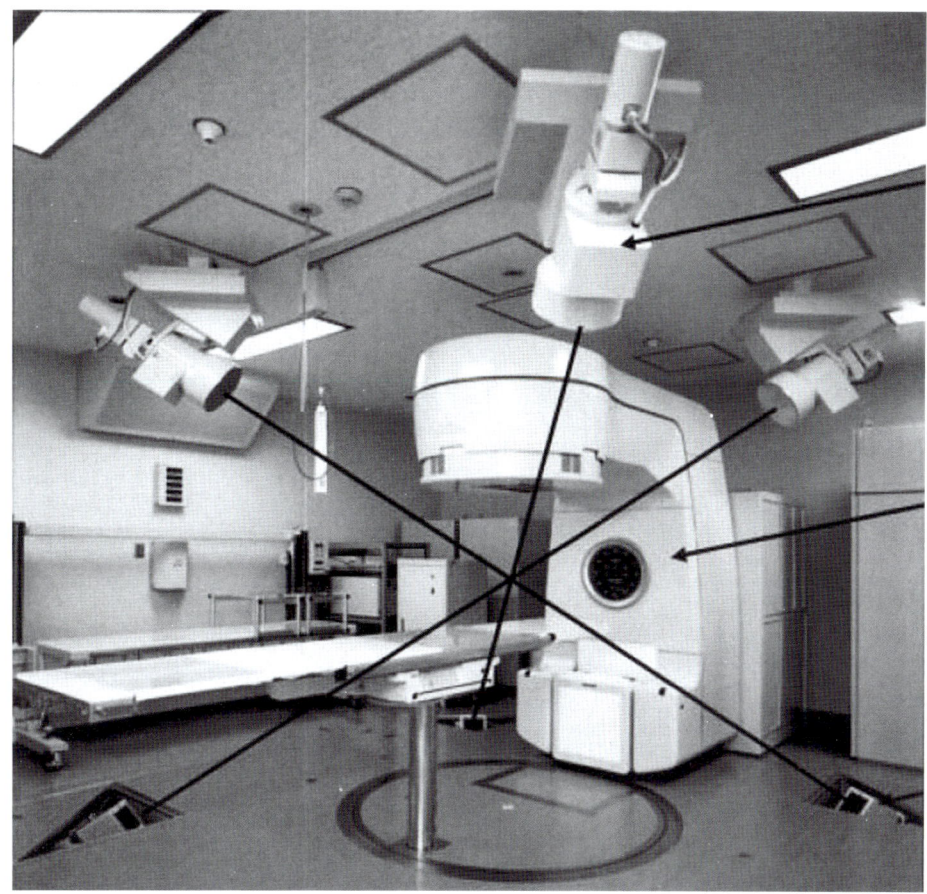

Fig. 81.6
Hokkaido University motion-gated linear accelerator system and fluoroscopic realtime tumor tracking system.
Reprinted from Int J Radiation Oncology Biol Phys, 48, Shirato et al, Four-dimensional treatment planning and fluoroscopic real-time tumor tracking radiotherapy for moving tumor, 435–442, 2000, with permission from Elsevier.

prognostic groups of patients with prostate cancer. Early randomized data is encouraging but long-term results are needed to confirm this outcome.

Further refinements in radiotherapy strategy for prostate cancer will include consideration of the radiobiologic rationale for hypofractionation in prostate cancer and the assessment of volumes appropriate to the prognostic group for high-dose irradiation. The utilization of biologic images to include functional, biochemical, metabolic, and physiologic data may aid in defining more appropriate treatment volumes. Technologic advances have ushered the capability to consider 4D treatment strategies for online realtime and/or gated treatments to further enhance accuracy and reliability of high-dose radiation schemes. Further developments for 4D treatments are expected into the next decade. This will substantially alter the way the practice of radiotherapy is perceived and influence the manner in which patients are treated with radiotherapy.

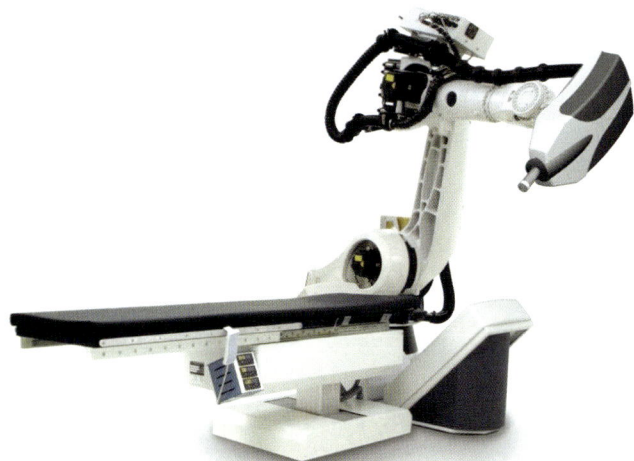

Fig. 81.7
CyberKnife.
Courtesy of Accuray Inc.

REFERENCES

1. Dearnaley DP, Melia J. Early prostate cancer—to treat or not to treat? Lancet 1997;349:892–893.
2. Chodak GW, Thisted RA, Gerber GS, et al. Results of conservative management of clinically localised prostate cancer. N Engl J Med 1994;330:242–248.
3. Partin AW, Kattan MW, Subong EN, et al. Combination of prostate-specific antigen, clinical stage, and Gleason score to predict pathological stage of localized prostate cancer. A multi-institutional update. JAMA 1997;277:1445–1451.
4. Roach M 3rd, Marquez C, Yuo HS, et al. Predicting the risk of lymph node involvement using the pre-treatment prostate specific antigen

and Gleason score in men with clinically localized prostate cancer. Int J Radiat Oncol Biol Phys 1994;28:33–37.

5. Parker CC, Norman AR, Huddart RA, et al. Pre-treatment nomogram for biochemical control after neoadjuvant androgen deprivation and radical radiotherapy for clinically localised prostate cancer. Br J Cancer 2002;86:686–691.

6. Kattan MW, Zelefsky MJ, Kupelian PA, et al. Pretreatment nomogram for predicting the outcome of three-dimensional conformal radiotherapy in prostate cancer. J Clin Oncol 2000;18:3352–3359.

7. Paulson DF, Lin GH, Hinshaw W, et al. Radical surgery versus radiotherapy for adenocarcinoma of the prostate. J Urol 1982;128:502–504.

8. Hanks GE. More on the Uro-Oncology Research Group report of radical surgery vs. radiotherapy for adenocarcinoma of the prostate. Int J Radiat Oncol Biol Phys 1988;14:1053–1054.

9. NIH Consensus Development Conference. Management of clinically localized prostate cancer. Oncology (Huntingt) 1987;1:46–49, 54.

10. D'Amico AV, Whittington R, Malkowicz SB, et al. Biochemical outcome after radical prostatectomy or external beam radiation therapy for patients with clinically localized prostate carcinoma in the prostate specific antigen era. Cancer 2002;95:281–286.

11. Kupelian PA, Elshaikh M, Reddy CA, et al. Comparison of the efficacy of local therapies for localized prostate cancer in the prostate-specific antigen era: a large single-institution experience with radical prostatectomy and external-beam radiotherapy. J Clin Oncol 2002;20:3376–3385.

12. Vicini FA, Martinez A, Hanks G, et al. An interinstitutional and interspecialty comparison of treatment outcome data for patients with prostate carcinoma based on predefined prognostic categories and minimum follow-up. Cancer 2002;95:2126–2135.

13. Morgan WR, Bergstralh EJ, Zincke H. Long-term evaluation of radical prostatectomy as treatment for clinical stage C (T3) prostate cancer. Urology 1993;41:113–120.

14. van den Ouden D, Davidson PJT, Hop W, Schroder FH. Radical prostatectomy as a monotherapy for locally advanced (stage T3) prostate cancer. J Urol 1994;151:646–651.

15. Gerber GS, Thisted RA, Chodak GW, et al. Results of radical prostatectomy in men with locally advanced prostate cancer: multi-institutional pooled analysis. Eur Urol 1997;32:385–390.

16. Zagars GK, von-Eschenbach AC, Johnson DE, et al. Stage C adenocarcinoma of the prostate. An analysis of 551 patients treated with external beam radiation. Cancer 1987;60:1489–1499.

17. Pilepich MV, Krall JM, Sause WT, et al. Prognostic factors in carcinoma of the prostate—analysis of RTOG study 75-06. Int J Radiat Oncol Biol Phys 1987;13:339–349.

18. Hanks GE, Hanlon AL, Hudes G, et al. Patterns-of-failure analysis of patients with high pretreatment prostate-specific antigen levels treated by radiation therapy: the need for improved systemic and locoregional treatment. J Clin Oncol 1996;14:1093–1097.

19. Shipley WU, Thames HD, Sandler HM, et al. Radiation therapy for clinically localized prostate cancer: a multi-institutional pooled analysis. JAMA 1999;281:1598–1604.

20. Hanlon AL, Hanks GE. Failure pattern implications following external beam irradiation of prostate cancer: long-term follow-up and indications of cure. Cancer J 2000;6(Suppl 2):S193–197.

21. Vicini FA, Kestin LL, Martinez AA. The correlation of serial prostate specific antigen measurements with clinical outcome after external beam radiation therapy of patients for prostate carcinoma. Cancer 2000;88:2305–2318.

22. RTOG-EORTC. LENT SOMA Tables: Tables of contents. Radiother Oncol 1995;35:17–60.

23. Duncan W, Warde P, Catton CN, et al. Carcinoma of the prostate: results of radical radiotherapy (1970–1985). Int J Radiat Oncol Biol Phys 1993;26:203–210.

24. Amdur RJ, Parsons JT, Fitzgerald LT, et al. Adenocarcinoma of the prostate treated with external-beam radiation therapy: 5-year minimum follow-up. Radiother Oncol 1990;18:235–246.

25. Mithal NP, Hoskin PJ. External beam radiotherapy for carcinoma of the prostate: a retrospective study. Clin Oncol (R Coll Radiol) 1993;5:297–301.

26. Leibel SA, Hanks GE, Kramer S. Patterns of Care outcome studies: results of the national practice in adenocarcinoma of the prostate. Int J Radiat Oncol Biol Phys 1984;10:401–409.

27. Hanks GE, Diamond JJ, Krall JM, et al. A ten year follow-up of 682 patients treated for prostate cancer with radiation therapy in the United States. Int J Radiat Oncol Biol Phys 1987;13:499–505.

28. Hanks GE. External beam irradiation for clinically localised prostate cancer: Patterns of Care studies in the United States. NCI Monogr 1988;7:75–84.

29. Shipley WU, Zietman AL, Hanks GE, et al. Treatment related sequelae following external beam radiation for prostate cancer: a review with an update in patients with stages T1 and T2 tumor. J Urol 1994;152:1799–1805.

30. Lawton CA, Won M, Pilepich MV, et al. Long-term treatment sequelae following external beam irradiation for adenocarcinoma of the prostate: analysis of RTOG studies 7506 and 7706. Int J Radiat Oncol Biol Phys 1991;21:935–939.

31. Pilepich MV, Asbell SO, Krall JM, et al. Correlation of radiotherapeutic parameters and treatment related morbidity—analysis of RTOG Study 77-06. Int J Radiat Oncol Biol Phys 1987;13:1007–1012.

32. Dewit L, Ang KK, Van der Schueren E. Acute side effects and late complications after radiotherapy of localized carcinoma of the prostate. Cancer Treat Rev 1983;10:79–89.

33. Roach M, Chin DM, Holland J, et al. A pilot study of sexual function and quality of life following 3D conformal radiotherapy for clinically localised prostate cancer. Int J Radiat Oncol Biol Phys 1996;35:869–874.

34. Pilepich MV, Krall JM, al-Sarraf M et al. Androgen deprivation with radiation therapy compared with radiation therapy alone for locally advanced prostatic carcinoma: a randomized comparative trial of the Radiation Therapy Oncology Group. Urology 1995;45:616–623.

35. Potosky AL, Legler J, Albertsen PC, et al. Health outcomes after prostatectomy or radiotherapy for prostate cancer: results from the Prostate Cancer Outcomes Study. J Natl Cancer Inst 2000;92:1582–1592.

36. Horwitz EM, Vicini FA, Ziaja EL, et al. Assessing the variability of outcome for patients treated with localized prostate irradiation using different definitions of biochemical control. Int J Radiat Oncol Biol Phys 1996;36:565–571.

37. Leibel SA, Ling CC, Kutcher GJ, et al. The biological basis for conformal three-dimensional radiation therapy. Int J Radiat Oncol Biol Phys 1991;21:805–811.

38. Fuks Z, Leibel SA, Wallner JE, et al. The effect of local control on metastatic dissemination in carcinoma of the prostate: long term results in patients treated with I-125 implantation. Int J Radiat Oncol Biol Phys 1991;21:537–547.

39. Perez CA, Walz BJ, Zivnuska FR. Irradiation of carcinoma of the prostate localized to the pelvis: Analysis of tumor response and prognosis. Int J Radiat Oncol Biol Phys 1980;6:555–563.

40. Hanks GE, Martz KL, Diamond JJ. The effect of dose on local control of prostate cancer. Int J Radiat Oncol Biol Phys 1988;15:1299–1305.

41. Hanks GE, Krall JM, Martz KL, et al. The outcome of 313 patients with T1 (UICC) prostate cancer treated with external beam irradiation. Int J Radiat Oncol Biol Phys 1988;14:243–248.

42. Smit WGJM, Helle PA, van Putten LJ, Wijnmaalen AJ, et al. Late radiation damage in prostate cancer patients treated by high dose external beam radiotherapy in relation to rectal dose. Int J Radiat Oncol Biol Phys 1990;18:23–29.

43. Goitein M, Wittenberg J, Mendiondo M, et al. The value of CT scanning in radiation therapy treatment planning: A prospective study. Int J Radiat Oncol Biol Phys 1979;5:1787–1798.

44. ICRU-50. International Commission on Radiation Units and Measurements. ICRU Report 50: Prescribing, recording, and reporting photon beam therapy. Bethesda, MD: International Commission on Radiation Units and Measurement 1993, pp 3–16.

45. ICRU-62. International Commission on Radiation Units and Measurements. ICRU Report 62: Prescribing, recording, and reporting photon beam therapy. Bethesda, MD: International Commission on Radiation Units and Measurement 1999, pp 3–20.

46. Khoo VS, Dearnaley DP, Finnigan DJ, et al. Magnetic resonance imaging (MRI): considerations and applications in radiotherapy planning. Radiother Oncol 1997;42:1–15.

47. Sannazzari GL, Ragona R, Ruo Redda MG, et al. CT-MRI image fusion for delineation of volumes in three-dimensional conformal radiation therapy in the treatment of localized prostate cancer. Br J Radiol 2002;75:603–607.

48. Pickett B, Vigneault E, Kurhanewicz J, Verhey L, Roach M. Static field intensity modulation to treat a dominant intra-prostatic lesion to 90 Gy compared to seven field 3-dimensional radiotherapy. Int J Radiat Oncol Biol Phys 1999;44:921–929.

49. Pouliot J, Kim Y, Lessard E, et al. Inverse planning for HDR prostate brachytherapy used to boost dominant intraprostatic lesions defined by magnetic resonance spectroscopy imaging. Int J Radiat Oncol Biol Phys 2004;59:1196–1207.

50. Dearnaley DP, Khoo VS, Norman A, et al. Comparison of radiation side-effects of conformal and conventional radiotherapy in prostate cancer: a randomised trial. Lancet 1999;353:267–272.

51. Bayley AJ, Catton CN, Haycocks T, et al. A randomized trial of supine vs. prone positioning in patients undergoing escalated dose conformal radiotherapy for prostate cancer. Radiother Oncol 2004;70:37–44.

52. Soffen EM, Hanks GE, Hwang CC, et al. Conformal static field therapy for low volume low grade prostate cancer with rigid immobilization. Int J Radiat Oncol Biol Phys 1991;20:141–146.

53. Fiorino C, Reni M, Bolognesi A, et al. Set-up error in supine-positioned patients immobilized with two different modalities during conformal radiotherapy of prostate cancer. Radiother Oncol 1998;49:133–141.

54. Nutting CM, Khoo VS, Walker V, et al. A randomized study of the use of a customized immobilization system in the treatment of prostate cancer with conformal radiotherapy. Radiother Oncol 2000;54:1–9.

55. Padhani AR, Khoo VS, Suckling J, et al. Evaluating the effect of rectal distension and movement on prostate gland position using cine MRI. Int J Radiat Oncol Biol Phys 1999;44:525–533.

56. D'Amico AV, Manola J, Loffredo M, et al. A practical method to achieve prostate gland immobilization and target verification for daily treatment. Int J Radiat Oncol Biol Phys 2001;51:1431–1436.

57. Wachter S, Gerstner N, Dorner D, et al. The influence of a rectal balloon tube as internal immobilization device on variations of volumes and dose–volume histograms during treatment course of conformal radiotherapy for prostate cancer. Int J Radiat Oncol Biol Phys 2002;52:91–100.

58. Fransson P, Bergstrom P, Lofroth PO, et al. Daily-diary evaluated side effects of dose-escalation radiotherapy of prostate cancer using the stereotactic BeamCath technique. Acta Oncol 2003;42:326–333.

59. Khoo VS, Padhani AR, Tanner SF, et al. Comparison of MRI sequences with CT for the radiotherapy planning of prostate cancer: a feasibility study. Br J Radiol 1999;72:590–597.

60. Ohori M, Scardino PT, Lapin SL, et al. The mechanisms and prognostic significance of seminal vesicle involvement by prostate cancer. Am J Surg Pathol 1993;17:1252–1261.

61. Kestin L, Goldstein N, Vicini F, et al. Treatment of prostate cancer with radiotherapy: should the entire seminal vesicles be included in the clinical target volume? Int J Radiat Oncol Biol Phys 2002;54:686–697.

62. Golimbu M, Morales P, Al-Askari S, et al. Extended pelvic lymphadenectomy for prostatic cancer. J Urol 1979;121:617–620.

63. Heidenreich A, Varga Z, Von Knobloch R. Extended pelvic lymphadenectomy in patients undergoing radical prostatectomy: high incidence of lymph node metastasis. J Urol 2002;167:1681–1686.

64. Khoo VS, Bedford JL, Webb S, et al. Comparison of 2D and 3D algorithms for adding a margin to the gross tumor volume in the conformal radiotherapy planning of prostate cancer. Int J Radiat Oncol Biol Phys 1998;42:673–679.

65. Khoo VS, Bedford JL, Webb S, et al. Class solutions for conformal external beam prostate radiotherapy. Int J Radiat Oncol Biol Phys 2003;55:1109–1120.

66. Rowbottom CG, Khoo VS, Webb S. Simultaneous optimization of beam orientations and beam weights in conformal radiotherapy. Med Phys 2001;28:1696–1702.

67. Bedford J, Henrys A, Dearnaley D, et al. Treatment planning evaluation of non-coplanar techniques for conformal radiotherapy of the prostate. Radiother Oncol 2005; 75:287–292.

68. De Meerleer GO, Vakaet LA, De Gersem WR, et al. Radiotherapy of prostate cancer with or without intensity modulated beams: a planning comparison. Int J Radiat Oncol Biol Phys 2000;47:639–648.

69. Fiorino C, Broggi S, Corletto D, et al. Conformal irradiation of concave-shaped PTVs in the treatment of prostate cancer by simple 1D intensity-modulated beams. Radiother Oncol 2000;55:49–58.

70. Bos LJ, Damen EM, de Boer RW, et al. Reduction of rectal dose by integration of the boost in the large-field treatment plan for prostate irradiation. Int J Radiat Oncol Biol Phys 2002;52:254–265.

71. Nutting CM, Convery DJ, Cosgrove VP, et al. Reduction of small and large bowel irradiation using an optimized intensity-modulated pelvic radiotherapy technique in patients with prostate cancer. Int J Radiat Oncol Biol Phys 2000;48:649–656.

72. Benk VA, Adams JA, Shipley WU, et al. Late rectal bleeding following combined x-ray and proton high dose irradiation for patients with stages T3-T4 prostate carcinoma. Int J Radiat Oncol Biol Phys 1993;26:551–7.

73. Lu Y, Song PY, Li SD, et al. A method of analyzing rectal surface area irradiated and rectal complications in prostate conformal radiotherapy. Int J Radiat Oncol Biol Phys 1995;33:1121–1125.

74. Boersma LJ, van den Brink M, Bruce AM, et al. Estimation of the incidence of late bladder and rectum complications after high-dose (70–78 Gy) conformal radiotherapy for prostate cancer, using dose–volume histograms. Int J Radiat Oncol Biol Phys 1998;41:83–92.

75. Storey MR, Pollack A, Zagars G, et al. Complications from radiotherapy dose escalation in prostate cancer: preliminary results of a randomized trial. Int J Radiat Oncol Biol Phys 2000;48:635–642.

76. Jackson A, Skwarchuk MW, Zelefsky MJ, et al. Late rectal bleeding after conformal radiotherapy of prostate cancer. II. Volume effects and dose–volume histograms. Int J Radiat Oncol Biol Phys 2001;49:685–698.

77. Wachter S, Gerstner N, Goldner G, et al. Rectal sequelae after conformal radiotherapy of prostate cancer: dose–volume histograms as predictive factors. Radiother Oncol 2001;59:65–70.

78. Fiorino C, Cozzarini C, Vavassori V, et al. Relationships between DVHs and late rectal bleeding after radiotherapy for prostate cancer: analysis of a large group of patients pooled from three institutions. Radiother Oncol 2002;64:1–12.

79. Fiorino C, Sanguineti G, Cozzarini C, et al. Rectal dose–volume constraints in high-dose radiotherapy of localized prostate cancer. Int J Radiat Oncol Biol Phys 2003;57:953–962.

80. Pollack A, Zagars GK, Starkschall G, et al. Prostate cancer radiation dose response: results of the M. D. Anderson phase III randomized trial. Int J Radiat Oncol Biol Phys 2002;53:1097–1105.

81. Gallagher MJ, Brereton HD, Rostock RA, et al. A prospective study of treatment techniques to minimize the volume of pelvic small bowel with reduction of acute and late effects associated with pelvic irradiation. Int J Radiat Oncol Biol Phys 1986;12:1565–1573.

82. Marks LB, Carroll PR, Dugan TC, et al. The response of the urinary bladder, urethra, and ureter to radiation and chemotherapy. Int J Radiat Oncol Biol Phys 1995;31:1257–1280.

83. Emami B, Lyman J, Brown A, et al. Tolerance of normal tissue to therapeutic radiation. Int J Radiat Oncol Biol Phys 1991;21:109–122.

84. Gildersleve J, Dearnaley DP, Evans PM, et al. Reproducibility of patient positioning during routine radiotherapy, as assessed by an integrated megavoltage imaging system. Radiother Oncol 1995;35:151–160.

85. Dearnaley DP, Khoo VS, Norman AR, et al. Comparison of radiation side-effects of conformal and conventional radiotherapy in prostate cancer: a randomised trial. Lancet 1999;353:267–272.

86. Williams MV, Denekamp J, Fowler JF. Dose response relationships for human tumours: implications for clinical trials of dose modifying agents. Int J Radiat Oncol Biol Phys 1984;10:1703–1707.

87. Thames HD, Schultheiss TE, Hendry JH, et al. Can modest escalations of dose be detected as increased tumor control? Int J Radiat Oncol Biol Phys 1992;22:241–246.

88. Hanks GE, Krall JM, Hanlon AL, et al. Patterns of Care and RTOG studies in prostate cancer: long-term survival, hazard rate observations, and possibilities of cure. Int J Radiat Oncol Biol Phys 1994;28:39–45.

89. Fiveash JB, Hanks G, Roach M, et al. 3D conformal radiation therapy (3DCRT) for high grade prostate cancer: a multi-institutional review. Int J Radiat Oncol Biol Phys 2000;47:335–342.

90. Zelefsky MJ, Leibel SA, Gaudin PB, et al. Dose escalation with three-dimensional conformal radiation therapy affects the outcome in prostate cancer. Int J Radiat Oncol Biol Phys 1998;41:491–500.

91. Valicenti R, Lu J, Pilepich M, et al. Survival advantage from higher-dose radiation therapy for clinically localized prostate cancer treated on the Radiation Therapy Oncology Group trials. J Clin Oncol 2000;18:2740–2746.

92. D'Amico AV, Chen MH, Oh-Ung J, et al. Changing prostate-specific antigen outcome after surgery or radiotherapy for localized prostate cancer during the prostate-specific antigen era. Int J Radiat Oncol Biol Phys 2002;54:436–441.

93. Dearnaley DP, Hall E, Lawrence D, et al. Phase III pilot study of dose escalation using conformal radiotherapy in prostate cancer: PSA control and side effects. Br J Cancer 2005;92:488–498.

94. Seddon B, Bidmead M, Wilson J, et al. Target volume definition in conformal radiotherapy for prostate cancer: Quality assurance in the MRC RT-01 trial. Radiother Oncol 2000;56:73–83.

95. Sydes MR, Stephens RJ, Moore AR, et al. Implementing the UK Medical Research Council (MRC) RT01 trial (ISRCTN 47772397): methods and practicalities of a randomised controlled trial of conformal radiotherapy in men with localised prostate cancer. Radiother Oncol 2004;72:199–211.

96. Lebesque J, Koper P, Slot A, Tabak H, et al. Acute and late GI and GU toxicity after prostate irradiation to doses of 68 Gy and 78 Gy: results of a randomized trial. Int J Radiat Oncol Biol Phys 2003;57:S152.

97. Beckendorf V, Bachaud JM, Bey P, et al. [Target–volume and critical-organ delineation for conformal radiotherapy of prostate cancer: experience of French dose-escalation trials]. Cancer Radiother 2002;6(Suppl 1):78s–92s.

98. Staffurth J, Dearnaley D, McNair H, et al. Early results of a phase 2 trial of pelvic nodal irradiation in prostate cancer IMRT. Clin Oncol 2003;15:S17.

99. Zelefsky MJ, Fuks Z, Hunt M, et al. High-dose intensity modulated radiation therapy for prostate cancer: early toxicity and biochemical outcome in 772 patients. Int J Radiat Oncol Biol Phys 2002;53:1111–1116.

100. Brenner DJ, Hall EJ. Fractionation and protraction for radiotherapy of prostate carcinoma. Int J Radiat Oncol Biol Phys 1999;43:1095–1101.

101. Fowler J, Chappell R, Ritter M. Is alpha/beta for prostate tumors really low? Int J Radiat Oncol Biol Phys 2001;50:1021–1031.

102. Haustermans KM, Hofland I, Van Poppel H, et al. Cell kinetic measurements in prostate cancer. Int J Radiat Oncol Biol Phys 1997;37:1067–1070.

103. Rew DA, Wilson GD. Cell production rates in human tissues and tumours and their significance. Part II: clinical data. Eur J Surg Oncol 2000;26:405–417.

104. Yeoh EE, Fraser RJ, McGowan RE, et al. Evidence for efficacy without increased toxicity of hypofractionated radiotherapy for prostate carcinoma: early results of a Phase III randomized trial. Int J Radiat Oncol Biol Phys 2003;55:943–955.

105. Lukka H, Hayter C, Warde P, et al. A randomized trial comparing two fractionation schedules for patients with localized prostate cancer. Int J Radiat Oncol Biol Phys 2003;57:S126.

106. Cheung R, Tucker SL, Dong L, et al. Dose–response for biochemical control among high-risk prostate cancer patients after external beam radiotherapy. Int J Radiat Oncol Biol Phys 2003;56:1234–1240.

107. Livsey JE, Cowan RA, Wylie JP, et al. Hypofractionated conformal radiotherapy in carcinoma of the prostate: five-year outcome analysis. Int J Radiat Oncol Biol Phys 2003;57:1254–1259.

108. Nahum AE, Movsas B, Horwitz EM, et al. Incorporating clinical measurements of hypoxia into tumor local control modeling of prostate cancer: implications for the alpha/beta ratio. Int J Radiat Oncol Biol Phys 2003;57:391–401.

109. Djemil T, Reddy CA, Willoughby TR, et al. Hypofractionated Intensity-Modulated Radiotherapy (70 Gy at 2.5 Gy per fraction) for localized prostate cancer. Int J Radiat Oncol Biol Phys 2003;57:S275–276.

110. Bergstrom P, Lofroth PO, Widmark A. High-precision conformal radiotherapy (HPCRT) of prostate cancer—a new technique for exact positioning of the prostate at the time of treatment. Int J Radiat Oncol Biol Phys 1998;42:305–311.

111. Shimizu S, Shirato H, Kitamura K, et al. Use of an implanted marker and real-time tracking of the marker for the positioning of prostate and bladder cancers. Int J Radiat Oncol Biol Phys 2000;48:1591–1597.

112. King CR, Lehmann J, Adler JR, Hai J. CyberKnife radiotherapy for localized prostate cancer: rationale and technical feasibility. Technol Cancer Res Treat 2003;2:25–30.

113. Perez CA, Pilepich MV, Garcia D, et al. Definitive radiation therapy in carcinoma of the prostate localized to the pelvis: experience at the Mallinckrodt Institute of Radiology. NCI Monogr 1988;7:85–94.

114. Goffinet DR, Bagshaw MA. Radiation therapy of prostate carcinoma: thirty year experience at Stanford University. In Schroder FH (ed): EORTC Genitourinary Group Monograph 8: Treatment of Prostate Cancer—Facts and Controversies. New York: Wiley–Liss, 1990, pp 209–222.

115. Shirato H, Shimizu S, Kitamura K, et al. Four-dimensional treatment planning and fluoroscopic real-time tumor tracking radiotherapy for moving tumor. Int J Radiation Oncol Biol Phys 2000;48:435–442.

Brachytherapy for the treatment of prostate cancer

82

Jamie A Cesaretti, Nelson N Stone, Johnny Kao, Richard G Stock

INTRODUCTION

In its modern form, transperineal brachytherapy using computer-based dosimetry is capable of both curing prostate cancer and decreasing the morbidity long associated with all definitive prostate cancer treatments.[1] The application of trans-rectal ultrasound guided transperineal technique using a two-dimensional (2D) probe, first reported by Holm in 1983, heralded the era of modern image-guided prostate brachytherapy.[2] Since that time, the implant technique has evolved to its present form, allowing the brachytherapist to visualize the dose distribution in real time while radioactive sources are placed, resulting in tumoricidal doses within the prostate and minimizing radiation dose to uninvolved normal anatomy. In addition to precise source placement, brachytherapy fully utilizes the innate advantage of radiation therapy in cancer treatment by allowing for preservation of normal anatomy and functional relationships in order to preserve physiologically complex functions such as orgasm, urination and ejaculation.[3]

The application of intraoperative radiation dosimetry allows the physician to directly visualize the dosing consequences of each seed placement. These innovations allow the prostate implant to become an interactive process reliant on the combined input of the multidisciplinary care team as the procedure progresses in the surgical suite.[4]

HISTORICAL CONTRIBUTIONS

Shortly after the discovery of radium by Marie Curie in 1898, Alexander Graham Bell suggested that inserting radioactive sources directly into a tumor might be a highly effective approach to cancer therapy.[5] The use of radioactive sources to treat patients with prostate cancer was pioneered early in the 20th century by such luminaries as Hugh Hampton Young at Johns Hopkins School of Medicine and Benjamin Stockwell Barringer at the Memorial Hospital in New York City.[6] These practitioners beginning with Young's acquisition of the then extremely valuable 102 mCi of refined radium, and the development of gold-encapsulated harvested radon seeds by the Memorial Hospital physicist Giocchino Failla, carried out numerous innovative brachytherapy applications over the following decades. Several of the concepts of therapeutic radiation usage have been consistently applied since its inception. In a paper in JAMA from 1917, Young revealed a prescient appreciation of normal tissue toxicity by noting the location, date, and dose of each treatment he delivered to the patient. He was careful to not repeat transrectal radiation treatments to the same position on the rectal mucosa, and used a technique that allowed the entire prostate to be treated over a period of several days. The combinations of several different treatments were intended to add to adequate treatment of the whole prostate[7] (Figure 82.1).

In the 1970s Whitmore et al developed retropubic iodine-125 (^{125}I) radioactive seed implantation at the time of laparotomy.[8] The placement of seeds was performed freehand and was not image guided resulting in significant underdosed areas. Long-term disease control was disappointing, particularly for patients with poor dosimetry.[9] Advances in imaging—notably 2D transrectal ultrasound, computed tomography (CT)-based post-implant dosimetry and, more recently, magnetic resonance imaging (MRI) using an endorectal coil—have contributed significantly to higher quality since the mid-1980s.

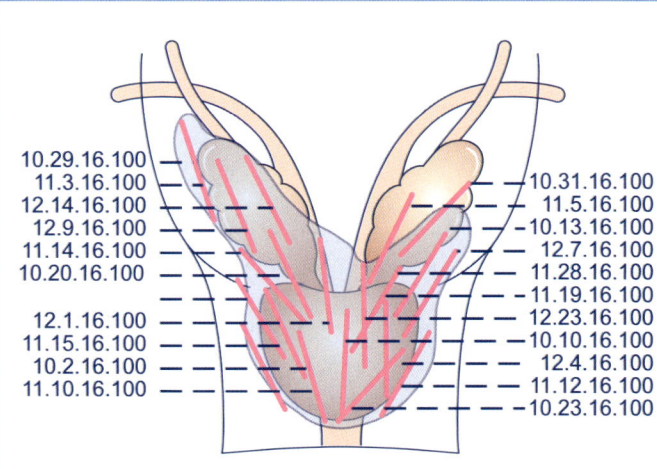

10.29.16.100
11.3.16.100
12.14.16.100
12.9.16.100
11.14.16.100
10.20.16.100

12.1.16.100
11.15.16.100
10.2.16.100
11.10.16.100

10.31.16.100
11.5.16.100
10.13.16.100
12.7.16.100
11.28.16.100
11.19.16.100
12.23.16.100
10.10.16.100
12.4.16.100
11.12.16.100
10.23.16.100

Fig. 82.1

An example of an early understanding of dose-volume and time relationships in the application of brachytherapy by Hugh Hampton Young, MD. Young used a single radium source to apply multiple treatments over several months. The dwell time of the application and the date of the treatment are noted relative to this patient's locally advanced prostate cancer (in the public domain).

From Young HH. The use of radium in cancer of the prostate and bladder: A presentation of new instruments and new methods of use. JAMA 1917;68:1174–1177.

PHYSICS OF BRACHYTHERAPY

Radioactive sources obey physical laws, several of which are useful for the practicing urologist to fully understand. The isotopes commonly used in therapy are manmade radioactive elements, which decay at a constant rate. The isotopes chosen to treat prostate cancer emit gamma ray energy. A gamma ray has no mass, travels at the speed of light, and can display both the properties of a wave or a particle. The energy spectra of the gamma rays emitted by the isotopes used in brachytherapy are well characterized. Of particular relevance to the brachytherapist is that the dose falloff from a radioactive source obeys the inverse square law, that is it is proportional to $1/r^2$, where r is the distance from the source. In general, high-energy gamma ray sources are used for temporary implants or high dose rate (HDR) applications and low-energy sources are used for low dose rate (LDR) permanent implants. The modern treatment planning systems used by radiation oncologists are programmed to obey these physical rules as they assist in determining optimal source placement.

IODINE-125

Iodine-125 has a physical half-life of 59.4 days and relatively low photon energy of 0.028 MeV. The implications of this are that the sources require less lead shielding to protect the operating room staff and that the actual physical geometry of the seed and its encasement significantly influence the dosimetry characteristics of the source. As the field continues to progress, new isotopes may prove to be useful, in addition to novel seed architecture.[10] The model 6711 seed (Oncura, Amersham, Buckinghamshire, England) is in common usage throughout the United States; the encapsulation consists of a 0.05-mm thick titanium tube welded at both ends forming a cylinder-like seed; the seed is 4.5 mm in length and 0.8 mm in diameter. A silver wire is at the center of the seed, making it readily identifiable during post-implant fluoroscopy. The initial dose rate of ^{125}I is lower than palladium-103 (^{103}P), but due to its longer half-life, the dose is given over a longer period of time. Clinical differences between ^{103}P and ^{125}I in terms of outcome and symptom spectrum are minimal.[11]

PALLADIUM-103

Palladium-103 has a physical half-life that is 17 days and photon energy of 0.021 MeV. In terms of shielding, 0.008 mm of lead thickness is required to reduce the amount of radiation emitted by 50% compared with 0.025 mm of lead for ^{125}I. ^{103}Pd has a much shorter half-life than ^{125}I, therefore, the initial dose rate of ^{103}Pd (20 cGy/h) must be higher than that for ^{125}I (7 cGy/h) in order for them to give approximately similar doses. In addition, the amount of radioactivity per seed must be more with ^{103}Pd than ^{125}I at the time of implant in order for the radiotherapist to be able to proscribe roughly similar levels of absorbed dose. It is important to also understand that there are significant variations in brachytherapy practice; some centers prefer to use fewer sources with a higher activity per seed, while others prefer to use a greater number of low energy sources to achieve the optimal absorbed dose. However, in most cases the total amount of activity prescribed, in mCi, is quite consistent for most centers.[12]

IRIDIUM-192

Iridium-192 (^{192}Ir) has a physical half-life of 73.8 days, which is much longer than ^{103}Pd and on par with ^{125}I. The important physical feature of ^{192}Ir is its relatively high gamma energy, which is much higher than the LDR isotopes at 0.38 MeV. The ^{192}Ir source is used for fractionated HDR brachytherapy by using temporary indwelling catheters. The ^{192}Ir source requires much more shielding in order to protect the operative staff—it requires over a centimeter of lead to decrease the transmitted dose by 96.9% of the source intensity. ^{192}Ir has become the preferred source for HDR temporary implants.[13] A potential advantage for HDR is improved dose distributions due to the ability to vary dwell times of radioactive sources.[14] A major disadvantage of the HDR technique is the need for inpatient hospitalization for the duration of the implant.

RADIOBIOLOGY

The characterization of the radiation sensitivity of cancer and human normal tissues has a long history from which many of the fundamental concepts of modern cancer biology have evolved. Fundamentally, the target of radiation in the cancer cell is DNA, resulting in potentially lethal double strand breaks. A complex cellular pathway is mobilized in order to maintain genomic integrity by repairing DNA lesions.[15] These DNA repair processes are able to successfully repair most types of DNA damage within a few hours. Unrepaired DNA double strand breaks will result in cell death.[16] The four major differences between the way cancer cells and normal cells respond to radiation are repair, reassortment, reoxygenation, and repopulation. Cancer cells are usually more sensitive than normal cells because they are less proficient at repairing DNA damage, are more likely to become synchronized in radiosensitive phases of the cell cycle, and become reoxygenated during the course of radiation therapy. Since the proliferative rate of prostate cancers are relatively slow, repopulation, the regrowth of tumor cells during a course of radiation, is considered a minor issue for prostate cancer. However, some clinicians choose to employ ^{103}Pd, with its higher initial dose rate, rather than ^{125}I to treat high grade tumors.[16,84]

Based on significant scientific and empirical evidence, the optimal approach to external beam radiation therapy (EBRT) has been to treat most cancers with standard fractions of radiation, 1.8 to 2 Gy, 5 days per week over several weeks. The alpha/beta model attempts to predict the effect of various dose-fractionation schemes on tumor and late toxicity. Most tumor cells and early reacting normal tissues (lymphocytes, gastrointestinal epithelium) have a high alpha/beta ratio (>10) whereas many types of late reacting normal tissues (skin, bone, bladder) have low alpha/beta ratios.[2-3] This model predicts that repeated small doses of radiation delivers a biologically more effective dose to tumor cells while allowing normal tissues to recover. There is some evidence that indicates that the alpha/beta ratio for prostate cancer cells may be very low, on the order of 1.5 to 2.[19] The implication of this finding is that

long courses of fractionated radiotherapy or permanent seed implantation may not be the best treatment strategy for men with prostate cancer. Several radiobiologists have made a persuasive case to treat prostate cancer with very large doses of radiation per fraction over a short time period.[20,21] This concept provides the radiobiologic rationale for the recent interest in HDR brachytherapy.[22]

It is important to note that not all radiation oncologists and radiation biologists agree about the alpha/beta ratio for prostate cancer, and its implications.[23] The most important counterargument to the widespread adaptation of HDR is the considerable clinical success obtained using both LDR brachytherapy and dose escalation with EBRT using standard radiation fraction sizes realized over the past decade.[24-26] Additionally, it is not known whether HDR will result in greater late toxicity than permanent seed implant, as predicted by the alpha/beta model. To date, follow up is too short to assess the rate of late toxicity in patients treated by HDR.[22,27]

TREATMENT PLANNING

Brachytherapy treatment planning is an anatomy-based concept that is entirely dependent upon properly measuring distance and volume relationships within and beyond the prostate gland. The placement of needles through a template into the prostate gland under ultrasound guidance, allows for markedly increased accuracy of seed placement compared with the obsolete retropubic freehand technique and has become the standard of care for brachytherapy.[14] Because the prostate gland has a characteristic barrel type shape, it is amenable to several different dosimetric solutions in terms of how to place radioactive sources to cover the volume.

Historically, brachytherapy planning was significantly influenced by two schools of thought, which evolved prior to the era of the modern computational power and 3D imaging. The Patterson–Parker method refers to a set of rules and tables developed in the 1940s in Manchester, UK.[28] The goal of the brachytherapy implant rules was to limit dose inhomogeneity within the implanted volume while treating the volume with a tumoricidal dose. In brief, the method places radioactive sources non-uniformly in order to achieve a uniform dose distribution. In terms of spherical shapes, such as an idealized prostate, this meant that most of the total activity of an implant was placed on the outer edges of the implanted volume. A competing system of interstitial implantation developed in the US was called the Quimby system. This system was characterized by placing all of the radioactive sources uniformly throughout the implanted structure. In general, this implant technique resulted in a non-uniform dose distribution with very high central region doses. However, with this geometry the risk of encountering an underdosed region or "cold spot" due to seed migration is low.

Modern brachytherapy treatment planning systems allow for preoperative images from either ultrasound or CT to be captured and manipulated as 3D objects. The current planning system known as the computer system calculates 3D doses to the implanted volume. However, our current philosophy of implanting 75% to 80% of the activity in the peripheral needles and 20% to 25% of the activity in the interior needles is reminiscent of the Patterson–Parker philosophy. When pursuing a preplanned strategy, details such as hip and leg position become very important in order to assure that, at the time of implant, the plan generated by the physicist can be successfully produced at the time of implant. This method has been well described and is widely used in the US.[29] Using the preplanned approach, seeds may be implanted by either preloaded needles or the Mick applicator.[14]

Another solution is to use intraoperative images captured at the time of implant to plan the procedure in real time.[4] This method also allows the operator to account for variations in patient set-up, intra- and interoperative prostate gland movement, and prostate swelling secondary to the trauma caused by needle placement. The seeds can be placed in the gland using the Mick applicator (Mick TP-200, Mick Radionuclear Instruments. Mount Vernon, NY), under the guidance of the biplanar transrectal ultrasound probe.[30] As the procedure progresses, the treating team can determine optimal placement of seeds in order to cover the prostate gland, and avoid the urethra and rectum[4] (Figure 82.2).

DOSING AND CONSTRAINTS

In radiation oncology the concept of radiation dosing and dose constraints are of fundamental importance to successful and optimal treatment. From a modern perspective when using 3D planning the dose of radiation can be defined for the entire 3D structure. Modern treatment planning systems require the user to delineate, by outlining, structures of interest on a computer screen. In prostate cancer treatment, these structures include the prostate, urethra, bladder wall, and rectal wall. The dose to these structures can be quantified and analyzed in a number of different ways that emphasize important concepts in radiation oncology: low-dose regions or "cold spots" may lead to tumor relapse, while high-dose regions or "hot spots" in normal tissues may result in late complications.

Dose using the Standard International (SI) unit Gray (Gy, equivalent to 100 rads) can be expressed in terms of a percentage of the volume of interest. For example, D90 for the prostate is the minimum dose received by at least 90% of the prostate gland. When a typical D90 is 144 Gy, the D100 (or dose to 100% of the prostate gland) for the implant could be markedly less—on the order of 80 to 100 Gy. The reason that the D90 is often chosen as a reference value is that it is representative of the quality of the implant; also clinical correlation has been made in terms of a dose-response relationship by several investigators.[31] If one were to prescribe a dose of 144 Gy to the D95 or D100; the D90 in such an implant would be significantly hotter than 144 Gy. Such an approach has the potential of allowing concern over dose to a relatively small portion of the gland drive up the dose to the entire gland. If one were to automate such an approach using a dose

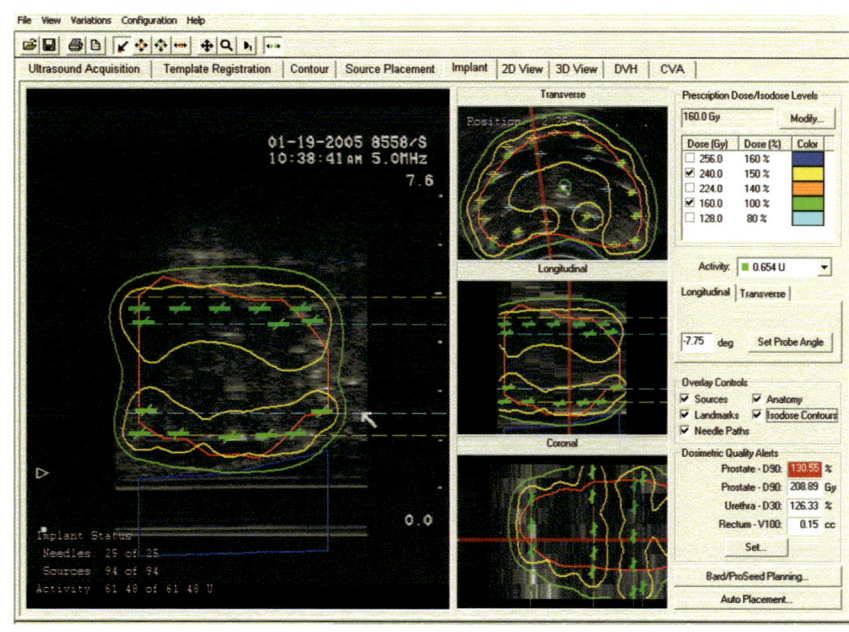

Fig. 82.2

Sagittal image of prostate and rectum encompassed by prescription dose. Seed placement (hashed rectangles) is continually modified throughout the case in order to conform prescription dose and limit high-dose regions (interior isodose clouds).

constraint prescribing 144 Gy to the D100, the D90 could be as high as 240 to 280 Gy. It is also important to pay special attention to the 10% not accounted for in the D90 dosing parameter. This is done by looking at each 2D slice of a prostate implant while it is being completed. If the 90% dosing line dips into the prostate where there is a known cancerous nodule then that part of the cancer will be underdosed even though the D90 might be within an acceptable range. Therefore, successful brachytherapy requires not only thoughtful consideration by the therapeutic physics staff; but also active participation by the brachytherapist with special attention given to such details.

Determination of the volume of normal tissue receiving the prescription dose is a useful way to quantify the effects of radiation toxicity. If we know that a patient is at a much higher risk of radiation proctitis when more than 2 cm^3 is exposed to the prescription dose, then this information can be incorporated into a treatment planning system and used as a dose constraint. For normal tissues, quantifying dose constraints in terms of tissue volume is advantageous relative to quantification in terms of percentage of a volume because a significant portion of any given volume can be at no or very little risk of being exposed to radiation from brachytherapy. The bladder and the rectum are good examples of tissues that are better analyzed in terms of radiation late effects based upon the amount of tissue in each cubic centimeter receiving the prescription dose; the posterior rectum and the superior bladder should not be included in dosing considerations because they receive minimal radiation doses after implant (unless of course the patient is also receiving EBRT). In contrast, the external radiation beam must traverse normal tissues to reach the prostate.

The V100 refers to the volume of a structure in percent receiving the prescription dose. For example, if the prescription dose for an ^{125}I implant is 144 Gy, and the post-implant dosimetry study shows that the entire prostate received 144 Gy, the V100 would be 100%. A common use for V is to help the brachytherapist determine the extent of the intraprostatic hot spots of an implant. If the V150 (the volume of the prostate receiving 150% of the prescription dose) is equal to 80% and the prescription dose was 144 Gy, then the majority of the gland would be covered by 216 Gy, putting the patient at considerable risk for urinary morbidity.[30,32] If the V150 of an implant was 40% and the D90 160 Gy, this would be an optimal use of brachytherapy sources, the brachytherapist, or the planning module, would have had significant success in decreasing the intraprostatic doses and still covering the entire gland with the target dose.

PATIENT SELECTION

There are several strategies one can use to decide which patients are best suited for prostate brachytherapy. Most clinicians recognize that the long-term cure rate is favorable with early stage prostate cancer regardless of the treatment strategy employed, and the selection of therapy often must be made based on expected toxicity profile and patient preferences.[33] Advice given to patients is often variable and usually represents components from the extremes of therapeutic philosophies.[34] The patients often welcome a frank discussion of tailored risks associated with the brachytherapy procedure. Certain clinical situations might require additional discussions, for example in patients with prior transurethral resection of the prostate (TURP) where there may be an increased risk of urinary toxicity and concerns of poor implant quality.[35,36] Other risks, including proctitis, incontinence, and erectile dysfunction are discussed, with a focus on our own institutional results.

Patients who present with localized prostate cancer may have a spectrum of diseases. Low-, moderate-, and high-risk prostate cancer should be recognized as different diseases that require different approaches. A patient with low-risk prostate cancer—defined as a prostate-specific antigen (PSA) of 10 ng/mL or less, a Gleason score of 6 or less, and clinical stage T2a or less—will do well with radical prostatectomy or brachytherapy. These patients have a high likelihood that disease is confined to the prostate.[37] Radical prostatectomy is not a cancer operation in which wide surgical margins are easily achieved, therefore, patients at risk for extracapsular disease are often not cured by a prostatectomy. A similar situation exists for brachytherapy. Due to the inverse square2 law, the radioactivity travels only a short distance from the sources. While brachytherapy adequately treats minimal (<3 mm) extracapsular extension typically seen in modern prostatectomy series, a seed implant in a high-risk patient is not likely to achieve an adequate peripheral radiation dose in a patient with significant extracapsular extension.[38] Thus, the ideal patient for brachytherapy monotherapy is the same as for radical prostatectomy.

Patients who present with more advanced features will require additional therapy if implantation is elected. Further work-up is required before the selection of therapy is made. Patients who present with a Gleason score of 7 or higher, or PSA above 10 ng/mL, or clinical stage greater than T2b should have a seminal vesicle biopsy to exclude extraprostatic extension to this area. Several investigators have shown that this biopsy can identify patients with disease in the seminal vesicles. Linzer et al compared a cohort of radical prostatectomy patients with those undergoing seminal vesicle biopsy.[39] In six biopsies performed of the seminal vesicle, no difference was found between these patients and the radical prostatectomy group in likelihood of positive biopsies. The chance of finding extension to the seminal vesicles was at least 20% in men with these high-risk features.

Physicians and patients who are considering brachytherapy as a treatment option do not often think about the indications for a pelvic lymph node dissection, because brachytherapy is considered a minor outpatient procedure, whereas the node dissection can have much more morbidity. High-risk patients, however, can be considered candidates for brachytherapy combined with either hormonal therapy or EBRT or both. Such patients may benefit from having the pelvic lymph nodes analyzed. Lymph node dissection can be limited to those patients with a positive seminal vesicle biopsy (33% positive) or with perineural invasion found in the biopsy specimen (27%). If the seminal vesicle biopsy is negative and the prostate biopsy specimen is free of perineural invasion, fewer than 2% will have nodal metastases.[40] An advantage of this approach is to obviate the need for nodal irradiation in patients with high-risk disease.[37,40]

In addition to disease-related selection criteria, other factors can influence the decision to offer brachytherapy. Many so-called inclusion or exclusion criteria were developed when the limitations of preplanning did not afford the flexibility of real-time planning to overcome certain technical problems, most often those related to patient anatomy. Prostate size was often limited to 50 cm³ or less because of the fear of pubic arch interference. Stone, however, has shown that patients with prostate volumes greater than 50 cm³ can have excellent results from implants when the real-time method is used.[41] Patients with prior TURP were also considered inappropriate candidates for brachytherapy because of the high risk of incontinence.[42] This complication is rare even in a patient with a prior TURP if a peripheral seed distribution is used and accurate urethral imaging guides seed deposition no closer than 5 mm to the urethra.[41] Some mistakenly call this method urethral-sparing and speculate that it is risky to place lower doses around the urethra where prostate cancer may exist. Others have likened this technique to cryoablation, where a warming catheter protects the urethra from freezing. In actuality, the urethra typically will still receive a higher dose than the prostate and is only spared the very high doses (>2× prescription dose) typically seen with a uniform seed placement.

HORMONAL THERAPY AND BRACHYTHERAPY

Androgen deprivation (AD) in conjunction with EBRT has gained widespread acceptance, especially in patients with locally advanced prostate cancer.[43–46] Androgen deprivation with brachytherapy has been less well studied, although it has become accepted clinical practice for some indications. Large prostate size is probably the most agreed-upon indication for the use of hormonal therapy. The absolute prostate size for which AD should be advocated, the type of AD to use (luteinizing hormone-releasing hormone [LHRH] agonists alone or in combination with an antiandrogen), or the length of time a patient should remain on AD are not known. Data from several studies seem to indicate that a minimum of 3 months of AD will result in a 30% to 45% volume reduction. Most trials used a combination of LHRH agonists plus an antiandrogen; two trials showed an advantage with the addition of an antiandrogen to the LHRH agonist. Several also showed that patients with larger glands had a greater degree of shrinkage than those with smaller glands. If a recommendation is to be made, patients with a prostate volume greater than 50 cm³ can be considered for a short course of AD to facilitate the implantation and reduce the likelihood of postimplantation voiding difficulties.[47]

More controversy exists concerning the use of AD in patients with locally advanced disease.[48-52] Several well-performed randomized studies with AD and EBRT have demonstrated the advantages of short- and long-term AD in improving both local and systemic disease control.[43-46] In patients receiving either ¹²⁵I or ¹⁰³Pd brachytherapy, Stone has shown a clear advantage in local control when high-risk patients are treated with 6 months of AD. Of 268 men who had biopsy 2 years after implantation, 2% of those receiving AD (n = 96) had a positive biopsy, compared with 16.3% of those treated with implants alone.[53] Lee, et al has demonstrated that only high-risk patients benefit from the addition of AD and that the local control rates for low-risk patients treated by implants alone are no different from for those treated with implants plus AD.[48]

TECHNOLOGY

There are many similarities between EBRT and brachytherapy. Both deliver radiation therapy from X-rays (photons), and both may result in acute and chronic late radiation injuries. While ¹²⁵I and ¹⁰³Pd emit low energy X-rays, modern linear accelerators deliver high energy, penetrating radiation beams (6–18 MV). The most conformal dose distributions are obtained by an inadequate implant because of the physical advantage of the inverse square law. While high-energy radiation beams must traverse normal tissues to treat the target volume, relative rectal and bladder sparing may be achieved by 3-D conformal radiation therapy (3D-CRT) and intensity modulated radiation therapy (IMRT). Doses from EBRT have increased over the last 10 years as treatment-planning systems have become more sophisticated (3D-CRT and IMRT), and dose response studies have shown the need for increased doses with longer follow-up, or in patients with more advanced local disease.[54,55] Treatment planning with EBRT usually includes a generous margin, although margins have been scaled back as doses have increased and setup accuracy has improved with widespread adoption of B-mode abdominal ultrasound, fiducial markers, or rectal balloons. The recommended doses for ^{125}I and [103]Pd are 145 Gy and 124 Gy, respectively. These recommendations came from the American Association of Physicists in Medicine guidelines and are based on physics work relating to the radiobiologic characteristics of these isotopes and constructing a biologic equivalent dose (BED) to that of EBRT.[56]

The best dosing recommendations are those that have been substantiated by clinical investigation. Although ample dosing data are available for EBRT, only a few studies have addressed proper doses for prostate brachytherapy. Stock et al published the first dose response study for ^{125}I implants.[31] One hundred thirty-four men treated with ^{125}I monotherapy and followed for biochemical failure (defined as PSA > 1.0 ng/mL) were analyzed. Computed tomographic scans of the prostate were taken within 1 month of implantation, and dose volume histograms of the prostate were analyzed. Patients who had received a D90 of 140 Gy had a 92% biochemical relapse-free survival rate, compared with 48% who received a dose less than 140 Gy. Potters found similar results in an evaluation of dose and biochemical outcomes using the definition of PSA failure promulgated by the American Society for Therapeutic Radiology and Oncology (ASTRO).[57]

Stone et al also demonstrated the importance of the delivered radiation dose and biopsy results.[53] With ^{125}I brachytherapy, a D90 of at least 160 Gy resulted in less than 5% with a positive biopsy. No patients treated with [103]Pd to a dose of at least 120 Gy had a positive biopsy. Long-term follow up of these patients show that most achieve complete eradication of local disease by 5 years. If the D90 was at least 140 Gy (^{125}I), 97.2% had a negative biopsy, compared with 88.8% if the delivered dose was less.[53]

Computed tomography-based postimplantation dosimetry at approximately 1 month after implantation (to allow for postimplantation edema to subside) is a mandatory component of a high quality implant program.[58,59] Detailed analysis of prostate, urethra, and rectal doses will yield prognostic information for both disease and quality-of-life outcomes. For example, early urinary morbidity (irritative voiding symptoms) is more likely to occur when prostate and urethral doses are high.[60] The risk of radiation proctitis have also been correlated with rectal doses. Snyder et al has shown that if the volume of the rectum irradiated by 160 Gy (^{125}I) is kept below 1.3 cm³, grade 2 radiation proctitis will occur in less than 5% of patients.[61] This information should be used prospectively when planning the implantation to reduce this complication.

TREATMENT RESULTS

Assessment of treatment success following prostate brachytherapy has usually been reported based on a non-rising PSA rather than a nadir value. Most investigators have adopted the ASTRO consensus definition of three consecutive PSA rises to classify a patient as having biochemical failure.[62] Critz et al suggested that a nadir value of 0.1 or 0.2 ng/mL is more appropriate, while other definitions of biochemical failure are currently undergoing evaluation.[63,65] A PSA decline can take as long as 5 years following ^{125}I implantation.[66] During this time, 35% of patients will experience a temporary rise of PSA of at least 0.2 ng/mL followed by sustained biochemical remission.[67] The average time to PSA bounce is 24 months. Grimm has shown that if patients are followed at least 7 years, the PSA nadir and ASTRO definitions yield the same results.[68]

Low-risk patients (PSA ≤ 10 ng/mL, Gleason score <7, and clinical stage ≤ T2a) are the best candidates for brachytherapy monotherapy. Most reports demonstrate prostate-specific antigen failure-free rates between 80 and 95% at 5 years[69,70] (Table 82.1). It should be emphasized that implant quality is strongly correlated to outcome. Several studies have established that biochemical relapse-free survival is highly correlated with implant dose.[31,57] Patients implanted with ^{125}I who received a D90 of at least 140 Gy had a significantly improved rate of disease-free survival over those implanted with a lower dose. Grimm stratified patients based on date of implantation.[26] Patients treated before 1988 had an inferior outcome compared with the more contemporary patients (65% versus 87% free of failure). Although no dosimetry data were available for those earlier patients, implant quality was no doubt inferior.

Emerging MR spectroscopy data from University of California, San Francisco demonstrate that 100% of patients treated by brachytherapy had metabolic resolution of disease compared with an 86% metabolic complete response for high dose (≥72 Gy) EBRT. These radiographic findings translated to lower nadir PSA levels in the brachytherapy group.[71] While these data suggest that a 144 Gy implant is biologically more potent than 72 Gy of EBRT, whether this will translate to a disease control or survival advantage is unknown. Due to limited numbers of events seen in the low-risk patient population, a sizeable randomized trial would be needed to definitively address this question. A randomized trial comparing prostate brachytherapy versus radical prostatectomy, known as the SPIRIT trial, sponsored by the American College of Surgical Oncologists has been closed due to lack of accrual.

Patients presenting with intermediate- or high-risk prostate cancer may also be candidates for permanent prostate brachytherapy, usually in combination with

Table 82.1 Freedom from prostate-specific antigen (PSA) failure among low-risk patients

Author	Patient (#)	Prognostic group (PSA, ng/mL)	Rate (%)	Time (years)	PSA definition of failure (ng/mL)
Stone[107]	146	PSA ≤ 10, Stage ≤ 2b, Gleason ≤ 6	91	10	ASTRO
Blasko[42]	NA	PSA 0–10	78	8	PSA > 1.0
Ragde[97]	98	Stage T1–2		10	PSA > 0.5
D'Amico[49]	123	PSA ≤ 10, Stage ≤ 2a, Gleason ≤ 6	88 (estimate from survival curve)	5	ASTRO
Grado[98]	114	Gleason 2–4	95	5	2 rises > nadir
Dattoli[99]	60	PSA 4.1–10	80	5	PSA > 1.0
Potters[100]	52	PSA ≤ 10, Stage T1–2, Gleason ≤ 6	91	5	ASTRO
Stokes[101]	72	PSA ≤ 10, Gleason ≤ 6, Stage ≤ 2a	76	5	ASTRO or PSA nadir > 1
Zelefsky[73]	146	PSA ≤ 10, Stage ≤ 2b, Gleason ≤ 6	82	5	ASTRO
Critz[102]*	451	PSA 4.1–10	93	5	PSA > 0.2
Beyer[104]	128	PSA 0–4	85	7	ASTRO or PSA > 10 or + biopsy
Lederman[105]*	164	PSA ≤ 20, Stage ≤ 2b, Gleason ≤ 6	88	6	PSA > 1.0
Sharkey[106]	528	PSA ≤ 10 and Gleason < 7	87	6	PSA > 1.5
Kwok[107]	41	PSA ≤ 10, Stage ≤ 2a, Gleason ≤ 6	85	5	ASTRO
Kollmeier[24]	75	PSA ≤ 6, Stage ≤ 2a, Gleason ≤ 6	88 94 (D90 >144)	8 8	ASTRO ASTRO
Wallner[108]	57 58	PSA 4–10, Stage ≤ 2a, Gleason ≤ 6	89(^{125}I) 91(^{103}Pd)	3 3	PSA > 0.5

*Indicates treatment with adjuvant EBRT.

ASTRO, definition of PSA failure promulgated by the American Society for Therapeutic Radiology and Oncology.

EBRT and/or hormonal therapy. This issue is still controversial, suggesting the need for randomized studies to determine the optimal regimen. In a widely quoted retrospective comparison of three selected databases, D'Amico et al reported inferior PSA control for patients treated with brachytherapy ± hormonal therapy compared with surgery or EBRT for intermediate- and high-risk patients.[72] Lack of dosimetric data, use of orthogonal films rather than CT for postimplant dosimetry, and a limited experience in implant technique contributed to the unusually poor results in the brachytherapy arm. In stark contrast, experienced brachytherapy teams from Mount Sinai, Seattle Prostate Cancer Center, and Memorial Sloan Kettering Cancer Center have reported results comparable or superior to surgery or definitive EBRT for intermediate- and high-risk patients.[48,69,73] Nonetheless, there has been significant interest in adding EBRT and/or hormonal therapy to interstitial brachytherapy with the goal of further improving outcomes in patients with intermediate- and high-risk disease by addressing regional and/or micrometastatic disease. Lee et al has demonstrated 94% biochemical control in men with intermediate-risk prostate cancer treated with either ^{125}I

or ^{103}Pd with 6 months of hormonal therapy and also receiving a high-dose implant (>140 Gy for ^{125}I and >100 Gy for ^{103}Pd).[48] For patients with high-risk disease, Stock reported 86% biochemical control at 5 years for patients treated by androgen ablation (9 months), brachytherapy, and external beam radiotherapy.[74]

Currently our approach is to treat patients with intermediate-risk disease with brachytherapy combined with either short-term hormonal therapy or EBRT. For high-risk disease, brachytherapy is combined with hormonal therapy and EBRT to maximize the likelihood of disease control. We prefer to deliver brachytherapy prior to EBRT, although there are no published data, to the authors' knowledge, addressing whether the sequence of treatment affects outcome. In addition to interstitial brachytherapy, temporary HDR-brachytherapy, 3D-CRT, IMRT, or proton therapies are methods of dose escalation in intermediate and high-risk patients.

Other centers using the combination therapy in high-risk patients also report promising results.[75,76]

In summary, brachytherapy alone is at least as effective as either surgery or high-dose EBRT for low-risk patients. For intermediate- and high-risk patients, brachytherapy in combination with EBRT and/or hormonal therapy is at least or more effective as surgery or external beam radiotherapy[70,75,77] (Tables 82.2 and 82.3).

TREATMENT MORBIDITY

The ideal treatment for prostate cancer would eradicate the tumor and would not severely alter the patient's quality of life. Brachytherapy, an organ-preserving approach, can accomplish these goals because the radiation is placed inside the prostate and travels only a short distance from the gland. However, both early and late complications can occur following the seed implantation and are related to both technical and patient factors.

Needle and seed placement during the procedure can result in edema and bleeding within the prostate, leading to obstructive symptoms and, in some cases, to urinary retention, especially in patients with some degree of obstructive prostatism. The incidence of urinary retention ranges is usually between 4% and 7%.[4,42,76,78] The need for catheterization is generally days to weeks. In a study of 451 patients, Terk et al found that a high urinary symptom score, rather than prostate size, is the most significant predictor of postimplant retention.[79] Patients who had an International Prostate Symptom Score (IPSS) greater than 15 had a 25%

likelihood of developing urinary retention. Pre- and post-treatment prostate volume and American Urological Association symptom score predicted for retention.[80]

Irritative voiding symptoms are quite common following permanent seed implantation. Patients treated with ^{125}I tend to develop urinary symptoms 1 to 2 months after implantation, whereas patients treated with [103]Pd may experience symptoms within 1 to 2 weeks of the implantation. Kleinberg reported urinary symptoms in 80% of patients, with complaints starting within 2 months of the implantation and lasting for 1 year in 45%.[81] Desai found that postimplantation urinary symptoms peak 1 month following implantation and gradually return to normal by 24 months.[60] Urinary symptoms were also highly correlated to the dose received by the prostate and urethra. Stone et al determined the late urinary morbidity of 250 men treated with ^{125}I who prospectively completed an IPSS assessment.[3] There were no significant changes between the pretreatment individual, total, and quality-of-life scores and post-treatment scores an average of 3 years following implantation.

Late urinary complications include stricture and incontinence. Patients who have had prior prostate surgery, such as a TURP, may be at greater risk for urinary incontinence. The Seattle group report an almost 20% rate of incontinence among patients that had a prior TURP.[36] The preplanned technique combined with a

Table 82.2 Freedom from prostate-specific antigen (PSA) failure among moderate risk patients

Author	Patient (#)	Prognostic group (PSA, ng/mL)	Rate (%)	Time (years)	PSA definition of failure (ng/mL)
Blasko[42]	NA	PSA 10–20	67	8	PSA > 1.0
Ragde[97]*	152	Stage T1–T3	66	10	PSA > 0.5
D'Amico[49]	53	(1 feature: PSA 10.1–20, Stage 2b, Gleason 7)	34	5	ASTRO
Grado[98]*†	262	Gleason 5–6	82	5	2 rises > nadir
Dattoli[99]*	29	PSA 10–20	75	5	PSA > 1.0
Potters[100]*	NA	PSA > 10, Stage > T2, Gleason > 6	85	5	ASTRO
Stokes[101]	75	PSA 10–20, Stage 2b, Gleason ≤ 6	64	5	ASTRO or PSA nadir > 1
Critz[102]*	144	PSA 10.1–20	75	5	PSA > 0.2
Singh[103]*	47	(1 feature: PSA > 10, Gleason ≥ 7)	85	3	ASTRO
Beyer[104]	345	PSA 4.1–10	66	7	ASTRO or PSA > 10 or + biopsy
Lederman[105]*	124	PSA ≥ 20, Stage ≥ 2c, Gleason ≥ 7	75	6	PSA > 1.0
Sharkey[106]	287	PSA > 10 or Gleason ≥ 7	77	6	PSA > 1.5
Kwok[107]	33	(1 feature: PSA >10, Stage ≥ 2b, Gleason ≥ 7)	63	5	ASTRO
Kollmeier[24]	70	(1 feature: PSA 10.1–20, Stage 2b, Gleason 7)	81	8	ASTRO

*Indicates treatment with adjuvant EBRT; †87% of reported patients were treated with adjuvant external beam radiation therapy.

ASTRO, definition of PSA failure promulgated by the American Society for Therapeutic Radiology and Oncology.

Table 82.3 Freedom from prostate-specific antigen (PSA) failure among high risk patients

Author	Patient (#)	Prognostic group (PSA, ng/mL)	Rate (%)	Time (years)	PSA definition of failure (ng/mL)
Blasko[42]	NA	PSA > 20	36	8	PSA >1.0
D'Amico[49]	42	(1 feature: PSA > 20, Stage 2c, Gleason > 7)	15(est)	2	ASTRO
Grado[98]*	114	Gleason ≥ 7	58	5	2 rises > nadir
Dattoli[99]*	35	PSA > 20	70	5	PSA >1.0
Potters[100]*	NA	(>1 feature: PSA >10, Stage > T2, Gleason > 6)	85	5	ASTRO
Stokes[101]	39	Stage 2c or 3, Gleason ≥ 7	36	5	ASTRO or PSA nadir > 1
Critz[102]*	44	PSA > 20	75	5	PSA > 0.2
Singh[103]*	18	(2 features: PSA > 10, Gleason > 6)	85	3	ASTRO
Beyer[104]	144	PSA 10.1–20 PSA > 20	53	7	ASTRO or PSA > 10
	73		33	7	or + biopsy
Lederman[105]*	59	(>1 feature: PSA ≥ 20, Stage ≥ 2c, Gleason ≥ 7)	51	5	PSA >1.0
Sharkey[106]	59	PSA > 10 and Gleason ≥ 7	40	6	PSA > 1.5
Kwok[107]	28	(>1 feature: PSA > 10, Stage ≥ 2b, Gleason > 6)	24	5	ASTRO
Stock[74]*	38	PSA > 20 Gleason 8–10	79	5	ASTRO
	37		76	5	

*Indicates treatment with adjuvant EBRT.

ASTRO, definition of PSA failure promulgated by the American Society for Therapeutic Radiology and Oncology.

uniform seed-loading pattern resulted in urethral doses higher than 400 Gy that led to significant urethral damage.[82] The incidence of urethral stricture is approximately 10% with the uniform seed-loading pattern. The peripheral loading technique with real-time seed placement avoids placing the sources too close to the urethra and has been shown to reduce the risk of incontinence greatly, to less than 1%, even after TURP.[83] Among patients without TURP, the incidence of incontinence after brachytherapy is less than 1% irrespective of the seed loading pattern.[14]

Radiation proctitis has been reported to occur in 2% to 12% of patient following seed implantation and results from the proximity of the anterior rectal wall to the posterior aspect of the prostate, where a large number of seeds are placed.[78,80,84,99] Although proctitis is usually mild, with most patients complaining of intermittent painless rectal bleeding, 1% to 2% of patients will develop more serious complications of ulceration and fistula.[87] Patients who are treated with the combined EBRT and implantation can be expected to have a higher rate of radiation proctitis. Snyder found a relationship between the volume of the rectum irradiated and the incidence of grade 2 proctitis.[61] If the rectal volume irradiated by 160 Gy was less than 1.3 cm^3, fewer than 5% of the patients developed grade 2 proctitis by 5 years after implantation. Han measured rectal surface area encompassed by the dose and determined that rectal bleeding is more common when larger surface areas are covered by the prescribed dose.[88]

More severe rectal complications such as ulcer (grade 3) or fistula formation (grade 4) have been more commonly reported in patients who have had rectal bleeding treated by some form of caustic therapy. Theodorescu reported 7 fistulas out of 724 men treated with implantation alone or in combination with EBRT.[89] Six of the seven patients had rectal bleeding managed by biopsy and electrocautery. Gelbum noted that 50% of the grade 3 rectal complications had an antecedent rectal biopsy and that the biopsied patients took twice as long to heal.[80] Most experienced brachytherapists caution patients against biopsy and fulguration of bleeding areas in the anterior rectal wall. It is prudent to caution the patients not to have any rectal procedures performed without getting clearance from the physicians who performed the implantation.

All forms of treatment for localized prostate cancer can cause erectile dysfunction. Brachytherapy has historically been associated with lower impotence rates than seen with radical prostatectomy or EBRT. Because the radiation dose from the seeds falls off so rapidly, the total dose of radiation delivered to the penile vessels and neurovascular bundles is less than that delivered with EBRT, and probably causes far less trauma than that caused by prostatectomy. The data for the newer ultrasound-guided implants tend to bear out this finding, with potency rates of 34% to 86%.[42,76,85,90,91] Stock demonstrated at 59% of patients with potency prior to implant retained erectile function.[91] Patients with good erectile function before implantation have much greater likelihood of maintaining an adequate erection following the implantation. Stock showed that age and hormonal therapy are less important than pretreatment erectile function in determining long-term potency.[91] Merrick found that the addition of EBRT also had a negative effect on erectile function.[92]

The introduction of sildenafil citrate has had a significant effect on treatment-related impotence. Incrocci performed a placebo-controlled study in patients receiving conformal EBRT.[93] Successful intercourse was reported by 55% of the patients after sildenafil citrate versus 18% after placebo (P < 0.001). When sildenafil citrate was included in Merrick's 6-year potency analysis, potency rates increased from 39% to 92%.[92] Potters found that 62% of the men who were impotent following brachytherapy had a favorable response to sildenafil citrate.[94]

Health-related quality-of-life (HRQOL) assessment for brachytherapy patients may provide additional quality-of-life information to help patients select the appropriate treatment for prostate cancer. Wei assessed 1400 men treated by brachytherapy, EBRT, or radical prostatectomy.[95] The RAND 36, functional assessment of cancer therapy—general (FACT-G), functional assessment of cancer therapy—prostate (FACT-P), and the Expanded Prostate Cancer Index (EPIC) were mailed to patients after initial therapy. These investigators found that long-term HRQOL domains for brachytherapy were no better than for radical prostatectomy or EBRT. Unfortunately, no baseline studies were available, and dosimetry data on the implants were not reported, making interpretation of this data problematic. Davis performed a similar study in more than 500 patients using five HRQOL instruments.[96] Little difference was found between the three treatments in general health assessment, although treatment-specific differences were noted for bowel, urinary, and sexual function.

SUMMARY

Prostate brachytherapy has become an accepted treatment modality for localized prostate cancer. Long-term biochemical and biopsy data confirm the early positive impressions that brachytherapy is as valid a treatment option as radical prostatectomy or EBRT. Quality-of-life data also look promising, but more follow-up data are needed. Is brachytherapy as good as or perhaps better than radical prostatectomy? This question cannot be answered yet. Well-controlled, randomized studies are needed. In the meantime, the clinician will have to rely on the available published data.

REFERENCES

1. Stone NN. Brachytherapy or radical prostatectomy: is there a preferred method for treating localized prostate cancer? BJU Int 2004;93:5.

2. Holm HH, Juul N, Pedersen JF, et al. Transperineal ^{125}iodine seed implantation in prostatic cancer guided by transrectal ultrasonography. J Urol 1983;130:283–286.

3. Stone NN, Stock RG. Prospective assessment of patient-reported long-term urinary morbidity and associated quality of life changes after ^{125}I prostate brachytherapy. Brachytherapy 2003;2:32–39.

4. Stock RG, Stone NN, Wesson MF, et al. A modified technique allowing interactive ultrasound-guided three-dimensional transperineal prostate implantation. Int J Radiat Oncol Biol Phys 1995;32:219–225.

5. Bell AG. The uses of radium. Am Med 1903;6:261.

6. Aronowitz JN. Dawn of prostate brachytherapy: 1915–1930. Int J Radiat Oncol Biol Phys 2002;54:712–718.

7. Young HH. The use of radium in cancer of the prostate and bladder: A presentation of new instruments and new methods of use. JAMA 1917;68:1174–1177.

8. Whitmore WF Jr, Hilaris B, Grabstald H, et al. Implantation of ^{125}I in prostatic cancer. Surg Clin North Am 1974;54:887–895.

9. Zelefsky MJ, Whitmore WF Jr. Long-term results of retropubic permanent ^{125}iodine implantation of the prostate for clinically localized prostatic cancer. J Urol 1997;158:23–29; discussion 29–30.

10. Nath R, Yue N. Dosimetric characterization of a newly designed encapsulated interstitial brachytherapy source of iodine-125-model LS-1 BrachySeed. Appl Radiat Isot 2001;55:813–821.

11. Wallner K, Merrick G, True L, et al. ^{125}I versus ^{103}Pd for low-risk prostate cancer: preliminary PSA outcomes from a prospective randomized multicenter trial. Int J Radiat Oncol Biol Phys 2003;57:1297–1303.

12. Bice WS Jr, Prestidge BR, Grimm PD, et al. Centralized multiinstitutional postimplant analysis for interstitial prostate brachytherapy. Int J Radiat Oncol Biol Phys 1998;41:921–927.

13. Mate TP, Gottesman JE, Hatton J, et al. High dose-rate afterloading ^{192}Iridium prostate brachytherapy: feasibility report. Int J Radiat Oncol Biol Phys 1998;41:525–533.

14. Blasko JC, Mate T, Sylvester JE, et al. Brachytherapy for carcinoma of the prostate: techniques, patient selection, and clinical outcomes. Semin Radiat Oncol 2002;12:81–94.

15. Shiloh Y. ATM and related protein kinases: safeguarding genome integrity. Nat Rev Cancer 2003;3:155–168.

16. Shiloh Y, Lehmann AR. Maintaining integrity. Nat Cell Biol 2004;6:923-8.

17. Ling CC, Li WX, Anderson LL. The relative biological effectiveness of I-125 and Pd-103. Int J Radiat Oncol Biol Phys, 1995. 32:373–378.

18. Ling CC. Permanent implants using Au-198, Pd-103 and I-125: radiobiological considerations based on the linear quadratic model. Int J Radiat Oncol Biol Phys 1992;23:81–87.

19. Brenner DJ, Martinez AA, Edmundson GK, et al. Direct evidence that prostate tumors show high sensitivity to fractionation (low alpha/beta ratio), similar to late-responding normal tissue. Int J Radiat Oncol Biol Phys 2002;52:6–13.

20. Fowler JF, Ritter JF, Chappell RJ, et al. What hypofractionated protocols should be tested for prostate cancer? Int J Radiat Oncol Biol Phys 2003;56:1093–1104.

21. Brenner DJ, Hall EJ. Fractionation and protraction for radiotherapy of prostate carcinoma. Int J Radiat Oncol Biol Phys 1999;43:1095–1101.

22. Martinez A, Gonzalez J, Spencer W, et al. Conformal high dose rate brachytherapy improves biochemical control and cause specific survival in patients with prostate cancer and poor prognostic factors. J Urol 2003;169:974–979; discussion 979–980.

23. Wang JZ, Guerrero M, Li XA. How low is the alpha/beta ratio for prostate cancer? Int J Radiat Oncol Biol Phys 2003;55:194–203.

24. Kollmeier MA, Stock RG, Stone N. Biochemical outcomes after prostate brachytherapy with 5-year minimal follow-up: importance of patient selection and implant quality. Int J Radiat Oncol Biol Phys 2003;57:645–653.

25. Zelefsky MJ, Fuks Z, Hunt M, et al. High dose radiation delivered by intensity modulated conformal radiotherapy improves the outcome of localized prostate cancer. J Urol 2001;166:876–881.

26. Grimm PD, Blasko JC, Sylvester JE, et al. 10-year biochemical (prostate-specific antigen) control of prostate cancer with ^{125}I brachytherapy. Int J Radiat Oncol Biol Phys 2001;51:31–40.

27. Gardner BG, Zietman AL, Shipley WU, et al. Late normal tissue sequelae in the second decade after high dose radiation therapy with combined photons and conformal protons for locally advanced prostate cancer. J Urol 2002;167:123–6.

28. Meredith J. Radium dosage. The Manchester System. London: Livington, 1967.

29. Blasko JC, Grimm PD, Ragde H. Brachytherapy and organ preservation in the management of carcinoma of the prostate. Semin Radiat Oncol 1993;3:240–249.

30. Stock RG, Stone NN, Lo YC, et al. Postimplant dosimetry for ^{125}I prostate implants: definitions and factors affecting outcome. Int J Radiat Oncol Biol Phys 2000;48:899–906.

31. Stock RG, Stone NN, Tabert A, et al. A dose-response study for I-125 prostate implants. Int J Radiat Oncol Biol Phys 1998;41:101–108.

32. Stone NN, Stock RG. Prospective assessment of patient-reported long-term urinary morbidity and associated quality of life changes after ^{125}I prostate brachytherapy. Brachytherapy 2003;2:32–39.

33. Jani AB, Hellman S. Early prostate cancer: clinical decision-making. Lancet 2003;361:1045–1053.

34. Fowler FJ Jr, McNaughton Collins M, Albertsen PC, et al. Comparison of recommendations by urologists and radiation oncologists for treatment of clinically localized prostate cancer. JAMA 2000;283:3217–3222.

35. Cesaretti JA, Stone NN, Stock RG. Does prior transurethral resection of prostate compromise brachytherapy quality: a dosimetric analysis. Int J Radiat Oncol Biol Phys 2004;60:648–653.

36. Blasko JC, Ragde H, Grimm PD. Transperineal ultrasound-guided implantation of the prostate: morbidity and complications. Scand J Urol Nephrol Suppl 1991;137:113–118.

37. Partin AW, Kattan MW, Subong EN, et al. Combination of prostate-specific antigen, clinical stage, and Gleason score to predict pathological stage of localized prostate cancer. A multi-institutional update. JAMA 1997;277:1445–1451.

38. Davis BJ, Pisansky TM, Wilson TM, et al. The radial distance of extraprostatic extension of prostate carcinoma: implications for prostate brachytherapy. Cancer 1999;85:2630–2637.

39. Linzer DG, Stock RG, Stone NN, et al. Seminal vesicle biopsy: accuracy and implications for staging of prostate cancer. Urology 1996;48:757–761.

40. Stone NN, Stock RG, Unger P. Laparoscopic pelvic lymph node dissection for prostate cancer: comparison of the extended and modified techniques. J Urol 1997;158:1891–1894.

41. Stone NN, Stock RG. Prostate brachytherapy in patients with prostate volumes >/= 50 cm³: dosimetric analysis of implant quality. Int J Radiat Oncol Biol Phys 2000;46:1199–1204.

42. Blasko JC, Ragde H, Luse RW, et al. Should brachytherapy be considered a therapeutic option in localized prostate cancer? Urol Clin North Am 1996;23:633–650.

43. Bolla M, Collette L, Blank L, et al. Long-term results with immediate androgen suppression and external irradiation in patients with locally advanced prostate cancer (an EORTC study): a phase III randomised trial. Lancet 2002;360:103–106.

44. D'Amico AV, Manola J, Loffredo M, et al. 6-month androgen suppression plus radiation therapy vs radiation therapy alone for patients with clinically localized prostate cancer: a randomized controlled trial. JAMA 2004;292:821–827.

45. Pilepich MV, Winter K, John MJ, et al. Phase III radiation therapy oncology group (RTOG) trial 86-10 of androgen deprivation adjuvant to definitive radiotherapy in locally advanced carcinoma of the prostate. Int J Radiat Oncol Biol Phys 2001;50:1243–1252.

46. Lawton CA, Winter K, Murray K, et al. Updated results of the phase III Radiation Therapy Oncology Group (RTOG) trial 85-31 evaluating the potential benefit of androgen suppression following standard radiation therapy for unfavorable prognosis carcinoma of the prostate. Int J Radiat Oncol Biol Phys 2001;49:937–946.

47. Marshall DT, et al. Hormonal therapy reduces the risk of post-implant urinary retention in symptomatic prostate cancer patients with glands larger than 50 cc. 2004;60(Suppl. 1):S451.

48. Lee LN, Stock RG, Stone NN. Role of hormonal therapy in the management of intermediate- to high-risk prostate cancer treated with permanent radioactive seed implantation. Int J Radiat Oncol Biol Phys 2002;52:444–452.

49. D'Amico AV, Whittington R, Malkowicz SB, et al. Biochemical outcome after radical prostatectomy, external beam radiation therapy, or interstitial radiation therapy for clinically localized prostate cancer. JAMA 1998;280:969–974.

50. Martinez A, Galalae R, Gonzalez J, et al. No apparent benefit at 5 years from a course of neoadjuvant/concurrent androgen deprivation for patients with prostate cancer treated with a high total radiation dose. J Urol 2003;170:2296–2301.

51. Potters L, Torre T, Ashley R, et al. Examining the role of neoadjuvant androgen deprivation in patients undergoing prostate brachytherapy. J Clin Oncol 2000;18:1187–1192.

52. Merrick GS, Butler WM, Galbreath RW, et al. Does hormonal manipulation in conjunction with permanent interstitial brachytherapy, with or without supplemental external beam irradiation, improve the biochemical outcome for men with intermediate or high-risk prostate cancer? BJU Int 2003;91:23–29.

53. Stone NN, Stock RG, Unger P, et al. Biopsy results after real-time ultrasound-guided transperineal implants for stage T1–T2 prostate cancer. J Endourol 2000;14:375–380.

54. Pollack A, Zagars GK, Starkschall G, et al. Prostate cancer radiation dose response: results of the M. D. Anderson phase III randomized trial. Int J Radiat Oncol Biol Phys 2002;53:1097–1105.

55. Zelefsky MJ, Fuks Z, Hunt M, et al. High dose radiation delivered by intensity modulated conformal radiotherapy improves the outcome of localized prostate cancer. J Urol 2001;166:876–881.

56. Nath R, Anderson LL, Luxton G, et al. Dosimetry of interstitial brachytherapy sources: recommendations of the AAPM Radiation Therapy Committee Task Group No. 43. American Association of Physicists in Medicine. Med Phys 1995;22:209–234.

57. Potters L, Huang D, Calugaru E, et al. Importance of implant dosimetry for patients undergoing prostate brachytherapy. Urology 2003;62:1073–1077.

58. Nag S, Bice W, DeWyngaert K, et al. The American Brachytherapy Society recommendations for permanent prostate brachytherapy postimplant dosimetric analysis. Int J Radiat Oncol Biol Phys 2000;46:221–230.

59. Stock RG, Stone NN. Importance of post-implant dosimetry in permanent prostate brachytherapy. Eur Urol 2002;41:434–439.

60. Desai J, Stock RG, Stone NN, et al. Acute urinary morbidity following I-125 interstitial implantation of the prostate gland. Radiat Oncol Investig 1998;6:135–141.

61. Snyder KM, Stock RG, Hong SM, et al. Defining the risk of developing grade 2 proctitis following ^{125}I prostate brachytherapy using a rectal dose-volume histogram analysis. Int J Radiat Oncol Biol Phys 2001;50:335–341.

62. Consensus statement: guidelines for PSA following radiation therapy. American Society for Therapeutic Radiology and Oncology Consensus Panel. Int J Radiat Oncol Biol Phys 1997;37:1035–1041.

63. Critz FA, Levinson AK, Williams WH, et al. Prostate specific antigen nadir achieved by men apparently cured of prostate cancer by radiotherapy. J Urol 1999;161:1199–1203; discussion 1203–1205.

64. Critz FA, Levinson AK, Williams WH, et al. Prostate-specific antigen nadir: the optimum level after irradiation for prostate cancer. J Clin Oncol 1996;14:2893–2900.

65. Thames H, Kuban D, Levy L, et al. Comparison of alternative biochemical failure definitions based on clinical outcome in 4839 prostate cancer patients treated by external beam radiotherapy between 1986 and 1995. Int J Radiat Oncol Biol Phys 2003;57:929–943.

66. Critz FA. Time to achieve a prostate specific antigen nadir of 0.2 ng/ml after simultaneous irradiation for prostate cancer. J Urol 2002;168:2434–2438.

67. Stock RG, Stone NN, Cesaretti JA. Prostate-specific antigen bounce after prostate seed implantation for localized prostate cancer: descriptions and implications. Int J Radiat Oncol Biol Phys 2003;56:448–453.

68. Grimm PD, Blasko JC, Sylvester JE, et al. 10-year biochemical (prostate-specific antigen) control of prostate cancer with ^{125}I brachytherapy. Int J Radiat Oncol Biol Phys 2001;51:31–40.

69. Blasko JC, Grimm PD, Sylvester JE, et al. Palladium-103 brachytherapy for prostate carcinoma. Int J Radiat Oncol Biol Phys 2000;46:839–850.

70. Sylvester J, Blasko JC, Grimm PD, et al. Neoadjuvant androgen ablation combined with external-beam radiation therapy and permanent interstitial brachytherapy boost in localized prostate cancer. Mol Urol 1999;3:231–236.

71. Pickett B, et al. Efficacy of external beam radiotherapy compared to permanent prostate implant in treating low risk prostate cancer based on endorectal magnetic resonance spectroscopy imaging and PSA. 2004;60(Suppl. 1):S185.

72. D'Amico AV, Whittington R, Malkowicz SB, et al. Biochemical outcome after radical prostatectomy, external beam radiation therapy, or interstitial radiation therapy for clinically localized prostate cancer. JAMA 1998;280:969–974.

73. Zelefsky MJ, Hollister T, Raben A, et al. Five-year biochemical outcome and toxicity with transperineal CT-planned permanent I-125 prostate implantation for patients with localized prostate cancer. Int J Radiat Oncol Biol Phys 2000;47:1261–1266.

74. Stock RG, Cahlon O, Cesaretti JA, et al. Combined modality treatment in the management of high-risk prostate cancer. Int J Radiat Oncol Biol Phys 2004;59:1352–1359.

75. Blasko JC, Grimm PD, Sylvester JE, et al. The role of external beam radiotherapy with I-125/Pd-103 brachytherapy for prostate carcinoma. Radiother Oncol 2000;57:273–278.

76. Dattoli M, Wallner K, Sorace R, et al. ^{103}Pd brachytherapy and external beam irradiation for clinically localized, high-risk prostatic carcinoma. Int J Radiat Oncol Biol Phys 1996;35:875–879.

77. Zelefsky MJ, Fuks Z, Hunt M, et al. High dose radiation delivered by intensity modulated conformal radiotherapy improves the outcome of localized prostate cancer. J Urol 2001;166:876–881.

78. Arterbery VE, Wallner K, Roy J, et al. Short-term morbidity from CT-planned transperineal I-125 prostate implants. Int J Radiat Oncol Biol Phys 1993;25:661–667.

79. Terk MD, Stock RG, Stone NN. Identification of patients at increased risk for prolonged urinary retention following radioactive seed implantation of the prostate. J Urol 1998;160:1379–1382.

80. Gelblum DY, Potters L, Ashley R, et al. Urinary morbidity following ultrasound-guided transperineal prostate seed implantation. Int J Radiat Oncol Biol Phys 1999;45:59–67.

81. Kleinberg L, Wallner K, Roy J, et al. Treatment-related symptoms during the first year following transperineal ^{125}I prostate implantation. Int J Radiat Oncol Biol Phys 1994;28:985–990.

82. Wallner K, Roy J, Harrison L. Dosimetry guidelines to minimize urethral and rectal morbidity following transperineal I-125 prostate brachytherapy. Int J Radiat Oncol Biol Phys 1995;32:465–471.

83. Stone NN, Ratnow ER, Stock RG. Prior transurethral resection does not increase morbidity following real-time ultrasound-guided prostate seed implantation. Tech Urol 2000;6:123–127.

84. Wallner K, Roy J, Zelefsky M, et al. Short-term freedom from disease progression after I-125 prostate implantation. Int J Radiat Oncol Biol Phys 1994;30:405–409.

85. Wallner K, Roy J, Harrison L. Tumor control and morbidity following transperineal iodine 125 implantation for stage T1/T2 prostatic carcinoma. J Clin Oncol 1996;14:449–453.

86. Merrick GS, Butler WM, Dorsey AT, et al. Rectal function following prostate brachytherapy. Int J Radiat Oncol Biol Phys 2000;48:667–674.

87. Stone NN, Stock RG. Complications following permanent prostate brachytherapy. Eur Urol 2002;41:427–433.

88. Han BH, Wallner KE. Dosimetric and radiographic correlates to prostate brachytherapy-related rectal complications. Int J Cancer 2001;96:372–378.

89. Theodorescu D, Gillenwater JY, Koutrouvelis PG. Prostatourethral-rectal fistula after prostate brachytherapy. Cancer 2000;89:2085–2091.

90. Kao J, Jani A, Vijayakumar S. Sexual functioning after treatment for early stage prostate cancer. Sexuality and Disability 2002;20:239–260.

91. Stock RG, Kao J, Stone NN. Penile erectile function after permanent radioactive seed implantation for treatment of prostate cancer. J Urol 2001;165:436–439.

92. Merrick GS, Bulter WM, Galbreath RW, et al. Erectile function after permanent prostate brachytherapy. Int J Radiat Oncol Biol Phys 2002;52:893–902.

93. Incrocci L, Koper PC, Hop WC, et al. Sildenafil citrate (Viagra) and erectile dysfunction following external beam radiotherapy for prostate cancer: a randomized, double-blind, placebo-controlled, cross-over study. Int J Radiat Oncol Biol Phys 2001;51:1190–1195.

94. Potters L, Torre T, Feam PA, et al. Potency after permanent prostate brachytherapy for localized prostate cancer. Int J Radiat Oncol Biol Phys 2001;50:1235–1242.

95. Wei JT, Dunn RL, Sandler HM, et al. Comprehensive comparison of health-related quality of life after contemporary therapies for localized prostate cancer. J Clin Oncol 2002;20:557–566.

96. Davis JW, Kuban DA, Lynch DF, et al. Quality of life after treatment for localized prostate cancer: differences based on treatment modality. J Urol 2001;166:947–952.

97. Ragde H, Elgamal AA, Snow PB, et al. Ten-year disease free survival after transperineal sonography-guided iodine-125 brachytherapy with or without 45-gray external beam irradiation in the treatment of patients with clinically localized, low to high Gleason grade prostate carcinoma. Cancer 1998;83:989–1001.

98. Grado GL, Larson TR, Balch CS, et al. Actuarial disease-free survival after prostate cancer brachytherapy using interactive techniques with biplane ultrasound and fluoroscopic guidance. Int J Radiat Oncol Biol Phys 1998;42:289–298.

99. Dattoli M, Wallner K, True L, et al. Prognostic role of serum prostatic acid phosphatase for ^{103}Pd-based radiation for prostatic carcinoma. Int J Radiat Oncol Biol Phys 1999;45:853–856.

100. Potters L, Cha C, Ashley R, et al. The role of external beam irradiation in patients undergoing prostate brachytherapy. Urol Oncol 2000;5:112–117.

101. Stokes SH. Comparison of biochemical disease-free survival of patients with localized carcinoma of the prostate undergoing radical prostatectomy, transperineal ultrasound-guided radioactive seed implantation, or definitive external beam irradiation. Int J Radiat Oncol Biol Phys 2000;47:129–136.

102. Critz FA, Williams WH, Levinson AK, et al. Simultaneous irradiation for prostate cancer: intermediate results with modern techniques. J Urol 2000;164:738–741.

103. Singh A, Zelefsky MJ, Raben A, et al. Combined 3-dimensional conformal radiotherapy and transperineal Pd-103 permanent implantation for patients with intermediate and unfavorable risk prostate cancer. Int J Cancer. 2000;90:275–280.

104. Beyer DC and Brachman DG. Failure free survival following brachytherapy alone for prostate cancer: comparison with external beam radiotherapy. Radiother Oncol. 2000;57:263–267.

105. Lederman GS, Cavanagh W, Albert PS, et al. Retrospective stratification of a consecutive cohort of prostate cancer patients treated with a combined regimen of external-beam radiotherapy and brachytherapy. Int Jnl Radiat Oncol Biol Phys 2001;49:1297–1303.

106. Sharkey J, Cantor A, Solc Z, et al. Brachytherapy versus radical prostatectomy in patients with clinically localized prostate cancer. Curr Urol Rep 2002;3:250–257.

107. Kwok Y, DiBiase SJ, Amin PP, et al. Risk group stratification in patients undergoing permanent ^{125}I prostate brachytherapy as monotherapy. Int J Radiat Oncol Biol Phys 2002;53:588–594.

108. Wallner K, et al. ^{125}I versus ^{103}Pd for low-risk prostate cancer: preliminary PSA outcomes from a prospective randomized multicenter trial. Int J Radiat Oncol Biol Phys 2003;57:1297–1303.

High dose rate ^{192}Ir as monotherapy or as a boost: the new prostate brachytherapy

83

*Alvaro Martinez, Jeffrey Demanes, Razvan Galalae, Jose Gonzalez,
Nils Nuernberg, Carlos Vargas, Rodney Rodriguez, Mitchell Hollander,
Gary Gustafson*

INTRODUCTION

Since the mid-1980s, surgery and radiotherapy have been the treatment modalities most frequently used to treat patients with prostate cancer. However, it is important to recognize the prominence brachytherapy treatments have achieved. To this respect, The American Urologic Society,[1] and the American College of Radiology[2] patterns of care of utilization have reported the significant increase of utilization of brachytherapy during the last decade. We will limit the extent of our data analysis and comments to a type of brachytherapy called high dose rate (HDR) brachytherapy, whether used as a monotherapy or as a boost therapy combined with pelvic external beam with or without androgen deprivation therapy (ADT).

Prostate brachytherapy has been performed using one of two treatment techniques, low dose rate (LDR) or high dose rate (HDR). Low dose rate brachytherapy involves the permanent implantation of multiple radioactive seeds into the prostate. This signifies that the patient remains radioactive and must comply with the state rules and regulations for patients harboring radioactive material. High dose rate brachytherapy, on the other hand, uses a single high-intensity radioactive source stored in a "robot-like machine" called a remote afterloader. The afterloader sends and retracts this single source of radiation in a very short period of time, typically 10 to 15 minutes. Hence, the patients are no longer radioactive after the completion of treatment.

ADVANTAGES OF HIGH DOSE RATE BRACHYTHERAPY

High dose rate brachytherapy has a number of advantages over LDR, which are both patient- and target-specific. They are summarized below:

1. The overall treatment time is reduced from many weeks with LDR to several minutes with HDR. This eliminates the uncertainties related to volume changes occurring over weeks (typical with LDR) due to trauma and swelling or subsequent shrinkage due to postradiation fibrosis.
2. HDR significantly improves the radiation dose distribution secondary to the ability to modulate and accurately control the spatial source position and vary the source dwell time during treatment.
3. The intraoperative (or real-time) optimization used with HDR allows ideal selection of needle placement in real-time and better source position targeting, hence modulating the intensity with the potential for limiting treatment toxicity.
4. HDR can significantly reduce the cost of treatment because the radioactive sources are not purchased per case treated, as is done with LDR.
5. There are advantages in radiation safety and protection with HDR, since the patient is not radioactive when he returns home. The HDR single radiation source is retracted into the robot at the completion of treatment.
6. There are multiple radiobiologic considerations favoring HDR since the treatment is given in several minutes for which repopulation, cell cycle, and recovery of sublethal damage cannot occur.

For patients with early-stage prostate cancer, radical prostatectomy, external beam radiotherapy (EBRT), and brachytherapy are commonly used treatment modalities. Although the most appropriate definition of biochemical failure may be controversial, the Cleveland Clinic Foundation,[3] and William Beaumont Hospital,

Michigan,[4] have reported similar outcomes for patients with favorable prognostic features undergoing either radical prostatectomy or EBRT at a single institution. In addition, several other investigators have reported excellent results with interstitial prostate brachytherapy,[6–11] with biochemical control rates comparable to those of patients treated with either radical prostatectomy or external beam irradiation. While most monotherapy series have utilized LDR technique with iodine-125 (^{125}I) seeds or palladium-103 (^{103}Pd) seeds, HDR brachytherapy with iridium-192 (^{192}Ir) is gaining popularity.[10–13]

A wide variety of treatment approaches has been used for patients with unfavorable prostate cancer. However, treatment remains a challenge. Survival rates from series in which radical prostatectomy is performed for stage C or T3 disease,[14–16] and/or low-dose EBRT are given remain suboptimal.[17] To improve on these results three radiotherapeutic strategies have been tested: 1) the addition of hormonal ablation before standard radiotherapy[18–20]; 2) the addition of particle beam as a boost to EBRT[21,22]; and 3) dose-escalating conformal radiotherapy. Dose escalation has been accomplished by using three-dimensional (3D) conformal EBRT,[23,24] or brachytherapy using a conformal HDR boost.[25,26]

ASSESSING HIGH DOSE RATE BRACHYTHERAPY

In 1991, the William Beaumont Hospital (WBH) Human Investigation Committee (HIC) approved a prospective clinical trial that was designed to test the hypothesis that for patients with intermediate and/or poor prognostic factors local failure is related to the large volume of cell mass and radioresistant cell clones, both of which require biologically higher radiation dosages, than those conventionally used. Thus, we selected a hypofractionated 3D conformal HDR brachytherapy boost as the method of dose escalation. We have published our results previously.[25,26] We reported an update combining the data from Kiel University and WBH, using a similar treatment program.[27] In this report, we are adding the data from the California Endocuritherapy Cancer Center (CET). In total, 1660 patients were treated with HDR brachytherapy as a boost or as monotherapy: CET treated 889 patients, WBH 527 patients, and Kiel 244 patients.

MATERIALS AND METHODS

HYPOFRACTIONATED TREATMENT PROGRAM

The radiotherapeutic approach at the three institutions involved a hypofractionated regimen delivering a very high biologic equivalent dose to EBRT. Our treatment

schedule (Figure 83.1) was designed for 5 weeks instead of the conventional 8-week course of EBRT

HIGH DOSE RATE BRACHYTHERAPY AS A BOOST

Our treatment technique has been previously described.[25,26,28,29] The pelvis was treated with an isocentric dose of 46 Gy in 23 fractions using a 4-field technique. All patients underwent pretreatment pelvic computed tomography (CT) with contrast to assist in defining the prostate and normal tissue volumes. Pelvic EBRT was interdigitated with transrectal ultrasound (TRUS)-guided transperineal conformal interstitial ^{192}Ir implants. The overall treatment time was compressed to only 5 weeks (see Figure 83.1). Patients with a prostate gland volume of more than 65 cm^3 or length of 5.5 cm were initially ineligible for the protocol. These patients underwent downsizing with a short course of hormonal therapy (<6 months) and were the subject of a separate analysis.[30] The dosimetry was done in real-time intraoperatively. The optimal needle positions within the reference plane were determined intraoperatively using our real-time, interactive optimization program.[28,29] After placement of all needles, cystoscopy was performed to reconfirm the prostate treatment length with adequate depth by virtue of bladder mucosa tenting. To reconfirm the gland apex during cystoscopy, the TRUS probe was placed in the sagittal plane. The veru montanum (1 cm behind) was used to correlate with the TRUS probe position in the longitudinal plane. On each transverse TRUS image, the 100% isodose line encompassed the contoured prostate volume (Figure 83.2). The urethra was limited to less than 125% of the prostate dose and a dose–volume histogram (DVH) was used to assess dosimetry quality as seen in Figure 83.3. The rectal dose was limited to 75% of the prostate dose.

When the trial began in 1991, the linear-quadratic formula was used to calculate the biologic effective dose (BED).[31] The α/β value ratio for tumor control probability was 10, and for normal tissue complications, 4. There is evidence now that the α/β ratio for prostate

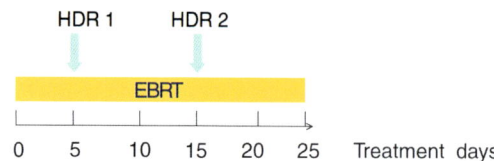

Fig. 83.1
Treatment schedule for prostate cancer patients treated with pelvic external beam radiotherapy (EBRT) and a high dose rate (HDR) brachytherapy boost. External beam radiotherapy: total dose 46 Gy in 23 fractions of 2 Gy/fraction; technique—pelvis 4-field 3D conformal radiotherapy, including pelvic nodes. High dose rate boost: 11.5 Gy on day 5 and day 15 of EBRT without interruption.

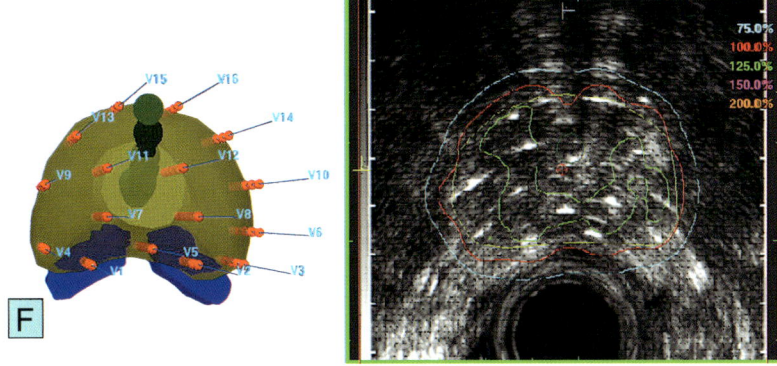

Fig. 83.2

Swift PTV rendering of the prostate, urethra and seminal vesicles with needle trajectory on the left. Real time transrectal ultrasound (TRUS) image with final implant dosimetry on the right. 100% isodose line in red, 125% in green.

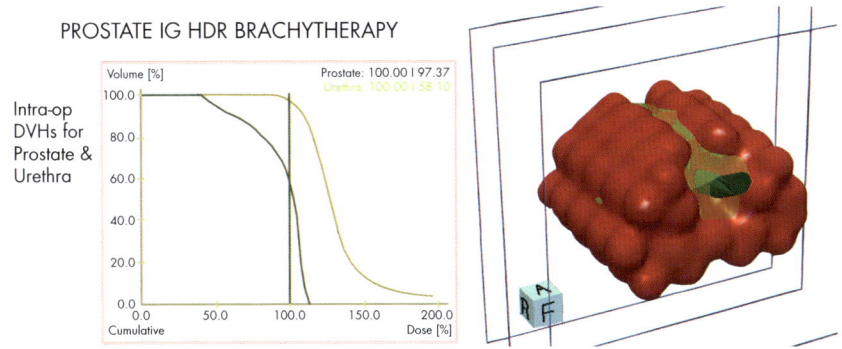

Fig. 83.3

Swift dose–volume histogram (DVH) for prostate and urethra on the left. Prostate 100% isodose cloud (red) rendering on the right with sparing of urethra (green)

cancer is much lower. In 1998, we published the validation of this low α/β value. The value 1.2 was derived from this EBRT and HDR clinical trial.[32] The WBH dose-escalation trial with the corresponding α/β ratios and length of follow up are depicted on Table 83.1.

Table 83.1 Biologic equivalent dose between an external beam radiotherapy (EBRT) alone versus a combined treatment with EBRT and high dose rate (HDR) prostate brachytherapy

Dose level, Gy (# sessions)	# of patients	Mean follow-up years	BED* (Gy) α/β = 10	α/β = 12
Low				
5.50 (3)	19	8.8	67.1	80.2
6.00 (3)	15	8.7	70.0	86.1
6.5 (3)	25	6.7	72.6	92.5
8.25 (2)	26	4.7	72.0	94.2
High				
8.75 (2)	25	4.6	74.2	99.9
9.5 (2)	38	4.5	78.0	108.9
10.50 (2)	46	3.3	82.9	122.0
11.5 (2)	32	1.9	87	136.3

*Biological equivalent dose to external beam.

HIGH DOSE RATE BRACHYTHERAPY AS MONOTHERAPY

The twice per day accelerated hypofractionated regimen was selected based on HDR favorable radiobiologic considerations described above and physical dose-delivery advantages of TRUS guidance,[10] with conformal intensity modulated real-time dosimetry of prostate HDR brachytherapy.[11,26,8,29] Figures 83.2 and 83.3 depict an HDR intraoperative implant using the Nucletron Swift guidance system. Patients with clinical stage II (T1c–T2a) disease, Gleason score less than 7, and pretreatment PSA of less than 12 ng/mL were treated with monotherapy. The majority of patients presented with what would be considered low-risk or favorable prostate cancer. Once it was determined that the patient met all clinical and anatomic criteria for monotherapy, the HDR and LDR brachytherapy treatment options were discussed and then the patient selected the brachytherapy modality. A short course of neoadjuvant androgen deprivation (<6 months) was utilized for downsizing the gland volume, in 31% of WBH patients in equal proportions between permanent seeds and HDR, and in 30% of the CET patients.[13] All procedures were done under spinal anesthesia.

WILLIAM BEAUMONT HOSPITAL EXPERIENCE

Between January 1996 and December 2002, 253 patients with clinically localized prostate cancer, were treated with accelerated hypofractionated brachytherapy as the sole treatment modality. Of the patients, 92 were treated with HDR brachytherapy alone using ^{192}Ir, and 161 patients were treated with LDR brachytherapy alone using ^{103}Pd.

For the implant procedure, as well as for pain control during the entire treatment time, spinal anesthesia was administered following placement of an epidural catheter. In the same manner as in the boost technique, using both transverse and sagittal views, TRUS was used to visualize and identify the base and apex of the prostate, as well as normal structures, such as urethra, rectum, and bladder. Images were captured, and the urethra was mapped at each 5 mm transverse slice from base to apex. The transverse image with the largest cross-sectional area was considered the "reference plane."

Dosimetry was continuously updated in real-time, based on the actual location of needles, to compensate for organ distortion and motion and to assure conformal coverage of the gland.[28] Gold seed markers were then placed under TRUS guidance at the base and at the apex of the prostate to assess and measure possible interfraction needle displacement. Before delivery of the radiation, the entire prostate was imaged again, with final needle and urethral positions captured by TRUS, and a final treatment plan was created.

The prescription dose was 950 cGy delivered four times for a total dose of 3800 cGy. Two fractions were delivered daily over 2 days, with at least 6 hours separating each fraction.

CALIFORNIA ENDOCURITHERAPY CANCER CENTER EXPERIENCE

Between January 1996 and December 2002, 77 patients with clinically localized prostate cancer were treated with interstitial brachytherapy as the sole treatment modality.[13] After recovery, the patient underwent a dual method of simulation radiography consisting of plain film localization for applicator adjustment and quality control and a CT scan was performed. The images were downloaded to the "treatment-planning" computer and a 3D reconstruction was carried out. The dose was prescribed to a point 5 to 6 mm beyond the prostate capsule laterally and 3 mm posteriorly. A dose-volume histogram and virtual images of the anatomy, clinical target volume (CTV), and planning target volume (PTV) were obtained. A series of six HDR fractions was administered twice per day in two separate procedures 1 week apart. Each fraction delivered 7 Gy for a total dose of 42 Gy. Postoperative management was similar to that described for the WBH experience.

RESULTS

HIGH DOSE RATE BRACHYTHERAPY AS A BOOST

For the WBH dose-escalation trial and stratifying the patients by dose level (low-dose level <95 Gy; high-dose level >95 Gy), the ASTRO 5-year biochemical control (BC) was 87% for high dose and 52% for low dose (Figure 83.4). Mean follow-up was 8.1 years (range 2–12 years) for the low dose level and 4.2 years (range 0.5–8.2 years) for the high dose level. The mean dose for the biochemically-controlled patients was 108.2 Gy versus 92.5 Gy for biochemical failures (t-test, $P = 0.001$).

The collaborative long-term outcome results with HDR brachytherapy as a boost with or without adjuvant/concurrent hormonal therapy are presented. A total of 1491 patients were treated at WBH, CET, and Keil University. The mean follow up was 4.9 years with a range of 0.5 to 15.7 years. At 5 years, 589 have been followed; at 8 years, 216 patients; and at more than 10 years, 97 patients were followed.

For all 1491 patients, the 5 and 10-year actuarial analysis of biochemical control, freedom from clinical failure, disease-free survival, cause-specific survival, and overall survival, are shown in Table 83.2. Of significance is that the percentage drop in outcome from 5 years to 10 years is very small for all the above tested categories.

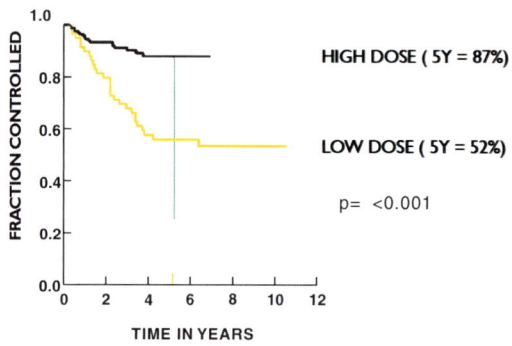

Fig. 83.4
Actuarial analysis of biochemical failure (ASTRO definition) stratified by high dose rate (HDR) brachytherapy dose level.

Table 83.2 Clinical outcome for patients with intermediate and high-risk prostate cancer treated with a combination of external beam radiotherapy (EBRT) with a high dose rate (HDR) brachytherapy boost (n = 1491)

	5 years (%)	10 years (%)
Biochemical no evidence of disease	85	82
Freedom from clinical failure	93	85
Disease free survival	85	69
Cause-specific survival	97	93
Overall survival	90	76

Also, the freedom from clinical failure of 85% at 10 years is very remarkable for these patients with intermediate- and high-risk prostate cancer.

For the three institutions collaborative group (n = 1491), the 10 year cause-specific survival (CSS) and overall survival are depicted in Figure 83.5. Despite the unfavorable group of patients treated, at 10 years only 16% have died of prostate cancer.

Since this is a long-term analysis, we want to emphasize clinical failures, CSS, and distant metastatic rates. In Figure 83.6, the clinical failure rate by poor risk factors is depicted. The risk factors were patients with a stage higher than T2b, PSA greater than 10 ng/mL and

Gleason score of more than 7. A clear spread of failures ($P < 0.001$) can be seen as risk factors increased. However, a remarkably low 10-year clinical failure rate of 27% was seen for those 204 patients with all three poor prognostic factors. The CSS by risk factors is illustrated in Figure 83.7. The number of risk factors has a significant influence in cancer death ($P < 0.001$). At 10 years, for those patients with all three poor risk factors, the cancer mortality rate was only 16%.

Figure 83.8 depicts the 5-year and 10-year distant metastatic rate for 934 patients, of whom 528 patients did not receive, and 406 patients did receive, a short course (<6 months) of total ADT. Only patients with a minimum follow up of 18 months, or three times the exposure to ADT were analyzed. A detrimental effect can be seen with the use of a short course of ADT ($P = 0.035$). We explain

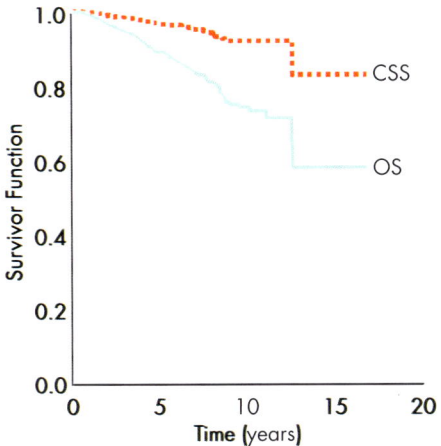

Fig. 83.5
Overall survival (OS) and cause-specific survival (CSS, cancer mortality) for all 1491 prostate cancer patients treated with a high dose rate (HDR) prostate brachytherapy boost.

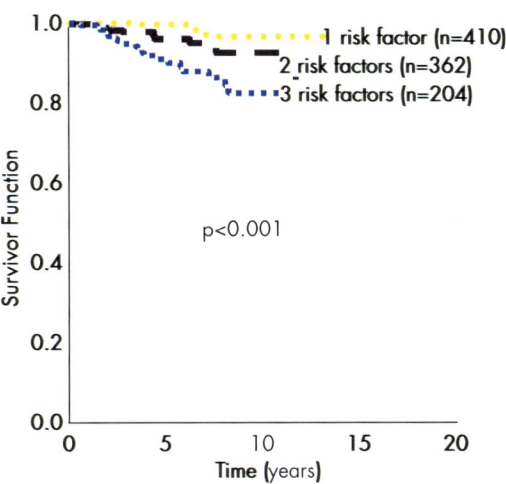

Fig. 83.7
Assessment of cause-specific survival (cancer mortality) stratified by patients harboring one, two, or all three poor prognostic factors for patients treated with a high dose rate (HDR) prostate brachytherapy boost.

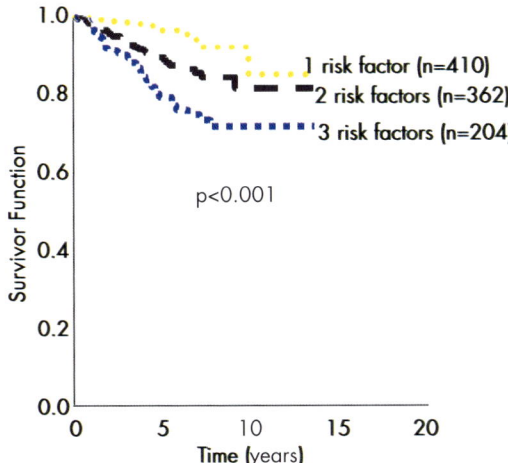

Fig. 83.6
Assessment of clinical failures stratified by patients harboring one, two or all three poor prognostic factors for patients treated with a high dose rate (HDR) prostate brachytherapy boost.

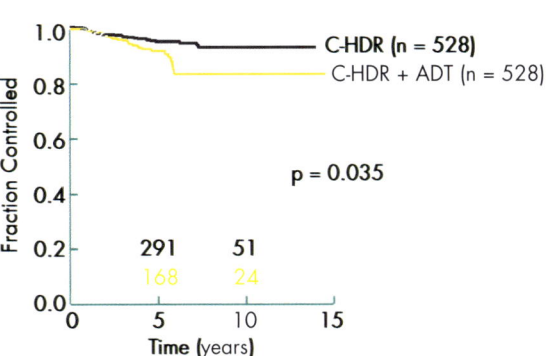

Fig. 83.8
Actuarial analysis of distant metastasis for patients with intermediate- and high-risk prostate cancer treated with a high dose rate (HDR) prostate brachytherapy boost with or without androgen deprivation therapy (ADT).

this finding as a negative impact of delaying the initiation of the curative treatment by high-dose radiation. Figure 83.9 and Table 83.3 are subset analysis of these patients. In Figure 83.9 we are demonstrating a very negative influence of less than 6 months of ADT for those 204 patients with all three poor prognostic factors (P = 0.02). Table 83.3 depicts a subset analysis of patients under 70 years of age to 1) be comparable in age with radical prostatectomy series; and 2) diminish the influence of elderly patients with significant co-morbidities affecting survival. If one looks at the worst group (Gleason score 8–10, PSA > 15 ng/mL, and palpable disease >T2a), there is a clear detrimental effect in terms of increased metastatic rate (P = 0.007), increased cancer mortality (P = 0.01), and decrease survival (P = 0.01). These findings are rather distressing and emphasize the importance of not delaying

curative treatment in these patients with a high probability of developing metastasis if not treated in a timely fashion.

To place our collaborative HDR boost results in perspective, we selected a recently published radical prostatectomy study by Hull et al.[33] They reported the results on 1000 consecutive patients treated with a radical retropubic prostatectomy. Gleason grade utilized for analysis was the one on the biopsy/transurethral resection of the prostate, and not the one at prostatectomy, and was assigned by one pathologist. This improves the validity of the comparison with our clinical data base.[34] The median follow-up for prostatectomy patients was 3.9 years, while our HDR series was 4.9 years. Table 83.4 depicts the 10-year freedom from distant metastasis stratified by Gleason score. While the 10-year results for Gleason scores up to 6 are equivalent in both studies, there is a clear superiority for Gleason 7 (58% versus 92%) and for Gleason 8 to 10 (58% versus 84%), favoring the EBRT with an HDR boost.

HIGH DOSE RATE BRACHYTHERAPY AS MONOTHERAPY

A total of 330 prostate cancer patients were treated with either HDR ^{192}Ir or LDR ^{103}Pd brachytherapy alone. The median follow-up for all patients was 4.1 years (range 0.8–12.3 years).

Acute toxicity

High dose rate brachytherapy alone was associated with statistically significant reductions in the acute rates of dysuria, from 65% with ^{103}Pd seeds to 38% with HDR monotherapy (P < 0.001), as well as urinary frequency and/or urgency, from 94% for ^{103}Pd to 53% for HDR (P < 0.001) and urinary retention from 43% for ^{103}Pd to 29% for HDR (P = 0.012). In addition to reduced acute

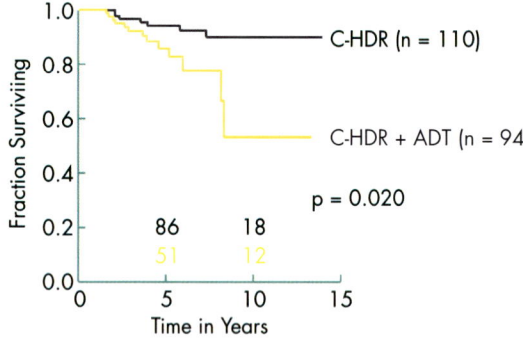

Fig. 83.9

Actuarial analysis of cause-specific survival (cancer deaths) for patients with all three poor prognostic factors treated with a high dose rate (HDR) prostate brachytherapy boost with or without androgen deprivation therapy (ADT).

Table 83.3 Outcome analysis in terms of distant metastasis, cause-specific survival and overall survival for the high-risk group in patients ≤ 70 years stratified by androgen deprivation therapy

		Cases	Mets, 5 year	Cause-specific survival, 5 year	Overall survival, 5 year
All cases	No AD	308	5%	98%	91%
P-value	AD	252	10%	93%	89%
			0.04	0.02	0.4
Gleason score 8–10 or PSA ≥ 15 ng/mL or ≥T2a	No AD	250	6%	98%	91%
P-value	AD	198	12%	92%	90%
			0.03	0.02	0.9
Gleason score 8–10 and ≥T2a	No AD	49	13%	93%	89%
P-value	AD	48	27%	78%	78%
			0.04	0.2	0.1
Gleason score 8–10 and PSA ≥ 15 ng/mL and ≥T2a	No AD	16	13%	93%	92%
P-value	AD	18	40%	65%	60%
			0.007	0.01	0.01

Table 83.4 Comparative outcome for prostate cancer treated patients, 10-year freedom from distant metastasis stratified by Gleason score, between radical prostatectomy versus external beam radiotherapy (EBRT) with a high dose rate (HDR) brachytherapy boost

| | 10-year freedom from distant metastasis | |
	Surgery* (n = 987)	Brachytherapy† (n = 528)
Gleason score:		
2–6	95% (n = 723)	99% (n = 194)
7	58% (n = 226)	92% (n = 236)
8–10	58% (n = 38)	84% (n = 98)
Median follow-up	3.9 years	4.9 years

*Hull et al. J Urol 2002;167:528–534.

†Martinez et al[34]

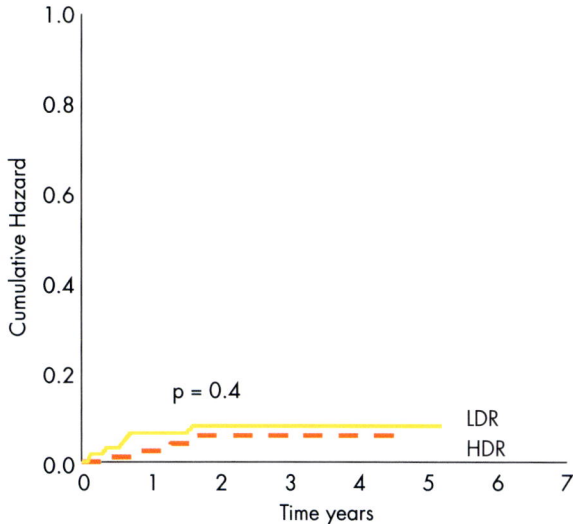

Fig. 83.10
Actuarial chronic genitourinary and gastrointestinal grade 3 toxicity comparison between high dose rate (HDR) and low dose rate (LDR, permanent seeds) monotherapy treated patients.

genitourinary symptoms, HDR was also associated with lower rates of rectal pain, 18% for LDR versus 7% for HDR ($P = 0.025$). The majority of acute toxicities in both groups were grade 1. Hormonal androgen ablation for gland downsizing was given to 31% of patients in both groups.

Chronic toxicity

Again, HDR brachytherapy alone was associated with reduced urinary frequency and urgency, 54% for ^{103}Pd versus 32% for HDR ($P < 0.001$). The majority of toxicities were grade 1. There were no differences in the remaining chronic toxicity rates of urinary incontinence or retention, hematuria, diarrhea, rectal pain, or rectal bleeding between the two treatment groups. The rate of urethral stricture requiring dilatation was 3% with HDR compared with 1% with ^{103}Pd ($P = 0.3$). The median time to development of urethral stricture was 17 months, with a range of 4 to 37 months. Figure 83.10 shows, the cumulative proportion of chronic grade 3 toxicity by treatment modality. No difference was noted between the two treatment types.

Potency

Regardless of the use of adjuvant hormonal therapy all cases were included. This included 51 patients treated with HDR brachytherapy alone and 71 patients treated with permanent ^{103}Pd. The 4-year probability of impotency was 38% for all patients with available data. As shown in Figure 83.11, the probability was 61% for LDR patients, and 21% for HDR patients ($P = 0.006$). The mean times to impotency for the HDR and LDR treatments were 3.9 years and 3.2 years, respectively.

Monotherapy outcomes

The 5-year actuarial outcomes for monotherapy can be seen in Table 83.5. No difference was noted in terms of ASTRO definition for biochemical control, cancer mortality, or overall survival.

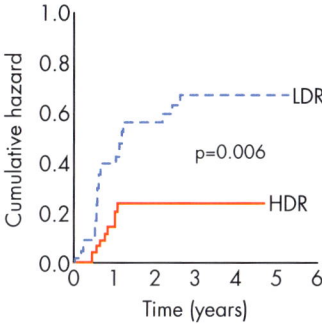

Fig. 83.11
Probability of erectile dysfunction stratified by treatment modality high dose rate (HDR) versus low dose rate (LDR, permanent seeds) for monotherapy treated patients with favorable prostate cancer.

Table 83.5 Actuarial 5-year outcome for the favorable group prostate cancer patients treated with monotherapy divided by high dose rate (HDR) versus low dose rate (LDR, permanent seeds) prostate brachytherapy

5-year actuarial	HDR brachytherapy, %WBH+CET (n = 169)	LDR brachytherapy, %WBH (n = 161)	p-value*
Overall survival	99	93	0.35
Cause-specific survival	100	100	–
Biochemical control	99	98	0.602

*Kaplan–Meier log rank.

Box 83.1 Summary of high dose rate (HDR) brachytherapy

HDR prostate brachytherapy

- Allows the delivery of very high doses of radiation (>95 Gy BED) to the prostate with significant sparing of radiation dose to rectum and urethra, therefore, decreasing toxicity.

- Similar results were obtained at three different institutions when used as a boost and at two institutions when utilized as monotherapy to replace permanent seeds.

- Does not leave the patient radioactive after the procedure, nor irradiate intraoperatively the urologists, radiation oncologists, anesthesiologists, and operating room personnel.

HDR as a boost

- Excellent long-term outcomes for patients with intermediate- and high-risk factors, particularly with Gleason scores >8.

- The use of a short course of neoadjuvant androgen deprivation therapy has a detrimental effect increasing distant metastasis and cancer related metastasis and decreasing survival. Most likely related to the delay in curative therapy by high dose radiation.

- When HDR boost was compared with retropubic prostatectomy, HDR improved the 10-year freedom from distant metastasis for patients harboring Gleason scores 7 and 8–10.

- There is an improved outcome with doses (BED) above 95 Gy.

HDR as monotherapy

- At 5 years, equal biochemical control, cause-specific survival, and overall survival when compared with permanent seeds.

- HDR produced less grade 1 chronic genitourinary toxicity compared with permanent seeds.

- Very large improvement in erectile dysfunction rates, from 41% with permanent seeds to 61% with HDR.

- Cost effective since the seeds do not have to be purchased for each patient.

ACKNOWLEDGMENT

This work is supported in part by the Department of Defense award PC031163.

REFERENCES

1. Mettlin CJ, Murphy GP, McDonald CJ, et al. The national Cancer Data Base Report on increased use of brachytherapy for the treatment of patients with prostate carcinoma in the USA. Cancer 1999;86:1877–1882.

2. Lee WR, Moughan J, Owen JB, et al. The 1999 patterns of care study of radiotherapy in localized prostate carcinoma. A comprehensive survey of prostate carcinoma. A comprehensive survey of prostate brachytherapy in the United States. Cancer 2003;98:1987–1994.

3. Kupelian P, Katcher J, Levin H, et al. External beam radiotherapy versus radical prostatecomy for clinical Stage T1-T2 prostate cancer: Therapeutic implications of stratification by pretreatment PSA levels and biopsy Gleason scores. Cancer J Sci Am 1997;3:78–87.

4. Martinez AA, Gonzalez JA, Chung AK, et al. A comparison of external beam radiation therapy versus radical prostatectomy for patients with low risk prostate carcinoma diagnosed, staged and treated at a single institution. Cancer 2000;88:425–432.

5. D'Amico AV, Whittington R, Malkowski SB, et al. Biochemical outcome after radical prostatectomy, external beam radiation therapy or interstitial radiation therapy for clinically localized prostate cancer. JAMA 1998;280:969–974.

6. Blaska JC, Grimm PD, Sylvester JE, et al. Palladium-103 brachytherapy for prostate carcinoma. Int J Radiat Oncol Biol Phys 2000;46:839–850.

7. Stock RG, Stone NN, Tabert A, et al. A dose-response study for I-125 prostate implants. Int J Radiat Oncol Biol Phys 1998;41:101–108.

8. Wallner K, Merrick G, True L, et al. I-125 versus Pd-103 for low risk prostate cancer. Morbidity outcomes from a perspective randomized multicenter trial. Cancer J Sci Am 2002;8:67–73.

9. Beyer DC, Priestley JB. Biochemical disease-free survival following I-125 prostate implantation. Int J Radiat Oncol Biol Phys 1997;37:559–563

10. Martinez AA, Pataki I, Edmundson G, et al. Phase II prospective study of the use of conformal high-dose rate brachytherapy as monotherapy for the treatment of favorable stage prostate cancer: A feasibility report. Int J Radiat Oncol Biol Phys 2001;49:61–69.

11. Grills IS, Martinez A, Hollander M, et al. High does rate brachytherapy as prostate cancer monotherapy reduces toxicity compared to low dose rate Palladium seeds. J Urol 2004;171:1098–1104.

12. Yoshioka Y, Nose T, Yoshida K, et al. High-dose rate interstitial brachytherapy as monotherapy as monotherapy for localized prostate cancer: Treatment description and preliminary results of phase I/II clinical trial. Int J Radiat Oncol Biol Phys 2000;48:675–681.

13. Demanes JD, Rodriguez RR, Altieri GA. Hose dose rate prostate brachytherapy the California Endocurietherapy (CET) Method. Radiother Oncol 2000;57:289–296.

14. Morgan WR, Bergstralh EJ, Zincke H. Long-term evaluation of radical prostatectomy as treatment for clinical state C (T3) prostate cancer. Urology 1993;41:113–120.

15. Gerber GS, Thisted RA, Chodak GW, et al. Results of radical prostatectomy in men with locally advanced prostate cancer: Multi-institutional pooled analysis. Eur Urol 1997;32:385–390.

16. Oefelein MG, Smith ND, Grayhack JT, et al. Long-term results of radical retropubic prostatectomy in men with high grade carcinoma of the prostate. J Urol 1997;158:1460–1465.

17. Hanks GE, Diamond JJ, Krall JM, et al. A ten-year follow-up of 682 patients treated for prostate cancer with radiation therapy in the United States. Int J Radiat Oncol Biol Phys 1987;13:499–505.

18. Pilepich MV, Caplan R, Byhardt CA, et al. Phase III trial of androgen suppression using goserelin in unfavorable-prognosis carcinoma of the prostate treated with definitive radiotherapy: Report of Radiation Therapy Oncology Group Protocol 85-35. J Clin Oncol 1997;15:1013–1021.

19. Bolla M, Gonzalez D, Warde P, et al. Improved survival in patients with locally advanced prostate cancer treated with radiotherapy and goserelin. N Engl J Med 1997;337:295–300.

20. Roach M, Lu J, Pilepich M, et al. Predicting survival and the role of androgen suppressive therapy (AST): Radiation Therapy Oncology Group (RTOG) phase III randomized prostate cancer trials. Int J Radiat Oncol Biol Phys 1998;42–177.

21. Shipley WU, Verhey JJ, Munzenrider JE, et al. Advanced prostate cancer: The results of a randomized comparative trial of high dose irradiation boosting with conformal protons compared with conventional dose irradiation using photons alone. Int J Radiat Oncol Biol Phys 1995;32:3–12.

22. Forman JD, Duclos M, Sharma R, et al. Conformal mixed neutron and photon irradiation in localized and locally advanced prostate cancer: Preliminary estimates of the therapeutic ratio. Int J Radiat Oncol Biol Phys 1996;35:259–266.

23. Zelefsky MJ, Leibel, SA, Gaudin, PB, et al. Dose escalation with three-dimensional conformal radiation therapy affects the outcome in prostate cancer. Radiology 1998;209:169–174.

24. Hanks GE, Lee WR, Hanlon Al, et al. Conformal technique dose escalation for prostate cancer: Biochemical evidence of improved cancer control with higher doses in patients with pretreatment prostate-specific antigen ≥ 10 ng/ml. Int J Radiat Oncol Biol Phys 1996;35:861–868.

25. Martinez AA, Kestin LL, Stromberg J, et al. Interim report of image-guided conformal high dose rate brachytherapy for patients with unfavorable prostate cancer. The William Beaumont phase II dose-escalating trial. Int J Radiat Oncol Biol Phys 2000;47:343–352.

26. Martinez AA, Gonzales J, Spencer W, et al. Conformal high dose rate brachytherapy improves biochemical control and cause specific survival in patients with prostate cancer and poor prognostic factors. J Urol 2003;169:974–980.

27. Galalae R, Martinez A, Mate T, et el. Long term outcome by risk factors using conformal HDR brachytherapy boost with or without

neoadjuvant androgen deprivation for localized prostate cancer. Int. J. Radiat. Oncol Biol. Phys 2004;58:1048–1055.

28. Edmundson G, Rizzo N, Teahan M, et al. Concurrent treatment planning for outpatient high dose rate prostate template implants. Int J Radiat Oncol Biol Phys 1993;27:1215–1223.

29. Edmundson GK, Yan D, Martinez A. Intraoperative optimization of needle placement and dwell times for conformal prostate brachytherapy. Int J Radiat Oncol Biol Phys 1995;33:1257–1263.

30. Martinez AA, Galalae R, Gonzalez J, et al. No apparent benefit at 5 years from a course of neoadjuvant/concurrent androgen deprivation for prostate cancer patients treated to a high total radiation dose. J Urol 2003;170:2296–2301.

31. Brenner DJ, Hall EJ. Fractionation and protraction for radiotherapy of prostate carcinoma. Int J Radiat Biol Phys 1999;43:1095–1101.

32. Brenner DJ, Martinez AA, Edmundson GK, et al. Direct evidence that prostate tumors show high sensitivity to fraction (low α/β ratio) comparable to late-responding normal tissues. Int J Radiat Oncol Biol Phys 2002;52:6–13.

33. Hull GW, Rabbani F, Abbas F, et al. Cancer control with radical prostatectomy alone in 1000 consecutive patients. J Urol 2202;167:528–534.

34. Martinez AA, Demanas J, Galalae R, et al. Lack of benefit from a short course of androgen deprivation for unfavorable prostate cancer patients treated with an accelerated Hypofractionated regime. Int J Radiat Oncol Biol Phys 2005;62:1322–1331.

MRI-guided partial prostatic irradiation in select patients with clinically localized adenocarcinoma of the prostate

84

Michele Albert, Mark Hurwitz, Clair Beard, Clare M Tempany,
Robert A Cormack, Anthony V D'Amico

INTRODUCTION

The introduction of the serum prostate-specific antigen (PSA) has changed the presentation of prostate cancer worldwide. Patients now present at a younger age, with lower grade disease, and are more likely to have organ-confined cancers found upon pathologic evaluation of the radical prostatectomy specimen.[1] This migration toward smaller volume disease raises the possibility of more tailored therapy.

Brachytherapy is the therapeutic delivery of radiation to a diseased site by the insertion, either temporarily or permanently, of sources containing radioactive material. The current method of prostate brachytherapy in the United States commonly uses transrectal ultrasound (TRUS) imaging to guide radioactive seed placement.[2] Using this approach, the goal is to deliver 100% of the prescription dose to the entire prostate gland.

Since the late 1990s, a real-time intraoperative magnetic resonance image (IMRI) guided prostate brachytherapy technique[3] has been designed and implemented. This utilized both MRI[4,5] and dose and volume histogram (DVH) analysis performed in real time, intraoperatively. Using this technique, regions of the prostate gland (i.e., peripheral zone [PZ], transition zone [TZ], periurethral, anterior base) can be delineated using MRI providing the opportunity to focus the radiation dose delivery to specific zone(s) of the prostate gland, based on the likelihood of cancer presence using the individual patient's pretreatment clinical characteristics. In particular, several investigators have identified a subset of patients—based on the pretreatment PSA level, biopsy Gleason score, and clinical T-category—in which the presence of cancer in the anterior base is rare.[6,7]

A direct correlation with the development of acute urinary morbidity and brachytherapy dose to the entire prostate gland has been documented.[8] Given that the IMRI technique limits dose to the anterior base and the transition zone anterior to the urethra to under 100%, while delivering 100% or more of the prescription dose to the peripheral zone of the prostate gland, this approach has permitted the treatment of patients with large prostate glands (>60 cm^3) with a resultant low risk of self-limited acute urinary retention,[9] and no need for neoadjuvant hormonal therapy to achieve prostate gland shrinkage. However, such an approach for patients with moderate prostate gland enlargement intentionally did not treat a portion of the prostate gland to high dose. Therefore, whether not treating part of the prostate gland in these patients to high dose led to a decrement in PSA outcome when compared at 5 years with patients treated with maximal therapy (i.e., radical prostatectomy [RP]) was the subject of this study.

PATIENT POPULATION, STAGING, AND TREATMENT

Between 1997 and 2002, of 406 and 227 patients who underwent RP or an IMRI-guided prostate brachy monotherapy procedure, repectively, at the Brigham and Women's Hospital (BWH) for the 2002 American Joint Commission on Cancer (AJCC),[10] and who had clinical category T1c, PSA less than 10 ng/mL and biopsy Gleason 3 + 4 or less, and who had perineural invasion biopsy negative adenocarcinoma of the prostate, 322 and 196 had a 2-year minimum follow up respectively.[11] No patient received neoadjuvant or adjuvant androgen suppression or radiation therapy. Patients who had a history of a transurethral resection of the prostate (TURP), urinary daytime frequency less than every 2 hours, and/or nocturia exceeding 4 that was not medically correctable with an α_{1A}-blocker were not eligible for brachytherapy. However, patients who had a previous abdominal perineal resection were not excluded because the IMRI-guided technique did not require a rectum to guide source placement because the imaging apparatus was extrinsic to the patient.[12] In addition, long-term quality-of-life data were available on 152 of the 196 patients who underwent brachytherapy and 50 patients who underwent external-beam radiation therapy to 45 Gy plus a brachytherapy boost to 77 Gy. Internal Review Board (IRB)-approved informed consent was obtained on all patients. All biopsy slides were reviewed by a single genitourinary pathology group at the BWH, and all patients had at least a sextant biopsy. The prostate gland volume (PG Vol) was determined in each case using a 1.5 tesla staging endorectal MRI study and an ellipsoid approximation where PG Vol = $\pi/6 \times$ length $\times$ width $\times$ height. The median age (range) of the surgical and IMRI brachytherapy patients at the time of initial therapy was 60 (44–75) and 62 (49–79) years respectively. Table 84.1 lists the pretreatment clinical characteristics of the RP and IMRI brachytherapy cohorts. The pretreatment medical management,[3] intraoperative magnetic resonance unit,[13] and IMRI technique[14] have been previously described and mandated that the end of operating-room dosimetry provided a V100 of at least 100%.

Table 84.1 Percent distribution of the pre-treatment clinical characteristics of the 406 surgery and 227 brachytherapy managed patients comprising the study cohort*

Clinical characteristic	Surgery (%)	Brachytherapy (%)	$P_{Chi-square}$
PSA (ng/mL)			0.0005
<4	9	91	
4–9.99	19	81	
Biopsy Gleason score			<0.0001
≤5	20	8	
6	65	81	
3 + 4	15	11	
Age (years)†			<0.0001
<60	48	32	
60–64	24	33	
65–69	21	17	
≥70	7	18	
% Positive biopsies			0.25
<34	73	78	
34–50	17	12	
>50	11	10	
Prostate volume (cm³)			<0.0001
<20	1	6	
20–44.9	26	58	
45–59.9	38	20	
60–99.9	30	15	
≥100	5	1	

PSA, prostate-specific antigen.

*Percentages may not sum to 100 due to rounding. †Age at the time of initial therapy.

FOLLOW-UP

For the 322 RP- and 196 brachytherapy-managed patients whose minimum follow-up was 2 years the median follow up was 4.2 and 3.95 years, respectively. Patients generally had a serum PSA measurement and digital rectal examination performed every 3 months for 2 years, then every 6 months for an additional 3 years, then annually thereafter. The median (range) number of PSA values per patient whose minimum follow up was 2 years was 14 (8–26). Prostate-specific antigen failure was defined using the American Society for Therapeutic Radiology and Oncology (ASTRO) consensus criteria.[15] Determinations of PSA were made no more frequently then every 3 months, and three consecutive increments were necessary to constitute a rise in order to avoid overcalling PSA failure in brachytherapy-managed patients due to the PSA bounce phenomenon.[16] A PSA level postoperatively was not considered detectable until it exceeded 0.2 ng/mL. No patient died of prostate cancer during the study period, and no patient was lost to follow-up.

ASSESSMENT OF LATE TOXICITY

RECTAL FUNCTION

Patients were asked whether they had experienced any rectal bleeding at each follow-up by a specialty oncology nurse. All rectal bleeding was analyzed with colonoscopy, and evidence of proctitis needed to be confirmed endoscopically before grading the rectal bleeding as an event related to radiation. In all cases, the date that the patient reported the first evidence of rectal bleeding was noted as the event date. The following scales were used to quantify the rectal bleeding: grade 1 (G1) no clinical evidence of rectal bleeding but with evidence of mild proctitis seen on screening colonoscopy; grade 2 (G2) cortisone enemas necessary for eradication of rectal bleeding; and grade 3 (G3) argon plasma coagulation (APC)[17,18] necessary for the eradication of bleeding. Other late gastrointestinal (GI) toxicity such as diarrhea and rectal urgency was not collected in this study.

ERECTILE FUNCTION

At baseline and then at each follow-up, patients were asked about their ability to have an erection sufficient for vaginal intercourse and, specifically, how this ability compared with their erectile function prior to treatment. Erectile function was noted as being the same as the baseline, worse than the baseline, or better than the baseline. Information on the use of erectile function aids and their efficacy was collected. A standardized questionnaire was not used.[19] The date that the patient reported the first evidence of any decrease in erectile function compared with baseline was noted as the event date.

URINARY FUNCTION

Prior to treatment and at the time of each follow-up, patients were asked whether they had noted any blood in the urine. All patients who presented with hematuria were evaluated with a urine analysis and culture to rule out a urinary tract infection (UTI).

Once a UTI had been excluded then a cystoscopy was performed to determine the etiology of the hematuria. In addition, patients were asked about the strength of their urinary stream and the frequency of voiding, nocturia, hesitancy, and urgency, as well as the presence of any urinary incontinence. In cases where a significant change had occurred in their voiding pattern, a cystoscopy and a urodynamic study was performed to assess for a urethral stricture or the need for a TURP.

STATISTICAL METHODS

A Cox regression multivariable analysis[20] was performed to evaluate the ability of the treatment received (RP versus brachytherapy), pretreatment PSA level (continuous), percent positive biopsies (continuous), prostate gland volume (continuous), and biopsy Gleason score (continuous but could only take on integer values from 2 to 7 inclusive) to predict time to post-treatment PSA failure. In addition, a Cox regression analysis was performed to evaluate the ability of the categorical variables of initial treatment received (RP versus brachytherapy), PSA level (≤4 ng/mL versus >4 and <10 ng/mL), biopsy Gleason score (3 + 4 versus ≤6), percent positive biopsies (≥34% versus <34%), and prostate gland volume (≥45 cm^3 versus <45 cm^3) to predict time to post-treatment PSA failure. The cut-points for the categorical variables were selected based on data suggesting their predictive value from previously reported studies for PSA, biopsy Gleason score, and the percent positive biopsies.[21] The cut-point for prostate gland volume was selected based on the currently accepted maximum prostate gland

volume recommended by the American Brachytherapy Society for a TRUS-guided brachytherapy procedure.[22]

A chi-square metric was used to evaluate whether the distribution in age, PSA level, biopsy Gleason score, and percent positive prostate biopsies at the time of treatment were significantly different between surgically and brachytherapy-managed patients. Estimates of PSA failure following RP or IMRI-guided brachytherapy were calculated using the method of Kaplan and Meier[23] and are graphically displayed for patients with a minimum follow-up of 2 years. Comparisons of PSA failure-free survival were made using a log rank test, and time zero was defined as the date of diagnosis for all patients.

Quality-of-life data are available on 152 and 50 patients who underwent IMRI-guided prostate brachytherapy as monotherapy or as a boost in conjunction with 45 Gy neoadjuvant external-beam radiation therapy, respectively. Freedom from rectal bleeding, freedom from radiation cystitis, freedom from urethral stricture, freedom from the need for a post-implant TURP, and freedom from any decrease in erectile function compared with the baseline were computed using the actuarial method of Kaplan and Meier.[23] Comparisons were made using a log rank test. One and four patients were not evaluable for rectal toxicity and erectile dysfunction respectively due to lack of information in the patient's chart.

PROSTATE-SPECIFIC ANTIGEN CONTROL

As shown in Table 84.1, there were statistically significant differences in the distribution of the PSA level ($P = 0.0005$), biopsy Gleason score ($P < 0.0001$), and the prostate gland volume ($P < 0.0001$) between surgically and brachytherapy-managed patients. However, only the percent positive prostate biopsies ($P_{Cox} = 0.02$) was a significant predictor of time to post-treatment PSA failure in the Cox regression multivariable analyses in which the pretreatment predictors were analyzed first as continuous and then categorical variables as noted in Table 84.2. Importantly, the distribution of the percent positive biopsies amongst RP- and brachytherapy-managed patients was not significantly different ($P_{chi\ square} = 0.25$) as shown in Table 84.1.

The median (range) PSA nadir for the brachytherapy managed patients was 0.5 (<0.2–1.2) ng/mL. Initial therapy received did not predict for time to post-therapy PSA failure ($P_{Cox} = 0.18$). Specifically, for patients with a minimum 2-year follow up and a median follow-up ranging from 3.95 to 4.2 years, Figure 84.1 illustrates that the 5-year estimates of PSA control were 93% versus 95% ($P_{log\ rank} = 0.16$) following RP or brachy monotherapy respectively.

A few points are worth noting. First, while a Cox proportional-hazards model was used to adjust for

Table 84.2 P-values from the Cox regression multivariable analyses evaluating the ability of the initial therapy received and pretreatment clinical characteristics to predict time to prostate-specific antigen (PSA) failure following treatment

Pretreatment predictor	P value	
	Continuous	Categorical*
Surgery vs brachytherapy	0.18†	0.18
Percent positive biopsies	0.02	0.02
PSA level	0.26	0.18
Biopsy Gleason score	0.42	0.57
Prostate gland volume	0.49	0.62

*Categories: percent positive biopsies (≥34% vs <34%); PSA (4–9.99 ng /mL vs <4 ng/mL); Gleason score (3 + 4 vs ≤6); prostate volume (≥45 cm³ vs <45 cm³). †evaluated as a categorical variable with surgery as the baseline.

significant predictors of the time to PSA failure following initial therapy when comparing the two treatment groups, factors not yet discovered that predict for time to PSA failure following RP or IMRI-guided brachytherapy may be imbalanced between the two treatment arms and can confound the results of this study. Therefore, the findings should be viewed as hypothesis generating and not conclusive.

Second, no matter what definition of PSA failure is used, there remains a bias in favor of radiation because of the time it takes to nadir before a rise can be scored compared with surgery where any value more than 0.2 ng/mL would be considered detectable. This bias has been previously described and noted,[21] and is also noted in this study. Specifically, careful examination of Figure 84.1 will reveal that the brachytherapy-managed patient's PSA control curve is slightly above the surgical control curve during the early years of follow-up reflecting this potential bias.

Third, following brachytherapy, PSA bouncing has been described and in this study population nearly two thirds of patients were reported to experience this effect.[16] As a result, PSA failure could potentially be overestimated in the brachytherapy group. To minimize this problem, PSA determinations were made no more frequently then every 3 months and three consecutive increments in the PSA of at least 0.2 ng/mL needed to be observed in order to define a PSA failure.

Interestingly however, the prostate gland volume was not a significant predictor of time to post-therapy PSA failure when considered as a continuous ($P_{Cox} = 0.49$) or categorical ($P_{Cox} = 0.62$) variable above and below a gland volume of 45 cm³ using a Cox regression multivariable analysis as shown in Table 84.2. Therefore, in the patients selected for implant monotherapy in this study who also had moderate benign prostatic hyperplasia (BPH; n = 81/227, 36% of all study patients had prostate gland volumes of at least 45 cm³), delivering radiation doses to regions of the TZ anterior to the urethra that were less than prescription dose did not appear to negatively impact on PSA outcome.

This lack of impact of prostate gland volume on PSA outcome may be explained by suggesting that patients with moderate BPH would also be expected to have smaller volume cancers compared with patients without BPH and the same PSA level, because some of the serum PSA in patients with BPH was contributed from the benign component of the prostate gland. Another potential explanation may be that for the select group of patients with low-risk disease treated in this study, prostate cancer residing in the TZ may be an infrequent finding. However, given the slow rate of progression expected for the low-risk patients selected for treatment in this study, further follow-up will be needed to evaluate whether these results are maintained.

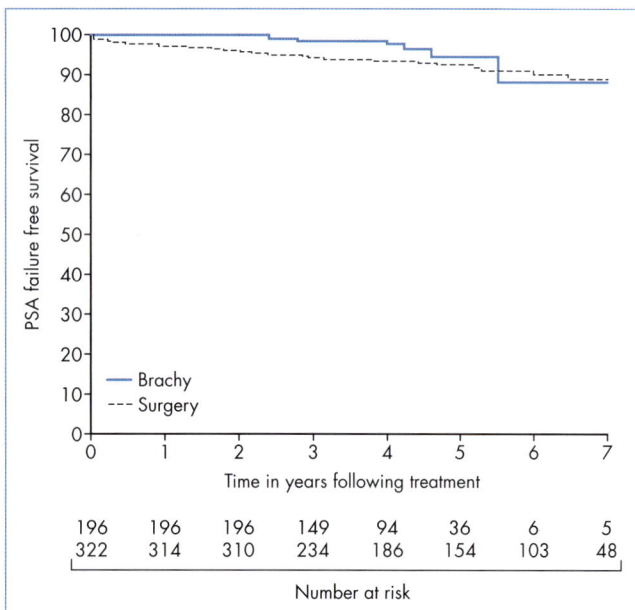

Fig. 84.1

Prostate-specific antigen (PSA) failure-free survival for patients with a minimum follow up of 2 years stratified by initial therapy received. Surgery versus brachytherapy: $P_{log\ rank} = 0.16$.

RADIATION PROCTOPATHY

Estimates of grade 3 rectal bleeding stratified by implant mono or combined modality therapy are shown in Figure 84.2. Four years following initial therapy, estimates of the rates of grade 1, 2, and 3 rectal bleeding were 80% versus 85% ($P_{\text{log rank}}$ = 0.88), 18% versus 22% ($P_{\text{log rank}}$ = 0.16), and 8% versus 30% ($P_{\text{log rank}}$ = 0.0001) for patients who received implant versus combined modality, respectively. All patients who sustained grade 2 or 3 rectal bleeding were controlled using cortisone enemas or APC.

ERECTILE DYSFUNCTION

Figure 84.3 illustrates the estimated rate of patients experiencing any decrease in their ability to have an erection sufficient for vaginal intercourse compared with baseline stratified by initial therapy. While there was a significant difference ($P_{\text{log rank}}$ = 0.03) in patients receiving mono as opposed to combined therapy in the estimate of erectile dysfunction, essentially all patients (82–93%) were estimated to experience some degree of erectile dysfunction compared with baseline within 4 years following therapy. However, as shown in Figure 84.4, when erectile function aids were utilized, which was sildenafil citrate (Viagra®) in 95% of the cases, at least two thirds of patients reported rates of erectile function comparable to or superior to baseline by 4 years following either implant or combined modality therapy ($P_{\text{log rank}}$ = 0.46).

RADIATION CYSTITIS

In two prior reports,[24,25] a decrease in acute urinary retention and urinary obstructive and irritative symptoms have been reported for IMRI-guided compared with TRUS-guided prostate brachytherapy. In this study, there were no events with regard to bladder or urethral dysfunction after implant monotherapy. Specifically, no patient required a post-implant TURP. In addition urethral strictures and radiation cystitis was not documented. However, two patients who received combined modality therapy presented with radiation cystitis. Specifically, cystoscopy performed after a single episode of gross hematuria confirmed this finding. The first patient presented in the setting of a UTI and the hematuria resolved and did not recur following administration of an antibiotic. The other patient's hematuria resolved after bladder irrigation. Neither patient has had recurrent symptoms 3 years following the initial presentation of gross hematuria. Figure 84.5 illustrates the 100% versus 95% ($P_{\text{log rank}}$ = 0.01) estimates of freedom from radiation cystitis at 4 years following treatment for patients who received mono or combined modality therapy respectively.

The quality-of-life results suggest that the ability of the IMRI-guided approach to keep the dose to any point on the urethra at less than 200 Gy was urethral sparing. In particular, urethral and/or bladder toxicity were rare. Specifically, there were no reports of gross hematuria or need for a post-implant TURP, or documentation of urethral stricture for patients treated with monotherapy, and only two patients (5%) were estimated to have radiation cystitis by 4 years following combined modality therapy, both of which were resolved with minimal intervention (antibiotics by mouth and bladder irrigation). These very low rates of late urinary toxicity coupled with the low rates of acute urinary retention[25] and need for post-implant Flomax support the urethral sparing effect of IMRI-guided brachytherapy.

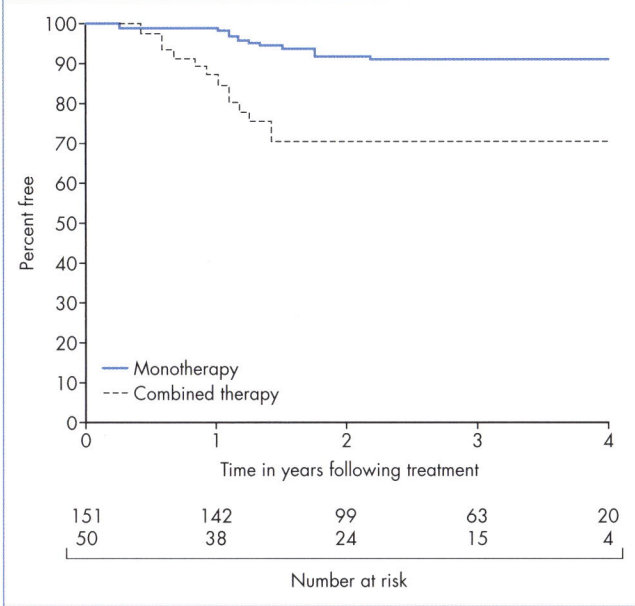

Fig. 84.2

Estimates of grade 3 rectal bleeding following magnetic resonance imaging (MRI)-guided implant monotherapy or combined modality therapy. $P_{\text{log rank}}$ = 0.0001.

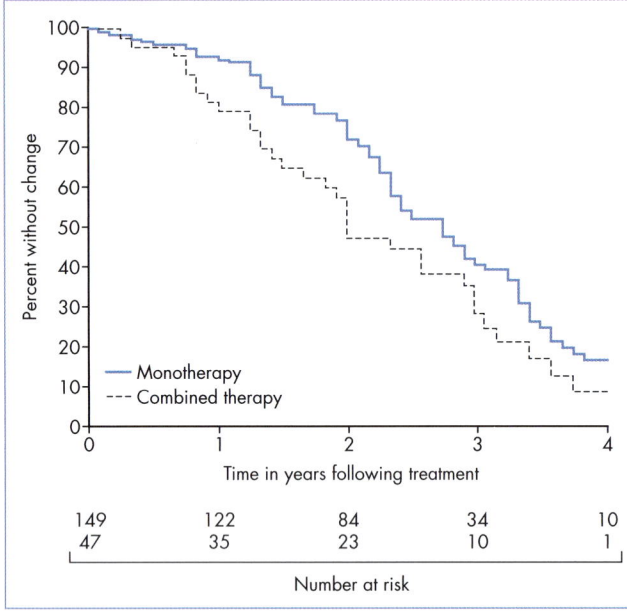

Fig. 84.3
Estimates of erectile function compared with baseline following magnetic resonance imaging (MRI)-guided implant monotherapy or combined modality therapy. $P_{\log rank} = 0.03$.

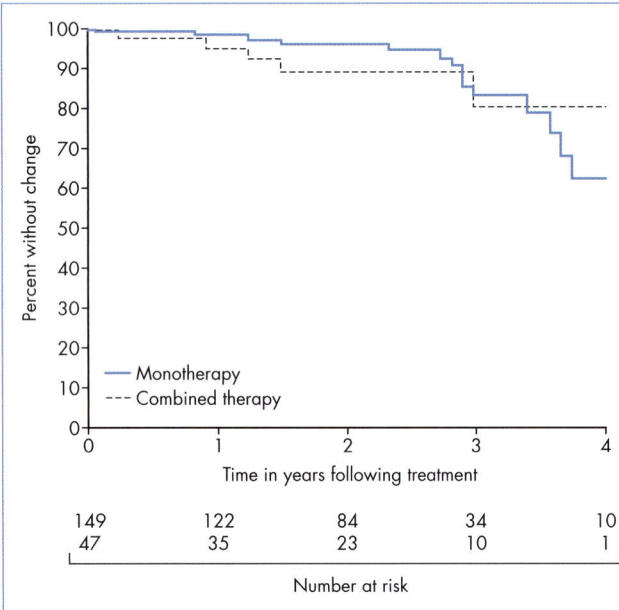

Fig. 84.4
Estimates of erectile function with sildenafil citrate (Viagra) compared with baseline following magnetic resonance imaging (MRI)-guided implant monotherapy or combined modality therapy. $P_{\log rank} = 0.46$.

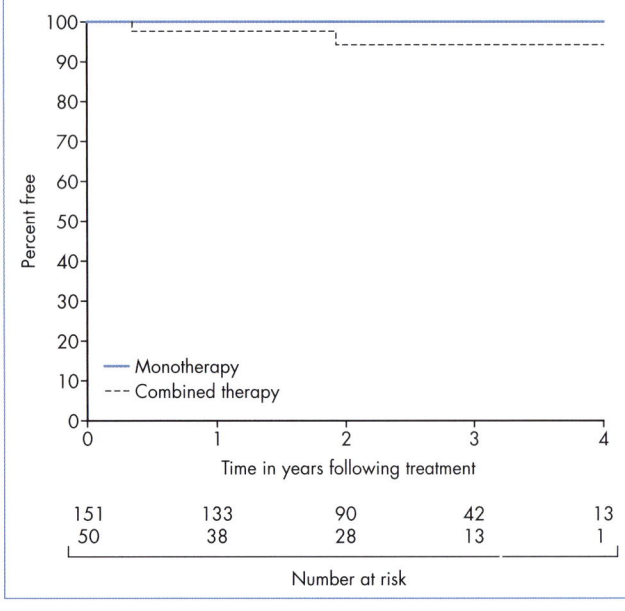

Fig. 84.5
Estimates of freedom from any late urinary dysfunction following magnetic resonance imaging (MRI)-guided implant monotherapy or combined therapy. $P_{\log rank} = 0.01$.

CONCLUSION

Five-year estimates of PSA control following either RP or partial prostatic irradiation using an IMRI-guidance technique[3] in select patients are not significantly different. Longer follow-up will determine if these results are maintained. While estimates of grade 3 rectal bleeding were low following implant monotherapy, they were significantly higher following combined modality therapy. Nearly all patients experienced a decrease in erectile function compared with the baseline, however, the vast majority of patients returned to at least baseline function with the use of sildenafil citrate (Viagra). Urethral and bladder toxicity were rare which may be attributed to the urethral sparing technique of the IMRI-guided approach.

REFERENCES

1. Catalona WJ, Smith DS, Ratliff TL, et al. Detection of organ-confined prostate cancer is increased through prostate-specific antigen-based screening. JAMA 1993;270:948–954.

2. Ragde H, Korb LJ, Elgamal AA, et al. Modern prostate brachytherapy. Prostate specific antigen results in 219 patients with up to 12 years of observed follow up. Cancer 2000;89:135–141.

3. D'Amico AV, Cormack R, Tempany CM, et al. Real time magnetic resonance image guided interstitial brachytherapy in the treatment of select patients with clinically localized prostate cancer. Int J Rad Oncol Biol Phys 1998;42:507–516.

4. Jolesz FA, Kikinis R. Intraoperative imaging revolutionizes therapy. Diagn Imaging 1995;17:62–68.

5. Silverman SG, Jolesz FA, Newman RW, et al. Design and implementation of an interventional MR imaging suite. AM J Roentgenol 1997;168:1465–1471.

6. D'Amico AV, Davis A, Vargas SO, et al. Defining the implant treatment volume for patients with low risk prostate cancer: does the anterior base need to be treated? Int J Radiat Oncol Phys 1999;43:587–590.

7. Takashima R, Egawa S, Kuwao S, et al. Anterior distribution of Stage T1c nonpalpable tumors in radical prostatectomy specimens. Urology 2002;59:692–697.

8. Desai J, Stock RG, Stone NN, et al. Acute urinary morbidity following I-125 interstitial implantation of the prostate gland. radiation oncology investigations. 1998;6:135–141.

9. Thomas MD, Cormack R, Tempany CM, et al. Identifying the predictors of acute urinary retention following magnetic-resonance image guided prostate brachytherapy. Int J Radiat Oncol Biol Phys 2000;47:905–908.

10. Greene FL, Page DL, Fleming ID, et al. American Joint Committee on Cancer, Manual for staging cancer, 6th ed. New York: Springer-Verlag, 2002, pp 337–346.

11. Gleason DF, and the Veterans Administration Cooperative Urological Research Group. Histologic grading and staging of prostatic carcinoma. In: Tannenbaum M (ed.): Urologic pathology. Philadelphia, PA: Lea & Febiger, 1977, pp 171–187.

12. D'Amico AV, Cormack RA, Tempany CM. MRI-guided diagnosis and treatment of prostate cancer. N Engl J Med 2001;344:776–777.

13. Hirose M, Bharatha A, Hata N, et al. Quantitative MR imaging assessment of prostate gland deformation before and during MR imaging-guided brachytherapy. Acad Radiol 2002;9:906–912.

14. Cormack RA, Tempany CM, D'Amico AV. Optimizing target coverage by dosimetric feedback during prostate brachytherapy. Int J Radiat Oncol Biol Phys 2000;48:1245–1249.

15. Cox JD, for the American Society for Therapeutic Radiology and Oncology Consensus Panel. Consensus Statement: Guidelines for PSA Following Radiation Therapy. Int J Radiat Oncol Biol Phys 1997;37:1035–1041.

16. Das P, Chen M, Valentine K, et al. Utilizing the magnitude of PSA bounce following magnetic resonance image guided prostate brachytherapy to distinguish recurrence, benign precipitating factors and idiopathic bounce. Int J Radiat Oncol Biol Phys 2002;54:698–703.

17. Smith S, Wallner K, Domonitz JA, et al. Argon plasma coagulation for rectal bleeding after prostate brachytherapy. Int J Rad Oncol Biol Phys 2001;51:636–642.

18. Venkatesh KS, Ramanujam P. Endoscopic therapy for radiation proctitis-induced hemorrhage in patients with prostatic carcinoma using argon plasma coagulator application. Surg Endosc 2002;16:707–710.

19. Rosen RC, Riley A, Wagner G, et al. The international index of erectile function (IIEF): a multidimension scale for assessment of erectile dysfunction. Urology 1997;49:822–830.

20. Neter J, Wasserman W, Kutner M. Simultaneous inferences and other topic in regression analysis-1. In Neter J, Wasserman W, Kutner M (eds): Applied Linear Regression Models. Homewood, Ill: Richard D Irwin Inc, 1983, pp 150–153.

21. D'Amico AV, Whittington R, Malkowicz SB, et al. Biochemical outcome following radical prostatectomy or external beam radiation therapy for clinically localized prostate cancer in the PSA era. Cancer 2002;95:281–286.

22. Nag S. Brachytherapy for prostate cancer: summary of American Brachytherapy Society recommendations. Semin Urol Oncol 2000;18:133–136.

23. Kaplan EL, Meier P. Non-parametric estimation from incomplete observations. J Am Stat Assoc 1958;53:457–500.

24. Thomas MD, Cormack R, Tempany CM, et al. Identifying the predictor of acute urinary retention following magnetic-resonance-guided prostate brachytherapy. Int J Rad Oncol Biol Phys 2000;47:905–908.

25. Seo PH, Clark JA, Mitchell SP, et al. Early symptoms and symptom distress after standard ultrasound guided brachytherapy or MRI-guided brachytherapy in early stage prostate cancer. Proc Am Soc Clin Oncol 2001;20:157b [abstract #2377].

Hyperthermia for treatment of localized prostate cancer

85

Serdar Deger

INTRODUCTION

Standard therapy for localized prostate cancer is radical prostatectomy. Experience since the mid-1990s has shown that radical surgery could not achieve local tumor control in patients with extracapsular extension of prostate cancer.[1] Looking at long-term results of radical prostatectomy, clinicopathologic parameters influence cancer-specific and overall survival.[2] Unfavorable risk factors like extraprostatic extension and seminal vesical involvement affect long-term biochemical recurrence-free survival.[3]

In the early 1990s radiation therapy was technically improved so that a dose increase within the prostate gland could be achieved.[4–6] Many institutions had suggested that better progression-free survival could be achieved with escalated treatment doses achieved by improvements in treatment planning and delivery technology.[7–11] Intensity modulated radiotherapy (IMRT) is a new form of external beam radiotherapy to achieve higher doses in the prostate without increasing side effects.[12]

Another possibility to raise the radiation dose in the prostate gland is high dose rate brachytherapy. Different institutions were able to demonstrate local tumor control in patients with unfavorable prognostic parameters.[13–15] These data suggested that increasing the intraprostatic dose while reducing side effects could be a treatment strategy for local advanced prostate cancer. To achieve higher doses in the prostate while reducing the nominal radiation brought hyperthermia into this concept. Adding hyperthermia to radiation therapy seems to be an additional strategy to effectively achieve a higher dose in the treatment of prostate cancer.

Cytotoxic effects of hyperthermia were first demonstrated in 1979 by Raaphorst. The extent of the

hyperthermic cytotoxicity depends on the thermal dose, which is a function of the administered amount of heat and the duration of the exposure to the heat.[16,17]

Hyperthermia has been the subject of several recent reviews on results of both phase I/II and randomized studies, demonstrating the benefit of adding hyperthermia.[18,19] Randomized studies have shown that the addition of hyperthermia to radiotherapy does improve the clinical outcome. Additional hyperthermia improved local tumor control rates, palliative effects, and/or overall survival rates for breast cancer,[20] cervical cancer,[21] head and neck tumors,[22] glioblastoma multiforme,[23] and melanoma.[24]

HYPERTHERMIA IN PROSTATE CANCER

Regarding prostate cancer, Ryu reported on radiosensitization using hyperthermia in 1996.[25] Li et al studied apoptosis in irradiated and heated PC-3 prostate cancer cells. They found that apoptosis was an important mode of death in heated cells, but not in irradiated cells. No significant apoptosis was observed when cells were heated to 42°C for 240 minutes; therefore, a heating temperature of 43°C and above may be required to induce significant apoptosis in a clinically feasible duration of time. They concluded that apoptosis-inducing modalities such as hyperthermia may supplement radiation therapy in the future management of prostate cancer.[26]

Peschke et al studied three different sublines (anaplastic, moderately differentiated, and well differentiated) of a Dunning rat prostate carcinoma R3327 model, in which local tumor hyperthermia alone induced growth delay in both differentiated tumors, while the anaplastic tumor subline did not respond. Combining hyperthermia with radiation intensified cell damage in anaplastic tumors.[28,29] This study group also worked on radiation dose rate, sequence, and frequency of heating. They found a clear thermal enhancement of low dose rate irradiation, with maximal sensitization when hyperthermia was given just before irradiation.[29] Mittelberg also reported synergistic effects between hyperthermia and radiation. He concluded that injury of heated and irradiated Dunning cells is likely to be induced by separate mechanisms, which may explain the observed synergy.[30]

It is difficult to achieve adequate hyperthermia temperatures within the prostate under clinical circumstances. Different forms of heat application have been published. The combination of hyperthermia with radiation therapy to treat prostate cancer has been investigated since the 1970s. Several single institution and collaborative group results were disappointing.[31–33] Anscher et al[31] reported 3-year disease-free survival rates of 25%. The main problem of this study was the inability to achieve adequate therapeutic temperatures within the prostate.

The option to overcome the limitations of external heating systems is interstitial hyperthermia. The interstitial application modality of hyperthermia seems to be interesting for urologist. In the early 1990s, a transrectal ultrasound device was developed specially for prostate hyperthermia.[34,35] A phase I trial combining transrectal hyperthermia using a transrectal ultrasound device with external beam radiation therapy was performed at the University of Arizona by Fosmire et al.[36] The ultrasound power is delivered from a water cooled 16-element partial-cylindrical intracavitary array. Fosmire et al measured an average temperature, using thermocouples, of only 41.9 ± 0.9∞C over 30 min. Using this device, a phase II trial of hyperthermia and external beam radiation therapy with or without hormonal therapy for locally advanced prostate cancer was performed by Hurwitz on nine patients with clinical T2b to T3b prostate cancer.[37] The total dose was 6660 cGy ± 5% of the prescribed target volume using a 3D conformal technique. Acute toxicity was limited to National Cancer Institute Common Toxicity Criteria grade 1. No excess toxicity was noted with full course of radiation therapy with or without hormonal therapy. This study group reported on approximately 30 patients having rectal toxicity using the described method in 2002.[38] A cooling water bolus was maintained between 33∞C and 37∞C to keep the maximum rectal wall temperature within treatment guidelines. Rectal toxicity was correlated with maximum allowable rectal wall temperature of >40∞C (7 of 11 patients had an acute grade 2 proctitis). Both papers, however, do not include oncologic data.

Using the same ultrasound device, long-term toxicities with the combination of hyperthermia and radiation for treatment of prostate cancer in 26 patients

with stage T3 or N+ prostate cancer with a median follow-up of 71 months were reported by Algan et al.[39] They had no additional toxicity. Disease free survival rate was 39% in a patient population with a median pretreatment prostate-specific antigen (PSA) level of 29 ng/mL.

Using regional radiofrequency systems resulted in relatively low temperatures in the tumor.[40] A phase I study was reported in 1994, which included 36 patients with prostate cancer (5 with locally recurrent, 15 with T2, and 16 T3 prostate cancer), treated with radiofrequency-induced hyperthermia and high dose rate brachytherapy from 1987 until 1992.[41] In this study 2D-steered 0.5-MHz radiofrequency-induced interstitial hyperthermia was administered in combination with 50 Gy external radiation for 5 weeks, followed by 30 Gy high dose rate brachytherapy using iridium-192 (^{192}Ir). Two hyperthermia sessions of 45 min were planned, immediately before and after brachytherapy. Between 7 and 32 1.5-mm steel trocar hyperthermia electrodes were positioned transperineally in the prostate. The treatment was well tolerated.

To overcome the problem of too low local temperatures in the prostate using a radiofrequency system, a multielectrode current source (MECS) interstitial hyperthermia system was developed. This system uses segmented radiofrequency electrodes. Each individual electrode controls the locally measured tissue temperature.[42,43]

In 2003, van Pulpen et al[44] published data from 26 patients, treated between 1997 and 2001 with T3 to T4, Nx prostate cancer. Of 14 patients, 5 received weekly regional hyperthermia treatments within a phase II study, using the coaxial transverse electrical magnetic system with a mean follow up of 3 years. Twelve patients received one interstitial hyperthermia treatment within a phase I trial, using the multielectrode current source system. Radiation therapy was administered to a total dose of 70 Gy in 2-Gy fractions over 7 weeks using a conformal three-field technique. There was no severe toxicity. All patients survived; 27% of patients had a biochemical relapse. Three of these patients were in the regional and four patients were in the interstitial group. The actuarial probability of freedom from biochemical relapse was 79% for the regional and 57% for the interstitial group. Actuarial probability of freedom from biochemical relapse was 70% at 36 months for all patients.

Kalapurakal et al reported a phase I/II study in 13 patients with locally advanced, hormone-refractory prostate cancer using thermoradiotherapy[45] between 1997 and 2002. Eight patients had a recurrence of the disease after radiotherapy and five had recurrence without having prior radiotherapy. All patients had clinical symptomatic disease. The patients with prior radiation received 39.6 Gy and those without prior external beam radiation received 66.6 Gy. Hyperthermia was applied in 8 to 10 sessions, using MECS. Despite the size of these large tumors, radiotherapy and hyperthermia resulted in significant tumor shrinkage, rapid serum prostate-specific antigen decline, durable treatment responses, and durable palliation of symptoms in a median follow-up of 13 to 14 months for both groups.

An innovative technique for interstitial hyperthermia is the use of implantable ferromagnetic thermoseeds. They are heated by induction in a magnetic field based on the so-called Curie temperature, at which the material loses its magnetic dipole momentum. Paramagnetism occurs when the temperature of an alloy rises above this level. Ferromagnetism is based on the quantum-mechanic nature of the inner electrons of a material and leads to the generation of a dipole. When the magnetic field oscillates and the ferromagnetic material is exposed to a surrounding field, atomic dipoles straighten out and heat is generated. The material heats up until the Curie temperature is reached and the ferromagnetic characteristics are lost. The selection of alloys allows for a self-regulating system according to the respective Curie temperatures.[46–48] As the thermoseeds remain in the prostate, hyperthermia induction can, therefore, be repeated as often as necessary, even in case of local tumor recurrence.

Different studies worked with animal models using ferromagnetic thermoseeds for prostate treatment.[49–51] Deger et al[52] described a combination of interstitial hyperthermia with external radiation therapy for prostate cancer patients. They used ferromagnetic cobalt–palladium alloy thermoseeds. This study group examined several alloys (e.g., nickel–copper) to come to the optimal biocompatibility, and cobalt–palladium was the most promising alloy.[47,53,54] Other investigators also reported palladium–nickel and ferrite core/metallic sheath thermoseeds.[55,56]

Using thermoseeds overcomes the problem of routine clinical application of hyperthermia. Advantages of thermoseeds are exactly defined energy application in the tumor with protection of benign tissue, more effective local therapy, homogeneous energy distribution and compact measure matrix, as well as better representation of invasively measured temperatures.

Deger et al used thermoseeds with a Curie temperature of 55°C in a phase II trial.[57,58] They added a 3D-conformal radiotherapy of 68.4 Gy given simultaneously to the hyperthermia in daily fractions of 1.8 Gy. A patented coil system of 50 kHz was utilized to establish the magnetic field. Patients received 1-hour hyperthermia at intervals of 1 week for 6 sessions. Temperatures were measured using thermocouples. The intraprostatic, urethral, and rectal temperatures were between 42°C and 48°C, between 38°C and 43°C, and between 37°C and 39.5°C, respectively.[59] A median follow-up of 36 months was published for this patient

population in 2004. There was no seed migration observed on follow-up X-rays and no major side effects during hyperthermia. The initial median PSA value was 11.6 ng/mL, which regressed after 12, 24, and 36 months to 1.1 ng/mL, 0.9 ng/mL, and 0.6 ng/mL, respectively. Forty-two percent of the patients reached a PSA nadir of 0.5 ng/mL in a median time of 12 months. Nine patients progressed at a median time of 20 months. Three patients had local and six patients had systemic progression.[60] Prostate-specific antigen follow-up data of this patient group were equal to the data of the patients who were treated with a high dose rate brachytherapy, and better than the data of those patients who received conformal radiation therapy in the same institution.[61]

Another exciting new tool for applying interstitial hyperthermia is nanoparticle technology. Jordan et al reported that magnetic fluid hyperthermia (MFH) selectively heats up tissue by coupling alternating current magnetic fields to targeted magnetic fluids, so that boundaries of different conductive tissues do not interfere with power absorption.[62]

This is a completely new approach to deep tissue hyperthermia application. It couples the energy magnetically to nanoparticles in the target region. A new aminosilan-type nanoparticle preparation (manufactured at the Institute of New Materials [INM] Saarbruecken, Germany) is taken up by prostate carcinoma cells but not by normal prostate cells. Preliminary data indicate that the malignant cells take up nine times more particles than normal cells do.[62] Johannsen et al[63] published the first experimental data using this technology on a rat model of prostate cancer. They used an orthotopic Dunning R3327 prostate cancer model on male Copenhagen rats. The animals either received MFH treatment following intratumoral administration of magnetic fluids or were used as either tumor growth controls to determine iron distribution in selected organs or as histologic controls without MFH treatment. The MFH treatments were carried out at 45°C or 50°C using an alternating current (AC) magnetic field applicator system. Sequential treatments with MFH were possible following a single intratumoral injection of magnetic fluid. Intratumoral temperatures of 50°C and more were obtained and were monitored online using fluoro-optic thermometry. Four days after MFH treatments, 79% of the injected dose of ferrites was still present in the prostate.

Interstitial hyperthermia in combination with conformal radiotherapy may be a powerful new method to improve the results of external radiation therapy for localized prostate cancer. Most studies describe feasibility and toxicity. Quality-of-life studies are urgently needed in this area. Van Pulpen et al[64] published a prospective quality-of-life study in patients with locally advanced prostate cancer, treated with radiotherapy with or without regional or interstitial hyperthermia. They concluded that after radiotherapy with or without hyperthermia only a temporary deterioration of quality of life occurs, concerning social, psychological, and disease-related symptoms. Additional hyperthermia does not seem to decrease quality of life.

Nevertheless, the addition of hyperthermia to different treatment strategies like chemotherapeutics[65,66] or thermo- or radiosensitizing modalities[67-69] has further research potential for the new treatment strategies of localized prostate cancer.

REFERENCES

1. Zietman AL, Shipley WU, Willet CG. Residual disease after radical surgery or radiation therapy for prostate cancer—clinical significance and therapeutic implications. Cancer 1993;71:959–969.
2. Roehl KA, Han M, Ramos CG, et al. Cancer Progression and survival rates following anatomical radical retropubic prostatectomy in 3478 consecutive patients: long term results. J Urol 2004;172:910–914.
3. Khan MA, Partin AW, Mangold LA, et al. Probability of biochemical recurrence by analysis of pathologic stage, Gleason score, and margin status for localized prostate cancer. Urology 2003;62:866–871.
4. Hanks GE, Schultheiss TE, Hunt MA, et al. Factors influencing incidence of acute grade 2 morbidity in conformal and standard radiation treatment of prostate cancer. Int J Radiat Oncol Biol Phys 1995;31:25–29.
5. Schultheiss TE, Hanks GE, Hunt MA, et al. Incidence of and factors related to late complications in conformal and conventional radiation treatment of cancer of the prostate. Int J Radiat Oncol Biol Phys 1995;32:643–650.
6. Hanks GE, Hanlon AL, Schultheiss TE, et al. Conformal beam treatment of prostate cancer. Urology 1997;50:87–92.
7. Pollack A, Zagars GK. External beam radiotherapy dose response of prostate cancer. Int J Radiat Oncol Biol Phys 1997;39:1011–1018.
8. Pollack A, Smith LG, von Eschenbach AC. External beam radiotherapy dose response characteristics of 1127 men with prostate cancer treated in the PSA era. Int J Radiat Oncol Biol Phys 2000;48:507–512.
9. Hanks GE, Hanlon AL, Schultheiss TE, et al. Dose escalation with 3D conformal treatment: five year outcomes, treatment optimization, and future directions. Int J Radiat Oncol Biol Phys 1998;41:501–510.
10. Zelefsky MJ, Leibel SA, Gaudin PB, et al. Dose escalation with three-dimensional conformal radiation therapy affects the outcome in prostate cancer. Int J Radiat Oncol Biol Phys 1998;41:491–500.
11. Lyons JA, Kupelian PA, Mohan DS, et al. Importance of high radiation doses (72 Gy or greater) in the treatment of stage T1-T3 adenocarcinoma of the prostate. Urology 2000;55:85–90.
12. Roach M 3rd. Reducing the toxicity associated with the use of radiotherapy in men with localized prostate cancer. Urol Clin North Am 2004;31:353–366.
13. Deger S, Boehmer D, Tuerk I, et al. High dose rate brachytherapy of localized prostate cancer. Eur Urol 2002;41:420–426.
14. Martinez A, Gonzalez J, Spencer W, et al. Conformal high dose rate brachytherapy improves biochemical control and causes specific survival in patients with prostate cancer and poor prognostic factors. J Urol 2003;169:974–980.
15. Galalae RM, Kovacs G, Schultze J, et al. Long term outcome after elective irradiation of the pelvic lymphatics and local dose escalation using high dose rate brachytherapy for locally advanced prostate cancer. Int J Radiat Oncol Biol Phys 2002;52:81–90.
16. Raaphorst GP, Romano SL, Mitchell JB, et al. Intrinsic differences in heat and/or x-ray sensitivity of seven mammalian cell lines cultured and treated under identical conditions. Cancer Res 1979;39:396–401.
17. Sapareto SA, Dewey WC. Thermal dose determination in cancer therapy. Int J Radiat Oncol Biol Phys 1984;10:787–800.
18. Hildebrandt B, Wust P, Ahlers O, et al. The cellular and molecular basis of hyperthermia. Crit Rev Oncol Hematol 2002;43:33–56.
19. Van der Zee J. Heating the patient: A promising approach? Ann Oncol 2002;13:1173–1184.
20. Vernon CC, Hand JW, Field SB, et al. Radiotherapy with or without hyperthermia in the treatment of superficial breast cancer: Results from five randomized controlled trials. International Collaborative Hyperthermia Group. Int J Radiat Oncol Biol Phys 1996;35:731–744.
21. Van der Zee J, Gonzalez Gonzalez D, Van Rhoon GC, et al. Comparison of radiotherapy alone with radiotherapy plus hyperthermia in locally advanced pelvic tumours: A prospective, randomised, multicentre trial. Lancet 2000;355:1119–1125.
22. Valdagni R, Amichetti M. Report of long-term follow-up in a randomized trial comparing radiation therapy and radiation therapy plus hyperthermia to metastatic lymph nodes in stage IV head and neck patients. Int J Radiat Oncol Biol Phys 1994;28:163–169.
23. Sneed PK, Stauffer PR, McDermott MW, et al. Survival benefit of hyperthermia in a prospective randomized trial of brachytherapy boost +/- hyperthermia for glioblastoma multiforme. Int J Radiat Oncol Biol Phys 1998;40:287–295.
24. Overgaard J, Gonzalez Gonzalez D, Hulshof MCCM, et al. Randomised trial of hyperthermia as adjuvant to radiotherapy for recurrent or metastatic malignant melanoma. Lancet 1995;345:163–169.
25. Ryu S, Brown SL, Khil MS, et al. Preferential radiosensitization of human prostatic carcinoma cells by mild hyperthermia. Int J Radiat Oncol Biol Phys 1996;34:133–138.
26. Li WX, Franklin WA. Radiation- and heat-induced apoptosis in PC-3 prostate cancer cells. Radiat Res 1998 Aug;150:190–194.
27. Peschke P, Hahn EW, Wenz F, et al. Differential sensitivity of three sublines of the rat Dunning prostate tumor system R3327 to radiation and/or local tumor hyperthermia. Radiat Res 1998;150:190–194.
28. Peschke P, Klein V, Wolber G, et al. Morphometric analysis of bromodeoxyuridine distribution and cell density in the rat Dunning prostate tumor R3327-AT1 following treatment with radiation and/or hyperthermia. Histol Histopathol 1999;14:461–469.
29. Peschke P, Hahn EW, Wolber G, et al. Interstitial radiation and hyperthermia in the Dunning R3327 prostate tumour model: therapeutic efficacy depends on radiation dose-rate, sequence and frequency of heating. Int J Radiat Biol 1996;70:609–616.
30. Mittelberg KN, Tucker RD, Loening SA, et al. Effect of radiation and hyperthermia on prostate tumor cells with induced thermal tolerance and the correlation with HSP70 accumulation. Urol Oncol 1996;2:146–151.
31. Anscher MS, Samulski TV, Dodge R, et al. Combined external beam irradiation and external regional hyperthermia for locally advanced adenocarcinoma of the prostate. Int J Radiat Oncol Biol Phys 1997;37:1059–1065.
32. Emami B, Scott C, Perez CA, et al. Phase III study of interstitial thermoradiotherapy compared with interstitial radiotherapy alone in the treatment of recurrent or persistent human tumors. A prospectively controlled randomized study by the Radiation Therapy Group. Int J Radiat Oncol Biol Phys 1996;34:1097–1104.
33. Myerson RJ, Scott CB, Emami B, et al. A phase I/II study to evaluate radiation therapy and hyperthermia for deep-seated tumours: a report of RTOG 89-08. Int J Hyperthermia 1996;12:449–459.
34. Hynynen K. Ultrasound heating technology. In Seegenschmiedt MH, Fessenden P, Vernon CC (eds): Thermo-Radiotherapy and Thermo-Chemotherapy, vol. 1. Berlin: Springer-Verlag, 1995, p 253.
35. Diederich CJ, Hynynen K. The development of intracavitary ultrasonic applicators for hyperthermia:a design and experimental study. Med Phys 1990;17:626–634.
36. Fosmire H, Hynynen K, Drach GW, et al. Feasibility and toxicity of transrectal ultrasound hyperthermia in the treatment of locally advanced adenocarcinoma of the prostate. Int J Radiat Oncol Biol Phys 1993;26:253–259.
37. Hurwitz MD, Kaplan ID, Svensson GK, et al. Feasibility and patient tolerance of a novel transrectal ultrasound hyperthermia system for treatment of prostate cancer. Int J Hyperthermia 2001;17:31–37.
38. Hurwitz MD, Kaplan ID, Hansen JL, et al. Association of rectal toxicity with thermal dose parameters in treatment of locally advanced prostate cancer with radiation and hyperthermia. Int J Radiat Oncol Biol Phys 2002;53:913–918.

39. Algan O, Fosmire H, Hynynen K, et al. External beam radiotherapy and hyperthermia in the treatment of patients with locally advanced prostate carcinoma. Cancer 2000;89:399–403.

40. Raaymakers BW, Van Vulpen M, Lagendijk JJ, et al. Determination and validation of the actual 3D temperature distribution during interstitial hyperthermia of prostate carcinoma. Phys Med Biol 2001;46:3115–3131.

41. Prionas SD, Kapp DS, Goffinet DR, et al. Thermometry of interstitial hyperthermia given as an adjuvant to brachytherapy for the treatment of carcinoma of the prostate. Int J Radiat Oncol Biol Phys 1994;28:151–162.

42. van der Koijk JF, Lagendijk JJ, Crezee J, et al. The influence of vasculature on temperature distributions in MECS interstitial hyperthermia: Importance of longitudinal control. Int J Hypertherm 1997;13:365–385.

43. Kaatee RS, Crezee J, Kanis AP, et al. Design of applicators for a 27 MHz multielectrode current source interstitial hyperthermia system; impedance matching and effective power. Phys Med Biol. 1997;6:1087–1108.

44. Van Vulpen M, De Leeuw AA, Raaymakers BW, et al. Radiotherapy and hyperthermia in the treatment of patients with locally advanced prostate cancer: preliminary results. BJU Int. 2004;93:36–41.

45. Kalapurakal JA, Pierce M, Chen A, et al. Efficacy of irradiation and external hyperthermia in locally advanced, hormone-refractory or radiation recurrent prostate cancer: a preliminary report. Int J Radiat Oncol Biol Phys. 2003;57:654–664.

46. Case JA, Tucker RD, Park JB. Defining the heating characteristics of ferromagnetic implants using calorimetry. J Biomed Mater Res 2000;53:791–798.

47. Le UT, Tucker RD, Park JB. The effects of localized cold work on the heating characteristics of thermal therapy implants. J Biomed Mater Res 2002;63:24–30.

48. Tucker RD, Ehrenstein T, Loening SA. Thermal ablation using interstitial temperature self regulating cobalt - palladium seeds. A new treatment alternative for localized prostate cancer ? In Schnorr D, Loening SA, Dinges S, Budach V (eds): Lokal fortgeschrittenes Prostatakarzinom. Berlin: Blackwell, 1995, 221–240.

49. Paulus JA, Tucker RD, Loening SA, et al. Thermal ablation of canine prostate using interstitial temperature self-regulating seeds:new treatment for prostate cancer. J Endourol 1997;11:295–300.

50. Tompkins DT, Vanderby R, Klein SA, et al. The use of generalized cell-survival data in a physiologically based objective function for hyperthermia treatment planning: a sensitivity study with a simple tissue model implanted with an array of ferromagnetic thermoseeds. Int J Radiat Oncol Biol Phys 1994;30:929–943.

51. Tompkins DT, Vanderby R, Klein SA, et al. Temperature-dependent versus constant-rate blood perfusion modelling in ferromagnetic thermoseed hyperthermia: results with a model of the human prostate. Int J Hyperthermia 1994;10:517–536.

52. Deger S, Boehmer D, Roigas J, et al. Interstitial hyperthermia using thermoseeds in combination with conformal radiotherapy for localized prostate cancer. Front Radiat Ther Oncol 2002;36:171–176.

53. Ferguson SD, Paulus JA, Tucker RD, et al. Effect of thermal treatment on heating characteristics of Ni-Cu alloy for hyperthermia: preliminary studies. J Appl Biomater 1993;4:55–60.

54. Paulus JA, Parida GR, Tucker RD, et al. Corrosion analysis of NiCu and PdCo thermal seed alloys used as interstitial hyperthermia implants. Biomaterials. 1997;18:1609–1614.

55. Cetas TC, Gross EJ, Contractor Y. A ferrite core/metallic sheath thermoseed for interstitial thermal therapies. IEEE Trans Biomed Eng 1998;45:68–77.

56. Meijer JG, van Wieringen N, Koedooder C, et al. The development of PdNi thermoseeds for interstitial hyperthermia. Med Phys 1995;22:101–104.

57. Deger S, Boehmer D, Tuerk I, et al. Thermoradiotherapy with interstitial thermoseeds in treatment of local prostatic carcinoma. Initial results of a phase II study. Urologe A 2001;403:195–198.

58. Deger S, Boehmer D, Tuerk I, et al. Interstitial hyperthermia using self-regulating thermoseeds combined with conformal radiation therapy. Eur Urol 2002;2:147–153.

59. Tucker RD, Loening SA, Huidobro C, et al. The use of permanent interstitial temperature self regulating rods for the treatment of prostate cancer. [Abstract] Rad Oncol 2000;55:132.

60. Deger S, Taymoorian K, Boehmer D, et al. Thermoradiotherapy using interstitial self-regulating thermoseeds: an intermediate analysis of a phase II trial. Eur Urol 2004;45:574–579.

61. Deger S, Boehmer D, Tuerk I, et al. High dose rate brachytherapy of localized prostate cancer. Eur Urol 2002;41:420–426.

62. Jordan A, Scholz R, Maier-Hauff K, et al. Presentation of a new magnetic field therapy system for the treatment of human solid tumors with magnetic fluid hyperthermia. J Magn Magn Mater 2001;225:118–126.

63. Johannsen M, Jordan A, Scholz R, et al. Evaluation of magnetic fluid hyperthermia in a standard rat model of prostate cancer. J Endourol 2004;18:495–500.

64. Van Vulpen M, De Leeuw JR, Van Gellekom MP, et al. Prospective quality of life study in patients with locally advanced prostate cancer, treated with radiotherapy with or without regional or interstitial hyperthermia. Int J Hyperthermia 2003;19:402–413.

65. Roigas J, Wallen ES, Loening SA, et al. Estramustine phosphate enhances the effects of hyperthermia and induces the small heat shock protein HSP27 in the human prostate carcinoma cell line PC-3. Urol Res 2002;30:130–155.

66. Roigas J, Wallen ES, Loening SA, et al. Effects of combined treatment of chemotherapeutics and hyperthermia on survival and the regulation of heat shock proteins in Dunning R3327 prostate carcinoma cells. Prostate 1998;34:195–202.

67. Asea A, Mallick R, Lechpammer S, et al. Cyclooxygenase inhibitors are potent sensitizers of prostate tumours to hyperthermia and radiation. Int J Hyperthermia 2000;17:401–414.

68. Asea A, Ara G, Teicher BA, et al. Effects of the flavonoid drug quercetin on the response of human prostate tumours to hyperthermia in vitro and in vivo. Int J Hyperthermia 2001;17:347–356.

69. Lee YJ, Lee H, Borrelli MJ. Gene transfer into human prostate adenocarcinoma cells with an adenoviral vector: Hyperthermia enhances a double suicide gene expression, cytotoxicity and radiotoxicity. Cancer Gene Ther 2002;9:267–274.

Initial management of high risk early stage prostate cancer: radiation

86

Eric M Horwitz, Steven J Feigenberg, Alan Pollack

INTRODUCTION

Because there are many treatment options for nonmetastatic prostate cancer, it is vitally important to define risk and determine a patient's prognosis to aid in the treatment design. Risk is defined many ways, although the single most important prognostic variable is a person's pretreatment PSA level.[1] Other important variables include Gleason score, T stage, and radiation dose.[2] At Fox Chase Cancer Center (FCCC) and elsewhere, these variables are used to categorize men into multiple risk groups.[3-5] Patients with low-risk disease include those with PSA (10 ng/mL, Gleason score 2 to 6 and T1c/T2a disease. The high-risk group consists of patients having one of the following high-risk features: Gleason score 8 to 10, PSA greater than 20 ng/mL, or T3/T4 disease. Intermediate-risk patients do not fit into either of the above risk groups. Treatment options for low- and high-risk disease are discussed elsewhere. The focus of this chapter is on radiation treatment options for men with intermediate risk prostate cancer.

Over the last few decades, the goal for radiation oncologists has been to improve the therapeutic index by increasing radiation dose to the cancer or target (prostate in this case) while restricting or decreasing dose to the surrounding normal tissue (bladder and rectum). This will allow the delivery of a lethal dose of radiation to the cancer while protecting the normal tissue and minimizing side effects. This can be accomplished using a variety of radiation techniques.

RADIATION TREATMENT TECHNIQUES

Planning for patients treated with conventional radiation therapy (RT) is the least complex of these techniques. These patients undergo simulation (planning) and treatment in the supine position. Custom immobilization devices are usually not utilized. Rectal and bladder contrast and retrograde urethrograms to aid in the localization of the prostate are not mandatory during the simulation. Treatment fields are based upon bony landmarks from orthogonal radiographs. Radiation dose distributions for conventional treatment plans are typically generated in a single plane, and the dose is prescribed at the isocenter and normalized at the 100% isodose line.

For patients treated with three-dimensional conformal radiation therapy (3DCRT), the planning begins first by defining treatment volumes including both the target (prostate) and the surrounding normal structures (bladder and rectum most importantly) based on a 3D data set. Target volumes are defined according to the International Commission on Radiation Units and Measurements (ICRU) report 50.[6] Three-dimensional conformal radiation therapy is the process where the radiation dose is planned and delivered so that the high-dose volume conforms to an accurately defined target volume. This process minimizes the volume of normal tissue receiving a clinically significant radiation dose, thereby reducing the probability of normal tissue complications.

As with 3DCRT, planning for treatment with intensity modulated radiation therapy (IMRT) begins by defining the target and normal tissues. This technique can achieve tighter dose distributions through the use of non-uniform intensity radiation beams. Each beam is divided into multiple segments or beamlets. The target volume and critical normal organs are defined and the upper and lower dose limits for the target and normal structures selected. The quality of the plan is assessed using dose–volume histograms (DVHs), which graphically represent the specific dose of radiation the volume an organ receives (Figure 86.1).

RADIATION DOSE ESCALATION

Beginning in the 1980s, prospective dose-escalation studies were conducted at Fox Chase Cancer Center (FCCC) and the University of Michigan and Memorial Sloan-Kettering Cancer Center (MSKCC).[7–9] At Fox Chase, the first patients to benefit from increased dose were those with intermediate features. Pinover et al reported the Fox Chase experience treating patients with pretreatment prostate-specific antigen (PSA) levels greater than 10 ng/mL. Patients were placed in good (T1–T2a, Gleason score 2–6, absence of perineural invasion) or poor risk strata based on palpation T stage, Gleason score and the presence of perineural invasion and biochemical non-evidence of disease (bNED) control was calculated based upon radiation dose received. Patients were stratified into three groups according to dose: less than 72.50 Gy; 72.50 to 75.99 Gy; and greater than or equal to 76 Gy. Median dose in these three groups was 70.67 Gy, 72.78 Gy, and 77.34 Gy, respectively. bNED control was 91% versus 76% at 5 years for good risk patients treated

with greater than or equal to 71.5 Gy and less than 71.5 Gy, respectively. The same trend was observed for the poor risk patients (98%, 79%, and 72% for ≥74.5, 71.5–74.5, and <71.5 Gy, respectively).[10]

The long-term results from the original group of prostate cancer patients treated in the first prospective FCCC radiation dose-escalation study with an 8 to 12 year follow-up was reported by Hanks et al.[7] Between 1989 and 1992, 232 patients with clinically localized prostate cancer were treated with 3DCRT alone at FCCC on a prospective dose-escalation study and 229 patients were evaluable. The median total dose for all patients was 74 Gy (range: 67–81 Gy). The median follow-up for patients alive was 110 months (range: 89–147 months). bNED control was defined using the American Society of Therapeutic Radiology and Oncology (ASTRO) definition and for all patients included in this series was 55% at 5 years, 48% at 10 years, and 48% at 12 years.[11] Only for patients with pretreatment PSA levels of 10 to 20 ng/mL were statistically significant differences in bNED control seen for all patients stratified by dose from less than 71.5, 71.5 to 75.6, and more than 75.6 Gy (19%, 31%, 84%, respectively; p = 0.0003) (Table 86.1). For the 229 patients with follow-up, 124 (54%) were clinically and biochemically free of disease. Sixty-nine patients were alive at the time of last follow-up and 55 patients were dead of intercurrent disease. On multivariate analysis, radiation dose was a statistically significant predictor of bNED control for all of the patients. Freedom from distant metastases (DM) for all patients was 89%, 83%, and 83% at 5, 10, and 12 years, respectively. For patients with pretreatment PSA levels less than 10 ng/mL, all four covariates (radiation dose, Gleason score, pretreatment PSA, and T stage) were significant predictors of DM. Based on the RTOG morbidity scale, there was no difference in the frequency of grade 2 and 3 genito-urinary (GU) and grade 3 gastrointestinal (GI) morbidity when patients in this dataset were stratified by radiation dose. There was, however, a significant increase in grade 2 GI complications as radiation dose increased.

Long-term data from institutions including FCCC, MSKCC, the Cleveland Clinic and M.D. Anderson Cancer Center (MDACC) show increased rates of bNED control, especially for patients with pretreatment PSA levels less than 10 ng/mL (Figures 86.2 and 86.3).[4,7,12,13] The 10-year update of the MSKCC dose comparison trial was reported by Zelefsky et al; MSKCC risk groups are similar to those at FCCC and are based on the presence or absence of the following parameters: PSA less than 10 ng/mL, stage T1 to T2, and Gleason score less than 7 disease. The favorable risk group has all three parameters present, the intermediate risk group has two parameters present, and the unfavorable risk group has none or only one parameter present. Eight hundred twenty

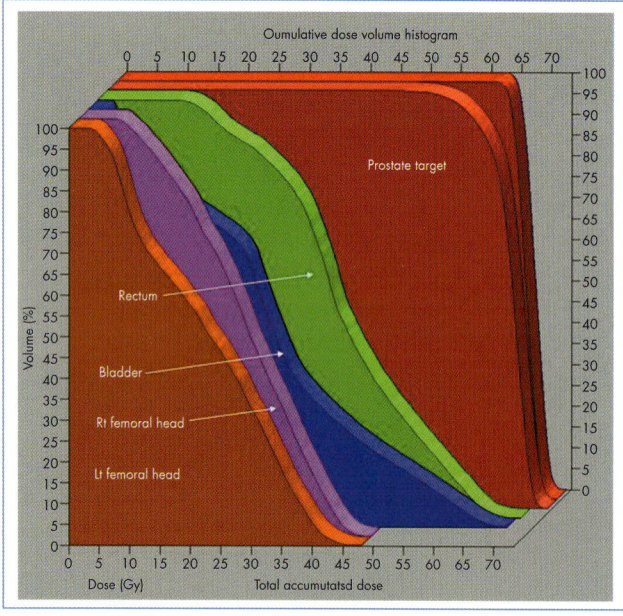

Fig. 86.1
Dose–volume histogram (DVH) for an intensity modulated radiotherapy (IMRT) treatment plan.

Table 86.1 Eight-year biochemical non-evidence of disease (bNED) control rates at Fox Chase Cancer Center stratified by pretreatment prostate-specific antigen (PSA) level, radiation dose, and prognostic group

Pretreatment PSA (ng/mL)	Dose group (Gy)	Median dose (Gy)	All patients	Favorable (events)	Unfavorable (events)
<10	<70	69	68%	5/23 (73%)	3/7 (44%)
	70–71.9	71	74%	3/22 (85%)	5/11 (51%)
	>72	76	69%	4/16 (75%)	5/15 (64%)
Significance			p = 0.9518	p = 0.7219	p = 0.7388
10–20	<71.5	70	19%	7/13 (30%)	6/8 (0%)
	71.5–75.75	72	31%	5/11 (37%)	6/10 (36%)
	>75.75	76	84%	1/17 (92%)	3/11 (73%)
Significance			p = 0.0003	p = 0.0065	p = 0.0265
>20	<71.5	70	8%	8/10 (13%)	8/9 (44%)
	71.5–75.75	73	23%	5/6 (17%)	10/15 (51%)
	>75.75	76	11%	4/7 (38%)	16/18 (64%)
Significance			p = 0.34	p = 0.3180	p = 0.3745

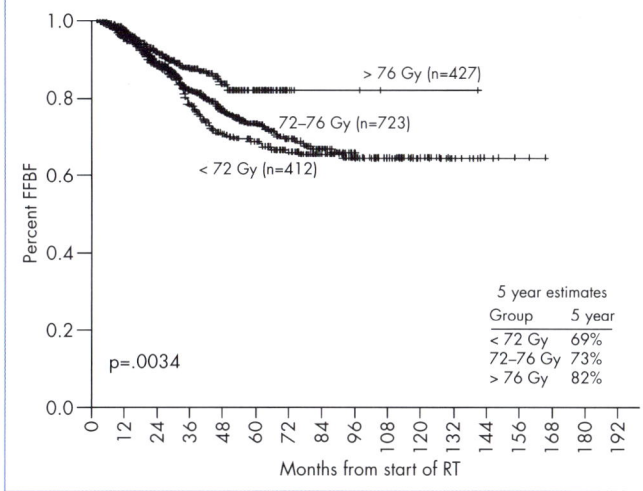

Fig. 86.2

Biochemical non-evidence of disease (bNED) control for all Fox Chase Cancer Center patients treated in the prostate-specific antigen (PSA) era with 3D conformal radiotherapy (3DCRT). They are subdivided into three dose groups: <72 Gy, 72–76 Gy, and >76 Gy. (FFBF, freedom from biochemical failure; RT, radiotherapy.)

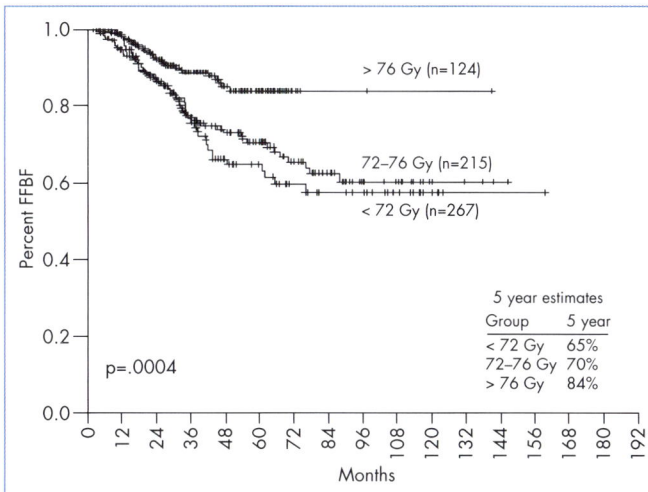

Fig. 86.3

Biochemical non-evidence of disease (bNED) control for the intermediate-risk patients treated at Fox Chase Cancer Center in the prostate-specific antigen (PSA) era with 3D conformal radiotherapy (3DCRT). They are subdivided into three dose groups: <72 Gy, 72 Gy–76 Gy, and >76 Gy. (FFBF, freedom from biochemical failure.)

eight patients were treated as part of this prospective study, and 10-year bNED control rates for good-, intermediate-, and poor-risk patients were 70%, 49%, and 35%, respectively. Differences in bNED control were associated with dose within each group. For low-risk patients, bNED control was 83% versus 57% for patients treated with 75.6 Gy versus less than 70.2 Gy. These rates were 50% versus 42% for intermediate-risk patients and 42% versus 24% for poor-risk patients (Table 86.2).[14]

Table 86.2 Sequential radiotherapy dose escalation studies

Institution	Dose (Gy)	Group	bNED control (length of follow-up)	p-value
CC[35]	<72	All	54% (5 year)	<0.001
	≥72	All	85% (5 year)	
FCCC[7]	<71.5	PSA 10–20	19% (8 year)	0.0003
	71.5–75.75	PSA 10–20	31% (8 year)	
	>75.75	PSA 10–20	84% (8 year)	
MDACC[36]	≤67	All	54% (4 year)	<0.0001
	>67–77	All	71% (4 year)	
	>77	All	77% (4 year)	
MSKCC[37]	64.8–70.2	Int risk*	55% (4 year)	0.04
	75.6–81.0	Int risk*	79% (4 year)	

*Intermediate risk—patients with prostate-specific antigen (PSA) >10 ng/mL, or Gleason score 7, or T2b/T2c disease.

bNED, biochemical non-evidence of disease; CC, the Cleveland Clinic; FCCC- Fox Chase Cancer Center; MDACC, M.D. Anderson Cancer Center; MSKCC, Memorial Sloan-Kettering Cancer Center.

In 1999, the results using external beam radiation therapy (EBRT) alone in 1765 men with T1 and T2 prostate cancer from six institutions (FCCC, Massachusetts General Hospital, Mallinckrodt Institute of Radiology, the University of Michigan, Eastern Virginia Medical School, and Stanford University) was summarized and reported. The biochemical durability of radiation therapy as well as the effect of prognostic factors on outcome was described.[15] As a follow-up to this experience, nine institutions (the original six along with MDACC, William Beaumont Hospital, and the Mayo Clinic College of Medicine) pooled data on nearly 5000 patients treated with EBRT alone between 1986 and 1995, with a median follow-up of more than 6 years. The results of this collaborative effort were first reported in 2003.[2,16] Kuban et al reported long-term biochemical and clinical outcomes for patients with stage T1 to T2 prostate cancer using the ASTRO definition. bNED control for the entire group was 59% at 5 years and 53% at 8 years. For patients who had received at least 70 Gy, bNED control was 61% and 55%. The greatest risk of failure was at 1.5 to 3.5 years post-treatment. In multivariate analysis for bNED failure, pretreatment PSA, Gleason score, radiation dose, T stage, and treatment year were all significant prognostic factors. The effect of radiation dose was most significant in the intermediate risk group.[2]

A more detailed analysis of the effect of dose on bNED control was reported by Kupelian using this same large dataset. Because differences in bNED control have been observed in some series attributed solely to differences in length of follow-up, the dose response was analyzed in patients treated during a 2-year period, 1994 and 1995; for this study, 1061 were treated with less than 72 Gy and 264 patients with greater than or equal to 72 Gy. The median follow-up for the first group

was 5.8 years and for the second group was 5.7 years. The median radiation doses for the 2 groups were 68.4 Gy and 75.6 Gy, respectively. For all 1325 patients, the 5- and 8-year bNED control rates were 64% and 62%, respectively. The 5-year bNED control rates for the low- and high-dose groups were 63% and 69%, respectively ($p = 0.046$). Pretreatment PSA ($p < 0.001$), Gleason score ($p < 0.001$), radiation dose ($p < 0.001$), and T stage ($p = 0.007$) were independent predictors of outcome on multivariate analysis. The authors concluded that while controlling for follow-up duration, higher than conventional radiation doses were associated with improved bNED control rates when controlling for pretreatment PSA, Gleason score, and clinical T stage.[17]

The first national prospective phase I/II study investigating dose escalation was completed in 2000. RTOG 94-06 enrolled 1055 analyzable patients from 34 institutions into five sequential dose levels—68.4 Gy, 73.8 Gy, 79.2 Gy, 74 Gy, and 78 Gy. Prostate-specific antigen failure was defined prior to the adoption of the ASTRO definition and included a failure to fall below 4 ng/mL by 1 year after the start of treatment or two consecutive rises at least 1 month apart during the first year after the start of treatment. The first long-term clinical results became available in 2004. The 5-year rates for the first three groups and 3-year rates for the last two groups for clinical and biochemical failure were 44%, 53%, 49%, 29%, and 26%, respectively. Local failure without PSA endpoints for the five groups was 5% for groups 1 to 3, 4% for group 4, and 2% for group 5. The 5-year clinical disease-free survival (DFS) for groups 1 to 3 was 86%, 82%, and 81%, respectively and 90% for groups 4 and 5 at 3 years. The results from this study support those seen in single institution studies.[18]

The strongest evidence to support a particular treatment is class I evidence from a randomized prospective trial. The first and most mature study in the PSA era was from M.D. Anderson Cancer Center.[19] In this study, 301 men were randomized between 70 Gy and 78 Gy. All were initially treated with a four-field box to 46 Gy, prescribed to the isocenter. The 150 patients randomized to 70 Gy received the remaining dose through a smaller volume using a four-field arrangement, while the 151 patients who received 78 Gy were treated with a six-field 3D conformal boost. The clinical target volume (CTV) consisted of the prostate and seminal vesicles. With 60 months median follow-up, patients with an initial pretreatment PSA greater than 10 ng/mL experienced the greatest benefit, whereas the additional 8 Gy had no effect on the more favorable patients (pretreatment PSA ≤ 10 ng/mL). Freedom from biochemical failure (FFBF) and clinical failures for patients with pretreatment PSA levels greater than 10 ng/mL are shown in Figure 86.4. The freedom from failure results (based on biochemical criteria) supported the conclusions of the sequential dose escalation trials. The FFBF rates were significantly higher for those randomized to 78 Gy (70% versus 64% at 6 years; p = 0.03). The greatest benefit was observed in men with a pretreatment PSA greater than 10 ng/mL who had a 19% absolute gain in FFBF at 6 years when treated to 78 Gy. This translated into a borderline reduction in distant metastasis (2% versus 12% at 6 years; p = 0.056); although there were only eight patients with distant metastasis at the time of the analysis. For patients with a pretreatment PSA less than or equal to 10 ng/mL, no dose-related difference in FFBF or any other endpoint were observed.

Results from the second phase III randomized prospective trial were reported by Zietman et al; in this study, 393 patients were randomized to receive a boost to the prostate of either 19.8 Gray equivalent (GyE) (70.2 GyE total) or 28.8 GyE (79.2 GyE total) using protons. All patients first received 50.4 Gy using 3DCRT techniques with photons. Patients eligible for treatment on this study included those with T1b to T2b tumors and a pretreatment PSA level less than 15 ng/mL. Fifteen percent of patients had Gleason score 7 tumors and 8% had Gleason score 8 to 10. The 5-year bNED failure rate was 37.3% for the low-dose arm and 19.1% for the high-dose group. This difference was statistically significant (p = 0.00001). When patients were stratified by risk group, this difference remained statistically significant for both low (34.9% versus 17.2%; p = 0.002) and intermediate groups (39.5% versus 21.3%; p = 0.01). Although this study used protons to deliver the radiation boost in the experimental arm, this study clearly demonstrated an improvement in clinical and biochemical outcome with higher radiation doses. This was the second randomized prospective trial to confirm that patients with both low- and intermediate-risk prostate cancer achieve higher rates of bNED control with high doses of radiation.[20]

Although no national prospective trial involving IMRT has been reported, several series utilizing this technique have been published. As with the 3DCRT data, patients with intermediate risk features benefit the most from an escalation of radiation dose. The largest published experience with the longest follow-up of biochemical outcome and toxicity using IMRT to treat prostate cancer comes from MSKCC. The 3-year bNED control rates for 772 patients treated with IMRT at MSKCC were 92%, 86%, and 81% for patients with low risk, intermediate risk and high risk, respectively (Figure 86.5).[21] The risk group stratification used for the MSKCC IMRT experience was the same as the system used with

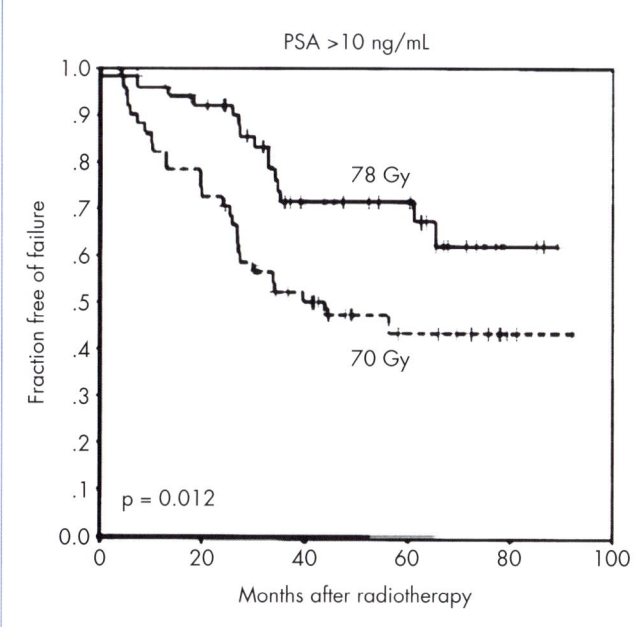

Fig. 86.4
The biochemical and clinical failures curves for patients in the M.D. Anderson Cancer Center randomized trial who had a pretreatment prostate-specific antigen (PSA) > 10 ng/mL and were treated to 70 or 78 Gy.
With permission from Pollack A, Zagars GK, Starkschall G, et al. Prostate cancer radiation dose response: Results of the M.D. Anderson phase III randomized trial. Int J Radiat Oncol Biol Phys 2002;53:1097–1105.

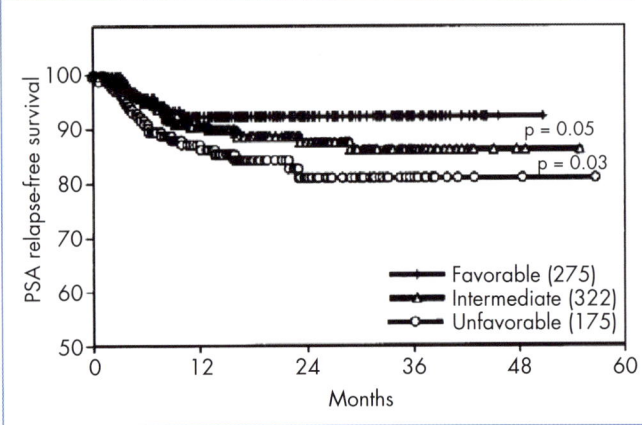

Fig. 86.5

Biochemical non-evidence of disease (bNED) control for favorable, intermediate- and high-risk patients treated with intensity modulated radiotherapy (IMRT) at Memorial Sloan-Kettering Cancer Center.

With permission from Zelefsky MJ, Fuks Z, Hunt M, et al. High-dose intensity modulated radiation therapy for prostate cancer: early toxicity and biochemical outcome in 772 patients. Int J Radiat Oncol Biol Phys 2002;53:1111–1116.

the 3DCRT experience. A subset of these patients treated between 1996 and 1998 with long follow-up was reported and confirmed the durability of results as well as low rate of complications. For this group of 171 patients, the median follow-up was 6.3 years and all these patients received 81 Gy. The 5-year bNED control rates for the low-, intermediate-, and high-risk disease were 91%, 73%, and 64%, respectively (p = 0.008).

TOXICITY

CONVENTIONAL AND 3D CONFORMAL RADIATION THERAPY TOXICITY

Normal tissue complication risk has been well-established and is related to radiation dose, volume,[19,22–24] and other dosimetric and clinical parameters. Bladder complications can manifest much later than rectal complications.[25] Several authors have reported on techniques to reduce rectal toxicity.[23,26]

The late GI and GU complications following treatment with conventional or 3DCRT at FCCC were reported by Schultheiss et al. Seven hundred twelve patients treated between 1986 and 1994 with conventional (150 patients) or conformal (562 patients) techniques were analyzed for factors using a modified RTOG/SWOG scoring system to predict late GI (rectal bleeding requiring ≥3 procedures to correct or proctitis) and GU (cystitis or stricture) morbidity. One hundred fifteen patients experienced grade 2 or higher GI toxicity a mean of 13.7 months after treatment. Fifteen of these patients experienced grade 3 or 4 toxicity. Forty three cases of grade 2 or higher late GU toxicity were observed a mean of 22.7 months after treatment. On multivariate analysis only radiation dose (>74 Gy) significantly predicted late grade 3 GI toxicity. Radiation dose, use of increased rectal shielding, hormone therapy before RT, history of obstructive symptoms, and acute GU symptoms significantly predicted for late grade 2 GU toxicity on multivariate analysis. After the presence of minor rectal bleeding was noted in 1993, techniques were developed to reduce the radiation dose to the anterior rectal wall.[23] The need for endoscopic coagulation for bleeding was reduced from 5% to 2% at 75 to 76 Gy.[27] In the MSKCC 3DCRT series, the risk of grade 2 and grade 3 or higher rectal toxicity at 10 years was 17% and 1.5%, respectively. For GU side effects, the 10 year rates were 17% and 1.5%, respectively (Figure 86.6).[14]

Michalski et al reported toxicity data from 3DOG/RTOG 94-06, the prospective phase I dose

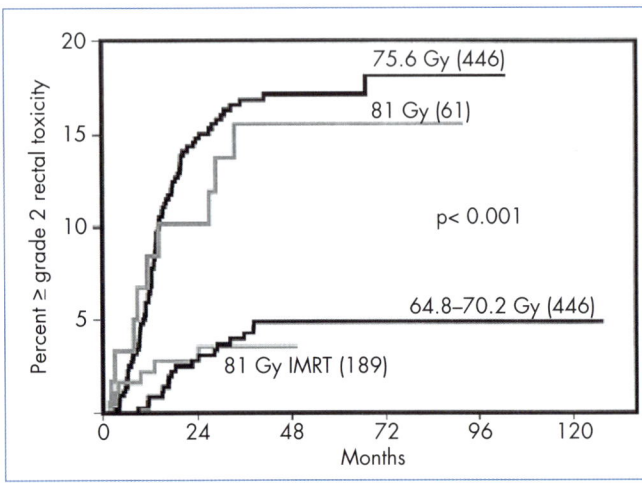

Fig. 86.6

Freedom from grade 2 or higher rectal complications for patients treated with 3D conformal radiotherapy (3DCRT) and intensity modulated radiotherapy (IMRT) at Memorial Sloan-Kettering Cancer Center.

Used with permission from Zelefsky MJ, Fuks Z, Hunt M, et al. High-dose intensity modulated radiation therapy for prostate cancer: early toxicity and biochemical outcome in 772 patients. Int J Radiat Oncol Biol Phys 2002;53:1111–1116.

escalation trial determining the maximally tolerated radiation dose in men treated with 3DCRT in a multi-institutional setting. Two hundred ninety two patients treated between 1994 and 1997 at the first two dose levels of 68.4 and 73.8 Gy were analyzed for rates of acute and chronic GI and GU toxicity. Acute and chronic grade 1 toxicity for both dose groups ranged from 30% to 46%. Rates of acute grade 2 toxicity ranged from 34% to 45%. Chronic grade 2 toxicity rates were 8% to 16%. Acute grade 3 rates were between 1% and 3%, while there were no acute grade 4 or 5, or chronic grade 3, 4, or 5 complications.[28] The first data from the final dose group (78 Gy, Level V), demonstrate that grade 3 acute effects were 2% for Group 1 and 4% for Group 2. No grade 4 or 5 complications were reported.[29]

Similar results were observed from two European randomized prospective trials that compared toxicity data with different radiation dose levels using 3D conformal techniques. In the first study, Lebesque et al described the acute and late GI and GU toxicity rates from a two arm phase III study, which randomized men between 68 and 78 Gy. Between 1997 and 2003, 669 men in the Netherlands were randomized to these two doses using 3DCRT. Data was available for 606 men and RTOG scoring was used to measure acute effects while RTOG/EORTC and SOMA/LENT scoring was used for late effects. No statistically significant differences in rates were observed for grade 2 and grade 3 GI and GU of complications between the two arms.[30] In the second study, 306 men with intermediate-risk prostate cancer were randomized in a French phase II prospective trial between 70 and 80 Gy from 1999 through 2002. There was also no statistically significant difference in acute toxicity between the two arms. Overall GU and GI grade 3 toxicity rates were 6% and 2%, respectively, for both groups. The target volume (prostate) size was the only independent predictor of acute grade 2 and 3 toxicity.[31]

In the MDACC randomized prospective trial, the 5-year actuarial freedom from a grade 2 or higher rectal complication was 26% for those in the 78 Gy arm and 12% for those in the 70 Gy arm. Dose–volume histogram analysis identified that exposure of more than 25% of the rectal volume to greater than or equal to 70 Gy resulted in a 5 year risk of grade 2 or higher rectal complications of 54%, as opposed to 84% when 25% or less was exposed. In a more detailed follow-up analysis of patients treated with 3DCRT at MDACC, Huang et al confirmed that the proportion of the rectum receiving over certain marker doses (e.g., 70 Gy) was found to be more significant than absolute rectal volume (Figure 86.7).[32] Kupelian et al, on the other hand, reported that the absolute rectal volume radiated was an independent predictor of grade 2 or higher complications. When more than 15 cm^3 of the rectal volume received the prescription dose, the 2-year rate of rectal bleeding was 22%, versus 5% for 15 cm^3 or less.[33]

INTENSITY MODULATED RADIOTHERAPY TOXICITY

The MSKCC group has had the most experience in the treatment of prostate cancer with IMRT. Zelefsky et al found that grade 2 or higher rectal complication rate at 3 years was 14% for 81 Gy (n = 189) using 3DCRT, compared with 2% using IMRT (n = 61) (see Figure 86.6). Seven patients developed grade 2 rectal bleeding. At 6 years there was a 4% risk of developing rectal bleeding, and two patients developed grade 3 rectal bleeding. Eighteen patients developed grade 2 urinary toxicity. At 6 years, the risk was 10%, and there were no cases of grade 4 toxicity. The results look promising, although the follow-up in the IMRT patients was shorter. The reduction in morbidity using IMRT seems to be related to a reduction in rectal complications and longer follow up is needed to confirm these results (Figure 86.8).[21,34]

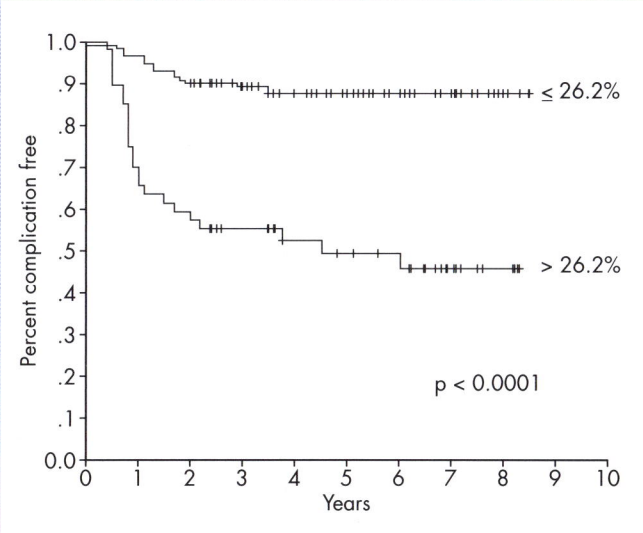

Fig. 86.7

Freedom from grade 2 or higher rectal complications for patients treated with 3D conformal radiotherapy (3DCRT) in the M.D. Anderson Cancer Center randomized trial. The patients are divided by <26.2% versus >26.2% of the rectal volume received ≥70 Gy in dose–volume histogram analysis.

With permission from Pollack A, Zagars GK, Starkschall G, et al. Prostate cancer radiation dose response: Results of the M.D. Anderson phase III randomized trial. Int J Radiat Oncol Biol Phys 2002;53:1097–1105.

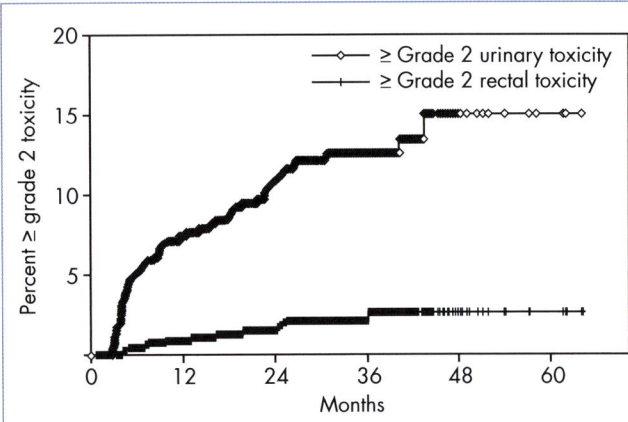

Fig. 86.8

Freedom from grade 2 or higher late rectal and urinary complications after intensity modulated radiotherapy (IMRT) to 81 and 86.4 Gy at Memorial Sloan-Kettering Cancer Center.

With permission from Zelefsky MJ, Fuks Z, Hunt M, et al. High-dose intensity modulated radiation therapy for prostate cancer: early toxicity and biochemical outcome in 772 patients. Int J Radiat Oncol Biol Phys 2002;53:1111–1116.

REFERENCES

1. Horwitz EM, Hanlon AL, Pinover WH, et al. Defining the optimal radiation dose with three-dimensional conformal radiation therapy for patients with nonmetastatic prostate carcinoma by using recursive partitioning techniques. Cancer 2001;92:1281–1287.

2. Kuban DA, Thames HD, Levy LB, et al. Long-term multi-institutional analysis of stage T1-T2 prostate cancer treated with radiotherapy in the PSA era. Int J Radiat Oncol Biol Phys 2003;57:915–928.

3. Chism DB, Hanlon AL, Horwitz EM, et al. A comparison of the single and double factor high-risk models for risk assignment of prostate cancer treated with 3D conformal radiotherapy. Int J Radiat Oncol Biol Phys 2004;59:380–385.

4. Khuntia D, Reddy CA, Mahadevan A, et al. Recurrence-free survival rates after external-beam radiotherapy for patients with clinical T1-T3 prostate carcinoma in the prostate-specific antigen era: what should we expect? Cancer 2004;100:1283–1292.

5. Kattan MW, Zelefsky MJ, Kupelian PA, et al. Pretreatment nomogram that predicts 5-year probability of metastasis following three-dimensional conformal radiation therapy for localized prostate cancer. J Clin Oncol 2003;21:4568–4571.

6. International Commission on Radiation Units and Measurements. ICRU Report 50: Prescribing, recording, and reporting photon beam therapy. Bethesda, MD: International Commission on Radiation Units and Measurements, 1993.

7. Hanks GE, Hanlon AL, Epstein B, et al. Dose response in prostate cancer with 8-12 years' follow-up. Int J Radiat Oncol Biol Phys 2002;54:427–435.

8. Symon Z, Griffith KA, McLaughlin PW, et al. Dose escalation for localized prostate cancer: substantial benefit observed with 3D conformal therapy. Int J Radiat Oncol Biol Phys 2003;57:384–390.

9. Zelefsky MJ, Ben-Porat L, Scher HI, et al. Outcome predictors for the increasing PSA state after definitive external-beam radiotherapy for prostate cancer. J Clin Oncol 2005;23:826–831.

10. Pinover WH, Hanlon AL, Horwitz EM, et al. Defining the appropriate radiation dose for pretreatment PSA < or = 10 ng/mL prostate cancer. Int J Radiat Oncol Biol Phys 2000;47:649–654.

11. American Society for Therapeutic Radiology and Oncology Consensus Panel. Consensus statement: Guidelines for PSA following radiation therapy. Int J Radiat Oncol Biol Phys 1997;37:1035–1041.

12. Zelefsky MJ, Marion C, Fuks Z, et al. Improved biochemical disease-free survival of men younger than 60 years with prostate cancer treated with high dose conformal external beam radiotherapy. J Urol 2003;170:1828–1832.

13. Cheung R, Tucker SL, Lee AL, et al. Assessing the impact of an alternative biochemical failure definition on radiation dose response for high-risk prostate cancer treated with external beam radiotherapy. Int J Radiat Oncol Biol Phys 2005;61:14–19.

14. Zelefsky M, Fuks Z, Chan H, et al. Ten-year results of dose escalation with 3-dimensional conformal radiotherapy for patients with clinically localized prostate cancer. Int J Radiat Oncol Biol Phys 2003;57:S149–150.

15. Shipley WU, Thames HD, et al. Radiation therapy for clinically localized prostate cancer: a multi-institutional pooled analysis. JAMA 1999;281:1598–1604.

16. Thames H, Kuban D, Levy L, et al. Comparison of alternative biochemical failure definitions based on clinical outcome in 4839 prostate cancer patients treated by external beam radiotherapy between 1986 and 1995. Int J Radiat Oncol Biol Phys 2003;57:929–943.

17. Kupelian P, Kuban D, Thames H, et al. Improved biochemical relapse-free survival with increased external radiation doses in patients with localized prostate cancer: The combined experience of nine institutions in patients treated in 1994 and 1995. Int J Radiat Oncol Biol Phys 2005;61:415–49.

18. Michalski JM, Winter K, Roach M, et al. Clinical outcome of patients treated with 3D conformal radiation therapy 3DCRT for prostate cancer on RTOG 94-06. Int J Radiat Oncol Biol Phys 2004;60:169.

19. Pollack A, Zagars GK, Starkschall G, et al. Prostate cancer radiation dose response: Results of the M.D. Anderson phase III randomized trial. Int J Radiat Oncol Biol Phys 2002;53:1097–1105.

20. Zietman AL, DeSilvio M, Slater JD, et al. A randomized trial comparing conventional dose (70.2 GyE) and high-dose (79.2 GyE) conformal radiation in early stage adenocarcinoma of the prostate: Results of an interim analysis of PROG 95-09. International Journal of Radiation Oncology Biology and Physics 2004;60:131–132.

21. Zelefsky MJ, Fuks Z, Hunt M, et al. High-dose intensity modulated radiation therapy for prostate cancer: early toxicity and biochemical outcome in 772 patients. Int J Radiat Oncol Biol Phys 2002;53:1111–1116.

22. Shipley WU, Verhey LJ, Munzenrider JE, et al. Advanced prostate cancer: The results of a randomized comparative trial of high dose irradiation boosting with conformal protons compared with conventional dose irradiation using photons alone. Int J Radiat Oncol Biol Phys 1995;32:3–12.

23. Lee WR, Hanks GE, Hanlon AL, et al. Lateral rectal shielding reduces late rectal morbidity following high dose three-dimensional conformal radiation therapy for clinically localized prostate cancer: further evidence for a significant dose effect. Int J Radiat Oncol Biol Phys 1996;35:251–257.

24. Boersma LJ, van den Brink M, Bruce AM, et al. Estimation of the incidence of late bladder and rectum complications after high-dose (70–78 GY) conformal radiotherapy for prostate cancer, using dose-volume histograms. Int J Radiat Oncol Biol Phys 1998;41:83–92.

25. Gardner BG, Zietman AL, Shipley WU, et al. Late normal tissue sequelae in the second decade after high dose radiation therapy with combined photons and conformal protons for locally advanced prostate cancer. J Urol 2002;167:123–126.

26. Dearnaley DP, Khoo VS, Norman AR, et al. Comparison of radiation side-effects of conformal and conventional radiotherapy in prostate cancer: a randomised trial. Lancet 1999;353:267–272.

27. Schultheiss TE, Lee WR, Hunt MA, et al. Late GI and GU complications in the treatment of prostate cancer. Int J Radiat Oncol Biol Phys 1997;37:3–11.

28. Michalski JM, Winter K, Purdy JA, et al. Preliminary evaluation of low-grade toxicity with conformal radiation therapy for prostate cancer on RTOG 9406 dose levels I and II. Int J Radiat Oncol Biol Phys 2003;56:192–198.

29. Michalski J, Winter K, Purdy JA, et al. Toxicity following 3D radiation therapy for prostate cancer on RTOG 9406 dose level V. Int J Radiat Oncol Biol Phys 2003;57:S151.

30. Lebesque J, Koper P, Slot A, et al. Acute and late GI and GU toxicity after prostate irradiation to doses of 68 Gy and 78 Gy; results of a randomized trial. Int J Radiat Oncol Biol Phys 2003;57:S152.

31. Beckendorf V, Guerif S, Le Prise E, et al. The GETUG 70 Gy vs. 80 Gy randomized trial for localized prostate cancer: feasibility and acute toxicity. Int J Radiat Oncol Biol Phys 2004;60:1056–1065.

32. Huang EH, Pollack A, Levy L, et al. Late rectal toxicity: dose-volume effects of conformal radiotherapy for prostate cancer. Int J Radiat Oncol Biol Phys 2002;54:1314–1321.

33. Kupelian PA, Reddy CA, Carlson TP, et al. Dose/volume relationship of late rectal bleeding after external beam radiotherapy for localized prostate cancer: absolute or relative rectal volume? Cancer J 2002;8:62–66.

34. Zelefsky MJ, Fuks Z, Hunt M, et al. High dose radiation delivered by intensity modulated conformal radiotherapy improves the outcome of localized prostate cancer. J Urol 2001;166:876–881.

35. Lyons JA, Kupelian PA, Mohan DS, et al. Importance of high radiation doses (72 Gy or greater) in the treatment of stage T1-T3 adenocarcinoma of the prostate. Urology 2000;55:85–90.

36. Pollack A, Smith LG, von Eschenbach AC. External beam radiotherapy dose response characteristics of 1127 men with prostate cancer treated in the PSA era. Int J Radiat Oncol Biol Phys 2000;48:507–512.

37. Zelefsky MJ, Leibel SA, Gaudin PB, et al. Dose escalation with three-dimensional conformal radiation therapy affects the outcome in prostate cancer. Int J Radiat Oncol Biol Phys 1998;41:491–500.

Management of biochemical recurrence following radiation therapy

87

Timothy S Collins, Daniel J George

INTRODUCTION

The introduction and use of the prostate-specific antigen (PSA) test has had a profound impact on the diagnosis and management of patients with prostate cancer. Prostate-specific antigen has gained wide acceptance as a screening tool for early detection of prostate cancer, yet it was originally developed as a tumor marker.[1] As a tumor marker, PSA has demonstrated exceptional sensitivity and specificity for disease progression. One of the most important applications of PSA is its use in patients following definitive local therapy.

Following radical prostatectomy (RP), radiation therapy is the second most common treatment modality chosen for clinically localized prostate cancer. According to the SEER database, approximately 30% of patients in the United States are treated with external-beam radiation, initially.[2] In addition, various forms of brachytherapy, either as monotherapy or in combination with external-beam radiation, have gained widespread acceptance and use as an alternative standard therapy. Unfortunately, despite early detection and risk stratification, a significant percentage of patients will relapse following primary therapy, with estimates ranging from 10% to 50% depending on pretreatment prognostic factors.[3] Often the first evidence of disease recurrence is detected by the PSA test. To better manage patients with rising PSA following local therapy, clinicians must have a thorough understanding of several important issues. This chapter will cover biochemical recurrence after primary radiation therapy including its definition, natural history, diagnostic considerations, and treatment options.

DEFINITION OF BIOCHEMICAL RECURRENCE

Unlike post-prostatectomy, the definition of biochemical failure post-radiation is less straightforward. Since the goal of a prostatectomy is to remove all prostate tissue, the PSA in most patients declines to undetectable levels soon after surgery. In contrast, the decline of PSA following radiation therapy is more gradual, and, frequently, it does not drop to undetectable levels. Following external-beam radiation therapy or brachytherapy, PSA levels decline over the first 12 months with more subtle decreases occurring over 12 to 24 months.[4,5] Confounding this parameter further is the incidence of false elevations of PSA following radiation therapy. In as many as 30% of cases, a transient rise in PSA level, or bounce, has been described following brachytherapy and external-beam radiation.[6,7] In addition, the use of adjuvant androgen-deprivation therapy (ADT) frequently suppresses PSA levels and may alter the kinetics of PSA progression as testosterone levels recover.[8,9] Overall, the interpretation of biochemical relapse following radiation therapy can be complex and ambiguous.

In order to standardize the definition of biochemical failure after radiation therapy, an expert committee was formed. From this effort, the American Society for Therapeutic Radiology and Oncology (ASTRO) issued a consensus statement detailing guidelines for PSA following radiation therapy[10] (Box 87.1). In addition to these guidelines, the authors presented recommendations for study publications. For publications, they recommended: 1) a minimum observation period of 24 months; 2) PSA levels should

Box 87.1 ASTRO guidelines for PSA following radiation therapy

- Biochemical failure is not justification per se to initiate additional treatment. It is not equivalent to clinical failure. It is, however, an appropriate early end point for clinical trials.
- Three consecutive increases in PSA is a reasonable definition of biochemical failure after radiation therapy. For clinical trials, the date of failure should be the midpoint between the post-irradiation nadir PSA and the first of the three consecutive rises.
- No definition of PSA failure has, as yet, been shown to be a surrogate for clinical progression or survival.
- Nadir PSA is a strong prognostic factor, but no absolute level is a valid cut point for separating successful and unsuccessful treatments. Nadir PSA is similar in prognostic value to pretreatment prognostic variables.

ASTRO, American Society for Therapeutic Radiology and Oncology

From Cox JD for the American Society for Therapeutic Radiology and Oncology Concensus Panel. Concensus Statement Guidelines for PSA following radiation therapy. Int J Radiat Oncol Biol Phys 1997;37:1035–41.

be measured every 3 to 4 months during the first 2 years and every 6 months thereafter; and 3) the results of patients who have had less than three consecutive rises should be reported separately from those with three or more. While such definitions still do not justify broad comparisons of nonrandomized studies, they do help in the extrapolation of data into clinical settings.

NATURAL HISTORY

A substantial proportion of patients will develop a biochemical recurrence following external-beam radiation. For example, Shipley et al demonstrated a 5-year estimate of freedom from biochemical failure rate of 65.8% in a multi-institutional pooled analysis.[11] Similarly, Kuban et al reported PSA disease-free survival (DFS) rates of 59% at 5 years and 53% at 8 years.[12] In addition, there is emerging evidence that longer term follow-up periods may be needed to fully appreciate the true rate of biochemical recurrence. In a recent long-term study with a minimum follow-up period of 22.9 years, it was found that recurrences developed throughout the length of the study.[13] In fact, over half of the recurrences occurred after 10 years and some even occurred after 20 years.

PREDICTORS OF BIOCHEMICAL RECURRENCE AND PATIENT OUTCOMES

Several clinical factors have been used to predict who is at risk for a biochemical recurrence following primary radiation therapy. It is important to recognize that biochemical recurrence will include patients with localized only relapse, microscopic metastatic disease progression, and

combinations of both. In almost all cases, PSA recurrence will precede symptoms by several years. Differentiating local recurrence only from distant relapse, and potentially more aggressive disease progression, is critical to determining the most appropriate treatment course.

PRIMARY TUMOR FEATURES

Several large reports have studied predictors of long-term outcomes following primary radiation therapy. Zagars et al analyzed the outcomes of 938 men treated with definitive external-beam radiation from 1987 to 1995.[14] In a multivariate regression model, pretreatment PSA, treatment stage, and Gleason scores were independent predictors of rising PSA, local recurrence, and incidence of metastases. Similarly, Kuban et al reported the long-term outcomes for patients treated for T1/T2 prostate cancer from 1986 to 1995 at nine institutions.[15] In multivariate analysis, several factors were found to be prognostic for biochemical failure including pretreatment PSA, Gleason score, radiation dose, tumor stage, and treatment year. Finally, Kupelian et al reviewed the biochemical relapse-free survival in 2991 patients receiving local therapy at two institutions.[16] In this group of patients, which included surgery, radiation, and brachytherapy, baseline PSA, Gleason score, and year of therapy were all found to be independent predictors of relapse.

PREDICTION MODELS

Numerous prostate cancer nomograms have been developed to help predict patient outcomes. For an excellent review on the topic, one should turn to a recent publication cataloging 42 published nomograms.[17] For the nomograms designed to predict PSA recurrence following external-beam radiation and brachytherapy, the three most common predictors used in the nomograms include the biopsy Gleason score, clinical stage, and pretreatment PSA.

PROSTATE-SPECIFIC ANTIGEN DOUBLING TIME

The prostate-specific antigen doubling time (PSADT) has emerged as an important prognostic tool in patients with a biochemical recurrence following local therapy. Following RP, Partin et al studied several clinical parameters to help predict PSA recurrence.[18] In an updated report from the same group, PSADT was shown to predict distant failure and prostate cancer specific survival.[19] At 10 years following RP, prostate cancer-specific survival was 85% in the group with PSADT of more than 10 months and 47% in the group with PSADT of less than 10 months.

Prostate-specific antigen doubling time has also been studied in patients following radiation therapy. For example, Lee et al reported an outcome study of 151 patients with a biochemical recurrence following radiation therapy.[20] In this study, multivariate analysis showed that the time to PSA elevation and post-treatment PSADT were important predictors of the development of distant metastases. Furthermore, in a second retrospective report, D'Amico et al demonstrated that patients with a short PSADT (defined as 3 months or less) following radiation therapy was an important predictor of prostate cancer specific death[21-23] (Figure 87.1).

In addition to its use as a prognostic tool, PSADT may also be used to help guide management decisions. For example, Pinover et al reported on their institutions' experience using PSADT to manage patients following radiation therapy.[24] In their report, the use of ADT in men with a PSADT of less than 12 months was associated with a statistically significant improvement in 5-year freedom from distant metastasis (FDM) rate (57% versus 78%; $P = 0.0026$). Furthermore, the FDM rates in patients with PSADT of more than 12 months were similar in both the ADT group (88%) and observation group (92%) lending support for the strategy of reserving early ADT for patients with high-risk features such as a short PSADT.

100-DAY PROSTATE-SPECIFIC ANTIGEN

Developing surrogate markers with shorter periods of follow-up allows researchers to study newer treatment strategies in shorter periods of time. Johnstone et al recently published the results of a study which looked at the PSA value of patients 100 days after definitive radiotherapy for localized prostate cancer.[25] Patients with a PSA at 100 days of less than 4 ng/mL had significantly greater 8-year biochemical no evidence of disease (bNED) rates compared with patients with 100-day PSA value greater than 4 ng/mL (62% versus 20%, respectively; $P < 0.001$). As the authors point out, these results will need to be followed up in order to validate the 100-day PSA as a surrogate marker for long-term disease outcomes.

DIAGNOSTIC CONSIDERATIONS

Once biochemical recurrence has been established, further clinical and radiographic staging may be indicated. Diagnostic options include digital rectal exam for localized recurrence, radionuclide bone scan, computed tomography (CT), magnetic resonance imaging (MRI), indium-111-labeled CYT-356 (ProstaScint) scan, and prostate re-biopsy. Decisions on which tests are needed are made based on an individual patient's PSA, symptoms, and further treatment goals. Clearly, one important goal of this work-up is to determine whether the cancer has recurred locally, in distant metastatic sites, or both.

BONE SCAN

Although the radionuclide bone scan is the most sensitive test to detect bone metastases, clinicians must remember that the yield of this study is often very low in patients with a biochemical recurrence following

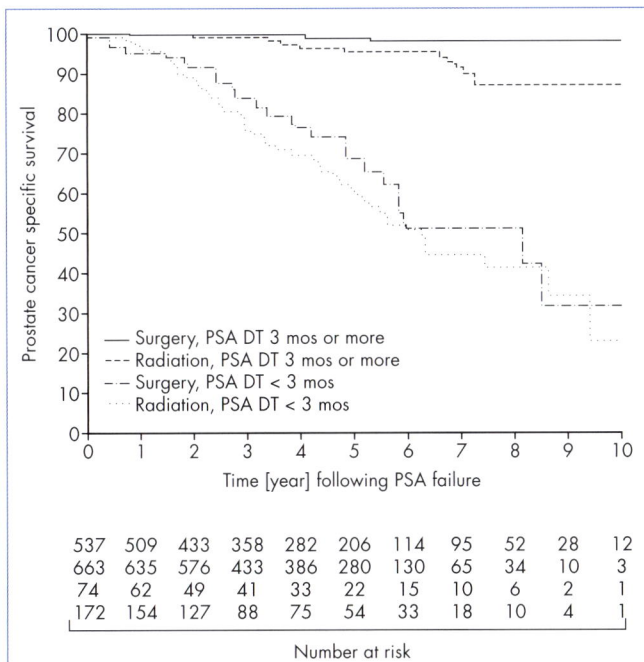

Fig. 87.1

Prostate cancer-specific survival after prostate-specific antigen (PSA) -defined recurrence stratified by treatment received and the value of the post-treatment PSA doubling time (PSADT). A pairwise two-sided log-rank test was used. P values are as follows: for a PSADT <3 months (surgery versus radiation), $P = 0.38$; for PSA-DT ≥3 months (surgery versus radiation), $P < 0.001$; for PSADT <3 months versus PSADT of ≥3 months (surgery), $P < 0.001$; for PSADT <3 months versus PSADT of ≥3 months (radiation), $P < 0.001$. Adapted from D'Amico AV, Moul JW, Carroll PR, Sun L, Lubeck D, Chen MH. Surrogate end point for prostate cancer-specific mortality after radical prostatectomy or radiation therapy. J Natl Cancer Inst 2003;95:1376–1383 (by permission of Oxford University Press).

radiation therapy. The yield of a bone scan in patients with biochemical recurrence has been better studied in the post-RP population. In one series of 132 patients, only 9.4% (12 of 127 patients who had bone scans) had a positive bone scan within 3 years of biochemical recurrence following RP.[26] In a second series, the probability of a positive bone scan was determined to be 5% or lower in patients until serum PSA levels reach the range of 30 to 40 ng/mL.[27]

Unfortunately, less data has been published in patients after radiation therapy. In one series of patients after either RP or radiation therapy, a PSA value of less than 8 ng/mL excluded bone metastases with a predictive value of a negative test of 98.5%.[28] A second retrospective study, studied the utility of bone scan in patients at time of biochemical failure after RP (n = 24) and radiotherapy (n = 20).[29] Bone scans were more commonly positive post-radiotherapy (6 of 20; 30%) than post-RP (1 of 20; 5%). In the post-radiation group, the PSA ranged from 1.31 to 23.6 ng/mL (median 13.9 ng/mL) in patients with a positive bone scan and from 1.02 to 9.53 ng/mL (median 5.5 ng/mL) in patients with a negative bone scan. Taken together, a rational approach would be to consider bone scan in patients who: 1) have bone pain symptoms; 2) are candidates for local salvage procedures; or 3) have a PSA over 5 ng/mL.[30,31]

COMPUTED TOMOGRAPHY AND MAGNETIC RESONANCE IMAGING

Abdominal and pelvic CT or MRI scan are other important imaging studies used to help determine the extent of spread of a patient's cancer at time of biochemical recurrence. Similar to the bone scan, the yield of CT or MRI can be expected to be quite low at the time of biochemical recurrence. In the Johnstone series, only 10 patients underwent CT imaging at time of biochemical recurrence following external-beam radiotherapy.[29] Of these 10 patients, three had positive findings including one with an abdominal wall metastasis, one with a positive pelvic lymph node, and one with bone metastases that were also seen with bone scan. Similar to the bone scan, CT or MRI imaging should be considered in patients with symptoms, those with higher PSA levels, and those who are candidates for potentially morbid local salvage procedures.

PROSTASCINT SCAN

The ProstaScint scan (Cytogen, Princeton, NJ) is a murine monoclonal antibody-based imaging modality that has been FDA approved for use in the staging of newly diagnosed prostate cancer patients who are at high risk for metastases, and for patients with a biochemical recurrence following prostatectomy. Although the ProstaScint scan has been used in patients following primary radiation therapy, the test has not been FDA approved for this indication.[32,33] Preliminary studies evaluating ProstaScint scan following definitive radiation therapy demonstrated positive prostatic uptake in 21 of 24 patients imaged and confirmed with positive biopsies in 10 of 15 patients.[34] Further studies are needed to evaluate the positive predictive value in this setting.

PROSTATE RE-BIOPSY

A consensus panel convened by ASTRO recommended that systematic prostate re-biopsy is not routinely necessary after radiation therapy.[35] One caveat is in patients being considered for local salvage therapy, such as salvage prostatectomy. Under these circumstances, confirmation of localized disease recurrence may be necessary prior to committing patients to a potentially morbid procedure.

MANAGEMENT STRATEGIES

The management of a biochemical recurrence requires a careful understanding of the nature of recurrence (local versus distant), prognostic features, and patient preferences. In patients suspected of local recurrence only, management options include observation, salvage prostatectomy, cryotherapy, brachytherapy, and hormonal therapy. For patients suspected of having microscopic metastatic disease, hormonal therapy is the most commonly employed initial treatment modality; however, alternative approaches using chemotherapy or investigational agents are being studied.

SURGERY

Salvage RP remains an option in a subset of patients with a local recurrence following radiation therapy. Traditionally, the use of salvage prostatectomy has been limited due to high reported rates of perioperative complications including incontinence rates of 40% to 50% and rectal injury rates of 10% to 15%.[36] Despite these limitations, salvage prostatectomy can result in long-term DFS in 30% to 47% of patients.[37-40]

Patients should be carefully selected prior to salvage prostatectomy. For example, Rogers et al studied PSA as a predictor of treatment outcome in patients who underwent prostatectomy following radiation.[41] In their report, 2 of the 13 patients (15%) with a PSA level below 10 ng/mL had an advanced pathologic stage (seminal vesicle invasion or lymph node metastasis) at time of surgery compared with 12 of 14 (86%) of patients with a PSA of 10 ng/mL or higher. Using prognostic factors including PSA below 10 ng/mL and Gleason score less than 7, salvage prostatectomy results approach those of RP in untreated patients with similar pathologic findings.[42]

Currently, a multicenter phase II study is ongoing (CALGB 9687) to gain an up-to-date understanding of the utility and side-effect profile of salvage prostatectomy for patients with a local recurrence following radiation therapy.

BRACHYTHERAPY

Brachytherapy has also been used for patients with a biochemical recurrence following primary radiation therapy (Figure 87.2). Grado et al reported the results of a retrospective study on the effectiveness and side effect profile of 49 patients who had undergone salvage brachytherapy.[43] The actuarial biochemical DFS at 3 and 5 years was 48% and 34%, respectively. In patients with a post-brachytherapy PSA nadir under 0.5 ng/mL, the actuarial biochemical DFS rates at 3 and 5 years were 77% and 56%, respectively. The reported serious complication rate was low. For example, although acute urinary symptoms (frequency, nocturia, urgency) were common, these symptoms were generally transient and often managed medically. More serious complications included persistent gross hematuria in two patients (4%), significant post-treatment pain in three patients (6%), and the development of rectal ulcers in two patients (4%). Nonetheless, salvage brachytherapy remains highly investigational. One caveat to these results is that this data represents a single institutional effort and should be replicated in a larger, multicenter setting before more standard application is considered.

CRYOTHERAPY

A further option for patients with a local recurrence of their prostate cancer is salvage cryoablation of the prostate. Pisters et al reported on 150 patients who underwent salvage cryotherapy for a biochemical recurrence following primary radiation.[44] In their first report, a double freeze-thaw cycle was found to be more effective than a single freeze-thaw cycle in achieving a negative post-cryotherapy biopsy and lower biochemical failure rates. Unfortunately, complication rates were high, including urinary incontinence (73% of patients), obstructive symptoms (67%), impotence (72%), and severe perineal pain (8%). A second analysis was later reported to better define predictive factors, such as pretreatment PSA and Gleason scores, which were associated with better outcomes.[45] The 2-year actuarial DFS rates were significantly higher in patients with pre-

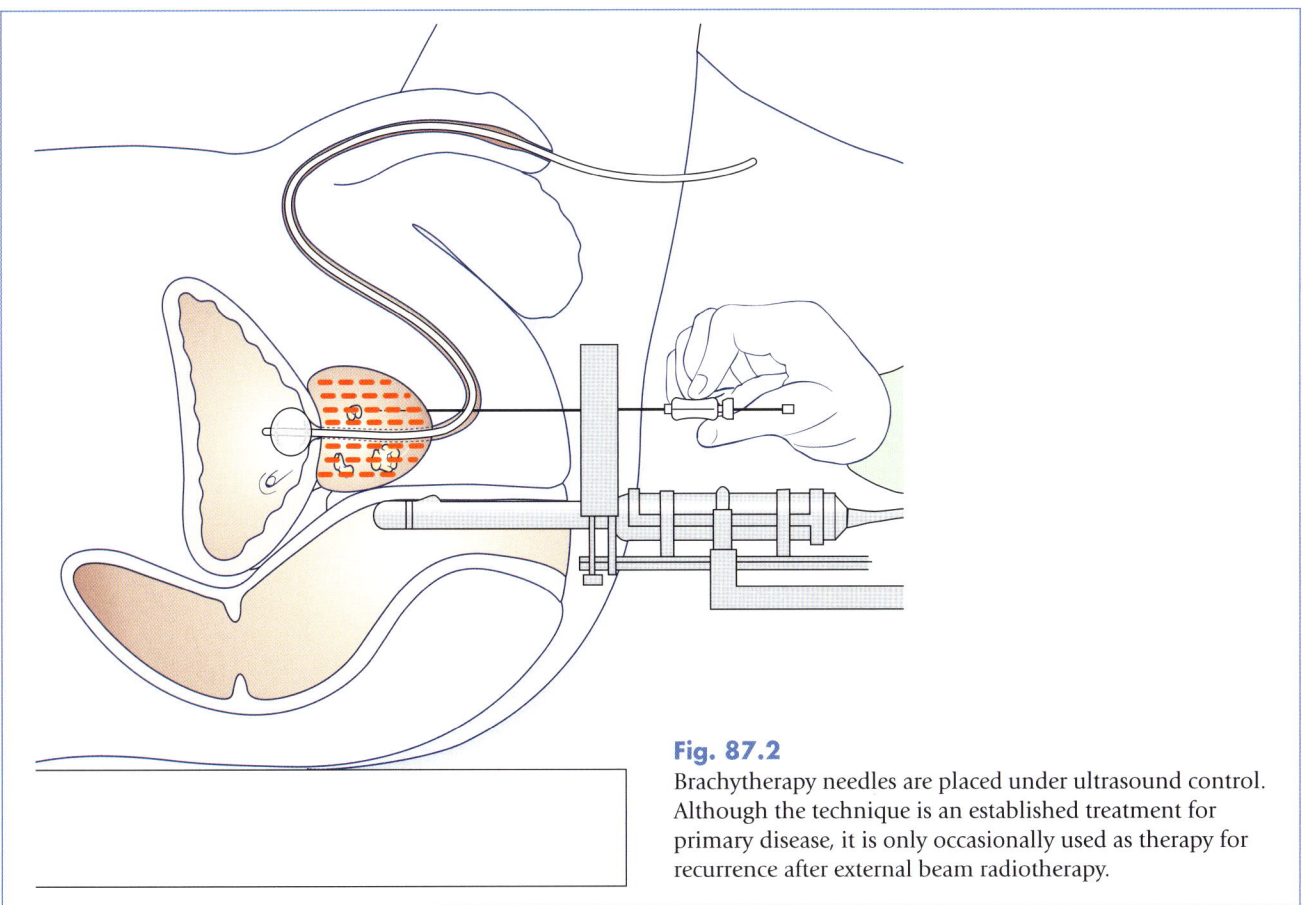

Fig. 87.2
Brachytherapy needles are placed under ultrasound control. Although the technique is an established treatment for primary disease, it is only occasionally used as therapy for recurrence after external beam radiotherapy.

cryotherapy PSA values of under 10 ng/mL compared with those above 10 ng/mL (74% versus 28%, respectively; $P < 0.00001$). Similarly, 2-year DFS rates were significantly higher in patients with a Gleason score of less than 8 compared with over 9 (58% versus 29%, respectively; $P < 0.004$). Chin et al reported on an additional 118 patients treated with salvage cryotherapy.[46] Similar to the above series, worse outcomes were seen in patients with either a PSA above 10 ng/mL or a Gleason score of 8 or more. While new-generation techniques may decrease the morbidity rates associated with salvage cryotherapy, these results would suggest that candidates for cryotherapy should have a Gleason score of their recurrent tumor below 8 and PSA value below 10 ng/mL.

HORMONAL THERAPY

TIMING

The decision of when to start ADT remains controversial, and currently there is wide variation in clinical practice patterns. However, several studies since the mid-1990s support the hypothesis that ADT started before overt bone metastases have formed is associated with improved disease-specific survival. In 1997, Bolla et al published results of an 8-year study of 415 patients with locally advanced prostate cancer treated with 50 Gy of pelvic irradiation with a 20 Gy boost to the prostate versus a combination of the same radiation therapy plus 3 years of continuous ADT.[47,48] Their results demonstrated a significant improvement in the 5-year local control rate (97% versus 77%; $P < 0.001$) and overall survival (79% versus 62%; $P = 0.001$), both in favor of the combination group. All but two patients received ADT at the time of disease progression in the radiotherapy alone arm, suggesting that the timing of ADT (immediate versus disease progression) contributed in part to the improved survival. Further support for early versus delayed androgen deprivation therapy comes from Messing et al, who demonstrated a survival advantage for men with N1 disease following prostatectomy who were treated with androgen deprivation therapy immediately versus at the time of disease progression.[49] However, both of these studies defined disease progression as radiographic evidence of either local regional or metastatic disease recurrence. Whether PSA recurrence alone would identify relapse early enough to negate any survival advantage seen in the groups receiving immediate ADT is unclear.

Recent studies have begun to evaluate the possible benefit of early versus delayed androgen deprivation therapy in the post-PSA era. In particular, investigators have used PSA parameters (velocity, doubling time, and various thresholds) to evaluate in which patients early treatment impacts outcome. For example, Moul et al

published results from the Department of Defense Center for Prostate Disease Research Database demonstrating that in 1352 men with PSA recurrence following RP early ADT resulted in a delay in clinical metastases in patients with a Gleason score greater than 7 and a PSA doubling time of less than 12 months (HR = 2.12; $P = 0.01$).[50] Conversely, no improvement in time to clinical metastases was detected for patients with Gleason score 7 or less tumors and PSA doubling times of more than 12 months. Unfortunately, further studies are needed to clarify the stratification of patients for intervention versus observation in this setting and currently this issue remains unresolved. In fact, a recent ASCO recommendation guideline report was unable to come up with specific recommendations on the issue of early versus deferred therapy.[51]

Clinicians must balance the side effects of ADT with the possibility for improved long-term outcomes. Potential side effects for ADT include hot flashes, muscle weakness, loss of libido, and erectile dysfunction. In addition, long-term complications include osteoporosis, depression, and anemia. Furthermore, the early use of ADT has financial considerations as these treatments are expensive and patients may remain on them for many years.

INTERMITTENT ANDROGEN DEPRIVATION

As an alternative to continuous androgen ablation, the strategy of intermittent androgen deprivation (IAD) has received considerable interest. Preclinical studies have demonstrated that IAD may delay the onset of androgen-independence in prostate cancer models.[52–54] Several nonrandomized studies have demonstrated the feasibility of different strategies of IAD.[55–60] Each of these studies demonstrated the ability of IAD to give patients time off of therapy and presumably freedom from some of the negative side effects of ADT. Specific improvements in quality of life have been reported in a few reports.[61,62] Preliminary results from two randomized studies comparing IAD with continuous ADT have been reported.[63,64] To further define the utility of IAD, two large, cooperative group phase III studies are currently open in two different populations.[65] In the first, JPR7, men with a PSA relapse without evidence of clinical metastases are being randomized to either intermittent or continuous androgen deprivation. In the second, SWOG-9346, men with distant metastatic disease will receive either intermittent or continuous combined androgen deprivation comprising bicalutamide and goserelin. Results of both of these trials will help clinicians gain a better understanding of the use of IAD as a hormonal strategy.

OTHER STRATEGIES

As a further way to avoid some of the side effects of total androgen ablation, other hormonal strategies are currently under investigation. One of these strategies is the combination of a 5α-reductase inhibitor with an antiandrogen. For example, finasteride has been combined with flutamide in at least three studies in men with advanced prostate cancer.[66-68] In all three reports, more than half of men with sexual potency at baseline maintained their erectile function on therapy. In a larger study, Barqawi et al studied the use of low-dose flutamide and finasteride in 71 men with a PSA-only recurrence following primary local therapy.[69] In this report, 45 patients (58%) achieved a nadir PSA of 0.1 ng/mL or less. Importantly, the therapy was well tolerated with the most common side effects being breast tenderness (90%), gynecomastia (72%), gastrointestinal disturbances (22%), and fatigue (10%). To date, these strategies have not been compared in a randomized study with standard ADT but, nonetheless, remain an option for some patients.

In a related approach, Scandinavian investigators performed a large, randomized, placebo-controlled trial randomizing patients to receive either high-dose bicalutamide (150 mg/day p.o.) versus placebo. Patients in this study also received standard care (RP, radiotherapy, or watchful waiting). With a 5.3 year median follow-up, bicalutamide improved overall survival (HR = 0.68; 95% CI 0.50–0.92) in patients with locally advanced disease (T3/4, M0, any N; or any T, M0, N+).[70] This type of approach may have utility in the setting of PSA relapse following local therapy in patients who wish to avoid the side effects of ADT.

Chemotherapy is actively being investigated in patients with biochemical relapse for prostate cancer. Recent studies have demonstrated a clear survival benefit to docetaxel-based chemotherapy regimens in men with metastatic hormone-refractory prostate cancer.[71,72] High-risk prognostic criteria, including PSADT of less than 3 months, may aid in patient selection for these studies, and combinations before, after, or concomitantly with ADT will need further evaluation. For the time being, chemotherapy is not considered a standard approach for management of hormone-naive prostate cancer patients with disease recurrence.

SUMMARY

The management of patients with a biochemical recurrence following primary radiation therapy requires a thoughtful and balanced approach from a multidisciplinary team of prostate cancer specialists. In discussing options of therapy, clinicians need to consider each individual clinical situation. Clinicians continue to be faced with questions such as:

- What is the preferred salvage therapy in patients with suspected local-only recurrence?

- When is the appropriate time to start hormonal therapy?
- What is the relative efficacy of intermittent versus continuous androgen deprivation therapy?
- Are there better tolerated alternatives to complete androgen deprivation?
- Is there benefit to combining chemotherapy to ADT in patients at risk for developing androgen-independent prostate cancer and prostate cancer-specific mortality?

Hopefully, the results of ongoing and future trials will investigate these areas and lead to a more evidenced-based clinical approach.

REFERENCES

1. Wang MC, Papsidero LD, Kuriyama M, et al. Prostate antigen: a new potential marker for prostatic cancer. Prostate 1981;2:89–96.

2. Stephenson RA. Prostate cancer trends in the era of prostate-specific antigen. An update of incidence, mortality, and clinical factors from the SEER database. Urol Clin North Am 2002;29:173–181.

3. D'Amico AV, Whittington R, Malkowicz SB, et al. Biochemical outcome after radical prostatectomy, external beam radiation therapy, or interstitial radiation therapy for clinically localized prostate cancer. JAMA 1998;280:969–974.

4. Iannuzzi CM, Stock RG, Stone NN. PSA kinetics following I-125 radioactive seed implantation in the treatment of T1-T2 prostate cancer. Radiat Oncol Investig 1999;7:30–35.

5. Critz FA. Time to achieve a prostate specific antigen nadir of 0.2 ng/ml after simultaneous irradiation for prostate cancer. J Urol 2002;168:2434–2438.

6. Stock RG, Stone NN, Cesaretti JA. Prostate-specific antigen bounce after prostate seed implantation for localized prostate cancer: descriptions and implications. Int J Radiat Oncol Biol Phys 2003;56:448–453.

7. Sengoz M, Abacioglu U, Cetin I, et al. PSA bouncing after external beam radiation for prostate cancer with or without hormonal treatment. Eur Urol 2003;43:473–477.

8. Tyldesley S, Coldman A, Pickles T. PSA doubling time post radiation: the effect of neoadjuvant androgen ablation. Can J Urol 2004;11:2316–2321.

9. Merrick GS, Butler WM, Wallner KE, et al. Temporal effect of neoadjuvant androgen deprivation therapy on PSA kinetics following permanent prostate brachytherapy with or without supplemental external beam radiation. Brachytherapy 2004;3:141–146.

10. Consensus statement: guidelines for PSA following radiation therapy. American Society for Therapeutic Radiology and Oncology Consensus Panel. Int J Radiat Oncol Biol Phys 1997;37:1035–1041.

11. Shipley WU, Thames HD, Sandler HM, et al. Radiation therapy for clinically localized prostate cancer: a multi-institutional pooled analysis. JAMA 1999;281:1598–1604.

12. Kuban DA, Thames HD, Levy LB, et al. Long-term multi-institutional analysis of stage T1-T2 prostate cancer treated with radiotherapy in the PSA era. Int J Radiat Oncol Biol Phys 2003;57:915–928.

13. Swanson GP, Riggs MW, Earle JD. Long-term follow-up of radiotherapy for prostate cancer. Int J Radiat Oncol Biol Phys 2004;59:406–411.

14. Zagars GK, Pollack A, von Eschenbach AC. Prognostic factors for clinically localized prostate carcinoma: analysis of 938 patients irradiated in the prostate specific antigen era. Cancer 1997;79:1370–1380.

15. Kuban DA, Thames HD, Levy LB, et al. Long-term multi-institutional analysis of stage T1-T2 prostate cancer treated with radiotherapy in the PSA era. Int J Radiat Oncol Biol Phys 2003;57:915–928.

16. Kupelian PA, Potters L, Khuntia D, et al. Radical prostatectomy, external beam radiotherapy <72 Gy, external beam radiotherapy > or

=72 Gy, permanent seed implantation, or combined seeds/external beam radiotherapy for stage T1-T2 prostate cancer. Int J Radiat Oncol Biol Phys 2004;58:25–33.

17. Ross PL, Scardino PT, Kattan MW. A catalog of prostate cancer nomograms. J Urol 2001;165:1562–1568.

18. Pound CR, Partin AW, Eisenberger MA, et al. Natural history of progression after PSA elevation following radical prostatectomy. JAMA 1999;281:1591–1597.

19. Partin AW, Eisenberger MA, Sinibaldi VJ, et al. Prostate specific antigen doubling time (PSADT) predicts for distant failure and prostate cancer specific survival (PCSS) in men with biochemical relapse after radical prostatectomy (RP). J Clin Oncol 2004;22:14S [abstract].

20. Lee WR, Hanks GE, Hanlon A. Increasing prostate-specific antigen profile following definitive radiation therapy for localized prostate cancer: clinical observations. J Clin Oncol 1997;15:230–238.

21. D'Amico AV, Cote K, Loffredo M, et al. Determinants of prostate cancer specific survival following radiation therapy during the prostate specific antigen era. J Urol 2003;170:S42–S46.

22. D'Amico AV, Moul JW, Carroll PR, et al. Surrogate end point for prostate cancer-specific mortality after radical prostatectomy or radiation therapy. J Natl Cancer Inst 2003;95:1376–1383.

23. D'Amico AV, Moul J, Carroll PR, et al. Prostate specific antigen doubling time as a surrogate end point for prostate cancer specific mortality following radical prostatectomy or radiation therapy. J Urol 2004;172:S42–S46.

24. Pinover WH, Horwitz EM, Hanlon AL, et al. Validation of a treatment policy for patients with prostate specific antigen failure after three-dimensional conformal prostate radiation therapy. Cancer 2003;97:1127–1133.

25. Johnstone PA, Williams SR, Riffenburgh RH. The 100-day PSA: usefulness as surrogate end point for biochemical disease-free survival after definitive radiotherapy of prostate cancer. Prostate Cancer Prostatic Dis 2004;7:263–267.

26. Kane CJ, Amling CL, Johnstone PA, et al. Limited value of bone scintigraphy and computed tomography in assessing biochemical failure after radical prostatectomy. Urology 2003;61:607–611.

27. Cher ML, Bianco FJ, Jr., Lam JS, et al. Limited role of radionuclide bone scintigraphy in patients with prostate specific antigen elevations after radical prostatectomy. J Urol 1998;160:1387–1391.

28. Freitas JE, Gilvydas R, Ferry JD, et al. The clinical utility of prostate-specific antigen and bone scintigraphy in prostate cancer follow-up. J Nucl Med 1991;32:1387–1390.

29. Johnstone PA, Tarman GJ, Riffenburgh R, et al. Yield of imaging and scintigraphy assessing biochemical failure in prostate cancer patients. Urol Oncol 1998;3:108–112.

30. Lee WR, Hanks GE, Hanlon A. Increasing prostate-specific antigen profile following definitive radiation therapy for localized prostate cancer: clinical observations. J Clin Oncol 1997;15:230–238.

31. Moul JW. Biochemical recurrence of prostate cancer. Curr Probl Cancer 2003;27:243–272.

32. Sodee DB, Malguria N, Faulhaber P, et al. Multicenter ProstaScint imaging findings in 2154 patients with prostate cancer. The ProstaScint Imaging Centers. Urology 2000;56:988–993.

33. Elgamal AA, Troychak MJ, Murphy GP. ProstaScint scan may enhance identification of prostate cancer recurrences after prostatectomy, radiation, or hormone therapy: analysis of 136 scans of 100 patients. Prostate 1998;37:261–269.

34. Fang DX, Stock RG, Stone NN, et al. Use of radioimmunoscintigraphy with indium-111-labeled CYT-356 (ProstaScint) scan for evaluation of patients for salvage brachytherapy. Tech Urol 2000;6:146–150.

35. Cox JD, Gallagher MJ, Hammond EH, et al. Consensus statements on radiation therapy of prostate cancer: guidelines for prostate re-biopsy after radiation and for radiation therapy with rising prostate-specific antigen levels after radical prostatectomy. American Society for Therapeutic Radiology and Oncology Consensus Panel. J Clin Oncol 1999;17:1155.

36. Russo P. Salvage radical prostatectomy after radiation therapy and brachytherapy. J Endourol 2000;14:385–390.

37. Brenner PC, Russo P, Wood DP, et al. Salvage radical prostatectomy in the management of locally recurrent prostate cancer after 125I implantation. Br J Urol 1995;75:44–47.

38. Rogers E, Ohori M, Kassabian VS, et al. Salvage radical prostatectomy: outcome measured by serum prostate specific antigen levels. J Urol 1995;153:104–110.

39. Gheiler EL, Tefilli MV, Tiguert R, et al. Predictors for maximal outcome in patients undergoing salvage surgery for radio-recurrent prostate cancer. Urology 1998;51:789–795.

40. Amling CL, Lerner SE, Martin SK, et al. Deoxyribonucleic acid ploidy and serum prostate specific antigen predict outcome following salvage prostatectomy for radiation refractory prostate cancer. J Urol 1999;161:857–862.

41. Rogers E, Ohori M, Kassabian VS, et al. Salvage radical prostatectomy: outcome measured by serum prostate specific antigen levels. J Urol 1995;153:104–110.

42. Stephenson AJ, Scardino PT, Bianco FJ, et al. Salvage therapy for locally recurrent prostate cancer after external beam radiotherapy. Curr Treat Options Oncol 2004;5:357–365.

43. Grado GL, Collins JM, Kriegshauser JS, et al. Salvage brachytherapy for localized prostate cancer after radiotherapy failure. Urology 1999;53:2–10.

44. Pisters LL, von Eschenbach AC, Scott SM, et al. The efficacy and complications of salvage cryotherapy of the prostate. J Urol 1997;157:921–925.

45. Pisters LL, Perrotte P, Scott SM, et al. Patient selection for salvage cryotherapy for locally recurrent prostate cancer after radiation therapy. J Clin Oncol 1999;17:2514–2520.

46. Chin JL, Pautler SE, Mouraviev V, et al. Results of salvage cryoablation of the prostate after radiation: identifying predictors of treatment failure and complications. J Urol 2001;165:1937–1941.

47. Bolla M, Gonzalez D, Warde P, et al. Improved survival in patients with locally advanced prostate cancer treated with radiotherapy and goserelin. N Engl J Med 1997;337:295–300.

48. Bolla M, Collette L, Blank L, et al. Long-term results with immediate androgen suppression and external irradiation in patients with locally advanced prostate cancer (an EORTC study): a phase III randomised trial. Lancet 2002;360:103–106.

49. Messing EM, Manola J, Sarosdy M, et al. Immediate hormonal therapy compared with observation after radical prostatectomy and pelvic lymphadenectomy in men with node-positive prostate cancer. N Engl J Med 1999;341:1781–1788.

50. Moul JW, Wu H, Sun L, et al. Early versus delayed hormonal therapy for prostate specific antigen only recurrence of prostate cancer after radical prostatectomy. J Urol 2004;171:1141–1147.

51. Loblaw DA, Mendelson DS, Talcott JA, et al. American Society of Clinical Oncology recommendations for the initial hormonal management of androgen-sensitive metastatic, recurrent, or progressive prostate cancer. J Clin Oncol 2004;22:2927–2941.

52. Akakura K, Bruchovsky N, Goldenberg SL, et al. Effects of intermittent androgen suppression on androgen-dependent tumors. Apoptosis and serum prostate-specific antigen. Cancer 1993;71:2782–2790.

53. Sato N, Gleave ME, Bruchovsky N, et al. Intermittent androgen suppression delays progression to androgen-independent regulation of prostate-specific antigen gene in the LNCaP prostate tumour model. J Steroid Biochem Mol Biol 1996;58:139–146.

54. Hsieh JT, Wu HC, Gleave ME, et al. Autocrine regulation of prostate-specific antigen gene expression in a human prostatic cancer (LNCaP) subline. Cancer Res 1993;53:2852–2857.

55. Higano CS, Ellis W, Russell K, et al. Intermittent androgen suppression with leuprolide and flutamide for prostate cancer: a pilot study. Urology 1996;48:800–804.

56. Crook JM, Szumacher E, Malone S, et al. Intermittent androgen suppression in the management of prostate cancer. Urology 1999;53:530–534.

57. Strum SB, Scholz MC, McDermed JE. Intermittent androgen deprivation in prostate cancer patients: factors predictive of prolonged time off therapy. Oncologist 2000;5:45–52.

58. Grossfeld GD, Chaudhary UB, Reese DM, et al. Intermittent androgen deprivation: update of cycling characteristics in patients without clinically apparent metastatic prostate cancer. Urology 2001;58:240–245.

59. De La Taille A, Zerbib M, Conquy S, et al. Intermittent androgen suppression in patients with prostate cancer. BJU Int 2003;91:18-22.

60. Youssef E, Tekyi-Mensah S, Hart K, et al. Intermittent androgen deprivation for patients with recurrent/metastatic prostate cancer. Am J Clin Oncol 2003;26:e119–e123.

61. Klotz LH, Herr HW, Morse MJ, et al. Intermittent endocrine therapy for advanced prostate cancer. Cancer 1986;58:2546–2550.

62. Rashid MH, Chaudhary UB. Intermittent androgen deprivation therapy for prostate cancer. Oncologist 2004;9:295–301.

63. Tunn U, Eckart O, Kienle E. Can intermittent androgen deprivation be an alternative to continuous androgen withdrawal in patients with a PSA relapse? First results of the randomized prospective phase III clinical trial EC 507. J Urol 2003;169:1481.

64. Schasfoort E, Heathcote P, Lock T. Intermittent androgen suppression for the treatment of advanced prostate cancer. J Urol 2003;169:1483 [abstract].

65. http://www.cancer.gov/search/ResultsClinicalTrials.aspx?protocolsearch=1850073.

66. Fleshner NE, Fair WR. Anti-androgenic effects of combination finasteride plus flutamide in patients with prostatic carcinoma. Br J Urol 1996;78:907–910.

67. Brufsky A, Fontaine-Rothe P, Berlane K, et al. Finasteride and flutamide as potency-sparing androgen-ablative therapy for advanced adenocarcinoma of the prostate. Urology 1997;49:913–920.

68. Ornstein DK, Rao GS, Johnson B, et al. Combined finasteride and flutamide therapy in men with advanced prostate cancer. Urology 1996;48:901–905.

69. Barqawi AB, Moul JW, Ziada A, et al. Combination of low-dose flutamide and finasteride for PSA-only recurrent prostate cancer after primary therapy. Urology 2003;62:872–876.

70. Iversen P, Johansson JE, Lodding P, et al. Bicalutamide (150 mg) versus placebo as immediate therapy alone or as adjuvant to therapy with curative intent for early nonmetastatic prostate cancer: 5.3-year median followup from the Scandinavian Prostate Cancer Group Study Number 6. J Urol 2004;172:1871–1876.

71. Petrylak DP, Tangen CM, Hussain MH, et al. Docetaxel and estramustine compared with mitoxantrone and prednisone for advanced refractory prostate cancer. N Engl J Med 2004;351:1513–1520.

72. Tannock IF, de Wit R, Berry WR, et al. Docetaxel plus prednisone or mitoxantrone plus prednisone for advanced prostate cancer. N Engl J Med 2004;351:1502–1512.

Cryotherapy as primary therapy for prostate cancer

88

Ulrich K Fr Witzsch

INTRODUCTION

Cryoablation of the prostate has been used clinically for more than half a century. Early results were unsatisfactory due to poor oncologic outcome and high morbidity. Technical evolution and clinical experience has led to improved results with less morbidity.

CRYOBIOLOGY

Generally there are five effects discussed that might be of importance in destroying the prostate cancer cells[1,2]:

1. As the temperature falls, extracellular ice is created. The unfrozen intracellular water flows into the extracellular space causing dehydration, which is reversed during thawing. Water inflow into the hyperosmolaric intracellular space leads to rupture of the cell.
2. At lower temperatures intracellular ice forms. The ice crystals are needle shaped if the speed of freezing is fast. The sharper the ice, the more likely it is to destroy the cell membranes and organelles. During thawing, shear forces also destroy cell membranes.
3. Ice clots obstruct the blood vessels. These emboli or thrombi interrupt blood and oxygen supply to the tissue.
4. Apoptosis is induced by freezing.
5. Immunologic processes are initiated. The exact role of immunology in cryotherapy is still under investigation.

Experimental data[3] proves that the velocity of freezing correlates with the temperatures which must be achieved to be 100% lethal. The higher the velocity of freezing, the higher the temperature that destroys all cells. It has also been shown experimentally that repeated freeze thaw cycles are more effective than a single cycle (Table 88.1).

Table 88.1 Temperature that has to be reached to kill 100% of prostate cancer cells depending on velocity of freezing (Tatsutani)

| | Velocity of freezing | | |
	1°C/min	5°C/min	25°C/min
One cycle	<−40°C	<−40°C	−40°C
Two cycles	−40°C	−35°C	−18°C

CRYOABLATION

Clinical experience and experimental data[4] show that maximum ablation occurs with: 1) fast freezing; 2) slow thawing; and 3) repetitive freeze thaw cycles.

The speed of freezing is dependent on the density and efficacy of the probes. Size wise the relation between effective (kill) zone and affected (side effect) zone is always the same. Creating big iceballs leads to a larger zone of morbidity than do small iceballs. Due to this fact, it is obvious that multiple small iceballs covering the prostate homogeneously leads to a smaller zone of possible morbidity than a few big iceballs. Also, it is obvious that due to the circular form of the iceballs in larger ones warm areas are more probable between the killing zones than with more and smaller ones. Coverage of the prostate with numerous small iceballs is, therefore, known as "high-resolution cryotherapy."

CRYOTECHNOLOGY

The aim of cryotherapy is to ablate the prostate cancer tissue precisely, predictably, and in a controlled fashion.[5] This is most likely achieved with multiple small iceballs created by cryoneedles rather than thicker probes.

Influenced by technical inventions, cryotechnology developed considerably over the last few decades. The technology can be divided into three generations according to cryogen and type of probes:

1. First generation technology used liquid nitrogen for freezing. The probes had to be surgically placed.
2. Second generation uses high-pressure argon. Probes are still thick and have to be placed surgically with an insertion kit.
3. The most recent advance has been third generation devices.[6] Cryoneedles, miniaturized 17G double lumen needles, replace cryoprobes. The needles can be easily inserted into the prostate. High-pressure argon gas is expanded in the tip of the needle leading to cooling. High-pressure helium gas can be alternated in the same needle to produce a warming effect. The expanded gas returns back via the second lumen of the needle.

The change of temperature of gases while expanding is known as the Joule–Thompson effect. Using cooling and warming at the same location leads to higher controllability of the procedure. The iceballs created are approximately 2 cm × 3 cm, and they extend 0.5 cm from the tip of the needle. The needle tips are echogenic and, therefore, visible with ultrasound.

PROCEDURE

Initially a cystoscopy is done to measure the distance between the ureteral orifices and the bladder neck. Then a suprapubic catheter (SPC) is placed, and an extrastiff (Amplat2-) guide wire is inserted via the cystoscope for placement of the transurethral warming catheter later on in the procedure.

The transrectal ultrasound probe (TRUS) is placed in the rectum, and the preoperative measurements and landmarks of the prostate are re-identified. The TRUS probe will remain in place until the end of procedure for continuous real-time monitoring.

NEEDLE PLACEMENT

On average, *14 cryoneedles* are placed homogeneously in the prostate (Figure 88.1). The density of needles is higher in the dorsal aspect of the prostate for more effective treatment and better control of the peripheral zone. Needle placement is constantly monitored with TRUS. The placement is guided by a grid-like template. Cryotherapy grids differ from brachytherapy grids because they offer the possibility of placing needles in Denonvilliers' space or outer rectal wall. This is achieved by a distance of less than 5 mm between the lower aspect of the grid and the TRUS probe. An inflatable stand off should be used over the TRUS probe to improve the image and position the prostate gland to facilitate needle placement.

Two needles are placed in Denonvilliers' space just above the rectal wall. These needles are used only in the warming mode to avoid freezing into the rectal wall while a sufficient temperature is reached in the dorsal aspect of the prostate.[7]

Temperature probes are placed in the prostate at positions where the cancer location is suspected. A temperature probe is placed between the *warming needles* just above the rectal wall.

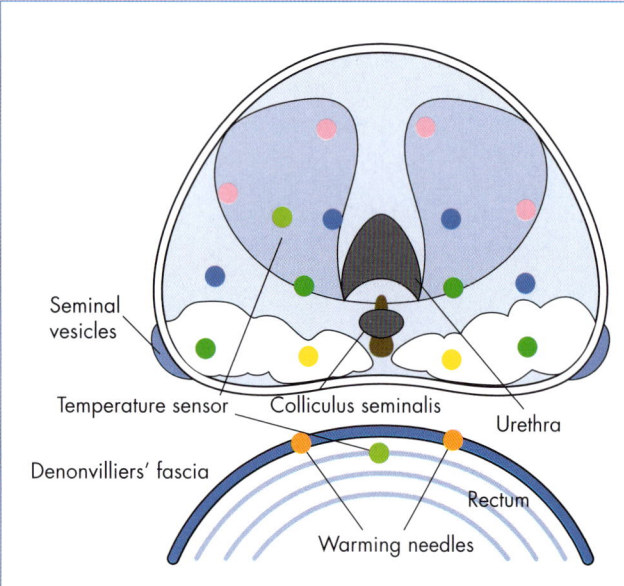

Fig. 88.1
Placement of the cryoneedles within the prostate.

A transurethral *warming catheter* is placed via the guide wire. This prevents urethral sloughing and also protects the external urethral sphincter area.

FREEZING AND THAWING

Reviewing the literature several modes of freezing and thawing are used.

We decided to freeze down to target temperature (–40°C) and keep this for 10 minutes. The prostate disappears in TRUS (blacked out). Then passive thawing (by switching the argon flow off) is started. When a plateau in temperature change is reached, active thawing (by turning helium flow on) is started. One minute of active thawing is interrupted by one of passive thawing—the so-called "barcode thawing". After reaching positive temperatures and regaining echoes in TRUS, the next cycle of freezing is started. Two freeze thaw cycles are performed at each location. It may be necessary to reduce the time of freezing or to keep the temperature above certain levels to protect sensitive areas. It may also be useful to keep the temperature below a certain level but not cool further. This ensures both cancer eradication and the minimization of side effects. All this is possible with the software of third generation technology.

PULL BACK

For prostates longer than 3 cm a pull-back maneuver is required. This means the needles have to be pulled back for the distance by which the prostate extends over 3 cm. After each repositioning of the needles, two more freeze thaw cycles are applied.

PROTECTION

Protection of sensitive areas is performed by special modes of operating. Warm water is applied to the perineal skin if the moisture in the operating room is frosting the needles. If the temperature in the rectal wall is falling too low, the inflatable stand off can be irrigated with warm water.

PERIOPERATIVE CARE

Preoperatively, a complete staging should be done. We prefer a full bowel preparation the day before the procedure and an enema on the morning of the procedure. Prophylactic antibiotics are prescribed as for transurethral resection of the prostate (TURP) with i.v. broad spectrum penicillin.

Postoperatively, we check the patient every second week for 6 weeks for urinary tract infections. If this occurs the patient receives antibiotic therapy according to the urine culture. Prostate-specific antigen (PSA) is checked every 3 months. The PSA nadir will be reached after 3 to 6 months after an significant rise on the first postoperative day. At postoperative visits, the patient is regularly checked for local side effects and residual urine after voiding. The SPC is removed once the residual urine is below 50 mL but not before the end of the first week.

SIDE EFFECTS

Antibiotic prophylaxis and therapy have made post-cryoablation infection a rare occurrence. Urethral sloughing also appears in a reduced percentage of cases. Perineal fistulas or fistulas between the urinary tract and the rectum are unknown in primary cryoablation of the prostate with third generation technology.

After early removal of the SPC, urinary retention may occur due to delayed swelling of the organ. If the residual urine remains high a TURP for removal of devitalized tissue is indicated. This should not be done before the third postoperative month because, until then, spontaneous improvement is still possible.

RESULTS

LONG-TERM RESULTS—FIRST AND SECOND GENERATION

Bahn et al[8] reported their 7-year experience. Five hundred and ninety patients were treated for localized or locally advanced prostate cancer. Thirty-two patients were retreated for recurrence. Patients were classified in three risk groups:

- Low risk: PSA <10 ng/mL, stage <T2b, and Gleason score <7.
- Medium risk if one risk factor was present.
- High risk if two or three risk factors were present.

Seven-year biochemical-free survival was 61%, 68%, and 61% in the low, medium, and high risk groups, respectively at a PSA threshold of 0.5 ng/mL; at a threshold of 1.0 ng/mL biochemical-free survival of 87%, 79%, and 71% was achieved, and using the ASTRO criteria 92%, 89%, and 89% maintained free of biochemical relapse.

After an average of 16 months 5.1% of patients regained potency. Incontinence (any leakage) was reported in 15.9% although only 4.3% used pads. Transurethral resection of the prostate was performed on 5.5 % of the patients and two fistulas occurred.

LONG-TERM RESULTS — SECOND GENERATION

Donnelly et al[9] report on results of a prospective nonrandomized clinical trial between December 1994 and February 1998. Eighty seven cryoprocedures were performed on 76 consecutive patients. All patients had histologically confirmed cancer of the prostate and PSA levels below 30 ng/mL. All patients had a negative bone scan. Patients with high risk for lymph node metastasis underwent laparoscopic lymph node dissection. Exclusion criteria were gland size greater than 60 mL, prior radiotherapy, and evidence of metastatic disease. After treating the first 30 patients, glands greater than 45 mL were downsized with 3 months of maximal androgen blockade.

Five probes were used. The first 10 patients only received a second freeze cycle if the prostate was longer than 4.5 cm. Starting with the eleventh patient, two freeze cycles were standard in all treatments. Eighty eight percent of the patients had T1 to T2 stage, Gleason score was less than 7 in 45% and 7 in 38%, and PSA was below 10 ng/mL in 62%. Transurethral resection of necrotic tissue due to sloughing was required in 3.9%. Incontinence was reported in 1.3% and testicular abscesses in 1.3%. The erectile dysfunction rate was 100%, initially, but five patients regained potency spontaneously and 13 with sexual aids.

Sixty five patients received one, ten patients received two, and one patient received three treatments. After all those treatments, 72 patients were negative for follow-up biopsies of the prostate area. One patient died of prostate cancer. At five years, PSA level was less than 0.3 ng/mL at 60% in the low-risk, 77% in the moderate-risk, and 48% in the high-risk group.

SHORT-TERM RESULTS — THIRD GENERATION

Cytron et al[7] first described results on 31 patients treated in a cryoablation technique with active rectal wall protection. The 12-month median PSA was 0.4 ng/mL, and no fistulas occurred. Potency was preserved in 20% of the patients who were potent preoperatively.

Prolonged catheterization was required in 10% of the patients, two cases of urinary tract infection had to be treated with antibacterial agents, and one patient suffered bulbar urethral trauma due to improper placement of the transurethral warming catheter.

PERSONAL RESULTS

Between September 2001 and October 2004 we treated 80 patients with cryotherapy for prostate cancer, 38 of whom were primary patients. Treatment was only considered primary in the absence of any other treatment for prostate cancer such as hormonal, radiation, or radical prostatectomy. A neoadjuvant treatment of less than 3 months was not considered as prior treatment.

All patients underwent a transrectal TRUS-guided biopsy, a bone scan, and, if the risk for lymph node metastases was high, either computed tomography (CT), magnetic resonance imaging (MRI), or a laparoscopic pelvic lymph node dissection. All patients treated were considered to have localized prostate cancer. The majority received cryotherapy because they had high comorbidity or were elderly, leading to a statistical life expectancy of less than 10 years. Two patients who were suitable for radical prostatectomy chose to have cryotherapy after receiving repetitively complete information on the outcome of all treatments for localized prostate cancer. Patients were categorized as favorable (n = 12) and unfavorable (n = 26) (Figure 88.2). Favorable patients had PSA <10 ng/mL, clinical stage less than T3, and combined Gleason score below 7.

Figure 88.3 shows the tumor stages based on clinical staging. Eight patients underwent a TURP unrelated to cryotherapy prior to the treatment. A prior TURP is not a contraindication for cryoablation of the prostate in experienced hands. Median preoperative PSA was 7.8 ng/mL, and median preoperative volume of the gland was 30 mL (12–80 mL).

Median treatment time was 135 minutes. A pull back was necessary in 85% due to length of the prostate being greater than 35 mm. The transurethral warming catheter remained in place for 20 minutes after finishing the last freeze cycle. Perioperative antibiotic prophylaxis was given for the time the SPC remained in place.

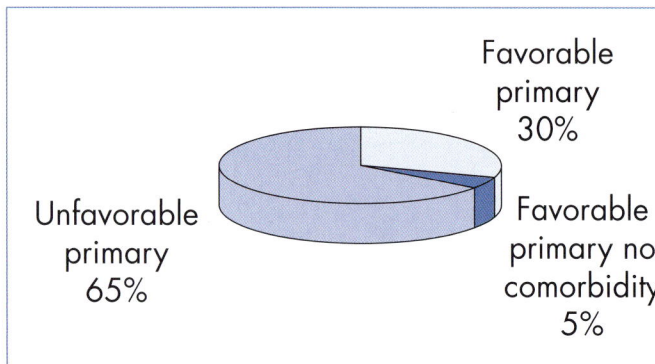

Fig. 88.2
Categorization of patients as favorable or unfavorable based on prostate-specific antigen level, tumor stage, and Gleason score.

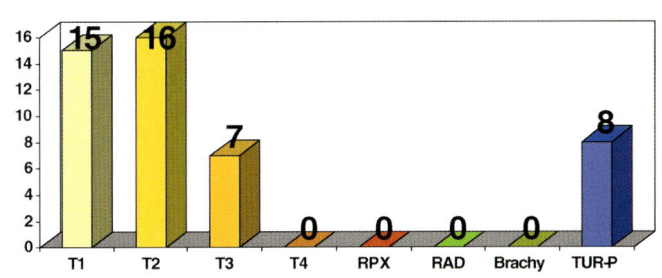

Fig. 88.3
Tumor stages based on clinical staging (T1–T4), and previous treatments undergone by the patients in Figure 88.2. (RAD, radiotherapy; RPX, radical prostatectomy; Brachy, brachytherapy; TUR-P, transurethral resection of the prostate.)

There were no serious adverse events. Especially, there were no perineal or rectal fistulas as described for earlier generation technology. Forty two percent of the patients had gross hematuria, which spontaneously subsided the next day without special therapy except increased fluid intake. The first two patients had a scrotal hematoma. This can be avoided by applying pressure to the perineum for at least 5 minutes after removal of the needles. Since then, only superficial hematomas of the perineal skin, if any, were observed.

The suprapubic catheter remained open until the gross hematuria has subsided (if present) and was clamped the next day so that the patient could perform a residual voiding chart. The SPC remained in place at least for 1 week or until the patients could void properly (residual volume <50 mL). In case of residual volume of more then 50 mL, a transurethral removal of necrotic tissue was performed in 13% of the patients not earlier than 6 weeks after the cryoablation. These patients all had a preoperative IPSS score of 16 or more. It is unlikely that patients with low preoperative IPSS score will not be able to void properly.

Urethral sloughing was not reported, to our knowledge. One patient reported a stress incontinence, which improved under medication and pelvic floor training. Two patients reported a prolonged time of incontinence after TURP.

At 3 months, 64% of the patients had achieved a PSA level below 0.1 ng/mL. Table 88.2 shows the postoperative median PSA level over time.

Table 88.2 Prostate-specific antigen (PSA) levels at intervals after cryotherapy

Time after cryotherapy (months)	3	6	12	18	24
PSA (ng/mL)	<0.1	0.4	0.2	0.1	0.2

INDICATIONS

Clinical experience gained during the last decades leads to several possible indications for primary cryoablation of the prostate:

- Primary patients with high comorbidity and increased anesthetic risk.
- Primary patients with suspected locally extended disease, which makes positive margins in radical prostatectomy probable. In these patients, an extended freezing may lead to good oncologic outcomes and minimizes the side effects, such as incontinence.
- Patients who are on hormone ablation for a while and their PSA is rising again. If the staging is negative, cryoablation may be an option for local tumor control even though there is not sufficient data on this subgroup available in the literature.
- Patients who definitely do not want radical surgery or other therapies.

DISCUSSION

The minimally invasive nature of cryoablation earns it a place in the range of therapeutic options for localized prostate cancer. Adhering to the concept of "nihil nocere" it is a good option if other therapeutic modalities have absolute or relative contraindications. Also, it opens a therapeutic option with curative possibilities if other modalities have a low probability of curative results such that the side effects of those other therapies would be more probable than cure. Clinical studies tend to suggest that even if there is a difference in the outcome regarding the risk of preoperative occult metastasis or postoperative progression this is lower for cryoablation in relation to other therapeutic options.[10,11]

The time of stay in the hospital is not comparable between centers. It depends very much on the structure of the health system, availability of facilities, and mentality of the patients. In Germany, for example, patients tend to stay longer in the hospital due to historical developments and patients demands. Also, numbers for presence of side effects are hard to compare due to inter-institutional and intercultural differences. It seems to be disappointing for European patients if the "bad tissue" is not passed out, whereas sloughing seems to bother patients in North America very much.

Clinical results improve with the development of the technology. The learning curve can be reduced with technical improvement and structured training programs including workshops, nurses training, proctoring sessions, and support by clinical application specialists.

CONCLUSION

Cryotherapy for primary prostate cancer is a minimally invasive alternative to other therapeutic options. Technical and clinical evolution has reduced the side effects and improved the results. It will not replace radical prostatectomy or other therapeutic modalities, but it closes a gap in the concept of local tumor control in well-selected patients.

REFERENCES

1. Hoffmann NE, Bischof JC. The cryobiology of cryosurgical injury. Urology 2002;60 (Suppl 2A):40–49.

2. Gage AA, Baust J. Mechanisms of tissue injury in cryosurgery. Cryobiology 1998;37:171–186.

3. Tatsutani K, Rubinsky B, Onik G, et al. Effect of thermal variables on frozen human primary prostatic adenocarcinoma cells. Urology 1996;48:441–447.

4. Larson T, Robertson D, Corica A, et al. In vivo interstitial temperature mapping of the human prostate during cryosurgery with correlation to histopathological outcomes. Urology 2000;55:547–552.

5. Patel B, Parsons C, Bidair M, et al. Cryoablation for carcinoma of the prostate. J Surg Oncol 1996;63:256–264.

6. Moore Y, Sofer P. Successful treatment of locally confined prostate cancer with the seed net™system—preliminary multicenter results. Clin Appl Notes 2001;June:1–7.

7. Cytron S, Paz A, Kravchick S, et al. Active rectal wall protection using direct transperitoneal cryo-needles for histologically proven prostate adenocarcinomas, Eur Urol 2003;44:315–321.

8. Bahn D, Lee F, Badalament R, et al. Targeted cryoablation of the prostate: 7-year outcomes in the primary treatment of prostate cancer. Urology 2002;60 (Suppl 2A):3–11.

9. Donnelly B, Saliken J, Ernst D, et al. Prospective trial of cryosurgical ablation of the prostate: five-year results. Urology 2002;60:645–649.

10. Zisman A, Pantuck A, Cohen J, et al. Prostate cryoablation using direct transperineal placement of ultrathin probes through a 17-gauge brachytherapy template—technique and preliminary results. Urology 2001;58:988–993.

11. Long J, Bahn D, Lee F, et al. Five-year retrospective, multi-institutional pooled analysis of cancer-related outcomes after cryosurgical ablation of the prostate. Urology 2001;57:518–523.

Cryotherapy as salvage therapy for prostate cancer

89

Dan Leibovici, Louis L Pisters

OVERVIEW

The routine use of prostate-specific antigen (PSA) analysis in men over 50 years of age since the early 1990s has revolutionized the diagnosis of prostate cancer. With the advent of PSA, early detection of prostate cancer is often possible before any symptoms or palpable abnormalities occur in the prostate. As a result, patients typically present for treatment with organ-confined disease, and are subjected to a primary therapy modality with curative intent.[1,2] Despite this, cancer recurrence following initial therapy is not uncommon. It has been estimated that each year in the USA alone, 50,000 men have PSA recurrence after either radical prostatectomy or radiation therapy.[3] This typically precedes any clinical finding by 3 to 5 years.[4] Although PSA elevation following primary therapy is a very sensitive predictor of subsequent clinical disease progression, it does not reliably distinguish between local recurrence and systemic (metastatic) disease. The distinction between these two entities is crucial in determining the next line of therapy and the patient's prognosis. Generally, systemic disease is not amenable to curative therapy, and the goals of treatment in that setting are to preserve quality of life and minimize morbidity. Conversely, an isolated local recurrence following primary treatment has the potential of being cured by salvage therapy.

Finding the source of PSA elevation following primary therapy for prostate cancer has been challenging. Digital rectal examination or transrectal ultrasound are neither sensitive nor specific in the detection of local recurrence.[5,6] Conversely, prostate biopsy may be the single most reliable test to confirm local recurrence of prostate cancer. Nevertheless, it provides no information about the presence or absence of systemic disease in conjunction with a local recurrence. Cross-sectional imaging with computerized tomography also lacks sensitivity in detecting local recurrence following initial therapy.[7] Conversely, magnetic resonance imaging (MRI) with an external and an endorectal coil provides high-resolution anatomic images and has been found to be more accurate in the diagnosis of local cancer recurrence than any other imaging modality.[8] However, the experience with MRI in this setting has been limited, and larger studies are needed to confirm its role in detection of local recurrence. Although any of the above modalities could diagnose local cancer recurrence, none of them can distinguish between isolated local recurrence, which might be amenable to salvage therapy, and a combination of local recurrence and microscopic metastasis. Radionuclide bone scan is rarely positive in the presence of serum PSA below 20 ng/mL and, potentially, would miss microscopic metastatic disease in its early phase.[9] Monoclonal antibody based radioisotope scans were developed with the purpose of locating the site of recurrent tumor. Despite its initial promise, this modality did not show the expected accuracy in ruling out metastatic disease, although the predictive value of a positive extrapelvic scan was high.[10,11] The velocity with which serum PSA increases after an initial failed primary treatment, specifically the PSA doubling time, may more reliably distinguish between an isolated localized tumor recurrence and metastatic disease.[12]

Recurrence of prostate cancer following initial therapy may reflect the aggressive biologic nature of the original tumor or, conversely, may be caused by a technical malfunction occurring at the time of the initial treatment procedure, leading to failure to eradicate an otherwise curable cancer. In the latter case, the residual cancer may still be curable if subjected to a salvage procedure. This curative prospect, albeit small, justifies the use of aggressive means that would not normally be applied to patients with metastasis. The decision to use a salvage procedure versus hormonal treatment largely depends on patient factors such as performance status, comorbidities, and personal preferences; but also depends on the type of initial therapy that has been given. Data from a national disease registry of patients with prostate cancer, (Cancer of the Prostate Strategic Urologic Research Endeavor [CaPSURE]) shows that the type of salvage therapy following initial radical prostatectomy is equally divided between androgen deprivation therapy (ADT) and radiation therapy, whereas ADT is applied as salvage therapy following radiation therapy in more than 90% of cases.[13] The available interventional procedures done in the other 10% of the patients who have failed radiation therapy include: salvage radical prostatectomy, salvage cystoprostatectomy or total pelvic exenteration, hyperthermia, and cryosurgery. The chapter will discuss cryosurgery as a post-radiation salvage procedure for prostate cancer.

GENERAL PRINCIPLES OF SALVAGE CRYOTHERAPY

Assuming that the prostate is the single site of tumor recurrence, any procedure resulting in complete ablation of the recurrent tumor has curative potential. Typically, this can be achieved either by surgical excision (i.e., salvage radical prostatectomy), or by in-situ ablation of the entire prostate, including the organ-confined tumor. Cryotherapy consists of in-situ tissue ablation by application of extremely cold temperature. This is accomplished by direct transperineal insertion of cryogenic probes into the prostate that are precisely positioned under transrectal ultrasound guidance. Cryogenic temperature is created inside and around the probe tip by flow of pressurized argon gas through a narrow nozzle over an abrupt pressure gradient. According to the Joule–Thompson principle, the flow of argon gas under such conditions is associated with a thermal sink. Following activation, an iceball is created around the tip of each probe, and sequentially additional cryogenic probes are activated until the freezing has encompassed the entire prostate. The number of probes used varies depending on the shape and size of the prostate. Typically, between 6 and 8 probes are used to conform the ice ball to the shape of the gland.[14] The freezing process is monitored in real time by transrectal ultrasound, and the temperature is

measured at specific sites, such as the external urinary sphincter. Caution is used to prevent cryogenic injury to the rectal wall and urinary sphincter, and the urethra is kept warm by a designated warming catheter, which prevents urethral sloughing and stricture. The cryogenic temperature within the coalescent iceball is not homogenous but follows a thermal gradient, and isotherms corresponding to different temperatures can be calculated.[15] The biologic ablative effect of freezing corresponds to the volume of tissue included within lethal isotherms. Cryogenic tissue injury is caused by several putative mechanisms, including osmotic changes as the result of extracellular water transforming into ice, shearing forces exerted upon the cell membrane by extracellular ice crystals, intracellular freezing, tissue ischemia, and immune responses targeting the ablated tumor cells.[16] To achieve cure in the patient with recurrent prostate cancer, the entire tumor must be included within the lethal isotherm. This implies that the tumor needs to be confined to the prostate on the one hand and cryosurgery needs to be adequately performed on the other. Previous exposure of the urethra, rectum, or bladder to radiation renders these organs more susceptible to cryogenic-induced injury; consequently, the side effects of cryosurgery in the salvage setting are more pronounced than in primarily treated patients.

CANCER CONTROL ACHIEVED BY CRYOSURGERY IN THE SALVAGE SETTING

SALVAGE CRYOSURGERY FOLLOWING PREVIOUS RADIATION THERAPY

The risk for recurrence of prostate cancer following initial radiation therapy depends on tumor factors such as Gleason grade, pretreatment PSA level, and T stage. In addition, the previously administered radiation dose appears to affect outcome, especially in patients in the intermediate- and high-risk groups.[17,18] Among patients who present for radiation therapy with T1 to T2 tumors 47% will experience biochemical progression at 8 years following treatment, and 14% to 34% will die of disease.[19,20] Furthermore, higher failure rates have been observed in high-risk patients (T3 or Gleason 8–10), who are most commonly treated with radiation therapy.[21] Following radiation therapy, tissue fibrosis occurs within the treated fields causing obliteration of anatomic planes, and making surgical dissection a major technical challenge and more prone to complications. As a result, many patients are left with the choices of watchful waiting or hormonal treatment, neither of which are curative approaches. Cryosurgery, on the other hand, offers the advantage of complete prostate ablation without the need to dissect through previously irradiated tissues. In comparison with salvage radical prostatectomy, salvage cryosurgery is much easier to perform, easier to learn, and more tolerable for the patient, making it a particularly appealing treatment approach in the patients who need a salvage procedure following radiation therapy.

The most important clinical endpoint in assessing the efficacy of cancer therapy is disease-specific survival. Because prostate cancer is a relatively slow growing malignancy, long follow-up is necessary to evaluate this endpoint. Surrogate endpoints such as serum PSA following therapy and post-cryosurgery prostate biopsy may not be as accurate as disease-specific survival in assessing the effect of therapy, because some of these patients may have been treated with hormone ablation leading to low PSA levels, and biopsies are often not specific. Most reported series on cryosurgery as salvage therapy for recurrent prostate cancer have a short follow-up, and consequently caution is needed in inferring the results to all patients.

As shown in Table 89.1, salvage cryosurgery following radiation therapy achieves a nadir PSA of less than 0.5 ng/mL and negative biopsies for most patients. With longer follow-up however, disease recurrence as evidenced by biochemical relapse occurs in some of the patients. The biochemical progression-free survival rate at 2 years after salvage cryosurgery ranges between 55% and 74%.[24,28,29] The risk of biochemical failure increases with higher pretreatment PSA levels and Gleason grades, and in patients with a PSA nadir greater than 0.1 ng/mL. Salvage cryosurgery may fail either due to incomplete ablation of the prostate reflecting technical limitations, or due to extraprostatic or seminal vesicle involvement beyond the reach of the freezing process. Ideally, a better staging method would improve patient selection leading to the restriction of this modality for the patients who are most likely to benefit from it.

There are limited long-term reports of the results of salvage cryosurgery. In 2002, Izawa et al reported on 131 patients who underwent salvage cryosurgery following initial radiation therapy.[30] In patients with Gleason grade 8 or less tumors, the 5-year disease-specific survival rate was 87% compared with 63% in patients with Gleason grade 9 or 10. Similarly, the disease-free survival rate was 57% versus 23% in patients with presalvage PSA level below or above 10 ng/mL, respectively. Although the results of salvage radical prostatectomy in terms of biochemical progression-free survival have been reported to exceed those of salvage cryosurgery, because there have been no randomized controlled trials directly comparing the two modalities, the comparison of efficacy between the two procedures remains inconclusive.[31,32]

Androgen deprivation therapy has been used in conjunction with cryosurgery in the salvage setting. Its main effect appears to be that of downsizing the prostate, which decreases the distance between cryogenic probes and may facilitate a more efficient tissue ablation. There is no evidence, however, that ADT improves disease-specific survival in patients who undergo salvage cryosurgery.

A specific technical difficulty may be encountered when performing salvage cryosurgery following initial brachytherapy. Because the prostate is loaded with seeds, their echogenic appearance on ultrasound may interfere with that of the cryogenic probes and may render the accurate positioning of the cryogenic probes difficult. This problem is manageable, however, and cryosurgery can be done safely in this setting. Many of the patients treated with external beam radiation therapy have poor risk and thereby may not be cured by a procedure targeting the primary tumor alone. In contrast, most of the patients undergoing brachytherapy have low-risk disease, and consequently, cancer recurrence in this subset is more likely to result from technical failure than from the adverse biology of the disease. Due to this inherent difference in patient selection, salvage cryosurgery after previously failed brachytherapy may prove particularly effective in achieving cure.

COMPLICATIONS

Performing cryosurgery in tissues that have been previously irradiated may be associated with increased

Table 89.1 Efficacy of cryosurgery in controlling recurrent prostate cancer after failure of radiation therapy

# of patients	Median FU (months)	Undetectable PSA [<0.05 ng/mL], n (%)	PSA <0.5 ng/mL, n (%)	Negative FU biopsies, n (%)	Patients receiving ADT, n (%)	Reference
33	16.8	NA	39	26 (79)	16 (48)	Miller[22]
150	17	47 (31)	63 (42)	116 (77)	40 (27)	Pisters[23]
106	43	NA	114 (97)	91 (86)	71 (67)	Chin[24,25]
43	21.9	NA	26 (60)*	NA	43 (100)†	De la Taille[26]
18	20	NA	13 (72)	NA	0	Han[27]

FU, follow-up duration; PSA, prostate specific antigen.

*These patients had a nadir PSA level <0.1 ng/mL. †All received 3 months of neoadjuvant hormonal therapy that was discontinued at the time of cryosurgery.

tissue damage and more frequent complications. The same complications occur following cryosurgery either in the primary treatment or salvage settings; however, their frequency is higher with salvage cryosurgery. Reported complications include urethral sloughing, which is manifested by obstruction, urinary incontinence, perineal pain, rectal injury, and fistula formation, osteitis pubis, and erectile dysfunction. Lee et al reported that the risk of rectal fistula was 8.7% in patients who had been previously treated with radiation, compared with less than 0.5% in patients for whom cryosurgery was done as primary therapy.[33] Others confirmed a higher prevalence of prostate-related symptoms in patients undergoing salvage versus primary cryosurgery of the prostate.[34] The risk for urinary incontinence is increased in patients who undergo salvage cryosurgery and varies between 7% and 8% compared with 1.3% and 4% in patients in whom cryosurgery was performed as primary treatment.[24,28,35,36] Ensuring a positive temperature in the external sphincter during cryosurgery can reduce the incidence of urinary incontinence.[27] The risk for complications increases in patients with locally invasive or high Gleason grade tumors, presumably due to the need of more aggressive cryosurgery to achieve tumor control.[24] Similarly, we reported incontinence and urethral sloughing rates of 72% and 67%, respectively in a cohort of 150 patients in whom 90% had T3 to T4 tumors and/or Gleason scores of 8 to 10.[23] In six of these patients, major extirpative surgery was necessary to control chronic debilitating symptoms, including refractory hematuria, osteitis pubis, recto-urethral fistula, bladder outlet obstruction, and chronic rectal pain.[37] It is important to note that this high complication rate was observed in patients whose treatment involved older equipment, including second-generation cryogenic probes, without the use of thermocouples. In order to maximize safety, we recommend using third-generation probes with judicious use of thermocouples particularly at Denonvilliers' fascia (to reduce the risk of rectal injury and fistula) as well as the external urinary sphincter (to reduce incontinence). Urethral protection is best achieved by the commercial designated warmer catheter, and its use is essential. The risk for urethral sloughing decreased significantly following the FDA approval of the designated warming catheter, and, consequently, the quality of life of patients who underwent salvage cryosurgery is better in contemporary series than in previous reports, and is comparable to that of patients undergoing primary cryosurgery.[34,38,39] Another feared complication is rectal fistula. In contemporary series, the incidence of this complication has been 1% to 3%.[22–26,34] Pelvic or rectal pain occurs in about 10% of the patients and typically subsides within 3 to 4 weeks. It is presumed that this is caused by cryogenic injury to sensory nerves. Ischemia of the rectal wall may be

another possible cause, and topical nitrates have been used anecdotally to prevent the pain. Erectile dysfunction has been reported in 80% to 100% of the patients who underwent cryosurgery as primary treatment for prostate cancer with some improvement over time after the procedure.[27] In the salvage setting, erectile dysfunction is the rule, and can be expected to occur in almost all patients.

SALVAGE CRYOSURGERY FOLLOWING PREVIOUS CRYOSURGERY

Radical prostatectomy aims to cure localized prostate cancer by en-bloc resection of the entire prostate gland, prostatic urethra, and seminal vesicles. Due to the multifocal nature of prostate cancer, there is no role for partial prostatectomy. Radical prostatectomy, therefore, provides one single surgical opportunity to cure the patient. Similarly, the cumulative lifetime tolerance to radiation limits the total dose that can safely be given without unacceptable morbidity. The maximal efficacy of radiation therapy is, therefore, achieved by delivering a maximally tolerated dose during one single radiation therapy course.

Conversely, cryosurgery is unique in that it can be repeated, if necessary, with no increased morbidity. Thus, this modality offers the patient a "second shot" to win the battle. Many of the series that report on cryosurgery as primary care for prostate cancer indicate that, in a subset of their patients, more than one cryosurgical session was necessary to achieve tumor control. As is the case with other circumstances of disease recurrence, the dilemma is whether the biochemical failure is caused by residual cancer that is confined to the prostate or represents metastatic disease. Because complete exposure of all prostate cells to two cycles of freezing to −40°C or below invariably results in necrosis and should lead to an undetectable PSA level, true localized cancer recurrence implies that such freezing conditions have not been achieved throughout the entire prostate.[40] Potential reasons of incomplete freezing include technical problems, the inability to include the entire prostate within the lethal isotherm without risking rectal injury, and the warming catheter that keeps a thin rim of viable prostatic tissue surrounding the urethra. A prostate biopsy may help to distinguish between a local source of PSA as viable glands within the prostate and extraprostatic disease. It has been our approach to perform an extensive (20-core) prostate biopsy in all patients with biochemical failure after cryosurgery. In the case that such biopsy demonstrates extensive coagulative necrosis with no viable glands, the PSA elevation should be attributed to extraprostatic sources, implying microscopic metastatic disease. When the biopsy shows viable glands, it supports the possibility of inadequate freezing. When the absolute PSA level is low (<2.0

ng/mL) and the PSA doubling time is long, localized disease can be assumed, and repeat cryosurgery can be reasonably elected. The chance of achieving a durable PSA response and of converting a positive biopsy to a negative one by repeat cryosurgery varies depending on patient selection. Overall, in patients with low-risk disease, there seems to be a 20% to 30% chance for a second cryosurgical ablation to achieve cancer control.[41-43] The risk for complications with repeated cryosurgery is equivalent to that of primary cryosurgery, although the occasional patients who remain potent after the first procedure are likely to lose erectile function following the salvage procedure.

SALVAGE CRYOSURGERY FOLLOWING RADICAL PROSTATECTOMY

A visible measurable target lesion into which cryogenic probes can be inserted is a prerequisite for cryosurgery performance. In the majority of patients who experience biochemical progression following radical prostatectomy, the disease is either outside the prostatic fossa or is only microscopic and cannot be treated by cryosurgery. In occasional patients, however, with histologically confirmed recurrence of prostate cancer and a measurable lesion at the anastomosis, salvage cryosurgery can be done. Cytron et al (Barzilai Medical Center, Israel) have performed salvage cryosurgery following radical prostatectomy on five patients (personal communication). In all patients, the target lesion was clearly visible by transrectal ultrasound, with a median volume of the treated lesions of 4.0 mL. A significant PSA decrease was observed in all patients after salvage cryosurgery. Undetectable PSA levels were achieved in three patients and were maintained for 2 years following the salvage procedure. Temporary urinary incontinence occurred following salvage cryosurgery; however, this resolved over the first 6 months. This probably represents the first series of salvage cryosurgery performed following initial radical prostatectomy. These preliminary results indicate that salvage cryosurgery may have a role in selected patients after failed radical prostatectomy and that this concept deserves further study.

PATIENT SELECTION FOR SALVAGE CRYOSURGERY

Accomplishing cure by salvage cryosurgery depends on adequate technical performance of the procedure, state-of-the-art equipment, and appropriate patient selection. The best results can be achieved in patients with low-volume, low-grade disease that is confined to the prostate. Because the available staging methods are not accurate enough to identify the ideal candidates, some auxiliary parameters should be used. A low PSA level at

the time of recurrence and a long doubling time (>12 months) have been associated with localized disease.[44,45] In addition, the grade and extent of extracapsular extension of cancer may be determined by staging biopsy with multiple cores. Magnetic resonance imaging may have a role in the detection of macroscopic extraprostatic tumor extension. Other important considerations include prostate volume (effective cryosurgery is usually limited to 50 mL or less), adequate patient performance status, and absence of bladder outlet obstruction.

SALVAGE RADIATION THERAPY AFTER FAILED CRYOSURGERY

Occasional patients, who have recurrent disease following repeated cryosurgery and are believed to have localized disease benefit from salvage radiation therapy. Burton et al reported on 49 patients who received 63 Gy on average following biopsy-confirmed recurrence of prostate cancer after primary cryosurgery. The average pretreatment PSA was 2.4 ng/mL and a nadir PSA level below 1.0 ng/mL was achieved in 42 (86%) patients. With an average follow-up duration of 32 months the biochemical progression free survival was 60%.[46] Complete resolution of palpable lesion was observed in 4 of 6 patients in another series treated with salvage radiation therapy following primary cryosurgery.[47] Urethral strictures and proctitis were reported in both series, but the numbers are too small to permit comparison with radiation therapy series done as primary treatment.

SUMMARY

Depending on the risk factors, patients with recurrent prostate cancer following primary therapy may have localized versus disseminated disease. In patients with localized cancer recurrence, salvage cryosurgery is a viable and effective treatment modality with efficacy comparable to that of salvage radical prostatectomy and a lower complication rate. Cryosurgery offers more flexibility in planning the treatment for prostate cancer by permitting repeated performance in the case of failure.

REFERENCES

1. Stephenson RA. Population based prostate cancer trends in the PSA-era: data from the Surveillance, Epidemiology, and End Results (SEER) program. Monogr Urol 1998;19:1–19.

2. Newcomer LM, Stanford JL, Blumenstein BA, et al. Temporal trends in rates of prostate cancer: declining incidence of advanced stage disease, 1974 to 1994. J Urol 1997;158:1427–1430.

3. Moul JW. Prostate specific antigen only progression of prostate cancer. J Urol 2000;163:1632–1642.

4. Paulson DF. Impact of radical prostatectomy in the management of clinically localized prostate cancer. J Urol 1994;152:1826–1830.

5. Pound CR, Christens-Barry OW, Gurganus RT, et al. Digital rectal examinations and imaging studies are unnecessary in men with undetectable prostate specific antigen following radical prostatectomy. J Urol 1999;162:1337–1340.

6. Johnstone PA, McFarland JT, Riffenburgh RH, et al. Efficacy of digital rectal examination after radiotherapy for prostate cancer. J Urol 2001;166:1684–1687.

7. Kramer S, Gorich J, Gottfried HW, et al. Sensitivity of computed tomography in detecting local recurrence of prostatic carcinoma following radical prostatectomy. Br J Radiol 1997;70:995–999.

8. Silverman JM, Krebs TL. MR imaging evaluation with a transrectal surface coil of local recurrence of prostatic cancer in men who have undergone radical prostatectomy. AJR Am J Roentgenol 1997;168:379–385.

9. Cher ML, Bianco FJ Jr, Lam JS, et al. Limited role of radionuclide bone scintigraphy in patients with prostate specific antigen elevations after radical prostatectomy. J Urol 1998;160:1387–1391.

10. Kahn D, Williams RD, Manyak MJ, et al. 111Indium - in the evaluation of patients with residual or recurrent prostate cancer after radical prostatectomy. The ProstaScint Study Group. J Urol 1998;159:2041–2046.

11. Kahn D, Williams RD, Haseman MK, et al. Radioimmunoscintigraphy with In-111 labeled capromab pendetide predicts prostate cancer response to salvage radiotherapy after failed radical prostatectomy. J Clin Oncol1998;16:284–289.

12. D'Amico AV, Cote K, Loffredo M, et al. Determinants of prostate cancer-specific survival after radiation therapy for patients with clinically localized prostate cancer. J Clin Oncol 2002;20:4567–4573.

13. Grossfeld GD, Stier DM, Flanders SC, et al. Use of second treatment following definitive local therapy for local prostate cancer: data from the CaPSURE database. J Urol 1998;160:1398–1404.

14. Zippe CD. Cryosurgery of the prostate technique and pitfalls. Urol Clin N Am 1996;23:147–163.

15. Rewcastle JC, Sandison GA, Hahn LJ, et al. A model for the time dependent thermal distribution within an iceball surrounding a cryoprobe. Med Phys 2001;28:1125–1137.

16. Gage AA, Baust J. Mechanisms of tissue injury in cryosurgery. Cryobiology 1998;37:171–186.

17. Jacob R, Hanlon AR, Horwitz EM, et al. The relationship of increasing radiotherapy dose to reduced distant metastases and mortality in men with prostate cancer. Cancer 2004;100:538–543.

18. Valicenti R, Lu J, Pielpich M, et al. Survival advantage from higher-dose radiation therapy for clinically localized prostate cancer treated on the Radiation Therapy Oncology Group trials. J Clin Oncol 2000;18:2740–2746.

19. Kuban DA, Thames HD, Levy LB, et al. Long-term multi-institutional analysis of stage T1-T2 prostate cancer treated with radiotherapy in the PSA era. Int J Radiation Oncol Biol Phys 2003;57:915–928.

20. Maartense S, Hermans J, Leer JW. Radiation therapy in localized prostate cancer: long-term results and late toxicity. Clin Oncol (Royal Col Radiol) 2000;12:222–228.

21. D'Amico AV. Radiation and hormonal therapy for locally advanced and clinically localized prostate cancer. Urology 2002;60:32–37.

22. Miller RJ, Cohen JK, Shuman B, et al. Percutaneous, transperineal cryosurgery of the prostate as salvage therapy for post radiation recurrence of adenocarcinoma. Cancer 1996;77:1510–1514.

23. Pisters LL, von Eschenbach AC, Scott SM, et al. The efficacy and complications of salvage cryotherapy of the prostate. J Urol 1997;157:921–925.

24. Chin JL, Pautler SE, Mouraviev V, et al. Results of salvage cryoablation of the prostate after radiation: identifying predictors of treatment failure and complications. J Urol 2001;165:1937–1942.

25. Chin JL, Touma N, Pautler SE, et al. Serial histopathology result of salvage cryoablation for prostate cancer after radiation failure. J Urol 2003;170:1199–1202.

26. De la Taille A, Hayek O, Benson MC, et al. Salvage cryotherapy for recurrent prostate cancer after radiation therapy: the Columbia experience. Urology 2000;55:79–84.

27. Han KR, Belldegrun AS. Third-generation cryosurgery for primary and recurrent prostate cancer. BJU international 2004;93:14–18.

28. Ghafar MA, Johnson CW, De la Taille A, et al. Salvage cryotherapy using an argon-based system for locally recurrent prostate cancer after radiation therapy: the Columbia experience. J Urol 2001;166:1333–1338.

29. Bales GT, Williams MJ, Sinner M, et al. Short-term outcomes after cryosurgical ablation of the prostate in men with recurrent prostate carcinoma following radiation therapy. Urology 1995;46:676–680.

30. Izawa JI, Madsen LE, Scott SM, et al. Salvage cryotherapy for recurrent prostate cancer after radiotherapy: variables affecting patient outcome. J Clin Oncol 2002;20:2664–2761.

31. Leibovich BC, Zincke H, Blute ML, et al. Recurrent prostate cancer after radiation therapy: Salvage prostatectomy versus salvage cryosurgery. American Urological Association, 96th Annual Meeting. 2001;165:1595.

32. Cheng L, Sebo TJ, Slejak J, et al. Predictors of survival for prostate carcinoma patients treated with salvage radical prostatectomy after radiation therapy. Cancer 1998;83:2164–2171.

33. Lee F, Bahn DK, McHugh TA, et al. Cryosurgery of prostate cancer. Use of adjuvant hormonal therapy and temperature monitoring a one year follow-up. Anticancer Res 1997;17:1511–1516.

34. Anastasiadis AG, Sachdev R, Salomon L, et al. Comparison of health related quality of life and prostate associated symptoms after primary and salvage cryotherapy for prostate cancer. J Cancer Res Clin Oncol 2003;129:676–682.

35. Bahn DK, Lee F, Badalament R, et al. Targeted cryoablation of the prostate:7-year outcomes in the primary treatment of prostate cancer. Urology 2002;60:3–11.

36. Donnelly BJ, Saliken JC, Ernst DS, et al. Prospective trial of cryosurgical ablation of the prostate: 5-year results. Urology 2002;60:645–649.

37. Izawa JI, Ajam K, McGuire E, et al. Major surgery to manage definitively severe complications of salvage cryotherapy for prostate cancer, J Urol 2000;64:1978–1981.

38. Perrotte P, Litwin MS, McGuire EJ, et al. Quality of life after salvage cryotherapy: the impact of treatment parameters. J Urol 1999;162:398–402.

39. Robinson JW, Donnelly BJ, Saliken JC, et al. Quality of life and sexuality of men with prostate cancer 3 years after cryosurgery. Urology 2002;60:12–18.

40. Larson TR, Robertson DW, Corica A, et al. In vivo interstitial temperature mapping of the human prostate during cryosurgery with correlation to histopathologic outcomes. Urology 2000;55:547–552.

41. Cohen JK, Miller RJ, Rooker GM, et al. Cryosurgical ablation of the prostate: two year prostate specific antigen and biopsy results. Urology 1996;47:395–401.

42. Wong WS, Chinn DO, Chinn M, et al. Cryosurgery as the treatment of prostate carcinoma. Cancer 1997;79:963–974.

43. Koppie TM, Shinohara K, Grossfeld GD, et al. The efficacy of cryosurgical ablation of prostate cancer: The University of California San Francisco experience. J Urol 1999;162:427–432.

44. D'Amico AV, Cote K, Loffredo M, et al. Determinants of prostate cancer specific survival following radiation therapy during the prostate specific antigen era. J Urol 2003;170:S42–S46.

45. D'Amico AV, Moul JW, Carroll PR, et al. Surrogate end point for prostate cancer-specific mortality after radical prostatectomy or radiation therapy. J Natl Cancer Inst 2003;95:1376–1383.

46. Burton S, Brown DM, Colonias A, et al. Salvage radiotherapy for prostate cancer recurrence after cryosurgical ablation. Urology 2000;56:833–838.

47. McDonough MJ, Feldmeier JJ, Parsai I, et al. Salvage external beam radiotherapy for clinical failure after cryosurgery for prostate cancer. Int J Radiat Oncol Biol Phys 2001;51:624–627.

Androgen deprivation for the treatment of prostate cancer: general principles

90

David G McLeod, Albaha Barqawi

HISTORICAL BACKGROUND

Hormonal manipulation for the treatment of prostate disease dates back more than 100 years. However, little was known of the effect of sex hormones on the initiation and progression of prostate cancer until the late 1930s. In 1941, Huggins and Hodges at the University of Chicago presented their Nobel prize-winning paper in which they demonstrated that, due to the dependence of the normal prostate gland on sex hormones for growth, either surgical castration or treatment with diethylstilbestrol (DES) had significant therapeutic implications for men with prostate cancer.[1] This discovery marked the beginning of modern hormonal manipulation in men with prostate cancer.

Since the 1940s, hormonal manipulation has been the mainstay of the systemic treatment of advanced prostate cancer. In the 1940s, estrogen treatments, primarily DES, became the primary alternative to orchiectomy. In the 1960s, trials initiated by the Veterans Administration Co-operative Urological Research Group (VACURG) found no statistically significant differences in median and in 2-, 5-, and 10-year survival rates in patients either receiving DES or undergoing orchiectomy.[2,3] A later review of three VACURG trials concluded that the use of either DES or orchiectomy provided a significant survival benefit in patients with locally advanced nonmetastatic prostate cancer.[4] However, estrogen therapy fell out of favor due to the increased risk of cardiovascular death after treatment with 5 mg/day DES in these studies. In addition, a more recent study showed that daily treatment with 3 mg DES as the primary hormonal therapy for stage D2 prostate cancer caused more serious cardiovascular or thromboembolic complications than occurred with the antiandrogen flutamide.[5]

A parenteral route of administration for estrogen therapy has been suggested as a way to minimize cardiovascular adverse events by avoiding the first-pass effect in the liver, thereby minimizing overproduction of coagulation factor VII.[6–8] However, in trials conducted to date, parenteral estrogens have not been shown to offer a survival advantage.[9] In a small study, Henriksson et al found that intramuscular injections of polyestradiol phosphate had clinical effects comparable with bilateral orchiectomy.[10] Although parenteral estrogens have been shown to be inferior to androgen blockade using luteinizing hormone-releasing hormone (LHRH) agonists, a recent large randomized study from Sweden reported that current parenteral estrogen therapy and complete androgen blockade using an LHRH agonist with an antiandrogen had comparable efficacy in terms of overall survival and cardiovascular safety.[11] Compared with LHRH agonists, synthetic estrogens have been shown to reduce testosterone production from extratesticular sites and to achieve a greater reduction in serum testosterone.[12]

In 1977, Schally won the Nobel Prize for Medicine and Physiology for his extensive research in hypothalamic regulatory hormones, including the isolation and synthesis of LHRH.[13] The emergence of synthetic LHRH agonists following the pioneering work by Schally and his colleagues led to the most dramatic changes in hormonal treatment of prostate cancer since the work of Huggins and Hodges.[14] The discovery of LHRH, which was well known by the mid-1980s,[15] marked the beginning of a new era in the manipulation of hormones in prostate cancer patients, and the use of LHRH agonists has become standard therapy for the treatment of metastatic prostate cancer. In their systematic meta-analysis of the literature, Seidenfeld et al found no difference in survival after either LHRH-agonist therapy or orchiectomy.[16] Nevertheless, LHRH-agonist therapy gained in popularity, primarily due to greater patient acceptance and tolerance of this medical approach compared with surgical castration.

Luteinizing hormone-releasing hormone agonist therapy greatly reduces testosterone levels.[17] Although less than 50 ng/dL is usually considered a castrate level of testosterone, the National Comprehensive Cancer Network has provisionally recommended setting a lower testosterone threshold (i.e., <20 ng/dL) to match the effect of orchiectomy.[18] This lower testosterone level can be achieved by an LHRH agonist alone or by combined androgen blockade. The latter approach utilizes an LHRH agonist to block testicular production of testosterone in combination with a nonsteroidal antiandrogen (e.g., flutamide, bicalutamide, or nilutamide) to achieve maximal binding of circulating adrenal androgens at the cellular level.[19]

Nonsteroidal antiandrogens can also be used as monotherapy in some patients. Monotherapy with flutamide or bicalutamide has been show to have a palliative effect on symptoms while preserving libido and sexual potency.[20] However, the American Society of Clinical Oncology recommends that monotherapy using steroidal antiandrogens, such as cyproterone acetate, not be offered to patients.[21] A number of trials have compared the outcome of using a combined total androgen blockade versus monotherapy with an LHRH agonist. In their meta-analysis, Samson et al found no statistical difference in long-term survival between patients receiving monotherapy and those receiving combined therapy.[22] In order for patients to make an informed decision about therapy, they must be fully informed about the cost and toxicity of combined hormonal treatment versus its marginal additional survival benefit. Nevertheless, combined androgen blockade should be considered in all men with spinal bony metastasis or in whom there is a high risk of voiding dysfunction in order to counteract the initial flare phenomenon[23] (i.e., the transitory rise in testosterone levels following treatment with an LHRH agonist). It is important to recognize that the risk of experiencing a testosterone flare effect is not totally eliminated with combined androgen blockade; close clinical observation of symptoms is warranted.

Recent evidence supports the role of LHRH antagonists (e.g., abarelix and ganirelix) in the treatment of prostate cancer and the benefit of applying hormonal manipulation in the early stages of disease.[24] Use of abarelix has been shown to result in rapid medical castration without a testosterone surge, thereby avoiding the initial testosterone flare observed with LHRH agonists.[25] However, any potential advantages associated with LHRH antagonist therapy have not yet been shown to extend survival.[26]

MECHANISM OF ACTION AND REGULATION OF PROSTATE HORMONE-SENSITIVE CELL GROWTH

EFFECT OF TESTOSTERONE

Testosterone, which is essential for the growth and differentiation of prostate cells and for the development and function of the prostate, is regulated by androgen activity.[27] In the male, testosterone is secreted primarily from the Leydig cells in the testis. In addition, the adrenals produce inactive testosterone precursors, including dehydroepiandrosterone (DHEA) and androstenedione, which can be converted to active testosterone both in the prostate and in most peripheral tissues. The adrenal glands are the source of approximately 10% of total testosterone, which contributes to intraprostatic dihydrotestosterone (DHT).

The enzyme 5α-reductase acts to convert testosterone to the more potent DHT in the prostate. Therefore, testosterone acts as both a hormone and a prohormone, exerting its action via the intracellular androgen receptor (AR), a ligand-dependent transcription activator. Testosterone is also converted to an estrogen in tissues that have a high level of aromatase via the estrogen receptor (ER). Numerous in-vitro studies have shown a synergistic activation of the ligand-independent AR by various growth factors and cytokines in the presence of smaller amounts of androgens.[28,29] The role of these observations in the long-term effect of hormonal treatment on prostate cancer remains unclear.

The hypothalamic-pituitary-testicular axis is responsible for the primary regulation of testosterone production by way of a negative feedback mechanism that is based on the release of LHRH from the pituitary gland under the influence of gonadotropin-releasing hormone from the hypothalamus (Figure 90.1). Agonists of LHRH suppress synthesis of endogenous testicular gonadotropin, and the chronic administration of LHRH agonists causes a hypogonadal condition, with suppression of luteinizing hormone and follicle-stimulating hormone levels. Thompson et al found that the testosterone flare phenomenon occurred in 11% of 765 patients within the first 1 to 2 weeks of LHRH agonist therapy.[30] The flare phenomenon may manifest as severe hot flashes and voiding dysfunction. In addition, there is concern about cord compression and ureteral obstruction in patients with widely disseminated metastases.

EFFECT OF HORMONAL DEPRIVATION ON APOPTOSIS

Most prostate cancers are a heterogeneous mixture of androgen-dependent and -independent cell colonies at

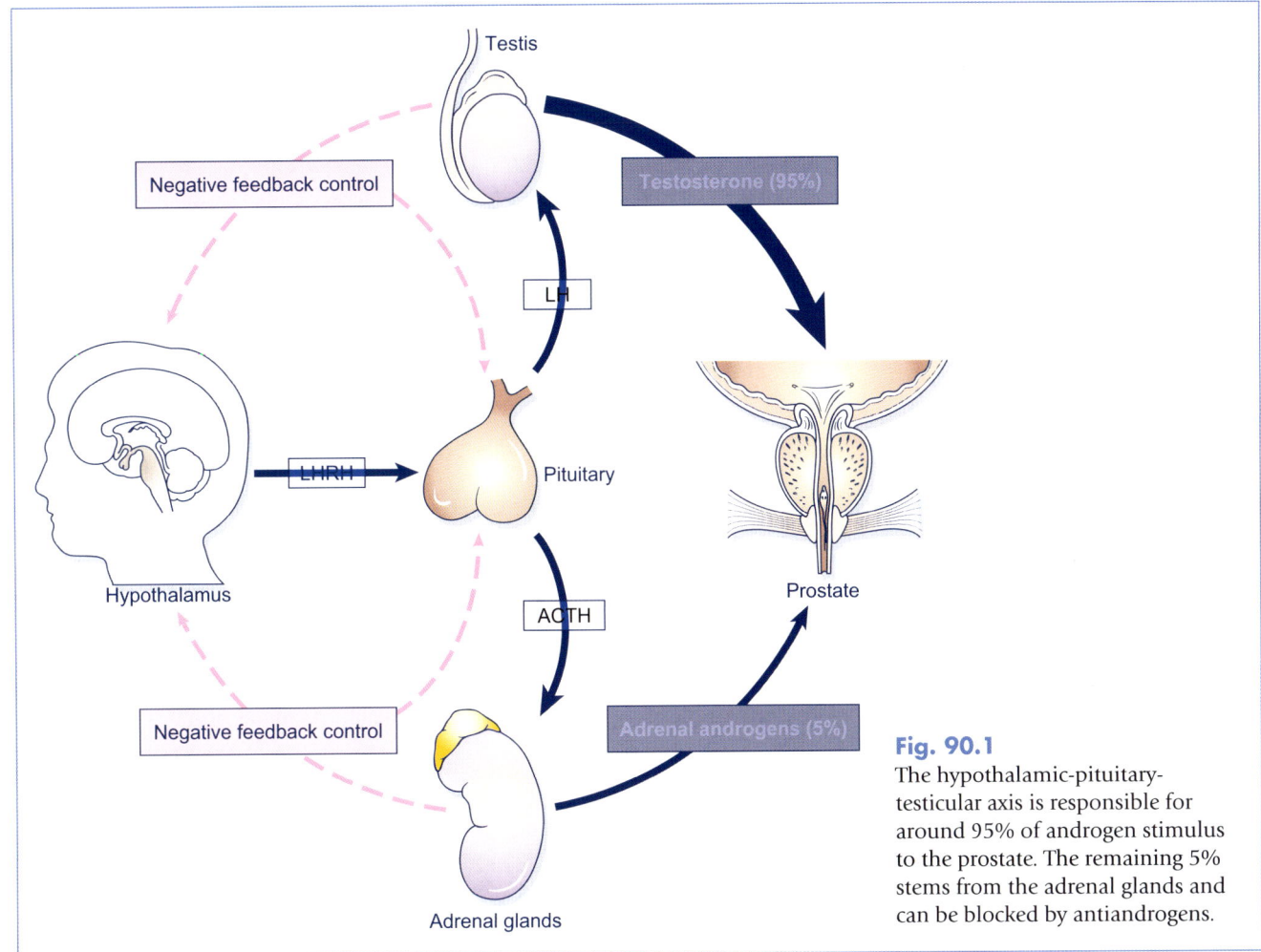

Fig. 90.1
The hypothalamic-pituitary-testicular axis is responsible for around 95% of androgen stimulus to the prostate. The remaining 5% stems from the adrenal glands and can be blocked by antiandrogens.

the time of diagnosis. Castration has been shown to promote an extensive apoptotic response both in normal prostate cells[31] and in androgen-dependent tumor cells.[32] In the early stages of the malignant transformation of prostate cancer, hormonal deprivation appears to have a reduction in or to lose its effect on the apoptotic response in androgen-independent cells in 80% of cases[33]; however, the effect is seen primarily in the reduction of cell proliferation rather than in an apoptotic response. Since most of these cells retain their molecular factors and mechanisms for apoptosis, they represent a potential target for new chemotherapeutic regimens currently under investigation.

It has been postulated that some androgen-dependent cells can evolve during therapy, transforming into androgen-independent cells. Although the mechanisms underlying this transformation are still poorly understood, it has been suggested that Bcl2, a suppressor of apoptosis, may play a pivotal role.[34] Some researchers are exploring the idea that androgen-dependent cancer cells that are sensitive to apoptosis may predominate in patients on androgen-deprivation therapy who maintain undetectable levels of prostate-specific antigen (PSA) for a prolonged period (i.e., >1

year). This subset of patients can receive the most benefit from intermittent hormonal manipulation.[35] To date, no prospective randomized trials have supported the use of intermittent LHRH agonist therapy in all patients with prostate cancer.

TREATMENT OF EARLY PROSTATE CANCER

RATIONALE FOR THE USE OF HORMONE THERAPY: A BRIEF OVERVIEW

Although the long-term benefit of hormone deprivation in advanced prostate cancer has been well established in clinical practice, the use of hormonal manipulation in early prostate cancer is still controversial. Numerous studies have shown a significant reduction in positive margin rates after prolonged neoadjuvant hormonal treatment before radical prostatectomy.[36] However, neoadjuvant therapy did not reduce PSA recurrence in these studies.[37] A study conducted by Messing et al showed a significant improvement in survival in patients with node-positive prostate cancer who received immediate hormonal therapy after radical prostatectomy and pelvic lymphadenectomy.[38] In addition, a therapeutic advantage was reported for the use of adjunctive (i.e., during or immediately following) and neoadjuvant androgen deprivation with radiation therapy.[39,40]

Nomograms and artificial neural network programs have been developed in an effort to identify those patients who will achieve a survival benefit from early hormonal treatment. These programs define predictors of poor outcome in a subgroup of patients with specific predictors (e.g., Gleason score, initial PSA, and clinical stage).[41] However, the optimal initiation time, duration, and continuity of hormonal manipulation in early prostate cancer remains unknown. Prostate-specific antigen doubling time appears to be the best basis for recommending early hormonal treatment; for example, it is advisable to start hormonal therapy as early as possible in men with a short PSA doubling time (i.e., <3 months). Although the effect of hormone therapy on long-term overall survival and PSA-free progression is still undetermined in early prostate cancer, this approach appears to offer the best advantage in the group of men at high risk based on Gleason score, extent of the tumor, and pretreatment initial PSA velocity.

DURATION OF ANDROGEN DEPRIVATION IN CONJUNCTION WITH PRIMARY THERAPY

Most patients diagnosed with clinically localized prostate cancer receive a recommendation for either surgery or radiation as primary treatment, and fewer patients are currently being put on a regimen of close observation, or "watchful waiting." Studies have shown that neoadjuvant androgen therapy dramatically reduces the rate of local recurrence after tumor excision. In a phase III randomized trial, the rate of PSA recurrence and positive margin were significantly reduced in patients treated intramuscularly with leuprolide 7.5 mg/month and oral flutamide 250 mg t.i.d for 3 or 8 months before radical prostatectomy.[42] In another study, patients who received neoadjuvant therapy for more than 3 months prior to surgery showed a significant reduction in the incidence of biochemical failure.[43] Numerous randomized trials have addressed the impact of using short-term (i.e., 4 months) versus long-term (i.e., 2 or more years) androgen deprivation with radiation therapy.[44-46] In patients with clinical stage T3 to T4 disease, cancer-specific survival was no better when the patient received 4 months of hormonal treatment than with no adjuvant hormonal therapy. Although patients receiving 2 years of hormonal therapy had better cancer-specific survival at 5 years than patients receiving 4 months of therapy, overall survival was similar in both groups. Longer term hormonal

manipulation was better than no treatment at 2 years and with lifelong treatment. It is interesting to note that overall survival was comparable between patients who received either 2 years or 4 months of hormonal treatment. However, it is important to wait until the cancer-specific survival-benefit results are known before judging short-term treatment to be beneficial. Today, the standard of practice in men with clinically advanced local prostate cancer remains long-term (i.e., 2–3 years) hormonal therapy in conjunction with radiation therapy.[40]

SIDE EFFECTS TO BE AWARE OF PRIOR TO INITIATING HORMONAL THERAPY

As studies continue to provide evidence supporting the use of androgen deprivation early in the management of prostate cancer, the toxicity associated with this treatment has become more of an issue. Table 90.1 lists the side effects most often associated with hormonal therapy.[47-54] Loss of libido, impotence, and erectile dysfunction are well recognized side effects of androgen deprivation.[55] Other side effects, including fatigue, hot flashes, muscle wasting, cognitive problems, and gynecomastia, can affect a patient's quality of life.[56] The metabolic changes resulting from hormonal therapy are associated with significant morbidity; they adversely affect the lipid profile and can result in anemia, osteoporosis, and liver toxicity.

Hot flashes, which are the most common symptom associated with androgen deprivation, are due to an alteration in the thermoregulatory center of the hypothalamus in response to an increase in catecholamine production following the positive feedback resulting from a lack of testosterone. Patients who find hot flashes to be intolerable may be treated with selective serotonin (5-hydroxytryptamine) reuptake inhibitors (e.g., venlafaxine).[57] These agents provide more effective treatment than estrogen preparations, megestrol acetate, DES, and soy

Table 90.1 Incidence of adverse events associated with androgen deprivation therapy

Adverse events	Frequency (%)
Fatigue[47]	14
Hot flashes	50–80
Erectile dysfunction	50–100
Decline in cognitive function[48,49]	0–50
Bone fracture[50,51]	6–9
Anemia[52]	81
Gynecomastia[53]	16
Increase in liver function test[54] *	22

*Antiandrogen therapy

supplements that are commonly used to control hot flashes in these patients.

The lack of testosterone following androgen deprivation therapy has been linked to muscle wasting and a net increase in body weight, primarily due to increased fat deposition.[58] These changes may have a profound effect on a patient's lipid profile and may theoretically increase the risk of cardiovascular complications. Currently, the use of LHRH agonists has not been linked to these complications in controlled studies. Nevertheless, since high doses of antiandrogens have been associated with increased mortality, clinicians should use caution when prescribing these drugs, particularly in high-risk patients. Long-term (i.e., >6 months) treatment with androgen deprivation therapy may be associated with impairments in memory, attention, and executive functions.[48] In contrast, Salminen et al found no such impairment in cognitive functions in a small cohort of 25 men after up to 12 months of androgen deprivation.[49] Further randomized controlled trials addressing the issue of side effects after long-term androgen deprivation are needed. Meanwhile, patients should be made aware of the risks associated with hormone therapy when treatment options are discussed in the early stage of their disease.

Downregulation of both the production and activity of nitric oxide is another side effect of androgen deprivation.[59] In addition, the effects of surgical or radiation treatment on the neurovascular conduction pathways can also affect symptoms. Therefore, the efficacy of sexual health-enhancing medications prescribed for these patients can vary from no effect to a return to satisfactory sexual intercourse.

Bone fractures—especially osteoporotic fractures of the hip and spine—are associated with significant morbidity and mortality (i.e., 20% mortality at 1 year after an osteoporotic hip fracture[60]), particularly in older men. Stepan et al first reported the association between castration in prostate cancer patients and a progressive loss of bone mineral density leading to fractures.[61] Increasing evidence has recently confirmed the effects of androgen deprivation on bone loss[62] and osteoporosis.[63] Prostate cancer patients with no apparent bone metastasis who were on androgen deprivation therapy are reported to have had a two-fold increase in fracture rate (after adjusting for age and preexisting osteoporosis).[64] African-American men and individuals with a high body mass index appear to be protected against skeletal fractures associated with androgen suppression.[65] All men who receive androgen deprivation therapy should be counseled about following a regular exercise regimen, using vitamin D and calcium supplements, and making other lifestyle changes to reduce their risk of osteoporosis. Various bisphosphonates have also been recommended as prophylactic agents in men receiving antiandrogen deprivation therapy for extended time periods.

Liver toxicity, including rising transaminase levels, has been associated mainly with antiandrogen therapy (i.e., flutamide).[54,66] There have also been sporadic reports in the literature linking liver necrosis and severe hepatitis to hormonal manipulation with antiandrogens.[67] Other less common side effects associated with androgen deprivation therapy include hair loss, dry eyes, depression, and vertigo.

CONCLUSIONS

Many questions about the use of androgen deprivation in early prostate cancer as yet remain unanswered. Should monotherapy or combined androgen blockade be used? What is the role of androgen deprivation as either neoadjuvant or adjuvant therapy? What effects do the adverse events associated with hormone therapy have on the quality of life of these patients? Only large, well-designed, randomized, controlled trials can provide the answers to these important questions.

REFERENCES

1. Huggins C, Hodges CV. Studies on prostatic cancer, 1. The effect of castration, of estrogen and of androgen injection of serum phosphatases in metastatic carcinoma of the prostate. Cancer Res 1941;1:293–297.

2. The Veterans Administration Co-operative Urological Research Group. Treatment and survival of patients with cancer of the prostate. Surg Gynecol Obstet 1967;124:1011–1017.

3. Jordan WP Jr, Blackard CE, Byar DP. Reconsideration of orchiectomy in the treatment of advanced prostatic carcinoma. South Med J 1977;70:1411–1413.

4. Byar DP, Corle DK. Hormone therapy for prostate cancer: Results of the Veterans Administration Cooperative Urological Research Group studies. NCI Monogr 1988;7:165–170.

5. Chang A, Yeap B, Davis T, et al, Double-blind, randomized study of primary hormonal treatment of stage D2 prostate carcinoma: flutamide versus diethylstilbestrol. J Clin Oncol 1996;14:2250–2257.

6. Henriksson P, Blomback M, Bratt G, et al. Effects of oestrogen therapy and orchidectomy on coagulation and prostanoid synthesis in patients with prostatic cancer. Med Oncol Tumor Pharmacother 1989;6:219–225.

7. Carlstrom K, Collste L, Eriksson A, et al, A comparison of androgen status in patients with prostatic cancer treated with oral and/or parenteral estrogens or by orchidectomy. Prostate 1989;2:177–182.

8. von Schoultz B, Carlstrom K, Collste L, et al. Estrogen therapy and liver function—metabolic effects of oral and parenteral administration. Prostate 1989;14:389–395.

9. Mikkola AK, Ruutu ML, Aro JL, et al. Parenteral polyoestradiol phosphate vs orchidectomy in the treatment of advanced prostatic cancer. Efficacy and cardiovascular complications: a 2-year follow-up report of a national, prospective prostatic cancer study, Finnprostate Group. Br J Urol 1998;82:63–68.

10. Henriksson P, Carlstrom K, Pousette A, et al. Time for revival of estrogens in the treatment of advanced prostatic carcinoma? Pharmacokinetics, and endocrine and clinical effects, of a parenteral estrogen regimen. Prostate 1999;40:76–82.

11. Hedlund PO, Henriksson P. Parenteral estrogen versus total androgen ablation in the treatment of advanced prostate carcinoma: effects on overall survival and cardiovascular mortality. The Scandinavian Prostatic Cancer Group (SPCG)-5 Trial Study. Urology 2000;55:328–333.

12. Kitahara S, Yoshida K, Ishizaka K, et al. Stronger suppression of serum testosterone and FSH levels by a synthetic estrogen than by castration or an LH-RH agonist. Endocr J 1997;44:527–532.

13. Schally AV. Aspects of hypothalamic regulation of the pituitary gland with major emphasis on its implications for the control of reproductive processes, Nobel Lecture, December 8, 1977, http://nobelprize.org/medicine/laureates/1977/schally-lecture.html

14. Schally AV, Redding TW, Comaru-Schally AM. Inhibition of prostate tumors by agonistic and antagonistic analogs of LH-RH. Prostate 1983;4:545–552.

15. Smith JA Jr, Glode LM, Wettlaufer JN, et al. Clinical effects of gonadotropin-releasing hormone analogue in metastatic carcinoma of prostate. Urology 1985;25:106–114.

16. Seidenfeld J, Samson DJ, Hasselblad V, et al. Single-therapy androgen suppression in men with advanced prostate cancer: a systematic review and meta-analysis, Ann Intern Med 2000;132:566–577.

17. Limonta P, Montagnani Marelli M, et al. LHRH analogues as anticancer agents: pituitary and extrapituitary sites of action. Expert Opin Investig Drugs 2001;10:709–720.

18. Oefelein MG, Feng A, Scolieri MJ, et al. Reassessment of the definition of castrate levels of testosterone: implications for clinical decision making. Urology 2000;56:1021–1024.

19. Crawford ED, Eisenberger MA, McLeod DG, et al. A controlled trial of leuprolide with and without flutamide in prostatic carcinoma. N Engl J Med 1989;321:419–424.

20. Boccon-Gibod L. Are non-steroidal anti-androgens appropriate as monotherapy in advanced prostate cancer? Eur Urol 1998;33:159–164.

21. Loblaw DA, Mendelson DS, Talcott JA, et al. American Society of Clinical Oncology recommendations for the initial hormonal management of androgen-sensitive metastatic, recurrent, or progressive prostate cancer. J Clin Oncol 2004;22:2927–2941.

22. Samson DJ, Seidenfeld J, Schmitt B, et al. Systematic review and meta-analysis of monotherapy compared with combined androgen blockade for patients with advanced prostate carcinoma. Cancer 2002;95:361–376.

23. Altwein JE, Complete androgen blockade versus monotherapy. Urologe A 1998;37:149–152 [Article in German].

24. Stricker HJ. Luteinizing hormone-releasing hormone antagonists in prostate cancer. Urology 2001;58 (2 Suppl 1):24–27.

25. Trachtenberg J, Gittleman M, Steidle C, et al. A phase 3, multicenter, open label, randomized study of abarelix versus leuprolide plus daily antiandrogen in men with prostate cancer. J Urol 2002;167:1670–1674.

26. Weckermann D, Harzmann R. Hormone therapy in prostate cancer: LHRH antagonists versus LHRH analogues. Eur Urol 2004;46:279–284.

27. Mooradian AD, Morley JE, Korenman SG. Biological actions of androgens. Endocr Rev 1987;8:1–28.

28. Huang ZQ, Li J, Wong J. AR possesses an intrinsic hormone-independent transcriptional activity. Mol Endocrinol 2002;16:924–937.

29. Dai J, Shen R, Sumitomo M, et al. Synergistic activation of the androgen receptor by bombesin and low-dose androgen. Clin Cancer Res 2002;8:2399–2405.

30. Thompson IM, Zeidman EJ, Rodriguez FR. Sudden death due to disease flare with luteinizing hormone-releasing hormone agonist therapy for carcinoma of the prostate. J Urol 1990;144:1479–1480.

31. English HF, Kyprianou N, Isaacs JT. Relationship between DNA fragmentation and apoptosis in the programmed cell death in the rat prostate following castration. Prostate 1989;15:233–250.

32. Isaacs JT, Lundmo PI, Berges R, et al. Androgen regulation of programmed death of normal and malignant prostatic cells. J Androl 1992;13:457–464.

33. Murphy WM, Soloway MS, Barrows GH. Pathologic changes associated with androgen deprivation therapy for prostate cancer. Cancer 1991;68:821-828.

34. Tang DG, Porter AT. Target to apoptosis: a hopeful weapon for prostate cancer. Prostate 1997;32:284–293.

35. Strum SB, Scholz MC, McDermed JE. Intermittent androgen deprivation in prostate cancer patients: factors predictive of prolonged time off therapy. Oncologist 2000;5:45–52.

36. Kollermann J, Caprano J, Budde A, et al. Follow-up of nondetectable prostate carcinoma (pT0) after prolonged PSA-monitored neoadjuvant hormonal therapy followed by radical prostatectomy. Urology 2003;62:476–480.

37. Gleave ME, La Bianca SE, Goldenberg SL, et al. Long-term neoadjuvant hormone therapy prior to radical prostatectomy: evaluation of risk for biochemical recurrence at 5-year follow-up. Urology 2000;56:289–294.

38. Messing EM, Manola J, Sarosdy M, et al. Immediate hormonal therapy compared with observation after radical prostatectomy and pelvic lymphadenectomy in men with node-positive prostate cancer. N Engl J Med 1999;341:1781–1788.

39. Pilepich MV, Caplan R, Byhardt RW, et al. Phase III trial of androgen suppression using goserelin in unfavorable-prognosis carcinoma of the prostate treated with definitive radiotherapy: report of Radiation Therapy Oncology Group Protocol 85-31. J Clin Oncol 1997;15:1013–1021.

40. Bolla M, Gonzalez D, Warde P, et al. Improved survival in patients with locally advanced prostate cancer treated with radiotherapy and goserelin. N Engl J Med 1997;337:295–300.

41. Crawford ED. Early versus late hormonal therapy: debating the issues. Urology 2003;61(2 Suppl 1):8–13.

42. Gleave ME, Goldenberg SL, Chin JL, et al. Randomized comparative study of 3 versus 8-month neoadjuvant hormonal therapy before radical prostatectomy: biochemical and pathological effects. J Urol 2001;166:500-506; discussion 506–507.

43. Meyer F, Bairati I, Bedard C, et al. Duration of neoadjuvant androgen deprivation therapy before radical prostatectomy and disease-free survival in men with prostate cancer. Urology 2001;58 (2 Suppl 1):71–77.

44. Hanks GE, Pajak TF, Porter A, et al. Phase III trial of long-term adjuvant androgen deprivation after neoadjuvant hormonal cytoreduction and radiotherapy in locally advanced carcinoma of the prostate: the Radiation Therapy Oncology Group Protocol 92-02. J Clin Oncol 2003;21:3972–3978.

45. Bolla M, Collette L, Blank L, et al. Long-term results with immediate androgen suppression and external irradiation in patients with locally advanced prostate cancer (an EORTC study): a phase III randomised trial. Lancet 2002;360:103–106.

46. Shipley WU, Lu JD, Pilepich MV, et al. Effect of a short course of neoadjuvant hormonal therapy on the response to subsequent androgen suppression in prostate cancer patients with relapse after radiotherapy: a secondary analysis of the randomized protocol RTOG 86-10. Int J Radiat Oncol Biol Phys 2002;54:1302–1310.

47. Stone P, Hardy J, Huddart R, et al. Fatigue in patients with prostate cancer receiving hormone therapy. Eur J Cancer 2000;36:1134–1141.

48. Green HJ, Pakenham KI, Headley BC, et al. Altered cognitive function in men treated for prostate cancer with luteinizing hormone-releasing hormone analogues and cyproterone acetate: a randomized controlled trial, BJU Int 2002;90:427–432.

49. Salminen E, Portin R, Korpela J, et al. Androgen deprivation and cognition in prostate cancer. Br J Cancer 2003;89:971–976.

50. Hatano T, Oishi Y, Furuta A, et al. Incidence of bone fracture in patients receiving luteinizing hormone-releasing hormone agonists for prostate cancer. BJU Int 2000;86:449–452.

51. Townsend MF, Sanders WH, Northway RO, et al. Bone fractures associated with luteinizing hormone-releasing hormone agonists used in the treatment of prostate carcinoma. Cancer 1997;79:545–550.

52. Asbell SO, Leon SA, Tester WJ, et al. Development of anemia and recovery in prostate cancer patients treated with combined androgen blockade and radiotherapy. Prostate 1996;29:243–248.

53. Rizzo M, Mazzei T, Mini E, et al. Leuprorelin acetate depot in advanced prostatic cancer: a phase II multicentre trial. J Int Med Res 1990;18 (Suppl 1):114–125.

54. Rosenthal SA, Linstadt DE, Leibenhaut MH, et al, Flutamide-associated liver toxicity during treatment with total androgen suppression and radiation therapy for prostate cancer, Radiology 1996;199:451–455.

55. Bokhour BG, Clark JA, Inui TS, et al. Sexuality after treatment for early prostate cancer: exploring the meanings of "erectile dysfunction." J Gen Intern Med 2001;16:649–655.

56. Basaria S, Lieb J 2nd, Tang AM, et al. Long-term effects of androgen deprivation therapy in prostate cancer patients. Clin Endocrinol (Oxf) 2002;56:779–786.

57. Loprinzi CL, Pisansky TM, Fonseca R, et al. Pilot evaluation of venlafaxine hydrochloride for the therapy of hot flashes in cancer survivors. J Clin Oncol 1998;16:2377–2381.

58. Tayek JA, Heber D, Byerley LO, Steiner B, Rajfer J, et al. Nutritional and metabolic effects of gonadotropin-releasing hormone agonist treatment for prostate cancer. Metabolism 1990;39:1314–1319.

59. Baba K, Yajima M, Carrier S, et al. Effect of testosterone on the number of NADPH diaphorase-stained nerve fibers in the rat corpus cavernosum and dorsal nerve. Urology 2000;56:533–538.

60. Osteoporosis Prevention, Diagnosis, and Therapy. NIH Consensus Statement. March 27-29, 2000;17:1-45. Available at http://consensus.nih.gov/cons/111/111_statement.pdf. Accessed 08-04.

61. Stepan JJ, Lachman M, Zverina J, et al. Castrated men exhibit bone loss: effect of calcitonin treatment on biochemical indices of bone remodeling. J Clin Endocrinol Metab 1989;69:523–527.

62. Diamond T, Campbell J, Bryant C, et al. The effect of combined androgen blockade on bone turnover and bone mineral densities in men treated for prostate carcinoma: longitudinal evaluation and response to intermittent cyclic etidronate therapy. Cancer 1998;83:1561–1566.

63. Daniell HW, Dunn SR, Ferguson DW, et al. Progressive osteoporosis during androgen deprivation therapy for prostate cancer. J Urol 2000;163:181–186.

64. Melton LJ 3rd, Alothman KI, Khosla S, Achenbach SJ, Oberg AL, Zincke H. Fracture risk following bilateral orchiectomy. J Urol 2003;169:1747–1750.

65. Oefelein MG, Ricchuiti V, Conrad W, et al. Skeletal fracture associated with androgen suppression induced osteoporosis: the clinical incidence and risk factors for patients with prostate cancer. J Urol 2001;166:1724–1728.

66. Gomez JL, Dupont A, Cusan L, et al. Incidence of liver toxicity associated with the use of flutamide in prostate cancer patients. Am J Med 1992;92:465–470.

67. Crownover RL, Holland J, Chen A, et al. Flutamide-induced liver toxicity including fatal hepatic necrosis. Int J Radiat Oncol Biol Phys 1996;34:911–915.

Neoadjuvant and adjuvant hormonal therapies for prostate cancer: data review and patient perspectives

91

William A See

INTRODUCTION

Hormonal therapy is being used increasingly in addition to primary therapies of curative intent, such as radiotherapy and radical prostatectomy, in patients with localized and locally advanced prostate cancer. The reason for the use of additional hormonal therapy is that a significant proportion of patients receiving these primary therapies alone will experience disease progression and may die from prostate cancer.

Improving overall survival remains the ultimate goal in the treatment of prostate cancer. However, other measurable endpoints in prostate cancer can also be relevant to treatment decisions, particularly, disease progression. Reducing the risk of disease progression is important for a number of reasons. Disease progression and concern about the risk of death from prostate cancer places a substantial emotional burden on patients and their families. There may also be serious clinical consequences for patients who experience disease progression, such as bone pain, spinal cord compression, pathologic fractures and urinary obstruction,[1] and the subsequent economic burden can be significant.[2] Whether considering disease progression or overall survival, a key question is whether additional hormonal therapy provides a positive balance between the benefits and risks of treatment. This balance is determined by the adverse effects of treatment relative to the beneficial effect on survival and quality of life. Regrettably few studies are able to provide insight into this risk:benefit ratio beyond the effect of treatment on progression or survival endpoints.

Options for patients receiving hormonal therapy in addition to their primary therapy include neoadjuvant hormonal therapy—short-term hormonal treatment used immediately before primary therapy—and adjuvant hormonal therapy—longer-term hormonal treatment given immediately after treatment of curative intent. The main aim of any additional hormonal therapy is usually to improve local control and overall survival compared with the primary therapy alone. Neoadjuvant hormonal therapy is also used to reduce the size of the prostate, with the intention of facilitating the primary therapy. For example, a reduction in prostate size before surgery or cryotherapy may reduce blood loss and operative difficulty. A reduction in prostate size before brachytherapy is intended to facilitate accurate seed implantation and allow a reduced radiation dose to be used. Similarly, neoadjuvant hormonal therapy given before external-beam radiotherapy may allow a smaller field size to be used.

Neoadjuvant or adjuvant hormonal therapies usually include luteinizing hormone-releasing hormone (LHRH) agonists, antiandrogens, or a combination of the two (combined androgen blockade [CAB]). Bilateral orchiectomy is also used occasionally.

Data from studies assessing additional hormonal therapies vary, in both quality and quantity, according to the different primary therapy modalities, hormonal therapies, and approaches (neoadjuvant or adjuvant) used. This chapter reviews the current role for neoadjuvant and adjuvant hormonal therapies in early prostate cancer and the supporting evidence. The focus is on published data relating to clinically important outcomes from prospective randomized controlled trials, subgroup analyses of such trials, and meta-analyses or systematic reviews of data from these studies. The level of evidence that supports the different treatment alternatives and the implications for patients and their urologists are discussed.

PRIMARY THERAPY: RADICAL PROSTATECTOMY

A number of patients treated with radical prostatectomy alone have a very low risk of disease progression and death from prostate cancer and, therefore, additional hormonal therapy has little or no role in their treatment. However, a significant proportion of patients with early stage prostate cancer treated with radical prostatectomy alone do subsequently experience disease progression, as a result of residual local disease or distant disease undetectable at diagnosis.

Several studies have investigated the clinical features that may help to predict disease progression following radical prostatectomy. A prospective, open-label trial in 1000 patients with localized (cT1–2) disease found that preoperative prostate-specific antigen (PSA) level, clinical stage, biopsy, postoperative Gleason score, extracapsular extension, seminal vesicle involvement, lymph node metastasis, and surgical margin status were all independent risk factors for metastatic progression (Figure 91.1).[3] Of the pretreatment characteristics examined, PSA level and Gleason score were the strongest predictive risk factors; for example, a pretreatment Gleason score of 8 to 10 was associated with a 42% risk of metastatic progression and an 18% risk of prostate cancer-related death within 10 years of radical prostatectomy.

The patient's risk profile is an important consideration when offering advice on treatment options; a key question is whether hormonal therapy can improve the prognosis of those patients identified as being at high risk of progression. To address this question, the following sections cover the evidence for neoadjuvant and adjuvant hormonal therapies in the surgical setting.

IS THERE A ROLE FOR NEOADJUVANT HORMONAL THERAPY PRIOR TO RADICAL PROSTATECTOMY?

A considerable number of randomized controlled trials of hormonal therapy neoadjuvant to radical prostatectomy have been conducted in patients with both localized and locally advanced prostate cancer. Overall, the available data do not show an improvement in clinical outcome with the use of neoadjuvant hormonal therapy prior to radical prostatectomy in terms of survival, disease progression, or postoperative morbidity. Indeed, the authors of one of these studies, using an LHRH agonist (triptorelin) as neoadjuvant hormonal therapy, concluded that 3 months of neoadjuvant hormonal therapy before radical prostatectomy offered no benefit to the patient and could not be recommended for routine clinical use.[4]

Of the studies conducted in this setting, some have only assessed characteristics such as tumor volume and surgical margin status,[5,6] while those with longer follow-up have also addressed PSA progression-free survival[4,7–13] (Table 91.1). The duration of these studies (longest follow-up median 7 years[4]) means that none of them is able to provide overall survival data.

In general, randomized controlled trials of neoadjuvant hormonal therapy in the surgical setting have demonstrated significant pathological down-staging of tumors, reduction in tumor volume, and reduction in the proportion of patients with positive surgical margins compared with surgery alone. However, none demonstrated any significant improvement in PSA progression-free survival with neoadjuvant hormonal

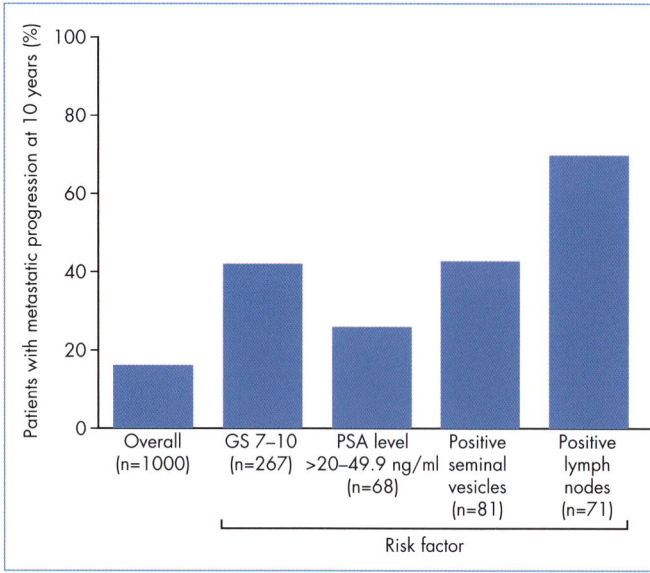

Fig. 91.1

Ten-year risk of metastatic progression following radical prostatectomy in patients with localized (cT1–T2) prostate cancer. (GS, Gleason score; PSA, prostate-specific antigen.)

Reproduced with permission from Hull GW, Rabbani F, Abbas F, Wheeler TM, Kattan MW, Scardino PT. Cancer control with radical prostatectomy alone in 1000 consecutive patients. J Urol 2002;167:528–534.

Table 91.1 Randomized controlled trials of 3 months' neoadjuvant hormonal therapy prior to radical prostatectomy compared with radical prostatectomy alone

Neoadjuvant hormonal therapy	Disease stage	No. patients randomized	Tumor volume	Patients with positive surgical margins	Follow-up, years	PSA progression-free survival
CAB (leuprorelin and CPA)[5]	cT1a–2b	183	Decreased in 31% of patients	39% vs 60% with RP alone (p = 0.01)	None	Not assessed
SAA (CPA)[7,9]	cT1b–2c	213	Decrease in mean volume from 42.8 cm^3 to 32.9 cm^3 (p = 0.0001)	27.7% vs 64.8% with RP alone (p = 0.001)	6 (median)	62.5% vs 66.4% with RP alone (p = NS)[a]
LHRH agonist (triptorelin)[4,8]	cT1b–3a	126	42% decrease in mean volume (from 36.9 cm^3 to 19.6 cm^3; p < 0.01)	23% vs 41% with RP alone (p = 0.013)	6.8 (median)	No difference (data not given; p = 0.588)[b]
CAB (leuprorelin and flutamide)[11,12]	cT2b	303	Decreased in 91% of patients	18% vs 48% with RP alone (p < 0.001)	5 (maximum)	64.8% vs 67.6% with RP alone (p = 0.663)[c]
CAB (goserelin and flutamide)[10,13]	cT2–3	402	Decrease in mean volume from 37.7 cm^3 to 26.8 cm^3 (p-value not given)	cT2 patients: 13% vs 37% with RP alone (p < 0.01) cT3 patients: 42% vs 61% with RP alone (p < 0.01)	4 (median)	74% vs 67% with RP alone (p = 0.18)[d]
CAB (leuprorelin and flutamide)[6]	B–C	161	Not given	7.8% vs 33.8% with RP alone (p < 0.001)	None	Not assessed

CAB, combined androgen blockade; CPA, cyproterone acetate; LHRH, luteinizing hormone-releasing hormone; NS, not significant; PSA, prostate-specific antigen; RP, radical prostatectomy; SAA, steroidal antiandrogen. PSA progression-free survival defined as: [a]time from randomization to the first of two consecutive occurrences of PSA >0.2 ng/ml ≥4 weeks apart, or death from prostate cancer; [b]time to detection of PSA >0.5 ng/ml or death from prostate cancer; [c]time from surgery to detection of PSA >0.4 ng/mL; [d]time from surgery to the first of two subsequent occurrences of PSA >1 ng/ml, distant metastases or local recurrence (confirmed by biopsy).

therapy compared with radical prostatectomy alone (see Table 91.1), although whether they were sufficiently powered to detect a difference was not always clear. Of the studies in Table 91.1 that did specify how they were powered, two were powered to detect differences in pathologic stage or surgical margin status[4,7] and only one was powered to detect a difference in terms of PSA progression.[10]

A subgroup analysis of 33 patients who had a baseline PSA level of more than 20 ng/mL, in a study assessing steroidal antiandrogen (cyproterone acetate [CPA]) neoadjuvant hormonal therapy in patients with clinically localized disease (median follow-up 6 years), identified a significant improvement in 7-year PSA progression-free survival compared with surgery alone (53% versus 35%; p = 0.015).[9] Prostate-specific antigen progression in this study was defined as a rise in PSA of more than 0.2 ng/mL on two consecutive occasions 4 weeks or more apart, or death from prostate cancer. However, given the lack of a significant difference in the overall population and the small number of patients analyzed, this result should be considered exploratory.

It seems contradictory that neoadjuvant hormonal therapy is associated with significant down-staging of tumors and a decrease in the rate of positive surgical margins but not an improvement in patient outcome. One possible reason for this is that hormonal deprivation leads to major histopathologic changes in the prostate, which may obscure evidence of residual tumor and result in the under-reporting of positive margins.[4,9,12] This reasoning is supported by a histologic study of androgen-ablated prostates, which showed that negative margins identified by hematoxylin–eosin staining may actually include residual tumor that can be detected by cytokeratin staining.[14] Incorrect information regarding margin status could have an adverse impact on treatment decisions following surgery, with consequent impairment of clinical outcomes.

To date, most studies have examined neoadjuvant hormonal therapy given for 3 months before radical prostatectomy; however, two randomized controlled trials have addressed whether longer periods of neoadjuvant hormonal therapy might lead to improved outcomes.

One study compared 3 and 6 months of CAB (bicalutamide plus goserelin) prior to radical prostatectomy in 431 men with localized or locally advanced (stage B or C) disease.[15] The results of this study showed that the additional 3 months of treatment improved the pathologic stage in patients with clinical stage C disease: organ-confined disease was seen in 32% and 63% of patients receiving 3 and 6 months of neoadjuvant hormonal therapy, respectively (p-value not given). However, similar improvements were not seen in patients with clinical stage B disease. The incidence of positive surgical margins following 3 or 6 months of neoadjuvant hormonal treatment was similar, irrespective of disease stage.

The second study compared 3 and 8 months of CAB (leuprorelin plus flutamide) in 547 men with localized (cT1c–2) disease.[16] Additional biochemical and pathologic regression of prostate tumors occurred between 3 and 8 months of neoadjuvant hormonal therapy, as demonstrated by significant increases in the numbers of patients with a preoperative PSA level of less than 0.1 ng/mL (43% versus 75% for 3 and 8 months, respectively; p < 0.0001) and decreases in the rates of positive surgical margins (23% versus 12% for 3 and 8 months, respectively; p = 0.0106).

Neither of these studies can offer the physician clear conclusions about the possible benefits of longer term neoadjuvant hormonal therapy in terms of PSA progression-free survival or overall survival, although this may be clarified with further follow-up.

Two systematic reviews of randomized controlled trials have assessed whether hormonal therapy neoadjuvant to radical prostatectomy offers any benefits in terms of reducing the difficulty of surgical dissection or surgical outcomes (e.g., operative time, blood loss, hospital stay, and postoperative complications).[17,18] Both reviews concluded there were no significant improvements in these parameters that would support the use of neoadjuvant hormonal therapy in this setting. The more recent review also found that neoadjuvant hormonal therapy might increase surgical difficulty and appears to increase post-operative patient morbidity as a consequence of the adverse effects of hormonal therapy in some patients.[18]

IS THERE A ROLE FOR ADJUVANT HORMONAL THERAPY WITH RADICAL PROSTATECTOMY?

Adjuvant hormonal therapy in the surgical setting has been studied in patients with localized and locally advanced prostate cancer; however, data from only a few randomized controlled trials are available at present.

PATIENTS WITH LOCALIZED PROSTATE CANCER

Only one randomized controlled trial currently provides data from patients with localized disease treated with hormonal therapy adjuvant to radical prostatectomy: the bicalutamide Early Prostate Cancer (EPC) program. Analyses of the subgroup of patients in this program with localized disease (T1–2, N0 or Nx, M0) who received radical prostatectomy (n = 2734) have been undertaken.[19] At a median 5.4 years' follow-up, there was no statistically significant difference in risk of objective progression (defined as objective progression confirmed by bone scan, computed tomography/ultrasound/magnetic resonance imaging, or histologic evidence of distant metastases or death from any cause without progression) between patients treated with bicalutamide 150 mg/day as adjuvant hormonal therapy, compared with radical prostatectomy alone within 16 weeks of treatment (hazard ratio [HR] 0.93; 95% confidence intervals [CI] 0.72–1.20). This suggests no benefit from adjuvant bicalutamide therapy for this patient group. Survival data for patients who underwent radical prostatectomy in this study are currently immature, with only 8% deaths.[20]

PATIENTS WITH LOCALLY ADVANCED PROSTATE CANCER

The available data from patients with locally advanced disease show that treatment with an LHRH agonist (goserelin) or orchiectomy adjuvant to radical prostatectomy offers a survival benefit for patients with lymph node metastases (pN+, M0). In addition, in a large study of bicalutamide, adjuvant hormonal therapy with a nonsteroidal antiandrogen has been shown to improve objective progression-free survival for patients with locally advanced disease, although overall survival data from this study are currently immature and a much smaller study of adjuvant flutamide treatment did not find a significant improvement in overall survival.

Messing et al compared immediate adjuvant with delayed hormonal therapy (with an LHRH agonist [goserelin] or orchiectomy) in 98 patients with clinically localized disease who were found to have lymph node metastases at surgery.[21,22] The most recent analysis, at a median follow-up of 10 years, showed that overall survival was significantly improved with immediate therapy compared with delayed hormonal therapy (72% versus 49%; p = 0.025).[22]

In another randomized controlled trial investigating 201 patients with locally advanced (T3–4) disease, treatment with an LHRH agonist (goserelin) adjuvant to radical prostatectomy resulted in a significant 25% advantage in terms of PSA progression-free survival (progression defined as PSA greater than 0.5 ng/mL or cytologic or histologic evidence of local or distant disease) compared with surgery alone (p < 0.05).[23] However, with a median follow-up of 5 years, overall survival data are not yet mature.

Analyses of the subgroup of patients with locally advanced disease (T3–4, any N, M0 or any T, N+, M0; n = 1719) who received radical prostatectomy in the EPC program show, at a median 5.4 years' follow-up, a significantly reduced risk of objective progression with bicalutamide 150 mg/day as adjuvant hormonal therapy, compared with radical prostatectomy alone (HR 0.71; 95% CI 0.57–0.89; p = 0.0034).[19] Current survival data for patients who underwent radical prostatectomy in this study are immature, with only 8% deaths.[20]

A smaller, open-label, randomized trial of another non-steroidal antiandrogen (flutamide) as adjuvant to radical prostatectomy has been conducted in 309 patients with locally advanced disease (pT3, N0).[24] At a median follow-up of 6.1 years, there was a significant

improvement in PSA progression-free survival (progression defined as PSA >5 ng/mL; or >2 ng/mL on two occasions; or PSA >1 ng/mL on three occasions >3 months apart; or any clinical progression) with adjuvant hormonal therapy compared with radical prostatectomy alone (p = 0.0041). However, there was no statistically significant difference in overall survival between the two treatment groups (p = 0.92).

COMPARATIVE STUDIES OF NEOADJUVANT AND ADJUVANT HORMONAL THERAPIES WITH RADICAL PROSTATECTOMY

To date there have been no studies of patients treated with radical prostatectomy that have directly compared outcomes with neoadjuvant and adjuvant hormonal therapy. It is unlikely that such comparative studies will be conducted as the current evidence suggests that, unlike adjuvant hormonal therapy, neoadjuvant hormonal therapy offers little benefit to patients treated with radical prostatectomy.

PRIMARY THERAPY: EXTERNAL-BEAM RADIOTHERAPY

As in the surgical setting, a proportion of patients with early prostate cancer treated with external-beam radiotherapy are at low risk of disease progression and death from prostate cancer. However, the incidence of disease progression in patients treated with radiotherapy is higher than for patients treated with surgery, as radiotherapy is generally considered suitable for patients who present at a higher clinical stage than those who are usually treated surgically.

Analyses of pretreatment characteristics demonstrate that outcomes following conventional doses of external-beam radiotherapy vary considerably and tend to be poorer for patients with locally advanced disease. Meta-analysis of four Radiation Therapy Oncology Group (RTOG) randomized trials of radiotherapy identified four prognostic groups based on the following factors: Gleason score, T-stage, and pathologic lymph node status.[25] Of these factors, Gleason score was identified as the strongest predictor of progression. Patients in the highest risk grouping (T3, Nx, Gleason score 8–10; or N+, Gleason score 8–10) had a 36% risk of disease-specific death at 5 years (Figure 91.2).

A more recent analysis of 927 patients with clinically localized disease, for whom pretreatment PSA values were available, compared the predictive nature of this factor with those described above.[26] The analysis found that pretreatment PSA level is a significant, independent prognostic factor for overall survival, but is not as important as Gleason score or T-stage.

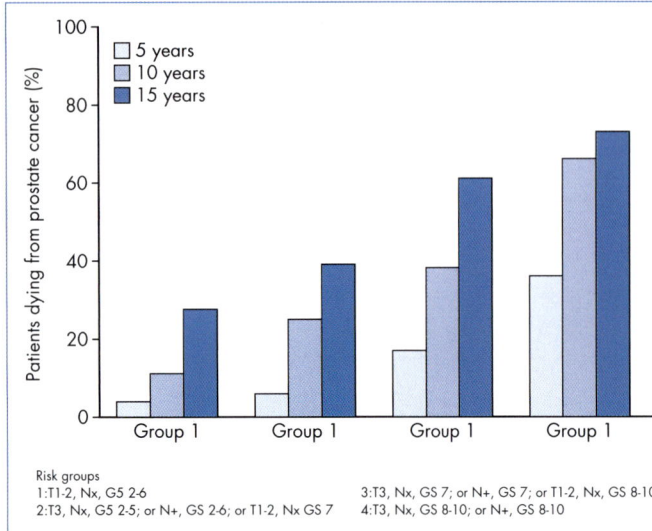

Risk groups
1: T1-2, Nx, G5 2-6
2: T3, Nx, G5 2-5; or N+, GS 2-6; or T1-2, Nx GS 7

3: T3, Nx, GS 7; or N+, GS 7; or T1-2, Nx, GS 8-10
4: T3, Nx, GS 8-10; or N+, GS 8-10

Fig. 91.2

Risk of prostate cancer death following conventional dose external-beam radiotherapy in patients with localized or locally advanced prostate cancer (n = 1557). (GS, Gleason score.)

Reproduced with permission from Roach III M, Lu J, Pilepich MV, et al. Four prognostic groups predict long-term survival from prostate cancer following radiotherapy alone on Radiation Therapy Oncology Group clinical trials. Int J Radiat Oncol Biol Phys 2000;47:609–615.

Once a patient's risk profile has been determined, it can be used in consultation with the patient to identify appropriate treatment options. As with patients treated surgically, the key question is whether hormonal therapy neoadjuvant or adjuvant to the primary therapy of curative intent can improve outcomes. To address this, the following sections cover the evidence for neoadjuvant and adjuvant hormonal therapies in patients receiving external-beam radiotherapy.

IS THERE A ROLE FOR NEOADJUVANT HORMONAL THERAPY PRIOR TO EXTERNAL-BEAM RADIOTHERAPY?

A limited number of randomized controlled trials have examined neoadjuvant hormonal therapy prior to external-beam radiotherapy in patients with localized or locally advanced disease. In these studies, the use of neoadjuvant hormonal therapy prior to external-beam radiotherapy reduced prostate volume and improved local control, progression-free survival, and disease-specific survival.

A large randomized controlled trial undertaken by the RTOG assessed neoadjuvant CAB (goserelin plus flutamide) given for 2 months prior to and 2 months during treatment with external-beam radiotherapy in 471 patients with localized or locally advanced (T2–4, N0 or N+ M0) disease.[27,28] Results at a median follow-up of 6.7 years showed a modest improvement in estimated 8-year clinical progression-free survival for patients receiving neoadjuvant hormonal therapy (33% versus 21% with radiotherapy alone; p = 0.004) and cause-specific mortality (23% versus 31% with radiotherapy alone; p = 0.05).[28] Subset analysis indicated that the beneficial effects specifically occurred in patients with a Gleason score of 2 to 6, for whom overall survival was significantly improved with neoadjuvant hormonal therapy compared with radiotherapy alone (70% versus 52%; p = 0.015). In patients with Gleason score 7 to 10 tumors, neoadjuvant hormonal therapy did not result in a statistically significant enhancement in either disease control or survival.

A smaller randomized controlled trial in 120 patients with localized or locally advanced (T2–4) prostate cancer compared local disease control with three different treatment regimens: external-beam radiotherapy alone; radiotherapy plus 3 months' neoadjuvant CAB (leuprorelin plus flutamide); and 3 months' neoadjuvant hormonal therapy plus adjuvant CAB for 6 months during and following radiotherapy.[29] The percentages of patients with positive biopsies at 24 months were 65% for external-beam radiotherapy alone, 28% for radiotherapy plus neoadjuvant CAB, and 5% for neoadjuvant hormonal therapy plus adjuvant CAB during and following radiotherapy (p-values not given). Laverdière et al have also reported a similar study in 161 patients with localized or locally advanced (T2–3) disease with a median follow-up of 5 years.[30] In this report, estimated 7-year PSA progression-free survival rates (progression defined as two consecutive increases in PSA level with at least one value of ≥1.5 ng/mL) were 42% with radiotherapy alone, 66% with neoadjuvant hormonal therapy (p = 0.009 versus radiotherapy alone), and 69% with neoadjuvant plus adjuvant hormonal therapy (p = 0.003 versus radiotherapy alone; not significant versus neoadjuvant hormonal therapy).

Neoadjuvant CPA has also been studied in a randomized controlled trial of 298 men with locally advanced (stage B2-C) prostate cancer.[31] Cyproterone acetate was given for 12 weeks prior to radiotherapy and patients were monitored for the following 18 to 36 months. Neoadjuvant hormonal therapy significantly reduced prostate volume (p = 0.0016) and increased the number of patients free from clinical (71% versus 49%; p = 0.019) or biochemical (47% versus 22%; p = 0.0001) evidence of disease compared with radiotherapy alone.

The outcomes summarized above contrast with neoadjuvant hormonal therapy in the surgical setting, where no clinical benefit is observed. One possible reason for this difference is that the effects of androgen ablation and radiotherapy may be synergistic in activating apoptosis in prostate cancer cells. Consequently the use of neoadjuvant hormonal therapy in the radiotherapy setting may result in an increased level of prostate cancer cell death relative to either treatment alone.[32]

IS THERE A ROLE FOR ADJUVANT HORMONAL THERAPY WITH EXTERNAL-BEAM RADIOTHERAPY?

A substantial amount of research has been conducted into hormonal therapy adjuvant to external-beam, conventional-dose radiotherapy, including a number of large randomized controlled trials in patients with localized or locally advanced prostate cancer (Table 91.2).[19,33–39] Data from these studies support the use of hormonal therapy adjuvant to external-beam radiotherapy in patients with locally advanced disease and those with high-risk localized disease.

PATIENTS WITH LOCALIZED PROSTATE CANCER

Two of the studies summarized in the next section included a small proportion of patients with localized disease in addition to those with locally advanced disease, but do not provide separate analyses of data from these patients. However, the bicalutamide EPC program does provide analysis of data from patients with localized disease treated with hormonal therapy adjuvant to radiotherapy.[19] Analysis of this subgroup of 1065 patients showed a small decrease in the risk of objective disease progression compared with radiotherapy alone (HR 0.80; 95% CI 0.62–1.03); however, this was not statistically significant, suggesting that bicalutamide 150 mg/day adjuvant to radiotherapy offers no clinical benefit in patients with localized disease. Currently, survival data for patients treated with radiotherapy in this study are immature, with 19% deaths.[40]

A recent randomized controlled trial has assessed the effect of 6 months CAB (leuprorelin or goserelin plus flutamide) adjuvant to radiotherapy in 206 patients with high-risk, clinically localized prostate cancer (PSA level ≥10 ng/mL, Gleason score ≥7 or radiographic evidence of extraprostatic disease).[33] At a median follow-up of 4.5 years overall survival was significantly higher for patients receiving adjuvant CAB, compared with radiotherapy alone, with 5-year estimates of survival of 88% and 78%, respectively (HR 2.07; 95% CI 1.02–4.20; p = 0.04).

PATIENTS WITH LOCALLY ADVANCED PROSTATE CANCER

Orchiectomy was studied as adjuvant hormonal therapy in a randomized controlled trial conducted in 91 patients with clinically localized (cT1–2 pN0; n = 37) or locally advanced (cT1–2 pN+ or cT3–4, any N; n = 54) prostate cancer.[39] After a median follow up of 9.3 years, there was a significant improvement in overall survival in patients who received adjuvant hormonal therapy compared with radiotherapy alone (62% versus 39%; p = 0.02); however, further subgroup analysis showed that the survival benefit was only significant for patients with lymph node metastases (p = 0.007).

An RTOG trial has examined long-term (indefinite duration) treatment with adjuvant LHRH agonist (goserelin) in 977 men with locally advanced disease (T1–2, N+ or T3, any N).[34–36] The most recent analysis of this study, at a median follow-up of 7.3 years, showed significant improvement in estimated 10-year overall survival with adjuvant hormonal therapy compared with radiotherapy alone (53% versus 38%; p < 0.0043).[36]

A European Organization for Research and Treatment of Cancer (EORTC) trial has also provided long-term follow-up data on the effect of an LHRH agonist (goserelin) adjuvant to radiotherapy in 415 men with high-risk localized (T1–2, Gleason score 3; 8% of the study population) or locally advanced (T3–4) tumors.[38,41] At a median follow-up of 5.5 years, 3 years' adjuvant hormonal therapy resulted in significant improvements in both 5-year disease-specific survival (94% versus 79%; p = 0.0001) and overall survival (78% versus 62%; p = 0.0002) compared with radiotherapy alone.

Analyses of the subgroup of patients with locally advanced disease who received radiotherapy in the bicalutamide EPC program have also been conducted.[19] At present, survival data for patients treated with radiotherapy in this study are immature, with 19% deaths.[40] However, at a median follow-up of 5.4 years, adjuvant bicalutamide 150 mg/day significantly decreased the risk of objective disease progression in the 305 patients with locally advanced disease by 42% compared with radiotherapy alone (HR 0.58; 95% CI 0.41–0.84; p = 0.00348).

COMPARATIVE STUDIES OF NEOADJUVANT AND ADJUVANT HORMONAL THERAPIES WITH EXTERNAL-BEAM RADIOTHERAPY

Relatively few studies have directly addressed whether neoadjuvant or adjuvant hormonal therapy offer the optimal outcome for a particular patient group. All such studies, however, have been undertaken in patients treated with external-beam radiotherapy as primary therapy. Overall, data from these studies provide no

Table 91.2 Randomised controlled trials of hormonal therapy adjuvant to external-beam radiotherapy compared with radiotherapy alone

Adjuvant hormonal therapy	Study	Disease stage	No. patients randomised	Treatment duration, years	Median follow-up, years	Progression-free survival	Overall survival
Orchiectomy	Granfors et al[39]	cT1–4, any N	91	Not applicable	9.3	69% vs 39% with RT alone (p = 0.005)[a]	62% vs 39% with RT alone (p = 0.02)
LHRH agonist (goserelin)	RTOG 85-31[34-36]	cT1–2, N+ or cT3, any N	977	Indefinite or until progression	7.3	Not given*	53% vs 38% with RT alone (p < 0.0043) [10-year estimate]
LHRH agonist (goserelin)	EORTC 22863[37,38]	cT1–2, Gleason grade 3 or cT3–4, any grade, N0–1	415	3 years	5.5	74% vs 40% with RT alone (p < 0.0001) [5-year estimate][b]	78% vs 62% with RT alone (p = 0.0002) [5-year estimate]
NSAA (bicalutamide)	EPC[19]	cT1b–2, N0/X or cT3–4, any N or cT1b–2, N+	1065 305	≥2 years	5.4 (whole study)	HR 0.80; 95% CI 0.62, 1.03; p = 0.088[c] HR 0.58; 95% CI 0.41–0.84; p = 0.0035[c]	Survival data immature (19% deaths in RT group)
CAB (leuprorelin or goserelin plus flutamide)	D'Amico et al[33]	cT1b–2, PSA ≥ 10 ng/mL, GS ≥ 7	206	6 months	4.5	82% vs 57% with RT alone; HR 2.30; 95% CI 1.36–3.89; p = 0.002 [5-year estimate][d]	88% vs 78% with RT alone; HR 2.07; 95% CI 1.02–4.20; p = 0.04 (5-year estimate)

*10-year estimates of local progression-free survival 77% vs 61% with RT alone, p<0.0001 and distant metastatic progression-free survival: 75% vs 61% with RT alone. Progression-free survival defined as: [a]time from randomization to the occurrence of clinically evident local tumor growth or bone or other distant metastases; [b]time to first clinical progression or death from any cause; [c]time from randomization to objective progression confirmed by bone scan, computed tomography/ultrasound/magnetic resonance imaging or histological evidence of distant metastases or death from any cause without progression; [d]time to initiation of salvage hormonal therapy.

CAB, combined androgen blockade; CI, confidence intervals; EPC, bicalutamide 150 mg early prostate cancer program; HR, hazard ratio; LHRH, luteinizing hormone-releasing hormone; NSAA, nonsteroidal antiandrogen; RT, external-beam radiotherapy.

clear evidence as to whether neoadjuvant or adjuvant hormonal therapy provide superior benefits for patients receiving radiotherapy, although subgroup analyses suggest that patients in particular risk groups may have better outcomes with one type of hormonal therapy.

One RTOG randomized controlled trial has compared 4 months of hormonal therapy neoadjuvant or adjuvant to external-beam radiotherapy in 1323 patients with clinically localized disease, elevated PSA levels, and a 15% estimated risk of lymph node metastases.[42] At a median follow-up of 5 years, there was no significant difference between patients receiving neoadjuvant or adjuvant CAB with goserelin or leuprorelin plus flutamide in terms of 4-year PSA progression-free survival (52% with neoadjuvant versus 49% with adjuvant, p = 0.56; PSA progression defined as two consecutive PSA rises of ≥20% from baseline or of ≥0.3 ng/mL from a baseline of ≤1.5 ng/mL, local or metastatic progression, or death from any cause). However, in this study, patients received either whole pelvic or prostate only external-beam radiotherapy and for those patients who received whole-pelvic radiotherapy, there was a significant improvement in PSA progression-free survival with neoadjuvant compared with adjuvant hormonal therapy (60% versus 49%; p-value not given).

A second RTOG trial, in 1554 patients with locally advanced or high-risk localized (T2c–4) disease, addressed the effects of 2 years' treatment with an LHRH agonist (goserelin) adjuvant to radiotherapy plus neoadjuvant CAB (goserelin plus flutamide) compared with radiotherapy plus neoadjuvant CAB alone.[43] At a median follow-up of 5.8 years, this study found no significant difference in 5-year estimates of overall survival between the two patient groups (p = 0.73). However, an exploratory subset analysis showed that adjuvant hormonal therapy significantly improved overall survival for patients with Gleason score 8 to 10 tumors compared with neoadjuvant CAB and radiotherapy alone (81% versus 71%; p = 0.044).

A smaller study, in 325 patients with localized or locally advanced (T2–3) prostate cancer, compared 5 months of hormonal therapy neoadjuvant to and concomitant with external-beam radiotherapy with 10 months of hormonal therapy neoadjuvant, concomitant and adjuvant to radiotherapy.[30] This study found no significant difference between the two treatment groups in terms of 4-year PSA progression-free survival (65% versus 68% with 5 and 10 months' hormonal therapy, respectively; p = 0.55). Prostate-specific antigen progression was defined as two consecutive increases in PSA level, with at least one value of 1.5 ng/mL or more.

A meta-analysis of data from five RTOG randomized controlled trials, using the risk groups defined in Figure 91.2, investigated which patients are most likely to benefit from either neoadjuvant or adjuvant hormonal therapy.[44] This analysis found that, in group 2, benefit in

terms of 8-year disease-specific survival was achieved with neoadjuvant CAB (goserelin and flutamide) for 2 months prior to, and for 2 months during, external-beam radiotherapy compared with radiotherapy alone (98% versus 83%; p = 0.003). Patients in groups 3 and 4 had an approximately 20% higher overall survival at 8 years with the addition of long-term adjuvant LHRH agonist (goserelin) following radiotherapy compared with radiotherapy alone (p ≤ 0.0004), while neoadjuvant hormonal therapy appeared to have no benefit in these risk groups.

OTHER PRIMARY THERAPIES

Brachytherapy and cryotherapy are alternatives to radical prostatectomy and external-beam radiotherapy for patients with early prostate cancer. For patients receiving brachytherapy or cryotherapy, addition of hormonal therapy is an option for the same reasons as other primary therapies. However, no randomized controlled studies have been conducted in which patients received hormonal therapy neoadjuvant or adjuvant to either brachytherapy or cryotherapy. For this reason, only limited conclusions can be drawn about the benefits of adding hormonal therapy to either brachytherapy or cryotherapy.

For brachytherapy, some data are available from retrospective or observational studies of additional hormonal therapy. Most of these studies focus on neoadjuvant hormonal therapy because, as with other primary therapies, any reduction in prostate volume induced by the neoadjuvant hormonal therapy may facilitate brachytherapy. However, a recent literature review reported that there was little evidence to indicate that biochemical or clinical progression-free survival is improved by hormonal therapy either neoadjuvant or adjuvant to brachytherapy.[45] Moreover, this review suggested that use of hormonal therapy might lead to increased acute urinary morbidity and decreased erectile function.

There are no published studies assessing clinical outcomes with hormonal treatment neoadjuvant or adjuvant to cryotherapy. The literature is limited to a few observational studies that assessed hormonal therapy neoadjuvant to salvage cryotherapy.

RISK: BENEFIT CONSIDERATIONS

Decisions regarding additional hormonal therapy should be based on an informed discussion between patient and urologist, in the same way as those relating to choice of primary therapy. Patients faced with a diagnosis of prostate cancer and a complex set of treatment options can experience strong emotional reactions, including depressive symptoms and feelings of overwhelming anxiety.[46] Their families can also be profoundly affected and may wish to have some input into treatment decisions. For example, a recent survey found that 88% of patients' partners reported an active involvement in the treatment decision-making process, with information gathering and emotional support as their primary roles.[47] The urologist guiding a patient through the treatment choices needs an understanding of the patient's, and their family's, concerns; the sources of information and support available to them; and the expectations they have. This will help to develop a positive patient–physician relationship and will contribute to a treatment decision the patient is happy with and, thus, more likely to adhere to.

While the focus of the preceding sections has been studies designed to determine the efficacy of hormonal therapy neoadjuvant or adjuvant to the primary therapy, there are a number of other important factors to consider when contemplating additional hormonal therapy. These include patient preference, age, life expectancy, comorbid disease, and level of sexual and physical activity. Such factors, plus a patient's risk profile, will impact on decisions relating to both the choice of neoadjuvant or adjuvant hormonal therapy and the specific agent used.

The overall impact of a treatment regimen on a patient's quality of life needs careful consideration in the context of that individual's circumstances. Likewise, the tolerability profile of the specific agent or agents used for neoadjuvant or adjuvant hormonal therapy is important, and the differing adverse event profiles of LHRH agonists or antiandrogens and any between-agent differences within each class of treatment need to be considered (Table 91.3).[48–56] In the case of CAB, side effects of both agents may occur, with a consequent increase in the overall incidence of adverse effects, although with gynecomastia and breast pain, the combination of an LHRH agonist and an antiandrogen reduces the incidence of this adverse effect compared with antiandrogen therapy alone.[57] As well as forming part of the treatment decision-making process, clear

Table 91.3 Common adverse events associated with hormonal therapies

Hormonal therapy	Adverse event	Agent	Reported frequency (%)
LHRH agonists	Hot flushes	All	52–84[48–53]
	Loss of libido	All	73–85[48–53]
	Impotence	All	76–84[48–53]
Non-steroidal antiandrogens	Gynecomastia	Bicalutamide	37–66[54]
		Flutamide	21–80[54]
		Nilutamide	50[54]
	Breast pain	Bicalutamide	13–73[54]
		Flutamide	22-69[54]
		Nilutamide	Not reported
	Hot flushes	All	<10[54]
	Diarrhea	Flutamide	10–20[55]
		Bicalutamide	2–6[54,55]
		Nilutamide	2–4[55]
	Serious/fatal hepatotoxicity	Flutamide	[Estimated risk 3 per 10,000[56]]
		Bicalutamide	Rare[54]
		Nilutamide	Rare[54]
	Interstitial pneumonitis	Nilutamide	1–3.8[54]
		Bicalutamide	Rare[54]
		Flutamide	Rare[54]
	Delayed adaptation to darkness	Nilutamide	Unique to nilutamide: 11–50[54]
	Alcohol intolerance	Nilutamide	Unique to nilutamide: 4–17[54]
	Loss of libido/impotence	All	~33[54]
Steroidal antiandrogens	Cardiovascular events	CPA	9.5–11[54]
	Adverse changes in serum lipids	CPA	Decreased HDL cholesterol and increased VLDL triglyceride levels[54]
	Impotence	CPA	87–92[54]

CAB, combined androgen blockade; CPA, cyproterone acetate; HDL, high-density lipoprotein; LHRH, luteinizing hormone-releasing hormone; VLDL, very-low-density lipoprotein.

Table 91.4 Summary of evidence for neoadjuvant and adjuvant hormonal therapeutic approaches

Therapeutic approach	Disease stage	Strength of evidence*	Randomised controlled trials reviewed	Comments
Neoadjuvant to radical prostatectomy	Localized/locally advanced	—	Aus et al[4]; Prezioso et al[5]; Labrie et al[6]; Goldenberg et al[7]; Hugosson et al[8]; Klotz et al[9]; Schulman et al[10]; Soloway et al[11,12]; Wirjes et al[13]	No overall survival data from randomized controlled trials PSA progression-free survival data available from randomized controlled trials in patients with localized or locally advanced disease show no significant difference compared with radical prostatectomy alone Studies of longer periods (>3 months) of neoadjuvant hormonal therapy required
Adjuvant to radical	Localized	–	Wirth et al[19]	Only randomized controlled study in patients with localized disease found no significant difference in risk of objective progression compared with radical prostatectomy alone Further randomized controlled studies required
Adjuvant to radical prostatectomy	Locally advanced	+	Messing et al[21,22]; Prayer-Galetti et al[23]; Wirth et al[24]	Improvements in overall survival demonstrated in patients with N+, M0 disease Improvements in PSA progression-free survival and risk of progression in T3–4 patients Overall survival data in N0 patients and additional randomized controlled trials required
Neoadjuvant to external-beam radiotherapy	Localised/locally advanced	+/–	Pilepich et al[27,28]; Laverdière et al[29,30]; Porter et al[31]	Improvements in disease-free survival in patients with T2–4 disease; improved overall survival in patients with GS 2–6, but not GS 7–10, tumors Improvements in PSA progression-free survival in patients with T2–3 and B2–C disease. Further overall survival data and additional randomized controlled trials required
Adjuvant to external-beam radiotherapy	Localized	+/–	D'Amico et al[33]; Granfors et al[39]	Improvements in overall survival seen in a study of adjuvant orchiectomy, but these were confined to N+ patients No significant difference in progression-free survival seen in a study of adjuvant non-steroidal antiandrogen therapy Significant improvements in overall survival with adjuvant CAB in patients with high risk localized disease (PSA ≥ 10 ng/mL, GS ≥ 7 or radiographic evidence of extraprostatic disease) Further randomized controlled studies required to establish optimal duration of adjuvant hormonal therapy
Adjuvant to external-beam radiotherapy	Locally advanced	++	Wirth et al[19]; Lawton et al[34]; Pilepich et al[35,36]; Bolla et al[38,41]	Improvements demonstrated in overall survival with an LHRH agonist (goserelin) and in risk of disease progression with a non-steroidal antiandrogen (bicalutamide) Studies required to clarify optimal duration of adjuvant hormonal therapy
Neoadjuvant to brachytherapy	Localized/locally advanced	–	No randomized controlled trials	Randomized controlled trials required
Adjuvant to brachytherapy	Localized/locally advanced	–	No randomized controlled trials	Randomized controlled trials required
Neoadjuvant to cryotherapy	Localised/locally advanced	–	No randomized controlled trials	Randomised controlled trials required
Adjuvant to cryotherapy	Localised/locally advanced	–	No randomised controlled trials	Randomised controlled trials required

*Summary of the strength of evidence for hormonal therapy in the setting described. ++, strong evidence of benefit (numerous large studies and consensus positive results); +, some evidence of benefit (limited overall survival data); +/–, mixed evidence (evidence of benefit in only certain patient groups) –, no strong supporting evidence (no randomized controlled trials or limited data suggesting no benefit); —, clear evidence of no benefit.

GS, Gleason score; LHRH, luteinizing hormone-releasing hormone; PSA, prostate-specific antigen.

communication of the possible side effects of treatments is important in promoting long-term adherence to the chosen treatment regimen.

Many of the studies outlined in this chapter show that some patients with early prostate cancer are at greater risk of a poorer outcome when primary treatment of curative intent is given alone. However, for those patients at low risk of progression, in the majority of cases, additional hormonal therapy is not advisable and these patients need to be counseled carefully about the potential benefit of neoadjuvant or adjuvant hormonal therapy compared with the impact of treatment on their quality of life.

Nomograms, which are designed to predict outcomes such as progression-free survival on the basis of a set of specific clinical parameters, are a helpful tool when assessing a patient's risk of progression. A variety of nomograms exist, not all of which have been validated; those developed by Partin et al and Kattan et al are among the better known.[58–61] When advising a patient about the balance between risks and benefits of a particular treatment, nomograms can provide useful additional input. The full complexity of the use and limitations of nomograms is discussed elsewhere in this book.

When weighing the potential risks and benefits of a treatment approach, an important part of the process is to examine the strength and quality of the evidence that supports the benefits provided by the therapy. Where fewer high-level data are available, or conclusions are not clear-cut, the decision may be weighted in favor of deferring hormonal therapy and thereby minimizing the risk of adverse events. Table 91.4 outlines the strength of data available for each therapeutic approach discussed in this chapter and highlights where additional research is needed to clarify the suitability of each treatment option.

SUMMARY

The range of neoadjuvant and adjuvant hormonal therapeutic approaches that may delay disease progression and improve survival for prostate cancer patients is outlined in Figure 91.3. At present, there are no data to indicate that neoadjuvant hormonal therapy prior to radical prostatectomy offers benefit to patients with localized or locally advanced disease in terms of overall survival or delaying disease progression. Hormonal therapy adjuvant to radical prostatectomy is of benefit to patients with lymph node metastases (both in terms of progression and survival) and also appears to offer benefits in terms of delaying disease progression for other patients with locally advanced disease, but survival data are currently immature. For patients with T2 to T4, Gleason score 2 to 6 disease, the current data indicate that hormonal therapy neoadjuvant to external-beam radiotherapy may offer benefits. There is also evidence of benefit for patients with locally advanced or high-risk localized disease receiving hormonal therapy adjuvant to external-beam radiotherapy.

Ultimately, assessing where the balance lies between the potential benefits and the possible risks associated with neoadjuvant or adjuvant hormonal therapy is an individual process, unique to each patient and their urologist. Treatment decisions should be based on clinical evidence as well as the patient's disease status, personal circumstances, and preferences.

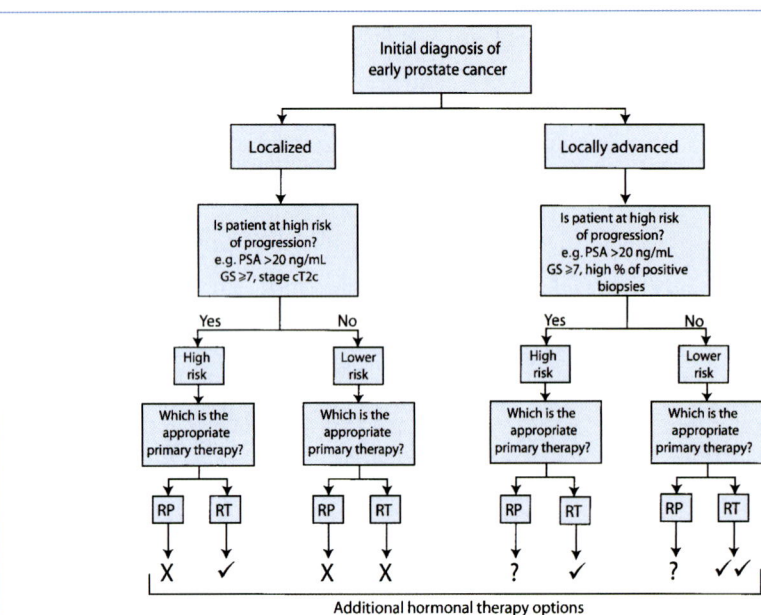

Fig. 91.3
Flow diagram outlining the decision-making process for patients with early prostate cancer. (GS, Gleason score; PSA, prostate-specific antigen; RP, radical prostatectomy; RT, external-beam radiotherapy.)

✓ Data support adjuvant hormonal therapy
✓✓ Data support adjuvant hormonal therapy and suggest there may be benefits from neoadjuvant hormonal therapy
X Data do not support adjuvant or neoadjuvant hormonal therapy
? Data suggest there may be benefits from adjuvant hormonal therapy

REFERENCES

1. Smith JA Jr, Soloway MS, Young MJ. Complications of advanced prostate cancer. Urology 1999;54 (Suppl 6A):8–14.

2. Penson DF, Moul JW, Evans CP, et al. The economic burden of metastatic and prostate specific antigen progression in patients with prostate cancer: findings from a retrospective analysis of health plan data. J Urol 2004;171:2250–2254.

3. Hull GW, Rabbani F, Abbas F, et al. Cancer control with radical prostatectomy alone in 1,000 consecutive patients. J Urol 2002;167:528–534.

4. Aus G, Abrahamsson P-A, Ahlgren G, et al. Three-month neoadjuvant hormonal therapy before radical prostatectomy: a 7-year follow-up of a randomized controlled trial. BJU Int 2002;90:561–566.

5. Prezioso D, Lotti T, Polito M, et al. Neoadjuvant hormone treatment with leuprolide acetate depot 3.75 mg and cyproterone acetate, before radical prostatectomy: a randomized study. Urol Int 2004;72:189–195.

6. Labrie F, Cusan L, Gomez J-L, et al. Neoadjuvant hormonal therapy: the Canadian experience. Urology 1997;49 (Suppl 3A):56–64.

7. Goldenberg SL, Klotz LH, Srigley J, et al. Randomized, prospective, controlled study comparing radical prostatectomy alone and neoadjuvant androgen withdrawal in the treatment of localized prostate cancer. J Urol 1996;156:873–877.

8. Hugosson J, Abrahamsson PA, Ahlgren G, et al. The risk of malignancy in the surgical margin at radical prostatectomy reduced almost three-fold in patients given neo-adjuvant hormone treatment. Eur Urol 1996;29:413–419.

9. Klotz LH, Goldenberg SL, Jewett MAS, et al. Long-term follow-up of a randomized trial of 0 versus 3 months of neoadjuvant androgen ablation before radical prostatectomy. J Urol 2003;170:791–794.

10. Schulman CC, Debruyne FMJ, Forster G, et al. 4-year follow-up results of a European prospective randomized study on neoadjuvant hormonal therapy prior to radical prostatectomy in T2-3N0M0 prostate cancer. Eur Urol 2000;38:706–713.

11. Soloway MS, Sharifi R, Wajsman Z, et al. Randomized prospective study comparing radical prostatectomy alone versus radical prostatectomy preceded by androgen blockade in clinical stage B2 (T2bNxM0) prostate cancer. J Urol 1995;154:424–428.

12. Soloway MS, Pareek K, Sharifi R, et al. Neoadjuvant androgen ablation before radical prostatectomy in cT2bNxMo prostate cancer: 5-year results. J Urol 2002;167:112–116.

13. Witjes WPJ, Schulman CC, Debruyne FMJ, for the European Study Group on Neoadjuvant Treatment of Prostate Cancer. Preliminary results of a prospective randomized study comparing radical prostatectomy versus radical prostatectomy associated with neoadjuvant hormonal combination therapy in T_{2-3} N_0 M_0 prostatic carcinoma. Urology 1997;49 (Suppl 3A):65–69.

14. Bazinet M, Zheng W, Begin LR, et al. Morphologic changes induced by neoadjuvant androgen ablation may result in underdetection of positive surgical margins and capsular involvement by prostatic adenocarcinoma. Urology 1997;49:721–725.

15. Bono AV, Pagano F, Montironi R, et al. Effect of complete androgen blockade on pathologic stage and resection margin status of prostate cancer: progress pathology report of the Italian PROSIT study. Urology 2001;57:117–121.

16. Gleave ME, Goldenberg SL, Chin JL, et al. Randomized comparative study of 3 versus 8-month neoadjuvant hormonal therapy before radical prostatectomy: biochemical and pathological effects. J Urol 2001;166:500–506.

17. Scolieri MJ, Altman A, Resnick MI. Neoadjuvant hormonal ablative therapy before radical prostatectomy: a review. Is it indicated? J Urol 2000;164:1465–1472.

18. Chun J, Pruthi RS. Is neoadjuvant hormonal therapy before radical prostatectomy indicated? Urol Int 2004;72:275–280.

19. Wirth M, See WA, McLeod DG, et al. Bicalutamide ("Casodex") 150 mg in addition to standard care in patients with localized or locally advanced prostate cancer: results from the second analysis of the Early Prostate Cancer program at 5.4 years' median follow-up. J Urol 2004;172:1865–1870.

20. Wirth M, Iversen P, McLeod D et al. Bicalutamide ("Casodex") 150 mg as adjuvant to radical prostatectomy significantly increases progression-free survival in patients with early non-metastatic prostate cancer: analysis at a median follow-up of 5.4 years. Eur Urol Suppl 2004;3:48 [abstract 181].

21. Messing EM, Manola J, Sarosdy M, et al. Immediate hormonal therapy compared with observation after radical prostatectomy and pelvic lymphadenectomy in men with node-positive prostate cancer. N Engl J Med 1999;341:1781–1788.

22. Messing E, Manola J, Sarosdy M, et al. Immediate hormonal therapy compared with observation after radical prostatectomy and pelvic lymphadenectomy in men with node positive prostate cancer: results at 10 years of EST 3886. J Urol 2003;169:396 [abstract 1480].

23. Prayer-Galetti T, Zattoni F, Capizzi A, et al. Disease free survival in patients with pathological "C STAGE" prostate cancer at radical retropubic prostatectomy submitted to adjuvant hormonal treatment. Eur Urol 2000;38.504 [abstract 48].

24. Wirth MP, Weissbach L, Marx FJ, et al. Prospective randomized trial comparing flutamide as adjuvant treatment versus observation after radical prostatectomy for locally advanced, lymph node-negative prostate cancer. Eur Urol 2004;45:267–270.

25. Roach III M, Lu J, Pilepich MV, et al. Four prognostic groups predict long-term survival from prostate cancer following radiotherapy alone on Radiation Therapy Oncology Group clinical trials. Int J Radiat Oncol Biol Phys 2000;47:609–615.

26. Roach III M, Weinberg V, McLaughlin PW, et al. Serum prostate-specific antigen and survival after external beam radiotherapy for carcinoma of the prostate. Urology 2003;61:730–735.

27. Pilepich MV, Krall JM, Al-Sarraf M, et al. Androgen deprivation with radiation therapy compared with radiation therapy alone for locally advanced prostatic carcinoma: a randomized comparative trial of the Radiation Therapy Oncology Group. Urology 1995;45:616–623.

28. Pilepich MV, Winter K, John MJ, et al. Phase III Radiation Therapy Oncology Group (RTOG) trial 86-10 of androgen deprivation adjuvant to definitive radiotherapy in locally advanced carcinoma of the prostate. Int J Radiat Oncol Biol Phys 2001;50:1243–1252.

29. Laverdière J, Gomez JL, Cusan L, et al. Beneficial effect of combination hormonal therapy administered prior and following external beam radiation therapy in localized prostate cancer. Int J Radiat Oncol Biol Phys 1997;37:247–252.

30. Laverdière J, Nabid A, De Bedoya LD, et al. The efficacy and sequencing of a short course of androgen suppression on freedom from biochemical failure when administered with radiation therapy for T2-T3 prostate cancer. J Urol 2004;171:1137–1140.

31. Porter AT, Elhilali M, Manji M, et al. A phase III randomized trial to evaluate the efficacy of neoadjuvant therapy prior to curative radiotherapy in locally advanced prostate cancer patients. A Canadian Urologic Oncology Group study. Proc Am Soc Clin Oncol 1997;16:315a [abstract 1123].

32. Pollack A, Zagars GK, Kopplin S. Radiotherapy and androgen ablation for clinically localized high-risk prostate cancer. Int J Radiat Oncol Biol Phys 1995;32:13–20.

33. D'Amico AV, Manola J, Loffredo M, et al. 6-month androgen suppression plus radiation therapy vs radiation therapy alone for patients with clinically localized prostate cancer: a randomized controlled trial. JAMA 2004;292:821–827.

34. Lawton CA, Winter K, Murray K, et al. Updated results of the Phase III Radiation Therapy Oncology Group (RTOG) trial 85-31 evaluating the potential benefit of androgen suppression following standard radiation therapy for unfavorable prognosis carcinoma of the prostate. Int J Radiat Oncol Biol Phys 2001;49:937–946.

35. Pilepich MV, Caplan R, Byhardt RW, et al. Phase III trial of androgen suppression using goserelin in unfavorable-prognosis carcinoma of the prostate treated with definitive radiotherapy: report of Radiation Therapy Oncology Group protocol 85-31. J Clin Oncol 1997;15:1013–1021.

36. Pilepich MV, Winter K, Lawton C, et al. Androgen suppression adjuvant to radiotherapy in carcinoma of the prostate. Long-term results of phase III RTOG study 85-31. Int J Radiat Oncol Biol Phys 2003;57:S172 [abstract 82].

37. Bolla M, Gonzalez D, Warde P, et al. Improved survival in patients with locally advanced prostate cancer treated with radiotherapy and goserelin. N Engl J Med 1997;337:295–300.

38. Bolla M, Collette L, Blank L, et al. Long-term results with immediate androgen suppression and external irradiation in patients with locally advanced prostate cancer (an EORTC study): a phase III randomised trial. Lancet 2002;360:103–108.

39. Granfors T, Modig H, Damber J-E, et al. Combined orchiectomy and external radiotherapy versus radiotherapy alone for nonmetastatic prostate cancer with or without pelvic lymph node involvement: a prospective randomized study. J Urol 1998;159:2030–2034.

40. McLeod D, Iversen P, See W, et al. Bicalutamide ("Casodex") 150 mg as adjuvant to radiotherapy significantly improves progression-free survival in early non-metastatic prostate cancer: results from the bicalutamide Early Prostate Cancer programme after a median 5.4 years' follow-up. Eur Urol Suppl 2004;3:48 [abstract 182].

41. Bolla M, Gonzalez D, Kurth J, et al. Adjuvant hormonal therapy with goserelin improves survival in patients with locally advanced prostate cancer treated with radiotherapy. Results of phase III randomized trial of the EORTC Radiotherapy and Genito-urinary tract Cancer Cooperative Groups. Eur Urol 1998;33 (Suppl 1):135 [abstract 537].

42. Roach III M, DeSilvio M, Lawton C, et al. Phase III trial comparing whole-pelvic versus prostate-only radiotherapy and neoadjuvant versus adjuvant combined androgen suppression: Radiation Therapy Oncology Group 9413. J Clin Oncol 2003;21:1904–1911.

43. Hanks GE, Pajak TF, Porter A, et al. Phase III trial of long-term adjuvant androgen deprivation after neoadjuvant hormonal cytoreduction and radiotherapy in locally advanced carcinoma of the prostate: the Radiation Therapy Oncology Group Protocol 92-02. J Clin Oncol 2003;21:3972–3978.

44. Roach III M, Jiandong L, Pilepich MV, et al. Predicting long-term survival and the need for hormonal therapy: a meta-analysis of RTOG prostate cancer trials. Int J Radiat Oncol Biol Phys 2000;47:617–627.

45. Lee WR. The role of androgen deprivation therapy combined with prostate brachytherapy. Urology 2002;60:39–44.

46. Manne SL. Prostate cancer support and advocacy groups: their role for patients and family members. Semin Urol Oncol 2002;20:45–54.

47. Srirangam SJ, Pearson E, Grose C, et al. Partner's influence on patient preference for treatment in early prostate cancer. BJU Int 2003;92:365–369.

48. Heyns CF, Simonin MP, Grosgurin P, et al. Comparative efficacy of triptorelin pamoate and leuprolide acetate in men with advanced prostate cancer. BJU Int 2003;92:226–231.

49. Kaisary AV, Tyrrell CJ, Peeling WB, et al. on behalf of Study Group, Comparison of LHRH analogue (Zoladex) with orchiectomy in patients with metastatic prostatic carcinoma. Br J Urol 1991;67:502–508.

50. Parmar H, Edwards L, Phillips RH, et al. Orchiectomy versus long-acting D-Trp-6-LHRH in advanced prostatic cancer. Br J Urol 1987;59:248–254.

51. Vogelzang NJ, Chodak GW, Soloway MS, et al. Goserelin versus orchiectomy in the treatment of advanced prostate cancer: final results of a randomized trial. Urology 1995;46:220–226.

52. Suprefact® prescribing information, 2004.

53. Lupron Depot 3.75 mg package insert, 2004.

54. Fourcade R-O, McLeod D. Tolerability of antiandrogens in the treatment of prostate cancer. UroOncology 2004;4:5–13.

55. McLeod DG. Tolerability of nonsteroidal antiandrogens in the treatment of advanced prostate cancer. Oncologist 1997;2:18–27.

56. Wysowski DK, Fourcroy JL. Flutamide hepatotoxicity. J Urol 1996;155:209–212.

57. Kaisary AV. Compliance with hormonal treatment for prostate cancer. Br J Hosp Med 1996;55:359–366.

58. Kattan MW, Eastham JA, Stapleton AMF, et al. A preoperative nomogram for disease recurrence following radical prostatectomy for prostate cancer. J Natl Cancer Inst 1998;90:766–771.

59. Kattan MW, Wheeler TM, Scardino PT. Postoperative nomogram for disease recurrence after radical prostatectomy for prostate cancer. J Clin Oncol 1999;17:1499–1507.

60. Partin AW, Yoo J, Carter HB, et al. The use of prostate specific antigen, clinical stage and Gleason score to predict pathological stage in men with localized prostate cancer. J Urol 1993;150:110–114.

61. Partin AW, Mangold LA, Lamm DM, et al. Contemporary update of prostate cancer staging nomograms (Partin Tables) for the new millennium. Urology 2001;58:843–848.

Controversies in hormone treatment for prostate cancer 92

Mario A Eisenberger

INTRODUCTION

For several decades, it has been well known that the growth and differentiation of prostate cancer cells is to a great extent under hormonal control.[1,2] Circulating testosterone (T) is converted to dihydrotestosterone (DHT) by the enzyme 5α-reductase. Dihydrotestosterone will bind to intracellular androgen receptor (AR) and subsequently induce intra nuclear transcriptional activity.[1] The AR is also activated by other androgens including T and adrenal androgens, which are converted peripherally to T or DHT.[3] Androgen deprivation for prostate cancer focuses primarily in maneuvers that will reduce circulating testosterone to levels around or below castrate levels (<50 ng/mL). Gonadal androgen deprivation is the standard therapeutic approach. It triggers the induction of a swift apoptotic cascade resulting in irreversible changes in the genomic DNA and, clinically, it represents one of the most effective systemic palliative treatments known for solid tumors in man.[1,3]

The biology of the AR has been the focus of significant attention over the past several years. Transcriptional activity of the AR can be induced by ligand dependent and ligand independent mechanisms as well as coactivators. Undoubtedly, the molecular and functional status of the AR play an important role in the endocrine dependence of prostate cancer and over the past years has also been focus of various therapeutic interventions.[4]

While androgen deprivation treatment for prostate cancer has been extensively applied in the clinic for many years, there are important remaining controversies regarding its optimal use. The focus of this chapter is not to review in any major detail the different approaches currently in clinical practice, but to highlight the background of some of the unresolved controversies associated with endocrine treatment for prostate cancer.

OPTIMAL TIMING FOR ANDROGEN ABLATION: THE IMMEDIATE VERSUS DEFERRED TREATMENT CONTROVERSY

At the present time there is a general consensus that immediate hormonal therapy improves the quality of life of patients with *metastatic disease* despite the fact that survival is not clearly better than treatment deferred until time of progression. The Veterans Administration Cooperative Research Group (VACURG) conducted important studies in patients with various stages of prostate cancer.[5–7] These studies have made a significant impact on various current issues related to endocrine treatment for this disease even though they were conducted approximately 4 decades ago. In VACURG study 1, patients with stage D2 and stage C were randomized to receive initial treatment with bilateral orchiectomy plus either placebo or 5 mg/day diethylstilbestrol (DES), or 5 mg/day DES alone, or a placebo alone. The data suggested that patients randomized to the placebo arm and subsequently crossed over to one of the three other study arms at the time of disease progression had a comparable survival to those randomized to initial treatment on the remaining three arms.[5,6] These data prompted the controversy that immediate androgen deprivation treatment for patients with metastatic disease was not associated with a survival benefit compared with treatment at the time of disease progression. While treatment with 5 mg/day DES was associated with comparable death rates due to prostate cancer as bilateral orchiectomy, there was a significant increase in deaths due to cardiovascular complications attributed to the use of DES. A subsequent study, VACURG study 2, was designed to evaluate the safety of different doses of DES (5.0, 1.0, or 0.2 mg/day) compared with a placebo initially. The final results of VACURG study 2, indicated that 1.0 mg/day was as effective as 5 mg/day DES in terms of deaths due to prostate cancer; however, there was a significant decrease in the incidence of severe and potentially fatal cardiovascular complications on the 1.0 mg/day arm. Both 5 mg/day and 1.0 mg/day DES had a lower incidence of deaths due to prostate cancer compared with a dose of 0.2 mg/day of DES or placebo. Unlike VACURG study 1, several patients on the placebo arm never received any treatment at the time of progression, and so study 2 is not perceived as an adequate test of the immediate versus deferred treatment question. Furthermore, VACURG study 2 was designed primarily to address the safety issue.

Several years later, the Medical Research Council (MRC) evaluated the survival of men receiving immediate treatment versus deferred treatment (at the time of progression) in patients with metastatic (M+; 434 patients) and nonmetastatic (M0; 500 patients) disease.[8,9] In the 434 patients with M+ disease there was no significant difference in prostate cancer-specific survival, however, the incidence of pathologic fractures, epidural cord compression, and renal failure was significantly lower in those receiving immediate treatment. While in the M0 group, the proportion of deaths due to prostate cancer was substantially lower in those receiving immediate treatment, a substantial number of patients randomized to deferred treatment never received any treatment at all. In the MRC studies, the criteria for initiating treatment on the deferred group was left at the discretion of the primary general physician. Despite the severe methodologic short-comings of these studies, which prevent definitive recommendations regarding survival advantages for immediate treatment, the choice of immediate treatment for patients with M+ disease or locally advanced disease (M0) disease is primarily aimed at the reduction of severe disease related morbidity. An overview analysis conducted by the agency for Health Care Policy and Research (AHCPR) evaluating various aspect on hormonal therapy for prostate cancer concluded that the survival benefits of early hormonal therapy were not statistically significant with a combined hazard ratio of 0.914.

ADJUVANT AND CONCOMITANT ANDROGEN SUPPRESSION WITH RADIATION AND SURGERY IN PATIENTS WITH CLINICALLY LOCALIZED PROSTATE CANCER

There is a growing amount of information on combined approaches employing hormonal therapy with concomitant radiation therapy for patients with palpable primary tumors. In one of the first studies reported by Pilepich et al[12] (RTOG 8531) patients with high-risk disease (M0) or with local recurrence after surgery were randomized to receive external-beam radiation therapy (EBRT) with or without permanent gonadal (medical or surgical) suppression. With a median follow-up of 13 years,[12] there was a statistically significant survival advantage for those receiving radiation plus permanent hormonal therapy. Of concern is that over the entire follow-up period of this study, the methodology used to evaluate patients and document progression changed significantly during the lifetime of the study. Furthermore no information regarding initiation of deferred treatment is available at this time. At the time of initiation of study (1985), the RTOG investigators did not count with the availability of PSA tests, which only became widely utilized much later during the conduct of the study. Two subsequent studies, RTOG 8610 and RTOG 9202,[10,11] have demonstrated a survival advantage for hormonal therapy on subsets only. RTOG 8610 demonstrated that a short course of 4 months adjuvant/neoadjuvant hormonal therapy is adequate for low-risk patients, whereas a 2-year hormonal therapy is effective in prolonging survival in high-risk patients on RTOG 9202. EORTC 22863 (Bolla et al) which included mostly high-risk patients, demonstrated that a 3-year androgen deprivation treatment plus EBRT was superior to EBRT alone in terms of local control, clinical and biochemical disease-free survival, and overall survival. Ongoing trials in the US are likely to provide additional information to support routine use of ADT plus radiation therapy in patients with palpable, clinically localized prostate cancer. Of importance is that none of these studies were designed to address the question of immediate versus deferred hormonal therapy. The primary hypothesis in these trials involves the biologic interaction between radiation and androgen deprivation, however, given the known effects of androgen deprivation in delaying the onset of distant metastatic disease, survival remains the key endpoint of clinical trials. Most North American studies (all except RTOG 8531) have only shown a survival benefit in subsets thus far, but despite this most physicians recommend a combined approach to patients with palpable primary tumors who are candidates for EBRT. It is hope that the ongoing RTOG studies will shed more light on the optimal duration of ADT on these patients and further characterized short- and long-term toxicities.

The Eastern Cooperative Oncology Group carried out a randomized prospective analysis of immediate hormonal therapy compared with observation in men following radical prostatectomy who had positive lymph nodes.[14] Ninety-eight men were randomized to either immediate hormonal ablation or followed until disease progression. After a median of 7.1 years of follow-up there was a significant difference in survival favoring immediate therapy. This result is rather surprising because there was a fairly large difference in survival within a relatively short period of observation.

In this study, cancer-specific survival in the observation group was 78% at 5 years. This is quite low compared with the rate of 91% in two contemporary series of patients with microscopic nodal metastasis who were treated with radical prostatectomy alone.[15–17] Furthermore, a series from the Mayo Clinic series, which represents the largest retrospective series with a nonrandomized control arm of patients and almost 3 decades of follow-up, found that the survival advantage in favor of immediate androgen deprivation was limited to DNA diploid tumors and did not become apparent until after 10 years.[16] Indeed, in that study of 790 men with lymph node-positive disease who underwent radical prostatectomy, androgen ablation therapy had no effect on cause-specific survival in nondiploid tumors. In the 57 men with diploid tumors who were followed for 10 years, there was also no significant difference in survival. At 15 years there were 14 patients with diploid tumors, 12 of whom received early hormonal therapy and 2 who did not. It is only in this small group where there was a statistical difference in survival (83.2 ± 4.1% versus 48.5 ± 13%). Thus, this finding is based on 14 patients out of 790 node positive men. Why is this ECOG study so different from the others? In an editorial, that accompanied the paper, a concern was raised that this study never realized its projected goal of 240 patients.[18] This is important because the outcome of patients with nodal metastasis is extremely variable and can be affected by a number of known and possibly unknown prognostic factors. Such effects on the outcome of trials can be minimized by randomization, but this ECOG trial was relatively small and might have been affected by imbalances of factors that had not been identified at the time the study began. The fact that 50% of the men in the deferred arm had progressed at 5 years and 22% were dead supports the argument that the control arm (deferred treatment) in the ECOG study most likely represented a high-risk group of patients composed of many high-grade tumors. These observations stress the importance of patient selection factors in the outcome of relatively small clinical studies in the adjuvant setting and highlight the complexities involved in the interpretation of results.

Another treatment explored in early stage prostate cancer is the use on antiandrogens as single agent. The most extensively developed drug in this setting is bicalutamide. Data in patients with metastatic disease suggest that bicalutamide (50 and 150 mg/day) as monotherapy is inferior to bilateral orchiectomy in prospective randomized trials.[19,20] The data in patients without metastasis is too preliminary for definitive conclusions. One large international placebo controlled study evaluated the adjuvant role of 150 mg/day of bicalutamide in high-risk patients treated with radical prostatectomy and radiotherapy or no treatment (watchful waiting). With a relatively short follow-up time, a statistically significant difference in progression

was observed in favor of bicalutamide, treatment was unblinded and the study was terminated. Toxicity (gynecomastia, gastrointestinal) was significant and because of the early unblinding of treatment, survival data may not be reliable. More recent evaluation ,with a median follow-up of 5.4 years, there were 25% of deaths on the bicalutamide arm compared with 20% on placebo (hazard ratio [HR] 1.2; 95% confidence interval [CI] 1.0–1.5).[1]

COMPLETE ANDROGEN BLOCKADE

While there is extensive data supporting a heterogeneity of cell populations with regard to androgen dependence[21,22] (androgen-dependent and -independent cell clones), it is increasingly recognized that the AR[3,4] albeit molecularly and functionally altered, continues to influence the progression of prostate cancer even after gonadal ablation. Transcriptional activity of the AR can be induced by ligand-dependent and ligand-independent mechanisms as well as coactivators. One of the earliest hypotheses focusing on a combined approach of gonadal androgen suppression and a blockade of AR, was promoted by Labrie et al[22,23] over 20 years ago. These authors suggested that following gonadal ablation prostate cancer cells continued a clinically significant hormone dependent tumor growth primarily due to the effects of androgens of adrenal origin. To neutralize the effects of adrenal androgens, a combined use of surgical or medical castration with a nonsteroidal antiandrogen was proposed and this approach was promoted as complete androgen blockade (CAB).[22] The concept generated a vigorous response from the urologic community in the world. A total of 27 prospectively randomized clinical trials involving more than 8000 patients were conducted to compare the efficacy of surgical or medical castration alone (monotherapy) to almost every possible combination of castration and antiandrogens. The first published large-scale prospectively randomized clinical trial was the NCI sponsored INT-0036, published by Crawford et al in 1989.[25] Six hundred and seventeen patients with stage D2 disease were randomly assigned to receive daily subcutaneous injections (1 mg/day) of leuprolide acetate plus flutamide versus leuprolide and placebo. The median overall survival with CAB and monotherapy was 35 and 29 months respectively (2 sided, p = 0.03). A number of factors, not directly related to the CAB concept, could not be excluded as alternative reasons for the outcome observations of INT-0036. One prevalent argument was that the difference in outcome could have been a result of the neutralizing effects of the antiandrogen on the flare phenomenon associated with leuprolide treatment alone. Indeed on NCI INT-0036, it was evident during the first 12 weeks of treatment that patients randomized to the CAB arm had a more favorable trend in the directions of pain control, performance status, and serum acid phosphatase. The second explanation related to possible compliance problems with the daily injections, which could result in inadequate testicular suppression, and consequently favor those receiving leuprolide with flutamide. In view of these two unresolved issues, a confirmatory trial employing surgical castration as the underlying method of gonadal ablation was subsequently conducted under the auspices of the National Cancer Institute (NCI INT-0105). NCI INT-0105 was a prospectively randomized, double-blinded, placebo-controlled trial comparing bilateral orchiectomy with and without flutamide in 1387 patients with stage D2 prostate cancer.[26] With a median follow-up time of approximately 50 months and with 70% deaths occurring at the time of the final analysis INT-0105 failed to confirm the initial findings of INT-0036. The median survival of patients on the CAB arm was 33 months compared with 30 months on the orchiectomy arm, which was not statistically significant (2 sided stratified, p = 0.14; HR, 0.91; 95% CI 0.81–1.01).[26] The Australian multicenter trial reported by Zalcberg et al[27] compared bilateral orchiectomy plus flutamide versus bilateral orchiectomy and placebo. This trial accrued 222 patients and was reported with a relatively short follow-up time. Interestingly, the Kaplan–Meier estimates of median survival favored the orchiectomy arm (31 and 23 months respectively) although the difference was not statistically significant (p = 0.21).

The second positive trial was reported by Dijkman et al[28] on a multinational prospectively randomized placebo-controlled study comparing orchiectomy plus nilutamide with orchiectomy alone. The results of this trial demonstrated a small but significant difference in median survival (27.3 versus 23.6 months, p = 0.032), observed after 8.5 years follow-up, in favor of the CAB regimen. Crawford et al subsequently reported the results of a prospective trial comparing the combination of leuprolide acetate plus nilutamide or leuprolide alone, which demonstrated no difference in survival.[29]

The third positive trial was conducted by the European Organization for Research and Treatment of Cancer (EORTC study 30853) comparing goserelin plus flutamide to bilateral orchiectomy in 327 patients mostly with stage D2 disease (M1 disease). EORTC 30853 demonstrated a 7 months difference in median overall survival (p = 0.04) in favor of the CAB arm.[30] The Danish Prostatic Cancer Group (DAPROCA) conducted a virtually identical study, with the same treatment arms and approximately the same number of patients. This study was completed around the same time as EORTC 30853 and showed a longer overall survival in favor of the monotherapy arm although the difference was not statistically significant.[31] The DAPROCA and EORTC-30853 trials had comparable populations and study

parameters. A combined analysis of both studies performed to enhance the power of comparisons did not show a significant survival difference.

In 1995, the Prostate Cancer Trialists' Collaborative Group (PCTCG)[32] reported on the first meta-analysis that was conducted as a measure to increase the statistical power of the observations of individual trials. Their report included data from 22 randomized trials comparing CAB to gonadal ablation alone in 5710 patients, which showed a 2.1% difference in mortality in favor of CAB treatment (6.4% reduction in annual odds of death, which is not statistically significant). The results were not influenced by the type antiandrogens (flutamide, nilutamide, or CPA) or the method of gonadal ablation.

The Agency for Health Care Policy and Research (AHCPR) published on the internet (*http://www.ahcpr.gov/clinic/index.html#evidence*—AHCPR report No.99-E012) the result of a comprehensive meta analysis based on all published CAB studies, which found no difference in 2-year survival rates (HR, 0.970; 95% CI 0.866–1.087). Only 10 of 27 trials reported both 2- and 5-year survival figures and in these 10 trials the preliminary results suggested a minimal 5-year survival difference in favor of CAB, which was considered of questionable clinical significance (HR, 0.871; 95% CI 0.805–0.9887). Quality of life was prospectively evaluated in patients undergoing CAB treatment on NCI INT-0105 in a companion study reported by Moinpour et al.[33] Patients on the CAB arm reported of a higher frequency of diarrhea and worsening of emotional functioning. It was concluded that the quality-of-life benefit resulting from orchiectomy in metastatic prostate cancer patients appeared to be offset by the addition of flutamide, primarily because of an increased incidence of adverse effects.

The lack of confirmatory results in trials of comparable design suggests that the most compelling explanation for the occasionally positive trial is that the overall CAB treatment effect size is indeed small (or perhaps minimal) and of questionable clinical significance.[34] The role of antiandrogens as second line treatment options for patients who demonstrate evidence of progression after gonadal ablation alone deserves further evaluation. The extensive clinical and laboratory investigation evolving from the initial reports on CAB have placed emphasis on AR biology research and added a new dimension on the consideration that progression after initial castration represents evidence of hormone resistance.

REFERENCES

1. Miyamoto H, Messing EM, Chang C. Androgen deprivation therapy for prostate cancer. Current status and future prospects. Prostate 2004;61:324–331.

2. Huggins C, Hodges CV. Studies on prostate cancer: effect of castration, of estrogen and of androgen injection on serum acid phosphatase in metastatic carcinoma of the prostate. Cancer Res 1941;1:293–297.

3. Feldman BJ, Feldman D. The development of androgen independent prostate cancer. Nature Rev Cancer 2001;1:34–45.

4. Gelman EP. Molecular Biology of the androgen receptor. J Clin Oncol 2002;20:3001–3015.

5. Byar DP. The Veterans Administration Cooperative Urological Research Groups studies of cancer of the prostate. Cancer 1973;32:1126–1130.

6. Veterans Administration Cooperative Urological Research Group. Factors in the prognosis of carcinoma of the prostate: A cooperative study. J Urol 1968;100:59–65.

7. Walsh PC, DeWeese T, Eisenberger MA. A structured debate: Immediate versus deferred androgen suppression in prostate cancer: evidence for deferred treatment. J Urol 2001;166:508–516.

8. Immediate versus deferred treatment for advanced prostatic cancer: initial results of the Medical Research Council. Prostate Cancer Working Party Investigators Group. Br J Urol 1997;79:235–246.

9. AHCPR report No. 99-E012. http://www.ahcpr.gov/clinic/index.html.

10. Pilepich MV, Caplan R, Byhardt RW, et al. Phase III trial of androgen suppression using goserelin in unfavorable-prognosis carcinoma of the prostate treated with definitive radiotherapy: report of Radiation Therapy Oncology Group Protocol 8531. J Clin Oncol 1997;15:1013–1021.

11. Pilepich MV, Winter K, John MJ, et al. Phase III radiation therapy oncology group (RTOG) study 8610 of androgen deprivation adjuvant to definitive radiation in locally advanced carcinoma of the prostate. Int J Rad Oncol Biol Phys 2001;50:1243–1252.

12. Pilepich MV, Winter K, Lawton RE. Phase III trial of androgen suppression adjuvant to definitive radiotherapy. Long term results of RTOG 8531. Proc ASCO 22 2003;381:1530 [abstract].

13. Bolla M, Gonzalez D, Warde P, et al. Improved survival in patients with locally advanced prostate cancer treated with radiotherapy and goserelin. N Engl J Med 1997;337:295–300.

14. Messing EM, Manola J, Sarosdy M, et al. Immediate hormonal therapy compared with observation after radical prostatectomy and pelvic lymphadenectomy in men with node-positive prostate cancer. N Engl J Med 1999;341:1781–1788.

15. deKernion JB, Neuwirth H, Stein A, et al. Prognosis of patients with stage D1 prostate cancer following radical prostatectomy with and without early endocrine therapy. J Urol 1990;144:700–703.

16. Sgrignoli AR, Walsh PC, Steinberg GD, et al. Prognostic factors in men with stage D1 prostate cancer: identification of patients less likely to have prolonged survival after radical prostatectomy. J Urol 1994;152:1077–1081.

17. Cheng L, Bergstralh E J, Cheville JC, et al. Cancer volume of lymph node metastasis predicts progression in prostate cancer. Am J Surg Pathol 1998;22:1491–1500.

18. Eisenberger MA, Walsh PC. Early androgen deprivation for prostate cancer? N Engl J Med 1999;341:1837–1838.

19. Tyrrel CJ, Kaisary AV, Iversen P, et al. A randomized comparison of casodex 150-mg monotherapy versus castration in the treatment of metastatic and locally advanced prostate cancer. Eur Urol 1998;33:447–456.

20. Iversen P, Tyrrell CJ, Karisary AV, et al. Casodex (bicalutamide) 150 mg monotherapy compared with castration in patients with previously untreated nonmetastatic prostate cancer: results from two multicenter randomized trials at a median follow-up of 4 years. Urology 1998;51:389.

21. DeMarzo A, Nelson WG, Isaacs WB, et al. Pathological and molecular aspects of prostate cancer. Lancet 2003;361:955–964.

22. Craft N, Sawyers CL. Mechanistics concepts in androgen- dependence of prostate cancer. Cancer Metastasis Rev 1998;17;421–427.

23. Labrie F, Veillux R, Fournier A. Low androgen levels induce the development of androgen-hypersensitive cell clones shionogi mouse mammary carcinoma cells in culture. J Natl Cancer Inst 1988;80:1138–1147.

24. Labrie F, Dupont A, Belanger A, et al. Combination therapy with flutamide and castration (LHRH agonists or orchiectomy) in advanced prostatic cancer: a marked improvement in response and survival. J Steroid Biochem 1985;23:833–841.

25. Crawford ED, Eisenberger MA, Mcleod DG, et al. A controlled trial of leuprolide with and without flutamide in prostatic carcinoma. N Eng J Med 1989;321:419–424.

26. Eisenberger MA, Blumenstein BA, Crawford ED, et al. A randomized and double-blind comparison of bilateral orchiectomy with or without flutamide for the treatment of patients with stage D2 prostate cancer: Results of NCI Intergroup Study 0105. N Eng J Med 1998;339:1036–1042.

27. Zalcberg JR, Raghhaven D, Marshall V, et al. Bilateral orchidectomy and flutamide versus orchidectomy alone in newly diagnosed patients with metastatic carcinoma of the prostate: an Australian multicentre trial. Br J Urol 1996;77:865–869.

28. Dijkman GA, Fernandez del Moral P, Debruyne FMJ, et al. Improved subjective response to orchiectomy plus nilutamide in comparison to orchiectomy plus placebo in metastatic prostate cancer. Eur Urol 1995;27:196–201.

29. Crawford ED, Kasimis BS, Gandara D, et al. A randomized controlled clinical trial of leuprolide and anandron vs. leuprolide and placebo for advanced prostate cancer. Proc Annu Meet Am Soc Clin Oncol 1990;9:A523.

30. Denis LJ, Keuppens F, Smith PH, et al. Maximal androgen blockade: final analysis of EORTC phase III trial 30853. Eur Urol 1998;33:144–151.

31. Iversen P, Ramussen F, Klarskov P, et al. Long-term results of Danish Prostatic Cancer Group Trial 86: Goserelin acetate plus flutamide versus orchiectomy in advanced prostate cancer. Cancer 1993;72:3851–3854.

32. Prostate Cancer Trialists Collaborative Group: Maximum androgen blockade in advanced prostate cancer: an overview of 22 randomized trials with 3283 deaths in 5710 patients. Lancet 1995;346:265–269.

33. Moinpour CM, Savage MJ, Troxel A, et al. Quality of life in advanced prostate cancer: Results of a randomized therapeutic trial. J Natl Cancer Inst 1998;90:1537–1544.

34. Laufer M, Denmeade S, Sinibaldi V, et al. Complete Androgen Blockade for Prostate Cancer. What went wrong? J Urol 2000;164:3–9.

Androgen deprivation therapy: the future 93

Marc B Garnick, Camille Motta

INTRODUCTION

Defining the future of androgen deprivation therapy (ADT) for prostate cancer can be best addressed by briefly reviewing the multitude of established uses, and then by evaluating the emerging utilities of hormonal therapy, which are not yet standard of practice. Box 93.1 presents an overview, with references, of existing and emerging uses of hormonal therapies in prostate cancer. Examples of the former include the use of ADT in patients with metastatic disease (N+, M+); use as a neoadjuvant and adjuvant therapy prior to, during, or after definitive radiation therapy; to downsize prostate gland volume prior to either external-beam radiation therapy (XRT) or brachytherapy. Emerging uses include ADT as an adjunct in the adjuvant setting for patients who have undergone radical prostatectomy and are found to harbor unfavorable pathologic characteristics (e.g., pT2 and pT3 with unfavorable histologies); use of hormonal therapies for those with a biochemical relapse following definitive therapy (so called rising prostate-specific antigen [PSA] following definitive therapy); use of ADT for intermittent hormonal therapy; use of ADT for primary therapy of clinically localized prostate cancer; use of sequences of hormonal therapies, either alone or in combination, in a sequential fashion such as "step-up" therapy; the use of therapies that induce androgen deprivation, either alone or in combination with cytotoxic chemotherapy for those with androgen independent prostate cancer; use of ADT, alone or in combination with cytotoxic chemotherapy for regionally advanced prostate cancer (e.g., cT3 or pT3 or greater) or those with intermediate or high risk characteristics (e.g., those with a ≤50% biochemical 5-year disease-free survival following definitive localized treatment).

While this list is probably not exhaustive, it does represent the vast majority of uses of hormonal therapy in current usage throughout the world. These uses—both established and emerging—utilize commercially available hormonal agents that induce states of actual or functional androgen deficiency, and represent

---

Box 93.1 Existing and emerging uses of hormonal therapy in prostate cancer

Existing

- Metastatic disease D_1, D_2, N+, M+; advanced stages T3, T4[27,48]
- Neoadjuvant—prior to surgery[19,49–51]
- Neoadjuvant—prior to radiotherapy[55,56]
- Adjuvant—post-external-beam radiation therapy for locally advanced prostate cancer[13,64]
- Neoadjuvant + adjuvant to external-beam radiation therapy[66]
- Prostate gland volume reduction[68–70]
- Sequential androgen blockade (anti-androgen + 5α-reductase inhibitor)[71–75]

Emerging

- Adjuvant—post-radical prostatectomy for unfavorable pathologic characteristics (seminal vesicle invasion and lymph node disease)[14,17]
- Adjuvant—post-radical prostatectomy in localized disease[21,52–54]
- Intermittent hormonal therapy[57–63]
- Androgen-independent prostate cancer alone or in combination with chemotherapy[43,65]
- Regionally advanced prostate cancer alone or in combination with chemotherapy[67]
- Rising prostate-specific antigen post definitive therapy; biochemical relapse[42]
- Primary therapy of local prostate cancer[76,77]

luteinizing hormone releasing hormone (LHRH) agonists; steroidal and nonsteroidal antiandrogens; progestational agents; estrogenic compounds; the recently introduced class of gonadotropin releasing hormone (GnRH) antagonists; and surgical removal (bilateral orchiectomy) of the main source of androgenic steroids.

Under development are a variety of additional compounds, including other LHRH analogs (both agonists and antagonists) and other classes of novel inhibitors of proliferation (that include both endocrine and non-endocrine mechanisms) that are being evaluated as both first- and second-line therapies for prostate cancer. As these therapies and usage patterns change, the potential for differing side effects also emerges. One example is bone mineral density loss associated with prolonged androgen deprivation therapies,[1,2] which can now be partially addressed with newer generation of bisphosphonates, zoledronic acid, in particular.[3,4] Another is the recent recognition that ADTs may be associated with non-thrombotic cardiovascular effects, such as prolongation of the electrocardiographic QT interval.[5] Thus, as the treatment programs that involve ADT evolve, the clinician will need to be aware of a spectrum of additional effects associated with these new treatments. Finally, the emergence of prostate cancers that have become "hormonally refractory" or androgen independent poses serious scientific and clinical challenges. Understanding the mechanisms underlying the transition to this more refractory state should help provide new directions in designing better and more targeted therapies.

HORMONAL THERAPY FOR PROSTATE CANCER

The use of ADT, also called hormonal therapy, endocrine therapy, castration therapy (either medical or surgical), or simply hormones, has for the past 65 years been the mainstay in the systemic management of advanced prostate cancer. Initially identified by the late Dr Charles Huggins,[6–8] the fundamental premise identified nearly 7 decades ago is that prostate cancer is under the tropic influence of the male hormones, including, but not limited to, testosterone and dihydrotestosterone. Indeed, under the influence of exogenous androgen administration, prostate cancer grows, and with this growth patients may experience worsening symptoms associated with proliferating cancer cells.[9] Conversely, the removal of androgenic sources, either by surgical removal of the testicles, a main source of androgens, or by medically abrogating the production of androgen via interruption of the hypothalamic-pituitary-gonadal axis, results in improvement in the signs and symptoms of a substantial proportion of patients.

Up until the more widespread introduction of the prostatic fraction of acid phosphatase, the majority of men who received ADT were those with extensive regional disease, leading to urinary obstruction, hydronephrosis, and pelvic adenopathy; or those with frank metastatic disease, in which patients presented with osseous disease, weight loss, anemia, and a generalized decrease in overall performance status. Thus, this population of patients who did not enjoy the advantage of earlier diagnosis of prostate cancer by currently available biochemical methods of diagnosis was identified later in the course of their disease. The use of ADT in these settings did lead to the palliation of both the signs and symptoms of disease advancement. Although the Veteran's Administration Cooperative Urological Research Group (VACURG) did study either single or combinations of hormonal therapies in earlier stage patients, the standard of practice usually dictated the use of ADT in more advanced patient populations.[10–12]

Since the 1980s, a series of clinical investigations has evaluated a multidisciplinary approach to prostate cancer. In addition, the introduction and widespread use of PSA-based methods of prostate cancer diagnosis has led to an ongoing dialog on the definition of the optimal treatment program that could include the disciplines of surgery, radiation, and systemic medical management. This chapter will evaluate the emerging uses of these combination approaches and discuss further strategies in which the role of ADT emerges as an integral part of both the regional and systemic management of patients with prostate cancer. With these novel uses of ADT, in which patients may be exposed to lowered testosterone for years, a new set of side effects have emerged, again requiring a deeper knowledge of the multitude actions of androgens on various tissues. This chapter will review some of these new adverse drug effects.

EMERGING USES

NEOADJUVANT AND ADJUVANT HORMONAL THERAPY

The uses of neoadjuvant or adjuvant hormonal therapy have been well covered in other chapters of this book. Several key studies, however, are worth emphasizing, as they may serve to chart the future of subsequent strategies that incorporate hormonal therapy into overall treatment programs.

ADJUVANT HORMONAL THERAPY

One randomized trial of 415 patients with locally advanced prostate cancer (T1/T2 tumors of World

Health Organization [WHO] grade 3 or T3/T4, N0/N1, M0 tumors) found that XRT combined with an analog of LHRH for 3 years (XRT + HT) conferred an improved 5-year disease-free survival over XRT alone of 74% versus 40% ($P = 0.0001$), as well as improved 5-year overall survival of 78% versus 62% ($P = 0.0002$); and a 5-year disease specific survival of 94% versus 79%.[13]

Another study of 98 men treated with radical prostatectomy and pelvic lymphadenectomy and nodal metastases were randomly assigned to receive immediate ADT (goserelin or bilateral orchiectomy) or no ADT. Both groups were followed until disease progression. After a median follow-up of 7.1 years, 7 of 47 in the ADT group had died, compared with 18 of 51 men in the control (no ADT) group ($P = 0.02$). The cause of death was prostate cancer in 3 ADT patients compared with 16 controls ($P < 0.01$).[14] This conclusion was recently validated by a new central pathology slide review, and evaluation and reassessment of Gleason scores. Revised results are in keeping with those published earlier. In addition to overall survival at median of 11.9 years follow-up, the advantages of immediate hormone therapy versus observation/delayed therapy include disease-specific survival (85% versus 51%), recurrence-free survival (62% versus 24%), and PSA progression-free survival (55% versus 14%).[15]

These two studies serve as the basis for combining hormonal therapy with either radiation therapy for men with both localized and regionally advanced prostate cancer, or radical prostatatectomy for men with nodal metastases. The first study evaluated the effect of 3 years of hormonal therapy and demonstrated that long-term adjuvant hormonal therapy is critical to improving survival, and the second study evaluated the utilization of immediate ADT. Anecdotally, many men do not tolerate such long-term androgen suppression well, and clinicians often treat with ADT for shorter periods of time.

A more recent study has evaluated the use of 6 months of ADT following 70 Gy 3D-conformal radiation therapy and suggested an overall survival advantage when added to patients with clinically localized prostate cancer treated with 3D-conformal radiation therapy.[16] These three studies serve as a basis for consideration of the timing, schedule, and duration of ADT associated with localized treatments in future trials.

Other less well-controlled studies also suggest advantages when ADT is added to localized treatments. A recent review of prospective randomized studies and of clinical information on stage pT3b cancer from a large single-institution prostate cancer database shows that early adjuvant hormonal therapy after radical prostatectomy has a significant impact on time to progression and causes specific survival in patients with seminal vesicle invasion and limited lymph node disease.[17]

NEOADJUVANT THERAPY—HOW LONG SHALL WE TREAT PATIENTS IN THE FUTURE?

There have been several recent investigations into the optimal treatment time for neoadjuvant hormonal therapy in an attempt to determine if longer is better. This remains an issue to be resolved in the future.

A recent Canadian study[18] evaluated the effect of 3 months versus 8 months of neoadjuvant hormonal therapy before conventional dose radiotherapy (RT) on disease-free survival using PSA and biopsies as end points for clinically localized prostate cancer. Three hundred seventy-eight men were randomized to either 3 or 8 months of flutamide and goserelin before conventional-dose RT (66 Gy) at four participating centers. The actuarial freedom from failure rate (biochemical by American Society for Therapeutic Radiology and Oncology definition), local or distant, for the 3-month versus 8-month arms at 3 years was 66% versus 68% and by 5 years was 61% versus 62%, respectively ($P = 0.36$). No statistically significant difference was noted in the types of failure between the two arms (crude final status): biochemical, 22.2% versus 22.3%; local, 10.2% versus 6.5%; and distant, 3.4% versus 4.4% ($P = 0.61$). A suggestion of improvement was found in the 8-month arm for disease-free survival at 5 years for high-risk patients (39% versus 52%) but did not achieve statistical significance. Results suggest that a longer period of neoadjuvant hormonal therapy before standard-dose RT does not appear to confer a benefit in terms of disease-free survival or to alter failure patterns. A suggested benefit was noted with a longer period of hormonal therapy for high-risk patients.

A prospective phase III trial[19] compared 8-month with 3-month neoadjuvant hormonal therapy prior to radical prostatectomy to determine reduction of PSA recurrence rates. Five hundred forty-seven men with organ-confined prostate cancer received either 7.5 mg leuprolide (i.m.) monthly and 250 mg flutamide (p.o.) 3 times/day for 3 months or for 8 months before radical prostatectomy. Mean serum PSA decreased 98% to 0.12 ng/mL after 3 months, with a further 57% to 0.052 ng/mL from 3 to 8 months. Prostate gland volume decreased by 37% from a mean of 40.6 to 25.4 cm³ after 3-month neoadjuvant hormonal therapy ($P = 0.0001$) and a further 13% to 22.2 cm³ after 8 months ($P = 0.03$). Five hundred men underwent radical prostatectomy. Positive margin rates were significantly lower in the 8-month than in the 3-month group (12% versus 23%, respectively; $P = 0.0106$). Since there appears to be ongoing regression, both biochemical and pathologic, of the prostate tumor that occurs between month 3 and month 8 of neoadjuvant therapy, results suggests that the optimal duration of neoadjuvant hormonal therapy is longer than 3 months. Additional patient follow-up is needed to determine whether longer therapy alters PSA recurrence rates.

ANTIANDROGEN MONOTHERAPY FOLLOWING TREATMENT OF CLINICALLY LOCALIZED PROSTATE CANCER

Because of complications associated with conventional ADT—loss of potency, libido, bone mineral density loss, and vasomotor hot flashes—several programs have addressed the utility of nonsteroidal, anti-androgen monotherapy, such as bicalutamide, to be administered as an adjunct to definitive localized therapies in an attempt to improve overall survival and progression-free survival. While preliminary results of these studies using 50 mg/day bicalutamide[20] were encouraging in prolonging disease free survival, and led to the marketing approval outside of the United States, when given to locally advanced patients at 150 mg/day (three times the conventional dose of 50 mg/day), although similar survival outcome to castration was observed, toxicity was also found, consisting of breast pain and gynecomastia, at times irreversible.[21-23] Further analyses demonstrated an overall survival disadvantage of antiandrogen monotherapy when compared with placebo. At 5-year follow-up, a trend was noted for an increase in the number of deaths in patients with localized prostate cancer receiving bicalutamide (Casodex) 150 mg compared with patients who received placebo (196 [25.2%] deaths versus 174 [20.5%] deaths.) This finding precipitated its removal from marketing authorization as a treatment for localized prostate cancer in Canada, the UK, and several other European countries.[24,25] The US FDA never granted marketing approval for this type of monotherapy.

NOVEL HORMONAL AGENTS

GONADOTROPIN RELEASING HORMONE ANTAGONISTS

Gonadotropin releasing hormone is a natural decapeptide. The synthetic GnRH antagonist decapeptide has five or more amino-acid substitutions; modifications involving position 6 hinder cleavage by serum proteases; substitutions at positions 2 and 3 affect gonadotropin release; and changes at positions 1, 6, and 10 affect receptor binding. In contrast to the LHRH agonists, GnRH antagonists bind immediately and competitively to GnRH receptors in the pituitary gland. Luteinizing hormone concentrations are reduced (51–84%) and follicle-stimulating hormone (FSH) concentrations are lessened (17–42%) within 8 to 24 hours following the first dose. The competitive blocking of the GnRH receptor results in a rapid, reversible decrease in LH, FSH, and testosterone, without any

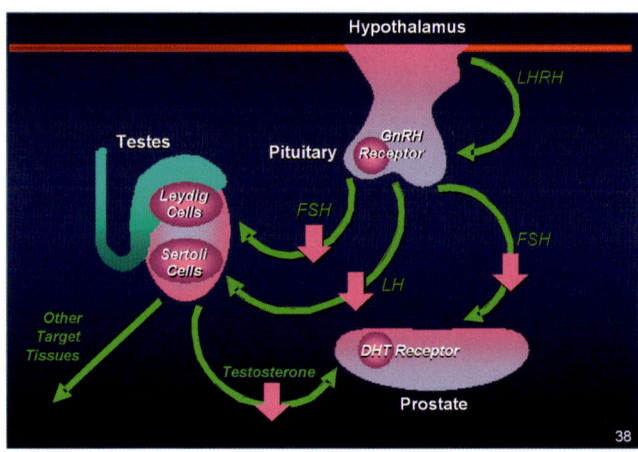

Fig. 93.1
Mechanism of action of gonadotropin-releasing hormone antagonist, abarelix. (DHT, dihydrotestosterone; FSH, follicle-stimulating hormone; GnRH, gonadotropin-releasing hormone; LHRH, luteinizing hormone releasing hormone.)

flare. Also, when GnRH antagonist therapy is stopped, a more rapid recovery of pituitary-gonadal function is possible.[26] Figure 93.1 portrays this mechanism of action.

Recently, the US FDA has approved abarelix for injectable suspension for the management of a subset of patients with advanced symptomatic prostate cancer in whom LHRH agonists are not appropriate and who refuse treatment with surgical castration. Abarelix is the first GnRH antagonist decapeptide formulated in a depot suspension indicated for prostate cancer. Other GnRH anatagonists (cetrorelix, ganirelix) are approved for shorter term administration for use in women for in-vitro fertilization.

EFFECTS OF ABARELIX IN ADVANCED SYMPTOMATIC PROSTATE CANCER PATIENTS

An open label, uncontrolled study[27] of abarelix was conducted in 72 evaluable men with advanced symptomatic prostate cancer who were at risk for clinical exacerbation ("clinical flare") if treated with an LHRH agonist. This study defined the approved patient population for use with of abarelix. The objective was to demonstrate that such patients could avoid surgical castration through at least 12 weeks of treatment. Patients were enrolled with bone pain from prostate cancer skeletal metastases; an enlarged prostate gland or pelvic mass causing bladder neck outlet obstruction; retroperitoneal adenopathy with ureteral obstruction; impending neurologic compromise from spinal, spinal cord, or epidural metastases. All patients were able to avoid the requirement for surgical castration throughout the study. Although the study was not designed to assess specific clinical outcomes, outcomes consistent with the expected benefits of castration and avoidance of adverse consequences of clinical flare were observed, and included relief of bladder outlet and ureteral obstruction; decreased bone pain and need for narcotic analgesics; avoidance of neurologic compromise, including spinal cord compression in those with vertebral or epidural metastases.

INVESTIGATIONAL THERAPIES WITH NOVEL HORMONAL MECHANISMS OF ACTION BEING STUDIED FOR PROSTATE CANCER

Table 93.1 lists other hormonal therapies recently introduced or under development for prostate cancer.

FOR HORMONALLY-SENSITIVE PROSTATE CANCER

ABIRATERONE ACETATE

Abiraterone acetate (CB7630) is a new compound that shows potential in the treatment of cancer and other hormonally-responsive, testosterone-related diseases. It is an orally active inhibitor (structurally related to ketoconazole) of the steroidal enzyme 17α-hydroxylase/C17,20-lyase, a cytochrome p450 complex that is involved in testosterone production (Figure 93.2). In preclinical studies, abiraterone has demonstrated the

Table 93.1 Hormonal therapies recently introduced or under development for prostate cancer[78,79]

Name	Mechanism of action	Route of admin	Phase	Notes	Refs
SARMs	Selective androgen receptor modulators	A-p.o.	Preclinical		80,81
Abiraterone acetate*	C17-20 Lyase inhibitor; Steroid synthesis inhibitor	A-p.o.	I (W)		28,29
Leuprolide inhalation	LHRH agonist	Inhaled 1×day	I (W)		82
NBI-42902	GnRH antagonist, 2nd generation	A-p.o.	I (USA)		
Izonsteride	5-alpha reductase inhibitor	p.o.	I (US)		83
Leuprorelin implant	LHRH agonist	Implant 4–6 mo. Depot	II (W)		84
Degarelix	GnRH antagonist	various	II (W)		85,86
D-63153	GnRH antagonist	P-i.m.	II (W)		87
Leupromaxx	LHRH agonist	P-varies 24 day & 84 day form.	II (W)	Extended release ProMaxx System	
Phenoxodiol*	Apoptosis stimulant; mitosis inhibitor; signal transduction pathway inhibitor	P-i.v. A-p.o.	II (W)		33
Teverelix LA	GnRH antagonist	P-s.c	IIa	Immed rel. & Sustained Rel.	88
Cetrorelix	GnRH antagonist	P-s.c	II	Already launched for other indications	89
Avorelin	LHRH agonist	P-s.c	II	6 month depot	90
Osaterone acetate (TZP 4238)	Androgen antagonist Steroidal antiandrogen	A-p.o.	II		91
PCK 3145 (PSP 94)	Apoptosis stimulant	i.v.	II (UK)	For AIPC	92,93
Tesmilifene (DPPE)	Estrogen antagonist; Intracellular histamine antagonist	P-i.v.	II (US & Can)	For AIPC combined with other drugs	34-37,94
Toremifene	Selective estrogen receptor modulator	A-p.o.	III	For AIPC	95,96
DN-101 (calcitriol)*	Vitamin D receptor agonist	A-p.o.	III (W)	For AIPC combined w/docetaxel	38-41
Vapreotide (RC-160)	Somatostatin (SST) analog Growth hormone antagonist	P-s.c P-i.v.	III	Also for AIPC	97-99
Histrelin (hydrogel implant)	LHRH agonist	P-s.c. 12 month depot (implant)	III (Can)		100,101
Altrasentan*	Endothelin A receptor antagonist	A-p.o.	III (USA)	For AIPC	46,47
Plenaxis*	GnRH antagonist	P-i.m.	IV	Launched 11/2003	27;45;102-104

*Discussed in this chapter.

AIPC, androgen-independent prostate cancer; GnRH, gonadotropin-releasing hormone; LHRH, luteinizing hormone releasing hormone. Phase: W, World; US, USA; Can, Canada. Rte Admin: A, alimentary; P, parenteral; i.m., intramuscular; i.v., intravenous; p.o., by mouth; s.c., subcutaneous.

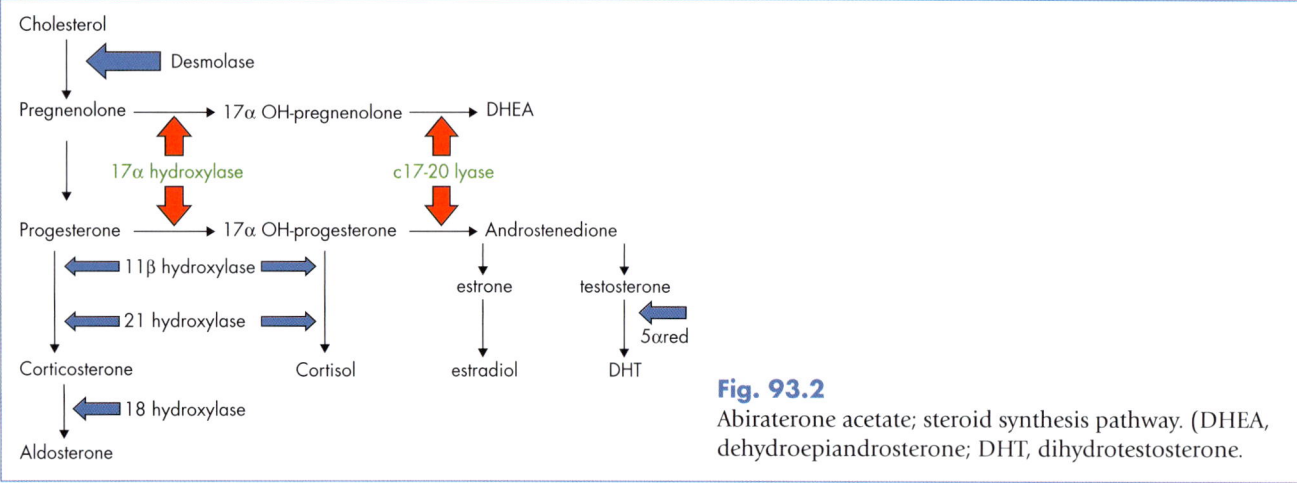

Fig. 93.2

Abiraterone acetate; steroid synthesis pathway. (DHEA, dehydroepiandrosterone; DHT, dihydrotestosterone.

ability to selectively inhibit the target enzyme, resulting in inhibition of testosterone production in both the adrenals and the testes. In phase I trials, abiraterone was administered to 26 patients with prostate cancer. These clinical studies demonstrated that the compound: 1) at a single oral dose of 800 mg, can successfully suppress testosterone levels to the castrate range; 2) can suppress testosterone produced by both the testes and the adrenals; 3) is well tolerated and non-toxic. This is the first report of the use of a specific 17α-hydroxylase[17,20] lyase inhibitor in humans. However, this level of testosterone suppression to the castrate range may not be sustained in all patients due to compensatory hypersecretion of luteinizing hormone. Adrenocortical suppression may necessitate concomitant treatment with replacement glucocorticoid.[28,29] Abiraterone acetate is currently under development as a second-line hormonal therapy for prostate cancer for patients who are refractory to first-line treatment with an LHRH agonist/antagonist and antiandrogen therapy.

PHENOXODIOL

Phenoxodiol belongs to a new class of anticancer drugs known as multiple signal transduction regulators (MSTRs) that show promise in the treatment of solid cancers, including prostate and breast, and benign prostatic hyperplasia. Phenoxodiol is the lead compound in a series of synthetic phenolic hormone analogues. Phenolic hormones are naturally occurring compounds produced in the human body from isoflavones in food.[30] Phenoxodiol is an effective inhibitor of three key enzymes involved in signal transduction processes; topoisomerase II, epidermal growth factor tyrosine kinase, and sphingosine kinase (primary target). It inhibits antiapoptotic proteins (c-FLIP and XIAP) and increases proapoptotic proteins (BAX). These MSTRs work by inducing programmed cell death in cancer cells (apoptosis), with little or no effect on normal cells.

In animal studies, phenoxodiol significantly inhibited the growth of transplanted human prostate tumors at nontoxic doses by induction of apoptosis and inhibition of cell division. Phenoxodiol caused cancer cells to differentiate into normal cells and inhibited growth of human leukemia, melanoma, breast, prostate, and bowel cancer cell cultures.[31,32] In phase Ib/IIa clinical trials with hormone-refractory prostate cancer patients, interim results show that two patients treated with the two highest dosages (200 and 400 mg) showed stabilization of their PSA levels after 3 months of therapy, while six (50%) showed a decrease in PSA levels. Two of these six responders showed a decline in PSA levels of greater than 75%.[33] Phenoxodiol is being developed as a monotherapy for early-stage and late-stage hormone-refractory prostate cancer patients, and as a combination therapy where it acts to enhance the efficacy of chemotherapeutic agents in chemosensitive patients and to restore sensitivity to those drugs in chemoresistant patients.

FOR HORMONE-REFRACTORY CANCER

TESMILIFENE

An intracellular histamine antagonist, tesmilifene (also known as DPPE), is being developed as a chemopotentiator for the treatment of malignant solid tumors. The compound is cytotoxic to tumor cells and cytoprotective to the gut and to normal bone marrow progenitor cells. Research suggests that it is able to augment the in-vivo antitumor activity of numerous cytotoxic drugs routinely used in the treatment of many types of cancers, such as doxorubicin, cyclophosphamide, fluorouracil, cisplatin, and mitoxantrone.[34,35] It has been shown to increase the cytotoxicity of fluorouracil and daunorubicin in cancer cell lines; and has increased the antitumour effects of doxorubicin and daunorubicin in mice.

The results of a study investigating the efficacy of tesmilifene plus cyclophosphamide in 20 patients with metastatic prostate cancer refractory to hormonal therapy have been reported. Tesmilifene and cyclophosphamide were both administered by i.v. infusion. Treatment was given for as long as the patient was deemed to benefit. Five of seven patients (71%) with measurable soft tissue disease had a partial remission. Three of 16 (19%) with assessable bone disease responded, one with complete remission and two partial remission. Nine of 18 (50%) with an elevated serum level of PSA had more than a 50% decrease. Eleven of 13 (85%) with bone pain had partial or complete resolution of this symptom; the PSA level and bone scan improved in six and two of these subjects, respectively.[36]

In a phase II trial in hormone-refractory prostate cancer, patients received mitoxantrone, prednisone, and tesmilifene, with mitoxantrone delivered during the last 20 min. Sixty-eight percent had both improved pain and reduced analgesia, 50% PSA reduction was seen in 13 patients (50%) and 75% PSA reduction in 11 patients (42%). Toxicity was the same as for mitoxantrone alone, except for three cases of transient hallucinations. Median survival was 18 months, and 38% survived more than 2 years[37]

CALCITRIOL

DN-101 contains high amounts of calcitriol (1,25 dihydroxycholecalciferol) a naturally occurring hormone and the biologically active form of vitamin D. In high doses, calcitriol is synergistic with many commonly used chemotherapeutic agents, producing antitumor activity as measured in laboratory and animal models. Until recently, the clinical use of calcitriol as an anticancer therapy has been limited by elevations in serum calcium (hypercalcemia) at doses thought to be required for antitumor activity. Available technology has overcome this problem and enables high-dose administration of calcitriol. Although the key physiologic function of calcitriol is maintenance of calcium homeostasis, it has potent growth inhibitory (antiproliferative) activities in multiple cancer cell lines and animal models of cancer (e.g., prostate, breast, colon, head and neck, lymphoma, and myeloma). Preclinical data indicate that transient high plasma levels are sufficient to effect antitumor activity in animals. Additionally, calcitriol is synergistic with many commonly used chemotherapeutic agents, such as taxanes, platinums, dexamethasone, mitoxantrone, and doxorubicin. While the exact mechanism for this synergy is not known, calcitriol has been shown in preclinical models to improve or restore the apoptosis pathway and cause cell cycle arrest during cell division. The pretreatment of a tumor with calcitriol and subsequent administration of a cytotoxin is hypothesized to significantly increase the proportion of cell kill via these mechanisms. In a phase II study, 22 prostate cancer patients, who had a recurrence as evidenced by a rising PSA level despite definitive local

therapy and who had not yet received hormonal therapy for recurrent disease, were treated with commercially available calcitriol on a high-dose pulse administration schedule. Patients received calcitriol until a four-fold increase in PSA or other evidence of disease progression was obtained. After a median treatment duration of 10 months, this therapy appeared to be well tolerated. No hypercalcemia or kidney stones were seen. Mild elevations in liver blood tests and mild anemia were the most common toxicities seen, and no severe toxicities related to the drug were reported. In an open-label phase II study of androgen-independent prostate cancer patients, the combination of weekly high doses of commercially available calcitriol and docetaxel (Taxotere) appeared active as measured by declines in PSA levels and tumor shrinkage. Of the 37 patients who received the combination treatment, 81% had a confirmed PSA reduction of 50% or more as compared to 36%–45% of patients in comparable previous studies of docetaxel alone. The PSA responses in this study persisted for a longer period of time (11.4 months) compared with patients who received docetaxel alone in other studies (5 months). Toxicity in this study was similar to toxicity seen in patients in other studies who received docetaxel alone. The most common severe toxicities in this study were lowering of the white blood cell counts and elevations in blood glucose.[38–41]

ABARELIX

Two clinical studies were conducted to evaluate the clinical efficacy of abarelix in hormone-refractory prostate cancer patients and to measure its effect on serum FSH levels. For the two studies, patients were identified as nonresponsive to hormonal therapy based on either disease progression during LHRH agonist therapy or progression after orchiectomy. The objective of the first study (n = 16)[42] was to determine the efficacy of abarelix in patients with androgen-independent prostate cancer progressing after orchiectomy and to measure its effect on serum FSH. Although none of the patients met the criteria for PSA response (50% reduction confirmed 4 weeks later), five patients experienced confirmed reductions in the PSA level ranging from 9.3% to 31.8% and six patients remained stable without PSA progression or other signs of disease progression. All patients had a decline in their FSH concentration. The mean FSH concentration declined from 45.1 IU/L to 5.3 IU/L after 4 weeks and to 5.6 IU/L after 8 weeks. The FSH concentration remained suppressed after 20 weeks (mean 3.6 IU/L).

The second study[43] elaborated on the clinical efficacy of abarelix in patients (n = 20) with androgen-independent prostate cancer and measured its effect on serum FSH and testosterone. No patients met the criteria for PSA response (50% reduction confirmed 4 weeks later), although two patients remained stable without PSA progression or other signs of disease progression. Median time to progression was 8 weeks. Mean serum FSH decreased by more than 50% from a baseline of 5.7 IU/L and remained suppressed throughout the observation period. Mean serum testosterone did not change after 4 and 8 weeks of therapy and remained in the anorchid range.

Since preclinical data[44] suggests that FSH may be an independent growth factor for hormone-refractory prostate cancers, it follows that potent suppressors of FSH may prove to be effective therapies for androgen-independent prostate cancers. Published clinical data demonstrates that LHRH agonist therapy results in only partial suppression of FSH levels in prostate cancer patients, while abarelix, a GnRH antagonist, has been shown to promptly and substantially reduce FSH to levels lower than LHRH agonists.[45]

ATRASENTAN

Atrasentan belongs to a class of oral drugs that block the activity of endothelin, a protein normally produced in the body that can stimulate the growth and spread of cancer cells. Both endothelin and its receptor are found in various cancers including prostate, non-small cell lung, colorectal, breast, and renal. There are two endothelin receptors, ETA and ETB. The ETA receptor, selectively targeted by atrasentan, appears to be important in prostate cancer progression.

Atrasentan was studied in two randomized, controlled phase II trials with a total population of 1097 hormone refractory prostate cancer patients. Patients were randomized to atrasentan or to placebo. Analyzed separately, the two studies demonstrated a trend toward delayed time to progression, but the difference was not statistically significant. The smaller of the two trials involved 288 patients. An analysis limited to 244 evaluable patients showed that the 10 mg dose of altrasentan significantly prolonged time to progression compared with placebo.[46]

Analysis of data from the phase III trials of hormone-refractory patients showed that atrasentan demonstrated statistically significant improvements in mean change of PSA levels versus placebo (175 ng/mL versus 257 ng/mL; $P = 0.045$); development of bone pain as an adverse event (24% versus 34%; $P = 0.003$); and improvements in mean change of biochemical markers of skeletal progression, although there was not a statistically significant improvement in time to disease progression.[47]

EMERGING ADVERSE EVENTS ASSOCIATED WITH HORMONAL THERAPY

Complications of ADT include those that primarily affect the patient's quality of life, such as hot flashes,

fatigue, weight gain, dry eyes, mood swings, muscle weakness, balance problems, insomnia, decreased libido, and impotence, as well as those that are associated with significant morbidity such as decrease in bone mineral density, cognitive dysfunction, and changes in lipid profiles.[105] Some side effects are associated with patient morbidity and mortality, such as anemia, blood glucose changes, liver enzyme changes, rare but potentially fatal hepatoxicity, and cardiac failure.[106,107] Box 93.2 outlines some recently reported adverse events associated with hormonal therapies, which are elaborated on briefly here.

BONE MINERAL DENSITY LOSS

Several reports have indicated a decrease in bone mineral density (BMD) in patients undergoing androgen deprivation therapy.[108,109] Since duration of treatment may lead to progressive bone loss,[110] it is prudent to investigate bone mineral density and the prediction of bone loss in patients undergoing continuing hormonal therapy.

There have been several recent studies that elucidate the nature of biochemical markers that are precursors of bone mineral loss. Biochemical markers represent the enzymes and skeletal component released into the circulating blood during bone formation or resorption. One study[1] elucidated the increase in biochemical markers during ADT as a reflection of the increase in the bone turnover rate and decrease in BMD. In 60 men with prostate cancer (19 men received LHRH agonist therapy and 41 did not) and 197 healthy controls of similar age, BMD, biochemical markers of bone turnover, and body composition were assessed. Bone mass density was assessed by dual energy X-ray absorptiometry and ultrasound. Biochemical markers of bone turnover included markers of bone resorption (urinary N-telopeptide) and bone formation markers (bone-specific alkaline phosphatase and osteocalcin). Body composition (total body fat and lean body mass) was assessed by dual energy X-ray absorptiometry. Significantly lower BMD was found at the lateral spine, total hip, and forearm in men receiving LHRH agonist therapy compared with those with prostate cancer who did not. Significant differences were also seen at the total body, finger, and calcaneus. The BMD

Box 93.2 Novel adverse events associated with hormonal therapies

- Decrease in bone mineral density / osteoporosis[1,2,108,109,126]
- Elongation of QT interval[5,114]
- Anemia[116,127]
- Cognitive dysfunction[120,121,128]
- Interstitial pneumonitis[123,124,129]

values in eugonadal men with prostate cancer and healthy controls were similar.

Markers of bone resorption (urinary N-telopeptide) and bone formation (bone-specific alkaline phosphatase) were elevated in men receiving LHRH agonist therapy compared with those in eugonadal men with prostate cancer. Men receiving LHRH agonist therapy also had a higher percent total body fat ($29 \pm 5\%$ versus $25 \pm 5\%$; $P < 0.01$) and lower percent lean body weight ($71 \pm 5\%$ versus $75 \pm 5\%$; $P < 0.01$) compared with eugonadal men with prostate cancer. The study concluded that men with prostate cancer receiving ADT have a significant decrease in bone mass and increase in bone turnover, thus placing them at increased risk of fracture.

Another study[2] used carboxy-terminal pro-peptide of human type I procollagen (PIPC) and pyridinoline cross-linked carboxy-terminal telopeptide of type I collagen (ICTP) as serum biochemical markers of bone metabolism; the former is released into the blood serving as a marker of the formation of type I collagen, a marker of bone formation, and the latter is released into the blood during degradation of type I collagen and thus serves as a marker of bone resorption. These specific markers were measured in 27 consecutive patients with prostate cancer without bone metastasis. The results showed that after 2 years of treatment, there was a statistically significant lowering of BMD from values measured immediately before the start of treatment. Immediately after start of treatment, ICTP began to increase and was significantly greater after 6 months of treatment. Immediately after the start of treatment, PICP showed a rise and after 6 months it was greater than before treatment, although this was not a statistically significant difference. Because a lowering of BMD was accompanied by changes in the markers of bone metabolism, the decrease in BMD can be attributed to the effects of hormonal therapy rather than being aging-related. Because PICP began to increase slightly later than ICTP increased, this suggests that LHRH agonists stimulate bone formation to compensate for lower bone mass and indicates a coupling between bone resorption and formation. Consequently, PICP and ICTP values might be predictors of bone loss in patients undergoing ADT.

Bisphosponates, particularly zoledronic acid, have been shown to increase bone mass in men undergoing ADT and is now an additional option that can provide benefits to patients with prostate cancer throughout the course of their disease. Zoledronic acid is the only bisphosphonate that has demonstrated efficacy in reducing objectively measurable skeletal complications in patients with bone metastases secondary to prostate cancer and appears to have potent activities against osteoclasts, which affect bone integrity.[3,4,111] Recently, however, spontaneous reports of osteonecrosis of the jaw, occurring mainly in cancer patients, has caused the manufacturer of zoledronic acid to revise its product labeling to include mention of this adverse reaction.

QT INTERVAL PROLONGATION

Since the mid-1990s, the single most common cause of the withdrawal or restriction of the use of drugs that have already been marketed has been the prolongation of the electrocardiographic QT interval associated with polymorphic ventricular tachycardia, or torsade de pointes, which can be fatal.[112,113] An association between hormonal therapy for prostate cancer and QT prolongation was demonstrated in three studies involving a total of 376 patients receiving initial hormonal treatment for prostate cancer.[5,114] In a trial comparing abarelix with goserelin plus bicalutamide,[115] QT intervals were evaluated prospectively at baseline and on days 84 and 336. In trials comparing abarelix to leuprolide monotherapy[102] and abarelix to leuprolide plus bicalutamide,[104] QT intervals were evaluated retrospectively at baseline and on day 169. The mean QT interval increased in all treatment groups, but the magnitude of the increase differed among the various hormonal therapies. With goserelin plus bicalutamide, baseline QT interval averaged 402 ms and increased by an average of 18 ms, which was significantly greater than the 13 ms increase from the 407 ms baseline mean in the abarelix group ($P = 0.018$). Baseline QT interval averaged 413 ms in patients treated with leuprolide monotherapy and increased by 21 ms. Patients treated with leuprolide plus bicalutamide had a mean baseline QT interval of 417 ms which increased by 9 ms. No patient developed torsades de pointes or ventricular tachycardia during the studies.

ANEMIA

The incidence and severity of anemia in patients on complete androgen blockade (CAB) was examined in a study of 142 patients receiving CAB.[116] Up to 90% of patients experienced at least a 10% decline in hemoglobin levels and in 13% of patients, hemoglobin declined by 25% or more. The anemia, occurring routinely in men receiving CAB, was characterized as normochromic, normocytic, and temporally-related to the initiation of androgen blockade, usually resolving after CAB is discontinued. This study led to the recommendation that patients receiving CAB undergo hematological testing at baseline, 1 to 2 months after initiating CAB, and periodically thereafter.

COGNITIVE DYSFUNCTION

There is considerable evidence suggesting that gonadal steroid hormones play an important role in the modulation of mood and cognitive function in women and in men. This has been physically observed in subjects taking LHRH agonists with or without estradiol replacement or progesterone replacement who have undergone positron-emission tomography scans during neuropsychological tests.[117] For women suffering from endometriosis, while LHRH agonists reduce the extent of the endometrial lesions and the occurrence of pelvic pain associated with the disease, agonists have been associated with physical and psychiatric side effects. Results of a prospective, double-blind placebo-controlled study and an open label trial indicate that depressive mood symptoms increase in women treated with LHRH agonist therapy for endometriosis.[118] There are case reports in the literature of women of reproductive age with no prior psychiatric history who were treated with a LHRH agonist for endometriosis. These women developed symptoms consistent with various psychiatric disorders, including panic disorder and major depression with and without psychotic features.[119]

Androgen suppression monotherapy for prostate cancer was found to be potentially associated with impaired memory, attention, and executive functions. Eighty-two men with extraprostatic prostate cancer were randomly assigned to receive either continuous leuprorelin, goserelin (both LHRH analogs), cyproterone acetate (a steroidal antiandrogen), or close clinical monitoring. These patients underwent cognitive assessments at baseline and before starting treatment, and then 6 months later. Compared with the baseline assessments, men receiving androgen suppression monotherapy performed worse in two of 12 tests of attention and memory; 24 of 50 men randomized to active treatment and assessed 6 months later had a clinically significant decline in one or more cognitive tests but not one patient randomized to close monitoring showed a decline in any test performance.[120,121]

INTERSTITIAL PNEUMONITIS

Pulmonary toxicities have been linked to treatment with antiandrogens, especially nilutamide, as is reflected in a black-box warning on its FDA-approved labeling. Interstitial pneumonitis has been reported in 2% of patients in controlled clinical trials in patients exposed to nilutamide. A small study in Japanese subjects showed that 8 of 47 patients (17%) developed interstitial pneumonitis. Reports of interstitial changes including pulmonary fibrosis that led to hospitalization and death have been reported rarely post-marketing. Symptoms included exertional dyspnea, cough, chest pain, and fever.[122] A class effect has been suggested, after a review of 3-years worth of records in the US FDA's adverse event reporting database.[123] All cases of pneumonitis associated with bicalutamide, flutamide, and nilutamide that were reported between 1998 and 2000 were reviewed. Pneumonitis occurred in 12 patients receiving bicalutamide, 16 patients receiving

flutamide, and 50 patients receiving nilutamide at a median of 7.5, 5, and 8 weeks of treatment. Deaths were reported from pulmonary toxicities in all three therapies. A note of caution, however, that incidence rates should not be calculated from spontaneously reported data because of extensive underreporting; fewer than 10% of serious reactions are reported to the FDA.[124]

IMMEDIATE ONSET SYSTEMIC ALLERGIC REACTIONS

The use of abarelix is accompanied by a black box warning indicating that immediate-onset systemic allergic reactions (occurring within 30 minutes of dosing), were observed in 1.1% of patients (15 of 1397) dosed with abarelix in clinical trials. Fourteen of these developed symptoms within 8 minutes of injection. Seven of the 15 experienced transient hypotension or syncope, representing 0.5% of all patients. The incidence was higher in patients with advanced symptomatic prostate cancer. The product label[125] further states that patients should be observed for at least 30 minutes after each injection of abarelix and that supportive measures such as leg elevation, oxygen, i.v. fluids, antihistamines, corticosteroids, and epinephrine (alone or in combination) should be employed if an allergic reaction occurs. Prescribing of abarelix will require adherence to a risk management plan that includes both a signed physician and patient attestation confirming that the risks and benefits of using abarelix are understood.

SUMMARY

This chapter has reviewed new hormonal therapies with their different mechanisms of action. As these therapies emerge, the following unanswered questions remain, which should be the subject of future research:

- What should be the role of neoadjuvant hormonal therapy?
  1. Which patients?
  2. Which therapies?
  3. How long should they be used?
- What should be the role of adjuvant hormonal therapy?
  1. Which patients?
  2. For which pathologic characteristics?
  3. What stages?
  4. How long should they be used?
- What is the role of hormonal therapy in patients with pathologically advanced features?
- How can we improve our understanding of the resistance to existing hormonal therapies in the hormone-refractory patient?

- Should hormonal therapy be used alone or in combination with chemotherapy?
- Can we induce second- or third-line response with novel therapies?
- What constitutes the optimal management for newly emerging adverse events associated with hormonal therapies?

DISCLOSURE

Dr Garnick is an officer of Praecis Pharmaceuticals Incorporated, from which he derives a salary and is a shareholder. Dr Motta is an employee of Praecis, from which she derives a salary and is a shareholder. Praecis markets Plenaxis® (abarelix for injectable suspension) for prostate cancer, which is mentioned in this chapter.

REFERENCES

1. Stoch SA, Parker RA, Chen L, et al. Bone loss in men with prostate cancer treated with gonadotropin-releasing hormone agonists. J Clin Endocrinol Metab 2001;86:2787–2791.

2. Miyaji Y, Saika T, Yamamoto Y, et al. Effects of gonadotropin-releasing hormone agonists on bone metabolism markers and bone mineral density in patients with prostate cancer. Urology 2004;64:128–131.

3. Smith MR, Eastham J, Gleason DM, et al. Randomized controlled trial of zoledronic acid to prevent bone loss in men receiving androgen deprivation therapy for nonmetastatic prostate cancer. J Urol 2003;169:2008–2012.

4. Saad F, Schulman CC. Role of bisphosphonates in prostate cancer. Eur Urol 2004;45:26–34.

5. Garnick MB, Pratt C, Campion M, et al. Increase in the electrocardiographic QTc interval in med with prostate cancer undergoing androgen deprivation therapy: results of three randomized controlled clinical studies [abstract]. European Association of Urology 19th Congress, Vienna, Austria March 24-27, 2004. 3-24-2004.

6. Huggins C, Hodges CV. Studies on prostate cancer I. The effect of castration, of estrogen and of androgen injection on serum phosphatases in metastatic carcinoma of the prostate. Cancer Res 1941;1:293–297.

7. Huggins C, Stevens RE, Jr., Hodges CV. Studies on prostatic cancer. II. The effects of castration on advanced carcinoma of the prostate gland. Arch Surg 1941;43:209–223.

8. Huggins C, Scott WW, Hodges CV. Studies on prostatic cancer. III. The effects of fever, of desoxycorticosterone and of estrogen on clinical patients with metastatic carcinoma. J Urol 1941;46:997–1006.

9. Fowler JE Jr, Whitmore WF Jr. The response of metastatic adenocarcinoma of the prostate to exogenous testosterone. J Urol 1981;126:372–375.

10. Bailar JC III, Byar DP. Estrogen treatment for cancer of the prostate. Early results with 3 doses of diethylstilbestrol and placebo. Cancer 1970;26:257–261.

11. Byar DP. Proceedings: The Veterans Administration Cooperative Urological Research Group's studies of cancer of the prostate. Cancer 1973;32:1126–1130.

12. Veterans Administration Cooperative Urological Research Group. Treatment and survival of patients with cancer of the prostate. The Veterans Administration Co-operative Urological Research Group. Surg Gynecol Obstet 1967;124:1011–1017.

13. Bolla M, Collette L, Blank L, et al. Long-term results with immediate androgen suppression and external irradiation in patients with locally advanced prostate cancer (an EORTC study): a phase III randomised trial. Lancet 2002;360:103–106.

14. Messing EM, Manola J, Sarosdy M, et al. Immediate hormonal therapy compared with observation after radical prostatectomy and pelvic lymphadenectomy in men with node-positive prostate cancer. N Engl J Med 1999;341:1781–1788.

15. Messing EM, Manola J, Yao J, et al. Immediate vs delayed hormonal therapy (HT) in patients with nodal positive (N+) prostate cancer who had undergone radical prostatectomy (RP) + pelvic lymphadenectomy (LND): results of central pathology review (CPR);[abstract #1455]. Annual Meeting of the American Urological Association, San Francisco, CA. 5-11-2004.

16. D'Amico AV, Manola J, Loffredo M, et al. 6-month androgen suppression plus radiation therapy vs radiation therapy alone for patients with clinically localized prostate cancer: a randomized controlled trial. JAMA 2004;292:821–827.

17. Zincke H, Lau W, Bergstralh E, et al. Role of early adjuvant hormonal therapy after radical prostatectomy for prostate cancer. J Urol 2001;166:2208–2215.

18. Crook J, Ludgate C, Malone S, et al. Report of a multicenter Canadian phase III randomized trial of 3 months vs. 8 months neoadjuvant androgen deprivation before standard-dose radiotherapy for clinically localized prostate cancer. Int J Radiat Oncol Biol Phys 2004;60:15–23.

19. Gleave ME, Goldenberg SL, Chin JL, et al. Randomized comparative study of 3 versus 8-month neoadjuvant hormonal therapy before radical prostatectomy: biochemical and pathological effects. J Urol 2001;166:500–506.

20. Chodak G, Sharifi R, Kasimis B, et al. Single-agent therapy with bicalutamide: a comparison with medical or surgical castration in the treatment of advanced prostate carcinoma. Urology 1995;46:849–855.

21. Kolvenbag GJ, Iversen P, Newling DW. Antiandrogen monotherapy: a new form of treatment for patients with prostate cancer. Urology 2001;58:16–23.

22. Iversen P. Bicalutamide monotherapy for early stage prostate cancer: an update. J Urol 2003;170:S48–S52.

23. Iversen P, Tyrrell CJ, Kaisary AV, et al. Bicalutamide monotherapy compared with castration in patients with nonmetastatic locally advanced prostate cancer: 6.3 years of followup. J Urol 2000;164:1579–1582.

24. Duff G. Casodex 150 mg (Bicalutamide): no longer indicated for treatment of localised prostate cancer; Broadcast to Directors of Public Health of PCTs. London, UK: Dept of Public Health, Committee on Safety of Medicines. Posted at http://www.info.doh.gov.uk/doh/embroadcast.nsf/. Ref CEM/CMO/2003/15. 10-28-2003.

25. Health Canada MHPD. Accelerated deaths in localized prostate cancer patients: Health Canada has withdrawn its approval for Casodex 150 mg for early (localized) prostate cancer. Ottawa, Canada: Health Canada. Available at http://www.hc-sc.gc.ca/hpfb-dgpsa/tpd-dpt/casodex_prof_e.html. 8-26-2003.

26. Weckermann D, Harzmann R. Hormone Therapy in Prostate Cancer: LHRH Antagonists versus LHRH Analogues. Eur Urol 2004;46:279–284.

27. Koch M, Steidle C, Brosman S, et al. An open-label study of abarelix in men with symptomatic prostate cancer at risk of treatment with LHRH agonists. Urology 2003;62:877–882.

28. Barrie SE, Potter GA, et al. Pharmacology of novel steroidal inhibitors of cytochrome P450(17 alpha) (17 alpha-hydroxylase/C17-20 lyase). J Steroid Biochem Mol Biol 1994;50:267–273.

29. O'Donnell A, Judson I, Dowsett M, et al. Hormonal impact of the 17alpha-hydroxylase/C(17,20) lyase inhibitor abiraterone acetate (CB7630) in patients with prostate cancer. Br J Cancer 2004;90:2317–2325.

30. Kelly GE, Husband AJ. Flavonoid compounds in the prevention and treatment of prostate cancer. Methods Mol Med 2003;81:377–394.

31. Constantinou AI, Mehta R, Husband A. Phenoxodiol, a novel isoflavone derivative, inhibits dimethylbenz[a]anthracene (DMBA)-induced mammary carcinogenesis in female Sprague-Dawley rats. Eur J Cancer 2003;39:1012–1018.

32. Constantinou AI, Husband A. Phenoxodiol (2H-1-benzopyran-7-0,1,3-(4-hydroxyphenyl)), a novel isoflavone derivative, inhibits DNA topoisomerase II by stabilizing the cleavable complex. Anticancer Res 2002;22:2581–2585.

33. Kelly G, Edwards M. Interim results of a phase Ib/IIa study of oral phenoxodiol in patients with late-stage, hormone-refractory prostate

cancer. 95th Annual Meeting of the American Association for Cancer Research: Late Breaker Abstracts 2004;103–104.

34. Brandes LJ, Bracken SP. The intracellular histamine antagonist, N,N-diethyl-2-[4-(phenylmethyl)phenoxy] ethamine.HCL, may potentiate doxorubicin in the treatment of metastatic breast cancer: Results of a pilot study. Breast Cancer Res Treat 1998;49:61–68.

35. Brandes LJ, LaBella FS, Warrington RC. Increased therapeutic index of antineoplastic drugs in combination with intracellular histamine antagonists. J Natl Cancer Inst 1991;83:1329–1336.

36. Brandes LJ, Bracken SP, Ramsey EW. N,N-diethyl-2-[4-(phenylmethyl)phenoxy]ethanamine in combination with cyclophosphamide: an active, low-toxicity regimen for metastatic hormonally unresponsive prostate cancer. J Clin Oncol 1995;13:1398–1403.

37. Raghavan D, Brandes KK, Snyder T, et al. Mitoxantrone plus DPPE in hormone-refractory prostate cancer (HR-CAP) with symptomatic metastases—response in 70% of cases: abstract # 786. American Society of Clinical Oncology, Annual Meeting. 2002.

38. Beer TM, Javle M, Henner W, et al. Pharmcokinetics (PK) and tolerability of DN-101, a new formulation of calcitriol, in patients with cancer [abstract]. American Association for Cancer Research Annual Meeting, Orlando, FL . 3-27-2004.

39. Beer TM. Development of weekly high-dose calcitriol based therapy for prostate cancer. Urol Oncol 2003;21:399–405.

40. Beer TM, Myrthue A. Calcitriol in cancer treatment: from the lab to the clinic. Mol Cancer Ther 2004;3:373–381.

41. Beer TM, Eilers KM, Garzotto M, et al. Quality of life and pain relief during treatment with calcitriol and docetaxel in symptomatic metastatic androgen-independent prostate carcinoma. Cancer 2004;100:758–763.

42. Beer TM, Garzotto M, Eilers KM, et al. Targeting FSH in androgen-independent prostate cancer: abarelix for prostate cancer progressing after orchiectomy. Urology 2004;63:342–347.

43. Beer TM, Garzotto M, Eilers KM, et al. Phase II study of abarelix depot for androgen independent prostate cancer progression during gonadotropin-releasing hormone agonist therapy. J Urol 2003;169:1738–1741.

44. Ben Josef E, Yang SY, Ji TH, et al. Hormone-refractory prostate cancer cells express functional follicle-stimulating hormone receptor (FSHR). J Urol 1999;161:970–976.

45. Garnick MB, Campion M. Abarelix Depot, a GnRH antagonist, v LHRH superagonists in prostate cancer: differential effects on follicle-stimulating hormone. Abarelix Depot study group. Mol Urol 2000;4:275–277.

46. Carducci MA, Padley RJ, Breul J, et al. Effect of endothelin-A receptor blockade with atrasentan on tumor progression in men with hormone-refractory prostate cancer: a randomized, phase II, placebo-controlled trial. J Clin Oncol 2003;21:679–689.

47. Carducci MA, Nelson JB, et al. Effects of altrasentan on disease progression and biological markers in men with metastatic hormone-refractory prostate cancer: phase 3 study;[abstract]. American Society of Clinical Oncology, 40th Annual Meeting, June 2004;4508.

48. Immediate versus deferred treatment for advanced prostatic cancer: initial results of the Medical Research Council Trial. The Medical Research Council Prostate Cancer Working Party Investigators Group. Br J Urol 1997;79:235–246.

49. Soloway MS, Pareek K, Sharifi R, et al. Neoadjuvant androgen ablation before radical prostatectomy in cT2bNxMo prostate cancer: 5-year results. J Urol 2002;167:112–116.

50. Schulman CC, Debruyne FM, Forster G, et al. 4-Year follow-up results of a European prospective randomized study on neoadjuvant hormonal therapy prior to radical prostatectomy in T2-3N0M0 prostate cancer. European Study Group on Neoadjuvant Treatment of Prostate Cancer. Eur Urol 2000;38:706–713.

51. Gleave ME, La Bianca SE, Goldenberg SL, et al. Long-term neoadjuvant hormone therapy prior to radical prostatectomy: evaluation of risk for biochemical recurrence at 5-year follow-up. Urology 2000;56:289–294.

52. Wirth M, Frohmuller H, Marz F, et al. Randomized multicenter trial on adjuvant flutamide therapy in locally advanced prostate cancer after radical surgery: Interim analysis of treatment effect and prognostic factors. Br J Urol 1997;80:263 [abstract].

53. See WA, McLeod D, Iversen P, et al. The bicalutamide Early Prostate Cancer Program. Demography. 2001;6:43–47.

54. Ditonno P, Battaglia M, Selvaggi FP. Adjuvant hormone therapy after radical prostatectomy: indications and results. Tumori 1997;83:567–575.

55. Roach M, III. Hormonal therapy and radiotherapy for localized prostate cancer: who, where and how long? J Urol 2003;170:S35–S40.

56. Pilepich MV, Winter K, John MJ, et al. Phase III radiation therapy oncology group (RTOG) trial 86-10 of androgen deprivation adjuvant to definitive radiotherapy in locally advanced carcinoma of the prostate. Int J Radiat Oncol Biol Phys 2001;50:1243–1252.

57. Sato N, Akakura K, Isaka S, et al. Intermittent androgen suppression for locally advanced and metastatic prostate cancer: preliminary report of a prospective multicenter study. Urology 2004;64:341–345.

58. Klotz LH, Herr HW, Morse MJ, et al. Intermittent endocrine therapy for advanced prostate cancer. Cancer 1986;58:2546–2550.

59. Sato N, Gleave ME, Bruchovsky N, et al. Intermittent androgen suppression delays progression to androgen-independent regulation of prostate-specific antigen gene in the LNCaP prostate tumour model. J Steroid Biochem Mol Biol 1996;58:139–146.

60. Wolf J, Tunn U. Intermittent androgen blockade in prostate cancer: rationale and clinical experience. Eur Urol 2000;38:365–371.

61. Bruchovsky N, Klotz LH, Sadar M, et al. Intermittent androgen suppression for prostate cancer: Canadian Prospective Trial and related observations. Mol Urol 2000;4:191–199.

62. Grossfeld GD, Small EJ, Carroll PR. Intermittent androgen deprivation for clinically localized prostate cancer: initial experience. Urology 1998;51:137–144.

63. Bales GT, Sinner MD, Kim.J.H., et al. Impact of intermittent androgen deprivation on quality of life. J Urol 2004;155:1069.

64. Lawton CA, Winter K, Murray K, et al. Updated results of the phase III Radiation Therapy Oncology Group (RTOG) trial 85-31 evaluating the potential benefit of androgen suppression following standard radiation therapy for unfavorable prognosis carcinoma of the prostate. Int J Radiat Oncol Biol Phys 2001;49:937–946.

65. Chao D, Harland SJ. The importance of continued endocrine treatment during chemotherapy of hormone-refractory prostate cancer. Eur Urol 1997;31:7–10.

66. D'Amico AV, Schultz D, Loffredo M, et al. Biochemical outcome following external beam radiation therapy with or without androgen suppression therapy for clinically localized prostate cancer. JAMA 2000;284:1280–1283.

67. Boccon-Gibod L, Bertaccini A, Bono AV, et al. Management of locally advanced prostate cancer: a European consensus. Int J Clin Pract 2003;57:187–194.

68. Merrick GS, Butler WM, Galbreath RW, et al. Five-year biochemical outcome following permanent interstitial brachytherapy for clinical T1-T3 prostate cancer. Int J Radiat Oncol Biol Phys 2001;51:41–48.

69. Stone NN, Stock RG, Unger P. Effects of neoadjuvant hormonal therapy on prostate biopsy results after (125)I and (103)Pd seed implantation. Mol Urol 2000;4:163–168.

70. Potters L, Torre T, Ashley R, et al. Examining the role of neoadjuvant androgen deprivation in patients undergoing prostate brachytherapy. J Clin Oncol 2000;18:1187–1192.

71. Fleshner NE, Trachtenberg J. Combination finasteride and flutamide in advanced carcinoma of the prostate: effective therapy with minimal side effects. J Urol 1995;154:1642–1645.

72. Ornstein DK, Rao GS, Johnson B, et al. Combined finasteride and flutamide therapy in men with advanced prostate cancer. Urology 1996;48:901–905.

73. Kirby R, Robertson C, Turkes A, et al. Finasteride in association with either flutamide or goserelin as combination hormonal therapy in patients with stage M1 carcinoma of the prostate gland. International Prostate Health Council (IPHC) Trial Study Group. Prostate 1999;40:105–114.

74. Brufsky A, Fontaine-Rothe P, Berlane K, et al. Finasteride and flutamide as potency-sparing androgen-ablative therapy for advanced adenocarcinoma of the prostate. Urology 1997;49:913–920.

75. Ornstein DK, Smith DS, Andriole GL. Biochemical response to testicular androgen ablation among patients with prostate cancer for whom flutamide and/or finasteride therapy failed. Urology 1998;52:1094–1097.

76. Dupont A, Labrie F, Giguere M, et al. Combination therapy with flutamide and [D-Trp6]LHRH ethylamide for stage C prostatic carcinoma. Eur J Cancer Clin Oncol 1988;24:659–666.

77. Labrie F. Androgen blockade in prostate cancer in 2002: major benefits on survival in localized disease. Mol Cell Endocrinol 2002;198:77–87.

78. Adis International Inc. Adis Clinical Trials Insight: DIALOG File 173; Database search. Langhorne, PA: Adis International Inc, 2004.

79. PJP Publications. Pharmaprojects: DIALOG file 128; Database search. Richmond, Surrey, UK: PJP Publications, 2004.

80. Chen J, Hwang DJ, Bohl CE, et al. A Selective Androgen Receptor Modulator (SARM) for hormonal male contraception. J Pharmacol Exp Ther 2004.

81. Gao W, Kearbey JD, Nair VA, et al. Comparison of the pharmacological effects of a novel selective androgen receptor modulator (SARM), the 5{alpha}-Reductase inhibitor finasteride, and the antiandrogen hydroxyflutamide in intact rats: New approach for benign prostate hyperplasia (BPH). Endocrinology 2004.

82. Inhale Therapeutic Systems Inc. Inhale announces positive phase I clinical results of inhaleable peptide, leuprolide. Media Release. Available from: URL: http://www.inhale.com 2001.

83. Laufer M, Thortone D, et al. Phase I study of escalating doses of the dual-action 5-alpha reductase inhibitor LY320236 in patients with advanced prostate cancer: preliminary clinical and hormonal results. Proceedings of 36th Annual Meeting of the American Society of Clinical Oncology 2000;19:369.

84. Periti P, Mazzei T, Mini E. Clinical pharmacokinetics of depot leuprorelin. Clin Pharmacokinet 2002;41:485–504.

85. Balchen T, Agerso H, et al. Single subcutaneous administration of a novel, fast-acting gonadotropin-releasing hormone antagonist degarelix (FE200486) with depot characteristics in healthy men. Clinical and Experimental Pharmacology and Physiology 2004;31 (Suppl.1):126.

86. Weston P, Hammonds J, Vaughton K, et al. Degarelix: a novel GnRH antagonist tested in a multicenter, randomized, dose-finding study in prostate cancer patients: [podium presentation, no. PD-4.03]. Congress of the Societe Internationale d'Urologie, 27th, Hawaii, October 5 2004.

87. Lorenzo A. Spectrum deals for rights to clinical-stage LHRH antagonist. Bioworld Today 2004;15:156.

88. Erb K, Pechstein B, Schueler A, et al. Pituitary and gonadal endocrine effects and pharmacokinetics of the novel luteinizing hormone-releasing hormone antagonist teverelix in healthy men—a first-dose-in-humans study. Clin Pharmacol Ther 2000;67:660–669.

89. Jungwirth A, Pinski J, Galvan G, et al. Inhibition of growth of androgen-independent DU-145 prostate cancer in vivo by luteinising hormone-releasing hormone antagonist Cetrorelix and bombesin antagonists RC-3940-II and RC-3950-II. Eur J Cancer 1997;33:1141–1148.

90. Kaisary AV, Bowsher WG, Gillatt DA, et al. Pharmacodynamics of a long acting depot preparation of avorelin in patients with prostate cancer. Avorelin Study Group. J Urol 1999;162:2019–2023.

91. Mieda M, Ohta Y, Saito T, et al. Antiandrogenic activity and endocrinological profile of a novel antiandrogen, TZP-4238, in the rat. Endocr J 1994;41:445–452.

92. Shukeir N, Arakelian A, Chen G, et al. A synthetic 15-mer peptide (PCK3145) derived from prostate secretory protein can reduce tumor growth, experimental skeletal metastases, and malignancy-associated hypercalcemia. Cancer Res 2004;64:5370–5377.

93. Shukeir N, Arakelian A, et al. Prostate secretory protein PSP-94 decreases tumor growth and hypercalcemia of malignancy in a syngenic in vivo model of prostate cancer. Cancer Res 2003;63:2072–2078.

94. Brandes LJ, Hogg GR. Study of the in-vivo antioestrogenic action of N,N-diethyl-2-[4-(phenylmethyl)phenoxy]ethanamine HCl (DPPE), a novel intracellular histamine antagonist and antioestrogen binding site ligand. J Reprod Fertil 1990;89:59–67.

95. Stein S, Zoltick B, Peacock T, et al. Phase II trial of toremifene in androgen-independent prostate cancer: a Penn cancer clinical trials group trial. Am J Clin Oncol 2001;24:283–285.

96. Steiner MS, Pound CR. Phase IIA clinical trial to test the efficacy and safety of Toremifene in men with high-grade prostatic intraepithelial neoplasia. Clin Prostate Cancer 2003;2:24–31.

97. Gonzalez-Barcena D, Schally AV, Vadillo-Buenfil M, et al. Response of patients with advanced prostatic cancer to administration of somatostatin analog RC-160 (vapreotide) at the time of relapse. Prostate 2003;56:183–191.

98. Pinski J, Schally AV, Halmos G, et al. Effect of somatostatin analog RC-160 and bombesin/gastrin releasing peptide antagonist RC-3095 on growth of PC-3 human prostate-cancer xenografts in nude mice. Int J Cancer 1993;55:963–967.

99. Pollak MN, Schally AV. Mechanisms of antineoplastic action of somatostatin analogs. Proc Soc Exp Biol Med 1998;217:143–152.

100. Chertin B, Spitz IM, Lindenberg T, et al. An implant releasing the gonadotropin hormone-releasing hormone agonist histrelin maintains medical castration for up to 30 months in metastatic prostate cancer. J Urol 2000;163:838–844.

101. Schlegel PN, Kuzma P, Frick J, et al. Effective long-term androgen suppression in men with prostate cancer using a hydrogel implant with the GnRH agonist histrelin. Urology 2001;58:578–582.

102. McLeod D, Zinner N, Tomera K, et al. A phase 3, multicenter, open-label, randomized study of abarelix versus leuprolide acetate in men with prostate cancer. Urology 2001;58:756–761.

103. Tomera K, Gleason D, Gittelman M, et al. The gonadotropin-releasing hormone antagonist abarelix depot versus luteinizing hormone releasing hormone agonists leuprolide or goserelin: initial results of endocrinological and biochemical efficacies in patients with prostate cancer. J Urol 2001;165:1585–1589.

104. Trachtenberg J, Gittleman M, Steidle C, et al. A phase 3, multicenter, open label, randomized study of abarelix versus leuprolide plus daily antiandrogen in men with prostate cancer. J Urol 2002;167:1670–1674.

105. Holzbeierlein JM, Castle E, Thrasher JB. Complications of androgen deprivation therapy: prevention and treatment. Oncology (Huntingt) 2004;18:303–309.

106. Hellerstedt BA, Pienta KJ. The current state of hormonal therapy for prostate cancer. CA Cancer J Clin 2002;52:154–179.

107. DIALOG. Diogenes Adverse Reaction Database. 2002.

108. Peters JL, Fairney A, Kyd P, et al. Bone loss associated with the use of LHRH agonists in prostate cancer. Prostate Cancer Prostatic Dis 2001;4:161–166.

109. Stepan JJ, Lachman M, Zverina J, et al. Castrated men exhibit bone loss: effect of calcitonin treatment on biochemical indices of bone remodeling. J Clin Endocrinol Metab 1989;69:523–527.

110. Kiratli BJ, Srinivas S, Perkash I, et al. Progressive decrease in bone density over 10 years of androgen deprivation therapy in patients with prostate cancer. Urology 2001;57:127–132.

111. Smith MR. The role of bisphosphonates in men with prostate cancer receiving androgen deprivation therapy. Oncology (Huntingt) 2004;18:21–25.

112. Lasser KE, Allen PD, Woolhandler SJ, et al. Timing of new black box warnings and withdrawals for prescription medications. JAMA 2002;287:2215–2220.

113. Roden DM. Drug-induced prolongation of the QT interval. N Engl J Med 2004;350:1013–1022.

114. Garnick MB, Pratt C, Campion M, et al. The effect of hormonal therapy for prostate cancer on the electrocardiographic QT interval: Phase 3 results following treatment with leuprolide and goserelin, alone or with bicalutamide, and the GnRH antagonist abarelix. J Clin Oncol 2004;22:4578 [abstract].

115. Debruyne FM. ABACAS 1: a comparison of the efficacy and safety of abarelix versus goserelin plus bicalutamide in patients with advanced or metastatic prostate cancer: a one year randomized open-label multicenter, Phase III trial [abstract]. Presented by P. Teillac at a workshop entitled "Advances in the Biology of Hormonal Therapy in the Treatment of Prostate Cancer". European Association of Urology 18th Congress, Madrid, Spain, 2003.

116. Strum SB, McDermed JE, Scholz MC, et al. Anaemia associated with androgen deprivation in patients with prostate cancer receiving combined hormone blockade. Br J Urol 1997;79:933–941.

117. Berman KF, Schmidt PJ, Rubinow DR, et al. Modulation of cognition-specific cortical activity by gonadal steroids: a positron-emission tomography study in women. Proc Natl Acad Sci USA 1997;94:8836–8841.

118. Warnock JK, Bundren JC, Morris DW. Depressive symptoms associated with gonadotropin-releasing hormone agonists. Depress Anxiety 1998;7:171–177.

119. Warnock JK, Bundren JC. Anxiety and mood disorders associated with gonadotropin-releasing hormone agonist therapy. Psychopharmacol Bull 1997;33:311–316.

120. Green HJ, Pakenham KI, Headley BC, et al. Quality of life compared during pharmacological treatments and clinical monitoring for non-localized prostate cancer: a randomized controlled trial. BJU Int 2004;93:975–979.

121. Green HJ, Pakenham KI, Headley BC, et al. Altered cognitive function in men treated for prostate cancer with luteinizing hormone-releasing hormone analogues and cyproterone acetate: a randomized controlled trial. BJU Int 2002;90:427–432.

122. Aventis Pharmaceuticals. Nilandron (Aventis) Nilutamide Tablets, Prescribing information as of July 2001 in Physician's Desk Reference Electronic Library. Thomson, Micromedex, 2004.

123. Bennett CL, Raisch DW, Sartor O. Pneumonitis associated with nonsteroidal antiandrogens: presumptive evidence of a class effect. Ann Intern Med 2002;137:625.

124. Ahmad SR, Graham DJ. Pneumonitis with antiandrogens. Ann Intern Med 2003;139:528–v529.

125. Praecis Pharmaceuticals Incorporated. Plenaxis [package insert]. Waltham, MA: PRAECIS PHARMACEUTICALS INCORPORATED, 2003.

126. Melton LJ, III, Alothman KI, Khosla S, et al. Fracture risk following bilateral orchiectomy. J Urol 2003;169:1747–1750.

127. Bogdanos J, Karamanolakis D, Milathianakis C, et al. Combined androgen blockade-induced anemia in prostate cancer patients without bone involvement. Anticancer Res 2003;23:1757–1762.

128. Almeida OP, Waterreus A, Spry N, et al. One year follow-up study of the association between chemical castration, sex hormones, beta-amyloid, memory and depression in men. Psychoneuroendocrinology 2004;29:1071–1081.

129. Shioi K, Yoshida M, Sakai N. Interstitial pneumonitis induced by bicalutamide and leuprorelin acetate for prostate cancer. Int J Urol 2003;10:625–626.

The assessment and management of urinary incontinence in patients with prostate cancer

94

Jane Dawoodi, Zach S Dovey, Mark R Feneley

INTRODUCTION

Urinary incontinence is defined by the International Continence Society as the complaint of any involuntary leakage of urine,[1] where patients are unable to hold their own urine and consequently wet themselves. In men with prostate cancer, urinary incontinence may arise from treatment of early stage disease, but it is also common in advanced prostate cancer. The effects of aging, concomitant age-related conditions, and other treatable factors may aggravate loss of urinary control and impair lower urinary tract function. Incontinence causes considerable distress and debility with a major negative effect on quality of life, impacting patients and their families.[2]

The pathophysiology of urinary incontinence is often complex. Assessment demands careful and comprehensive evaluation of a patient's habits, performance status, comorbidity and age-related factors, pharmacotherapy, and previous iatrogenic interventions. As a rule every patient should have a careful history, physical examination, and basic laboratory investigations. Urinary infection and urinary retention must always be excluded or treated. Guided by a patient's presentation, investigations may include urine flow studies, ultrasound imaging, urodynamic testing, and cystoscopy. Once a full assessment has been made, a clear diagnosis can direct appropriate treatment, with close cooperation between urologic nurses and physicians.

Prostate cancer may cause incontinence through a variety of mechanisms. Tumor growth causes bladder outflow obstruction and may directly involve the bladder base, compromising normal detrusor and bladder neck function. Local invasion may compromise the integrity of the urinary sphincters and pelvic neurological pathways, and metastases may give rise to spinal cord and nerve root compression. The treatment of prostate cancer may also cause or contribute to urinary incontinence. Although incontinence is usually treatable, iatrogenic incontinence is sometimes feared more than prostate cancer itself, particularly when an excellent oncologic prognosis following treatment of early-stage disease can be anticipated.

For the purposes of this chapter, urinary incontinence associated with prostate cancer will be discussed first in relation to lower urinary tract pathophysiology (disease-associated incontinence), and then in relation to the effects of potentially curative treatment for localized disease (iatrogenic incontinence). Functional and pathologic conditions primarily affecting systems outside the lower urinary tract may also influence continence, lower urinary tract function, and related measures of quality of life, but their full consideration is beyond the scope of this chapter.

DISEASE-ASSOCIATED INCONTINENCE

Urinary continence is maintained by passive and active mechanisms acting on the bladder outlet and proximal urethra, coordinated with detrusor regulation of filling, storage, and voiding of urine. The pathophysiology of incontinence acquired in association with prostate cancer relates to variable abnormalities in components of the lower urinary tract and their integrated functionality, including sphincteric insufficiency, bladder outflow obstruction, and changes in detrusor function.

Urinary leakage, therefore, indicates underlying changes in lower urinary tract function and its control. Incontinence may occur as a result of urinary overflow with chronic urinary retention in those patients with or without prostate cancer. Leakage may also occur as a result of detrusor overactivity[2] when this overcomes existing continence mechanisms. Prostate cancer may compromise bladder neck and/or external sphincter function by direct invasion of these structures or their innervation. Structural changes in the bladder wall may arise from secondary effects of outflow obstruction, from invasion by prostate cancer itself, or from other intrinsic disease of the bladder including aging. By affecting bladder capacity, compliance, storage, sensation, and contraction, bladder dysfunction may compromise overall lower urinary tract function and continence, particularly where there is coexisting sphincteric dysfunction. The local effects of invasive prostate cancer may, therefore, contribute to many aspects of lower urinary tract dysfunction.

Overflow incontinence arises from chronic urinary retention and progressive deterioration in bladder emptying. Chronic retention may be low-pressure retention with low detrusor contractility, or high-pressure retention with high detrusor contractility. These conditions may develop insidiously, sometimes without the patient's awareness of voiding difficulty. High-pressure retention may present with nocturnal incontinence or impaired renal function, and is then usually associated with voiding symptoms. In patients with overflow incontinence and low-pressure urinary retention, incomplete bladder emptying is associated with detrusor underactivity or an acontractile detrusor, and when intravesical pressure exceeds maximum urethral pressure (such as on body movement), urine leakage occurs. Studies of outflow obstruction in the rat[3] and the pig,[4] confirming a deterioration in detrusor function, have demonstrated increasing residual urine volumes in association with impairment of voiding pressure, and increases in smooth muscle cell number and total detrusor collagen content. It is not clear why detrusor acontractility develops in some patients and detrusor overactivity in others. It is possible that there is an additional variable neurologic element. Parys et al[5] found that 73% of their patients with chronic urinary retention demonstrated a sensory suprasacral abnormality with intact sacral reflex pathways. They proposed this as an adaptive mechanism in higher neurological centers to bladder outflow obstruction that results in low-pressure retention and renal protection.

Urinary incontinence may occur in association with detrusor overactivity. In men with prostate cancer, this generally develops secondary to bladder outflow obstruction, but it may be acquired independently with aging. The pathophysiology of detrusor overactivity due to outflow obstruction is the same for prostate cancer as for benign prostatic hyperplasia or any other cause of bladder outflow obstruction.[6] About 75% to 80% of men with prostatic obstruction develop detrusor overactivity and irritative bladder symptoms, including urinary frequency, urgency, nocturia, and urge incontinence.[6] There are quite marked ultrastructural changes that occur in conjunction with this, including collagenous infiltration of detrusor smooth muscle bundles combined with smooth muscle hypertrophy.[7,8] There is also a reduction in acetylcholine-positive nerve profiles in association with an increase in the ratio of abnormal to normal myoneural junctions,[8] both of which is in keeping with a muscular denervation response to the increase in bladder pressure. These changes may be caused by repeated episodes of detrusor ischemia that have been demonstrated in bladder outflow obstruction,[9] and they lend support to the belief that detrusor overactivity results from a post-junctional hypersensitivity phenomenon due to denervation.[10,11] Overactivity in other transmitter systems, such as non-cholinergic activation via purinergic receptors, has also been suggested as an etiological factor.[12] Studies have shown that relief of obstruction restores detrusor stability in about three quarters of patients; in the remaining quarter, it persists.[13]

IATROGENIC INCONTINENCE

Iatrogenic incontinence refers to incontinence that arises as a direct result of medical intervention or treatment. Primary treatment modalities for clinically localized prostate cancer include radical prostatectomy, external-beam radiotherapy, and brachytherapy. Cryotherapy is emerging as an alternative treatment option but tends to be reserved for patients with locally advanced cancer or those with recurrent disease after radiotherapy. The incidence and pathophysiology of incontinence following each of these treatments will be considered separately. Transurethral resection of the prostate (TURP) may sometimes cause or contribute to incontinence, and will be considered within the following sections.

RADICAL PROSTATECTOMY

Radical prostatectomy is undertaken as curative therapy for men with localized prostate cancer. By removing the whole prostate, the bladder neck and prostatic smooth muscle mechanisms that normally contribute to continence are lost. Following removal of the urethral catheter after surgery, some degree of immediate incontinence may be anticipated. In the majority of patients, this will be followed by gradual improvement in urinary control and continence. Nocturnal incontinence tends to resolve first, before daytime stress incontinence. Continence on standing from sitting tends to be reestablished last, and retraining contributes considerably to full recovery. In most patients, continence will continue to improve during the first 2 years after surgery. Persistent and troublesome incontinence beyond 2 years is unusual (see below), but may have a significant impact on the individual's quality of life.[14]

Post-prostatectomy incontinence is usually associated with an incompetent urethral closure mechanism. The clinician should be aware, however, that anastomotic stricture, detrusor dysfunction, or reduced bladder compliance may also contribute to the clinical picture.[15] Detrusor overactivity may have been present preoperatively (see above) or may result from bladder denervation injury acquired at the time of surgery. Functional recovery of continence that generally follows radical prostatectomy implies significant reversibility in the immediate postoperative dysfunction. Alongside resolution of neuropraxia and neuromuscular inactivity, healing, tissue repair, and regeneration may contribute to the function of remaining continence mechanisms. Factors that may promote their functional recovery include the vascularization, innervation, and viability of remaining normal tissues; potential for revascularization, re-innervation, functional tissue regeneration (particularly sphincteric), and mechanisms for compensatory neurologic control are currently poorly understood but may be important in the early postoperative period. Conversely, fibrosis, apoptosis, and ischemia may adversely affect recovery. Similar healing processes may influence recovery of erectile function. The importance of surgical technique and experience for functional recovery has been emphasized by Walsh in his description of the "anatomic radical retropubic prostatectomy"[16] (see Chapter 80).

Operative injury to the rhabdosphincter or its nerve supply is probably the most common factor in post-prostatectomy incontinence.[17] Continence following radical prostatectomy requires a functional distal urinary sphincter, and both active and passive mechanisms contribute to sphincteric competence. Components responsible for passive continence include opposing urethral mucosa for assuring a watertight seal, and fibroelastic and smooth muscle tissue within the wall of the urethra and the rhabdosphincter. The puborectalis part of the levator ani is responsive to sudden rises in intra-abdominal pressure, thereby also contributing to continence. Fibrosis or rigidity of the membranous urethra may compromise mucosal apposition and sphincteric function. Anastomotic stricture associated with sphincteric deficiency must be excluded. On clinical and urodynamic assessment of 88 patients with post prostatectomy incontinence, Groutz et al[18] reported that in 88% intrinsic sphincter

deficiency was the cause. One third of men with sphincteric deficiency were associated with detrusor overactivity, whereas isolated detrusor overactivity was present in only 6%; another 6% had outflow obstruction associated with stricture. Other authors have suggested that impaired posterior urethral sensation may contribute to postoperative incontinence by preventing the afferent loop of a guarding reflex of the periurethral striated sphincter.[19]

Reports of incidence for incontinence vary widely in the literature due to differences in definition, method of patient assessment (by physicians, patient questionnaires, or third parties), variations in surgical technique and length of follow-up.[20] Depending on the definition of incontinence (including the wearing of pads), reported prevalence rates after 1 year range from 8%[21] to 69%.[22] Predicting patients who are at risk has also proved problematic. Age is certainly a factor and a number of studies have shown that men over the age of 70 years are more likely to develop urinary incontinence postoperatively.[23,24] The continence index developed by Marsh and Lepor[25] attributes a score based on a clinical assessment of continence, bladder distention volume at the time of urine leakage, and the ability of the patient to stop and start the urinary stream. This score, measured by a clinician at the time of catheter removal post radical prostatectomy, has been shown to be valuable in predicting men who will regain continence and those in whom urinary incontinence will remain permanent. They suggest those men with low scores (a negative indication) should start treatment and biofeedback early in the postoperative period to facilitate recovery.

Surgical factors that contribute to long-term continence rates include meticulous operative technique in preserving the external striated sphincter mechanism, operative experience, and case selection. For individual cases where oncologic control will not be compromised, bilateral preservation of the neurovascular bundles (supplying the membranous urethra as well as penile corpora) may contribute to higher continence rates.[21,26] This effect, however, decreases with increasing age.[27] Employing two pubo-urethral suspension stitches may also contribute to postoperative continence and, by increasing the Valsalva leak point pressure, may reduce the severity of incontinence if it occurs.[28] Bladder neck preservation does not improve the long-term recovery of continence, but in those patients who will be continent, their recovery has been shown to be quicker.[29] The choice of either the perineal or retropubic route has not been shown to effect postoperative urinary incontinence rates.[30] Laparoscopic or robotic radical prostatectomy allows precise construction of the urethrovesical anastomosis in the hands of surgeons who are skilled and experienced in these techniques, and continence may be acquired quickly following (generally earlier) catheter removal. Overall, long-term continence rates appear to be comparable between different surgical approaches.[31]

EXTERNAL-BEAM RADIOTHERAPY

External-beam radiotherapy provides an alternative primary treatment for clinically localized prostate cancer that leaves irradiated prostate and sphincter mechanisms in situ. Side effects may be early (within the first 6 months of treatment) or late (acquired months or years later). In the early post-treatment period, urinary side effects relate to inflammation and may induce a transient clinical syndrome of acute cystitis, with or without prostatitis, including urgency and sometimes urge incontinence. There have been reported incidences from 70% to 90% for mild, 20% to 45% for moderate and 1% to 4% for severe reactions.[32-34] Acute side effects are expected to settle in 4 to 6 weeks, and they are dependent on the volume of tissue treated (pelvis or prostate) as well as radiation dose. Late complications are associated with ongoing chronic inflammation and tissue fibrosis with sequelae that may include chronic cystitis, bladder ulcer, urethral stricture, urinary urgency, incontinence, and impotence. In this late situation, incontinence can arise from a variety of mechanisms: overflow incontinence associated with a fibrotic shrunken bladder, stress incontinence with sphincteric insufficiency, urgency with detrusor overactivity and combinations of these. The incidence of late urinary complications is believed to be dose-dependent and reported in 5% to 12% of cases.[35,36] The overall incidence of urinary incontinence after radiotherapy has been reported as between 1.3% and 7%.[37,38] Patients are at higher risk of urinary incontinence if they have undergone previous TURP, especially if this is performed after radiotherapy.[27] Interestingly, radiotherapy for biochemical failure after radical prostatectomy does not increase the risk of urinary incontinence,[39] but salvage prostatectomy after radiation therapy can have a very high incontinence rate, with reports of as many as 58% to 64% of patients affected.[40,41]

BRACHYTHERAPY

In suitable patients, prostate brachytherapy is emerging as an alternative to radical prostatectomy and external-beam radiotherapy for clinically localized prostate cancer.[42] Side effects relate to intervention that manipulates the prostate and leaves it in situ, including prostatitis, urethritis, retention, stricture, and irritative voiding symptoms. Reported rates of urinary incontinence vary from 0% to 6%,[43-51] but, again, interpretation is difficult owing to variations in data collection and dosimetry.

Previous TURP is often considered a contraindication to brachytherapy, and may increase substantially the risk of incontinence, but with recent developments in brachytherapy technique, the risk of damage to

sphincter function may be minimized (see Chapter 82). Previous studies where urinary incontinence was not used as a specific end-point have suggested there may be a relationship between urethral morbidity and urethral dose.[52-55] Other reports have suggested the risk of incontinence is increased by combined external-beam radiotherapy and brachytherapy, affecting as many as 41% of patients at 4 years.[56] More recently, McElveen et al[42] demonstrated that high urethral doses and pre-implant (International-Prostate Symptom Score) I-PSS are predictive factors for the development of urinary incontinence, which in their patients was a mild form of stress incontinence. They recommended limiting the urethral dose to as close to the prescription dose as possible and selecting patients with an I-PSS less than 15.

CRYOTHERAPY

Cryosurgery has gained some favor since the mid-1990s as local treatment after failure of primary radiation therapy for prostate cancer or for locally advanced clinical stage disease. Incidence rates for urinary incontinence vary depending on definition and technology, with reported rates around 5% for primary cryosurgery, and 10% for secondary salvage cryosurgery.[57] The risk may be increased in those patients who have previously had TURP.[57] Since urethral-warming catheters have been introduced, the incidence of stress incontinence has declined. Thermocouples allow the temperature around the sphincter to be monitored and maintained at a healthy level throughout the procedure. Urethral fistula should be a rare complication with third-generation cryo-therapy delivering a precisely controlled freeze zone and real time monitoring.

CLINICAL ASSESSMENT

On the basis of a medical history, incontinence can be described as stress, urge, or mixed—unfortunately, these descriptions do not necessarily correlate with underlying pathophysiology and urodynamic findings. Patients with overflow incontinence tend to complain of complete loss of bladder sensation with repeated, and at times constant, dribbling of urine with no significant urinary stream or volume. Enuresis may raise suspicion of high-pressure chronic retention with overflow. The history will also identify previous interventions and management strategies that may have significant bearing on etiology and further treatment.

Urgency is an almost irresistible desire to pass urine because of fear of wetting oneself or pain. It is usually sudden in onset, felt in the perineum or suprapubic region, and is not the same as the normal sensation of bladder fullness. Sometimes it may be associated with incontinence if the patient is unable to relieve himself. The presence of urgency resulting in incontinence is strongly linked with detrusor overactivity. In some cases, if the patient has lost awareness of bladder sensation, detrusor overactivity will cause incontinence and leakage without any discomfort. Other symptoms that complete the urge syndrome include frequency (voiding more than once every 2 hours or more than 7 times a day) and nocturia when the desire to pass urine wakes the patient.[58]

With stress incontinence, urine leakage occurs on coughing or with other physical efforts associated with a rise in intra-abdominal pressure. Importantly, there may be concomitant detrusor overactivity (so called "mixed incontinence") that may complicate the clinical picture. Under these circumstances it is imperative that the clinical assessment includes urodynamic investigation and anastomotic stricture is excluded (see below).

Physical signs are not a major part of the clinical picture, but a complete examination should be undertaken in all patients. There may be systemic signs of urinary tract infection or uremia. The bladder may be palpable with urinary retention, but, in some situations, retention can be difficult to detect clinically. Spinal cord compression may be suspected from neurologic examination of the lower limbs. Digital rectal examination (DRE) will assess the extent of local cancer spread. Examination will also contribute to the assessment of a patient's overall health and fitness, an important consideration when planning future treatment.

Initial investigations will be guided by the medical history and examination findings. Urinary tract infection is not only commonly associated with incontinence, but may aggravate it and should be treated. Urine culture will identify infecting organisms and provide antibiotic sensitivities. Ultrasound scans can assess or exclude urinary retention, incomplete bladder emptying, and hydronephrosis. Renal function and prostate specific antigen profile may need to be monitored in particular cases. Pain or dysuria in the absence of infection may require further assessment with imaging (such as computed tomography [CT] or magnetic resonance imaging [MRI]) and cystoscopy.

Uroflow studies showing poor flow in spite of adequate voided volumes suggest underlying bladder outflow obstruction (including the possibility of anastomotic stricture) or detrusor acontractility. An acontractile detrusor may be associated with chronic retention, and it may be due to longstanding bladder outflow obstruction or surgical denervation injury. Where the diagnosis is uncertain and would influence treatment, or a trial of therapy has been unsuccessful, urodynamic assessment is imperative.[18,59] Cystometry may establish the pathophysiology of bladder filling, storage, and emptying.[60] Video-urodynamic studies may demonstrate incontinence and pressure-flow dynamics, and characterise the underlying pathophysiology.

Management of urinary incontinence in men with prostate cancer requires assessment of both sphincteric and detrusor components. Sphincteric insufficiency may coexist with detrusor overactivity, and it may conceal instability where the functional capacity of the bladder is compromised by incontinence; this may also apply during urodynamic assessment. Stress incontinence generally implies a degree of sphincteric insufficiency that may reflect disease or iatrogenic factors. Transurethral resection of the prostate involves resection of the bladder neck mechanism contributing to continence, along with prostate tissue that provides passive resistance to urine flow. Radical prostatectomy, radiotherapy, and TURP may also contribute specifically to weakness of the external striated sphincter.

The number of pads used per day gives a rather unreliable idea of degree of incontinence and its impact on the individual. It is sometimes helpful for the patient to complete a fluid intake/voiding/incontinence diary for a period of days and weigh pads daily. A quality-of-life questionnaire can be used to assess and monitor individual patients.

TREATMENT

Interventions for incontinence include general advice and conservative measures, with pharmacotherapy and surgery reserved for appropriately selected patients. Attention to fluid intake, diet, and voiding habit may be sufficient for some patients, or will at least reduce extraneous exacerbating factors. Conservative interventions including physiotherapy, bladder retraining, biofeedback, and electrical stimulation can be beneficial alone or in combination with pharmacotherapy. Surgical options are usually reserved for cases in which these measures have failed and troublesome incontinence persists beyond a period necessary for improvement.

Urinary infection should be treated with appropriate antibiotics. Infection must be excluded before invasive urologic investigations or procedures. Urinary retention should also be treated according to its etiology and circumstances. Both infection and retention may exacerbate other causes of incontinence.

CONSERVATIVE MEASURES

Patients with urinary incontinence may benefit from advice on fluid and dietary intake, identifying those factors that aggravate incontinence due to diuretic effects, bladder irritation, or bowel disturbance. Generally, one and a half liters per day are sufficient for hydration and an adequate urine output. Moderate quantities of tea, coffee, and soft drinks have mild diuretic and irritative effects on the bladder that can be avoided. Specific additives that can be avoided include caffeine and artificial sweeteners. Spicy foods and excessive alcohol consumption should be avoided and a regular bowel habit maintained. Pharmacotherapy for unrelated conditions may aggravate incontinence through effects on lower urinary tract pathophysiology and warrant review. Many of these considerations and other conservative approaches (below) are used in post radical prostatectomy rehabilitation, to be discussed later in this chapter.

For patients with urge incontinence, bladder retraining is a useful initial approach and is often undertaken by continence nurse specialists. Frequency–volume charting gives a starting point for the training, and the patient will have a base line of how frequently he is passing urine (Figure 94.1). The aim is for the patient to suppress the urge to void in order to expand functional bladder capacity, improve the volumes held, and increase continence. Additional pelvic floor exercises may also be helpful.[61] Anticholinergics can be used as a "crutch" until the patient has made some progress with retraining, after which the drug therapy can be discontinued.

Other conservative interventions include electrical stimulation, delivered via a rectal probe or perineal surface electrodes, and may both increase the contractility of the pelvic floor muscles and inhibit detrusor overactivity.[20] There have been studies proposing effective treatment of overflow incontinence outside the context of prostate cancer with electrical stimulation.[62] Other modalities that may be helpful in particular circumstances include hypnotherapy[63] and acupuncture.[64]

For incontinent patients with prostate cancer in whom continence cannot be restored, penile compression devices, urinary collection devices, or absorbent pads can be used provided there is not a significant degree of retention.[65] There may be concerns, however, with safety of long-term penile clamp usage. In refractory cases, an indwelling urethral catheter may become unavoidable, particularly where there is otherwise significant retention or renal function is compromised by bladder outflow obstruction. Pelvic tumors including prostate cancer relatively contraindicate suprapubic catheter placement, particularly when local disease is extensive or uncontrolled. Difficulties may arise in relation to their placement and ongoing-care; and a permanent tract can become a conduit for tumor invasion.

Continence

Frequency – volume chart

Name: ______________________ Week commencing: __________

[ ] In the blank column please record with (i) a tick each time you pass urine, or (ii) an "IE" for each incontinent episode.

[ ] In the shaded column please record the amount and type of fluid intake e.g. cup/tea, glass/juice etc.

	Sunday		Monday		Tuesday		Wednesday		Thursday		Friday		Saturday	
6am														
7am														
8am														
9am														
10am														
11am														
Mid-day														
1pm														
2pm														
3pm														
4pm														
5pm														
6pm														
7pm														
8pm														
9pm														
10pm														
11pm														
Mid-night														
1am														
2am														
3am														
4am														
Total														

Fig. 94.1
Frequency–volume and continence chart: patients are asked to document fluid intake (including time, volume, and type of beverage), voided urine (time and volume), and episodes of incontinence (if any). This enables the patient and their advisor to relate the voiding pattern to fluid intake, and measures total daily volumes taken and voided over several days.

PHARMACOTHERAPY

Pharmacotherapy targeting specific mechanisms of lower urinary tract function may contribute to urinary continence and bladder control, either alone or in combination with other conservative or surgical interventions. For instance, sphincter tone may be increased by alpha-adrenergic agonists (e.g., imipramine, pseudoephedrine, and phenylpropanolamine). Such drugs have been shown to improve mild stress incontinence, but cardiovascular side effects can limit their use. Imipramine also has some potentially beneficial anticholinergic activity, acting also in the bladder.

Anticholinergic pharmacotherapy with muscarinic antagonists is the first-line medical treatment for detrusor instability. There are a number of different anticholinergics available each with different efficacy and pharmacokinetics (oxybutinin, tolterodine, trospium). New compounds are being developed, such as solifenacin and darifenacin,[66] that are more selective, theoretically limiting the side effect profile (dry mouth, constipation, and blurred vision). These drugs, in spite of sometimes adverse effects on bladder emptying, surprisingly rarely precipitate urinary retention. It is important to try different anticholinergics and controlled release preparations in individual patients, as their suitability will vary according to efficacy and side effects profile.

Alpha-blockers (e.g. alfuzosin, tamsulosin, terazosin, and doxazosin) relax the smooth muscle fibers of bladder neck and prostatic smooth muscle. These drugs improve lower urinary tract symptoms and quality of life in men with symptomatic benign prostatic hyperplasia, but in men with prostate cancer whose prostate remains in situ, they have an extremely limited role. They have no role after radical prostatectomy, by which the target tissues are removed, and indeed this class of drugs should be avoided (for instance as treatment for unrelated conditions such as hypertension), owing to their pharmacological action that relaxes sphincteric smooth muscle.

CHANNEL TRANSURETHRAL RESECTION OF THE PROSTATE

Urinary retention, symptomatic bladder outflow obstruction and symptomatic detrusor acontractility may be relieved by channel TURP in men with prostate cancer who have not had radical prostatectomy. Particular care should be exercised in those patients with detrusor overactivity, as relieving obstruction can exacerbate symptoms of detrusor overactivity, especially urgency and urge incontinence. Coexisting sphincter weakness will increase this tendency, and some previously continent patients can be rendered incontinent. Channel TURP restores the lumen of the prostatic urethra and may be performed (with the patient's prior consent) after diagnostic cystoscopy and bimanual examination. It is a palliative procedure that does not attempt complete resection of the tumor bulk. Prostatic stents (e.g., Prostakath, Prostacoil, and Memotherm permanent prostatic stent systems) represent alternatives to channel TURP with advantages over indwelling catheters and repeated TURP procedures. They can also remain in situ if further radiotherapy is required.[67–69]

POST RADICAL PROSTATECTOMY REHABILITATION

Since sphincter function usually recovers following radical prostatectomy, physiotherapy, bladder retraining, and pharmacotherapy are mainstays of early postoperative rehabilitation. These approaches have been introduced in the above discussion. Electrical pelvic floor stimulation and biofeedback techniques may also be considered for individual patients. Conservative and supportive measures remain important during the phase of functional recovery[70];

these include attention to good skin care, fluid intake (both content and volume), diet, bowel function, and pharmacotherapy. Penile compression devices and condom catheters must be avoided in post-radical prostatectomy patients to facilitate restoration of pelvic floor, sphincter musculature, and reflexes necessary for urinary control and continence.

Stress incontinence may be considerably improved by pelvic floor (Kegal) exercises. These exercises help to strengthen the voluntary urinary sphincter and pelvic floor; bladder control may also improve. They should be practiced every day, and it is important that an individual program for each patient is developed. Both slow and fast contractions should be performed, and this should involve not holding the pelvic floor muscles for more than 10 seconds. It is also important to teach "the knack" (when a pelvic floor contraction is encouraged during an increase in intra-abdominal pressure, for example, with sneezing or coughing). The best positions for patients to be in for performing these exercises are lying on their back with their knees bent up or sitting on a chair with the knees apart. The exercises can then be taught in two parts. First the patient should learn to tighten the anus as though trying to control flatus or diarrhea and second he should imagine trying to stop the flow of urine midstream. This can be taught by suggesting the patient looks in a mirror, whilst standing, to see the base of the penis move nearer to the abdomen and the testicles rise. The patient is then taught to tighten these muscles and hold on, for example, for the count of five, then gently let go and repeat this series of contractions five times. He should also do 20 short sharp contractions once a day. This involves tightening the pelvic floor and immediately letting go. Pelvic floor exercises may be taught prior to radical prostatectomy, and this may facilitate an individual's appreciation of pelvic floor and sphincter control; studies have suggested this may contribute to earlier achievement of continence, but is unlikely to influence persistent or severe incontinence.[71]

Other techniques may be used in conjunction with pelvic floor exercises to improve an individual's exercise technique and stimulate normal pelvic floor function. Biofeedback can be achieved with a small anal probe or skin surface electrodes and either visual display or audio equipment to register pelvic floor activity.[72–74] Specifically, it may promote control and strength of the levator ani muscle. Electrical stimulation may also be used to stimulate the pelvic floor with either an anal probe or surface electrodes.[19,75,76]

If conservative approaches fail the treatment options include collagen injection therapy, implantation of an artificial urinary sphincter, or a bulbourethral sling procedure. Collagen injection therapy tends to give short-term success in 20% to 62% of patients,[77–80] may require repeated injections and is most effective in milder forms of stress incontinence.[16] A study of over

250 patients with over 2 years follow-up showed 20% were dry and 39% were significantly improved with a mean number of injections of 4.4 (range 1–11).[81] Patients with milder incontinence (less than 6 pads/day) had much higher success rates, but often four injections were required for cure. Cespedes[82] also emphasized that more than four treatments may be worthwhile, using injections of 2.5 to 7.5 mL to avoid mucosal ulceration, not less than 1 month apart. Attempts to inject collagen in an antegrade fashion on the basis of better visualization have not yielded significantly better results,[83] and collagen injection is known to be less effective in patients who have a bladder neck contracture or who have undergone radiation, cryotherapy, or bladder neck incision.[16] Collagen injections should be reserved for patients with mild stress incontinence who have failed conservative treatment and who would not be suitable for an artificial sphincter. Allergy to collagen should be ruled out by a prior skin test.

Artificial urinary sphincter placement offers the best opportunity for cure in suitable patients with persistent and troublesome incontinence, with 90% achieving a socially adequate degree of continence, and 30% to 50% achieving dryness.[84,85] A periurethral cuff inserted around the bulbar urethra maintains continence and, when the patient chooses to pass urine, he applies pressure to a pump placed in the scrotum to shift fluid out of the cuff into a reservoir. The cuff opens, the patient voids, the cuff then re-fills with fluid and continence is regained[16] (Figure 94.2). The revision rate after insertion is of the order of one-third, and between

4.5% and 23% will require removal of prosthesis within 10 years due to infection.[86] In the context of previous radiotherapy reports are conflicting; some studies have suggested the continence rate is lower (66%),[87] whereas others have found the outcomes to be similar.[88] In view of these success rates, some urologists would recommend using the artificial sphincter as first line treatment for post-prostatectomy incontinence.[16] Management of incontinence with an artificial sphincter may, however, be complicated by coexisting anastomotic stricture (see below).

The bulbourethral sling procedure is emerging as a third surgical treatment option, originally proposed by Clemens in 1976.[89] There are a number of variations on the technique, but generally a sling is placed transperineally around the bulbar urethra and fixed to the medial aspect of the descending pubic rami using titanium bone screws[90] (Figure 94.3). Sling tension is adjusted intraoperatively in relation to urethral and leak-point pressure. Although initial reports were guarded and perineal discomfort was a persistent complication, more recently reports have been favorably compared to artificial sphincters, with up to 67% of patients becoming pad free and 92% showing some improvement.[90]

The management of post-prostatectomy incontinence may be complicated by coexisting anastomotic stricture. The management of anastomotic stricture depends upon lower urinary tract function and factors that include stricture length and caliber; detailed discussion is beyond the scope of this chapter. Surgical interventions include dilatation, optical incision, or

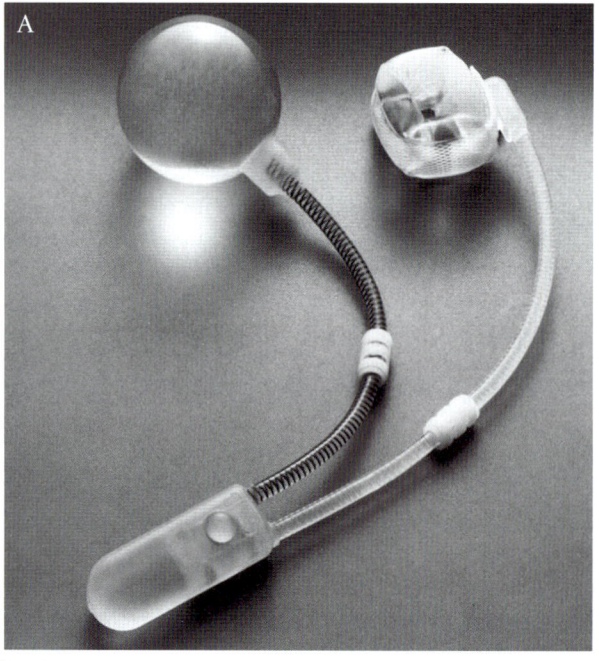
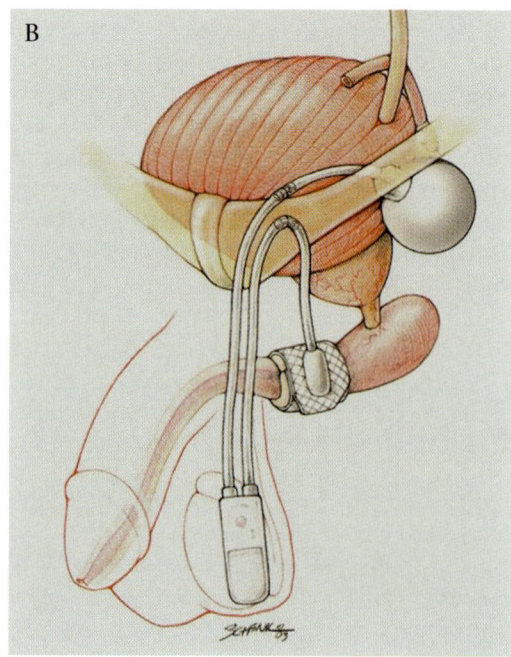

Fig. 94.2
A, AMS 800 Artificial Urinary Sphincter™ (American Medical Systems, MN, USA) device for stress urinary incontinence due to sphincter weakness, including inflatable cuff, pump chamber, and reservoir. B, Drawing showing placement of AMS 800 artificial urinary sphincter with inflatable cuff around bulbar urethra, pump chamber in scrotum, and reservoir in preperitoneal space.

A

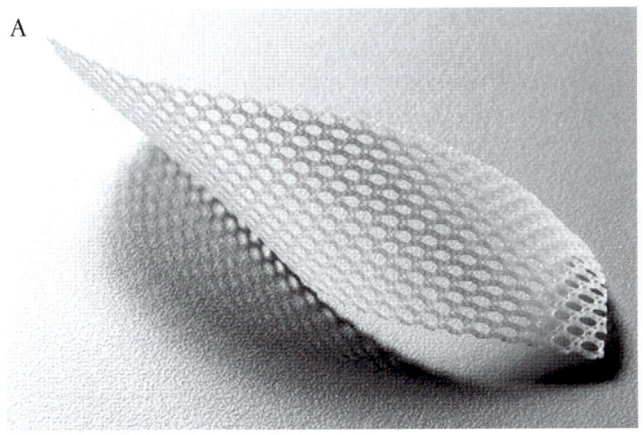

B

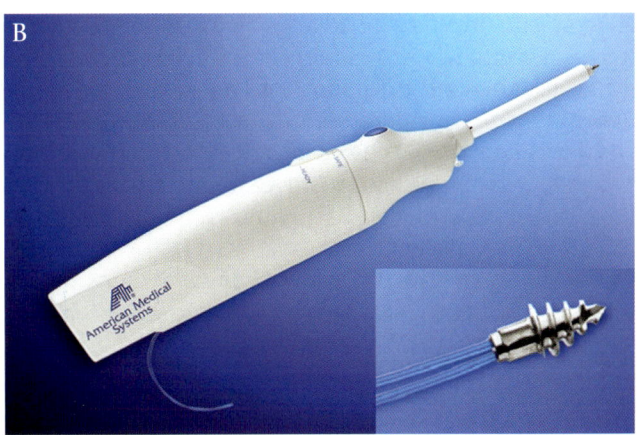

C

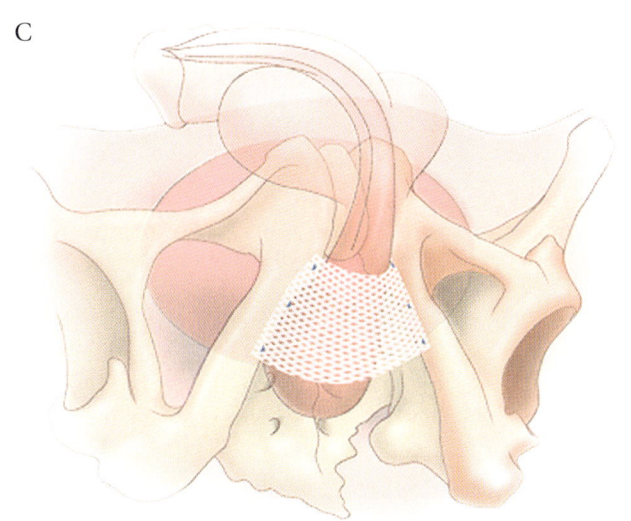

Fig. 94.3
Invance™ (American Medical Systems, MN, USA) male urethral sling system for minimally invasive treatment of stress urinary incontinence. A, Intemesh™ biocompatible silicone-coated multifilament polyester knitted weave mesh allowing for tissue ingrowth. B, Screw inserter and 5 mm self-tapping screw (inset). C, Drawing showing mesh in position, anchored with six bone screws inserted into inferior aspect of pubic rami.

transurethral resection; and patients may be required to carry out regular clean intermittent self-catheterization to prevent recurrence. Continence may improve or recover following treatment of stricture depending on detrusor and sphincter function. In those patients with persistent incontinence, artificial sphincter placement should be deferred until further recovery of sphincter function is unlikely and the anastomosis is sufficiently healthy and mature that further intervention and intermittent catheterization are not required. In some circumstances where there is a recurrent contracture, an artificial sphincter can be combined with a urethral stent for symptomatic improvement.[91] In severe cases, urethral obliteration by fibrosis may be permitted to restore continence where an alternative continent conduit can be established surgically for intermittent catheterization. A long-term catheter is an undesirable alternative, with its inevitable complications, and ileal loop urinary diversion is a very last resort. Surgical interventions for incontinence other than those for anastomotic stricture and overflow incontinence should generally be deferred for at least 1 year and usually longer to allow sufficient opportunity for functional recovery and healing processes to mature.

QUALITY OF LIFE

Clinicians must appreciate the impact of urinary incontinence, uncontrolled urinary leakage, and urinary wetness for the patient and his family, including their potential effects on quality of life, lifestyle, social behavior, and employment. Studies have repeatedly confirmed that a physician's estimation of urinary incontinence is more favorable than that of the patient.[20,92] The impact on quality of life is measurable and can be substantial. Poor communication by healthcare professionals also adversely affects quality of life, particularly in the early post-treatment period.[93,94] The concept of urinary "bother" has also developed, referring to the annoyance and interference caused by the impairment in lower urinary tract function. Bother may not, however, correlate with the degree of incontinence.[95] Despite observations showing that use of pads is greater and urinary leak after treatment is more common with radical prostatectomy than radiation,[92,96] most patients are satisfied with their treatment decision with no significant difference in bother score between treatments.[95] Attending support groups, and meeting patients with similar experience may encourage individuals, and improve their understanding and access to local resources, and some will in time become active in helping others through similar experiences. Psychological adjustment by patients, and the possibility of changing attitudes with time and experience contribute to the complexity of the relationship between medical decision-making, urinary incontinence, quality of life and bother. These issues are addressed in detail in Chapters 61, 69, and 70.

SUMMARY

Urinary incontinence is extremely debilitating to patients with prostate cancer. When associated with advanced-stage disease, management can become extremely difficult, particularly after conservative, pharmacologic, and surgical methods become ineffective or inappropriate. In such circumstances, attention to hygiene, skin care, and infection is mandatory, and devices to control urinary drainage such as a penile clamp, convene, or long-term catheterization must be considered according to an individual patient's needs and circumstances.

Fortunately, long-term iatrogenic incontinence is uncommon. With effective treatment strategies and growing numbers of patients having treatment for early-stage disease, iatrogenic incontinence may be a significant problem for individual patients, and faced increasingly by urologists. Incontinence may be due to overflow, detrusor overactivity, incompetent urethral closure, stricture, or a combination of these factors. It is manifest clinically as overflow incontinence, urge or stress or mixed incontinence, and, rarely, continuous incontinence. In the face of such varied underlying pathophysiology, the use of urodynamic assessment should not be underestimated, particularly in those patients with unexplained or persistent refractory incontinence. Patient communication and education should be emphasized and can have a direct positive influence on patient quality of life. Conservative management includes medical treatment, advice about diet and fluid intake, physiotherapy techniques such as pelvic floor exercises, and bladder retraining. Biofeedback, electrical stimulation, and other specific or supervised interventions may contribute to functional recovery in individual patients. Supportive measures such as skin care and use of absorbent pads are important in all patients, whereas a penile clamp or convene should be avoided during post-prostatectomy rehabilitation and advised only according to individual circumstances. Surgical options for persistent post-radical prostatectomy incontinence include collagen injections, bulbourethral sling procedure, placement of an artificial sphincter, and occasionally complex urologic reconstruction. Urinary incontinence following treatment of early stage prostate cancer is overall an uncommon complication that can usually be treated or managed effectively according to the underlying pathophysiology and individual patient factors.

REFERENCES

1. Abrams P, Cardiozo L, et al. The standardisation of terminology of lower urinary tract function report from the Standardisation Sub-Committee of the International Continence Society. Neuro Urodyn 2002;21:167–178.

2. Herr HW. Quality of life of incontinent men after radical prostatectomy. J Urol 1994;151:652–654.

3. Parys BT, Machin DG, Woolfenden KA, et al. Chronic urinary retention – a sensory problem? BJU 1988;62:546–549.

4. Nielsen KK, Andersen CB, Petersen LK, et al. Morphological, stereological and biochemical analysis of the mini-pig urinary bladder after chronic outflow obstruction and after recovery from obstruction. Neurourol Urodyn 1996;15:167.

5. Saito M, Ohmura M, Kondo A. Effects of long term partial outflow obstruction on bladder function in the rat. Neurol Urodyn 1996;15:157–165.

6. Chapple C, Turner-Warwick R. Bladder outflow obstruction in the male. In AR Mundy, TP Stephenson, AJ Wein (eds): Urodynamics: Principles, practice and application. Churchill Livingstone. 1984, pp 233–257.

7. Gosling JA, Dixon JS. Structure of trabeculated detrusor smooth muscle in cases of prostatic hypertrophy. Urologia Internationalis 1980;35:351–355.

8. Tse V, Wills E, Szonyi G, et al. The application of ultrastuctural studies in the diagnosis of bladder dysfunction in a clinical setting. J Urol 2000;163:535–539.

9. Greenland JE, Brading AF. The effect of bladder outflow obstruction on detrusor blood flow changes during the voiding cycle in conscious pigs. J Urol 2001;165:245–248.

10. Andersson KE. Changes in bladder tone during filling: Pharmocological aspects. Scand J Urol Nephrol Suppl 1999;201:67–72.

11. Sibley GN. The pathophysiological response of the detrusor muscle to experimental bladder outflow obstruction in the pig. BJU 1987;60:332–336.

12. Andersson, KE. Overactive bladder – pharmacological aspects. Scand J Urol Nephrol Suppl 2002;210:72–81.

13. Turner-Warwick R. Observations on the function and dysfunction of the sphincter and detrusor mechanisms. Urol Clin N Am 1979;6:13–30.

14. Fowler FJ, Barry MJ, Lu-Yao G, et al. Effect of radical prostatectomy on patient quality of life: results from a Medicare survey. Urology 1995;45:1007–1013.

15. MacDiarmid SA. Incontinence after radical prostatectomy: pathophysiology and management. Curr Urol Rep 2001;2:209–213.

16. Walsh PC. Anatomic radical retropubic prostatectomy. In Walsh PC, Retik AB, Vaughan ED, Wein AJ (eds): Campbell's Urology, 8th ed. Philadelphia: WB Saunders, 2002.

17. Feneley MR, Walsh PC. Incontinence after radical prostatectomy. Lancet 1999;353:2091–2092.

18. Groutz A, Blaivas JG, Chaikin DC, et al. The pathophysiology of post-radical prostatectomy incontinence: a clinical and video urodynamics study. J Urol 2000;163:1767–1770.

19. John H, Sullivan MP, Bangerter U, et al. Effect of radical prostatectomy on sensory threshold and pressure transmission. J Urol 2000;163:1761–1766.

20. Grise P, Thurman S. Urinary incontinence following treatment of localised prostate cancer. Cancer Control 2001;8:532–539.

21. Catalona WJ, Carvalhal GF, Mager DE, et al. Potency, continence and complication rates in 1870 consecutive radical retropubic prostatectomies. J Urol 1999;162:433–438.

22. Bates TS, Wright MP, Gillat DA. Prevalence and impact of incontinence and impotence following total prostatectomy assessed anonymously by the ICS-male questionnaire. Eur Urol 1998;33:165–169.

23. Eastham JA, Kattan MW, Rogers E, et al. Risk factors for urinary incontinence after radical prostatectomy. J Urol 1996;156:1707–1713.

24. Stanford JL, Feng Z, Hamilton AS, et al. Urinary and sexual function after radical prostatectomy for clinically localised prostate cancer: the Prostate cancer outcomes study. JAMA 2000;283:354–360.

25. Marsh DW, Lepor H. Predicting continence following radical prostatectomy. Curr Urol Rep 2001;2:248–252.

26. O'Donnell PD, Finan BF. Continence following nerve sparing prostatectomy. J Urol 1989;142:1227–1229.

27. Smith JA. Outcome after radical prostatectomy depends on surgical technique but not approach. Curr Urol Rep 2002;3:179–181.

28. Campenni MA, Harmon JD, Ginsberg PC, et al. Improved Continence after radical retropubic prostatectomy using two pubo-urethral suspension stitches. Urol Int 2002;68;109–112.

29. Selli C, De Antoni P, Moro U, et al. Role of bladder neck preservation in urinary incontinence following radical retropubic prostatectomy. Scand J Urol Nephrol 2004;38:32–37.

30. Gray M, Petroni GR, Theodorescu D. Urinary function after radical prostatectomy: a comparison of retropubic and perineal approaches. Urology 1999;53:881–891.

31. Herrel SD, Smith JA. Laparoscopic and robotic radical prostatectomy: what are the real advantages? BJU Int 2005;95:3–4.

32. Duncan W, Warde P, Catton CN, et al. Carcinoma of the prostate: results of radical radiotherapy, 1970–1985. Int J Radiat Oncol Biol Phys 1993;26:203–210.

33. Amdur RJ, Parsons JT, Fitzgerald LT, et al. Adenocarcinoma of the prostate treated with external beam radiation therapy: 5 year minimum follow up. Radiother Oncol 1990;18:235–246.

34. Mithal NP, Hoskin PJ. External beam radiotherapy for carcinoma of the prostate: a retrospective study. Clin Oncol1993;5:297–301.

35. Schellhammer PF, El-Mahdi AM. Pelvic complications after definitive treatment of prostate cancer by interstitial or external beam radiation. Urology 1983;21:451–457.

36. Lawton CA, Won M, Pilepich MV, et al. Long-term treatment sequelae following external beam irradiation for adenocarcinoma of the prostate: analysis of RTOG studies 7506 and 7706. Int J Radiat Oncol Biol Phys 1991;21:935–939.

37. Griffiths TR, Neal DE. Localised prostate cancer: early intervention or expectant therapy? J R Soc Med 1997;90:665–669.

38. Lee WR, Schultheiss TE, Hanlon AL, et al. Urinary Incontinence following external beam radiotherapy for clinically localised prostate cancer. Urology 1996;48:95–99.

39. Van Cangh PJ, Richard F, Lorge F, et al. Adjuvant radiation therapy does not cause urinary incontinence after radical prostatectomy: results of a prospective randomised study. J Urol 1998;159:164–166.

40. Pontes JE, Montie J, Klein E. Salvage surgery for radiation failure in prostate cancer. Cancer 1993;71:976–980.

41. Rogers E, Ohori M, Kassabian VS. Salvage radical prostatectomy: outcome measured by serum prostate specific antigen levels. J Urol 1995;153:104–110.

42. McElveen TL, Waterman FM, Kim H, et al. Factors predicting for urinary incontinence after prostate brachytherapy. Int J Radiat Oncol Biol Phys 2004;59:1395–1404.

43. Ragde H, Blasko JC, Grimm PD, et al. Brachytherapy for clinically localised prostate cancer: results at 7 and 8 year follow up. Semin Surg Oncol 1997;13:438–443.

44. Ragde H, Elgamal AA, Snow PB, et al. Ten year disease free survival after transperineal sonography guided iodine 125 brachytherapy with or without 45 gray external beam irradiation in the treatment of patients with clinically localised, low to high Gleason grade prostate carcinoma. Cancer 1998;83:989–1001.

45. Talcott JA, Clark JA, Starck PC, et al. Long term treatment related complications of brachytherapy for early prostate cancer. A survey of patients previously treated. J Urol 2001;166:494–499.

46. Gelblum DY, Potters L, Ashley R, et al. Urinary morbidity following ultrasound guided transperineal prostate seed implantation. Int J Radiat Oncol Biol Phys 1999;45:59–67.

47. Kaye KW, Olsen DJ, Payne JT. Detailed preliminary analysis of 125 iodine implantation for localised prostate cancer using the percutaneous approach. J Urol 1995;153:1020–1025.

48. Brown D, Colonias A, Miller R, et al. Urinary morbidity with a modified peripheral loading technique of transperineal 125 I prostate implantation. Int J Radiat Oncol Biol Phys 2000;47:353–360.

49. Stokes SH, Real JD, Adams PW, et al. Transperineal ultrasound guided radioactive seed implantation for organ confined carcinoma of the prostate. Int J Radiat Oncol Biol Phys 1997;37:337–341.

50. Benoit RM, Naslund M, Cohen JL. Complications after prostate brachytherapy in the medicare population. Urology 2000;55:91–96.

51. Wallner K, Lee H, Wasserman S, et al. Low risk of urinary incontinence following prostate brachytherapy in patients with prior transurethral prostate resection. Int J Radiat Oncol Biol Phys 1997;37:565–569.

52. Desai J, Stock RG, Stone NN, et al. Acute urinary morbidity following I 125 interstitial implantation of the prostate gland. Radiat Oncol Investig 1998;6:135–141.

53. Wallner K, Roy J, Harrison L. Dosimetry guidelines to minimise urethral and rectal morbidity following transperineal I 125 prostate brachytherapy. Int J Radiat Oncol Biol Phys 1995;32:465–471.

54. Merrick GS, Butler WM, Tollenaar BG, et al. The dosimetry of prostate brachytherapy-induced urethral strictures. Int J Radiat Oncol Biol Phys 2002;52:461–468.

55. Zelefsky MJ, Yamada Y, Marion C, et al. Improved conformality and decreased toxicity with intraoperative computer-optimised transperineal ultrasound guided prostate brachytherapy. Int J Radiat Oncol Biol Phys 2003;55:956–963.

56. Joly F, Brune D, Couette JE, et al. Health-related quality of life and sequelae in patients treated with brachytherapy and external beam irradiation for localised prostate cancer. Ann Oncol 1998;9:751–757.

57. Ahmed S, Davies J. Managing the complications of prostate cryosurgery. BJU Int 2005;95:480–481

58. Stephenson T, Mundy AR. The urge syndrome. In AR Mundy, TP Stephenson, AJ Wein (eds): Urodynamics: Principles, practice and application. Churchill Livingston, 1984.

59. Leach GE, Trockman B, Wong A, et al. Post-prostatectomy incontinence: urodynamic findings and treatment outcomes. J Urol 1996;155:1256–1259.

60. Abrams P. Urodynamics, 2nd ed. Springer, 1997.

61. Frewem WM. The management of urgency and frequency of micturition. BJU 1980;52:367–369.

62. Moore KN. Treatment of urinary incontinence in men with electrical stimulation: is practice evidence based? J Wound Ostomy Continence Nurse 2000;27:20–31.

63. Freeman RM, Baxby K. Hypnotherapy for incontinence caused by the unstable detrusor. Br Med J 1982;284:1831–1834.

64. Philp T, Shar PRJ, Worth PHL. Acupuncture in the treatment of bladder instability. BJU 1988;61:490–493.

65. Richardson DA. Overflow incontinence and urinary retention. Clin Obstet Gynecol 1990;33:378–381.

66. Kershen RT, Hsieh M. Preview of new drugs for overactive bladder and incontinence: darifenacin, solifenacin, trospium, and duloxetine. Curr Urol Rep 2004;5:359–367.

67. Aridogan IA, Yachia D. Relief of bladder outlet obstruction caused by prostate cancer using a long term urethral stent (Prostacoil), In Yachia D, Paterson PJ (eds). Stenting in the Urinary System. 2004, pp 435–439.

68. Gottfried HW. Permanent prostatic stent in the management of obstructive prostate cancer in high risk patients. In Yachia D, Paterson PJ (eds). Stenting in the Urinary System. 2004, pp 439–445.

69. Gez E, Cederbaum M. External Irradiation for prostate cancer in patients with urethral stents. In Yachia D, Paterson PJ (eds). Stenting in the Urinary system. 2004, pp 445–453.

70. Hunter KF, Moore KN, Cody DJ, et al. Conservative management for postprostatectomy urinary incontinence. Cochrane Database Syst Rev. 2004:CD001843.

71. Parekh AR, Feng MI, Kirages D, et al. The role of pelvic floor exercises on post-prostatectomy incontinence. J Urol 2003;170:130–133.

72. Jackson J, Emerson L, Johnston B, et al. Biofeedback: a noninvasive treatment for incontinence after radical prostatectomy. Urol Nurs 1996;16:50–54.

73. Bales GT, Gerber GS, Minor TX, et al. Effect of preoperative biofeedback/pelvic floor training on continence in men undergoing radical prostatectomy. Urology 2000;56:627–630.

74. Franke JJ, Gilbert WB, Grier J, et al. Early post-prostatectomy pelvic floor biofeedback. J Urol 2000;163:191–193.

75. Wille S, Sobottka A, Heidenreich A, et al. Pelvic floor exercises, electrical stimulation and biofeedback after radical prostatectomy: results of a prospective randomized trial. J Urol 2003;170:490–493.

76. Moore KN, Griffiths D, Hughton A. Urinary incontinence after radical prostatectomy: a randomized controlled trial comparing pelvic muscle exercises with or without electrical stimulation. BJU Int 1999;83:57–65.

77. Faerber GJ, Richardson TD. Long term results of transurethral collagen injection in men with intrinsic sphincter deficiency. J Endourol 1997;11:273–277.

78. Cummings JM, Boullier JA, Parra RO. Transurethral collagen injection in the therapy of post radical prostatectomy stress incontinence. J Urol 1996;155:1011–1013.

79. Cespedes RD, O'Connell HE, McGuire EJ. Collagen injection therapy for the treatment of male urinary incontinence. J Urol 1996;155:1458A.

80. Politano VA, Stanisic TH, Jennings CE, et al. Transurethral polytef injection for post-prostatectomy urinary incontinence. A urodynamic and fluoroscopic point of view [Surgical therapy of urinary incontinence in the male]. A bladder behavior clinic for post prostatectomy patients. Br J Urol 1992;69:26–28.

81. Bevan-Thomas R, Wesley OL, Cespedes RD, et al. Long term follow up of periurethral collagen injection for male intrinsic deficiency. J Urol 1999;166:257.

82. Cespedes RD. Collagen injection or artificial sphincter for post-prostatectomy incontinence. Urology 1999;55:5–7.

83. Wainstein MA, Klutke CG. Antegrade techniques of collagen injection for post-prostatectomy stress urinary incontinence: the Washington University experience. World J Urol 1997;15:310–315.

84. Marks JL, Light JK. Management of urinary incontinence after prostatectomy with the artificial urinary sphincter. J Urol 1989;142:145–1461.

85. Fishman IJ, Shabsigh R, Scott FB. Experience with the artificial sphincter AS800 in 148 patients. J Urol 1989;141:307.

86. Venn SN, Greenwell TJ, Mundy AR. The long term outcome of artificial urinary sphincters. J Urol 2000;164:702–707.

87. Manunta A, Guille F, Patard JJ et al. Artificial sphincter insertion after radiotherapy: is it worthwhile? BJU Int 2000;85:490.

88. Gomha MA, Boone TB. Artificial urinary sphincter for post-prostatectomy incontinence in men who had prior radiotherapy: a risk and outcome analysis. J Urol 2002;167:591–596.

89. Clemens JQ, Bushman W, Schaeffer AJ. Questionnaire based results of the bulbourethral sling procedure. J Urol 1999;162:1972–1976.

90. Ullrich NFE, Comiter CV. The male sling for stress urinary incontinence: 24 month follow up with questionnaire based assessment. J Urol 2004;172:207–209.

91. Elliot DS, Boone TB. Combined stent and artificial urinary sphincter for management of severe recurrent bladder neck contracture and stress incontinence after prostatectomy: a long term evaluation. J Urol 2001;165:413–415.

92. McCammon KA, Kolm P, Main B, et al. Comparative quality of life analysis after radical prostatectomy or external beam radiation for localised prostate cancer. Urology 1999;54:509–516.

93. Moore KN, Estey A. The early postoperative concerns of men after radical prostatectomy. J Adv Nurs 1999;29:1121–1129.

94. Brockopp DY, Hayko D, Davenport W, et al. Personal control and the needs for hope and information among adults diagnosed with cancer. Cancer Nurs 1989;12:112–116.

95. Moul JW, Mooneyhan RM, Kao TC, et al. Preoperative and operative factors to predict incontinence, impotence and stricture after radical prostatectomy. Prostate Cancer Prostatic Dis 1998;1:242–249.

96. Shrader-Bogen CL, Kjellberg JL, McPherson CP, et al. Quality of life and treatment outcomes: prostate carcinoma patients' perspectives after prostatectomy or radiation therapy, Cancer 1997;79:1977–1986.

Rehabilitation of sexual function following definitive treatment of local prostate cancer

95

Francesco Montorsi, Alberto Briganti, Andrea Salonia, Patrizio Rigatti

INTRODUCTION

Radical prostatectomy is an increasingly used therapeutic option for patients with clinically localized prostate cancer and a life expectancy of at least 10 years.[1] The pioneering work by Walsh and Donker[2] significantly contributed to the understanding of the surgical anatomy of the prostate and posed the bases for the subsequent development of the anatomic radical prostatectomy technique, i.e., a surgical approach aimed at completely excising the prostate providing optimal cancer control while maintaining the integrity of the anatomic structures devoted to the functions of urinary continence and sexual potency.[3–5] Since the initial reports on this technique, an increasing number of studies have reported very satisfactory postoperative rates of urinary continence, while the preservation of erectile function after surgery has clearly been shown to be a major challenge for most urologists.[6–8] This finding contributed to the development of an increasing interest in the elucidation of the pathophysiology of postoperative erectile dysfunction (ED) and on its potential prophylaxis and treatment.[9,10] Furthermore ED after radical prostatectomy shows a profound effect on quality of life (QoL). Indeed, it has been shown that more than 70% of patients who had undergone radical retropubic prostatectomy had a moderately or severely affected QoL because of their postoperative ED, when investigated.[11] Moreover, although the International Index of Erectile Function (IIEF)[12] has been widely accepted as a validated instrument to assess ED, it has it has been demonstrated that different definitions of potency after surgery yield different results when applied to the same patients in the same time. This underlines the observation that sexual function entails more than penile erection as the classic definition of potency firm enough for intercourse in fact demonstrated variable agreement.[13]

PATIENT SELECTION

The anatomic nerve-sparing approach to the prostate is considered for patients with clinically localized prostate cancer. Patients with clinical stages T1 and T2, as defined following digital rectal examination and/or transrectal ultrasonography of the prostate, are the best candidates. As clinical stage is often correlated to both prostate-specific antigen (PSA) values and the biopsy Gleason sum, it has been suggested that a nerve-sparing approach may be considered in patients with PSA less than 10 ng/mL and a Gleason sum of 7 or less.[14]

Patients being considered for a nerve-sparing radical prostatectomy should be potent prior to the procedure. This is of major importance as patients who report some degree of ED or patients who use phosphodiesterase type 5 inhibitors (PDE5Is) prior to the procedure are more likely to develop severe ED after the procedure itself.[15] The use of validated questionnaires such as the IIEF[12] may facilitate the diagnosis of preoperative ED during the initial patient assessment. This questionnaire assesses various domains of male sexuality, including erectile and ejaculatory function, orgasm, desire, and intercourse satisfaction, and by reviewing the results of this patient self-assessment interesting baseline information are always obtained. Morphology of the corpora cavernosa deteriorates with aging, and this may be correlated with the high prevalence of ED seen in the aging men.[16] Rates of recovery of erectile function after a nerve-sparing radical prostatectomy are inversely correlated with the patient's age, i.e., best postoperative potency rates are obtained in the younger patient population, and it seems reasonable to consider patients of 65 years of age or less as candidates for a nerve-sparing procedure.[3] Patient age seems to be one of the most important factors for the recovery of sexual potency also after unilateral nerve sparing surgery. Indeed, in a group of 46 patients who received unilateral nerve-sparing radical retropubic prostatectomy, 14 (30.4%) regained full potency after surgery and, in the vast majority of them, recovery occurred within a period of 18 months. Of these patients, those aged less than 60 years reported the highest rate of recovery of potency, sufficient for vaginal penetration, after a mean of 13 months after surgery.[17] Comorbid conditions seem also to affect the recovery of spontaneous erections postoperatively as they may impact on the baseline penile hemodynamics. Therefore, a concomitant diagnosis of diabetes mellitus, hypertension, ischemic heart disease, hypercholesterolemia, or history of cigarette smoking identified at the time of the preoperative patient assessment should be taken into account as a potential negative predictive factor for potency recovery after surgery.[15] Although a higher prostate volume could be associated with higher intraoperative bleeding, it does not seem to influence postoperative potency rate.[18,19] Nevertheless, body weight does not seem to be related with the feasibility of a nerve-sparing approach, even in clinically obese patients.[19]

SURGICAL TECHNIQUE

In suitable candidates, radical excision of the prostate should be performed with the objective of achieving total cancer control (i.e., removing all cancer present in the prostatic tissue), while maintaining the integrity of the anatomic structures on which urinary continence and erectile function are based (i.e., the corpora cavernosa receive the innervation responsible for erections through the cavernosal nerves which branch out from the pelvic plexus). This latter structure is located adjacent to the tip of the seminal vesicles on the anterolateral wall of the rectum and may be damaged during radical prostatectomy. The cavernous nerves course adjacent to small vessels forming the so-called neurovascular bundle along the posterolateral margin of the prostate, bilaterally, and are located between the visceral layer of the endopelvic fascia and the prostatic fascia. The neurovascular bundles are located at the 5 and 7 o'clock positions at the level of the membranous urethra and, after piercing the urogenital diaphragm, they enter the corpora cavernosa where they innervate

the smooth muscle cells of the penile vessel walls and sinusoids.[20]

Based on the better understanding of the surgical anatomy of the prostate, Walsh has clearly described the technique of anatomic radical prostatectomy in a step-by-step fashion.[20] The use of a frontal xenon light and of magnifying loupes significantly improves vision during the procedure, and I feel that this armamentarium should be always used when performing nerve-sparing radical prostatectomies. Some crucial surgical steps deserve particular attention. Following pelvic lymphadenectomy, the endopelvic fascia is incised to allow the dissection of the prostatic apex. Care should be taken to ligate small branches of pudendal vessels, which are located just underneath the endopelvic fascia in the area of the prostatic apex; cautery should not be used to secure these vessels in order to avoid damage to pudendal nerve branches also located there. Ligation of the Santorini's plexus is a fundamental step in the procedure as it must guarantee perfect hemostasis in order to obtain the best visualization of the surgical field during the excision of the prostate. Walsh has suggested ligation of the Santorini's plexus distally first, with its subsequent division with scissors; control of the proximal stump of the venous plexus is then achieved with a V-shaped suture, which avoids a central retraction of the neurovascular bundles, thus facilitating the nerve sparing procedure. After controlling and dividing the Santorini's plexus, the visceral layer of the endopelvic fascia should be bluntly incised on the lateral side of the prostate to allow for the gentle lateral displacement of the neurovascular bundles, which is achieved with the use of small sponge sticks. If this maneuver is performed correctly, the neurovascular bundles become clearly visible along their entire course from the membranous urethra and the seminal vesicles in most patients. It is of mandatory importance to avoid the use of the cautery during every step of the prostatic excision as this can facilitate a definitive damage of the neurovascular bundles. As the pelvic plexus is located adjacent to the posterolateral tips of the seminal vesicles, particular care should be taken while excising them. The possible advantage of partially excising of the seminal vesicles to reduce the risk of damaging the pelvic plexus has been reported.[21] Hemostasis must be accurate, and this is usually obtained with small-sized clips. When pelvic hematomas occur, it is advisable to drain them surgically as the fibrosis occurring after the slow spontaneous resolution of any blood collection significantly lengthens the duration of cavernosal neuropraxia. Reviewing the videotapes of one's own nerve-sparing radical prostatectomies and comparing the surgical technique with the results seen in terms of margins status, urinary continence, and erectile function may be of significant importance, as it allows to identify the parts of the operation that are at higher risks for surgical errors from the surgeon.[22]

PATHOPHYSIOLOGY OF ERECTILE DYSFUNCTION FOLLOWING NERVE SPARING RADICAL PROSTATECTOMY

Patients undergoing nerve-sparing radical prostatectomy often experience impairment of erections in the early postoperative period. This has been related to the development of neuropraxia, which is believed to be caused by some damage to the cavernosal nerves that inevitably occurs during the excision of the prostate, even in the hands of most experienced surgeons. Absence of early postoperative erections is associated with poor corporeal oxygenation, which may facilitate the development of corporeal fibrosis, ultimately leading to veno-occlusive dysfunction.[23] Recently, the role of apoptosis has been considered in the pathophysiology of post-prostatectomy ED. Apoptosis, or programmed cell death, is essential for the normal development of multicellular organism as well as for physiologic cell turnover. Morphologically this phenomenon is characterized by chromatin condensation, membrane blebbing, and cell volume loss. In the penis, chronic hypoxia and denervation have been shown to stimulate apoptosis: it is possible that cellular apoptosis leads to increased deposition of connective tissue, which may finally lead to a decrease in penile distensibility.[24–27] Recently, User et al[28] have elegantly elucidated the role of apoptosis in the pathophysiology of post-prostatectomy ED in the rat model. Post-pubertal rats were randomized to bilateral or unilateral cavernous nerve transection versus a sham operation. At different time intervals following the procedure, penile wet weight, DNA content, and protein content were measured. Tissue sections of the penis were stained for apoptosis, and the apoptotic index was calculated. Finally, staining for endothelial and smooth muscle cells was done to identify the apoptotic cell line. Wet weight of the denervated penises was significantly decreased after bilateral cavernous neurotomy, while unilateral cavernous neurotomy allowed much greater preservation of penile weight. DNA content was also significantly reduced in bilaterally denervated penises, while no difference was found between unilaterally denervated penises and controls. Bilateral cavernous neurotomy induced significant apoptosis, which peaked on postoperative day 2. In addition, it was found that most apoptotic cells were located just beneath the tunica albuginea of the corpus cavernosum, i.e., the anatomical area where the subtunical venular plexus is located. Finally, the authors found that apoptotic cells were smooth muscle cells and not endothelial cells. The subsequent hypothesis suggested by the authors was that the bilateral injury to the cavernous nerves may induce significant apoptosis of smooth muscle cells, particularly in the subtunical area, thus causing an abnormality of the veno-occlusive mechanism of the corpus cavernosum. Apoptosis seems to play a role also in the genesis of ED seen in the aging population (which is clearly of crucial importance in the radical prostatectomy patient group) as it has been shown that antiapoptotic genes and proteins are expressed in young rats but not in aging rats.[24] These findings on apoptosis following radical prostatectomy confirm the known fact that most patients reporting postoperative ED develop massive corporeal venous leaks in the long term.[29] However, a reduction of the arterial inflow to the corpora cavernosa in patients with post-prostatectomy ED has been reported by several authors as a significant etiological cofactor.[30,31] In conclusion, the postoperative combination of reduced penile arterial inflow and excessive venous outflow due to the apoptosis-induced damage of the veno-occlusive mechanism leads to reduced oxygen transport and increased production of transforming growth factor-β. This subsequently causes significant tissue damage, i.e., increased corporeal fibrosis, which not only is at the root of the known penile hemodynamic abnormality but also is probably causing the postoperative decrease of penile length, recently reported in an interesting study.[32]

PHARMACOLOGIC PROPHYLAXIS AND TREATMENT OF POSTOPERATIVE ERECTILE DYSFUNCTION

PROPHYLAXIS

The better understanding of pathophysiology of post-prostatectomy ED, including the concept of tissue damage induced by poor corporeal oxygenation, paved the way for the application of pharmacologic regimens aimed at improving early postoperative corporeal blood filling. Montorsi et al[33] showed that by using intracorporeal injections of alprostadil early after a bilateral nerve-sparing radical prostatectomy the rate of recovery of spontaneous erections was significantly higher than observation alone. In the author's experience, alprostadil injection therapy should be started as soon as possible after the procedure, usually at the end of the first postoperative month. The initial dose is alprostadil 5 µg. Patients should be instructed to use injections 2 or 3 times per week in order to obtain penile tumescence; injections are not necessarily associated with sexual intercourse, but it is clear that if the patient desires, he may be able to resume satisfactory sexual intercourse with penetration as soon as he is able to identify the correct dosing of the drug. Brock et al[34] have also shown that the continuous use of intracavernous alprostadil injection therapy was able to significantly improve penile hemodynamics and the return of spontaneous erections (either partial or total) in patients with arteriogenic ED, thus confirming a potential curative role of this therapeutic modality in selected patients. The early postoperative use of intracavernosal injection therapy may exert also a significant psychological role. Commonly, after a nerve sparing radical prostatectomy with the slow return of spontaneous erections, a dysfunctional sexual dynamic may develop in couples. The patient withdraws sexually as he is increasingly discouraged with his lack of erectile function, which is a constant reminder of his cancer. The female partner, relieved that the patient has survived the surgery, may be satisfied with his companionship and is not anxious to upset him by making sexual overtures that may frustrate him. Successful intracorporeal injection therapy early after radical prostatectomy may contribute to breaking this negative cycle.[15]

The advent of PDE5Is in the treatment of ED has clearly revolutionized the management of this medical condition. This class of agents acts within the smooth muscle cell by inhibiting the enzyme phosphodiesterase type 5, which naturally degrades cyclic guanosine monophosphate (cGMP) an intracellular nucleotide which acts as second messenger in the process smooth muscle cell relaxation. The cascade of intracellular events that leads to the relaxation of the smooth muscle cell is initiated by the release of nitric oxide, which follows sexual stimulation. Both intracorporeal cavernous nerve terminals and endothelium release nitric oxide, which as a gas diffuses into the smooth muscle cells and activates the enzyme guanylate cyclase, which ultimately catalyzes the reaction from guanosine triphosphate (GTP) to cGMP. Increased levels of cGMP lead to the activation of cGMP-specific protein kinases that activate further intracellular events leading to the final reduction of intracellular calcium—this being associated with smooth muscle cell relaxation. At present, sildenafil, tadalafil, and vardenafil are approved for clinical use in the European Union and have been utilized also to treat post-prostatectomy ED. The rationale for the use of these drugs as prophylaxics is not yet well understood. The basic concept would be to administer a PDE5I at bedtime in order to facilitate the occurrence of nocturnal erections, which are believed to have a natural protective role on the baseline function of the corpora cavernosa. Montorsi et al showed that when sildenafil citrate 100 mg is administered at bedtime in patients with ED of various etiologies, the overall quality of nocturnal erections as recorded with the RigiScan device is significantly better than those obtained after the administration of placebo.[35] Padma-Nathan et al[36] recently reported on the prospective administration of sildenafil 50 and 100 mg versus placebo, daily and at bedtime, in patients undergoing bilateral nerve sparing radical prostatectomy who were potent preoperatively. Four weeks after surgery, patients were randomized to sildenafil or placebo which were administered for 36 weeks. Eight weeks after

discontinuation of treatment, erectile function was assessed with the question "Over the past 4 weeks, have your erections been good enough for satisfactory sexual activity?" and by IIEF and nocturnal penile tumescence assessments. Responders were defined as those having a combined score of 8 or more for IIEF questions 3 and 4, and a positive response to the above question. Twenty seven percent of the patients receiving sildenafil were responders (i.e., demonstrated a return of spontaneous normal erectile function) compared with 4% in the placebo group ($P = 0.0156$). Postoperative nocturnal penile tumescence (NPT) assessments were supportive. I believe that in the hands of experienced surgeons, a 27% overall rate of return to normal erectile function after a bilateral nerve-sparing procedure is far from being impressive but the important message from this study is that daily bedtime administration of sildenafil 50 or 100 mg after this procedure should be able to improve every surgeon's baseline results. Although similar data are not available yet for tadalafil and vardenafil, I believe there is no reason not to expect similar findings with these drugs. In practical terms, I feel that the need for postoperative prophylactic therapy should be discussed with the patient when counseling him about radical prostatectomy as one of the treatment options for prostate cancer. Patients must also have the chance to guide their choice by being informed of the pharmacologic approaches needed to recover a normal postoperative erectile function.

TREATMENT

PHOSPHODIESTERASE TYPE 5 INHIBITORS

Phosphodiesterase type 5 inhibitors have acquired an established role in the treatment of post-prostatectomy ED. As the mechanism of action of this class of drugs implies the presence of nitric oxide within the corporeal smooth muscle cells, only patients undergoing a nerve-sparing procedure should be expected to respond to these agents. Sildenafil is the drug that has been studied more extensively in this patient subgroup as it has been on the market worldwide since 1998. In general terms, it is now known that sildenafil gives the best results in young patients (those less than 60-years-old responding the best), in patients treated with a bilateral nerve-sparing procedure, and in patients who show some degree of spontaneous postoperative erectile function. Sildenafil is usually administered at the largest available dose, although it is common experience to have post-prostatectomy patients responding to the 25 and 50 mg doses. Typically the response to sildenafil has been shown to improve with time after the procedure: best results are seen from 12 to 24 months postoperatively.[5,37-41] Unfortunately, no data from multicenter, randomized, placebo controlled trials assessing sildenafil in patients undergoing nerve-sparing radical prostatectomy are available to date. It has been suggested that the early postoperative prophylactic administration of alprostadil injections allowed a subsequent better response rate for sildenafil, with lower doses of the drug being necessary.[42] Raina et al recently reported the long-term results of sildenafil use in patients affected by ED after radical prostatectomy.[43] This study enrolled 91 patients stratified according to the type of nerve-sparing procedure they had undergone: bilateral nerve sparing (n = 53), unilateral nerve sparing (n = 12) and non-nerve-sparing (n = 26) radical retropubic prostatectomy. All patients, at least 3 months after surgery, were prescribed sildenafil with the starting dose of 50 mg, which was titrated up to 100 mg in cases with unsatisfactory responses. At the 12-month assessment, performed by completion of Sexual Health Inventory of men (SHIM) and Erectile Dysfunction Inventory for Treatment Satisfaction (EDITS) questionnaires, 48 out of the 91 patients enrolled (52.7%) reported successful vaginal intercourse. This percentage increased to 71.7% (38 out of 53) if only those who had had the bilateral nerve-sparing approach were considered. Moreover, at the 3-year follow-up assessment, 31 out of 43 (72%) patients who returned the questionnaires were still using sildenafil for sexual intercourse, with a variable degree of partial erections. Interestingly, when the responses were stratified according to the neurovascular bundle status, the magnitude of improvement in SHIM score over time was greater in the bilateral nerve-sparing group than unilateral nerve-sparing and non-nerve-sparing groups. This data suggests how the vast majority of the patients affected by ED after radical prostatectomy who initially respond to sildenafil continue to do so and are satisfied with the treatment regimen. Furthermore, early use of high-dose sildenafil after radical prostatectomy seems to be associated with preservation of smooth muscle content within human corpora cavernosa. Indeed, Schwartz et al enrolled 40 potent patients affected by localized prostate cancer who underwent radical retropubic prostatectomy at a single institution and were subsequently treated either with daily sildenafil 50 mg (group 1) or 100 mg (group 2) for 6 months starting from the day of catheter removal.[44] Patients underwent percutaneous penile biopsy both preoperatively (under general anesthesia prior to surgical incision) and 6 moths after surgery (using local anesthesia). Interestingly, while in group 1 there was no statistically significant difference change in the mean intracavernosal smooth muscle content between the preoperative and postoperative measurements (51.1% and 52.6%, respectively), in group 2 a statistically significant increase in mean smooth muscle content after surgery (42.8% versus 56.8%; $P < 0.05$) was found. Therefore, although it remains unclear how the chronic administration of sildenafil could increase the intracavernosal smooth muscle content after surgery, daily high-dose administration of PDE5Is may be a key factor in the cavernosal smooth muscle preservation, thus reinforcing the idea of the clinical application of sexual pharmacologic prophylaxis after surgery.

Vardenafil has been tested in patients treated with ED following a unilateral or bilateral nerve-sparing prostatectomy in a multicenter, prospective, placebo-controlled, randomized study done in the US and Canada. This was a 12-week parallel-arm study comparing placebo to vardenafil 10 and 20 mg. In this study, sildenafil failures were excluded. Seventy-one percent and 60% of patients treated with a bilateral nerve-sparing procedure reported an improvement of erectile function following the administration of vardenafil 20 mg and 10 mg, respectively. A positive answer to SEP question 2 ("Were you able to insert your penis into your partner's vagina?") was seen in 47% and 48% of patients using vardenafil 10 and 20 mg, respectively. A positive answer to the more challenging SEP question 3 ("Did your erections last long enough to have successful intercourse?") was seen in 37% and 34% of patients using vardenafil 10 and 20 mg, respectively[45]

Tadalafil was also evaluated in a large multicenter trial conducted in Europe and in the US involving patients with ED following a bilateral nerve sparing procedure. Seventy-one percent of patients treated with tadalafil 20 mg reported the improvement of their erectile function compared with 24% of those treated with placebo ($P < 0.001$). The erectile function domain score of the IIEF was significantly higher after treatment with tadalafil 20 mg compared with placebo, and this difference was clinically significant (21.0 versus 15.2; $P < 0.001$).[12] Tadalafil 20 mg allowed a 52% rate of successful intercourse attempts, which was significantly higher than the 26% obtained with a placebo ($P < 0.001$).[46]

The adverse event profile of the three PDE5Is was very similar in this patient population, and I feel that discontinuation from treatment with one of the PDE5Is is usually caused by lack of efficacy, while tolerability is overall more than satisfactory. There is a necessity to obtain comparative data between the three drugs in terms of efficacy, safety, tolerability, and overall patient preference also in this challenging patient population . Well-designed head-to-head trials are ongoing at present, and this information will become available soon.

OTHER MEDICAL TREATMENTS

Patients either who do not respond to or who cannot use PDE5Is are typical candidates for second-line pharmacologic treatments, which currently include the intraurethral and the intracorporeal administration of alprostadil. The most recent information on the use of intraurethral alprostadil use suggests that its combination with oral sildenafil may salvage a significant proportion of sildenafil failures.[47,48] Intracorporeal injection therapy with alprostadil is effective in the majority of post-prostatectomy patients, regardless of the status of their cavernosal nerves (Figure 95.1). Recently, Gontero et al have shown that the best clinical and hemodynamic response with alprostadil injection therapy is seen 1 month after the procedure, but that the attrition rate for this approach is high when it is started early after surgery. They proposed that, in order to optimize long-term success with intracavernous injections of alprostadil, this treatment should be started 3 months after surgery.[49] In my experience, the use of alprostadil monotherapy should be matched against the use of the combination of alprostadil, papaverine, and phentolamine mesilate. Patients treated with the three-drug combination obtain very high response rates, and report penile pain, the typical adverse event related to alprostadil, only rarely.[50] The major disadvantage of the use of the three-drug combination is caused by its non-availability on the market, which obliges the urologist to prepare the solution and then distribute it to the patient. This off-label use requires the approval of the Ethics Committee of the hospital and a signed informed consent from the patient. In a retrospective study conducted by Raina et al, 102 patients using intracorporeal injections for ED following radical prostatectomy, were assessed by means of preoperative and postoperative SHIM administration a mean of 4 ± 2.2 years after surgery.[51] Of these 102 patients, 40 had a bilateral nerve-sparing, 19 a unilateral nerve-sparing, and 43 a non-nerve-sparing procedure. Injection therapy, based on use of either PGE1 alone (10 or 20 μg/mL in normal saline; 61%) or high-dose (20 μg/mL PGE1 + 1 μg/mL phentolamine + 30 μg/mL papaverine; 19%) or low-dose (5.88 μg/mL PGE1 + 0.59 μg/mL phentolamine + 17.65 μg/mL papaverine) (20%) triple therapy, was started a mean of 9 months (range: 6–12) after surgical procedure. Overall, 68% (69/102) of the patients achieved and maintained an erection sufficient for sexual intercourse and 48% (49/102) of the patients continued a long-term therapy. This excellent long-term efficacy, despite the type of the intracavernosal compound used, has also been associated with a high compliance that reached up to 70% of patients. Although no statistically significant differences have been reported between the three-drug formulations, no mention has been made by the authors regarding eventual differences in local or systemic side effects.

CAVERNOUS NERVE RECONSTRUCTION

Cavernous nerve reconstruction has generated great interest recently for preserving erectile function after radical prostatectomy. The interest is guided by the premise that nerve grafts provide a scaffold for autonomic nerve regrowth and reconnection with targets that mediate erectile function. Original preclinical studies by Quinlan et al[52] and Ball et al[53] using the genitofemoral nerve as a replacement for resected cavernous nerves in rats introduced the possibility of interposition nerve grafting for the recovery of erectile function after injury of the penile innervation. The surgical application was extended to the human level in the context of radical prostatectomy initially by Walsh who used the genitofemoral nerve as an autologous nerve graft[54] and subsequently by Kim et al[55] who applied the sural nerve as a conduit.

Kim et al described definite promise for cavernous nerve interposition grafting based on their success.[55–60] Among several reports by this group, they described their extended experience involving 28 men undergoing bilateral sural nerve grafting at radical prostatectomy (with a mean follow up of 23 months), of whom 6 of 23 (26%) men completing IIEF questionnaires had

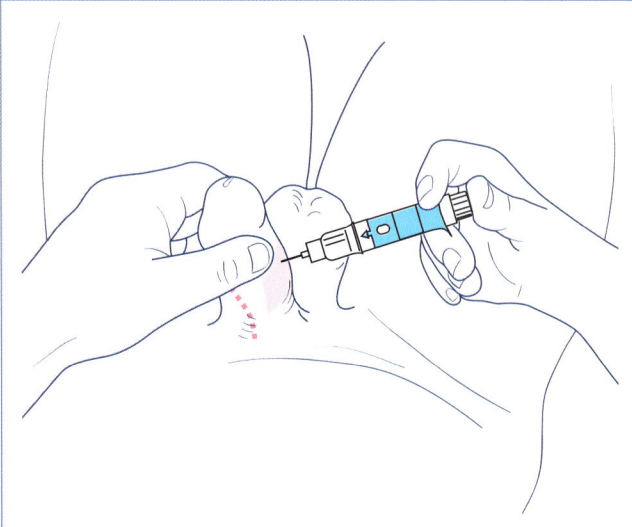

Figure 95.1
The intracavernosal injection of alprostadil is usually effective regardless of the status of the cavernosal nerves.

spontaneous, medically unassisted erections sufficient for sexual intercourse and an IIEF erectile function domain score of 20.[56] Their inclusion of 4 additional men whose partial erections were enhanced sufficiently to allow sexual intercourse using sildenafil resulted in an overall potency rate of 43% (10 of 23).[56] They also identified the benefit of unilateral sural nerve grafting based on a 78% erectile function rate with this treatment (compared with the 30% rate without grafting), which approximated the level of recovery observed in their hands for men having undergone bilateral nerve-sparing surgery (79%).[55,56]

Other groups have also described their early experiences with sural nerve grafting after radical prostatectomy. Anastasiadis et al described 4 of 12 (33%) men who achieved spontaneous erections sufficient for intercourse based on an IIEF erectile function domain score of 20 (with a mean follow up of 16 months) after unilateral nerve grafting (including one man recovering erections who required bilateral cavernous nerve excision).[61] Chang et al determined that 18 of 30 (60%) patients who underwent bilateral autologous sural nerve grafting achieved spontaneous erectile ability and 13 of these 30 (43%) were able to have intercourse (with a mean follow-up of 23 months).[62]

The evolution of the procedure has related to the application of a variety of technical modifications. One such modification is the use of electrical stimulation to confirm the function and location of the recipient nerve.[58-62] Additional recommendations include the use of microsurgical instruments and loupe magnification, and attention to such procedural details as maintenance of hemostasis within the surgical field and completion of grafting without tension. The feasibility of sural nerve grafting by a laparoscopic approach has also been demonstrated.[63]

Before assigning the fundamental utility of cavernous nerve interposition grafting as for any innovation, the procedure must withstand a critical process of evaluation. Clearly, advantages of sural nerve grafting include the autogenous basis for the nerve conduit, which confers biocompatibility without apparent immunogenicity, as well as support from earlier demonstrations that autonomic nerve replacement grafting succeeds.[64-66] The reportedly negligible functional compromise or consequence from the donor site also represents a favorable consideration. However, concerns persist along the primary grounds that the procedure may be technically impracticable and infrequently useful. The first consideration relates to the difficulty in identifying and performing grafting in humans in which the cavernous nerve is contained within a heterogeneous structure of nerve fibers and blood vessels, unlike the rat in which the cavernous nerve is easily identifiable as a large, discrete cable-like structure. Of greater concern is the issue that the

majority of candidates for radical prostatectomy in the modern era of early prostate cancer detection are likely to be satisfactorily treated with nerve-sparing techniques that do not compromise the intent of cancer control. On this basis, the widespread applicability of this procedure may be questioned. Quite likely, the candidate selected for nerve grafting will have high-stage disease that is associated with a low probability of sexual function recovery after surgery and likely will require adjuvant therapy, further reducing the likelihood of the graft preserving erectile function.[54] A fair statement at this time may well be that this innovation requires further investigation, particularly through clinical trials, before establishing its optimal role.

CONCLUSIONS

Radical prostatectomy is an increasingly performed procedure in patients with prostate cancer. As the mean age of this patient subgroup is progressively declining due to the advent of prostate cancer screening programs, the demand for optimal postoperative quality of life is becoming more important. Erectile function can be preserved in patients undergoing a nerve sparing radical prostatectomy provided that the patient is rigorously selected prior to surgery and that an anatomic radical prostatectomy following the most modern templates is precisely performed. Pharmacologic prophylaxis, either with oral or intracavernosal drugs, may potentially have a significantly expanding role in the future strategies aimed at preserving postoperative erectile function. The advent of the on demand use of PDE5Is has clearly improved the overall postoperative potency rate also in this challenging subgroups of patients. Future management avenues including cavernous nerve reconstruction and neuroprotection strategies are based on interesting rationales but need to undergo the test of time.

REFERENCES

1. Holmberg L, Bill-Axelson A, Helgesen, et al. A randomised trial comparing radical prostatectomy with watchful waiting in early prostate cancer. N Engl J Med 200;2347:781–789.

2. Walsh PC, Donker PJ. Impotence following radical prostatectomy: insight into etiology and prevention. J Urol 1982;128:492–497.

3. Walsh PC, Marschke P, Ricker D, et al. Patient-reported urinary continence and sexual function after anatomic radical prostatectomy. Urology 2000;55:58–61.

4. Walsh PC. Radical prostatectomy for localized prostate cancer provides durable cancer control with excellent quality of life: a structured debate. J Urol 2000;163:1802–1807.

5. Rabbani F, Stapleton AM, Kattan MW, et al. Factors predicting recovery of erections after radical prostatectomy. J Urol 2000;164:1929–1934.

6. Stanford JL, Feng Z, Hamilton AS, et al. Urinary and sexual function after radical prostatectomy for clinically localized prostate cancer: The Prostate Cancer Outcomes Study. JAMA 2000;283:354–360.

7. Mulcahy JJ. Erectile function after radical prostatectomy. Semin Urol Oncol, 2000;18:71–75.

8. Lepor H. Practical considerations in radical retropubic prostatectomy. Urol Clin North Am 2003;30:363–368.

9. Montorsi F, Salonia A, Zanoni M, et al. Counselling the patient with prostate cancer about treatment-related erectile dysfunction. Curr Opin Urol 2001;11:611–617.

10. Meuleman EJ, Mulders PF. Erectile function after radical prostatectomy: a review. Eur Urol 2003;43:95–101.

11. Meyer JP, Gillat DA, Lockyer R, et al. The effect of erectile dysfunction on the qulity of life of men after radical prostatectomy. BJU Int 2003;92:929–931.

12. Rosen RC, Cappelleri JC, Gendrano N 3rd. The International Index of Erectile Function (IIEF): a state-of-the-science review. Int J Impot Res 2002;14:226–244.

13. Krupski TL, Saigal CS, Litwin MS. Variation in continence and potency by definition. J Urol 2003;170:1291–1294.

14. Aus G, Abbou CC, Pacik D, et al. Guidelines on prostate cancer. EAU Guidelines, 2005 (in Press).

15. McCullough AR. Prevention and management of erectile dysfunction following radical prostatectomy. Urol Clin North Am 2001;28:613–627.

16. Wespes E. Erectile dysfunction in the ageing man. Curr Opin Urol 2000;10:625–628.

17. Van der Aa F, Joniau S, De Ridder D, et al. Potency after unilateral nerve sparing surgery: a report on functional and oncological results of unilateral nerve sparing surgery. Pros Can Pros Dis 2003;6:61–65.

18. Foley CL, Bott SRJ, Parkinson MC, et al. A large prostate at radical retropubic prostatectomy does not adversely affect cancer control, continence or potency rate. BJU Int 2003;92:370–374.

19. Hsu EI, Hong EK, Lepor H. Influence of body weight and prostate volume on intraoperative, perioperative and postoperative outcomes after radical prostatectomy. Urology 2003;61.601–606.

20. Walsh PC. Anatomic radical retropubic prostatectomy. In: Walsh PC, Retik AB, Vaughan ED Jr, Wein AJ (eds): Campbell's Urology, 8th ed. Philadelphia: WB Saunders, 2002, pp 3107–3129.

21. Sanda MG, Dunn R, Wei JT, et al. Sexual function recovery after prostatectomy based on quantified pre-prostatectomy sexual function and use of nerve-sparing and seminal-vesicle-sparing surgical technique. J Urol 2003;4(Suppl):181.

22. Walsh PC, Marschke P, Ricker D et al. Use of intraoperative video documentation to improve sexual function after radical retropubic prostatectomy. Urology 2000;55:62–67.

23. Moreland RB. Is there a role of hypoxemia in penile fibrosis: a viewpoint presented to the Society for the Study of Impotence. Int J Impotence Res 1998;10:113–120.

24. Yamanaka M, Shirai M, Shiina H, et al. Loss of anti-apoptotic genes in aging rat crura. J Urol 2002;168:2296–2300.

25. Yao KS, Clayton M, O'Dwyer PJ. Apoptosis in human adenocarcinoma HT29 cells induced by exposure to hypoxia. J Natl Cancer Inst 1995;158:656–659.

26. Chung WS, Park YY, Kwon SW. The impact of aging on penile hemodynamics in normal responders to pharmacological injection: a Doppler sonographic study. J Urol 1997;157:2129–2131.

27. Klein LT, Miller MI, Buttyan R, et al. Apoptosis in the rat penis after penile denervation. J Urol 1997;158:626–630.

28. User HM, Hairston JH, Zelner DJ, et al. Penile weight and cell subtype specific changes in a post-radical prostatectomy model of erectile dysfunction. J Urol 2003;169:1175–1179.

29. De Luca V, Pescatori ES, Taher B, et al. Damage to the erectile function following radical pelvic surgery: prevalence of veno-occlusive dysfunction. Eur Urol 1996;29:36–40.

30. Mulhall JP, Slovick R, Hotaling J, et al. Erectile dysfunction after radical prostatectomy:hemodynamic profiles and their correlation with the recovery of erectile function. J Urol 2002;167:1371–1375.

31. Mulhall JP, Graydon RJ. The hemodynamics of erectile dysfunction following nerve-sparing radical retropubic prostatectomy. Int J Impot Res 1996;8:91–94.

32. Savoie M, Kim SS, Soloway MS. A prospective study measuring penile length in men treated with radical prostatectomy for prostate cancer. J Urol 2003;169:1462–1464.

33. Montorsi F, Guazzoni G, Strambi LF, et al. Recovery of spontaneous erectile function after nerve-sparing radical retropubic prostatectomy with and without early intracavernous injections of alprostadil: results of a prospective, randomised trial. J Urol 1997;158:1408–1410.

34. Brock G, Tu LM, Linet OI. Return of spontaneous erection during long-term intracavernosal alprostadil (Caverject) treatment. Urology 2001;57:536–541.

35. Montorsi F, Maga T, Strambi LF, et al. Sildenafil taken at bedtime significantly increases nocturnal erections: results of a placebo-controlled study. Urology 2000;20;56:906–911.

36. Padma-Nathan E, McCullough AR, Giuliano F, et al. Postoperative nightly administration of sildenafil citrate significantly improves the return of normal spontaneous erectile function after bilateral nerve-sparing radical prostatectomy. J Urol 2003;4(Suppl):375.

37. Zippe CD, Jhaveri FM, Klein EA, et al. Role of Viagra after radical prostatectomy. Urology 2000;55:241–245.

38. Lowentritt BH, Scardino PT, Miles BJ, et al. Sildenafil citrate after radical retropubic prostatectomy. J Urol 1999;162:1614–1617.

39. Hong EK, Lepor H, McCullough AR. Time dependent patient satisfaction with sildenafil for erectile dysfunction (ED) after nerve-sparing radical retropubic prostatectomy (RRP). Int J Impot Res1999;11 Suppl 1:S15–22.

40. Feng MI, Huang S, Kaptein J, et al. Effect of sildenafil citrate on post-radical prostatectomy erectile dysfunction. J Urol 2000;164:1935–1938.

41. Blander DS, Sanchez-Ortiz RF, Wein AJ, et al. Efficacy of sildenafil in erectile dysfunction after radical prostatectomy. Int J Impot Res. 2000;12:165–168.

42. Montorsi F, Salonia A, Barbieri L, et al. The subsequent use of I.C. alprostadil and oral sildenafil is more efficacious than sildenafil alone in nerve sparing radical prostatectomy. J. Urol 2002;167:279 [abstract 1098].

43. Raina R, Lakin MM, Agarwal A, et al. Long-term effect of sildenafil citrate on erectile dysfunction after radical prostatectomy: 3-year follow-up. Urology 2003;62:110–115.

44. Scwartz EJ, Wong P, Graydon J. Sildenafil preserves intracorporeal smooth muscle after radical retropubis prostatectomy. J Urol 2004;171:771–774.

45. Brock G, Nehra A, Lipshultz LI, et al. Safety and efficacy of vardenafil for the treatment of men with erectile dysfunction after radical retropubic prostatectomy. J Urol 2003;170:1278–1283.

46. Montorsi F, Nathan HP, McCullough A, et al. Tadalafil in the treatment of erectile dysfunction following bilateral nerve sparing radical retropubic prostatectomy: a randomized, double-blind, placebo controlled trial. J Urol 2004;172:1036–1041.

47. Nehra A, Blute ML, Barrett DM, et al. Rationale for combination therapy of intraurethral prostaglandin E1 and sildenafil in the salvage of erectile dysfunction patients desiring noninvasive therapy. Int J Impot Res 2002;14 Suppl 1:S38–42.

48. Raina R, Oder M, Afarwal A, et al. Combination therapy: muse enhances sexual satisfaction in sildenafil citrate failures following radical prostatectomy (RP). J Urol 2003;4(Suppl):354.

49. Gontero P, Fontana F, Bagnasacco A, et al. Is there an optimal time for intracavernous prostaglandin E1 rehabilitation following nonnerve sparing radical prostatectomy? Results from a hemodynamic prospective study. J Urol 2003;169:2166–2169.

50. Montorsi F, Guazzoni G, Bergamaschi F, et al. Effectiveness and safety of multidrug intracavernous therapy for vasculogenic impotence. Urology 1993;42:554–558.

51. Raina R, Lakin MM, Thukral M, et al. Long-term efficacy and compliance of intracorporeal (ICI) injection for erectile dysfunction following radical prostatectomy: SHIM (IIEF-5) analysis. Int J Impot Res 2003;15:318–322.

52. Quinlan DM, Nelson RJ, Walsh PC. Cavernous nerve grafts restore erectile function in denervated rats. J Urol 1991;145:380–383.

53. Ball RA, Richie JP, Vickers MA Jr. Microsurgical nerve graft repair of the ablated cavernosal nerves in the rat. J Surg Res 1992;53:280–286.

54. Walsh PC. Nerve grafts are rarely necessary and are unlikely to improve sexual function in men undergoing anatomic radical prostatectomy. Urology 2001;57:1020–1024.

55. Kim ED, Scardino PT, Hampel O, et al. Interposition of sural nerve restores function of cavernous nerves resected during radical prostatectomy. J Urol 1999;161:188–192.

56. Kim ED, Scardino PT, Kadmon D, et al. Interposition sural nerve grafting during radical retropubic prostatectomy. Urology 2001;57:211–216.

57. Kim ED, Nath R, Kadmon D, et al. Bilateral nerve graft during radical retropubic prostatectomy: 1-year followup. J Urol 2001;165:1950–1956.

58. Scardino PT, Kim ED. Rationale for and results of nerve grafting during radical prostatectomy. Urology 2001;57:1016–1019.

59. Kim ED, Nath R, Slawin KM, et al. Bilateral nerve grafting during radical retropubic prostatectomy: extended follow-up. Urology 2001;58:983–987.

60. Canto EI, Nath RK, Slawin KM. Cavermap-assisted sural nerve interposition graft during radical prostatectomy. Urol Clin North Am 2001;28:839–848.

61. Anastasiadis AG, Benson MC, Rosenwasser MP, et al. Cavernous nerve graft reconstruction during radical prostatectomy or radical cystectomy: safe and technically feasible. Prostate Cancer Prostatic Dis 2003;6:56–60.

62. Chang DW, Wood CG, Krol, SS, et al. Cavernous nerve reconstruction to preserve erectile function following non-nerve-sparing radical retropubic prostatectomy: a prospective study. Plast Reconstr Surg 2003;111:1174–1181.

63. Turk IA, Deger S, Morgan WR, et al. Sural nerve graft during laparoscopic radical prostatectomy. Initial experience. Urol Oncol 2002;7:191–194.

64. Hammerschlag PE. Facial reanimation with jump interpositional graft hypoglossal facial anastomosis and hypoglossal facial anastomosis: evolution in management of facial paralysis. Larynogoscope 1999;109:1–23.

65. Hogikyan ND, Johns MM, Kileny PR, et al. Motion-specific laryngeal reinnervation using muscle-nerve-muscle neurotization. Ann Otol Rhinol Laryngol 2001;110:801–810.

66. Golub DM, Kheinman FB, Novikov II, et al. Reinnervation of internal organs and vessels by the neuropexy technic. Arkh Anat Gistol Embriol 1979;76:5–16.

The limitations of evidence-based comparisons of treatment for localized prostate cancer

96

Lars Ellison

INTRODUCTION

The primary goal of evidence-based medicine (EBM) is the rapid and efficient diffusion of new medical findings in order to effect rational changes in clinical practice patterns. To achieve this goal, analytic techniques for EMB rely heavily on the use of standard measures of patient outcome. For many disease states, reliance on patient outcome measures is not an impediment: for example, viral load counts and low-density lipoproteins (LDL) levels are effective outcome measures in human immunodeficiency virus (HIV) infection and cardiac disease, respectively.

However, measures of outcome for patients with localized prostate cancer are not standardized: there is no agreement on the use of prostate-specific antigen (PSA) as a biomarker, nor is there an accepted gold standard for the measurement of quality-of-life issues. In this chapter, I argue that the failure of the prostate cancer research community to identify standard endpoints for reporting treatment outcomes has resulted in a heterogeneous literature that defies the application of EMB techniques to comparisons of treatment for localized prostate cancer. Until such time as standard endpoints are agreed upon the development of best practice guidelines for treatment of localized prostate cancer using EBM will remain highly problematic.

BACKGROUND

The challenge of translating bench research to bedside patient care has always been difficult. Often the findings of basic science require multiple refinements prior to the development of meaningful and practical clinical applications. Since the end of World War II and the sudden expansion of medical funding in the United States, the guiding principal of medical practice has been the integration of detailed understanding of pathophysiology combined with "expert" interpretation regarding the best methods for treatment.[1] This marriage of scientific method and opinion thus form the nexus at which the practice of medicine becomes an "Art."

Expert opinion is intended to provide objective and informed practice recommendations. The strengths of this approach are self-evident. Experts tend to have a strong basic science background and, therefore, work at the interface between bench research and clinical application. Their broad knowledge as thought leaders gives them unique perspective regarding the relative value of new findings. In addition, these same individuals often are involved with key regulatory, policy and research funding decisions.

The problem with reliance of this form of analysis is that it is subject to a number of significant biases that, in the estimation of many, far outweigh the relative benefits.[2] The primary concern is that opinion may not represent the full spectrum of data. Often, these thought pieces reflect an aspect of the research agenda of the author and may not incorporate the findings of other lines of inquiry. The resulting unstructured analysis of the literature is subject to both intentional and unintentional omissions.[3] Second, not every important clinical observation has an *a priori* set of basic science findings. What is more, at times the underlying basic science may stand in stark contrast to the observed outcomes at the clinical level. While this may seem obvious, it is just this type of discordance that is subject to omission in an opinion-based system. When studies contradict basic science, or stand alone as observation, they tend to receive minimal attention.[4]

EVIDENCE-BASED MEDICINE CONCEPTS

It is from these criticisms of "expert opinion" that the competing concept of "evidence-based medicine" was born. In the late 1980s, individuals at Macallister University began to discuss the limitations of developing medical practice patterns in the face of an ever-increasing volume of scientific findings.[5] The primary concern was that the rapid expansion of medical literature was far outpacing the rate of change in medical practice. As a result of this expansion, it became necessary to develop systems for analyzing the quality of studies reported, and then rank ordering and aggregating data when possible.[6] While the concepts of meta-analysis and structured literature reviews had been described previously, these have served as the cornerstones for this new movement.

The accepted definition of EBM is "the explicit, judicious and conscientious use of current best evidence from health care research in decisions about the care of individuals and populations."[5] To achieve this end, three broad elements from the principals of clinical epidemiology arise for grading studies. First, the research question must be clearly identified and must address a clinically relevant issue. Unfortunately, for many peer reviewed journals this most basic of premises is not rigorously upheld.[7] Second, the study design must be concise, reproducible, and free of inherent biases. Many studies suffer from failure to use validated quality-of-life instruments or standard clinical endpoints. Third, the study population must resemble the usual clinical population. Highly selected subgroups modify treatment effect and result in blunted outcomes when applied to the general population. Finally, the outcomes measured must be relevant to patients. While biochemical measures may appease patient's anxiety, ultimately, the hard outcomes of morbidity and mortality are what drive patient adherence and compliance.

Rank ordering the importance of studies is the second step in this process. One particularly appealing ranking system is that used by the American Society of Clinical Oncology (ASCO).[8] Within this hierarchy, the randomized trial retains its position as the gold standard for study design. However, combining the data from multiple comparable studies in a scientific manner, the meta-analysis provides greater accuracy for point estimates of true clinical effect. Interestingly, it is important to note that committee reports and expert opinion hold a ranking below that of a clinical case series. This serves as a rather scathing indictment of what has traditionally been considered the preeminent method of disseminating new recommendations for clinical practice.

As the 1990s progressed, the EBM concept became the driving force behind efforts to take the lessons from published studies and, where appropriate, implement the findings into usual practice. The guiding principal is that scientific observations should define best practices. This necessitates that the system of evaluating studies for scientific and clinical merit is reliable and reproducible. On the surface, this appears as a perfectly reasonable application of sound epidemiologic and applied research analysis of study design and outcome.

FLUID ENDPOINTS ARE THE FAILURE OF PROSTATE CANCER RESEARCH

Prostate cancer is clearly a disease that has significant associated morbidity and mortality. There is mounting evidence that active treatment has beneficial effect on survival.[9] However, the indolent course of the disease means that survival, the one true hard outcome, requires years of observation.[10] Consequently, even large well-designed studies suffer from low event rates, loss of participants, and confounding medical conditions.

In order to circumvent this limitation, there has been a long and to date fruitless search for surrogate primary endpoints.[11-17] Prostate-specific antigen has been the obvious primary target of this search. The correlation with long-term survival and trends in PSA after definitive local therapy is weak at best. To be sure, recent findings regarding PSA velocity hold promise as prognostic indicators for specific subgroups of prostate cancer patients.[18] Indeed, the failure to predict recurrence has provided quality-of-life advocates fertile ground for active commentary regarding the relative value of the available primary treatments. The net result has been a slow but steady transition of the debate regarding the value of these treatments from that of "cancer control" and "survival" to that of preservation of "quality of life."

The primary failure of prostate cancer research is the absence of accepted standards for assessing and reporting outcomes after definitive therapy. It appears that the success of population-based prostate cancer screening has served as the primary driver in reductions in prostate cancer mortality since the mid-1990s. While the screening issue has not been without debate, the actual practice of screening when performed is relatively uniform, with set protocols prompting further evaluation of the patient. However, once initial treatment has been delivered, broad consensus on follow-up intervals and thresholds for definition of cancer control are lacking. This disconnect is a function of the failure of the radiation therapists and urologists to identify common biochemical trends shared by the competing treatment modalities.

Health-related quality of life (HRQOL) has also suffered from a lack of consensus of definitions. This is, in large part, due to the limitations of previously available instruments. As more accurate instruments have been developed, application of these to ever larger cohorts of men have been attempted.[19] To date, studies have been primarily limited to single institutions.[20]

I would argue that the inability to identify standard methods for assessing patient outcome has precluded prostate cancer from the benefits of widespread application of EBM analysis. Essentially, there is minimal capacity for comparisons of different treatments (radical prostatectomy [RP], external-beam radiotherapy [EBRT], and brachytherapy) because the various stakeholders have been incapable of agreeing on standard reporting schemes of patient outcomes.

UROLOGY

The plausibility that PSA is a biochemical surrogate for disease status after initial treatment of prostate cancer is in large part based on the observed performance of PSA as a screening tool. This argument is supported by multiple observational studies that have correlated the changes in serum concentration of PSA after RP with subsequent patient outcomes (local recurrence, development of metastases, and disease-specific mortality).

Partin et al reported a retrospective review of PSA trends in 955 men treated with RP over a 10-year period (1982–1991).[21] Of those men whose PSA became detectable, 28% developed evidence of local or metastatic disease. In addition, when stratified by postoperative year of failure, men with detectable PSA within the first year had significantly higher rates of progression than men with detectible PSA found after the first year.

The threshold for the definition of "detectible PSA" has been examined by a number of authors.[22,23] While a consensus on the critical absolute serum concentration of "detectible" PSA has not been reached (<0.1 ng/mL versus 0.2 ng/mL versus 0.4ng/mL), it has been accepted that the postoperative level should be very low and remain as such.

A rising PSA is accepted as a poor prognostic sign. Pound analyzed 1997 men treated with RP between 1982 and 1997.[24] In this case series 15% of men developed a rising PSA. Of these 304 men, the median time to metastasis was 8 years. The median survival from the time of the development of distant metastasis was 5 years. Furthermore, the authors identified time of biochemical recurrence, pathologic grade (Gleason score), and PSA doubling time as predictors of progression to metastatic disease.

The net result is that there are as many competing surveillance strategies as "thought leaders." As a result, the heterogeneity of study design precludes systematic aggregation of data and EBM-type generation of best practice guidelines.

RADIATION ONCOLOGY

In contrast to single institution reports and competing proposed criteria for cancer control in the urologic literature, the American Society for Therapeutic Radiology and Oncology (ASTRO) convened a consensus panel to develop a set of criteria for patients treated with radiation therapy for prostate cancer.[25] The report outlined the salient characteristics of PSA and a set of guidelines for post-treatment surveillance. Among the guiding principals were two key concepts. First, that post-treatment PSA nadir should be used in place of an absolute serum threshold. Second, that time of failure should be determined from backdating a sequentially rising PSA. The guidelines were intended to unify management within radiation oncology, and to set standards for reporting outcomes. Since the publication of the ASTRO criteria, a number of studies have critically appraised and offered refinement to the guidelines.

Reports in the radiation therapy literature have generally provided evidence that early trends in PSA using the ASTRO criteria predict general measures of disease control. Horwitz reported correlation between biochemical failure and 5-year actuarial distant metastasis-free survival, disease-free survival, cause-specific survival, and local control.[26] Despite the short follow-up, the authors determined that ASTRO defined biochemical failure appropriately predicted clinical outcome at 5 years. Following on this study, Shipley conducted a pooled analysis of 1765 men with clinically localized disease, treated at six different institutions between 1988 and 1995.[27] Using the ASTRO criteria, the PSA failure rate for a subset of men whose presentation PSA was less than 10 ng/mL was 22% at 5 years and 27% at 7 years.

More recently, others have suggested that PSA velocity may be a better predictor than consecutive rises, and alternatively that the threshold nadir of 1.0 ng/mL may provide better discrimination of probability of progression.[28]

ASTRO CRITERIA APPLIED TO SURGERY COHORTS

A number of researchers have attempted to apply the ASTRO criteria to post-RP patients. D'Amico reported trends in PSA failure using the ASTRO criteria as applied to a pooled two-institution data set of surgery, eternal-beam radiotherapy, and brachytherapy patients.[11] Relative risks of PSA failure by treatment modality and pretreatment risk groups were reported. Amling applied ASTRO criteria to RP patients.[29] While the analysis suggested a higher threshold for the definition of PSA recurrence might be more appropriate, they found the radiation therapy standard provided poor accounting of disease progression.

The definition of cancer control is critical. The absence of an accurate and broadly applicable yardstick for the assessment of prostate cancer treatment is a major problem. Urologists have attempted to use PSA thresholds as critical indicators of cancer control. Radiation therapists have applied PSA trends as the defining characteristics of cancer control. Either approach in isolation has significant limitations and biases one treatment over the other. Ultimately, the goal of a biochemical definition of cancer control is to guide appropriate initiation of adjuvant therapy. Currently, a single definition of cancer control does not exist. As long as there are heterogeneous definitions of cancer control, accurate evidence-based comparisons of treatments for localized prostate cancer will not be possible.

HEALTH-RELATED QUALITY-OF-LIFE INSTRUMENTS

While a single definition of cancer control has remained elusive, health-service researchers have begun to standardize the measurement of the known complications associated with the treatment of localized prostate cancer (e.g., urinary incontinence and impotence). The quality-of-life field has moved from simple studies measuring cross-sectional or retrospective HRQOL after treatment, to elegant longitudinal prospective models. Along with increased sophistication of study design, the instruments for measurement of quality of life have improved.

With the introduction of the University of California Los Angeles Prostate Cancer Index (UCLA-PCI), assessment of prostate cancer-specific HRQOL took a significant leap forward.[19] Prior instruments incorporated crude measures of general urinary and sexual function and were intended for use in men with advanced prostate cancer. The UCLA-PCI has been recently modified.[20] The new Expanded Prostate Cancer Index (EPIC) allows for accurate discrimination between the domains of urinary incontinence and irritative symptoms. In addition, the instrument quantifies the impact of hematuria, provides an expanded assessment of bowel function, and measures the impact of hormone ablation. These are critical domains when comparing the effects of surgery versus those of radiation therapy.

Application of the EPIC instrument to a retrospective cohort of patients treated either with RP or brachytherapy from a single institution was recently reported.[30] The results suggest that 1 year after treatment, brachytherapy patients have preponderance of irritative urinary symptoms, whereas surgery patients are more likely to have problems with urinary incontinence. In addition, the impact of hormonal symptoms on HRQOL appears much greater than previously appreciated.

It has been assumed that RP, EBRT, and brachytherapy each have an associated constellation of potential complications. The development and acceptance of a single instrument for measuring HRQOL is an important contribution. Application of such an instrument in a multi-institutional and multi-treatment longitudinal setting would provide robust benchmark data to which future trials data could be compared.

CONCLUSION

Prostate cancer is an important medical condition that has fallen victim to the tradition model of medical education in the United States. "Expert opinion" has failed to identify common standard endpoints to measure the performance of the various initial treatments for localized disease. The result is a heterogeneous body of literature that in large part does not lend itself to analysis using evidence-based measures. What is more, there is no will on the part of the treating stakeholders (urologists and radiation therapists) to accept that true equipoise exists regarding radical surgery and radiation therapy. The failures of the SPIRIT Trial to achieve recruitment goals, and my own personal experience attempting to initiate a cohort study comparing high-volume treatment centers underscores these barriers to change.

If prostate cancer patients are to benefit from rapid acceptance and diffusion of important clinically relevant medical advances, the treating community must first identify standard and well-defined outcome measures for biochemical cancer control as well as HRQOL. These standards must become the core of prostate cancer clinical trials. Additionally, the editors of major medical journals must embrace these as minimum standards to manuscripts entering into the peer review process. Until this happens EBM will remain an outsider to the debates that surround the treatment of localized prostate cancer.

REFERENCES

1. Haynes RB. What kind of evidence is it that Evidence-Based Medicine advocates want health care providers and consumers to pay attention to? BMC Health Serv Res 2002;2:3.

2. Woolf SH, Grol R, Hutchinson A, et al. Clinical guidelines: potential benefits, limitations, and harms of clinical guidelines. BMJ 1999;318:527–30.

3. Haynes RB, Wilczynski NL. Optimal search strategies for retrieving scientifically strong studies of diagnosis from Medline: analytical survey. BMJ 2004;328:1040.

4. Bornstein BH, Emler AC. Rationality in medical decision making: a review of the literature on doctors' decision-making biases. J Eval Clin Pract 2001;7:97–107.

5. Haynes RB. Evidence-based medicine and healthcare: advancing the practice. Singapore Med J 2004;45:407–409.

6. Upshur RE. Seven characteristics of medical evidence. J Eval Clin Pract 2000;6:93–97.

7. Seigel D. Clinical trials, epidemiology, and public confidence. Stat Med 2003;22:3419–3425.

8. Smith TJ, Somerfield MR. The ASCO experience with evidence-based clinical practice guidelines. Oncology (Huntingt) 1997;11:223–227.

9. Johansson JE, Andren O, Andersson SO, et al. Natural history of early, localized prostate cancer. JAMA 2004;291:2713–2719.

10. Neugut AI, Grann VR. Waiting time in prostate cancer. JAMA 2004;291:2757–2758.

11. D'Amico AV, Desjardin A, Chung A, et al. Assessment of outcome prediction models for patients with localized prostate carcinoma managed with radical prostatectomy or external beam radiation therapy. Cancer 1998;82:1887–1896.

12. de Reijke TM, Collette L. EORTC prostate cancer trials: what have we learnt? Crit Rev Oncol Hematol 2002;43:159–165.

13. Eisenberger M, Partin A. Progress toward identifying aggressive prostate cancer. N Engl J Med 2004;351:180–181.

14. Lieberman R, Nelson WG, Sakr WA, et al. Executive Summary of the National Cancer Institute Workshop: Highlights and recommendations. Urology 2001;57:4–27.

15. Scher HI, Mazumdar M, Kelly WK. Clinical trials in relapsed prostate cancer: defining the target. J Natl Cancer Inst 1996;88:1623–1634.

16. Schroder FH, Kranse R, Barbet N, et al. Prostate-specific antigen: A surrogate endpoint for screening new agents against prostate cancer? Prostate 2000;42:107–115.

17. Woolf SH, Rothemich SF. Screening for prostate cancer: the roles of science, policy, and opinion in determining what is best for patients. Annu Rev Med 1999;50:207–221.

18. D'Amico AV, Moul JW, Carroll PR, et al. Surrogate end point for prostate cancer-specific mortality after radical prostatectomy or radiation therapy. J Natl Cancer Inst 2003;95:1376–1383.

19. Litwin MS, Hays RD, Fink A, et al. The UCLA Prostate Cancer Index: development, reliability, and validity of a health-related quality of life measure. Med Care 1998;36:1002–1012.

20. Wei JT, Dunn RL, Litwin MS, et al. Development and validation of the expanded prostate cancer index composite (EPIC) for comprehensive assessment of health-related quality of life in men with prostate cancer. Urology 2000;56:899–905.

21. Partin AW, Pound CR, Clemens JQ, et al. Serum PSA after anatomic radical prostatectomy. The Johns Hopkins experience after 10 years. Urol Clin North Am 1993;20:713–725.

22. Patel A, Dorey F, Franklin J, et al. Recurrence patterns after radical retropubic prostatectomy: clinical usefulness of prostate specific antigen doubling times and log slope prostate specific antigen. J Urol 1997;158:1441–1445.

23. Zincke H, Oesterling JE, Blute ML, et al. Long-term (15 years) results after radical prostatectomy for clinically localized (stage T2c or lower) prostate cancer. J Urol 1994;152:1850–1857.

24. Pound CR, Partin AW, Eisenberger MA, et al. Natural history of progression after PSA elevation following radical prostatectomy. JAMA 1999;281:1591–1597.

25. Consensus statement: guidelines for PSA following radiation therapy. American Society for Therapeutic Radiology and Oncology Consensus Panel. Int J Radiat Oncol Biol Phys 1997;37:1035–1041.

26. Horwitz EM, Vicini FA, Ziaja EL, et al. The correlation between the ASTRO Consensus Panel definition of biochemical failure and clinical outcome for patients with prostate cancer treated with external beam irradiation. American Society of Therapeutic Radiology and Oncology. Int J Radiat Oncol Biol Phys 1998;41:267–272.

27. Shipley WU, Thames HD, Sandler HM, et al. Radiation therapy for clinically localized prostate cancer: a multi-institutional pooled analysis. JAMA 1999;281:1598–1604.

28. Critz FA, Williams WH, Holladay CT, et al. Post-treatment PSA < or = 0.2 ng/mL defines disease freedom after radiotherapy for prostate cancer using modern techniques. Urology 1999;54:968–971.

29. Amling CL, Bergstrath EJ, Blute ML, et al. Defining prostate specific antigen progression after radical prostatectomy: what is the most appropriate cut point? J Urol 2001;165:1146–1151.

30. Wei JT, Dunn RL, Sandler HM, et al. Comprehensive comparison of health-related quality of life after contemporary therapies for localized prostate cancer. J Clin Oncol 2002;20:557–566.

Treatment of locally advanced and metastatic prostate cancer

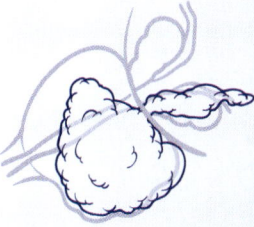

Hormonal therapy for prostate cancer: optimization and timing

97

David Kirk

INTRODUCTION

Hormone therapy is an effective treatment for prostate cancer and continues to have a key role in the management of the disease.[1] It is the only initial systemic treatment available for the man with advanced disease. Despite prostate-specific antigen (PSA) testing, many men still have incurable disease at diagnosis, and failure of curative treatment is often seen as an indication for hormonal treatment.[2] Disease presenting at an advanced stage where hormonal treatment is the only option continues to be common in many countries. Paradoxically, there may well now be more men who are candidates for hormonal treatment than ever before. There is also considerable interest in exploring the merits of adjuvant treatment[3] (Chapter 91)[CN]—the urologic equivalent of tamoxifen in breast cancer.

The effect of hormonal therapy on survival continues to be debated. However, doubts about the value of immediate versus deferred treatment are not confined to survival issues alone. With earlier diagnosis, many could be on treatment for many years. There is an increasing awareness of the toxicity of hormonal therapy, which has to be balanced against any benefits. The decision when to start therapy and which treatment to use depends on the balance of benefit and risk.

CLINICAL TRIALS

Although trials in prostate cancer are dealt with in Chapters 91 and 93 and other chapters in this book, some important issues are relevant here.

1. Meaningful data can only come from randomized trials, analyzed on an intention to treat basis. Due to potential bias "statistical significance" from nonrandomized data is meaningless—the difference may be significant, but not necessarily for the reason being investigated.

2. Demonstration of equivalence between two treatment strategies requires substantially more patients than are included in most trials. Although a difference with $P > 0.05$ may not be significant in the statistical sense, it should not be concluded that there is *not* a difference. It often means simply that insufficient numbers have been included to rule out the *possibility* of chance. Also, statistical significance does not always equate with clinical significance.

3. In assessing survival differences, "snapshots" of data can be misleading. Even where survival curves show a highly significant difference, the difference in numbers alive at any one point is often small. Also, absolute numbers surviving on a particular date will include patients who have been in the study for varying lengths of time.

4. An issue of particular importance, and regularly discussed in prostate cancer, is the relationship between disease-specific versus overall survival. Interventions that reduce or delay mortality from prostate cancer are often perceived not to affect overall survival. In the Medical Research Council (MRC) study PR03, comparing immediate versus deferred hormonal treatment, current survival curves (Figure 97.1) confirm that the highly significant improvement in disease-specific survival in those treated immediately in earlier reports[4] persists. However, although overall survival is longer in those

treated immediately, the difference is not significant. This apparent discrepancy is a familiar finding, and was also seen in the recently published Scandinavian Radical Prostatectomy Study.[5] In both instances, it has been concluded that the intervention, be it early hormone treatment or radical prostatectomy does not increase the patient's life span. This is an example of the erroneous assumption that, although there was a difference in overall survival, because it was not significant (i.e., $P > 0.05$) there was actually *no* difference.

SURVIVAL IN MEN WITH PROSTATE CANCER

Prostate cancer occurs in an elderly population, who will experience co-morbidity, and as they get older have a reducing life expectation (Tables 97.1 and 97.2). The actual proportion of men surviving is the product of life expectation and prostate cancer survival. Even where survival from prostate cancer is similar, as men get older, fewer will survive because of comorbid deaths. Therefore, an intervention which will significantly extend prostate cancer survival will clearly improve the survival of a group of 60-year-olds but will have a negligible effect on that of men in their 80s. It is this effect of age and comorbidity that reduces the statistical significance of overall survival—the coincidental deaths diluting any overall benefit from improved prostate cancer survival.

If an intervention improving prostate cancer survival was genuinely associated with an unchanged overall mortality then that intervention should be associated with a treatment-related mortality. This was indeed the case in patients treated with estrogens, due to an increased risk of cardiovascular death,[6] but no such effect is apparent in trials using orchiectomy or luteinizing hormone releasing hormone (LHRH) analogs (unpublished meta-analysis), nor is such an effect apparent in MRC PR03 (see Figure 97.2). In

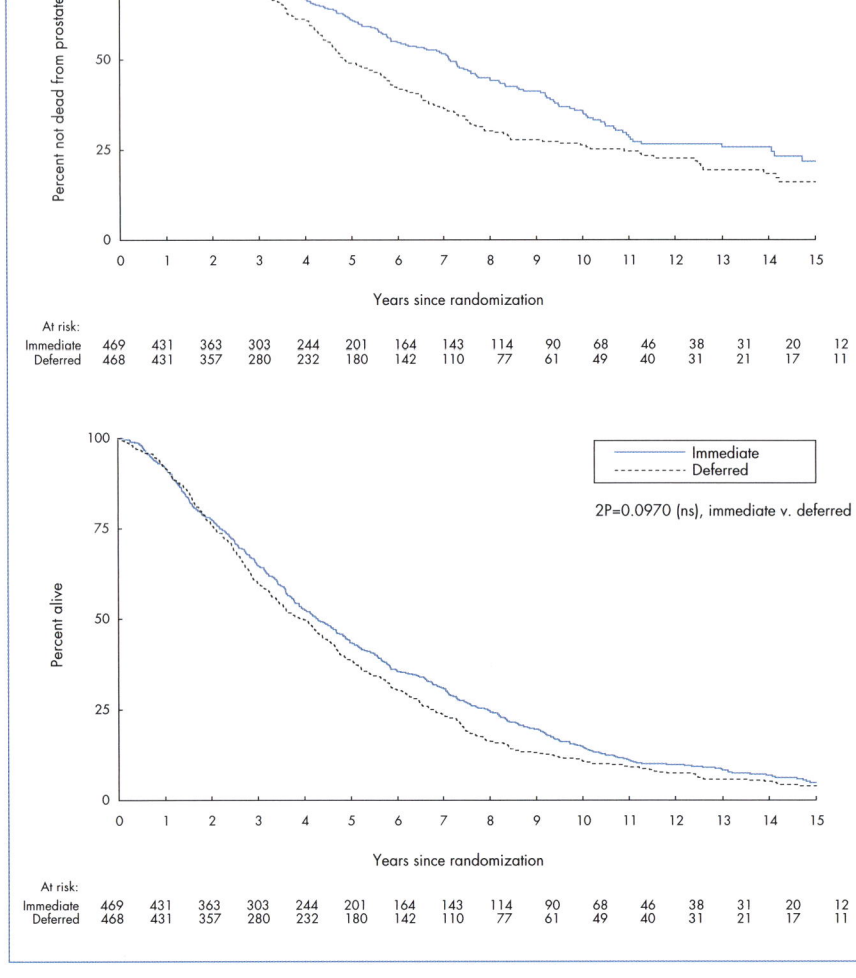

Fig. 97.1
Medical Research Council (MRC) trial of immediate versus deferred hormone treatment—survival curves for all patients, by randomization group. *A*, Disease-specific survival. Time to death from prostate cancer, showing statistical significance. *B*, Overall survival. Time to death from any cause, not significant.

Table 97.1 Cause specific versus overall survival; overall survival is the product of the 10 year mortality from prostate cancer and the age related survival for other causes of death

Age	Expected 10-year survival, %	Prostate cancer survival, %	Overall survival, %
60	75	60	45
70	50	60	30
80	25	60	15

Table 97.2 Effect of treatment which reduces prostate cancer mortality from 40% to 28%, related to age

Age (years)	Expected 10 year survival, %	Prostate cancer survival, %	Overall survival, %
60	75	72 vs 60	54 vs 45
70	50	72 vs 60	36 vs 30
80	25	72 vs 60	18 vs 15

comments on the Scandinavian Radical Prostatectomy study[5] it has been stated "there was no difference in overall mortality",[7] but there *was* a difference, numerically almost the same as the difference in prostate cancer survival (there was one postoperative death). It was not statistically significant because of "dilution" by deaths from other causes, but it was a difference none the less.

In other words, improved survival from prostate cancer should be seen as a bonus on top of the patients' other risks of dying, but one which will only be realized by a small proportion of men in their 80s. The real issue is whether sufficient men will benefit to justify the intervention, something which may well apply in men with age and comorbidity that severely reduces life expectation.

IMMEDIATE VERSUS DEFERRED TREATMENT

The issue of immediate versus deferred treatment has been discussed since the inception of hormonal therapy.[8] The results of MRC trial PR03, first published in 1996,[4] which demonstrated a disease-specific survival benefit from immediate treatment, have been controversial. The main concern[9] was that there were a number of patients who apparently died from prostate cancer without treatment. The number was not as great as initially reported, and the suggestion that failure to treat these patients explained the difference does not stand up to analysis.[10] This was an example of the misuse of the "snapshot," as, even if their survival had been increased by treatment, it is likely they still would have died before that date.

The current status of MRC PR03 is indicated in Table 97.3. Since the majority of patients have now died, the data is mature and unlikely to change significantly in future. From other studies, including those of adjuvant hormone treatment in patients receiving radiotherapy,[11] a consistent pattern is emerging that hormonal treatment improves survival in advanced prostate cancer. The issue of survival should finally be resolved by a meta-analysis of all studies involving immediate versus deferred treatment, although this is awaiting the outcome of an EORTC study.

OTHER BENEFITS FROM HORMONE TREATMENT

In 1996, results from PR03 demonstrated a reduction in complications in those treated immediately. Although in many cases, the complications, particularly spinal cord compression, occurred in the deferred treatment

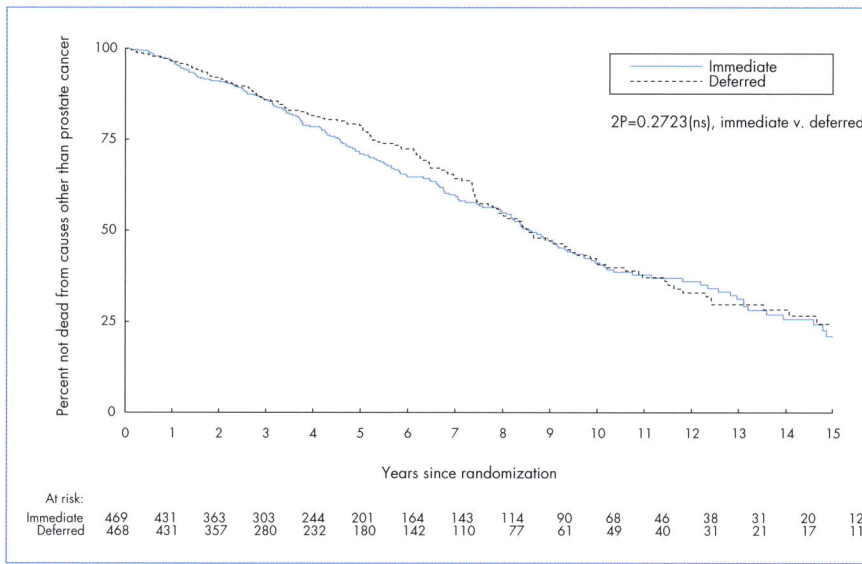

Fig. 97.2
Medical Research Council (MRC) trial of immediate versus deferred hormone treatment—survival curves for all patients, by randomization group. Time to death from causes other than prostate cancer. No excess deaths apparent in the immediate group.

Table 97.3 Medical Research Council (MRC) PR03, comparison of immediate versus deferred hormone treatment in advanced prostate cancer—current status (2004)

	Immediate, n (%)	Deferred, n (%)
Entered	469	469
No with follow-up data	469	468
Died	446 (95.1)	449 (95.9)
Patients with metastases	126/130 (96.9)	130/131 (99.2)

group *after* treatment had already been started for another unrelated cause, it did seem likely that, as the data matured, these complications would appear more frequently in the immediate treatment group, who would "catch up." Except for the incidence of ureteric obstruction, this does not seem to have happened (Table 97.4), and suggests that tumor progression, taking place during the period for which treatment is deferred, may not be fully reversible. Clearly, the reduction in these events has clear quality-of-life benefits, albeit for a minority of patients, to set against the disadvantages of hormone therapy.

ANDROGEN DEPRIVATION—THE DISADVANTAGES

Hormonal therapy conventionally involves androgen deprivation, whether achieved by orchiectomy or use of LHRH analogs. Reduction in serum testosterone has a number of adverse effects. In addition to the immediate problems with sexual dysfunction[12] and hot flushes,[13] in the medium term, patients experience weight increase and loss of muscle mass.[14] Patients can become anemic, and recently, it has been recognized that there can also be a loss of cognitive function.[15] Perhaps the most serious problem is osteoporosis,[16] with an increased incidence of pathologic fractures not due to metastases;

most significant, in view of the trend towards earlier use of hormonal treatment, is its relation to duration of treatment.

The principle trials of immediate versus deferred treatment did not have access to modern quality-of-life measurements. Thus, a recent study by Gardiner et al[17] is of particular importance. This small, randomized study, has shown a clear loss of quality of life up to 1 year after starting treatment. However, patients for whom this period represents a significant portion of their survival will probably have had a mandatory indication for treatment with symptomatic disease. In others with longer expectation of survival, later benefits from delay in progression might compensate for the earlier loss of quality of life. This study does give pause for thought before commencing hormonal treatment in those for whom the benefits are unproven, and the results should be introduced into the discussion of treatment options with the patient. There will be some for whom short-term quality of life is more important than maximum longevity.

CHOICE OF TREATMENT

Whereas once the only choice available was between orchiectomy and estrogen treatment, there are now several options. These produce different endocrine changes (Table 97.5), which influence their potential side effects, and possibly their relative efficacy.

It is generally accepted that LHRH analogs are equivalent therapeutically to earlier methods of hormone treatment—but is this really the case? The clinical trials on which this is based[18–22] involved from 80 to less than 300 patients—too small a number to conclusively exclude a difference that might be clinically significant. In these studies, the survival curves were far from coincident, and, again, an assumption of equivalence was made because the differences did not reach clinical significance. The

Table 97.4 Medical Research Council (MRC) PR03 incidence of complications (all patients by randomization group)

Complication	Results in 1996		Results in 2004	
	Immediate, n	Deferred, n	Immediate, n	Deferred, n
Spinal cord compression	9	23	10	24
Pathologic fracture	11	21	14	22
Extraskeletal metastases	37	55	47	63
Ureteric obstruction	33	55	50	65
Transurethral resection of the prostate* (*>6/52 after entry)	65	141	88	152
Number of patients reported with pain from metastases				
Number died from prostate cancer	–	–	249	295
Number with pain	–	–	138	223

Table 97.5 Hormone therapies: effects on luteinizing hormone releasing hormone (LHRH), luteinizing hormone (LH), follicle stimulating hormone (FSH), and testosterone

Therapy	LHRH	LH	FSH	Testosterone
Orchiectomy	↑	↑	↑	↓
LHRH analog	↑	↓	↓	↓
Cyproterone acetate	↓	↓	↓	↓R
Nonsteroidal antiandrogen	↑ or →	↑ or →	↑ or →	↑ or →
Estrogens	↓	↓	↓	↓R

R = testosterone replaced by non androgen steroid hormone.

large randomized trial necessary to prove this point will never be done, so likely equivalence in efficacy must be accepted. However, the possibility that testosterone may not have been suppressed to castrate levels should be considered if a patient does not respond to LHRH analog treatment as expected

ORCHIECTOMY VERSUS LUTEINIZING HORMONE RELEASING HORMONE ANALOG TREATMENT

Accepting the therapeutic equivalence of orchiectomy and luteinizing hormone releasing hormone analog treatment, the decision as to which to use relates to the practical and other consequences of the treatment. Orchiectomy involves an operation and potential surgical complications. Whether "castration" produces the psychological problems often assumed is less clear. Most urologists will do a subcapsular orchiectomy, which reduces the size of the testis rather than removing it. There are clear advantages in terms of compliance, and, although the procedure is irreversible, there must be few occasions when this will matter. Luteinizing hormone releasing hormone analogs have the problem of tumor flare,[23] and most users will recommend flare prevention with an antiandrogen. The need for continuing injections may, over a long period, cancel out the disadvantage of an operation, and occasional drug idiosyncrasies can occur. In practice, although in the author's practice a few patients do opt for orchiectomy, LHRH analog treatment is the current standard, whether as monotherapy or as part of a combined regime.

REDUCING MORBIDITY FROM HORMONE TREATMENT

Deferred treatment is essentially a strategy to reduce morbidity. If deferment involved no loss of therapeutic benefit, there would be no issue. If earlier treatment does improve survival, a complex equation emerges. Perhaps some of the concern about quality of life ignores the fact that throughout medicine, and especially in oncology, there is always a price to pay, both in terms of potential side effects and of cost. Why should prostate cancer be different? Unlike chemotherapy, which produces severe short-term complications but is given for a defined period, hormonal therapy is an ongoing treatment for which the risk of significant toxicity increases with time. Hormonal therapy is a form of disease control, not a cure, and, until we can elucidate the problem of hormone refractory relapse, will ultimately fail. Add to this the fact that many men will not die from prostate cancer and a picture emerges which, for example, contrasts strongly with the treatment of testicular cancer in young men.

Alternatively, to maximize any survival advantage, there are alternative strategies to reduce toxicity of treatment, some of which are discussed in other chapters of this book.

THE USE OF OTHER DRUGS

There is some evidence that nonsteroidal antiandrogens may have less toxicity.[24] Bicalutamide 150 mg/day, licensed for use as monotherapy in locally advanced disease, may be appropriate for selected patients and can be discussed as an alternative option. Were it not for cardiovascular toxicity, estrogens would have much to commend them.[25] Toxicity could be reduced either by use in low dosage combined with aspirin, or by parenteral administration avoiding the initial metabolism in the liver, believed to be the source of the toxicity. The depot injection estrodurin was used in a Scandinavian study,[26] which demonstrated equivalent efficacy. However, the number of cardiovascular adverse events was increased and although there was no excess in cardiovascular mortality, this may have been the result of the small numbers involved.

OTHER REGIMENS

Particularly in early disease (i.e., PSA relapse after radical treatment) there is interest in drug escalation,[27] perhaps commencing with a 5α-reductase inhibitor, then an antiandrogen, with the medical or surgical castration only as relapse occurs. This approach is probably not appropriate in advanced disease. Intermittent therapy is discussed in detail in another chapter. It may not only reduce the impact of toxicity but also delay the onset of hormone-refractory disease.[28] Complications might be preempted by therapy such as bisphophonate treatment, which, although principally to modify the development of metastatic disease, may also help prevent osteoporosis.[29]

COMBINED ANDROGEN BLOCKADE

If this book had been written in the mid-1990s, it would certainly have contained a whole chapter devoted to combination treatment with androgen deprivation (be it orchiectomy or LHRH analog) and antiandrogens. Although the Prostate Cancer Trialist's Collaborative Group's second meta-analysis published in 2000[30] did show a statistically significant survival benefit, this was small, and generally seems not to be thought clinically worthwhile. Certainly in the UK, after over a decade of intense investigation, interest in routine use of combined androgen blockade as primary hormone treatment has waned. In patients in whom there has been a good response to primary monotherapy with androgen deprivation, addition of an antiandrogen may produce a further response,[31] and the author's practice is to start an LHRH analog for patients relapsing on antiandrogen monotherapy.

HORMONAL TREATMENT IN 2006

There seems a general consensus that treatment is indicated on diagnosis of M1 disease. Deferred treatment is likely to be needed early, and these are the patients most at risk from serious complications like spinal cord compression. Trial data on survival after deferred treatment is inconclusive, and is likely to remain so, partly because treatment is delayed for such a short time (Peto, personal communication). In most cases, an LHRH analog will be indicated, although the need for a speedy effect makes disease presenting with actual or impending spinal cord compression an indication for orchiectomy.[32]

In locally advanced disease, although the debate about immediate versus deferred treatment continues, the following points can be made:

- Hormone treatment does have an impact on advanced prostate cancer.
- Immediate treatment may reduce, not simply delay, significant complications.
- Disease progression during deferred period may not be completely reversible.
- Disease-specific survival is improved.
- The lack of statistically significant overall survival benefit in individual trials may simply reflect the expected mortality from other diseases in men surviving longer from prostate cancer.
- Even if a reduction in prostate cancer mortality is at the expense of an increase in deaths from other causes, it might be better to die from a myocardial infarct than from prostate cancer.

However, although in M0 disease, immediate treatment seems to improve local and distant disease control and may produce a survival advantage, this has to be balanced against the risk of toxicity in what may be a prolonged period of treatment. In practice, each patient has to be considered individually and should be involved himself in the decision. His age, health, and aspirations are all important. Deferred treatment remains an option in many, selected patients, but the patient's compliance is essential, with careful follow-up and responding to rapid PSA rises, which may be the best indicator of aggressive disease, with prompt treatment. The balance in this equation changes as the stage of the disease reduces and the length of time for which treatment is likely to continue increases. Failure of curative treatment is dealt with elsewhere in this book. Although there is randomized study suggesting survival benefit from hormone treatment in patients with node positive disease,[33] it should be interpreted with caution because of its small size. The adverse implications of early initiation of hormonal treatment must be carefully considered until the benefits of treatment at this stage of the disease become clearer.

REFERENCES

1. Rabbini F, Gleave ME. Treatment of metastatic prostate cancer: endocrine therapy. In: Hamdy FC, Basler JW, Neal DE, Catalona WJ (eds): Management of Urologic Malignancies. Edinburgh: Churchill Livingstone, 2002, pp 210–226.
2. Davis NB, Jani AB, Vogelzang NJ. Selecting a treatment. Urol Clin N Am 2003;30:403–414.
3. See WA. Wirth MP, Mcleod DG, et al, Bicalutamide as immediate therapy either alone or as adjuvant to standard care of patients with localised or locally advanced prostate cancer: first analysis of the early prostate cancer program. J Urol 2002;168:429–435.
4. Medical Research Council Prostate Cancer Working Party Investigators Group. Immediate versus deferred treatment for advanced prostatic cancer: initial results of the Medical Research Council Trial. Brit J Urol 1997;79:235–246.
5. Holmberg L, Bill-Axelson A, Helgesen F, et al. A randomised trial comparing radical prostatectomy with watchful waiting in early prostate cancer. New Eng J Med 2002;347:781–789.
6. Byar DP. The Veterans Administration Cooperative Research Group's studies of cancer of the prostate. Cancer 1973;32:1126–1130.
7. Kirby RS, Fitzpatrick JM. Radical prostatectomy or watchful waiting? Br J Urol International 2003;91:5.
8. Nesbit RM, Baum WC. Endocrine control of prostatic cancer. Clinical survey of 1818 cases. JAMA 1950;143:1317–1320.
9. Schröder FH. Endocrine treatment of prostate cancer – recent developments and the future. Part 1: maximal androgen blockade. Early vs delayed endocrine treatment and side effects. Br J Urol Intl 1999;83:161–170.
10. Kirk D. Medical Research Council immediate versus deferred treatment study; patients dying without treatment. Br J Urol 1998;81:31.
11. Bolla M, Gonzalez D, Warde P, et al. Improved survival in patients with locally advanced prostate cancer treated with radiotherapy and goserelin. N Engl J Med 1997;337:295–300.
12. Ellis WJ, Grayhack JT, Sexual function in aging males after orchiectomy and estrogen therapy. J Urol 1963;89:895–899.
13. Radlmier A, Bormacher K, Neumann F. Hot flushes: mechanism and prevention. Prog Clin Biol Res 1990;359:131–140.
14. Morley JE, Kaiser FE, Hajjar R, Perr HM III. Testosterone and frailty. Clin Geriat Med 1997;13:655–695.
15. Gardiner RA, Green H, Yaxley J, et al. Cognition and hormonal manipulation in prostate cancer. Br J Urol Intl 2000;86:218–219.
16. Daniell HW. Osteoporosis after orchiectomy for prostate cancer. J Urol 1997;157:439–444.

17. Green HJ, Pakenham KI, Headley, BC, et al. Quality of life compared during pharmacological treatments and clinical monitoring for non-localised prostate cancer: a randomised controlled trial. Br J Urol Intl 2004;93:975–979.

18. Mahler C. Is disease flare a problem? Cancer 1993;72:3799–3802.

19. Soloway MS, et al. Zoladex versus orchiectomy in treatment of advanced prostate cancer: a randomised trial. Urology 1991;37:46–51.

20. Kaisary AV, Tyrell CJ, Peeling WB, et al on behalf of Study Group. Comparison of LHRH analogue (Zoladex) with orchiectomy in patients with metastatic prostate cancer. Br J Urol 1991;67:502–508.

21. Botto H, Richard F, Mathieu F, Camey M. Decapeptyl in the treatment of metastatic prostatic cancer. Comparative study with pulpectomy. In Liss AR: Prostate Cancer, Part A: Research, Endocrine Treatment, and Histopathology. 1987, pp 199–296.

22. The Leuprolide Study Group. Leuprolide vs diethylstilbestrol for metastatic prostate cancer. N Eng J Med 1984;311:1281–1286.

23. Mahler C. Is disease flare a problem? Cancer 1993;72:3799–3802.

24. Anderson J. The role of antiandrogen monotherapy in the treatment of prostate cancer. Br J Urol Intl 2003;91:455–61.

25. Bishop MC, Experience with low-dose oestrogen in the treatment of advanced prostate cancer: a personal view. Br J Urol 1996;78:921–928.

26. Hedlund PO, Ala-Opas M, Brekkan E, et al. Parenteral estrogen versus combined androgen deprivation in the treatment of metastatic prostate cancer. Scand J Urol Nephrol 2002;36:405–413.

27. Fleshner NE, Trachtenberg J. Sequential androgen blockade: a biological study in the inhibition of prostatic growth. J Urol 1992;148:1928–1931.

28. Goldenberg SL, Bruchovsky N, Gleave ME, et al. Intermittent androgen suppression in the treatment of prostate cancer: a preliminary report. Urology 1995;45:839–844.

29. Ernst DS. The role of bisphosphonates in prostate cancer. In: Bangma CH, Newling DWW (eds): Prostate and renal cancer, benign prostatic hyperplasia, erectile dysfunction and basic research an update. New York: Parthenon, 2003, pp 414–420.

30. Prostate Cancer Trialists' Collaborative Group. Maximum androgen blockade in advanced prostate cancer: an overview of the randomised trials. Lancet 2000;355:1491–1498.

31. Fujikawa, Matsui Y, Fukuzawa S, Takeuchi H. Prostate-specific antigen levels and clinical response to flutamide as a second hormone therapy for hormone-refractory prostate carcinoma. Eur Urol 2000;37:218–222.

32. Basler JW, Werschman J. Prostate cancer: management of sequelae, voiding dysfunction and renal failure In Hamdy FC, Basler JW, Neal DE, Catalona WJ (eds): Management of Urologic Malignancies Edinburgh Churchill Livingstone, 2002, pp 261–269.

33. Messing E, Manola J, Sarosdy M, et al. Immediate hormonal therapy vs observation for node positive prostate cancer following radical prostatectomy and pelvic lymphadenectomy. N Engl J Med 1999;314:1781–1788.

Intermittent androgen suppression for prostate cancer: rationale and clinical experience

98

Martin Gleave, S Larry Goldenberg

ABSTRACT

Since the mid-1980s, research on hormonal treatments for prostate cancer have focused on maximizing androgen ablation through combination therapy. Unfortunately, maximal androgen ablation increases treatment-related side effects and expense and has not significantly prolonged time to androgen-independent (AI) progression. The rationale behind intermittent androgen suppression (IAS) is based on: 1) observations that androgen ablation delays tumor progression but is rarely curative in most patients, and hence quality of life must be considered; 2) the assumption that immediate androgen ablation is superior to delayed therapy in improving survival of patients with prostate cancer; and 3) the hypothesis that if tumor cells surviving androgen withdrawal can be forced along a normal pathway of differentiation by androgen replacement, then apoptotic potential might be restored, androgen dependence may be prolonged, and progression to androgen independence may be delayed. Observations from animal model studies suggest that progression to androgen independence involves adaptive responses to androgen deprivation, which are, in turn, modulated by intermittent androgen replacement.

Supported by these animal model observations, several centers have now tested the feasibility of IAS therapy in nonrandomized groups of patients with prostate cancer using serum prostate-specific antigen (PSA) as trigger points. Experimental and clinical data suggest that prostate cancer is amenable to control by IAS, and so IAS may offer clinicians an opportunity to improve quality of life in patients with prostate cancer by balancing the benefits of immediate androgen ablation (delayed progression and prolonged survival) while reducing treatment-related side effects and expense. Whether time to progression and survival is affected in a beneficial or adverse way is being studied in randomized, prospective protocols. This chapter will review the rationale behind IAS, compare observations from published series, and discuss potential indications and treatment strategies using IAS.

INTRODUCTION

More than 80% of men with advanced prostate cancer have symptomatic and objective responses following androgen suppression, and serum PSA levels decrease in almost all patients. Surgical or medical castration results in a median progression-free survival of 12 to 33 months and a median overall survival of 23 to 37 months in patients with stage D2 disease.[1,2] However, for reasons that are only partly defined, the apoptotic process induced by androgen ablation fails to eliminate the entire malignant cell population. Another limitation of conventional androgen ablation is that it accelerates the rate of progression of prostate cancer to an androgen-independent state,[3] and after a variable period of time averaging 24 months, progression inevitably occurs with rising serum PSA levels and androgen-independent growth. Since the mid-1980s, many efforts have focused on maximizing the degree of androgen suppression therapy by combining agents that inhibit or block both testicular and adrenal androgens. Unfortunately, maximal androgen ablation (i.e., the addition of an antiandrogen to medical or surgical castration) increases treatment-related side effects and expense and has not significantly prolonged time to androgen-independent progression in most patients.[2,4,5]

The idea of intermittent cycling of endocrine therapies arose through a realization that treatment resistance emerges from a Darwinian interplay of genetic and epigenetic factors and selective pressures of treatment. Early observations that prostatic involution after castration is an active process involving rapid elimination of most epithelial cells led to the postulate that replacement of androgens, even in small amounts, would have a conditioning effect on surviving cells and allow them to conserve or regain desirable traits of differentiation.[6,7] In the case of tumors, several lines of evidence obtained by Foulds[7] and Noble[8] implied that long periods of hormone deprivation simply accelerated progression towards autonomous growth and thus were better avoided. Although, no practical method of countering progression by hormonal means emerged from this work, the subsequent demonstration that consecutive episodes of testosterone-induced regeneration of involuted prostate completely restored the susceptibility of the epithelium to further androgen withdrawal,[9] was an incentive to try similar experiments on tumors. The potential benefits of intermittent, rather than continuous, therapy include improved quality of life through reduced therapy-induced side effects, decreased costs, and possibly improved control over progression to androgen-independence. However, IAS is a feasible treatment option only if immediate hormone therapy is superior to delayed, and if adaptive mechanisms help mediate androgen-independent progression. The following section will review evidence that supports this rationale.

RATIONALE FOR INTERMITTENT ANDROGEN SUPPRESSION

BALANCING THE BENEFITS OF "EARLY" ANDROGEN ABLATION

While early diagnosis and treatment is a long-held paradigm in oncology, the controversy surrounding optimal time to initiate hormone therapy in prostate cancer remains relevant considering how wide the spectrum of advanced prostate cancer has become. Although androgen ablation has been the standard therapy for advanced prostate cancer for over 60 years, the optimal time to begin this treatment in asymptomatic patients remains controversial: whether to start treatment early after diagnosis or wait until the disease burden is larger and causes symptoms. This issue is especially relevant in the PSA era, with its expanding proportion of PSA-relapses after failed local therapy, many of whom may be candidates for androgen ablation therapy.

The rationale for IAS would be weak if time to disease progression and overall survival were similar between early (i.e., at the time of diagnosis of metastatic or recurrent disease) and delayed (i.e., waiting for the development of symptoms) androgen ablation. Measuring serum PSA after radical prostatectomy or radiotherapy would be a waste of time and resources, and only patients with clinical symptomatic recurrences would require hormonal therapy. Accumulating theoretical, preclinical, and clinical evidence support treatment at the time of diagnosis of locally advanced or metastatic disease. The Goldie–Coldman[10] hypothesis of increasing somatic genomic alterations and tumor heterogeneity over time provides a theoretical basis to support initiation of therapy as early as possible. Also, data from several xenograft models support initiation of androgen ablation when tumor burden is small.[11,12] For example, using the androgen-dependent Shionogi mouse model, So et al[12] reported that large tumor volume and corresponding delay of castration reduced the time to androgen-independent recurrence and death. Earlier androgen ablation, at time of subclinical (nonpalpable) disease, significantly delayed the rate and time to androgen-independent recurrence compared with delayed therapy when tumor burden was high.

Many clinical studies also report prolonged time to androgen-independence and improved survival with early therapy in men with advanced prostate cancer. While the first Veterans Administration Cooperative Urological Research Group (VACURG) study[13] reported that delayed endocrine therapy was equivalent to immediate treatment, reanalysis by Byar[14] indicated that earlier therapy, when corrected for the cardiovascular mortality associated with diethylstilbestrol (DES), was more effective. The Medical Research Council (MRC) study from the UK randomized over 800 men with advanced M0 or M1 disease to immediate or deferred therapy and showed that palliative surgery for bladder outlet or ureteral obstruction was reduced by almost 50% and disease-specific survival improved with immediate therapy.[15] Another, more recent study from the European Organisation for Research and Treatment of Cancer (EORTC) also demonstrated significant improvement in time to disease progression, and 5-year survival (58% versus 78%) in patients with locally advanced disease treated with radiotherapy and either immediate androgen ablation for 3 years or delayed therapy until symptomatic progression.[16] In an Eastern Collaborative Oncology Group (ECOG) trial, Messing et al[17] reported dramatically improved overall and recurrence-free survival in patients with node-positive disease that underwent radical prostatectomy treated with immediate androgen ablation compared with deferred therapy. Finally, recent data from the Early Prostate Cancer (EPC) trials demonstrates that those patients treated immediately with the antiandrogen bicalutamide had a lower risk of progression of disease.[18] Importantly, however, data from Trial 25 (Scandinavia) also reported that time to death is accelerated in men with T1/T2 prostate cancer treated with bicalutamide compared with watchful waiting alone (hazard ratio [HR] 1.47; P = 0.0195). This decrease in overall survival in T1/T2 watchful waiting patients treated with bicalutamide is significant, appears to be drug related, and is biologically plausible. While the effects may be due to bicalutamide itself and not be related to androgen receptor blockade, the effects are most plausibly due to androgen blockade. In contrast, in Trial 25 in T3/T4 prostate cancer patients, time to death was significantly longer (HR 0.67; P = 0.0125) in bicalutamide- compared with placebo-treated men. Accelerated rate of death in watchful waiting T1/T2 tumors with a reverse trend in watchful waiting T3/T4 patients is consistent with the hypothesis that bicalutamide treatment improved survival in men at high risk of progression, but worsened survival in men at low risk of progression.

Coincident with accumulating evidence supporting immediate therapy is a shift in the target population eligible to receive androgen ablation from metastatic disease to PSA failures after radical prostatectomy or radiotherapy. Use of PSA for early detection has produced a stage migration and 50% decrease in the incidence of stage D2 disease over the last 2 years.[19] Because the median survival in hormone-naive M+ disease is only 2 to 3 years, the long-term side-effects of androgen ablation do not become apparent and are, therefore, not clinically relevant. However, use of PSA and stage migration has resulted in earlier diagnosis at younger ages and earlier stages of disease, with the prospect of much longer therapy and risk of chronic complications. Furthermore, the use of PSA to detect biochemical recurrences following radical prostatectomy or radiotherapy identifies men at risk to recur and who may benefit from early adjuvant therapy but who have life expectancies exceeding 10 years. Hence, combinations of stage migration, earlier diagnosis of PSA recurrences, longer life expectancies, and trend towards immediate therapy will force clinicians to balance the potential benefits of early adjuvant therapy with risks of development of metabolic complications, as well as the increased expense, associated with long-term continuous androgen withdrawal therapy. These metabolic complications include loss of bone mass (osteoporosis) and fractures, loss of muscle mass, anemia with easy fatigue and decreased energy levels, changes in lipid profile with increased risk of cardiovascular complications, glucose intolerance, and depressive and/or irritable personality changes.[20] Decreased overall survival in low risk watchful waiting patients treated with bicalutamide in the EPC trials further emphasize the need to carefully select patients at high risk of disease progression who are most likely to benefit from early hormone therapy. In this regard, IAS may offer clinicians an opportunity to improve quality of life in patients with prostate cancer by balancing the benefits of immediate androgen ablation (delayed progression and prolonged survival) while reducing treatment-related side effects and expense.

MODULATING ADAPTIVE RESPONSES MEDIATING ANDROGEN INDEPENDENCE

The development of therapeutic resistance, after hormone- or chemotherapy, for example, is the underlying basis for most cancer deaths. Therapeutic resistance and tumor progression result from multiple, stepwise changes in DNA structure and gene expression—a Darwinian interplay of genetic and epigenetic factors, many arising from selective pressures of treatment. This highly dynamic process cannot be attributed to singular genetic events, involving instead cumulative changes in gene expression that facilitate escape from normal regulatory control of cell growth and survival. Prostate cancer initially progresses as an androgen-dependent tumor, manifested by apoptosis, cell cycle arrest, and changes in androgen-regulated gene expression after androgen ablation.[21] Unfortunately, progression to androgen-independence nearly always occurs in prostate cancer after androgen ablation. It is somewhat ironic that the very same agents used to kill or control cancer cells also trigger cascades of events that lead to a hormone-resistant phenotype.

Progression to androgen independence is a multifactorial process by which cells acquire the ability to both survive in the absence of androgens and proliferate using non-androgenic stimuli for mitogenesis, and involves variable combinations of clonal selection, adaptive upregulation of antiapoptotic cytoprotective genes (e.g., *BCL2*, clusterin *HSP27*), androgen receptor transactivation in the absence of androgen from mutations or increased levels of coactivators and alternative growth factor pathways, including HER2/NEU, epidermal growth factor receptor (EGFR), transforming growth factor-β (TGFβ), and insulin-like growth factor 1 (IGF1).[3,23–31] A complete review of these mechanisms is beyond the scope of this review, but likely all variably operate in heterogenous tumors like prostate cancer.

Bruchovsky et al[3] described a model whereby prostate cancer cells surviving androgen withdrawal are derived from adaptive cell survival mechanisms in a small number of initially androgen-dependent stem cells. High-throughput bioprofiling using gene and tissue microarrays is used by many research groups to characterize genetic and signaling networks that enable tumors to progress and adapt to treatments. In general, there is a reproducible, programmatic drift in gene expression in prostate tissues after androgen ablation.

Of interest, while clusterin, BCL2, BCLXL, HSP27, insulin-like growth factor binding proteins 2 and 5 (IGFBP2, IGFBP5) are expressed at very low levels in androgen-dependent tumors, they are all upregulated after castration and remain constitutively overexpressed in recurrent androgen-independent tumors. Increased expression of BCL2,[25,27] androgen receptor,[26] clusterin,[28,32] IGFBP5,[29] IGFBP2,[30] and HSP27[31] after castration help confer androgen resistance and represent adaptive responses by malignant cells to activate survival and mitogenic pathways to compensate for androgen withdrawal.

Based on the above observations, it is reasonable to postulate that the adaptive changes in gene expression precipitated by androgen ablation may be modulated by re-exposure to the differentiating effects of androgen. The ability of benign or malignant prostate cells to undergo apoptosis, and to express PSA, is acquired as a feature of differentiation of prostatic cells under the influence of androgens. Even in malignancy, the ability to undergo apoptosis is acquired as a feature of differentiation under the influence of androgens. Therefore, in the absence of androgens, dividing cells cannot differentiate and become pre-apoptotic (to androgen withdrawal) again, which explains why recurrent tumor growth after castration is characterized by androgen independence.[3] The rationale behind IAS is based on the hypothesis that if tumor cells surviving androgen withdrawal are forced along a pathway of differentiation by androgen replacement, then apoptotic potential might be restored and progression to androgen independence delayed. It follows that, if androgens are replaced soon after regression of tumor, it should be possible to bring about repeated cycles of androgen-stimulated growth, differentiation, and androgen-withdrawal regression of tumor.

PRECLINICAL STUDIES OF INTERMITTENT ANDROGEN SUPPRESSION

DUNNING R3327 RAT PROSTATIC ADENOCARCINOMA

Using the Dunning rat carcinoma as a model of progression to androgen-independence, Isaacs et al[11,22] emphasized the importance of genetic instability, which increases tumor heterogeneity by increasing the number of distinctly different clones of cells, analogous to the Goldie–Coldman hypothesis of tumor progression.[10] Androgen-independent progression results from selective outgrowth of one or more androgen resistant clones after androgen ablation. Trachtenberg et al[33] reported no significant growth reduction in Dunning R3327 tumors treated with IAS, and concluded that IAS

was inferior to early castration in inhibiting tumor growth. Similarly, Russo et al[34] reported that Dunning R3327 tumors treated with continuous or intermittent DES had tumor volumes at death smaller than control or castrate rats, but a survival advantage was achieved only in the castrate or continuous DES groups. Although the intermittent regimen was successful in delaying tumor growth, it did not yield a survival advantage and in this respect was inferior to castration. The foregoing experiments using the Dunning R3327 model draw attention to the importance of using cyclic androgen deprivation only for the treatment of androgen-dependent cancer. Dunning tumors are androgen-sensitive, not androgen-dependent, and apoptotic regression does not occur following castration. Hence, the failure to improve outcome with IAS in Dunning tumors is not an unexpected result. Indeed, IAS may be detrimental because of stimulation of androgen-sensitive cells when testosterone levels increase. Androgen ablation with the addition of cytotoxic agents appears to be the most effective therapy in this model.[22]

SHIONOGI MOUSE CARCINOMA

Intermittent androgen suppression of the androgen-dependent Shionogi carcinoma has been carried out experimentally by transplanting tumors into a succession of male mice. The cycle of transplantation and castration-induced apoptosis was successfully repeated four times before growth became androgen-independent during the fifth cycle.[3,35] The mean time to androgen independence increased three-fold compared with one-time castration, consistent with a retarding effect of cyclic therapy on tumor progression. Some caution is required in the interpretation of these results since the procedure of transplanting a regressing tumor from a castrated to a noncastrated animal temporarily may reduce the rate of cell division and give rise to an apparent delay in progression. However, in addition to tumor growth, other markers of androgen dependence such as castration-induced apoptosis and *TRPM2* (clusterin) gene expression were maintained three times longer with IAS compared with continuous therapy, paralleling and supporting the changes in tumor volume.

LNCaP XENOGRAFT MODEL

As in human prostate cancer, serum PSA levels in LNCaP xenografts are androgen-regulated and proportional to tumor volume.[36,37] After castration, serum and tumor-cell PSA levels decrease by 80% and remain suppressed for 3 to 4 weeks before increasing again. With intermittent testosterone withdrawal and replacement in castrated mice bearing LNCaP tumors, androgen-independent regulation of the PSA gene was delayed three-fold.[38] Taking an alternative approach, Thalmann et al[39] reported evidence suggesting that continuous androgen suppression may facilitate development of androgen-independent osseous metastasis. Characterization of androgen-independent-LNCaP cell lines produced a subline (C4-2) that metastasized to bone, and, interestingly, the incidence of osseous metastases appeared higher in castrated than in intact male hosts. Additional indirect evidence supporting the concept of IAS come from two independent reports that isolated androgen-repressed LNCaP cell lines that grew faster in castrated than in intact hosts, and exhibited growth rates that were actually suppressed by androgens.[40,41] Taken together, these data emphasize the potentially diverse biologic effects that androgens have on a heterogeneous and adapting tumor population and supports the concept that progression to androgen-independence involves loss of androgen-induced differentiation and/or upregulation of androgen-repressed growth regulatory pathways.

CLINICAL STUDIES OF INTERMITTENT ANDROGEN SUPPRESSION

The intermittent regulation of serum testosterone levels for therapeutic purposes in prostate cancer was first attempted with cyclic administration of estrogenic hormone.[42] Nineteen patients with advanced prostate cancer received DES until a clinical response was clearly demonstrated, and then it was withheld until symptoms recurred. One additional patient was treated with flutamide using a similar schedule. The mean duration of initial therapy was 30 months (range 2–70 months). Subjective improvement was noted in all patients during the first 3 months of treatment. When therapy was stopped, 12 of 20 patients relapsed after a mean interval of 8 months (range 1–24 months) and all subsequently responded to re-administration of drug. Therapy-induced impotency was reversed in 9 of 10 men within 3 months of the break in treatment. An improved quality of life was achieved owing to the reduced intake of DES, and no adverse effects on survival were apparent.

The first nonsteroidal antiandrogens became available around the same time as this study, and subsequently most clinical research focused on the combined use of luteinizing hormone releasing hormone (LHRH) agonists and antiandrogens. Little attention has been given to the reversibility of action of LHRH agonists, the significance of which is far-reaching. The potential for a full recovery from therapy makes it possible to alternate a patient between periods of treatment and no treatment. Furthermore, serial serum PSA measurements, which were not available at the time

of the study by Klotz et al,[42] permit accurate monitoring of disease activity and serve as trigger points for stopping and restarting therapy. In response to this androgenic stimulus, atrophic cells are recruited into a normal pathway of differentiation where the risk of progression to androgen-independence is reduced. With the associated movement through the division cycle, the cells become pre-apoptotic again making it possible to repeat therapy.

Preliminary results of IAS in 47 patients using reversible medical castration and serum PSA as trigger points were reported by Goldenberg et al[43] in 1995, and updated to include 80 patients in 1999[44] and 2002.[45] Patients with a minimum follow-up of 12 months and either recurrent or metastatic disease were followed for a mean of 46 months. Mean initial serum PSA was 110 ng/mL. Treatment was initiated with combined androgen blockade and continued for an average of 9 months. Because prognosis is poor in patients who do not achieve normal PSA levels after androgen ablation, only patients with PSA nadir levels below 4 ng/mL were candidates for this IAS protocol. Medication was withheld after 9 months of therapy until serum PSA increased to mean values between 10 and 20 ng/mL. This cycle of treatment and no treatment was repeated until the regulation of PSA became androgen independent (Figure 98.1).

Thirty-two men are currently in their second cycle and 24 are in their third or higher cycle. The mean time to PSA nadir during the first three cycles was 5 months. The first two cycles averaged 18 months in length with 45% of the time off therapy, while the third cycle averaged 15.5 months. Serum testosterone returned to the normal range within a mean of 8 weeks of stopping treatment. The off-treatment period in all cycles was associated with an improvement in sense of well-being, and the recovery of libido and potency in the men who reported normal or near-normal sexual function before the start of therapy. Androgen-independent progression occurred in 10 of 29 stage D patients and 7 of 41 with localized disease after a mean follow-up of 43 months (Table 98.1). Of 21 stage D2 patients, 12 remained on study with stable disease. Nine patients died, three from noncancer-related illness, with median time to progression and overall survival of 26 and 42 months, respectively.

Since these initial reports, other investigators have confirmed the feasibility of IAS in patients with advanced or recurrent prostate cancer. Higano et al[46] reported their experience in Seattle using IAS with a cohort of 22 patients (7 stage D2, 3 stage D1, 2 stage T2/T3, and 10 biochemical failures after definitive local therapy). The median follow-up was 26 months, and all patients remained alive, with two patients (1 biochemical relapse and 1 D1) progressing to androgen-independence at 33 and 22 months, respectively. Time off therapy for stage D2 patients was 35%, slightly less than the percentage of

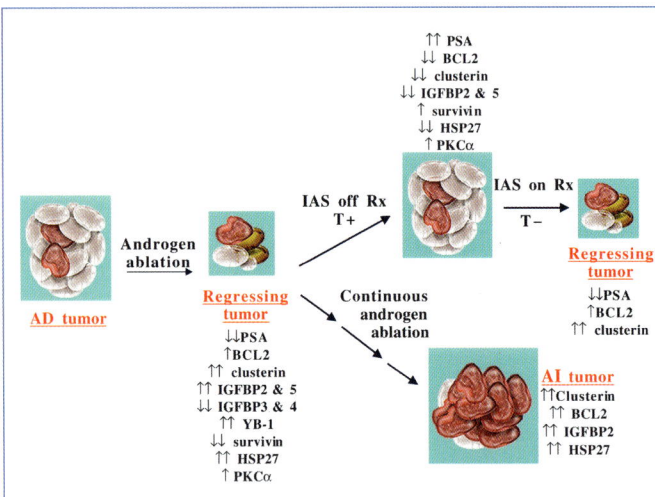

Fig. 98.1

Androgen ablation results in apoptosis and upregulation of previously androgen-repressed genes (e.g., Bcl-2, clusterin). However, not all cells are eliminated and, in the absence of androgens, proliferating cells do not differentiate to become pre-apoptotic again, which results in development of the androgen-independent phenotype and constitutive overexpression of resistance-associated genes like *BCL2*, clusterin, and HSP27. With intermittent re-exposure to testosterone (T+), proliferating cells differentiate, expression of resistance associated genes decrease, and cells become pre-apoptotic again, permitting another round of androgen ablation-induced apoptosis and tumor regression (T–). (IAS, intermittent androgen suppression; IGFBP, insulin-like growth factor binding protein; PKC, protein kinase C; PSA, prostate-specific antigen;

Table 98.1 Clinical studies of intermittent androgen suppression (IAS)

Investigator	Sample size	Clinical stage	Mean follow-up (months)	Cycle 1 start PSA (μg/L)	Cycle 2 start PSA, μg/L	Cycle 3 start PSA, μg/L	Mean cycle length (months),* cycle 1, 2, 3	Mean time off therapy (%)	Mean time to PSA nadir (months)
Goldenberg[43]	47	local + metastatic	30	128	15 (n = 30)	18 (n = 15)	18, 18, 16	47	5
Oliver[46]	20	local + metastatic	n/a	n/a	n/a	n/a	n/a	n/a	n/a
Grossfeld[48]	47	local	24	21	7.0 (n = 17)	20.5 (n = 3)	16, 11, n/a†	50	4
Higano[47]	22	local + metastatic	26	25	7.7 (n = 12)	n/a (n = 0)	15, 18	38	3.5
Crook[55]	54	Local	33	43	n/a	n/a	18	46	5
Hurtado-Coll[45]	70	local + metastatic	46	110	16 (n = 56)	12 (n = 24)	18, 18, 16	47	5

PSA, prostate-specific antigen.

*Length of time spent on drug therapy and off therapy during each cycle of IAS; †Treatment was continued for 1–2 months after nadir PSA reached.

time off for biochemical failures (44%). All patients cycled off therapy for three or more months noted some improvement in overall quality of life.

Oliver et al[47] in London reviewed 20 patients with localized or metastatic prostate cancer who elected to stop androgen ablation therapy after median of 12 months (range 3–48 months). After a median of 9 months off therapy, 13 patients progressed and were restarted on androgen ablation, and 10 of these remain progression-free after 2 years. Of particular interest were 7 patients who were on therapy for 3, 3, 3, 16, 12, 5, and 12 months and subsequently off hormone therapy for 33, 43, 36, 36, 36, 40, and 42 months, respectively. These authors commented on trends in their small series for better duration off therapy in older patients and in those with nonmetastatic disease.

Carrol et al[48] in San Francisco reported on their initial experience with 47 patients with clinically localized prostate cancer treated with an IAS protocol. Patients were followed for a mean of 24 months and completed on average two treatment cycles. Only one patient failed to respond to reinstitution of treatment, and no other patients demonstrated progression during the follow-up period, illustrating the ability of reversible medical castration to induce repeated cycles of therapeutic response. Average cycle length was 16 months for the first cycle and 11 months for the second, and patients averaged 50% of their time off therapy.

A prospective phase II study in post-radiotherapy recurrences accrued over 100 men at 4 centers across Canada.[49] Patients were treated for 9 months and cycled off therapy until serum PSA rose back to levels between 8 and 15 ng/mL (Figure 98.2). Study endpoints included monitoring length of time off therapy, quality-of-life measurements, and time to androgen-independent progression. First cycle analysis

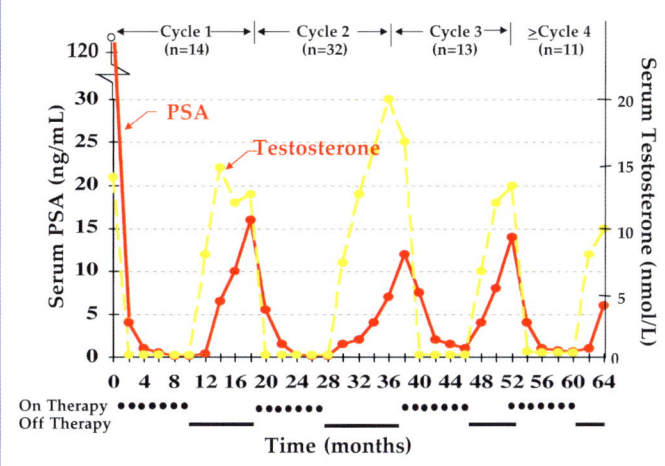

Fig. 98.2

Composite results on 70 patients with prostate cancer treated with intermittent androgen suppression, of whom 14 are in their first cycle of treatment, 32 in their second cycle, 13 in their third, 5 in their fourth cycle, and 6 in their fifth cycle. Mean serum prostate-specific antigen (PSA) at the start of the first, second, third and fourth cycles was 110, 16, 12, and 14 ng/mL, respectively. The first three cycles averaged 18, 18, and 15.5 months in length, respectively.

demonstrated improved quality-of-life measurements when men were cycled off therapy.

Observations from these series, as well as those from recently published studies[50–52] add to and are consistent with the initial reports from Vancouver[42–44] in terms of response rates and time off therapy. Each of these small series collectively illustrate that relatively short on-therapy periods may result in off-therapy intervals of several years in some men, which suggests that continuous androgen ablation may represent overtreatment in a proportion of men. These IAS series use serum PSA as the marker of response to therapy and tumor progression, as well as a guide for when to restart therapy. Serum PSA increases before evidence of tumor progression becomes apparent in more than 90% of patients with progressive disease treated with continuous therapy.[53] As a result, bone scans for monitoring disease progression are used in patients with new symptoms or biochemical progression. Dissociation between biochemical and clinical progression occasionally occurs, however, and stopping therapy with IAS in this scenario would likely accelerate progression. Although unusual, dissociation between biochemical and clinical progression emphasizes the need for phase III controlled data to better characterize the risks and benefits of IAS.

CANDIDATES FOR INTERMITTENT ANDROGEN SUPPRESSION

Failure of serum PSA to nadir below 4 ng/mL after 6 months of therapy is associated with a short duration of response to androgen ablation and poor prognosis,[54] and IAS is not offered to these patients. Men with TxN1–3M0 who are sexually active, compliant to close follow-up, or who do not tolerate the side effects of androgen ablation can be considered for IAS as long as they realize it is investigational. Biochemical failures after radiotherapy or surgery are groups most likely to benefit from IAS, which permits flexibility in applying

and achieving survival benefits of immediate therapy[48,49,55] while balancing potential long-term side effects and costs of continuous therapy. The authors believe that most men with TxNxM1 should be treated with continuous therapy and not be offered IAS except when enrolled in a clinical trial.

LENGTH OF TREATMENT CYCLE

Conceptually, a cycle of androgen ablation should continue until maximal castration-induced apoptosis and tumor regression is induced, but stopped before constitutive development of an androgen-independent phenotype. Premature termination of therapy may permit some cancer cells destined to undergo apoptosis to survive upon re-exposure to testosterone. Some investigators treated for 1 to 2 months past PSA nadir, which results in shorter "on" cycles and shorter "off" cycles, but similar percentages of time spent off therapy. The definition of nadir must be consistent, however, and should be the lowest, plateau serum PSA level attained following initiation of androgen ablation. Standardization of treatment regimens is necessary for comparison of future series.

A 9 month treatment on cycle is used in most series for the following reasons. First, PSA nadir and maximal soft tissue regression is not reached until 8 or 9 months in many patients on IAS.[44,45] Similarly, the duration of time necessary for PSA to reach its nadir in clinically confined disease after institution of neoadjuvant hormone therapy is often longer than 6 months.[56,57] Using a lower limit of sensitivity of 0.2 ng/mL, PSA nadir was reached in only 34% after 3 months, 60% after 5 months, 70% after 6 months, and 84% at 8 months.[56] The initial rapid decrease in PSA results from cessation of androgen-regulated PSA synthesis and apoptosis, while the ongoing slower decline reflects decreasing tumor volume. Second, immunostaining for proliferation markers (Ki67 and proliferating cell nuclear antigen [PCNA]) showed minimal or reduced activity in radical prostatectomy specimens after 8 months of neoadjuvant therapy compared to pretreatment biopsy specimens.[58,59] Third, levels of the antiapoptotic cytoprotective proteins like BCL2 and clusterin, increase beginning during the first 3 months of neoadjuvant hormone therapy (NHT), and remain elevated after 8 months of therapy, consistent with their role in prevention of castration-induced apoptosis.[25,32,59] These observations indicate that stress-induced increases in BCL2 and clusterin occur early after castration and that concerns regarding constitutively elevated levels that are indicative of developing androgen independence are less likely. Interestingly, androgen can downregulate BCL2 expression in LNCaP cells in vitro[27] and clusterin levels in Shionogi tumors in vivo,[60] observations that may be significant when considering mechanisms by which IAS delays time to androgen-independent progression. Based on time to PSA nadir, reduced proliferation marker staining, and early upregulation of cytoprotective proteins, treatment duration of 9 months is recommended prior to stopping therapy, as illustrated in Figure 98.3.

WHEN TO RESTART

Trigger points for reinstitution of androgen withdrawal therapy are similar among investigators reporting on their IAS experience.[43–49] Although the optimal time remains undefined and empirical, time off therapy should be long enough to permit normalization of improved quality of life and testosterone-induced tumor cell differentiation. Re-exposure of tumor cells to testosterone during the off-treatment cycles of IAS is critical to the underlying hypothesis and rationale behind IAS. Furthermore, recovery of testosterone between treatment cycles is necessary for recovery of sexual function, reduced side

effects, and normal sense of well-being. Until more information is obtained, PSA trigger points are regarded as tentative settings only. Trigger points are individualized and factors that are considered include pretreatment PSA levels, stage, PSA velocity, presence of symptoms, and tolerance of androgen ablation therapy. In general, in patients with metastatic disease and high pretreatment PSA levels, therapy is restarted when PSA increases to 20 ng/mL; in patients with locally recurrent disease and moderately elevated pretreatment PSA levels, therapy is restarted when PSA reaches 6 to 15 ng/mL, and earlier for post-radical prostatectomy recurrences.

PHASE III TRIALS

Several trials are underway comparing continuous versus intermittent therapy. Both quality of life and cancer outcome events are being measured. These studies include:

- NCIC CTG (PR.7)—for patients with *biochemical failure* following radiotherapy and without radiographic evidence of metastatic disease. Target sample size is 1360 patients, with over 800 accrued by the end of 2004.
- SWOG 9346 (NCIC PR.8)—for newly diagnosed *metastatic* prostate cancer. This group recently reported some early data on PSA normalization rates. 84% of 527 patients had their PSA fall to within the normal range during the induction (first) cycle. This was more likely to occur in men who had: a younger age, a lower initial PSA, no weight change, no bone pain, no visceral metastases or distant nodal metastases. 96% of men whose PSA normalized, did so within 180 days. Target enrollment of 1360 patients should be met by 2006.

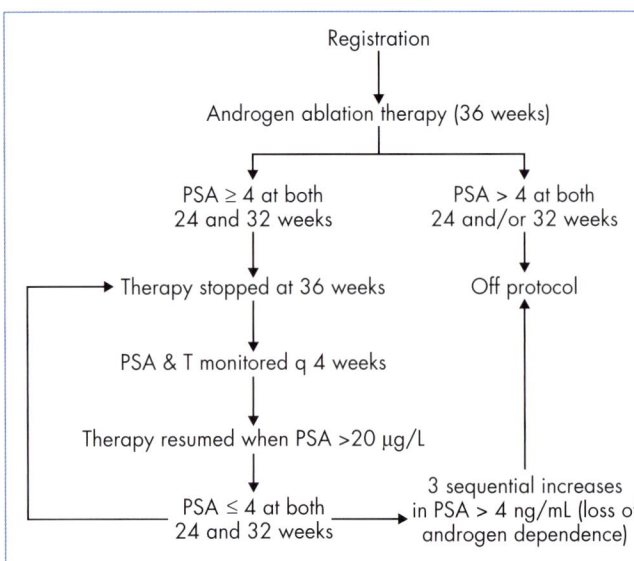

Fig. 98.3
Schema of intermittent androgen suppression therapy for patients with biochemical recurrences following radiation therapy for clinically localized prostate cancer. (PSA, prostate-specific antigen; T, testosterone.)

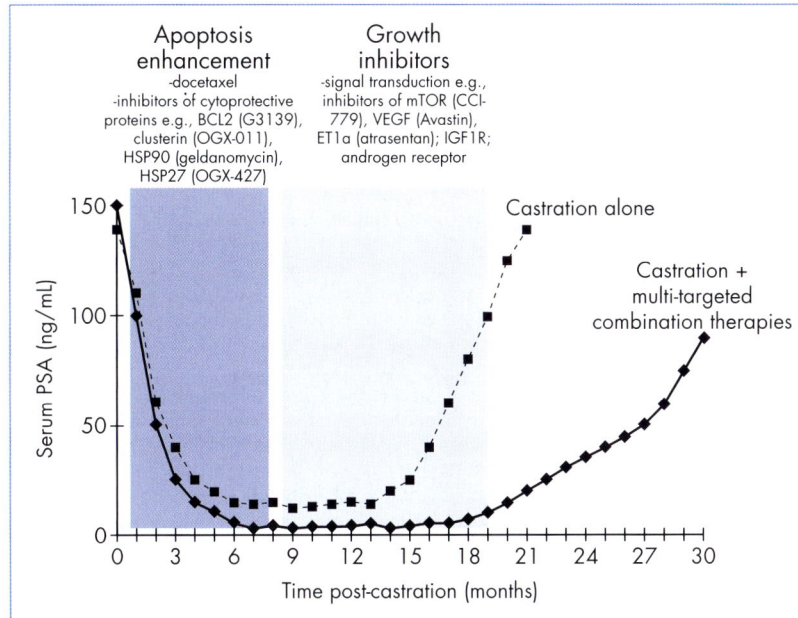

Apoptosis enhancement
-docetaxel
-inhibitors of cytoprotective proteins e.g., BCL2 (G3139), clusterin (OGX-011), HSP90 (geldanomycin), HSP27 (OGX-427)

Growth inhibitors
-signal transduction e.g., inhibitors of mTOR (CCI-779), VEGF (Avastin), ET1a (atrasentan); IGF1R; androgen receptor

Fig. 98.4

Illustrative example of how integration of targeted biologic agents with active cytotoxic agents like docetaxel into cycles of intermittent androgen suppression (IAS) may prolong the length of each IAS cycle by enhancing castration-induced apoptosis and/or inhibiting activation of alternative growth factor signaling pathways. (ET, endothelin; IGF1R, insulin-like growth factor 1 receptor; VEGF, vascular endothelial growth factor.)

The mature results of these trials will be keenly awaited and hopefully will determine the role of IAS in the treatment of prostate cancer.

FUTURE DIRECTIONS

Observations from phase II studies suggest that IAS does not have a negative impact on time to progression or survival, both of which appear similar to continuous combined therapy. However, the available information about IAS remains limited and leaves several questions unanswered. The issue of survival is the most important and phase III randomized studies are required to accurately assess the effects of IAS on this critical parameter. Intermittent androgen suppression appears to improve quality of life by permitting recovery of libido and potency, increasing energy levels, and enhancing sense of well-being during off-treatment periods. Preclinical and preliminary clinical studies have identified groups of patients who are most likely to benefit from IAS, trigger points on when to restart therapy, and determined optimal duration of treatment. It is important to look for other signs of progressive disease when serum PSA is used to monitor disease activity, in case of the unusual scenario of PSA-negative disease progression.

The possibility of expanding the use of IAS to earlier stage disease should be examined in greater detail. Conceivably, IAS may become an alternative to radical prostatectomy or irradiation for the primary treatment of localized prostate cancer in some men with life expectancies of less than 15 years. The prospect of improving the results of IAS by increasing the length and number of cycles is attractive. Prolongation of the length of each off treatment cycle may be possible with 5α-reductase inhibitors like finasteride. As illustrated in Figure 98.4, augmentation of intermittent therapy might be accomplished by the administration of apoptotic-enhancing agents, like cytotoxic agents (docetaxel) or targeted biologic agents (e.g., antisense clusterin, angiogenesis inhibitors, atrasentan), administered at specific times during a cycle of treatment when the modality-of-choice would have its maximum effect.

REFERENCES

1. Miyamoto H, Messing EM, Chang C. Androgen deprivation therapy for prostate cancer: current status and future prospects. Prostate 2004;61:332–53.

2. Denis L, Murphy GP. Overview of phase III trials on combined androgen treatment in patients with metastatic prostate cancer. Cancer 1993;72:3888–3895.

3. Bruchovsky N, Rennie PS, Coldman AJ, et al. Effects of androgen withdrawal on the stem cell composition of the Shionogi carcinoma. Cancer Res 1990;50:2275–2282.

4. Crawford ED, Eisenberger M, McLeod DG, et al. Comparison of bilateral orchiectomy with or without flutamide for the treatment of patients with stage D2 adenocarcinoma of the prostate: Results of NCI intergroup study 0105 (SWOG and ECOG). Br J Urol 1997;80:278 [Abstract].

5. Prostate Cancer Trialists' Collaborative Group. Maximum androgen blockade in advanced prostate cancer: an overview of 22 randomised trials with 3283 deaths in 5710 patients. Lancet 1995;346:265–269.

6. Bruchovsky N, Lesser B, Van Doorn E, et al. Hormonal effects on cell proliferation in rat prostate. Vitamin Horm 1975;33:61–102.

7. Foulds L. Neoplastic Development 1. New York, Academic Press, 1969.

8. Noble RL. Hormonal control of growth and progression in tumors of Nb rats and a theory of action. Cancer Res 1977;37:82–94.

9. Sanford NL, Searle JW, Kerr JFR. Successive waves of apoptosis in the rat prostate after repeated withdrawal of testosterone stimulation. Pathology 1984;16:406–410.

10. Goldie JH, Coldman AJ. A mathematical model for relating the drug sensitivity of tumours to their spontaneous mutation rate. Cancer Treat Rep 1979;63:1727–1733.

11. Isaacs JT. The timing of androgen ablation therapy and / or chemotherapy in the treatment of prostatic cancer. Prostate 1984;5:1–17.

12. So AI, Bowden M, Gleave M. Effect of time of castration and tumour volume on time to androgen-independent recurrence in Shionogi tumours. BJU Int 2004;93:845–850.

13. Mellinger GT. Veterans Administration Cooperative Urological Research Group. Carcinoma of the prostate: a continuing co-operative study. J Urol 1964;91:590–594.

14. Byar DP. Proceedings: The Veterans Administration Cooperative Urological Research Group's studies of cancer of the prostate. Cancer 1973;32:1126–1130

15. Immediate vs deferred treatment for advanced prostate cancer: Initial results of the MRC trial. The Medical Research Council Prostate Cancer Working Party Investigators Group. Br J Urol 1997;79:235–246.

16. Bolla M, Gonzalez MD, Warde P, et al. Improved survival in patients with locally advanced prostate cancer treated with radiotherapy and goserilin. N Engl J Med 1997;337:295–300.

17. Messing EM, Manola J, Sarosdy M, et al. Immediate hormonal therapy compared with observation after radical prostatectomy and pelvic lymphadenectomy in men with node-positive prostate cancer. N Engl J Med 1999;341:1781–1788

18. Iversen P, Johansson JE, Lodding P, et al. Scandinavian Prostatic Cancer Group. Bicalutamide (150 mg) versus placebo as immediate therapy alone or as adjuvant to therapy with curative intent for early nonmetastatic prostate cancer: 5.3-year median followup from the Scandinavian Prostate Cancer Group Study Number 6. J Urol 2004;172:1871–1876.

19. Stanford JL, Blumenstein BA, Brawer MK. Temporal trends in prostate cancer rates in the Pacific Northwest. J Urol 1996;155:604A.

20. Townsend MF, Sanders WH, Northway RO, et al. Bone fractures associated with luteinizing hormone-releasing hormone agonists used in the treatment of prostatic carcinoma. Cancer 1997;79:545–550.

21. Tenniswood M. Apoptosis, tumour invasion and prostate cancer. Br J Urol 1997;79:27–34.

22. Isaacs JT, Wake N, Coffey DS, et al. Genetic instability coupled to clonal selection as a mechanism for progression in prostatic cancer. Cancer Res 1982;42:2353–2361.

23. Craft N, Shostak Y, Carey M, et al. A mechanism for hormone-independent prostate cancer through modulation of androgen receptor signaling by the HER-2/neu tyrosine kinase. Nat Med 1999;5:280–285.

24. Feldman BJ, Feldman D. The development of androgen-independent prostate cancer. Nature Rev 2001;1:34–45.

25. Raffo AJ, Periman H, Chen MW, et al. Overexpression of bcl-2 protects prostate cancer cells from apoptosis in vitro and confers resistance to androgen depletion in vivo. Cancer Res 1995;55:4438–4445.

26. Chen CD, Welsbie DS, Tran C, et al. Molecular determinants of resistance to antiandrogen therapy. Nat Med 2004;10:33–39.

27. Gleave ME, Tolcher A, Miyake H, et al. Progression to androgen-independence is delayed by antisense Bcl-2 oligodeoxynucleotides after castration in the LNCaP prostate tumor model. Clinical Cancer Res 1999;5:2891–2898.

28. Miyake H, Rennie P, Nelson C, et al. Testosterone-repressed prostate message-2 (TRPM-2) is an antiapoptotic gene that confers resistance to androgen ablation in prostate cancer xenograft models. Cancer Res 2000;60:170–176.

29. Miyake H, Nelson C, Rennie P, et al. Overexpression of Insulin-Like Growth Factor Binding Protein-5 helps accelerate Progression to Androgen-Independence in the human prostate LNCaP tumor model through activation of phosphatidylinositol 3'-kinase pathway. Endocrinology 2000;141:2257–2265.

30. Kiyama S, Morrison K, Zellweger T, et al. Castration-induced increases in insulin-like growth factor-binding protein-2 promotes proliferation of androgen-independent human prostate LNCaP tumors. Cancer Res 2003;63:3575–3584.

31. Rocchi P, So A, Kojima S, et al. Heat shock protein 27 increases after androgen ablation and plays a cytoprotective role in hormone refractory prostate cancer. Cancer Research, 2004;64:6595–6602

32. July LV, Akbari M, Zellweger T, et al. Clusterin expression is significantly enhanced in prostate cancer cells following androgen withdrawal therapy. Prostate 2002;50:179–188.

33. Trachtenberg J. Experimental treatment of prostatic cancer by intermittent hormonal therapy. J Urol 1987;137:785–788.

34. Russo P, Liguori G, Heston WDW, et al. Effects of intermittent diethylstilbestrol diphosphate administration on the R3327 rat prostatic carcinoma. Cancer Res 1987;47:5967–5970.

35. Akakura K, Bruchovsky N, Goldenberg SL, et al. Effects of intermittent androgen suppression on androgen-dependent tumours: apoptosis and serum prostate specific antigen. Cancer 1993;71:2782–2790.

36. Gleave ME, Hsieh JT, Wu H-C, et al. Serum PSA levels in mice bearing human prostate LNCaP tumors are determined by tumor volume and endocrine and growth factors. Cancer Res 1992;52:1598–1605.

37. Sato N, Gleave M, Bruchovsky N, et al. A metastatic and androgen-sensitive human prostate cancer model using intraprostatic inoculation of LNCaP cells in SCID mice. Cancer Res 1997;57:1584–1589.

38. Sato N, Gleave ME, Bruchovsky N, et al. Intermittent androgen suppression delays time to non-androgen regulated prostate specific antigen gene expression in the human prostate LNCaP tumour model. J Steroid Biochem Molec Biol 1996;58:139–146.

39. Thalmann, GN, Anezinis, PE, Chang SH, et al. Androgen-independent cancer progression and bone metastasis in the LNCaP model of human prostate cancer. Cancer Res 1994;54:2577–2581.

40. Umekita Y, Hiipakka RA, Kokontis JM, et al. Human prostate tumor growth in athymic mice: inhibition by androgens and stimulation by finasteride. Proc Natl Acad Sci USA 1996;93:11802–11807.

41. Zhou HYE, Chang S-H, Chen B-Q, et al. Androgen-repressed phenotype in human prostate cancer. Proc Natl Acad Sci USA 1996;93:15152–15157.

42. Klotz LH, Herr HW, Morse MJ, et al. Intermittent endocrine therapy for advanced prostate cancer. Cancer 1986;58:2546–2250.

43. Goldenberg SL, Bruchovsky N, Gleave ME, et al. Intermittent androgen suppression in the treatment of prostate cancer: a preliminary report. Urology 1995;45:839–845.

44. Goldenberg SL, Gleave ME, Taylor D. Clinical experience with intermittent androgen suppression for prostate cancer: Minimum 3 years of follow-up. Molecular Urology 1999;3:287–292.

45. Hurtado-Coll A, Goldenberg SL, Gleave ME, et al. Intermittent androgen suppression in prostate cancer: the Canadian experience. Urology 2002;60:52–56.

46. Oliver RT, Williams G, Paris AM, et al. Intermittent androgen deprivation after PSA-complete response as a strategy to reduce induction of hormone-resistant prostate cancer. Urology 1997;49:79–82.

47. Higano CS, Ellis W, Russell K, et al. Intermittent androgen suppression with leuprolide and flutamide for prostate cancer. A pilot study. Urology 1996;48:800–804.

48. Grossfeld GD, Small EJ, Lubeck DP, et al. Androgen deprivation therapy for patients with clinically localized (stages T1 to T3) prostate cancer and for patients with biochemical recurrence after radical prostatectomy. Urology 2001;58:56–64.

49. Bruchovsky N, Klotz LH, Sadar M, et al. Intermittent androgen suppression for prostate cancer: Canadian prospective trial related observations. Mol Urol 2002;4:191–199.

50. Sato N, Akakura K, Isaka S, et al. Chiba Prostate Study Group. Intermittent androgen suppression for locally advanced and metastatic prostate cancer: preliminary report of a prospective multicenter study. Urology 2004;64:341–345.

51. Albrecht W, Collette L, Fava C, et al. Intermittent maximal androgen blockade in patients with metastatic prostate cancer: an EORTC feasibility study. Eur Urol 2003;44:505–511.

52. Lane TM, Ansell W, Farrugia D, et al. Long-term outcomes in patients with prostate cancer managed with intermittent androgen suppression. Urol Int 2004;73:117–122.

53. Stamey TA, Kabalin JN, Ferrari M, et al. Prostate specific antigen in the diagnosis and treatment of adenocarcinoma of the prostate. IV. Anti-androgen treated patients. J Urol 1989;141:1088–1090.

54. Miller JI, Ahmann FR, Drach GW, et al. The clinical usefulness of serum prostate specific antigen after hormonal therapy of metastatic prostate cancer. J Urol 1992;147:956–961.

55. Crook JM, Szumacher E, Malone S, et al. Intermittent androgen suppression in the management of prostate cancer. Urology 1999;53:530–534.

56. Gleave ME, Goldenberg SL, Jones EC, et al. Maximal biochemical and pathological downstaging requires 8 months of neoadjuvant hormonal therapy prior to radical prostatectomy. J Urol 1996;155:213–219.

57. Gleave ME, Goldenberg SL, Chin J, et al. Phase III randomized comparative study of 3 vs 8 months of neoadjuvant hormone therapy prior to radical prostatectomy: Biochemical and pathologic endpoints. J Urol 2001;166:500–506.

58. Patterson R, Gleave M, Jone E, et al. Immunohistochemical analysis of radical prostatectomy specimens after 8 months of neoadjuvant hormone therapy. Mol Urol 1999;3:277–286.

59. Tsuji M, Murakami Y, Kanayama H, et al. Immunohistochemical analysis of Ki-67 antigen and Bcl-2 protein expression in prostate cancer: effect of neoadjuvant hormonal therapy. Br J Urol 1998;81:116–121.

60. Rennie PS, Bruchovsky N, Akakura K, et al. Effect of tumour progression on the androgenic regulation of the androgen receptor, TRPM-2 and YPT1 genes in the Shionogi carcinoma. J Steroid Biochem Mol Biol 1994;50:31–40.

99

Antiandrogen withdrawal syndromes: pathophysiology and clinical implications

Kathleen W Beekman, Grant Buchanan, Wayne D Tilley,
Howard I Scher

INTRODUCTION

The "antiandrogen withdrawal syndrome" describes the anti-prostate cancer effects following the selective discontinuation of an antiandrogen such as flutamide, bicalutamide, or nilutamide in a patient with progressive prostate cancer treated with a combination of an antiandrogen and testicular androgen ablation. The effects, when they occur, do so in castrate patients with rising prostate-specific antigen (PSA) and/or clinical metastatic disease-points in the illness where the tumor is considered by many to be "hormone-refractory" (Figure 99.1)[1]. While the withdrawal syndrome was originally described with flutamide by three groups including our own in 1993,[2–4] it was soon recognized that withdrawal responses could occur following the selective discontinuation of other hormones including estrogens, progestational agents, and glucocorticoids (reviewed by Kelly et al[5]). The responses were similar to what had been observed previously in breast cancer patients following discontinuation of tamoxifen.[6,7] It would thus appear that designating these prostate tumors as "hormone-refractory" is a misnomer.

Since the original description of the antiandrogen withdrawal syndrome, much has been learned about the mechanisms associated with prostate cancer progression. Indeed, in retrospect, a "bedside to bench" observation helped to focus researchers on the clinical significance of continued signaling through the androgen receptor (AR) in tumors that progress following castration. The antiandrogen withdrawal syndromes provides an in-vivo demonstration of how a specific treatment influences both the biology and clinical behavior of the disease. This phenomenon, now termed "therapy-mediated selection pressure,"[8] illustrates why localised prostate cancers at the time of diagnosis may have different molecular profiles than tumors than metastatic tumors that progress following castration. As such, when considering a targeted therapy, it is essential to understand the targets that are present within the context of the specific clinical state[1] in which the therapy will be utilized or studied.[9]

HISTORICAL PERSPECTIVE

The original descriptions of the palliative effects of diethylstilbestrol or surgical orchiectomy on progressive prostate cancer, made over 6 decades ago,[10,11] highlighted an important management principle that is still valid today: blocking the production or action of testicular androgens by medical or surgical means does not eliminate all of the malignant cells within a tumor mass, and as such is not curative. Reports of the palliative benefits of surgical[12] or medical[13] adrenalectomy to eliminate androgens from non-testicular sources followed, which, coupled with studies showing incomplete suppression of intratumoral dihydrotestosterone with medical castration alone,[14] suggested that strategies to eliminate both testicular and adrenal androgens as the initial therapeutic approach might be more beneficial than the elimination of testicular androgens alone. Estimates were that androgens from adrenal sources might represent 5% to 45% of the residual androgens present in tumors after surgical castration alone.[15]

The anti-prostate cancer effects of androgen ablative therapies include an apoptotic response in a proportion

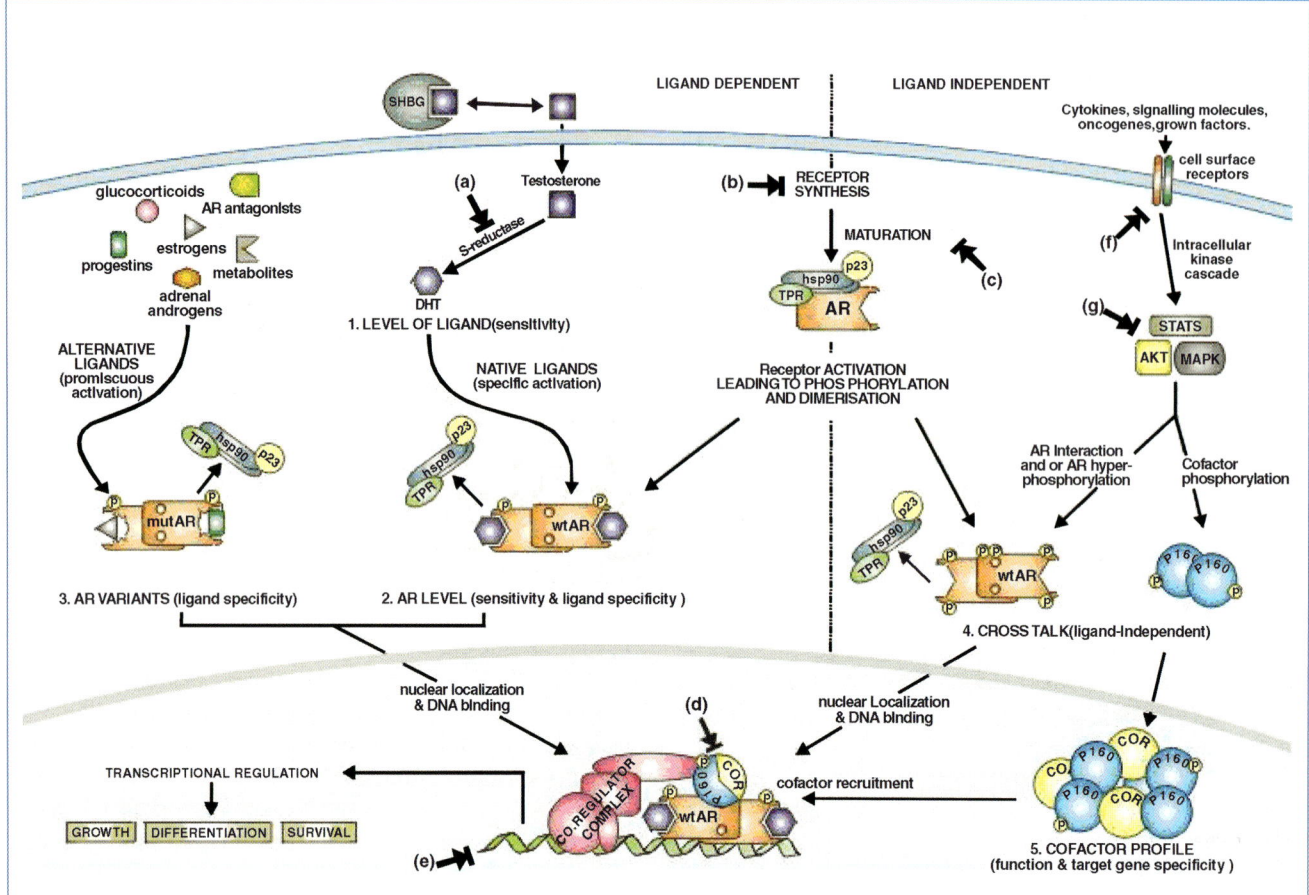

Figure 99.1

Mechanisms by which signaling through the androgen receptor (AR) continues following castration. Following synthesis, the AR exists in dynamic equilibrium between an immature state and an active form capable of binding high affinity androgenic ligands via association/dissociation with a complex that includes heat-shock proteins. (*a*) Receptor-dependent, ligand-mediated signaling. Ligand binding results in the dissociation of this complex, receptor dimerization and phosphorylation, nuclear transport, DNA binding, the recruitment of components of the transcription machinery and other cofactor molecules, such as the p160 coactivators, and ultimately, the activation of particular gene pathways. (*b*) Receptor-dependent, ligand-independent. The AR can also be activated in the absence of ligand by membrane bound tyrosine kinase receptors such as HER2/neu, as well as by signaling molecules, growth factors and cytokines. Intracellular kinase cascades result in receptor activation, transport, binding to androgen response elements and the transactivation of target genes. *1 to 5*, Mechanisms of continued androgen signaling implicated in maintaining prostate cancer growth in a castrate environment following androgen ablation therapy. *1*, Tumor cells may acquire mechanisms to accumulate androgens, such as sequestration by steroid hormone binding globulin or altered regulation of enzymes involved in the synthesis and metabolism of androgens. *2*, Castrate-resistant clinical prostate cancer samples often exhibit increased AR levels compared with early stage tumors or normal prostate cells. This may result from amplification or overexpression of the AR gene. *3*, AR gene mutations can allow promiscuous activation of the AR by alternative ligands, such as glucocorticoids, estrogens, adrenal androgens, progestins and traditional receptor antagonists such as hydroxyflutamide. Other mutations may alter the recruitment of cofactors. *4*, Cross-talk with other signaling pathways may activate the AR in the absence of native ligands. *5*, An altered profile of AR coregulators (coactivators and corepressors) may facilitate ligand-independent AR signaling, or enhance AR activation by low levels of ligand. (i) to (vii), Represent potential new points of therapeutic intervention.
Reproduced with permission from Scher et al[53]

of cells within a mass, producing a decrease in size but not the complete elimination of the tumor; followed by a period of apparent stability in which PSA levels do not change and the tumor is viable but not proliferating; followed by a period of regrowth as a castration resistant lesion. Because ablation of testicular androgens alone was not curative, an important clinical question in the 1980s was whether an approach designed to ablate both testicular and adrenal androgens as initial hormone therapy would prove to be superior to those directed solely at testicular sources. It was postulated that superiority would be demonstrated in several ways:

1) an increase in the proportion of patients who are cured; 2) a delay in time to progression as assessed by post-therapy PSA changes (after 1990 when the test became available), new metastases on an imaging study, or the development of prostate cancer related symptoms; 3) prolongation of life; and 4) an improved safety profile.

It was also during this era that a range of medical approaches became available that obviated the need for both a surgical orchiectomy and surgical adrenalectomy to ablate androgens from these sources. Among the medications introduced and subsequently approved for use were the gonadotropin-releasing hormone (GnRH) agonists and antagonists, steroidal and nonsteroidal antiandrogens, 5α-reductase inhibitors, and inhibitors of adrenal androgen synthesis. With surgical orchiectomy the least preferred method by patients to ablate testicular androgens,[16] and the recognized morbidity of surgical adrenalectomy, medical therapies soon replaced surgery (both adrenalectomy and orchiectomy) as the so-called "treatment of choice." It was at this point that prospective, randomized trials comparing GnRH agonists/antagonists (leuprolide acetate and goserelin) and antiandrogens (flutamide and later bicalutamide and nilutamide) to gonadrotropin-releasing hormone agonists/antagonists alone were begun. Similar trials were designed and initiated with surgical orchiectomy as the method of testicular androgen ablation. Using a variety of combinations of medical and surgical approaches, over 27 prospective randomized comparisons were initiated and completed. Two in particular were perhaps the most influential on clinical practice: SWOG Intergroup 1, which compared the combination of leuprolide acetate plus flutamide to leuprolide acetate plus placebo[17]; and EORTC 30893, which compared goserelin plus flutamide to surgical orchiectomy.[18] Both trials showed a survival benefit for the combined or maximal androgen blockade approach relative to a monotherapy approach that reduced testicular androgens alone. However, despite the survival benefit, the combined androgen blockade was not curative for the majority of men. Consequently, a large number of men with progressive disease who had either undergone an orchiectomy or who received GnRH hormone agonists/antagonists in combination with flutamide presented for further therapy.

CLINICAL OBSERVATION OF ANTIANDROGEN WITHDRAWAL RESPONSE

The antiandrogen withdrawal syndrome was first described when clinical responses were observed following selective discontinuation of flutamide in combination with a GnRH analog or surgical orchiectomy. No additional therapy was added at the

point that flutamide was stopped, and those patients who had not undergone surgical castration were continued on medical therapies to maintain testosterone levels in the castrate range.[2-4] At the University of Michigan and Memorial Sloan-Kettering Cancer Center (MSKCC), the observation was the result in part of our focus on how to reduce the methodologic difficulties associated with drug development in this disease, and in particular how to base eligibility and outcomes on pre- and post-therapy changes in PSA.[19] In the first patient, a withdrawal response was observed, and flutamide was discontinued to avoid the potential hepatic toxicities associated with an investigational agent prior to enrollment on an experimental protocol we were conducting for the palliation of pain secondary to osseous metastases. Following flutamide discontinuation, and prior to protocol enrollment, the PSA level was observed to decline and bone pain decreased. A repeat PSA performed 2 weeks later showed a further PSA reduction, and protocol therapy was not administered.[4] Suspecting this might be an effect similar to what had been reported with tamoxifen,[6,7] flutamide was selectively discontinued in additional patients and additional responses were observed.[20] A most important finding was that effects were not limited to declines in PSA, as objective tumor regressions were documented. Tumor sites in which objective regressions were observed included the epidural space, nodal disease, and in the viscera visceral sites such as the liver. The responses to flutamide withdrawal, when they occurred, did so rapidly, consistent with the short half-life of the drug. As shown in Table 99.1, a range of response rates were reported, with estimates that up to 40% of patients would experience subjective and objective benefits.[2,3,20-23]

Predictive factors for a response to flutamide discontinuation included high baseline alkaline phosphatase and prolonged drug exposure.[24,25] Factors associated with prolonged drug exposure, included the disease extent at the start of therapy, clinical characteristics associated with minimal disease burdens (such as a good performance status), and low PSA levels. For example, in study INT-0105, in which men with non-castrate metastatic tumor with or without prior local therapy were randomized to receive an orchiectomy plus flutamide versus orchiectomy alone, progression-free survival times were 20.4 months in the flutamide arm versus 18.6 months in the placebo arm ($P = 0.2$).[26] These results contrasted with those of another study, in which 309 men in the rising PSA state following prostatectomy had a median response duration of 10.8 years.[27] This contrast in response reflects differences between the two studies in the extent of disease.

It is important to note that at the time withdrawal responses to flutamide were first described, flutamide was the only antiandrogen in general use. Currently, there are two general classes of antiandrogens in clinical

Table 99.1 Responses to antiandrogen withdrawal

Reference	Antiandrogen	Median exposure (months)	>50% PSA decline, n (%)	Time to progression (months)
Scher HI 1993[20]	Flutamide	NA	10/25 (40)	5+
Dupont 1993[2]	Flutamide	57	32/40 (80)	14.5
Sartor 1994[22]	Flutamide	27	14/29 (48)	8
Figg 1995[36]	Flutamide	28	7/21 (33)	3.7
Scher 1995[101]	Flutamide	16	16/57 (28)	4
Small 1995[29]	Flutamide	21.5	12/82 (15)	3.5
Herrada 1996[23]	Flutamide	19	11/39 (28)	3.3
Sella 1988[102]	Cyproterone acetate	10.5	4/12 (33)	7.2
Small 1997[103]	Flutamide	NA	4/8 (50)	NA
Nieh J Urol 1997[31]	Bicalutamide	26	1/3 (33)	6
Schelhammer 1997[32]	Flutamide	NA	4/8 (50)	NA
Schelhammer 1997[32]	Bicalutamide	NA	4/14 (29)	NA
Small 2004[43]	Bicalutamide 59%	NA	15/132 (11)	5.9

use: steroidal and nonsteroidal. Steroidal antiandrogens, which have progestational as well as antiandrogenic effects, include cyproterone acetate (available primarily in Europe) and megestrol acetate. In addition to differences in clearance and side effect profiles, the agents have variable affinity for the androgen receptor and the exact site of binding to the receptor, as evidenced by the effectiveness of these agents in second and third-line settings. It was hypothesized that patients that progressed while receiving bicalutamide or nilutamide in combination with a GnRH analog or orchiectomy would exhibit a withdrawal response as well, and reports soon followed of withdrawal responses to the selective discontinuation of bicalutamide[28–32] and nilutamide,[33] thus establishing the "antiandrogen withdrawal syndrome" as a clinical entity.[29,34] In addition, similar withdrawal responses were observed with the progestational agents megestrol acetate,[35–37] diethylstilbestrol,[38] and chlormadinone acetate.[39]

The paradox of the antiandrogen withdrawal response is that both the steroidal and nonsteroidal agents used initially to inhibit tumor growth could, in certain situations, stimulate tumor growth to the point where discontinuation of the agent became a "therapeutic intervention" for the individual patient. The range of agents associated with this phenomenon, and the fact that most of them acted through the AR, suggested promiscuity in ligand binding and receptor activation. Additional evidence of the agonist effect of these agents is the clinical flare of disease associated with the use of progestational agents administered to treat cachexia, consistent with aberrant receptor activation.[40]

An obvious consideration is that a withdrawal response cannot be observed in a patient who is not receiving the drug, which implies that under the "selection pressure" of prolonged exposure a drug initially used to antagonize androgen action transforms into an agonist that promotes tumor growth. The withdrawal response occurs only in patients who are otherwise medically or surgically castrated and serum testosterone levels are low (<50 ng/mL). It is not observed in patients who are receiving nonsteroidal antiandrogens as monotherapy—when testosterone levels are elevated due to increased hypothalamic release of GnRH and consequent increased luteinizing hormone release from the anterior pituitary gland. The response is rarely seen when the antiandrogen is added at the time of progression following an initial response to orchiectomy or GnRH analog. Overall, the frequencies of response to bicalutamide or nilutamide discontinuation are less than observed with flutamide.[29,41] In addition, withdrawal responses to bicalutamide and nilutamide may not occur for as long as 10 to 12 weeks following discontinuation of the drug, reflecting the long half-life (greater than 7 days) of the two agents.[29,34] This presents a dilemma for the clinician as to whether there is sufficient time to wait for a withdrawal response that occurs infrequently, or whether to simply start a new therapy immediately. There is no straightforward answer.

COMBINED ANTIANDROGEN WITHDRAWAL AND ADRENAL ANDROGEN ABLATION

Several studies reported even more "dramatic" responses to flutamide discontinuation when combined with a direct inhibitor of adrenal androgen synthesis such as aminoglutethimide[22] or ketoconazole.[42] This ultimately led to a prospective, randomized comparison of the combination of antiandrogen discontinuation and ketoconazole to antiandrogen discontinuation alone.[43] In this trial, patients who received the combination of antiandrogen withdrawal and ketoconazole had a higher PSA response (27%; 95% confidence interval [CI] 20–35%) and longer median time to progression (8.6 months) than patients who received antiandrogen alone (11%; 95% CI 7–17% and 6 months) ($P = 0.0002$). There was no survival difference. The lower overall PSA decline rate may reflect the fact that over two-thirds of the patients in the population received bicalutamide and one-third flutamide. Whether a survival difference would have been observed if only flutamide was used is unknown.

SECOND-LINE ANTIANDROGENS THERAPY

The role of second- and third-line hormonal therapy for patients who progress despite castration and antiandrogen withdrawal is largely undefined. As many trials of second- and third-line therapy were conducted prior to PSA based standards of reporting,[44] interpreting the literature is difficult. Flutamide has been the most widely studied in the second-line setting, primarily following castration alone, with response rates ranging from 35% to 45%.[45,46] Similar results have been demonstrated with other nonsteroidal antiandrogens. Retrospective analyses of patients treated with nilutamide after progression on another antiandrogen resulted in PSA declines in up to 50% of patients.[47,48] In addition, several studies have suggested that the response rate to an antiandrogen increases following exposure to another antiandrogen,[25,49] and that different antiandrogens can be non-cross-resistant even though they are all directed toward the AR and represent the same class of drug. Large studies testing the utility of flutamide after antiandrogen withdrawal have not been conducted. However, one small study reported a response rate of 50% (5 of 10) in patients treated with flutamide following progression with a GnRH and bicalutamide.[50]

Currently, it is not known whether the survival advantage observed with taxotere-based chemotherapy is affected by the number of prior hormonal manipulations a patient has experienced. A phase III trial which sought to clarify this issue by testing whether docetaxel is superior to ketoconazole (ECOG 1899),[51] was closed secondary to poor accrual, most likely because many physicians feel that maximizing hormonal therapy, especially for asymptomatic patients, is preferable to initiating chemotherapy. Although we agree with this approach, there has been no prospectively designed trial that has shown a survival benefit for second-line hormonal therapy.

BIOLOGY OF ANTIANDROGEN WITHDRAWAL RESPONSE

Studies to understand the mechanisms contributing to withdrawal responses have been limited in part by the lack of appropriate tumor tissue for study. It is compounded by the nature of progressive prostate cancers which are often manifest by a rising PSA or bony metastases, neither of which are conducive to tissue acquisition. As noted previously, the change in the clinical behavior of the disease under the selection pressure of a drug mandates characterization of the tumor both at the time of relapse and at the time therapy is first initiated. The results of these studies, along with the characterization of prostate cancer cell lines and xenografts, show that androgen receptor signaling is maintained or enhanced in the majority of tumors that are progressing despite castrate levels of testosterone. The result is an altered androgen signaling pathway that has enhanced sensitivity to castrate levels of dihydrotestosterone, is promiscuous for activation by alternative ligands, or is activated by cross talk with cytokine and/or growth factor pathways.

ANDROGEN RECEPTOR STRUCTURE

The cellular mediator of androgen action is the AR, a transcription factor that modulates expression of genes involved in differentiation, homeostasis, and angiogenesis. The AR has a modular structure, consisting primarily of a large amino-terminal transactivation domain (NTD), a centrally located DNA-binding domain (DBD), and a carboxy-terminal ligand binding domain (LBD) that confers high affinity and specificity for androgen binding.

Mutations of the AR gene have been reported in prostate cancer at frequencies of 5% to 50%, depending upon disease stage and prior treatment. The majority involve a small number of discrete regions of the LBD.[52] Most of these mutations confer promiscuity or sensitivity for receptor activation by other steroid hormones and/or by the specific antiandrogen used in clinical management of the disease.[52,53] The concept of "therapy-mediated selection pressure" is exemplified by the detection of AR variants in tumors from patients treated with hydroxyflutamide, as part of a combined androgen blockade strategy, which confers enhanced receptor activity in response to flutamide, but which retains sensitivity to other antiandrogens.[54,55] This has been observed clinically, as patients who have progressed on flutamide do respond to bicalutamide. This has also been described for several other antiandrogens, and can be recapitulated in vitro. Culture of LNCaP cells with bicalutamide resulted in outgrowth of a subline containing a mutation at codon 741, which conferred increased cell growth and PSA secretion in response to bicalutamide but not flutamide.[56] These data suggest that each antiandrogen may elicit a specific mechanism that can lead to a withdrawal response, consistent with clinical observations that second-line therapy with antiandrogens often results in tumor regression. Studies of the autochthonous TRAMP model of prostate cancer[57,58] demonstrate that therapy mediated selection of AR mutations is not limited to antiandrogen treatment. Whereas noncastrate mice develop mutations in the AR LBD, mice castrated at 12 weeks of age developed mutations in the NTD.[59] Importantly, mutations in the NTD can affect the AR function in a manner distinct from those in the LBD. Enforced expression in the mouse prostate of the AR-NTD variant, Gln231Glu, conferred rapid development of prostatic intraepithelial neoplasia that progressed to invasive and metastatic disease in 100% of mice.[60] In contrast, enforced expression of the wild-type AR or a common LBD AR variant responsive to other steroid hormones had no discernible effect.[60] This study highlights the potential functional significance of mutations in the AR-NTD, and demonstrates that specific mutations can turn the AR into a potent oncogene sufficient to promote metastatic prostate cancer.

While AR gene mutations likely are an important part of antiandrogen agonist activity and subsequent withdrawal responses, they cannot be detected in all patients.[61] Although this may be due to technical issues, differences in patient populations, stage of disease, tumor burden, and/or time on antiandrogen therapy,[61] it is likely that multiple mechanisms will play a role in antiandrogen agonist activity and subsequent withdrawal response, with AR mutations being only one contributing mechanism.

ANDROGEN RECEPTOR EXPRESSION

Xenograft models of human prostate cancer are useful models in which to study the AR, as most grow initially in an androgen-dependent state, undergo regression upon castration, and subsequently regrow in the castrate environment. In support of the hypothesis that AR continues to play an important role in growth of progressive castrate prostate cancer, several studies have demonstrated an increase in the level of AR and/or AR-regulated genes in xenograft tumors with castrate levels of testosterone in comparison to untreated tumors.[62–66] In particular, comprehensive gene expression profiling determined that the AR was the only gene upregulated in the progression from androgen-sensitive to castration-resistant growth in all 7 human prostate cancer xenograft models analyzed.[67] In clinical disease, recent studies have show an analogous increase in both AR mRNA and protein levels in metastatic castrate-resistant prostate cancer compared with localized disease.[53] Moreover, increased AR levels in the prostate of clinically localized disease has been shown to predict relapse following radical prostatectomy, suggesting that increased AR may predispose to castrate resistance and/or metastatic spread.[68] Importantly, increased levels of AR may be all that is required to switch antagonists such as bicalutamide to receptor agonists,[67] providing a mechanism distinct from AR mutations to explain disease progression and antiandrogen withdrawal.

There are likely to be several mechanisms that contribute to increased AR levels, including AR gene amplification (as demonstrated in up to 29% of tumors)[69–71] and increased stability or reduced degradation of the AR protein in progressive disease.[72] However, not all progressive tumors demonstrate an increase in AR, and some may have actually shown a decrease.[73] These differences highlight that the AR alone is probably not sufficient to ensure continued signaling, but is probably dependent upon multiple factors that impact on its pathway.

Increased levels of androgenic steroids, combined with an increase in the amount of receptor protein (see below), could contribute to maintenance of AR signaling despite castrate levels of testosterone in the blood.[71] A recent study using laser capture mass spectrometry documented levels of androgenic steroids in tumors from men with progressive disease after hormonal therapy that were sufficient to induce signaling.[63]

ROLE OF COREGULATORY MOLECULES

Transcriptional activity of the AR is mediated, in part, by the recruitment of coregulator proteins that enhance (coactivators) or repress (corepressors) receptor function. An increase in coactivator proteins has been shown to develop in the setting of castrate disease,[62,74,75] coinciding with an increase in AR expression during the growth phase of prostate cancer cells following androgen deprivation.[72] The clinical consequence of an increase in coactivator proteins may be manifested as an increased sensitivity of the AR to lower concentrations of androgen or an alteration in AR specificity. In support of this hypothesis, several studies have shown that AR coactivators, such as ARA70 and ARA55, selectively enhance the ability of 17-β-estradiol and hydroxyflutamide to activate the AR.[60,76,77] Important coactivators include transcriptional intermediary factor (TIF2) and steroid receptor co-activator-1 (SRC1), which have been shown to be increased in prostate tumors following castration. TIF2 broadens the ligand-binding specificity of certain AR mutants to include activation of the receptor by adrenal androgens.[72] Nuclear corepressors mediate transcriptional repression and may play an important role in prostate cancer growth as well. Nuclear hormone receptor corepressor (NCoR) is recruited to the ligand-bound AR and can mediate the antagonist action of bicalutamide, flutamide, and mifepristone on the AR; the lack of NCoR may allow for an increase in the agonist activity of these agents on the AR.[78,79]

Although a large array of nuclear coregulators has been described thus far, the exact mechanism of how coregulators affect transcription is still being elucidated. Aberrant regulation of coregulators may result in androgen independent growth and provide a mechanism for agonist activity of antiandrogens resulting in therapy-mediated alterations of progressive prostate cancers. Disruption of coregulator-mediated growth may prove to be an important therapeutic target.

CROSSTALK WITH OTHER SIGNALING PATHWAYS

Activation of the AR by tyrosine kinase receptors, growth factors, or cytokines is thought to provide a mechanism by which prostate cancer growth can bypass the requirement for native ligand.[77,80-86] Activation of the AR by these factors results in the proliferation of prostate cancer cells, and increased tumor cell survival during androgen deprivation.[87,88] Indeed, several studies have reported increased HER2/NEU expression in prostate cancer at all stages of disease.[89-91] In a recent study analyzing radical prostatectomy specimens obtained at surgery for clinically organ-confined prostate cancer, 90% of patients who subsequently developed extensive metastatic disease requiring androgen ablation therapy already expressed high levels of both HER2/NEU and AR (Dr Camela Ricciardelli, University of Adelaide; personal communication). It is currently thought that HER2/NEU can promote DNA binding and stability of the AR through activation of MAPK and AKT, which can bind to and activate the AR.[88,92] Other mechanisms that directly activate MAPK and AKT elicit a similar effect.[88] Hydroxyflutamide has been shown to potentiate this pathway by allowing rapid phosphorylation of MAPK, possibly via RAS/RAF association.[87]

CLINICAL SIGNIFICANCE OF ANTIANDROGEN WITHDRAWAL RESPONSE

While the antiandrogen withdrawal response has been critical in propelling an improved understanding of the biology of prostate cancer, it is important not

to overstate the clinical significance of withdrawal response for patients with castration resistant disease. As noted earlier in the chapter, an obvious consideration is that a withdrawal response cannot be observed in a patient who is not receiving the drug. One potential reason that the antiandrogen withdrawal response is less prominent in clinical practice than would be predicted is the use of bicalutamide over flutamide. The approval of bicalutamide on the basis of a prospective, randomized trial demonstrating similar anti-prostate cancer effects, similar survival times, and an improved safety profile relative to flutamide, when each was combined with a GnRH agonist,[93] led to a dramatic decrease in flutamide use. Although never studied on a comparative basis, cumulative reports suggest that withdrawal responses occur more frequently following flutamide discontinuation relative to bicalutamide. It can, therefore, be anticipated that, on a cumulative basis, the frequency of responses to antiandrogen withdrawal will decrease.

Nevertheless, it is still reasonable to consider a trial of antiandrogen withdrawal alone at the time of progression in the appropriate setting because the degree and duration of response when it occurs in the individual patient can be significant. In this context, subsequent therapy is withheld until progression is documented after the steroidal or nonsteroidal antiandrogen is discontinued, allowing a sufficient observation period for a response to occur as a function of the half-life of agent that was discontinued.[94]

The clinical significance of the antiandrogen withdrawal response is also affected by a decrease in the duration of antiandrogen treatment when combined with a GnRH analog. A number of randomized trials have been conducted comparing different hormonal approaches as monotherapy and/or as a part of so-called combined androgen blockade strategies. A meta-analysis of trials evaluating LHRH agonists/antagonists, orchiectomy, DES, or choice of DES or orchiectomy as monotherapy showed that, in general, hormonal interventions that lower serum testosterone levels to castrate levels result in similar survival times.[95] Other meta-analyses have repeatedly shown a modest survival benefit at 5 years with combined androgen blockade.[96-99] One report included 21 trials with 6871 patients and showed a modest but significant survival advantage at 5 years for combined therapy (hazard ratio 0.87; 95% CI 0.80–0.94), favoring combined therapy. The analysis was most influenced by three trials in which a 3.7- to 7-month median survival difference was observed.[100] These findings are in direct contrast, however, to the results of the INT-0105 comparing orchiectomy alone with orchiectomy and flutamide, which did not show any benefit with combined therapy. Based on the knowledge that GnRH analogs produce a rise in testosterone for the first few weeks of administration, and that no difference is observed when the antiandrogen is combined with a surgical orchiectomy, the authors suggested that the likely benefit of the approach is elimination of the negative effects of the testosterone surge on prostate cancer growth observed in the first 2 to 3 weeks of treatment with GnRH agonist/antagonist, rather than the superiority of the combination approach itself. The result has led many physicians to change their practice to limit the total duration of antiandrogen treatment (e.g., 1–3 months), as opposed to long-term continuous therapy. Given that one of the predictive factors for response to antiandrogen withdrawal is the duration of antiandrogen treatment, this likely will result in fewer patients progressing on antiandrogen based combination therapy, further reducing the frequency of withdrawal responses that are observed.

CONCLUSIONS

Until recently, patients with progressive prostate cancer in the setting of castrate levels of testosterone were considered to have "hormone-refractory" disease. However, this notion is not supported by recent evidence that the AR continues to play an important role in the growth of castration resistant prostate cancers. Moreover, the observations that the AR has increased sensitivity for activation and may be activated by non-classical ligands in the castrate state, makes a compelling case for the development of AR targeted strategies that are effective, even in the progressive castrate state. Such new therapies are necessary for significant therapeutic advances for the majority of patients with advanced prostate cancer who will ultimately fail androgen ablation. Elucidation of the mechanisms contributing to the antiandrogen withdrawal response provides a window into this process.

REFERENCES

1. Scher HI, Heller G. Clinical states in prostate cancer: towards a dynamic model of disease progression. Urology 2000;55:323–327.
2. Dupont A, Gomez J, Cusan L, et al. Response to flutamide withdrawal in advanced prostate cancer in progression under combination therapy. J Urol 1993;150:908–913.
3. Collinson MP, Daniel F, Tyrell CJ, et al. Response of carcinoma of the prostate to withdrawal of flutamide. Br J Urol 1993;72:662–663.
4. Kelly WK, Scher HI. Prostate specific antigen decline after antiandrogen withdrawal: the flutamide withdrawal syndrome. J Urol 1993;149:607–609.
5. Kelly WK, Slovin S, Scher HI. Steroid hormone withdrawal syndromes: pathophysiology and clinical significance. Urol Clin North Am 1997;24:421–433.
6. Belani CP, Pearl P, Whitley ND, et al. Tamoxifen withdrawal response. Arch Intern Med 1989;149:449–450.
7. Howell A, Dodwell DJ, Anderson H, et al. Response after withdrawal of tamoxifen and progestins in advanced breast cancer. Ann Oncol 1992;3:611–617.
8. Buchanan G, Greenberg NM, Scher HI, et al. Collocation of androgen receptor gene mutations in prostate cancer. Clin Cancer Res 2001;7:1273–1281.
9. Scher H, Shaffer D. Prostate cancer: a dynamic disease with shifting targets. Lancet Oncology 2003;4:407–414.
10. Huggins C, Hodges CV. Studies on prostatic cancer. I. The effect of castration, of estrogen and of androgen injection on serum phosphatases in metastatic carcinoma of the prostate. Cancer Res 1941;1:193–197.
11. Huggins C, Stevens RE Jr, Hodges CV. Studies on prostatic cancer. II. The effect of castration on advanced carcinoma of the prostate gland. Arch Surg 1941;43:209–223.
12. Huggins C, Bergenstal DM. Effect of bilateral adrenalectomy on certain human tumors. Proc Natl Acad Sci USA 1952;38:73–76.
13. Robinson MR, Shearer RJ, Fergusson JD. Adrenal suppression in the treatment of carcinoma of the prostate. Br J Urol 1974;46:555–559.
14. Geller J, Albert JD, Nochstein DA, et al. Comparison of prostatic cancer tissue dehydrotestosterone levels at the time of relapse following orchiectomy or estrogen therapy. J Urol 1984;132:693–696.
15. Labrie F, Dupont A, Belanger A, et al. New approach in the treatment of prostate cancer: complete instead of partial withdrawal of androgens. Prostate 1983;4:579–594.
16. Cassileth BR, Soloway MS, Vogelzang NJ, et al. Patients' choice of treatment in stage D prostate cancer. Urology 1989;33:57–62.
17. Crawford ED, Eisenberger MA, McLeod DG, et al. A controlled trial of leuprolide with and without flutamide in prostatic carcinoma. N Engl J Med 1989;321:419–424.
18. Denis LJ, Keuppens F, Smith PH, et al. Maximal androgen blockade: final analysis of EORTC phase III trial 30853. EORTC Genito-Urinary Tract Cancer Cooperative Group and the EORTC Data Center. Eur Urol 1998;33:144–151.
19. Scher HI, Mazumdar M, Kelly WK. Clinical trials in relapsed prostate cancer: defining the target. J Natl Cancer Inst 1996;88:1623–1634.
20. Scher HI, Kelly WK. The flutamide withdrawal syndrome: its impact on clinical trials in hormone-refractory prostatic cancer. J Clin Oncol 1993;11:1566–1572.
21. Scher H, Kelly WK, Cohen L, et al. Flutamide withdrawal response in patients with metastatic prostate cancer (PC) progressing on hormonal therapy. Proc Am Soc Clin Oncol 1993;12:723.
22. Sartor O, Cooper M, Weinberger M, et al. Surprising activity of flutamide withdrawal, when combined with aminoglutethimide, in treatment of "hormone-refractory" prostate cancer. J Natl Cancer Inst 1994;86:222–227.
23. Herrada J, Dieringer P, Logothetis CJ. Characterization of patients with androgen-independent prostatic carcinoma whose serum prostate specific antigen decreased following flutamide withdrawal. J Urol 1996;155:620–623.
24. Scher HI, Zhang ZF, Kelly WK. Hormone and anti-hormone withdrawal therapy: implications for management of androgen independent prostate cancer. Urology 1996;47:61–69.
25. Scher HI, Kolvenbag GJ. The antiandrogen withdrawal syndrome in relapsed prostate cancer. Eur Urol 1997;31:3–7; discussion 24–27.
26. Eisenberger MA, Blumenstein BA, Crawford ED, et al. Bilateral orchiectomy with or without flutamide for metastatic prostate cancer. N Engl J Med 1998;339:1036–1042.
27. Bianco FJ, Dotan ZA, Kattan MW, et al. Duration of response to androgen deprivation therapy and survival after subsequent biochemical relapse in men initially treated with radical prostatectomy. Proc Am Soc Clin Onc 2004;23:393 [Abstract #4552].
28. Small EJ, Carroll PR. Prostate-specific antigen decline after casodex withdrawal: evidence for an antiandrogen withdrawal syndrome. Urology 1994;43:408–410.
29. Small EJ, Srinivas S. The antiandrogen withdrawal syndrome: experience in a large cohort of unselected patients with advanced prostate cancer. Cancer 1995;76:1428–1434.
30. Schellhammer P, Kolvenbag GJCM. Serum PSA decline after casodex withdrawal. Urology 1994;44:790–791.
31. Nieh PT. Withdrawal phenomenon with the antiandrogen casodex. J Urol 1995;153:1070–1072.
32. Schellhammer PF, Venner P, Haas GP, et al. Prostate specific antigen decreases after withdrawal of antiandrogen therapy with bicalutamide or flutamide in patients receiving combined androgen blockade. J Urol 1997;157:1731–1735.

33. Haun SD, Gerridzen RG, Yau JC, et al. Antiandrogen withdrawal syndrome with nilutamide. Urology 1997;49:632–634.

34. Wirth MP, Froschermaier SE. The antiandrogen withdrawal syndrome. Urol Res 1997;25:S67–71.

35. Dawson NA, McLeod DG. Dramatic prostate specific antigen decrease in response to discontinuation of megestrol acetate in advanced prostate cancer: expansion of the antiandrogen withdrawal syndrome. J Urol 1995;153:1946–1947.

36. Figg WD, Sartor O, Cooper MR, et al. Prostate specific antigen decline following the discontinuation of flutamide in patients with stage D2 prostate cancer. Am J Med 1995;98:412–414.

37. Burch PA, Loprinzi CL. Prostate-specific antigen decline after withdrawal of low-dose megestrol acetate. J Clin Oncol 1999;17:1087–1088.

38. Bissada NK, Kaczmarek AT. Complete remission of hormone refractory adenocarcinoma of the prostate in response to withdrawal of diethylstilbesterol. J Urol 1995;153:1944–1945.

39. Akakura K, Akimoto S, Furuya Y, et al. Incidence and characteristics of antiandrogen withdrawal syndrome in prostate cancer after treatment with chlormadinone acetate. Eur Urol 1998;33:567–571.

40. Tassinari D, Fochessati F, Panzini I, et al. Rapid progression of advanced "hormone-resistant" prostate cancer during palliative treatment with progestins for cancer cachexia. J Pain Symptom Manage 2003;25:481–484.

41. Small E, Schellhammer P, Venner P, et al. A double-blind assessment of antiandrogen withdrawal from casodex (C) or eulexin (E) therapy while continuing luteinizing hormone releasing hormone analogue (LHRH-A) therapy for patients (pts) with stage D2 prostate cancer (PCA). Proc Am Soc Clin Oncol 1996;15.

42. Small EJ, Baron A, Apodaca D. Simultaneous anti-androgen withdrawal (AAWD) and treatment with ketoconazole (KETO)/hydrocortisone (HD) in patients with advanced "hormone-refractory" prostate cancer (HRPC). Proc Am Soc Clin Oncol 1997;16:313a.

43. Small EJ, Halabi S, Dawson NA, et al. Antiandrogen withdrawal alone or in combination with ketoconazole in androgen-independent prostate cancer patients: a phase III trial (CALGB 9583). J Clin Oncol 2004;22:1025–1033.

44. Bubley GJ, Carducci M, Dahut W, et al. Eligibility and response guidelines for phase II clinical trials in androgen-independent prostate cancer: recommendations from the PSA Working Group. J Clin Oncol 1999:3461–3467.

45. Labrie F, Dupont A, Giguere M, et al. Benefits of combination therapy with flutamide in patients relapsing after castration. Br J Urol 1988;61:341–346.

46. Fossa SD, Slee PH, Brausi M, et al. Flutamide versus prednisone in patients with prostate cancer symptomatically progressing after androgen-ablative therapy: a phase III study of the European organization for research and treatment of cancer genitourinary group. J Clin Oncol 2001;19:62–71.

47. Kassouf W, Tanguay S, Aprikian AG. Nilutamide as second line hormone therapy for prostate cancer after androgen ablation fails. J Urol 2003;169:1742–1744.

48. Desai A, Stadler WM, Vogelzang NJ. Nilutamide: possible utility as a second-line hormonal agent. Urology 2001;58:1016–1020.

49. Joyce R, Fenton MA, Rode P, et al. High dose bicalutamide for androgen independent prostate cancer: effect of prior hormonal therapy. J Urol 1998;159:149–153.

50. Kojima S, Suzuki H, Akakura K, et al. Alternative antiandrogens to treat prostate cancer relapse after initial hormone therapy. J Urol 2004;171:679–683.

51. Walczak JR, Carducci MA. Phase 3 randomized trial evaluating second-line hormonal therapy versus docetaxel-estramustine combination chemotherapy on progression-free survival in asymptomatic patients with a rising prostate-specific antigen level after hormonal therapy for prostate cancer: an Eastern Cooperative Oncology Group (E1899), Intergroup/Clinical Trials Support Unit study. Urology 2003;62:141–146.

52. Buchanan G, Yang M, Nahm SJ, et al. Mutations at the boundary of the hinge and ligand binding domain of the androgen receptor confer increased transactivation function. Mol Endocrinol 2000;15:46–56.

53. Scher HI, Buchanan G, Gerald W, et al. Targeting the androgen receptor: improving outcomes for castration-resistant prostate cancer. Endocrine Rel Cancer 2004;11:459–476.

54. Taplin ME, Bubley GJ, Ko YJ, et al. Selection for androgen receptor mutations in prostate cancers treated with androgen antagonist. Cancer Res 1999;59:2511–2515.

55. Fenton MA, Shuster TD, Fertig AM, et al. Functional characterization of mutant androgen receptors from androgen-independent prostate cancer. Clin Cancer Res 1997;8:1383–1388.

56. Hara T, Miyazaki J, Araki H, et al. Novel mutations of androgen receptor: a possible mechanism of bicalutamide withdrawal syndrome. Cancer Res 2003;63:149–153.

57. Greenberg NM, DeMayo F, Finegold MJ, et al. Prostate cancer in a transgenic mouse. Proc Natl Acad Sci USA 1995;92:3439–3443.

58. Gingrich JR, Barrios RJ, Kattan MW, et al. Androgen-independent prostate cancer progression in the TRAMP model. Cancer Res 1997;57:4687–4691.

59. Han G, Foster BA, Mistry S, et al. Hormone status selects for spontaneous somatic androgen receptor variants that demonstrate specific ligand and cofactor dependent activities in autochthonous prostate cancer. J Biol Chem 2001;276:11204–11213.

60. Han G, Buchanan G, Ittmann M, et al. Mutation of the androgen receptor causes oncogenic transformation of the prostate. Proc Natl Acad Sci USA 2005;102:1151–1156.

61. Taplin ME, Rajeshkumar B, Halabi S, et al. Androgen receptor mutations in androgen-independent prostate cancer: Cancer and Leukemia Group B Study 9663. J Clin Oncol 2003;21:2673–2678.

62. Gregory CW, Hamil KG, Kim D, et al. Androgen receptor expression in androgen-independent prostate cancer is associated with increased expression of androgen-regulated genes. Cancer Res 1998;58:5718–5724.

63. Mohler JL, Gregory CW, Ford 3rd OH, et al. The androgen axis in recurrent prostate cancer. Clinical Cancer Res 2004;10:440–448.

64. Culig Z, Hobisch A, Hittmair A, et al. Expression, structure, and function of androgen receptor in advanced prostatic carcinoma. Prostate 1998;35:63–70.

65. Takeda H, Akakura K, Masai M, et al. Androgen receptor content of prostate carcinoma cells estimated by immunohistochemistry is related to prognosis of patients with stage D2 prostate carcinoma. Cancer 1996;77:934–940.

66. Sadi MV, Barrack ER. Image analysis of androgen receptor immunostaining in metastatic prostate cancer. Cancer 1993;71:2574–2580.

67. Chen CD, Welsbie DS, Tran C, et al. Molecular determinants of resistance to antiandrogen therapy. Nat Med 2004;10:33–39.

68. Ricciardelli C, Choong CS, Buchanan G, et al. Androgen receptor levels in prostate cancer epithelial and peritumoral stromal cells identify non-organ confined disease. Prostate 2005;63:19–28.

69. Bubendorf L, Kolmer M, Konenen J, et al. Hormone therapy failure in human prostate cancer: analysis by complementary DNA and tissue microarrays. J Natl Cancer Inst 1999;91:1758–1764.

70. Koivisto P, Visakorpi T, Kallioniemi OP. Androgen receptor gene amplification: a novel molecular mechanism for endocrine therapy resistance in human prostate cancer. Scand J Clin Lab Invest Suppl 1996;226:57–63.

71. Holzbeierlein J, Lal P, LaTulippe E, et al. Gene expression analysis of human prostate carcinoma during hormonal therapy identifies androgen-responsive genes and mechanisms of therapy resistance. Am J Pathol 2004;164:217–227.

72. Gregory CW, He B, Johnson RT, et al. A mechanism for androgen receptor-mediated prostate cancer recurrence after androgen deprivation therapy. Cancer Res 2001;61:4315–4319.

73. Kinoshita H, Shi Y, Sandefur C, et al. Methylation of the androgen receptor minimal promoter silences transcription in human prostate cancer. Cancer Res 2000;60:3623–3630.

74. Debes JD, Schmidt LJ, Huang H, et al. P300 mediates androgen-independent transactivation of the androgen receptor by interleukin 6. Cancer Res 2002;62:5632–5636.

75. Fujimoto N, Yeh S, Kang HY, et al. Cloning and characterization of androgen receptor coactivator, ARA55, in human prostate. J Biol Chem 1999;274:8316–8321.

76. Yeh S, Miyamoto H, Shima H, et al. From estrogen to androgen receptor: A new pathway for sex hormones in prostate. Proc Natl Acad Sci USA 1998;95:5527–5532.

77. Yeh S, Chang HC, Miyamoto H, et al. Differential induction of the androgen receptor transcriptional activity by selective androgen receptor coactivators. Keio J Med 1999;48:87–92.

78. Berrevoets CA, Umar A, Trapman J, et al. Differential modulation of androgen receptor transcriptional activity by the nuclear receptor corepressor (N-CoR). Biochem J 2004;379:731–738.

79. Hodgson MC, Astapova I, Cheng S, et al. The androgen receptor recruits nuclear receptor CoRepressor (N-CoR) in the presence of mifepristone via its N and C termini revealing a novel molecular mechanism for androgen receptor antagonists. J Biol Chem 2005;280:6511–6519.

80. Kim D, Gregory CW, French FS, et al. Androgen receptor expression and cellular proliferation during transition from androgen-dependent to recurrent growth after castration in the CWR22 prostate cancer xenograft. Am J Pathol 2002;160:219–226.

81. Culig Z, Hobisch A, Cronauer MV, et al. Androgen receptor activation in prostatic tumor cell lines by insulin-like growth factor-I, keratinocyte growth factor, and epidermal growth factor. Cancer Res 1994;54:5474–5478.

82. Nazareth LV, Weigel NL. Activation of the human androgen receptor through a protein kinase: A signaling pathway. J Biol Chem 1996;271:19900–19907.

83. Craft N, Chhor C, Tran C, et al. Evidence for clonal outgrowth of androgen-independent prostate cancer cells from androgen-dependent tumors through a two-step process. Cancer Res 1999;59:5030–5036.

84. Grossmann ME, Huang H, Tindall DJ. Androgen receptor signaling in androgen-refractory prostate cancer. J Natl Cancer Inst 2001;93:1687–1697.

85. Ueda T, Mawji NR, Bruchovsky N, et al. Ligand-independent activation of the androgen receptor by interleukin-6 and the role of steroid receptor coactivator-1 in prostate cancer cells. J Biol Chem 2002;277:38087–38094.

86. Ueda T, Bruchovsky N, Sadar MD. Activation of the androgen receptor N-terminal domain by interleukin-6 via MAPK and STAT3 signal transduction pathways. J Biol Chem 2002;277:7076–7085.

87. Lee SO, Lou W, Hou M, et al. Interleukin-6 promotes androgen-independent growth in LNCaP human prostate cancer cells. Clin Cancer Res 2003;9:370–376.

88. Wen Y, Hu MC, Makino K, et al. HER-2/neu promotes androgen-independent survival and growth of prostate cancer cells through the AKT pathway. Cancer Res 2000;60:6841–6845.

89. Shi Y, Brands FH, Chatterjee S, et al. Her-2/neu expression in prostate cancer: high level of expression associated with exposure to hormone therapy and androgen independent disease. J Urol 2001;166:1514–1519.

90. Reese DM, Small EJ, Magrane G, et al. HER2 protein expression and gene amplification in androgen-independent prostate cancer. Am J Clin Pathol 2001;116:234–239.

91. Lara PN Jr, Meyers FJ, Gray CR, et al. HER-2/neu is overexpressed infrequently in patients with prostate carcinoma. Results from the California Cancer Consortium Screening Trial. Cancer 2002;94:2584–2589.

92. Mellinghoff IK, Vivanco I, Kwon A, et al. HER2/neu kinase-dependent modulation of androgen receptor function through effects on DNA binding and stability. Cancer Cell 2004;6:517–527.

93. Schellhammer P, Sharifi R, Block N, et al. A controlled trial of bicalutamide versus flutamide, each in combination with luteinizing hormone-relapsing hormone analogue therapy, in patients with advanced prostate cancer. Urology 1995;45:745–752.

94. Carducci M, Nelson BJ, Saad F, et al. Effects of atrasentan on disease progression and biological markers in men with metastatic hormone-refractory prostate cancer: Phase 3 study. Proc Am Soc Clin Onc 2004;23:383 [Abstract # 4058].

95. Seidenfeld J, Samson DJ, Hasselblad V, et al. Single-therapy androgen suppression in men with advanced prostate cancer: a systematic review and meta-analysis. Ann Intern Med 2000;132:566–577.

96. Bennett CL, Tosteson TD, Schmitt B, et al. Maximum androgen-blockade with medical or surgical castration in advanced prostate cancer: A meta-analysis of nine published randomized controlled trials and 4128 patients using flutamide. Prostate Cancer Prostatic Dis 1999;2:4–8.

97. Caubet J, Tosteson TD, Dong EW, et al. Maximum androgen blockade in advanced prostate cancer: a meta-analysis of published randomized controlled trials using nonsteroidal antiandrogens. Urology 1997;49:71–78.

98. Schmitt B, Bennett C, Seidenfeld J, et al. Maximal androgen blockade for advanced prostate cancer. Cochrane Database Sys Rev; 2000 CD001526.

99. Group PCTC. Maximum androgen blockade in advanced prostate cancer: an overview of 22 randomized trials with 3283 deaths in 5711 patients. Lancet 1995;346:265–269.

100. Samson DJ, Seidenfeld J, Schmitt B, et al. Systematic review and meta-analysis of monotherapy compared with combined androgen blockade for patients with advanced prostate carcinoma. Cancer 2002;95:361–376.

101. Scher HI, Zhang Z-F, Cohen L, et al. Hormonally relapsed prostatic cancer: lessons from the flutamide withdrawal syndrome. Adv Urol 1995;8:61–95.

102. Sella A, Flex D, Sulkes A, et al. Antiandrogen withdrawal syndrome with cyproterone acetate. Urology 1998;52:1091–1093.

103. Small EJ, Baron A, Bok R. Simultaneous and antiandrogen withdrawal and treatment with ketoconazol and hydrocortisone in patients with advanced prostate carcinoma. Cancer 1997;80:1755–1759.

Chemotherapy for advanced prostate cancer 100

Andrew J Armstrong, Michael A Carducci

INTRODUCTION

Prostate cancer will result in approximately 30,000 annual deaths in men in the United States in 2005 and is the second leading cause of cancer deaths in men after lung cancer.[1,2] While the death rate from prostate cancer has been declining due to a number of factors such as earlier diagnosis and effective, less morbid local treatment options, approximately 6% of men will present with distant metastases and approximately 40% to 60% will relapse following local treatments.[2–4] In general, androgen suppression leads to the response and stabilization of metastatic hormone-sensitive disease for approximately 18 to 24 months with a historic median survival from the time of diagnosis of metastases ranging from 24 to 30 months.[5,6] A recent update of select patients from the Pound database from Johns Hopkins has demonstrated a median survival from development of metastases to death of 6.5 years.[7] Prostate-specific antigen (PSA) doubling time at relapse following radical prostatectomy, time to recurrence, and original Gleason score were predictive of metastasis-free survival, illustrating the heterogeneity of this disease.[7] However, eventually these patients will develop progressive hormone-refractory metastatic prostate cancer and these patients have a median survival of approximately 12 to 18 months.[8–11]

The concept that hormone-refractory metastatic prostate cancer is a chemo-resistant disease has been challenged by recent clinical trials. The use of surrogate outcomes such as PSA response has led to the more rapid identification of novel agents with activity in hormone-refractory metastatic prostate cancer (HRPC). Docetaxel (Taxotere), a taxoid with a more manageable benefit-to-toxicity ratio than historic cytotoxic agents used in prostate cancer, has demonstrated a clinical benefit and overall survival advantage in recent multi-institutional trials. Further refinements of the definitions of hormone independence, quality-of-life outcomes, and surrogate markers of response have led to improved standardization across clinical trials that allow for head to head comparisons of active agents.[12,13] The earlier detection of biochemical recurrence and asymptomatic metastatic disease with the use of serum PSA measurements and improved imaging techniques may also translate into the earlier initiation of therapy before disease burden and pain become overwhelming factors. While hormone-refractory metastatic prostate cancer remains an incurable disease, chemotherapy has come to play a role in prolonging patient survival with meaningful quality-of-life endpoints and has generated optimism about progress among both clinicians and patients.

Currently, approved chemotherapy regimens in hormone refractory metastatic prostate cancer include docetaxel, mitoxantrone, and estramustine but these agents have not yet demonstrated consistent clinical benefits in earlier stages of disease. The use of chemotherapy in high-risk patients either as neoadjuvant treatment or adjuvant to local therapy, as well as in nonmetastatic high-risk patients with PSA-only recurrence, is an active area of clinical investigation and these patients should be encouraged to enroll in clinical trials to answer these questions.

DEFINITION OF HORMONE-REFRACTORY PROSTATE CANCER

The most widely accepted criteria for the hormone-refractory state has been the demonstration of progressive, measurable, or evaluable disease in the face of castrate levels of serum testosterone (<50 ng/dL).[12] Biochemical progression after antiandrogen (bicalutamide, flutamide, nilutamide) withdrawal, as measured consecutively over a 4 to 6 week period, has been proposed for eligibility into clinical trials for HRPC. Patients are usually continued on luteinizing hormone releasing hormone (LHRH) agonists during this time if tolerable. There is at this time no universally accepted definition of progression of hormone-refractory disease, however, and patients may have no measurable or evaluable disease with PSA-only progression and be termed hormone refractory. These PSA-only hormone refractory patients represent a heterogeneous group depending on when hormonal therapy was initiated, and, therefore, time to progression is highly variable. Survival in this group that is increasingly encountered in the clinic is generally better when compared with patients with metastatic hormone-refractory disease, and chemotherapy trials such as ECOG 1899 attempted to define this population prospectively (see below).

The demonstration of progressive disease in the face of continuous androgen suppression with gonadotropin releasing hormone (GnRH) agonists often leads to the introduction of combined androgen blockade with antiandrogens, followed shortly by antiandrogen withdrawal and trials of third-line hormonal therapy, often with the combination of ketoconazole and hydrocortisone. The response time to each of these manipulations is brief, on the order of several months, with likely survival benefits for responders.[14] Eventually, prostate cancer growth becomes refractory to these manipulations. Consequently, until recently, the indication for chemotherapy in practical terms has generally been progression despite the utilization of all hormonal options, manifested generally by clinically measurable disease. This paradigm is likely to shift as new chemotherapeutic and biologic agents are shown to be more active.

CHEMOTHERAPY FOR EARLY ADVANCED PROSTATE CANCER

The use of chemotherapy for high-risk patients following local therapy, or in high-risk patients with a rising PSA following local therapy, is an active area of clinical investigation. Modeling therapy after adjuvant or neoadjuvant therapy for localized breast cancer, several groups are using combination chemotherapy before and after radical prostatectomy or external-beam radiation therapy. CALGB trial 90203 is examining pre-radical prostatectomy estramustine and docetaxel in high-risk men with a predicted 5-year survival of less than 60%.[15] SWOG 9921 will look at adjuvant androgen

deprivation with or without mitoxantrone in high-risk men following radical prostatectomy.[16] RTOG P-0014 is a multicenter trial examining the role of chemotherapy in the adjuvant setting for high-risk men who have failed local therapy or are at high risk for recurrence (Gleason >7, or >6 with positive lymph nodes or capsular penetration). Four cycles of chemotherapy in this trial will be selected from one of a number of trial approved regimens, including docetaxel and combination regimens, and will be given either upfront with androgen ablation or at progression after androgen ablation.[17] In addition ECOG 1899 randomized men with biochemical progression after androgen suppression to either second line hormonal manipulation with ketoconazole and hydrocortisone or to chemotherapy with docetaxel and estramustine (closed in 2005 due to poor accrual).[18] Until these studies are complete and confirmed, it is difficult to recommend the use of chemotherapy in these settings outside of a clinical trial.

HISTORICAL PERSPECTIVE OF CHEMOTHERAPY FOR METASTATIC PROSTATE CANCER

Objective, measurable response rates of metastatic prostate cancer to single agent chemotherapy has ranged from 10% to 30%, while multi-agent chemotherapy response rates have ranged from 20% to 60%.[19,20] Trials reporting PSA declines of greater than 50% for single agents have ranged from 4% to 48%, and for combination therapies from 25% to 82% (see Tables 100.1 and 100.2). These objective response rates are similar in magnitude to the response rates of other advanced, metastatic malignancies such as colon and breast cancer.[21,22] Historically, however, the demonstration of improved survival and time to progression was not demonstrated with chemotherapy for metastatic prostate cancer. Until recently, approval of the major active agents, estramustine and mitoxantrone, were based on response rates and quality of life outcomes, respectively, rather than quantity of life gained. Only in the last several years have newer docetaxel-based approaches demonstrated both improved response rates and prolonged survival.[8,9]

BIOLOGY OF CHEMORESISTANCE IN PROSTATE CANCER

During the progression of human prostate cancer, multiple steps leading to drug resistance, resistance to apoptosis, and increased growth fraction, as well as immune evasion lead to the general concept of treatment resistance. Many of these changes may be related to genomic instability and acquired somatic mutations, possibly as a result of increased susceptibility of prostate cancer cells to environmental toxins and oxidative damage.[23] The methylation and subsequent loss of expression of glutathione S-transferase-π, a phase II detoxification enzyme likely involved in genome protection from carcinogens, is one of the earliest changes seen during prostate cancer progression.[24] Increased expression of multidrug resistance protein (MRP), BCL2, vascular endothelial growth factor (VEGF), cyclin-D1, and p53 have all been correlated with progression to the androgen-independent state, as have diminished levels of the tumor suppressors phosphatase and tensin homolog deleted on chromosome ten (PTEN), and P27KIP1.[24–28] *BCL2* is a unique protooncogene expressed in the basal regenerating compartment of the prostate that extends cell viability in the absence of cell proliferation, by preventing programmed cell death, or apoptosis.[25] While the cell of origin in prostate cancer is unclear, these basal cells are typically androgen independent and may contain the putative prostate cancer stem cell responsible for relapse following androgen ablation.[23] Destruction of the more differentiated compartment of luminal type cells that are androgen dependent would not be expected to eradicate these stem cells. Whether these regenerating cells are present from the beginning of prostate cancer development or acquired during progression remains to be determined. However, BCL2 was found to be expressed in 6 of 19 androgen-dependent carcinomas compared with 9 of 12 androgen-independent patient samples, with overexpression generally correlating with androgen independence.[25] Currently, therapies are under evaluation that target BCL2 and examine the impact of chemotherapy on global markers of apoptosis.

Resistance to cytotoxic therapy-induced programmed cell death may also be related to the relative inactivation of the *PTEN* tumor suppressor gene during the progression to the hormone refractory state.[29] Loss of heterozygosity of *PTEN* is seen in approximately 60% of prostate metastases, compared with 15% of early malignancies.[30,31] This tumor suppressor gene regulates the activity of the AKT/PI3K survival pathway, which is important in contributing to apoptotic resistance to cytotoxic agents, cell-anchorage independent growth, angiogenesis, and nutrient-driven proliferation.[32,33] Inhibition of this overactive pathway in conjunction with cytotoxic therapy may correct this resistance seen in prostate cell lines exposed to long-term androgen deprivation.[31]

Resistance to cytotoxic therapy may be related to concurrent resistance to androgen deprivation and progression to HRPC. Upregulation of the androgen receptor has been observed during progression to the androgen refractory state.[34] Alterations in coactivators and corepressors of the androgen receptor may function as a biologic signal amplification switch associated with

increased androgen receptor expression, and may explain some of the lack of benefit, and even paradoxical growth, seen during treatment with antiandrogens.[34] Androgen receptor mutations, about 45% of which are activating mutations, have been observed in a minority of patients with HRPC and may lead to increased sensitivity to estrogens, progestins, and other non-androgen ligands.[35–37] Increased sensitivity to local autocrine and paracrine stromal growth factors (i.e. epidermal growth factor [EGF], heregulin, insulin-like growth factor 1 [IGF1], interleukin 6 [IL6]) that act either through the androgen receptor or bypass it downstream have been reported.[35,38] Transition to the hormone-refractory state may thus be accompanied by an amplification of androgen signaling, the transition to codependence on growth factor pathways, and a resistance to apoptotic death due to the overactivity of these survival pathways, such as AKT/PI3K. Prostate-specific antigen production may also become driven by non-androgen signals.[31,38] These changes may also lead to chemoresistance, and so represent novel targets for combination therapies.

EARLY CHEMOTHERAPY TRIALS

In the pre-PSA era, the first cytotoxic agents tested in metastatic prostate cancer were nitrogen mustard (1947), thio-tepa (1959), diphenylthiocarbazone (1960), and mithramycin (1963), with some objective and subjective responses in small numbers of patients.[39] In the 1960s, cyclophosphamide (1965), fluorouracil (1968), and vinblastine, often in combination with nitrogen mustards, demonstrated anecdotal responses but no large studies were conducted until 1976.[39,40] The first randomized trial was conducted with cyclophosphamide and fluorouracil showing a 41% and 36% objective response respectively (7% and 12% partial responses with stable disease excluded) in 74 patients.[41] In the 1970s, multiple randomized trials compared single and combination agents often in comparison to standard treatment with glucocorticoids and second line hormonal agents.[39,42] Several agents, such as diethylstilbestrol in the 1960s, had initial high response rates, but were later categorized into hormonal therapies.

Before 1976, few agents were systematically studied, due to the difficulties of defining measurable disease and the relative biochemical success of hormonal therapy, which relegated chemotherapy trials to those patients with the poorest prognosis and most advanced stages.[39] The initial National Prostatic Cancer Projects (NPCP) in the 1970s found between a 10-40% response rate among multiple single agents, if stabilized disease was excluded. Highest objective response rates on the order of 30% to 40% were seen in lomustine (CCNU), cisplatin, and cyclophosphamide, while the lowest responses (<10%) were seen with fluorouracil, melphalan, and prednimustine.[39] Combination regimens involving cyclophosphamide and fluorouracil, as well as doxorubicin-based regimens, improved on response rates and subjective pain measures, but did not demonstrate overall cohort survival superiority.[39,43] In all of these early chemotherapy trials, the control groups received what was then standard therapy, including synthetic estrogens and secondary hormonal manipulations, radiation, and steroids. Baseline characteristics of the groups were not uniform in terms of prior treatment, making results difficult to interpret. Response rates in the 1980s were reported most often as measurable disease response, but were not standardized and generally had wide 95% confidence intervals and inter-investigator variability, and, therefore, conclusions about relative efficacy were difficult.[43] In general, no single agent or combination of agents was shown to improve survival, despite response rates that ranged from 10% to 70%. In their review of the current status of chemotherapy for prostate cancer in 1985, Eisenberger et al concluded that no single agent or combination of agents changed the overall downward slope of the survival curve, and that most trials were difficult to interpret due to non-uniformity, the use of stable disease as a response criteria, crossover, and the lack of power in the studies to demonstrate small survival benefits.[43] The overall complete remission (CR) and partial remission (PR) rates of 17 randomized trials combined in this review in 1985, based on variable response criteria, was 4.5%, with no change in survival compared with standard palliative care.[43] It was felt that even a potential small incremental benefit in survival at the expense of chemotherapy toxicity was not clinically useful, thus contributing to the therapeutic nihilism of the era.

A 1992 review by Yagoda et al found a similarly disappointing 8.7% overall CR/PR rate among different chemotherapy agents ranging from 2% to 10% for cyclophosphamide, 10% for cisplatin and continuous fluorouracil, and 21% for vinblastine.[44] The notion that prostate cancer was intrinsically chemoresistant has been questioned, however, as less toxic, more active agents became available, notably docetaxel and other microtubule targeted therapies. The development of PSA as a surrogate marker of response has certainly contributed to our ability to select for active agents.

outcomes was mitoxantrone in 1996, although many of the above chemotherapy agents studied in the past demonstrated anecdotal and even some randomized data in temporarily improving pain from prostate cancer.[39] Kantoff et al studied 242 men with HRPC randomized to mitoxantrone and hydrocortisone, or hydrocortisone alone, with survival, response, and QoL parameters as primary outcomes.[45] While no survival benefit was observed (12.3 months versus 12.6 months), there was a trend to symptomatic pain improvement in terms of severity and frequency. This was similar to the Canadian trial by Tannock et al that demonstrated a 29% palliative response with mitoxantrone and prednisone compared with 12% in the prednisone only group, with a longer duration of pain control and overall improved cost-effectiveness in the chemotherapy arm (43 weeks versus 18 weeks).[46] Since these publications in the 1990s, newer agents have been examined with QoL outcomes among the secondary measured outcomes, notably docetaxel in the TAX327 trial (vida infra).

Quality-of-life outcomes are subjective and determined by the patient, and are consequently difficult to quantify and standardize across groups and among different instruments for measurement. The QoL outcomes are unlikely to change clinical practice if the survival of two comparison groups are significantly disparate. However, prostate cancer-specific questionnaires and instruments such as the functional assessment of cancer therapy for prostate cancer (FACT-P), the EORTC quality-of-life questionnaire (QLQ), the functional living index in cancer (FLIC) and other validated measures of prostate cancer-specific QoL scales may be useful in helping clinicians and patients determine the appropriate individualized therapies, especially when two comparison agents have similar survival endpoints.[46-49] Importantly, QoL outcomes should ideally be considered as a primary endpoint in phase III trials, in addition to survival, and measured at baseline and serially throughout treatment and follow-up as for other standard measured variables. Emphasis by physicians to patients on the importance of these QoL questionnaires may lead to more compliance and the development of less toxic, effective therapies based on outcomes that are important to the patient.

CLINICAL ENDPOINTS IN MANAGEMENT OF ANDROGEN-INDEPENDENT PROSTATE CANCER

QUALITY-OF-LIFE OUTCOMES

The first chemotherapy agent to be USFDA approved in prostate cancer based on quality-of-life (QoL)

PROSTATE-SPECIFIC ANTIGEN DECLINES AS SURROGATE MARKER

Prostate-specific antigen levels are a sensitive indicator of response to multiple modalities of treatment, including radical prostatectomy, external-beam radiation, brachytherapy, and hormonal manipulation. After hormonal treatment of metastatic prostate cancer, a greater than 90% decline in the serum PSA has correlated with progression-free survival.[50] A greater than 90% decline corresponded to a probability of progression at 1 year of 25%, compared with a probability of 80% to 90% progression for smaller percent declines.[50] The use of this surrogate endpoint for disease activity in the setting of chemotherapy for HRPC has also been validated as a predictor of objective disease progression and survival. A greater than 50% decline in serum PSA in the absence of clinical or radiographic evidence of disease progression, and confirmed 4 weeks later, was established in 1999 by the Prostate Specific Antigen Working Group (NCI) as clinical guidelines for HRPC trials.[12,51,52] In general, these recommendations were made as a guide to the design of larger, randomized, survival-based trials, rather than as a true surrogate for survival. Expression of PSA is generally regulated by autocrine, paracrine, and hormonal activity, and levels may be altered independent of disease activity if this activity is affected by the investigational agent.[53,54] Generally, cytotoxic agents have not been shown to alter PSA levels independently of their clinical responses, but it has been recommended that new agents examine the effect on PSA expression independently before entering into large-scale trials. Multiple analyses have demonstrated a correlation between a greater than 50% serum PSA decline at 8 weeks and overall survival, with some demonstrating a three-fold increase in survival compared with smaller responses.[51,52] Thus for most cytotoxic agents, serum PSA declines of greater than 50% may be a useful surrogate outcome in early clinical trials until larger, randomized trials are able to be conducted to examine progression-free and overall survival. For biologic agents, PSA changes are generally considered in the context of the independent effects of these agents on secretion of PSA.

SURVIVAL AND DISEASE PROGRESSION

The natural history of untreated metastatic hormone-refractory prostate cancer is heterogeneous but generally that of progressive disease, skeletal metastases, and impairment in quality of life related to bony pain, fractures, and deterioration in functional status. Prior to the recent USFDA approval of docetaxel, no agents had been shown to alter the natural history of this progression and thus extend life. Median survival of untreated symptomatic disease has generally been less than 12 months, with 6 to 10 months median survival.[43,45,55] Recently, a CALGB prognostic model for predicting survival in HRPC has been developed and validated.[55] Four risk groups were identified using the following factors: lactate dehydrogenase (LDH); Prostate specific antigen (PSA), alkaline phosphatase, Gleason score, ECOG performance status, hemoglobin, and presence of visceral metastases (Box 100.1). Median survival by quartiles for each of these four groups were 8.8, 13.4, 17.4, and 22.8

months, illustrating the heterogeneity of this disease and the need for standardization among potential treatment groups.[55] A similar nomogram has been developed and validated at Memorial Sloan-Kettering Cancer Center.[10] Prostate-specific antigen kinetics have not yet been validated as a surrogate marker for survival in the hormone refractory state, unlike the utility of PSA doubling time in men with rising PSA preceding and following local treatment.[56,57] However, larger scale studies are anticipated to show a correlation of overall survival and the rate of rise of PSA. Thus, men with HRPC are a diverse group whose survival is affected by multiple variables that have confounded the search for therapeutic agents in the past.

Measurable disease has been difficult to quantify in metastatic HRPC, given that many patients have bone-only metastases that may change over time, independently of treatment effect. Initial clinical trials of cytotoxic agents, therefore, included stable disease as a measure of response, clouding the ability to assess the efficacy of these agents.[43] The criteria for evaluating objective responses to therapy have been updated to include the RECIST (response evaluation criteria in solid tumors) criteria, but bony disease remains an unmeasurable quantity.[58] Survival as a primary endpoint has become an indisputable and necessary approach to advancing newer agents toward approval and into the clinic. The plenary sessions of the American Society of Clinical Oncology (ASCO) 2004 demonstrated for the first time that chemotherapy is able to prolong survival in this population, with TAX327 demonstrating a 2.5 month survival advantage of docetaxel over mitoxantrone, and SWOG 9916 demonstrating a similar increment with the combination of docetaxel and estramustine.[8,9] Both studies correlated improved PSA responses and objective response rates with overall survival. Progression-free survival was improved in both trials by similar magnitudes, and tended to correlate with improved QoL scores and pain outcomes. Thus, these two large scale phase III trials demonstrate the feasibility, tolerability, and improved outcomes of doceaxel based chemotherapy, and should serve as a new baseline with which to compare new agents.

Box 100.1 Adverse prognostic variables in metastatic hormone refractory prostate cancer[10,53]

- Poor performance status
- Elevated lactate dehydrogenase
- Liver metastases
- Low hemoglobin
- Elevated alkaline phosphatase
- Less than 2 year interval from onset of hormonal therapy to chemotherapy initiation
- PSA kinetics (likely)

PIVOTAL TRIALS OF CHEMOTHERAPY IN METASTATIC HORMONE-REFRACTORY PROSTATE CANCER

Tables 100.1 and 100.2 present a selected comparison of modern PSA-era trials of single agent and combination therapies examined in phase II and III trials. A further historical review is well summarized by Yagoda et al in 1992[44] and by Beer in 2004.[19] The major pivotal trials that have changed clinical practice are discussed below.

ESTRAMUSTINE

The oral microtubule inhibitor estramustine sodium phosphate (EMP) was the first cytotoxic chemotherapy agent to be approved for use in metastatic prostate cancer, receiving FDA approval in 1981. Estramustine was conceived as a novel targeted agent and is a conjugate of estradiol and nitrogen mustard, and its principle mechanism has been felt to be microtubule disassembly.[57,59] In addition to estrogenic effects, it may additionally cause disruption to the nuclear matrix and chromatin structure independently. Its use as monotherapy has generally been disappointing in terms of response rate (see Table 100.1), and limited by systemic toxicity, notably thromboembolic events seen in about 6% to 7% of patients.[9,60] Response rates in combination regimens have been higher but also limited by these toxicities.[61-63] The recent SWOG 9916 trial of estramustine and docetaxel was unable to reduce this risk with an adult aspirin and low dose coumadin given concurrently.[9]

Table 100.1 Selected single agent activity in high-risk prostate cancer

Agent	References	Number of patients	Survival (months)	Time to progression (months)	Measurable RR (%)	PSA RR (95% CI)
Docetaxel	8, 56–59	810	9–18.9	4.6–5.1	12–28	38–48
Paclitaxel	60–62	126	9–13.5	NR	17	4–39
Mitoxantrone	43, 44, 63	255	12.3-23	3.7–8.1	13	33–48
Epirubicin	64–67	260	9–13	NR	31	24–32
Vinorelbine	68–71	154	10.2–17	2.9–7	7	4–28
Estramustine	72	113	NR	NR	40	21
Cyclophosphamide	73–74	53	8–12.7	NR	14	4
Doxorubicin	65, 75	135	9–13	NR	22	NR
Gemcitabine	76	50	14.7	2.7	NR	NR
Cisplatin	77	29	NR	NR	10	NR

Table 100.2 Selected combination chemotherapy activity in high-risk prostate cancer

Agents	Refs	No. of patients	Survival (months) (months)	Time to progression	Clinical response (%)	PSA response (%)
Paclitaxel, estramustine, etoposide, and carboplatin (TEEC)	78	19	14.2	5.5	58	58
Docetaxel/estramustine	9, 79–83	619	12–20	6–10	17–42	50–82
Paclitaxel/estramustine	84–87	119	13–17.3	4.6–5.6	49	53–62
Vinorelbine/estramustine	88–90	72	10.5–15.1	3.5–5.8	6	24–71
Vinblastine/estramustine	91	95	11.9	3.7	20	25
Ketoconazole, doxorubicin, vinblastine, estramustine (KAVE)	92–93	80	19–23.4	NR	61	56–67
Estramustine/etoposide	93–97	211	11–14	NR	48	14–58
Docetaxel/vinorelbine	98	21	NR	NR	60	66
Docetaxel/capecitabine	99	23	NR	NR	30	71
Mitoxantrone, Estramustine, vinorelbine	100	70	18.4	NR	20	50
Cyclophosph., Dexamethasone, Vincristine	101	52	10.6	2.5	25	29

Combination therapy with estramustine and other microtubule inhibitors in phase II trials has demonstrated additive PSA declines (greater than 50%) on the order of 60%–70%, with a median survival of 20 months (see Table 100.1). The recent phase III trial of docetaxel and estramustine given every 3 weeks with low dose prednisone confirmed the efficacy of this regimen. This trial, SWOG 9916, examined 770 men with progressive HRPC, and randomized to two 21-day regimens: estramustine 280 mg orally on days 1 to 5 with docetaxel 60 mg/m^2 i.v. day 2 and dexamethasone given 20 mg t.i.d. on day 1; versus mitoxantrone 12 mg/m^2 i.v. day 1 with prednisone 5 mg b.i.d. continuously.[9] The estramustine/docetaxel combination demonstrated a 20% improvement in overall survival and a 27% improvement in progression-free survival. Overall median survival improved from 16 to 18 months favoring estramustine/docetaxel with an improved time to progression from 3 to 6 months. This modest improvement, however, has been counterbalanced by the similar results obtained in phase III trials of docetaxel alone (*vida infra*), thus likely limiting the clinical utility of estramustine in combination regimens. Additionally, the 7% risk of thromboembolic complications in a recent meta-analysis, and the cumulative gastrointestinal toxicities of estramustine/docetaxel combinations likely preclude this combination therapy from standard of care.[19,60]

MITOXANTRONE/PREDNISONE

Mitoxantrone is an anthracenedione with cytotoxic activity, and was the first drug to be tested in phase III trials for HRPC in which clinically meaningful QoL parameters were used as an assessment of response.[45,46] Monotherapy PSA response rates (RRs) have ranged from 33% to 48%, with measurable RRs of 13%, without demonstrable improvements in overall survival. The USFDA approval of mitoxantrone in 1996 was the result of two large phase III randomized trials that showed a clinically beneficial response measured in pain ratings and palliative response.[45,46] Tannock et al demonstrated a significantly longer duration of palliation with mitoxantrone and prednisone versus prednisone alone (43 versus 18 weeks), but no difference in overall survival.[46] Kantoff et al confirmed this in a large CALGB trial reported in 1999, which showed improved secondary QoL outcomes and delayed disease progression of about 2 months.[45] Toxicity with mitoxantrone has been primarily hematologic including about a 40% to 50% incidence of grade 3 and 4 neutropenia. However, neutropenic fever has been reported in less than 1% of cases, and no toxic deaths have been reported in the large phase III trials. Cardiac toxicity, mostly congested heart failure (CHF) has been observed in less than 5% of patients. Mitoxantrone has additionally been studied in a large phase II trial of men with HRPC and asymptomatic metastatic disease.[64]

While no overall difference in survival was seen, men on the chemotherapy arm had a prolonged disease-free period and time to progression as compared with prednisone alone (8.1 months versus 4.1 months). Toxicity in these trials have mostly consisted of hematologic toxicity (grade 3/4 neutropenia in about 60–70%) and cardiac toxicity (5%).

DOCETAXEL

Docetaxel is a cytotoxic agent and member of the taxoid family. It induces apoptosis in cancer cells through p53-independent mechanisms that are felt to be due to its inhibition of microtubule depolymerization and inhibition of antiapoptotic signaling.[65,66] The induction of microtubule stabilization intracellularly through β-tubulin interactions causes GTP-independent polymerization and cell cycle arrest at G2/M, and some have reported a two-fold greater microtubule affinity compared with paclitaxel.[65,67] Additionally, docetaxel has been found to induce BCL2 phosphorylation in vitro, a process which has been correlated with caspace activation and loss of its normal antiapoptotic activity.[68] Unable to inhibit the proapoptotic molecule BAX, phosphorylated BCL2 may also induce apotosis through this independent mechanism. However, additional mechanisms may be important such as P27KIP1 induction and repression of BCLXL.[67,69]

Weekly docetaxel has been studied in several phase II trials and the phase III TAX327 trial with favorable results and toxicity profiles. Berry et al conducted a multi-institutional phase II study that gave 36 mg/m^2 docetaxel weekly for 6 out of 8 weeks per cycle with dexamethasone premedication, which demonstrated a 9.4 month survival and 46% PSA response (greater than 50% decline) among men with HRPC, 25% of whom were previously treated with mitoxantrone.[70] Likewise, a trial by Beer et al in previously untreated men demonstrated improved pain outcomes in 48% and a 46% PSA "response" using a similar regimen.[71] The every 3-week schedules of docetaxel were developed in two large randomized trials[72,73] that demonstrated a 38% to 46% PSA-response rate and median survival of 9 months using docetaxel at 75 mg/m^2 every 21 days with dexamethasone premedication. Responders had a median survival of 27 months with favorable quality of life outcomes. It has generally been felt that the every 3-week schedule has had more neutropenia (43–71% versus 3–25%) compared with the weekly regimens, but all regimens have been well tolerated without any significant clinical differences.

Docetaxel has become the agent of choice as of 2004 for metastatic HRPC, based on a large phase III randomized trial, TAX 327, which demonstrated its superiority to the past standard, mitoxantrone and prednisone.[8] TAX 327 built on the work of the above four phase II trials,[72,73] which demonstrated the safety and efficacy of weekly and every 3-week schedules of docetaxel. TAX-327 enrolled 1006 patients with progressive HRPC, no prior chemotherapy, and stable pain scores to one of three arms, all with concomitant prednisone at 5 mg p.o. b.i.d.: mitoxantrone 12 mg/m² i.v. q21 days; docetaxel 75 mg/m² i.v. q21 days; and docetaxel 30 mg/m² i.v. weekly. Patents remained on gonadal suppression but had all other hormonal agents discontinued within 4 to 6 weeks. Treatment duration was 30 weeks in all arms, or a maximum of 10 cycles in the every 3-week arms, with more patients completing treatment in the every 3-week docetaxel arm than the mitoxantrone arm due mostly to differences in disease progression (46% versuss 25%).[8] After a median 20.7 month follow-up, overall survival in the every 3-week docetaxel arm was 18.9 months with a pain response rate of 35% and a PSA response of 45%, contrasted with weekly docetaxel at 17.3 months, 31%, and 48% respectively. This translated into a 24% relative risk reduction in death (95% CI 6–48%; p = 0.0005) with every 3-week docetaxel (Figure 100.1).[8] The mitoxantrone arm performed favorably against historic mitoxantrone-treated patients, with a median survival of 16.4 months, a pain response of 22%, and a PSA response of 32%.[8]

Toxicity in the every 3-week versus weekly docetaxel arms was notable for more hematologic toxicity in the every 3-week arm (3% neutropenic fever versus 0%; 32% grade 3/4 neutropenia versus 1.5%), but slightly lower rates of nausea and vomiting, fatigue, nail changes, hyperlacrimation, and diarrhea. Neuropathy was slightly more common in the every 3-week arm (grade 3/4 in 1.8% versus 0.9%).[8] Quality of life as measured by the FACT-P scores did not differ significantly among the docetaxel schedules but were more favorable than the mitoxantrone arm.[8] In extrapolating the use of docetaxel to large populations of men with HRPC, it is also important to be point out significant reports of interstitial pneumonitis, extravasation injuries, colitis, excess tearing, and maculopapular rash that may occur with docetaxel but were not seen in TAX327.[65]

Of note, paclitaxel has been studies in several phase II trials with similar response rates to docetaxel using prolonged 24-hour infusion schedules.[74–76] However, no phase III trials of paclitaxel have been advanced nor any head-to-head comparisons with docetaxel and are unlikely to be performed given the likely minor differences in clinical outcomes expected.

COMBINATION CHEMOTHERAPY

DOCETAXEL/ESTRAMUSTINE

Based on the success of multiple phase II studies with the combination of docetaxel and estramustine, SWOG conducted the large phase III trial SWOG 99-16, the results of which were reported in 2004.[9,61–63,77,78] The rationale for the addition of two microtubule targeted therapies has been the in-vitro synergism observed in some hormone-sensitive cell lines between estramustine and docetaxel, the clinical experience of improved PSA, and objective response rates historically and when compared with docetaxel alone.[62,79]

SWOG 99-16 randomized 770 patients with progressive HRPC to oral estramustine 280 mg p.o. t.i.d. with docetaxel 60 mg/m² every 21 days or mitoxantrone 12 mg/m² every 21 days with low dose prednisone. The protocol was amended due to a high rate of cardiovascular thromboembolic events to include prophylactic low dose coumadin and aspirin, which unfortunately was unable to demonstrate a reduction in thromboembolism. While the docetaxel/estramustine arms demonstrated improvement over the control group in terms of overall survival by 2 months and progression-free survival by 3 months, the clinical utility of the regimen suffered as a result of the excessive grade 3 and 4 gastrointestinal and cardiovascular toxicities (20% and 15%, respectively).[9] Given the similar magnitude of

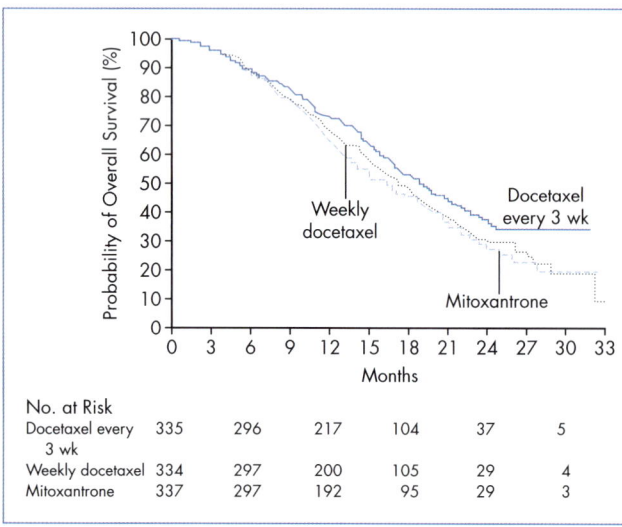

No. at Risk

Docetaxel every 3 wk	335	296	217	104	37	5
Weekly docetaxel	334	297	200	105	29	4
Mitoxantrone	337	297	192	95	29	3

Fig. 100.1

Kaplan–Meier estimates of overall survival in the three arms of the TAX 327 trial involving 1006 men with hormone-refractory metastatic prostate cancer randomized to prednisone plus docetaxel (every 3 weeks or weekly) versus mitoxantrone and prednisone.

survival benefit and response rates with single agent docetaxel with substantially less toxicity than estramustine regimens, it is likely that the use of estramustine combinations will drop off considerably. While head-to-head comparisons of separate phase III trials are impossible due to differences in schedule, patient populations, and docetaxel dosing (60 mg/m² in SWOG 9916 and 75 mg/m² in TAX 327), it is unlikely that a large survival benefit with estramustine will be missed despite the combination's improved response rate.

While multiple other chemotherapy agents have been studied in phase II clinical trials, none have advanced into phase III trials or demonstrated improved survival over the currently approved drugs: docetaxel, estramustine, and mitoxantrone. Table 100.1 lists selected active combination regimens with phase II and III activity in HRPC. In general, combination therapies with active single agents, such as paclitaxel, etoposide, estramustine, and carboplatin (TEEC), or ketoconazole, doxorubicin, vinblastine, and estramustine (KAVE), have shown improved response rates and increased toxicity but comparable survival times to single agent docetaxel, precluding their use as standard therapy.[80–82] Doublets of microtubule-based therapies, including vinorelbine and vinblastine with docetaxel or estramustine, have not demonstrated significantly improved response or progression-free survival rates.[61–63,77,78,81–95]

Certain agents, such as oral continuous "metronomic" cyclophosphamide and dexamethasone in combination have shown activity in a retrospective trial of a mixed population of men with HRPC.[96] A decline of more than 50% PSA was seen in 78% of 34 men, 13 of whom had been treated with prior chemotherapy, with a 9-month duration of response. This appealing well-tolerated oral treatment may be a reasonable alternative in select patients who have progressed despite chemotherapy, suffered adverse reactions to standard chemotherapy, or, given the nearly 10% cerebrospinal-fluid bioavailability of cyclophosphamide, have central nervous system or leptomeningeal disease.[96] Dividing doses into more frequent, or metronomic fractions, such as weekly docetaxel, has not been shown to be less toxic and has not demonstrated improved durable responses prospectively; however, continued prospective study of this low toxicity, patient friendly approach with new agents is warranted.[97]

MODIFYING CHEMOTHERAPY RESPONSE

ANDROGEN PRIMING

Given the theoretical sensitivity of rapidly dividing cells to cytotoxic therapy, the rationale for the addition of androgen to chemotherapy as a way of inducing cell cycle turnover was tested in 1988 by Manni et al.[98] They theorized that priming with the androgen fluoxymesterone 3 days prior to and concurrent with chemotherapy administration would synchronize tumor growth and lead to a greater response rate than placebo. Eight-five patients with prostate cancer who had progressed despite orchiectomy were treated initially with aminoglutethamide and hydrocortisone to induce androgen depletion and then with cyclophosphamide, fluorouracil, and doxorubicin every 3 weeks. Randomization was to androgen or no androgen. Median response and duration of response was no different, and median survival was shorter in the androgen arm (10 versus 15 months).[98] There were significant toxicities related to tumor growth during androgen administration, including cord compression, increased bone pain, and worsening liver function. While this does not address androgen priming in the modern era with active cytotoxic M-phase specific agents, it has not currently been shown to be more effective than no treatment or continued hormonal ablation.[99]

ANDROGEN DEPRIVATION

While metastatic HRPC may remain androgen responsive, it is unclear if continued androgen suppression in the face of disease progression and trials of cytotoxic therapy has clinical utility. The specific question of whether clinicians should continue GnRH agonists while initiating chemotherapy has not been addressed in modern randomized clinical trials. However, retrospective and anecdotal reports have documented progressive disease and inferior outcomes on discontinuation of androgen suppression during chemotherapy with resumption of response on restarting hormonal therapy.[100,101] In one small series, PSA progression was documented during chemotherapy for HRPC, with resumption of PSA response with reinstitution of hormone ablation.[100] This may indicate that HRPC is not truly androgen independent, but rather maintains features of androgen driven growth. However, androgen ablation alone is insufficient to maintain responses in HRPC, and antiandrogen withdrawal remains a therapeutic measure in a fraction of patients. Currently, the PSA working group has recommended that patients stay on LHRH agonists during chemotherapy and chemotherapy trials and all recently reported studies maintain this level of hormonal therapy.

ROLE OF CORTICOSTEROIDS

The role of glucocorticoids as adjunctive treatment to chemotherapy in HRPC is controversial, based on the fact that most current clinical trials have allowed the use of these agents in both treatment and control arms. Prednisone or hydrocortisone alone have demonstrated more than 50% PSA declines on the order of 20% and relief of QoL parameters such as pain control in 20% to 50% of patients.[102] Time to progression in men with symptomatic metastatic HRPC treated with low dose prednisone alone has been comparable to flutamide, with a time to progression of 3.4 months and 56% subjective response rate.[103] As glucocorticoids suppress pituitary adrenocorticotrophic hormone (ACTH) production and thus adrenal androgen levels, one mechanism may be this third-line antiandrogen effect. However, glucocorticoids also have direct cytopathic effects and immunomodulatory effects that may interfere with intracellular growth and survival pathways. For example, dexamethasone has been shown to reduce IL–6 and nuclear factor κB (NFκB) levels, factors which may be important in hormone refractory prostate cancer cell growth.[104] Alternatively, one potential mechanism wherein glucocorticoids may worsen outcome in men with HRPC has been the demonstration of androgen receptor mutations that lead to steroidal agonism and tumor growth rather than growth inhibition.[105] It may continue to be difficult to separate out these effects due to the approval of recent agents that included low dose prednisone as part of the treatment arm.

NOVEL BIOLOGIC AGENTS IN COMBINATION WITH CHEMOTHERAPY

Novel targeted combination therapies of biologic agents to enhance the efficacy chemotherapy are being extensively investigated, and include such agents as EGF receptor tyrosine kinase inhibitors (gefitinib, erlotinib), platelet-derived growth factor (PDGF) receptor tyrosine kinase inhibitors (imatinib), thalidomide and other immunomodulatory agents, differentiating agents such as DN101 (calcitriol), radioimmunotherapies, antiangiogenic agents such as bevacizumab, proapoptotic agents, and others. These will be discussed extensively in subsequent chapters, as primary first-line therapy and for relapsed progressive disease after chemotherapy. However, a brief discussion of the more active agents is warranted here, and these are listed in Box 100.2.

Thalidomide in combination with docetaxel was investigated in a recent phase II study based on the principle that an immunomodulatory and anti-angiogenic molecule would enhance the efficacy of a traditional cytotoxic agent.[106] Thalidomide inhibits IL6 and tumor necrosis factor-α (TNF-α), and has other immunostimulatory effects, while metabolites of thalidomide have been found to have antiangiogenic

---

Box 100.2 Novel biologic agents in development for advanced prostate cancer in combination with chemotherapy

- Thalidomide
- CC5013 (Revlimid) and CC-4047 (Actimid)
- DN-101 (calcitriol)
- Imatinib (Gleevec)
- Bortezomib (Velcade)
- Bevacizumab (Avastin)
- Proapoptotic agents, i.e., BCL2 antisense oligonucleotides (oblimersen sodium)
- CCI-779 and inhibitors of AKT and mTOR pathways
- Lapatinib and other EGFR, PDGFR, HER2/HER3 inhibitors
- Bisphosphonates (pamidronate, clodronate, zoledronic acid)
- Atrasentan (Xinlay)
- Radiolabeled isotopes and monoclonal antibodies (samarium, strontium, lutetium, yttrium)
- Vaccine strategies

EGFR, epithelial growth factor receptor; PDGFR, platelet-derived growth factor receptor

---

activity in rat aortic ring assays.[107,108] This trial randomized patients with chemotherapy naive metastatic HRPC to either weekly docetaxel alone or in combination with 200 mg/day of oral thalidomide. Prostate-specific antigen and objective responses were seen in 53% and 35% of the combined group, respectively, compared with 37% and 27% in the docetaxel alone arm. Progression-free survival was improved from 3.7 months to 5.9 months in the combined group, and at 26 months of follow-up, overall survival was improved from 14.7 months to 28.9 months, the longest seen yet of any combination therapy in HRPC.[106] Adverse effects in the thalidomide group included the expected sedation and dizziness seen in 43%, grade 1 and 2 peripheral neuropathy in 76%, thrombosis in 18%, and slightly more constipation. Although this trial was underpowered, with only 75 patients, it is suggestive of an incremental benefit in disease progression and stabilization. Other novel immunomodulatory and potentially anti-angiogenic agents such as Revlimid and CC-4047 that are structurally based on thalidomide but without the neurotoxicity and sedative properties are currently moving into phase II studies after initial studies demonstrated their activity and safety.[109,110]

DN101 represents a new formulation of calcitriol, a vitamin D analog that has demonstrated preclinical synergy with docetaxel and improved PSA responses and median survival in phase II trials when used in combination with docetaxel.[111] In 37 patients treated on this trial with weekly docetaxel and pretreatment with oral calcitriol 0.5 μg/kg, median time to progression was 11.4 months, and median survival was 19.5 months, comparing favorably with historic controls. The phase II/III ASCENT trial will examine the combination of

DN101, a high-dose oral calcitriol formulation, and weekly docetaxel, in a larger population compared with the current docetaxel standard.

Other agents such as imatinib (Gleevec) as a targeted therapy of the PDGF receptor pathway, bortezomib (Velcade) as a novel proteasome inhibitor, and bevacizumab (Avastin) as a VEGF inhibitor have demonstrated preclinical and phase I activity and are moving forward to larger scale trials currently, such as the CALGB trial 90006 of estramustine and docetaxel in combination with Avastin in men with HRPC.[112–114] The antiapoptotic protein BCL2 is a rational target of therapy and is being investigated as a predictor of clinical response. The inhibitory antisense oligonucleotide oblimersen sodium is being tested in phase II/III trials in combination with docetaxel and has shown some promising early results.[115] Correlation of antiapoptotic gene protein levels with response has not yet been clinically correlated, and this theory is being examined by ECOG 1899, discussed earlier in this chapter. Epidermal growth factor receptor (EGFR) and other growth factor receptor inhibitors hold some promise in combination with cytotoxic agents based on responses seen in NSCLC; however only modest PSA responses and no clinical activity has been demonstrated with single agent use of gefitinib in HRPC.[116] Improved responses with multitargeted tyrosine kinase inhibition (i.e., lapatinib) or inhibition of additional cell survival pathways important to prostate cancer such as mTOR (i.e., CCI-779) or AKT/PI3K remain to be demonstrated but are eagerly anticipated.[115] Bone targeted agents such as bisphosphonates and atrasentan, a novel endothelin receptor antagonist, have also shown clinical activity in HRPC and will be discussed in subsequent chapters.[114]

THERAPY FOR PROGRESSIVE DISEASE FOLLOWING CHEMOTHERAPY

To date, there remains no FDA approved therapies for second- or third-line treatment of metastatic prostate cancer that has progressed after chemotherapy, and this unfilled niche represents an active area of clinical investigation that should encourage enrollment on clinical trials. Overall survival in this group of patients is approximately 12 months based on time to progression and overall survival in large phase III trials.[8,9] As stated above, combination therapies may result in higher response rates but at increased toxicity, especially in heavily pretreated individuals, with lower response rates generally seen in those who have failed first line chemotherapy.

One agent that is currently under evaluation as second line therapy is the oral platinum agent, Satraplatin, which has shown in vivo activity against taxane and cisplatin

refractory prostate cell lines. A small phase III trial has shown improved response rates and progression free survival of Satraplatin 100 mg/m^2 × 5 days in combination with prednisone every 28 days, with a trend toward improved overall survival, although the study was not powered to detect a difference.[118] Median progression-free (5.2 versus 2.5 months) and overall survival (14.9 versus 11.9 months) were slightly better compared with prednisone alone, and has led to the initiation of the SPARC trial (Satraplatin and prednisone against refractory cancer) for second line HRPC chemotherapy. It remains to be seen if this agent has improved toxicity and survival data over standard palliative care or currently available well tolerated agents, such as oral cyclophosphamide and dexamethasone or other active agents.

The epothilones are a class of microtubule targeting cytotoxic agents in development for second line HRPC as well, and their activity in this scenario is an area of active investigation. The epothilones are derived from the myxobacterium *Sorangium cellulosum*, and in preclinical models they demonstrated a wide range of clinical activity, including taxane-resistant models, with a mechanism similar to the taxanes.[119] By suppressing microtubule depolymerization, these agents induce G2/M arrest and apoptosis. However, while taxanes are susceptible to P-glycoprotein-induced drug efflux, the epothilones are not.[119] One such agent, Epothilone-B analog BMS-247550 (Ixabepilone) has been studied in a phase II trial of men with HRPC. Initial results demonstrate a 34% PSA response and 30% objective response, with a progression-free survival of 8 months, comparable to the best results seen with taxane based therapy.[16] The use of BMS 247550 in taxane-resistant HRPC is being investigated currently by Rosenberg et al in NCI protocol 6046 compared with mitoxantrone and prednisone.[120] Additional schedules are being evaluated in other phase II studies that may be less neurotoxic than the initial phase II trials.

It is worth mentioning that studies of chemotherapy in combination with radiolabeled antibodies or radioisotopes for metastatic prostate cancer are also under development for progressive disease following chemotherapy. The most advanced of these approaches involves strontium-89 (^{89}Sr) given with doxorubicin as consolidation following induction chemotherapy on the MD Anderson KAVE regimen. This approach has shown significant palliation of pain (>50%), prolongation of survival (from 17 to 28 months), and improved time to progression with ^{89}Sr as consolidation with doxorubicin compared with doxorubicin alone in a randomized phase II trial.[17] While involving a fairly toxic, nonstandard chemotherapy regimen and a small number[57] of patients that require confirmation testing, this trial demonstrated the potential additive benefits of radioisotopes such as samarium-153 (^{153}Sm)or ^{89}Sr to chemotherapy. Whether these agents can add benefit following or in combination with docetaxel chemotherapy remains unanswered. The use of these agents as salvage therapy for symptomatic metastases has been studied in several randomized trials and will be discussed in a subsequent chapter. While survival benefits have not been demonstrated to date, radioisotopes have been shown to reduce analgesic requirements in symptomatic men with multiple metastatic sites at the expense of myelosuppression.[121] Prostate-specific membrane antigen (PSMA) monoclonal antibody-tagged radioisotopes such as Yttrium-90 (^{90}Y) or Lutetium-177 (^{177}Lu) are also in development and have begun to enter phase II trials.[122]

CURRENT INDICATIONS FOR CHEMOTHERAPY

In conclusion, chemotherapy with docetaxel or mitoxantrone for metastatic HRPC has become the standard of care given the improved survival demonstrated in recent phase III trials. The benefits or the addition of estramustine is likely offset by its toxicity profile and lack of demonstrable survival benefit over docetaxel alone. Treatment with docetaxel seems to favor an every 3-week schedule, given up to 10 cycles, but may be continued as long as objective responses are seen. The use of chemotherapy in earlier phases of advanced disease, such as biochemical only HRPC, asymptomatic metastatic HRPC subgroups, and as adjuvant or neoadjuvant to definitive local therapies remains to be proven but these clinical trials are moving forward quickly to change the treatment paradigms in high-risk men.[123,124] Surrogate markers such as PSA doubling time and changes in PSA velocity are under investigation to facilitate the development of these therapies in a more rapid manner.[125,126] A large number of novel agents with diverse mechanisms of action that target many of the critical checkpoints in prostate cancer growth, invasion, apoptosis, and metastasis are additionally bringing a great deal of excitement to this rapidly changing field. Whether these agents will replace chemotherapy or be used in conjunction with cytotoxic chemotherapy remains to be seen.

CONFLICT-OF-INTEREST STATEMENT

Funding for some of the studies described in this article was provided by Aventis Pharmaceuticals and Abbott Laboratories. Dr Carducci is on the Speakers Bureau for Aventis Pharmaceuticals and is a consultant to Abbott Laboratories. The terms of this arrangement are being managed by the Johns Hopkins University in accordance with its conflict of interest policies.

REFERENCES

1. Weir, HK, Thun MJ, Hankey BF, et al. Annual Report to the Nation on the Status of Cancer 1975-2000, Featuring the Uses of Surveillance Data for Cancer Prevention and Control. J Natl Cancer Inst 2003;95:1276–1299.

2. Jemal A, Murray T, Ward E, et al. Cancer Statistics 2005. CA Cancer J Clin 2005;55:10–30.

3. Han M, Partin AW, Piantadosi S, et al. Era Specific Biochemical Recurrence-Free Survival Following Radical Prostatectomy for Clinically Localized Prostate Cancer. J Urol 2001;166:416–419.

4. Zietman AL, Coen JJ, Dallow KC, et al. The Treatment of Prostate Cancer by Conventional Radiation Therapy:an Analysis of Long-Term Outcome. Int J Radiat Oncol Biol Phys 1995;32:287–292.

5. Goktas S, Crawford ED. Optimal Hormonal Therapy for Advanced Prostatic Carcinoma. Semin Oncol 1999;26:162–173.

6. Eisenberger MA, Partin AW, Pound C, et al. Natural History of Progression of Patients with Biochemical (PSA) Relapse Following Radical Prostatectomy: Update. Proc Am Soc Clin Oncol 2003;22:280 [abstract 1527].

7. Eisenberger MA, Blumenstein BA, Crawford ED, et al. Bilateral Orchiectomy with or without Flutamide for Metastatic Prostate Cancer. N Engl J Med 1998;339:1036–1042.

8. Eisenberger MA, de Wit R, Berry W, et al. A Multicenter Phase III Comparison of Docetaxel (D) + Prednisone (P) and Mitoxantrone (M) + P in Patients with Hormone-Refractory Prostate Cancer. Proc Am Soc Clin Oncol 2004 [abstract 4].

9. Petrylak D, Tangen C, Hussain M, et al. SWOB 99-16:Randomized Phase III Trial of Docetaxel (D)/Estramustine (E) versus Mitoxantrone (M)/Prednisone (P) in Men with Androgen-Independent Prostate Cancer. Proc Am Soc Clin Oncol 2004 [abstract 3].

10. Smaletz O, Scher HI, Small EJ, et al. Nomogram for Overall Survival of Patients with Progressive Metastatic Prostate Cancer After Castration. J Clin Oncol 2002;20:3972–3982.

11. Kantoff PW, Halabi S, Conaway M, et al. Hydrocortisone with or without Mitoxantrone in Men with Hormone-Refractory Prostate Cancer: Results of the Cancer and Leukemia Group B 9182 Study. J Clin Oncol 1999;17:2506–2513.

12. Bubley GJ, Carducci MA, Dahut W, et al. Eligibility and Response Guidelines for Phase II Clinical Trials in Androgen-Independent Prostate Cancer: Recommendations from the Prostate-Specific Antigen Working Group. J Clin Oncol 1999;17:3461–3467.

13. Scher HI, Eisenberger M, D'Amico AV, et al. Eligibility and Outcomes Reporting Guidelines for Clinical Trials for Patients in the State of a Rising Prostate Specific Antigen: Recommendations from the Prostate-Specific Antigen Working Group. J Clin Oncol 2004;22:537–556.

14. Small EJ, Halabi S, Dawson NA, et al. Antiandrogen Withdrawal Alone or in Combination with Ketoconazole in Androgen-Independent Prostate Cancer Patients: A Phase III Trial (CALGB 9583). J Clin Oncol 2004;22:1025–1033.

15. Eastham JA, Kelly WK, Grossfeld GD, et al. Cancer and Leukemia Group B (CALGB) 90203:a Randomized Phase 3 Trial of Radical Prostatectomy Alone versus Estramustine and Docetaxel Before Radical Prostatectomy for Patients with High Risk Localized Disease. Urology 2003;62 Suppl 1:55–62.

16. Hussain M, Faulkner J, Vaishampayan U, et al. Epothilone B Analogue BMS-247550 Administered Every 21 Days in Patients with Hormone Refractory Prostate Cancer. A Southwest Oncology Group Study (S0111). Proc Am Soc Clin Oncol 2004 [abstract 4510].

17. Tu SM, Millikan RE, Mengistu RE, et al. Bone Targeted Therapy for Advanced Androgen-Independent Carcinoma of the Prostate: a Randomized Phase II Trial. Lancet 2001;357:336–341.

18. Walczak JR, Carducci MA. Phase III Randomized Trial Evaluating Second Line Hormonal Therapy versus Docetaxel-Estramustine Combination Chemotherapy on Progression-Free Survival in Asymptomatic Patients with a Rising PSA After Hormonal Therapy for Prostate Cancer:an Eastern Cooperative Oncology Group (E1899), Intergroup/Clinical Trials Support Unit Study. Urology 2003;62 Suppl 1:141–146.

19. Beer TM. Advances in Systemic Therapy for Prostate Cancer: Chemotherapy for Androgen-Independent Prostate Cancer. Proc Am Soc Clin Oncol 2004;225–232.

20. Martel CL, Gumerlock PH, Meyers FJ, et al. Current Strategies in the Management of Hormone Refractory Prostate Cancer. Cancer Treat Rev 2003;29:171–187.

21. Fosati R, Confalonieri C, Torri V, et al. Cytotoxic and Hormonal Treatment for Metastatic Breast Cancer:A Systematic Review of Published Randomized Trials Involving 31, 510 Women. J Clin Oncol 1998;16:3439–3460.

22. Goldberg RM, Sargent DJ, Morton RF, et al. A Randomized Controlled Trial of Fluorouracil Plus Leukovorin, Irinotecan, and Oxaliplatin Combinations in Patients with Previously Untreated Metastatic Colorectal Cancer. J Clin Oncol 2004;22:23–30.

23. Isaacs JT. The Biology of Hormone Refractory Prostate Cancer: Why does it Develop? Urol Clin NA 1999;26:263–273.

24. Lee WH, Morton RA, Epstein JI, et al. Cytidine Methylation of Regulatory Sequences near the P-class Glutathione-S-Transferase Gene Accompanies Human Prostate Cancer Carcinogenesis. Proc Natl Acad Sci USA 1994;91:11733–11737.

25. McDonnell TJ, Troncoso P, Brisbay SM, et al. Expression of the Protooncogene bcl-2 in the Prostate and its Association with Emergence of Androgen-Independent Prostate Cancer. Cancer Res 1992;52:6940–6944.

26. Sullivan GF, Amenta PS, Villanueva JD, et al. The Expression of Drug Resistance Gene Products during the Progression of Human Prostate Cancer. Clin Cancer Res 1998;4:1393–1403.

27. Apakama I, Robinson MC, Walter NM, et al. Bcl-2 Overexpression Combined with p53 Protein Accumulation Correlates with Hormone-Refractory Prostate Cancer. Br J Cancer 1996;74:1258–1262.

28. Graff JR. Emerging Targets in the AKT Pathway for Treatment of Androgen-Independent Prostatic Adenocarcinoma. Expert Opin Ther Targets 2002;6:103–113.

29. Whang YE, Wu X, Suzuki H, et al. Inactivation of the Tumor Suppressor PTEN/MMAC1 in Advanced Human Prostate Cancer Through Loss of Expression. Proc Natl Acad Sci USA 1998;95:5246–5250.

30. McMenamin ME, Soung P, Perera S, et al. Loss of PTEN Expression in Paraffin-Embedded Primary Prostate Cancer Correlates with High Gleason Score and Advanced Stage. Cancer Res 1999;59:4291–4296.

31. Pfeil K, Eder IE, Putz T, et al. Long Term Androgen-Ablation Causes Increased Resistance to PI3K/Akt Pathway Inhibition in Prostate Cancer Cells. Prostate 2004;58:259–168.

32. Cantley LC, Neel BG. New Insights into Tumor Suppression: PTEN Suppresses Tumor Formation by Restraining the Phosphoinositide 3-kinase/AKT Pathway. Proc Natl Acad Sci USA 1999;96:4240–4245.

33. Ramaswamy S, Nakamura N, Vazquez F et al. Regulation of the G1 Progression by the PTEN Tumor Suppressor Protein is Linked to Inhibition of the Phosphatidylinositol 3-kinase/akt Pathway. Proc Natl Acad Sci USA 1999;96:2110–2115.

34. Chen CD, Welsbie DS, Tran C, et al. Molecular Determinants of Resistance to Antiandrogen Therapy. Nature Medicine 2004;10:33–38.

35. Tilley WD, Buchanan G, Hickey TE, et al. Mutations in the Androgen Receptor Gene are Associated with Progression of Human Prostate Cancer to Androgen Independence. Cancer Res 1996;2:277–285.

36. Taplin ME, Bubley GJ, Chuster TD, et al. Mutation of the Androgen-Receptor Gene in Metastatic Androgen-Independent Prostate Cancer. N Engl J Med 1995;332:1393–1398.

37. Marcelli M, Ittman M, Mariani S, et al. Androgen Receptor Mutations in Prostate Cancer. Cancer Res 2000;60:944–949.

38. Culig Z, Hobisch A, Cronauer MV, et al. Androgen Receptor Activation in Prostatic Tumor Cell Lines by Insulin-Like Growth Factor-I, Keratinocyte Growth Factor, and Epidermal Growth Factor. Cancer Res 1994;54:5474–5478.

39. Torti, FM, Carter SK. The Chemotherapy of Prostatic Adenocarcinoma. Ann Int Med 1980;92:681–689.

40. Schmidt, JD. Chemotherapy of Hormone-Resistant Stage D Prostatic Cancer. J Urol 1980;123:797–805.

41. Scott W, Johnson DE, Schmidt JE, et al. Chemotherapy of Advanced Prostatic Carcinoma with Cyclophosphamide or 5-Fluorouracil: Results of First National Randomized Study. J Urol 1976;114:909–911.

42. Klein LA. Prostatic Carcinoma. N Eng J Med 1979;300:824–833.

43. Eisenberger MA, Simon R, O'Dwyer PJ, et al. A Reevaluation of Nonhormonal Cytotoxic Chemotherapy in the Treatment of Prostatic Carcinoma. J Clin Oncol 1985;3:827–841.

44. Yagoda A, Petrylak D. Cytotoxic Chemotherapy for Advanced Hormone-Resistant Prostate Cancer. Cancer 1993;71 Supp 3:1098–1109.

45. Kantoff PW, Halabi S, Conaway M, et al. Hydrocortisone with or without Mitoxantrone in Men with Hormone-Refractory Prostate Cancer: Results of the Cancer and Leukemia Group B 9182 Study. J Clin Oncol 1999;17:2506–2513.

46. Tannock IF, Osoba D, Stocklet MR. Chemotherapy with Mitoxantrone plus Prednisone or Prednisone Alone for Symptomatic Hormone-Resistant Prostate Cancer: a Canadian Randomized Trial with Palliative Endpoints. J Clin Oncol 1996;14:1756–1764.

47. Esper P, Fei M, Chodak G, et al. Measuring Quality of Life in Men with Prostate Cancer using the Functional Assessment of Cancer Therapy-Prostate Instrument. Urology 1997;50:920–928.

48. Schipper CJ, McMurray A, Levitt M. Measuring the Quality of Life of Cancer Patients: The Functional Living Index-Cancer: Development and Validation. J Clin Oncol 1984;2:472–483.

49. Fossa S, Aaronson N, Newling D. Quality of Life and Treatment of Hormone-Resistant Metastatic Prostate Cancer. Eur J Cancer 1990;26:1133–1136.

50. Matzkin, H, Eber P, Todd B, et al. Prognostic Significance of Changes in Prostate-Specific Markers after Endocrine Treatment of Stage D2 Prostatic Cancer. Cancer 1992;70:2302–2309.

51. Scher HI, Kelly WK, Zhang ZF, et al. Post-Therapy Serum Prostate-Specific Antigen Level and Survival in Patients with Androgen-Independent Prostate Cancer. J Natl Cancer Inst 1999;91:244–251.

52. Smith DC, Dunn RL, Strawderman MS, et al. Change in Serum Prostate-Specfic Antigen as a Marker of Response to Cytotoxic Therapy for Hormone-Refractory Prostate Cancer. J Clin Oncol 1998;16:1835–1843.

53. Horti J, Dixon SC, Logothetis C, et al. Increased Transcriptional Activity of PSA in the Presences of TNP-470, an Angiogenesis Inhibitor. Br J Cancer 1999;79:1588–1593.

54. Wasilenkko WJ, Palad AJ, Somers KD, et al. Effect of the Calcium Influx Inhibitor Carboxyamido-triazole on the Proliferation and Invasiveness of Human Prostate Tumor Cell Lines. Int J Cancer 1996;68:259–264.

55. Halabi S, Small EJ, Katoff PW, et al. Prognostic Model for Predicting Survival in Men with Hormone-Refractory Metastatic Prostate Cancer. J Clin Oncol 2003;21:1232–1237.

56. Loberg, RD, Fielhauer JR, Peinta BA, et al. Prostate-Specific Antigen Doubling Time and Survival in Patients with Advanced Metastatic Prostate Cancer. Urology 2003;62 Suppl 6B:128–133.

57. Eklov S, Nilsson S, Larson A. Evidence for a Non-Estrogenic Cytostatic Effect of Estramustine on Human Prostatic Carcinoma Cells In Vivo. Prostate 1992;20:43–50.

58. Therasse P, Arbuck SG, Eisenhauer EA, et al. New Guidelines to Evaluate the Response to Treatment in Solid Tumors. J Natl Cancer Inst 2000;92:205–216.

59. Hartley-Asp B. Estramustine-Induced Mitotic Arrest in Two Human Prostatic Carcinoma Cell Lines DU 145 and PC-3. Prostate 1984;5:93.

60. Lubiniecki GM, Berlin JA, Weinstein RB, et al. Risk of Thromboembolic Events (TE) with Estramustine-Based Chemotherapy in Hormone-Refractory Prostate Cancer: Results of a Meta-analysis. Proc Am Soc Clin Oncol 2003 [abstract 1581].

61. Savarese DM, Halabi S, Hars V, et al. Phase II Study of Docetaxel, Estramustine, and Low-Dose Hydrocortisone in Men with Hormone-Refractory Prostate Cancer: A Final Report of CALGB 9780. J Clin Oncol 2001;19:2509–2515.

62. Eymard JC, Joly F, Priou F, et al. Phase II Randomized Trial of Docetaxel plus Estramustine (DE) versus Docetaxel (D) in Patients with Hormone Refractory Prostate Cancer: A Final Report. Proc Am Soc Clin Oncol 2004 [abstract 4603].

63. Petrylak D, Shelton G, England-Owen C, et al. Response and Preliminary Survival Results of a Phase II Study of Docetaxel and Estramustine in Patients with Androgen-Independent Prostate Cancer. Proc Am Soc Clin Oncol 2000 [abstract 1312].

64. Berry W, Dakhil S, Modiano M, et al. Phase III Study of Mitoxantrone plus Low Dose Prednisone versus Low Dose Prednisone Alone in Patients with Asymptomatic Hormone Refractory Prostate Cancer. J Urol 2002;168:2539–2443.

65. Khan MA, Carducci MA, Partin AW. The Evolving Role of Docetaxel in the Management of Androgen Independent Prostate Cancer. J Urol 2003;170:1709–1716.

66. Ringel I, Horwitz SB. Studies with RP 56976 (Taxotere): A Semisynthetic Analogue of Taxol. J Natl Cancer Inst 1991;83:288–291.

67. Stein CA. Mechanisms of Action of Taxanes in Prostate Cancer. Semin Oncol 1999;26:3–7.

68. Haldar S, Chintapalli J, Croce CM. Taxol Induces Bcl-2 Phosphorylation and Death of Prostate Cancer Cells. Cancer Res 1996;56:1253–1255.

69. Lara PN Jr, Kung HJ, Gumerlock PH, et al. Molecular biology of prostate carcinogenesis. Crit Rev Oncol Hematol 1999;32:197–208

70. Berry W, Rohrbaugh T. Phase II Trial of Single Agent, Weekly Taxotere in Symptomatic, Hormone-Refractory Prostate Cancer. Proc Am Soc Clin Oncol 1999 [abstract 1290].

71. Beer T, Pierce W, Lowe B, et al. Phase II Study of Weekly Docetaxel (Taxotere) in Hormone Refractory Metastatic Prostate Cancer. Proc Am Soc Clin Oncol 2000 [abstract 1368].

72. Picus J, Schultz M. Docetaxel (Taxotere) as Monotherapy in the Treatment of Hormone-Refractory Prostate Cancer: Preliminary Results. Semin Oncol 1999;26:14–18.

73. Friedland D, Cohen J, Miller R, et al. A Phase II Trial of Docetaxel (Taxotere) in Hormone Refractory Prostate Cancer: Correlation of Antitumor Effect to Phosphorylation of Bcl-2. Semin Oncol 1999;26:19–23.

74. Roth BJ, Yeap BY, Wilding G, et al. Taxol in Advanced Hormone-Refractory Carcinoma of the Prostate: A Phase II Trial of the Eastern Cooperative Oncology Group. Cancer 1993;72:2457–2460.

75. Trivedi C, Redman B, Flaherty LE, et al. Weekly 1-hour Infusion of Paclitaxel: Clinical Feasibility and Efficacy in Patients with Hormone Refractory Prostate Carcinoma. Cancer 2000;89:431–436.

76. Berry W, Gregurich M, Dakhil S, et al. Phase II Randomized Trial of Weekly Paclitaxel with or without Estramustine Phosphate in Patients with Symptomatic Hormone Refractory, Metastatic Carcinoma of the Prostate. Proc Am Soc Clin Oncol 2001 [abstract 696].

77. Sinibaldi VJ, Carducci MA, Moore-Cooper S, et al. Phase II Evaluation of Docetaxel plus One-Day Oral Estramustine Phosphate in the Treatment of Patients with Androgen Independent Prostate Carcinoma. Cancer 2002;94:1457–1465.

78. Birch R, Kalman L, Holt L, et al. Randomized Phase IIb Trial Comparing Two Schedules of Docetaxel (D) plus Estramustine (E) for Metastatic Hormone Refractory Prostate Cancer. Proc Am Soc Clin Oncol 2004 [abstract 4622].

79. Kreis W, Budman DR, Calabro A. Unique Synergism or Antagonism of Combinations of Chemotherapeutic and Hormonal Agents in Human Prostate Cancer. Br J Urol 1997;79:196–202.

80. Smith DC, Chay CH, Dunn RL. Phase II Trial of Paclitaxel, Estramustine, Etoposide, and Carboplatin in the Treatment of Patients with Hormone-Refractory Prostate Carcinoma. Cancer 2003;98:269–276.

81. Ellerhorst JA, Tu SM, Amato RJ, et al. Phase II Trial of Alternating Weekly Chemohormonal Therapy for Patients with Androgen-Independent Prostate Cancer. Clin Cancer Res 1997;3:2371–2376.

82. Millikan R, Thall PF, Lee SJ, et al. Randomized Multicenter Phase II Trial of Two Multicomponent Regimens in Androgen-Independent Prostate Cancer. J Clin Oncol 2003;21:878–883.

83. Hudes GR, Nathan F, Khater C, et al. Phase II Trial of 96-Hour Paclitaxel plus Oral Estramustine Phosphate in Metastatic Hormone-Refractory Prostate Cancer. J Clin Oncol 1997;15:3156–163.

84. Vaishampayan U, Fontana J, Du W, et al. An Active Regimen of Weekly Paclitaxel and Estramustine in Metastatic Androgen-Independent Prostate Cancer. Urology 2002;60:1050–1054.

85. Athanasiadis A, Tsavdaridis D, Rigatos SK, et al. Hormone Refractory Prostate Cancer Treated with Estramustine and Paclitaxel Combination. Anticancer Res 2003;23:3085–3088.

86. Ferrari AC, Chachoua A, Singh H, et al. A Phase I/II Study of Weekly Paclitaxel and 3 Days of High Dose Oral Estramustine Phosphate in Metastatic Androgen-Independent Prostate Cancer. Cancer 2001;91:2039–2045.

87. Smith MR, Kaufman D, Oh W, et al. Vinorelbine and Estramustine in Androgen-Independent Metastatic Prostate Cancer: a Phase II Study. Cancer 2000;89:1824–1828.

88. Sweeney CJ, Monaco FJ, Jung SH, et al. A Phase II Hoosier Oncology Group Study of Vinorelbine and Estramustine Phosphate in Hormone-Refractory Prostate Cancer. Ann Oncol 2002;13:435–440.

89. Carles J, Domenech M, Gelabert-Mas A, et al. Phase II Study of Estramustine and Vinorelbine in Hormone-Refractory Prostate Carcinoma Patients. Acta Oncol 1998;37:187–191.

90. Hudes G, Einhorn L, Ross E, et al. Vinblastine versus Vinblastine plus Oral Estramsutine Phosphate for Patients with Hormone-Refractory Prostate Cancer: A Hoosier Oncology Group and Fox Chase Phase III Trial. J Clin Oncol 1999;17:3160–3166.

91. Pienta KJ, Redman B, Hussain M, et al. Phase II Study of Oral Estramustine and oral Etoposide in Hormone-Refractory Adenocarcinoma of the Prostate. J Clin Oncol 1994;12:2005–2012.

92. Pienta KJ, Redman B, Bandekar R, et al. A Phase II Study of Oral Estramustine and Oral Etoposide in Hormone-Refractory Prostate Cancer. Urology 1997;50:401–406.

93. Pienta KJ, Fisher EI, Eisenberger MA, et al. A Phase II Trial of Estramustine and Etoposide in Hormone Refractory Prostate Cancer: A Southwest Oncology Group Trial (SWOG 9407). Prostate 2001;46:257–261.

94. Dimopoulos MA, Panopoulos C, Bamia C, et al. Oral Estramustine and Oral Etoposide for Hormone-Refractory Prostate Cancer. Urology 1997;50:754–758.

95. Koletsky AJ, Guerra ML, Kronish L. Phase II Study of Vinorelbine and Low Dose Docetaxel in Chemotherapy-Naïve Patients with Hormone-Refractory Prostate Cancer. Cancer J 2003;9:286–292.

96. Glode LM, Barqawi A, Crighton F. Metronomic Therapy with Cyclophosphamide and Dexamethasone for Prostate Carcinoma. Cancer 2003;98:1643–1648.

97. DiPaola RS, Durvage HJ, Kamen BA. High Time for Low-Dose Prospective Clinical Trials. Cancer 2003;98:1559–1561.

98. Manni A, Bartholomew M, Caplan R, et al. Androgen Priming and Chemotherapy in Advanced Prostate Cancer: Evaluation of Determinants of Clinical Outcome. J Clin Oncol 1988;6:1456–1466.

99. Morris MJ, Kelly WK, Slovin S, et al. Phase I Trial of Exogenous Testosterone for the Treatment of Castrate Metastatic Prostate Cancer. Proc Am Soc Clin Oncol 2004 [abstract 4560].

100. Chao D, Harland SJ. The Importance of Continued Endocrine Treatment during Chemotherapy of Hormone-Refractory Prostate Cancer. Eur Urol 1997;31:7–10.

101. Taylor CD, Elson P, Trump DL. Importance of Continued Testicular Suppression in Hormone-Refractory Prostate Cancer. J Clin Oncol 1993;11:2167–2172.

102. Tannock I, Gospodarowicz M, Meakin W, et al. Treatment of Metastatic Prostate Cancer with Low Dose Prednisone: Evaluation of Pain and Quality of Life as Pragmatic Indices of Response. J Clin Oncol 1989;7:590–597.

103. Fossa SD, Slee PH, Brausi M, et al. Flutamide versus Prednisone in Patients with Prostate Cancer Symptomatically Progressing After Androgen-Ablative Therapy: a Phase III Study of the European Organization for Research and Treatment of Cancer Genitourinary Group. J Clin Oncol 2001;19:62–71.

104. Nishimura K, Nonomura N, Satoh E, et al. Potential Mechanism for the Effects of Dexamethasone on Growth of Androgen-Independent Prostate Cancer. J Natl Cancer Inst 2001;93:1739–1746.

105. Matias PM, Carrondo MA, Coelho R, et al. Structural Basis for the Glucocorticoid Response in a Mutant Human Androgen Receptor Derived from an Androgen-Independent Prostate Cancer. J Med Chem 2002;45:1439–1446.

106. Dahut WL, Gulley JL, Arlen PM, et al. Randomized Phase II Trial of Docetaxel Plus Thalidomide in Androgen-Independent Prostate Cancer. J Clin Oncol 2004;22:2532–2539.

107. Bauer KS, Dixon SC, Figg WD. Inhibition of Angiogenesis by Thalidomide Requires Metabolic Activation, which is Species-Dependent. Biochem Pharmacol 1998;55:1827–1834.

108. Bartlett JB, Dredge K, Dalgleish AG. The Evolution of Thalidomide and its IMiD Derivatives as Anticancer Agents. Nat Rev Cancer 2004;4:314–322.

109. Liu Y, Tohnya TM, Figg WD, et al. Phase I Study of CC-5013 (Revlimid), a Thalidomide Derivative in Patients with Refractory Metastatic Cancer. Proc Am Soc Clin Oncol 2003;22 [abstract 927].

110. Sison B, Bond T, Amato RJ, et al. Phase II Study of CC-4047 in Patients with Metastatic Hormone-Refractory Prostate Cancer. Proc Am Soc Clin Oncol 2004 [abstract 4701].

111. Beer TM, Eilers KM, Garzotto M, et al. Weekly High Dose Calcitriol and Doceteaxel in Metastatic Androgen-Independent Prostate Cancer. J Clin Oncol 2003;21:123–128.

112. Chatta GS, Fakih M, Ramalingam S, et al. Phase I Pharmacokinetic Study of Daily Imatinib in Combination with Docetaxel for Patients with Advanced Solid Tumors. Proc Am Soc Clin Oncol 2004 [abstract 2047].

113. Papandreou CN, Daliani DD, Nix D, et al. Phase I Trial of the Proteasome Inhibitor Bortezomib in Patients with Advanced Solid Tumors with Observations in Androgen-Independent Prostate Cancer. J Clin Oncol 2004;22:2108–2121.

114. Picus J, Halabi S, Rini B, et al. The Use of Bevacizumab with Docetaxel and Estramustine in Hormone Refractory Prostate Cancer:Initial Results of CALGB 90006. Proc Am Soc Clin Oncol 2003;22:393 [abstract 1578]

115. Schroder FH, Wldhagen MF. ZD1839 (Gefitinib) and Hormone Resistant Prostate Cancer-Final Results of a Double Blind Randomized Placebo-Controlled Phase II Study. J Clin Oncol 2004;22 [abstract 4698].

116. Tolcher AW, Chi K, Juhn K, et al. A phase II, pharmacokinetic, and biological correlative study of oblimersen sodium and docetaxel in patients with hormone-refractory prostate cancer. Clin Cancer Res 2005;11:3854–3861.

117. Carducci M, Nelson JB, Saad F. Effects of atrasentan on disease progression and biological markers in men with metastatic hormone-refractory prostate cancer: Phase 3 study. Proc Am Soc Clin Oncol 2004 [abstract 4508].

118. Sternberg CN, Hetherington J, Paluchowska PHTJ, et al. Randomized Phase III Trial of a New Oral Platinum, Satraplatin (JM-216) plus Prednisone or Prednisone Alone in Patients with Hormone Refractory Prostate Cancer. Proc Am Soc Clin Oncol 2003;22:395 [abstract 1586].

119. Goodin S, Kane MP, Rubin EH. Epothilones: Mechanism of Action and Biologic Activity. J Clin Oncol 2004;22:2105–2125.

120. Rosenberg JE, Galsky MD, Weinberg V, et al. Response to second-line taxane based therapy after first-line epothdone B analogue BMS 247550(BMS) therapy in hormone refractory prostate cancer (HRPC). Proc Am Soc Clin Oncol 2004 [abstract 4564].

121. Porter AT, McEwan AJ, Powe JE, et al. Results of a Randomized Phase III Trial to Evaluate the Efficacy of Strontium-89 Adjuvant to Local Field External Beam Irradiation in the Management of Endocrine Resistant Metastatic Prostate Cancer. Int J Radiat Oncol Biol Phys 1993;25:805–813.

122. Glode LM. Phase III Randomized Study of Adjuvant Androgen Deprivation Therapy with or without Mitoxantrone and Prednisone after Prostatecomy in Patients with High Risk Adenocarcinoma of the Prostate. Retrieved Aug 17, 2004 from NCI Clinical Trials website:http://cancer.gov/search/viewclinicaltrials.aspx?version=healthprofessional&cdrid=67352.

123. Bander N, Milowsky MI, Nanus DM, et al. Phase I trail . 177 Lutetium-labeled J591, a monoclonal antibody to prostate-specific membrane antigen, in patients with androgen-independent prostate cancer. J Clin Oncol 2005;23:4591–4601.

124. Pienta KJ. Radiation Therapy Oncology Group P-0014:A Phase 3 Randomized Study of Patients with High Risk Hormone-Naïve Prostate Cancer: Androgen Blockade with 4 Cycles of Immediate Chemotherapy versus Androgen Blockade with Delayed Chemotherapy. Urology 2003;62:95–101.

125. D'Amico AV, Halabi S, Vogelzang NJ, et al. A Reduction in the Rate of PSA Rise Following Chemotherapy in Patients with Metastatic Hormone Refractory Prostate Cancer Predicts Survival:Results of a Pooled Analysis or CALGB HRPC Trials. Proc Am Soc Clin Oncol 2004 [abstract 4506].

126. Crawford ED, Pauler DK, Tangen CM, et al. Three-month Change in PSA as a Surrogate Endpoint for Mortality in Advanced Hormone-Refractory Prostate Cancer: Data from SWOG 9916. Proc Am Soc Clin Oncol 2004 [abstract 4505].

Danny Y Song, Salma K Jabbour, Theodore L DeWeese

RADIOTHERAPY IN THE MANAGEMENT OF LOCALLY ADVANCED PROSTATE CANCER

INTRODUCTION

The value of radiotherapy in the treatment of prostate cancer has been recognized for nearly a century. The use of transurethral radium was first described in 1911 by Pasteau and Degrais.[1] In 1930, Smith and Pierson described the utility of high voltage X-ray therapy in the treatment of prostate cancer, and, in 1930, Widmann subsequently noted an improvement in survival for patients with advanced prostate cancer treated with kilovoltage X-rays.[2,3] Prior to the advent of prostate-specific antigen (PSA), the majority of patients were diagnosed based on clinically evident disease, which was often more advanced than the presentations commonly seen today. The activity of radiation in prostate cancer was evident by its effect on large palpable tumors that resolved following treatment. Widespread screening for prostate cancer has led to an increasing frequency of the disease being detected in its early stages, but there remains a significant proportion of patients who are diagnosed with locally advanced or even metastatic disease.

The historical definition of locally advanced prostate cancer refers to patients with advanced clinical stage based on direct extension of disease beyond the prostatic capsule either felt on digital rectal examination or seen on imaging—i.e., stage T3 or T4. Such patients are at high risk for disease recurrence following surgical or nonsurgical treatment. In addition to tumor stage, a number of studies have correlated histologic tumor grade and pretreatment PSA with not only extracapsular extension of disease found at radical prostatectomy, but also risk of disease recurrence following any therapy.[4–7] Therefore, a more contemporary and commonly used method of defining locally advanced disease also includes patients who have biologically more aggressive and, therefore, higher risk disease as predicted by prognostic factors such as PSA level and tumor grade. High-risk patients are generally considered to be those who have advanced clinical stage disease, high presenting PSA, and/or poorly differentiated histology (Gleason 8–10).[8] In addition, patients with involvement of regional pelvic lymph nodes are also frequently included in the category of locally advanced disease. As a result, patients seen in modern clinical practice who are classified as having locally advanced disease differ significantly from those termed to have locally advanced disease in prior eras, and this should be kept in mind when reviewing older data. Although the optimal treatment of this group of patients remains undefined, radiation is a commonly utilized primary modality. Historical results with either radical prostatectomy or radiation therapy alone are suboptimal, with biochemical control rates of less than 40% at 5 years.[9–12] We describe the innovations in radiation oncology that have been developed in an attempt to improve on these results via the use of dose escalation (using either external-beam radiation therapy [EBRT] or brachytherapy as a boost), whole pelvic radiation therapy (WPRT), and androgen suppression (AS).

DOSE-ESCALATED RADIOTHERAPY

RATIONALE

Although many patients with locally advanced prostate cancer develop metastatic disease as the first sign of failure, local control with standard radiotherapy is poor and intraprostatic tumor may serve as a reservoir for metastatic dissemination.[11,13] Coen et al analyzed 1469 patients treated with radiation therapy who had more than 2 years of follow-up data. Gleason score of 7 or more, PSA greater than 15 ng/mL, and T3/T4 stage predicted a higher incidence of distant failure. On multivariate analysis, local failure was the strongest predictor for distant metastasis, with 77% versus 61% distant metastasis-free survival at 10 years for patients with locally controlled versus uncontrolled disease.[14] Several retrospective studies of long-term data in patients treated with conventional techniques in the 1970s and 1980s describe a direct relationship between radiation dose and local control in men with locally advanced prostate cancer. Valicenti et al reviewed the data from Radiation Therapy Oncology Group (RTOG) phase III trials of EBRT, and on multivariate analysis found that a dose of more than 66 Gy significantly reduced the relative risk of prostate cancer-related death in men with Gleason scores of 8 to 10.[15] Data from the American College of Radiology Patterns of Care study on 624 patients with stage T3 disease revealed the actuarial 7-year local recurrence rate was 36% with doses of 60 to 64.9 Gy, 32% for 65 to 69.9 Gy, and 24% for 70 Gy and over.[16] Multivariate analysis of the MD Anderson experience in 1127 patients with stage T1 to T4 disease treated with radiotherapy from 1987 to 1997 found radiation dose to be an independent predictor of biochemical control in addition to pretreatment PSA, Gleason score, and palpable stage. The patients who benefited most from higher doses were those with pretreatment PSA greater than 10 ng/mL.[17]

The radiotherapy technique utilized in the majority of patients in these studies relied on estimations of prostate boundaries based on surrogate landmarks such as the pubic bones and rectal and bladder contrast media. The ability to escalate radiation dose to greater than 70 Gy with such conventional radiotherapy techniques was limited by rectal and bladder complications. In the Patterns of Care study, the rate of grade 3 or 4 complications increased from 3.5% to 6.9% when doses exceeding 70 Gy were delivered.[18] Smit et al reported up to 30% incidence of late proctitis after conventional prostate radiation therapy to 70 Gy, with the incidence of proctitis correlating with the maximum rectal dose.[19] Schultheiss et al attempted to identify factors predictive of late genitourinary (GU) and gastrointestinal (GI) morbidity in patients treated with doses above 65 Gy. Central axis dose was the only independent variable significantly related to the incidence of late GI morbidity.[20]

The past two decades have witnessed the development of innovative radiotherapy techniques including three-dimensional conformal radiation therapy (3DCRT), which utilizes computed tomography (CT)-based targeting as well as more sophisticated beam delivery and treatment plan assessment techniques. In conjunction with the development of 3DCRT, improvements in the accuracy of patient positioning and the quantitation of prostate motion have created the ability to more accurately as well as conformally target the shape and location of the prostate while minimizing treatment of surrounding tissues.[21] These benefits have resulted in the ability to decrease toxicity of treatment at iso-effective dose levels. A randomized trial of 64 Gy conventional radiotherapy versus similar doses delivered with 3DCRT demonstrated grade 1 or higher proctitis occurring in 37% of the 3DCRT group versus 56% of the conventional group ($P = 0.004$). Grade 2 proctitis was also significantly lower at 5% in the 3DCRT group versus 15% in the conventional group. There were no significant differences in bladder function after treatment between the groups.[22] A similar study by Koper et al utilizing doses of 66 Gy found a significant reduction in grade 2 GI toxicity with the use of 3DCRT compared to conventional techniques (19 versus 32%; $P = 0.02$). Again, there was similar grade 2 or higher GU toxicity between the arms, despite a significant reduction in bladder volumes treated in patients receiving 3DCRT.[23]

TRIALS

The combination of the enhanced therapeutic ratio of 3DCRT and evidence of a dose response effect in prostate cancer have led to clinical trials of dose escalated radiotherapy in an attempt to improve on the results seen with conventional treatment.

Long-term, 12-year follow-up of the initial Fox Chase dose escalation study cohort of 232 patients has been reported by Hanks. Doses ranged from 67 to 81 Gy, with median total dose (at the center of the prostate) being 74 Gy. The American Society for Therapeutic Radiology and Oncology (ASTRO) consensus definition of three consecutive rises in PSA was used to determine biologic no evidence of disease (bNED) status.[24] For purposes of analysis, patients were divided into six prognostic subgroups by pretreatment PSA, clinical stage, Gleason score, and presence of perineural invasion. Patients with pretreatment PSA levels of 10 to 20 ng/mL had statistically significant differences in bNED control when stratified by dose on univariate analysis. On multivariate analysis, radiation dose was a statistically significant predictor of bNED control for all patients and for unfavorable patients with a pretreatment PSA less than 10 ng/mL. No radiation dose response was seen for patients with pretreatment PSA greater than 20 ng/mL, but only 44 patients were in this group. No difference was noted in the frequency of Grade 2 and 3 GU and Grade 3 GI morbidity when patients were stratified by radiation dose, although a significant increase in Grade 2 GI complications occurred as the dose increased.[25]

Pollack recently updated the Fox Chase experience, reporting on 839 patients treated to doses from 63 to 84 Gy (median 74 Gy) with a median follow-up of 63 months. Multivariate analysis found radiotherapy dose and pretreatment PSA to be the most significant factors prognostic for bNED survival, followed by Gleason score and T stage. Perineural invasion was no longer a significant predictor of PSA outcome. Within six prognostic groups, higher radiotherapy dose was significantly associated with outcome in all but the most favorable (PSA < 10 ng/mL and Gleason 2–6) and least favorable (PSA > 20 ng/mL and T3/T4) groups. However, there were only 22 patients available for analysis within the latter group. For patients with PSA over 20 ng/mL and T1/T2 clinical stage, dose was significant for bNED survival when analyzed by the Wilcoxon test.[26]

Preliminary results of a multi-institutional, prospective dose escalation study performed by a collaboration of French centers has been reported by Bey et al. Eligible patients had T1b-T3 disease: Gleason score and PSA were not criteria for study entry. Thirty-one percent of patients had stage T3 disease, and 9% had pretreatment PSA greater than 20 ng/ml. The inital cohort received 66 Gy prescribed to the center of the prostate, with subsequent cohorts receiving escalating doses to a maximum of 80 Gy. With mean follow-up time of 32 months, no statistical differences were observed in Grade 2 or higher GI or GU late toxicity between the 66–70 Gy vs. 74–80 Gy groups. The probabilty of achieving a post-treatment PSA nadir of 1 ng/ml or more was significantly greater in the 74–80 Gy group, and directly related to the dose of radiation given.

Investigators at Memorial Sloan-Kettering have also performed a dose-escalation trial using 3DCRT in patients with clinical stage T1–T3 disease. Doses were 64.8 to 75.6 Gy prescribed at the prostate periphery, with isocenter doses approximately 5% to 7% higher than the stated dose. Patients were stratified into three risk groups based on PSA level, Gleason score, and clinical stage. At 10 years, bNED survival (ASTRO definition) was significantly better with higher doses in all three risk groups. For intermediate risk patients, 10-year bNED survival was 50% in patients receiving 75.6 Gy, versus 42% in patients receiving 70.2 Gy (P = 0.05); for unfavorable risk patients, the corresponding rates were 42% versus 24% (P = 0.04). Grade 2 and grade 3 or higher rectal toxicity was 17% and 1.5%, respectively, while grade 2 and grade 3 or higher urinary toxicity were 15% and 2.5%.[28]

COOPERATIVE GROUP TRIAL

Preliminary toxicity results of a prospective phase I/II 3DCRT dose-escalation study performed by the RTOG have been reported. RTOG 94-06 enrolled patients with T1–T3 tumors to sequentially escalated dose levels beginning at 68.4 Gy at 1.8 Gy per fraction, to 78 Gy at 2 Gy per fraction daily. Patients were grouped into three categories based on risk of seminal vesicle invasion greater than or less than 15% and presence of T3 disease. Patients with more than 15% risk of seminal vesicle involvement were treated to both prostate and seminal vesicles to 55.8 Gy, followed by a reduction in target volume to the prostate alone. Patients with T3 disease received the full dose to both prostate and seminal vesicles. Doses were prescribed as a minimum dose to a target volume. Michalski et al evaluated late effects in 424 patients treated on the first two dose levels of 68.4 Gy (level I) and 73.8 Gy (level II). Average months at risk after completion of therapy ranged from 21.4 to 40.1 months for patients on dose level I, and 10.0 to 34.2 months for patients on dose level II. The incidence of RTOG grade 2 or higher GU toxicity was 10% to 13%, and RTOG grade 2 or higher GI toxicity was 7% to 8%, with most toxicity occurring within the first 2 years after therapy. When compared with historical RTOG data derived from prior studies using pre-3DCRT techniques, the incidence of grade 3 or higher toxicity was reduced for all groups (despite the administration of higher doses), but this was associated with an increase in the rate of grade 1 complications. This resulted in an overall statistically significant increase in the number of patients with any late effects when compared with expected complications derived from the historical data. These data implied a reduction of higher grade toxicity occurred with the toxicity being shifted to lower grades, as well as an overall increase in low-grade toxicity presumably due to dose escalation.[29] Results in 173 patients with stage T1 and T2 disease treated on dose level III (79.2 Gy) have also been reported (T3 patients were excluded due to poor accrual). No patients experienced grade 3 or higher acute toxicity. The incidences of late grade 1 and 2 GU toxicity were 31% and 11%, respectively, while the rates of grade 1 and 2 GI toxicity were 24% and 7%. The overall rate of toxicity was comparable to previous dose levels. With a median follow-up of 3.3 years, 4 patients (2.4%) experienced grade 3 late toxicity, with 3 GU events and one related to the rectum. There were no grade 4 or 5 late complications. Again, comparison with historical controls revealed that the observed rate of grade 3 or higher late effects was significantly lower than expected.[30]

RANDOMIZED TRIALS

In order to validate the hypothesis that dose escalation results in improved outcomes in prostate cancer, Shipley et al at the Massachusetts General Hospital carried out a phase III randomized study of dose escalation using proton beam irradiation as method of delivering higher doses to the prostate. Unlike the more commonly utilized photon beams, proton beams penetrate surrounding tissues depositing only a small amount of energy until they reach a specified distance, at which point the dose is delivered. This gives the ability to minimize doses to the tissues around the target. Currently, proton beam for routine clinical use is available at only two centers within the United States, although construction is underway at additional facilities. The study enrolled only patients with locally advanced (stages T3/T4) disease, randomizing them to either 67.2 Gy with conventional radiotherapy, or 75.6 Gy equivalent with the last 25.2 Gy delivered by proton beam. The trial was performed from 1982 to 1992, and, therefore, used older definitions of treatment effectiveness, namely disease-specific survival was defined as PSA less than 4 ng/mL, negative digital rectal exam, and negative rebiopsy (if performed). With a median follow-up of 61 months, there were no significantly differences in disease-specific survival, overall survival, or local control between the two arms. The only statistically significant benefit seen was in the planned subgroup analysis of patients with poorly differentiated tumors (Gleason 4 or 5 of 5), where the rates of local control were 19% versus 84% at 8 years ($P = 0.0014$). For the entire group, the incidence of grades 1 and 2 rectal bleeding was greater in the high dose arm (32 versus 12%; $P = 0.002$).[31] It must be noted that, due to stage migration from the widespread adoption of PSA screening, the patients treated in the era when this study was performed are significantly different from the majority of patients seen today, even within the same category of T3/T4 disease, and, therefore, the applicability of this study to current practice is uncertain.

A more contemporary dose-escalation study utilizing proton beam irradiation was recently reported by researchers at Massachusetts General Hospital and Loma Linda University. This study randomized 393 patients with stages T1b–T2b prostate cancer and PSA less than 15 ng/mL to either 19.8 GyE (photon Gy equivalents) or 28.8 GyE, followed by a 3DCRT dose of 50.4 Gy (total doses 70.2 GyE versus 79.2 GyE, respectively). Only 2% of patients receiving 70.2 GyE and 1.5% receiving 79.2 GyE had acute RTOG morbidity greater than grade 2. At a median follow-up of 4 years, the 5-year biochemical failure rate was significantly lower in the patients receiving higher dose radiation (19.1% versus 37.3%; $P = 0.00001$); this difference also held true when patients with intermediate risk disease were analyzed. The majority of the patients treated on this study had low- to intermediate-risk disease (only 8.4% had Gleason grade ≥ 8), but this study deserves mention because it strongly supports the concept of dose escalation in prostate cancer.[32]

Pollack et al have also performed a phase III randomized trial at the MD Anderson Cancer Center comparing 70 Gy versus 78 Gy radiotherapy using 3DCRT. A total of 305 patients with stage T1 to T3

tumors were treated using 2 Gy daily fractions prescribed to the isocenter; androgen ablation was not given as part of initial therapy. Treatment failure was defined by the ASTRO consensus definition or the initiation of salvage treatment. For the entire cohort, the freedom-from-failure (FFF) rates at 5 years were 64% and 70% for the 70 Gy and 78 Gy arms, respectively ($P = 0.03$). The patients who benefited most from the dose escalation were the subgroup with PSA greater than 10 ng/mL, where the FFF rates were 43% and 62% ($P = 0.01$). Within this subgroup there was also a significant difference in the rates of metastasis-free survival (98% versus 88%; $P = 0.056$), although no differences in overall survival were seen during the follow-up period to date. Among patients with stage T3 disease, there were also statistically significant differences in FFF (36% versus 61%; $P = 0.047$). The data did not indicate a difference in FFF for the patients with Gleason scores of 7 through 10, where FFF rates were 64% and 68%, respectively ($P = 0.39$). Although bladder toxicity was not increased in the high-dose group, there was an increase in the rate of grade 2 or higher late rectal toxicity with a significant, direct correlation between the extent of treated rectal volume and grade 2 or higher rectal toxicity. Among patients with detailed dose–volume histogram information available, 8 of 9 patients with grade 3 or higher rectal toxicity had more than 25% of rectum receiving at least 70 Gy, and the majority of grade 2 or higher rectal toxicity was also in patients with more than 25% of rectum receiving at least 70 Gy.[33,34]

NONRANDOMIZED DATA FOR HIGH-GRADE TUMORS

A retrospective analysis of a larger number of patients with high grade (Gleason 8–10) tumors is available from Roach et al at the University of California-San Francisco. Fifty patients with T1 to T4 clinical stage and median PSA of 22.7 ng/mL were treated with a variety of doses of external-beam radiation. Biochemical failure was defined as increase in PSA of 0.5 ng/mL per year, PSA level more than 1.0 ng/mL, or positive post-treatment biopsy. The overall actuarial probability of freedom from biochemical failure at 4 years was 23%. Multivariate analysis of all patients revealed pretreatment PSA to be the only predictor of PSA failure. In a multivariate analysis restricted to patients with PSA less than 20 ng/mL, 83% of those treated to more than 71 Gy were free of progression compared with none of those treated to lower doses ($P = 0.03$).[35] Fiveash et al reported on the combined results of a group of 180 patients treated at the University of Michigan, University of California-San Francisco, and Fox Chase Cancer Center. Patients had T1 to T4 N0 to Nx adenocarcinoma with a pretreatment PSA; 27% received adjuvant or neoadjuvant hormonal therapy. The total dose received was less than 70 Gy in 30%, 70 to 75 Gy in 37%, and more than 75 Gy in 33%. At a median follow-up of 3.0 years, the 5-year freedom from PSA failure was 62.5% for all patients and 79.3% in T1/T2 patients. Univariate analysis revealed T-stage, pretreatment PSA, and radiotherapy (RT) dose predictive of freedom from PSA failure. Univariate analysis of likelihood of 5-year overall survival revealed RT dose to be the only significant predictive factor. When Cox proportional hazards model was performed separate for T1/2 and T3/4 tumors, none of the prognostic factors achieved statistical significance for overall survival or freedom from biochemical progression in the T3/4 group, but lower RT dose and higher pretreatment PSA did predict for PSA failure within the T1/2 patients.[36]

In summary, the available randomized evidence suggests that dose escalation with 3DCRT results in significant improvements in PSA-defined disease control in patients with "intermediate-risk" prostate cancer. The impact on disease control in patients with higher risk features such as stage T3/T4, Gleason 8 to 10, and PSA greater than 20 ng/mL in these studies is unclear, although most suffer from low accrual within this subgroup. However, retrospective data suggest that patients with high-grade, low-stage tumors benefit from dose escalation. It remains to be seen whether these improvements will result in differences in overall survival. Only with very long-term follow-up will these differences become evident. While the use of 3DCRT results in improvements in toxicity profile compared to conventional radiotherapy, escalated doses with these techniques do seem to result in increased rectal toxicity, although mostly limited to grade 2 or less. Further study will allow for development of better estimates of late toxicity associated with higher doses, as well as agreement on what constitutes an acceptable level of toxicity.

The "next" technologic advancement beyond 3DCRT is intensity-modulated radiotherapy (IMRT). Compared with 3DCRT, IMRT gives the ability to create steeper dose gradients around the target, thereby reducing the volume of surrounding tissues receiving high doses of radiation. It also allows for even greater conformality of the treatment volume to the target. Since IMRT is a more recently developed technique than 3DCRT, there is less available data regarding clinical experience with dose escalation. However, it offers the possibility of reduced toxicity and thus dose escalation to even higher levels without concomitant increase in risk.[37] Investigators at Memorial Sloan-Kettering have reported 6-year results in a cohort of 171 patients with T1c to T3 prostate cancer treated with 81 Gy using IMRT. Doses were prescribed to the isodose line encompassing the target volume. Fifty-four percent of patients received neoadjuvant androgen deprivation therapy prior to radiation. The 6-year PSA relapse-free survival rates for favorable, intermediate, and unfavorable risk disease were 91%, 73%, and 64%

using the ASTRO consensus definition. Notably, the 6-year likelihood of grade 2 rectal bleeding was 4%, and 1.1% of patients developed grade 3 rectal toxicity. The 6-year risk of grade 2 GU toxicity was 10%. There were no grade 4 toxicities. These results appear favorable when compared with the toxicity profiles described previously for 3DCRT treatment.[38]

DOSE ESCALATION VIA HIGH-DOSE RATE BRACHYTHERAPY

The use of brachytherapy is another means by which it is possible to increase local dose to the prostate. Conformal high dose rate brachytherapy (HDR) is an alternative means of dose escalation, which offers a potential advantage over EBRT in that a steep dose gradient between the prostate and adjacent normal tissues can be generated. Other theoretical advantages are the elimination of inter- and intrafraction motion of the prostate gland, random and systemic treatment setup errors, gland edema, and imprecise target localization.[39,40] Briefly, the technique utilizes catheters placed into the prostate under intraoperative transrectal ultrasound guidance. The catheters are subsequently attached to an afterloading unit that sequentially feeds a high-activity (iridum-192) source into predetermined positions within the catheters. The dwell times within each position can be adjusted, thus allowing for development of a treatment plan which optimally conforms to the target volume. Typically, the patient receives HDR in one to three fractions (separated by 4–6 hours) after each intraoperative catheter placement session, with the catheters remaining in place between fractions. Between one and three sessions may take place during a treatment course, either following or interdigitated with conformal EBRT.

There may be radiobiologic advantages to the use of large doses per HDR fraction. Traditionally, tumors have been considered to be less sensitive to large doses per fraction than normal tissues, and, therefore, delivering an increased number of fractions to the same total dose was associated with decreased normal tissue late effects. More recent analyses of clinical and laboratory data suggest that prostate cancer is more sensitive to large doses per fraction relative to normal tissues.[41,42] If true, this would also mean that iso-effective doses of hypofractionated HDR could be delivered with less acute toxicity than possible with smaller fractions.

One of the largest published experiences to date comes from Deger et al, who analyzed 230 patients with T2 (35%) and T3 (58%) tumors. The median PSA was 12.8 ng/mL; 60% and 16% of patients had Grade 2 and Grade 3 histologic grade, respectively. The mean time to PSA nadir was 15 months, and 47% of patients reached a nadir less than 0.5 ng/mL. The 5-year biochemical progression-free survival rate was 75% for T2 and 60% for T3 tumors. Following modifications to technique and a decrease in the HDR fractional dose to 9 Gy, complications were reported to decrease from 16.4% to a rate of 6.9%.[43]

Investigators at William Beaumont Hospital have described their experience in a dose escalation trial of HDR with EBRT in 207 patients with poor prognostic factors of PSA 10 ng/mL or higher, Gleason 7 or above, or clinical stage T2b or higher. No patient received hormonal therapy, and the ASTRO consensus definition was used for determining biochemical failure. Treatment consisted of EBRT 46 Gy to the prostate, with a total of two HDR treatments given during the first and third weeks of treatment. The majority of patients (57%) had T2b/T2c disease; 19.8% had Gleason 8 to 10 tumors, and most patients had pretreatment PSA between 4 and 10 ng/mL. At a mean follow-up of 4.7 years, the 5-year actuarial biochemical control rate was 74%. The 5-year biochemical control rate was 85% for one poor prognostic factor, 75% for two and 50% for all three. On Cox regression analysis, lower HDR dose and higher Gleason score were associated with biochemical failure.[44] Table 101.1 summarizes several institutional reports on HDR.

Due to the heterogeneity of patient groups treated in many of the reported experiences, it is difficult to draw conclusions about the efficacy of HDR relative to other treatments. However, the biochemical control rates appear favorable compared to historic results.[9–12] Given the comparably short median follow-up times, longer observation will be needed to better determine the incidence of late complications.

DOSE ESCALATION VIA PERMANENT INTERSTITIAL SEED IMPLANTATION

A similar means of performing dose escalation is by performing permanent interstitial seed implantation (low dose rate brachytherapy) in addition to EBRT. The vast majority of the low dose rate brachytherapy experiences reported have not included patients with high-risk disease due to concerns about extraprostatic involvement or microscopic systemic disease minimizing the impact of increased local dose. D'Amico et al retrospectively analyzed outcomes with radical prostatectomy, permanent interstitial seed implantation, or EBRT in 1872 men treated at two institutions. High-risk patients were defined as those with stage T2c or PSA greater than 20 ng/mL or Gleason score of 8 or above. Within the 590 patients in this category, those treated with seed implantation or seed implantation combined with AS had significantly inferior PSA outcomes compared with patients receiving radical prostatectomy or EBRT (relative risk of failure 3.0 and 3.1, respectively).[45] Potential criticisms of this study include the relatively small cohort of patients in the implant group and the fact that no EBRT was utilized as is more commonly practiced today. However, if improved disease control in locally advanced disease via dose escalation is a valid concept, then permanent interstitial implantation may offer a method of achieving safe dose escalation when used in addition to EBRT. Stock et al treated 139 patients with high-risk features (defined as Gleason score 8–10, PSA ≥ 20 ng/mL, stage T2b, or positive seminal vesicle biopsy) with 9 months of AS, seed implantation, and 45 Gy EBRT. Negative laparoscopic pelvic lymph node dissections were performed in 44% of patients. At 5 years, the actuarial overall freedom from PSA failure rate was 86%. Post treatment prostate biopsies performed in 47 patients were negative in 100% at last biopsy.[46] Sylvester et al reported results of combined EBRT and seed implantation in 232 patients and evaluated the subset of high-risk patients as defined by the D'Amico risk criteria (Gleason 8–10, PSA > 20 ng/mL, or stage T2c).[8] The 10-year biochemical relapse-free survival in these patients was 48%.[47] Dattoli et al reported results using 41 Gy EBRT followed by palladium-101 (^{101}Pd) seed implantation in a more favorable group of patients (Gleason ≥ 7 and/or PSA > 10 ng/mL). The 10-year freedom from biochemical progression rate was 79% using a strict PSA failure criteria of a nadir greater than 0.2 ng/mL.[48] These results may come at a cost of increased morbidity compared with brachytherapy alone. Brandeis et al prospectively evaluated quality of life following combined modality therapy or seed implantation alone, and found urinary, bowel, and sexual function as well as American Urological Association symptom score to be all statistically worse in patients receiving combined treatment.[49] Others have not found combined modality treatment to be more toxic than seed implantation alone.[50]

ANDROGEN DEPRIVATION THERAPY

IN CONJUNCTION WITH RADIATION IN LOCALLY ADVANCED PROSTATE CANCER

Human prostate cancer cells vary in their in-vitro sensitivity to both acute radiation (like that delivered as EBRT) and low dose rate radiation (like that used in prostate brachytherapy). The radiosensitivity does not appear to be dependent on p53 status or the ability of the cell to initiate G1 cell cycle arrest—both previously thought to be important to radiation response. These studies also do not reveal dependence on androgen responsiveness.[51] Androgen-responsive prostate cells undergo programmed cell death (apoptosis) when deprived of androgens.[52,53] Like radiation, this death does not seem to be p53-dependent.[52] Several authors have performed in-vivo analyses of radiation combined with androgen deprivation on androgen-responsive tumors of both prostate and nonprostate origin.[54,55] None of these studies have conclusively demonstrated synergy between radiation and androgen deprivation but do suggest that timing of the androgen deprivation

Table 101.1 Reports from several institutions on high dose rate brachytherapy (HDR)

Group	# Patients	T-Stage	Mean (median) PSA, ng/mL	Median FU, months	Biochem. control, %	HDR fractional dose, Gy	# Fractions	GU toxicity	GI Toxicity
William Beaumont	207	T1c–T3c	11.5	52.8	74 @ 5 yrs	5.5–11.5	2–3	8% late grade 3	1% late Grade 3-4
Seattle	104	T1b–T3c	(8.1)	45	84 @ 5 yrs	3–4	4	6.7% stricture	2% spotty bleeding
Kiel	144	T1b–T3	25.6	96	69 @ 8 yrs	9.0	2	2.1% late grade 3	4.1% late Grade 3
Goteburg	50	T1b–T3b	Not stated	45	78 @ 5 yrs	10	2	8% acute; 4% chronic dysuria	26% mild diarrhea, 8% moderate diarrhea
Berlin	230	T2–T3	(12.8)	40	T2: 75	9–10	2	10% frequency/dysuria @ 3 months	1.7% recto-urehtral fistula
Munich	40	T2–T3	40.7	74	79.5	9	2	5% prostate necrosis	2.5% recto-vesical fistula
Lahey Clinic	52	T1–T2	10.4	11.8	92.2	6	3	11% Grade 2	18% Grade 2
Long Beach	200	T1c–T3b	10	30	93 @ 25 months	5–6.5	3–4	10% acute grade 3–4	20% acute grade 3–4
Offenbach	102	T1–T3	(15.3)	31	82 @ 3 yrs	5–7	4	27% acute grade 2–3	8% Acute Grade 2
Gothenburg	214	T1–T3	(9.6)	48	Low risk 92 @ 5 yrs	10	2	6% urethral stricture	
Kawasaki, Japan	98	T1c–T3b	(11.7)	43	T1–T2 95.9 @ 5 yrs	6	4	29.6% cystourethritis or proctitis	29.6% cystourethritis or proctitis
California Endocurietherapy	491	T1c–T3b	Not stated	Not stated	Not stated	6	4	0.6% incontinence	0.2% rectal bleeding

FU, follow-up; PSA, prostate-specific antigen.

may be critical. In one study of androgen withdrawal in the Shionogi breast tumor model, Zietman et al found that a lower dose of radiation was required to control 50% of the tumors if androgens were used in combination with radiation. Specifically, animals treated with radiation following maximal androgen withdrawal-mediated tumor regression required 42.1 Gy of radiation to control 50% of the tumors compared with 89.0 Gy in animals treated with radiation only. The most direct interpretation of these data is that following androgen withdrawal, there is a smaller number of tumor clonogens for the radiation to eradicate.

As early as 1967, hormonal therapy was being added to radiation therapy in an attempt to modify the outcome of patients with stage C (T3) prostate cancer.[56] Historically, the rationale for the treatment of these patients was based on the knowledge that these patients had an inferior outcome compared with patients with earlier stage prostate cancer treated with radiation therapy. In addition, these T3 tumors were quite large, and it was thought that a course of cytoreductive therapy might provide a more favorable geometry for external irradiation, as well as reduce tumor burden.[57]

In the early 1980s, two institutional series reported encouraging results with the use of AS and EBRT in this group of patients.[57,58] Pilepich et al also found that patients with histologically unfavorable lesions who had been treated on the Radiation Therapy Oncology Group (RTOG) 75-06 trial receiving AS and EBRT had a similar disease-free survival and overall survival as patients with more favorable tumors who did not receive the AS.[59] In part, these studies provided the basis for the next series of RTOG phase II studies designed to test the efficacy of combined EBRT and AS, with the hypothesis that preradiation cytoreduction as well as concomitant radiation- and AS-induced cell death would improve local control in patients with locally advanced prostate tumors.[60,61] Based on this experience, RTOG study 86-10 was initiated.[62] This was a randomized, phase III trial of EBRT alone (standard treatment arm) versus neoadjuvant and concomitant total androgen suppression (TAS) and EBRT (experimental treatment arm). Eligible patients were those with bulky, locally advanced tumors (>25 cm²), stage T2b to T4, N0 to N1, M0. Those patients randomized to receive TAS were treated with goserelin acetate 3.6 mg every 28 days and flutamide 250 mg t.i.d. for 2 months prior to the start of radiation and during radiation therapy. A total of 471 patients were enrolled and randomized to one of the two treatment arms. Analysis of this series revealed that those patients treated with TAS and radiation had a statistically significant improvement in local control at 5 years compared with those patients treated with radiation only ($P < 0.001$). An update of this study at a median follow-up of 6.7 years for all patients and 8.6 years for patients who were still alive continued to show statistically significant

differences in local control (42% versus 30%), biochemical disease-free survival (24% versus 10%), and cause-specific mortality (23% versus 31%). Subset analysis indicated a preferential effect in patients with Gleason score 2 to 6, where there was a significant difference in overall survival between the arms (70% versus 52%).[63] To date, there is no difference in the overall survival of the two groups of patients. This may have several possible explanations. It is possible that there may not be an overall survival benefit to patients when TAS is added to EBRT in this fashion and/or this patient population. However, it is important to note that this study was limited in that it did not routinely collect serum PSA on all patients prior to entry, a parameter that is now recognized to be an extremely important prognostic factor and indicator of disease extension. Therefore, there likely were a large number of patients with elevated serum PSA in the range frequently associated with a high risk of micrometastatic disease. The study also included patients with node-positive disease, also recognized as a poor risk factor, and one in which the value of any treatment modality to overall survival can be debated. Nonetheless, this is an important study, performed in a rigorous fashion, revealing important and measurable benefit with the addition of AS to radiation therapy for this high-risk group of patients.

A concurrent study, the RTOG 85-31, trial compared EBRT alone with EBRT followed by adjuvant goserelin indefinitely for patients with clinical or pathologic stage T3 or node-positive prostate cancer. At a median follow-up of 6 years, investigators reported statistically significant differences in rates of local failure (23% versus 37%), distant metastasis (27% versus 37%), and disease-free survival (36% versus 25%). However, these differences did not translate into improvements in cause-specific or overall survival for the cohort as a whole. In contrast to RTOG 86-10, subset analysis did reveal that patients with Gleason 8 to 10 tumors who had not undergone prostatectomy received a significant improvement in absolute survival with the addition of immediate and long-term goserelin ($P = 0.036$).[64]

Bolla et al have published a long-term analysis of the EORTC 22863 trial.[65] This phase III trial enrolled 415 patients with stage T3/T4 any grade, or stage T1/T2 WHO grade 3, prostate cancer with no evidence of nodal or metastatic disease. Patients were randomized to receive either EBRT alone (control arm) or AS plus EBRT (experimental arm). Androgen suppression consisted of oral cyproterone acetate (50 mg t.i.d.) for 4 weeks prior to radiation and an luteinizing hormone releasing hormone (LHRH) agonist started on the first day of radiation and continued every month for 3 years. A total of 401 patients were analyzed with a median follow-up of 66 months. The 5-year locoregional recurrence-free survival was 98% in the experimental arm versus 84% in the control arm ($P < 0.001$), and clinical relapse-free survival 74% in the experimental arm versus 40% in the control arm ($P < 0.001$). There was also a difference in favor of AS in the 5-year incidence of distant metastases (29% versus 9.8%; $P < 0.0001$). Most significantly, this study was the first to report that there was an overall survival advantage with the addition of AS to radiation with an estimated 5-year survival of 78% in the experimental arm versus 62% in the control arm ($P = 0.001$). It still remains to be determined whether the intriguing results generated in the EORTC 22863 trial regarding improved overall survival using 3 years of adjuvant AS are reproducible and broadly applicable.

A more recent study from Harvard is the only other trial to demonstrate an overall survival advantage with the addition of AS to EBRT. This was a phase III randomized study comparing 70 Gy of 3DCRT alone versus 3DCRT and 6 months of LHRH agonist and flutamide. Eligible patients had PSA of at least 10 ng/mL, Gleason score of 7 or higher, or radiographic evidence of extraprostatic disease. Patients also underwent cardiac stress testing prior to enrollment to rule out competing causes of mortality. Although the majority of these patients had "intermediate-risk" disease, 13% had PSA values of 20 to 40 ng/mL, and 64% had Gleason score of 7 or higher. Patients who developed biochemical failure (PSA > 1.0 ng/mL with two consecutive PSA) received salvage AS when PSA reached approximately 10 ng/mL. The trial was stopped after interim analysis at median follow-up of 4.5 years revealed an overall survival benefit in favor of the AS arm (5-year survival 88% versus 78%, $P = 0.04$).[66]

DURATION OF TREATMENT

The EORTC series and others raise several significant issues. One in particular concerns the optimum duration of androgen deprivation administration. Although results of the EORTC study and RTOG 85-31 suggest that long-term AS may be beneficial for disease control, prolonged AS has been associated with other causes of patient morbidity including osteopenia, anemia, muscle wasting, and impotence.[67] These toxicities are especially worthy of consideration given that patients treated for prostate cancer tend to be older.

The study by Laverdiere et al provided important information in this regard. In this study, patients with stage T2a to T4 disease were randomized to receive either EBRT alone, 3 months of neoadjuvant AS (LHRH-agonist plus flutamide) followed by EBRT, or 3 months of TAS then AS plus EBRT followed by another 6 months of adjuvant AS. Interestingly, the addition of 3 months of TAS prior to radiation reduced the two year positive prostate biopsy rate from 65% (radiation only) to 28%. Those patients receiving neoadjuvant, concomitant and adjuvant TAS and radiation had only a 5% positive prostate biopsy rate. These data would seem to confirm

the idea that a more protracted course of AS is important, at least in terms of local control. While impressive, the length of follow-up is too short to determine if the addition of AS to radiation has made any significant impact on other meaningful endpoints such as disease-free survival (DFS) or overall survival.[68] In contrast to the above results, Laverdiere et al. have also reported an analysis based on patients with T2-T3 disease enrolled in 2 studies of AS with EBRT, including the study described above. The second study randomized patients to neoadjuvant and concomitant AS (total 5 months) versus neoadjuvant, concomitant and short-course adjuvant (total 10 months) AS; both groups received EBRT. At a median follow-up of 5 years, there was a significant advantage in bNED survival rate with the addition of neoadjuvant and concomitant AS, but no advantage with the addition of short-course adjuvant AS after EBRT.[69]

The RTOG has also performed a phase III randomized study (RTOG 92-02) to ascertain the benefit of prolonged AS following neoadjuvant and concomitant AS with EBRT. Patients with locally advanced (T2c–T4) prostate cancers with PSA of less than 150 ng/mL received 4 months of goserelin and flutamide, 2 months before and 2 months during RT. A dose of 65 to 70 Gy was given to the prostate, and 44 to 50 Gy to the pelvic lymph nodes. Randomization was between no additional AS therapy following completion of RT, versus 24 months of additional goserelin; 1554 patients entered the study. The 5-year rate of biochemical DFS was 46.4% versus 28.1% in the long-term and short-term AS arms, respectively ($P < 0.0001$). The long-term AS arm showed significant improvement in all end points except overall survival (80% versus 78.5% at 5 years, $P = 0.73$), although an unplanned subset analysis revealed a significant survival benefit for patients with Gleason 8 to 10 tumors as determined by the institution (but not on central pathology review). Despite a statistically significant reduction in the rate of prostate cancer-related deaths in the long-term arm (38% versus 24%, $P = 0.001$), there was an absolute increase in the number of deaths as a result of other causes, resulting in a similar rate of overall survival. Cardiovascular disease at the time of enrollment was more prevalent in the patients treated on the long-term arm (55% versus 44%, respectively), but a detrimental effect of long-term AS therapy on other causes of death cannot be excluded.[70]

Other data also suggest that the benefit of long-term AS may be greater in patients with high Gleason scores. Roach et al analyzed patients enrolled on five randomized RTOG studies that treated patients with radiotherapy and AS. Patients with stage T3 disease, nodal involvement, or Gleason 7 grade had a disease-specific survival benefit with the addition of 4 months of goserelin and flutamide, whereas patients with Gleason 8 to 10 disease or multiple high-risk factors had an approximately 20% higher survival at 8 years with the use of up-front, long-term hormonal therapy.[71] However, it is unclear how much of this conclusion overlaps with that from RTOG 85-31, since it was included in the analysis. Another re-analysis of RTOG data comes from Horwitz et al, who assessed the benefit of long-term versus short-term androgen deprivation in studies 85-31 and 86-10. The benefit in bNED control, distant metastasis-free survival, and cause-specific survival from long-term AS was limited to those patients with centrally reviewed Gleason score of 7 to 10; multivariate analysis demonstrated Gleason score and the use of long-term AS to be independent predictors for all three outcome measures.[72]

Related data comes from a number of surgical series investigating the use of AS therapy prior to radical prostatectomy. Several of these series have shown reduction in the positive margin rate, inferring AS-induced cell death. Relevant to this discussion is that a longer course of AS (i.e., 8 months) resulted in the greatest reduction in serum PSA, and only a 12% incidence of positive surgical margins compared with 23% in the 3-month AS arm.[73]

While these data are not conclusive and the studies assess differing endpoints, they provide some useful information. Taken together, they would seem to support the theory that a longer course of AS may very well lead to improved locoregional control of large tumors or high-risk tumors that possess an elevated risk of extraprostatic extension. However, although differences have been shown in biochemical and clinical disease control, so far there is no demonstrated overall survival advantage of prolonged versus short-course AS.

SEQUENCING OF ANDROGEN DEPRIVATION AND RADIATION THERAPY

The question of optimal sequencing of AS and radiation is similarly unanswered. As will be discussed later, it is not clear whether the effects of AS on tumor control are merely additive to the tumoricidal effects of radiation or whether they are synergistic, providing an enhancement of tumor killing that cannot be simply explained by the killing of each modality individually.

In order to assess the importance of AS timing in relation to EBRT, the RTOG performed a phase III trial (RTOG 94-13) where patients were randomized to either 2 months of neoadjuvant AS followed by AS and EBRT (control arm) or EBRT followed by 4 months of adjuvant AS.[74] Patients were also randomized in a 2 × 2 factorial design to receive WPRT versus prostate-only radiation. Eligibility included localized prostate cancer with risk of lymph node involvement of 15% or more (based on an equation using pretreatment PSA, Gleason score, and stage).[75] At a median follow-up of 59 months, patients treated with neoadjuvant and concomitant AS

experienced a similar 4-year progression-free survival compared with those receiving adjuvant AS (52% versus 49%; P = 0.56). However, the group that received WPRT and neoadjuvant and concomitant AS had a significantly improved progression-free survival rate compared with the other three arms (60% versus 44–50%; P = 0.008). Further information regarding the most effective duration of neoadjuvant treatment will be provided by RTOG 99-10, which randomized patients to either 6 months or 2 months of neoadjuvant AS followed by concurrent AS and radiation.

ALTERATION OF TOXICITY

In addition to improved tumor control, androgen deprivation therapy adds its own side-effect profile but may also alter possible radiation-induced side effects. In the randomized study by D'Amico et al, patients receiving AS with 3DCRT had statistically significant increases in grade 3 impotence (26% versus 21%) as well as gynecomastia, but no other significant differences in late toxicity were noted in this trial.[66] In contrast, Chen et al found no significant differences in 1-year potency rates between men receiving 3DCRT with AS versus 3DCRT alone, and patients treated in RTOG 86-10 had no differences in frequency or time to return of sexual potency.[63,76]

Reductions in prostatic volume after neoadjuvant AS can result in smaller treatment fields and consequent reductions in the amount of surrounding normal tissue that is secondarily irradiated. Reduction in the volume of irradiated rectum, for example, is associated with a significant decrease in long-term rectal injury.[77] Comparisons of dose–volume histograms from 3DCRT plans generated on patients pre- and post-neoadjuvant AS reveal a median reduction in prostate volume of 27% to 42%. This was also correlated with a decrease in the amount of irradiated rectum, bladder, and bowel.[78–80] Despite this expected benefit of AS, most studies do not support such a hypothesis. Late grade 1 to 3 incontinence was increased within the combined therapy group in the Bolla study (29% versus 16%; P = 0.002).[81] In a retrospective analysis by Sanguineti et al, rectal dose and the use of adjuvant AS were both significantly associated with higher risk of late rectal toxicity. The 2-year estimates of grade 2 to 4 late rectal toxicity were 30.3% versus 14.1% in patients receiving or not receiving AS, respectively.[82] The RTOG 94-13 study found the acute and 2-year rates of late grade 3 or higher GU/GI toxicity to be higher on the arm receiving whole pelvic EBRT with neoadjuvant and concomitant AS, but these differences did not reach statistical significance.[74] Valicenti et al compared toxicity rates in patients enrolled in RTOG 94-06, where approximately half of men received neoadjuvant AS (with variable dose levels of radiation). On univariate analysis, AS significantly increased the incidence of grade 2 acute GU complications, but was not significant in the multivariate analysis when volume of bladder treated was taken into account. The use of AS did increase risk of acute GU effects in men with preexisting obstructive symptoms.[83] Long-term AS may increase toxicity in and of itself. In RTOG 92-02, there was a small but statistically significant increase in the frequency of late grade 3 to 5 GI toxicity in the long-term compared with the short-term AS arm (2.6% versus 1.2% at 5 years; P = 0.037), although there is no clear explanation for this difference.[70]

The combination of AS and EBRT for the treatment of locally advanced prostate cancer results in an apparent increase in local control and disease-free survival as supported by several prospective, randomized trials. There are conflicting data from such trials as to the benefit in overall survival, and the most favorable duration as well as timing of AS in relation to radiation is not yet known. These are important questions to answer because of the potential added toxicity of AS, especially when administered long-term. Besides the well-recognized side effects of AS such as hot flashes and decreased libido, there are other important physiologic changes that occur with long-term use, including anemia, loss of muscle mass, decreased bone density, and depression.[67] Consideration of these potentially limiting side effects is required before instituting therapy.

WHOLE PELVIC RADIATION THERAPY FOR OCCULT NODAL METASTASIS

A significant proportion of patients with locally advanced prostate cancer will have clinically occult pelvic lymph node spread. The primary nodes at risk for involvement include the external iliac, hypogastric, presacral, and obturator nodes.[84] Theoretically, treatment of these nodal areas in patients with meaningful risk of nodal involvement might be of therapeutic benefit if sufficient doses of radiation are given to eradicate microscopic tumor.

Partin et al developed predictive nomograms for lymph node involvement as well as other surgical findings based on multi-institutional data from radical prostatectomy specimens. Using these tables, it is possible to estimate the risk of lymph node involvement based on a patient's preoperative Gleason score, clinical stage, and PSA.[85] Roach et al developed an equation that estimates the risk of lymph node involvement based on the Partin tables[86]:

$$\text{Lymph node risk} = \{2/3\}\ \text{PSA} + ([\text{Gleason score} - 6] \times 10) \qquad [101.1]$$

The true incidence of nodal involvement is most likely underestimated in data based on surgical series, due to the inherent false-negative rate of lymph node

dissections as typically performed in modern surgical practice. Heidenreich et al compared results in patients with similar risk characteristics undergoing extended pelvic lymphadenectomy versus standard pelvic lymphadenectomy. The incidence of lymph node detection was significantly higher in the extended lymphadenectomy group (26% versus 12%), and 42% of nodal metastases in the extended lymphadenectomy group were outside of areas dissected in a standard pelvic lymphadenectomy, including external iliac and obturator nodes. All except one patient with lymph node involvement had PSA greater than 10.5 ng/mL and Gleason score of 7 or higher.[87] Therefore, a larger proportion of patients may benefit from pelvic nodal irradiation than might be estimated by using the Partin nomograms.

Several retrospective, single institutional analyses have shown conflicting results as to the benefit of WPRT. Some of these studies are flawed by the fact that they are from the pre-PSA era, making the determination of patients at risk of nodal involvement as well as evaluation of treatment efficacy more difficult. They also suffer from low patient numbers and use of dated radiotherapy techniques.[88–90] However, some studies did find a benefit to the use of larger treatment fields that encompassed pelvic nodal areas.[91] Ploysongsang et al reported statistically significant improvements in 5-year survival rates amongst stage B and stage C patients receiving WPRT in comparison with stage-matched controls treated to prostate only.[92] Seaward et al analyzed a group of 506 patients treated at the University of California San Francisco who had a 15% or greater risk of nodal involvement (based on the Roach equation: Eq. 101.1). The median biochemical progression-free survival was significantly higher (34 months versus 21 months; P = 0.0001) in patients who received initial WPRT followed by prostate boost as opposed to prostate only radiation.[93]

Three randomized trials have been performed to evaluate the benefit of WPRT. Bagshaw reported a series of 57 patients with surgically staged, node-negative prostate cancer who were randomized to either WPRT and prostate boost versus prostate-only radiotherapy. Although the disease-free survival was improved with the use of WPRT, the results were not statistically significant, possibly due to the small sample size.[94] The RTOG has reported results of two randomized studies performed to date on the value of WPRT in prostate cancer. RTOG 77-06 evaluated WPRT in patients with stage A2 and stage B prostate cancer with no evidence of lymph node involvement on lymphangiogram or biopsy. Randomization was to either 65 Gy to the prostate alone or to 45 Gy WPRT with 20 Gy prostatic boost. At a median follow-up of 7 years, there was no beneficial effect of WPRT on local control, distant metastases, disease-free or overall survival.[95] Given that the patients on this study were at low risk of lymph node involvement, it is inconclusive in determining whether patients at moderate to high risk of nodal metastasis benefit from WPRT.

As discussed above in the section on AS, RTOG 94-13 also looked at the role of WPRT in patients with either risk of nodal involvement of 15% or greater (based on the Roach equation: Eq. 101.1) or with T2c to T4 disease; the maximum allowable pretreatment PSA was 100 ng/mL. Whole pelvic radiation therapy was associated with a 4-year progression-free survival of 54%, compared with 47% in the arms treated with prostate-only radiation. Interestingly, when comparing all four treatment arms there was a progression-free survival advantage for WPRT plus neoadjuvant/concurrent AS compared with the other arms (60% versus 44–50%; $P = 0.008$). No overall survival differences were seen.[74]

The positive results in this study for WPRT may be attributed to the use of AS in addition to WPRT, which has been shown to be synergistic with radiation.[54] The optimal dose of WPRT associated with durable control of microscopic nodal disease has not been determined, but doses beyond 50 to 55 Gy have not been utilized due to the limited radiation tolerance of small bowel which is often in whole pelvic radiotherapy fields. In a retrospective analysis on 963 patients performed by Perez et al, patients receiving whole pelvic doses of 50 to 55 Gy had fewer pelvic failures compared with those receiving 40 to 45 Gy ($P = 0.07$). A statistically significant reduction in pelvic failures was noted in stage C poorly differentiated tumors when the pelvic nodes received doses greater than 50 Gy compared with lower doses (23% versus 46%; $P = 0.01$).[96] In RTOG 94-13, the addition of AS to an otherwise modest dose of radiation may have allowed the WPRT to cross a threshold of efficacy.

Another factor that may enhance the benefit of WPRT is the use of CT-based treatment planning, which allows for better targeting of lymphatic regions at risk. The "standard" 4-field pelvic radiation portal as practiced in the conventional radiotherapy era (including RTOG 94-13) often underdosed or missed portions of at-risk nodal chains entirely. With CT, the location of the pelvic vasculature can be used as approximations of the lymph node locations, with margin added to cover the associated lymph nodes.[97,98]

CONCLUSIONS

Radiation therapy is the current standard of care for patients with locally advanced prostate cancer. The addition of AS to EBRT results in increased local control and disease-free survival, and data are emerging to show an improvement in overall survival as well. The optimal sequencing and duration of AS when combined with radiotherapy remains to be determined, and

considerations must be made for the impact of prolonged AS on overall health and quality of life. The use of dose-escalated radiotherapy using modern treatment planning and delivery techniques results in increased biochemical control rates in patients with "intermediate-risk" disease, but further study is needed regarding its impact on patients with "high-risk" prognostic features. The use of WPRT combined with AS in patients at meaningful risk of lymph node involvement is now supported by prospective randomized data. Finally, radiotherapy delivered either by external beam or radioisotope remains an important adjunct in the management of patients with metastatic prostate cancer, especially in the palliation of bony metastases.

RADIATION THERAPY IN THE TREATMENT OF METASTATIC PROSTATE CANCER

BACKGROUND

Fortunately, relatively few men now present with metastatic disease. According to Jemal et al, currently, only 6% of men present at the time of diagnosis with distant metastases, whereas between 1984 and 1990, up to 25% of men presented with distant metastases.[99,100] Unfortunately, a number of men who are diagnosed with prostate cancer and receive definitive therapy for their disease still ultimately progress to and die of metastatic cancer. A recent study from a large Midwestern hospital found that 8.9% of a cohort of 2056 patients had metastatic progression at a mean follow-up of 3.6 years.[101] Another study found that after 21 years of follow-up for patients who underwent an observational approach for T0 to T2 disease, 17% of patients experienced metastatic disease.[102] Pound et al reported that up to one quarter of men who demonstrated biochemical recurrence after prostatectomy had a recurrence after 5 years.[103]

Prostate cancer has a proclivity to spread to bone, causing predominantly osteoblastic metastases with frequent components of osteosclerosis. Hematogenous dissemination of prostate cancer cells tends to favor the axial skeleton, where red marrow is abundant, likely because blood flow to these areas is high.[104] In a meta-analysis of autopsies of 1589 patients who died of prostate cancer from 1967 to 1995, it was found that hematogenous metastases were present in one third of patients. The site of most frequent involvement was bone (90%), followed by lung (46%), liver (25%), pleura (21%), and adrenals (13%).[105] The previously held concept that Batson's venous plexus acts as a direct conduit of spread of prostate cancer[106] was disproved in a study that analyzed the distribution of bone metastases using technicium-99 whole-body scans. The distribution of metastases in patients with prostate cancer were largely identical to those of patients with other cancers, and one quarter of prostate cancer patients had lesions exclusively outside of the pelvis, sacrum or lumbar spine.[107] A more contemporary theory is that tumors with propensity to metastasize to bone possess the ability to not only survive but also proliferate and colonize in bone and bone marrow.[108] It has been shown that tumor cells produce cell adhesion molecules that allow them to bind to and penetrate bone marrow sinusoids.[109] Bone also harbors inactive but multiple important growth factors, which are thought to support metastatic cell deposit growth.[110] In turn, the presence of tumor cells causes reactions of bone destruction and new bone formation, and the resulting products from bone resorption may act as chemoattractants for more tumor cells.[111-114] Prostate-specific antigen, a serine protease with trypsin-like activity, has also been implicated in the development of prostate cancer bone metastases. It has been shown to be a protease for insulin-like growth factor binding protein, a molecule that can inhibit the osteoblastic activity of insulin-like growth factors.[115,116]

Patients who experience bone metastases may suffer from pain, fractures, and spinal cord compression (Figure 101.1), all of which may require hospitalization, affect patient functionality and independence, and contribute to increased healthcare costs.[117] Many patients with bone metastases will develop other medical complications or become bed-ridden. Not surprisingly, the presence of skeletal metastases is associated with a significant reduction in quality of life.[118]

CLINICAL ASSESSMENT OF BONE METASTASES

Any patient with a diagnosis of prostate cancer who presents with new complaints of bone pain must have a full history and physical exam performed. Important components of the history of review include the patient's disease status (last PSA, androgen sensitivity, and prior treatments) and pain characteristics such as onset, location, duration, radiation, and alleviating or exacerbating factors. Metastatic bone pain may have an insidious and nonspecific onset and typically increases in severity at a focal or referred location over weeks to months. However, a pathologic fracture may cause acute pain, and spinal cord compression may present with acute onset of pain with paresthesias, weakness, or bladder or bowel incontinence. The pain is most typically somatic in nature. The differential diagnosis of bone pain should include nonmalignant causes such as arthritis, muscle strain or spasm, hyperparathyroidism, or osteopenic vertebral body collapse.

A general physical examination should be performed, including palpation and percussion of the painful sites and full neurologic exam. Laboratory data should be obtained including serum PSA (although poorly differentiated prostate cancer may not produce PSA) and alkaline phosphatase. Occasionally urinary hydroxyproline, a collagen metabolite, can also be useful.

Radiographic assessment of a patient with presumed bone metastases should include a radionuclide bone scan to evaluate the presence and distribution of metastases. Plain X-rays are useful in evaluating a specific, symptomatic area or as part of further

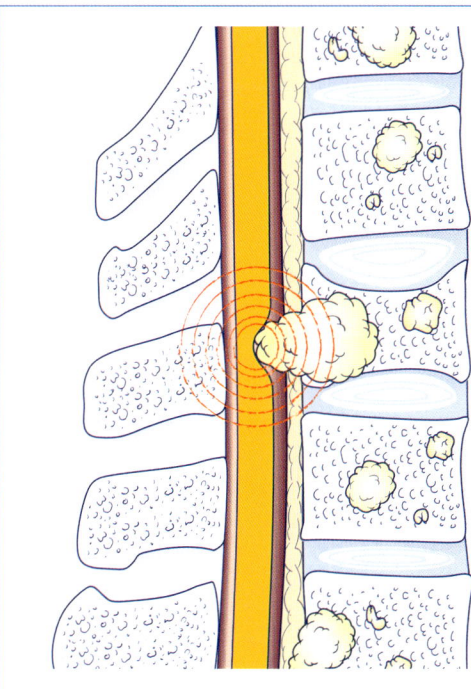

Fig. 101.1
Spinal cord compression resulting from metastatic involvement of the spine by prostate cancer may require treatment by radiotherapy.

evaluation of a lesion seen by bone scan, but are generally less sensitive than bone scans for detecting new, metastatic foci of disease. X-rays do, however, remain particularly helpful in evaluating a bone risk for the risk of pathologic fracture and whether prophylactic fixation is required.

RADIATION THERAPY FOR PALLIATION OF BONE METASTASES

For patients with hormone-naive metastatic disease, initial management with AS will often provide substantial symptom relief.[119] However, patients may present with pain not completely alleviated by AS, or may develop painful metastases in the setting of androgen-unresponsive disease. Focal EBRT is a well-established modality for palliation of bone pain occurring in one or several sites. Studies have shown that up to 90% of patients receiving EBRT for painful bony metastases obtain some degree of pain relief, and more than half of patients experience complete pain relief.[120,121]

The mechanism of the pain-modulating effects of EBRT are not well elucidated and not completely explained by reduction in tumor size, as pain relief may be rapid and precede the onset of tumor response.[122] The goals of palliative radiotherapy are to alleviate pain, prevent pathologic fracture, and improve quality of life by increasing mobility and functional status. Also, patients experiencing side effects from large doses of opioids may be treated with EBRT in order to minimize pain medication requirements. Acute morbidities related to skeletal radiation are usually modest and can include local erythema, lowered blood counts, and tiredness. Nausea and vomiting can occur if the abdomen is in the treatment portal, but effective prophylaxis is achievable with antiemetic agents.[123] No significant differences have been noted in the toxicities associated with single fraction or multifraction regimens. Pathologic fractures occur in approximately 5% of patients, probably due to unresponsive or recurrent disease.[129,131]

EXTERNAL-BEAM RADIATION THERAPY FRACTIONATION SCHEDULES FOR BONE METASTASES

Controversy surrounds the optimal dose and fractionation schedule for palliating bone metastases with radiation. RTOG 74-02 was an early, randomized clinical trial that assessed the difference in pain relief among various fractionation schemes in 1000 patients. The fractionation schemes were 40.5 Gy in 15 fractions versus 20 Gy in 5 fractions for solitary metastases, and 30 Gy in 10 fractions versus 25 Gy in 5 fractions for

multiple metastases. All of the schedules appeared equally effective in initially alleviating pain, but patients receiving higher doses of radiation appeared to have better outcome with less need for re-treatment and less narcotic use.[120,124] Twice daily treatment done three times per week (2 Gy per fraction) was found to have no advantage over conventional schedules of 30 Gy in 15 fractions and 22.5 Gy in 5 fractions.[125] Therefore, most palliative fractionation schemes appear reasonable and have a high probability of achieving adequate pain relief.[126–129]

SINGLE FRACTION VERSUS MULTIPLE FRACTION REGIMENS

In a trial from the UK, 765 patients with painful skeletal metastases were randomly assigned to receive either 8 Gy in a single fraction, 20 Gy in 5 fractions, or 30 Gy in 10 fractions and were followed for 1 year after treatment. Overall survival at 12 months was 44%, and no survival differences were seen among the three groups. There were no differences in time to first improvement in pain, with more than 50% of patients achieving pain relief by 1 month after the start of treatment, time to complete pain relief with a two-thirds chance of having no pain by one year, or time to first increase in pain up to 12 months from EBRT. Re-treatment was twice as common after 8 Gy than after multifraction radiotherapy, but may have been due to a greater readiness to prescribe additional radiotherapy after a single fraction.[130]

In the Dutch Bone Metastases Study, 1171 patients were randomized to receive either 8 Gy in one fraction or 24 Gy in six fractions. A median survival of 7 months was observed. Seventy one percent of patients experienced a response at some time during the first year. No difference between the two groups were found with regard to pain medication, quality of life, and side effects. Re-treatment was needed in 25% of the 8 Gy group and 7% of the 24 Gy group. More pathologic fractures also were observed in the single fraction group.[131] Both the Dutch and British multicenter trials reaffirmed the palliative benefit both of single and fractionated schedules but suggested that re-treatment was required more frequently with single dose EBRT.

A large North American trial, RTOG 97-14, has also investigated the question of single (8 Gy in one fraction) versus multiple (30 Gy in 10 fractions) fractions in the palliative management of painful prostate and breast cancer bone metastases and enrolled 949 patients. Preliminary results at 3 months follow-up has demonstrated no difference in partial or complete pain relief between the two groups (65% versus 66%), and one-third no longer required narcotic medications.[132] Quality-of-life analyses showed little differences between the two treatment arms. The increased utility in changes of emotion in the 30 Gy arm was hypothesized to be due to a benefit from increased social support gained with longer treatment time.[133]

Two meta-analyses, each evaluating over 3000 patients, showed that re-irradiation rates were consistently different between low-dose and high-dose arms, with more frequent re-irradiation required in the lower dose arms. No dose response relationships could be detected.[134] Re-treatment rates and pathologic fracture rates were higher with single fraction EBRT compared with multifraction EBRT (21%, 3% versus 7.4%, 1.6%). Both single and multifraction EBRT were effective in achieving pain relief.[135] Single-fraction EBRT was found to be most cost-effective palliative treatment when compared with pain medication, chemotherapy, and multifraction RT.[136] Nevertheless, further studies prospectively evaluating quality of life and cost are warranted.

There is variation among patterns of care among physicians. When American radiation oncologists were questioned about four hypothetical clinical scenarios concerning painful osseous metastases, the most commonly used schedule was 30 Gy in 10 fractions.[137] Canadian radiation oncologists were more likely to recommend treatment with 20 Gy in 5 fractions.[138] In deciding on the optimal palliative EBRT dosing for any single patient, the physician must consider multiple factors for each individual patient including the patient's life expectancy, extent of disease, volume of the treatment field, rate of disease progression, performance status, and cost of therapy. For those cases in which the patient is estimated to have a one- to two-year survival or more, doses of 40 to 50 Gy over 4 to 5 weeks should be considered to maximize duration and response to treatment. In patients whose life expectancies are less than 1 year, 30 Gy in 10 fractions are typically given and in instances where survival is estimated to be 3 months or less, 8 Gy in one fraction may be appropriate.[119]

SYSTEMIC RADIONUCLIDES

The reactive bone formation that frequently occurs in the presence of metastatic bone involvement from prostate cancer results in new bone, which has increased avidity for bone-seeking molecules such as bisphosphonates.[139] This is the basis by which radionuclides such as samarium-153 and rhenium-186, when complexed to bone-avid molecules, may be selectively delivered to sites of metastatic bone involvement. Other radionuclides (including strontium-89) have a natural affinity for metabolically active bone.[140] The advantage of radionuclide treatment is the ability to simultaneously target multiple sites of involvement with a single intravenous administration. After administration with ^{153}Sm chelated to ethylenediaminetetramethylene phosphonic acid (EDTMP) , 65% to 80% of patients report pain relief, and symptom response usually occurs within 1 week of treatment. The average duration of response is 2 to 3 months. An initial pain flare may occur in approximately 10% of patients, and the major toxicity of treatment is myelosuppression.[141–143] A detailed discussion of radionuclide therapy is presented elsewhere in this text.

WIDE-FIELD RADIATION THERAPY/ HEMIBODY RADIATION THERAPY

Hemibody radiation therapy (HBRT) was first developed in the 1960s for patients with multiple sites of painful bone metastases. Although blood counts are lowered with wide-field radiation therapy (WFRT), the body can regenerate the marrow supply when at least 10% of the bone marrow is spared from radiation. Ordinarily, sequential treatments to the upper and lower halves were possible provided that the treatments were separated by 4 to 6 weeks. These treatments could be used alone or as an adjunct to local-field irradiation. The optimal single doses were found to be 6 Gy to the upper hemibody and 8 Gy for the middle or lower segment, with increasing doses showing no benefit in pain response.[149] The maximum tolerated dose of fractionated (2.5 Gy) HBRT was found to be 17.5 Gy; however it was found that pain from prostate cancer osseous metastases is sufficiently treated with 3 Gy on 2 consecutive days and was as effective as 3 Gy for 5 days.[144,145] Fractionated schedules allow for a higher total dose without increased toxicity. Fractionated schemes may also give longer duration of relief and more complete relief, as well as improved overall and progression free survival with less toxicity.[146] RTOG 82-06 sought to explore the possibility that HBRT (8 Gy in one fraction) added to local-field radiotherapy (30 Gy in 10 fractions) might delay the onset of metastases in the affected hemibody and decrease the frequency of further treatment. The addition of HBRT to local-field EBRT was found to delay the progression of existing disease and prolong the median time to new disease (12.6 versus 6.3 months). Time to new treatment within the hemibody segment was delayed and 16% fewer patients were retreated. There was also a trend to improved survival in prostate cancer patients treated with HBRT. These findings suggest that hemibody irradiation may eradicate micrometastases.[147]

Despite these potential advantages, the morbidity of HBRT is greater than localized radiotherapy. Patients may experience thromboleukopenia, emesis, rigors and fevers, pneumonitis, xerostomia, and cataracts. Nowadays, WFRT/HBRT is used in 1% to 2% of cases since patients with widespread painful bone metastases can usually be palliated with radioisotopes.[137] However, unlike radioisotopes, HBRT can palliate both osseous and extraosseous metastases. Moreover, in those cases in which systemic radioisotopes cannot be given, HBRT may be a reasonable alternative. Hemibody radiation therapy is thought to provide more rapid relief of pain compared with radioisotope therapy.[148,149] Pain relief with HBRT is rapid in onset, and 50% of patients were found to have pain relief within 48 hours, 80% had pain relief within 1 week, and all had pain relief within 2 weeks. One fifth of all patients had a complete response in their pain.

IRRADIATION OF PREVIOUSLY TREATED AREAS

Although most patients have a good initial response to radiotherapy, approximately 10% to 25% of patients will have pain relapse necessitating retreatment.[32,33] Local-field radiation may need to be repeated at the same site and can generally be recommended with a similar probability of response. Overall response rates with re-treatment are reported to be 84% to 87%.[150] The patients who benefit most from re-irradiation are those who relapse 4 months or more beyond initial treatment, have good performance status, and have a solitary metastasis.[151] In patients with vertebral metastases, the risk of re-irradiation must be carefully considered against the risk of radiation-induced myelopathy if the re-irradiation dose would exceed the normal tolerance of the spinal cord.[152] Nevertheless, because of the short life expectancy of most patients considered for this therapy, the immediate benefits of re-irradiation may outweigh the potential for long-term toxicities.

In an attempt to increase the safety and efficiency of vertebral body re-irradiation by limiting dose to the spinal cord, intensity-modulated radiotherapy and stereotactic body radiation therapy have been utilized. Stereotactic body radiation therapy refers to a variety of techniques that have in common the ability to increase the precision of radiation delivery.[153] One series evaluated 19 patients retreated for recurrent spinal cord metastases with IMRT or fractionated conformal RT with a maximal re-treatment dose of less than 20 Gy. Most patients achieved an improvement in pain. Although there were no significant late toxicities after a median follow-up of 1 year, 12 patients had died within this timeframe.[154] Another series of 125 patients treated with stereotactic body radiation therapy included 78 who had received prior spinal radiation. Patients received a mean dose of 17.5 Gy in a single fraction to the 80% isodose line. No acute radiation toxicity or new neurological deficits occurred during a median follow-up of 18 months. Axial and radicular pain improved in 74 of 79 patients who were symptomatic before treatment.[155]

POSTOPERATIVE RADIATION THERAPY

Pathologic fractures occur in approximately 10% to 20% of cancer patients with bony metastatic disease, and orthopedic stabilization is frequently performed either prophylactically or after the occurrence of fracture.[156] Postoperative radiotherapy has been shown to help patients attain an improved functional status and use of the extremity following orthopedic stabilization. For patients who do not initially receive postoperative radiation therapy, 15% require a second orthopedic procedure after an average of 1 year, compared with 3% in patients receiving radiotherapy. Postoperative radiation therapy may also contribute to an increase in overall survival.[157]

For patients with spinal cord compression due to metastatic disease, a combined surgical and radiotherapeutic approach is warranted. Regine et al randomized patients with spinal cord compression to either radical decompressive surgical resection followed by radiation therapy or radiation therapy alone. Surgery was performed within 24 hours of study entry with the intent in all cases to remove as much tumor as possible, provide immediate decompression, and stabilize the spine. Radiation therapy in both groups was given to a total dose of 30 Gy in fractions of 3 Gy. The combined modality group required fewer steroids and narcotics, and was able to maintain ambulatory ability and functional status longer than the patients receiving radiotherapy alone.[158]

CONCLUSIONS

Radiotherapy is an important therapeutic modality in the management of metastatic prostate cancer, and should be used to alleviate symptoms from bone pain or in the postoperative setting. It has been shown that the use of EBRT for metastatic bone lesions provides pain relief regardless of the fractionation scheme chosen, although the data also suggest that a more prolonged course of radiotherapy may be associated with reduced risk of fracture and less relapse of pain. Radiation therapy should be considered as a first line treatment for the palliation of a few symptomatic bone metastases. For diffuse bony metastases causing widespread pain, for areas that have been treated with previous EBRT to maximal normal tissue tolerances, or for painful areas that have recurred, patients should be considered for treatment with radionuclides or wide-field radiation.[27] Patients undergoing surgical treatment of bone metastases should receive postoperative radiation to maximize functional recovery and limit risk of recurrence.

REFERENCES

1. Pasteau O, Degrais J. The radium treatment of cancer of the prostate. Rev Malad Nutr 1911;363–367.
2. Smith GS, Pierson EL. The value of high voltage x-ray therapy in carcinoma of the prostate. J Urol 1930;23:331.
3. Widmann BP. Cancer of the prostate. The result of radium and roentgen ray treatment. Radiology 1934;22:153.

4. Kupelian P, Katcher J, Levin H, et al. Stage T1-2 prostate cancer. Int J Radiat Oncol Biol Phys 1997;37:1043–1052.

5. Partin A, Mangold L, Lamm D, et al. Contemporary update of prostate cancer staging nomograms (Partin tables) for the new millennium. Urology 2001;58:843–848.

6. Roach M, Lu J, Pilepich M, et al. Four prognostic groups predict long-term survival from prostate cancer following radiotherapy alone on Radiation Therapy Oncology Group clinical trials. Int J Radiat Oncol Biol Phys 2000;47:609–615.

7. D'Amico AV, Whittington R, Malkowicz SB, et al. Biochemical outcome after radical prostatectomy, EBRT, or interstitial radiation therapy for clinically localized prostate cancer. JAMA 1998;280:969–974.

8. D'Amico AV. Combined-modality staging for localized adenocarcinoma of the prostate. Oncology (Huntington) 2001;15:49 59.

9. Zietman AL, Coen JJ, Shipley WU, et al. Radical radiation therapy in the management of prostatic adenocarcinoma: the initial prostate specific antigen value as a predictor of treatment outcome. J Urol 1994;151:640–645.

10. Kuban DA, el-Mahdi AM, Schellhammer PF. Prostate-specific antigen for pretreatment prediction and posttreatment evaluation of outcome after definitive irradiation for prostate cancer. Int J Radiat Oncol Biol Phys 1995;32:307–316.

11. Hanks GE, Hanlon AL, Hudes G, et al. Patterns-of-failure analysis of patients with high pretreatment prostate-specific antigen levels treated by radiation therapy: the need for improved systemic and locoregional treatment. J Clin Oncol 1996;1093–1097.

12. Shipley WU, Thames HD, Sandler HM, et al. Radiation therapy for clinically localized prostate cancer. JAMA 1999;281:1598–1604.

13. Coen JJ, Zietman AL, Thakral H, et al. Radical radiation for localized prostate cancer: local persistence of disease results in a late wave of metastases. J Clin Oncol 2002;20:3199–3205.

14. Kuban DA, el-Mahdi AM, Schellhammer PF. Potential benefit of improved local tumor control in patients with prostate carcinoma. Cancer 1995;75:2373–2382.

15. Valicenti R, Lu J, Pilepich M. Survival advantage from higher-dose radiation therapy for clinically localized prostate cancer treated on the radiation therapy oncology group trials. J Clin Oncol 2000;18:2740–2746.

16. Hanks GE, Martz KL, Diamond JJ. The effect of dose on local control of prostate cancer. Int J Radiat Oncol Biol Phys 1988;15:1299–305.

17. Pollack A, Smith LG, von Eschenbach AG. External beam radiotherapy dose response characteristics of 1127 men with prostate cancer treated in the PSA era. Int J Radiat Oncol Biol Phys 2000;48:57–512.

18. Leibel SA, Hanks GE, Kramer S. Patterns of care outcome studies: results of the national practice in adenocarcinoma of the prostate. Int J Radiat Oncol Biol Phys 1984;10:401–409.

19. Smit WG, Helle PA, Van Putten WL. Late radiation damage in prostate cancer patients treated by high dose external radiotherapy in relation to rectal dose. Int J Radiat Oncol Biol Phys 1990;18:23–29.

20. Schultheiss TE, Lee WR, Hunt MA, et al. Late GI and GU complications in the treatment of prostate cancer. Int J Radiat Oncol Biol Phys 1997;37:3–11.

21. Roach M. Reducing the toxicity associated with the use of radiotherapy in men with localized prostate cancer. Urol Clin N Am 2004;31:353–366.

22. Dearnaley DP, Khoo VS, Norman AR, et al. Comparison of radiation side-effects of conformal and conventional radiotherapy in prostate cancer: a randomised trial. Lancet 1999;23:267–272.

23. Koper PC, Stroom JC, van Putten WL, et al. Acute morbidity reduction using 3DCRT for prostate carcinoma: a randomized study. Int J Radiat Oncol Biol Phys 1999;43:727–734.

24. American Society for Therapeutic Radiology and Oncology Consensus Panel. Consensus statement: Guidelines for PSA following radiation therapy. Int J Radiat Oncol Biol Phys 1997;37:1035–1041.

25. Hanks GE, Hanlon AL, Epstein B, et al. Dose response in prostate cancer with 8-12 years' follow-up. Int J Radiat Oncol Biol Phys 2002;54:427–435.

26. Pollack A, Hanlon AL, Horwitz EM, et al. Prostate cancer radiotherapy dose response: an update of the Fox Chase experience. J Urol 2004;171:1132–1136.

27. Bey P, Carrie C, Beckendorf V, et al. Dose escalation with 3D-CRT in prostate cancer: French study of dose escalation with conformal 3D radiotherapy in prostate cancer-preliminary results. Int J Radiat Oncol Biol Phys 2000,48:513–517.

28. Zelefsky M, Fuks Z, Chan H, et al. Ten-year results of dose escalation with 3-dimensional conformal radiotherapy for patients with clinically localized prostate cancer. Int J Radiat Oncol Biol Phys 2003;57S:149–150.

29. Michalski JM, Winter K, Purdy JA, et al. Preliminary evaluation of low-grade toxicity with conformal radiation therapy for prostate cancer on RTOG 9406 dose levels I and II. Int J Radiat Oncol Biol Phys 2003;56:192–198.

30. Ryu JK, Winter K, Michalski JM, et al. Interim report of toxicity from 3D conformal radiation therapy for prostate cancer on 3DOG/RTOG 9406, level III (79.2 Gy). Int J Radiat Oncol Biol Phys 2002;54:1036–1046.

31. Shipley WU, Verhey LJ, Munzenrider JE, et al. Advanced prostate cancer: the results of a randomized comparative trial of high dose irradiation boosting with conformal protons compared with conventional dose irradiation using photons alone. Int J Radiat Oncol Biol Phys 1995;32:3–12.

32. Zietman AL, DeSilvio M, Slater JD, et al. A randomized trial comparing conventional dose (70.2GyE) and high-dose (79.2GyE) conformal radiation in early stage adenocarcinoma of the prostate: results of an interim analysis of PROG 95-09. Int J Radiat Oncol Biol Phys 2004;60:S131.

33. Pollack A, Zagars GK, Smith LG, et al. Preliminary results of a randomized radiotherapy dose-escalation study comparing 70 Gy with 78 Gy for prostate cancer. J Clin Oncol 2000;18:3904–3911.

34. Pollack A, Zagars GK, Starkschall G, et al. Prostate cancer radiation dose response: results of the M.D. Anderson phase III randomized trial. Int J Radiat Oncol Biol Phys 2002;53:1097–1105.

35. Roach M 3rd, Meehan S, Kroll S, et al. Radiotherapy for high grade clinically localized adenocarcinoma of the prostate. J Urol 1996;156:1719–1723.

36. Fiveash JB, Hanks G, Roach M 3rd, et al. 3D conformal radiation therapy (3DCRT) for high grade prostate cancer: a multi-institutional review. Int J Radiat Oncol Biol Phys 2000;47:335–342.

37. Luxton G, Hancock SL, Boyer AL. Dosimetry and radiobiologic model comparison of IMRT and 3D conformal radiotherapy in treatment of carcinoma of the prostate. Int J Radiat Oncol Biol Phys 2004;59:267–284.

38. Chan HM, Zelefsky MJ, Fuks Z, et al. Long-term outcome of high dose intensity modulated radiotherapy for clinically localized prostate cancer. Int J Radiat Oncol Biol Phys 2004;60:S169–S170.

39. Ghilezan M, Yan D, Liang J, et al. Online image-guided intensity-modulated radiotherapy for prostate cancer: how much improvement can we expect? A theoretical assessment of clinical benefits and potential dose escalation by improving precision and accuracy of radiation delivery. Int J Radiat Oncol Biol Phys 2004;60:1602–1610.

40. Yan D, Xu B, Lockman D. The influence of interpatient and intrapatient rectum variation on external beam treatment of prostate cancer. Int J Radiat Oncol Biol Phys 2001;51:1111.

41. Fowler J, Chappell R, Ritter M. Is alpha/beta for prostate tumors really low? Int J Radiat Oncol Biol Phys 2001;50:1021–1031.

42. Duchesne GM, Peters LJ. What is the alpha/beta ratio for prostate cancer? Rationale for hypofractionated high-dose-rate brachytherapy. Int J Radiat Oncol Biol Phys 1999;44:747–748.

43. Deger S, Boehmer D, Turk I, et al. High dose rate brachytherapy of localized prostate cancer. Eur Urol 2002;41:420–426.

44. Martinez A, Gonzalez J, Spencer W, et al. Conformal high dose rate brachytherapy improves biochemical control and cause specific survival in patients with prostate cancer and poor prognostic factors. J Urol 2003;169:974–980.

45. D'Amico AV, Whittington R, Malkowicz B, et al. Biochemical outcome after radical prostatectomy, external beam radiation therapy, or interstitial radiation therapy for clinically localized prostate cancer. JAMA 1998;280:969–974.

46. Stock RG, Cahlon O, Cesaretti JA, et al. Combined modality treatment in the management of high-risk prostate cancer. Int J Radiat Oncol Biol Phys 2004;1352–1359.

47. Sylvester JE, Blasko JC, Grimm PD, et al. Ten-year biochemical relapse-free survival after external beam radiation and brachytherapy for localized prostate cancer: the Seattle experience. Int J Radiat Oncol Biol Phys 2003;57:944–952.

48. Dattoli M, Wallner K, True L, et al. Long-term outcomes after treatment with external beam radiation therapy and palladium 103 for patients with higher risk prostate carcinoma. Cancer 2003;97:979–983.

49. Brandeis JM, Litwin MS, Burnison CM, et al. Quality of life outcomes after brachytherapy for early stage prostate cancer. J Urol 2000;163:851–857.

50. Gelblum DY, Potters L. Rectal complications associated with transperineal interstitial brachytherapy for prostate cancer. Int J Radiat Oncol Biol Phys 2000;48:119–124.

51. DeWeese TL, Shipman JM, Dillehay LE, et al. Sensitivity of human prostatic carcinoma cell lines to low dose rate radiation exposure. J Urol 1998;159:591–598.

52. Furuya Y, Lin XS, Walsh JC, et al. Androgen ablation-induced programmed death of prostatic glandular cells does not involve recruitment into a defective cell cycle or p53 induction. Endocrinology 1995;136:1898–1906.

53. Denmeade SR, Lin XS, Isaacs JT. Role of programmed (apoptotic) cell death during the progression and therapy for prostate cancer. Prostate 1996;28:251–265.

54. Zietman AL, Nakfoor BM, Prince EA, et al. The effect of androgen deprivation and radiation therapy on an androgen-sensitive murine tumor: an in vitro and in vivo study. Cancer J Sci Am 1997;3:31–36.

55. Joon DL, Hasegawa M, Sikes C, et al. Supraadditive apoptotic response of R3327-G rat prostate tumors to androgen ablation and radiation. Int J Radiat Oncol Biol Phys 1997;38:1071–1077.

56. Del Regato J. Radiotherapy for carcinoma of the prostate. A report from the Committee for the Cooperative Study of Radiotherapy for Carcinoma of the Prostate. Colorado Springs, Colo: Penrose Cancer Hospital, 1968.

57. Green N, Bodner H, Broth E, et al. Improved control of bulky prostate carcinoma with sequential estrogen and radiation therapy. Int J Radiat Oncol Biol Phys 1984;10:971–976.

58. Mukamel E, Servadio C, Lurie H. Combined external radiotherapy and hormonal therapy for localized carcinoma of the prostate. Prostate 1983;4:283–287.

59. Pilepich MV, Krall JM, Johnson RJ, et al. Prognostic factors in carcinoma of the prostate-analysis of the RTOG 75-06. Int J Radiat Oncol Biol Phys 1987;13:339–349.

60. Pilepich MV, Krall JM, John MJ, et al. Hormonal cytoreduction in locally advanced carcinoma of the prostate treated with definitive radiotherapy: Preliminary results of RTOG 83-07. Int J Radiat Oncol Biol Phys 1989;16:813–817.

61. Pilepich MV, John MJ, Krall JM, et al. Phase II Radiation Therapy Oncology Group study of hormonal cytoreduction with flutamide and zoladex in locally advanced carcinoma of the prostate treated with definitive radiotherapy. Am J Clin Oncol 1990;13:461–464.

62. Pilepich MV, Krall JM, al-Sarraf M, et al. Androgen deprivation with radiation therapy alone for locally advanced prostatic carcinoma: a randomized comparative trial of the Radiation Therapy Oncology Group. Urology 1995;45:616–623.

63. Pilepich MV, Winter K, John MJ, et al, Phase III radiation therapy oncology group (RTOG) trial 86-10 of androgen deprivation adjuvant to definitive radiotherapy in locally advanced carcinoma of the prostate. Int J Radiat Oncol Biol Phys 2001;50:1243–1252.

64. Lawton CA, Winter K, Murray K, et al. Updated results of the phase III radiation therapy oncology group (RTOG) trial 85-31 evaluating the potential benefit of androgen suppression following standard radiation therapy for unfavorable prognosis carcinoma of the prostate. Int J Radiat Oncol Biol Phys 2001;49:937–946.

65. Bolla M, Collette L, Blank L, et al. Long-term results with immediate androgen suppression and external irradiation in patients with locally advanced prostate cancer (an EORTC study): a phase III randomized trial. Lancet 2002;360:103–108.

66. D'Amico AV, Manola J, Loffredo M, et al. 6-month androgen suppression plus radiation therapy vs radiation therapy alone for patients with clinically localized prostate cancer. JAMA 2004;292:821–827.

67. Holzbeierlein JM, Castle E, Thrasher JB. Complications of androgen deprivation therapy: prevention and treatment. Oncology 2004;18:303–309.

68. Laverdiere J, Gomez JL, Cusan L, et al. Beneficial effect of combination hormonal therapy administered prior and following external beam radiation therapy in localized prostate cancer. Int J Radiat Oncol Biol Phys 1997;37:247–252.

69. Laverdiere J, Nabid A, de Bedoya LD, et al. The efficacy and sequencing of a short course of androgen suppression on freedom from biochemical failure when administered with radiation therapy for T2-T3 prostate cancer. J Urol 2004;171:1137–1140.

70. Hanks GE, Pajak TF, Porter A, et al. Phase III trial of long-term adjuvant androgen deprivation after neoadjuvant hormonal cytoreduction and radiotherapy in locally advanced carcinoma of the prostate: the Radiation Therapy Oncology Group protocol 92-02, J Clin Oncol 2003;21:3972–3978.

71. Roach M, Lu J, Pilepich MV, et al. Predicting long-term survival and the need for hormonal therapy: a meta-analysis of RTOG prostate cancer trials. Int J Radiat Oncol Biol Phys 2000;47:617–627.

72. Horwitz EM, Winter K, Hanks GE, et al. Subset analysis of RTOG 85-31 and 86-10 indicates an advantage for long-term vs. short-term adjuvant hormones for patients with locally advanced nonmetastatic prostate cancer treated with radiation therapy. Int J Radiat Oncol Biol Phys 2001;49:947–956.

73. Gleave ME, Goldenberg SL, Chin JL, et al. Randomized comparative study of 3 versus 8-month neoadjuvant hormonal therapy before radical prostatectomy: biochemical and pathological effects. J Urol 2001;166:500–507.

74. Roach M 3rd, DeSilvio M, Lawton C, et al. Phase III trial comparing whole-pelvic versus prostate-only radiotherapy and neoadjuvant versus adjuvant combined androgen suppression: radiation therapy oncology group 9413. J Clin Oncol 2003,21:1904–1911.

75. Roach M 3rd, Marquez C, Yuo HS, et al. Predicting the risk of lymph node involvement using the pre-treatment prostate specific antigen and Gleason score in men with clinically localized prostate cancer. Int J Radiat Oncol Biol Phys 1994;28:33–37.

76. Chen CT, Valicenti RK, Lu J, et al. Does hormonal therapy influence sexual function in men receiving 3D conformal radiation therapy for prostate cancer? Int J Radiat Oncol Biol Phys 2001;50:591–595.

77. Dearnaley DP, Khoo VS, Norman AR, et al. Comparison of radiation side-effects of conformal and conventional radiotherapy in prostate cancer: a randomised trial. Lancet 1999;353:267–272.

78. Zelefsky MJ, Harrison A. Neoadjuvant androgen ablation prior to radiotherapy for prostate cancer: Reducing the potential morbidity of therapy. Urology 1997;49:38–45.

79. Forman JD, Kumar R, Haas G, et al. Neoadjuvant hormonal downsizing of localized carcinoma of the prostate: Effects on the volume of normal tissue irradiation. Cancer Invest 1995;13:8–15.

80. Yang FE, Chen GTY, Ray P, et al. The potential for normal tissue dose reduction with neoadjuvant hormonal therapy in conformal treatment planning for stage C prostate cancer. Int J Radiat Oncol Biol Phys 1995;33:1009–1017.

81. Bolla M, Gonzalez D, Warde P, et al. Improved survival in patients with locally advanced prostate cancer treated with radiotherapy and goserelin. N Eng J Med 1997;337:295–300.

82. Sanguineti G, Agostinelli S, Foppiano F, et al. Adjuvant androgen deprivation impacts late rectal toxicity after conformal radiotherapy of prostate carcinoma. Br J Cancer 2002;86:1843–1847.

83. Valicenti RK, Winter K, Cox JD, et al. RTOG 94-06: is the addition of neoadjuvant hormonal therapy to dose-escalated 3D conformal radiation therapy for prostate cancer associated with treatment toxicity? Int J Radiat Oncol Biol Phys 2003;57:614–620.

84. Gray H. Anatomy of the Human Body. Philadelphia: Lea & Febiger, 1985.

85. Partin AW, Mangold LA, Lamm DM, et al. Contemporary update of prostate cancer staging nomograms (Partin Tables) for the new millennium. Urology 2001;58:843–848.

86. Roach M 3rd, Marquez C, Yho HS, et al. Predicting the risk of lymph node involvement using the pre-treatment prostate specific antigen and Gleason score in men with clinically localized prostate cancer. Int J Radiat Oncol Biol Phys 1994;28:33–37.

87. Heidenreich A, Varga Z, Von Knobloch R. Extended pelvic lymphadenectomy in patients undergoing radical prostatectomy: high incidence of lymph node metastasis. J Urol 202;167:1681–1686.

88. Rosen E, Cassady JR, Connolly J, et al. Radiotherapy for prostate carcinoma: the JCRT experience (1968–1978). II. Factors related to tumor control and complications. Int J Radiat Oncol Biol Phys 1985;11:723–730.

89. Aristizabal SA, Steinbronn D, Heusinkveld RS. External beam radiotherapy in cancer of the prostate. The University of Arizona experience. Radiother Oncol 1984;1:309–315.

90. Zagars GK, von Eschenbach AC, Johnson DE, et al. Stage C adenocarcinoma of the prostate. An analysis of 551 patients treated with external beam radiation. Cancer 1987;60:1489–1499.

91. McGowan DG. The value of extended field radiation therapy in carcinoma of the prostate. Int J Radiat Oncol Biol Phys 1981;7:1333–1339.

92. Ploysongsang SS, Aron BS, Shehata WM. Radiation therapy in prostate cancer: whole pelvis with prostate boost or small field to prostate? Urology 2002;40:18–26.

93. Seaward SA, Weinberg V, Lewis P, et al. Improved freedom from PSA failure with whole pelvic irradiation for high-risk prostate cancer. Int J Radiat Oncol Biol Phys 1998;42:1055–1062.

94. Bagshaw M. Radiotherapeutic treatment of prostatic carcinoma with pelvic node involvement. Urol Clin N Am 1984;11:297–304.

95. Asbell SO, Krall JM, Pilepich MV, et al. Elective pelvic irradiation in Stage A2, B carcinoma of the prostate: analysis of RTOG 77-06. Int J Radiat Oncol Biol Phys 1988;15:1307–1316.

96. Perez CA, Michalski J, Brown KC, et al. Nonrandomized evaluation of pelvic lymph node irradiation in localized carcinoma of the prostate. Int J Radiat Oncol Biol Phys 1996;36:573–584.

97. Forman JD, Lee Y, Robertson P, Montie JE, et al. Advantages of CT and beam's eye view display to confirm the accuracy of pelvic lymph node irradiation in carcinoma of the prostate. Radiology 1993;186:889–892.

98. Taylor A, Rockall AG, Usher C, et al. Delineation of a reference target volume for pelvic lymph node irradiation using MR imaging with ultrasmall superparamagnetic iron oxide particles. Int J Radiat Oncol Biol Phys 2004;60:S225.

99. Jemal A, Tiwari RC, Murray T, et al. Cancer statistics 2004. CA Cancer J Clin 2004;54:8–29.

100. Guinan P, Stewart AK, Fremgen AM, et al. Patterns of care for metastatic carcinoma of the prostate gland: results of the American College of Surgeons' patient care evaluation study. Prostate Cancer Prostatic Dis 1998;1:315–320.

101. Penson DF, Moul JW, Evans CP, et al. The economic burden of metastatic and prostate specific antigen progression in patients with prostate cancer: findings from a retrospective analysis of health plan data. J Urol 2004;161:2250–2254.

102. Johansson JE, Andren O, Andersson SO, et al. Natural history of early, localized prostate cancer. JAMA 2004;291:2713–2719.

103. Pound CR, Partin AW, Eisenberger MA, et al. Natural history of progression after PSA elevation following radical prostatectomy. JAMA 1999;281:1591–1597.

104. Kahn D, Weiner GJ, Ben-Haim S, et al. Positron emission tomographic measurement of bone marrow blood flow to the pelvis and lumbar vertebrae in young normal adults. Blood 1994;83:958–963. Erratum in Blood 1994;84:3602.

105. Bubendorf L, Schopfer A, Wagner U, et al. Metastatic patterns of prostate cancer: an autopsy study of 1,589 patients. Hum Pathol 2000;31:578–583.

106. Batson OV. The role of the vertebral veins in metastatic processes. Ann Intern Med 1942;16:38–45.

107. Dodds PR, Caride VJ, Lytton B. The role of the vertebral veins in the dissemination of prostatic carcinoma. J Urol 1981;126:753–755.

108. Roodman GD. Mechanisms of bone metastasis. N Engl J Med 2004;350:1655–1664.

109. Cooper CR, Pienta KJ. Cell adhesion and chemotaxis in prostate cancer metastasis to bone: a minireview. Prostate Cancer Prostatic Dis 2000;3:6–12.

110. Hauschka PV, Mavrakos AE, Iafrati MD, et al. Growth factors in bone matrix: isolation of multiple types by affinity chromatography on heparin-sepharose. J Biol Chem 1986;261:12665–12674.

111. Galasko CSB. Mechanisms of lytic and blastic metastatic disease of bone. Clin Orthop 1982;169:20–27.

112. Jacob K, Webber M, Benayahu D, et al. Osteonectin promotes prostate cancer cell migration and invasion: a possible mechanism for metastasis to bone. Cancer Res 1999;59:4453–4457.

113. Dodwell DJ. Malignant bone resorption: cellular and biochemical mechanisms. Ann Oncol 1992;3:257–267.

114. Schneider A, Kalikin LM, Mattos AC, et al. Bone turnover mediates preferential localization of prostate cancer in the skeleton. Endocrinology 2005;146:1727–1736.

115. Watt KW, Lee PJ, M'Timkulu T, et al. Human prostate-specific antigen: structural and functional similarity with serine proteases. Proc Natl Acad Sci USA 1986;83:3166–3170.

116. Fielder PJ, Rosenfeld RG, Graves HC, et al. Biochemical analysis of prostate specific antigen-proteolyzed insulin-like growth factor finding protein-3. Growth Regul 1994;4:164–172.

117. Coleman RF. Skeletal complications of malignancy. Cancer 1997;80:1588–1594.

118. Jonler M, Nielsen OS, Groenvold M, et al. Quality of life in patients with skeletal metastases of prostate cancer and status prior to start of endocrine therapy: results from the Scandinavian Prostate Cancer Group study 5. Scan J Urol Nephrol 2005;39:42–48.

119. Sartor OA, DiBiase SJ. Management of bone metastases in advanced prostate cancer. UpToDate Online 12.3, http://www.uptodate.com.

120. Tong D, Gillick L, Hendrickson FR. The palliation of symptomatic osseous metastases: final results of the Study by the Radiation Therapy Oncology Group. Cancer 1982;50:893–899.

121. Arcangeli G, Giovinazzo G, Saracino B, et al. Radiation therapy in the management of symptomatic bone metastases: the effect of total dose and histology on pain relief and response duration. Int J Radiat Oncol Biol Phys 1998;42:1119–1126.

122. Zelefsky MJ, Scher HI, Forman JD, et al. Palliative hemiskeletal irradiation for widespread metastatic prostate cancer: a comparison of single dose and fractionated regimens. Int J Radiat Oncol Biol Phys 1989;17:1281–1285.

123. Franzen L, Nyman J, Hagberg H, et al. A randomised placebo controlled study with ondansetron in patients undergoing fractionated radiotherapy. Ann Oncol 1996;7:587–592.

124. Blitzer PH. Reanalysis of the RTOG study of the palliation of symptomatic osseous metastasis. Cancer 1985;55:1468–1472.

125. Okawa T, Kita M, Goto M, et al. Randomized prospective clinical study of small, large and twice-a-day fraction radiotherapy for painful bone metastases. Radiother Oncol 1988;13:99–104.

126. Madsen EL. Painful bone metastasis: efficacy of radiotherapy assessed by the patients: a randomized trial comparing 4 Gy × 6 versus 10 Gy × 2. Int J Radiat Oncol Biol Phys 1983;9:1775–1779.

127. Martin WM. Multiple daily fractions of radiation in the palliation of pain from bone metastases. Clin Radiol 1983;34:245–249.

128. Cole DJ. A randomized trial of a single treatment versus conventional fractionation in the palliative radiotherapy of painful bone metastases. Clin Oncol 1989;1:59–62.

129. Nielsen OS, Bentzen SM, Sandberg E, et al. Randomized trial of single dose versus fractionated palliative radiotherapy of bone metastases. Radiother Oncol 1998;47:233–240.

130. Yarnold JR. 8 Gy single fraction radiotherapy for the treatment of metastatic skeletal pain: randomised comparison with a multifraction schedule over 12 months of patient follow-up. Bone Pain Trial Working Party. Radiother Oncol 1999;52:111–121.

131. Steenland E, Leer JW, van Houwelingen H, et al. The effect of a single fraction compared to multiple fractions on painful bone metastases: a global analysis of the Dutch Bone Metastasis Study. Radiother Oncol 1999;52:101–109.

132. Hartsell WF, Scott C, Bruner CW, et al. Phase III randomized trial of 8 Gy in 1 fraction vs 30 Gy in 10 fractions for palliation of painful bone metastases: preliminary results of RTOG 97-14. Int J Radiat Oncol Biol Phys 2003;57:S124.

133. Bruner DW, Winter K, Hartsell A. Prospective Health-Related Quality of Life Valuations (Utilities) of 8 Gy in 1 fraction vs 30 Gy in 10 fractions for palliation of painful bone metastases: preliminary results of RTOG 97-14. Int J Radiat Oncol Biol Phys 2004;60:S142.

134. Wu JS, Wong R, Johnston M, et al. Meta-analysis of dose-fractionation radiotherapy trials for the palliation of painful bone metastases. Int J Radiat Oncol Biol Phys 2003;55:594–605.

135. Wai MS, Mike S, Ines H, et al. Palliation of metastatic bone pain: single fraction versus multifraction radiotherapy – a systematic review of the randomised trials. Cochrane Database Syst Rev 2004;2:CD004721.

136. Konski A. Radiotherapy is a cost-effective palliative treatment for patients with bone metastasis from prostate cancer. Int J Radiat Oncol Biol Phys 2004;60:1373–1378.

137. Ben-Josef E, Shamsa F, Williams AO, et al. Radiotherapeutic management of osseous metastases: a survey of current patterns of care, Int J Radiat Oncol Biol Phys 1998;40:915–921.

138. Chow E, Danjoux C, Wong R. Palliation of bone metastases: a survey of patterns of practice among Canadian radiation oncologists. Radiother Oncol 2000;56:305–314.

139. Fleisch H. Bisphosphonates: pharmacology and use in the treatment of tumor-induced hypercalcaemic and metastatic bone disease. Drugs 1991;42:919–944.

140. Lewington VJ. Bone-seeking radionuclides for therapy. J Nucl Med 2005;46:38S–47S.

141. Collins C, Eary JF, Donaldson G, et al. Samarium-153 -EDTMP in bone metastases of hormone refractory prostate carcinoma: a phase I/II trial. J Nucl Med 1993;34:1839–1844.

142. Farhanghi M, Holmes RA, Volkert WA, et al. Samarium-153-EDTMP: pharmacokinetic, toxicity and pain response using an escalating dose schedule in treatment of metastatic bone cancer. J Nucl Med 1992;33:1451–1458.

143. Dickie GJ, Macfarlane D. Strontium and samarium therapy for bone metastases from prostate carcinoma. Australas Radiol 1999;43:476–479.

144. Scarantino CW, Caplan R, Rotman M, et al. A phase I/II study to evaluate the effect of fractionated hemibody irradiation in the treatment of osseous metastases—RTOG 88-22. Int J Radiat Oncol Biol Phys 1996;36:37–48.

145. Salazar OM, Sandhu T, da Motta NW, et al. Fractionated half-body irradiation (HBI) for the rapid palliation of widespread, symptomatic, metastatic bone disease:a randomized Phase III trial of the International Atomic Energy Agency. Int J Radiat Oncol Biol Phys. 2001;50:765–775.

146. Salazar OM, DaMotta NW, Bridgman SM, et al. Fractionated half-body irradiation for pain palliation in widely metastatic cancers: comparison with single dose. Int J Radiat Oncol Biol Phys 1996;36:49–60.

147. Poulter CA, Cosmatos D, Rubin P. A report of RTOG 8206: a phase III study of whether the addition of single dose hemibody irradiation to standard fractionated local field irradiation is more effective than local field irradiation alone in the treatment of symptomatic osseous metastases. Int J Radiat Oncol Biol Phys 1992;23:207–214.

148. Dearnaley DP, Bayly RJ, A'Hern RP, et al. Palliation of bone metastases in prostate cancer. Hemibody irradiation or strontium-89? Clin Oncol 1992;4:101–107.

149. Salazar OM, Rubin P, Hendrickson FR. Single-dose half-body irradiation for palliation of multiple bone metastases from solid tumors. Final Radiation Therapy Oncology Group report. Cancer. 1986;58:29–36.

150. Mithal NP, Needham PR, Hoskin PJ. Retreatment with radiotherapy for painful bone metastases. Int J Radiat Oncol Biol Phys 1994;29:1011–1014.

151. Hayashi S, Hoshi H, Iida T. Reirradiation with local-field radiotherapy for painful bone metastases. Radiat Med 2002;20:231–236.

152. Grosu AL, Andratschke N, Nieder C, et al. Retreatment of the spinal cord with palliative radiotherapy. Int J Radiat Oncol Biol Phys 2002;52:1288–1292.

153. Song DY, Kavanagh BD, Benedict SH, Schefter TA. Stereotactic Body Radiation Therapy: rationale, techniques, application, and optimization. Oncology (Huntington), 2004;18:1419–1430.

154. Milker-Zabel S, Zabel A, Thilmann C, et al. Clinical results of retreatment of vertebral bone metastases by stereotactic conformal radiotherapy and intensity-modulated radiotherapy. Int J Radiat Oncol Biol Phys 2003;55:162–167.

155. Gerszten PC, Ozhasoglu C, Burton SA. CyberKnife frameless stereotactic radiosurgery for spinal lesions: clinical experience in 125 cases. Neurosurgery 2004;55:89–98.

156. Harrington KD. Orthopaedic management of pelvic and extremity lesions. Clin Orthop Relat Res 1995;312:136–147.

157. Townsend PW, Smalley SR, Cozad SC, et al. Role of postoperative radiation therapy after stabilization of fractures caused by metastatic disease. Int J Radiat Oncol Biol Phys 1995;31:43–49.

158. Regine WF, Tibbs PA, Young A, et al. Metastatic spinal cord compression: a randomized trial of direct decompressive surgical resection plus radiotherapy vs. radiotherapy alone. Int J Radiat Oncol Biol Phys 2003;57S:S125.

Use of bisphosphonates in the management of osseous metastases 102

Roger S Kirby, Jonathan P Coxon

INTRODUCTION

Bone is by far the most common site for metastases in prostate cancer, accounting for considerable morbidity (Figure 102.1). Until recently, there have been few viable options for the treatment of the patient with hormone-refractory metastatic disease. This chapter examines the pathophysiology underlying the development of bone metastases. It also summarizes some of the clinical approaches for the management of this common condition, focusing on recent evidence supporting the use of one of the most promising groups of pharmacological agents, the third-generation bisphosphonates.

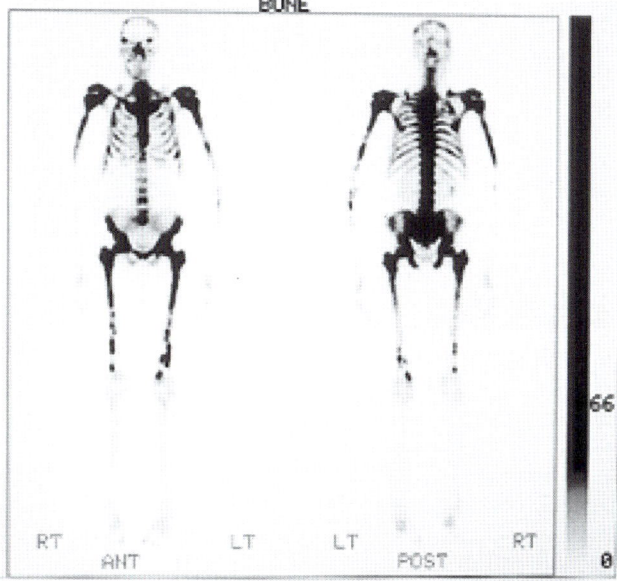

Fig. 102.1
Bone metastases from prostate cancer shown on radionuclide bone scan.

ETIOLOGY AND IMPACT OF PROSTATE CANCER-RELATED BONE METASTASES

Prostate cancer is the most commonly diagnosed malignancy in males in the UK, with nearly 25,000 cases being reported in 1999.[1] Prostate cancer-related morbidity and mortality are closely associated with the formation of metastases. Bone is the preferred site for these metastases, and estimates indicate that bone metastases are present in more than 80% of men with advanced prostate cancer.[2,3] A UK study has shown that bone metastases are present in up to 50% of men at the time of first presentation.[4]

Considerable morbidity arises from the various complications from bone metastases, and it is estimated that the average frequency of a "skeletal related event" in patients with bone metastases is 3 to 4 months, with these events invariably leading to a reduced quality of life.[5] Common presentations include pain, spinal cord compression, pathologic fracture, and abnormalities in serum calcium levels.[6] Patients with hormone-refractory metastatic prostate cancer are particularly prone to incapacitating progressive bone disease.[7]

The normal resculpturing of bone is governed by the coupled processes of bone resorption and formation. Modeling occurs in localized areas of cortical and trabecular bone known as bone metabolic units. Osteoclast-mediated resorption usually takes approximately 7 to 10 days, while the subsequent formation phase, governed by osteoblasts, lasts approximately 3 months (Figure 102.2). Local "coupling" factors produced in the bone marrow regulate the remodeled bone.[8]

The rich milieu of growth factors in the bone environment provide an attractive "soil" for the seeding of certain tumor cells. In the presence of such cells, factors from tumor-induced breakdown of bone stimulate growth of further cancer cells, which in turn leads to further increases in bone resorption (Figure 102.3). This has been described as the vicious cycle.[8] As an example, tumor cells have been shown to release parathyroid hormone-related peptide (PTHrP), which stimulates osteoclastic resorption, via messaging from the osteoblast.[9] Resultant osteolysis releases several bone-derived growth factors, such as transforming growth factor-β (TGFβ). Normally, TGFβ serves to limit bone resorption via a negative feedback mechanism, but in the bone metastasis TGFβ stimulates invading tumor cells, partly accounting for this vicious cycle.[10]

Prostate cancer bone metastases usually appear on radiographs as areas of increased bone density, being principally sclerotic in nature. This suggests the occurrence of osteoblast-mediated excessive bone formation, in response to the presence of tumor cells. However, biochemical and histomorphometric studies indicate that osteolysis (excessive bone destruction) is also concurrently increased, and probably represents a vital initial step in the establishment of the metastases.[6,7,11,12] For example, recent studies using biochemical indices of bone turnover in patients with prostate cancer have found that, although the disease is characterized by osteoblastic metastases, there is also a direct correlation between skeletal metastases and bone resorption markers.[13,14] Indeed, the excretion of these indices was better correlated than plasma alkaline phosphatase, which is an accepted index of bone formation. The classic sclerotic bone lesions seen in prostate cancer represent an uncoupling of normal bone resorption and deposition shifting the balance towards new matrix formation and mineralization. It is now largely accepted that osteolysis is an important component of the influence of malignancy on bone, even when profound increases in new bone formation are also observed.[15] Therefore, it follows that interfering with the process of osteolysis could have an important influence on the development of prostate cancer metastases.

CURRENT TREATMENT OPTIONS FOR BONE METASTASES

Given the nature of the vicious cycle described above, options that can be considered for the treatment of metastatic bone disease are: 1) directly reducing tumor cell proliferation, for example, by direct inhibition of growth factors and cytokines; 2) antagonizing the effect of tumor cells on the host; or 3) a combination of these. Direct antitumor treatment options include chemotherapy, surgery, endocrine therapy, or radiotherapy. In practice, chemotherapy has for many years had no established role in prostate cancer, but encouraging results are

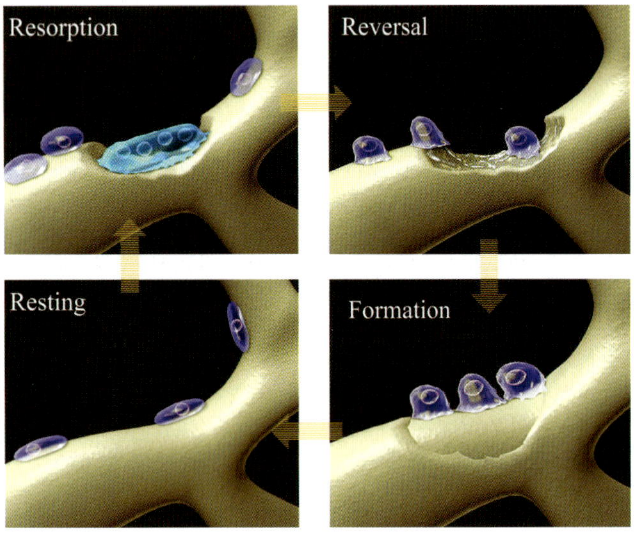

Fig. 102.2

Normal bone remodeling. Resorption—stimulated osteoblast precursors release factors that induce osteoclast differentiation and activity. Osteoclasts remove bone mineral and matrix, creating an erosion cavity. Reversal—mononuclear cells prepare bone surface for new osteoblasts to begin forming bone. Formation—successive waves of osteoblasts synthesize an organic matrix to replace resorbed bone and fill the cavity with new bone. Resting—bone surface is covered with flattened lining cells. A prolonged resting period follows with little cellular activity until a new remodeling cycle begins.

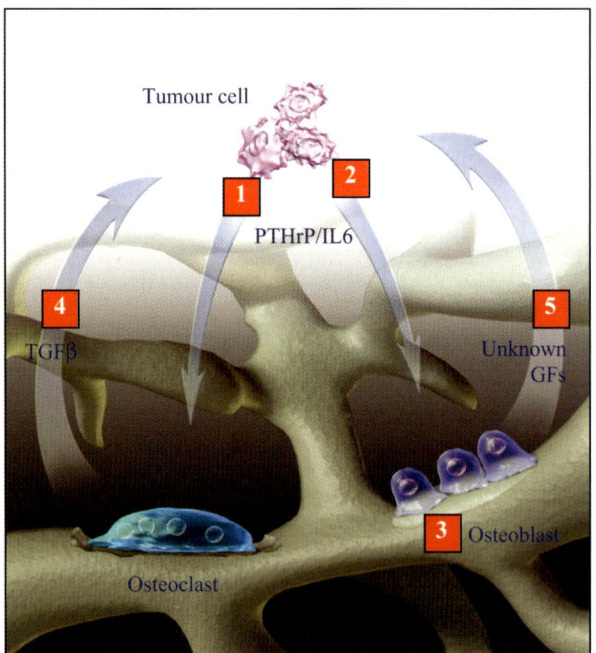

Fig. 102.3

Pathogenesis of bone metastases. Factors are released by tumor cells that stimulate both osteoclast (1) and osteoblast (2) activity. Excessive new bone formation (3) occurs around tumor cell deposits, resulting in low bone strength and potential vertebral collapse. Osteoclastic (4) and osteoblastic (5) activity releases growth factors that stimulate tumor cell growth, perpetuating the cycle of bone resorption and abnormal bone growth. (GFs, growth factors; IL6, interleukin 6; PTHrP, parathyroid hormone-related peptide; TGFβ, transforming growth factor-β.)

now indicating some benefit in the most advanced cases, with agents such as mitoxantrone,[16,17] estramustine,[18,19] and in particular, docetaxel,[20–24] thalidomide.[25] Surgical tumor removal is not appropriate in the metastatic setting. For many years, endocrine therapy has represented the mainstay of treatment for the patient with advanced prostate cancer. When the hormone-refractory state has been reached though, a palliative approach is often sought. Radiotherapy and radiopharmaceuticals can provide local control of symptoms. Calcitonin or gallium nitrate, as indirect antitumor treatments, are occasionally used in a palliative setting for medical control of hypercalcemia, though this condition is rare in prostate cancer.[5] Otherwise, there have been very few options that have proved beneficial in this setting. There is, therefore, a great deal of interest in seeking out alternative therapies for the large number of men suffering with metastatic prostate cancer.

BISPHOSPHONATES: EVOLUTION OF A THERAPEUTIC THEORY

Bisphosphonates are a well-established class of drugs that have been known for many years to inhibit bone turnover, and have become established therapeutic options in the treatment of diseases such as Paget's disease, osteoporosis, and general tumor-associated bone disease (such as hypercalcemia).

The structure of these drugs is characterized by a central P-C-P bond, which promotes their binding to the mineralized bone matrix, and two variable R chains that determine the relative potency, side effects, and the precise mechanism of action (Figure 102.4). Following administration, bisphosphonates bind strongly to

exposed bone mineral around resorbing osteoclasts, leading to very high local concentrations (possibly up to 1000 µM) in the resorption lacunae.[26]

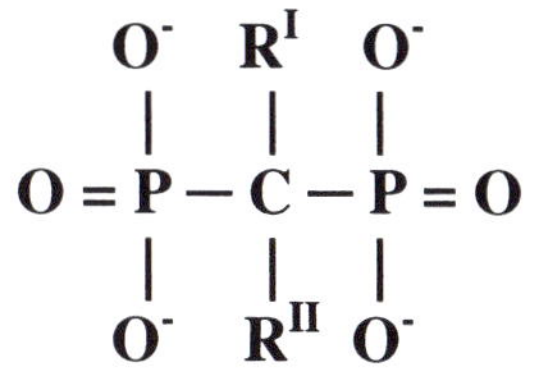

Bisphosphonates have been shown to reduce bone turnover by primarily inhibiting osteoclast function. It has been proposed that these drugs can be thought of as working at three levels.[27] At the tissue level, they decrease bone turnover via initial inhibition of bone resorption, with suppressed bone formation following as a consequence of this. At the cellular level, bisphosphonates exert their activity principally via actions on osteoclasts, inhibiting their formation, migration, and osteolytic activity, as well as directly inducing apoptosis. It has been shown that bisphosphonates also act partly via modulation of signaling from osteoblasts to osteoclasts (Figure 102.5).[28] At the molecular level, the mode of action of bisphosphonates depends on their structure. Non-nitrogen-containing bisphosphonates (in which the R chains contains no N atoms) are metabolized to non-hydrolysable ATP analogs, which become toxic as they accumulate.[29] The more recently developed and more potent nitrogen-containing bisphosphonates act via inhibition of the mevalonate pathway.[30,31] This pathway usually provides the cell with lipids that are required for the normal post-translational modification of GTP-binding proteins, the functions of which are essential for many normal cellular processes.

The action of bisphosphonates on osteoclasts alone represented an initial rationale for investigating their potential use in prostate cancer-associated bone disease, as a reduction in osteoclast activity would reduce the release of growth factors in the bone environment and make it a less fertile soil for the seeding of tumor cells, as indicated above.[32]

Early animal work in the 1980s demonstrated that the bisphosphonates clodronate and etidronate inhibited tumor-mediated osteolysis induced by implanted prostate cancer cells.[33–35] A later exciting development came when in-vitro work established that bisphosphonates also act directly on tumor cells themselves. They have been shown to inhibit cell proliferation and viability, and induce apoptosis in a number of cancer cell lines, including prostate cancer.[36–40] Work in our center with breast cancer cells provided early evidence that inhibition of the mevalonate pathway was again central to the observed apoptotic

$$O=P-C-P=O$$

with structure:

$$
\begin{array}{ccccc}
O^- & & R^I & & O^- \\
| & & | & & | \\
O= & P & - C & - P & =O \\
| & & | & & | \\
O^- & & R^{II} & & O^-
\end{array}
$$

Fig. 102.4
Schematic molecular structure of bisphosphonates.

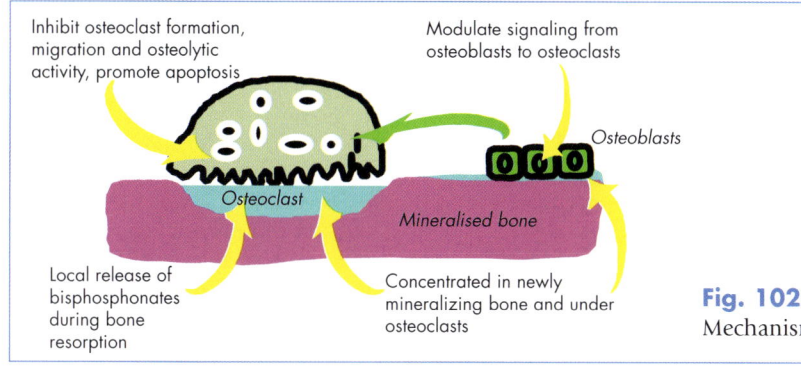

Inhibit osteoclast formation, migration and osteolytic activity, promote apoptosis

Modulate signaling from osteoblasts to osteoclasts

Osteoblasts

Osteoclast

Mineralised bone

Local release of bisphosphonates during bone resorption

Concentrated in newly mineralizing bone and under osteoclasts

Fig. 102.5
Mechanisms of action of bisphosphonates.

effects.[41] We recently published similar results for various prostate cancer cell lines,[38] and provided evidence that the resultant apoptosis was dependent on the activation of caspases. Work in our laboratory has confirmed an apoptotic effect on prostate cancer cells at concentrations that are likely to be physiologically relevant.[42] Other work has shown bisphosphonates to inhibit the adhesion of cancer cells to bone slices,[43,44] and to inhibit their invasion through extracellular matrices.[45,46]

In addition to the work outlined above, a number of clinical studies have investigated the usefulness of bisphosphonates in various settings. The results of several small pilot studies encouraged breast cancer investigators to evaluate early-generation bisphosphonates, using either regular intravenous infusions of pamidronate, enteric-coated oral pamidronate, or either oral or parenteral clodronate. A reduction in skeletal morbidity was usually reported. There were initially rather fewer studies in the prostate cancer setting, though some early work showed reductions in bone pain with clodronate,[47,48] though was not later borne out in randomized studies with this drug.[49,50] Early small-scale studies with pamidronate provided encouraging signs of its potential benefit,[51,52] but it was several years before a well-designed randomized study was published on the use of later-generation bisphosphonates in prostate cancer.

DEVELOPMENT OF MORE MODERN BISPHOSPHONATES

Pharmacologic advances have led to several newer bisphosphonates being developed in recent years. The question of whether bisphosphonate potency is directly associated with therapeutic efficacy was investigated in work by van der Pluijm et al.[44] They demonstrated that the relative order of potency of six bisphosphonates (etidronate, clodronate, pamidronate, olpadronate, alendronate, and ibandronate) in inhibiting the adhesion of cancer cells to cortical and trabecular bone corresponded to their relative antiresorptive potencies in vivo as well as their ranking in in-vitro bone resorption assays, with predictive value for their clinical efficacy.

It is, therefore, reasonable to suggest that using more potent bisphosphonates could simplify treatment and possibly improve the therapeutic effectiveness of bisphosphonate therapy. Potencies of various bisphosphonates discovered to date are shown in Table 102.1.[53]

The most recent group of bisphosphonates to be developed is the so-called third-generation, the most potent of which is zoledronic acid. Recent large targeted studies indicate that this agent could help clinicians to effectively manage bone metastases in prostate cancer patients.

The most noteworthy trial, whose first results were published by Saad et al in 2002, investigated 643 patients with hormone-refractory prostate cancer and a history of bone metastases. These subjects were randomized to receive a double-blind treatment regimen of intravenous zoledronic acid at either 8 mg (n = 221) or 4 mg (n = 214), or placebo (n = 208), every 3 weeks for 15 months. Infusions were given over 15 minutes. During the trial, renal safety concerns merited the reduction of the 8 mg dose to doses of 4 mg.[54] Primary efficacy measures included proportion of patients with skeletal-related events, time to first event, skeletal morbidity rate, pain and analgesic scores, and disease progression. Safety analyses were also performed.

Results have recently been presented with follow-up extended to 24 months.[55] The study showed that patients receiving 4 mg zoledronic acid experienced 11% fewer skeletal-related events than the placebo cohort (38% versus 49%; p = 0.028). Median time to first skeletal event was 488 days with placebo, and 321 days for patients receiving zoledronic acid 4 mg (p = 0.009). This represents a difference of more than 5 months. The placebo group also witnessed higher increases in pain and analgesic scores. Median survival was extended by 77 days in patients treated with 4 mg zoledronic acid compared with placebo, a non-significant difference. Zoledronic acid was well tolerated, and, although renal function deterioration was seen in approximately 20% of patients in the 8 mg cohort compared with placebo, the 4 mg group showed a relative risk ratio of only 1.07 (p = 0.882).

The authors concluded that in patients with metastatic prostate cancer, treatment with 4 mg zoledronic acid every 3 weeks reduces skeletal-related events, compared with placebo. Further, they confirmed that at this recommended dose and regimen, the benefit-to-risk ratio is acceptable for patients with hormone-refractory prostate cancer metastatic to bone. They proposed that further work is warranted to investigate earlier intervention with zoledronic acid, such as in patients with advanced prostate cancer and rising PSA on endocrine therapy, who have not yet developed metastases. It should be noted though that one such study (Novartis Protocol 704) had to be prematurely closed when an unexpected low frequency of events was observed. Other trials are proposed or underway, under the auspices of the European

Table 102.1 Relative potencies of bisphosphonates. Measured on a molar basis in an in-vivo assay, namely the inhibitory activity on bone resorption induced by 1,25-dihydroxyvitamin D3 in the thyroparathyroidectomized rat[50]

Bisphosphonate	Relative potency
Clodronate	0.05
Pamidronate	1
Olpadronate	2.8
Alendronate	7.4
Risedronate	35.9
Ibandronate	43.6
Zoledronate	847

Organisation for Research and Treatment of Cancer (EORTC), European Association of Urology (EAU) and the Medical Research Council (MRC). These look at the potential benefit of zoledronic acid in hormone-naïve patients who have not developed metastases but who are at high risk of doing so. The MRC trial ("STAMPEDE," looking in addition at celecoxib and docetaxel) is also recruiting those who have had adjuvant or neo-adjuvant hormonal therapy, and those with metastases.

That reducing skeletal-related events (SREs) in prostate cancer patients with bone metastases may well also be economically beneficial is suggested by work that has shown, in the Netherlands at least, around 50% of the total cost of care for such patients is directly attributable to the treatment of SREs.[56]

The results of the study by Saad et al compare favorably to those recently published from the MRC Pr05 trial.[57] This looked at the use of oral clodronate, a first-generation bisphosphonate, in patients with bone metastases who had just started or were responding to first-line therapy. While a tendency towards increased bone progression-free survival was seen with 2080 mg/day clodronate, this difference was not statistically significant. The clodronate group reported significantly more gastrointestinal problems and increased lactate dehydrogenase levels, prompting a significant number of dose adjustments in this group.

A further potential benefit of bisphosphonate treatment is related to the bone loss that is known to occur in prostate cancer patients. It has been shown that many patients with advanced prostate cancer have a low bone mineral density at diagnosis, even before commencing androgen deprivation therapy.[58,59] This is of course compounded by the known osteoporotic effects of luteinizing hormone releasing hormone (LHRH) analogs, to which many patients are now being exposed for longer durations. Recently published results showed that, in patients without bone metastases receiving androgen deprivation therapy, 4 mg zoledronic acid significantly increased the bone mineral density, while a decrease was seen in the placebo group (p < 0.001).[60] A previous study using the second-generation bisphosphonate pamidronate failed to show an increase in bone mineral density,[61] though it did reduce bone loss when compared to placebo.

Zoledronic acid is the only bisphosphonate with the clinically proven indication for use in patients with bone metastases to prevent skeletal related events. Its ease of administration, as a short 15-minute intravenous infusion, is especially important considering that previous-generation bisphosphonates, such as pamidronate, have a standard infusion time of 2 to 4 hours. Such longer infusion times would clearly incur costs in terms of clinical staff time and healthcare resources. The simpler mode of administration with zoledronic acid means that clinicians may shortly be able to offer community-based bisphosphonate treatment, which should benefit health-care budgets and patients alike. However, further research is required until this can become the standard of care.

CONCLUSIONS

- Bone is the most important metastatic site in prostate cancer.
- Skeletal complications, including fractures, are relatively common in prostate cancer.
- Accelerated bone resorption is an important component of the pathophysiology of bone metastases.
- Bisphosphonates are potent, safe, and well-tolerated inhibitors of bone resorption.
- Skeletal morbidity is significantly reduced by administration of bisphosphonates.
- Studies suggest that potent, third-generation bisphosphonates could play a vital role in the management of bone metastases from prostate cancer.

REFERENCES

1. www.cancerresearchuk.org/statistics/.
2. Carlin BI, Andriole GL. The natural history, skeletal complications, and management of bone metastases in patients with prostate carcinoma. Cancer 2000;88:2989–2994.
3. Pentyala SN, Lee J, Hsieh K, et al. Prostate cancer: a comprehensive review. Med Oncol 2000;17:85–105.
4. George NJ. Natural history of localised prostatic cancer managed by conservative therapy alone. Lancet 1988;1:494–497.
5. Coleman RE. Uses and abuses of bisphosphonates. Ann Oncol 2000;11 Suppl 3:179–184.
6. Scher HI, Chung LW. Bone metastases: improving the therapeutic index. Semin Oncol 1994;21:630–656.
7. Berruti A, Dogliotti L, Bitossi R, et al. Incidence of skeletal complications in patients with bone metastatic prostate cancer and hormone refractory disease: predictive role of bone resorption and formation markers evaluated at baseline. J Urol 2000;164:1248–1253.
8. Mundy GR. Bone resorption and turnover in health and disease. Bone 1987;8 Suppl 1:S9–16.
9. Thomas RJ, Guise TA, Yin JJ, et al. Breast cancer cells interact with osteoblasts to support osteoclast formation. Endocrinology 1999;140:4451–4458.
10. Guise TA, Mundy GR. Cancer and bone. Endocr Rev 1998;19:18–54.
11. Clarke NW, McClure J, George NJ. Morphometric evidence for bone resorption and replacement in prostate cancer. Br J Urol 1991;68:74–80.
12. Garnero P, Buchs N, Zekri J, et al. Markers of bone turnover for the management of patients with bone metastases from prostate cancer. Br J Cancer 2000;82:858–864.
13. Ikeda I, Miura T, Kondo I. Pyridinium cross-links as urinary markers of bone metastases in patients with prostate cancer. Br J Urol 1996;77:102–106.
14. Takeuchi S, Arai K, Saitoh H, et al. Urinary pyridinoline and deoxypyridinoline as potential markers of bone metastasis in patients with prostate cancer. J Urol 1996;156:1691–1695.
15. Goltzman D. Mechanisms of the development of osteoblastic metastases. Cancer 1997;80:1581–1587.
16. Kantoff PW, Halabi S, Conaway M, et al. Hydrocortisone with or without mitoxantrone in men with hormone-refractory prostate cancer: results of the cancer and leukemia group B 9182 study. J Clin Oncol 1999;17:2506–2513.
17. Tannock IF, Osoba D, Stockler MR, et al. Chemotherapy with mitoxantrone plus prednisone or prednisone alone for symptomatic

hormone-resistant prostate cancer: a Canadian randomized trial with palliative end points. J Clin Oncol 1996;14:1756–1764.

18. Savarese DM, Halabi S, Hars V, et al. Phase II study of docetaxel, estramustine, and low-dose hydrocortisone in men with hormone-refractory prostate cancer: a final report of CALGB 9780. Cancer and Leukemia Group B. J Clin Oncol 2001;19:2509–2516.

19. Smith PH, Suciu S, Robinson MR, et al. A comparison of the effect of diethylstilbestrol with low dose estramustine phosphate in the treatment of advanced prostatic cancer: final analysis of a phase III trial of the European Organization for Research on Treatment of Cancer. J Urol 1986;136:619–623.

20. Beer TM, Pierce WC, Lowe BA, et al. Phase II study of weekly docetaxel in symptomatic androgen-independent prostate cancer. Ann Oncol 2001;12:1273–1279.

21. Berry W, Dakhil S, Gregurich MA, et al. Phase II trial of single-agent weekly docetaxel in hormone-refractory, symptomatic, metastatic carcinoma of the prostate. Semin Oncol 2001;28:8–15.

22. Picus J, Schultz M. Docetaxel (Taxotere) as monotherapy in the treatment of hormone-refractory prostate cancer: preliminary results. Semin Oncol 1999;26:14–18.

23. Eisenberger MA, De Wit R, Berry W, et al. A multicenter phase III comparison of docetaxel (D) + prednisone (P) and mitoxantrone (MTZ) + P in patients with hormone-refractory prostate cancer (HRPC). ASCO 2004;Abstract 4.

24. Petrylak DP, Tangen C, Hussain M, et al. SWOG 99–16: Randomized phase III trial of docetaxel (D)/estramustine (E) versus mitoxantrone (M)/prednisone(P) in men with androgen-independent prostate cancer (AIPCA). ASCO 2004;Abstract 3.

25. Figg WD, Arlen P, Gulley J, et al. A randomized phase II trial of docetaxel (taxotere) plus thalidomide in androgen-independent prostate cancer. Semin Oncol 2001;28:62–66.

26. Sato M, Grasser W, Endo N, et al. Bisphosphonate action. Alendronate localization in rat bone and effects on osteoclast ultrastructure. J Clin Invest 1991;88:2095–2105.

27. Fleisch H. Bisphosphonates: mechanisms of action. Endocr Rev 1998;19:80–100.

28. Vitte C, Fleisch H, Guenther HL. Bisphosphonates induce osteoblasts to secrete an inhibitor of osteoclast-mediated resorption. Endocrinology 1996;137:2324–2333.

29. Frith JC, Monkkonen J, Blackburn GM, et al. Clodronate and liposome-encapsulated clodronate are metabolized to a toxic ATP analog, adenosine 5′-(beta, gamma-dichloromethylene) triphosphate, by mammalian cells in vitro. J Bone Miner Res 1997;12:1358–1367.

30. Amin D, Cornell SA, Gustatson SK, et al. Bisphosphonates used for the treatment of bone disorders inhibit squalene synthase and cholesterol biosynthesis. J Lipid Res 1992;33:1657–1663.

31. Luckman SP, Hughes DE, Coxon FP, et al. Nitrogen-containing bisphosphonates inhibit the mevalonate pathway and prevent post-translational prenylation of GTP-binding proteins, including Ras. J Bone Min Res 1998;13:581–589.

32. Green JR, Clezardin P. Mechanisms of bisphosphonate effects on osteoclasts, tumor cell growth, and metastasis. Am J Clin Oncol 2002;25:S3–S9.

33. Nemoto R, Kanoh S, Koiso K, et al. Establishment of a model to evaluate inhibition of bone resorption induced by human prostate cancer cells in nude mice. J Urol 1988;140:875–879.

34. Pollard M, Luckert PH. Effects of dichloromethylene diphosphonate on the osteolytic and osteoblastic effects of rat prostate adenocarcinoma cells. J Natl Cancer Inst 1985;75:949–954.

35. Pollard M, Luckert PH. The beneficial effects of diphosphonate and piroxicam on the osteolytic and metastatic spread of rat prostate carcinoma cells. Prostate 1986;8:81–86.

36. Aparicio A, Gardner A, Tu Y, et al. In vitro cytoreductive effects on multiple myeloma cells induced by bisphosphonates. Leukemia 1998;12:220–229.

37. Lee MV, Fong EM, Singer FR, et al. Bisphosphonate treatment inhibits the growth of prostate cancer cells. Cancer Res 2001;61:2602–2608.

38. Oades GM, Senaratne SG, Clarke JA, et al. Nitrogen containing bisphosphonates induce apoptosis and inhibit the mevalonate pathway, impairing Ras membrane localization in prostate cancer cells. J Urol 2003;170:246–252.

39. Senaratne SG, Pirianov G, Mansi JL, et al. Bisphosphonates induce apoptosis in human breast cancer cell lines. Br J Cancer 2000;82:1459–1468.

40. Shipman CM, Rogers MJ, Apperley JF, et al. Bisphosphonates induce apoptosis in human myeloma cell lines: a novel anti-tumour activity. Br J Haematol 1997;98:665–672.

41. Senaratne SG, Mansi JL, Colston KW. The bisphosphonate zoledronic acid impairs Ras membrane (correction of impairs membrane) localisation and induces cytochrome c release in breast cancer cells. Br J Cancer 2002;86:1479–1486.

42. Coxon JP, Oades GM, Kirby RS, et al. Zoledronic acid induces apoptosis and inhibits adhesion to mineralized matrix in prostate cancer cells via inhibition of protein prenylation. BJU Int 2004;94:164–170.

43. Boissier S, Magnetto S, Frappart L, et al. Bisphosphonates inhibit prostate and breast carcinoma cell adhesion to unmineralized and mineralized bone extracellular matrices. Cancer Res 1997;57:3890–3894.

44. van der Pluijm G, Vloedgraven H, van Beek E, et al. Bisphosphonates inhibit the adhesion of breast cancer cells to bone matrices in vitro. J Clin Invest 1996;98:698–705.

45. Boissier S, Ferreras M, Peyruchaud O, et al. Bisphosphonates inhibit breast and prostate carcinoma cell invasion, an early event in the formation of bone metastases. Cancer Res 2000;60:2949–2954.

46. Denoyelle C, Hong L, Vannier JP, et al. New insights into the actions of bisphosphonate zoledronic acid in breast cancer cells by dual Rhoα-dependent and -independent effects. Br J Cancer 2003;88:1631–1640.

47. Adami S, Salvagno G, Guarrera G, et al. Dichloromethylene-diphosphonate in patients with prostatic carcinoma metastatic to the skeleton. J Urol 1985;134:1152–1154.

48. Cresswell SM, English PJ, Hall RR, et al. Pain relief and quality-of-life assessment following intravenous and oral clodronate in hormone-escaped metastatic prostate cancer. Br J Urol 1995;76:360–365.

49. Elomaa I, Kylmala T, Tammela T, et al. Effect of oral clodronate on bone pain. A controlled study in patients with metastatic prostatic cancer. Int Urol Nephrol 1992;24:159–166.

50. Kylmala T, Taube T, Tammela TL, et al. Concomitant i.v. and oral clodronate in the relief of bone pain—a double-blind placebo-controlled study in patients with prostate cancer. Br J Cancer 1997;76:939–942.

51. Clarke NW, Holbrook IB, McClure J, et al. Osteoclast inhibition by pamidronate in metastatic prostate cancer: a preliminary study. Br J Cancer 1991;63:420–423.

52. Pelger RC, Nijeholt AA, Papapoulos SE. Short-term metabolic effects of pamidronate in patients with prostatic carcinoma and bone metastases. Lancet 1989;2:865.

53. Green JR, Muller K, Jaeggi KA. Preclinical pharmacology of CGP 42′446, a new, potent, heterocyclic bisphosphonate compound. J Bone Miner Res 1994;9:745–751.

54. Saad F, Gleason DM, Murray R, et al. A randomized, placebo-controlled trial of zoledronic acid in patients with hormone-refractory metastatic prostate carcinoma. J Natl Cancer Inst 2002;94:1458–1468.

55. Saad F, et al. Zoledronic acid is well tolerated for up to 24 months and significantly reduces skeletal complications in patients with advanced prostate cancer metastatic to the bone. Presented at: American Urological Association Annual Meeting 2003 [abstract 1472].

56. Groot MT, Boeken Kruger CG, Pelger RC, et al. Costs of prostate cancer, metastatic to the bone, in the Netherlands. Eur Urol 2003;43:226–232.

57. Dearnaley DP, Sydes MR, Mason MD, et al. A double-blind, placebo-controlled, randomized trial of oral sodium clodronate for metastatic prostate cancer (MRC PR05 Trial). J Natl Cancer Inst 2003;95:1300–1311.

58. Smith MR, McGovern FJ, Fallon MA, et al. Low bone mineral density in hormone-naive men with prostate carcinoma. Cancer 2001;91:2238-2245.

59. Hussain SA, Weston R, Stephenson RN, et al. Immediate dual energy X-ray absorptiometry reveals a high incidence of osteoporosis in patients with advanced prostate cancer before hormonal manipulation. BJU Int 2003;92:690–694.

60. Smith MR, Eastham J, Gleason DM, et al. Randomized controlled trial of zoledronic acid to prevent bone loss in men receiving androgen deprivation therapy for nonmetastatic prostate cancer. J Urol 2003;169:2008–2012.

61. Smith MR, McGovern FJ, Zietman AL, et al. Pamidronate to prevent bone loss during androgen-deprivation therapy for prostate cancer. N Engl J Med 2001;345:948–955.

Managing the complications of advanced prostate cancer 103

Roger S Kirby

INTRODUCTION

The most commonly encountered complications of prostate cancer result from either obstructive uropathy or the effects of metastatic spread. Since the favored site of secondary spread is the skeleton, the majority of problems stem from that source. Pathologic fractures may affect the long bones, spine, or pelvis. If the spinal cord is compressed urgent action may be required to prevent permanent paralysis. The first step in management is to accurately establish the diagnosis, treatment selection will depend on whether the cancer is hormone naive or whether one is dealing with a hormone-resistant prostate cancer (HRPC). In the latter situation the prognosis is significantly worse. Recent data suggests that some skeletal-related events may be prevented or delayed by the judicious use of the bisphosphonate zoledronic acid (See Chapter 102).

LOWER URINARY TRACT SYMPTOMS AND OBSTRUCTIVE UROPATHY

LOWER URINARY TRACT SYMPTOMS

Lower urinary tract symptoms (LUTS) are common among men suffering from locally advanced prostate cancer.[1] Patients often present with symptoms of frequency and poor flow, as well as a sensation of incomplete emptying. Other problems include hematuria, anorexia, and weight loss; these may indicate incipient renal failure and/or widespread metastases. Urinary retention is signified by a palpable bladder.

DIAGNOSIS

A digital rectal examination is mandatory and a palpable nodule, hardening, or irregular asymmetry requires further evaluation. Normally the lateral and upper borders and the median sulcus are identifiable, and the seminal vesicles impalpable. Loss of the median sulcus and irregularity of the seminal vesicle suggests malignant infiltration, which may be confirmed by transrectal ultrasound-guided biopsy. The upper and lower urinary tract is best evaluated by ultrasound and flow studies. A computed tomography (CT) or magnetic resonance imaging (MRI) scan may be required to determine the location and extent of lymphatic metastases, or other soft tissue metastases. A bone scan is the most frequently utilized way of determining the presence of bone metastases (see Figure 102.1). Local MRI can be used to confirm these and to evaluate whether or not spinal cord compression is present.

MANAGEMENT AND TREATMENT OPTIONS

In many patients with metastatic prostate cancer who present with severe LUTS, hormone treatment (usually with an luteinizing hormone releasing hormone [LHRH] analog) will improve voiding function. In patients with acute or chronic retention who fail to void, androgen ablation therapy will generally facilitate voiding and also make a transurethral resection of the prostate (TURP) easier by reducing tumor bulk and vascularity. If voiding does not occur after 8 weeks or so of hormone therapy, a TURP should be considered, although it is associated with a higher incidence of stress incontinence when performed for malignant rather than benign bladder outflow obstruction, and the patient should be informed of this before surgery.

Alpha blockers, such as doxazosin, alfuzosin, or tamsulosin, are less effective in malignant prostatic obstruction than in benign prostatic hyperplasia (BPH). However, external-beam radiotherapy to the prostate should be considered even in the presence of bone metastases, as it may arrest local progression and can also control bleeding.

OBSTRUCTION OF THE UPPER URINARY TRACTS

Obstructive uropathy, caused either by direct compression of the ureterovesical junction, or through invasion of the ureteric orifice and/or the intramural ureter by tumor tissue, can lead to deterioration in renal function, and ultimately, kidney failure if left untreated. In patients with prostate cancer, urinary tract obstruction secondary to the local extension and lymphatic spread of disease is a common finding at both diagnosis, and at later stages of disease,[2] with an incidence varying between 2% and 51%.[3]

Upper and lower urinary tract obstruction may lead to troublesome complications causing significant morbidity, and often indicates a poor prognosis in patients with prostate cancer.[2,4] Recently, the prognosis for patients with advanced-stage disease has been significantly improved through a number of endoscopic interventions,[2] with survival ranging from 4 to 24 months, depending on whether hormone-naive or hormone-resistant prostate cancer is present.[5–9]

PRESENTATION

Patients may sometimes present acutely with ureteric colic.[3] However, patients typically present insidiously either with deranged blood chemistry or the incidental finding of renal cortical atrophy or ureteric dilatation on an upper abdominal imaging study.[4] Both acute and chronic bilateral ureteric obstruction are associated with a decreased urine output, as well as symptoms of uremia, and may lead to renal failure.[4] In cases where upper urinary tract obstruction leads to infection, fever, and urosepsis, this necessitates emergency decompression or percutaneous drainage.[4] Chronic or acute urinary retention should be excluded clinically/sonographically in a patient presenting with bilateral hydronephrosis, and may be treated by the simple measure of urethral or suprapubic catheterization of the bladder.

INVESTIGATION OF RENAL FAILURE

When an alteration in serum creatinine is present and obstructive uropathy is suspected, immediate further investigation is indicated. In patients with previously confirmed prostate cancer, possible urologic complications should be anticipated and the patient monitored accordingly.[2] In the majority of cases, initial workup includes serum chemistry and urinary tract ultrasound to check for both lower and upper urinary tract obstruction.[2] Further investigation may include CT to determine the extent of local/nodal disease. Assessment of peak urinary flow rate, symptom scores, or ultrasound of the prostate may be appropriate in some patients.[2] Other imaging modalities available for the diagnosis of obstructive uropathy include intravenous urography, MRI, and radionuclide renography (Figure 103.1).

Ultrasound

Ultrasound is the most commonly employed of investigation in suspected cases of urinary tract obstruction, whether the renal function is normal or abnormal.[2] Ultrasound of the abdomen may show hydronephrosis or hydroureter, suggesting the probable level of an obstruction.

Intravenous urography

While ultrasound has to a large extent replaced the intravenous urogram (IVU), an IVU can provide useful additional information,[10] provided there is adequate renal function (generally a serum creatinine <200 mmol/L). In acute obstruction, a hydronephrosis may not be visible on an early ultrasound and the IVU might then be more informative. A retrograde ureterogram is often technically difficult in locally advanced prostate cancer, and seldom yields information of therapeutic value unless performed as a prelude to attempted ureteric stent insertion.

Computed tomography

Computed tomography plays an important role in determining the etiology of obstructive uropathy when ultrasound and other modalities are not conclusive, and may help to inform subsequent management strategies.[10] A prospective study by Bosniak et al[10] investigated 36 patients with hydronephrosis secondary to obstructive uropathy of uncertain etiology. Abdominal CT was performed following intravenous contrast to establish the cause of ureteric obstruction, and proved to be of value in 92% of cases. In addition, extrinsic masses were demonstrated in 20 patients with metastatic disease.[10]

Ideally, CT is performed with intravenous contrast, but non-contrast-enhanced CT, in particular spiral CT, may still be useful in patients who have an indeterminate ultrasound, or have an allergy to the contrast medium or ureamia.[10]

Radionuclide renography

Radionuclide renography is a nuclear imaging technology for the evaluation of renal function. Radionuclides are injected to provide a noninvasive measure of renal split-function.[11] In general,

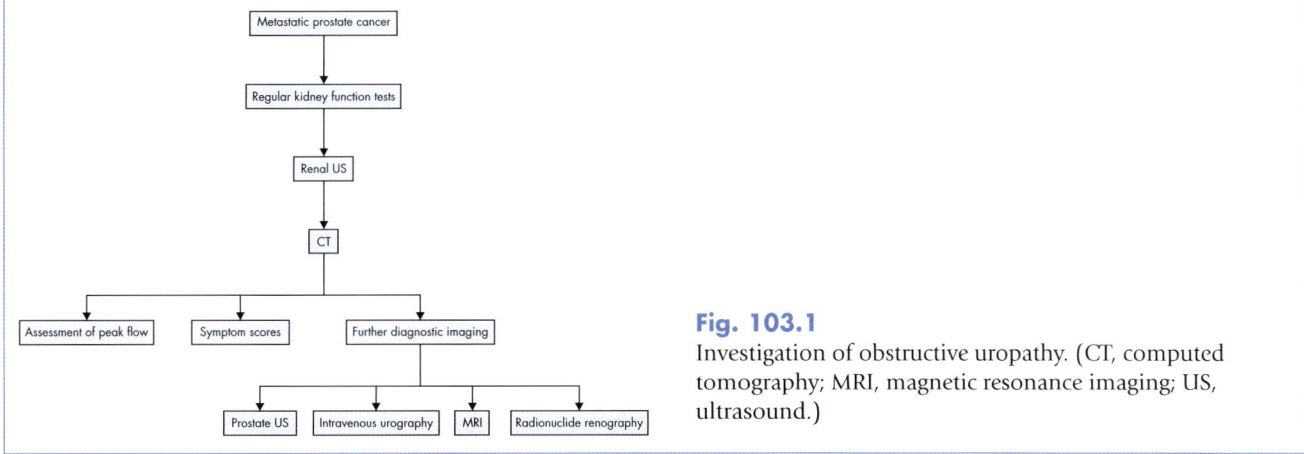

Fig. 103.1
Investigation of obstructive uropathy. (CT, computed tomography; MRI, magnetic resonance imaging; US, ultrasound.)

radionuclides establish renal function at the time of examination and not the potential for renal recovery.

MANAGEMENT AND TREATMENT

The management of obstructive uropathy is directed by two principles: first, treatment of the causative lesion; second, diagnosis and treatment of the underlying obstructive uropathy. The approach to treatment of obstructive uropathy is dependent on the site of obstruction.[12] In the emergency setting, patients with acute urinary retention resulting from lower tract obstruction can be managed simply by passing a urethral or suprapubic catheter into the bladder.[4] In patients with upper tract obstruction, the placement of a nephrostomy tube, or, more rarely, the retrograde introduction of a ureteric stent, may be necessary.[12] Following drainage, the diagnosis and treatment of the underlying obstructive uropathy can commence. In patients with low-grade acute obstruction or partial chronic obstruction, intervention may be delayed.[12] However, bilateral obstruction and unilateral obstruction accompanied by symptoms of pyonephrosis require prompt management and drainage[12] to prevent irreversible renal damage.

In patients with previously confirmed locally advanced prostate cancer, the choice of treatment for upper tract obstruction is additionally influenced by whether the patient is hormone-naive or has HRPC. Ureteric obstruction in the hormone-naive individual can be treated with androgen blockade or orchidectomy,[7] while in patients with HRPC decompression of ureteric obstruction provides temporary urinary diversion.[2] Lower urinary tract obstruction in patients with significant residual urine and recurrent bouts of urosepsis can be alleviated through the establishment of clean intermittent catheterization.[12] This approach to managing urinary retention requires patient acceptance and training,[4] but can preserve kidney function.[12]

The diagnosis of obstructive uropathy in patients with advanced prostate cancer sometimes raises difficult ethical questions for the treating urologist/oncologist. Although palliative treatment may improve renal function in the short-term, the patient's suffering may be prolonged.[4] Palliative urinary diversion or decompression is usually justified where improvement in renal function facilitates effective treatment options for the primary disease, for example, taxane-based chemotherapy, or for the alleviation of pain.[4] However, the decision to proceed with urinary diversion may not always be in the patient's best interests in end-stage HRPC, particularly if there is advanced symptomatic pelvic disease. Therefore, an individual approach to treatment is required, based on patient age, history, evolution of cancer, as well as ethical and social considerations.[13]

Intervention

Decompression of the urinary tract can help to prolong survival and significantly decrease morbidity in patients with ureteric obstruction.[7,14] Minimally invasive interventions including percutaneous needle nephrostomy (PCNN), long-term ureteric stenting, and endoscopic ureteroneocystostomy have largely replaced traditional open surgical procedures.[7,15] The placement of a stent can provide immediate relief in cases of urinary tract obstruction, but in malignant obstruction urinary flow is via the stent lumen and any blockage of the lumen will cause further obstruction. Percutaneous needle nephrostomy provides direct drainage from the kidneys. If ureteric stenting via the antegrade or retrograde routes is not achievable, extra-ureteric stenting may be indicated. The role of TURP is only to achieve voiding after retention, or to improve lower urinary tract symptoms. It does not have a principal role in the management of prostate cancer or the management of upper urinary tract obstruction.

Percutaneous needle nephrostomy

Percutaneous needle nephrostomy offers both immediate relief and long-term improvement, with minimum inconvenience if followed by antegrade stenting. In a study[16] of 22 patients with advanced pelvic cancer, 24 nephrostomies were performed (bilateral in 2 patients) for malignant ureteric obstructions. Indications for nephrostomy in this group included renal failure, urosepsis, or pre-treatment before chemotherapy. Sixty-eight percent of patients were able to achieve a useful lifestyle after the procedure, with a survival time ranging from 3 months to 2 years. Similarly, in a study[17] of 77 patients with obstructive uropathy secondary to pelvic malignant disease, a successful nephrostomy insertion rate resulted in an overall median patient survival of over 6 months.

However, although percutaneous drainage via an antegrade or retrograde approach provides a reliable method of renal recovery, the impact of treatment on patient quality of life remains controversial. The studies referred to previously[12,16] included various primary tumor types and the situation in advanced prostate cancer is less clear cut unless the patient is hormonally-naive. A study[5] of 22 HRPC patients with both unilateral (n = 5) and bilateral (n = 17) obstructions, reported that 18 of the patients died with a median survival time of just under 4 months following percutaneous urinary diversion; less than that expected for similar patients without ureteric obstruction. On average, patients spent 41% of their remaining lifetime after PCNN in hospital. The authors concluded that PCNN did not improve the quality of life of these patients.[5]

Conversely, in a later study[7] of 36 patients with bilateral ureteric obstruction and renal failure, the mean survival period for patients in whom androgen depletion had been undertaken after ureteric obstruction was around 21.5 months. In these patients, for whom hormonal therapy remained an option, urinary tract decompression offered a worthwhile improvement in terms of increased survival and reduced in-patient time.[7] However, in patients where androgen depletion had been carried out prior to the diagnosis of ureteric obstruction, survival was significantly worse, at only 2.7 months.[7] The authors of this study concluded that in patients with bilateral ureteric obstruction secondary to prostate cancer who have not undergone hormone manipulation there should be little hesitation in the use of upper tract decompression in either short-term or long-term disease management.[7]

Similar findings were observed by Chiou et al,[6] who reported longer survival rates in 15 prostate cancer patients with both unilateral and bilateral obstructive uropathy following percutaneous nephrostomy, prior to hormone therapy. The 1- and 2-year survival rates of these patients were 73% and 47%, respectively, while those of patients who had previously undergone hormone therapy were lower at 48% and 19%, respectively.[6] However, the authors of this study did not advocate withholding PCNN from patients who had previously undergone hormone manipulation, due to the significant number of patients in this group who survived for longer than a year following treatment.[6]

Ureteric stenting

In patients with prostate cancer, stents provide a palliative and attractive alternative to PCNN in acute relief from ureteric obstruction.[15] Inserted percutaneously or endoscopically into the ureter, longer-term stents may be placed for up to 6 months in patients with obstruction and end-stage disease. However, planned replacement is essential to prevent fractures within the stent wall, or build-up of encrustation.

Endoscopic ureteroneocystostomy

Endoscopic ureteroneocystostomy can restore ureterovesical continuity through the resection of the ureteric meatus following either PCNN or ureteric stent placement. Chefchaouni et al[13] performed endoscopic ureteroneocystostomy in 31 patients with renal failure resulting from advanced unilateral (n = 12) or bilateral (n = 18) obstructive uropathy secondary to prostate cancer, in an attempt to restore continuity of the ureteric orifice. Eleven patients were hormone-naive, whilst 18 had HRPC. All patients underwent PCNN prior to ureteroneocystostomy. Under fluoroscopic guidance the position of the obstruction was then determined, and deep resection of the lateral part of the trigone was performed, enabling the reopening of the ureteric lumen. The nephrostomy tube was removed after normalization or stabilization of renal function. Continuity of the ureteric orifice was achieved in 76% of patients, and a median survival after surgery of 8 months was achieved. Additionally, the average time in hospital was reduced from 27.5 days to 6.8 days following ureteroneocystostomy. The hormonal status of patients had no effect on survival. The authors concluded that ureteroneocystostomy provided an attractive option for patients with obstructive uropathy, due to the short hospital stay and high success rate of this treatment.

CONCLUSIONS

Obstructive uropathy is not an uncommon complication among prostate cancer patients.[2] An algorithm for the diagnosis and management of this condition is set out in Figure 103.2. All patients with progressive disease should have their serum creatinine monitored regularly and undergo renal ultrasound if their creatinine becomes deranged. If obstructive uropathy is suspected, an ultrasound or CT scan will assist the diagnosis. The management of obstructive uropathy by urgent upper urinary tract decompression through PCNN or ureteric stenting can significantly reduce patient morbidity and prolong patient survival,[7,14] and is almost always indicated in patients who are hormonally-naive. In patients with HRPC, a palliative approach may sometimes be more appropriate, although the recent publication of data suggesting that taxane-based chemotherapy with docetaxol can prolong survival by several months provides a rationale for a more interventional approach.

MANAGEMENT OF SPINAL CORD COMPRESSION DUE TO PROSTATE CANCER

As previously mentioned symptomatic spinal cord metastases occur in around 5% to 10% of prostate cancer patients; however, asymptomatic lesions are probably much more common.[18,19] The most common site for spinal metastasis to occur is the vertebral bodies of the thoracic and lumbar regions (See Figure 103.1).[20,21] The most frequent site of symptomatic neural compression is the thoracic region (67%), with 27% in the lumbar spine and 6% in the cervical spine, in part reflecting the narrower volume of the spinal canal in this region.[22,23]

Ninety per cent of prostatic spinal metastases are osteoblastic.[24] Spinal deformity is, therefore, unusual although epidural compression is not uncommon, being the initial sign of malignancy in 36% of patients with epidural metastasis.[25] By contrast, only 7% of breast metastases are osteoblastic, 30% are mixed and 63% are osteolytic.[26] The majority of spinal metastases from other sites are also osteolytic. Osteolytic metastases weaken bone resulting in pathologic fracture with the potential for neurologic compromise as a result of bony compression rather than tumor compression. Recognition of this difference is axiomatic to under-

standing the difference in clinical presentation and management strategies for prostatic epidural spinal cord compression (ESCC) compared with metastasis from other primary sites. This applies particularly to surgical management, except, in the unusual circumstance (<10%) of osteolytic prostatic metastasis resulting in pathologic fracture with the potential for neurologic compromise.

Several reviews[27–29] emphasize the clinical impact of ESCC, which is defined as a compression at any level of the spinal canal (including cauda equina). Epidural spinal cord compression is, in itself, not fatal; nevertheless, incapacitating pain and subsequent neurologic compromise, such as paraplegia and loss of sphincter control, have major social and clinical implications (Figure 103.3). Complete loss of neurologic function is irretrievable, and, therefore, prevention of ESCC is desirable whenever possible. Several clinically relevant algorithms have been developed to aid the clinician in their early diagnosis and management strategies.[30,31]

CLINICAL FEATURES OF PRESENTATION

Patients may present via a variety of different routes: as an acute admission, as a referral from a clinic with unexplained musculoskeletal pain or as an existing patient referred by an oncologist or member of the prostate care team.[32] Osborn et al[33] investigated symptoms at presentation in a retrospective study of four large series of spinal metastases from prostate cancer. It was concluded that patients at risk or with actual ESCC, present with four main initial symptoms: back pain, weakness, and autonomic and sensory loss.

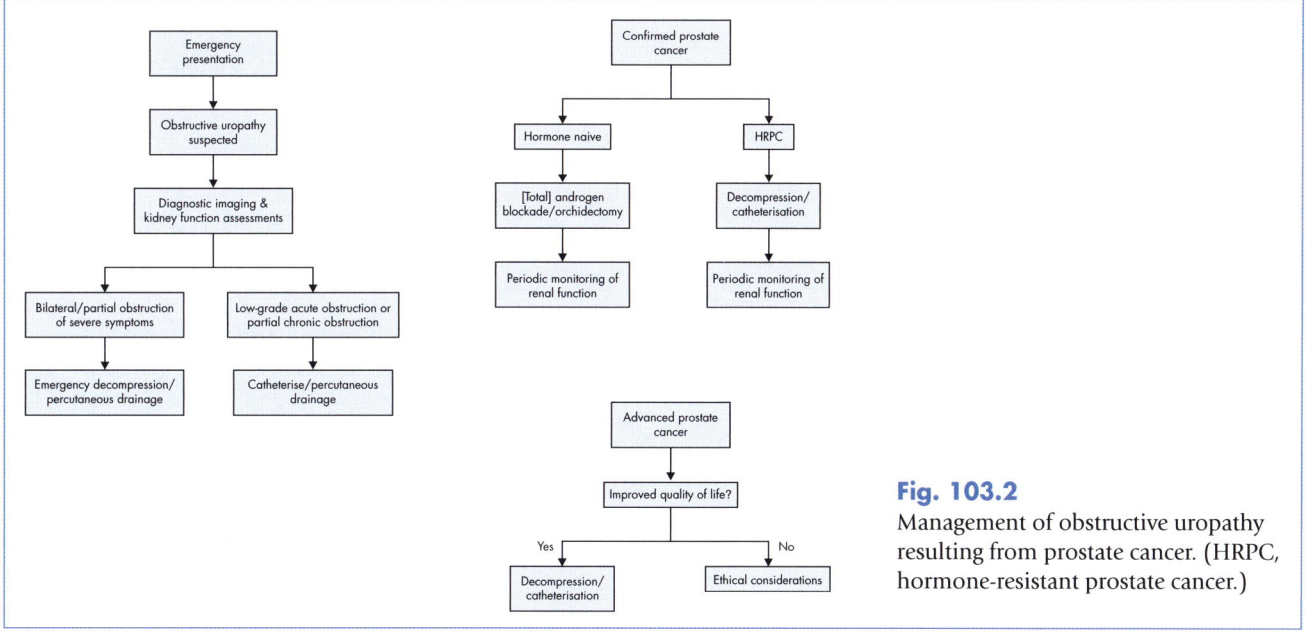

Fig. 103.2
Management of obstructive uropathy resulting from prostate cancer. (HRPC, hormone-resistant prostate cancer.)

Back pain

The most frequent symptom reported in up to 100% of adult ESCC patients is back pain resulting mainly from the involvement of bone with the metastatic tumour[34–38] (Table 103.1).

A recent retrospective analysis by Cereceda et al[35] analyzed 119 patients who had 212 significant episodes of prostatic osseous spinal metastases and confirmed that pain was almost universal (93%). The type of pain and the relieving and aggravating factors reflect the underlying local pathologic process. At first, pain may be local in origin due to periosteal stretching as the metastasis enlarges, sometimes accompanied by somatic referred pain. Radicular pain may also develop with incipient root compression.[33] Prostate cancer patients may suffer this pain for a median duration of 12 months before the onset of ESCC.[39] Localized pain may be relentless and be exacerbated by anything that raises cerebrospinal fluid pressure, such as straining, coughing, or sneezing.[27,33] With increasing occlusion of the spinal canal pain may be aggravated by lying down, in contrast to degenerative spinal disease which is often relieved by recumbency.

Patients often recognize the pain as different to their more longstanding, mechanical, low back pain of degenerative origin, and it is often more proximal given the predilection for the thoracic spine. A retrospective survey of 131 patients with spinal metastases by Stark et al[40] found localized vertebral tenderness in 74% of patients. Care should be taken when attributing pain to degenerative spinal disease in patients with a history of prostate cancer who should be carefully evaluated for spinal metastases.[27,31] Symptomatic neurologic compromise in the form of sensory loss, weakness, and autonomic dysfunction typically develop after pain, commonly but not always in this sequence.

The neurologic presentation differs with the level of neural compression and its direction. Cord compression above T12 typically results in an upper motor neuron (UMN) picture, while at the conus and below, a lower motor neuron (LMN) picture results. If compression is initially anterior, weakness, loss of pain, and temperature sensitivity may precede compromise of light touch and proprioception (dissociated sensory loss). Conversely, if compression is initially posterior the reverse may apply.

Weakness

Weakness is usually bilateral and frequently involves the muscle groups below the lesion[33] (Table 103.2). The degree of weakness and ambulatory ability at diagnosis are important clinical predictors of outcome.[34,40] Smith et al[36] reported that in patients with prostate cancer and ESCC, 93% of ambulatory patients, 83% of paraparetic patients, and 0% of paraplegic patients were ambulatory after appropriate treatment. Once weakness is present, progression to ESCC in prostate cancer patients is relatively swift.

Autonomic and sensory dysfunction

According to Gilbert et al,[34] autonomic dysfunction in a cancer patient is an unfavorable prognostic sign. Symptoms of bowel and bladder problems, such as incontinence and urinary retention are frequent in these patients at diagnosis (57%) depending on the level of the compression.[27] In addition, Cereceda et al[35] reports that 3% of prostate patients suffered with bladder dysfunction. Over half of patients (51%) report symptoms of numbness and paresthesia, while on examination a sensory loss is found in 78%[27] (Table

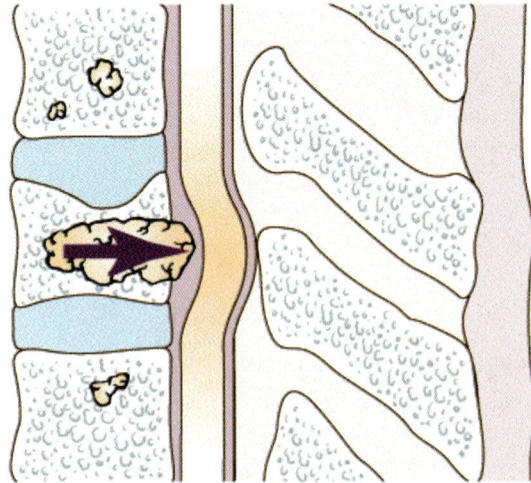

Fig. 103.3
Epidural spinal cord compression: neurological complications result from pressure on the spinal cord.

Table 103.1 Pain as a symptom of epidural spinal cord compression in patients with prostate cancer in four retrospective studies

Author	Episodes of spinal metastases	Patients with pain, n (%)
Smith et al[36]	26	25 (96)
Shoskes et al[37]	28	21 (75)
Zelefsky et al[23]	50	48 (96)
Rosenthal et al[38]	31	31 (100)

Table 103.2 Weakness as a symptom of epidural spinal cord compression in patients with prostate cancer in four retrospective studies

Author	Episodes of spinal metastases	Patients with weakness, n (%)
Smith et al[36]	26	14 (54)
Shoskes et al[37]	28	23 (82)
Zelefsky et al[23]	50	25 (50)
Rosenthal et al[38]	31	30 (97)

103.3). Past medical history may be of importance when considering ESCC; previous radiotherapy, injury, vascular disease, and disk disease may also be indicative of a future risk of ESCC.[27]

CLINICAL ASSESSMENT

A complete history and examination with particular attention to neurologic status is necessary in a patient presenting with any combination of these symptoms.[32]

EXAMINATION

In addition to a routine general examination with particular attention to excluding visceral metastasis, neurologic examination should assess mental status, cranial nerves, motor and sensory examination, reflexes, and cerebellar function.[31] Posture, stance, and gait in particular, represent an integration of these functions. Assessment in the vertical position, in particular, the ability to tiptoe walk, heel-walk and do single-knee dips will often reveal latent weakness or proprioceptive loss not apparent on bed assessment. If there is a significant history of mechanical spinal pain, plain radiographs of the painful area to exclude incipient spinal collapse should be obtained prior to standing and walking assessment. Precise definition of complete/incomplete neurologic deficit and time after which neurologic recovery cannot be anticipated is not easy to achieve.

IMAGING AND DIAGNOSIS

Magnetic resonance imaging

Magnetic resonance imaging is considered the gold standard diagnostic test for imaging spinal metastases.[33] It is noninvasive, gives excellent anatomical detail of the spinal cord, and is able to image the desired spinal segments irrespective of spinal block. Several studies[41-43] have demonstrated that spinal MRI is as sensitive as other modalities for detecting spinal epidural metastases. However, one potential disadvantage is that it has not been routine to image the whole spinal column, which potentially misses other asymptomatic lesions. In line with other guidelines,[32] it is recommended that all patients should ideally receive an urgent MRI of the entire spine and other affected bones.

Radiography

Prior to the availability of MRI, definitive diagnosis of ESCC required myelography, a highly invasive test for patients who are already in pain. Consequently, routine investigations, such as conventional radiography, were used to determine those patients at low risk of ESCC in whom myelography would not be required. Conventional radiography has the ability to demonstrate vertebral abnormalities in up to 85% of patients with ESCC from both osteoblastic and osteolytic lesions or vertebral collapse.[34,40] Portenoy et al[44] studied the probability of epidural metastatic disease based on the presence of symptoms and radiographic or bone scan changes. It was reported that if there was a localized sign and the radiograph was abnormal the probability of epidural disease was 0.9; however, if the radiograph was normal it was only 0.1 (this was not, however, controlled with MRI). This was increased to 0.95 if both the radiograph and bone scan were abnormal and reduced to 0.02 if the radiograph and bone scan were normal.

For osteolytic metastases, lesions need to be greater than 1 cm and more than 50% of the bone has to be destroyed before these are necessarily evident using conventional radiography. In addition, in HRPC patients, the multiplicity of bony metastases and that the majority are osteoblastic rather than osteolytic means that a high number of false negatives result. It is, therefore, unlikely that radiographs alone have enough predictive value to warrant their routine use in predicting prostate cancer patients at risk from ESCC.

Myelography

Although MRI has largely replaced myelography, there are still some circumstances in which myelography is useful. Magnetic resonance imaging is contraindicated in those with pacemakers, intracardiac stents and with intraocular metallic foreign bodies. In addition, MR images of the spine are usually grossly distorted by the presence of ferrous implants from previous spinal surgery. If a second episode of ESCC has developed despite prior surgery with implants, myelography combined with CT will usually provide sufficient information on which to base management decisions.

Radionuclide bone scans

Radionuclide bone scans are a useful single test for staging prostate cancer and are more sensitive than radiographs at detecting vertebral metastases.[45,46] A recent study by Soerdjbalie-Maikoe et al,[47] using a new method of evaluating bone scintigraphy concluded that radionuclide bone scans performed at the time of development of

Table 103.3 Nervous dysfunction as a symptom of epidural spinal cord compression in patients with prostate cancer in four retrospective studies

Author	Episodes of spinal metastases	Patients with autonomic dysfunction, n (%)	Patients with sensory loss, n (%)
Smith et al[36]	26	9 (35)	6 (23)
Shoskes et al[37]	28	14 (50)	19 (68)
Zelefsky et al[23]	50	1 (2)	n/a
Rosenthal et al[38]	31	18 (58)	18 (58)

hormone refractoriness in HRPC patients is of high predictive value for the inherent risk of ESCC. It does not, however, provide sufficient detail to be of surgical value in discriminating which of the often multiple vertebral site(s) is responsible for neural compression and the direction of that compression. In the context of spinal metastatic disease in practice, isotope bone scans are used only to define extraspinal osseous disease and its extent, and this can usually be delayed until after spinal surgery, if this is necessary. However, if neurology is deteriorating appropriate surgical intervention should not be delayed.

Computed tomography

Computed tomography has for practical purposes been replaced by MRI. This is on the basis of the higher sensitivity of MRI and lack of ionizing radiation. However, there are circumstances in which MRI is contraindicated or the presence of ferrous implants may render it useless.

The usefulness of spinal CT in predicting epidural tumor was investigated by Weissman et al[48] in 30 cancer patients, including four men with prostate cancer. Twenty-one of 23 patients (91%) with cortical disruption at more than one vertebral level on spinal CT had epidural tumor. Spinal CT can, therefore, be a useful test to define a high risk of ESCC if MRI cannot be used. It may also provide additional bony detail to answer particular anatomical questions, for example, bony dimensions for instrumentation or the course of the vertebral artery.

Summary of imaging requirements

Although each case will require a thorough individual assessment the initial assessment of spinal metastases from prostate cancer should include: a neurologic and general assessment, plain radiographs of the spine, an urgent MRI and a chest X-ray. Chest and abdominal CT and radionuclide bone scans are desirable staging investigations, but these should not impede surgical intervention, if neurological status is deteriorating.

Biopsy of spinal lesions

A spinal biopsy is recommended if the lesion is a solitary bony lesion and there is doubt as to the underlying pathology. In these cases imaging with scintigraphy, MRI of the lesion and percutaneous bone biopsy need to be performed before surgery to prevent inappropriate procedures.[32] Experienced surgeons should generally perform percutaneous biopsies, under X-ray control.[32]

TREATMENT OPTIONS

RADIOTHERAPY

The response of epidural metastases to radiotherapy is well documented.[49,50] Radiotherapy is the preferred first-line treatment for ESCC in known prostate cancer patients as it is the optimal treatment for what are usually radiosensitive tumors. In 1978 before the advent of modern spinal surgical methods, Gilbert et al[34] reviewed 235 cases of ESCC: 170 patients were treated with radiotherapy alone and 65 patients underwent radiotherapy and decompressive laminectomy. There was no significant difference in functional outcome of the two groups. Zelefsky et al[23] reported similar findings in their analysis of 42 patients with spinal metastases from prostate cancer who had been treated with external-beam radiation. At completion of treatment, it was reported that 92% of patients experienced pain relief, and 67% had significant or complete improvement on neurologic examination. In a further study,[36] which analyzed 35 patients with prostate cancer and suspected spinal cord compression; 26 patients were found to have ESCC. All patients were initially treated with radiation, steroids, and androgen deprivation therapy. In ambulatory or paraparetic patients, radiation, androgen deprivation therapy and steroids can be effective palliative therapy. However, patients who present with paraplegia or in whom paraplegia developed secondary to recurrent compression are often not palliated by this combination of therapies. Surgery is recommended for these patients.[36]

The Radiation Therapy Oncology Group (RTOG) evaluated different dose fractionation irradiation schedules in a randomized, controlled trial[51] to determine their palliative effectiveness in patients with osseous metastases. The frequency, promptness, and duration of pain relief were utilized as measures of response. Ninety percent of patients experienced some relief of pain and 54% achieved eventual complete pain relief. However, the optimal dose fractionation scheme for treating ESCC is still unknown. Most radiation oncologists adhere to standard schedules of 25 to 36 Gy, with an average of 30 Gy over 10 fractions being chosen because it is considered to be a relatively well-tolerated dose for the spinal cord.[27] There may be no optimal plan for every metastatic prostate cancer patient because each plan constructed will represent a compromise between delivery of the highest dose possible to control progression of the tumor and palliate pain effectively, whilst limiting the effect on the spinal cord.

Radiotherapy has minimal side effects in metastatic prostate cancer patients and is efficacious in terms of preventing further tumor growth and ameliorating pain. The neurologic outcome of radiotherapy depends on two factors. Firstly, the degree of functional limitation at initiation of radiotherapy will alter the outcome of therapy. Neurologic status at initiation is important as it has been reported that radiotherapy may preserve the ability to ambulate in 80% to 100% of patients who initiate treatment while still ambulatory.[34,50,52] Secondly, the extent of subarachnoid impingement will also affect the outcome of treatment. Epidural metastases that produce a minor impression on the thecal sac will have a better outcome than a large mass that completely obliterates the subarachnoid space. This has been confirmed in clinical studies, but is the weakest of the two prognostic indicators.[53,54]

In the era of MRI, the response of spinal metastases to radiotherapy has not been thoroughly investigated. Median survival for patients undergoing radiotherapy for ESCC is between 3 and 6 months. Survival rates are higher in patients who were ambulatory when treatment was initiated and in radiosensitive tumors, such as prostate with a single metastasis. The risk of recurrence increases with the length of survival, and 50% of 2-year survivors will develop recurrence.[34] In line with results from other studies, Leviov et al,[55] concluded that a radiotherapeutic success ceiling of 80% existed for metastatic ESCC patients and, in view of this, future investigative studies should focus on educating clinicians in the early detection and diagnosis of this complication. Indications for radiotherapy are given in Box 103.1.

CHEMOTHERAPY

Chemotherapy is a reasonable treatment option in patients with ESCC who have undergone previous radiotherapy and are not candidates for surgery when the underlying tumor is likely to be chemosensitive.[27]

HORMONE DEPRIVATION THERAPY

Hormonal manipulation has been successfully employed in hormone-naive patients with ESCC from prostate cancer, and there is a definite relationship between neurologic deficit at presentation and response to hormone therapy. Bilateral orchiectomy is the most expeditious method of achieving castrate levels of serum testosterone. If LHRH analogs are utilized, they should be combined with an antiandrogen, as the well-described flare phenomenon may exacerbate the ESCC. However, in patients who have complete paraplegia at the time of presentation, hormone therapy has little benefit.[56] It should not be forgotten that patients with HRPC may respond to second-line therapy, such as estrogens, or taxane-based chemotherapy.

Box 103.1 Indications for radiotherapy for spinal metastases[32]

- No spinal instability
- Radiosensitive tumor
- Stable or slow neurological progression
- Multi-level disease
- Surgery precluded by general condition
- Poor prognosis
- Postoperative adjuvant treatment

SURGERY

A variety of surgical strategies can be employed for neoplastic spinal disease. Appropriate selection is dependent upon the individual case and requires tailoring accordingly. The objectives from a patient perspective are to minimize pain and to maximize or maintain neurologic function with the minimum procedure adequate to the prognosis. From a spinal perspective, the objectives are to ensure adequate decompression; to ensure the maintenance of, or restoration of, spinal cord or nerve root function, and to eliminate actual or potential spinal instability with preservation of as many normal motion segments as possible.[32]

In the majority of patients with ESCC resulting from prostatic metastases, the clinical problem is local tumor-related pain with accompanying radicular or cord compression syndrome pain rather than spinal instability. In the absence of symptoms or imaging evidence of instability, neural compression symptoms may be adequately managed by decompression alone often in the form of laminectomy with, as necessary, specific root decompression in isolation.

Unusually, if osteolytic metastases are present, or if there is significant instability pain, and/or there is other imaging evidence of potential or actual progressive deformity, techniques of stabilization may be required. They may also be necessary if adequate decompression in itself results in iatrogenic destabilization. For example, distal to T10, if posterior decompression requires removal of one or both facet joints, stabilization would be appropriate. Proximal to this in the thoracic spine, it may be judged that the rib cage may provide adequate stability.

Surgery may also be required if the tumor is found to be radioresistant or is progressing despite adequate radiotherapy.[57] A variety of surgical strategies and techniques are available for treatment of metastatic disease of the spine. Metastatic and HRPC patients may benefit from specific techniques of surgical decompression and stabilization dependent upon the location of their metastases.

Box 103.2 summarizes the indications for and objectives of surgery.

SUPPORTIVE MEASURES

Analgesics

A systematic approach to regular assessment, review, and treatment needs to be adopted. It is important to elicit the type, nature, and intensity of pain together with the impact on the patient and quality of life. Treatment should be in line with the World Health Organization (WHO) guidance, with medication given regularly (to prevent pain), and by the "ladder": a stepwise progression from non-opioids, to weak opioids, to strong opioids, with appropriate adjuncts.[58]

Steroid treatment

Corticosteroids are an integral part of the therapy of ESCC.[33] Steroids initiated immediately after diagnosis may benefit the prostate cancer patient by relieving pain and improving neurologic function. Corticosteroids such as dexamethasone perform a principle role in supportive treatment and have also been demonstrated to improve outcomes. A randomized trial of dexamethasone in patients undergoing radiotherapy for ESCC from solid tumors found that a significantly higher percentage were ambulatory on dexamethasone at the long-term follow-up.[59] Dexamethasone is the most frequently used agent in the clinical environment; however, no prospective studies have investigated the optimal dose and schedule for patients with ESCC and this remains an area for debate. Supportive evidence of daily doses ranging from 16 to 96 mg is available.[50,60] In the absence of data, an initial dose within this range is justifiable; however, regardless of the dose used, dexamethasone should be tapered as tolerated, since complications can arise rapidly.

Prevention of skeletal related events with bisphosphonates

As well as being a major cause of morbidity, it has now been shown that skeletal fractures correlate negatively with overall survival in men with prostate cancer and are an independent and adverse predictor of survival.[35] It is, therefore, important that skeletal fractures and skeletal morbidity are kept at a minimum. Bisphosphonates seem a promising way ahead in this respect (See Chapter 102).

Biochemical and histomorphometric studies indicate that osteolysis (excessive bone destruction) is present in prostate cancer metastases despite the sclerotic appearance on X-rays. In this respect bisphosphonates, which are pyrophosphate analogs that block osteolysis, may be useful for the treatment of patients with osteoblastic metastases as well as those with osteolytic metastases.

Zoledronic acid is a new nitrogen-containing bisphosphonate that has been evaluated in patients with metastatic HRPC. It has previously been shown to be at least as effective as pamidrinate 90 mg infusion in reducing skeletal complications in patients with myeloma or breast cancer.[36]

In a randomized controlled trial zoledronic acid (4 mg) given intravenously was evaluated against a placebo in patients with metastatic HRPC. A greater proportion of patients who received placebo had skeletal-related events than those who received zoledronic acid at 4 mg (44.2% versus 33.2%; difference, 11.0%; p = 0.021). Median time to first skeletal-related event was 321 days for patients who received placebo, compared with 420 days for patients who received zoledronic acid at 4 mg (p = 0.011 versus placebo) (Figure 103.4). Zoledronic acid 4 mg given as a 15 minute infusion was well tolerated. The main side effect was influenza-like malaise at the time of and shortly after the infusion.

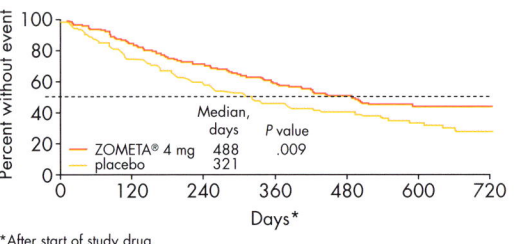

*After start of study drug.

Fig. 103.4
Impact of zoledronic acid (Zometa©) on time to first event. The onset of skeletal complications is significantly delayed by more than 5 months.

CONCLUSIONS

The treatment of metastatic prostate cancer to the spine differs from that of other spinal metastases, and, in many cases, there is debate as to the optimal management of these patients. Early diagnosis and appropriate imaging are essential. It is imperative to involve spinal surgeons to evaluate neural compromise before deciding on the appropriateness or otherwise of surgical intervention, and the opinion of an experienced radiotherapist should also be sought. Androgen ablation therapy should be urgently instituted in hormone-naive patients; in men with HRPC, second-line therapy should be considered. Early institution of appropriate therapy can make the crucial difference between an independent existence and wheelchair-bound paraplegia.

Box 103.2 Surgery for neoplastic spinal disease

Indications
- Spinal instability
- Clinically significant neurologic compression, in particular by bone
- Unresponsive tumor (to radiotherapy, chemotherapy or androgen ablation)

Objectives
- Maintenance or restoration of spinal cord function
- Correction of spinal instability

REFERENCES

1. Hamilton W, Sharp D. Symptomatic diagnosis of prostate cancer in primary care: a structured review. Br J Gen Prac 2004;54:617–621.
2. Colombel M, Mallame W, Abbou CC. Influence of urological complications on the prognosis of prostate cancer. Eur Urol 1997;31(suppl 3):21–24.
3. Villavicencio H. Quality of life of patients with advanced and metastatic prostatic carcinoma. Eur Urol 1993;24:118–121.
4. Russo P. Urologic emergencies in the cancer patient. Semin Oncol 2000;27:284–298.

5. Dowling RA, Carrasco CH, et al. Percutaneous urinary diversion in patients with hormone-refractory prostate cancer. Urology 1991;37:89–91.

6. Chiou RK, Chang WY, Horan JJ. Ureteral obstruction associated with prostate cancer: the outcome after percutaneous nephrostomy. J Urol 1990;143:957–959.

7. Paul AB, Love C, Chisholm. The management of bilateral ureteric obstruction and renal failure in advanced prostate cancer. Br J Urol 1994;74:642–645.

8. Sandhu DP, Mayor PE, Sambrook PA, et al. Outcome and prognostic factors in patients with advanced prostate cancer and obstructive uropathy. Br J Urol 1992;70:412–416.

9. Oefelein MG. Prognostic significance of obstructive uropathy in advanced prostate cancer. Urology 2004;63:1117–1121.

10. Bosniak MA, Megibow AJ, Ambos MA, et al. Computed tomography of ureteral obstruction. AJR Am J Roentgenol 1982;138:1107–1113.

11. Thomsen HS, Hvid-Jacobsen K, Meyhoff HN, et al. Combination of DMSA-scintigraphy and hippuran renography in unilateral obstructive nephropathy. Improved prediction of recovery after intervention. Acta Radiol 1987;28:653–655.

12. Chevalier RL, Klahr S. Therapeutic approaches in obstructive uropathy. Semin Nephrol 1998;18:652–658.

13. Chefchaouni MC, Flam TA, Pacha K, et al. Endoscopic ureteroneocystostomy: palliative urinary diversion in advanced prostate cancer. Tech Urol 1998;4:46–50.

14. Ortlip SA, Fraley EE. Indications for palliative urinary diversion in patients with cancer. Urol Clin North Am 1982;9:79–84.

15. Lang EK. Antegrade ureteral stenting for dehiscence, strictures, and fistulae. AJR Am J Roentgenol 1984;143:795–801.

16. Hoe JW, Tung KH, Tan EC. Re-evaluation of indications for percutaneous nephrostomy and interventional uroradiological procedures in pelvic malignancy. Br J Urol 1993;71:469–472.

17. Lau MW, Temperley DE, Mehta S, et al. Urinary tract obstruction and nephrostomy drainage in pelvic malignant disease. Br J Urol 1995;76:565–569.

18. Sorensen S, Borgesen SE, Rhode K, et al. Metastatic epidural spinal cord compression. Results of treatment and survival. Cancer 1990;65:1502–1508.

19. Rodichok LD, Ruckdeschel JC, Harper GR, et al. Early detection and treatment of spinal epidural metastases: the role of myelography. Ann Neurol 1986;20:696–702.

20. Schiff D. Spinal cord compression. Neuro Clin N Am 2003;21:67–86.

21. Jacobs SC. Spread of prostatic cancer to bone. Urology 1983;2:337–344.

22. Flynn DF, Shipley WU. Management of spinal cord compression secondary to metastatic prostatic carcinoma. Urol Clin North Am 1991;18:145.

23. Zelefsky MJ, Scher HI, Krol G, et al. Spinal epidural tumour in patients with prostate cancer: Clinical and radiographic predictors of response to radiation therapy. Cancer 1992 70:2319–2325.

24. Cook GB, Watson FR. Events in the natural history of prostate cancer: using salvage curves, mean age distributions and contingency coefficients. J Urol 1968;99:87.

25. Liskow A, Chang CH, DeSanctis P, et al. Epidural cord compression in association with genitourinary neoplasms. Cancer 1986;59:949–954.

26. Arseni CN, Simionescu MD, Horwarth L. Tumours of the spine. A follow up study of 350 patients with neurosurgical considerations. Acta Psychiatr Scand 1959;34:398.

27. Grant R, Papadopoulos SM, et al. Metastatic epidural spinal cord compression. Neurol Clin 1991;9:825–841.

28. Byrne TN. Spinal cord compression from epidural metastases. N Engl J Med 1992;327:614–619.

29. Ratanatharathorn V, Powers WE. Epidural spinal cord compression from metastatic tumor: diagnosis and guidelines for management. Cancer Treat Rev 1991;18:55–71.

30. Redmond J, Friedl KE, et al. Clinical usefulness of an algorithm for the early diagnosis of spinal metastatic disease. J Clin Oncol 1988;6:154–157.

31. Chen TC. Prostate cancer and spinal cord compression. Oncology (Huntington) 15:841–861.

32. British Orthopaedic Association and British Orthopaedic Oncology Society. Metastatic Bone Disease. A guide to good practice. Available at www.boa.ac.uk.

33. Osborn JL, Getzenberg RH, et al. Spinal cord compression in prostate cancer. J Neurooncol 1995;23:135–147.

34. Gilbert RW, Kim JH, et al. Epidural spinal cord compression from metastatic tumor: diagnosis and treatment. Ann Neurol 1978;3:40–51.

35. Cereceda LE, Flechon A, et al. Management of vertebral metastases in prostate carcinoma: a retrospective analysis in 119 patients. Clin Prostate Cancer 2003;2:34–40.

36. Smith EM, Hampel N, et al. Spinal cord compression secondary to prostate carcinoma: treatment and prognosis. J Urol 1993;149:330–333.

37. Shoskes DA, Perrin RG. The role of surgical management for symptomatic spinal cord compression in patients with metastatic prostate cancer. J Urol 1989;142:337–339.

38. Rosenthal MA, Rosen D, et al. Spinal cord compression in prostate cancer. A 10-year experience. Br J Urol 1992;69:530–583.

39. Schaberg J, Gainor BJ. A profile of metastatic carcinoma of the spine. Spine 1985 10:19–20.

40. Stark RJ, Henson JA, et al. Spinal metastases. A retrospective survey from a general hospital. Brain1982;105:189–213.

41. Godersky JC, Smoker WR, Knutson R. Use of magnetic resonance imaging in the evaluation of metastatic spinal disease. Neurosurgery 1987;21:676–680.

42. Carmody RF, Yang PJ, et al. Spinal cord compression due to metastatic disease: diagnosis with MR imaging versus myelography. Radiology 1989;173:225–259.

43. Li KC, Poon PY. Sensitivity and specificity of MRI in detecting malignant spinal cord compression and in distinguishing malignant from benign compression fractures of vertebrae. Magn Reson Imaging 1988;6:547–556.

44. Portenoy RK, Galer BS et al. Identification of epidural neoplasm. Radiography and bone scintigraphy in the symptomatic and asymptomatic spine. Cancer 1989;64:2207–2213.

45. Pollen JJ, Gerber K, Ashburn WL, et al. The value of nuclear bone imaging in advanced prostate cancer. J Urol 1981;125:222–223.

46. Merrick MV, Stone AR, Chisolm GD. Prostatic cancer. Nuclear medicine. Recent Res Cancer Res 1981;78:108–118.

47. Soerdjbalie-Maikoe V, Pelger RCM, Lycklama GA, et al. Bone scinigraphy predict the risk of spinal cord compression in hormone refractory prostate cancer. Eur J Nucl Med Mol Imaging 2004;31:958–963.

48. Weissman DE, Gilbert M, Wong H, et al. The use of computed tomography of the spine to identify patients at high risk of epidural metastases. J Clin Oncol 1985;3:1541–1544.

49. Martenson JA, Evans RG, et al. Treatment outcome and complications in patients treated for malignant epidural spinal cord compression (SCC). J Neurooncol 1985;3:77-84.

50. Greenberg HS, Kim JH et al. Epidural spinal cord compression from metastatic tumor: results with a new treatment protocol. Ann Neurol 1980;8:361–366.

51. Tong D, Gillick L, et al. The palliation of symptomatic osseous metastases: final results of the Study by the Radiation Therapy Oncology Group. Cancer 1982;50:893–899.

52. Findlay GF. The role of vertebral body collapse in the management of malignant spinal cord compression. J Neurol Neurosurg Psychiatry 1987;50:151–154.

53. Tomita TJ, Galicich H, et al. Radiation therapy for spinal epidural metastases with complete block. Acta Radiol Oncol 1983;22:135–143.

54. Helweg-Larsen S Johnsen A, et al. Radiologic features compared to clinical findings in a prospective study of 153 patients with metastatic spinal cord compression treated by radiotherapy. Acta Neurochir (Wien)1997;139:105–111.

55. Leviov M, Dale J, et al. The management of metastatic spinal cord compression: a radiotherapeutic success ceiling. Int J Radiat Oncol Biol Phys 1993;27:231–234.

56. Sasagawa I, Gotoh H et al. Hormonal treatment of symptomatic spinal cord compression in advanced prostatic cancer. Int Urol Nephrol 1991;23:351–356.

57. McLain RF, Bell GF. Newer management options in patients with spinal metastasis. Cleve Clin J Med 1998;65:359–366.

58. World Health Organization. Cancer pain relief and palliative care. Report of a WHO Expert Committee. World Health Organization Technical Report Series, 804. Geneva, Switzerland, World Health Organization, 1990;1–75.

59. Soresen PS, Helweg-Larsen S, Mouridsen H, et al. Effect of high dose dexamethasone in carcinomatous metastatic spinal cord compression treated with radiotherapy: a randomised trial. Eur J Cancer 1994;30A:22–27.

60. Heimdal K, Hirschberg H, et al. High incidence of serious side effects of high-dose dexamethasone treatment in patients with epidural spinal cord compression. J Neurooncol 1992;12:141–144.

61. Oefelein MG, Ricchiuiti V, Conrad W, et al. Skeletal fractures negatively correlate with overall survival in men with prostate cancer. J Urol 2002;1687:1005–1007.

62. Rosen LS, Gordon D, Antonio BS, et al. Zoledronic acid versus pamidronate in the treatment of skeletal metastases in patients with breast cancer or osteolytic lesions of multiple myeloma: a phase III, double-blind, comparative trial. Cancer J 2001;7:377–387.

Principles of palliative care and psychosocial support of the metastatic prostate cancer patient

104

Donald Newling

INTRODUCTION

The principal problem in the management of far advanced prostate cancer is the provision of the best palliative and psychosocial care for those patients who, because of metastatic disease, have a limited longevity and impending reduction of their quality of life.

There are a number of clearly defined problems, which are:

- The management of pain
- The management of urinary obstruction—upper or lower tract
- Skeletal-related events
- Rectal involvement
- Bone marrow failure
- Lymph edema
- Incontinence
- Psychosocial problems

CONTINUING ANTICANCER THERAPY

Patients with far advanced metastatic prostate cancer will almost certainly have been medically or surgically castrated and there is evidence to suggest that it is important that the castrate levels of testosterone are maintained even in this advanced state. In addition to hormonal therapy, there is an increasing role for cytotoxic treatment with docetaxel (Taxotere) or mitoxanthrone plus steroids.[1] These treatments, although having minimal effects on survival, can undoubtedly reduce the symptoms of advanced, and advancing, prostate cancer.

The recent demonstration that high-dose estrogens can also exert a cytotoxic effect at this stage of the disease has led to their increasing use systemically, via plasters or by intramuscular injections.[2] In addition, corticosteroids on their own have been shown on a number of occasions to have a beneficial effect on subjective progression and symptomatology in this advanced metastatic stage.[3]

MANAGEMENT OF PAIN IN ADVANCED PROSTATE CANCER

The majority of pain is caused by skeletal metastases. However, patients may experience severe pain from upper or lower urinary tract obstruction, rectal involvement, or direct involvement of the nerve plexuses in the pelvis. The cause of pain needs to be identified, in order that adequate analgesia may be given. The World Health Organization (WHO) have issued a pain ladder for the management of cancer-related pain and in this respect, prostate cancer is no different from other cancers and the general principles should be followed[4] (Figure 104.1).

The first step on this so-called pain ladder is the use of simple analgesics such as paracetamol or aspirin, or other nonsteroidal anti-inflammatory drugs. If pain persists, or increases, the second step would be the use of a weak opioid plus a non-opioid. For persistent pain after that then a strong opioid such as morphine itself plus a non-opioid should be used. Cancer related pain is continuous, and analgesia should be given in a continuous manner. Once the top rung of the ladder is reached, there is probably little point in increasing the

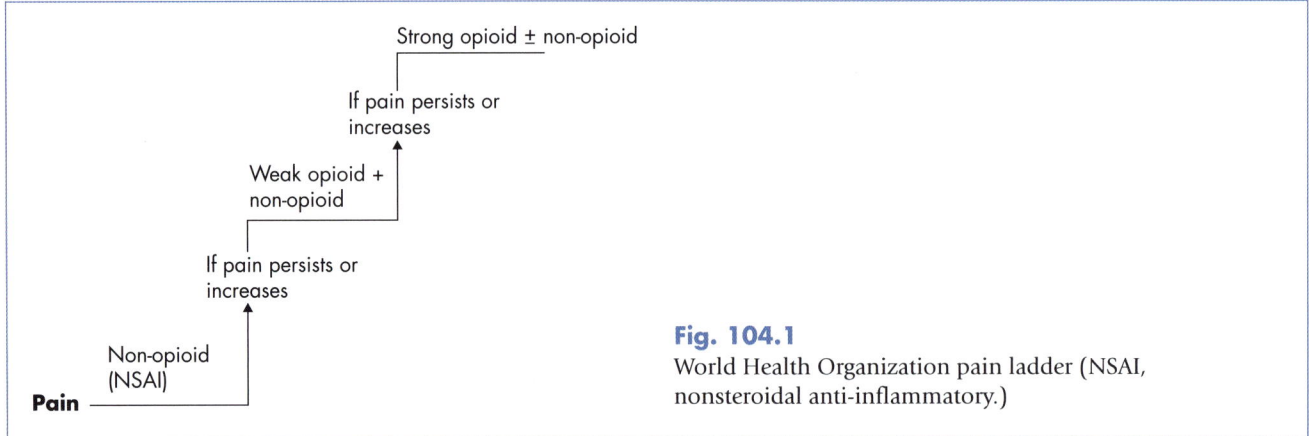

Fig. 104.1
World Health Organization pain ladder (NSAI, nonsteroidal anti-inflammatory.)

dose of morphine by less than 30% of the existing dose. Only then will the analgesia be adequate.[5] In the presence of excess nausea and/or vomiting, thought should be given to administering the opioid by a systemic or intrathecal route. The giving of opioids should be accompanied by the administration of suitable laxatives.

Ancillary therapy—such as the use of radiotherapy for individual sites of bone pain, the use of systemic radiotherapy via radioactive nucleotides such as strontium-89 (^{89}Sr), and if necessary the use of nerve blocks or rhizotomy—should be considered.[6,7]

The adequacy of analgesia can be improved by the treatment of related disorders such as muscle spasm. The use of anticonvulsants and muscle relaxants, the use of anxiolytics and antidepressants, which can relieve the distress caused by the pain, can also potentiate the activity of many analgesic drugs. For pain caused by a rising intracranial pressure or spinal cord compression, dexamethasone is an important and necessary adjunct.

The various contributing factors to the pain felt by prostate cancer sufferers is summarized in Figure 104.2.

URINARY TRACT OBSTRUCTION

UPPER URINARY TRACT

Local advancement of prostate cancer will frequently involve compression of the lower ureters, dilatation of the upper tract, and impending uremia. With the advent of JJ stents and the simplicity of bringing in nephrostomy tubes, it is tempting to suggest that upper urinary tract obstruction should always so be treated. However, if the general condition of the patient is deteriorating rapidly, and particularly if he has severe pain from other metastatic lesions, the dulling of the sensorium consequent upon the onset of uremia may be a blessing and diminish the need for large doses of strong analgesics and other similar drugs.[10] JJ stents can usually only be left in situ for 6 months and very frequently will block earlier. It may then be necessary to substitute these internal splints for external nephrostomies with accompanying deterioration in the patient's mobility and quality of life. Recently metal stents have been

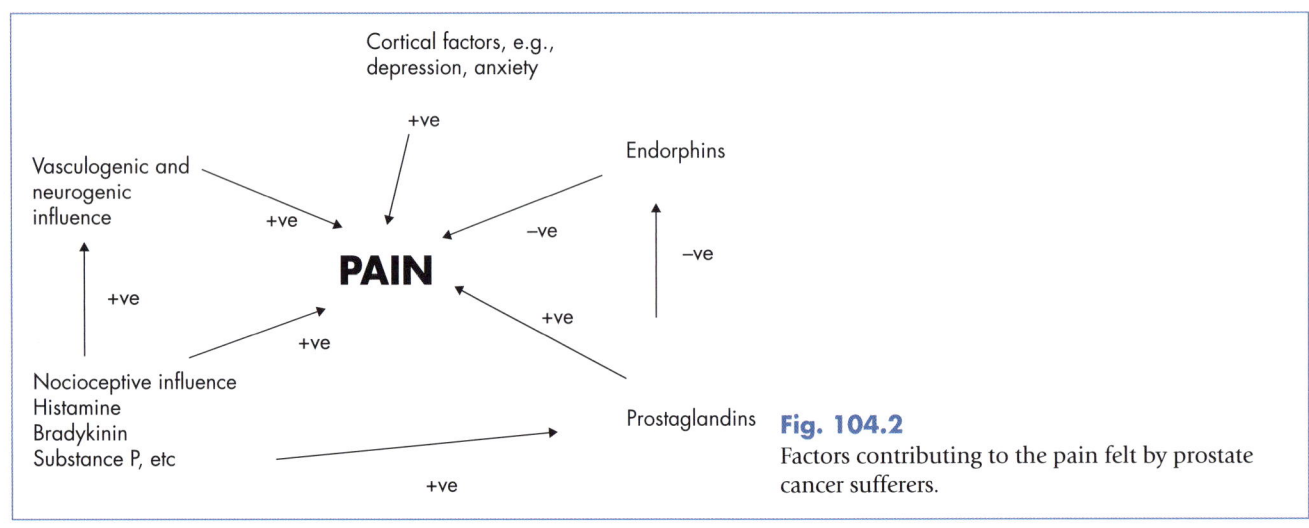

Fig. 104.2
Factors contributing to the pain felt by prostate cancer sufferers.

developed that can be inserted into the renal pelvis at the one end and into the bladder at the other end. These can be brought in via a laparoscopy and do not necessarily mean a long operative procedure. They can frequently be left in for longer than 6 months.[11]

LOWER URINARY TRACT

If the patient's general condition is good, lower urinary tract obstruction may be relieved by a simple transurethral procedure. Removing large quantities of malignant tissue may often impair sphincter activity and lead to incontinence. The alternative is the use of a transurethral catheter or suprapubic catheter if incontinence is not a problem.[12]

SKELETAL-RELATED EVENTS

Skeletal-related events such as fracture are associated with pain and the danger of neurologic damage involving spinal cord compression and paralysis. The greatest hazard exists in the lower thoracic cord where the spinal canal is narrower than elsewhere. When a skeletal-related event such as fracture or nerve compression occurs, it is important that action is taken as quickly as possible in order to diminish the long-term effects. This may require local radiotherapy or surgery with or without radiotherapy. The use of high-dose steroids such as dexamethasone is recommended. Recently the incidence of skeletal related events in bony metastases has been shown to be lessened by the use of second and third generation bisphosphonates. These can be given in an intermittent manner once every 3 weeks until the situation is under control, and possibly in smaller doses than have been used in the recent past. In addition to bisphosphonates, endothelium A receptor antagonists diminish the activity of osteoblasts and can, therefore, limit new bone formation stimulated by prostate cancer metastases.[13]

RECTAL SYMPTOMS

Direct invasion from the primary prostate tumor into the rectum is not an infrequent occurrence. Occasionally the tumor can cause obstruction of the rectum. A transanal resection of the tumor is sometimes necessary under these circumstances.[14] If the tumor encircles the rectum causing complete obstruction, then a diverting colostomy may become necessary. This is also a useful palliative tool in the presence of a fistula or fecal incontinence caused by direct involvement of the nerves involved in anal sphincter control. Occasionally the local spread of tumor is so ferocious that the sacral plexus is involved, giving rise to very severe pain and often necessitating the placement of a colostomy, a suprapubic catheter, and neurolysis.[13]

BONE MARROW FAILURE

In prostatic cancer, bone marrow failure is caused by direct infiltration of the marrow with depletion of myeloid and erythroid lines. There may also be severe platelet reduction and dysfunction. Apart from direct infiltration by tumor cells, the castrate levels of testosterone give rise to a reduction of at least 10% in the average hemoglobin of patients with prostate cancer. The platelet dysfunction can be so severe as to give rise to disseminated intravascular coagulation, and this may necessitate the paradoxical use of anticoagulants in the short term.[15] For total bone marrow failure blood transfusion will be necessary, but again the use of transfusions must be weighed against the likely prognosis for individual patients. Where the predominance is of anemia, the use of recombinant erythropoietin is an attractive, though expensive, substitute for blood transfusion.[16]

LYMPH EDEMA

In the first instance, lymph edema, which is often very troublesome in the genital region, may be relieved by elevation of the bed at night and of a settee during the day. Sometimes the edema is so severe that it is necessary to pass a catheter to enable adequate voiding to take place. Graduated compression with stockings of the lower limbs is an alternative, and intermittent pneumatic compression is recommended if the lower-limb edema is very severe. Lymph edema may occur together with venous edema. Where there is a clear indication that venous obstruction plays a significant role, then anticoagulant therapy may be indicated.[17]

INCONTINENCE

Diagnosis of incontinence must be adequately made. The differentiation between overflow incontinence due to outflow obstruction and incontinence caused by neurogenic or muscular damage either caused iatrogenically or by the disease process itself must be made. If overflow incontinence is the problem and the patient's general condition is good, then a transurethral resection is the best alternative. Neurogenic incontinence or incontinence caused by direct involvement via the tumor should probably be managed by a transurethral catheter. A suprapubic catheter is not to be recommended apart from in the management of overflow incontinence.[18]

PSYCHOSOCIAL DISORDERS AND THEIR MANAGEMENT

There are four stages during the development and progression of prostate cancer where there is major psychosocial trauma, frequently accompanied by the appearance of psychological or even psychiatric disturbance.[19]

The diagnosis of a malignancy is always a life-shattering event. At the beginning of the disease, the patient and his family must be given realistic prognoses and a logical and clear description of the various treatment options at their disposal. If the initial therapy, as is most frequent, is to be carried out with curative intent then the next psychological blow will occur when the patient develops rising prostate-specific antigen (PSA) levels or can be clearly told that the disease has recurred. The decision, at this point in time, of whether to introduce palliative therapy in the form of hormonal treatment will vary from patient to patient and from one tumor to another. Once the second line treatment has been started, there will probably be a period of 18 months to 2 years before "hormone escape" occurs. Ultimately, the tumor will progress, and this will be the third blow to the patient's psyche and that of his family. In the past, the fourth shock came when patients were told that we had no further therapeutic options. In the present treatment climate, this is never to be said. It is almost always possible for the symptoms of the disease to be controlled even if the disease itself is rampant.

Prostate cancer is a disease that affects the whole family and, therefore, the decision process, if the patient so wishes, should be shared. From the beginning, it is often wise to involve the patient and his family in the care process whether by modifications of diet or physical activity or simply by broadening the consultation process.

Sadly, the psychiatric care of the elderly with psychiatric disturbances has often been inadequate because of the fear of side effects of treatment.[20,21] The patient with prostate cancer who develops psychological or psychiatric disturbances should be treated exactly the same way as someone who does not have the cancer. If the disturbance is iatrogenic then modification of their medication is the first and most important step. Depression, anxiety, and fear are the three most common psychological disturbances, and each should be managed on its own merit. The use of anxiolytic drugs and antidepressants is to be encouraged, not only to relieve the psychological disturbance, but also to improve the effectiveness of analgesia and other therapeutic maneuvers. Care must be taken with the use of some antidepressants, such as the tricyclics, which can have a deleterious effect on urinary control.[22] It is important to remember that, because many of the patients at this stage of their disease are elderly, communication may become increasingly difficult, particularly in the presence of psychotropic or neurotropic drugs and in the presence of strong analgesia. It is important that a clinician knows the patient has received and understood the messages and suggestions.

The patient sits in the middle of a circle of carers including the primary care team, palliative care team, the lead care team (Urology) and the oncology team (Figure 104.3). Just as important in this circle is the family and the needs of the family before, during and after the death of the patient must be considered.[23]

Patients with an advancing malignancy often go through a number of psychological disturbances throughout the course of the disease. There is always an element of confusion at the beginning, associated with a certain amount of resentment and often attempts to find a cause involving other people or his environment. Once progression of the disease has been confirmed, there is often a tacit acceptance, which may lead to a reluctance to try further therapeutic measures. As the end approaches, the patient often experiences considerable fear, which may include fear of the method

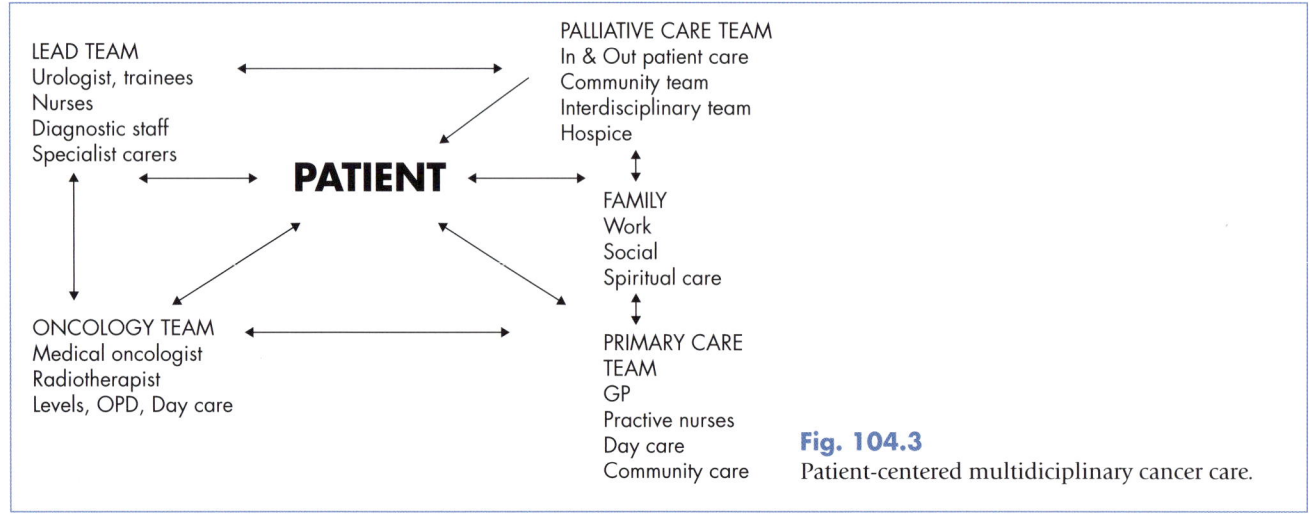

Fig. 104.3
Patient-centered multidiciplinary cancer care.

of his demise, fear of losing control either physically, of bowel or bladder, or mentally, with an inability to control his emotions and other thought processes, but also an intense fear for those that he is leaving behind who may also be elderly and infirm. These factors must all be addressed appropriately by members of the teams, and the patient and his family must know that, at the end, his symptoms will be adequately controlled and his family and those others he leaves behind will be adequately looked after.[24]

CONCLUSIONS

The progress of prostate cancer is much slower than with other malignant tumors, and, therefore, the prognosis is longer and sometimes more complicated. This means that the quality of care for the patient needs to be carefully maintained throughout, involving multidisciplinary teams and sensible and logical use of the therapeutic modalities available. Although the greatest responsibility for the management of these patients lies with the lead team, that team must be prepared at all stages to involve other teams who could help individual aspects of the patients condition. The Association of Palliative Medicine defines palliation as the appropriate medical care of patient's with advanced and progressive disease for whom the focus of care is quality of life and in whom the prognosis is limited. In the case of prostate cancer this prognosis may be limited but may last many years giving the clinician and those who work with him/her the opportunity at all stages to optimize therapy ensuring the best quality of life, where the quantity cannot be increased, and the highest possible quality of death for the patient and those around him.

REFERENCES

1. Petrylak DP. Chemotherapy for androgen independent prostate cancer. Semin Urol Oncol 2002;3:31–35.
2. Ockrim JL, Lalani E-N, Laniado ME, et al. Transdermal Estradiol Therapy for Advanced Prostate Cancer – Forward to the Past?, Departments of Surgical Oncology and Technology, Histopathology, Faculty of Medicine, Imperial College and Department Urology, Hammersmith Hospitals NHS Trust.
3. Hanks GW, Trueman T, Twycross RG. Corticosteroids in terminal cancer – a prospective analysis of current practice. Postgrad Med J 1983;59:702–706.
4. World Health Organization, Cancer Pain Relief. Geneva: WHO, 1994.
5. Hanks G, Expert Working Group EAPC. Morphine in cancer pain: modes of administration. Br Med J 1996;312:823–826.
6. Soerdjbalie-Maikoev V, Pelger RC, Lycklama A, et al. Strontium-89 (Metastron) and the bisphosphonate olpadronate reduce the incidence of spinal cord compression in patients with hormone-refractory prostate cancer metastatic to the skeleton. Eur J Nucl Med Imaging 2002;29:494–498.
7. Lacovou J, Marks JC, Abrams PH, et al. Cord compression and carcinoma prostate: is laminectomy justified. Br J Urol 1985;57:733–736.
8. Holland JC. Psycho-oncology: overview, obstacles and opportunities. Pscyho Oncol 1992;1:1–13.
9. Moorey S, Greer S, Bliss J, et al. Comparison of adjuvant psychological therapy and supportive counselling in patients with cancer. Psycho Oncol 1998;7:218–228.
10. Paul AB, Love C, Chisholm GD. The management of bilateral ureteric obstruction and renal failure in advanced prostate cancer. Br J Urol 1994;5:642–645.
11. Jabour ME, Desgrandchamps F, Angelscu E, et al. Percutaneous implantation of subcutaneous prosthetic ureters: long term outcome. J Endo Urol 2001;15:611–614.
12. Mazur AW, Thompson IM. Efficacy and morbidity of 'channel' TURP. Urology 1991;38:562–628.
13. Clarke NW. The management of hormone-relapsed prostate cancer, Christie Hospital NHS Trust and Salford Royal Hospitals NHS Trust, Manchester, UK. BJU Intl 2003;92:860–868.
14. Chen TF, Eardley I, Doyle PT, et al. Rectal obstruction secondary to carcinoma of the prostate treated by trans-anal resection of the prostate. Br J Urol 1992;70:643–647.
15. Gobel BH. Bleeding disorders. In Groenwald S, Grogge M, Goodman M, Yarbro C eds, Cancer Nursing—Principles and Practice. Boston, MA: Jones Bartlett, 1993, pp 575–607.
16. Albers PH, Cappell R, Schwaibold H, et al. Erythropoietin in urologic oncology. Eur Urol 2001;39:1–8.
17. Brennan MJ. Lymphoedema following the surgical management of breast cancer. J Pain Sympt Manage 1992;2:110–116.
18. Fossa SD. Quality of life in advanced prostate cancer. Semin Oncol 1996;23:32–34.
19. Derogatis LR. The prevalence of psychiatric disorders among cancer patients. J Am Med Assoc 1983;249:751–757.
20. Cleary JF, Carbonne PP. Palliative medicine in the elderly. Cancer 1997;80:1335–1347.
21. Lynch M. The assessment and prevalence of affective disorders in advanced cancer. J Palliat Care 1995;11:10–18.
22. Massie MJ, Holland JC. Depression and the cancer patient. J Clin Psychiatry 1990;51:12–17.
23. Grzybowska P. What are the palliative care needs of prostate cancer patients? In Bowsher W (ed.): Challenges in Prostate Cancer. Oxford: Blackwell Science, 2000.
24. Stjernswald J. Palliative medicine: a global perspective, In Doyle D, Hanks GWC, MacDonald N (eds): Oxford Textbook of Palliative Medicine. Oxford: Oxford University Press, 1996, pp 805–816.

The promise of immunotherapy in prostate cancer: from concept to reality

105

Vasily J Assikis, William Jonas, Jonathan W Simons

INTRODUCTION

Significant progress has been made since the mid 1990s in our ability to treat patients with advanced prostate cancer. Most prostate cancer patients now present with localized disease and mortality rates are dropping.[1] Despite the fact that the vast majority of men with prostate cancer are diagnosed with localized disease, current therapies for localized disease will cure only 50% to 85% of patients.[2–4] For patients with widespread prostate cancer the disease remains incurable with the currently available agents. Historically, metastatic disease has been treated with androgen deprivation therapy. Despite the extremely high response rates with this modality (>85%), patients universally progress once the cancer transitions to a castration-independent phenotype. Castration-independent prostate cancer (CIPC) is currently treated with cytotoxic chemotherapy. Work done over the past decade has clearly established that: 1) chemotherapy offers superior palliation (over steroids alone) and improvement of quality of life[5]; and 2) taxane-based chemotherapy offers a statistically significant, albeit modest, overall survival benefit.[6–7] This minor survival benefit achieved with taxanes has been met with great enthusiasm—since it is the first time ever any systemic therapy has been shown to affect overall survival in the CIPC setting. Nonetheless, a median survival of 1.5 years (as reported in the phase III registration trials with docetaxel) can not be seen as the goal but, rather, the starting line for further improvement. New concepts for treatment of advanced prostate cancer are urgently needed.

Currently, over 200 novel therapies are being tested in patients with prostate cancer. In addition to novel cytotoxic agents, interest has also focused on immunologic modulation (vaccines), targeted therapies (based on prostate-specific antigen [PSA] or prostate-specific membrane antigen [PSMA]), overcoming antiapoptotic and proliferative signaling (vitamin D analogs, PPARγ agonists, anti-BCL2), and disruption of key intracellular circuitry (signaling through epidermal growth factor receptor [EGFR], PI3/Akt, insulin-like growth factor 1 receptor [IGF1R], mitogen-activated protein kinase [MAPK], and interleukin 6 [IL6], just to name a few).[8] An expanding body of literature is developing over the merit and clinical benefits of targeting the host for metastatic prostate cancer, namely the bone. We now have well-described pairs of targets/therapeutic agents: osteoclasts/bisphosphonates, osteoblasts/endothelin 1 inhibitors, cancer-stroma interface/radiopharmaceuticals. Finally, targeting of the prerequisite new blood vessel formation, namely angiogenesis, has led to a number of investigational options currently tested in large scale trials.

It is the scope of this chapter to review recent advances in emerging therapies with a special focus on immunotherapy for prostate cancer.

IMMUNOTHERAPY

The origins of immunotherapy as a treatment for cancer were first given credence when surgeons in the late nineteenth century observed spontaneous tumor regressions in patients. Noting that these were often preceded by infections, Coley et al were challenged in reproducing this phenomenon by treating patients with bacterial extracts.[9] Spontaneous remissions following intense inflammatory reactions are a known phenomenon reported in current literature as well.[10] In the early 1970s, the hypothesis of immune surveillance was presented. At its crux, the hypothesis held that the immune system maintained a role in protecting the host against tumors.[11] This hypothesis was later discounted with observations that the incidence of cancer in athymic mice was no different than that observed in wild-type mice.[12] In support of the above preclinical finding is the epidemiologic observation that immunosuppressed individuals do not appear to be more susceptible to common malignancies including prostate, colon, breast, and lung cancer, (although there is a higher incidence of Epstein–Barr virus-associated lymphomas, Kaposi's sarcoma and cervical cancer[13]). Subsequent research has demonstrated that tumors are not lacking potential antigens, but rather fail to activate the immune system to respond to them.[14] Tumors are, therefore, successful in inducing immune tolerance, hence circumventing the innate mechanisms of defense. It is now felt that it is not lack of appropriate nonself antigens that prevents a robust activation of the immune effector arm against tumor, but rather an unsuccessful discrimination between self and nonself.[15] Therefore, there is a role for the immune system in surveillance. In fact, the goal of therapy has shifted towards how to 1) most effectively present antigens to T cells; 2) enhance activation of cytotoxic immune effector cells as well as maximize humoral response; and 3) optimize delivery/trafficking of immune effector cells/cytokines to the tumor.

Pertinent issues to prostate cancer, with regard to immunomodulatory approaches, include the type and number of antigens employed as targets, various methods to generate either an in-vivo or an ex-vivo activation of specific anti-prostate immunity. A unique advantage is the lack of need for specificity for malignant prostate tissue: attack of benign prostatic tissue by use of antigens not restricted to cancer cells is, by and large, without clinical implications (of note, inflammation of benign prostatic tissue secondary to immune activation may lead to PSA elevation). In the following paragraphs we will review several methods of active and passive immunotherapy that have been tested in clinical trials.

ACTIVE IMMUNOTHERAPY

PROSTATE CANCER VACCINES

In designing a vaccine, there are two basic categories of antigens to take advantage of, those that have been identified and those that have not.[16] As one would expect, there are numerous antigens that have not been identified and there are over 500 sequences, unique to prostate cancer, known already. When a vaccine is developed from a whole cancer cell lysate, the underlying principle is that myriads of antigens, both known and unknown, would be present. This, in turn, would present more antigens for priming to the immune system and, as prostate cancer cells are known to downregulate antigens to evade immune recognition, it would make it more difficult for them to do so. There are advantages and disadvantages to approaches using defined and undefined antigens; some of these are listed in Table 105.1.

Since the mid-1990s, one of the preferred platforms for active immunotherapy has been the use of autologous dendritic cells. Such an approach has a number of advantages. Dendritic cells (DCs) are the most efficient antigen-presenting cells (APCs) that initiate an antigen-specific immune response via uptake, processing, and presentation of antigens to T cells. Dendritic cells migrate to draining lymph nodes, where they present antigens to resting lymphocytes. When fully activated, DCs express high levels of cell surface major histocompatibility antigen complexes (MHC). For optimal activation of the effector arm it is crucial that co-stimulatory molecules (CD80,86/CD28; or the CD40 ligand/CD40 pairs) bind as well. Autologous dendritic cells can be harvested by leukapheresis, treated ex vivo with protocols that maximize maturation and activation, and then used as vehicles for carrying antigens to selected targets.[17] Antigen delivery to DCs can employ peptides, whole proteins, or even tumor mRNA; or, alternatively, viral vector systems can be used to transfect DCs with DNA encoding tumor associated antigens. In the next paragraphs we will provide a review of some DC-based vaccines for prostate cancer that have been tested in the clinic.

Table 105.1 Comparison of defined and undefined antigens for prostate cancer

	Defined antigens (e.g., PSA, PSMA)	Undefined cell-based vaccine antigens
Advantages	Potential to monitor immune response Easier biotechnology for manufacture and FDA review Prostate specificity	Available to larger patient population Enhance tumor immune surveillance Polyclonal immune responses Prostate specificity
Disadvantages	Genetically unstable tumors can easily evade immune surveillance through single antigenic loss Expression of antigen only in a fraction of cancer cells	Difficulty in assessing specific immune response in trials Requires autologous or allogeneic cells More complex biotechnology for manufacture and FDA review

PSA, prostate-specific antigen; PMSA, prostate-specific membrane antigen.

PROSTATE-SPECIFIC MEMBRANE ANTIGEN VACCINES

The first published report on a DC vaccine in prostate cancer involved the intravenous administration of autologous DCs pulsed with synthetic PSMA peptides. A phase I trial using DCs looked at human leukocyte antigen A2 (HLA-A2)-specific PSMA peptides (PSM-P1 and PSM-P2). Autologous DCs pulsed with these PSMA peptides were administered to 51 patients with CIPC.[18] All patients received four infusions of the preparations at 6-week intervals. There was no dosing limit achieved, and there were no significant toxicities. Cellular responses to the appropriate PSMA peptides were monitored. Subjects who were positive for HLA-A2 and who received DCs pulsed with PSM-P1 and PSM-P2 had increased cellular responses. There were 7 patients who achieved a greater than 50% reduction in their serum PSA levels; and 11 patients had stable disease. A subsequent phase II trial recruited 95 men with either locally recurrent (n = 37) or metastatic (n = 58) CIPC.[19] Six infusions of dendritic cells pulsed with either PSM-P1 or P2 were administered at 6-week intervals. This time, half of the patients also received 7 days of subcutaneous granulocyte-macrophage colony-stimulating factor (GM-CSF) with each infusion. Using the same response criteria as in the phase I study, three complete and 16 partial responses were reported; 11 responses were still ongoing at the time of the report. The addition of GM-CSF was not reported to significantly improve the clinical or immune response to vaccination. One of the major criticisms of the early work with this approach was the lack of correlation of peptide specific T-cell cytotoxicity with favorable outcome.[20] Furthermore, many patients were not HLA-A2-positive, and five of the responders were in fact HLA-A2-negative, an observation that called into question the specificity of the response to this peptide-based intervention. More recently, preliminary clinical data with a modification of the initial PSMA-targeted vaccine were presented. In a phase I/II trial, 24 patients with metastatic CIPC underwent a dose escalation of DCVax™ (Northwest Biotherapeutics), an autologous DC vaccine loaded with recombinant whole PSMA.[21] While only two patients had a greater than 50% reduction in their PSA, a total of 38% (nine) had an improvement in their post-treatment PSA slope. Of note, favorable clinical outcome was correlated with humoral response (development of anti-PSMA antibodies) but not with markers of cellular response.

PROVENGE

Provenge™ (Dendreon, Seattle, Washington) is a vaccine consisting of autologous dendritic cells exposed ex vivo to PA-2024 (a recombinant fusion protein of human prostatic acid phosphatase and GM-CSF). In a phase I/II study, 31 men with metastatic CIPC received escalating doses of intravenous Provenge during weeks 0, 4, 8, and 24.[22] There were no significant adverse events and the only toxicity reported was minor infusional reactions (fever, chills). Three of 19 men treated on the phase II portion had a decline in PSA of more than 50%, and time to progression was significantly longer in immune responders compared with non-responders (34 versus 13 weeks).These promising results led to a placebo-controlled phase III trial that randomized 127 men with asymptomatic metastatic CIPC to Provenge or placebo every 2 weeks for three doses.[23] In a preliminary report, the longer time to progression in the treated group did not reach the level of statistical significance (16 versus 9 weeks; p = 0.085), but those receiving the vaccine had a significantly higher chance of remaining free of cancer-related pain. A subset analysis found a significant clinical benefit for patients with Gleason score 7 or less and led the foundation for a second randomized phase III trial that is currently ongoing. Provenge is currently being tested also in the setting of PSA rise after prostatectomy in a prospective fashion.

PROSTATE-SPECIFIC ANTIGEN VACCINES

There are many reasons to consider using mRNA as a basis of a DC vaccine strategy including: 1) the generation of mRNA is relatively easy; 2) there is very little risk of the mRNA inserting itself into the host DNA; and 3) the production of an antigen by RNA will present multiple epitopes.[24] This approach will also be available to a wider range of patients as HLA-typing will not be necessary. In a phase I clinical trial, autologous DCs transfected with mRNA encoding PSA were used to treat 13 patients with metastatic CIPC.[25] They were treated with escalating doses of the vaccine, with the maximum dose being determined by the level of obtained DCs. There were no dose limiting toxicities with only grade 1 toxicity being reported including four patients with fever and influenza-like symptoms and four patients with injection site erythema. Nine patients had PSA-reactive T-cells measured pre- and post-treatment, all of whom initially had low or undetectable levels of PSA-reactive T-cells, and all had measurable levels after vaccination. There was no cross-reactivity against negative control proteins including human serum kallikrein or keyhole limpet hemocyanin (KLH). Prostate-specific antigen serum levels were also monitored. Seven patients were evaluable (the other 6 proceeded with therapies that could affect PSA levels including radiation for progressive disease or use of herbal medications). One of seven patients had a minor decrease in PSA. Interestingly, five additional patients were observed to have a decrease in their PSA velocity. While this does not provide evidence for clinical benefit, the measurable immune responses are promising.

CARBOHYDRATE VACCINES

Taking a very different approach, Slovin et al, have worked on vaccines that target epithelial surface carbohydrates: the idea is based on the observation that malignant cells express a different carbohydrate pattern on their cell surfaces than normal cells.[26]

Alpha-*N*-acetylgalactosamine-*O*-serine/threonine (Tn), is a monosaccharide that is found to be highly expressed by mucins on most epithelial cancers. Slovin et al conjugated the mucin-related *O*-linked glycopeptide Tn to KLH to give Tn(c)-KLH and to palmitic acid (PAM) to give Tn(c)-PAM, both with the saponin adjuvant QS21 so as to boost immune response. In a phase I study, they treated 25 patients with biochemically relapsed prostate cancer.[27] Three groups of five patients received separate dosing regimens of the Tn(c)-KLH vaccine and, in the fourth group, 10 patients received Tn(c)-PAM. Administration was at random sites subcutaneously on patients' extremities at weeks 1, 2, 3, 7, 19, and a booster at week 50. All patients were able to complete the series. Side effects were mainly limited to pain and irritation at the injection sites. As the target here was not isolated to malignant cells only, there was a concern for autoimmunity, which was not observed. Interestingly, the lower dose of Tn(c)-KLH appeared to be optimal, with the suggestion that higher doses may in fact confer a suppression of antibody responses. At 50 weeks, of the 15 patients treated with Tn(c)-KLH, 5 had a greater than 50% decrease in their PSA slopes. Of the 10 Tn(c)-PAM recipients, only one had a greater than 50% PSA slope reduction.

HUMAN TELOMERASE REVERSE TRANSCRIPTASE VACCINES

Human telomerase reverse transcriptase (hTERT) is overexpressed in more than 85% of solid tumors.[28] Due to its presence in solid tumors and its role in tumor growth, hTERT is an attractive molecular target.[29] It has been demonstrated that autologous DCs transfected with mRNA encoding hTERT are potent inducers of cytotoxic T lymphocytes (CTLs) and antitumor immunity.[30] Having established antitumor efficacy in models, a phase I trial was undertaken in 18 patients with CIPC.[31] Patients were vaccinated with DCs trandsfected with either hTERT or both hTERT and lysosome-associated membrane protein (LAMP) RNA. Lysosome-associated membrane protein was included as it has been shown previously that it leads to a greater stimulation of CD4+ T cells without negatively affecting the CTL response.[32] All 18 patients were found to have high frequencies of hTERT-specific CD8+ and CD4+ T cells. The vaccine was associated with clearance of circulating tumor cells and a positive impact on PSA velocity in a few patients. Those receiving hTERT/LAMP were found to have higher frequencies of CD4+ T cells and, additionally, their CTLs were found to exhibit a greater cytolytic activity against their targets.

Another group investigating hTERT conducted a phase I trial evaluating cancer patients.[33] Seven patients, five with hormone refractory prostate cancer and two with metastatic breast cancer resistant to conventional cytotoxic therapy, were vaccinated with HLA-A2-restricted hTERT 1540 peptide presented with keyhole limpet hemocyanin by ex-vivo generated DCs. Researchers recognized that certain normal cells, including the bone marrow, express telomerase activity and, therefore, followed the bone marrow by aspirations at the initial and at the third vaccine. There were no grade 3 or 4 adverse events, and no histologic changes were noted in the marrow. Serum immunoglobulin levels and absolute peripheral B-lymphocyte counts were monitored with no significant changes observed. Four of the prostate cancer patients had stable disease by standard radiographic assessment post-vaccination whereas one patient with breast cancer had progressive disease. Prostate-specific antigen levels were found to fall slightly during the vaccine schedule in two patients, before rising again. Important in this study was the demonstration of the induction of hTERT-specific CD8+ T cells without significant toxicity. In addition, after vaccination, there was one patient who experienced partial tumor regression, and with biopsy demonstrated infiltrating CD8+ lymphocytes.

MISCELLANEOUS VACCINES

Utilizing identified antigens for a peptide vaccine, a phase I trial was conducted with 10 patients with CIPC who were positive for HLA-A2.[34] After a prevaccination measurement of peptide-specific CTL precursors, a vaccine was individually designed based on each patient's positivity to a panel of 16 identified peptides. The median number of positive peptides administered was three (range 1–5). There were no major adverse reactions, but all developed grade I or II local erythema/edema at the injection site. Of the 10 patients, three were found to have a minor (<50%) PSA response. Recognizing that immune response did not translate into clinical benefit, Noguchi et al combined their vaccine with chemotherapy (estramustine).[35] Release of antigens by cells dying due to chemotherapy should allow cross-priming and, thus, enhance the activation of the effector arm. Results were very promising with 10 of 11 patients experiencing a decrease in PSA level, with eight of them experiencing a reduction of more than 50%. Six patients had an augmentation of peptide-specific CTL precursors, while peptide-specific IgG was observed in 10 of 11. There are plans for phase II studies.

GENE TRANSFER BIOTECHNOLOGIES FOR PROSTATE CANCER IMMUNOTHERAPY

Gene therapy involves the insertion of DNA into a cell to replace, or otherwise affect, gene expression of that cell. The goal of gene therapy, as it relates to cancer, is to reverse the malignant phenotype of the cell, trigger apoptosis, or for the altered cell to be marked for immune disposal by way of increasing the tumor cell's immunogenicity and/or by increasing the immune system's responsiveness to the tumor cell. Great strides in the field of gene therapy research have been made since the first human gene therapy trial was performed in 1990.[36] While the simplicity of the concept is elegant, it is a complex process.

Gene therapy requires a delivery vehicle (vector) to carry the therapeutic genetic information. A vector needs only to contain the gene of interest and a promoter to drive its expression.[37] There are many considerations when choosing the optimal vector: the ideal vector would be able to deliver its product specifically to the target cell, deliver it efficiently, not be toxic to the host, not be immunogenic, and not be mutagenic. On top of that, it would need to be reproducible, widely applicable, and of a reasonable cost. Vectors can be separated into two general categories: viral and nonviral (liposomes, naked DNA, DNA polymer complexes). Viral vectors are further subdivided to either DNA- or RNA-based platforms. Viral vectors utilize the inherent ability of viruses to carry foreign DNA into cells, and they are known to deliver genes much more efficiently than their nonviral counterparts. DNA vaccines are often preferable because they are easier to make, are not pathogenic, and the vectors are nonreplicating.[38] In the early experience with viral vectors, modified replication-deficient adenoviruses were employed: in an effort to curtail uncontrolled pathogenic replication, the price was transient expression of the therapeutic gene. More recently, replication-competent viruses (such as retroviruses) have been employed; they have the unique advantage of incorporating into the DNA of rapidly dividing (i.e., cancer) cells so that they are continuously expressed in the original target cell, and in any subsequent cells after mitosis. The efficiency of this approach is hindered by the low proliferative rates typically seen in prostate cancer.[38]

While the technology of DNA transporters continues to advance, some of the issues remain unresolved:

- Should the vector require a synthesizing target cell for integration of the delivered gene?
- If the vector provides incorporation of the delivered gene into the DNA of the target cell or into its cytoplasm, is it necessary for the gene to be expressed transiently or continuously?
- In a viral vector, is the desired effect for the vector to be replication deficient, attenuated, such that it enters only permissive cells, or competent?

Table 105.2 lists various vectors with their advantages and disadvantages. Additional considerations include whether the vector is used to deliver DNA into cells removed from the patient (ex-vivo approach) that are subsequently re-administered upon genetic manipulation, or delivered to the subject directly

---

Table 105.2 Advantages and disadvantages of some vectors for gene therapy

Vector	Advantage	Disadvantage
RNA retroviruses		
Oncovirus	Transmit to offspring, possible long-term expression	Only infects actively dividing cells, risk of insertional mutagenesis, low efficiency, inactivated by complement
Lentivirus	Can infect nondividing cells, long-term expression, not inactivated by complement	Possible recombination with other viruses
Human foamy virus	Can infect nondividing cells, not inactivated by complement, nonpathogenic	Low titers
DNA viruses		
Vaccinia virus	Large size, replicates	Low efficiency, immunity develops
Herpes simplex virus	Large size, can infect nondividing cells, episomal therefore no risk for insertional mutagenesis	Low titers, transient expression
Adenovirus	Can infect nondividing cells, episomal therefore no risk for insertional mutagenesis	Transient expression
Adeno-associated viruses	Can infect nondividing cells, nonpathogenic	Limited size, insertional mutagenesis
Synthetic vectors		
Naked DNA	Low cost, simple preparation, nontoxic	Poor efficiency
Liposomes	Large insertion size, safe for repeated use, low cost, nontoxic	Poor efficiency, short expression
DNA–protein complex	Large insertion size, safe for repeated use, low cost, nontoxic	Poor efficiency, short expression

Adapted from Mabjeesh NJ, Zhong H, Simons JW. Gene therapy of prostate cancer: current and future directions. Endocrine-related cancer 2002;9:115–139.

(in-vivo approach). In the next paragraphs we will review some approaches that have been of particular interest to prostate cancer

GRANULOCYTE-MACROPHAGE COLONY-STIMULATING FACTOR GENE THERAPY

Initial investigations in gene therapy for prostate cancer consisted of ex-vivo approaches, in which the patient's own prostate cancer cells (typically obtained at the time of prostatectomy) were manipulated to overexpress the cytokine GM-CSF via retroviral transfer. When the irradiated cells were then reintroduced into the patient, in-vivo secretion of GM-CSF was postulated to promote the uptake of tumor antigens by the patient's dendritic cells.[39]

Granulocyte-macrophage colony-stimulating factor is a cytokine that regulates granulocyte and macrophage stimulation, proliferation, differentiation, and survival. Mulligan et al used a relatively nonimmunogenic tumor model to identify specific gene products that could

induce antitumor immunity that could not be achieved with the tumor cells alone.[40] They found GM-CSF to be the most potent product they studied, later attributed to its most potent stimulation and activation of antigen uptake by DCs.[41] This laid the framework for using GM-CSF as vaccine therapy. Using an ex-vivo approach, as demonstrated in Figure 105.1, a vaccine was generated where a patient's own prostate cancer cells, usually collected at the time of prostatectomy, were engineered by way of a retrovirus to incorporate a gene, which led to the overexpression of GM-CSF. The cells were then irradiated and reintroduced into the patient: in-vivo secretion of GM-CSF should promote uptake of antigens by DCs. In a phase I trial, eight patients, who underwent a radical prostatectomy with curative intent but at surgery were found to have metastatic disease to the regional lymph nodes, were treated with an autologous, GM-CSF-secreting, and irradiated tumor vaccine prepared ex vivo from surgically obtained autologous prostate cancer cells.[39] The number of administered courses was limited to the amount of prepared vaccine. The main side effects

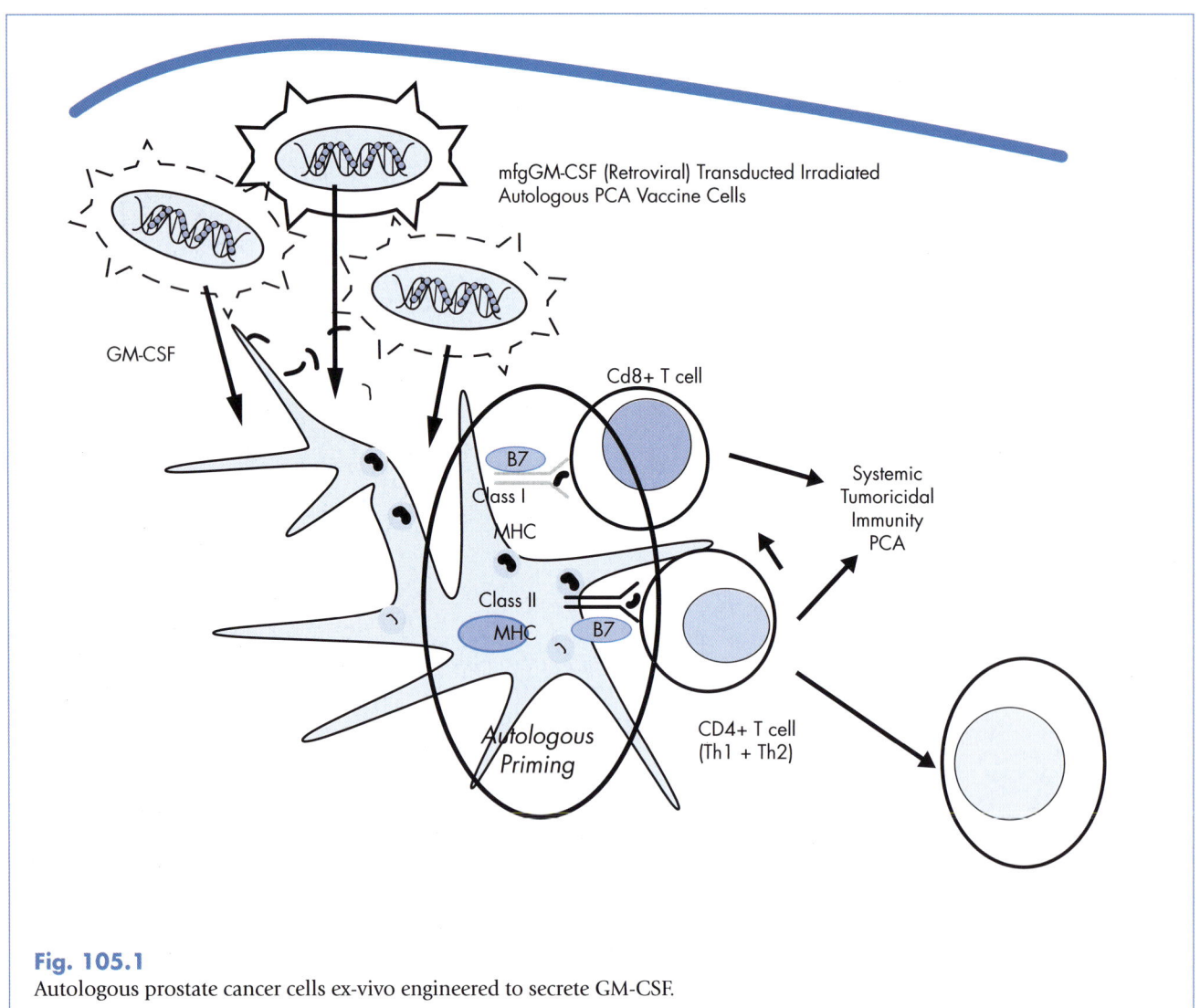

Fig. 105.1
Autologous prostate cancer cells ex-vivo engineered to secrete GM-CSF.

were limited to local irritation at the injection site. Using untransduced autologous prostate cancer cells, a delayed-type hypersensitivity (DTH) reaction, only present in 2 of 8 patients prior to vaccination, was present in 7 of 8 patients after treatment. In addition, biopsies of reactive DTH sites demonstrated degranulated eosinophils consistent with both helper 1 and 2 T-cell activation. This phase I proof-of-concept trial was able to demonstrate an inducible immune response against the patient's own prostate cancer cells.[39] An attempt to broaden the applicability of this approach involved the ex-vivo transduction of the GM-CSF gene into allogeneic rather than autologous prostate cancer cells. In a phase II trial, 96 men (55 with castration-independent and 41 hormone-naive metastatic prostate cancer) were treated with the prostate cancer vaccine GVAX™(Cell Genesys), which consists of irradiated allogeneic human prostate cancer cell lines PC-3 and LNCaP ex-vivo transduced to secrete human GM-CSF.[42] Eighty-six patients received a priming dose of 500 million cells followed by 12 booster doses (100 million cells each) at 2-week intervals, while the remaining 10 patients (all with CIPC) received higher booster doses (300 million cells each). Toxicity was restricted to minor local skin reactions at the injections site, and there was no autoimmunity. Only two patients met NCI Consensus PSA Panel criteria for biochemical response.[43] In the group of CIPC patients there was a trend towards a prolonged median time to progression (defined by radiologic imaging criteria) in the 10 patients who received the higher booster doses (140 days versus 85 days, p = 0.095). A follow-up presentation on the 34 CIPC patients with asymptomatic bone metastases showed a median overall survival of 26 months.[44] To increase the efficacy of GM-CSF transduction, the retroviral vector was substituted by a an adeno-associated viral vector and another phase I/II study was done investigating different schedules and various doses of vaccination. At the time of presentation, 80 patients had been treated on this study and median overall survival had not been reached at a median follow up of 12 months.[45] In this study, there was a correlation of escalating dose of vaccine with humoral response. Of interest there was stabilization or improvement in the serum levels of type I carboxyterminal telopeptide (ICTP), a known marker of osteolytic activity, raising the possibility of the vaccine targeting the bone microenvironment as well as the prostate cancer cells. These exciting preliminary results led to a currently ongoing phase III trial that randomizes men with asymptomatic metastatic CIPC to the bone to either GVAX or cytotoxic chemotherapy.

INTERLEUKIN 2 GENE THERAPY

Another gene-therapy vaccine designed to enhance the immune system's response, utilizes interleukin 2 (IL2). A phase I trial treated 24 patients with locally advanced prostate cancer with Leuvectin, a DNA–lipid complex encoding for the IL2 gene.[46] Leuvectin was directly injected into the prostate twice, 1 week apart. Biopsies were obtained at baseline and again after Leuvectin administration. There was demonstrable response in the injected sites by way of increased intensity of T-cell infiltration. In addition, there were some transient decreases in PSA.

PROSTATE-SPECIFIC ANTIGEN-BASED GENE THERAPY

Prostate-specific antigen is, by and large, a protein specific to the prostate, and thus offers itself as a prime antigen for vaccination. A number of approaches have been investigated with this platform. PVAX/PSA is a plasmid vector DNA vaccine encoding recombinant PSA. In a phase I trial of pVAX/PSA, three cohorts of three patients received separate doses of the vaccine (100, 300, or 900 μg), maintained for five cycles. Granulocyte-macrophage colony-stimulating factor and IL2 were provided as vaccine adjuvants.[47] Two of three patients who received the highest dose had a measurable cellular immune response against recombinant PSA. Given that PSA is a secreted protein, it would follow that PSA is a target for the activation of cellular immunity rather than the humoral arm of the immune system. While not membrane bound, (thus negating the conventional activation of the humoral arm), the expression of PSA by MHC class I on APCs would trigger the cellular immune response. This hypothesis has been eloquently demonstrated in mice, where the expression of human PSA by a mouse tumor cell line was able to elicit a PSA-specific CTL response and effect tumor cell death.[48] In the initial phase I study, a recombinant vaccinia virus encoding human PSA (Prostvac [Therion Biologics]) in metastatic prostate cancer was administered to five groups of patients.[49] The first two groups received Prostvac by dermal scarification; however, the remaining groups received the vaccine subcutaneously due to the increased dose levels. They all received GM-CSF subcutanesously as an adjuvant. Complications were mainly related to injection site irritation and vesicle formation with additional complications of fatigue, grades 2 and 3, in 5 (12%) patients, 2 patients (5%) with grade 2 elevated liver function tests, and 6 patients (14%) with grades 2 and 3 fevers. Evidence of an increased proportion of PSA-specific T cells after vaccination combined with the fairly safe toxicity profile are expected to lead to further studies. In another study, 33 men with biochemical progression received Prostvac along with GM-CSF.[50] There were only minor local skin reactions and promising clinical activity. Currently, Prostvac has been modulated to add costimulatory molecules (B7.1 ICAM1, LFA3) and as PROSTVAC-VF/TRICOM™ (Therion Biologics) is currently in phase II trials in metastatic CIPC. In a similar strategy, an

ECOG phase II clinical trial was conducted to evaluate the feasibility and tolerability of a prime/boost vaccine strategy using vaccinia virus and fowlpox virus expressing human PSA in patients with biochemical progression after local therapy for prostate cancer.[51] The induction of PSA-specific immunity was also evaluated. The endpoint was PSA progression. Twenty-nine (45.3%) patients remained free of PSA progression at 19.1 months and 78.1% patients were found to have clinical progression-free survival. Of the subset of patients who were HLA-A2-positive, 46% were found to have an increase in PSA-specific T-cell response. Currently, an ongoing trial is addressing the question of optimal sequencing of the two pox viral vectors (fowlpox and vaccinia) and the role of adjuvant GM-CSF.

SUICIDE GENE THERAPY

Suicide gene therapy, as the name implies, involves altering of the prostate cancer cell so that a newly incorporated gene, when expressed, will lead the cancer cell to apoptosis. *BCL2* (an antiapoptotic gene) overexpression has been shown to be associated with resistance to radiation therapy and androgen deprivation.[52] *BAX* is a proapoptotic gene that counteracts the *BCL2* antiapoptotic effects. Using an adenoviral vector, *BAX* was combined with a prostate-specific promoter.[53] Cancer cell lines treated with the vector had high levels of Bax expression and an 85% reduction in cell viability. Apoptosis was confirmed, as was specificity as cancer cells other than prostate were subjected to the vector. This study demonstrated tissue specificity for the vector and confirmed apoptosis of prostate cancer cells.

Adenoviruses have received much unfavorable attention after the death of a study patient with ornithine transcarbamylase deficiency when he received intravascular administration of an adenoviral agent.[54] This has served notice that, while most common side effects of vaccines are related to the injection site, serious reactions can still occur. Injecting the adenovirus-based therapy construct directly into the tumor may alleviate some of these concerns. Adenoviruses can be used as vectors for tumor-specific gene therapy that will impart apoptosis. Such oncolytic viruses have been produced by inserting a prostate-specific enhancer and a promoter coupled to the E1A gene, into a replication-competent adenovirus.[55] Expression of the E1A viral gene allows the virus to reproduce and enter the lytic cycle. Proof of specificity is provided by the observation that the oncolytic construct replicates 100 times better in PSA-positive than in PSA-negative cells. A phase I trial was performed to evaluate the safety and activity of CV706, a PSA selective replication-competent adenovirus.[56] Twenty patients who had locally recurrent prostate cancer after radiation therapy were treated in five groups with various doses of

viral particles delivered intratumorally under guidance by TRUS. CV706 was found to be safe. Post-treatment biopsies as well as circulating virus copies demonstrated intraprostatic replication. The five patients who received the highest dose of CV706 achieved more than a 50% reduction in PSA. CV706 has also been studied in combination with radiation therapy in animal models yielding a synergistic effect.[57]

A similar oncolytic virus was constructed in an effort to further enhance affinity for prostatic tissue. CV787 is a replication-competent adenovirus that contains the prostate-specific rat probasin promoter, driving the adenovirus type 5 (Ad5) E1A gene, and the human prostate-specific enhancer/promoter, driving the E1B gene. CV787 was shown to destroy PSA-expressing prostate cancer cells 10,000 times more efficiently than PSA negative cells.[58] CG7870, a replication-selective, PSA-targeted oncolytic adenovirus, was administered to 23 patients with CIPC as a single intravenous infusion.[59] The treatment was well tolerated with flu-like symptoms being the most common adverse event. All patients developed antibodies to CG7870. Five patients had a minor decrease in serum PSA (25%–49%). This vaccine will be studied in combination with a taxane-based chemotherapy.

The most conventional approach to suicide gene therapy has been to deliver the herpes simplex virus–thymidine kinase (HSV-TK) gene: when expressed in the target cells it allows for targeted kill with ganciclovir. In a phase I/II study, 36 patients with local recurrence after radiotherapy were treated with doses of a replication-deficient adenoviral vector that coded for HSV-TK followed by ganciclovir.[60] Just one cycle of treatment caused a statistically significant prolongation of the PSA doubling time from 15.9 months to 42.5 months. Additionally, in 28 (77.8%) of the patients there was a mean reduction in PSA of 28%. An additional cycle of the therapy did not significantly alter the PSA doubling time; however, it did cause modest further decline PSA levels. The investigators also noted a correlation between the density of tumor infiltrating post-treatment CD8+ cells in biopsies with the number of apoptotic cells. The difficult question for future research is: what will be the most appropriate setting for this therapy as described? Besides the trial of 36 patients who had failed radiotherapy, two additional trials were conducted with this approach: one that enrolled 22 patients who received gene therapy prior to radical prostatectomy, and another that treated 27 patients concurrently with radiotherapy.[61] Activated CD8+ cells were measured as the endpoint. All three trials had significant elevations of CD8+ cells most prominently seen in conjunction with radiation therapy.

A novel approach of the same concept is to fuse HSV-TK with the gene for cytosine deaminase.[62] Cytosine deaminase activates the prodrug flucytosine (5-fluorcytosine) to fluorouracil. In a phase I trial, 16 patients, in four cohorts, with locally recurrent prostate cancer received under TRUS visualization an intraprostatic injection of replication-competent adenovirus containing the fused gene in an escalating dose fashion.[62] Two days after injection with the gene therapy, patients were given flucytosine and ganciclovir for 1 week (cohorts 1–3) or 2 weeks (cohort 2). There were no dose limiting toxicities and the maximum tolerated dose was not defined. Seven of the 16 (44%) patients demonstrated a 25% or more decrease in PSA and three experienced a reduction of 50% or more. Transgene expression and tumor destruction were confirmed by biopsy of the prostate at 2 weeks. Two patients were negative for prostate cancer at 1 year. Although the transgene DNA could be detected in blood as far out as 76 days, there was no adenovirus detected in serum or urine.

In an effort to regain control of cell cycling, another approach focused on reintroducing wild-type p53 in prostate cancer cells. INGN 201 (Ad-p53) (Introgen Therapeutics) is a replication-defective adenoviral vector that encodes a wild-type p53 gene. Thirty patients with clinical stage T3, or T1c to T2a with a Gleason score of 8 to 10, or T2a to T2b with a Gleason score of 7 and a PSA of more than 10 ng/mL, were administered TRUS-guided intraprostatic injections of INGN 201.[63] There were no grade 3 or 4 adverse events. Twenty-six patients went on to have a prostatectomy. Ten of 11 patients who had negative immunostaining for p53 protein at baseline were subsequently positive for p53 after the first injection of INGN 201.

Clearly, this line of investigation carries great promise. As the technology continues to mature we hope to see various platforms of oncolytic gene therapy being further developed.

ACTIVE CYTOKINE IMMUNOTHERAPY

GRANULOCYTE-MACROPHAGE COLONY-STIMULATING FACTOR

There have been studies that demonstrated that IL2 can induce prostate tumor cell regression in animals.[64] Granulocyte macrophage colony-stimulating factor has also been demonstrated to have antitumor properties and has been shown to cause a reduction in PSA.[65] In a phase II trial that comprised 36 patients who had progressive disease after androgen deprivation and antiandrogen withdrawal, 23 patients received a subcutaneous dose of GM-CSF at 250 μg/m^2/day for 14 days of a 28 day cycle.[66] Declines in PSA were seen during the first 2 weeks on therapy, but they dissipated in the 2 weeks following GM-CSF. Based on the observed oscillating PSA responses in the first cohort, the second cohort (n = 13) also received GM-CSF 250 μg/m^2 3-times weekly maintenance doses. In cohort 1, 10 patients (45%) had a decline in PSA while on therapy, with a resultant rise

while off treatment. In cohort 2, 12 of 13 patients had a response with a median decline of 32%. Of note, no evidence that GM-CSF was interfering with PSA measurement or secretion was detected. The same type of therapy has been investigated in men with biochemical, non-metastatic prostate cancer (D0).[67] Thirty patients with rising PSA after failure to be cured with either surgery or radiation therapy received GM-CSF at 250 μg/m^2/day for 14 days of a 28 day cycle. Only three (10%) patients achieved a reduction in PSA of 50%.[67] The biologic effect was reflected by an increase in the PSA doubling time (PSA-DT): the median PSA-DT increased from 8.4 to 15 months (p = 0.001).

PASSIVE (ANTIBODY-BASED) IMMUNOTHERAPY

PROSTATE-SPECIFIC MEMBRANE ANTIGEN

Tissue-specific targeting for prostate cancer has been achieved with monoclonal antibodies against a prostate-specific, nonshed surface antigen: PSMA. A second generation antibody (J591), targeting the extracellular domain of PSMA has been employed either as a single agent or as a platform for radioimmunotherapy (RIT) or targeted cytotoxic therapy. Use of J591 as single agent is based on the potential benefits from activation of antibody-dependent cellular cytotoxicity (ADCC). Early reports of clinical use with anti-PSMA single agent antibody have not shown very promising results.[68,69] On the other hand, when PSMA is used as a platform for targeted therapy, results appear to be more promising. MLN-2704 (Millenium) is an immunoconjugate consisting of the chemotherapeutic agent DM1 (Drug Maytansinoid-1) linked to the monoclonal antibody J591. MLN-2704 binds to the external portion of PSMA, is rapidly internalized, delivering DM1 directly to prostate cancer cells. DM1 inhibits microtubule formation, disrupting cell division and other cellular survival processes. MLN-2704 is currently being investigated in a phase I/II trial at Memorial Sloan-Kettering Cancer Center. As mentioned earlier, PSMA can also be employed to guide RIT to prostate cancer cells. Lutetium-177 and yttrium-90 are two radiopharmaceuticals that have been investigated in combination to J591 antibodies.[70] Both have shown promising clinical activity in pilot studies and are currently actively investigated.

CYTOTOXIC T-LYMPHOCYTE ANTIGEN 4-BASED THERAPY

One of the primary mechanisms of failure of CTLs to eradicate tumor cells is the inability to express adequate amounts of co-stimulatory molecules. When specific epitopes are presented by the MHC complex of the APCs to the T-cell receptor (TCR) optimal activation requires the expression of additional co-stimulatory molecules CD80,86 which will bind to CD28 on the TCR or signaling through the CD40/CD40-ligand pathway. The TCR also expresses CTLA-4 that may bind to CD80,86. The function of the CD28/CD80,86 pair is to promote activation of T-cell stimulation, whereas CTLA-4 mediates inhibitory signals. By preventing binding to CTLA-4 through the use of a neutralizing monoclonal antibody, it may be possible to sustain and augment immune responses.[71] A recent phase I trial reported on 14 men with metastatic CIPC treated with a single dose of a human anti-CTLA-4 antibody (MDX-101, Medarex).[72] Two patients sustained grade 3 toxicities (pruritus, rash) while two patients had a decline of more than 50% PSA. In a follow up study, MDX-101 was combined with GM-CSF and eight men with CIPC were treated in a phase I study without any clinical or laboratory evidence of autoimmunity[73]

CONCLUSIONS

Immunotherapy for prostate cancer offers much promise. The field has gone from no publications in 1993 to global clinical trials. New concepts are being integrated into immunotherapy clinical development, for example, the activation of DCs with prostate-associated antigens followed by the treatment of patients with co-stimulatory molecules such as the CTLA-4a antibody. As Eli Gilboa pointed out "from early excitement to total disillusionment" immunotherapy is gaining the momentum again.[14] Review of results outlined above suggests that several techniques can lead to relevant immune responses. Correlation of immunologic surrogates to clinical outcome has been problematic. Measurement of clinical response has traditionally been based on PSA measurements. While criteria of an association of PSA with clinical outcome have been defined for response to cytotoxic chemotherapy, they may not apply to immunotherapy. Early clinical experience suggests that activation of immune effector mechanisms initially leads to a deceleration of cancer growth followed by stabilization of disease progression, which, in select patients, may be followed by a conventionally measurable response. Also, it should be pointed out that, although most early clinical work has been in the androgen independent setting (proof-of concept and assessment of safety), immunotherapy is most likely to be successful in lower tumor burden states as therapy aiming to eradicate micrometastatic disease. The evolution of technology and the ever better understanding of the mechanisms governing an effective and sustainable immune response will pave the way for more efficacious

applications of immunotherapy principles. It may be that combination of different approaches may be superior to any single modality. "Co-targeting" DC antigen presentation and augmentation of B-cell and T-cell anti-neoplastic immune responses are likely to have the highest probability of favorably increasing time to progression, overall survival. Lessons on the immunobiology of prostate cancer immune response learned from patients who participated in early clinical trials need to be integrated in the design of future translational investigations to further refine selection of patients, administration of therapy, and assessment of outcome.

REFERENCES

1. Jemal A, Murray T, Ward E, et al. Cancer Statistics 2005. CA Cancer J Clin 2005;55:10–30.

2. Han M, Partin AW, Zahurak M, et al. Biochemical (prostate specific antigen) recurrence probability following radical prostatectomy for clinically localized prostate cancer. J Urol. 2003;169:517–523.

3. Roehl KA, Han M, Ramos CG, et al. Cancer progression and survival rates following anatomical radical retropubic prostatectomy in 3,478 consecutive patients: long-term results. J Urol 2004;172:910–914.

4. Kattan MW, Wheeler TM, Scardino PT. Postoperative nomogram for disease recurrence after radical prostatectomy for prostate cancer. J Clin Oncol 1999;17:1499–1507.

5. Tannock IF, Osoba D, Stockler MR, et al. Chemotherapy with mitoxantrone plus prednisone or prednisone alone for symptomatic hormone-resistant prostate cancer: a Canadian randomized trial with palliative end points. J Clin Oncol 1996;14:1756–1764.

6. Petrylak DP, Tangen CM, Hussain MH, et al. Docetaxel and estramustine compared with mitoxantrone and prednisone for advanced refractory prostate cancer. N Engl J Med 2004;351:1513–1520.

7. Tannock IF, de Wit R, Berry WR, et al. Docetaxel plus prednisone or mitoxantrone plus prednisone for advanced prostate cancer. N Engl J Med 2004;351:1502–1512.

8. Assikis VJ, Simons JW. Novel therapeutic strategies for androgen-independent prostate cancer: an update. Semin Oncol 2004;31:26–32.

9. Nauts HC. Bacteria and cancer: antagonisms and benefits. Cancer Surv 1989;7:713–723.

10. Krikorian J, Portlock C, Conney D, et al. Spontaneous regression of non-Hodgkin's lymphoma. A report of nine cases. Cancer 1980;46:2093–2099.

11. Burnet FM. The concept of immunological surveillance. Prog Exp Tumor Res 1970;13:1–27.

12. Rygaard J, Povlsen CO. The mouse mutant nude does not develop spontaneous tumors. An argument against immunological surveillance. Acta Pathol Microbiol Scand Microbiol Immunol 1974;82:89–98.

13. DeVita Jr V. Principles of chemotherapy. Cancer principles & practice of oncology. Philadelphia: Lippincott, 1997, p 276.

14. Gilboa E. The promise of cancer vaccines. Nature Rev Cancer 2004;4:401–411.

16. Hurwitz AA, Yanover P, Markowitz M, et al. Prostate cancer, advances in immunotherapy. Biodrugs 2003;17:131–138.

17. Ragde H, Cavanagh WA, Tjoa BA, et al. Dendritic cell based vaccines: progress in immunotherapy studies for prostate cancer. J Urol 2004;172:2532–2538.

18. Murphy G, Tjoa B, Ragde H, et al. Phase I clinical trial: T cell therapy for prostate cancer using autologous dendritic cells pulsed with HLA-A0201-specific peptides from prostate-specific membrane antigen. Prostate 1996;29:371–380.

19. Tjoa BA, Simmons SJ, Elgamal A, et al. Follow-up evaluation of a phase II prostate cancer vaccine trial. Prostate 1999;40:125–129.

20. Lodge PA, Jones LA, Bader RA, et al. Dendritic cell-based immunotherapy of prostate cancer: immune monitoring of a phase II clinical trial. Cancer Res 2000;60:829–833.

21. Assikis VJ, Elgamal AA, Daliani D, et al. Immunotherapy for androgen independent prostate cancer: results of a Phase I trial with a tumor vaccine of autologous dendritic cells loaded with r-PSMA Proc AACR 2002 [abstract 3352].

22. Small EJ, Fratesi P, Reese DM, et al. Immunotherapy of hormone-refractory prostate cancer with antigen-loaded dendritic cells. J Clin Oncol 2000;18:3894–3903.

23. Small EJ, Rini B, Higano C, et al. A randomized, placebo-controlled phase III trial of APC8015 in patients with androgen-independent prostate cancer. Proc ASCO 2003 [abstract 1534].

24. Gilboa E, Vieweg J. Cancer immunotherapy with mRNA-transfected dendritic cells. Immunol Rev 2004;199:251–263.

25. Heiser A, Coleman D, Dannull J, et al. Autologous dendritic cells transfected with prostate-specific antigen RNA stimulate CTL responses against metastatic prostate tumors. J Clin Inv 2002;109:409–417.

26. Slovin SF, Kelly WK, Scher HI. Immunological approaches for the treatment of prostate cancer. Semin Urol Oncol 1998;16:53–59.

27. Slovin S, Govindaswami R, Musselli C, et al. Fully synthetic carbohydrate-based vaccines in biochemically relapsed prostate cancer: Clinical trial results with a-N-Acetylgalactosamine-O-Serine/Threonine conjugate vaccine. J Clin Oncol 2003;21:4292–4298.

28. Kim NW, Piatyszek MA, Prowse KR, et al. Specific association of human telomerase activity with immortal cells and cancer. Science 1994;266:2011–2015.

29. Shay JW, Wright WE. Telomerase: a target for cancer therapeutics. Cancer Cell 2002;2:257–265.

30. Nair SK, Heiser A, Boczkowski D, et al. Induction of cytotoxic T cell responses and tumor immunity against unrelated tumors using telomerase reverse transcriptase RNA transfected dendritic cells. Nat Med 2000;6:1011–1101.

31. Su Z, Vieweg W, Dannull J, et al. Vaccination of metastatic prostate cancer patients using mature dendritic cells transfected with mRNA encoding hTERT or an MHC class II targeted hTERT/LAMP fusion protein: Results from a phase I clinical trial. Proc ASCO 2004 [abstract 2507].

32. Su Z, Vieweg J, Weizer AZ, et al. Enhanced induction of telomerase-specific CD4+ T cells using dendritic cells transfected with RNA encoding a chimeric gene product. Cancer Res 2002;62:5041–5048.

33. Vonderheide RH, Domchek SM, Schultze JL, et al. Vaccination of cancer patients against telomerase induces functional antitumor CD8+ T lymphocytes, Clin Cancer Res 2004;10:828–839.

34. Noguchi M, Itoh K, Suekane S, et al. Phase I trial of patient-oriented vaccination in HLA-A2-positive patients with metastatic hormone-refractory prostate cancer. Cancer Sci 2004;95:77–84.

35. Noguchi M, Itoh K, Suekane S, et al. Immunological monitoring during combination of patient-oriented peptide vaccination and estramustine phosphate in patients with metastatic hormone refractory prostate cancer. Prostate 2004;60:32–45.

36. Anderson WF. Human gene therapy. Nature 1998;392:25–30.

37. Mahzar D, Waxman J. Gene therapy for prostate cancer. BJU Intern 2004;93:465–469.

38. Mabjeesh NJ, Zhong H, Simons JW. Gene therapy of prostate cancer: current and future directions. Endocr Relat Cancer 2002;9:115–139.

39. Simons JW, Mikhak B, Chang J, et al. Induction of immunity to prostate cancer antigens: Results of a clinical trial of vaccination with irradiated autologous prostate tumor cells engineered to secrete granulocyte-macrophage colony-stimulating factor using ex vivo gene transfer. Cancer Res 1999;59:5160–5168.

40. Mulligan RD. The basic science of gene therapy. Science 1993;260:926–932.

41. Nelson WG, Simons JW, Mikhak B, et al. Cancer cells engineered to secrete granulocyte-macrophage colony-stimulating factor using ex vivo gene transfer as vaccines for the treatment of genitourinary malignancies. Cancer Chemother Pharmacol 2000;46:S67–S72.

42. Simons JW, Small E, Nelson W, et al. Phase II trials of a GM-CSF gene-transduced prostate cancer cell line vaccine (GVAX®) demonstrate anti-tumor activity. Proc ASCO 2001 [abstract 1073].

43. Bubley GJ, Carducci M, Dahut W, et al. Eligibility and response guidelines for phase II clinical trials in androgen-independent prostate cancer: recommendations from the Prostate-Specific Antigen Working Group. J Clin Oncol 1999;17:3461–3467.

44. Simons J, Nelson W, Nemunaitis J, et al. Phase II trials of a GM-CSF gene-transduced prostate cancer cell line vaccine (GVAX) in hormone refractory prostate cancer. Proc ASCO 2002 [abstract 729].

45. Small EJ, Higano C, Smith D, et al. A phase 2 study of an allogeneic GM-CSF gene-transduced prostate cancer cell line vaccine in patients with metastatic hormone-refractory prostate cancer. Proc ASCO 2004 [abstract 4565].

46. Belldegrun A, Tso CL, Zisman A, et al. Interleukin 2 gene therapy for prostate cancer: phase I clinical trial and basic biology. Hum Gene Ther 2001;12:883–892.

47. Pavlenko M, Roos AK, Lundqvist A, et al. A phase I trial of DNA vaccination with a plasmid expressing prostate-specific antigen in patients with hormone-refractory prostate cancer. Br J Cancer 2004;91:688–694.

48. Wei C, Storozynsky E, McAdam AJ, et al. Expression of human prostate-specific antigen (PSA) in a mouse tumor cell line reduces tumorigenicity and elicits PSA-specific cytotoxic T lymphocytes. Cancer Immunol Immunother 1996;42:362–368.

49. Gulley J, Chen AP, Dahut W, et al. Phase I study of a vaccine using recombinant vaccinia virus expressing PSA (rV-PSA) in patients with metastatic androgen-independent prostate cancer. Prostate 2002;53:109–117.

50. Eder JP, Kantoff PW, Roper K, et al. A phase I trial of a recombinant vaccinia virus expressing prostate-specific antigen in advanced prostate cancer. Clin Cancer Res 6:1632–1638.

51. Kaufman HL, Wang W, Manola J, et al. Phase II randomized study of vaccine treatment of advanced prostate cancer (E7897): A trial of the Eastern Cooperative Oncology Group. J Clin Oncol 2004;22:2122–2132.

52. Mackey TJ, Borkowski A, Amin P, et al. Bcl-2/bax ratio as a predictive marker for therapeutic response to radiotherapy in patients with prostate cancer. Urology 1998;52:1085–1090.

53. Lowe SL, Rubinchik S, Honda T, et al. Prostate-specific expression of Bax delivered by an adenoviral vector induces apoptosis in LNCaP prostate cancer cell. Gene Ther 2001;8:1363–1371.

54. Reid T, Warren R, Kirn D. Intravascular adenoviral agents in cancer patients: lessons from clinical trials. Cancer Gene Therapy 2002;9:979–986.

55. Rodriguez R, Schuur ER, Lim HY, et al. Prostate attenuated replication competent adenovirus (ARCA) CN706: a selective cytotoxic for prostate-specific antigen-positive prostate cancer cells. Cancer Res 1997;57:2559–2563.

56. DeWeese Tl, van der Poel H, Li S, et al. A phase I trial of CV706, a replication-competent PSA selective oncolytic adenovirus, for the treatment of locally recurrent prostate cancer following radiation therapy. Cancer Res 2001;61:7464–7472.

57. Chen Y, DeWeese T, Dilley J, et al. CV706, a prostate cancer-specific adenovirus variant in combination with radiotherapy produces synergistic antitumor efficacy without increasing toxicity. Cancer Res 2001;61:5453–5460.

58. Yu DC, Chen Y, Seng M, et al. The addition of adenovirus type 5 region E3 enables calydon virus 787 to eliminate distant prostate tumor xenografts. Cancer Res 1999;59:4200–4203.

59. Wilding G, Carducci M, Yu DC, et al. A phase I/II trial of IV CG7870, a replication-selective, PSA-targeted oncolytic adenovirus, for the treatment of hormone-refractory, metastatic prostate cancer. Proc ASCO 2004 [abstract 3036].

60. Miles BJ, Shalev M, Aguilar-Cordova E, et al. Prostate-specific antigen response and systemic T-cell activation after in situ gene therapy in prostate cancer patients failing radiotherapy. Hum Gene Ther 2001;12:1955–1967.

61. Satoh T, Teh BS, Timme TL, et al. Enhanced systemic T-cell activation after in situ gene therapy with radiotherapy in prostate cancer patients. Int J Rad Oncol 2004;59:562–571.

62. Freytag SO, Khil M, Stricker H, et al. Phase I study of replication-competent adenovirus-mediated double suicide gene therapy for the treatment of locally recurrent prostate cancer. Cancer Res 2002;62:4968–4976.

63. Pisters LL, Pettaway CA, Troncoso P, et al. Evidence that transfer of functional p53 protein results in increased apoptosis in prostate cancer. Clinical Cancer Res 2004;10:2587–2593.

64. Triest JA, Grignon DJ, Cher ML, et al. Systemic interleukin 2 therapy for human prostate tumors in a nude mouse model. Clin Cancer Res 1998;4:2009–2014.

65. LeBlanc G, Small EJ, Bok RA, et al. Granulocyte Macrophage Colony-Stimulating Factor (GM-CSF) therapy for prostate cancer patients with serologic progression after definitive local therapy. Proc ASCO 2001;20:724.

66. Small EJ, Reese DM, Um B, et al. Therapy of advanced prostate cancer with granulocyte macrophage colony-stimulating factor. Clin Cancer Res 1999;5:1738–1744.

67. Rini BI, Weinberg V, Bok R, et al. Prostate-specific antigen kinetics as a measure of the biologic effect of granulocyte-macrophage colony-stimulating factor in patients with serologic progression of prostate cancer. J Clin Oncol 2003;21:99–105.

68. Bander NH, Nanus D, Goldsmith S, et al. Phase I trial of humanized monoclonal antibody (mAb) to prostate specific membrane antigen/extracellular domain (PSMAext). Proc ASCO 2001 [abstract 722].

69. Morris MJ, Pandit-Tasker N, Divgi C, et al. Pilot trial of anti-PSMA antibody J591 for prostate cancer. Proc ASCO 2003 [abstract 1634].

70. Milowsky MI, Nanus DM, Kostakoglu L, et al. Phase I trial of yttrium-90-labeled anti-prostate-specific membrane antigen monoclonal antibody J591 for androgen-independent prostate cancer. J Clin Oncol 2004;22:499–500.

71. Thompson CB, Allison JP. The emerging role of CTLA-4 as an immune attenuator. Immunity 1997;7:445–450.

72. Davis TA, Tchekmedyian S, Korman A, et al. MDX-010 (human anti-CTLA4): a phase I trial in hormone refractory prostate carcinoma (HRPC). Proc ASCO 2002 [abstract 74].

73. Fong L, Rini B, Kavanaugh B, et al. CTLA-4 blockade-based immunotherapy for prostate cancer. Proc ASCO 2004 [abstract 2590]

Index

References to genes, genetic loci, and studies, trials and projects have been grouped.